THE COMPLETE RESOURCE GUIDE
FOR PEOPLE WITH
CHRONIC ILLNESS

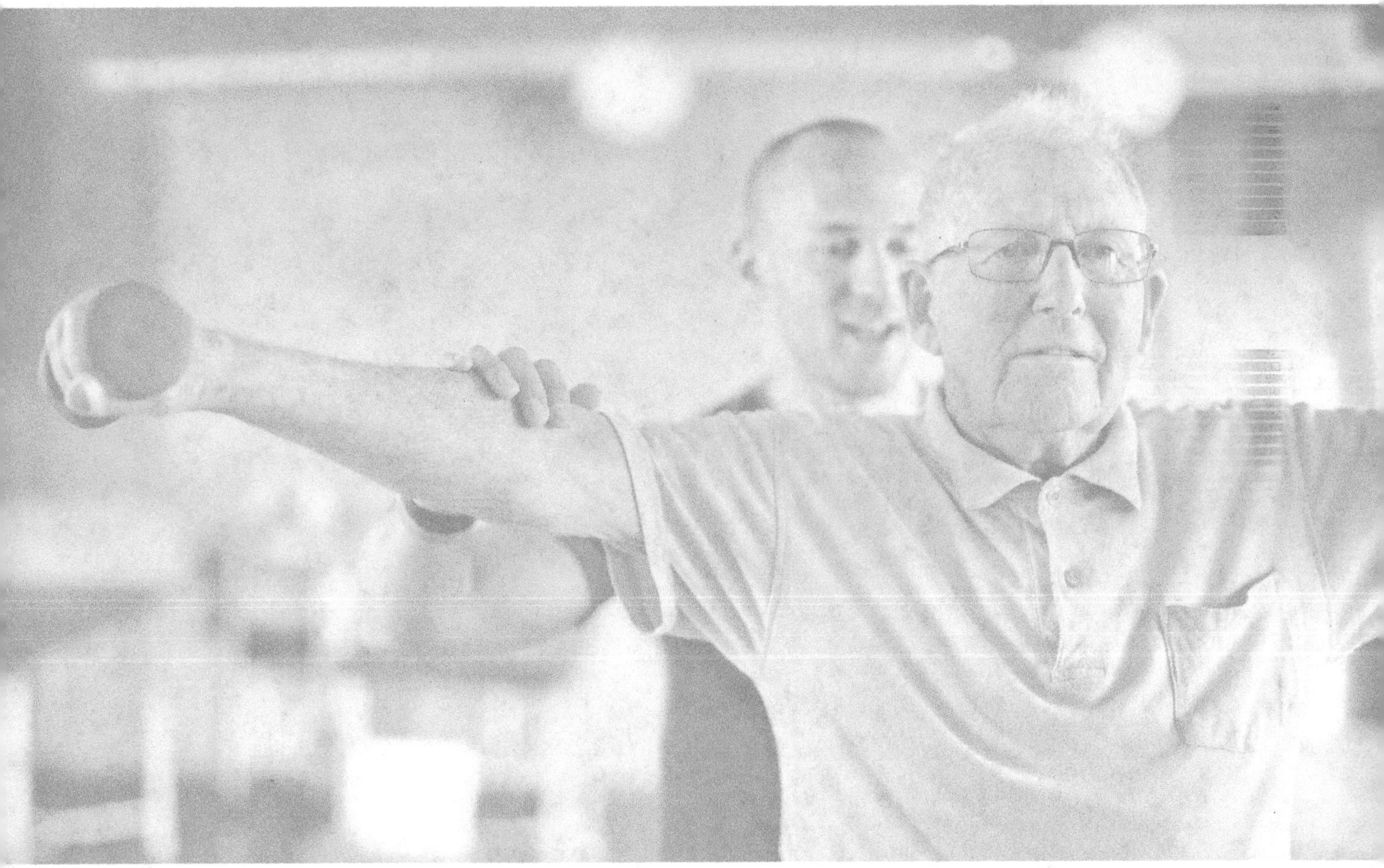

2019/20
FOURTEENTH EDITION

THE COMPLETE RESOURCE GUIDE FOR PEOPLE WITH
CHRONIC ILLNESS

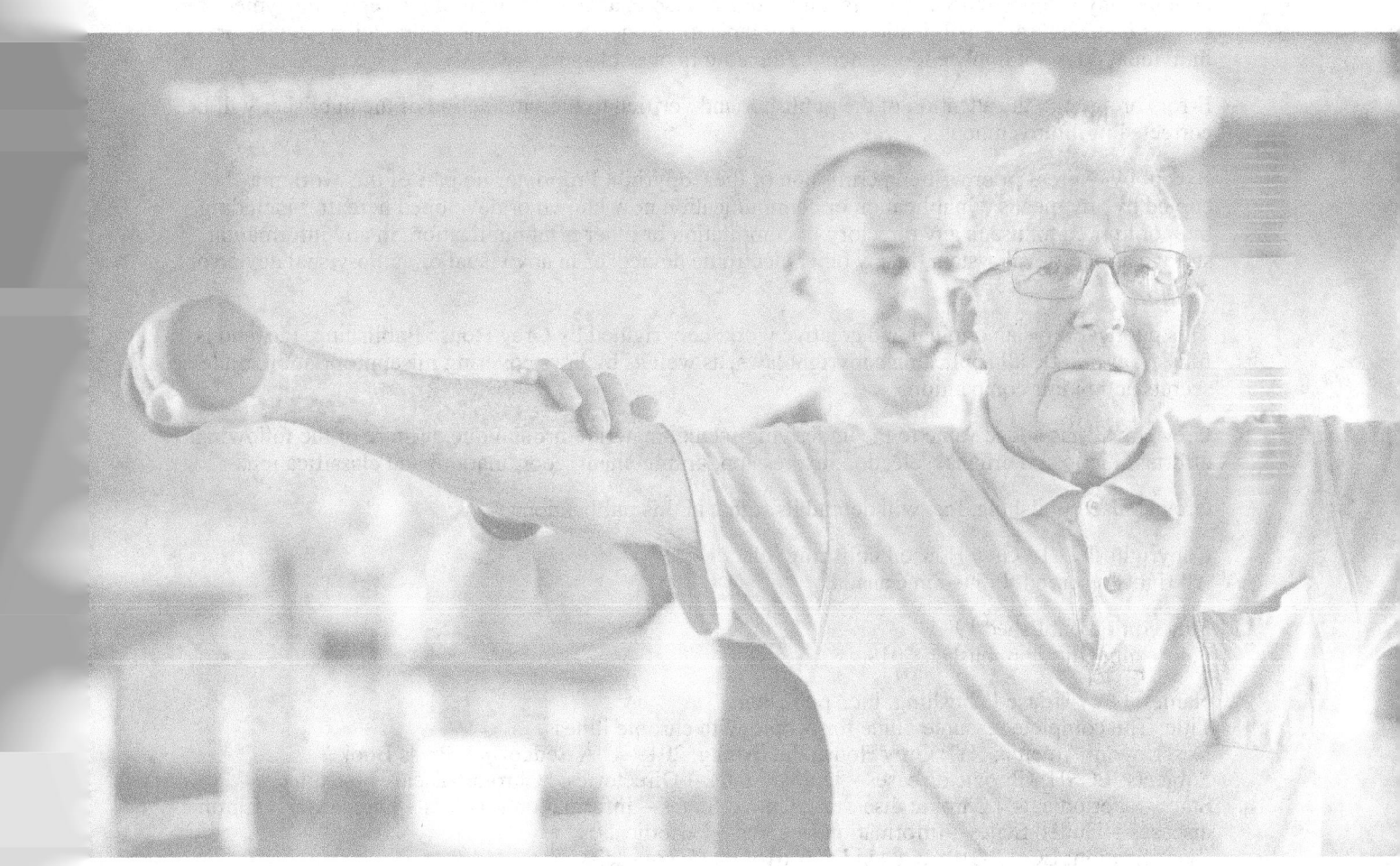

GREY HOUSE PUBLISHING

PRESIDENT: Richard Gottlieb
PUBLISHER: Leslie Mackenzie
EDITORIAL DIRECTOR: Laura Mars
PRODUCTION MANAGER & COMPOSITION: Kristen Hayes
MARKETING DIRECTOR: Jessica Moody

Grey House Publishing, Inc.
4919 Route 22
Amenia, NY 12501
518.789.8700
Fax: 845.373.6390
www.greyhouse.com
books@greyhouse.com

First edition published 1994
Fourteenth edition published 2019

Names: Grey House Publishing, Inc., publisher.
Title: The complete resource guide for people with chronic illness.
Description: Amenia, NY : Grey House Publishing, 2019- | "A Sedgewick Press Book."
Subjects: LCSH: Chronic diseases—United States—Directories. | Chronic diseases—United States—Periodicals. | Chronic diseases—United States—Information services—Directories. | Chronic diseases—United States—Information services—Periodicals.
Classification: LCC RC108 .C645 | DDC 616/.0025/73—dc23

Table of Contents

Introduction ix
Chronic Illness—Body Systems xi
"An Empirical Study of Chronic Diseases in the United States: A Visual
    Analytics Approach to Public Health" xv
Next Steps After Your Diagnosis: Finding Information and Support xxxix

Addison Disease and Adrenal Insufficiency 1
Aging 3
AIDS/HIV 19
Alcoholism, *see* Substance Abuse Disorder
Allergies 47
Alzheimer's Disease 56
Amyotrophic Lateral Sclerosis 80
Anorexia Nervosa, *see* Eating Disorders
Arthritis 89
Asthma 102
Ataxia 112
Attention Deficit Hyperactivity Disorder 117
Autistic Spectrum Disorders 122
Birth Defects 135
Blindness, *see* Visual Impairments
Brain Tumors 140
Bulimia, *see* Eating Disorders
Cancer 151
Carpal Tunnel Syndrome 191
Celiac Disease 193
Cerebral Palsy Syndromes 196
Chronic Bronchitis, *see* Lung Disease
Chronic Fatigue Syndrome 209
Chronic Obstructive Pulmonary Disorder (COPD), *see* Lung Disease
Chronic Pain 215
Congenital Heart Defects 218
Cooley's Anemia (Thalassemia) 220
Crohn Disease 224
Cystic Fibrosis 231
Deafness, *see* Hearing Impairment
Diabetes Mellitus 240
Down Syndrome 263
Drug Abuse, *see* Substance Abuse Disorder
Eating Disorders (Anorexia Nervosa, Bulimia) 273
Eczema, *see* Skin Disorders
Endometriosis 282
Fabry Disease 286
Fibromyalgia Syndrome 288
Gastrointestinal Disorders 292
Gaucher Disease 299

Table of Contents

Geriatric Disorders, *see* Aging; Alzheimer's Disease
Growth Disorders. 301
Head Injuries 304
Hearing Impairment. 319
Heart Disease. 363
Hemophilia 370
Hepatitis. 383
Hydrocephalus 388
Hypertension 392
Impotence 396
Incontinence. 398
Infertility 402
Kidney Disease 414
Liver Disease 424
Lung Disease 430
Lyme Disease, *see* Tick-Borne Disease
Mental Illness/General. 438
Mental Illness/Depression 457
Mental Illness/Schizophrenia 462
Migraine. 465
Multiple Sclerosis 470
Muscular Dystrophy 482
Myasthenia Gravis. 488
Neurofibromatosis 494
Obesity. 498
Obsessive Compulsive Disorder, *see* Mental Illness
Osteogenesis Imperfecta 503
Osteoporosis 506
Paget Disease. 510
Parkinson Disease 512
Post-Polio Syndrome. 521
Post-Traumatic Stress Disorder. 523
Prader-Willi Syndrome 532
Psoriasis, *see* Skin Disorders
Raynaud's Disease. 537
Retinitis Pigmentosa, *see* Visual Impairment
Sarcoidosis. 539
Scleroderma. 544
Scoliosis. 550
Seizure Disorders. 555
Sexually Transmitted Diseases 563
Sickle Cell Disease 566
Sjogren's Syndrome 569
Skin Disorders 571
Sleep Disorders 578
Spina Bifida. 585
Spinal Cord Injuries. 592
Stroke. 599
Substance Abuse Disorder 604

Sudden Infant Death Syndrome.................................645
Systemic Lupus Erythematosus................................656
Tay-Sachs Disease...664
Thyroid Disease...667
Tick-Borne Disease..669
Tourette Syndrome 673
Transplant-Related Conditions 680
Tuberculosis..688
Tuberous Sclerosis Complex..................................693
Turner Syndrome...695
Ulcerative Colitis..698
Visual Impairment...700
War Syndromes...750
Wilson Disease 766
General Resources...768
Wish Foundations 791
Death and Bereavement.......................................794

Entry Index 799
Geographic Index..849

Introduction

This fourteenth edition of *The Complete Resource Guide for People with Chronic Illness* offers a comprehensive overview of 90 specific chronic illnesses from Addison to Wilson Disease, including chapters on Aging, Allergies, Cancer, Chronic Pain, Post-Traumatic Stress Disorder, and Sleep Disorders. Each chapter includes a current, easy-to-understand description, plus a wide range of condition-specific support services and information resources to help not only those living with a chronic illness, but also those who support the chronic illness community.

A chronic condition is a physical or mental health condition that lasts more than one year and causes functional restrictions or requires ongoing monitoring or treatment. Nearly 45% of all Americans suffer from a chronic disease and that number is growing. In fact, according to the *International Journal of Environmental Research and Public Health*, persistent conditions are the nation's leading cause of death and disability. This new edition will prove invaluable in dealing with the multiple issues involved with living with a chronic illness.

Support Material

The Complete Resource Guide for People with Chronic Illness starts with an article from the IJERPH, "An Empirical Study of Chronic Diseases in the United States: A Visual Analytics Approach to Public Health." Using data from the Centers for Disease Control and Prevention, detailed tables and maps, this 24-page article discusses five main categories: chronic disease conditions; behavioral health; mental health; demographics, and overarching conditions.

Following this article is a reprint of *Next Steps After Your Diagnosis*, from the Agency for Healthcare Research and Quality, a 23-page booklet that offers general advice for people with almost any disease or condition. It covers five broad categories: Take the time you need; Get the support you need; Talk with your doctor; Seek out information; and Decide on a treatment plan.

Next is a **Chronic Illness-Body Systems Chart** — a two-part table includes first a list of chronic illnesses and their relevant body systems, and then a list of body systems and the chronic illnesses that affect it.

Chapter Content

After these extremely helpful front matter sections, *The Complete Resource Guide for People with Chronic Illness* includes, in 90 chapters that are arranged alphabetically by condition, associations, state agencies, libraries & resource centers, research centers, magazines, newsletters, audio & video, hot lines, support groups and valuable web sites. This new edition includes more than 200 new listings. Plus, in addition to chapters dealing with specific chronic conditions, this work includes several chapters designed to support the chronic illness community as a whole, including wish foundations, and death and bereavement groups.

This longstanding resource guide is designed for both those dealing with the stress, uncertainty and need-to-know issues that accompany a new chronic illness diagnosis, as well as those already coping with chronic disease. ...*How can I connect with others with heart disease? ...Which cancer treatment is best for me? ...What do I need to know about living with a 7-year old with hemophilia? ...How do I protect my chronically ill child without causing resentment among other family members?* You'll find answers to these questions and more in these pages. In addition to resources crucial for people with chronic illness as they transition from diagnosis to home, work, and community life, *The Complete Resource Guide for People with Chronic Illness* is also invaluable to hospital and medical center personnel, especially discharge planners, social service workers, and disability coordinators. It provides, in one source, comprehensive, critical, immediate information—from national associations to children's books. It is the answer for those who find navigating the Internet overwhelming, and those who are uncomfortable asking critical questions during visits with doctors and other professionals.

Format

The 90 chronic condition chapters are arranged alphabetically by name of the disorder. Each chapter begins with a brief description of the illness, written in layman's terms, with probable causes, symptoms and treatment options. These descriptions include the most current medical thinking and treatments.

Following each description are disease-specific resources. Most chapters contain the following: National Associations; State Agencies; Libraries & Resource Centers; Magazines, Newsletters, Pamphlets; Research Centers; Books for Adults; Books for Children; Support Groups & Hotlines; Audio & Video Resources; Web Sites. This reference work profiles 10,743 listings. This edition includes 6,988 fax numbers, 5,693 e-mails, 8,919 web sites, and 11,178 key executives. Brief descriptions and other details are included depending on the type of listing; Associations may include year founded and yearly dues, while Magazines may include frequency and number of pages.

In addition to the 90 chapters of chronic illnesses, *The Complete Resource Guide for People with Chronic Illness* includes several supplemental chapters in the back of the book designed to provide value to individuals with chronic illness and their families: General Resources – information relevant to the general chronic illness community; Wish Foundations – organizations devoted to granting wishes of chronically and terminally ill individuals; and Death & Bereavement – support services for those who find themselves or a loved one close to death or grieving a loss. Rounding out this directory are two indexes that allow users additional access to the information: Entry Name Index and Geographic Index.

Praise for previous editions:

" ..a solid purchase for any library needing to provide information to users on chronic illness ..particularly well suited for consumer health and public libraries."
—**ARBA**

"...among the most useful of directories, with its goal of helping people with long-term medical conditions find helpful resources..Recommended"
—**Choice**

"...logically organized and offers an extensive range of information resources and support services."
—**Doody's Notes**

The Complete Resource Guide for People with Chronic Illness is also available for subscription on G.O.L.D. – Grey House OnLine Database. Subscribers to G.O.L.D. can access their subscription via the Internet and do customized searches that make finding information quicker and easier. Visit http://gold.greyhouse.com for more information.

Chronic Illness — Body Systems

The following chart lists the chronic illness and its body system(s) or disorder category. Chronic conditions not listed do not fall into a specific system(s). A cross-reference chart that lists the information in reverse follows — body system or disorder categories followed by chronic illnesses.

CHRONIC ILLNESS	BODY SYSTEM/DISORDER CATEGORY
Addison Disease and Adrenal Insufficiency	Endocrine
Aging	Cells & Tissues
AIDS/HIV	Immune, Infectious Disease
Allergies	Immune
Alzheimer's Disease	Nervous
Amyotrophic Lateral Sclerosis	Nervous
Arthritis	Muscular, Skeletal
Asthma	Respiratory
Ataxia	Nervous
Attention Deficit Hyperactivity Disorder	Behavioral, Developmental
Autistic Spectrum Disorders	Behavioral, Developmental
Brain Tumors	Nervous
Carpal Tunnel Syndrome	Muscular, Skeletal, Nervous
Celiac Disease	Gastrointestinal
Cerebral Palsy Syndromes	Nervous, Muscular
Chronic Fatigue Syndrome	Immune
Chronic Pain	Nervous
Cooley's Anemia (Thalassemia)	Blood
Congenital Heart Defects	Cardiovascular
Crohn Disease	Gastrointestinal
Cystic Fibrosis	Respiratory, Gastrointestinal
Diabetes Mellitus	Endocrine
Down Syndrome	Developmental
Eating Disorders (Anorexia Nervosa, Bulimia)	Behavioral
Endometriosis	Reproductive
Fabry Disease	Gastrointestinal
Fibromyalgia Syndrome	Muscular, Skeletal
Gastrointestinal Disorders	Gastrointestinal
Gaucher Disease	Gastrointestinal
Growth Disorders	Developmental
Head Injuries	Nervous
Hearing Impairment	Sensory
Heart Disease	Cardiovascular
Hemophilia	Blood
Hepatitis	Infectious Disease
Hydrocephalus	Nervous
Hypertension	Cardiovascular
Impotence	Reproductive
Incontinence	Urinary
Infertility	Reproductive
Kidney Disease	Gastrointestinal

CHRONIC ILLNESS	BODY SYSTEM/DISORDER CATEGORY
Liver Disease	Gastrointestinal
Lung Disease	Respiratory
Mental Illness: General	Behavioral
Mental Illness: Depression	Behavioral
Mental Illness: Schizophrenia	Behavioral
Migraine	Cardiovascular, Nervous
Multiple Sclerosis	Nervous
Muscular Dystrophy	Nervous
Myasthenia Gravis	Nervous
Neurofibromatosis	Nervous, Dermatologic
Osteogenesis Imperfecta	Skeletal
Osteoporosis	Skeletal
Paget Disease	Skeletal
Parkinson Disease	Nervous
Post-Polio Syndrome	Muscular, Skeletal
Post-Traumatic Stress Disorder	Nervous
Prader Willi Syndrome	Endocrine
Raynaud's Disease	Cardiovascular
Sarcoidosis	Cells & Tissues, Respiratory
Scleroderma	Cells & Tissues, Dermatologic
Scoliosis	Skeletal
Seizure Disorders	Nervous
Sexually Transmitted Diseases	Reproductive, Infectious Disease
Sickle Cell Disease	Blood
Sjogren's Syndrome	Cells & Tissues
Skin Disorders	Dermatologic
Sleep Disorders	Nervous
Spina Bifida	Nervous, Skeletal
Spinal Cord Injuries	Nervous
Stroke	Nervous
Substance Abuse Disorder	Behavioral
Systemic Lupus Erythematosus	Cells & Tissues
Tay-Sachs Disease	Nervous
Thyroid Disease	Endocrine
Tick-Borne Disease	Infectious Disease
Tourette Syndrome	Nervous
Tuberculosis	Respiratory, Infectious Disease
Tuberous Sclerosis Complex	Nervous, Dermatologic
Turner Syndrome	Endocrine
Ulcerative Colitis	Gastrointestinal
Visual Impairment	Sensory
War Syndromes	Nervous
Wilson Disease	Gastrointestinal

By Body System/Disorder Category

Behavioral
Attention Deficit Disorder; Autism; Eating Disorders; Mental Illness; Substance Abuse Disorder

Blood
Cooley's Anemia; Hemophilia; Sickle Cell Disease

Cardiovascular
Heart Disease; Hypertension; Migraine; Raynaud's Disease

Cells & Tissues
Aging; Scleroderma; Sjogren's Syndrome; Systemic Lupus Erythematosus

Dermatologic
Neurofibromatosis; Scleroderma; Skin Disorders; Tuberous Sclerosis Complex

Developmental
Attention Deficit Disorder; Autism; Down Syndrome; Growth Disorders

Endocrine
Addison Disease and Adrenal Insufficiency; Diabetes; Turner Syndrome

Gastrointestinal
Celiac Disease; Crohn Disease; Cystic Fibrosis; Fabry Disease; Gastrointestinal Disorders; Gaucher's Disease; Kidney Disease; Liver Disease; Ulcerative Colitis

Immune
AIDS; Allergies; Chronic Fatigue Syndrome

Infectious Disease
AIDS; Hepatitis; Sexually Transmitted Diseases; Tick-Borne Disease; Tuberculosis

Muscular
Arthritis; Carpal Tunnel Syndrome; Cerebral Palsy; Fibromyalgia Syndrome; Post-Polio Syndrome

Nervous
Agent Orange Related Injuries; Alzheimer's Disease; Amyotrophic Lateral Sclerosis; Ataxia; Brain Tumors; Carpal Tunnel Syndrome; Cerebral Palsy; Charcot-Marie-Tooth Disorder; Chronic Pain; GulfWar Syndrome; Head Injuries; Hydrocephalus; Multiple Sclerosis; Muscular Dystrophy; Myasthenia Gravis; Neurofibromatosis; Parkinson Disease; Post-Traumatic Stress Disorder; Seizure Disorders; Spina Bifida; Spinal Cord Injuries; Stroke; Tourette Syndrome; Tuberous Sclerosis Complex

Reproductive
Endometriosis; Impotence; Infertility; Sexually Transmitted Diseases

Respiratory
Asthma; Cystic Fibrosis; Lung Disease; Tuberculosis

Skeletal
Arthritis; Carpal Tunnel Syndrome; Fibromyalgia Syndrome; Osteognesis Imperfecta; Osteoporosis; Paget Disease; Post-Polio Syndrome; Scoliosis; Spina Bifida

Sensory
Hearing Impairment; Visual Impairment

Urinary
Incontinence

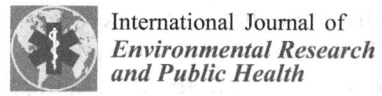
International Journal of
*Environmental Research
and Public Health*

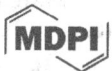

Article

An Empirical Study of Chronic Diseases in the United States: A Visual Analytics Approach to Public Health

Wullianallur Raghupathi [1] and Viju Raghupathi [2,*

[1]   Gabelli School of Business, Fordham University, New York, NY 10023, USA; Raghupathi@fordham.edu
[2]   Koppelman School of Business, Brooklyn College of the City University of New York,
      Brooklyn, NY 11210, USA
*   Correspondence: Vraghupathi@brooklyn.cuny.edu; Tel.: +1-(718)-951-5000

Received: 12 January 2018; Accepted: 27 February 2018; Published: 1 March 2018

Abstract: In this research we explore the current state of chronic diseases in the United States, using data from the Centers for Disease Control and Prevention and applying visualization and descriptive analytics techniques. Five main categories of variables are studied, namely chronic disease conditions, behavioral health, mental health, demographics, and overarching conditions. These are analyzed in the context of regions and states within the U.S. to discover possible correlations between variables in several categories. There are widespread variations in the prevalence of diverse chronic diseases, the number of hospitalizations for specific diseases, and the diagnosis and mortality rates for different states. Identifying such correlations is fundamental to developing insights that will help in the creation of targeted management, mitigation, and preventive policies, ultimately minimizing the risks and costs of chronic diseases. As the population ages and individuals suffer from multiple conditions, or comorbidity, it is imperative that the various stakeholders, including the government, non-governmental organizations (NGOs), policy makers, health providers, and society as a whole, address these adverse effects in a timely and efficient manner.

Keywords: behavioral health; chronic disease; comorbidity; overarching condition; population health; preventive health

---

1. Introduction

A chronic condition "is a physical or mental health condition that lasts more than one year and causes functional restrictions or requires ongoing monitoring or treatment" [1,2]. Chronic diseases are among the most prevalent and costly health conditions in the United States. Nearly half (approximately 45%, or 133 million) of all Americans suffer from at least one chronic disease [3–5], and the number is growing. Chronic diseases—including, cancer, diabetes, hypertension, stroke, heart disease, respiratory diseases, arthritis, obesity, and oral diseases—can lead to hospitalization, long-term disability, reduced quality of life, and death [6,7]. In fact, persistent conditions are the nation's leading cause of death and disability [6].

Globally, chronic diseases have affected the health and quality of life of many citizens [8,9]. In addition, chronic diseases have been a major driver of health care costs while also impacting workforce patterns, including, of course, absenteeism. According to the Centers for Disease Control, in the U.S. alone, chronic diseases account for nearly 75 percent of aggregate healthcare spending, or an estimated $5300 per person annually. In terms of public insurance, treatment of chronic diseases comprises an even larger proportion of spending: 96 cents per dollar for Medicare and 83 cents per dollar for Medicaid [4,10–12]. Thus, the understanding, management, and prevention of chronic diseases are important objectives if, as a society, we are to provide better quality healthcare to citizens and improve their overall quality of life.

An Empirical Study of Chronic Diseases in the United States

More than two thirds of all deaths are caused by one or more of these five chronic diseases: heart disease, cancer, stroke, chronic obstructive pulmonary disease, and diabetes. Additional statistics are quite stark [5,13]: chronic diseases are responsible for seven out of 10 deaths in the U.S., killing more than 1.7 million Americans each year; and more than 75% of the $2 trillion spent on public and private healthcare in 2005 went toward chronic diseases [5]. What makes treating chronic conditions (and efforts to manage population health) particularly challenging is that chronic conditions often do not exist in isolation. In fact, today one in four U.S. adults have two or more chronic conditions [5], while more than half of older adults have three or more chronic conditions. And the likelihood of these types of comorbidities occurring goes up as we age [5]. Given America's current demographics, wherein 10,000 Americans will turn 65 each day from now through the end of 2029 [5], it is reasonable to expect that the overall number of patients with comorbidities will increase greatly.

Trends show an overall increase in chronic diseases. Currently, the top ten health problems in America (not all of them chronic) are heart disease, cancer, stroke, respiratory disease, injuries, diabetes, Alzheimer's disease, influenza and pneumonia, kidney disease, and septicemia [14–18]. The nation's aging population, coupled with existing risk factors (tobacco use, poor nutrition, lack of physical activity) and medical advances that extend longevity (if not also improve overall health), have led to the conclusion that these problems are only going to magnify if not effectively addressed now [19].

A recent Milken Institute analysis determined that treatment of the seven most common chronic diseases coupled with productivity losses will cost the U.S. economy more than $1 trillion dollars annually. Furthermore, compared with other developed nations, the U.S. has ranked poorly on cost and outcomes. This is predominantly because of our inability to effectively manage chronic disease. And yet the same Milken analysis estimates that modest reductions in unhealthy behaviors could prevent or delay 40 million cases of chronic illness per year [11]. If we learn how to effectively manage chronic conditions, thus avoiding hospitalizations and serious complications, the healthcare system can improve quality of life for patients and greatly reduce the ballooning cost burden we all share [10].

The success of population health and chronic disease management efforts hinges on a few key elements: identifying those at risk, having access to the right data about this population, creating actionable insights about patients, and coaching them toward healthier choices. Methods such as data-driven visual analytics help experts analyze large amounts of data and gain insights for making informed decisions regarding chronic diseases [10,20]. According to the U.S.-based Institute of Medicine and the National Research, the vision for 21st century healthcare includes increased attention to cognitive support in decision making [21]. This encompasses computer-based tools and techniques that aid comprehension and cognition. Visualization techniques offer cognitive support by offering mental models of the information through a visual interface [22]. They combine statistical methods and models with advanced interactive visualization methods to help mask the underlying complexity of large health data sets and make evidence-based decisions [23]. Chronic diseases are characterized by high prevalence among populations, rising complication rates, and increased incidence of people with multiple chronic conditions, to name a few. In this scenario, visualization can represent association between preventive measures and disease control, summary health dimensions across diverse patient populations and, timeline of disease prevalence across regions/populations, to offer actionable insights for effective population management and national development [24]. Additionally, visual techniques offer the ability to analyze data at multiple levels and dimensions starting from population to subpopulation to the individual [25]. This paper addresses the challenge of understanding large amounts of data related to chronic diseases by applying visual analytics techniques and producing descriptive analytics. Our overall goal is to gain insight into the data and make policy recommendations.

Given that large segments of the U.S. population suffer from one or more chronic disease conditions, a data-driven approach to the analysis of the data has the potential to reveal patterns of association, correlation, and causality. We therefore studied the variables extracted from a highly reliable source, the Centers for Disease Control. Data for variables pertaining to several categories, namely chronic condition ("condition" is used interchangeably with "disease"), behavioral health, mental health, preventive health, demographics, overarching conditions, and location for several years (typically 2012 to 2014). We analyzed relationships within each category and across categories to obtain multi-dimensional views and insight into the data. The analytics provide insights and implications that suggest ways for the healthcare system to better manage population health.

This paper is organized as follows: Section 1 offers an introduction to the research, Section 2 discusses the methodology, Section 3 presents and discusses the visual charts and results, Section 4 contains the scope and limitations of the research, Section 5 describes the policy implications and future research, and Section 6 presents our conclusions.

2. Materials and Methods

This study analyzes the characteristics of chronic diseases in the U.S. and explores the relationships between demographics, behavior habits, and other health conditions and chronic diseases, thereby revealing information for public health practice at the state-specific level. In this data-driven study we use visual analytics [26], conducting primarily descriptive analytics [20] to obtain a panoramic insight into the chronic diseases data set pulled from the Centers for Disease Control and Prevention web site. The discipline of visual analytics aims to provide researchers and policymakers with better and more effective ways to understand and analyze large data sets, while also enabling them to act upon their findings in real time. Visual analytics integrates the analytic capabilities of the computer and the abilities of human analysts, thus inviting novel discoveries and empowering individuals to take control of the analytical process. It sheds light on unexpected and hidden insights, which may lead to beneficial and profitable innovation [27,28]. Driving visual analytics is the aim of turning information overload into opportunity; just as information visualization has changed our view on databases, the goal of visual analytics is to make our way of processing data and information transparent and accessible for analytic discourse. The visualization of these processes provides the means for examining the actual processes and not just the results. Visual analytics applies such technology as business intelligence (BI) tools to combine human analytical skill with computing power. Clearly, this research is highly interdisciplinary, involving such areas as visualization, data mining, data management, data fusion, statistics, and cognitive science, among others. One key understanding of visual analytics is that the integration of these diverse areas is a scientific discipline in its own right [29,30].

Historically, automatic analysis techniques, such as statistics and data mining, were developed independently of visualization and interaction techniques. One of the most important steps in the direction of visual analytics research was the need to move from confirmatory data analysis (using charts and other visual representations to present results) to exploratory data analysis (interacting with the data), first introduced to the statistics research community by John W. Tukey in his book, *Exploratory Data Analysis* [31].

With improvements in graphical user interfaces and interaction devices, the research community devoted its efforts to information visualization [27]. Eventually, this community recognized the potential of integrating the user's perspective into the knowledge discovery and data mining process through effective and efficient visualization techniques, interaction capabilities, and knowledge transfer. This led to visual data exploration and visual data mining [29] and widened considerably the scope of applications of visualization, statistics, and data mining—the three pillars of analytics. In visual analytics is defined as "the science of analytical reasoning facilitated by interactive human-machine interfaces" [29]. A more current definition says "visual analytics combines automated analysis techniques with interactive visualizations for an effective understanding reasoning and decision-making on the basis of very large and complex data sets" (both reported in [27]). In their book *Illuminating the Path*, Thomas and Cook define visual analytics as the science of analytical reasoning facilitated by interactive visual interfaces.

One application of visualization is descriptive analytics, the most commonly used and most well understood type of analytics. It was the earliest to be introduced and the easiest by far to implement and understand in that it describes data "as is" without complex calculations. Descriptive analytics is more data-driven than other models. Most health data analyses start with descriptive analytics, using data to understand past and current health patterns and trends and to make informed decisions [20]. The models in descriptive analytics categorize, characterize, aggregate, and classify data, converting it into information for understanding and analyzing business decisions, outcomes, and quality. Such data summaries can be in the form of meaningful charts and reports, and responses to queries using SQL. Descriptive analytics uses a significant amount of visualization. One could, for example, obtain standard and customized reports and drill down into the data, running queries to better understand, say, the sales of a product [20]. Descriptive analytics helps answer such questions as: How many patients with diabetes also have obesity? Which of the chronic diseases are more prevalent in different regions of the country? What behavioral habits are correlated to the chronic diseases? Which groups of patients suffer from more than one chronic condition? Is there an association between health insurance (and lack thereof) and chronic diseases? What are cost trade-offs between chronic disease prevention and management? What are typical patient profiles for various chronic diseases?

This study concentrates on chronic condition indicators and related demographics, behavior habits, preventive health, and oral health factors. As mentioned, the data source for this study is the Center for Disease Control and Prevention (CDC) [32]. The CDC's Division of Population Health offers a crosscutting set of 124 indicators that were developed by consensus. Those indicators are integrated from multiple resources, with the help of the Chronic Disease Indicator web site, which serves as a gateway to additional information and data sources. In this research we downloaded secondary data for the United States from the CDC dataset, for the years 2012 to 2014. The data is for states, territories, and large metropolitan areas in the U.S., including the 50 states and District of Columbia, Guam, Puerto Rico, and the U.S. Virgin Islands. Data cleaning, integration, and transformation were conducted on the raw data set. The main categories of variables included—chronic condition, mental health, behavior habits, preventative health, and demographics. In addition, overarching conditions and location were also studied. Table 1 summarizes the categories and variables.

Table 1. Chronic diseases and related indicators.

Category	Sub-Category	Variables (Measure)	Definition
Chronic condition	Diabetes	Diabetes (%)	Prevalence of diagnosed diabetes among adults aged ≥18 years—2012–2014
		Hospital diabetes (number)	Hospitalization with diabetes as diagnosis; 2010 and 2013
		Mortality diabetes (per 100,000)	Mortality rate due to diabetes listed as cause of death, 2010–2014
	Arthritis	Arthritis (%)	Prevalence of arthritis among adults aged ≥18 years; 2013–2014
		Fair or poor health—arthritis (%)	Prevalence of fair or poor health among adults aged ≥18 years with arthritis—2013–2014
		Obesity—arthritis (%)	Prevalence of Arthritis among adults aged ≥18 years who are obese—2013–2014
	Asthma	Asthma (%)	Current asthma prevalence among adults aged ≥18 years, through 2012–2014
		Mortality—asthma (case per 100,000)	Asthma mortality rate through 2010–2014
		Hospital—asthma (case per 100,000)	Hospitalizations for Asthma
	Chronic Kidney Disease	Kidney (%)	Prevalence of chronic kidney disease among adults aged ≥18 years—2012–2014
		Mortality—kidney (case per 100,000)	Mortality with end stage renal disease, through 2010 to 2014
	Chronic Obstructive Pulmonary Disease	Pulmonary (%)	Prevalence of chronic obstructive pulmonary disease among adults aged ≥18 years, through 2012 to 2014
		Hospital—pulmonary (case per 100,000)	Hospitalization for chronic obstructive pulmonary disease as any diagnosis of 2010 and 2013
		Mortality—pulmonary (case per 100,000)	Mortality with chronic obstructive pulmonary disease as underlying cause among adults aged ≥45 years, through 2010 and 2014.

Table 1. *Cont.*

Category	Sub-Category	Variables (Measure)	Definition
Mental health	Mental health	Mental—women (%)	The crude prevalence rate of at least 14 recent mentally unhealthy days among women aged 18–44 years, through 2012 to 2014
		Postpartum (%)	The crude prevalence rate of Postpartum depressive symptoms in 2011
		Mental (number)	The aged-adjusted mean of recently mentally unhealthy days among adults aged $\geq$18 years, through 2012 to 2014
Behavioral Habits	Alcohol	Binge drink (%)	Binge drinking prevalence among adults aged $\geq$18 years, through 2012 to 2014
		Heavy drink (%)	Heavy drinking among adults aged $\geq$18 years, through 2012 to 2014
	Nutrition, Physical Activity, and Weight Status	Physical activity (%)	No leisure-time physical activity among adults aged $\geq$18 years, through 2012 to 2014
		Tobacco—smokeless (%)	Current smokeless tobacco use among adults aged $\geq$18 years, through 2012 to 2014
		Tobacco (%)	Current smoking among adults aged $\geq$18 years, through 2012 to 2014
		Obesity (%)	Obesity among adults aged $\geq$18 years, through 2012 to 2014
Preventive health	Pneumococcal vaccination	Pneumonia—smoke (%)	Pneumococcal vaccination among noninstitutionalized adults aged 18–64 years who smoke, through 2012 to 2014
		Pneumonia—heart (%)	Pneumococcal vaccination among noninstitutionalized adults aged 18–64 years with a history of coronary heart disease, through 2012 to 2014
		Pneumonia—asthma (%)	Pneumococcal vaccination among noninstitutionalized adults aged 18–64 years with asthma, through 2012 to 2014
		Pneumonia—diabetes (%)	Pneumococcal vaccination among noninstitutionalized adults aged 18–64 years with diagnosed diabetes, through 2012 to 2014
	Immunization	Influenza—asthma (%)	Influenza vaccination among noninstitutionalized adults aged 18–64 years with asthma, through 2012 to 2014;
		Influenza—diabetes (%)	Influenza vaccination among noninstitutionalized adults aged 18–64 years with diagnosed diabetes, through 2012 to 2014
		Influenza—heart (%)	Influenza vaccination among noninstitutionalized adults aged 18–64 years with a history of coronary heart disease or stroke
		Influenza (%)	Influenza vaccination among noninstitutionalized adults aged $\geq$18 years, through 2012 to 2014
	Smoke	Quit (number)	Quit attempts in the past year among current smokers, through 2012 to 2014
Demographics	Gender	Gender (character)	Male and female
	Ethnicity	Race (character)	Race
Location	State location	Location (character)	50 states and District of Columbia, Guam, Puerto Rico, Virgin Islands
Overarching Conditions	Overarching Conditions	Insurance (%)	Current lack of health insurance among adults aged 18–64 years, through 2012 to 2014
		Poor—self rate (%)	Fair or poor self-rated health status among adults aged $\geq$18 years
		Sleep (%)	Prevalence of sufficient sleep among adults aged $\geq$18 years

3. Results

We use visualization and descriptive analytics to explore chronic conditions, preventive healthcare, mental health, and overarching conditions, with the objective of deciphering relationships and patterns that emerge from the visualization. We would like to point out that since our sample includes adults aged 18 and over our results are applicable for adults in that age group.

Figure 1 models the average prevalence of diagnosed diabetes among adults aged $\geq$18 years in the period 2012 to 2014. Puerto Rico leads the pack, followed by Mississippi.

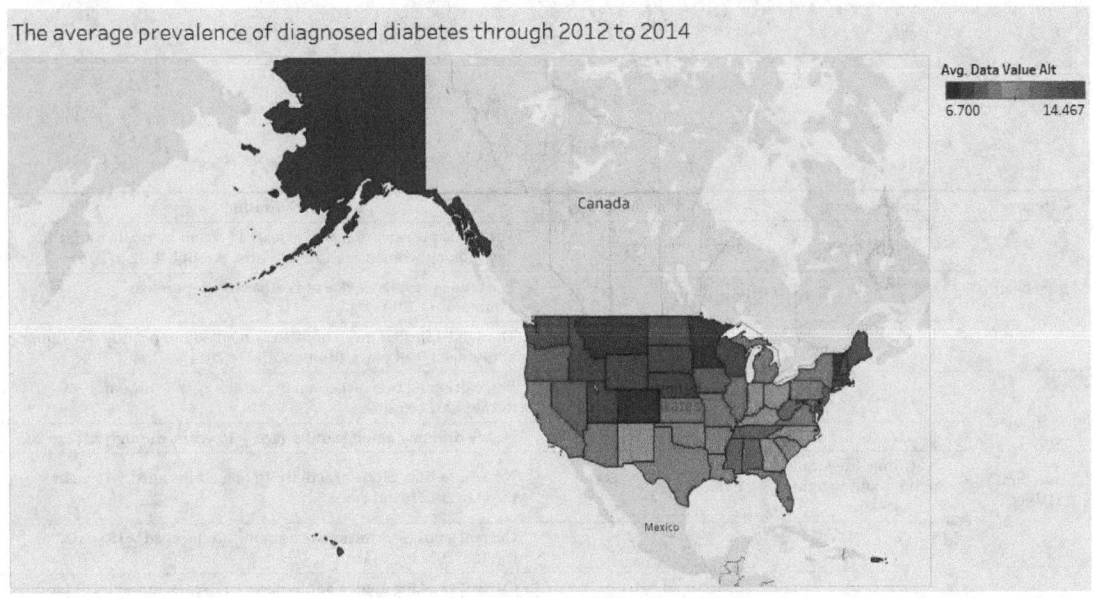

Figure 1. Diabetes by state.

As Figure 2 below shows, Puerto Rico has the highest number of citizens among adults aged ≥18 years, in fair or poor health with arthritis for the period 2013 to 2014. Puerto Rico is followed by Tennessee and Mississippi.

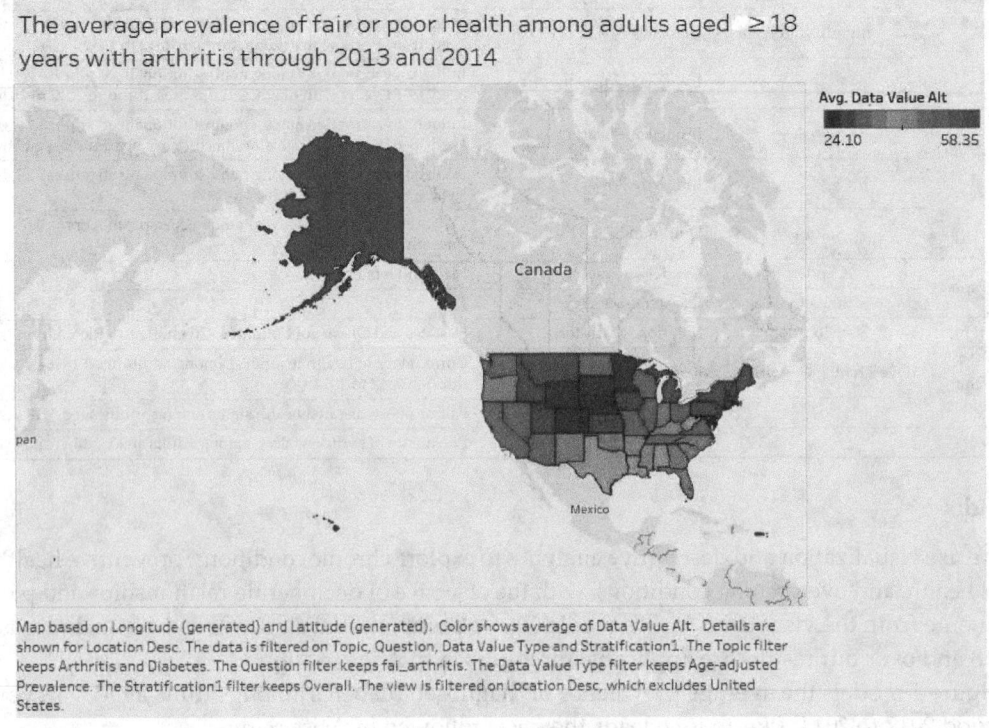

Figure 2. Arthritis by state.

The current asthma prevalence among adults aged ≥18 years for the period 2012 to 2014 is indicated in Figure 3. West Virginia has a higher prevalence of the condition compared to other states.

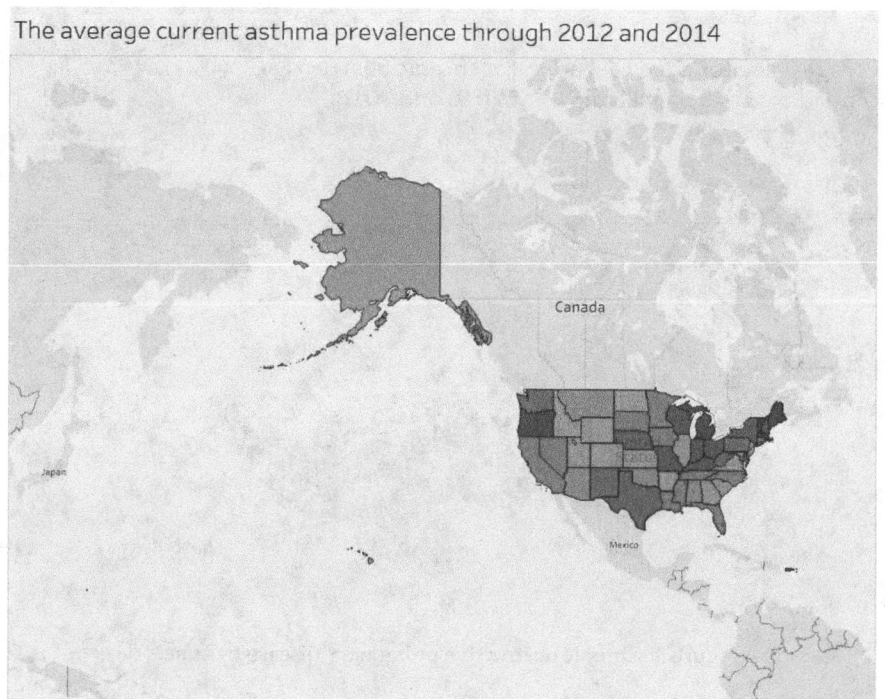

The average current asthma prevalence through 2012 and 2014

Figure 3. Asthma by state.

With regard to end-stage renal disease, Figure 4 shows that the condition is dispersed widely among various areas.

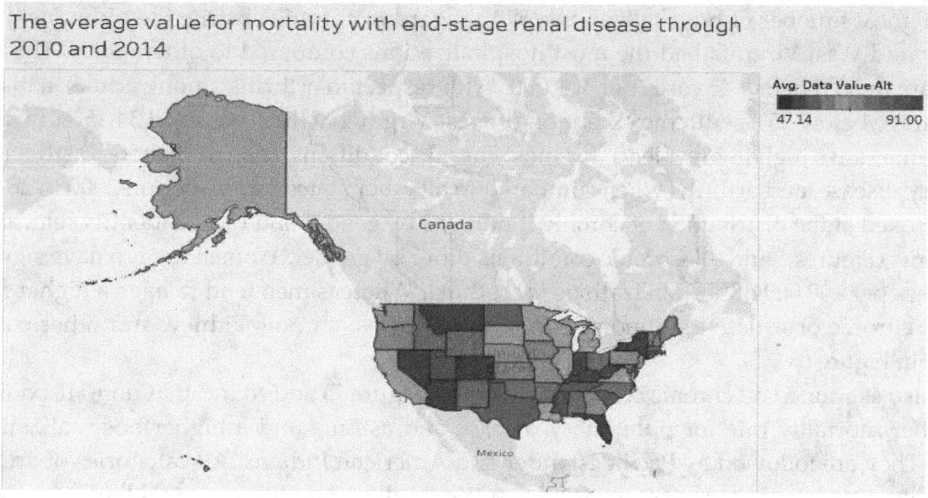

The average value for mortality with end-stage renal disease through 2010 and 2014

Avg. Data Value Alt
47.14   91.00

Figure 4. End-stage renal disease by region.

The average value for hospitalization for chronic obstructive pulmonary disease for all diagnoses between 2010 and 2013 is shown in Figure 5. Kentucky and West Virginia have higher hospitalizations compared to other states. Most of the areas are below 45 cases per 100,000.

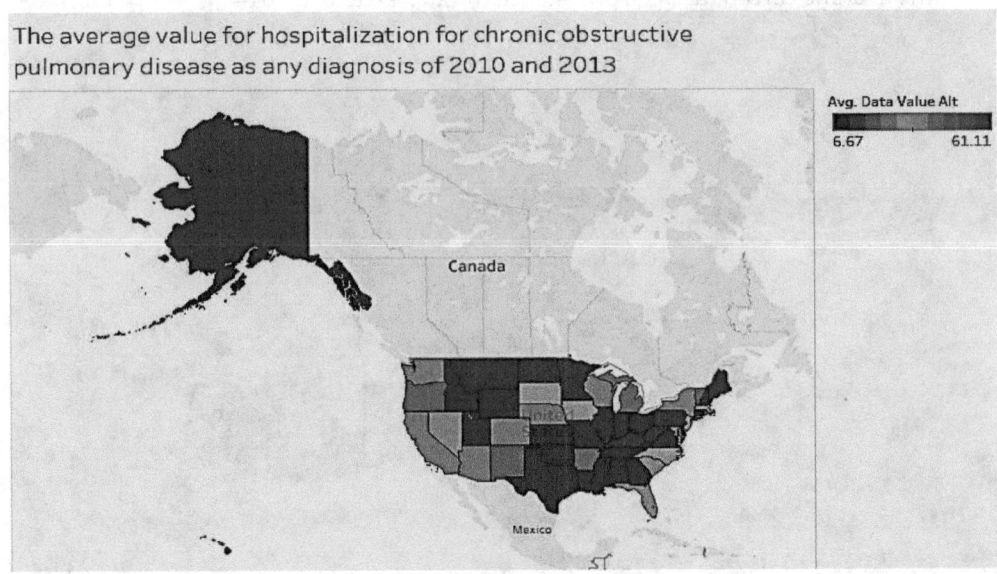

The average value for hospitalization for chronic obstructive pulmonary disease as any diagnosis of 2010 and 2013

Avg. Data Value Alt
6.67   61.11

Canada

Mexico

Figure 5. Chronic obstructive pulmonary disease by state.

In exploring chronic conditions by location in the U.S., we see that some conditions, such as diabetes, arthritis, and obstructive pulmonary diseases, are more prevalent in eastern states, while others, such as asthma, occur more often in northeastern states. For diabetes, listed as a cause of death for the years 2010 to 2014, the states of Oklahoma and West Virginia had the relatively high average threshold of over 100 (age adjusted rate per 100,000). In the case of asthma, West Virginia has the highest prevalence of the condition (among adults), while Maryland, Massachusetts, and New York had the highest number of hospitalizations. With regard to chronic obstructive pulmonary disease, Kentucky and West Virginia had the most hospitalizations compared to other states. The majority of states are indeed below 45 cases per 100,000. With respect to arthritis among adults, a majority of states average below 25%, with the exception of West Virginia, which averaged 34.15%. In summary, West Virginia ranks high in prevalence for most chronic conditions, such as diabetes, asthma, chronic pulmonary disease, and arthritis when compared to all other states for the period 2000 to 2014.

We looked at the distribution of chronic conditions by gender and race to identify relevant trends and patterns (Figures 6 and 7). Chronic conditions differ by gender. Women tend to have significantly higher cases per 100,000 of hospitalizations for asthma. Whereas men tend to have a higher mortality rate from chronic obstructive pulmonary disease, diabetes, chronic kidney, and other conditions, as shown in Figure 6.

We also examined all chronic conditions by race (Figure 7) and found that non-Hispanic Blacks have higher mortality rate for pulmonary disease and asthma and a higher hospitalization from diabetes. They are followed by Pacific Islander and American Indians. All categories of arthritis are fairly evenly distributed among Black, non-Hispanic, Multiracial, Whites, and other.

Females have a higher hospitalization rate for asthma (per 100,000), while in terms of mortality rate for chronic obstructive pulmonary disease, diabetes, and chronic kidney disease, males have the higher hospitalization rate. Again, American Indian or Alaskan Natives have higher mortality rate for chronic obstructive pulmonary disease, diabetes, and kidney disease. They're followed by Blacks and non-Hispanics.

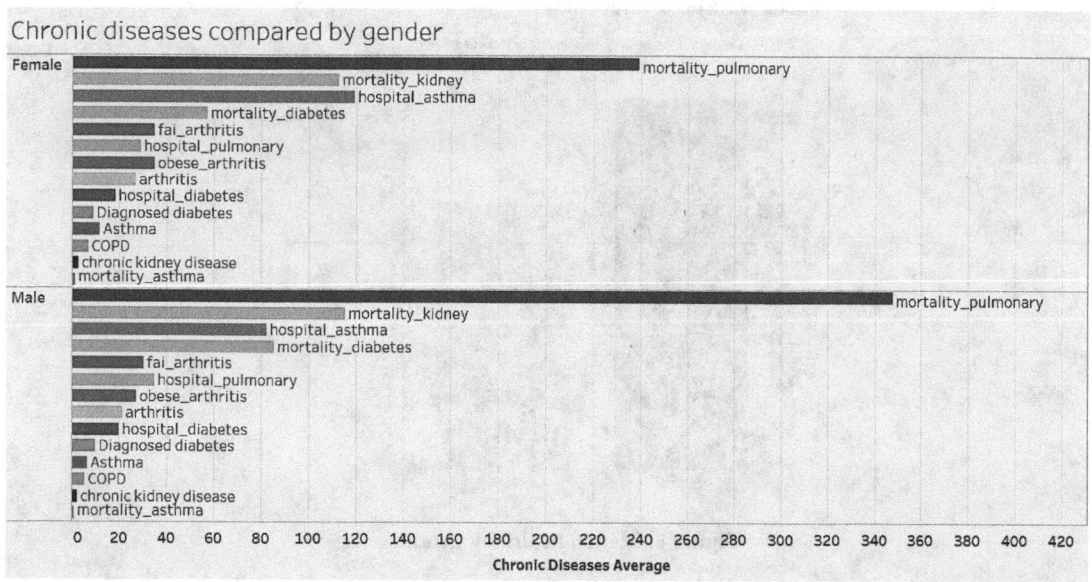

Figure 6. Chronic condition by gender.

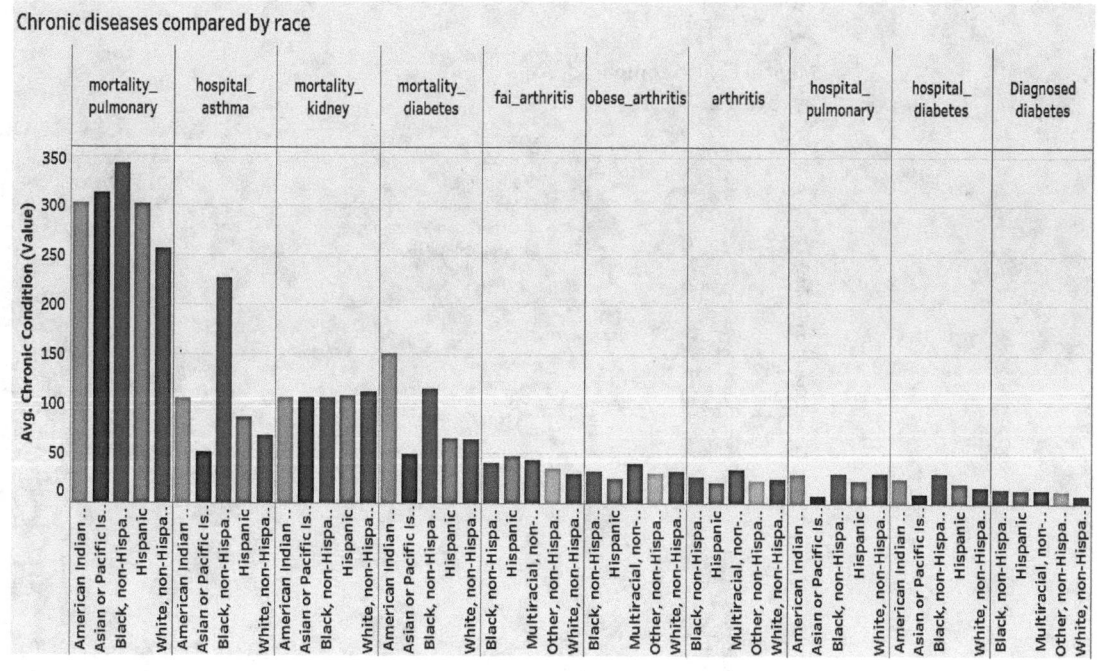

Figure 7. Chronic conditions by race.

3.1. Mental Health by Gender and Race

Mental health is an important aspect of national healthcare impacting chronic diseases. We analyzed mental health by gender (Figure 8) and by race (Figure 9). When we examine how many days an individual feels "mentally unhealthy" for the years 2012 to 2014, women are more likely to have more unhealthy days than men, as shown in Figure 8.

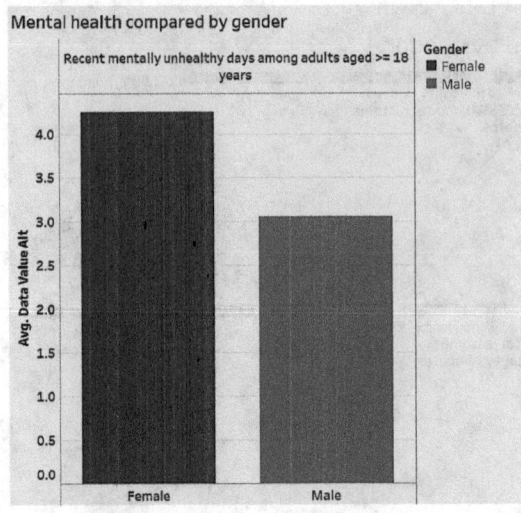

Figure 8. Mental health by gender.

Simultaneously, multi-racial, non-Hispanic women in the age group 18 to 44 have a higher crude prevalence rate of at least 14 recent "mentally unhealthy" days. This group is followed by black non-Hispanics.

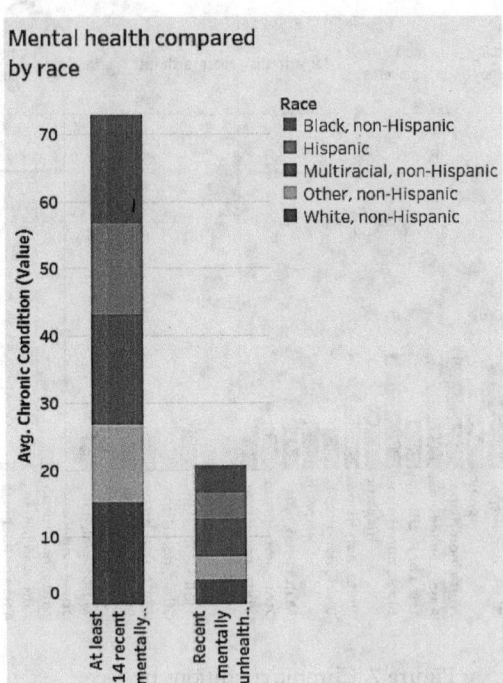

Figure 9. Mental health by race.

We then studied behavioral habits in the data set to gain insight into noticeable patterns, if in fact any exist.

3.2. Behavioral Habits by Gender and Race

Figure 10 charts behavioral habits by gender.

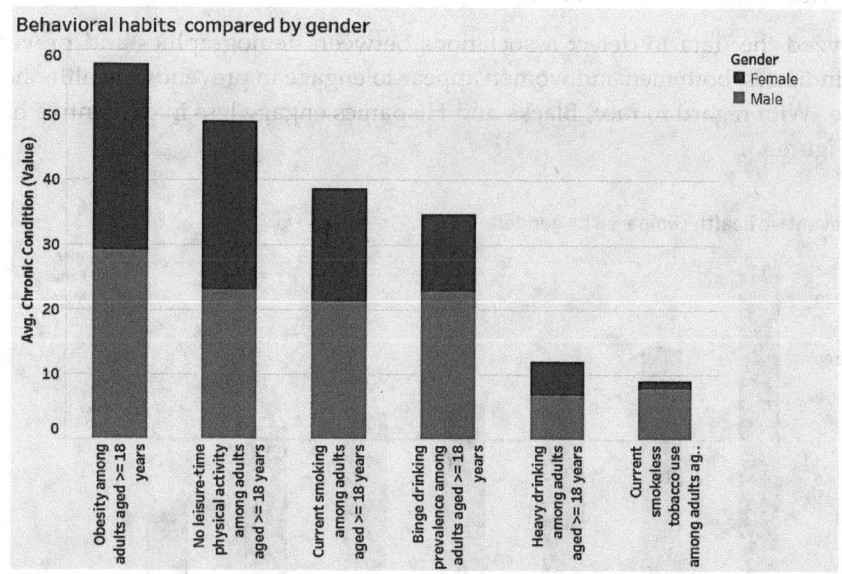

Figure 10. Behavioral habits by gender.

As seen in the chart above, men display higher numbers in the alcohol categories of "binge drinking" and "heavy drinking", as well as in "current smokeless" tobacco use among adults. In terms of engaging in "current smoking", "obesity", and "no leisure-time" physical activity, both men and women experience similar complications, that highlights the need for positive behavior modification.

Figure 11 illustrates the analysis of behavioral habits by race.

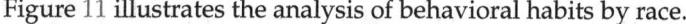

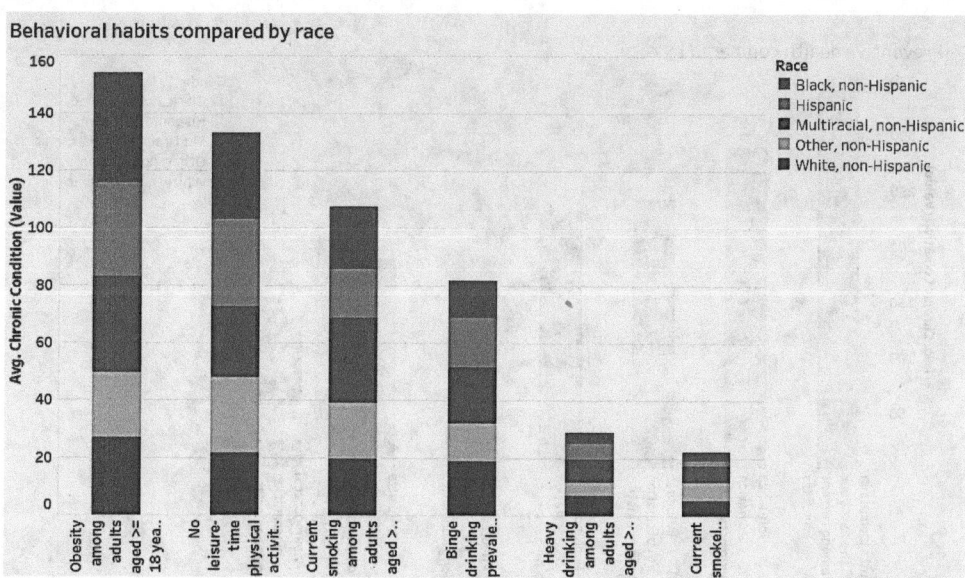

Figure 11. Behavioral habits by race.

Figure 11 reveals that for the behavioral habits of "obesity" and "no leisure-time" physical activity among adults aged 18 and over, the black non-Hispanic and Hispanic races have the highest frequency, while white non-Hispanics have the lowest. By and large, in most behavioral habits, the other non-Hispanics have the lowest frequency.

3.3. Preventive Health and Chronic Conditions

We analyzed the data to detect associations between demographics and preventive health. As Figure 12 indicates, both men and women appear to engage in preventive health, though women have the edge. With regard to race, Blacks and Hispanics engage less in preventive health overall, as shown in Figure 13.

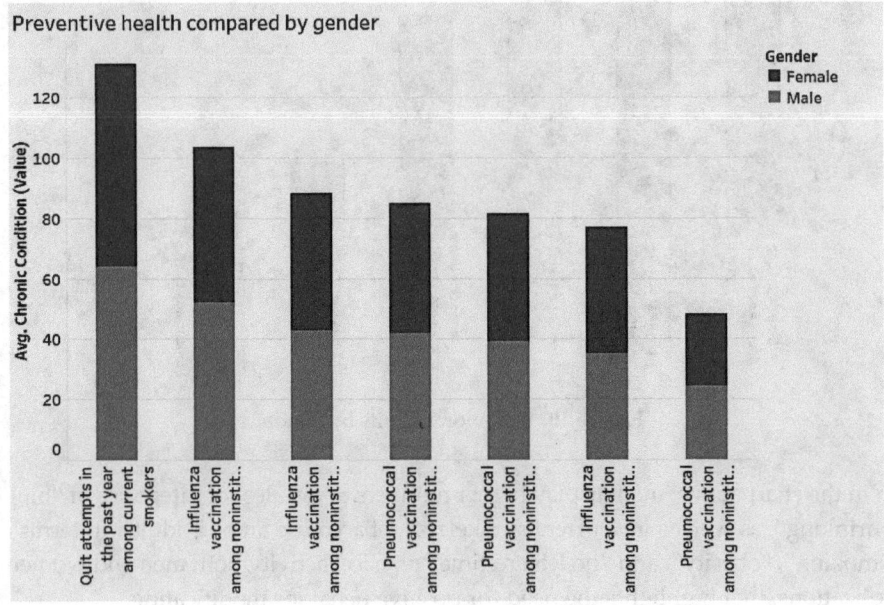

Figure 12. Preventive health by gender.

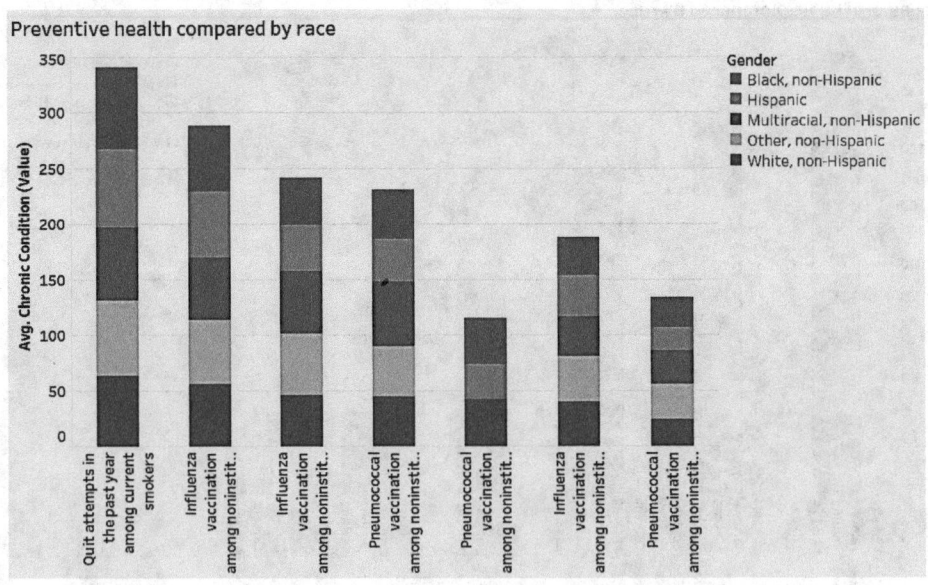

Figure 13. Preventive health by race.

While all chronic conditions are debilitating on the economy, for the sake of scope, we selectively analyze the influence of a few conditions such as diabetes and asthma. By 2034, the population with diabetes is expected to increase by 100% and the cost expected to increase by 53% [33]. Figure 14 depicts the association between diabetes and pneumococcal vaccination for diabetes.

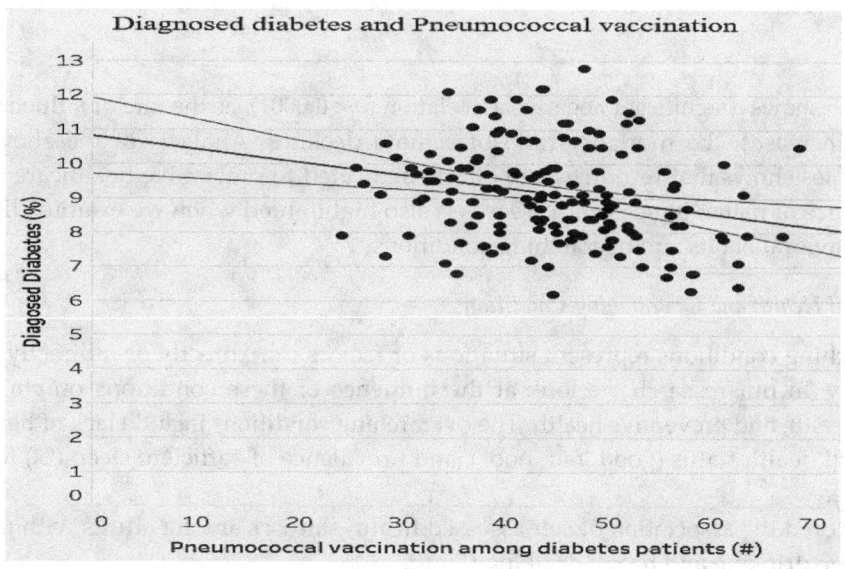

Figure 14. Diagnosed diabetes ratio by pneumococcal vaccination ratio. (#: number).

As indicated in Figure 14, there is a significant negative relationship between the average pneumococcal vaccination among diabetes patients and the average diagnosed diabetes ratio among the population ($p < 0.0001$). As the average pneumococcal vaccination among diabetes patients increases, the average diagnosed diabetes ratio decreases (fewer cases of diabetes). Given the importance of asthma as another prevalent chronic condition, we decided to analyze the relationship between the mortality ratio and influenza vaccinations for asthma to determine the efficiency of preventive measures (Figure 15).

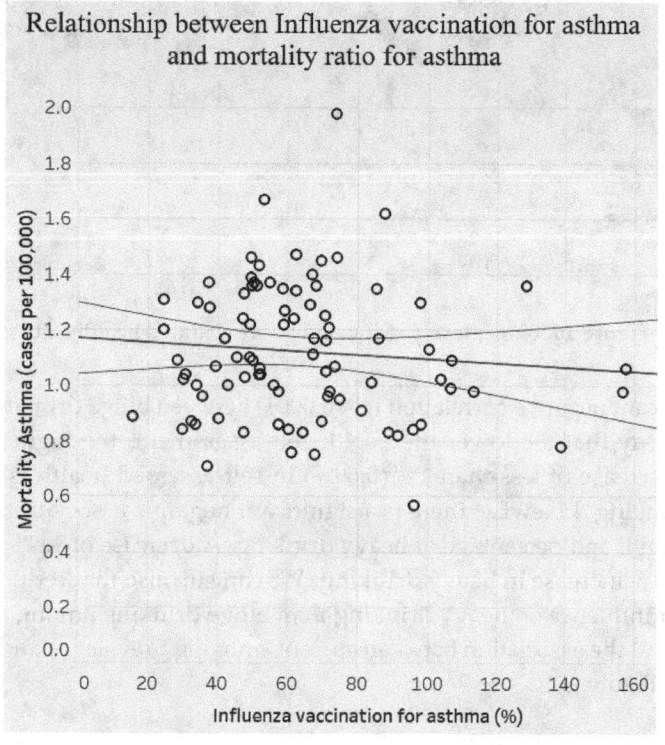

Figure 15. Mortality ratio for asthma and influenza vaccination for asthma.

Figure 15 shows a significant negative association ($p < 0.0001$): as the rate of influenza vaccination for asthma increases, the mortality ratio of asthma declines. Analysis of the above preventive health variables shows that resources and efforts dedicated to preventive healthcare offer promise. The importance of managing chronic diseases is also highlighted when we examine the association between behavioral habits and overarching conditions.

3.4. Behavioral Health and Overarching Conditions

Overarching conditions represent situations or factors that directly or indirectly influence the area of study. In our research we look at the influence of these conditions on chronic diseases, behavioral health, and preventive health. The overarching conditions include lack of health insurance (%), self-rated health status (good, fair, poor), and prevalence of sufficient sleep (%) for which data was available.

We explored the association of self-assessed health statuses among adults with the behavioral habits of binge drinking and heavy drinking (Figure 16).

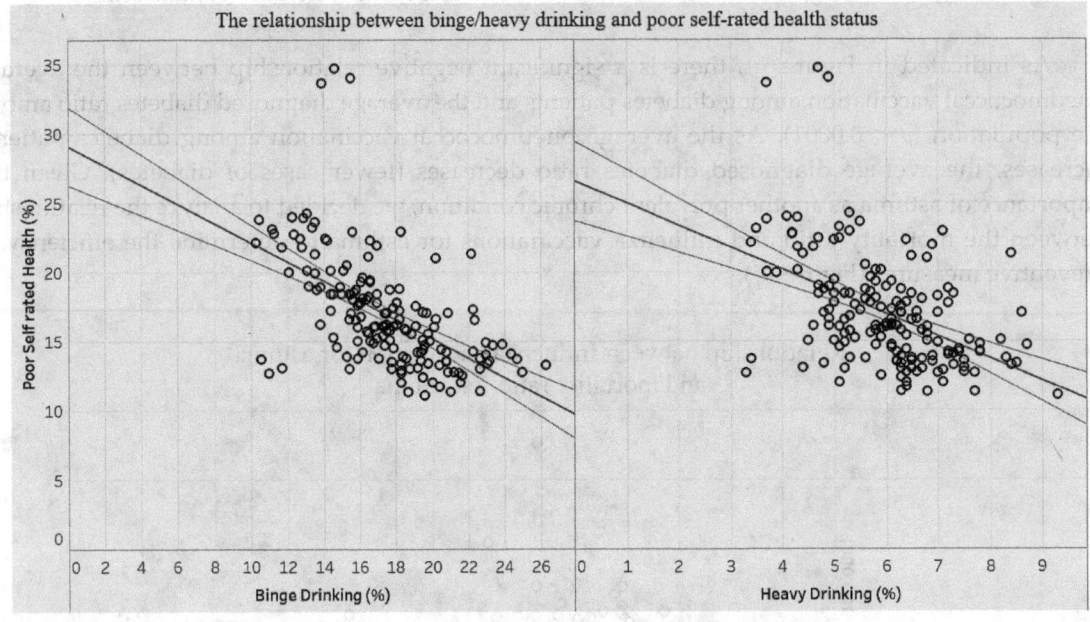

Figure 16. Binge/heavy drink and poor self-rated health status.

There is a significant negative correlation ($p < 0.0001$) between binge drinking and self-assessment of health. That is to say that the lower the health self-assessment, the higher is the percentage of binge drinking. A decrease of less than 1% (0.69%) in self-assessed health is associated with a 1% increase in binge drinking. Likewise, there is a significant negative association ($p < 0.0001$) between self-assessment of health and percentage of heavy drinking. A decrease of 1.6% in self-assessed health is associated with a 1% increase in heavy drinking. We can surmise that reduced self-assessment of health has a stronger influence on heavy drinking than binge drinking among adults.

Next, we looked at the association between current smoking prevalence and presence of sufficient sleep among adults (Figure 17).

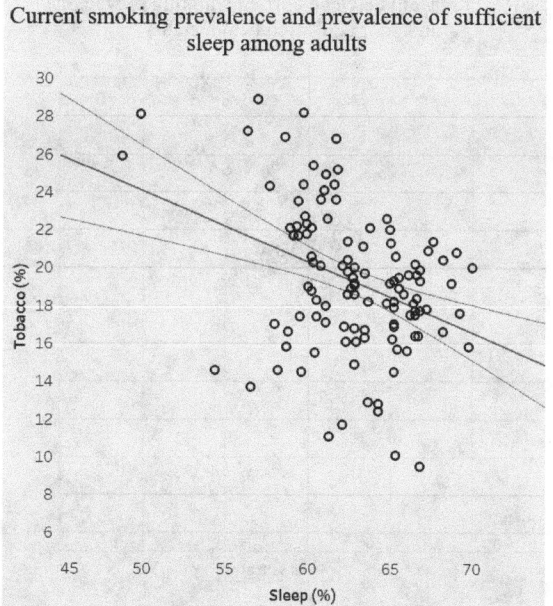

Figure 17. Current smoking prevalence by presence of sufficient sleep among adults.

Figure 17 above shows a significant negative association ($p < 0.0001$) between prevalence of current smoking and prevalence of sufficient sleep. When current smoking prevalence decreases by less than 1% (0.38%), the prevalence of sufficient sleep increases by 1%.

The relationship between poor self-rated health status and obesity is positive (Figure 18). The higher the prevalence of fair or poor self-rated health, the higher is the prevalence of obesity. When poor self-rated health increases by 1%, the prevalence of obesity increases by 0.468779%.

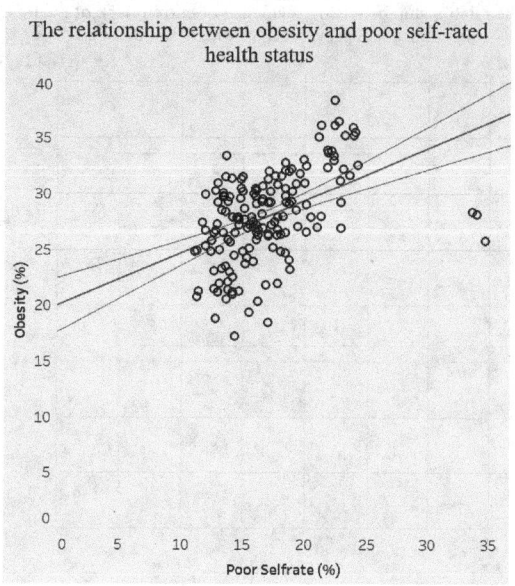

Figure 18. Obesity by poor self-rated health status.

Similarly, poor self-rated health has a positive association with current smoking, as indicated in Figure 19. As the prevalence of poor self-rated health increases by 1%, the prevalence of current smoking increases by 0.30425%.

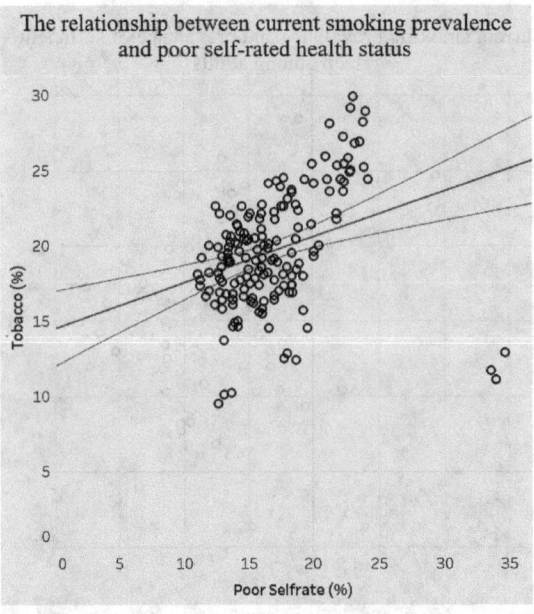

Figure 19. Smoking by self-rated health status.

3.5. Chronic Conditions and Overarching Conditions

In the analysis of various chronic conditions, there are significant clusters of conditions among men and women, such as the prevalence of asthma, with the women tending to have a higher prevalence of asthma than men. Regarding such chronic conditions as diabetes, there is a significant positive relationship ($p < 0.001$) between lack of health insurance and prevalence of diagnosed diabetes (Figure 20).

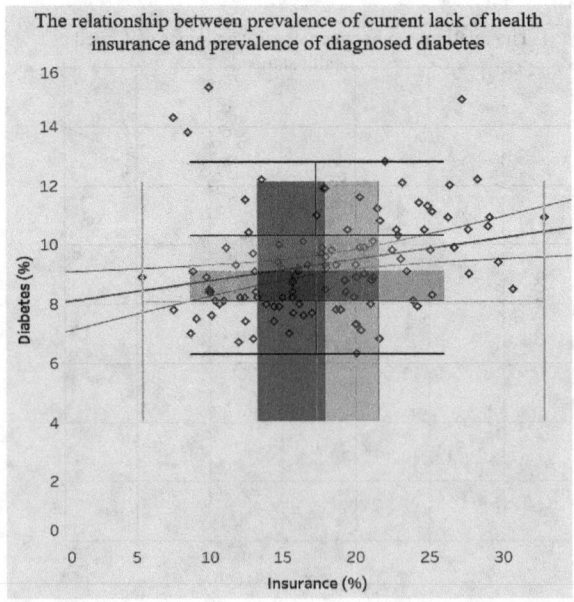

Figure 20. Current lack of health insurance by diagnosed diabetes.

We notice in Figure 20 that the distribution of lack of health insurance is sparse compared to that of diagnosed diabetes among adults aged 18 and older. Likewise, for chronic kidney disease (Figure 21) there is a significant positive relationship ($p < 0.0001$) with lack of health insurance.

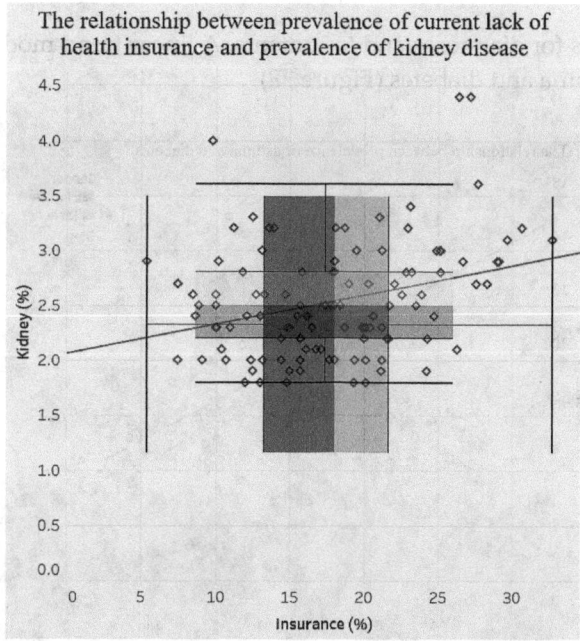

Figure 21. Lack of insurance by chronic kidney disease.

The relationship between lack of insurance and hospitalization for chronic pulmonary disease is positive and significant ($p < 0.0001$), as shown in Figure 22. An increase in the lack of insurance is associated with an increase in hospitalization for chronic pulmonary disease.

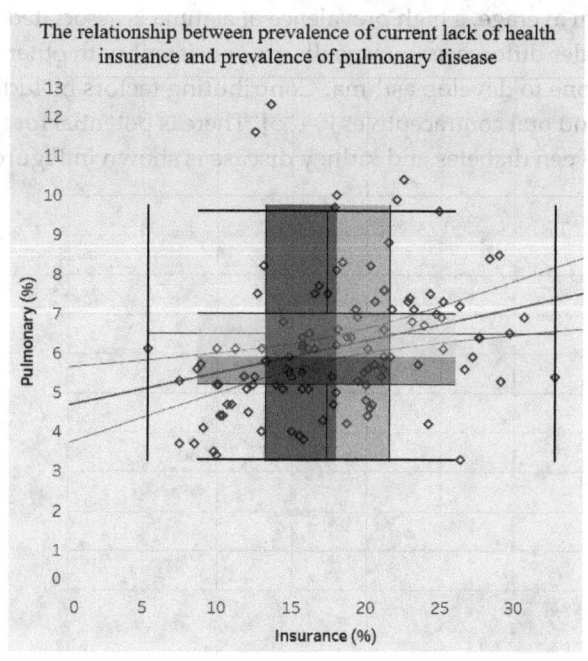

Figure 22. Lack of insurance by pulmonary disease.

3.6. Association between Chronic Conditions

We analyzed for any associations between different chronic conditions. It is important to incorporate gender as a factor in the association and prevalence of chronic diseases, so as to develop customized plans for diagnoses and treatments. A linear trend model was developed for the relationship between asthma and diabetes (Figure 23).

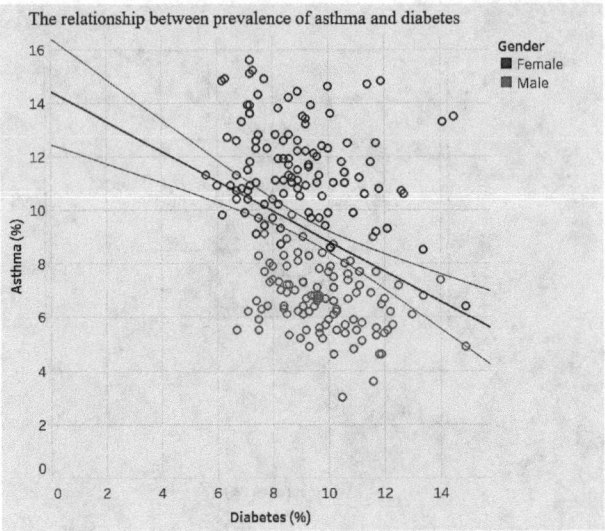

Figure 23. Asthma by diabetes.

The model in Figure 23 shows a significant negative relationship ($p < 0.01$) between asthma and diabetes. We can see gender clusters for the prevalence of asthma. Women tend to have higher prevalence of asthma compared to men. Overall, prevalence of asthma is negatively related to the prevalence of diabetes. On average, a high prevalence of asthma is associated with a low prevalence of diabetes. In terms of gender differences our results are consistent with other studies that have shown that women are more prone to develop asthma. Contributing factors include puberty, menstruation, pregnancy, menopause, and oral contraceptives [34,35]. There is potential for more research in this area.

The association between diabetes and kidney disease is shown in Figure 24.

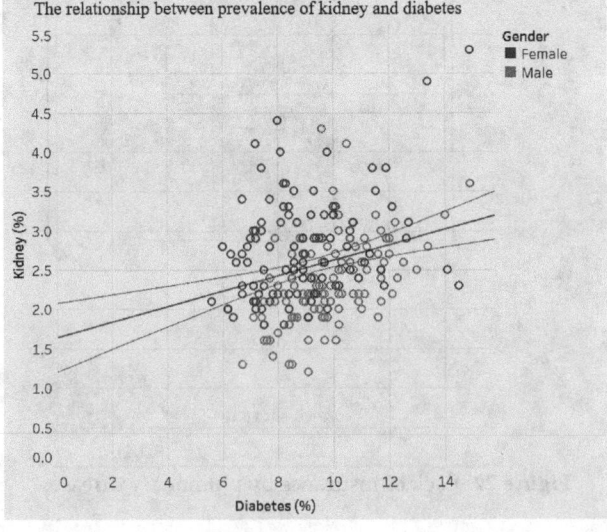

Figure 24. Diabetes by kidney disease.

Figure 24 shows a moderate, positive association ($p < 0.01$) between prevalence of kidney disease and diabetes. As the prevalence of diagnosed diabetes increases by 1%, the prevalence of chronic kidney disease increases by 0.09%. There are no obvious differences in gender here.

The association between diabetes and chronic pulmonary disease is shown in Figure 25, and that between arthritis and asthma is shown in Figure 26.

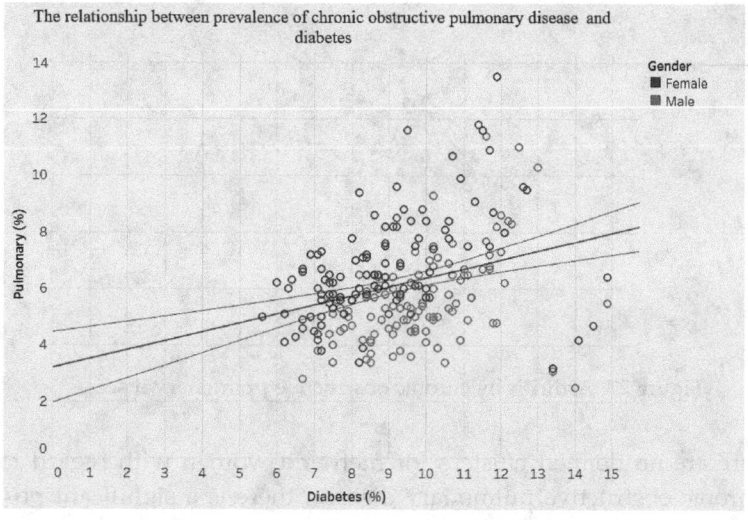

Figure 25. Diabetes by obstructive pulmonary disease.

In Figure 25, we find a significant positive association between diabetes and chronic pulmonary disease ($p < 0.001$).

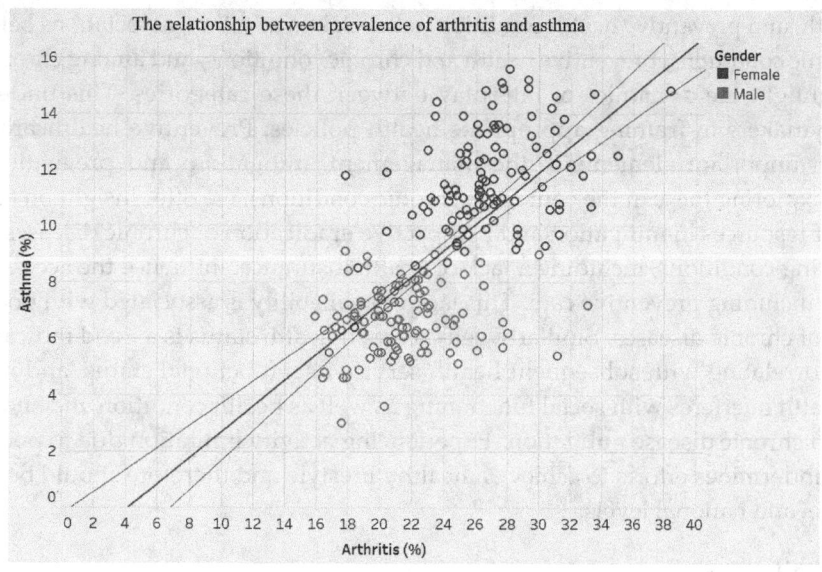

Figure 26. Arthritis by asthma.

When it comes to prevalence of arthritis and asthma, there clearly are clusters for men and women, as shown in Figure 26. There is a positive association such that an increase of 1% in prevalence of arthritis is associated with a 0.4% increase in prevalence of asthma.

Figure 27 shows the association between arthritis and chronic pulmonary disease.

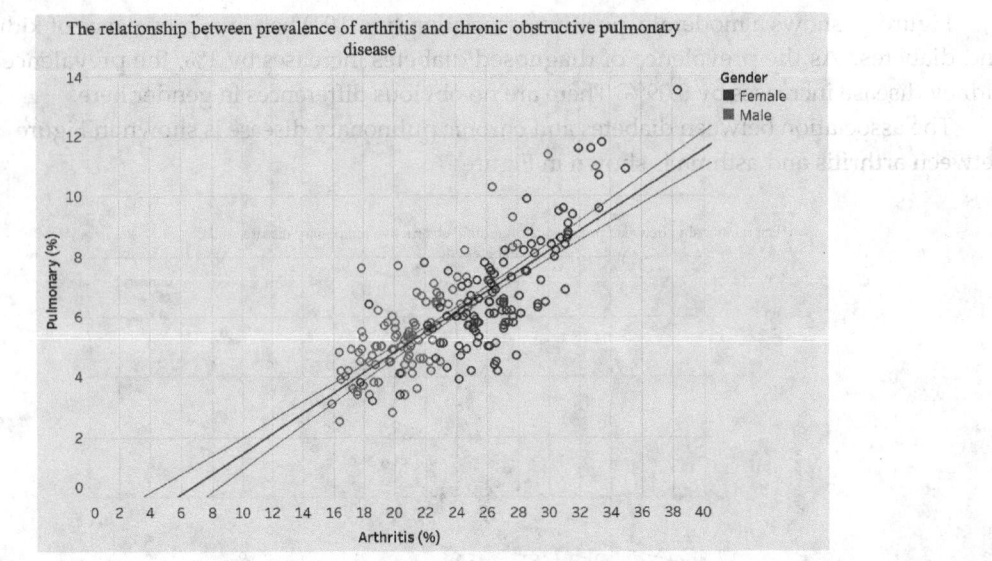

Figure 27. Arthritis by chronic obstructive pulmonary disease.

Although there are no defined clusters for men and women with regard to the prevalence of arthritis and chronic obstructive pulmonary disease, there is a significant positive association ($p < 0.0001$), as Figure 27 illustrates. An increase of 1% in prevalence of arthritis is associated with an increase of 0.3% in chronic obstructive pulmonary disease.

3.7. Summary of Results

The visual analytics figures above offer insight into a representative cross section of the data. They provide a bird's eye view of the dimensions and correlations of chronic diseases "conditions", behavioral health, and preventive health condition in the U.S. In addition, associations between mental health and chronic conditions, preventive health and chronic conditions, and among chronic conditions themselves highlight the dynamics of interplay between these categories. This understanding is useful to policymakers in framing appropriate health policies. Preventive healthcare and mental health are both important elements in the management, mitigation, and prevention of chronic conditions. By exploring these in the context of chronic conditions, we offer insight on allocation and prioritization of resources in mitigation and prospective eradication of chronic diseases at a national level. Overarching conditions, including a lack of health insurance, influence the access to necessary health services, including preventive care. This lack of availability is associated with poor health and the prevalence of chronic diseases. Similarly, self-assessed health status is a good indicator of overall health status, correlating with subsequent health service use, functional status, and mortality [36]. Poor mental health interferes with social functioning as well as health condition and should therefore be monitored in chronic disease mitigation. Experiencing activity limitation due to poor physical or mental health undermines efforts to achieve a healthy lifestyle and therefore should be addressed at individual, state, and national levels.

4. Scope and Limitations

Our research has a few limitations. First, our study is cross-sectional and covers only the years 2012 to 2014, the years for which data is available. Second, we included only a limited set of variables (indicators) from the large data repository on the CDC website. A more comprehensive study could draw from other sources and a larger set of variables. Third, as population and public health have emerged as key disciplines in the contemporary health ecosystem, more scalable, macro-level, and drill-down studies would inform greater understanding of chronic diseases. Fourth, one would assume that the quality of publicly available data is high and error-free. Lastly, the study is limited to examining associations and correlations and does not investigate causality. Furthermore, we only apply visual analytics and descriptive analytics, which have limitations in and of themselves.

5. Implications

This study has analyzed chronic conditions in conjunction with several demographic variables, including gender and race. There are widespread variations in the prevalence of diverse chronic diseases, the number of hospitalizations for specific diseases, and the diagnosis and mortality rates for different states. For some chronic diseases—such as diabetes, arthritis, and obstructive pulmonary —the prevalence in the east is higher than in other regions, while, there is higher prevalence for other conditions, such as asthma, in the northeast. The south and midwest also show their own prevalence of chronic diseases. Likewise, there are variations for hospitalization and mortality rates. In addition, there are gender differences related to chronic conditions. For example, women tend to have higher cases per 100,000 for asthma-related hospitalizations. Men, on the other hand, appear to have higher mortality rates for chronic obstructive pulmonary disease, diabetes, chronic kidney, and others. Also, when we examined chronic conditions by race, we noticed that American Indian or Alaska Natives had higher mortality rates for chronic obstructive pulmonary disease, diabetes, chronic kidney, and so on, followed by Black and non-Hispanic groups.

In addition, the study analyzed demographics of mental health, behavior habits, and preventive health. The associations between behavioral health and chronic conditions and between preventive health and chronic conditions were also analyzed. There is a positive relationship between average female coronary heart disease mortality ratio and average female tobacco use ratio. There is a negative relationship between the average pneumococcal vaccination among diabetes patients and the average diagnosed diabetes ratio among the population. Referring to the relationship between behavioral health and overarching conditions, the study found a negative correlation between age-adjusted prevalence percentage of fair or poor self-rated health status among adults aged ≥18 years and binge drinking adults. The current smoking prevalence and sufficiency of sleep among adults is negatively related. The current lack of health insurance is negatively related to both prevalence of current smoking and that of current smokeless tobacco use. The relationship between obesity and poor self-rated health status is positively related. Similarly, current smoking prevalence has a strong, positive correlation with fair or poor self-rated health status. There are different negative or positive correlations between overarching conditions and chronic conditions. For instance, there is a significant positive relationship between the prevalence of a lack of health insurance and that of diagnosed diabetes. But the relationship between prevalence of a lack of health insurance and prevalence of asthma is negatively related.

Finally, we conducted analyses of the differences among chronic conditions. There are obvious clusters between men and women for asthma, although women tend to have a higher prevalence of asthma than men. Overall, prevalence of asthma is negatively related to the prevalence of diabetes. There is a moderate, positive correlation between prevalence of kidney and diabetes, which is akin to the positive correlation between the prevalence of chronic obstructive pulmonary disease and diabetes, arthritis and asthma, arthritis and chronic obstructive pulmonary disease, and asthma and chronic obstructive pulmonary.

6. Conclusions

The study makes multiple essential contributions to chronic disease analysis at the patient/ physician and the state levels. At the patient level, analysis of chronic conditions and related behavioral factors allows patients to be proactive in managing their conditions as well as modifying behavioral health. In this day and age, patients are eager to assimilate health information from various sources [37,38]. Being informed allows patients to self-monitor and seek appropriate and timely medical care [39,40], contributing to an ultimate care model that is increasingly personalized.

Similar to patients, physicians too have varying information needs in healthcare that need to be satisfied [41]. To physicians, information on chronic conditions and more importantly, associations between multiple conditions and between categories of healthcare, enable developing personalized treatment plans based on patient-specific profiles that integrate various symptoms with environmental and other health data [42]. Additionally, the array of information increases their ability to guide patients in towards lifestyle medicine (making lifestyle changes in healthy diet, exercise etc.) in the management of chronic diseases [43]. The road from sickness to wellness requires integrated efforts from physicians and patients—physicians can coach and guide the patients but the ultimate cross-over to wellness lies in the patients' hands.

Whereas most studies on chronic diseases focus on specific chronic diseases and are somewhat limited, this study offers comprehensive analysis over multiple categories of chronic diseases at the state-level. By utilizing visual analytics and descriptive analytics, our study offers methods for gaining insight into the relationships between behavior habits, preventative health and demographics, and chronic conditions. Moreover, this study contributes in terms of the methodology of analytics used in the research. It demonstrates the efficacy of data-driven analytics, which can help make informed decisions on chronic diseases.

Going forward, more theoretical and empirical research is needed. Additional studies can address the relationship between chronic disease conditions and other indicators, such as economic, financial, and social. While chronic disease management has become the focus in modern medicine as our population ages and medical costs continue to rise, research should focus on preventive and mitigating policies. The benefits of prevention and its potential to reduce costs and improve outcomes have received the attention of insurance companies, health care plans, and the U.S. Congress. Healthcare systems are now incentivized to reduce readmissions and physicians are encouraged to meet evidence-based quality measures to provide the best outcomes for patients with chronic disease states.

Author Contributions: Both the authors contributed equally to the data analysis, design, and development of the manuscript.

Conflicts of Interest: The authors declare no conflict of interest.

References

1. Basu, J.; Avila, R.; Ricciardi, R. Hospital readmission rates in U.S. States: Are readmissions higher where more patients with multiple chronic conditions cluster? *Health Serv. Res.* **2016**, *51*, 1135–1151. [PubMed]
2. Buttorff, C.; Ruder, T.; Bauman, M. Multiple Chronic Conditions in the United States. Available online: https://www.rand.org/pubs/tools/TL221.html (accessed on 1 January 2018).
3. American Association of Retired Persons. Chronic Conditions among Older Americans. Available online: https://assets.aarp.org/rgcenter/health/beyond_50_hcr_conditions.pdf (accessed on 1 January 2018).
4. Fried, L. America's Health and Health Care Depend on Preventing Chronic Disease. Available online: https://www.huffingtonpost.com/entry/americas-health-and-healthcare-depends-on-preventing_us_58c0649de4b070e55af9eade (accessed on 31 December 2017).
5. Tinker, A. How to Improve Patient Outcomes for Chronic Diseases and Comorbidities. Available online: http://www.healthcatalyst.com/wp-content/uploads/2014/04/How-to-Improve-Patient-Outcomes.pdf (accessed on 30 December 2017).
6. Comlossy, M. *Chronic Disease Prevention and Management*; National Conference of State Legislatures: Denver, CO, USA, 2013.
7. Centers for Disease Control. The Power of Prevention: Chronic Disease the Public Health Challenge of the 21st Century. Available online: www.cdc.gov/chronicdisease/pdf/2009-Power-of-Prevention.pdf (accessed on 31 December 2017).

8. O'Grady, M.J.; Capretta, J.C. Health-Care Cost Projections for Diabetes and Other Chronic Diseases. Available online: http://www.civicenterprises.net/MediaLibrary/Docs/HR%20-%20health%20care%20cost%20projections%20for%20diabetes%20and%20other%20chronic%20diseases.pdf (accessed on 30 December 2017).

9. World Health Organization. Ten Facts about Chronic Disease. Available online: http://www.who.int/features/factfiles/chp/10_en.html (accessed on 31 December 2017).

10. Becker's Hospital Review. The Key to Population Health: Know Your Chronic Disease Patients and Coach Them. Available online: https://www.beckershospitalreview.com/healthcare-information-technology/the-key-to-population-health-know-your-chronic-disease-patients-and-coach-them.html (accessed on 31 December 2017).

11. National Association of Chronic Disease Directors. Why Public Health is Necessary to Improve Healthcare. Available online: http://www.chronicdisease.org/?page=whyweneedph2imphc (accessed on 31 December 2017).

12. Trotter, P.; Lobelo, F.; Heather, A.J. Chronic Disease Is Healthcare's Rising Risk. Available online: https://www.healthitoutcomes.com/doc/chronic-disease-is-healthcare-s-rising-risk-0001 (accessed on 31 December 2017).

13. The Growing Crisis of Chronic Disease in the United States. Available online: https://www.fightchronicdisease.org/sites/default/files/docs/GrowingCrisisofChronicDiseaseintheUSfactsheet_81009.pdf (accessed on 31 December 2017).

14. Anderson, G.; Horvath, J. The growing burden of chronic disease in America. *Public Health Rep.* **2004**, *119*, 263–270. [CrossRef] [PubMed]

15. Beaton, T. Top 10 Most Expensive Chronic Diseases for Healthcare Payers 2017. Available online: https://healthpayerintelligence.com/news/top-10-most-expensive-chronic-diseases-for-healthcare-payers (accessed on 1 January 2018).

16. Guidestone. The Cost of Chronic Disease and Obesity 2011. Available online: https://www.guidestone.org/-/media/Insurance/WorksiteWellness/CostOfChronicDiseaseAndObesity.pdf?la=en (accessed on 30 December 2017).

17. Healthcare Information and Management Systems Society. Keeping Communities Healthy: Wellness and Chronic Disease Management Initiatives. Available online: http://www.himssanalytics.org/news/top-pop-health-initiatives-essentials-brief-update (accessed on 1 January 2018).

18. U.S. Department of Labor, Bureau of Labor Statistics. Consumer Expenditure Survey. Available online: http://www.bls.gov/cex/#overview (accessed on 1 January 2018).

19. U.S. Department of Health and Human Services. *Multiple Chronic Conditions—A Strategic Framework: Optimum Health and Quality of Life for Individuals with Multiple Chronic Conditions*; U.S. Department of Health and Human Services: Washington, DC, USA, 2010.

20. Raghupathi, W.; Raghupathi, V. An overview of health analytics. *J. Health Med. Inform.* **2013**, *4*, 1–11. [CrossRef]

21. Committee on Engaging the Computer Science Research Community in Health Care Informatics; Nat'l Research Council. *Computational Technology for Effective Healthcare: Immediate Steps and Strategic Directions*; Stead, W.W., Lin, H.S., Eds.; National Academies Press: Washington, DC, USA, 2009.

22. Khan, M.; Khan, S.S. Data and information visualization methods, and interactive mechanisms: A survey. *Int. J. Comp. Appl.* **2011**, *34*, 1–14.

23. Caban, J.J.; Gotz, D. Visual analytics in healthcare—Opportunities and research challenges. *J. Am. Med. Assoc.* **2015**, *22*, 260–262. [CrossRef] [PubMed]

24. Gotz, D.; Borland, D. Data-driven healthcare: Challenges and opportunities for interactive visualization. *IEEE Comp. Graphic Appl.* **2016**, *36*, 90–96. [CrossRef] [PubMed]

25. Harle, C.; Neill, D.; Padman, R. Development and evaluation of an information visualization system for chronic disease risk assessment. *IEEE Intell. Syst.* **2012**, *27*, 81–85. [CrossRef]

26. Sun, G.-D.; Wu, Y.-C.; Liang, R.-H.; Liu, S.-X. A survey of visual analytics techniques and applications: State-of-the-art research and future challenges. *J. Comput. Sci. Technol.* **2013**, *28*, 852–867. [CrossRef]

27. Keim, D.; Kohlhammer, J.; Ellis, G.; Mansman, F. Solving Problems with Visual Analytics. Available online: http://www.vismaster.eu/wp-content/uploads/2010/11/VisMaster-book-lowres.pdf (accessed on 1 January 2018).

28. Thomas, J.; Cook, K. *Illuminating the Path: Research and Department Agenda for Visual Analytics*; United States Department of Homeland Security: Washington, DC, USA, 2005.

29. Keim, D.A. Visual exploration of large data sets. *Commun. ACM* **2001**, *44*, 38–44. [CrossRef]

30. Wong, P.C.; Thomas, J. Visual analytics—Guest editors' introduction. *IEEE Trans. Comput. Graphics Appl.* **2004**, *24*, 20–21. [CrossRef]

31. Tukey, J.W. *Exploratory Data Analysis*; Addison-Wesley: Boston, MA, USA, 1977.

32. Centers for Disease Control and Prevention. Leading Indicators for Chronic Diseases and Risk Factors. Available online: https://chronicdata.cdc.gov/ (accessed on 30 December 2017).

33. Bodenheimer, T.; Chen, E.; Bennett, H.D. Confronting the growing burden of chronic disease: Can the U.S. health care workforce do the job? *Health Aff.* **2016**, *28*, 64–74.

34. Keselman, A.; Heller, N. Estrogen signaling modulates allergic inflammation and contributes to sex differences in asthma. *Front. Immunol.* **2015**, *6*, 568. [CrossRef] [PubMed]

35. Zein, J.G.; Erzurum, S.C. Asthma is different in Women. *Curr. Allergy. Asthma Rep.* **2015**, *15*, 28. [CrossRef] [PubMed]

36. Centers for Disease Control and Prevention. MMWR Recommendations and Reports. Available online: https://www.cdc.gov/mmwr/preview/mmwrhtml/rr5311a6.htm (accessed on 7 February 2018).

37. Amante, D.J.; Hogan, T.P.; Pagoto, S.L.; English, T.M.; Lapane, K.L. Access to care and use of the Internet to search for health information: Results from the U.S. National Health Interview Survey. *J. Med. Internet Res.* **2015**, *17*, 106. [CrossRef] [PubMed]

38. Eysenbach, G.; Köhler, C. How do consumers search for and appraise health information on the world wide web? Qualitative study using focus groups, usability tests, and in-depth interviews. *Br. Med. J.* **2002**, *324*, 573–577.

39. Bodenheimer, T.; Wagner, E.H.; Grumbach, K. Improving primary care for patients with chronic illness. *J. Am. Med. Assoc.* **2002**, *288*, 1775–1779. [CrossRef]

40. Himes, B.E.; Weitzman, E.R. Innovations in health information technologies for chronic pulmonary diseases16. *Respir. Res.* **2016**, *17*, 1–7. [CrossRef] [PubMed]

41. Kourouthanassis, P.E.; Mikalef, P.; Ioannidou, M.; Pateli, A. Exploring the online satisfaction gap of Medical doctors: An expectation-confirmation investigation of information needs. *Springer* **2014**, *820*, 217–228.

42. Mikalef, P.; Kourouthanassis, P.E.; Pateli, A.G. Online information search behaviour of physicians. *Health Inf. Lib. J.* **2017**, *34*, 58–73. [CrossRef] [PubMed]

43. Hayes, C.; West, C.; Egger, G. *Chapter 22—Rethinking Chronic Pain in a Lifestyle Medicine Context*; Academic Press: Cambridge, MA, USA, 2017; pp. 339–353.

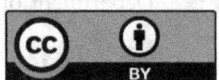
Raghupathi, Wullianallur, and Viju Raghupathi. "An Empirical Study of Chronic Diseases in the United States: A Visual Analytics Approach." International journal of environmental research and public health vol. 15,3 431. 1 Mar. 2018, doi:10.3390/ijerph15030431.

Next Steps After Your Diagnosis: Finding Information and Support

Introduction

Your doctor* gave you a diagnosis that could change your life. This booklet can help you take the next steps.

Every person is different, of course, and every person's disease or condition will affect them differently. But research shows that after getting a diagnosis, many people have some of the same reactions and needs.

About this Booklet

Next Steps After Your Diagnosis offers general advice for people with almost any disease or condition. And it has tips to help you learn more about your specific problem and how it can be treated.

The information in this booklet is presented in a simple way to help you scan the material and read only what you need right now. Organizations, publications, and other resources are included if you would like to know more. The on-line version www.ahrq.gov/consumer/diaginfo.htm has many additional resources and their Internet links.

Five Basic Steps

This booklet describes five basic steps to help you cope with your diagnosis, make decisions, and get on with your life.

Step 1: Take the time you need.
Do not rush important decisions about your health. In most cases, you will have time to carefully examine your options and decide what is best for you.

Step 2: Get the support you need.
Look for support from family and friends, people who are going through the same thing you are, and those who have "been there." They can help you cope with your situation and make informed decisions.

---

* Your medical care might come from a doctor, nurse, physician assistant, or another kind of clinician or health care practitioner. To keep it simple, in this booklet we use the term "doctor" to refer to any of these professionals with whom you might interact.

Step 3: Talk with your doctor.
Good communication with your doctor can help you feel more satisfied with the care you receive. Research shows it can even have a positive effect on things such as symptoms and pain. Getting a "second opinion" may help you feel more confident about your care.

Step 4: Seek out information.
When learning about your health problem and its treatment, look for information that is based on a careful review of the latest scientific findings published in medical journals.

Step 5: Decide on a treatment plan.
Work with your doctor to decide on a treatment plan that best meets your needs.

As you take each step, remember this: Research shows that patients who are more involved in their health care tend to get better results and be more satisfied.

Although most of the published research referred to in this publication focuses on cancer, it likely is relevant to people with other diseases and conditions as well.

Step 1:
Take the time you need.

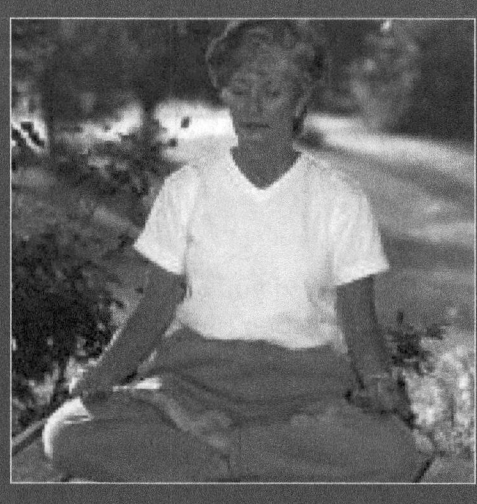

Take time to breathe. Don't panic, and don't feel pressured into making a rush decision.

Alexis, cancer survivor

A diagnosis can change your life in an instant.

Like so many other people in your situation, you might be feeling one or more of the following emotions after getting your diagnosis:

- Afraid
- Alone
- Angry
- Anxious
- Ashamed
- Confused
- Depressed
- Helpless
- In denial

- Numb
- Overwhelmed
- Panicky
- Powerless
- Relieved (that you finally know what's wrong)
- Sad
- Shocked
- Stressed

It is perfectly normal to have these feelings. It is also normal, and very common, to have trouble taking in and understanding information after you receive the news – especially if the diagnosis was a surprise. And it can be even harder to make decisions about treating or managing your disease or condition.

Take time to make your decisions.

No matter how the news of your diagnosis has affected you, do not rush into a decision. In most cases, you do not need to take action right away. Ask your doctor how much time you can safely take.

Taking the time you need to make decisions can help you:

- Feel less anxious and stressed.

- Avoid depression.

- Cope with your condition.

- Feel more in control of your situation.

- Play a key role in decisions about your treatment.

Step 2:
Get the support you need.

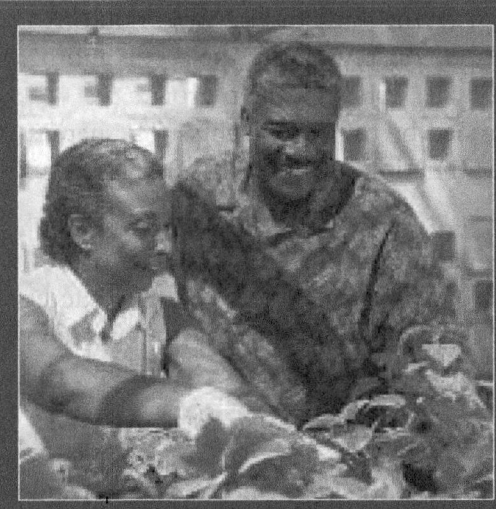

I was shocked when I was diagnosed with diabetes. The extra support I got from my friends and support group really helped me adjust to the new lifestyle I had to adopt.

Richard, person with diabetes

You do not have to go through it alone.

Sometimes the emotional side of illness can be just as hard to deal with as the physical side. You may have fears or concerns. You may feel overwhelmed. No matter what your situation, having other people to turn to will help you know you are not alone.

Here are the kinds of support you might want to seek:

▉ Family and friends.

Talking to family and friends you feel close to can help you cope with your illness or condition. Just knowing that someone is there can be a comfort.

Sometimes it is hard to ask for help. And sometimes your family and friends want to help, but they do not want to intrude, or they do not know how to ask or what to offer. Think about specific ways people can help you. One idea is to ask someone to come with you to a doctor's appointment to help ask questions, take notes, and talk with you afterward.

If you do not have family or friends who can provide support, other people or groups can.

Support or self-help groups.

Support groups are made up of people with the same disease or condition who get together to share information and concerns and to help one another. Support groups may or may not be led by experts. Self-help groups are similar to support groups but usually are led by the participants. The names "support group" and "self-help group" sometimes are used to refer to either kind.

Research on support groups shows that participants feel less anxious, experience less depression, have a better quality of life, and have more success coping with their disease or condition. Similar findings have been reported for self-help groups.

On-line support or self-help groups.

The Internet has support or self-help groups for people whose concerns and situations may be similar to yours. You can also find "message boards," where you can post questions and get answers. These on-line communities can help you connect with people who can give you support and provide information.

But be careful. Not every idea or treatment you come across in these groups will be scientifically proven to be safe and effective. If you read about something interesting and new, check it out with your doctor.

Counselor or therapist.

A good counselor or therapist can help you cope with sadness, depression, and feelings of being overwhelmed. If you think this kind of help might be right for you, ask your doctor or other health care professional to recommend someone in your area.

People like you.

You might want to meet and talk with someone in your own situation. Someone who has "been there" can talk about the real-life outcomes of their treatment choices as well as how they have learned to live with their disease or condition. Some advocacy or support groups can help you make this kind of contact.

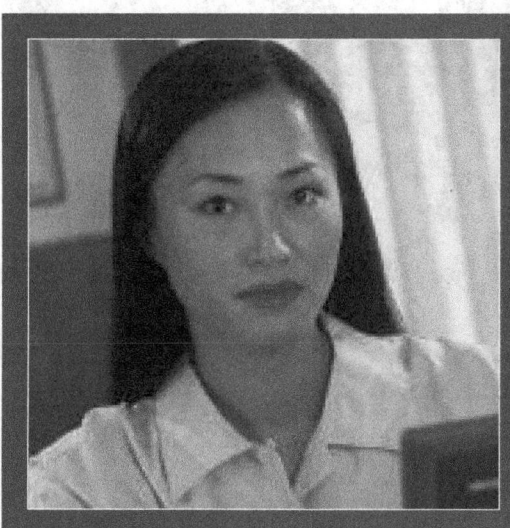

If only I had known what it would be like to live with the after-effects of this type of surgery, I might have chosen a different kind.

Susan, who underwent surgery for a digestive disease

Help is available.

Take advantage of the support that is available to you. See "Where to Find More Information" on page lvi for specific places to find support. An expanded list appears in the on-line version of this booklet at www.ahrq.gov/consumer/diaginfo.htm.

Step 3:
Talk with your doctor.

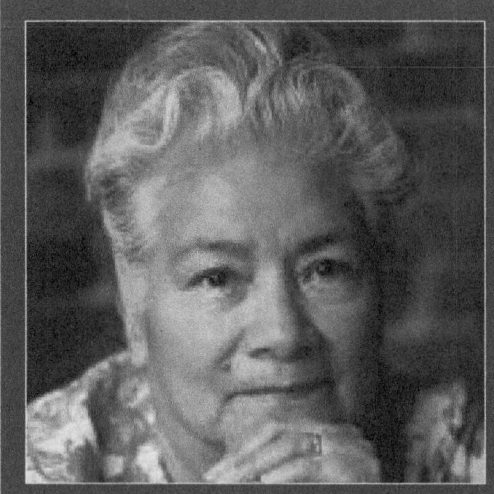

I had trouble under-standing what my doctor was telling me. The words were too technical, and there was too much to absorb. I finally asked her to slow down and keep it simple. That helped a lot.

Dana, person with heart disease

Your doctor is your partner in health care.

You probably have many questions about your disease or condition. The first person to ask is your doctor.

It is fine to seek more information from other sources; in fact, it is important to do so. But consider your doctor your partner in health care—someone who can discuss your situation with you, explain your options, and help you make decisions that are right for you.

It is not always easy to feel comfortable around doctors. But research has shown that good communication with your doctor can actually be good for your health. It can help you to:

• Feel more satisfied with the care you receive.

• Have better outcomes (end results), such as reduced pain and better recovery from symptoms.

Being an active member of your health care team also helps to reduce your chances of medical mistakes, and it helps you get high-quality care.

Of course, good communication is a two-way street. Here are some ways to help make the most of the time you spend with your doctor.

Prepare for your visit.

- Think about what you want to get out of your appointment. Write down all your questions and concerns. Some suggested questions are listed on page il.

- Prepare and bring to your doctor visit a list of all the medicines you take.

- Consider bringing along a trusted relative or friend. This person can help ask questions, take notes, and help you remember and understand everything once you leave the doctor's office.

Give information to your doctor.

- Do not wait to be asked.

- Tell your doctor everything he or she needs to know about your health—even the things that might make you feel embarrassed or uncomfortable.

- Tell your doctor how you are feeling—both physically and emotionally.

- Tell your doctor if you are feeling depressed or overwhelmed.

Get information from your doctor.

- Ask questions about anything that concerns you. Keep asking until you understand the answers. If you do not, your doctor may think you understand everything that is said.

- Ask your doctor to draw pictures if that will help you understand something.

- Take notes.

- Tape record your doctor visit, if that will be helpful to you. But first ask your doctor if this is okay.

- Ask your doctor to recommend resources such as Web sites, booklets, or tapes with more information about your disease or condition.

Also see "Ten Important Questions to Ask Your Doctor After a Diagnosis," on page il.

Do not hesitate to seek a second opinion.

A second opinion is when another doctor examines your medical records and gives his or her views about your condition and how it should be treated. You might want a second opinion to:

- Be clear about what you have.

- Know all of your treatment choices.

- Have another doctor look at your choices with you.

It is not pushy or rude to want a second opinion. Most doctors will understand that you need more information before making important decisions about your health.

Check to see whether your health plan covers a second opinion. In some cases, health plans require second opinions.

Here are some ways to find a doctor for a second opinion:

- Ask your doctor. Request someone who does not work in the same office, because doctors who work together tend to share similar views.

- Contact your health plan or your local hospital, medical society, or medical school.

- Use the Doctor Finder on-line service of the American Medical Association at www.ama-assn.org.

Get information about next steps.

- Get the results of any tests or procedures. Discuss the meaning of these results with your doctor.

- Make sure you understand what will happen if you need surgery.

- Talk with your doctor about which hospital is best for your health care needs.

Finally, if you are not satisfied with your doctor, you can do two things: (1) talk with your doctor and try to work things out, and/or (2) switch doctors, if you are able to. It is very important to feel confident about your care.

To learn more, see "Where to Find More Information" on page lvi. The on-line version of this booklet includes additional resources.

Ten Important Questions to Ask Your Doctor After a Diagnosis

These 10 basic questions can help you understand your disease or condition, how it might be treated, and what you need to know and do before making treatment decisions.

1. What is the technical name of my disease or condition, and what does it mean in plain English?

   _____

2. What is my prognosis (outlook for the future)?

   _____

3. How soon do I need to make a decision about treatment?

   _____

4. Will I need any additional tests, and if so what kind and when?

   _____

5. What are my treatment options?

   _____

6. What are the pros and cons of my treatment options?

   _____

7. Is there a clinical trial (research study) that is right for me? (See page 13.)

   _____

8. Now that I have this diagnosis, what changes will I need to make in my daily life?

   _____

9. What organizations do you recommend for support and information?

   _____

10. What resources (booklets, Web sites, audiotapes, videos, DVDs, etc.) do you recommend for further information?

    _____

Step 4:
Seek out information.

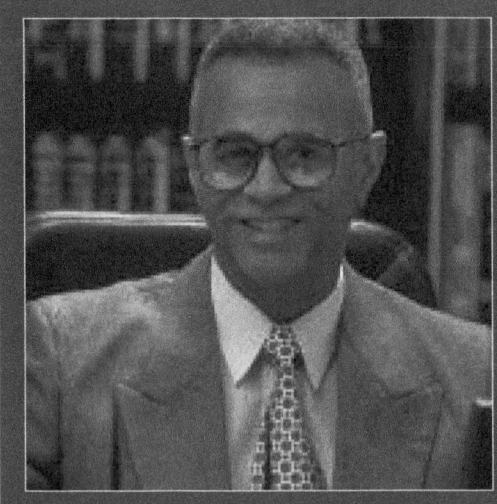

I'm really glad I took the time to research my options. It stopped me from jumping into a treatment that would have been completely wrong for me.

Seth, prostate cancer survivor

Now that you know your treatment options, you can learn which ones are backed up by the best scientific evidence. "Evidence-based" information—that is, information that is based on a careful review of the latest scientific findings in medical journals—can help you make decisions about the best possible treatments for you.

Evidence-based information comes from research on people like you.

Evidence-based information about treatments generally comes from two major types of scientific studies:

- **Clinical trials** are research studies on human volunteers to test new drugs or other treatments. Participants are randomly assigned to different treatment groups. Some get the research treatment, and others get a standard treatment or may be given a placebo (a medicine that has no effect), or no treatment. The results are compared to learn whether the new treatment is safe and effective.

- **Outcomes research** looks at the impact of treatments and other health care on health outcomes (end results) for patients and populations. End results include effects that people care about, such as changes in their quality of life.

Take advantage of the evidence-based information that is available.

Health information is everywhere—in books, newspapers, and magazines, and on the Internet, television, and radio. However, not all information is good information. Your best bets for sources of evidence-based information include the Federal Government, national nonprofit organizations, medical specialty groups, medical schools, and university medical centers.

Some resources are listed below, grouped by type of information. See "Where to Find More Information" on page lvi for additional ideas. The on-line version of *Next Steps After Your Diagnosis* lists many more, and includes links to Internet sites.

■■■ Information.

Information about your disease or condition and its treatment is available from many sources. Here are some of the most reliable:

- **healthfinder®:** www.healthfinder.gov/organizations/OrgListing.asp
  The healthfinder® site—sponsored by the U.S. Department of Health and Human Services—offers carefully selected health information Web sites from government agencies, clearinghouses, nonprofit groups, and universities.

- **Health Information Resource Database:**
  www.health.gov/nhic/#Referrals
  Sponsored by the National Health Information Center, this database includes 1,400 organizations and government offices that provide health information upon request. Information is also available over the telephone at 800-336-4797.

- **MEDLINEplus®:** www.nlm.nih.gov/medlineplus
  MedlinePlus® has extensive information from the National Institutes of Health and other trusted sources on over 650 diseases and conditions. The site includes many additional features.

- **National nonprofit groups** such as the American Heart Association, American Cancer Society, and American Diabetes Association can be valuable sources of reliable information. Many have chapters nationwide. Check your phone book for a local chapter in your community. The Health Information Resource Database (www.health.gov/nhic/#Referrals) can help you find national offices of nonprofit groups.

- **Health or medical libraries** run by government, hospitals, professional groups, and other reliable organizations often welcome consumers. For a list of libraries in your area, go to the MedlinePlus® "Find a Library" page at http://www.nlm.nih.gov/medlineplus/libraries.html.

▇ Current medical research.

You can find the latest medical research in medical journals at your local health or medical library, and in some cases, on the Internet. Here are two major online sources of medical articles:

- **MEDLINE/PubMed®:** http://www.ncbi.nlm.nih.gov/entrez/query.fcgi PubMed® is the National Library of Medicine's database of references to more than 14 million articles published in 4,800 medical and scientific journals. All of the listings have information to help you find the articles at a health or medical library. Many listings also have short summaries of the article (abstracts), and some have links to the full article. The article might be free, or it might require a fee charged by the publisher.

- **PubMed Central:** http://www.pubmedcentral.nih.gov/ PubMed Central is the National Library of Medicine's database of journal articles that are available free of charge to users.

▇ Clinical trials.

Perhaps you wonder whether there is a clinical trial that is right for you. Or you may want to learn about results from previous clinical trials that might be relevant to your situation. Here are two reliable resources:

- **ClinicalTrials.gov:** http://clinicaltrials.gov/ct/g ClinicalTrials.gov provides regularly updated information about federally and privately supported clinical research on people who volunteer to participate. The site has information about a trial's purpose, who may participate, locations, and phone numbers for more details. The site also describes the clinical trial process and includes news about recent clinical trial results.

- **Cochrane Collaboration:** www.cochrane.org The Cochrane Collaboration writes summaries ("reviews") about evidence from clinical trials to help people make informed decisions. You can search and read the review abstracts free of charge at http://www.cochrane.org/

reviews/index.htm. Or you can read plain-English consumer summaries of the reviews at www.informedhealthonline.org.

The full Cochrane reviews are available only by subscription. Check with your local medical or health library (see page lviii) [link back to library section in on-line version] to see whether you can access the full reviews there.

■ Outcomes research.

Outcomes research provides research about benefits, risks, and outcomes (end results) of treatments so that patients and their doctors can make better informed decisions. The U.S. Agency for Healthcare Research and Quality (AHRQ) supports improvements in health outcomes through research, and sponsors products that result from research such as:

- **Guidelines and Measures:** https://www.ahrq.gov/gam/index.html
  This AHRQ microsite, Guidelines and Measures (GAM), was set up by AHRQ to provide users a place to find information about its legacy guidelines and measures clearinghouses, National Guideline Clearinghouse (NGC) and National Quality Measures Clearinghouse (NQMC). This information was previously available on guideline.gov and qualitymeasures.ahrq.gov, respectively.

Steer clear of deceptive ads and information.

While searching for information either on or off the Internet, beware of "miracle" treatments and cures. They can cost you money and your health, especially if you delay or refuse proper treatment. Here are some tip-offs that a product truly is too good to be true:

- Phrases such as "scientific breakthrough," "miraculous cure," "exclusive product," "secret formula," or "ancient ingredient."

- Claims that the product treats a wide range of ailments.

- Use of impressive-sounding medical terms. These often cover up a lack of good science behind the product.

- Case histories from consumers claiming "amazing" results.

- Claims that the product is available from only one source, and for a limited time only.

- Claims of a "money-back guarantee."
- Claims that others are trying to keep the product off the market.
- Ads that fail to list the company's name, address, or other contact information.

To learn more about finding evidence-based information, see "Where to Find More Information," page lvi. The on-line edition of this booklet has many additional resources.

Step 5:
Decide on a treatment plan.

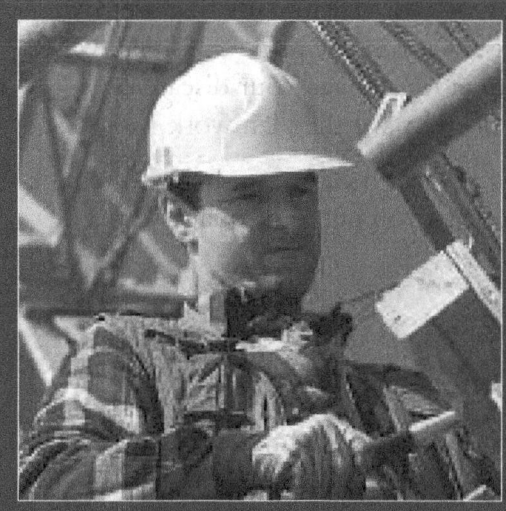

My doctor told me I had done one of the hardest but most important things a patient has to do: Face up to the diagnosis and make decisions. It feels good to be where I am now.

Bob, person with a neurological disorder

At this point, you have learned about your disease or condition and how it can be treated or managed. Your information may have come from the following sources:

- Your doctor.

- Second opinions from one or more other doctors.

- Other people who are or were in the same situation as you.

- Information sources such as Web sites, health or medical libraries, and nonprofit groups.

Work with your doctor to make decisions.

When you are ready to make treatment decisions, you and your doctor can discuss:

- Which treatments have been found to work well, or not work well, for your particular condition.

- The pros and cons of each treatment option.

Make sure that your doctor knows your preferences and feelings about the different treatments – for example, whether you prefer medicine over surgery.

Once you and your doctor decide on one or more treatments that are right for you, you can work together to develop a treatment plan. This plan will include everything that will be done to treat or manage your disease or condition—including what you need to do to make the plan work.

Remember, being an active member of your health care team helps to reduce your chances of medical mistakes, and it helps you get high-quality care.

Take another deep breath.

You have taken important steps to cope with your diagnosis, make decisions, and get on with your life. Remember two things:

* Call on others for support as you need it.

* Make use of evidence-based information for any future health decisions.

Where to Find More Information

Get the support you need.

American Self-Help Group Clearinghouse
http://mentalhelp.net/selfhelp/

National Board for Certified Counselors (NBCC)
3 Terrace Way, Suite D
Greensboro, NC 27403-3660
336-547-0607.
www.nbcc.org

National Institute of Mental Health
Public Information and Communications Branch
6001 Executive Boulevard, Room 8184, MSC 9663
Bethesda, MD 20892-9663
Phone: 866-615-6464 (toll-free)
TTY: 301-443-8431
http://www.nimh.nih.gov/HealthInformation/GettingHelp.cfm

Talk to your doctor.

Be an Active Member of Your Health Care Team. Food and Drug Administration. 2004. http://www.fda.gov/cder/consumerinfo/ active_member.htm. Phone: 888-INFO-FDA (888-463-6332).

Be Informed: Questions to Ask Your Doctor Before You Have Surgery. Agency for Healthcare Quality and Research. 1995. http://www.ahrq.gov/consumer/surgery.htm. Phone: 800-358-9295.

Five Steps to Safer Health Care. Agency for Healthcare Research and Quality. 2003. http://www.ahrq.gov/consumer/5steps.htm. Phone: 800-358-9295.

Getting a Second Opinion Before Surgery. Centers for Medicare & Medicaid Services. 2004. www.medicare.gov/Publications/Pubs/pdf/02173.pdf. Phone: 800-MEDICARE (800-633-4227).

How to Get a Second Opinion. National Women's Health Information Center. 2003. http://www.4woman.gov/pub/secondopinion.htm. Phone: 1-800-994-WOMAN.

Quick Tips – When Planning for Surgery. Agency for Healthcare Research and Quality. 2002. http://www.ahrq.gov/consumer/quicktips/ tipsurgery.htm. Phone: 800-358-9295.

Quick Tips – When Talking with Your Doctor. Agency for Healthcare Research and Quality. 2002. http://www.ahrq.gov/consumer/quicktips/ doctalk.htm. Phone: 800-358-9295.

Talking with Your Doctor: A Guide for Older People. National Institute on Aging. 2002. www.niapublications.org/pubs/talking/index.asp. Phone: 800-222-2225. |

Seek out information.

2005 Toll-Free Numbers for Health Information. National Health Information Center. www.health.gov/nhic/pubs/tollfree.htm. Phone: 800-336-4797.

AARP Health Guide. AARP. 2004. www.aarp.org/health/healthguide. Phone: 888-OUR-AARP (888-687-2277).

HON Code of Conduct (HONcode) for Medical and Health Web Sites Health on the Net Foundation. http://www.hon.ch/HONcode/

How to Evaluate Health Information on the Internet: Questions and Answers. National Cancer Institute. 2003. http://cis.nci.nih.gov/fact/ 2_10.htm. Phone: 800-4-CANCER (800-422-6237).

How to Find Medical Information. National Institute of Arthritis and Musculoskeletal and Skin Diseases. 2001. http://www.niams.nih.gov/hi/ topics/howto/howto.htm. Phone: 877-22-NIAMS (877-226-4267) (toll-free).

JAMA Patient Page: Health Information on the Internet. The Medem Network. http://www.medem.com/medlb/ article_detaillb.cfm?article_ID=ZZZLJLLLTMC&sub_cat=603

Guidelines and Measures. Agency for Healthcare Research and Quality. https://www.ahrq.gov/gam/index.html

NOAH: New York Online Access to Health. http://www.noah-health.org/

A User's Guide to Finding and Evaluating Health Information on the Web. Medical Library Association. 2003. http://www.mlanet.org/resources/ userguide.html#1

Virtual Treatments Can Be Real-World Deceptions. Federal Trade Commission. 2001. http://www.ftc.gov/bcp/conline/pubs/alerts/ mrclalrt.htm

Your Guide to Choosing Quality Health Care. Agency for Healthcare Research and Quality. 2002. http://www.ahrq.gov/consumer/qntool.htm. Phone: 800-358-9295.

AHRQ consumer publications:

20 Tips to Help Prevent Medical Errors—Practical tips and questions to ask. (AHRQ 00-P038)

20 Tips to Help Prevent Medical Errors in Children (AHRQ 02-P034)

Five Steps to Safer Health Care—Shorter version of 20 Tips. (AHRQ 03-M007)

Ways You Can Help Your Family Prevent Medical Errors!—Easy-to-read version, with drawings. (AHRQ 01-0017)

Your Guide to Choosing Quality Health Care—Based on research about the information people want and need when choosing health plans, doctors, treatments, hospitals, and long-term care. (AHRQ 99-012)

Improving Health Care Quality: A Guide for Patients and Their Families—Short version of *Your Guide to Choosing Quality Health Care*. (AHRQ 01-0004)

Quick Checks for Quality—Checklist to use when choosing health plans, doctors, treatments, hospitals, and long-term care. (AHRQ 99-R027)

Quick Tips:
　　When Getting Medical Tests (AHRQ 01-0040b)
　　When Getting a Prescription (AHRQ 01-0040c)
　　When Planning for Surgery (AHRQ 01-0040d)
　　When Talking with Your Doctor (AHRQ 01-0040a)

For electronic copies of these publications, go to the AHRQ Web site at https://www.ahrq.gov/patients-consumers/

Next Steps After Your Diagnosis. Content last reviewed July 2018. Agency for Healthcare Research and Quality, Rockville, MD. https://www.ahrq.gov/patients-consumers/diagnosis-treatment/diagnosis/diaginfo/index.html.

Description

1 Addison Disease and Adrenal Insufficiency

Adrenal insufficiency results from inadequate hormone production by the adrenal glands. The adrenal glands, which are located just above the kidneys, produce two main types of steroid hormones in their outer layer or cortex; glucocorticoids, which regulate energy metabolism, and mineralocorticoids, which regulate the salt balance in the body. Adrenocorticotropin (ACTH) secretion by the anterior lobe of the pituitary gland regulates adrenal hormone production and release. ACTH release by the pituitary gland is controlled by corticotropin-releasing hormone (CRH) production by the hypothalamus, which is located just above the pituitary in the brain. Direct damage to adrenal glands. as a result of adrenal gland tumors, surgery, bleeding, or developmental disorders, causes primary adrenal insufficiency, which is also known as Addison disease. Conditions that diminish ACTH production by the pituitary gland, such as pituitary tumors, infections (e.g., tuberculosis), or bleeding, traumatic brain injury, surgical removal of the pituitary, or development abnormalities of the pituitary gland cause secondary adrenal insufficiency. Other disorders that affect CRH production by the hypothalamus cause tertiary adrenal insufficiency. At least half of all cases of Addison disease result from destruction of the adrenal glands by the patient's own immune system (autoimmune process).

The symptoms of Addison disease can show a gradual onset and increase with the progression of the disease. EEarly signs may include fatigue, loss of appetite, low blood pressure (hypotension), weakness and significant loss from the kidneys of water and minerals. Other symptoms may include darkened scars and skin folds, as well as dark freckles on the head and shoulders. In the later stages, nausea may develop, as well as dizziness, further dehydration, low blood sugar (hypoglycemia) and mental changes including depression, confusion, and sleep disturbances.

Patients who are treated early have an excellent prognosis, but it is imperative that treatment be instituted immediately and vigorously. To treat the adrenal steroid hormonal inadequacy, physicians prescribe oral steroid hormone replacement therapy, which includes hydrocortisone, and, sometimes, fludrocortisone. Hormone doses need to be increased during times of illness and surgery. Treatment should never be stopped, even for a day, without the advice of a physician. Persons on treatment should wear an alert bracelet to let emergency medical providers know of their diagnosis.

National Agencies & Associations

2 American Association of Endocrine Surgeons
201 E Main Street   859-402-9810
Lexington, KY 40507   Fax: 859-514-9166
info@endocrinesurgery.org
www.endocrinesurgery.org
The American Association of Endocrine Surgeons (AAES) is dedicated to the advancement of endocrine surgery, which includes diseases of the thyroid, parathyroid, and adrenal glands, as well as neuroendocrine tumors of the pancreas and GI tract.
Lauren Santangelo, Executive Director
Ashley Peter, Project Coordinator

3 Canadian Addison Society
2 Palace Arch Drive   888-550-5582
Etobicoke, Ontario, M9A-2S1   info@addisonsociety.ca
www.addisonsociety.ca
A registered charitable organization devoted to providing information on Addison's disease, and organizing support groups for Addisonians.
Harold Smith, President
Derek Burpee, Vice-President

4 Endocrine Society
2055 L Street NW   202-971-3636
Washington, DC 20036   888-363-6274
Fax: 202-736-9705
info@endocrine.org
www.endocrine.org
Source of state-of-the-art research and clinical advancements in endocrinology and metabolism. Dedicated to promoting excellence in research education and clinical practice in the field of endocrinology. Prime advocate and integrative force for clinicians.
Barbara Byrd Keenan, Chief Executive Officer
Robert Lash, Chief Prof. and Clinical Affairs Officer

5 HypoPARAthyroidism Association
695 Montecito Ct   208-524-3857
Lemoore, CA 93245   866-213-0394
dmurphy@hypopara.org
www.hypopara.org
The HypoPARAthyroidism Association is an non-profit patient organization working to improve lives touched by hypoparathyroidism, a rare medical disorder in which the parathyroid glands fail to produce sufficient amounts of the parathyroid hormone.
Dana Crumpton, Chair
Deb Murphy, Vice-Chair

6 National Institute of Diabetes & Digestive & Kidney Diseases
Office Of Communications and Public Liaison, NIH
31 Center Drive   800-860-8747
Bethesda, MD 20892-2560   TTY: 866-569-1162
healthinfo@niddk.nih.gov
www.niddk.nih.gov
Research areas include diabetes, digestive diseases, endocrine and metabolic diseases, hematologic diseases, kidney disease, liver disease, urologic diseases, as well as matters relating to nutrition and obesity.
Griffin P. Rodgers, MD, MACP, Director
Gregory Germino, MD, Deputy Director

7 Pediatric Endocrine Society
6728 Old McLean Vg. Dr.   703-556-9222
McLean, VA 22101   Fax: 703-556-8729
info@pedsendo.org
www.pedsendo.org
The Pediatric Endocrine Society aims to assist children and adolescents with endocrine disorders through the advancement and promotion of research, as well as promoting the continuing education of its membership.
Madhusmita Misra, President
Peter A. Lee, Treasurer

Foundations

8 National Adrenal Diseases Foundation
P.O. Box 566   847-726-9010
Lake Zurich, IL 60047   nadfmail@nadf.us
                                  www.nadf.us
Nonprofit organization dedicated to offering support information and research for individuals with diseases of the adrenal glands. Goals of the organization include assisting patients through informational and educational activities, as well as support programs in states across the country.
Paul Margulies, Medical Director
Melanie G. Wong, Executive Director

Support Groups & Hotlines

9 National Health Information Center
Office of Disease Prevention & Health Promotion
1101 Wootton Pkwy   Fax: 240-453-8281
Rockville, MD 20852   odphpinfo@hhs.gov
                                  www.health.gov/nhic
Supports public health education by maintaining a calendar of National Health Observances; helps connect consumers and health professionals to organizations that can best answer questions and provide up-to-date contact information from reliable sources; updates on a yearly basis toll-free numbers for health information, Federal health clearinghouses and info centers.
Don Wright, MD, MPH, Director

Magazines

10 Endocrine News
Endocrine Society
2055 L Street NW   202-971-3636
Washington, DC 20036   888-363-6274
                                  Fax: 202-971-3646
                          societyservices@endo-society.org
                                  www.endo-society.org
Endocrine News is the source of trends and insights for members of the endocrine community.
Monthly
Kelly E Mayo PhD, President
Scott Hunt, Executive Director

Newsletters

11 Addison News
6142 Territorial   www2.dmci.net/users/hoffmanrj
Pleasant Lake, MI 49272

12 NADF News
National Adrenal Diseases Foundation
505 Northern Boulevard   516-487-4992
Great Neck, NY 11021   Fax: 516-829-5710
                                  nadfsupport@nadf.us
                                  www.nadf.us
Contains information on the latest research, question and answer column by an endocrinologist and helpful hints for those with Addison's Disease.
Quarterly Monthly
Melanie G Wong, Executive Director
Debbie Benish, Editor

Web Sites

13 Healing Well
                                  www.healingwell.com
An online health resource guide to medical news, chat, information and articles, newsgroups and message boards, books, disease-related web sites, medical directories, and more for patients, friends, and family coping with disabling diseases, disorders, or chronic illnesses.

14 Health Finder
                                  www.healthfinder.gov
A government Web site where you will find information and tools to help you and those you care about stay healthy.

15 Health Link USA
                                  www.healthlinkusa.com
Discussion forum for treatments, symptoms and causes of 700 health conditions, diseases and topics.

16 Hormone Foundation
                                  www.hormone.org
Educational resource for you, your loved ones, and your health professionals on the prevention, treatment, and cure of hormone-related conditions.

17 MedicineNet
                                  www.medicinenet.com
An online resource for consumers providing easy-to-read, authoritative medical and health information.

18 Medscape
                                  www.medscape.com
Search engine providing links to websites with information on illnesses, diseases and disorders.

19 National Adrenal Diseases Foundation
                                  www.nadf.us
Nonprofit organization dedicated to offering support information and research for individuals with diseases of the adrenal glands. Goals of the organization include assisting patients through informational and educational activities, as well as support programs in states across the country. Website features research, links & resources, articles, medical tools, & information on specific adrenal diseases.

20 WebMD
                                  www.webmd.com
Provides credible information, supportive communities, and in-depth reference material about health subjects. A source for original and timely health information as well as material from well known content providers.

Description

21 Aging

The elderly population in the United States is growing faster than any other segment of the population, and has done so since 1900. It is estimated that this trend will continue at least through the year 2050. In 2004, there were 36.3 million people in the U.S. One in eight persons is over 85 years, and is classified as 'old-old.' By 2040, as a result of baby boomer aging, it is projected that one person in five (~88 million) will exceed 65 years of age, and the number of people over 85 will increase to four times their number today (~19 million). By 2030, 74 million people will be over the age of 65, representing about 21 percent of the population. The female to male sex ratio increases with age, ranging from 114 women for every 100 men for the 65-69 age cohort to a high of 216 women for every 100 men among persons aged 85 and older.

Aging is not a disease, but part of the normal life cycle, and many seniors retain good health and live independently for long past the traditional age of retirement. In time, however, most will develop one or more chronic conditions; for those over 75 years of age, the most common conditions are hypertension, heart disease, hearing loss, arthritis, and cataracts. By the year 2030, 150 million Americans are expected to have a chronic condition, and 42 million will be limited in their ability to work or live independently. Psychological and social components of well-being are also integral components of healthy aging. Approximately 15 percent of women 65 and older and 10 percent of men 65 and older have clinically relevant symptoms of depression. Additionally, older adults are at risk for social isolation. Treating this population will require many medical and nonmedical services, integrated to provide a comprehensive continuum of care. See also *Alzheimer's Disease*.

National Agencies & Associations

22   ABA Commission on Law and Aging
1050 Connecticut Avenue   202-662-8690
Washington, DC 20003   Fax: 202-662-8698
aging@americanbar.org
www.americanbar.org/aging
The Commission examines the issues that affect the elderly as victims of abuse, dispute resolution, international rights, medicare, voting, health care decision-making and other issues arising from the aging prisons populations.
Charles P. Sabatino, JD, Director
Erica F. Wood, JD, Assistant Director

23   Academy for Gerontology in Higher Education
1220 L Street NW   202-289-9806
Washington, DC 20005   membership@geron.org
www.aghe.org
Membership organization comprised of more than 130 colleges and universities that offer education and research program in the field of aging. Affiliated with the Gerontological Society of America.
Judith L. Howe, President
Lisa Hollis-Sawyer, Treasurer

24   American Association of Retired Persons
601 E Street NW   202-434-3525
Washington, DC 20049   888-687-2277
TTY: 877-434-7598
member@aarp.org
www.aarp.org
AARP is the nation's leading organization for people age 50 and older. It serves their needs and interests through information and education, advocacy and community services provided by a network of local chapters and experienced volunteers.
Jo Ann Jenkins, Chief Executive Officer
Scott Frisch, Executive Vice-President and COO

25   Canadian National Seniors Council
Ottawa, Ontario,   canada.ca/en/national-seniors-council
The council works with older Canadians, stakeholders and experts to advise the Canadian government on matters relating to the health, well-being and quality of life of seniors.
Suzanne Dupuis-Blanchard, PhD, Chair

26   Commission on Accreditation of Rehabilitation Facilities
6951 E Southpoint Road   888-281-6531
Tucson, AZ 85756-9407   Fax: 520-318-1129
TTY: 520-495-7077
www.carf.org
CARF reviews and grants accreditation services nationally and internationally at the request of a facility or program. Standards are applied to service areas and business practices, and accreditation is ongoing in an effort to encourage service providers to continuously improve services. The CARF group also includes CARF Canada and CARF Europe.
Brian J. Boon, PhD, President & CEO
Christine MacDonnell, Managing Director, Int'l Aging Services

27   Family Caregiver Alliance/National Center on Caregiving
101 Montgomery Street   415-434-3388
San Francisco, CA 94104   800-445-8106
www.caregiver.org
Caregiver information and assistance via phone or e-mail; fact sheets and publications describing and documenting caregiver needs and services.
Jacquelyn Kung, PhD, Chief Executive Officer
Wyatt Ritchie, MBA, Managing Director

28   Gerontological Society of America
1220 L Street NW   202-842-1275
Washington, DC 20005   Fax: 202-842-1150
geron@geron.org
www.geron.org
Nonprofit professional organization with more than 5,500 members in the field of aging. Provides researchers, educators, practitioners and policy makers with opportunities to understand, advance, integrate and use basic and applied research on aging populations. Also runs the National Adult Vaccination Program (www.navp.org).
James Appleby, Chief Executive Officer
Karen Tracy, VP, Strategic Alliances & Communications

29   Goodwill Industries International, Inc.
15810 Indianola Drive   800-466-3945
Rockville, MD 20855   contactus@goodwill.org
www.goodwill.org
A nonprofit, community-based organization whose mission is to help people achieve self-sufficiency through the dignity and power of work, serving people who are disadvantaged, disabled or elderly. The mission is accomplished through providing independent living skills, affordable housing, and training and placement in community employment. The GoodWill Network includes 160 independent, local locations across the U.S. and Canada.
S. Dale Jenkins, Chair
Steven C. Preston, President & CEO

30   Heart Touch Project™
3400 Airport Avenue   310-391-2558
Santa Monica, CA 90405   Fax: 310-391-2168
executive@hearttouch.org
www.hearttouch.org

Non-profit, educational and service organization devoted to the delivery of compassionate and healing touch to home or hospital-bound men, women, and children.
Shawnee Isaac Smith, Co-Founder
Rene Russo, Co-Founder

31   Institute for Life Course and Aging
246 Bloor Street W.   416-978-0377
Toronto, Ontario, M5S-1V4   Fax: 416-978-4771
                                                          aging@utoronto.ca
                                                www.grandparentfamily.com
The Institute is a research center under the auspices of the Faculty of Social Work at the University of Toronto.
Esme Fuller-Thomson, Director
Susan Murphy, Administration

32   International Federation on Ageing
1 Bridgepoint Drive   416-342-1655
Toronto, Ontario, M4M-2B5   Fax: 416-639-2165
                                                          jbarratt@ifa-fiv.org
                                                          www.ifa-fiv.org
The IFA seeks to inform, educate and promote policies and practice to improve the quality of life of older persons around the world.
Greg Shaw, Director, Int'l & Corporate Relations
Dr. Jane Barratt, Secretary General

33   Leading Age
2519 Connecticut Avenue NW
Washington, DC 20008-1520   202-783-2242
                                                          info@LeadingAge.org
                                                          www.leadingage.org
National association of more than 6,000 nonprofit nursing homes, continuing care retirement communities, independent living centers and community service providers serving more than 60,000 older Americans each year.
Katie Smith Sloan, President & CEO
Nicole Fallon, Vice President, Health Policy

34   National Adult Day Services Association
11350 Random Hills Road   877-745-1440
Fairfax, VA 22030   info@nadsa.org
                                                          www.nadsa.org
Aims to be the leading voice of the Adult Day Services industry, representing providers, associations of providers, corporations, educators, students, and retired workers.
Donna Hale, Executive Director
Lance Roberts, Associate Director, Membership

35   National Alliance for Caregiving
4720 Montgomery Lane   301-718-8444
Bethesda, MD 20814   Fax: 301-951-9067
                                                          info@caregiving.org
                                                          www.caregiving.org
Advocates on behalf of caregivers, as well as conducting research and offering support services.
C. Grace Whiting, JD, President & CEO
Michael Wittke, BSW, MPA, Senior Director, Public Policy

36   National Council for Aging Care
1200 G Street NW   877-664-6140
Washington, DC 20005   www.aging.com
Seeks to provide older adults with information and resources on health & well-being, caregiving, money and financial planning, and lifestyle, through their Aging.com website.

37   National Council on Aging
251 18th Street S.   571-527-3900
Arlington, VA 22202   Fax: 202-479-0735
                                                 TTY: 202-479-6674
                                                          info@ncoa.org
                                                          www.ncoa.org
The nation's first charitable organization dedicated to promoting the dignity, independence, well-being and contributions of older Americans. The council has a goal of improving the health and economic well-being of 10 million older adults by 2020.
James P. Firman, EdD, President & CEO
Howard Bedlin, VP, Public Policy & Advocacy

38   National Hospice & Palliative Care Organization (NHPCO)
1731 King Street   703-837-1500
Alexandria, VA 22314   800-646-6460
                                                   Fax: 703-837-1233
                                                          www.nhpco.org
The organization seeks to improve end-of-life care, widen access to hospice care, and improve quality of life for the dying and their loved ones.
Edo Banach, JD, President & CEO
Hannah Yang Moore, MPH, Chief Advocacy Officer

39   National Institute on Aging
31 Center Drive, MSC 2292   800-222-2225
Bethesda, MD 20892   TTY: 800-222-4225
                                                          niaic@nia.nih.gov
                                                          www.nia.nih.gov
Seeks to understand the nature of aging, and to extend healthy, active years of life. Free resources are available on topics such as Alzheimer's & dimentia, caregiving, cognitive heath, end of life care, and more.
Richard J. Hodes MD, Director
Marie A. Bernard, MD, Deputy Director

40   National Seniors Council
1100 North Glebe Road   571-425-4153
Arlington, VA 22201   nationalseniorscouncil.org
The council seeks to serve the needs of the new generation of retirees, as an alternative to organizations such as the AARP.
Carole Rhodes, National Director

41   Senior Resource LLC
                                                 questions@seniorresource.com
                                                          www.seniorresource.com
The company operates Seniorresource.com, which provides information to older adults on needed facilities and services, including through internet directories and an archive of E-zines.
1995 pages

42   US Administration on Aging
330 C Street SW   202-401-4634
Washington, DC 20201   aclinfo@acl.hhs.gov
                                          acl.gov/about-acl/administration-aging
The Administration on Aging, an agency in the US Department of Health and Human Services, and under the Administration for Community Living, is one of the nation's largest providers of home and community-based care for older persons and their caregivers.
Lance Robertson, Administrator & Assistant Secretary
Edwin Walker, Deputy Assistant Secretary

State Agencies & Associations

Alabama

43   AARP Alabama
400 South Union Street   866-542-8167
Montgomery, AL 36104   alaarp@aarp.org
                                                states.aarp.org/region/alabama
Provides information, events, news, and resources to Alabamians over 50 years of age, and to a membership of over 430,000.
Candi Williams, State Director
Lisa Billingsley, Senior Operations Administrator

Alaska

44   AARP Alaska
3601 C Street   866-227-7447
Anchorage, AK 99503   Fax: 907-341-2270
                                                          ak@aarp.org
                                                states.aarp.org/region/alaska
Serves 95,000 members in Alaska, providing information, resources, news, and advocacy on matters relevant to individuals aged 50 years and older.
Ken Helander, Advocacy Director
Ann Secrest, Media Contact

Arizona

45 **AARP Arizona**
7250 N 16th Street   866-389-5649
Phoenix, AZ 85020   aarpaz@aarp.org
                                           states.aarp.org/region/arizona
The chapter seeks to enhance the quality of life for all Arizonans, with an emphasis on individuals 50 years and older.
David Parra, Director, Community Outreach
Alex Suarez, Communications Contact

Arkansas

46 **AARP Arkansas**
1701 Centerview Drive   866-544-5379
Little Rock, AR 72211   Fax: 501-227-7710
                                                         araarp@aarp.org
                                          states.aarp.org/region/arkansas
Seeks to redefine and improve life for Arkansans over the age of 50.
Charlie Wagener, State President

California

47 **AARP California: Pasadena**
200 S Los Robles Avenue   866-448-3614
Pasadena, CA 91101-2422   Fax: 626-583-8500
                                                         caaarp@aarp.org
                                         states.aarp.org/region/california
Provides news, tools, resources, and research to Californians 50 years and older.
Nancy McPherson, State Director
Joy Hepp, Media Contact, Southern California

48 **AARP California: Sacramento**
1415 L Street   866-448-3614
Sacramento, CA 95814   Fax: 916-446-2223
                                                         caaarp@aarp.org
                                         states.aarp.org/region/california
Provides news, tools, resources, and research to Californians 50 years and older.
Nancy McPherson, State President
Mark Beach, Media Contact, Northern California

Colorado

49 **AARP Colorado**
303 E 17th Avenue   866-554-5376
Denver, CO 80203-5012   Fax: 303-764-5999
                                                         coaarp@aarp.org
                                          states.aarp.org/region/colorado
The Colorado chapter seeks to keep Coloradans 50 years and older informed, engaged, and active.
Bob Murphy, State Director
Angela Cortez, Media Contact

Connecticut

50 **AARP Connecticut**
21 Oak Street   866-295-7279
Hartford, CT 06106   ctaarp@aarp.org
                                        states.aarp.org/region/connecticut
With nearly 600,000 members, the chapter provides recent news, information, and events for residents of Connecticut who are 50 years and older, as well as advocating for positive social change.
Nora Duncan, State Director
Anna Doroghazi, Assoc. State Dir., Advocacy & Outreach

Delaware

51 **AARP Delaware**
222 Delaware Avenue   866-227-7441
Wilmington, DE 19801   kiapalucci@aarp.org
                                          states.aarp.org/region/delaware
Provides news, advocacy, education, and lifestyle information for residents of Delaware who are 50 years and older.
Lucretia Young, State Director
Kimberly Iapalucci, Media Contact

District of Columbia

52 **AARP Washington DC**
100 M Street SE   866-554-5384
Washington, DC 20003   Fax: 202-434-7946
                                                          dcaarp@aarp.org
                                    states.aarp.org/region/washington-dc
Provides information, advocacy, and a variety of services to 87,000 members aged 50 and over.
Louis Davis, Jr., State Director
Peter Rankin, Associate State Director, Advocacy

Florida

53 **AARP Florida: Doral**
3750 Nw 87th Avenue   866-595-7678
Doral, FL 33178   Fax: 786-804-4544
                                                          flaarp@aarp.org
                                           states.aarp.org/region/florida
The chapter provides information, research, and events to 2.7 million members, and Floridians 50 years and older.
Donna L. Ginn, State President
Jeff Johnson, State Director

54 **AARP Florida: St. Petersburg**
360 Central Avenue   866-595-7678
St. Petersburg, FL 33701   Fax: 727-369-5191
                                                          flaarp@aarp.org
                                           states.aarp.org/region/florida
The chapter provides information, research, and events to 2.7 million members, and Floridians 50 years and older.
Donna L. Ginn, State President
Jeff Johnson, State Director

55 **AARP Florida: Tallahassee**
200 West College Avenue   866-595-7678
Tallahassee, FL 32301   Fax: 850-222-8968
                                                          flaarp@aarp.org
                                           states.aarp.org/region/florida
The chapter provides information, research, and events to 2.7 million members, and Floridians 50 years and older.
Donna L. Ginn, State President
Jeff Johnson, State Director

56 **Goodwill Industries-Suncoast**
10596 Gandy Boulevard   727-523-1512
St. Petersburg, FL 33702   888-279-1988
                                                      TTY: 727-579-1068
                                               www.goodwill-suncoast.org
A nonprofit, community-based organization whose mission is to help people achieve self-sufficiency through the dignity and power of work, serving people who are disadvantaged, disabled or elderly. The mission is accomplished through providing independent living skills, affordable housing, and training and placement in community employment.
Heather Ceresoli, CPA, Chair
Deborah A. Passerini, President & CEO

Georgia

57 **AARP Georgia**
999 Peachtree Street NE   866-295-7281
Atlanta, GA 30309   Fax: 404-815-7940
                                                          gaaarp@aarp.org
                                           states.aarp.org/region/georgia
The chapter strives to help Georgians 50 years and older.
Debra Tyler-Horton, State Director
Alisa Jackson, Media Contact

Hawaii

58 **AARP Hawaii**
1132 Bishop Street   866-295-7282
Honolulu, HI 96813   Fax: 808-537-2288
                                                          hiaarp@aarp.org
                                            states.aarp.org/region/hawaii
With 150,000 members, the chapter advocates at the state level, and provides information, resources, and volunteer opportunities.
Jessica Wooley, Director, Advocacy

59   **AARP Idaho**
250 S 5th Street   866-295-7284
Boise, ID 83702   Fax: 208-288-4424
                                                    aarpid@aarp.org
                                       states.aarp.org/region/idaho
The chapter advocates for and seeks to improve the lives of residents aged 50 years and older.
Lupe Wissel, Idaho AARP State Media Relations
Randy Simon, Media Contact

60   **AARP Illinois: Chicago**
222 N LaSalle Street   866-448-3613
Chicago, IL 60601   Fax: 312-372-2204
                                                    aarpil@aarp.org
                                     states.aarp.org/region/illinois
Advocates for and provides recent news, events, and lifestyle tips to Illinois residents aged 50 years and older.
Bob Gallo, State Director
Dina Anderson, Media Contact

61   **AARP Illinois: Springfield**
300 W Edwards Street   866-448-3613
Springfield, IL 62704   Fax: 217-522-7803
                                                    aarpil@aarp.org
                                     states.aarp.org/region/illinois
Legislative office of the Illinois chapter.
Bob Gallo, State Director
Dina Anderson, Media Contact

62   **Legal Council for Health Justice**
17 N State Street   312-427-8990
Chicago, IL 60602   Fax: 312-427-8419
                                                    legalcouncil.org
Provides legal advice and services for persons who are HIV positive or have AIDS, as well as their families. Also serves individuals with disabilities and chronic illnesses, senior citizens, and the homeless.
Tom Yates, Executive Director
Ruth Edwards, Senior Director, Program Services

63   **AARP Indiana**
One N Capitol Avenue   866-448-3618
Indianapolis, IN 46204-2025   Fax: 317-423-2211
                                                    inaarp@aarp.org
                                     states.aarp.org/region/indiana
The chapter seeks to improve life for residents of Indiana aged 50 years and older.
Sarah Waddle, State Director
Jason Tomcsi, Media Contact

64   **AARP Iowa**
600 E Court Avenue   866-554-5378
Des Moines, IA 50309   Fax: 515-244-7767
                                                    ia@aarp.org
                                       states.aarp.org/region/iowa
Provides news, information, and resources to Iowans aged 50 years and older.
Brad Anderson, State Director
Jeremy Barewin, Media Contact

65   **AARP Kansas**
6220 SW 29th Street   866-448-3619
Topeka, KS 66614   Fax: 785-232-1465
                                                    ksaarp@aarp.org
                                     states.aarp.org/region/kansas
The chapter provides news, events, and more to Kansans aged 50 years and older.
Maren Turner, Kansas AARP State Media Relations
Mary Tritsch, Media Contact

66   **AARP Kentucky**
10401 Linn Station Road   866-295-7275
Louisville, KY 40223   kyaarp@aarp.org
                                   states.aarp.org/region/kentucky
Provides news and resources for Kentuckians over the age of 50.
Scott Wagenast, Associate State Director

67   **AARP Louisiana: Baton Rouge**
301 Main Street   866-448-3620
Baton Rouge, LA 70825   la@aarp.org
                                  states.aarp.org/region/louisiana
The office seeks to advocate for and provide resources to residents of Louisiana aged 50 and over.
Denise Bottcher, State Director
Andrew Muhl, Director, Advocacy

68   **AARP Louisiana: New Orleans**
3502 S Carrollton Avenue   866-448-3620
New Orleans, LA 70118   la@aarp.org
                                  states.aarp.org/region/louisiana
AARP Louisiana's Community Resource Center.
Denise Bottcher, State Director
Andrew Muhl, Director, Advocacy

69   **AARP Maine**
53 Baxter Boulevard   866-554-5380
Portland, ME 04101   me@aarp.org
                                      states.aarp.org/region/maine
Seeks to enhance the lives of Mainers aged 50 years and over through advocacy, information sharing, volunteer opportunities, and service. The chapter counts 230,000 members.
Lori Parham, State Director
Amy Gallant, Director, Advocacy and Outreach

70   **AARP Maryland**
200 St. Paul Place   866-542-8163
Baltimore, MD 21202   Fax: 410-837-0269
                                                    md@aarp.org
                                   states.aarp.org/region/maryland
The chapter seeks to enhance the lives of Maryland residents aged 50 and over, as well as caregivers, through resources and a variety of social opportunities.
Jim Campbell, State President
Nancy Carr, Assoc. State Director, Communications

71   **AARP Massachusetts**
1 Beacon Street   866-448-3621
Boston, MA 02108   Fax: 617-723-4224
                                                    ma@aarp.org
                               states.aarp.org/region/massachusetts
Provides news, events, and resources to Massachusetts residents aged 50 and over.
Mike Festa, State Director
Cindy Campbell, Director, Communications

72   **AARP Michigan**
309 N Washington Square   866-227-7448
Lansing, MI 48933   Fax: 517-482-2794
                                                    TTY: 8
                                                    miaarp@aarp.org
                                   states.aarp.org/region/michigan
The chapter seeks to enhance the quality of life for aging residents of Michigan through information, advocacy, and services.
Paula D. Cunningham, State Director

73 AARP Minnesota
1919 University Avenue   866-554-5381
St. Paul, MN 55104   aarpmn@aarp.org
                        states.aarp.org/region/minnesota
Aims to connect aging residents of Minnesota with financial and
other resources to enhance quality of life.
Will Phillips, State Director
Maro Jo George, Associate State Director, Advocacy

74 AARP Mississippi
141 Township Avenue   866-554-5382
Ridgeland, MS 39157   Fax: 601-898-5429
                        msaarp@aarp.org
                        states.aarp.org/region/mississippi
Seeks to improve the lives of Mississippians, particularly those
over 50 years of age, through events, news, resources, and advo-
cacy.
John McDonald, AARP Missouri State Director
Ronda Gooden, Media Contact

75 AARP Missouri
9200 Ward Parkway   866-389-5627
Kansas City, MO 64114   Fax: 816-561-3107
                        aarpmo@aarp.org
                        states.aarp.org/region/missouri
Provides information to Missourians aged 50 and over on health,
finances, and lifestyle, as well as providing advocacy.
Craig Eichelman, State Director
Jamayla Long, Media Contact

76 AARP Montana
30 W 14th Street   866-295-7278
Helena, MT 59601   mtaarp@aarp.org
                        states.aarp.org/region/montana
With 150,000 members, the chapter provides advocacy, education,
information, resources, and collaborative projects for Montana
residents aged 50 and over.
Tim Summers, State Director
Stacia Dahl, Media Contact

77 AARP Nebraska: Lincoln
301 S 13th Street   866-389-5651
Lincoln, NE 68508   Fax: 402-323-6908
                        neaarp@aarp.org
                        states.aarp.org/region/nebraska
Works on behalf of over 200,000 members and their families to
provide news, services, information, resources, and advocacy for
individuals 50 years and older.
Connie Benjamin, AARP Nebraska State President
Devorah Lanner, Media Contact

78 AARP Nebraska: Omaha
1941 S 42nd Street   402-398-9568
Omaha, NE 68105   omnebraska@aol.com
                        states.aarp.org/region/nebraska
AARP Nebraska's Information Center.
Connie Benjamin, AARP Nebraska State President
Devorah Lanner, Media Contact

79 AARP Nevada
5820 S Eastern Avenue   866-389-5652
Las Vegas, NV 89119   aarpnv@aarp.org
                        states.aarp.org/region/nevada
Provides news, information, and resources to 320,000 members,
on matters affecting the lives of individuals aged 50 and over.
Maria Dent, State Director
Scott Gulbransen, Media Contact

80 AARP New Hampshire
45 South Main Street   866-542-8168
Concord, NH 03301   Fax: 603-224-6211
                        nh@aarp.org
                        states.aarp.org/region/new-hampshire
Provides information, resources, and advocacy services to
228,000 members, on matters relevant to individuals aged 50 years
and older.
Todd Fahey, State Director
Doug McNutt, Associate State Director, Advocacy

81 AARP New Jersey
303 George Street   866-542-8165
New Brunswick, NJ 08901   Fax: 609-987-4634
                        aarpnJ@aarp.org
                        states.aarp.org/region/new-jersey
The chapter seeks to educate and advocate for New Jersey resi-
dents aged 50 and over, and their families.
Stephanie Hunsinger, State Director
Jeff Abramo, Media Contact

82 AARP New Mexico
535 Cerrillos Road   866-389-5636
Santa Fe, NM 87501   Fax: 505-820-2889
                        aarpnm@aarp.org
                        states.aarp.org/region/new-mexico
The chapter advocates on behalf of individuals 50 years and older,
monitoring seniors' services, utility rates, transportation services,
as well as providing financial planning services to members.
Jennifer Baier, Interim State Director
DeAnza Valencia, Associate State Director, Advocacy

83 AARP New York: Albany
1 Commerce Plaza   866-227-7442
Albany, NY 12260   nyaarp@aarp.org
                        states.aarp.org/region/new-york
Provides information, resources, news, and advocacy services to
residents of New York who are 50 years and older.
Beth Finkel, State President
Erik Kriss, Media Contact

84 AARP New York: New York City
750 Third Avenue   866-227-7442
New York, NY 10017   nyaarp@aarp.org
                        states.aarp.org/region/new-york
Provides information, resources, news, and advocacy services to
residents of New York who are 50 years and older.
Beth Finkel, State President
Erik Kriss, Media Contact

85 AARP New York: Rochester
435 E Henrietta Road   866-227-7442
Rochester, NY 14620   nyaarp@aarp.org
                        states.aarp.org/region/new-york
Provides information, resources, news, and advocacy services to
residents of New York who are 50 years and older.
Beth Finkel, State President
Erik Kriss, Media Contact

86 AARP North Carolina
5511 Capital Center Drive   866-389-5650
Raleigh, NC 27606   ddickerson@aarp.org
                        states.aarp.org/region/north-carolina
Advocates for community issues such as health care, employ-
ment/income security, retirement planning, utilities, and protection from financial abuse, on behalf of a membership 1.1 million
strong.
Doug Dickerson, State Director
Michael Oldender, Manager, Outreach and Advocacy

North Dakota

87   **AARP North Dakota**
107 W Main Avenue
Bismarck, ND 58501
866-554-5383
Fax: 701-255-2242
aarpnd@aarp.org
states.aarp.org/region/north-dakota
Provides news, information, resources, events, advocacy, and more to North Dakotans aged 50 and over.
Josh Askvig, State Director
Doreen Redman, Assoc. State Dir., Community Outreach

Ohio

88   **AARP Ohio**
17 S High Street
Columbus, OH 43215
866-389-5653
Fax: 614-224-9801
ohaarp@aarp.org
states.aarp.org/region/ohio
The chapter shares information, advocates, and performs community services for 1.5 million members, 50 years and older, across the state.
Barbara Sykes, State Director

Oklahoma

89   **AARP Oklahoma**
126 N Bryant Avenue
Edmond, OK 73034
866-295-7277
Fax: 405-844-7772
ok@aarp.org
states.aarp.org/region/oklahoma
Assists individuals aged 50 and over through advocacy, news, information, resources, and more.
Sean Voskuhl, State Director
Chad Mullen, Associate State Director, Advocacy

Oregon

90   **AARP Oregon**
9200 SE Sunnybrook Boulevard
Clackamas, OR 97015
866-554-5360
oraarp@aarp.org
states.aarp.org/region/oregon
Strives for social change for its 500,000 members, and all individuals 50 years and over, through advocacy and community services.
Ruby Haughton-Pitts, State Director
Joyce DeMonnin, Media Contact

Pennsylvania

91   **AARP Pennsylvania: Harrisburg**
30 N 3rd Street
Harrisburg, PA 17101
866-389-5654
Fax: 717-236-4078
aarpa@aarp.org
states.aarp.org/region/pennsylvania
Seeks to enhance the quality of life for 1.8 million members across the state.
Bill Johnston-Walsh, State Director
Steve Gardner, Media Contact

92   **AARP Pennsylvania: Philadelphia**
1650 Market Street
Philadelphia, PA 19103
866-389-5654
Fax: 215-665-8529
aarpa@aarp.org
states.aarp.org/region/pennsylvania
Seeks to enhance the quality of life for 1.8 million members across the state.
Bill Johnston-Walsh, State Director
Steve Gardner, Media Contact

Rhode Island

93   **AARP Rhode Island**
10 Orms Street
Providence, RI 02904
866-542-8170
Fax: 401-272-0596
ri@aarp.org
states.aarp.org/region/rhode-island

Provides news, information, resources, advocacy, and community services to those aged 50 and older in the state.
Kathleen Connell, State Director
John Martin, Director, Communications

South Carolina

94   **AARP South Carolina**
1201 Main Street
Columbia, SC 29201
803-765-7381
866-389-5655
scaarp@aarp.org
states.aarp.org/region/south-carolina
Seeks to enhance the quality of life for members and individuals aged 50 and older, through information, resources, education, advocacy, and more.
Teresa Arnold, State Director
Nikki Hutchison, Associate State Director, Advocacy

South Dakota

95   **AARP South Dakota**
5101 S Nevada Avenue
Sioux Falls, SD 57108
866-542-8172
sdaarp@aarp.org
states.aarp.org/region/south-dakota
Provides news, information, resources, advocacy, and community services to 110,000 members and those aged 50 and older in the state.
Erik Gaikowski, State Director

Tennessee

96   **AARP Tennessee**
150 4th Avenue N
Nashville, TN 37219
866-295-7274
tnaarp@aarp.org
states.aarp.org/region/tennessee
Strives for positive social change for 660,000 members and individuals aged 50 and over.
Rebecca Kelly, State Director
Rob Naylor, Director, Communications

Texas

97   **AARP Texas: Austin**
1905 Aldrich Street
Austin, TX 78723
866-227-7443
states.aarp.org/region/texas
The chapter offers news, information, research, and events for individuals aged 50 and over, as well as conducting advocacy on their behalf.
Bob Jackson, State Director
Junita Jiminez-Soto, Associate State Director, Communications

98   **AARP Texas: Dallas**
8140 Walnut Hill Lane
Dallas, TX 75231
866-227-7443
states.aarp.org/region/texas
The chapter offers news, information, research, and events for individuals aged 50 and over, as well as conducting advocacy on their behalf.
Bob Jackson, State Director
Junita Jiminez-Soto, Associate State Director, Communications

99   **AARP Texas: Houston**
2323 S Shepherd Drive
Houston, TX 77019
866-227-7443
states.aarp.org/region/texas
The chapter offers news, information, research, and events for individuals aged 50 and over, as well as conducting advocacy on their behalf.
Bob Jackson, State Director
Junita Jiminez-Soto, Associate State Director, Communications

100   **AARP Texas: San Antonio**
1314 Guadalupe Street
San Antonio, TX 78207
866-227-7443
states.aarp.org/region/texas
The chapter offers news, information, research, and events for individuals aged 50 and over, as well as conducting advocacy on their behalf.
Bob Jackson, State Director
Junita Jiminez-Soto, Associate State Director, Communications

Utah

101 AARP Utah
6975 Union Park Center
Midvale, UT 84047

866-448-3616
Fax: 801-561-2209
utaarp@aarp.org
states.aarp.org/region/utah

Serves 211,000 members in 10 regions across the state, with advocacy, communications, programming, and outreach.
Alan Ormsby, State Director
Danny Harris, Director, Advocacy

Vermont

102 AARP Vermont
199 Main Street
Burlington, VT 05401

866-227-7451
Fax: 802-651-9805
vtaarp@aarp.org
states.aarp.org/region/vermont

Seeks to represent the concerns and interests of Vermonters aged 50 and over.
Greg Marchildon, State Director

Virginia

103 AARP Virginia
707 E Main Street
Richmond, VA 23219

866-542-8164
Fax: 804-819-1923
vaaarp@aarp.org
states.aarp.org/region/virginia

Serves Virginians aged 50 and older, and their families, through advocacy, information, resources, and outreach.
Jim Dau, State Director

Washington

104 AARP Washington
18000 International Blvd.
SeaTac, WA 98188

866-227-7457
Fax: 206-517-9350
waaarp@aarp.org
states.aarp.org/region/washington

Serves 950,000 members through information, advocacy, and a variety of services.
Doug Shadel, State Director

West Virginia

105 AARP West Virginia
300 Summers Street
Charleston, WV 25301

866-227-7458
Fax: 304-344-4633
wvaarp@aarp.org
states.aarp.org/region/west-virginia

Provides information, resources, advocacy, and more to individuals aged 50 and over in West Virginia.
Gaylene Miller, State Director
Tom Hunter, Associate State Director, Communications

Wisconsin

106 AARP Wisconsin
222 W Washington Avenue
Madison, WI 53703

866-448-3611
Fax: 608-251-7612
wistate@aarp.org
states.aarp.org/region/wisconsin

The chapter advocates for, and provides a variety of services to, its 840,000 members, aged 50 years and over.
Sam Wilson, State Director
Jim Flaherty, Media Contact

Wyoming

107 AARP Wyoming
2020 Carey Avenue
Cheyenne, WY 82009

866-663-3290
wyaarp@aarp.org
states.aarp.org/region/wyoming

Provides resources, information, and advocates for indviduals in Wyoming aged 50 and older, with an emphasis on health care, retirement, and utility issues.
Sam Shumway, State Director
Tom Lacock, Assoc. State Dir., Advocacy & Comm.

Foundations

108 AARP Foundation
American Association of Retired Persons
601 E Street NW
Washington, DC 20049

800-775-6776
TTY: 877-434-7598
www.aarp.org/aarp-foundation

The foundation seeks to assist seniors living in poverty through economic opportunities and social connectedness. Legal services and grants are also offered.
Lisa Marsh Ryerson, President
Emily Allen, Senior Vice President, Programs

109 Aging In America
2975 Westchester Avenue
Purchase, NY 10577

914-205-5030
contact@aginginamerica.org
www.aginginamerica.org

Previously a community-based, social service agency, Aging in America is transitioning into a foundation funding technological innovations in Gerontology.
William T. Smith, PhD, President & CEO
Kathleen Bufano, Executive Assistant

110 American Federation for Aging Research
55 W 39th Street
New York, NY 10018

212-703-9977
888-582-2327
Fax: 212-997-0330
info@afar.org
www.afar.org

AFAR supports the science of healthier aging through grants to 4,100 scientists to date.
Stephanie Lederman, Executive Director
Richard W. Besdine, MD, Medical Officer

111 Archstone Foundation
301 E Ocean Boulevard
Long Beach, CA 90802

506-590-8655
Fax: 506-495-0317
archstone@archstone.org
archstone.org

The foundation funds initiatives that meet the needs of an aging population, including stopping elder abuse, preventing falls, and compassionate end-of-life care.
Christopher Langston, PhD, President & CEO
Tanisha Davis, MAG, Grants Manager

112 John A. Hartford Foundation
55 E 59th Street
New York, NY 10022-1713

212-832-7788
Fax: 212-593-4913
terry.fulmer@johnahartford.org
www.johnahartford.org

The foundation is dedicated to improving care of older adults, including funding in areas such as age-friendly health systems, family caregiving, serious illness and end-of-life, and communications and special projects.
Terry Fulmer, PhD, RN, FAAN, President
Rani E. Snyder, MPA, Program Director

Research Centers

113 Academy for Gerontology in Higher Education
1220 L Street NW
Washington, DC 20005

202-289-9806
membership@geron.org
www.aghe.org

Membership organization comprised of more than 130 colleges and universities that offer education and research program in the field of aging. Affiliated with the Gerontological Society of America.
Judith L. Howe, President
Lisa Hollis-Sawyer, Treasurer

114   American Institutes for Research Center on Aging
1000 Thomas Jefferson Street NW   202-403-5000
Washington, DC 20007   Fax: 855-459-6213
                                          TTY: 877-334-3499
                             www.air.org/center/center-aging
Seeks to improve the lives of the disadvantaged through attention
to aging issues, connected to existing work at AIR, and examining
emerging issues.
Marilyn Moon, Director

115   Case Western Reserve University: Center on Aging and Health
10900 Euclid Avenue   216-368-6472
Cleveland, OH 44106   800-825-2540
                                          dlm5@case.edu
                                   case.edu/nursing/ucah
Research organization conducting, supporting and facilitating re-
search into gerontology and geriatrics.
Diana L Morris, PhD, RN, Executive Director
Evelyn Duffy, DNP, ANP/GNP-BC, Associate Director

**116   Center for Aging Research and Education at the UW-Madison
School of Nursing**
Signe Skott Cooper Hall
701 Highland Avenue   608-265-4330
Madison, WI 53705   care@son.wisc.edu
                                          care.nursing.wisc.edu
CARE seeks to prepare healthcare professionals to work with
older adults, as well as encouraging inter-professional and cam-
pus-community collaborations.
Barbara Bowers, Founding Director
Barbara King, Executive Director

117   Columbia University Robert N. Butler Aging Center
Mailman School Of Public Health
722 W 168th Street   212-305-0424
New York, NY 10032   ColumbiaAgingCenter@cumc.columbia.edu
                                          aging.columbia.edu
Clinical research in geriatric/gerontology and long-term care, and
promotes the study of aging across the university.
Linda P. Fried, MD, MPH, Interim Co-Director
Kavita Sivaramakrishnan, Interim Co-Director, PhD

**118   Duke University Center for the Study of Aging and Human
Development**
Box 3003 DUMC   919-660-7500
Durham, NC 27710   Fax: 919-668-0453
                                   sites.duke.edu/centerforaging
The center's research focuses on age-related decline, biomarkers
of aging, exercise, osteoporosis, Alzheimer's disease, cancer as it
relates to aging, viral diseases of aging, later-life depression, care-
giver stress, and spirituality and health.
Harvey Jay Cohen, MD, Director
Heather E. Whitson, Deputy Director

**119   George Washington University Center for Aging, Health and
Humanities**
1919 Pennsylvania Avenue NW   202-994-7901
Washington, DC 20006   Fax: 202-296-1229
                                          aging@gwu.edu
                                          nursing.gwu.edu
An interdisciplinary space for university faculty to collaborate on
aging research, education, scholarship, and innovations.
Melissa Batchelor-Murphy, PhD, Director
Elizabeth Cobbs, MD, Co-Director

120   Harvey A Friedman Center for Aging Washington University
Institute for Public Health
600 S Taylor   314-747-9192
St. Louis, MO 63110   centerforaging@wustl.edu
                                          publichealth.wustl.edu/aging
Seeks to provide older adults with the greatest opportunity for
health, security, and engagement.
Nancy L. Morrow-Howell, PhD, Director
Natalie Galucia, MSW, Center Manager

**121   Home Instead Center for Successful Aging University of
Nebraska Medical Center**
730 S 38th Avenue
Omaha, NE 68105   402-559-9600
                                          webmaster@unmc.edu
                                          www.unmc.edu/homeinsteadcenter

Provides patient care, as well as patient education, and research
into promoting independence and aging in place.
Bradley Britigan, MD, Dean, College Of Medicine

**122   Indiana University School of Medicine Center for Aging
Research**
545 Barnhill Drive   317-274-8438
Indianapolis, IN 46202   Fax: 317-274-1437
                                          medicine.iu.edu
Research on aging includes brain health, decision-making, physi-
cal fitness, transitional and nursing home care, and medication.
Mark Geraci, MD, Chair, Department of Medicine
Samir Gupta, MD, Vice Chair, Research

**123   Jean Mayer USDA Human Nutrition Research Center on Aging
at Tufts University**
711 Washington Street   617-556-3000
Boston, MA 02111   hnrca.tufts.edu
Makes research contributions to U.S. and international nutrition
and physical activity recommendations for older adults.
Sarah L. Booth, PhD, Director
Xiang-Dong Wang, MD, PhD, Associate Director

124   Johns Hopkins Center on Aging and Health
2024 E Monument Street   410-955-0491
Baltimore, MD 21205-2223   Fax: 410-614-9625
                                          coah.jhu.edu
Sponsored by the Johns Hopkins Schools of Medicine and Public
Health, COAH is an interdisciplinary group of research faculty
seeking to optimize the health of older adults.
David L. Roth, PhD, Director
Brian Buta, MHS, Program Manager

125   Kansas State University Center on Aging
1324 Lovers Lane   785-532-5945
Manhattan, KS 66506   Fax: 785-532-5504
                                          gerontology@k-state.edu
                                          www.he.k-state.edu/aging
Focused on education, research, & outreach in the field of geron-
tology.
Gayle Doll, Director
Migette Kaup, Chair, Research Committee

126   Landon Center on Aging University of Kansas Medical Center
University of Kansas Medical Center
3901 Rainbow Boulevard   913-588-5000
Kansas City, KS 66160   800-766-3777
                                          Fax: 913-588-1201
                                          mchandler@kumc.edu
                                          www2.kumc.edu/coa
Provides support for interdisciplinary research on the issue of age
and aging.
Matt Chandler, MBA, Program Director
Diane Clark, Assistant Director

127   Medical University of South Carolina Center on Aging
280 Calhoun Street   843-792-0712
Charleston, SC 29425   education.musc.edu/colleges/medicine
Engages in research, services, and education with the aim of pro-
moting health, quality of life, and longevity for seniors.
Heather Boger, Interim Director

128   National Academy on an Aging Society
1220 L Street NW   202-842-1275
Washington, DC 20005   Fax: 202-842-1150
                                          geron@geron.org
                                          www.geron.org
The policy branch of the Gerontological Society of America, the
NAAS is a non-partisan institute conducting research on popula-
tion aging.
James Appleby, Chief Executive Officer
Judie Lieu, VP, Publishing & Professional Resources

**129   Purdue University: Center for Research on Aging and the Life
Course**
1202 W. State Street   765-494-9692
W Lafayette, IN 47907-2055   Fax: 765-494-2180
                                          calc@purdue.edu
                                          www.purdue.edu/aging

Social science research on aging, health and health care delivery.
Kenneth F. Ferraro, PhD, Director
Paige Ebner, Assistant Director

130   Roy M and Phyllis Gough Huffington Center on Aging
Baylor College of Medicine
One Baylor Plaza   713-798-5804
Houston, TX 77030   fincher@bcm.edu
                                          www.hcoa.org
Internal unit of Baylor College representing research into the biology of aging.
Hui Zheng , PhD, Director
Ruth Andrea Reeves, MBA, BA, AAS, Center Administrator

131   Sanders-Brown Center on Aging University of Kentucky
800 S Limestone Street   859-323-6040
Lexington, KY 40536-0230   Fax: 859-323-2866
                                          linda.vaneldik@uky.edu
                                          www.uky.edu/coa
Investigates healthy brain aging and neurodegenerative disorders through research, education and outreach, and clinical programs.
Linda J. Van Eldik, PhD, Director
Gregory A. Jicha, MD, PhD, Associate Director

132   Sanford Center for Aging University Of Nevada, Reno
Center for Molecular Medicine
1664 North Virginia Street   775-784-4774
Reno, NV 89557   Fax: 775-784-1814
                                          sanford@unr.edu
                                          med.unr.edu/aging
Aims to enhance the quality of life and well-being among older adults through education, research, and outreach.
Peter Reed, PhD, MPH, Director
Heather Haslem, Director, Wellness

133   Stanford Center on Longevity
Littlefield Center, Stanford University
365 Lasuen Street   650-736-8643
Stanford, CA 94305-6053   info-longevity@stanford.edu
                                          longevity.stanford.edu
Seeks to advance scientific discoveries, advances in technology, and behavioral and social norms with the goal of enhancing century-long lives.
Laura Carstensen, PhD, Director
Nancy Easterbrook, Director, External Affairs

134   Stein Institute for Research on Aging UC San Diego School of Medicine
9500 Gilman Drive   858-534-6299
La Jolla, CA 92093-0012   Fax: 858-534-5475
                                          aging@ucsd.edu
                                          medschool.ucsd.edu/research/aging
Develops and applies recent advances in biomedical and behavioral science to issues of healthy aging, and reducing the burden of disease and disability in later life.
Dilip V. Jeste, MD, Director
Deborah Kado, MD, MS, Deputy Director, Clinical Research

135   The Center on Aging and Work at Boston College
140 Commonwealth Avenue   617-552-9195
Chestnut Hill, MA 02467   agework@bc.edu
                                          www.bc.edu/research/agingandwork
Conducts research into quality of employment for a multi-generational workforce.
Jacquelyn B. James, PhD, Interim Co-Director
Tay K. McNamara, PhD, Interim Co-Director

136   Tulane University Center For Aging
1430 Tulane Avenue   504-988-3369
New Orleans, LA 70112   aging-studies@tulane.edu
                                          medicine.tulane.edu
Dedicated to enhancing the quality of life of aging adults through research, education, and innovation.
S. Michal Jazwinski, PhD, Director

137   University Of North Carolina School of Medicine Center for Aging and Health
5003 Old Clinic   919-966-5945
Chapel Hill, NC 27599   www.med.unc.edu/aging

Provides care for older patients, provides community resources to families and caregivers, and trains not only geriatricians, but other medical professionals in geriatric medicine.
Jan Busby-Whitehead, Director
Ben Blomberg, Assistant Clinical Professor

138   University Of Wyoming Center on Aging
1000 E University Avenue   307-766-2829
Laramie, WY 82071   wycoa@uwyo.edu
                                          www.uwyo.edu/wycoa
Seeks to optimize the health and well-being of older adults and caregivers in Wyoming through partnerships, research, community education, and clinical training.
Christine McKibbin, PhD, Director
Catherine Phillips Carrico, PhD, Associate Director

139   University of Connecticut Center on Aging
135 Dowling Way   860-679-8400
Farmington, CT 06030   health.uconn.edu/aging
Provides care for older adults, as well as conducting research into the aging process in order to promote health and quality of life.
George A. Kuchel, MD, Director

140   University of Florida Institute on Aging
2004 Mowry Road   352-294-5800
Gainesville, FL 32611   lcrump@ufl.edu
                                          aging.ufl.edu
The IOA operates interdisciplinary teams in research, education and health care, dedicated to improving the health, independence, and quality of life for older adults.
Marco Pahor, MD, Director
Lauren Crump, MPH, Associate Director

141   University of Maryland School of Public Health Center on Aging
4200 Valley Drive   301-405-2438
College Park, MD 20742-2611   Fax: 301-405-8397
                                          asmaa@umd.edu
                                          sph.umd.edu
An interdisciplinary institution conducting applied and policy research, education, and public service into human aging.
Luisa Franzini, PhD, Director
Jim Hagberg, PhD, Associate Director

142   University of Pennsylvania Institute on Aging
3615 Chestnut Street   215-898-7801
Philadelphia, PA 19104-2676   aging@pennmedicine.upenn.edu
                                          www.med.upenn.edu/aging
The mission of the IOA is to improve the health of the elderly by increasing the quality and quantity of clinical and basic research as well as educational programs focusing on normal aging and age-related diseases at the UPSM and across the entire Penn campus.
John Q. Trojanowski, MD, PhD, Director
F. Bradley Johnson, MD, PhD, Associate Director

143   University of Vermont Larner College of Medicine Center on Aging
89 Beaumont Avenue   802-656-0292
Burlington, VT 05405   Fax: 802-656-8380
                                          Jeanne.Hutchins@uvm.edu
                                          www.med.uvm.edu/centeronaging
Aims to promote well-being and a high quality of life for older adults, through university collaboration.
William Pendlebury, MD, Director
Jeanne M. Hutchins, MA, Executive Director

144   Virginia Commonwealth University Virginia Center on Aging
730 East Broad Street   804-828-1525
Richmond, VA 23219   804-828-7905
                                          vcoa@vcu.edu
                                          vcoa.chp.vcu.edu
Interdisciplinary center for the study and research of the aged and the aging process.
Edward F. Ansello, PhD, Director
Constance L. Coogle, PhD, Associate Director, Research

145   de Tornyay Center For Healthy Aging at University of Washington
School of Nursing

PO Box 357260   206-616-4276
Seattle, WA 98195-7260   206-616-3064
agingctr@u.washington.edu
nursing.uw.edu
Supports gerontology research and education to promote healthy aging.
Basia Belza, PhD, RN, FAAN, Director
Heather Wicklein-Sanchez, Manager

Support Groups & Hotlines

146   **American Association of Caregiving Youth**
1515 N Federal Hwy.   561-391-7401
Boca Raton, FL 33432   800-508-9618
info@aacy.org
www.aacy.org
Seeks to raise awareness of and provide services for youth who act as caregivers for their parents and grandparents.
Connie Siskowski, RN, PhD, President

147   **Caregiver Action Network**
1150 Connecticut Avenue NW   202-454-3970
Washington, DC 20036-3904   info@caregiveraction.org
caregiveraction.org
Aims to improve quality of life for Americans who care for loved ones facing chronic illnesses, disabilities, diseases, or old age.
John Schall, Chief Executive Officer
Chance Browning, Senior Director, Programs

148   **Caregiver Support Services**
PO Box 4291   866-201-6896
Omaha, NE 68104   egreen@caregiversupportservices.org
caregiversupportservices.com
Provides guidance and resources to caregivers.
Eboni Green, President & CEO
Terrence Green, Vice President, Business Development

149   **Children of Aging Parents**
PO Box 167   215-355-6611
Richboro, PA 18954   800-227-7294
Fax: 215-355-6824
info@caps4caregivers.org
www.caps4caregivers.org
A nonprofit, charitable organization that assists the nation's nearly 54 million caregivers of the elderly or chronically ill with reliable information, referrals and support, and to heighten public awareness.

150   **Hospice and Homecare**
3801 Vanesta Drive   785-537-0688
Manhattan, KS 66503   Fax: 785-537-1309
info@hcandh.org
www.homecareandhospice.org
Aims to be the premier non-profit Homecare & Hospice provider of compassionate, affordable health, wellness and support services.

151   **National Alliance for Caregiving**
4720 Montgomery Lane   301-718-8444
Bethesda, MD 20814   301-951-9067
info@caregiving.org
www.caregiving.org
Advocates on behalf of caregivers, as well as conducting research and offering support services.
C. Grace Whiting, JD, President & CEO
Michael Wittke, BSW, MPA, Senior Director, Public Policy

152   **National Health Information Center**
Office of Disease Prevention & Health Promotion
1101 Wootton Pkwy   Fax: 240-453-8281
Rockville, MD 20852   odphpinfo@hhs.gov
www.health.gov/nhic
Supports public health education by maintaining a calendar of National Health Observances; helps connect consumers and health professionals to organizations that can best answer questions and provide up-to-date contact information from reliable sources; updates on a yearly basis toll-free numbers for health information, Federal health clearinghouses and info centers.
Don Wright, MD, MPH, Director

153   **Well Spouse Association**
63 W Main Street   732-577-8899
Freehold, NJ 07728   www.wellspouse.org
This association is a nonprofit national self-help organization serving the well spouse of the chronically ill. Members help each other develop coping and survival skills through local support groups (including bereavement), letter and telephone networks, and personal outreach and a quarterly newsletter.
Marilyn Kamp, Executive Director

Books

154   **Activities for the Disabled, Elderly and Adults**
Haworth Press
10 Alice Street   607-722-5857
Binghamton, NY 13904-1580   800-429-6784
Fax: 607-722-0012
www.haworthpress.com
Learn how to effectively plan and deliver activities for a growing number of older people with developmental disabilities. It aims to stimulate interest and continued support for recreation program development and implementation among developmental disability and aging service systems.
136 pages Hardcover
ISBN: 1-560240-92-X

155   **Adult Children and Aging Parents**
American Counseling Association
6101 Stevenson Ave.   703-823-9800
Alexandria, VA 22304-3302   800-347-6647
Fax: 703-823-0252
webmaster@counseling.org
www.counseling.org
Provides effective intervention strategies and suggestions for counselors who work with older persons, individually and with the family. Offers information on many vital topics such as Alzheimer's Disease, retirement, elder abuse and suicide.
216 pages
ISBN: 0-840354-48-7

156   **Aging and Family Therapy**
Haworth Press
10 Alice Street   607-722-5857
Binghamton, NY 13904-1580   800-429-6784
Fax: 607-722-0012
www.haworthpress.com
Here are creative strategies for use in therapy with older adults and their families. This book provides practitioners with information, insight, reference tools, and other sources that will contribute to more effective intervention with the elderly and their families.
244 pages Hardcover
ISBN: 0-866567-78-3

157   **Aging and Our Families**
Human Sciences Press
233 Spring Street   212-620-8000
New York, NY 10013-1522   800-221-9369
www.springer.com
Handbook for family caregivers.
132 pages Paperback
ISBN: 0-898854-41-5

158   **Caregivers' Roller Coaster**
Loyola University Press
3441 N Ashland Avenue   773-281-1818
Chicago, IL 60657-1355   800-621-1008
Fax: 773-281-0555
marketing@loyolapress.com
www.loyolapress.com
A simply written self-help guide for caregivers of the frail elderly. Offers support for men and women, not trained professionals, who find themselves caring for aging family members in their own homes. Offers practical advice and information on Alzheimer's, Medicare, insurance and community services for the elderly.
150 pages
ISBN: 0-829407-45-6

159 Caring for Those You Love: A Guide to Compassionate Care for the Aged
Bethany Chaffin, author
Horizon Publishers & Distributors, Inc.
191 N 650 East   801-295-9451
Bountiful, UT 84010-3628   Fax: 801-298-1305
                              hpservice09@hotmail.com
Includes helpful information on identifying the problems of the aged. It explains the best and most frequently used treatments prescribed for these problems, and tells how family members can help to meet the physical, emotional, and spiritual needs of aging parents and other loved ones.
108 pages
ISBN: 0-882902-70-9
Duane S Crowther, Owner/CEO
Jean D Crowther, Owner/CEO

160 Continuing Care Retirement Community Directory
American Assoc. of Homes & Services for the Aging
901 E Street NW   800-508-9442
Washington, DC 20004-2037   Fax: 301-206-9789
A national consumer's directory of continuing care retirement communities. This directory is a vital tool for individuals searching and evaluating a community for themselves or a loved one.

161 Court-Related Needs of the Elderly and Persons with Disabilities
Commission on the Mentally Disabled
1800 M Street NW   202-331-2240
Washington, DC 20036-5802   www.statejustice.org/
Report of the National Conference, examines the barriers of the judicial system impeding access for the elderly and persons with disabilities.

162 Creative Movements for Older Adults
Human Sciences Press
233 Spring Street   212-620-8000
New York, NY 10013-1522   800-221-9369
                                    www.springer.com
Exercises for the elderly.
172 pages Cloth
ISBN: 0-898854-14-8

163 Diagnosis and Treatment of Old Age
S Karger Publishers
26 W Avon Road   860-675-7834
Farmington, CT 06085-1162   800-828-5479
                                    Fax: 860-675-7302
These papers furnish a concise update on the diagnosis and treatment of Alzheimer's disease.
112 pages Hardcover
ISBN: 3-805548-44-3

164 Elder Care
Center For Public Representation
975 Bascom Mall   608-262-2240
Madison, WI 53706-0049   800-369-0388
                                    Fax: 608-251-1263
                                    law.wisc.edu
A compendium of alternatives for providing and financing long-term care. This practical guide provides the most comprehensive and comforting information to help navigate a number of consumer minefields.
224 pages
ISBN: 0-873371-13-5

165 Elderly in Modern Society
Vance Bibliographier
PO Box 229   217-762-3831
Monticello, IL 61856-0229
A bibliography of laws and human rights for the elderly.
15 pages
ISBN: 0-792001-10-9

166 Falling in Old Age
Reing Tideiksaar PhD, author
Springer Publishing Company

11 W 42nd Street   212-431-4370
New York, NY 10036   877-687-7476
                                    Fax: 212-941-7842
                                    cs@springerpub.com
                                    www.springerpub.com
This book provides an enormous body of fall-related research that has been organized by the author into easy, digestible information for geriatric health professionals. Extensively updated and revised for its second edition, the book has direct clinical applications and strategies for preventing and managing falls. It also contains new information on the physical, psychological, and social complications of falling.
412 pages Hardcover
ISBN: 0-826152-91-6

167 Family Carebook
CAREsource Program Development
505 Seattle Tower   206-625-9080
Seattle, WA 98101-3021
Guide to aging, the special needs of older adults, and the demands of providing care and support. Experts explain potential conflicts, planning opportunities and strategies for success.
475 pages Paperback
ISBN: 1-878866-12-5

168 From Theory to Therapy: The Development of Drugs for Alzheimer's Disease
Alzheimer's Association
225 N Michigan Avenue   800-272-3900
Chicago, IL 60611-1696   Fax: 866-699-1246
                                    TDD: 312-335-8700
                                    media@alz.org
                                    www.alz.org
Provides a layman's explanation of how experimental drugs are being developed and tested for Alzheimer's disease, and information about patient participation in clinical drug trials.

169 Geriatric Rehabilitation Preview
RTC on Aging
7601 E Imperial Highway   310-940-7402
Downey, CA 90242-4155
Covers research, training activities, and other issues pertaining to the rehabilitation of elderly persons with disabilities.

170 Health Care of the Aged
Abraham Monk, PhD, author
Haworth Press
10 Alice Street   607-722-5857
Binghamton, NY 13904-1580   800-429-6784
                                    Fax: 607-722-0012
                                    www.haworthpress.com
Focusing on the need for developing new service delivery models for the aged, this book examines fiscal, political, and social criteria influencing this challenge of the 1990s. The aged are caught in the sweeping changes currently occurring in the financing, organizing and delivery of human health care services.
183 pages Hardcover
ISBN: 1-560240-65-5

171 Healthy Aging: Good Investment & Together We Care: Helping Caregivers Find Supp.
National Council on Aging
1901 L Street NW   202-479-1200
Washington, DC 20036   800-677-1116
                                    Fax: 202-479-0735
                                    TDD: 202-479-6674
                                    info@ncoa.org
                                    www.ncoa.org
Describes seven model programs that could be used in community-based organizations serving older adults.
2 Book Set
James P Firman, EdD, President/CEO

172 International Health Guide for Senior Citizen Travelers
Pilot Books
103 Cooper Street   516-422-2225
Babylon, NY 11702-2368   Fax: 516-669-4173

Covers essential pre-departure health planning such as advice on specific health concerns, disease prevention, specific travel problems, medical preparedness and assistance.
70 pages Paperback
ISBN: 0-875761-39-9
Anne Small, President

173 Living Well in a Nursing Home
Lynn Dickinson, Xenia Vosen, author
Hunter House Publishing
445 Park Avenue   646-291-8961
New York, NY 10022   800-266-5592
                                         Fax: 646-291-8962
                                         ordering@hunterhouse.com
                                         www.turnerpublishing.com
This book concentrates on the positive aspects of nursing homes, providing tips, support and reassurance.
256 pages Paperback
ISBN: 0-897934-60-2

174 Mentally Impaired Elderly
Ellen D Taira, author
Haworth Press
10 Alice Street   607-722-5857
Binghamton, NY 13904-1580   800-429-6784
                                         Fax: 607-722-0012
                                         www.haworthpress.com
Provides effective support and sensitive care for the most vulnerable segment of the elderly population, those with mental impairment.
191 171 pages
ISBN: 1-560241-68-1

175 Mirrored Lives
Greenwood Publishing Group, Inc/Praeger Publishers
130 Cremona Drive   800-225-5800
Santa Barbara, CA 93117-6926   Fax: 877-231-6980
                                         service@greenwood.com
                                         www.abc-clio.com/ABC-CLIOGreenwood
Discusses geriatric decline connected to nonterminal illness in old age. Koch takes a sensitive but thorough look at the declining years of his father.
240 pages
ISBN: 0-275936-71-6

176 Nursing Home Information Services
925 15th Street NW   202-347-8800
Washington, DC 20005-2301
Lists acceptable nursing homes across the nation and provides information about their costs, admission requirements, standards and programs.

177 Nursing Home and You: Partners in Caring
American Assn. of Homes & Services for the Aging
901 E Street NW   800-508-9442
Washington, DC 20004-2037   Fax: 301-206-9789
Offers information to nursing home staff and family members about caring for persons with Alzheimer's Disease.

178 Older Americans Information Directory
Grey House Publishing
4919 Route 22   518-789-8700
Amenia, NY 12501   800-562-2139
                                         Fax: 518-789-8700
                                         books@greyhouse.com
                                         www.greyhouse.com
An invaluable resource that offers up-to-date information on the prevalent social, health and financial issues facing older Americans in the 21st century, as well as recreational and educational opportunities to enrich their lives.
1200 pages
ISBN: 1-592375-43-X
Leslie Mackenzie, Publisher

179 On Your Behalf
CAREsource Program Development
505 Seattle Tower
Seattle, WA 98101   206-625-9080
This book takes the mystery out of very important sets of legal options. It gives lay people as well as advisors, service providers, and

caregivers the information they need to understand their options and the importance of individual choice.
16 pages Books & Video
ISBN: 1-878866-14-1

180 Physical Activity and the Aging
Human Kinetic Publishers
1607 N Market Street   800-747-4457
Champaign, IL 61820-5076   Fax: 217-351-1549
                                         info@hkusa.com
                                         www.humankinetics.com
North America's leading scholars examine the effects of aging on motor function, cardiovascular function, balance, the nervous system, changes in activity level, and possible reasons for activity level changes.
208 pages
ISBN: 0-873222-20-2

181 Planning for Long-Term Care
National Council on Aging
1901 L Street NW   202-479-1200
Washington, DC 20036   800-677-1116
                                         Fax: 202-479-0735
                                         TDD: 202-479-6674
                                         info@ncoa.org
                                         www.ncoa.org
Identify the various long-term care resources within your family and in your community using this thorough and readable guide.
160 pages
James P Firman, EdD, President/CEO

182 Read Easy
CAREsource Program Development
505 Seattle Tower   206-625-9080
Seattle, WA 98101
If books, audio tapes and computers can spark the imagination of the young adult and the middle aged, why not seniors as well? All it takes is commitment to make quality library resources and programs accessible and user-friendly to older readers. Read Easy is an invaluable planning and operations guide, explaining senior needs to library professionals and librarianship principles to senior care professionals.
95 pages
ISBN: 1-878866-13-3

183 Resources for Elders with Disabilities
Resources for Rehabilitation
22 Bonad Road   781-368-9080
Winchester, MA 01890   Fax: 781-368-9096
                                         info@rfr.org
                                         www.rfr.org
Provides information that enables elders, family members and other caregivers, and service providers to locate appropriate services. Includes information about rehabilitation, laws that affect elders with disabilities, and self-help groups. Published in large print.
ISBN: 0-929718-31-3

184 Senior Center Self: Assessment & National Accreditation Manual
National Council on Aging
1901 L Street NW   202-479-1200
Washington, DC 20036   800-677-1116
                                         Fax: 202-479-0735
                                         TDD: 2024796674
                                         info@ncoa.org
                                         www.ncoa.org
Based upon compliance with standards (best practices) developed by the National Institutes of Senior Centers. This program was developed under the auspices of NCOA's National Institute of Senior Centers (NISC).
Book & CD Set
James P Firman, EdD, President/CEO

185 Senior Citizens and the Law
Center for Public Representation
PO Box 260049   608-251-4008
Madison, WI 53726-0049   800-369-0388
                                         Fax: 608-251-1263
An introduction to legal problems facing the elderly in Wisconsin. This edition discusses legal problems associated with Social Secu-

rity, Medicare, SSI, guardianship and its alternatives, community-based services, probate, taxes, private health insurance and consumer protection.
176 pages
ISBN: 0-932622-29-1

186   Successful Models of Community Long Term Care Services for the Elderly
Haworth Press
10 Alice Street   607-722-5857
Binghamton, NY 13904-1580   800-429-6784
                                Fax: 607-722-0012
                            www.haworthpress.com
Experienced practitioners provide examples of successful community-based long term care service programs for the elderly.
174 pages
ISBN: 0-866569-87-9

187   Unloving Care
Harper Collins Publishers/Basic Books
195 Broadway   212-207-7000
New York, NY 10007-5299   800-242-7737
                                Fax: 212-207-7203
                    tmpcorrections@harpercollins.com
                            www.harpercollins.com
A leading public health expert gives his account of the negative aspects of nursing homes.
305 pages
ISBN: 0-465088-81-3

Magazines

188   AARP Magazine
American Association of Retired Persons
601 East Street NW   202-434-3525
Washington, DC 20049   888-687-2277
                                TTY: 877-434-7598
                                member@aarp.org
                                www.aarp.org
Celebrity interviews. Features on health and finance. Movie reviews and more. All with an eye toward the topics and issues you care about most.
A Barry Rand, CEO

189   Abstracts in Social Gerontology
National Council on Aging
1901 L Street NW   202-479-1200
Washington, DC 20036   800-677-1116
                                Fax: 202-479-0735
                                TDD: 202-479-6674
                                info@ncoa.org
                                www.ncoa.org
Detailed abstracts are provided for recent major journal articles, books, reports and other materials on many facets of aging, including adult education, demography, family relations, institutional care and work attitudes.
Quarterly
James P Firman, EdD, President/CEO

190   Innovations
National Council on Aging
1901 L Street NW   202-479-1200
Washington, DC 20036   800-677-1116
                                Fax: 202-479-0735
                                TDD: 2024796674
                                info@ncoa.org
                                www.ncoa.org
Explores significant developments in the field of aging through opinion articles, profiles and research summaries. Features articles on social trends, articles on specific aging programs and information on NCOA's activities. Members are free.
Quarterly
James P Firman, EdD, President/CEO

191   International Journal of Technology and Aging
Human Sciences Press

233 Spring Street   212-620-8000
New York, NY 10013-1522   800-221-9369
                                Fax: 212-463-0742
                                www.springer.com
Designed to serve health-care professionals, researchers, academicians and industries concerned with the convergence of two recent trends, the dramatic advances in technology and the rapidly growing elderly population.

192   Modern Maturity
AARP
601 E Street NW   202-434-3525
Washington, DC 20049-0003   800-424-3410
                                TTY: 877-434-7598
                                member@aarp.org
                                www.aarp.org
Offers news and information of concern to those 50 and older. Features articles on current events, health, recreation, housing, family life, legislation and other issues.
6x Year

Newsletters

193   AARP Bulletin
American Association of Retired Persons
601 East Street NW   202-434-3525
Washington, DC 20049   888-687-2277
                                TTY: 877-434-7598
                                member@aarp.org
                                www.aarp.org
Get daily news about the issues that matter to you.
Bill Novelli, AARP CEO

194   Best Practices
American Assoc. of Homes & Services for the Aging
2519 Connecticut Ave NW   202-783-2242
Washington, DC 20008-1520   Fax: 202-783-2255
                                info@aahsa.org
                                www.aahsa.org
Keeps nonprofit aging service providers informed of new trends and developments in quality of care for older persons.

195   Bulletin
AARP
601 E Street NW   202-434-3525
Washington, DC 20049   800-424-3410
                                TTY: 877-434-7598
                                member@aarp.org
                                www.aarp.org
Get daily news about the issues that matter to you.
11x Year

196   CAPSule
Children of Aging Parents
PO Box 167   215-355-6611
Richboro, PA 18954-0167   800-227-7294
                                Fax: 215-355-6824
                            www.caps4caregivers.org
Newsletter devoted to assisting caregivers of the elderly.
12 pages Quarterly
Lenore Sherman, Executive Director
Karen Rosenberg, Director Senior Services

197   Capital Advantage
Capital Advantage Publishing
3708 Mount Diablo Blvd   925-299-1500
Lafayette, CA 94549   Fax: 925-299-1599
                            www.capitaladvantage.com
Publishes articles on all aspects of aging including legislation, innovative programs and services.
Monthly

198   Center for the Study of Aging Newsletter
University of Pennsylvania Center for Aging Study
3615 Chestnut Street   215-898-7801
Philadelphia, PA 19104-4205   Fax: 215-573-8684
                            ageweb@mail.med.upenn.edu
                            www.med.upenn.edu/aging

News and information concerning the University and Center aging activities, programs and seminars.

199 Elderly Health Services Letter
American Business Publishing
3100 Highway 138   732-681-1133
Wall Township, NJ 0771
Information on trends and developments in the expanding field of health services for the elderly.
Monthly
Robert Jenkins, Publisher

200 Geriatric Care News
DRS Geriatric Publishing Company
7435 SE 71st Street   206-232-9689
Mercer Island, WA 98040-5314
Newsletter for the elderly and their families.
Monthly
Denise Schramke, Publisher

201 Geriatrics
7500 Old Oak Boulevard   440-243-8100
Cleveland, OH 44130-3343
Articles for physicians and laypersons relating to care of middle-aged and elderly persons.
Monthly

202 Gerontology News
Gerontological Society of America
1220 L Street NW   202-842-1275
Washington, DC 20005   Fax: 202-842-1150
                                 geron@geron.org
                                  www.geron.org
It reports on policy issues, legislative actions, Society events, research results, and recently released major reports on aging. Regular features include Washington Updates; Research Highlights; Grants Available; New Resources and Reports; Data Updates; and Calls for Papers, Nominations, and Manuscripts.
Carol Ann Schutz, Executive Director

203 Health After 50: Johns Hopkins Medical Letter
Johns Hopkins Medical Institutions
550 Broadway   410-955-3182
Baltimore, MD 21205-2011   800-829-9170
Health newsletter for people over 50.
10 pages Monthly
ISBN: 1-042188-2 -
Rodney Friedman, Publisher

204 Lifelong Health and Fitness
Center for the Study of Aging
706 Madison Avenue   518-465-4927
Albany, NY 12208-3604   Fax: 518-462-1339
                                  iapaas@aol.com
A quarterly newsletter published by the Center for the Study of Aging.
8 pages Quarterly
Sara Harris, Executive Director

205 NCOA Week
National Council on Aging
1901 L Street NW   202-479-1200
Washington, DC 20036   800-677-1116
                               Fax: 202-479-0735
                               TDD: 202-479-6674
                                  info@ncoa.org
                                  www.ncoa.org
Breaking news of NCOA initiatives, crucial legislative and policy issues, research studies, developments in work and volunteering for older adults, benefits for seniors, trends in aging, grant opportunities, and more. Members only.
Weekly
James P Firman, EdD, President/CEO

206 Senior Focus
National Council on Aging
1901 L Street NW   202-479-1200
Washington, DC 20036   800-677-1116
                               Fax: 202-479-0735
                               TDD: 202-479-6674
                                  info@ncoa.org
                                  www.ncoa.org
Timely, objective, and practical information on health and wellness, lifestyle, and financial issues for seniors and people who work with them.
Bi-Monthly
James P Firman, EdD, President/CEO

207 Vital Aging Report
National Council on Aging
1901 L Street NW   202-479-1200
Baltimore, MD   800-677-1116
                               Fax: 202-479-0735
                               TDD: 202-479-6674
                                  info@ncoa.org
                                  www.ncoa.org
Packed with news about health and financial matters as well as United Senior's Health Council's innovative programs and research. The USHC is a program of the National Council on the Aging. Member price $17.50.
Quarterly
James P Firman, EdD, President/CEO

Pamphlets

208 American Perceptions of Aging in the 21st Century
National Council on Aging
1901 L Street NW   202-479-1200
Washington, DC 20036   800-677-1116
                               Fax: 202-479-0735
                               TDD: 2024796674
                                  info@ncoa.org
                                  www.ncoa.org
There are many interesting and important findings related to aging in America as reported by over 3000 respondents. This chartbook is intended as a handy reference for scholars, the press and advocates.
James P Firman, EdD, President/CEO

209 Care of the Elderly in America
Vance Bibliographies
PO Box 229   217-762-3831
Monticello, IL 61856-0229
A bibliography of aged care in America.
11 pages
ISBN: 1-555905-59-5

210 Exploring Care Options for a Relative with Alzheimer's Disease
American Assoc. of Homes & Services for the Aging
2519 Connecticut Ave NW   202-783-2242
Washington, DC 20008-1520   800-508-9442
                               Fax: 202-783-2255

211 Medicare Health Plan Choices: Consumer Update
National Council on Aging
1901 L Street NW   202-479-1200
Washington, DC 20036   800-677-1116
                               Fax: 202-479-0735
                               TDD: 202-479-6744
                                  info@ncoa.org
                                  www.ncoa.org
Annually updated report contains important information about options that are available to Medicare beneficiaries. Medicare is changing, Medigap premiums are going up, and many Medicare HMOs are dropping service to seniors. Pamphlets available in single copies or packs of 50.
James P Firman, EdD, President/CEO

212 Nonprofit Housing and Care Options for Older People
American Assoc. of Homes & Services for the Aging
901 E Street NW   800-508-9442
Washington, DC 20004-2037   Fax: 301-206-9789
Offers information on continuing care facilities, retirement communities and more for the elderly and relatives caring for Alzheimer's patients.

213 Time Out!
Alzheimer's Association
225 N Michigan Avenue   800-272-3900
Chicago, IL 60611-1696   Fax: 866-669-1246
                                          TDD: 312-335-8700
                                              media@alz.org
                                                www.alz.org
Details the Association's position supporting a national respite care policy and recommends actions for federal and state policy makers.
1991 14 pages

Audio & Video

214 Aphasia: Struggling for Understanding
Filmakers Library
3212 Duke Street   212-808-4980
Alexandria, VA 22314-1798   Fax: 212-808-4983
                                     sales@alexanderstreet.com
                                            www.filmakers.com
What if your ability to speak or understand speech was taken away without warning, and you struggled to find words that just won't come? This film is about two people faced with the daunting task of learning to speak again, of regaining their humanity. DVD or VHS, Classroom Rental VHS also available for $65. 14 minutes in length.
DVD or VHS
Sue Oscar, Co-President

Web Sites

215 Alliance for Aging Research
                                        www.agingresearch.org
Improving the health and independence of Americans as they age. Promotes medical and behavioral research into the aging process.

216 American Association of Retired Persons
                                                www.aarp.org
AARP is the nation's leading organization for people age 50 and older. It serves their needs and interests through information and education, advocacy and community services provided by a network of local chapters and experienced volunteers. The website features lifestyle and health information for retired persons, as well as entertainment, music, podcasts, and more.

217 American Society on Aging
                                              www.asaging.org
An association of diverse individuals bound together by a common goal: to support the commitment and enhance the knowledge and skills of those who seek to improve the quality of life of older adults and their families.

218 Canadian National Seniors Council
                                  canada.ca/en/national-seniors-council
The council works with older Canadians, stakeholders and experts to advise the Canadian government on matters relating to the health, well-being and quality of life of seniors. The website provides links to reports and other publications featuring research on aging and senior citizens.

219 Caring.com
                                              www.caring.com
Online portal for family caregivers who are caring for aging loved ones.

220 Eldercare Locator
                                             eldercare.acl.gov
Public service run by the U.S. Administration on Aging connecting older adults and their families to services and resources.

221 Gerontological Society of America
                                               www.geron.org
Nonprofit professional organization with more than 5000 members in the field of aging. Provides researchers, educators, practitioners and policy makers with opportunities to understand, advance, integrate and use basic and applied research on aging populations. The website provides access to publications, includ-

ing journals, as well as meetings, programs and services, and member benefits.

222 Healing Well
                                            www.healingwell.com
An online health resource guide to medical news, chat, information and articles, newsgroups and message boards, books, disease-related web sites, medical directories, and more for patients, friends, and family coping with disabling diseases, disorders, or chronic illnesses.

223 Health Finder
                                            www.healthfinder.gov
Searchable, carefully developed web site offering information on over 1000 topics. Developed by the US Department of Health and Human Services, the site can be used in both English and Spanish.

224 Healthlink USA
                                           www.healthlinkusa.com
Health information concerning treatment, cures, prevention, diagnosis, risk factors, research, support groups, email lists, personal stories and much more. Updated regularly.

225 LongTermCare.gov
                                            longtermcare.acl.gov
Provides information on long-term care for patients and caregivers.

226 Lotsa Helping Hands
                                           lotsahelpinghands.com
Platform for creating communities that assist in caring for loved ones, intended for caregivers, friends and family, and volunteers.

227 MedicineNet
                                            www.medicinenet.com
An online resource for consumers providing easy-to-read, authoritative medical and health information.

228 Medscape
                                              www.medscape.com
Medscape offers specialists, primary care physicians, and other health professionals the Web's most robust and integrated medical information and educational tools.

229 National Council for Aging Care
                                                www.aging.com
Seeks to provide older adults with information and resources on health & well-being, caregiving, money and financial planning, and lifestyle, through their Aging.com website.

230 National Council on Aging
                                                www.ncoa.org
The nation's first charitable organization dedicated to promoting the dignity, independence, well-being and contributions of older Americans. The council has a goal of improving the health and economic well-being of 10 million older adults by 2020. The website provides tools and resources for older adults and caregivers.

231 National Hospice & Palliative Care Organization (NHPCO)
                                               www.nhpco.org
The organization seeks to improve end-of-life care, widen access to hospice care, and improve quality of life for the dying and their loved ones. NHPCO's website offers information on regulations, advocacy, quality and performance, education, and a variety of other resources.

232 National Institute of Aging
                                               www.nia.nih.gov
Conducts research on aging, behavioral and social research, neuroscience and neuropsychology, geriatrics, and clinical gerontology.

233 Next Step in Care
                                           www.nextstepincare.org
Online platform with videos and guides for family caregivers and healthcare providers, as well as other resources.

234 Research Center
Online center offering information on consumer issues, demographics, independent living and other items of interest to senior citizens.

235 Seniorresource.com

www.seniorresource.com

Provides information to older adults on needed facilities and services, including through internet directories and an archive of E-zines.

236 US Administration on Aging

acl.gov/about-acl/administration-aging

An agency in the US Department of Health and Human Services, and under the Administration for Community Living, is one of the nation's largest providers of home and community-based care for older persons and their caregivers.

237 WebMD

www.webmd.com

Provides credible information, supportive communities, and in-depth reference material about health subjects. A source for original and timely health information as well as material from well known content providers.

Description

238 AIDS/HIV

AIDS (Acquired Immune Deficiency Syndrome) is an infectious disorder that suppresses the normal function of the human body's immune system. AIDS is a result of HIV (Human Immunodeficiency Virus) infection, which destroys the body's ability to fight infections. Specifically, the virus infects and later destroys helper T-cells, which are a part of the body's immune system that responds to invading organisms. This destructive process is slow and silent, which means that HIV can be contracted years before any symptoms appear. When enough T-cells have been destroyed, the body is invaded by organisms that wouldn't ordinarily be able to cause serious disease. An early symptom of HIV infection is usually an increasing number of infections. Weight loss, fever and night sweats are common. Certain cancers, especially lymphoma and Kaposi's sarcoma, also take advantage of the body's lowered resistance.

HIV transmission requires contact with body fluids and is usually spread from an infected person to a noninfected person by unprotected sexual intercourse, or by sharing needles. Mothers can give HIV infection to their children before and during childbirth and while breastfeeding.

Prevention of HIV infection is the best way to stop the AIDS epidemic. Unfortunately, progress on a vaccine has been disappointing, so avoiding contact with the virus is the primary method of prevention. Avoiding the riskier types of sexual intercourse will reduce one's risk, as will the use of a condom during vaginal and anal sex. Injecting drug users should not share needles. The use of needle exchange programs has decreased the spread of HIV infection. Women with HIV are encouraged to avoid pregnancy. If pregnant, HIV-positive women should stay on medicine directed against HIV and should not breastfeed, since HIV is transmitted in breastmilk. In certain situations, expectant HIV-positive women have scheduled cesarean deliveries. Today, infants born to HIV women are treated with medication immediately after birth for 4-6 weeks, which greatly reduces the incidence of vertical transmission of the infection from mother to child. Until anti-HIV drugs became available, infected persons usually had a rapid downhill course. Today, combination drug treatment or HAART (Highly Active Anti-Retroviral Therapy) can offer most infected persons a long period of relatively good health. However, the treatment regimen is often complex and expensive, involving three or four drugs which must be taken several times a day. Since skipping doses encourages growth of virus that is resistant to the drugs, it is very important to take the drugs exactly as directed.

National Agencies & Associations

239 AIDS Coalition of Cape Breton
150 Bentinck Street   902-567-1766
Sydney, Nova Scotia, B1P-4W4   Fax: 902-567-1766
christine.porter@bellaliant.com
www.aidscoalitionofcapebreton.ca
Provides support and advocacy services for PLW HIV/AIDS (people living with HIV/AIDS). Services provided deal with social, legal, ethical and spiritual issues.
Christine Porter, Executive Director
Jo-Anne Rolls, PHA Program Coordinator

240 AIDS Committee of Durham Region
115 Simcoe Street South   905-576-1445
Oshawa, Ontario, L1H-4G7   info@aidsdurham.com
www.aidsdurham.com
To provide HIV/AIDS related services to the infected or affected and the general community in the region of Durham.
Adrian Betts, Executive Director
Michael Morgan, Manager of Operations

241 AIDS Committee of North Bay & Area
269 Main Street W   705-497-3560
North Bay, Ontario, P1B-2T8   800-387-3701
Fax: 705-497-7850
oaacnba@vianet.ca
www.aidsnorthbay.com
To assist and support all persons infected or affected by HIV/AIDS and to limit the spread of the virus through education and outreach strategies.
Stacey Mayhall, PhD, Executive Director
Steve Lamb, Support Services Coordinator

242 AIDS Committee of Ottawa
19 Main Street   613-238-5014
Ottawa, Ontario, K1S-1A9   Fax: 613-238-3425
info@aco-cso.ca
www.aco-cso.ca
Works to empower people living with HIV/AIDS and the PLWHA (persons living with HIV/AID) community in Ottawa through promoting the well being and quality of life of those living with, or close affected by HIV/AIDS.
Khaled Salam, Executive Director
Cory Wong, Manager, Support Services

243 AIDS Committee of Toronto
543 Yonge Street   416-340-2437
Toronto, Ontario, M4Y-1Y5   Fax: 416-340-8224
ask@actoronto.org
www.actoronto.org
Delivers responsive, effective, and valued community-based HIV support services and education, prevention, outreach and fundraising programs that promote health, well-being, worth and rights of individuals and communities living with, affected by and at risk for HIV/AIDS, and increase awareness of HIV/AIDS.
John Maxwell, Executive Director
Jocelyn Watchorn, Director, Support Services

244 AIDS Committee of York Region
10909 Yonges Street   905-884-0613
Richmond Hill, Ontario, L4C-3E3   800-243-7717
Fax: 905-884-7215
info@acyr.org
www.acyr.org
The AIDS Committee of York Region envisions an informed and compassionate society, which is supportive of people living with HIV/AIDS who are striving to overcome social and service challenges, working with them towards a healthy and empowered lifestyle.
Vibhuti Mehra, Executive Director
Monica Meza-Opazo, Manager, Support Services

245 AIDS New Brunswick
65 Brunswick Street   800-561-4009
Fredericton, NB, E3B-1G5   Fax: 888-501-6301
info@aidsnb.com
www.aidsnb.com
A provincial organization committed to facilitating community-based responses to the issues of HIV/AIDS. The aim is to pro-

mote and support the health and well-being of persons living with and affected by HIV/AIDS and to reduce the spread of HIV/AIDS in New Brunswick.
Matthew Smith, Executive Director
Keri-Ann Scott, Operation Coordinator

246 AIDS United
1101 14th Street NW
Washington, DC 20005
202-408-4848
Fax: 202-408-1818
www.aidsunited.org
National organization dedicated to the development, analysis, cultivation, and encouragement of sound policies and programs through the dissemination of information and the building and use of advocacy.
Jesse Milan, Jr., President & CEO
John E. Roane, Jr., Vice President, Operations

247 AIDSinfo
PO Box 4780
Rockville, MD 20849-6303
301-315-2816
800-448-0440
Fax: 301-315-2818
TTY: 888-480-3739
contactus@aidsinfo.nih.gov
www.aidsinfo.nih.gov
AIDSinfo is a U.S. Department of Health and Human Services (DHHS) project that offers the latest federally approved information on HIV/AIDS clinical research, treatment and prevention, and medical practice guidelines for people living with HIV/AIDS, their families and friends, health care providers, scientists, and researchers.

248 ANKORS: Kootenay & Boundary HIV/AIDS and Hepatitis C Support Services
101 Baker Street
Nelson, BC, V1L-4H1
250-505-5506
800-421-2437
Fax: 250-505-5507
frontdesk@gmail.com
www.ankors.bc.ca
ANKORS' mission is to respond to the evolving needs of those living with and affected by HIV/AIDS and Hepatitis C.
Cheryl Dowden, Executive Director
Laura Buchanan, Support Services

249 Act Against AIDS
Centers for Disease Control
1600 Clifton Road
Atlanta, GA 30333
800-232-4636
877-242-9760
Fax: 301-562-1050
TTY: 888-232-6348
www.cdc.gov/actagainstaids
A program of the Centers for Disease Control and Prevention and the White House, aimed at raising awareness about HIV/AIDS among all Americans, and particularly among hardest-hit groups, such as gay and bisexual men, African Americans, Latinos, and other at-risk communities.

250 Alberta Reappraising AIDS Society
Box 61037
Calgary, Alberta, T2N-4S6
403-289-6609
Fax: 403-206-7717
aras@aras.ab.ca
www.aras.ab.ca
Promote critical discussion of the HIV/AIDS dogma.
David R. Crowe, President
Roger Swan, Treasurer

251 American Autoimmune Related Diseases Association
22100 Gratiot Avenue
Eastpointe, MI 48021
586-776-3900
800-598-4668
Fax: 586-776-3903
aarda@aarda.org
www.aarda.org
Awareness, education, referrals for patients with any type of autoimmune disease.
Virginia T. Ladd, President & Executive Director
Laura Simpson, Assistant Director

252 American Chronic Pain Association
PO Box 850
Rocklin, CA 95677
800-533-3231
ACPA@theacpa.org
www.theacpa.org

The ACPA facilitates peer support and education for individuals with chronic pain in its many forms, in order to increase quality of life. Also raises awareness among the healthcare community, and with policy makers.
Penney Cowan, Founder & CEO
Daniel Galia, Director, Global Support

253 American Civil Liberties Union LGBT & AIDS Project
125 Broad Street
New York, NY 10004
212-549-2500
www.aclu.org/other
Offers legislative and employment information public awareness materials and support for persons with HIV/AIDS and their families, as well as laws and rights specializing in gender identity and sexual orientation.
Susan Herman, President
Anthony D. Romero, Executive Director

254 Black Coalition for AIDS Prevention
20 Victoria Street
Toronto, M5C-2N8
416-977-9955
Fax: 416-977-7664
info@black-cap.com
www.blackcap.ca
A volunteer-driven, charitable, not-for-profit, community-based organization. Works in partnership with organizations and individuals who support in principle and practice our mission, philosophy and activities.
Andrew B. Campbell, PhD, Chair
Alexander Joseph, MSc, BEd, CertEd, Treasurer

255 CDC National Prevention Information Network
1600 Clifton Road
Atlanta, GA 30329
800-232-4636
TTY: 888-232-6348
NPIN-info@cdc.gov
npin.cdc.gov
The CDC National Prevention Information Network (NPIN) is the U.S. reference, referral, and distribution service for information on HIV/AIDS, sexually transmitted diseases (STDs), and tuberculosis (TB). NPIN produces, collects, catalogs, processes, stocks, and disseminates materials and information on HIV/AIDS, STD's, and TB to organizations and people working in those disease fields in international, national, state, and local settings.

256 Children's AIDS Fund International
PO Box 16433
Washington, DC 20041
703-433-1560
Fax: 703-433-1561
info@childrensaidsfund.org
www.childrensaidsfund.org
The Children's AIDS Fund aims to limit the suffering of children and their families caused by HIV, by providing care, services, resources, referrals, and education. The fund operates in the U.S. and abroad.
Anita Smith, President

257 Committee of Ten Thousand
71 Winfield Street
Needham, MA 02492
202-681-2351
cott.east@gmail.com
www.cott1.org
Represents people with hemophilia who contracted HIV/AIDS and Hepatitis C from tainted factory concentrates in the 1970s and 1980s. The only national advocacy, and support agency for this seriously disabled community.
Carl Weixler, President
Ray Dattoli, Vice President

258 Elevate NWO
102-106 Cumberland Street N.
Thunder Bay, Ontario, P7A-4M2
807-345-1516
Fax: 807-345-2505
info@elevatenwo.org
www.elevatenwo.org
Provides support, education and advocacy around HIV and AIDS, and related issues.
Shawn Hebert, Chair

259 HIV West Yellowhead Services
152 Athabasca Avenue
Hinton, Alberta, T7V-1X3
780-740-0066
877-291-8811
director@hivwestyellowhead.com
www.hivwestyellowhead.com

Services include harm reduction, needle exchange, overdose prevention, free safe sex supplies, care and support, prevention, and education.
Lori Phillips, Executive Director
Lisa Schwing, Outreach/Support

260 Health Information Network
PO Box 30762   206-784-5655
Seattle, WA 98113   information@healthinfonetwork.org
                                    healthinfonetwork.org
Offers information, public awareness and support for women with HIV/AIDS and the public in general.
Kathi Knowles, Executive Director

261 Heart Touch Project™
3400 Airport Avenue   310-391-2558
Santa Monica, CA 90405   Fax: 310-391-2168
                              executive@hearttouch.org
                                    www.hearttouch.org
Non-profit, educational and service organization devoted to the delivery of compassionate and healing touch to home or hospital-bound men, women, and children.
Shawnee Isaac Smith, Co-Founder
Rene Russo, Co-Founder

262 Housing Works
57 Willoughby St.   347-473-7400
Brooklyn, New York, NY 11201   877-296-9264
                                    TTY: 212-925-9560
                                 info@housingworks.org
                                 www.housingworks.org
Housing Works provides advocacy services for those living with HIV/AIDS, as well as housing, healthcare, nutrition, counseling, mental health and substance abuse treatment, job training, and legal assistance. Also runs thrift shops and bookstores that raise money for the organization's services.
Charles King, Chief Executive Officer
Matthew Bernardo, Executive Director

263 International Council of AIDS Service Organization
120 Carlton Street   416-921-0018
Toronto, Ontario, M5A-4K2   Fax: 416-921-9979
                                       icaso@icaso.org
                                        www.icaso.org
A global network of non-governmental and community-based organizations.
Mary Ann Torres, Executive Director
Galina Godovanny, Financial Manager

264 Keep A Child Alive
17 State Street   646-762-8200
New York, NY 10004   info@keepachildalive.org
                               www.keepachildalive.org
To make a positive difference in the lives of children infected with HIV and affected by AIDS.
Antonio Ruiz-Giminez, Jr., Executive Chair & CEO

265 Living Positive
9912-106 Street NW   780-424-2214
Edmonton, Alberta, T5K-1C5   Fax: 780-424-2215
                               living-positive@telus.net
                                      living-positive.net
Dedicated to providing emotional, spiritual and psychological support to all those living with HIV.

266 Medical Library Association
65 E Wacker Place   312-419-9094
Chicago, IL 60601-7246   Fax: 312-419-8950
                             websupport@mail.mlahq.org
                                         www.mlanet.org
Non-profit, educational organization comprised of more than 400 institutions and 3,000 individual members in the health sciences information field, committed to educating health information professionals, supporting health information research and promoting access to information.
Barry Grant, Director, Education
Kevin Baliozian, Executive Director

267 National AIDS Treatment Advocacy Project
580 Broadway   212-219-0106
New York, NY 10012   888-266-2827
                                     Fax: 212-219-8473
                                        info@natap.org
                                        www.natap.org
Seeks to eudcate by sending out literature, e-mail lists, and host forums on how to prevent HIV, or how to live with it.
Jules Levin, Executive Director
Jessica Gibson Schilling, Chief Operating Officer

268 National Hospice & Palliative Care Organization (NHPCO)
1731 King Street   703-837-1500
Alexandria, VA 22314   800-646-6460
                                     Fax: 703-837-1233
                                        www.nhpco.org
The organization seeks to improve end-of-life care, widen access to hospice care, and improve quality of life for the dying and their loved ones.
Edo Banach, JD, President & CEO
Hannah Yang Moore, MPH, Chief Advocacy Officer

269 National Native American AIDS Prevention Center
4710 Nome Street   todd@nnaapc.org
Denver, CO 80239   www.nnaapc.net
Aims to eliminate HIV/AIDS, HCV, and other STI's in Native communities, including American Indian, Alaska Native, Native Hawaiian, and other Indigenous peoples.
Todd Theringer, Chair
Bernadette Wolfe, Vice Chair

270 Ontario HIV Treatment Network
1300 Yonge Street   416-642-6486
Toronto, Ontario, M4T-1X3   877-743-6486
                                     Fax: 416-640-4245
                                     info@ohtn.on.ca
                                     www.ohtn.on.ca
To optimize the quality of life of people living with HIV in Ontario and to promote excellence and innovation in treatment, research, education and prevention through a collaborative network of excellence representing consumers, providers, researchers and other stakeholders.
Jean Bacon, Executive Director
Barry Adam, Senior Scientist, Prevention Research

271 PEERS Alliance
161 St. Peters Road   902-566-2437
Charlottetown, PE, C1A-5P7   Fax: 902-626-3400
                                 info@peersalliance.ca
                                 www.peersalliance.ca
Previously known as AIDS PEI, the organization aims to create a supportive environment for Persons Living with AIDS/HIV, to increase public understanding of the impact of HIV/AIDS, and to reduce the incidence of HIV/AIDS in Prince Edward Island.
Cybelle Rieber, Executive Director
Angela DesRoches, Program Coordinator

272 Peel HIV/AIDS Network
7700 Hurontario Street   905-361-0523
Brampton, Ontario, L6Y-4M3   866-896-8700
                                     Fax: 905-595-1443
                                         info@phan.ca
                                         www.phan.ca
Committed to serving people living with and affected by HIV/AIDS and to limit the spread of the virus through support, education, advocacy, and volunteerism.
Nilda Patey, Executive Director
Adam Chalcraft, Supervisor, Harm Reduction Program

273 Positive Living British Columbia
1101 Seymour Street   604-893-2200
Vancouver, BC, V6B-0R1   800-994-2437
                                     Fax: 604-893-2251
                               info@positivelivingbc.org
                               www.positivelivingbc.org
Exists to enable persons living with HIV/AIDS to empower themselves through mutual support and collective action. Its board of directors is composed of HIV-positive individuals.
Victor Elkins, Executive Director
Mike Hedges, Director, Operations

274 Positive Living Niagara
120 Queenston Street
St. Catharines, Ontario, L2R-2Z3
905-984-8684
800-773-9843
Fax: 905-988-1921
info@positivelivingniagara.com
positivelivingniagara.com
AIDS Niagara is dedicated to improving the quality of life for those infected and/or affected by HIV/AIDS.
Glen Walker, BA, BSW, RSW, Executive Director
Cathie Rogers, Chair

275 Positive Women's Network - USA
436 14th Street
Oakland, CA 94612
510-698-3811
info@pwn-usa.org
www.pwn-usa.org
Aims to empower women living with HIV through social justice and human rights.
Naina Khanna, Executive Director
Jennie Smith-Camejo, Communications Director

276 Project Inform
25 Taylor Street
San Francisco, CA 94102
415-558-8669
877-435-7443
Fax: 415-558-0684
www.projectinform.org
Runs an HIV Infoline, as well as a Hepatitis C helpline, while engaging in advocacy on behalf of individuals living with HIV/AIDS.
David Evans, Interim Executive Director

277 Regional HIV/AIDS Connection
186 King Street
London, Ontario, N6A-1C7
519-434-1601
866-920-1601
Fax: 519-434-1843
info@hivaidsconnection.ca
www.hivaidsconnection.ca
A community-based, charitable organization providing HIV-related services to people living with and concerned about HIV/AIDS in London and the surrounding area.
Brian Lester, Executive Director
Kelly Wright, Director, HIV/HCV Support Services

278 Reseau ACCESS Network
111 Larch Street
Sudbury, Ontario, P3C-4T5
705-688-0500
800-465-2437
Fax: 705-688-0423
www.reseauaccessnetwork.com
A non-profit, community-based charitable organization, promoting wellness, education, harm and risk reduction.
Richard Rainville, Executive Director

279 The AIDS Network
140 King Street East
Hamilton, ON, L8N-1B2
905-528-0854
866-563-0563
Fax: 905-528-6311
info@aidsnetwork.ca
www.aidsnetwork.ca
Providing services and education to Hamilton and the surrounding areas.
Tim McClemont, Executive Director
Karyn Cooper, Director, Programs & Services

280 The Well Project
update@thewellproject.org
www.thewellproject.org
The Well Project is a not for profit corporation and an initiative conceived, developed, and administered by HIV+ women and those who are affected by the disease.
Krista Martel, Executive Director
Juliana Hawawini Johnson, Director, Operations & Online Resources

281 Turning Point Society of Central Alberta
4611-50th Avenue
Red Deer, T4N-3Z9
403-346-8858
877-346-8858
Fax: 403-346-2352
info@turningpoint-ca.org
www.turningpoint-ca.org
Turning Point (formerly Central Alberta AIDS Network Society) is a local charity and agency offering support to individuals who

are infected or affected by HIV/AIDS, and also provides prevention and education throughout Central Alberta.
Stacey Carmichael, Executive Director

282 UNICEF USA
125 Maiden Lane
New York, NY 10038
212-686-5522
800-367-5437
Fax: 212-779-1679
www.unicefusa.org
Supports child survival, protection and development worldwide through education, advocacy, and fundraising for AIDS and other conditions.
Caryl M. Stern, President & CEO
Barron Segar, EVP & Chief Development Officer

283 Women Alive
1301 N. Willowbrook Avenue
Compton, CA 90222
310-605-1365
info@women-alive.org
www.women-alive.org
Coalition of, by and for women living with HIV/AIDS. Created ways to help women connect with each other, bring others out of isolation, exchange information about HIV treatments, and take charge of their lives.

State Agencies & Associations

Alabama

284 Alabama Department of Public Health
201 Monroe Street
Montgomery, AL 36104-3000
334-206-5364
800-228-0469
Fax: 334-206-2092
www.adph.org/aids
Offers health education and risk education activities, including a mobile app called Know Your Status, Manage Your Health, and Live Your Best Life (KML AL), intended to inform, prevent HIV/AIDS transmission, and assist those who have the disease.
Sharon Jordan, MPH, Director
Jora T. White, MA, Program Dir., Prevention & Development

Alaska

285 Alaska Department of Health and Social Services: HIV/STD Program
Section Of Epidemiology
3601 C Street
Anchorage, AK 99503-0249
907-269-8000
800-478-0084
Fax: 907-561-4239
hiv-std@alaska.gov
dhss.alaska.gov/dph/Epi/hivstd
The HIV/STD Program addresses public health issues and activities with the goal of preventing sexually transmitted diseases (STDs) and HIV infection in Alaska as well as their impact on health. AIDS program offers education to providers and organizations.
Merry Carlson, Director, Public Health
Joe McLaughlin, MD, State Epidemiologist

Arizona

286 Arizona Department of Health Services: HIV Prevention Program
150 N 18th Avenue
Phoenix, AZ 85007
602-542-1025
Fax: 602-542-0883
www.azdhs.gov
Provides HIV and AIDS seropositive surveillance, case investigation, and analysis, as well as AIDS health education and training for the public.
John Sapero, Office Chief
Alyssa Guido, MPH, Program Director

287 Southwest Center For HIV/AIDS
1101 North Central Avenue
Phoenix, AZ 85004
602-307-5330
Fax: 602-307-5021
swhiv.org
Formerly The Phoenix Body Positive, the organization is a non-profit created by and for people infected and affected by HIV/AIDS, that provides the community with the knowledge, re-

sources and collective strength necessary for individuals to live long and well with HIV and to prevent the spread of the disease.
Dolph Goldenburg, Interim Executive Director
Lisa M. Fontes, PhD, Director, Development

288 Tucson Interfaith HIV/AIDS Network (TIHAN)
2660 North 1st Avenue   520-299-6647
Tucson, AZ 85719   www.tihan.org
Serving interfaith communities of Tucson through compassionate care education training and spiritual support so that we can make more people aware of the health crisis which affects all of us. Also provide non-medical in-home help.
Scott Blades, Executive Director
Deidre Demers, Program Manager

Arkansas

289 Arkansas Department of Health: HIV Prevention Program
AIDS Prevention Program
4815 West Markham Street   501-661-2408
Little Rock, AR 72205-3867   800-462-0599
                                    Fax: 501-661-2082
                                    www.healthyarkansas.com
Engages in policy development, grants, training, and collaboration with community organizations and state agencies to prevent and control the spread of HIV, as well as monitoring cases across the state.
Nathaniel Smith, MD, MPH, Director & State Health Officer

California

290 California Collaborative Treatment Group
AntiViral Research Center
220 Dickinson Street   619-543-8080
San Diego, CA 92103-8208   avrc.ucsd.edu/programs/cctg
The CCTG is a multi-center clinical trials organization whose primary mission is to improve the scientific basis for HIV patient care and HIV prevention. CCTG develops treatment protocols and drug therapies.
Jill Kunkel, RN, Director, Operations
Adiba Hassan, Data Manager

291 California Department of Public Health: Office of AIDS
Office of AIDS
PO Box 997426   916-558-1784
Sacramento, CA 95899-7426   www.cdph.ca.gov
Works to develop strategies and implement programs for education and prevention, testing and counseling, supportive care and treatment and research to control the spread of HIV infection.
Karen Smith, MD, MPH, Director

292 County of Los Angeles Public Health: Division of HIV And STD Programs
AIDS Programs
600 S Commonwealth Avenue   213-351-8000
Los Angeles, CA 90005   800-243-7889
                                    Fax: 213-387-0912
                                    dhsp@ph.lacounty.org
                                    publichealth.lacounty.gov/dhsp
Responsible for planning, coordinating, and implementing county wide HIV/AIDS and sTD efforts.
Mario J. Perez, Director

293 Pacific AIDS Education and Training Center (PAETC)
University Of California San Francisco
550 16th Street, 3rd Floor   415-476-6153
San Francisco, CA 94158-2549   paetcmail@ucsf.edu
                                    paetc.org
Provides educational programs about HIV infection for healthcare providers to Arizona, California, Hawaii, Nevada, and the 6 U.S.-affiliated Pacific Jurisdictions.
E. Michael Reyes, MD, MPH, Principal Investigator
Monica Hahn, MD, Regional Clinical Director

294 San Francisco AIDS Foundation (SFAF)
1035 Market Street   415-487-3000
San Francisco, CA 94103   info@sfaf.org
                                    www.sfaf.org

SFAF provides confidential array of services-including financial benefits counseling, client advocacy, housing assistance, HIV prevention efforts, and needle exchange.
Joe Hollendoner, MSW, Chief Executive Officer
Lara Brooks, Chief Program Officer

295 San Francisco Community Health Center: HHOME/GTZ-ICM
730 Polk Street   415-292-3400
San Francisco, CA 94109   Fax: 415-292-3404
                                    TTY: 415-292-3410
                                    sfcommunityhealth.org
HIV Homeless Outreach and Mobile Engagement (HHOME) is a mobile program operating throughout San Francisco, serving homeless people living with HIV/AIDS. Getting to Zero Intensive Case Management (GTZ-ICM) aims to end new HIV infections across the city by 2020.
Lance Toma, Chief Executive Officer
Ruby Koger, Senior Medical Case Manager

Colorado

296 Mountain West AIDS Education and Training Center (MWAETC)
325 9th Avenue   206-543-2704
Seattle, WA 98104   aetcinfo@uw.edu
                                    mwaetc.org
Provides educational programs about HIV infection for healthcare providers to Alaska, Colorado, Idaho, Montana, Oregon, North and South Dakota, Utah, Washington, and Wyoming.
David Spach, MD, Principal Investigator/Clinical Director
Laurie Sylla, MHSA, Director

Connecticut

297 Connecticut Department of Health Services AIDS Programs
410 Capitol Avenue   860-509-7806
Hartford, CT 06134   webmaster.dph@ct.gov
                                    portal.ct.gov/DPH
Operates a speakers bureau, provides training, workshops, seminars, and counseling services, and conducts meetings and offers information and referral services.
Kate McEvoy, Director

Delaware

298 Delaware Department of Health and Social: Services HIV Prevention Program
Division of Public Health
540 S DuPont Highway   302-744-1050
Dover, DE 19901   Fax: 302-739-2548
                                    www.dhss.delaware.gov/dhss/dph/index.htm
Provides HIV counseling and testing prevention education and AIDS surveillance and studies.
Kara Odom Walker, Secretary

District of Columbia

299 Washington DC Department of Health: HIV/AIDS, Hepatitis, STD and TB Admin.
899 North Capitol Street NE   202-442-5955
Washington, DC 20002   Fax: 202-442-4796
                                    TTY: 711
                                    doh@dc.gov
                                    dchealth.dc.gov/service/hivaids
Mission is to reduce the incidence of HIV/AIDS and number of deaths related to HIV/AIDS in the District of Columbia by the application of sound public health practices and initiatives through HIV disease surveillance, tracking, monitoring, and intervention.
LaQuandra Nesbitt, Director
Michael Kharfen, Senior Deputy, HIV/AIDS

Florida

300 Florida Department of Health: HIV/AIDS Section
4052 Bald Cypress Way   850-245-4422
Tallahassee, FL 32399   DiseaseControl@flhealth.gov
                                    www.floridahealth.gov
Seeks to eliminate HIV transmission by making voluntary HIV testing a routine part of medical care, implementing new models

for diagnosing HIV infections outside medical settings, and preventing new infections by working with persons diagnosed with HIV and their partners.
Tom Liberti, Bureau Chief
Janell Clemons, Administrative Assistant

301   Pridelines
6360 NE 4th Court   305-571-9601
Miami, FL 33138   info@pridelines.org
                                     pridelines.org
The organization seeks to support, educate, and empower LGBTQ youth and the community as a whole in South Florida, including providing HIV/AIDS-related health services and support.
Victor Diaz Herman, Chief Executive Officer
Lisa Hayeem Carver, MPH, Director, HIV Services

Georgia

302   Georgia Department of Public Health: Office Of HIV/AIDS
AIDS Section
2 Peachtree Street NW   404-657-3100
Atlanta, GA 30303   dph.georgia.gov
Partners with local health districts, hospitals, colleges/universities, community-based organizations, and other stakeholders to provide prevention and care services.
Kathleen E. Toomey, MD, MPH, Commissioner
L. William Lyons, Director

Hawaii

303   Hawaii Department of Health: Harm Reduction Services Branch
728 Sunset Avenue   808-733-8443
Honolulu, HI 96816   health.hawaii.gov/harmreduction/hiv-aids
Offers research, education, surveillance and testing components. AIDS information and guidelines about the placement of infants, children and adolescents who test positive for HIV in nursery or school settings are also available.
Peter Whiticar, Branch Chief

Idaho

304   Idaho Department of Health and Welfare: The STD/AIDS Program
The STD/AIDS Program
450 W State Street 1st Floor   208-334-6527
Boise, ID 83720-0036   Fax: 208-332-7346
                                 DPHinquiries@dhw.idaho.gov
                                 www.healthandwelfare.idaho.gov
Program receives federal funding to support testing treatment and prevention services for Idaho's reportable sexually transmitted infections.

Illinois

305   Chicago Department of Public Health
333 S State Street   312-747-9884
Chicago, IL 60604   Fax: 312-747-9765
                                 TTY: 312-747-2374
                          www.chicago.gov/city/en/depts/cdph.html
Offers core medical and support services via funding from the federal Ryan White HIV/AIDS Program.
Julie Morita, MD, Commissioner
David Kern, Deputy Commissioner, HIV/STI Bureau

306   Illinois Department of Public Health: Division of Infectious Diseases
525-535 W Jefferson Street   217-782-4977
Springfield, IL 62761   800-243-2437
                                 TTY: 800-547-0466
                                 www.dph.illinois.gov
Provides HIV/AIDS initiatives, surveillance, training, and care services.
Ngozi O. Ezike, MD, Director

307   Legal Council for Health Justice
17 N State Street   312-427-8990
Chicago, IL 60602   Fax: 312-427-8419
                                 legalcouncil.org

Provides legal advice and services for persons who are HIV positive or have AIDS, as well as their families. Also serves individuals with disabilities and chronic illnesses, senior citizens, and the homeless.
Tom Yates, Executive Director
Ruth Edwards, Senior Director, Program Services

308   Midwest AIDS Education and Training Center (MATEC)
1919 West Taylor   312-996-1373
Chicago, IL 60612   312-413-4184
                                     matec@uic.edu
                                     www.matec.info
Provides educational programs about HIV infection for healthcare providers.
Ricardo A. Rivero, MD, MPH, Executive Director
Renslow Sherer, MD, Regional Clinical Director

309   Test Positive Aware Network (TPAN)
5537 N Broadway Street   773-989-9400
Chicago, IL 60640-1405   Fax: 773-989-9494
                                     tpan@tpan.com
                                     www.tpan.com
Empowers people living with HIV through peer-led programming support services, information dissemination, and advocacy. Provides services to the broader community to increase HIV knowledge and sensitivity and to reduce the risk of infection.
Christopher Clark, Chief Executive Officer
Julie Supple, MA, LCSW, Director, Client Services

Kansas

310   Kansas Department of Health & Environment: STI/HIV Section
1000 SW Jackson   785-296-6174
Topeka, KS 66612   kdhe.info@ks.gov
                                     www.kdheks.gov
Conducts surveillance of HIV/AIDS in Kansas. Conducts Prevention Program with training for counselors and educators, partial funding of counseling test sites and distribution of educational materials. Provides medications and primary care.
Laura Kelly, Governer
Lee A. Norman, MD, Secretary

Louisiana

311   Louisiana Department of Health: STD/HIV Program
1450 Poydras Street   504-568-7474
New Orleans, LA 70112   Fax: 504-568-7044
                                 DeAnn.Gruber@la.gov
                                 ldh.la.gov/index.cfm/page/919
The SHP runs statewide programs intended to prevent the transmission of STDs and HIV, track current cases, and provide medical services to those who have STDs and HIV.
DeAnn Gruber, Program Director
Chaquetta Johnson, Program Deputy Director

Maine

312   Maine Dept. of Health & Human Services: HIV, STD, & Viral Hepatitis Program
Division of Disease Surveillance
221 State Street   207-287-3747
Augusta, ME 04333   Fax: 207-287-3498
                                     TTY: 711
                                 Sheila.Krouse@maine.gov
                                 www.maine.gov/dhhs/mecdc
The program seeks to stop the spread of STDs, viral hepatitis, and HIV, and by doing so reduce the prevalence of illness and death. The proigram also promotes the health and well-being of individuals who have, or are at risk of contracting, these diseases.
Ann Farmer, Division Director
Sheila Krouse, Program Support

Massachusetts

313 Massachusetts Department of Public Health: Office Of HIV/AIDS
250 Washington Street
Boston, MA 02108
617-624-6000
Fax: 617-624-6001
TTY: 617-624-5206
www.mass.gov/hiv
The Massachusetts Department of Public Health coordinates HIV/AIDS response with the Bureau of Infectious Disease and Laboratory Services. Resources are provided for the public and healthcare professionals, including treatment guidelines, epidemiologic profiles, educational materials, and other resources.
Monica Bharel, MD, MPH, Commissioner
Lindsey Tucker, Associate Commissioner

314 New England AIDS Education and Training Center
Center for Health Policy and Research
333 South Street
Shrewsbury, MA 01545
617-262-5657
Fax: 617-502-1701
aidsed@neaetc.org
www.neaetc.org
NEAETC serves health care professionals in New England with consultation, technical assistance, and resource materials.
Philip Bolduc, MD, Clinical Director
Jennifer Daly, MD, Co-Clinical Director

Michigan

315 Michigan Department of Health & Human Services: Division of HIV & STD Programs
333 S Grand Avenue
Lansing, MI 48909
517-241-0855
www.michigan.gov/mdch
The divison focuses on prevention, care, and treatment of HIV and STDs. It also administers the Ryan White HIV/Aids Program in the state.
Mary-Grace Brandt, Acting Division Director
Dawn Lukomski, Section Manager

Minnesota

316 Minnesota Department of Health
PO Box 64975
St. Paul, MN 55164-0975
612-373-2437
800-248-2437
www.health.state.mn.us/diseases/hiv
The Infectious Disease Epidemiology, Prevention and Control Division oversees HIV/AIDS response in the state. The focus is on prevention and care, with resources offered to the public and to healthcare professionals.
Stefani Kloiber, Director, Communications & Operations

Mississippi

317 Mississippi State Department of Health: STD/HIV Office
570 E Woodrow Wilson Drive
Jackson, MS 39216
601-576-7723
800-826-2961
msdh.ms.gov
The STD/HIV Program aims to reduce incidents of death as a result of STDs and HIV through services for disease prevention and control.
Thomas Dobbs, State Health Officer
Melody M. Winston, Communicable Diseases

Missouri

318 Missouri Department of Health & Senior Services: Bureau of HIV, STD & Hepatitis
PO Box 570
Jefferson City, MO 65102
573-751-6439
Fax: 573-751-6447
info@health.mo.gov
health.mo.gov
The department offers a range of programs and services for individuals and communities affected by HIV/AIDS, with a focus on prevention, counseling and testing, and healthcare for those living with the disease.
Randall W. Williams, MD, FACOG, Director
D. Adam Crumbliss, Chief Dir., Community & Public Health

Montana

319 Montana Deptartment of Public Health & Human Services: HIV/STD/HepC Program
1400 Broadway
Helena, MT 59620
406-444-3565
dfejes@mt.gov
dphhs.mt.gov/publichealth/hivstd
Provides services and resources for the prevention and treatment of HIV, STDs, and Hepatitis C.
Sheila Hogan, Director
Dana Fejes, Section Supervisor

Nevada

320 Nevada Department of Health & Human Services: Office Of HIV Prevention
Division of Public & Behavioral Health
4126 Technology Way
Carson City, NV 89706
775-684-4200
Fax: 775-684-4056
dpbh@health.nv.gov
dhhs.nv.gov
Works to promote health and reduce the impact of HIV/AIDS, through the lens of public health and social justice.
Richard Whitley, Director
Tory Johnson, MMgt, Section Manager

New Hampshire

321 New Hampshire Department of Health and Human Services
29 Hazen Drive
Concord, NH 03301
603-271-4502
800-852-3345
Fax: 603-271-0545
TTY: 800-735-2964
nhbidc@dhhs.nh.gov
www.dhhs.nh.gov/dphs/std
The Infectious Disease Prevention, Investigation and Care Services Section focuses on HIV and STD prevention, including Ryan White Care for the state, as well as viral hepatitis, tuberculosis prevention and control, and more.
Jeffrey A. Meyers, Commissioner
Lisa M. Morris, Director, Public Health

New Jersey

322 New Jersey AIDS Services
44 South Street
Morristown, NJ 07960
973-285-0006
Fax: 973-285-0067
www.njas-inc.org
Provides support services, housing, prevention techniques, and community education to counter the HIV/AIDS crisis in New Jersey.
Laurie Litt, Chief Executive Officer
Joann McEniry, Chief Operating Officer

323 New Jersey Department of Health: Division of HIV, STD And TB Services
PO Box 360
Trenton, NJ 08625-0360
800-624-2377
www.nj.gov/health/hivstdtb
Focuses on pevention and care for those affected by HIV, STDs, and tuberculosis.
Shereef Elnahal, MD, MBA, Commissioner

New Mexico

324 New Mexico Department of Health: HIV Services Program
1190 S St. Francis Drive
Santa Fe, NM 87505
505-476-3628
nmhealth.org/about/phd/idb/hats
Provides a range of resources for those living with HIV/AIDS, as well as promoting professional development for healthcare providers, and coordinating with community-based organizations.
Kathy Kunkel, Secretary
Laine Snow, Program Manager

New York

325 New York Department of Health: AIDS Institute
AIDS Institute

Empire State Plaza
Albany, NY 12237

800-541-2437
dohweb@health.ny.gov
www.health.ny.gov/diseases/aids

Awards grants and maintains relationships with regional AIDS service groups, crisis intervention, psychosocial counseling and legal, financial and housing assistance. The Institute also offers preventive education, risk reduction education, HIV counseling and testing and patient care.
Johanne Morne, Director
S. Scully, Dep. Dir., Health Care, Grants & Data

326   Northeast/Caribbean AIDS Education and Training Center (NECAAETC)
Columbia University, HIV Center
601 West 168th Street
New York, NY 10032

646-774-6978
Fax: 212-568-3060
nynjaetc@columbia.edu
necaaetc.org

Provides educational programs about HIV infection for healthcare providers to New Jersey, New York, Puerto Rico and the U.S. Virgin Islands.
Francine Cournos, MD, Principal Investigator
Daria Boccher-Lattimore, DrPH, Director & Co-Investigator

North Carolina

327   North Carolina Department of Health and Human Services
Communicable Disease Branch
1902 Mail Service Center
Raleigh, NC 27699-1902

919-733-3419
Fax: 919-733-0490
epi.dph.ncdhhs.gov/cd/diseases/aids.html

Oversees the AIDS surveillance program, HIV counseling, testing, partner notification, health education, risk reduction, and public information efforts in North Carolina.
Mandy Cohen, Secretary
Mark Benton, Deputy Secretary, Health Services

Ohio

328   Ohio Department of Health: HIV/AIDS Surveillance Program
246 N High Street
Columbus, OH 43215-0118

614-387-2722
odh.ohio.gov

Consists of AIDS surveillance, seroprevalence programs, health care worker education, health education and risk reduction projects.
Amy Acton, MD, MPH, Director, Health
William McHugh, Assistant Director, Health

Oklahoma

329   Oklahoma Department of Health: HIV/STD Service
Office of The State Epidemiologist
1000 NE 10th
Oklahoma City, OK 73117

405-271-4636
www.ok.gov/health

Services include prevention and intervention, care delivery, and surveillance and analysis.
Tom Bates, Commissioner of Health
Laurence Burnsed, MPH, State Epidemiologist

Oregon

330   Oregon Health Authority: HIV Prevention Program
Health Division, HIV Program
800 NE Oregon Street
Portland, OR 97232

971-673-0153
Fax: 971-673-0178
TTY: 711
joshua.s.ferrer@state.or.us
www.oregon.gov/DHS/ph

The program focuses on prevention, training, and resources for the public and healthcare providers.
Patrick Allen, Director
Josh Ferrer, HIV/STD Prevention Manager

Pennsylvania

331   MidAtlantic AIDS Education and Training Center (MAAETC)
University of Pittsburgh

130 DeSoto Street
Pittsburgh, PA 15261

412-624-1895
Fax: 412-624-4767
www.maaetc.org

Provides educational programs about HIV infection for healthcare providers to Delaware, District of Columbia, Maryland, Pennsylvania, Virginia, and West Virgina.
Linda Rose Frank, PhD, Principal Investigator & Exec. Dir.

332   Pennsylvania Department of Health: Division Of HIV Disease
Bureau of Communicable Diseases
625 Forster Street
Harrisburg, PA 17120

717-783-0572
Fax: 717-772-6975
www.health.pa.gov

The division seeks to develop and implement a multi-dimensional, coordinated strategy to prevent disease and change high-risk behaviors, as well as provide resources and direction for sustaining preventive behavior and avoiding infection. HIV/AIDS Surveillance and Epidemiology is also run by the Bureau of Epidemiology.
Rachel Levine, Secretary
Loren Robinson, Deputy Secretary, Health Promotion

333   Philadelphia Department of Public Health: STD Control Program
AIDS Activities Coordinating Office (AACO)
1101 Market Street
Philadelphia, PA 19107

215-685-5600
www.phila.gov/health

Works to stop the spread of STDs, including HIV, in Philadelphia. Other city programs include: Club 1509, providing resources for men and transpeople of color; Take Control Philly, offering free condoms; and Do You, Philly, providing sexual information and resources to young men.
Thomas Farley, MD, Health Commissioner
Raynard Washington, Chief Epidemiologist

Rhode Island

334   Rhode Island Department of Health
3 Capitol Hill
Providence, RI 02908

401-222-5960
www.health.ri.gov/diseases/hivaids

The Division of Preparedness, Response, Infectious Disease and Emergency Medical Services oversees a number of programs related to controlling the spread of STDs, including HIV.
Nicole Alexander-Scott, MD, MPH, Director
Steven Boudreau, Chief Administrative Officer

South Carolina

335   South Carolina Department of Health & Environmental Control
Bureau of Preventive Health Services
2600 Bull Street
Columbia, SC 29201

803-898-3432
info@dhec.sc.gov
www.scdhec.gov

Provides services to prevent the spread of sexually transmitted diseases (STD's) and HIV infection, to reduce associated illness and death, and to provide care and support resources for persons with HIV.
Rick Toomey, Director

Tennessee

336   Southeast AIDS Education and Training Center (SEAETC)
Vanderbilt Health
719 Thompson Lane
Nashville, TN 37204

615-875-7873
Fax: 615-936-1583
www.seaetc.com

Provides educational programs about HIV infection for healthcare providers to Alabama, Florida, Georgia, Kentucky, Mississippi, North Carolina, South Carolina, and Tennessee.
Stephen P. Raffanto, MD, MPH, Principal Investigator
Anna Person, MD, Clinical Director

337   Tennessee Department of Health: HIV Prevention Services
710 James Robertson Parkway
Nashville, TN 37243

615-741-7500
www.tn.gov/health

Provides HIV/STD education and information, as well as collecting monitoring and distributing data. Provides assistance to individuals, and intervention and treatment services.
Lisa Piercey, MD, MBA, FAAP, Commissioner
David R. Reagan, MD, PhD, Chief Medical Officer

Texas

338 AIDS Outreach Center (AOC)
400 North Beach Street   817-335-1994
Fort Worth, TX 76111   info@aoc.org
                                       www.aoc.org
The staff and volunteers of the AIDS Outreach Center (AOC) provide a wide range of social services, outreach activities, testing and counseling, prevention education programs and public policy advocacy for men, women and children living with HIV, and their loved ones.
Shannon Hilgart, Executive Director
Mel LeRoy, Associate Executive Director

339 Houston Health Department: HIV-STD Viral Hepatitis Prevention
Houston HIV Prevention Community Planning Group
190 Heights Blvd.   832-393-4675
Houston, TX 77007   Chanda.Phanhphongsane@houstontx.gov
                     www.houstontx.gov/health/HIV-STD
Plans and implements public health strategies to reduce the spread of HIV and other STDs in Houston.
Stephen L. Williams, Director
David Persse, Health Authority

340 South Central AIDS Education and Training Center (SCAETC)
Parkland Health and Hospital System
8435 North Stemmons Freeway   214-590-2181
Dallas, TX 75247   877-275-2382
                                       Fax: 214-590-2184
                                       sc.aetc@phhs.org
                                       aidseducation.org
Provides educational programs about HIV infection for healthcare providers to Arkansas, Louisiana, New Mexico, Oklahoma, and Texa.
Henry Pacheco, MD, Project Director
Amneris Luqye, MD, Regional Clinical Director

341 Texas Department of State Health Services: HIV-STD Program
PO Box 149347   512-533-3000
Austin, TX 78714   800-255-1090
                                       Fax: 512-533-3171
                                       hivstd@dshs.texas.gov
                                       www.dshs.state.tx.us
Mission is to prevent, treat, and/or control the spread of HIV, STD, and other communicable diseases to protect the health of the citizens of Texas.
John Hellerstedt, MD, Commissioner
Felipe Rocha, TB/HIV/STD Contact

Utah

342 Utah Department of Health: Bureau of Epidemiology
Division of Epidemiology & Laboratory Services
288 N 1460 W   801-538-6191
Salt Lake City, UT 84114-2104   888-374-8824
                                       Fax: 801-538-9913
                                       epi@utah.gov
                              health.utah.gov/epi/diseases/hivaids
Secures and distributes funds for HIV/AIDS prevention services, provides educational programs and counseling to the general public, HIV/AIDS service organizations, health workers and groups at risk.
Joseph Miner, MD, Executive Director
Heather Borski, Director, Disease Control & Prevention

Vermont

343 Vermont Department of Health: Health Surveillance Division
PO Box 70   802-863-7240
Burlington, VT 05402   Fax: 802-865-7701
                              healthvermont.gov/disease-control/hiv

Focuses on HIV prevention, care, and surveillance, as well as providing resources for healthcare providers and the public.
Mark Levine, MD, Commissioner
Tracy Dolan, Deputy Health Commissioner

Virginia

344 Virginia Department of Health: Division of Disease Prevention
109 Governor Street   804-864-7964
Richmond, VA 23219   800-533-4148
                                       TTY: 888-232-6348
                              hiv-stdhotline@vdh.virginia.gov
                                       www.vdh.virginia.gov
Supports local health departments and community-based organizations in the prevention, surveillance and treatment of HIV and other STDs, including their complications, through provision of education, information, and health care services.
Laurie Forlano, DO, MPH, Director, Office of Epidemiology

Washington

345 Washington Department of Health: HIV Program
PO Box 47840   360-236-3444
Olympia, WA 98504-7840   800-272-2437
                                       Fax: 360-236-3470
                              Emalie.Huriaux@doh.wa.gov
                                       www.doh.wa.gov
Provides information and referrals to local, state and national resources relating to HIV/AIDS, provides informational and educational materials to individuals, agencies and organizations and actively works with print and broadcast media to promote HIV/AIDS awareness.
Emalie Huriaux, STD Program Manager
Zandt Bryan, Coordinator, Infectious Diseases

West Virginia

346 West Virginia Department of Health & Human Resources: Division of STD and HIV
350 Capitol Street   800-642-8244
Charleston, WV 25301   oeps.wv.gov
A division of the West Virginia Office of Epidemiology and Prevention Services, it seeks to prevent and control the spread of disease through surveillance, intervention, testing, education, and care.
Bill J. Crouch, Secretary

Wisconsin

347 AIDS Resource Center of Wisconsin
600 Williamson Street   608-252-6540
Madison, WI 53703   800-359-9272
                                       Fax: 608-252-6559
                                       feedback@arcw.org
                                       www.arcw.org
Provides critical AIDS care and prevention services. Sustained in these efforts by the resources, expertise and passion of hundreds of volunteers and donors.
Mike Gifford, President & CEO
Debra J. Endean, PhD, Vice President & COO

348 Wisconsin Department of Health Services: Wisconsin HIV Program
1 W Wilson Street   608-267-9005
Madison, WI 53703   877-865-3432
                                       TTY: 711
                              dhswebmaster@dhs.wisconsin.gov
                                       www.dhs.wisconsin.gov/hiv
Coordinates counseling and testing sites activities and services to HIV-infected persons, produces a report that contains information and recommendations for health care workers, emergency medical technicians and food service workers.
Timothy Pilcher, Supervisor, HIV Prevention Unit
Ryan Rohde, Project Development Coordinator

349 **Wyoming Department of Health: Communicable Disease Unit**
401 Hathaway Building   307-777-7529
Cheyenne, WY 82002   debi.anderson@wyo.gov
                                      health.wyo.gov/publichealth
Provides services for individuals living with HIV and their loved
ones, plus healthcare providers and case managers.
Debi Anderson, Unit Manager
Shelley Hood, Treatment Manager

Foundations

350 **AIDS Healthcare Foundation**
6255 Sunset Blvd.   323-860-5200
Los Angeles, CA 90028   www.aidshealth.org
The AHF is a non-profit organization that provides state-of-the-art
medicine and advocacy services to over 1,177,000 people in 43
countries. Funding is derived from a network of organization-run
pharmacies, thrift stores, healthcare agreements, and other
partnerships.
Michael Weinstein, President
Peter Reis, Senior Vice President

351 **American Foundation for AIDS Research**
120 Wall Street   212-806-1600
New York, NY 10005-3908   Fax: 212-806-1601
                                        TTY: 800-243-7889
                                            info@amfar.org
                                            www.amfar.org
Supports research in basic, clinical, prevention and public policy
and publishes the HIV/AIDS Treatment Directory.
Kevin Robert Frost, Chief Executive Officer
Annmari Shannahan, Vice President, Public Information

352 **American Foundation for Children with AIDS**
1520 Greening Lane   888-683-8323
Harrisburg, PA 17110   info@afcaids.org
                                            www.afcaids.org
A nonprofit organization founded to improve the quality of life for
drug-effected and HIV-infected children and their families in Africa. The foundation raises funds for family and community-based
services for children and their families affected by HIV.
Tanya Weaver, Executuve Director
Michelle Miller, Finance Director/Executive Assistant

353 **Canadian Foundation for AIDS Research**
2200 Yonge Street   416-361-6281
Toronto, Ontario, M4S-2C6   844-422-6327
                                            info@canfar.com
                                            canfar.ca
CANFAR is a national charitable foundation whose goal is to raise
awareness in order to generate funds for research into all aspects of
HIV infection and AIDS.
Alex Filiatrault, Chief Executive Officer
Logan Thayalan, Senior Manager, Development

354 **Clinical Focus on Primary Immune Deficiency Diseases**
Immune Deficiency Foundation
110 West Rd, Ste 300
Towson, MD 21204   410-321-6647
                                            800-296-4433
                                        Fax: 410-321-9165
                                      info@primaryimmune.org
                                          primaryimmune.org
Educational monograph is designed specifically for health care
professionals and focuses on topics relevant to primary immune
deficiency diseases.
Marcia Boyle, President & Founder
Christine Belser, Senior VP, Programs & Communications

355 **Elizabeth Glaser Pediatric AIDS Foundation**
1140 Connecticut Avenue NW   202-296-9165
Washington, DC 20036   Fax: 202-296-9185
                                          info@pedaids.org
                                          www.pedaids.org
Creates a future of hope for children and families worldwide by
eradicating pediatric AIDS, providing care and treatment to people

with HIV/AIDS, and accelerating the discovery of new treatments
for other serious and life-threatening pediatric illnesses.
Charles Lyons, President & CEO
Brad Kiley, Chief Operating Officer

356 **Fondation quebecoise du sida**
1 Sherbrooke Street East   514-642-4004
Montreal, QC, H2X-3V8   Fax: 514-844-2498
                                            info@fqsida.org
                                            fqsida.org
Fqsida seeks to support the fight against HIV/AIDS in Quebec, and
as of 2007, in French-speaking Africa as well through a partnership with Coalition PLUS. In early 2017 Farha Foundation merged
with Fondation quebecoise du sida.
Baya Toure, Director
Sabrina Boughlali, Donor Relations

357 **Immune Deficiency Foundation**
110 West Road   800-296-4433
Towson, MD 21204-4841   Fax: 410-321-9165
                                      info@primaryimmune.org
                                      www.primaryimmune.org
A national charitable organization aimed at fighting the primary
immune deficiency diseases. The founders included parents of
children with primary immune deficiency, immunologists who
treat immune deficient patients, and other individuals with an
immune deficiency.
John G. Boyle, President & CEO
Kara Moran, Vice President, Communications

358 **NAMES Project Foundation AIDS Memorial Quilt**
AIDS Memorial Quilt
117 Luckie Street NW   404-688-5500
Atlanta, GA 30303   Fax: 404-688-5552
                                          info@aidsquilt.org
                                          www.aidsquilt.org
International, non-governmental, non-profit organization that is
the custodian of the AIDS Memorial Quilt, a poignant memorial
and powerful tool for use in preventing new HIV infections.
Julie Rhoad, President & CEO
Roddy Williams, Director, Operations

359 **National Hemophilia Foundation**
7 Penn Plaza   212-328-3700
New York, NY 10001   800-42H-ANDI
                                        Fax: 212-328-3777
                                      handi@hemophilia.org
                                      www.hemophilia.org
The National Hemophilia Foundation is dedicated to finding better
treatments and cures for bleeding and clotting disorders and to preventing the complications of these disorders through education,
advocacy and research.
Val Bias, CEO
Neil Frick, VP, Research & Medical Information

360 **Toronto People with AIDS Foundation**
200 Gerrard Street E   416-506-1400
Toronto, Ontario, M5A-2E6   Fax: 416-506-1404
                                      info@pwatoronto.org
                                      www.pwatoronto.org
Promotes the health and well-being of all people living with
HIV/AIDS by providing accessible, direct, and practical support
services.
Suzanne Paddock, Executive Director
Gareth Henry, Director, Programs & Services

Libraries & Resource Centers

361 **AIDS Library of Philadelphia**
1233 Locust Street   215-985-4851
Philadelphia, PA 19107   Fax: 215-985-4492
                                      library@aidslibrary.org
                                      www.aidslibrary.org
Improving access to health and support services, preventing HIV
transmission, and raising the public awareness of HIV/AIDS re-
lated issues.
Allie Frase, Collection Management Librarian
Ben Remsen, Public Services

362 National Library of Medicine
8600 Rockville Pike
Bethesda, MD 20894
301-594-5983
888-346-3656
Fax: 301-402-1384
TDD: 800-735-2258
custserv@nlm.nih.gov
www.nlm.nih.gov/
The National Library of Medicine (NLM), on the campus of the National Institutes of Health in Bethesda, Maryland, is the world's largest medical library. The Library collects materials in all areas of biomedicine and health care, as well as works on biomedical aspects of technology, the humanities, and the physical, life, and social sciences.
Dr Donald Lindberg, Director
Betsy L Humphreys, Deputy Director

Research Centers

Alabama

363 Centers for AIDS Research: University of Alabama at Birmingham
BBRB 256
Birmingham, AL 35294-1150
205-934-4011
http://www.uab.edu
Provides expertise, resources, and services not otherwise readily obtained through traditional funding mechanisms.
Robert P. Kimberly, Director
Cheryl A. Perry, Deputy Director

364 General Clinical Research Center: UAB
Room 907 Medical Education Building
Birmingham, AL 35294
205-934-4852
ccts@uab.edu
AIDS and genetics research.
Burt Nabors, MD, Director
Stuart Frank, Co-Principal Investigator

365 University of Alabama at Birmingham: National Cooperative Drug/AIDS
UAB Center for AIDS Research
BBRB 256
Birmingham, AL 35294-1150
205-934-4011
http://www.uab.edu
Robert P. Kimberly, Director
Cheryl A. Perry, Deputy Director

California

366 AIDS Clinical Trials Unit CARES Clinic
CARES Clinic
2315 Stocktown blvd.
Sacramento, CA 95817
916-734-2011
800-2 U- DAV
Fax: 916-325-1955
actu@ucdavis.edu
www.ucdmc.ucdavis.edu/actu
The ACTU at Davis Medical Center is dedicated to offering the latest in research clinical trials to HIV/AIDS patients throughout Northern Central California.
Thomas S. Nesbitt, Vice Chancellor
david A Acosta, Associate Vice Chancellor

367 Adult Research Opportunities
220 Dickinson Street
San Diego, CA 92103-8208
619-543-8080
Fax: 619-543-5066
www.avrctrials.org
A university-based nonprofit clinical trials unit. Conduct's patient-oriented research and educational programs on HIV and other chronic infections. Studies have pioneered the development of treatments that continue to change the course of the HIV epidemic.
Constance Benson, Director
Richard S Garfein, Professor and Chairman

368 Center for AIDS Prevention Studies AIDS Research Institute University of C
AIDS Research Institute, University of California
50 Beale Street
San Francisco, CA 94105
415-597-9100
Fax: 415-597-9213
CAPS.Web@ucsf.edu
www.caps.ucsf.edu
The mission of the Center for AIDS Prevention Studies is to conduct domestic and international research to prevent the acquisition of HIV and to optimize health outcomes among HIV-infected individuals.
Stephen F Morin, Director
Susan Kegeles, Co-Director

369 Center for Interdisciplinary Research in Immunology and Diseases at UCLA
UCLA School of Medicine
924 Westwood Blvd. #545
Los Angeles, CA 90095
310-825-6373
Research into immunology and blood disorders with special focus on AIDS and HIV infections.
Albert Glover, Director, Academic Affairs

370 Centers for AIDS Research: North-Central California
UC Davis, Division of Infectious Diseases
4150 V Street
Sacramento, CA 95817
916-734-8033
Fax: 916-734-7766
nccfar@ucdavis.edu
www.ucdmc.ucdavis.edu/nccfar
Provides expertise resources and services not otherwise readily obtained through more traditional funding mechanisms.
Richard B Pollard, Division Chief
Krystin E Cheung, Director

371 Centers for AIDS Research: USCD Center for AIDS Research
Center for AIDS Research
9500 Gilman Drive
La Jolla, CA 92093-0716
858-534-5545
Fax: 858-822-5840
cfar@ucsd.edu
cfar.ucsd.edu
Provides expertise resources and services and services not otherwise readily obtained through traditional funding mechanisms.
Douglas Richman, Director
Kim Schafer, Administrative Director

372 Centers for AIDS Research: University of California, Los Angeles
UCLA AIDS Institute
10940 Wilshire Blvd.
Los Angeles, CA 90024-1678
310-794-4419
Fax: 310-794-3955
Provides expertise, resources, and services not otherwise readily obtained through traditional funding mechanisms.
Irvin S.Y. Chen, Director
Dr. Thomas Coates, Associate Director

373 City of Hope National Medical Center Drug Discover/AIDS Group
City of Hope
1500 E Duarte Road
Duarte, CA 91010
626-256-4673
www.cityofhope.org
Developmental research into the treatment of AIDS.
Michael A Friedman MD, CEO
Robert Stone, President

374 Kaiser Foundation Research Institute
2000 Broadway
Oakland, CA 94612
510-891-3400
www.dor.kaiser.org
Tracy A Lieu, Director
Alyce Adams, Health Care Delivery and policy

375 Pacific AIDS Education and Training Center (PAETC)
University Of California San Francisco
550 16th Street, 3rd Floor
San Francisco, CA 94158-2549
415-476-6153
paetcmail@ucsf.edu
paetc.org
Provides educational programs about HIV infection for healthcare providers to Arizona, California, Hawaii, Nevada, and the 6 U.S.-affiliated Pacific Jurisdictions.
E. Michael Reyes, MD, MPH, Principal Investigator
Monica Hahn, MD, Regional Clinical Director

376 Stanford University General Clinical Research Center
GCRC Administration
300 Pasteur Drive
Stanford, CA 94305-5251
650-723-4000
Fax: 650-725-6698
gcrcstanford@stanford.edu
The Stanford General Clinical Research Center (GCRC) is the major clinical research facility for Stanford University School of Medicine. With patient care units in Stanford University Hospital

and Lucile Packard Children's Hospital the center plays a crucial role in the school's bench-to-bedside research mission.
Ellen Jo Baron, Director
Branimir I Sikic, Program Director

377 Stanford University National Cooperative Drug Discovery/AIDS Group
School of Medicine
300 Pasteur Drive   650-723-4000
Stanford, CA 94305   Fax: 650-725-6698
                                     www.med.stanford.edu

Ellen Jo Baron, Director
Branimir I Sikic, Program Director

378 UCLA AIDS Clinical Research Center
1399 S Roxbury Drive   310-557-2273
Los Angeles, CA 90035   Fax: 310-557-3450
                                     www.uclacarecenter.org

Dr.A Eugene, Chancellor
David T Feinberg, President

379 UCSD Antiviral Research Center
220 Dickinson Street   619-543-8080
San Diego, CA 92103-8208   Fax: 619-543-5066
Develops treatment protocols and drug therapies and recruits research volunteers for AIDS studies and HIV related disorders.
Jill Kunkel, Director
Michael Giancola, Screening Co-ordinator

380 USC Internal Medicine
1520 San Pablo Street   800-872-2273
Los Angeles, CA 90033-1034   Fax: 213-224-6687
                                     www.usc.edu/health/internal
Research into internal medicine with specialties in cardiovascular endocrinology and diabetes gastrointestinal and liver disease geriatric medicine hematology infectious diseases nephrology oncology pulmonary and critical care and rheumatology and immunology.
Alexandra Levine, Head

381 University of California San Francisco Center for AIDS Prevention
Center for AIDS Prevention Studies (CAPS)
50 Beale Street   415-597-9100
San Francisco, CA 94105-3411   Fax: 415-597-9213
                                     CAPS.web@ucsf.edu
                                     www.caps.ucsf.edu
The mission of the Center for AIDS Prevention Studies is to conduct domestic and international research to prevent the acquisition of HIV and to optimize health outcomes among HIV- infected individuals.
Stephen F Morin, Director
Susan Kegeles, Co-Director

382 University of California: Institute of Health Policy Studies
513 Parnassus Avenue   415-476-9000
San Francisco, CA 94143-410   Fax: 415-476-0705
                                     claire.brindis@ucsf.edu
                                     www.ihps.medschool.ucsf.edu
Health policy and AIDS research.
Susan Desmond-Hellman, Chancellor
Phillip R. Lee, director

Colorado

383 Centers for AIDS Research: University of Colorado Health Sciences Center
Colorado Center for AIDS Research
4200 East 9th Avenue   303-315-7233
Denver, CO 80262   Fax: 303-315-8681
Describes forms and patterns of use of complimentary and alternative medicine (CAM) for the treatment of HIV/AIDS.
Robert T. Schooley, Director

384 Mountain West AIDS Education and Training Center (MWAETC)
325 9th Avenue   206-543-2704
Seattle, WA 98104   aetcinfo@uw.edu
                                     mwaetc.org

Provides educational programs about HIV infection for healthcare providers to Alaska, Colorado, Idaho, Montana, Oregon, North and South Dakota, Utah, Washington, and Wyoming.
David Spach, MD, Principal Investigator/Clinical Director
Laurie Sylla, MHSA, Director

District of Columbia

385 George Washington National Cooperative: Drug Discovery/AIDS Treatment
Department of Pharmacology & Physiology
2300 Eye Street NW   202-994-3541
Washington, DC 20037-2336   Fax: 202-994-2870
                                     www.gwumc.edu/pharm
Studies and researches natural products and synthetic anti-AIDS agents.
Susan Ceryak, Associate Research Professor
Jian-Zhong Guo, Associate Research Professor

386 Whitman Walker Clinic AIDS/Medical Services Programs
1701 14th Street NW   202-745-7000
Washington, DC 20009-3840   Fax: 202-745-0238
                                     info@wwc.org
                                     www.wwc.org
A non-profit community-based health organization serving the Washington D.C. metropolitan region. Established by and for the gay and lesbian community our clinic is comprised of diverse volunteers and staff who provide or facilitate the delivery of high quality comprehensive accessible health care and community services. Especially committed to ending the suffering of all those infected and affected by HIV/AIDS.
Adam Falcone, Chair
June Crenshaw, Vice Chair

Florida

387 Department of Epidemiology and Health Policy Research: University of Florida
1329 SW 16th Street   352-265-8035
Gainesville, FL 32608   Fax: 352-265-8047
                                     www.ehpr.ufl.edu
Studies into child and adolescent health financing and organization of health care delivery systems community health chronic conditions transition from pediatric to adult health care access to health care for vulnerable populations quality of life and outcomes research.
Clifford J Crook, Chair
John C Bierly, Program Assistant

388 Tampa Bay Research Institute
10900 Roosevelt Boulevard N   727-576-6675
Saint Petersburg, FL 33716-2308   Fax: 727-577-9862
                                     development@tampabayresearch.org
                                     www.tampabayresearch.org
TBRI is the first independent biomedical research organization of its kind in Florida. Our scientists dedicate their lives work to conquering chronic and infectious diseases while gaining a better understanding of the immune system.
Clifford J Crook, Chair
John C Bierly, Program Assistant

389 University of South Florida Center for HIV Education and Research
13301 Bruce B Downs Boulevard   813-974-4430
Tampa, FL 33612-3807   866-352-2382
                                     Fax: 813-974-8451
                                     Contact@FCAETC.org
Serves health care professionals throughout Florida by providing education and information on the transmission control treatment and prevention of HIV and AIDS and by conducting related research and community outreach.
jeffery beal, Director
Debbie Cestaro, Project Co-ordinator

Georgia

390 AIDS School Health Education Database Centers for Disease Control
Centers for Disease Control

1600 Clifton Road
Atlanta, GA 30333

404-639-3534
800-232-4636
TTY: 888-232-6348
cdcinfo@cdc.gov
www.cdc.gov

An information awareness resource produced by the Division of Adolescent and School Health. The database offers descriptions of various educational resources for professionals relevant to the education of children and youth about HIV infection and AIDS.
Thomas R. Frieden, Director
Ileana Arias, Principal Deputy Director

391 CDC National Prevention Information Network
1600 Clifton Road
Atlanta, GA 30329

800-232-4636
TTY: 888-232-6348
NPIN-info@cdc.gov
npin.cdc.gov

The CDC National Prevention Information Network (NPIN) is the U.S. reference, referral, and distribution service for information on HIV/AIDS, sexually transmitted diseases (STDs), and tuberculosis (TB). NPIN produces, collects, catalogs, processes, stocks, and disseminates materials and information on HIV/AIDS, STD's, and TB to organizations and people working in those disease fields in international, national, state, and local settings.

392 Center for AIDS Research: Emory University Rollins School of Public Health
1518 Clifton Road NE
Atlanta, GA 30322-4201

404-727-2924
Fax: 404-727-9853
cfar@emory.edu
www.cfar.emory.edu

Provides expertise resources and services not otherwise readily obtained through more traditional funding mechanisms.
James W Curran, Director
Carlos del Rio, Co-Director for Clinical Science

393 Educational Materials Database Centers for Disease Control
Centers for Disease Control
1600 Clifton Road
Atlanta, GA 30333-4201

404-639-3534
800-232-4636
TTY: 888-232-6348
cdcinfo@cdc.gov
www.cdc.gov

An information awareness resource produced by the Division of Adolescent and School Health. The database offers descriptions of various educational resources for professionals relevant to the education of children and youth about HIV infection and AIDS.
Thomas R. Frieden, Director
Ileana Arias, Principal Deputy Director

394 Emory University: National Cooperative Drug Discovery for AIDS Treatment
Emory Healthcare Pediatrics Department
201 Dowman Drive
Atlanta, GA 30322

404-727-6123
Fax: 404-727-5737
www.pediatrics.emory.edu

Barbara J Stoll MD, Professor, Chair
James W Wagner, President

395 Funding Database Centers for Disease Control
Centers for Disease Control
1600 Clifton Road
Atlanta, GA 30329

404-639-3534
800-232-4636
TTY: 888-232-6348
cdcinfo@cdc.gov
www.cdc.gov

A listing of HIV and AIDS related funding opportunities for community-based and HIV and AIDS service organizations.
Thomas Friedman MD, Director
Harold Jaffe, MD, MA, Associate Director of Science

Illinois

396 Clinical Research Center Northwestern Center for Clinical Researc
Northwestern Center for Clinical Research

633 Clark Street,
Chicago, IL 60611

312-503-8649
nucats@northwestern.edu
www.nucats.northwestern.edu
Colleen De Luca, Associate Director, Administration
Philip Greenland, Director

397 Midwest AIDS Education and Training Center (MATEC)
1919 West Taylor
Chicago, IL 60612

312-996-1373
312-413-4184
matec@uic.edu
www.matec.info

Provides educational programs about HIV infection for healthcare providers.
Ricardo A. Rivero, MD, MPH, Executive Director
Renslow Sherer, MD, Regional Clinical Director

Indiana

398 Purdue University Center for AIDS Research
School of Pharmacy and Pharmaceutical Sciences
575 Stadium Mall Drive
W Lafayette, IN 47907-2091

765-494-1361
Fax: 765-494-7880
oss@pharmacy.purdue.edu
www.pharmacy.purdue.edu

Steve Byrn, Department Head
Stanley L Hem, Associate Department Head

Maryland

399 Center for AIDS Research: Johns Hopkins University School of Medicine
733 N. Broadway
Baltimore, MD 21205-2196

410-955-3182

Provides expertise resources and services not otherwise readily obtained through more traditional funding mechanisms.
Ronald R Peterson, ,President, JHH/HS
Edward D Miller, MD, Dean, CEO

400 Johns Hopkins University: Center for Communication Programs
Johns Hopkins Bloomberg School of Public Health
111 Market Place
Baltimore, MD 21202

410-659-6300
Fax: 410-659-6266
info@jhuccp.org
www.jhuccp.org

Health communications family planning and AIDS prevention research.
Susan Krenn, Director
James bon tempo, Associate Director of Communican Science

401 University of Maryland Center for Research, Grants & Contracts
Family Studies Depatrment
1142 School of Public Health
College Park, MD 20742

301-405-3672
Fax: 301-314-9161
fmst@umd.edu

Erin McClure, Co-ordinator
Doris Richardson, business Manager

402 University of Maryland Center for Studies Family Studies Depatrment
1142 School of Public Health
College Park, MD 20742

301-405-3672
Fax: 301-314-9161
fmsc@umd.edu
www.sph.umd.edu/fmsc

Erin McClure, Co-ordinator
Doris Richardson, business Manager

403 University of Maryland: Medical Biotechnology Center
701 E. PRATT ST,
Baltimore, MD 21202-1513

410-706-8802
Fax: 410-706-8184
hill@UMCES.edu
www.umbi.umd.edu

Offers research into AIDS and HIV infection including vaccine development.
W Jonathan Lederer, Director
Kadir Aslan, Assistant Professor

AIDS/HIV / Research Centers

Massachusetts

404 Center for AIDS Research: Harvard Medical School, Division of AIDS
The Landmark Buiding
104 Mt. Auburn Street   617-384-9039
Cambridge, MA 02138   Fax: 617-495-8231
aids@hms.harvard.edu
aids.med.harvard.edu/cfar.htm
Provides expertise resources and services not otherwise readily obtained through traditional funding mechanisms.
Bruce Walker, Director
Myron Essex, Associate Director

405 Center for Blood Research Harvard Medical School/CBR
Harvard Medical School/CBR
200 Longwood Avenue   617-278-3140
Boston, MA 02115   Fax: 617-278-3131
kirchhausen@crystal.harvard.edu
Offers research into blood disorders including multidisciplinary studies on AIDS and hemophilia cancer and diabetes research as well.
Fredrick Alt, President/ Director
Stephen Carriuolo, Financial Manager

406 Centers for AIDS Research: University of Massachusetts Medical School
364 Plantation Street   508-856-3159
Worcester, MA 01605   publicaffairs@umassmed.edu
www.umassmed.edu/cfar
Provides expertise, resources, and services not otherwise readily obtained through traditional funding mechanisms.
celia Schiffer, Director
Shan Lu, Co-Director

407 Dana Farber Cancer Institute National Drug Discovery Group for AIDS Treatment
Dana-Farber Cancer Institute
450 Brookline Avenue   617-632-3000
Boston, MA 02215-5450   800-408-3324
TTY: 617-632-5330
TDD: 617-632-5330
dana-farbercontactus@dfci.harvard.edu
www.dana-farber.org
Edward Benz, President and CEO
Dorthy E Puhy, Executive Vice President and COO

408 Developmental Medicine Center Children's Hospital Boston
Children's Hospital Boston
300 Longwood Avenue   617-355-6000
Boston, MA 02115   Fax: 617-730-0633
TTY: 617-730-0152
www.childrenshospital.org
Studies developmental effects of infants at risk and development effects of congenital HIV infection.
James Mandell, CEO
Sandra Fenwick, President, COO

409 New England AIDS Education and Training Center
Center for Health Policy and Research
333 South Street   617-262-5657
Shrewsbury, MA 01545   Fax: 617-502-1701
aidsed@neaetc.org
www.neaetc.org
NEAETC serves health care professionals in New England with consultation, technical assistance, and resource materials.
Philip Bolduc, MD, Clinical Director
Jennifer Daly, MD, Co-Clinical Director

Michigan

410 University of Michigan: National Cooperative Drug/AIDS Group
School of Dentistry
1011 N University Avenue   734-763-6933
Ann Arbor, MI 48109-1078   Fax: 734-763-3453
paulk@umich.edu
www.dent.umich.edu
Focuses on the design of new drugs to fight AIDS.
John C Drach PhD, Director
Paul H Krebsbach, Department Chair

411 Wayne State University Center for Health Research
College of Nursing
Center for Health Research   313-577-4082
Detroit, MI 48202   888-837- 08
Fax: 313-577-6949
nursinginfo@wayne.edu
www.nursing.wayne.edu/CHR
Facilitates interdisciplinary health research across diverse settings where nursing is practiced and healthcare is provided.
Nancy T Artinian, Director
Barbara K Redman, Dean

New York

412 Aaron Diamond AIDS Research Center
455 First Avenue   212-448-5000
New York, NY 10016   Fax: 212-725-1126
webinfo@adarc.org
www.adarc.org
Committed to finding solutions to end the AIDS epidemic. In the decade and a half since HIV was identified researchers have learned more about this virus than about any other in history.
David Ho, Director & CEO
Gerald Friedland MD, Chairman

413 Centers for AIDS Research: Albert Einstein College of Medicine
Albert Einstein College of Medicine
Jack and Pearl Resnick Campus   718-430-2000
Bronx, NY 10461   Fax: 718-430-2374
information@einstein.yu.edu
www.aecom.yu.edu/cfar
Provides consultation and support to the medical and research community in the scientific evaluation of CAM therapies.
Allen M Spiegel MD, Dean
Matthew Scharff MD, CFAR Investigator

414 Centers for AIDS Research: Columbia University College of Physicians
Center for AIDS Research
630 W 168th Street   212-305-1296
New York, NY 10032   jka8@columbia.edu
www.cumc.columbia.edu
Provides a comprehensive framework for training educational programs and research which addresses health promotion disease prevention symptom management and quality of life for individuals with HIV. The goal of the Center is to create innovative research and service approaches for the prevention and management of HIV. This objective is fulfilled through research program development and program evaluations.
Lee Goldman MD, Executive Vice President
Lee Bollinger, JD, President of the University

415 Centers for AIDS Research: NYU School of Medicine
522 First Avenue   212-263-8527
New York, NY 10016   www.hivinfosource.org/hivis/cfar
Provides expertise resources and services not otherwise readily obtained through traditional funding mechanisms.
Derya Unutmaz MD, Director
David levy, Associate Dean

416 General Clinical Research Center Mount Sinai School of Medicine
Mount Sinai School of Medicine
One Gustave L Levy Place   212-241-6500
New York, NY 10029-6574   Fax: 212-348-5811
hugh.sampson@mssm.edu
www.mssm.edu/gcrc
Focuses on AIDS education and prevention.
Dennis S Charney, Executive Vice President
Kennith Davis, President

417 HIV Center for Clinical and Behavioral Studies
1051 Riverside Drive   212-543-5969
New York, NY 10032   Fax: 212-543-6003
www.hivcenternyc.org
Interdisciplinary research center that investigates the behavioral causes and consequences of HIV/AIDS. Focusing on the intersections of HIV infection gender and sexuality; treatment strategies

32

for infected populations; and innovative dissemination of scientific findings.
Anke A Ehrhardt, Director
Heino F L Meyer-Bahlbur, Associate Director

418   Institute for Clinical Research Weill Cornell Medical College
Weill Cornell Medical College
1300 York Avenue   212-746-5454
New York, NY 10065   Fax: 212-746-8970
                                                        cto@med.cornell.edu
                                                          www.med.cornell.edu
The mission of the ICR is to support, advance and promote clinical and translational research enterprises at WCMC. As part of Research and Sponsored Programs (RASP) the ICR streamlines the clinical research process and offers a wide range of services, resources and training.
David J Skorton MD, President of the University
Michelle A Lewis, MS, Director (Research and Sponsored Program

419   Northeast/Caribbean AIDS Education and Training Center (NECAAETC)
Columbia University, HIV Center
601 West 168th Street   646-774-6978
New York, NY 10032   Fax: 212-568-3060
                                                       nynjaetc@columbia.edu
                                                               necaaetc.org
Provides educational programs about HIV infection for healthcare providers to New Jersey, New York, Puerto Rico and the U.S. Virgin Islands.
Francine Cournos, MD, Principal Investigator
Daria Boccher-Lattimore, DrPH, Director & Co-Investigator

420   SUNY at Buffalo National Cooperative Drug Discovery Group for AIDS Treatment
Department of Biochemistry
140 Farber Hall   716-829-2727
Buffalo, NY 14214-3000   Fax: 716-829-2725
                                                           jluck@buffalo.edu
                                                              www.buffalo.edu
Kenneth M Blumenthal, Professor and Chairman
Elizabeth O'Brocta, Assistant to the Chairman

421   Spellman Center for HIV Related Disease The Spellman Center
The Spellman Center
415 W Fifty-First Street   212-459-8130
New York, NY 10019
David Kaufman, Director

422   State University of New York: SUNY Stony HIV Treatment Development Center
Center for Infectious Diseases
101 Nicolls Road   631-444-4000
Stony Brook, NY 11794-5120   Fax: 631-444-2493
                                                rsteigbigel@notes.cc.sunysb.edu
                                                www.stonybrookmedicalcenter.org
Human immunodeficiency virus research.
Joyce Klien, Director
Laura Coppola, Assistant Director

North Carolina

423   Centers for AIDS Research: Univeristy of North Carolina at Chapel Hill
UNC Center For AIDS Research
Lineberger Cancer Center   919-966-8645
Chapel Hill, NC 27599   cfar@med.unc.edu
                                                            cfar.med.unc.edu
Administrative and shared research support to synergistically enhance and coordinate high quality AIDS research projects.
Ronald Swanstrom, Director
Myron S Cohen, Associate Director

Ohio

424   Centers for AIDS Research: Case Western University
Department of Medicine
Division of Infectious Diseases   216-368-0271
Cleveland, OH 44106-5029   Fax: 216-368-3055
                                                             mxl6@case.edu
                                                         www.clevelandactu.org

Provides administrative and shared research support to enhance and coordinate high quality AIDS research projects.
Michael M Lederman, Co-Director
Jonathan Karn, Associate Director

Pennsylvania

425   Centers for AIDS Research: University of Pennsylvania
Penn Center for AIDS Research
295 John Morgan Building   215-573-7354
Philadelphia, PA 19104-6140   Fax: 215-573-7356
                                                     oliviere@mail.med.upenn.edu
                                                          www.med.upenn.edu
Also the Children's Hospital and the Wistar Institute provides important services and research for high quality projects.
James A Hoxie, Director
Ronald G Collman, Co-Director

426   MidAtlantic AIDS Education and Training Center (MAAETC)
University of Pittsburgh
130 DeSoto Street   412-624-1895
Pittsburgh, PA 15261   Fax: 412-624-4767
                                                              www.maaetc.org
Provides educational programs about HIV infection for healthcare providers to Delaware, District of Columbia, Maryland, Pennsylvania, Virginia, and West Virgina.
Linda Rose Frank, PhD, Principal Investigator & Exec. Dir.

427   Temple University Clinical Research Center Office of Clinical Research
Office of Clinical Research
Medical Education and Research Buil   215-707-7000
Philadelphia, PA 19140   Fax: 215-201-2684
                                                            tusm@temple.edu
                                                       www.temple.edu/medicine
CRC Unit provides space to perform clinical research on 4 West of Temple University Hospital. The CRC Unit has the potential for three rooms for inpatient/outpatient studies and an additional room for outpatient studies.
Antonio Giorgio MD, President

428   Thomas Jefferson University: Center for Research in Medical Education
Jefferson Medical College
1020 Walnut Street   215-955-6000
Philadelphia, PA 19107   Fax: 215-923-7583
                                                    Joseph.Gonnella@jefferson.edu
                                                         www.jefferson.edu/jmc
Joseph Gonne MD, Director
Robert L Barchi MD, President

Rhode Island

429   Centers for AIDS Research: Brown University
The Miriam Hospital
CFAR/RISE Building   401-793-4068
Providence, RI 02906   Fax: 401-793-4704
                                                         vgodleski@lifespan.org
Provides expertise resources and services not otherwise readily obtained through traditional funding mechanisms.
Charles C J Carpenter, Director
Susan Cu-Uvin, HIV and Women Core Co-Director

South Carolina

430   Medical University of South Carolina Health Services Administration
Medical University of South Carolina
171 Ashley Avenue   843-792-1414
Charleston, SC 29425   800-424-6872
                                                        Fax: 843-792-2601
                                                               www.musc.edu
Devoted to public health policy and health care management including AIDS research.
Raymond S Greenburg, President
Dr. Mark Sothman, Vice President

Tennessee

431   **Centers for AIDS Research: Vanderbilt University Medical Center**
Division of Infectious Disease
1161 21st Avenue S   615-322-8972
Nashville, TN 37232-2582   richard.daquila@vanderbilt.edu
                                           www.mc.vanderbilt.edu/cfar
Provides expertise resources and services not otherwise readily
obtained through more traditional funding mechanisms.
Richard D'Aquila, Director
G Fatima Lima Ph.D., Associate Director

432   **Southeast AIDS Education and Training Center (SEAETC)**
Vanderbilt Health
719 Thompson Lane   615-875-7873
Nashville, TN 37204   Fax: 615-936-1583
                                                 www.seaetc.com
Provides educational programs about HIV infection for healthcare
providers to Alabama, Florida, Georgia, Kentucky, Mississippi,
North Carolina, South Carolina, and Tennessee.
Stephen P. Raffanto, MD, MPH, Principal Investigator
Anna Person, MD, Clinical Director

Texas

433   **Centers for AIDS Research: Baylor College of Medicine**
Department of Molecular Virology & Microbiology
One Baylor Plaza   713-798-3006
Houston, TX 77030   Fax: 713-798-5019
                                                  jbutel@bcm.edu
                                               www.bcm.edu/cfar
A research center that is a branch of the Centers for AIDS Re-
search.
Janet S Butel, Director
William T Shearer, Co-Director

434   **South Central AIDS Education and Training Center (SCAETC)**
Parkland Health and Hospital System
8435 North Stemmons Freeway   214-590-2181
Dallas, TX 75247   877-275-2382
                                         Fax: 214-590-2184
                                               sc.aetc@phhs.org
                                               aidseducation.org
Provides educational programs about HIV infection for healthcare
providers to Arkansas, Louisiana, New Mexico, Oklahoma, and
Texa.
Henry Pacheco, MD, Project Director
Amneris Luqye, MD, Regional Clinical Director

Vermont

435   **University of Vermont: Office of Health Promotion Research**
1 S Prospect Street   802-656-4187
Burlington, VT 05401   Fax: 802-656-8826
                                                   ohpr@uvm.edu
                                               www.uvm.edu/~ohpr
Research done into public policy and human health including
AIDS information and evaluation.
Anne L Dorwaldt, Assistant Director
Rachael Chicoine, AAS, Research Project Assistant

Washington

436   **Centers for AIDS Research: University of Washington, Harborview Medical Center**
Center For AIDS & STDs
325 Ninth Avenue   206-744-4239
Seattle, WA 98104-2499   Fax: 206-744-3693
                                           worthy@u.washington.edu
                                         www.depts.washington.edu/cfas
Provides administrative and shared research support to synergisti-
cally enhance and coordinate high quality AIDS research projects.
CFARs accomplish this through core facilities that provide exper-
tise resource and services not otherwise readily obtained through
more traditional funding mechanisms.
King K Holmes, Director
Mary Fielder, Assistant to the Director

437   **HIV Prevention Trials Unit University of Washington/Seattle HPTU Si**
University of Washington/Seattle HPTU Site
Cabrini Medical Tower 901 Boren Av   206-520-3800
Seattle, WA 98104   Fax: 206-520-3801
                                           www.depts.washington.edu
A worldwide collaborative clinical trials network established by
the National Institutes of Health (NIH) to evaluate the safety and
efficacy of non-vaccine prevention interventions alone or in com-
bination using HIV incidence as the primary endpoint.
Connie Celum, Principal Investigator

Support Groups & Hotlines

438   **AEGIS AIDS Education Global Information System**
PO Box 184   949-495-1952
San Juan Capistrano, CA 92693   Fax: 949-443-1755
                                                    www.aegis.org
A not-for-profit, tax-exempt, educational corpoation that adds
more than 3000 documents each month. Reach more than 10 mil-
lion users annually, including: the US Federal Government, US
Educational Institutions, and Nonprofit organizations both here
and abroad.
Vanessa Robison, President
Sister Mary Elizabeth, Assistant Operations Director

439   **AIDS Alabama**
3521 7th Avenue S   205-324-9822
Birmingham, AL 35222   800-592-2437
                                         Fax: 205-324-9311
                                           maryanne@aidsalabama.org
                                               www.aidsalabama.org
Devotes its energy and resources statewide to helping people with
HIV/AIDS live healthy, independent lives and works to prevent
the spread of HIV. It is our goal to provide housing for those with
HIV in the Birmingham area, secure and administer grants for care
of persons with HIV statewide, and specialize in targeted preven-
tion education programs.
Elaine Cottle, Executive Director

440   **AIDS Hotline of Central New York**
AIDS Community Resources
627 W Genesee Street   315-475-2430
Syracuse, NY 13204   800-475-2430
                                         Fax: 315-472-6515
                                     information@aidscommunityresources.com
                                       www.aidscommunityresources.com
A not-for-profit, community-based organization providing pre-
vention, education and support services to those infected with and
affected by HIV/AIDS Serves Cayuga, Herkimer, Jefferson,
Lewis, Madison, Oneida, Onondaga, Oswego and St. Lawrences
counties in New York State.
Michael Crinnin, Executive Director

441   **AIDS Support Group of Cape Cod**
428 S Street   508-778-1957
Hyannis, MA 02610   866-990-2437
                                         Fax: 508-778-4501
                                                    info@asgcc.org
                                                    www.asgcc.org
Our mission is to provide services that maintain and enhance the
quality of life for persons living with HIV and AIDS on Cape Cod
and Martha's Vineyard and to provide health education, prevention and harm reduction outreach via timely and accurate information about HIV/AIDS, STIs and viral hepatitis.
Krystin St. Onge, Interim Director

442   **AIDSinfo**
US Department of Health and Human Services
PO Box 6303   301-315-2816
Rockville, MD 20849-6303   800-448-0440
                                         Fax: 301-315-2818
                                             TTY: 888-480-3739
                                           contactus@aidsinfo.nih.gov
                                               www.aidsinfo.nih.gov
Offers the latest federally approved information on HIV/AIDS
clinical research, treatment and prevention, and medical practice
guidelines for people living with HIV/AIDS, their families and
friends, health care providers, scientists, and researchers.

443 Alaskan Statewide AIDS Helpline
1057 W Fireweed   907-263-2050
Anchorage, AK 99503   800-478-AIDS
                                               Fax: 907-263-2051
                                               www.alaskanaids.org
A key collaborator within the state of Alaska in the provision of
supportive services to persons living with HIV/AIDS and their
families and in the elimination of the transmission of HIV infection and its stigma.
Heather Davis, Executive Director
Maureen Suttman, Client Resource Services

444 BABES Network-YWCA
1118 Fifth Ave   206-720-5566
Seattle, WA 98101   888-292-1912
                                               Fax: 206-720-5901
                                               the_staff@babesnetwork.org
                                               www.babesnetwork.org
A peer-based program, a sisterhood of women facing HIV together.
Reduces isolation, promotes self-empowerment, enhances quality
of life and serves the needs of women facing HIV and their families
through peer support, advocacy, education and outreach
Rhonda Kimm, Advocacy Coordinator
Amelia Vader, Program Manager

445 COMPASS Program
c/o Institute for Urban Family Health
16 East 16th Street   212-924-7744
New York, NY 10003   Fax: 212-691-4610
                                               info@institute2000.org
Medical services include HIV testing and specialized HIV medical
care for adults in addition to women's health services including gynecology, PAP tests, family planning and birth control methods.
Mental health services includes individual, couples, and family
counseling and psychiatric evaluations and monitoring.
Neil Calman MD/ABFP/FAAFP, President/Chief Executive Officer
Weston Willett, Chief Information Officer

446 Cascade AIDS Project Hotline
200 SW Fifth Avenue   503-223-5907
Portland, OR 97204   Fax: 503-223-6437
                                               info@cascadeaids.org
                                               www.cascadeaids.org
Provides HIV prevention and services information by phone and
internet to youth and adults across Orgeon and the Northwest.
Charles Washington, President
warren Jimanez, Vice President

447 Dunshee House
303-17th Avenue East   206-322-2437
Seattle, WA 98112   Fax: 206-322-1779
                                               josh@dunsheehouse.org
A non-profit organization, builds community and cultivates powerful, healthy lives by providing emotional support and personal
development services to those affected by HIV/AIDS, the Queer
communities, and those who love them.
Michael Kann, President
Adrienne Miller, Vice President

448 HEAL
Sidney Hillman Family Pracitce
16 E 16th Street   212-924-7744
New York, NY 10003-3105   healweb@thorup.com
The Health Education AIDS Liaison provides alternative and ho-
listic support groups and resources for people with HIV.

449 HIV/AIDS Prevention Program
Centers for Disease Control and Prevention
1600 Clifton Road   404-639-3534
Atlanta, GA 30333   800-232-4636
                                               TTY: 888-232-6348
                                               cdcinfo@cdc.gov
                                               www.cdc.gov
An information awareness resource produced by the Division of
Adolescent and School Health. The database offers descriptions of
various educational resources for professionals relevant to the ed-
ucation of children and youth about HIV infection and AIDS.
Thomas R. Frieden, Director
Ileana Arias, Principal Deputy Director

450 Immunization Division Centers for Disease Control
1600 Clifton Road   404-639-3534
Atlanta, GA 30333-2303   800-232-4636
                                               TTY: 888-232-6348
                                               cdcinfo@cdc.gov
                                               www.cdc.gov
An information awareness resource produced by the Division of
Adolescent and School Health. The database offers descriptions of
various educational resources for professionals relevant to the ed-
ucation of children and youth about HIV infection and AIDS.
Thomas R. Frieden, Director
Ileana Arias, Principal Deputy Director

451 King County Crisis Clinic
9725 3rdAvenue NE   206-461-3210
Seattle, WA 98115   866-427-4747
                                               Fax: 206-461-8368
                                               TDD: 206-461-3219
                                               info@crisisclinic.org
                                               www.crisisclinic.org
A non-profit organization, we offer an array of support services
available to everyone in King County, Washington.
Kathleen Southwick, Executive Director
Susan Gemmel, Director

452 Minnesota AIDS Project AIDSLine
1400 Park Avenue   612-341-2060
Minneapolis, MN 55404   800-248-7321
                                               Fax: 612-341-4057
                                               TTY: 888-820-2437
                                               mapaidsline@mnaidsproject.org
                                               www.mnaidsproject.org
A statewide, toll-free information and referral service that can answer your questions about HIV and connect you to resources that
can help
Bill Tiedmann, Executive Director

453 National Health Information Center
Office of Disease Prevention & Health Promotion
1101 Wootton Pkwy   Fax: 240-453-8281
Rockville, MD 20852   odphpinfo@hhs.gov
                                               www.health.gov/nhic
Supports public health education by maintaining a calendar of National Health Observances; helps connect consumers and health
professionals to organizations that can best answer questions and
provide up-to-date contact information from reliable sources; updates on a yearly basis toll-free numbers for health information,
Federal health clearinghouses and info centers.
Don Wright, MD, MPH, Director

454 Project Inform Hiv Health InfoLine
273 Ninth Street   415-558-8669
San Francisco, CA 94103-2621   800-822-7422
                                               Fax: 415-558-0684
                                               web@projectinform.org
                                               www.projectinform.org
Runs an HIV Infoline, as well as a Hepatitis C helpline, while en-
gaging in advocacy on behalf of individuals living with
HIV/AIDS.
Ferdinand Garcia, President
Dana Van Gorder, Executive Director

Books

455 ABC of AIDS
Michael W. Adler, author
BMJ Publishing Group
PO Box 281   800-2FO-NBMJ
Annapolis, MD 20701-0281   Fax: 800-2FA-XBMJ
                                               bmjpg@pmds.com

118 pages Paperback
ISBN: 0-727915-03-7

456 AIDS & HIV Related Diseases
Harper Collins Publishers
195 Broadway   212-207-7000
New York, NY 10007   tmpcorrections@harpercollins.com
                                               www.harpercollins.com

An education guide for professionals and the public which covers such topics as: Understanding HIV and its effect on the immune system; HIV transmission; The history of AIDS and HIV; HIV testing; The natural course of an HIV infection; Medical treatment and those who administer them; The people who have AIDS; AIDS education.
1996 246 pages
ISBN: 0-306450-85-2

457 AIDS & Other Manifestations of HIV Infection
Academic Press (Elsevier)
1183 Westline Indus Drive   800-545-2522
St Louis, MO 63146   Fax: 800-535-9935
    usbkinfo@elsevier.com
    www.elsevier.com
An essential reference resource providing a comprehensive overview of the biological properties of this etiologic viral agent, its clinicopathological manifestations, the epidemiology of its infection, and present and future therapeutic options.
2004-4th Edi 1000 pages
ISBN: 0-127640-51-7
Gary Wormser, Editor

458 AIDS Alert
American Health Consultants
3525 Piedmont Road   404-262-5476
Atlanta, GA 30355   800-688-2421
    Fax: 800-284-3291
    www.ahcmedia.com
The definitive source of AIDS news and advice for health care professionals. Covers up-to-the-minute developments and guidance on the entire spectrum of AIDS challenges, including treatment, education, precaustion, screening, diagnosis and policy.

459 AIDS and HIV Related Diseases
Josh Powell, author
Plenum Publishing Corporation
233 Spring Street   212-620-8000
New York, NY 10013   800-221-9369
    Fax: 212-463-0742
    books@plenum.com
    www.springer.com
An education guide for professionals and the public which covers such topics as: Understanding HIV and its effect on the immune system; HIV transmission; The history of AIDS and HIV; HIV testing; The natural course of an HIV infection; Medical treatment and those who administer them; The people who have AIDS; AIDS education.
1996 243 pages
ISBN: 0-306450-85-2

460 AIDS and Persons with Developmental Disabilities
Commission on the Mentally Disabled
1800 M Street NW   202-331-2240
Washington, DC 20036
A discussion of federal and state laws that defines the rights and responsibilities of individuals with disabilities and service providers with respect to HIV infection.

461 AIDS in the Twenty-First Century: Disease and Globalization
Tony Barnett, Alan Whiteside, author
Palgrave Macmillan
175 Fifth Avenue   212-982-3900
New York, NY 10010   800-221-7945
    Fax: 212-777-6359
    authors@palgrave.com
    www.palgrave.com
Presents compelling data and research which reveals the shocking social and economic impact of HIV/AIDS on a global scale
432 pages
ISBN: 1-403900-05-0

462 AIDS, Revised Edition
Alan E. Nourse, M.D., author
Franklin Watts c/o Grolier

90 Old Sherman Tpke   203-797-3500
Danbury, CT 06816   800-621-1115
    Fax: 203-797-6986
    www.grolier.com
This bestselling book has been updated with the latest findings and research into the AIDS epidemic. Includes new statistical information and findings on HIV and AIDS.
144 pages
ISBN: 0-531106-62-4

463 AIDS: A Communication Perspective
Lawrence Erlbaum Associates Publishers
10 Industrial Avenue   201-236-9500
Mahwah, NJ 07430-2262   Fax: 201-236-6396
    www.erlbaum.com
ISBN: 0-805809-98-8

464 AIDS: Distinguishing Between Fact and Opinion
Teresa Opheim, author
Greenhaven Press
PO Box 9187   800-877-GALE
Farmington Hills, MI 48333-9187   Fax: 800-414-5043
    solutions.cengage.com/greenhaven/
For beginning debaters, reports and classroom use this book offers three debates: Can AIDS be spread by casual contact? Should the Food and Drug Administration make AIDS drugs more available? Is AIDS a moral issue?.
36 pages
ISBN: 0-899086-33-0

465 AIDS: How it Works in the Body
Lorna Greenberg, author
Franklin Watts
96 Leonard Street   www.wattspub.co.uk
London EC2A 4XD,
For readers ages 9-12
64 pages School Binding

466 AIDS: Trading Fears for Facts: A Guide for Young People
Karen Hein, Theresa Foy Digernimo, author
Consumer Reports Books
101 Truman Avenue   www.consumerreports.org
Yonkers, NY 10703-1057
Listed for young adult readers.
232 pages Paperback
ISBN: 0-890437-21-1

467 Amfar AIDS Handbook: The Complete Guide to Understanding HIV and AIDS
Darrell Ward, author
W.W. Norton & Company, Inc.
500 Fifth Avenue   212-354-5500
New York, NY 10110   Fax: 212-869-0856
    in.norton.com
Gives a greater understanding of HIV/Aids. The causes and effects, what new treatment options are being developed.
360 pages
ISBN: 0-393316-36-X

468 Black Death: AIDS in Africa
Susan Hunter, author
Macmillan
175 Fifth Avenue   646-307-5151
New York, NY 10010   us.macmillian.com
The untold story of AIDS in Africa, home to 80 percent of the 40 million people in the world currently infected with HIV. Brings the staggering statistics to life and paints for the first time a stunning picture of the most important political issue today.
256 pages
ISBN: 1-403967-17-2

469 Children and the AIDS Virus: A Book for Children, Parents, and Teachers
Rosmarie Hausherr, author
Clarion Books
For readers ages 4-8.
48 pages Library Binding
ISBN: 0-899198-34-1

470 Community Service Delivery for Children with HIV Infection and Families
Geneva, Woodruff & Christopher Hanson, author
South Shore Mental Health Center
500 Victory Road
Quincy, MA 02171
617-847-1950
800-852-2844
Fax: 617-786-9894
contactus@ssmh.org
www.ssmh.org
A manual providing guidelines for developing community-based, family-centered services for children with HIV infection and their families. Describes how services can be planned and delivered using guiding principles and practices of transagency case management.

471 Coping When You or a Friend is HIV-Positive
Pat Kelly, author
Hazelden Publishing & Educational Services
15251 Pleasant Valley Rd
Center City, MN 55012-0176
651-213-4200
800-328-9000
Fax: 651-213-4793
info@hazelden.org
www.hazelden.org
Provides compassionate counsel for teens who have been diagnosed with the virus.
136 pages Paperback
ISBN: 1-568381-77-8

472 Dancing Against the Darkness: A Journey Through America in the Age of AIDS
Steven Petrow, author
Rowman & Littlefield Publishing Group
4501 Forbes Blvd.
Lanham, MD 20706
301-459-3366
800-462-6420
Fax: 301-429-5748
custserv@rowman.com
www.lexingtonbooks.com
218 pages Hardcover
ISBN: 0-669243-09-4

473 Everything You Need to Know About AIDS
Katherine White, author
Rosen Publishing Group
29 E 21st Street
New York, NY 10010
212-777-3017
800-237-9932
Fax: 888-436-4643
customerservice@rosenpub.com
www.rosenpublishing.com
Without proper information, our teens remain at risk for AIDS. This volume presents balanced information on the disease and on safer sex precautions, in a language that readers can understand.
64 pages Library Binding
ISBN: 0-823933-14-8
Barbara Taylor, Author

474 Everything You Need to Know About Being HIV Positive
Amy Shire, author
Rosen Publishing Group
29 E 21st Street
New York, NY 10010
212-777-3017
800-237-9932
Fax: 888-436-4643
customerservice@rosenpub.com
www.rosenpublishing.com
To teens who need to understand what thier options are when living with HIV on a day-to-day basis. This book explains the facts about HIV.
Hardcover
ISBN: 0-823926-14-1
Amy Shire, Author

475 Everything You Need to Know When a Parent has AIDS
Barbara Hermie Draimin, author
Rosen Publishing Group
29 E 21st Street
New York, NY 10010
212-777-3017
800-237-9932
Fax: 888-436-4643
customerservice@rosenpub.com
www.rosenpublishing.com

More and more teens have a parent who has AIDS. Teens must learn where they can turn for help in dealing with this difficult situation. By presenting stories of teens in the same situation, this book helps readers deal with their anger and grief.
64 pages Library Binding
ISBN: 0-823916-90-1
Barbara Hermie Draimin DSW, Author

476 Global AIDS: Myths and Facts, Tools for Fighting the AIDS Pandemic
Alexander Irwin, Joyce Millen, author
South End Press
7 Brookline Street
Cambridge, MA 02139-4146
718-874-0089
info@southendpress.org
www.southendpress.org
10 myths about HIV/AIDS treatment and prevention while calling for an international movement to fight the disease.
296 pages
ISBN: 0-896086-73-9

477 Guide to Living With HIV Infection
John G. Bartlett, Ann K. Finkbeiner, author
John's Hopkins University Press
2715 N Charles Street
Baltimore, MD 21218-4363
410-516-6900
800-537-5487
Fax: 410-516-6968
webmaster@jhupress.jhu.edu
www.press.jhu.edu
The most complete source of medical, emotional, social, and practical advice available for those infected with HIV and their loved ones. Provides essential information for making decisions about treatment and testing in a world transformed by new research and pharmacotherapy.
1996 408 pages Paperback
ISBN: 0-801884-85-6

478 Invisible People: How the U.S. Has Slept Through the Global AIDS Pandemic
Greg Behrman, author
Free Press Publishing Co.
1010 W Cass St
Tampa, FL 33606-1307
813-254-5888
368 pages
ISBN: 0-743257-55-3

479 Living Well With HIV and AIDS
Allen L Gifford MD, Kate Loring RN, author
Bull Publishing Company
PO Box 1377
Boulder, CO 80306
303-545-6350
800-676-2855
Fax: 303-545-6354
www.bullpub.com
Offers the latest information based on the HIV care guidelines from the Department of Health & Human Services and the Center for Disease Control. Disscuses a shift in treatments emphasis to the ways of managing side effects such as lypodystrophy, redistribution of body fat, cardiac risks, and concerns with vulnerability to other ailments called comorbidities
2005 328 pages Papberback
ISBN: 0-923521-86-8

480 Living on the Edge
Michael Kelly, author
HarperCollins Canada Limited/Order Department
1995 Markham Road
Ontario, Canada M1 B 5M8,
800-387-0117
Fax: 800-668-5788
A gritty, honest, biographical account of one young man's experience from the original diagnosis via the development of the illness, how Michael has learned to live with his illness and how it has affected him and all his friends who support him.
160 pages
ISBN: 0-551027-49-5

481 Local AIDS Sercices: The National Directory
US Conference of Mayors
1620 I Street NW
Washington, DC 20006
202-293-7330
Fax: 202-293-2352
info@usmayors.org
www.usmayors.org

2,500 organizations that provide various information and services for AIDS coordinates and other health-related professionals.

482 Lynda Madaras Talks to Teens About AIDS
Lynda Madaras, author
Waterfront Books
98 Brookes Avenue   802-658-7477
Burlington, VT 05401   800-639-6063
www.waterfrontbooks.com
An informative book about the HIV virus and AIDS.
128 pages

483 Night Kites
M.E. Kerr, author
HarperCollins Children's Books
1350 Ave of the Americas   212-261-6500
New York, NY 10019
For young adults.
224 pages Paperback
ISBN: 0-064470-35-0

484 No Longer Immune: A Counselor's Guide to AIDS
American Counseling Association
6101 Stevenson Ave.   703-823-9800
Alexandria, VA 22304   800-347-6647
Fax: 703-823-0252
webmaster@counseling.org
www.counseling.org
Covers a broad range of issues such as working with specific populations, handling pre- and posttesting situations, coping with fear, grief and survivor guilt, preventing caregiver burnout and dealing with countertransference.
295 pages Paperback
ISBN: 1-556200-64-1

485 Parent Education Program-HIV/AIDS: A Challenge to Us All
Pediatric AIDS Foundation
1140 Connecticut Ave, NW   202-296-9165
Washington, DC 20036-3092 800-499-4673
Fax: 202-296-9185
www.pedaids.org
This parent meeting kit with a guide book and two videos will help any adult set up a parent meeting on the subject of AIDS. This kit provides accurate information to parents about HIV/AIDS, allows parents to voice concerns and fears, gives examples of appropriate answers to your child's questions about HIV/AIDS and replaces fear with knowledge and compassion.

486 Predicting AIDS and Other Epidemics
Christopher Lampton, author
Franklin Watts
96 Leonard Street   www.wattspub.co.uk
London EC2A 4XD,
144 pages S & L Binding

487 Scarlet Letters
AIDS Project Los Angeles
The David Geffen Center   213-201-1600
Los Angeles, CA 90005   info@apla.org
www.apla.org
A bilingual (Spanidh/English) journal targeted at HIV prevention providers in the U.S. The Scarlet Letters features opinion pieces and research-based essays by invited HIV/STD prevention experts.

488 Teen Guide to AIDS Prevention
Alan E. Nourse, author
Franklin Watts
96 Leonard Street   www.wattspub.co.uk
London EC2A 4XD,
For young adult readers.
61 pages S & L Binding

489 We Have AIDS
Elaine Landau, author
Franklin Watts
96 Leonard Street   www.wattspub.co.uk
London EC2A 4XD,

For young adult readers.
S & L Binding

490 What Is AIDS?
Anna Forbes, author
The Rosen Publishing Group
PowerKids Press   212-777-3017
New York, NY 10010   800-237-9932
Fax: 888-436-4643
customerservice@rosenpub.com
www.rosenpublishing.com
For reader levels ages 4-8.
1st Edition 24 pages Hardcover

491 Women & AIDS
Diane Richardson, author
Methuen
35 Hospital Fields Road   190-462-4730
York, YO10 4DZ,   Fax: 190-462-4733
www.methuen.co.uk
The first sourcebook to provide the information women need by identifying the most accurate sources and providing valuable statistical data.
183 pages Paperback
ISBN: 0-416017-51-7

492 Women and AIDS: A Practical Guide for Those Who Help Others
Continuum Publishing Corporation
370 Lexington Avenue   212-532-3650
New York, NY 10017-6503
Tailored to women, this book grapples with attitudes and realities of AIDS.

493 Women and Aids: Coping and Caring
Plenum Publishing Corportation
233 Spring Street   212-620-8000
New York, NY 10013-1522   800-221-9369
Fax: 212-463-0742
info@plenum.com
www.springer.com
1996 263 pages
ISBN: 0-306452-58-8
Ann O'Leary, Editor

494 You Have HIV: A Day at a Time
Lynn S. Baker, author
W.B. Saunders Company
www.elsevierhealth.com
258 pages paperback
ISBN: 0-721636-06-3

Children's Books

495 AIDS Overview Series
Lucent Books
Thomson Gale
Farmington Hills, MI 48333-9187   800-877-4253
Fax: 800-414-5043
gale.customerservice@thomson.com
www.gale.com/lucent
A straightforward account that teaches young adults all about the growing problem of AIDS.
1998 112 pages
ISBN: 1-560061-93-6

496 AIDS Awareness Library
Rosen Publishing Group
29 E 21st Street   800-237-9932
New York, NY 10010   Fax: 888-436-4643
customerservice@rosepub.com
www.rosenpublishing.com
For reader levels ages 4-8.
1996 24 pages
ISBN: 0-823974-06-1

497 AIDS To the Point: Confronting Youth Issues
Diana L. Hynson, author
Abingdon Press

201 8th Avenue S
Nashville, TN 37202-0801
615-749-6347
800-251-3320
Fax: 615-749-6577
www.abingdonpress.com
A resource that offers a practical means of talking with teens, individually or in a group, about AIDS. This volume offers teaching articles, ready-to-go programs for teens, leader's guides, worship resources, facts and figures, where to go for help and a section exclusively in Spanish. This is a volume in the To The Point: Confronting Youth Issues series of books.
96 pages Paperback
ISBN: 0-687782-20-1

498   AIDS: How it Works in the Body
Franklin Watts Grolier
90 Old Sherman Turnpike
Danbury, CT 06816-0001
203-797-3500
Fax: 203-797-6986
www.grolier.com
Focuses on the physiological effects AIDS has on the body, explains the causes of the disease, how the immune system works to defend the body and how the HIV virus affects the immune system.
64 pages Grades 5-7
ISBN: 0-531200-74-4

499   AIDS: Trading Fears for Facts a Guide for Teens
Consumer Reports Books
9180 La Saint Drive
Fairfield, OH 45014
914-378-2567
Fax: 914-378-2907
www.consumerreports.com
Written specifically for teenage readers and filled with illustrations, this book includes the current facts about AIDS, discusses how the virus is transmitted and precautions that should be taken.

500   AIDS: Trading Fears for Facts: A Guide for Young People
Consumer Reports Books
9180 La Saint Drive
Fairfield, OH 45014
914-378-2567
Fax: 914-378-2907
www.consumerreports.com
Written specifically for teenage readers and filled with illustrations, this book includes the current facts about AIDS, discusses how the virus is transmitted and precautions that should be taken.
1993
ISBN: 0-890432-62-4

501   Dancing Against the Darkness: A Journey Through America in the Age of AIDS
Heath Publishing
125 Spring Street
Lexington, MA 02421-7801
617-822-6650
A professional in the field, this author has chosen people across the nation to interview and use as examples for how the AIDS epidemic has struck America and what kind of lives it has affected.
Grades 7-12

502   Everything You Need to Know When a Parent Has AIDS
Barbara Hermie Draimin, DSW, author
Rosen Publishing Group
29 E. 21st Street
New York, NY 10010
212-777-3017
800-237-9932
Fax: 888-436-4643
www.rosenpublishing.com
For reader levels ages 4-8.
ISBN: 0-823916-90-1

503   Impact of AIDS
Franklin Watts Grolier
90 Old Sherman Turnpike
Danbury, CT 06816-0001
203-797-3500
800-621-1115
Fax: 203-797-6986
www.grolier.com
Examines the effects of the HIV infection and discusses the efforts in finding a cure for AIDS.
64 pages Grades 5-7
ISBN: 0-531172-25-2

504   Night Kites
Harper Collins
195 Broadway
New York, NY 10007
212-207-7000
tmpcorrections@harpercollins.com
www.harpercollins.com

This book focuses on two brothers, one of whom is homosexual and how they interact in the face of AIDS and the intolerance of homosexuality among the many people they know.
Grades 8-12

505   Our Immune System
Sara LeBien, author
Immune Deficiency Foundation
110 West Road
Towson, MD 21204-4841
410-321-6647
800-296-4433
Fax: 410-321-9165
idf@primaryimmune.org
www.primaryimmune.org
This storybook educates children about primary immunodeficiency diseases through delightful, eye-catching illustrations. The characters explain how the immune system works and describe the treatments for pediatric patients. Children will understand their own bodies and be better prepared to deal with their own primary immunodeficiency.   Available in English & Spanish.
Marcia Boyle, President & Founder
Christine Belser, Senior VP, Programs & Communications

506   Predicting AIDS and Other Epidemics
Franklin Watts Grolier
90 Old Sherman Turnpike
Danbury, CT 06816-0001
203-797-3500
800-621-1115
Fax: 203-797-6986
www.grolier.com
Surveys the efforts of scientists and researchers to predict the spread of epidemic diseases, including AIDS.
128 pages Grades 7-12
ISBN: 0-531107-85-0

507   Problem of AIDS
Franklin Watts Grolier
90 Old Sherman Turnpike
Danbury, CT 06816-0001
203-797-3500
800-621-1115
Fax: 203-797-6986
www.grolier.com
Part of the Let's Talk About series, this book addresses the questions and answers children and young adults have about AIDS.
32 pages Grades 3-5
ISBN: 0-531171-91-4

508   Teen Guide to AIDS Prevention
Franklin Watts Grolier
90 Old Sherman Turnpike
Danbury, CT 06816-0001
203-797-3500
800-621-1115
Fax: 203-797-6986
www.grolier.com
Directly addresses the questions and fears of teenagers by explaining clearly and simply what AIDS is, how it is spread, and the preventive measures young persons should take.
64 pages Grades 9-12
ISBN: 0-531109-66-6

509   We Have AIDS
Franklin Watts Grolier
90 Old Sherman Turnpike
Danbury, CT 06816-0001
203-797-3500
800-621-1115
Fax: 203-797-6986
www.grolier.com
This book goes beyond statistics and facts and focuses on the personal side of the disease. Offers source notes, a bibliography and an index.
128 pages
ISBN: 0-531108-98-8

510   What's a Virus, Anyway? The Kid's Book About AIDS
Waterfront Books
98 Brookes Avenue
Burlington, VT 05401-3326
802-658-7477
A simple introduction to help adults talk with children about the subject of AIDS.
67 pages

Magazines

511 AIDS Alert
American Health Consultants
3525 Piedmont Road   404-262-5476
Atlanta, GA 30355   800-688-2421
                                                Fax: 404-262-5560
                                                www.ahcmedia.com
Covers up-to-the-minute developments and guidance on the entire
spectrum of AIDS challenges, including treatment, education, precautions, screening, diagnosis and policy.

512 AIDS Clinical Care
New England Journal of Medicine
860 Winter Street   781-893-4610
Waltham, MA 02451-1413   800-322-2303
                                                Fax: 781-893-3800
                                                www.massmed.org
Up to date information specifically targeted at physicians with
AIDS patients.
Monthly

513 AIDS: A Year In Review
Lippincott Williams & Wilkins
16522 Hunters Green Pkwy   301-223-2300
Hagerstown, MD 21740   800-638-3030
                                                Fax: 301-223-2400
                                                orders@lww.com
                                                www.lww.com
An interdisciplinary journal providing a synthesis of AIDS-related
information from all relevant clinical and basic sciences.

514 AIDS: International Monthly Journal
Lippincott Williams & Wilkins
16522 Hunters Green Pkwy   301-223-2300
Hagerstown, MD 21740   800-638-3030
                                                Fax: 301-223-2400
                                                orders@lww.com
                                                www.lww.com
An interdisciplinary journal providing a synthesis of AIDS-related
information from all relevant clinical and basic sciences.

515 AIDS: The Disease State Management Resource
American Health Consultants
PO Box 550669   404-262-5476
Atlanta, GA 30355   800-688-2421
                                                Fax: 800-284-3291
                                                www.ahcmedia.com
Covers up-to-the-minute developments and guidance on the entire
spectrum of AIDS challenges, including treatment, education, pre-
cautions, screening, diagnosis and policy.

516 Critical Path AIDS Project
2062 Lombard Street   215-545-2212
Philadelphia, PA 19146-1315   www.critpath.org
Articles and reprints on experimental treatments and alternative
therapies, and a listing of Philadelphia-area resources.
Monthly

**517 Institute on Health Care for the Poor and Underserved at
Meharry Medical College**
Sage Publications
1005 DB Todd Boulevard   615-327-6819
Nashville, TN 37208   800-669-1269
                                                Fax: 615-327-6362
                                                vbrennan@mmc.edu
Offers health care and public health policy research focusing on
poor and underserved populations.
100pages 4x a year
Dr. Amy Cato, Director
Dr. Virginia Brennan, Editor

518 Journal of Acquired Immune Deficiency Syndrome
Lippincott Williams & Wilkins
16522 Hunters Green Pkwy   301-223-2300
Hagerstown, MD 21740-2601   800-638-3030
                                                Fax: 301-223-2400
                                                orders@lww.com
                                                www.lww.com

An interdisciplinary journal providing a synthesis of AIDS-related
information from all relevant clinical and basic sciences.
Monthly
ISBN: 0-894925-5 -
William A Hazeltine, Editor

519 Journal of the Medical Library Association
Medical Library Association
65 E Wacker Place   312-419-9094
Chicago, IL 60601-7246   Fax: 312-419-8950
                                                info@mlahq.org
An international, peer-reviewed journal that aims to advance the
practice and research knowledgebase of health science librarian-
ship.
Quarterly
Kevin Baliozian, Executive Director
Susan C.T. Talmage, Managing Editor, Publications

520 POZ Magazine
POZ Publishing
462 Seventh Avenue   212-242-2163
New York, NY 10018-7424   Fax: 212-675-8505
                                                www.poz.com
A magazine for people living with, and affected by, HIV/AIDS.
60 pages BiMonthly
Regan Hofmann, Editor in Chief
Jennifer Morton, Managing Editor

521 Risky Business
San Francisco AIDS Foundation Materials Dept.
333 Valencia Street   415-861-3397
San Francisco, CA 94103-3547
A comic book style magazine providing accurate information
about AIDS using humor and real-life situations. Contains stories
that stress the importance of knowing how AIDS is transmitted and
prevented.

522 Straight Talk: A Magazine for Teens About AIDS
Custom Publishing Division of Rodale Press
33 E Minor Street   610-967-5171
Emmaus, PA 18098-0001
A lively magazine that includes articles about teens with AIDS,
teens involved in peer education and teens at risk for getting infected. Good information is presented in an interesting format for
young adults.

523 Washington Update
Committee of Ten Thousand
500 Belmont Street   508-587-2512
Brockton, MA 02301   cott-dc@earthlink.net
                                                www.cott1.org
Is a primer on government related issues of importance to COTT's
constituency. From health care legislation, to regulatory affairs to
Administration policy for chronic diseases. A hands-on journal for
grass roots health care advocacy in our Nation's capital.
Bi-Monthly
John Rider, Contact

Newsletters

524 AIDS Alert
American Health Consulants
3525 Piedmont Road   404-262-5476
Atlanta, GA 30355   800-688-2421
                                                Fax: 404-262-5560
                                                www.ahcmedia.com
Covers up-to-the-minute developments and guidance on the entire
spectrum of AIDS challenges, including treatment, education, precautions, screening, diagnosis and policy.

525 AIDS Link
University of Cincinnati-Medical Center Info.
231 Bethesda Avenue   513-558-5661
Cincinnati, OH 45267-0001   Fax: 513-558-3136
                                                medcenter.uc.edu/
Aimed at healthcare professionals working with HIV/AIDS in-
flicted patients.
Rebecca Atterrin, Editor

526 AIDS News
Northern California Chapter of the NHF
7700 Edgewater Drive   510-568-6243
Oakland, CA 94621-3023
Provides current information for people who need to cope mentally and physically with the issues of virus infection and transmission. Provides answers to questions about AIDS, ARC, HIV infection and transmission prevention.
BiMonthly

527 AIDS Policy and Law
LRP Publications
747 Dresher Road   www.lrp.com
Horsham, PA 19044-0980
A report on AIDS policy and law developments from the courts, NIH, federal and state AIDS agencies and advocacy organizations.
24 year

528 AIDS Treatment Data Network
611 Broadway   212-260-8868
New York, NY 10012   800-734-7104
                                          Fax: 212-260-8869
                                          www.atdn.org
Information bulletins covering new treatments, clinical trials, and more.

529 AIDS Treatment News
ATN Publications
PO Box 411256   800-873-2812
San Francisco, CA 94141-1256   www.atnonline.org
Reports on the developments in treatments for HIV disease and related infections. Also covers issues relating to research.
BiMonthly

530 AIDS Update
Dallas Gay Alliance
PO Box 190812   214-528-4233
Dallas, TX 75219-0812   Fax: 214-521-6424
                                          www.divanet.com/dgla/
Includes general information on AIDS issues and treatments.

531 AIDS Weekly Plus
Charles Henderson
Po Box 5528   info@hendersonnet.atl.ga.us
Atlanta, GA 31107-0528
All aspects of AIDS epidemic coverage, including research, treatments, vaccine development, political and public policy.
46 year

532 AIDS/STD News Report
CD Publications
2222 Sedwick Drive   301-588-6380
Durham, NC 27713   800-666-6380
                                          Fax: 301-588-6385
                                          info@cdpublications.com
                                          www.cdpublications.com
Formerly AIDS News Alert, provides grant listings from federal, private, and corporate sources; proposal writing tips; updates on successful programs, and the latest news on AIDS/STD federal/state legislation, research, and successful programs.

533 APICHA News
Asian & Pacific Islander Coalition on HIV/AIDS
400 Broadway   212-334-7940
New York, NY 10013   866-274-2429
                                          Fax: 212-334-7956
                                          apicha@apicha.org
                                          www.apicha.org
Provides information on prevention education, client services and advocacy for Asians and Pacific Islanders.
Quarterly
Therese R Rodriguez, CEO

534 APLA Update
AIDS Project Los Angeles
3550 Wilshire Boulevard   213-201-1600
Los Angeles, CA 90010   www.apla.org
Presents news about AIDS and programs of AIDS Project Los Angeles to people affected by the disease.
20 pages

535 BETA
San Francisco AIDS Foundation
1035 Market Street   415-487-3000
San Francisco, CA 94103   feedback@sfaf.org
                                          www.sfaf.org
Medical information.
Quarterly

536 Being Alive
Being Alive People with HIV/AIDS Action Coalition
7531 Santa Monica Blvd   323-874-4322
West Hollywood, CA 90046   Fax: 323-969-8753
                                          info@beingalivela.org
                                          www.beingalivela.org
Medical updates, plus information on AIDS advocacy, a calendar of local events and listings of AIDS support groups.

537 Being Alive Newsletter
Being Alive-People with HIV/AIDS Action Coalition
7531 Santa Monica Blvd   323-874-4322
West Hollywood, CA 90040   Fax: 323-969-8753
                                          kevin@beingalivela.org
                                          www.beingalivela.org
A regularly-published source of information and education for our peers living with HIV/AIDS and for the greater community. Standing articles cover timely issues such as HIV/AIDS treatment options, mental health, substance abuse, nutrition, advocacy, community referrals, and a variety of other topics. Additionally, we feature information on Being Alive events alongside other relevant community events.
Quarterly
Kevin Kurth, Executive Director/Editor

538 CORPUS
AIDS Project Los Angeles
The David Geffen Center   213-201-1600
Los Angeles, CA 90005   www.apla.org
A journal that uses art, cultural criticism, poetry, short stories and humor to reveal the challenges of HIV prevention in gay and bisexual communities.
Annually
Craig E Thompson, Executive Director

539 COTT News
Committee on Ten Thousand
500 Belmont Street   508-587-2512
Brockton, MA 02301   www.cott1.org
A range of information, reportage and viewpoints regarding issues and events of importance to grass roots health care advocacy and support.
John Rider, Contact

540 Center for AIDS Prevention Studies
AIDS Research Institute
550 16th Street   415-476-6288
San Francisco, CA 94158   Fax: 415-597-9213
                                          capsweb@psg.ucsf.edu
                                          www.caps.ucsf.edu
Local, national, and international interdisciplinary research.

541 Clinical Focus on Primary Immune Deficiency Diseases
Immune Deficiency Foundation
110 West Rd, Ste 300   410-321-6647
Towson, MD 21204   800-296-4433
                                          Fax: 410-321-9165
                                          info@primaryimmune.org
                                          primaryimmune.org
Educational monograph is designed specifically for health care professionals and focuses on topics relevant to primary immune deficiency diseases.
Marcia Boyle, President & Founder
Christine Belser, Senior VP, Programs & Communications

542 Community Health Funding Report
CD Publications
2222 Sedwick Drive   301-588-6380
Durham, NC 27713-4571   800-666-6380
                                          Fax: 301-588-6385
                                          info@cdpublications.com
                                          www.cdpublications.com

Covers grants for AIDS and sexually transmitted disease related programs from federal and private sources. Includes news on national and local issues affecting AIDS and STD's and case studies of successful fundraising programs. This biweekly newsletter describes changes in funding streams for community based health programs, including AIDS programs. It lists available federal and private grant opportunities, along with Washington News Medicare/Medicaid.
18 pages BiMonthly
Mike Gerecht, Publisher
Amy Bernstein, Editor

543   Cott Washington Update
Committee of Ten Thousand
236 Massachusetts Ave NE   202-543-0988
Washington, DC 20002-4971   800-488-2688
                                        Fax: 202-543-6720
                                        www.cott1.org
Offers legislative updates, information on clinical trials, therapies, book reviews, business and politics, a readers forum and resources pertaining to HIV/AIDS.
10 pages Monthly
Corey Dubin, President
Dave Cavenaugh, Government Relations

544   FOCUS
UCSF AIDS Health Project
1930 Market Street   415-476-3902
San Francisco, CA 94102   TTY: 415-476-3587
                                        ahpinfo@ucsf.edu
                                        www.ucsf-ahp.org
Reviews the counseling aspects of AIDS: how HIV-related counseling is affected by the medical, epidemiological, and social realities of AIDS, as well as the emotional response to the disease. It is written for mental health and health care providers working on the front lines and is of interest to researchers, policy makers, and program administrators.
10x/year
James W Dilley MD, Executive Director

545   Gay Men's Health Crisis
119 West 24th Street   212-367-1000
New York, NY 10011   www.gmhc.org
Not-for-profit, voluteer-supported and community-based organization committed to national leadership in the fight against AIDS.

546   HIV Counselor PERSPECTIVES
UCSF AIDS Health Project
1930 Market Street   415-476-3902
San Francisco, CA 94102   TTY: 415-476-3587
                                        ahpinfo@ucsf.edu
                                        www.ucsf-ahp.org
An educational resource for HIV antibody test counselors, prevention case managers, and other health and mental health professionals, particularly those working in brief counseling venues.
4 year
James W Dilley MD, Executive Director

547   HIV Frontline
Center for AIDS Prevention Studies
University of California   415-476-6288
San Francisco, CA 94158   Fax: 415-597-9213
                                        CAPSweb@psg.ucsf.edu
                                        www.caps.ucsf.edu
Monthly newsletter aimed at mental health and healthcare professionals who counsel people living with HIV/AIDS.
Monthly
Dr. Leon McKusick

548   IDF Advocate
Immune Deficiency Foundation
110 West Road   800-296-4433
Towson, MD 21204   idf@primaryimmune.org
                                        www.primaryimmune.org
Mailed to patients, family members, physicians, nurses, industry, government and interested individuals.
3x/year
Marcia Boyle, President/Founder

549   Immune Deficiency Foundation Newsletter
Immune Deficiency Foundation
110 West Road   410-321-6647
Towson, MD 21204-4841   800-296-4433
                                        Fax: 410-321-9165
                                        idf@primaryimmune.org
                                        www.primaryimmune.org
Offers medical updates and technology news on the latest services, products and treatments for persons with immune diseases.
Tamara Brown, Medical Programs Manager

550   In Focus
Project Inform
273 Ninth Street   415-558-8669
San Francisco, CA 94103-2461   877-435-7443
                                        Fax: 415-558-0684
                                        web@projectinform.org
                                        www.projectinform.org
The organizational newsletter of Project Inform.
20+ pages 3x/year
Skip Emerson, Executive Assistant

551   Just Kids
3 Corners
5th Avenue   212-634-4879
New York, NY 10014
Covers medical and social issues faced by HIV-positive children, teens and their parents.
Annual

552   MLA News
Medical Library Association
65 East Wacker Place   312-419-9094
Chicago, IL 60601-7246   Fax: 312-419-8950
                                        www.mlanet.org
Keeps you at the forefront of association matters and the profession as a whole. Regular departments include calendar, continuing education, employment opportunities, international news, Internet resources, personals, professional development, and technology. Columns include consumer health, expert searching, hospital librarianship, leadership and management, and new members. Members only.
Jean P Shipman, President

553   NMAC Update
National Minority AIDS Council
1931 13th Street, NW   202-483-6622
Washington, DC 20009-4389   Fax: 202-483-1135
                                        www.nmac.org
A newsletter reporting on public policy issues and information on subjects in organizational management.
BiMonthly

554   OUTReach
The San Francisco AID Foundation
1035 Market Street   415-487-3000
San Francisco, CA 94103   Fax: 415-487-8009
                                        TDD: 415-487-8099
                                        feedback@sfaf.org
                                        www.sfaf.org
Features concise articles on a wide range of HIV/AIDS topics.

555   PAACNOTES
101 W Grand Avenue   312-222-1326
Chicago, IL 60610-4272   800-243-3059
A news journal of the Physicians Coalition for AIDS Care featuring articles on clinical management, scientific research and a diverse range of legal, ethical and economic issues directly affecting the care of persons with HIV disease.

556   PWA Rag
Prisoners With AIDS Rights Advocacy Group
1626 Wilcox Avenue   770-946-9346
Loa Angeles, CA 90028   RAGNEWS@aol.com
Contains articles, treatment updates, and resources for prisoners.

557   Positive Living
APLA

3550 Wilshire Boulevard 213-201-1600
Los Angeles, CA 90010 800-922-2438
Monthly

558 Positive Outlook
2655 Swann Avenue 813-877-5696
Tampa, FL 33609
Focuses on local people and issues in West Central Florida.
Quarterly

559 Positive Social Support Newsletter
Lambda Center
4228 Wisconsin Avenue NW 202-965-8434
Washington, DC 20016 877-252-6232
Sponsored by and for people with HIV.

560 Positive Voice Newsletter
National Association of People with AIDS (NAPWA)
8401 Colesville Road 240-247-0880
Silverspring, MD 20910 866-846-9366
Fax: 240-247-0574
Frank J Oldham Jr, President/CEO
Peter Kronenberg, VP Communications/Editor

561 Positive Woman
PO Box 34372 202-898-0372
Washington, DC 20043-4372
Provides medical information, including alternative and holistic therapies for HIV-positive women.
BiMonthly

562 Positively Aware
Test Positive Aware Network
5537 N Broadway Street 773-989-9400
Chicago, IL 60640-1405 Fax: 773-989-9494
publications@tpan.com
www.positivelyaware.com
An internationally known and respected magazine devoted to HIV treatment, wellness, and optimum quality of life for those living with HIV, as well as those who care for them.
Bi-monthly
Jeff Berry, Publications Director

563 RAP* Time
Rural Center for AIDS/STD Prevention
Indiana University 812-855-7974
Bloomington, IN 47405-3085 800-566-8644
Fax: 812-855-3936
aids@indiana.edu
www.indiana.edu/~aids/
Summarizes current research concerning HIV/STD prevention, particularly in rural settings.
William L Yarber HSD, Senior Director

564 STEP Perspective
Seattle Treatment Exchange Project
750 3rd Avenue 206-329-4857
New York, NY 10017-5711 800-869-7837
www.thebody.com
Updates on treatments for HIV and related diseases condensed from journals, conferences and databases by the scientific review committee.

565 Seasons
National Native American AIDS Prevention Center
1031 33rd Street 510-444-2051
Denver, CO 80205-2011 Fax: 510-444-1593
Features articles and artwork by Native Americans impacted by HIV/AIDS.
Quarterly

566 Treatment Issues
Dep of Medical Info 212-337-1950
New York, NY 10011-3601
The gay men's health crisis newsletter of experimental AIDS therapies.
10x Year

567 Up Front Drug Information
5701 Biscayne Boulevard 305-757-2566
Miami, FL 33137-2601

Provides information on drugs and drug referrals.

568 Walk Talk
AIDS Coalition Silicon Valley
Walk For AIDS Silicon Vly 408-451-WALK
San Jose, CA 95154 Fax: 408-248-7423
The AIDS Coalition Silicon Valley Newsletter highlighting Walk for AIDS Silicon Valley fundraising events, issues and articles about HIV/AIDS service providers in the County.

569 Wisconsin AIDS Update
Wisconsin AIDS/HIV Program, Department of Health
1 West Wilson Street 608-266-1865
Madison, WI 50703-0309 888-701-1251
www.dhs.wisconsin.gov
Includes epidemiological and clinical care articles, selections from the most important current abstracts in ATIN and a statewide list of events and resources.
Quarterly

570 World/Mundo
PO Box 11535 415-658-6930
Oakland, CA 94611-0535
Contains letters, advice, events calendar, and information on support groups in Northern California.

Pamphlets

571 AIDS Medicines in Development
Pharmaceutical Research & Manufacturers of America
950 F Street NW 202-835-3400
Washington, DC 20004 Fax: 202-835-3414
www.phrma.org
An annual chart of antivirals, as well as information on diagnostics and vaccines.

572 AIDS and Hemophilia: Protecting Yourself and Others
Hemophilia Council of California: Bay Area Office
7700 Edgewater Drive 510-568-7074
Oakland, CA 94621 Fax: 510-568-2048
hccoak@aol.com
Lori Drake, Mental Health Counselor/Health Educator

573 AIDS, the Law & You
AIDS Action Committee
75 Amory Street 617-437-6200
Boston, MA 02119-5145 800-424-2634
Fax: 617-437-6445
webmaster@aac.org
www.aac.org
Discusses legal protection against AIDS-related discrimination, HIV testing and the law.

574 Americans with Disabilities Act: What it Means for People with AIDS
American Civil Liberties Union AIDS Project
125 Broad Street 212-549-2500
New York, NY 10004-6503 www.aclu.org

575 Basics of HIV Disease: Questions and Answers
National Hemophilia Foundation
7 Penn Plaza 212-328-3700
New York, NY 10001-3212 800-424-2634
Fax: 212-328-3777
handi@hemophilia.org
www.hemophilia.org
This publication contains basic information about hemophilia and HIV disease.
1992 28 pages
Alan Kinniburgh, PhD, CEO

576 Be Smart About HIV
American Red Cross
8550 Arlington Blvd. 703-584-8400
Fairfax, VA 22031-3100 Fax: 703-312-8738
www.redcross.org
This brochure offers very simple and informative information on the HIV virus, in both English and Spanish.
1996
Sandra L Mertz, Product Manager

577   Children with AIDS: Guidelines for Parents and Caregivers
AIDS Task Force of Central New York
627 W Genesee Street   315-415-2430
Syracuse, NY 13204-2347
Offers general information on AIDS, diet and feeding, household
chores, and coping with the illness.

578   Clinical Focus
Immune Deficiency Foundation
110 West Road   410-321-6647
Towson, MD 21204-4841   800-296-4433
                                             Fax: 410-321-9165
                                         info@primaryimmune.org
                                           www.primaryimmune.org
Biannual publication for medical professionals covering current
issues and information regarding clinical approaches to primary
immune deficiencies.
BiAnnual
Marcia Boyle, Founder/Chair

579   Clinical Focus on Primary Immune Deficiency Diseases
Immune Deficiency Foundation
110 West Rd   410-321-6647
Towson, MD 21204-4841   800-296-4433
                                             Fax: 410-321-9165
                                         info@primaryimmune.org
                                             primaryimmune.org
educational mongraph is designed specifically for health care professionals and focuses on topics relevant to primary immune deficiency diseases.
Marcia Boyle, Founder/Chair
Christine Belser, Senior VP, Programs & Communications

580   Clinical Presentation of the Primary Immunodeficiency Diseases
Immune Deficiency Foundation
110 West Road   410-321-6647
Towson, MD 21204-4841   800-296-4433
                                             Fax: 410-321-9165
                                         info@primaryimmune.org
                                           www.primaryimmune.org
A primer for physicians.
Tamara Brown, Medical Programs Manager

581   Clinical Trials: Talking it Over
NIAID, Office of Communications
200 Independence Avn, SW   301-496-5717
Washington, DC 20201-0001   877-696-6775
                                                   www.hhs.gov
Educational pamphlet pertaining to clinical trials.
Sylvia M. Burwell, HHS Secretary
Mary K. Wakefield, HHS Acting Deputy Secretary

582   Condoms and Sexually Transmitted Diseases, Especially AIDS
Department of Health and Human Services
Nat Institutes of Health   202-673-7700
Bethesda, MD 20892-0001
Offers information on condoms and how various forms of protec-
tion can be used to prevent sexually transmitted diseases, espe-
cially HIV/AIDS.

583   Eating Defensively: Food Safety Advice for Persons with AIDS
AIDSinfo
PO Box 4780   301-315-2816
Rockville, MD 20849-6303   800-448-0440
                                             Fax: 301-315-2818
                                            TTY: 888-480-3739
                                       ContactUs@aidsinfo.nih.gov
                                           www.aidsinfo.nih.gov
The food safety advice in this brochure is intended to help persons
with HIV infection to reduce the risk of food poisoning, thereby
avoiding an illness that could worsen their condition or even cause
death.
1992

584   HIV Infection and AIDS
NAID Office of Communications
31 Center Drive   301-496-1653
Bethesda, MD 20892-0001   Fax: 301-402-0779
                                       bettends@ficod.fic.nih.gov
                                            www.grants.nih.gov

Offers information on transmission, treatment, early symptoms,
diagnosis, prevention and research.

585   HIV and AIDS During Pregnancy
March of Dimes
233 Park Avenue South   212-353-8353
New York, NY 10003   Fax: 212-254-3518
                                       NY639@marchofdimes.com

586   HIV/AIDS in the Workplace
New York Business Group on Health
386 Park Avenue S   212-252-7440
New York, NY 10016-8804
Offers information on federal law and state law regarding
HIV/AIDS in the workplace, universal risks, health insurance and
other business costs.

587   Hope for Children with AIDS
Pediatric AIDS Foundation
16130 Ventura Blvd.   818-338-6361
Los Angeles, CA 91436-3092   888-499-4673
                                             Fax: 818-906-6951
                                              info@pedaids.org
                                                www.pedaids.org
A brochure offering information on the latest research and ad-
vances in the area of pediatric AIDS.

588   How to Keep an Infusion Log
Immune Deficiency Foundation
110 West Road   800-296-4433
Towson, MD 21204   info@primaryimmune.org
                                           www.primaryimmune.org
This brochure explains the value of keeping an immune globulin
infusion log, as well as practical information on how to set up your
personal records.
Marci Boyle, President/Founder

**589   IDF Guide for Nurses on Immune Globulin Therapy for Primary
Immunodeficiency**
Immune Deficiency Foundation
110 West Road   800-296-4433
Towson, MD 21204   info@primaryimmune.org
                                           www.primaryimmune.org
This guide provides direction for nurses to administer immune
globulin replacement therapy in the safest and most effective way.
Information includes: clinical uses for immune globulin replacement therapy; product selection and characteristics; infusions,
complications and adverse events of IVIG and SCIG; concomitant
medications; nursing interventions and responsibilities and
helpful references and resources.
Marcia Boyle, President/Founder

590   IDF Patient and Family Handbook
Immune Deficiency Foundation
110 West Road   800-296-4433
Towson, MD 21204   info@primaryimmune.org
                                           www.primaryimmune.org
For patients and family members, contains information about the
diagnosis and treatment of primary immunodeficiency diseases,
the immune system, specific diseases, therapies, general care,
health insurance and issues specific to adult, adolescent and
pediatric patients.
R Michael Blaese MD, Editor
E. Richard Stiehm MD, Editor

591   Immune Deficiency Foundation
110 West Road   800-296-4433
Towson, MD 21204   info@primaryimmune.org
                                           www.primaryimmune.org
Your partner for living with primary immune deficiency diseases.
This brochure describes the IDF and its activities and services.

592   Infections Linked to AIDS
NAID Office of Communications
31 Center Drive   301-496-5717
Bethesda, MD 20892-0001   www.hhs.gov
Offers information on infections related to HIV/AIDS and referral
numbers of where to receive help.

593 Our Immune System
Sara LeBien, author
Immune Deficiency Foundation
110 West Road   410-321-6647
Towson, MD 21204-4841   800-296-4433
                                                            Fax: 410-321-9165
                                                            info@primaryimmune.org
                                                            www.primaryimmune.org
This storybook educates children about primary immunodefi-ciency diseases through delightful, eye-catching illustrations. The characters explain how the immune system works and describe the treatments for pediatric patients. Children will understand their own bodies and be better prepared to deal with their own primary immunodeficiency.
Marcia Boyle, President & Founder
Christine Belser, Senior VP, Programs & Communications

594 Taking the HIV (AIDS) Test: How to Help Yourself
NAID Office of Communications
31 Center Drive   301-496-5717
Bethesda, MD 20892-0001
Offers information on the AIDS test, how it works, how it can help and should it be taken.

595 Teeens, Sexually Transmitted Diseases & HIV/AIDS
4 Brighton Road   info@avert.org
West Sussex, RH13 5BA UK,   www.avert.org
Designed for teens, and contains information on what STD's are, how to avoid becoming infected, safer sex, how to spot symptoms of STD's, STD treatment, information about HIV/AIDS, informa-tion about testing and treatment, and advice helplines.

596 Testing Positive for HIV
NAID Office of Communications
31 Center Drive   301-496-5717
Bethesda, MD 20892-0001
Information on what a positive HIV test means, how not to spread the disease to others, and various health and dieting tips.

597 Testing for HIV Infection
American Red Cross
1616 Fort Myer Drive   703-312-8724
Arlington, VA 22209-3100   Fax: 703-312-8738
1996
Sandra L Mertz, Product Manager

598 Women, Sex, and HIV
American Red Cross
1616 Fort Myer Drive   703-312-8724
Arlington, VA 22209-3100   Fax: 703-312-8738
1992
Sandra L Mertz, Product Manager

599 Your Job and HIV: Are There Risks?
American Red Cross
1616 Fort Myer Drive   703-312-8724
Arlington, VA 22209-3100   Fax: 703-312-8738
1992
Sandra L Mertz, Product Manager

Audio & Video

600 AIDS Work: Six Healthcare Workers Face the AIDS Crisis
Fanlight Productions
32 Court Street   718-488-8900
Brooklyn, NY 11201   800-876-1710
                                                            Fax: 718-488-8642
                                                            info@fanlight.com
                                                            www.fanlight.com
Two physicians and four nurses reflect on several decades of com-bined experiences in caring for patients with HIV/AIDS. They dis-cuss facing fear, frustration, burnout and grief as they struggle to deliver compassionate care, as well as the rewards of caring for this population. This inspirational program is invaluable for stress management programs, and in preparing students and new workers for the realities they will face.
VHS
ISBN: 1-572952-20-2
Steve Guy, Producer

601 Does Anyone Die of AIDS Anymore?
Louise Hogarth, author
Fanlight Productions
32 Court Street   718-488-8900
Brooklyn, NY 11201   800-876-1710
                                                            Fax: 718-488-8642
                                                            info@fanlight.com
                                                            www.fanlight.com
The answer to this disturbing film's title question is a resounding yes! Despite the much-hyped advances in treatment which, for some patients, have transformed HIV from a death sentence to a chronic illness, tens of thousands of people are still dying of AIDS in the United States. And tens of thousands more will die, even in this rich and medically advanced nation, because of ignorance and denial which have resulted in a 'third wave' of HIV infection.
26 Minutes
ISBN: 1-572958-48-0
Gregory A. Freeman, Author
Louise Hogarth, Producer

602 Roger's Story: For Cori
Howard Shepps, author
Fanlight Productions
32 Court Street   718-488-8900
Brooklyn, NY 11201   800-876-1710
                                                            Fax: 718-488-8642
                                                            info@fanlight.com
                                                            www.fanlight.com
Forty-four year-old Roger shares the harrowing story of his 20-year struggle against heroin, and his recent diagnosis with AIDS.
1989 28 Minutes
ISBN: 1-572950-47-1

603 Too Little, Too Late
Micki Dickoff, author
Fanlight Productions
32 Court Street   718-488-8900
Brooklyn, NY 11201   800-876-1710
                                                            Fax: 718-488-8642
                                                            info@fanlight.com
                                                            www.fanlight.com
In this moving video, family members of people with AIDS share their pain and frustration, as well as the solace they have derived from having been able to help their loved one to a peaceful death.
1987 49 Minutes
ISBN: 1-572950-27-7

604 Undetectable: The New Face of AIDS
Jay Corcoran, author
Fanlight Productions
32 Court Street   718-488-8900
Brooklyn, NY 11201   800-876-1710
                                                            Fax: 718-488-8642
                                                            info@fanlight.com
                                                            www.fanlight.com
This gripping documentary follows six women and men, straight and gay, of different ethnic and cultural backgrounds, over a three-year period as they deal for the first time with hope. Though the new multi-drug therapies for HIV disease offer a possible re-prieve from what was once a death sentence, those who are lucky enough to respond to the drugs nonetheless face both a grueling treatment regimen, and the complex physical and psychological challenges of rebuilding their lives.
2001 56 Minutes
ISBN: 1-572958-45-6

Web Sites

605 AIDS Education and Training Center National Multicultural Center
                                                            www.aetcnmc.org
Located at Howard University College of Medicine, AETC-NMC acted as an HIV/AIDS training and technical resource for provid-ers of minority HIV-infected patients throughout the country. It functioned as the training arm of the Ryan White HIV/AIDS Pro-

gram. Funding ceased in 2014, but the Center maintains its website as an archive of information.

606 AIDS United
www.aidsunited.org
To end the AIDS epidemic in the United States. We will achieve this goal through national, regional and local policy/advocacy, strategic grantmaking, and organizational capacity building. With partners throughout the country, we will work to ensure that people living with and affected by HIV/AIDS have access to the prevention and care services they need and deserve.

607 AIDS.ORG
www.aids.org
The mission of AIDS.ORG is to help prevent HIV infections and to improve the lives of those affected by HIV and AIDS by providing education and facilitating the free and open exchange of knowledge at any easy-to-find centralized website.

608 AIDSVu
aidsvu.org
Interactive maps of the AIDS epidemic across the states, including downloadable data sets and a services directory.

609 Children Affected by AIDS Foundation
keepachildalive.org
There mission is to realize the end of AIDS for children and families, by combating the physical, social and economic impacts of HIV.

610 Committee of Ten Thousand
www.cott1.org
Represents people with hemophilia who contracted HIV/AIDS and Hepatitis C from tainted factory concentrates in the 1970s and 1980s. The only national advocacy, and support agency for this seriously disabled community. Website includes a digital archive of photos, gatherings, and events.
Carl Weixler, President
Ray Dattoli, Vice President

611 HIV/Hepatitis C in Prison (HIP) Committee
www.prisons.org/hivin.htm
Fighting for consistent access to quality medical care including access to all new HIV and Hepatitis C medications, diagnostic testing and combination therapies.

612 Healing Well
www.healingwell.com
A social network and support community for patients, caregivers, and families coping with the daily struggles of diseases, disorders and chronic illness.

613 Health Finder
www.healthfinder.gov
Searchable, carefully developed web site offering information on over 1000 topics. Developed by the US Department of Health and Human Services, the site can be used in both English and Spanish.

614 Healthlink USA
www.healthlinkusa.com

Health information concerning treatment, cures, prevention, diagnosis, risk factors, research, support groups, email lists, personal stories and much more. Updated regularly.

615 Hiv.gov
www.hiv.gov
Online portal for HIV/AIDS-related resources, managed by the U.S. Department of Health & Human Services and supported by the Secretary's Minority AIDS Initiative Fund (SMAIF).

616 Immune Deficiency Foundation
www.primaryimmune.org
The national patient organization dedicated to improving the diagnosis, treatment and quality of life of persons with primary immunodeficiency diseases through advocacy, education and research.

617 MedicineNet
www.medicinenet.com
An online resource for consumers providing easy-to-read, authoritative medical and health information.

618 Medscape
www.medscape.com
Medscape offers specialists, primary care physicians, and other health professionals the Web's most robust and integrated medical information and educational tools.

619 National AIDS Information Clearinghouse
www.cdc.gov
Provides information and materials for employers on national, state and local resources related to HIV/AIDS in the workplace.

620 National Hospice & Palliative Care Organization (NHPCO)
www.nhpco.org
The organization seeks to improve end-of-life care, widen access to hospice care, and improve quality of life for the dying and their loved ones. NHPCO's website offers information on regulations, advocacy, quality and performance, education, and a variety of other resources.

621 People with AIDS Health Group
www.Aidsinfonyc.org
PWA is a non-profit buyers club organized to assist people with AIDS in obtaining medications — as well as provide support groups committed to the self-empowerment of people living with AIDS. They offer three programs: Treatment Education and Support, Advocacy and Public Policy, and Early Treatment Access.

622 Smart & Strong
www.smartstrong.com
A healthcare education company that supports providers and empowers HIV positive patients through publications, seminars and innovative educational programs.

623 WebMD
www.webmd.com
Provides credible information, supportive communities, and in-depth reference material about health subjects. A source for original and timely health information as well as material from well known content providers.

Description

624 # Allergies

Allergy means altered reactivity. Allergies are usually characterized by a hypersensitivity to substances, such as pollens, pet dander, certain foods, some medications and molds. Such substances (allergens) can trigger an allergic response in susceptible individuals. Symptoms of allergies may present in a wide spectrum ranging from the mild sneezing, runny nose and congestion of hay fever to life-threatening reactions, known as anaphylaxis. Additional allergic reactions include itchy, watery eyes, skin rashes and asthma. More severe symptoms may include a tingling sensation in the mouth, swelling of the tongue and throat, difficulty breathing, hives, vomiting abdominal cramps, diarrhea, drop in blood pressure, loss of consciousness, and cardiovascular collapse leading to death. Allergic symptoms typically appear within minutes to two hours after the person has been exposed to the allergen.

Approximately 35 million people suffer from allergies in the United States. The cause of allergies is unclear, although there may be a genetic link in some people. Treatment for allergies depends upon the specific substance, beginning with avoidance. Strict avoidance of the allergy-causing food is the only way to avoid a food allergy reaction. There are no medications that cure food allergies. Most people outgrow their food allergies, although peanuts, nuts, fish and shellfish are often considered life-long allergies.

For non-food allergies, medications such as antihistamines and inhaled bronchodilators and steroids, oral leukotriene receptor antagonists, as well as allergy shots to reduce the allergic response, may be prescribed by health care providers. Epinephrine, also called adrenaline, is the medication of choice for controlling a severe reaction. Individuals at risk of an anaphylactic reaction should have a bracelet or necklace with that information. Those who are allergic to insect stings should carry and use a pre-filled syringe of epinephrine (EpiPen) for prompt self-treatment. For food-based allergies, many younger and older children respond to Oral Immunotherapy (OIT), in which the allergenic food is gradually reintroduced to the child, little-by-little. Some OIT-treated children can eventually reincorporate the formerly-offending food into their diets.

National Agencies & Associations

625 **Academy of Nutrition & Dietetics**
120 South Riverside Plaza
Chicago, IL 60606-6995
312-899-0040
800-877-1600
media@eatright.org
www.eatright.org
Offers information and support to allergy sufferers. Serves the public through the promotion of optimal nutrition, health, and well-being. Formerly the American Dietetic Association.
Mary Russell, President
Patricia M. Babjak, Chief Executive Officer

626 **Agency for Healthcare Research and Quality**
5600 Fishers Lane
Rockville, MD 20857
301-427-1104
www.ahrq.gov
The Agency for Healthcare Research and Quality's (AHRQ) mission is to produce evidence to make health care safer, higher quality, more accessible, equitable, and affordable, and to work within the U.S. Department of Health and Human Services and with other partners to make sure that the evidence is understood and used.
Gopal Khanna, MBA, Director
Howard E. Holland, Director, Communications

627 **Agency for Toxic Substances and Disease Registry**
4770 Buford Hwy NE
Atlanta, GA 30341-3717
770-488-0736
800-232-4636
Fax: 770-488-1547
TTY: 888-232-6348
jah8@cdc.gov
www.atsdr.cdc.gov
The Agency for Toxic Substances and Disease Registry (ATSDR), based in Atlanta, Georgia, is a federal public health agency of the U.S. Department of Health and Human Services. ATSDR serves the public by using the best science, taking responsive public health actions, and providing trusted health information to prevent harmful exposures and diseases related to toxic substances.
Patrick Breysse, PhD, CIH, Director
Jack Hanley, Acting Branch Chief, Central Branch

628 **Allergy & Asthma Network**
8229 Boone Boulevard
Vienna, VA 22182
800-878-4403
Fax: 703-288-5271
info@aanma.org
www.allergyasthmanetwork.org
Non-profit membership organization dedicated to eliminating suffering and death due to asthma, allergies and related conditions through education, advocacy, community outreach, and research.
Tonya Winders, President & CEO
Marcela Gieminiani, Director, Outreach

629 **American Academy of Allergy, Asthma & Immunology**
555 East Wells Street
Milwaukee, WI 53202-3823
414-272-6071
Fax: 414-272-6070
info@aaaai.org
www.aaaai.org
Strives to serve the public through information on asthma and allergies, as well as referrals to allergists.
Mary-Beth Fasano, President
Giselle S. Mosnaim, Secretary-Treasurer

630 **American Academy of Environmental Medicine**
6505 E Central Avenue
Wichita, KS 67206
316-684-5500
Fax: 888-411-1206
defox@aaemonline.org
www.aaemonline.org
The AAEM Promotes the education of healthcare professionals in the interaction between humans and the environment. Offers names of Clinical Ecologists and Allergy Specialists in the United States.
De Rodgers-Fox, Executive Director

631 **American College of Allergy, Asthma & Immunology**
85 West Algonquin Road
Arlington Heights, IL 60005
847-427-1200
Fax: 847-427-9656
mail@acaai.org
www.acaai.org
Focuses on research and public awareness of allergies, asthma, and immunology. Distributes informational brochures and pamphlets, offers referrals and counseling services, as well as patient care.
Rick Slawny, Executive Diector
Nancy Ryan, Associate Executive Director

632 **Asthma Canada**
124 Merton Street
Toronto, Ontario, M4S-2Z2
416-787-4050
866-787-4050
Fax: 416-787-5807
info@asthma.ca
www.asthma.ca

National, volunteer-led organization devoted to enhancing the quality of life for individuals with asthma and respiratory allergies.
Vanessa Foran, President & CEO
Jenna Reynolds, Director, Programs & Services

633 Birth Defect Research for Children, Inc.
976 Lake Baldwin Lane   407-895-0802
Celebration, FL 32814   staff@birthdefects.org
                                              www.birthdefects.org/allergies
A non-profit organization providing parents and soon-to-be parents with information resources about birth defects, and support services for their children. Offers fact sheets on allergies.
Betty Mekdeci, Executive Director

634 Canadian Society of Allergy and Clinical Immunology
PO Box 51045   613-986-5869
Orleans, K1E-3W4   Fax: 866-839-7501
                                                      info@csaci.ca
                                                      www.csaci.ca
Promotes the advancement of the knowledge and practice of allergy, clinical immunology, and asthma for optimal patient care.
Harold Kim, President
Louise Tremblay, Executive Director

635 Centers for Disease Control & Prevention: Division of Adolescent & School Health
1600 Clifton Road   800-232-4636
Atlanta, GA 30329-4027   TTY: 888-232-6348
                                              www.cdc.gov/HealthyYouth
CDC promotes the health and well-being of children and adolescents to enable them to become healthy and productive adults.

636 Centers for Medicare & Medicaid Services
7500 Security Boulevard   410-786-3000
Baltimore, MD 21244   877-267-2323
                                              TTY: 866-226-1819
                                                      www.cms.gov
U.S. federal agency which administers Medicare, Medicaid, and the State Children's Health Insurance Program.
Seema Verma, Administrator
Tom Corry, Director

637 Food Allergy Research & Education
7901 Jones Branch Drive   703-691-3179
McLean, VA 22102   800-929-4040
                                              Fax: 703-691-2713
                                                      www.foodallergy.org
FARE aims to increase public awareness about food allergies and anaphylaxis, advance research, and provide education, emotional support and coping strategies to patients. It also serves as the communication link between the food industry, the government and the airline industry.
Lisa Gable, Chief Executive Officer
Thomas B. Casale, Chief Medical Advisor, Operations

638 Food Safety and Inspection Service
U.S. Department Of Agriculture
1400 Independence Avenue SW   202-720-9113
Washington, DC 20250-3700   fsis.webmaster@usda.gov
                                                      www.fsis.usda.gov
The Food Safety and Inspection Service (FSIS) is the public health agency in the U.S. Department of Agriculture responsible for ensuring that the nation's commercial supply of meat, poultry, and egg products is safe, wholesome, and correctly labeled and packaged.
Carmen M. Rottenberg, Administrator
Paul Kiecker, Deputy Administrator

639 National Center for Complementary and Integrative Health
9000 Rockville Pike   888-644-6226
Bethesda, MD 20892   TTY: 866-464-3615
                                                      info@nccih.nih.gov
                                                      nccih.nih.gov
The National Center for Complementary and Integrative Health (NCCIH) is the Federal Government's lead agency for scientific research on the diverse medical and health care systems, practices, and products that are not generally considered part of conventional medicine.
Helene M. Langevin, MD, Director
David Shurtleff, Ph.D., Deputy Director

640 National Eczema Association
505 San Marin Drive   415-499-3474
Novato, CA 94945   www.nationaleczema.org
Engages in research, support, and education to better the lives of individuals with eczema, including information on allergies.
Julie Block, President & CEO
Tim Smith, Vice President, Advocacy & Access

641 National Human Genome Research Institute
Building 31, Room 4B09   301-402-0911
Bethesda, MD 20892-2152   Fax: 301-402-2218
                                                      www.genome.gov
The National Human Genome Research Institute began as the National Center for Human Genome Research (NCHGR), which was established in 1989 to carry out the role of the National Institutes of Health (NIH) in the International Human Genome Project (HGP).
Eric D. Green, M.D., Ph.D., Director
Lawrence Brody, Ph.D., Director, Division of Genomics & Society

642 National Institute for Occupational Safety and Health
Patriots Plaza 1
395 E Street SW   202-245-0625
Washington, DC 20201   800-232-4636
                                              Fax: 513-533-8347
                                              TTY: 888-232-6348
                                                      www.cdc.gov/niosh
The National Institute for Occupational Safety and Health (NIOSH) is the U.S. federal agency that conducts research and makes recommendations to prevent worker injury and illness.
John Howard, MD, Director
Frank Hearl, PE, Chief of Staff

643 National Institute of Allergy and Infectious Diseases
NIAID Office of Communications & Govt Relations
5601 Fishers Lane   301-496-5717
Bethesda, MD 20892-9806   866-284-4107
                                              Fax: 301-402-3573
                                              TDD: 800-877-8339
                                              ocpostoffice@niaid.nih.gov
                                                      www.niaid.nih.gov
Conducts and supports research on allergies; focused on understanding what happens to the body during the allergic process. Educates patients and health care workers in controlling allergic disease; offers various research centers that conduct and evaluate educational programs focused on methods to control allergic diseases.
Anthony S. Fauci, MD, Director

644 National Institute of Biomedical Imaging and Bioengineering
9000 Rockville Pike   301-496-8859
Bethesda, MD 20892   info@nibib.nih.gov
                                                      www.nibib.nih.gov
The mission of the National Institute of Biomedical Imaging and Bioengineering (NIBIB) is to improve health by leading the development and accelerating the application of biomedical technologies.
Bruce J. Tromberg, PhD, Director
Jill Heemskerk, PhD, Deputy Director

645 National Institute of Environmental Health Sciences
105 T.W. Alexander Drive   919-541-3345
Research Triangle Park, NC 27709   webcenter@niehs.nih.gov
                                                      www.niehs.nih.gov
The mission of the NIEHS is to discover how the environment affects people in order to promote healthier lives.
Linda S. Birnbaum, PhD, Director
Richard Woychik, PhD, Deputy Director

646 National Institute of Food and Agriculture
Waterfront Centre
800 9th Street SW   nifa.usda.gov
Washington, DC 20024

National Institute of Food and Agriculture (NIFA) provides leadership and funding for programs that advance agriculture-related sciences.
J. Scott Angle, Director
William Hoffman, Chief of Staff

647 National Institute of General Medical Sciences
45 Center Drive MSC 6200   301-496-7301
Bethesda, MD 20892-6200   info@nigms.nih.gov
                                             www.nigms.nih.gov
The National Institute of General Medical Sciences (NIGMS) supports basic research that increases understanding of biological processes and lays the foundation for advances in disease diagnosis, treatment and prevention.
Jon R. Lorsch, PhD, Director
Judith H. Greenberg, PhD, Deputy Director

648 U.S. Food and Drug Administration
10903 New Hampshire Avenue   301-796-8240
Silver Spring, MD 20993-0002   888-463-6332
                                             www.fda.gov
FDA is responsible for protecting the public health by assuring the safety, efficacy and security of human and veterinary drugs, biological products, medical devices, the nation's food supply, cosmetics, and products that emit radiation.
Norman E. Sharpless, MD, Commissioner
Denise Hinton, Chief Scientist

State Agencies & Associations

Alaska

649 Asthma and Allergy Foundation of America: Alaska Chapter
PO Box 201927   907-349-0637
Anchorage, AK 99520-1927   800-651-4914
                                             Fax: 907-349-0637
                                             aafaalaska@gci.net
                                             www.aafaalaska.com
Serves patients of all ages in Alaska who are affected by asthma and allergies, and also provides resources to healthcare professionals, caregivers and childcare providers.
Dale Knutsen, Executive Director

Massachusetts

650 Asthma and Allergy Foundation of America: New England Chapter
25 Braintree Hill Office Park   781-444-7778
Braintree, MA 02184   david@aafane.org
                                             www.asthmaandallergies.org
Serves patients of all ages in Connecticut, Maine, Massachusetts, New Hampshire, Rhode Island and Vermont, who are affected by asthma and allergies, and also provides resources to healthcare professionals, caregivers and childcare providers.
David Guydan, Executive Director

Michigan

651 Asthma and Allergy Foundation of America: Michigan Chapter
26111 West 14 Mile   248-406-4254
Franklin, MI 48025   888-444-0333
                                             aafamich@sbcglobal.net
                                             www.aafamich.org
Serves patients of all ages in Michigan who are affected by asthma and allergies, and also provides resources to healthcare professionals, caregivers and childcare providers.
Kathleen Felice Slonager, Executive Director

Missouri

652 Asthma and Allergy Foundation of America: St. Louis Chapter
1500 S Big Bend   314-645-2422
St. Louis, MO 63117   Fax: 314-692-2022
                                             aafa@aafastl.org
                                             www.aafastl.org
Serves patients of all ages in St. Louis and surrounding counties who are affected by asthma and allergies, and also provides resources to healthcare professionals, caregivers and childcare pro-

viders. Offers the BREATH asthma and allergy management program for children.
Marjorie Moore, Executive Director

Foundations

653 American Academy of Allergy, Asthma & Immunology Foundation
555 East Wells Street   414-272-6071
Milwaukee, WI 53202-3823   Fax: 414-272-6070
                                             lwiensch@aaaai.org
                                             www.aaaaifoundation.org
Funds research in an effort to prevent and cure asthma and allergic/immunologic diseases.
Lee Wiensch, Executive Director
Anne Koenings, Development Manager

654 American College of Allergy, Asthma & Immunology Foundation
85 West Algonquin Road   847-427-1200
Arlington Heights, IL 60005   Fax: 847-427-9656
                                             mail@acaai.org
                                             college.acaai.org/acaai-foundation
Funds faculty research grants and travel scholarships.
Richard Weber, President
Stanley Fineman, Vice President

655 Asthma and Allergy Foundation of America
8201 Corporate Drive   202-466-7643
Landover, MD 20785   800-727-8462
                                             Fax: 202-466-8940
                                             info@aafa.org
                                             www.aafa.org
The AAFA is a non-profit patient organization dedicated to improving the quality of life for people with asthma and allergies and their caregivers, through education, advocacy, funding, and research.
Richard Murray, Chair
Kenneth Mendez, Chief Executive Officer

656 Immune Deficiency Foundation
110 West Road   800-296-4433
Towson, MD 21204-4841   Fax: 410-321-9165
                                             info@primaryimmune.org
                                             www.primaryimmune.org
A national charitable organization aimed at fighting the primary immune deficiency diseases. The founders included parents of children with primary immune deficiency, immunologists who treat immune deficient patients, and other individuals with an immune deficiency.
John G. Boyle, President & CEO
Kara Moran, Vice President, Communications

657 Kids with Food Allergies
4259 W Swamp Road   215-230-5394
Doylestown, PA 18902   Fax: 215-340-7940
                                             awaldron@aafa.org
                                             www.kidswithfoodallergies.org
A division of the Asthma and Allergy Foundation of America, KFA provides support to families with children suffering from food allergies.
Angel Waldron, Senior Communications Manager

Research Centers

658 Columbus Children's Research Institute
700 Children's Drive   614-722-2000
Columbus, OH 43205   Fax: 614- 35- 079
                                             John.Barnard@NationwideChildrens.org
                                             www.nationwidechildrens.org
Research institute dedicated to enhancing the health of children by engaging in the high quality cutting-edge research according to the highest scientific and ethical standards.
John A Barnard, Research Institute President
Steve Allen MD, CEO

659   Creighton University Allergic Disease Center
601 N 30th Street   402-280-4403
Omaha, NE 68131-0001   Fax: 402-280-4803
                                                    casalej@creighton.edu
                              medicine.creighton.edu/allergy/homepage.

Robert G Townley, Investigator
Thomas B Casale, Chief

660   Institute for Rehabilitation and Research
21720 Kingsland Blvd.   800-447-3422
Katy, TX 77450   Fax: 713-874-1798
                                    tirr.referrals@memorialhermann.org
                                          www.tirr.memorialhermann.org

Carl Josehart, Chief Executive Officer
Gerard E. Francisco, Chief Medical Officer

661   Mayo Clinic and Foundation: Division of Allergic Diseases
Department of Immunology
200 First Street SW   507-284-2511
Rochester, MN 55905   Fax: 507-284-0161
                                                  TTY: 507-284-9786
                                                    www.mayoclinic.org

Provides a focus for research into the causes prevention and management of allergic diseases.
John H Noseworthy MD, President
William C Rupp MD, Vice President, CEO

662   National Jewish Center for Immunology and Respiratory Medicine
Goodman Building Room 611   303-398-1287
Denver, CO 80206   800-423-8891
                                                  Fax: 303-398-1806
                                                    www.nationaljewish.org

Basic and clinical research into the causes and treatments of asthmatic disorders.
Tom Gart, Chairman
Michael Salem, President & CEO

663   Research Institute of Palo Alto Medical Foundation
795 El Camino Real   650-326-8120
Palo Alto, CA 94301-2302   www.pamf.org/research

Clinical and general medical sciences research including allergy and immunology disorders.
Jane Risser, Director
Andrea Norcia, Assistant Director

664   Scripps Research Institute
10550 N Torrey Pines Road   858-784-1000
La Jolla, CA 92037   www.scripps.edu

William Burfitt, President
Alex Bruner, Executive Vice President and Chief Opera

665   Texas Children's Allergy and Immunology Clinic
Clinical Care Center
6701 Fannin Street   832-824-1000
Houston, TX 77030   800-364-5437
                                                  Fax: 832-825-3072
                                    pediai@texaschildrenshospital.org
                                          www.texaschildrenshospital.org

Mark A Wallace, President & CEO
Mark W Kline MD, Physician In Chief

666   University of Florida: General Clinical Research Center
University of Florida
1600 SW Archer Road   352-273-5500
Gainesville, FL 32610-0322   888-635-0763
                                                  Fax: 352-273-5541
                                                    thomprd@ufl.edu
                                                    www.med.ufl.edu

Studies on allergies and immunology.
Robert Thompson, Program Director

667   University of Kansas Allergy and Immunology Clinic
University of Kansas Medical Center
3901 Rainbow Boulevard   913-588-5000
Kansas City, KS 66160   TTY: 913-588-7963
                                                  TDD: 913-588-7963
                                                    dstechsc@kumc.edu
                                                    www.kumc.edu

This service provides complete evaluation of patients with allergic diseases such as rhinitis and asthma immunological deficiencies food and drug intolerances and autoimmune dysfunctions.
Barbara F Atkinson MD, Executive Vice Chancellor
Shelley Gebar, RN, MHA, Chief of Staff

668   University of Michigan Montgomery: John M. Sheldon Allergy Society
Alllergy & Clinical Immunology
24 Frank Lloyd Wright Drive   734-232-2154
Ann Arbor, MI 48106-0380   Fax: 734-647-6263
                                                    echoreed@med.umich.edu
                                          www.med.umich.edu/sheldonsociety

Travis A Miller, President

669   University of Texas Southwestern Medical Center at Dallas
University of Texas Southwestern Medical Center
5323 Harry Hines Boulevard   214-648-3111
Dallas, TX 75390   Fax: 214-648-9119
                                                    news@utsouthwestern.edu
                                                    www.utsouthwestern.edu

Immunodermatology department researching allergies and immune disorders.
Daniel K Podolsky MD, President

670   Warren Grant Magnuson Clinical Center
National Institute of Health
9000 Rockville Pike   301-496-2563
Bethesda, MD 20892   800-411-1222
                                                  Fax: 301-402-2984
                                                  TTY: 866-411-1010
                                                    prpl@mail.cc.nih.gov
                                                    www.cc.nih.gov

Established in 1953 as the research hospital of the National Institutes of Health. Designed so that patient care facilities are close to research laboratories so new findings of basic and clinical scientists can be quickly applied to the treatment of patients. Upon referral by physicians, patients are admitted to NIH clinical studies.
Michael J Klag MD, Chair
David K Henderson MD, Clinical Director

Support Groups & Hotlines

671   ASTHMA Hotline
American Academy of Allergy, Asthma and Immunology
2275 East Bayshore Road   650-328-3123
Palo Alto, CA 53202   800-822-2762
                                                  Fax: 650-321-4457
                                                    www.aaai.org

Referral line offering information on allergy and asthma treatments, referrals to an allergy/immunology specialist, lay organization or support groups across the country.

672   National Health Information Center
Office of Disease Prevention & Health Promotion
1101 Wootton Pkwy   Fax: 240-453-8281
Rockville, MD 20852   odphpinfo@hhs.gov
                                                    www.health.gov/nhic

Supports public health education by maintaining a calendar of National Health Observances; helps connect consumers and health professionals to organizations that can best answer questions and provide up-to-date contact information from reliable sources; updates on a yearly basis toll-free numbers for health information, Federal health clearinghouses and info centers.
Don Wright, MD, MPH, Director

Books

673   Allergies A to Z
Facts on File
132 W 31st Street   212-967-8800
New York, NY 10001   800-322-8755
                                                  Fax: 800-678-3633
                                                    custserv@factsonfile.com
                                                    www.infobasepublishing.com

This vital resource for the one in five Americans who suffer from allergies provides reliable, up-to-date information on every aspect of this condition.
Paperback

674 Allergy Alerts from Living with Allergies
American Allergy Association
PO Box 7273   650-322-1663
Menlo Park, CA 94026-7273
These alerts cover a wide range of areas from dyes in medications to medication interactions, food additives like sulfites, spelt, situations that could trigger asthma, problems with collagen and even fabric softeners.

675 Allergy Plants that Cause Sneezing and Wheezing
Asthma and Allergy Foundation of America
8201 Corporate Drive   202-466-7643
Landover, MD 20785-2330   800-727-8462
                                               Fax: 202-466-8940
                                               info@aafa.org
                                               www.aafa.org
Destined to be displayed on coffee tables, the spectacular photographs in this book actually show allergy sufferers what causes their sneezing and wheezing.
64 pages Paperback

676 Complete Book of Children's Allergies
Allergy Central Products
1620-D Satellite Blvd   203-438-9580
Duluth, GA 30097-4053   800-422-3878
                                               Fax: 203-431-8963
                                               www.allergycontrol.com
Major childhood allergies, recommendations for treatment.
Softcover

677 Cooking for the Allergic Child
Allergy Central Products
1620-D Satellite Blvd   203-438-9580
Duluth, GA 30097-4053   800-442-3878
                                               Fax: 203-431-8963
                                               www.allergycontrol.com
More than 300 recipes with nutrients analysis.
Softcover

678 Diets to Help Gluten and Wheat Allergy
HarperCollins Canada Limited/Order Department
1995 Markham Road   800-387-0117
Scarborough, M1B 5M8,   Fax: 800-668-5788
This book offers sound and practical advice on gluten allergy wheat sensitivity and Celiac disease.
96 pages
ISBN: 0-722529-10-4

679 Food Allergy: A Primer for People
Asthma and Allergy Foundation of America
8201 Corporate Drive   202-466-7643
Landover, MD 20785-2330   800-727-8462
                                               Fax: 202-466-8940
                                               info@aafa.org
                                               www.aafa.org
Food allergies demystified.
66 pages Hardcover

680 Human Exposure Assessment for Airborne Pollutants: Advances & Opportunity
National Academies Press
500 5th Street NW   202-334-3313
Washington, DC 20001   888-624-8373
                                               Fax: 202-334-2451
                                               customer_service@nap.edu
                                               www.nap.edu
Explores the need for strategies to address indoor and outdoor exposures and examines the methods and tools available for finding out where and when significant exposures occur.
344 pages
ISBN: 0-309042-84-0
Sandy Adams, Publishing Operations Director
Dottie Lewis, Publishing Services Director

681 Indoor Allergens: Assessing & Controlling Adverse Health Effects
National Academies Press
500 5th Street NW   202-334-3313
Washington, DC 20055   888-624-8373
                                               Fax: 202-334-2793
                                               customer_service@nap.edu
                                               www.nap.edu
This comprehensive and practical volume will be important to allergists and other health care providers; public health professionals; specialists in building design, construction, and maintenance; faculty and students in public health; and interested allergy patients.
350 pages
ISBN: 0-309048-31-6
Andrew M. Pope, Author
Roy Patterson, Author

682 Infant Formulas for Allergic Infants and Dietetic Concerns for Toddlers
American Allergy Association
PO Box 7273   650-322-1663
Menlo Park, CA 94026-7273
Offers information on reliable food labels, evaluations of infant formulas, FDA labeling requirements under the new law and more.

683 New Food Labels
American Allergy Association
PO Box 7273   650-322-1663
Menlo Park, CA 94026-7273
Offers clear-cut and precise information on new label word definitions.

684 Pollen Times: By State, By Month
American Allergy Association
PO Box 7273   650-322-1663
Menlo Park, CA 94026-7273
A comprehensive guide offering information on how to plan vacations while avoiding pollen problems.

685 Traveling with Allergies: Prepare and Avoid Problems
American Allergy Association
PO Box 7273   650-322-1663
Menlo Park, CA 94026-7273
Prepare for travel, recognize and minimize the risk, sidestep smoke, food allergies, pollen, mold, dander, weather and emergencies.

Children's Books

686 All About Allergies
Susan Terkel, author
Dutton Children's Books
375 Hudson Street   212-366-2000
New York, NY 10014-3658   Fax: 212-366-2262
                                               www.penguin.com
1993 64 pages
ISBN: 0-525674-10-1

687 Allergies
Franklin Watts Grolier
90 Old Sherman Turnpike   203-797-3500
Danbury, CT 06816-0001   800-621-1115
                                               Fax: 203-797-3197
                                               www.grolier.com
Covers the major types of allergies, including those of the respiratory and gastrointestinal tracts.
112 pages Grades 7-12
ISBN: 0-531125-16-5

688 Living with Allergies
Franklin Watts Grolier
90 Old Sherman Turnpike   203-797-3500
Danbury, CT 06816-0001   800-621-1115
                                               Fax: 203-797-3197
                                               www.grolier.com

Shows how people with allergies are able to overcome their handicap to lead full and productive lives.
32 pages Grades 5-7
ISBN: 0-531108-57-0

Provides up-to-date medical news, emotional support and practical strategies for overcoming asthma and allergies.
8 pages 8x Year
Mary McGowan, Executive Director
Nancy Sander, Editor-in-Chief

Magazines

689 Allergy & Asthma Today
Allergy & Asthma Network
8229 Boone Boulevard   800-878-4403
Vienna, VA 22182   Fax: 703-288-5271
                                               info@aanma.org
                                   www.allergyasthmanetwork.org
Medically reviewed magazine for people living with asthma, allergies and other respiratory conditions. Free with Allergy & Asthma Network membership.
40 pages
Gary Fitzgerald, Managing Editor

690 Food & Nutrition
120 South Riverside Plaza   312-899-0040
Chicago, IL 60606-6995   800-877-1600
                                   foodandnutrition@eatright.org
                                               www.eatright.org
Formerly the ADA Times, Food & Nutrition is the member and professional magazine of the Academy of Nutrition & Dietetics.

691 Journal of the Academy of Nutrition and Dietetics
120 South Riverside Plaza   312-899-4831
Chicago, IL 60606-6995   journal@eatright.org
                                               www.eatright.org
Official research publication of the Academy of Nutrition and Dietetics.
Joe Skey, Advertising Contact

692 Understanding Anaphylaxis
Allergy & Asthma Network
8229 Boone Boulevard   800-878-4403
Vienna, VA 22182   Fax: 703-288-5271
                                               info@aanma.org
                                   www.allergyasthmanetwork.org
Magazine focusing on how to recognize and prevent anaphylaxis.
40 pages
Gary Fitzgerald, Managing Editor

Newsletters

693 Advice From Your Allergist
American College of Allergy & Immunology
85 W Algonguin Road   847-359-2800
Alrlington Heights, IL 60005
Offers information on the effects, triggers and causes of allergies including house dust, pets, hay fever, hives and exercise.

694 Food Allergy News
Food Allergy and Anaphylaxis Network
7901 Jones Branch Dr.   703-691-3179
McLean, VA 22102-2208   800-929-4040
                                            Fax: 703-691-2713
                                            faan@foodallergy.org
                                            www.foodallergy.org
Contains allergy free recipes, practical tips such as birthday party, trick-or-treating and travel tips, a dietitian's column, medical information and product information.
12 pages BiMonthly
James R. Baker, Jr., MD, CEO
Donna McKelvey, Senior VP and Chief Development Officer

695 MA Report
Allergy and Asthma Network/Mothers of Asthmatics
8229 Boone Boulevard   703-641-9595
Vienna, VA 22182   800-878-4403
                                            Fax: 703-288-5271
                                               editor@aanma.org
                                   www.allergyasthmanetwork.org

Pamphlets

696 Adverse Reactions to Foods
American Academy of Allergy, Asthma and Immunology
555 East Wells Street   414-272-6071
Milwaukee, WI 53202-3889   800-822-2762
                                            Fax: 414-272-6070
                                               www.aaaai.org
A patient's guide to problem foods, food additives, diagnosis, and treatment.

697 Allergic Diseases
National Institute of Allergy & Infectious Disease
5601 Fishers Lane   301-496-3204
Bethesda, MD 20892-9806   Fax: 301-480-4137
                                          domingug@mail.nih.gov
                                              www.niaid.nih.gov
Offers information on allergies, who gets them, diagnosis and treatments for various types of allergic diseases.

698 Allergies and You
American Lung Association
1740 Broadway   212-315-8700
New York, NY 10019-4315
Answers basic questions about allergy, particularly as it relates to asthma.

699 Allergies to Animals
American Academy of Allergy, Asthma and Immunology
555 East Wells Street   414-272-6071
Milwaukee, WI 53202-3889   800-822-2762
                                            Fax: 414-272-6070
                                               www.aaaai.org

700 Anaphylaxis
American Academy of Allergy, Asthma and Immunology
555 East Wells Street   414-272-6071
Milwaukee, WI 53202-3889   800-822-2762
                                            Fax: 414-272-6070
                                               www.aaaai.org

701 Eating Without Packet
American Allergy Association
PO Box 7273   650-322-1663
Menlo Park, CA 94026-7273
Twelve information sheets describing the most common food allergens, specific problems with common foods and supplements, and the facts on milk ingredient labeling, milk allergies, and milk sensitivity. Included in the packet is a 16-page handbook, Understanding Calcium and Osteoporosis.

702 FAAN Flashbacks
Food Allergy and Anaphylaxis Network
7901 Jones Branch Dr.   703-691-3179
McLean, VA 22102-2208   800-929-4040
                                            Fax: 703-691-2713
                                            faan@foodallergy.org
                                            www.foodallergy.org
Series of reprints on specific topics of Food Allergy News. Specific pamphlets offer information on wheat, milk, soy, egg, fish, peanuts, managing food allergy in schools and anaphylaxis.
James R. Baker, Jr., MD, CEO
Donna McKelvey, Senior VP and Chief Development Officer

703 Food Allergy and Atopic Dermatitis
Food Allergy and Anaphylaxis Network
7901 Jones Branch Dr.   703-691-3179
McLean, VA 22102-2208   800-929-4040
                                            Fax: 703-691-2713
                                            faan@foodallergy.org
                                            www.foodallergy.org

The purpose of this booklet is to provide tips and other sources of information to help parents raise a child who is afflicted with atopic dermatitis.
12 pages
James R. Baker, Jr., MD, CEO
Donna McKelvey, Senior VP and Chief Development Officer

704 Guide to Gluten-Free Diets
American Allergy Association
PO Box 7273   650-322-1663
Menlo Park, CA 94026-7273
Offers information on safe substitutes for baking and cooking. Differentiates celiac disease from wheat allergy. Sources of gluten in diet with warnings on when to check with the manufacturer.

705 Helpful Hints for the Allergic Patient
American Academy of Allergy, Asthma and Immunology
555 East Wells Street   414-272-6071
Milwaukee, WI 53202-3889   800-822-2762
                                                    Fax: 414-272-6070
                                                        www.aaaai.org
An informational brochure good for someone who has just been diagnosed with allergies.
8 pages

706 Immunitherapy
American Academy of Allergy, Asthma and Immunology
555 East Wells Street   414-272-6071
Milwaukee, WI 53202-3889   800-822-2762
                                                    Fax: 414-272-6070
                                                        www.aaaai.org
This brochure offers information on administration, benefits, and potential side effects of immune therapy.

707 Just One Little Bite Can Hurt! Important Facts About Anaphylaxis
Food Allergy and Anaphylaxis Network
7901 Jones Branch Dr.   703-691-3179
McLean, VA 22102-2208   800-929-4040
                                                    Fax: 703-691-2713
                                                 faan@foodallergy.org
                                                    www.foodallergy.org
Offers information on what anaphylaxis is, what the patient should do if they have a reaction and important medical safety tips regarding the illness.
8 pages Booklet
James R. Baker, Jr., MD, CEO
Donna McKelvey, Senior VP and Chief Development Officer

708 Latex Allergy
American Academy of Allergy, Asthma and Immunology
555 East Wells Street   414-272-6071
Milwaukee, WI 53202-3889   800-822-2762
                                                    Fax: 414-272-6070
                                                        www.aaaai.org

709 Nutrition Guide to Food Allergies
Food Allergy and Anaphylaxis Network
7901 Jones Branch Dr.   703-691-3179
McLean, VA 22102-2208   800-929-4040
                                                    Fax: 703-691-2713
                                                 faan@foodallergy.org
                                                    www.foodallergy.org
Offers answers to the most commonly asked questions about food allergies, common allergy causing foods and resources for the patient.
24 pages
James R. Baker, Jr., MD, CEO
Donna McKelvey, Senior VP and Chief Development Officer

710 Pollen and Spores Around the World
American Academy of Allergy, Asthma and Immunology
555 East Wells Street   414-272-6071
Milwaukee, WI 53202-3889   800-822-2762
                                                    Fax: 414-272-6070
                                                        www.aaaai.org
Multi-paged brochure offering graphes and tables of pollen levels and different times of the year in different parts of the country.
10 pages

711 Removing House Dust and Other Allergic Irritants From Your Home
American Academy of Allergy, Asthma and Immunology
555 East Wells Street   414-272-6071
Milwaukee, WI 53202-3889   800-822-2762
                                                    Fax: 414-272-6070
                                                        www.aaaai.org
This brochure covers some good ideas on how to reduce dust in the home.

712 Role of the Allergist & Clinical Immunologist in Patient Care
American Academy of Allergy, Asthma and Immunology
555 East Wells Street   414-272-6071
Milwaukee, WI 53202-3889   800-822-2762
                                                    Fax: 414-272-6070
                                                        www.aaaai.org
An informational brochure containing definitions and addresses for further information.

713 Something in the Air: Airborne Allergens
National Institute of Allergy & Infectious Disease
5601 Fishers Lane   301-496-5717
Bethesda, MD 20892-9806   www.niaid.nih.gov
Offers information on the symptoms to airborne substances, pollen, mold, dust, animal, chemical allergies and treatments for them.

714 Tips to Remember Brochures
American Academy of Allergy, Asthma and Immunology
555 East Wells Street   414-272-6071
Milwaukee, WI 53202-3889   800-822-2762
                                                    Fax: 414-272-6070
                                                        www.aaaai.org
Thirty three colorful brochures offered on numerous topics in allergy, asthma, and immunology.

715 Understanding the Pollen and Mold Season
American Academy of Allergy, Asthma and Immunology
555 East Wells Street   414-272-6071
Milwaukee, WI 53202-3889   800-822-2762
                                                    Fax: 414-272-6070
                                                        www.aaaai.org

716 Use of Steroids for Asthma and Allergies
American Academy of Allergy, Asthma and Immunology
555 East Wells Street   414-272-6071
Milwaukee, WI 53202-3889   800-822-2762
                                                    Fax: 414-272-6070
                                                        www.aaaai.org

717 What Every Patient Should Know About Asthma & Allergy Medications
American Academy of Allergy, Asthma and Immunology
555 East Wells Street   414-272-6071
Milwaukee, WI 53202-3889   800-822-2762
                                                    Fax: 414-272-6070
                                                        www.aaaai.org

718 What is an Allergic Reaction?
American Academy of Allergy, Asthma and Immunology
555 East Wells Street   414-272-6071
Milwaukee, WI 53202-3889   800-822-2762
                                                    Fax: 414-272-6070
                                                        www.aaaai.org
This brochure gives helpful information on what will cause an allergic reaction.

Audio & Video

719 Alexander, the Elephant Who Couldn't Eat Peanuts
Food Allergy and Anaphylaxis Network
7901 Jones Branch Dr.   800-929-4040
McLean, VA 22102-3309   Fax: 703-691-2713
                                                    www.foodallergy.org
Helps children cope with their own allergies and teach other children about tolerance. Both videos combine colorful animation with interviews of real-life children with food allergies who talk about their experiences.
James R. Baker, Jr., MD, CEO
Donna McKelvey, Senior VP and Chief Development Officer

720 Allergic Rhinitis
American Academy of Allergy, Asthma and Immunology
555 East Wells Street   414-272-6071
Milwaukee, WI 53202-3889   800-822-2762
                                    Fax: 414-272-6070
                                         www.aaaai.org
Allergic rhinitis, often called hay fever, affects the quality of life of millions of Americans. This video covers the causes and symptoms of seasonal and chronic allergic rhinitis, as well as environmental controls and treatments.
10-13 minutes

721 Allergic Rhinitis: Nothing to Sneeze At!
Asthma and Allergy Foundation of America
8201 Corporate Drive   202-466-7643
Landover, MD 20785-2330   800-727-8462
                                    Fax: 202-466-8940
                                         info@aafa.org
                                         www.aafa.org
The basics of allergic rhinitis, with a touch of humor. Common allergens, environmental control, skin testing and immunotherapy medications.
Videotape

722 Allergic Skin Reactions
American Academy of Allergy, Asthma and Immunology
555 East Wells Street   414-272-6071
Milwaukee, WI 53202-3889   800-822-2762
                                    Fax: 414-272-6070
                                         www.aaaai.org
In some people, allergy symptoms include itching redness, rashes, or hives. This video describes the symptoms, triggers, and treatment for common skin reactions such as dermatitis, hives and angioedema.
10-13 minutes

723 An Overview of Allergy
American College of Allergy & Immunology
800 E NW Highway   847-359-2800
Palatine, IL 60067-6580
Strengthen relationships with patients by providing them with the essential information they need.

724 Immunotherapy
American Academy of Allergy, Asthma and Immunology
555 East Wells Street   414-272-6071
Milwaukee, WI 53202-3889   800-822-2762
                                    Fax: 414-272-6070
                                         www.aaaai.org
Immunotherapy, of allergy shots, is a long-term allergy and asthma treatment program that helps control allergic symptoms and reduces the need for medications. Learn more about immunotherapy through this video, which includes information on allergy testing and how your allergist determines if immunotherapy is right for you.
10-13 minutes

725 Sinusitis and Sinus Surgery
Milner-Fenwick
119 Lakefront Drive   410-252-1700
Hunt Valley, MD 21030-3100   800-432-8433
                                    Fax: 410-252-6316
                                         mail@milner-fenwick.com
                                         www.milner-fenwick.com
Discusses sinusitis symptoms, causes, evaluation and treatments. Animation depicts how sinuses function and how irritants, allergies, colds or structural abnormalities cause sinus blockages. Also explains the role of medical therapy and irrigation in managing acute sinusitis.
14 minutes
Dolores McKee, Advertising Director

726 Stinging Insect Allergy
American Academy of Allergy, Asthma and Immunology
555 East Wells Street   414-272-6071
Milwaukee, WI 53202-3889   800-822-2762
                                    Fax: 414-272-6070
                                         www.aaaai.org
Although many people are afraid of stinging insects such as bees, the stings of these insects actually cause some people to have serious allergic reactions. This video tells how to recognize and avoid stinging insects, what to do if you are stung and how to identify symptoms of an allergic reaction and get medical help.
10-13 minutes

727 Understanding Allergic Reactions
American Academy of Allergy, Asthma and Immunology
555 East Wells Street   414-272-6071
Milwaukee, WI 53202-3889   800-822-2762
                                    Fax: 414-272-6070
                                         www.aaaai.org
During an allergic reaction, your body responds to a substance generally considered harmless to most people. This video portrays what happens in you body's immune system during an allergic reaction, how to avoid allergic substances, and methods your allergist uses to treat your allergies.
10-13 minutes

Web Sites

728 Academy of Nutrition & Dietetics
                                         www.eatright.org
Offers information and support to allergy sufferers. Serves the public through the promotion of optimal nutrition, health, and well-being. Formerly the American Dietetic Association.

729 Allergy & Asthma Network
                                         www.allergyasthmanetwork.org
Non-profit membership organization dedicated to eliminating suffering and death due to asthma, allergies and related conditions through education, advocacy, community outreach, and research.

730 American Academy of Allergy, Asthma & Immunology
                                         www.aaaai.org
Strives to serve the public through information on asthma and allergies, as well as referrals to allergists.

731 American College of Allergy, Asthma & Immunology
                                         www.acaai.org
Focuses on research and public awareness of allergies, asthma, and immunology. Distributes informational brochures and pamphlets, offers referrals and counseling services, as well as patient care.

732 Asthma and Allergy Foundation of America
                                         www.aafa.org
The AAFA is a non-profit patient organization dedicated to improving the quality of life for people with asthma and allergies and their caregivers, through education, advocacy, funding, and research.

733 Birth Defect Research for Children, Inc.
                                         www.birthdefects.org
Provides parents and expectant parents with information about birth defects and support services for their children

734 Food Allergy Research & Education
                                         www.foodallergy.org
FARE aims to increase public awareness about food allergies and anaphylaxis, advance research, and provide education, emotional support and coping strategies to patients. It also serves as the communication link between the food industry, the government and the airline industry.

735 Healing Well
                                         www.healingwell.com
A social network and support community for patients, caregivers, and families coping with the daily struggles of diseases, disorders and chronic illness.

736 Health Finder
                                         www.healthfinder.gov
Government website where individuals can find information and tools to hel you and those you care about stay healthy.

737 Healthlink USA
                                         www.healthlinkusa.com
Health information concerning treatment, cures, prevention, diagnosis, risk factors, research, support groups, email lists, personal stories and much more. Updated regularly.

738   Immune Deficiency Foundation

www.primaryimmune.org

The national patient organization dedicated to improving the diagnosis, treatment and quality of life of persons with primary immunodeficiency diseases through advocacy, education and research.

739   MedicineNet

www.medicinenet.com

An online resource for consumers providing easy-to-read, authoritative medical and health information.

740   Medscape

www.medscape.com

Medscape offers specialists, primary care physicians, and other health professionals the Web's most robust and integrated medical information and educational tools.

741   WebMD

www.webmd.com

Provides credible information, supportive communities, and in-depth reference material about health subjects. A source for original and timely health information as well as material from well known content providers.

Description

742 Alzheimer's Disease

Alzheimer's disease is a degenerative neurologic disease that attacks the brain and impairs memory, thinking faculties and behavior. As the most common form of dementing illness, it afflicts 5.8 million adults and is twice as common in women as in men. It primarily affects older people.

In spite of diligent research, the cause of Alzheimer's disease is unknown. The disease runs in families in about 15 to 20 percent of cases, although the remainder may have some genetic component. There are multiple symptoms of Alzheimer's disease, the most pronounced being gradual memory loss. Other symptoms include the inability to perform routine tasks, loss of language skills, disorientation and personality changes. The diagnosis is largely based on an interview with the patient and family members and an examination of the patient, although brain imaging tests and blood tests may add helpful information.

The brain's cells communicate with each other through various chemicals called neurotransmitters. In Alzheimer's disease, levels of the neurotransmitter acetylcholine are decreased. Drugs that enhance acetylcholine neurotransmission, such as donepezil, galantamine, and rivastigmine, can modestly improve memory during the early stages of Alzheimer's disease, but do not delay the overall progression of the disease. Another drug, memantine, modulates glutamate neurotransmission and can improve cognition over short periods of time, but also does not delay the progression of the disease. The antipsychotic drug, quetiapine, can control some of behavioral symptoms associated with dementia.

In general, nonpharmacological interventions, such as social support networks, community, and participation in hobbies are better treatments for Alzheimer disease. Because Alzheimer's disease severely affects both the patient and the family, proper planning, as well as medical and social programs tailored to the individual and to family members are essential. A well-structured and safe living environment is the best way to preserve the welfare and dignity of the person with Alzheimer's disease. See also *Aging*.

National Agencies & Associations

743 Alzheimer Society of Alberta and Northwest Territories
10430 - 61 Avenue 780-761-0030
Edmonton, Alberta, T6H-2J3 866-950-5465
Fax: 780-488-3055
reception@alzheimer.ab.ca
www.alzheimer.ca/en/ab
Provides support, education, and advocacy for all those affected by Alzheimer's disease in Alberta and the Northwest Territories, including patients, caregivers, patients' families, and the community.
Michele Mulder, Chief Executive Officer
Brenda Burrell, Provincial Lead, Operations

744 Alzheimer Society of B.C.
828 W 8th Avenue Street 604-681-6530
Vancouver, BC, V5C-1E2 800-667-3742
Fax: 604-669-6907
info@alzheimerbc.org
www.alzheimer.ca/en/bc
Provides support, education, and advocacy for all those affected by Alzheimer's disease in British Columbia, including patients, caregivers, patients' families, and the community.
Maria Howard, Chief Executive Officer
Cathryn France, Director, Resource Development

745 Alzheimer Society of Canada
20 Eglinton Avenue W 416-488-8772
Toronto, Ontario, M4R-1K8 800-618-8816
Fax: 416-322-6656
info@alzheimer.ca
www.alzheimer.ca
Identifies, develops and facilitates national priorities that enable its members to effectively alleviate the personal and social consequences of Alzheimer's disease and related disorders; promotes research and leads the search for a cure.
Pauline Tardif, Chief Executive Officer

746 Alzheimer Society of Manitoba
10 - 120 Donald Street 204-943-6622
Winnipeg, Manitoba, R3C-4G2 800-378-6699
alzmb@alzheimer.mb.ca
alzheimer.mb.ca
Provides support, education, and advocacy for all those affected by Alzheimer's disease in Manitoba, including patients, caregivers, patients' families, and the community.
Wendy Schettler, Chief Executive Officer
Norma Kirkby, Program Director

747 Alzheimer Society of New Brunswick
320 Maple Street 506-459-4280
Fredericton, NB, E3B-5G2 800-664-8411
Fax: 506-452-0313
info@alzheimernb.ca
alzheimer.ca/en/nb
Provides support, education, and advocacy for all those affected by Alzheimer's disease in New Brunswick, including patients, caregivers, patients' families, and the community.
Chandra MacBean, Executive Director

748 Alzheimer Society of Newfoundland & Labrador
835 Topsail Road 709-576-0608
Mount Pearl, NL, A1N-3J6 877-776-0608
Fax: 709-576-0798
info@alzheimernl.ca
alzheimer.ca/en/nl
Provides support, education, and advocacy for all those affected by Alzheimer's disease in Newfoundland and Labrador, including patients, caregivers, patients' families, and the community.
Shirley Lucas, Chief Executive Officer
Jessica Flynn, Coordinator, Education Development

749 Alzheimer Society of Nova Scotia
2719 Gladstone Street 902-422-7961
Halifax, Nova Scotia, B3K-4W6 800-611-6345
Fax: 902-422-7971
alzheimer@asns.ca
alzheimer.ca/en/ns
Provides support, education, and advocacy for all those affected by Alzheimer's disease in Nova Scotia, including patients, caregivers, patients' families, and the community.
Lloyd Brown, Executive Director
Linda Bird, Director, Programs & Services

750 Alzheimer Society of Ontario
20 Eglinton Avenue W 416-967-5900
Toronto, Ontario, M4R-1K8 800-879-4226
Fax: 416-967-3826
staff@alzon.ca
alzheimer.ca/en/on
Provides support, education, and advocacy for all those affected by Alzheimer's disease in Ontario, including patients, caregivers, patients' families, and the community.
Cathy Barrick, Chief Executive Officer

751 Alzheimer Society of Prince Edward Island
166 Fitzroy Street   902-628-2257
Charlottetown, PE, C1A-1S1   society@alzpei.ca
                                      alzheimer.ca/en/pei
Provides support, education, and advocacy for all those affected
by Alzheimer's disease in Prince Edward Island, including patients, caregivers, patients' families, and the community.
M. Lynn Murray, QC, President

752 Alzheimer Society of Saskatchewan
2550 - 12th Avenue   306-949-4141
Regina, Saskatchewan, S4P-3X1   800-263-3367
                                      Fax: 306-949-3069
                                      info@alzheimer.sk.ca
                                      www.alzheimer.ca/en/sk
Provides support, education, and advocacy for all those affected
by Alzheimer's disease in Saskatchewan, including patients, care-
givers, patients' families, and the community.
Joanne Bracken, Chief Executive Officer
Leslie Quennell, Manager, Communications & Marketing

753 Alzheimer's & Related Dementias Education & Referral Center
National Institute on Aging
31 Center Drive   800-438-4380
Bethesda, MD 20892   TTY: 800-222-4225
                                      adear@nia.nih.gov
                                      www.nia.nih.gov/health/alzheimers
A service of the National Institute on Aging, the center distributes
information on Alzheimer's disease, on current research activities
and on services available to patients and family members. Offers a
free list of publications available upon request.

754 Alzheimer's Association
225 N. Michigan Avenue   800-272-3900
Chicago, IL 60601   info@alz.org
                                      www.alz.org
Dedicated to research for the prevention, cure, and treatment of
Alzheimer's disease and related disorders, and to providing sup-
port and assistance to the afflicted patients and their families.
Harry Johns, President & CEO
Glenda Berry, Area Leader

755 Federation of Quebec Alzheimer Societies
5165 Sherbrooke Street W   514-369-7891
Montreal, Quebec, H4A-1T6   888-636-6473
                                      Fax: 514-369-7900
                                      info@alzheimerquebec.ca
                                      alzheimer.ca/en/federationquebecoise
Provides support, education, and advocacy for all those affected
by Alzheimer's disease in Quebec, including patients, caregivers,
patients' families, and the community.
Luc Pinard, President

756 John Douglas French Alzheimer's Foundation
11620 Wilshire Boulevard   323-930-6228
Los Angeles, CA 90025-1781   800-477-2243
                                      Fax: 310-479-0516
                                      bwelch@alz.org
                                      www.jdfaf.org
Provides seed money for promising research including the cause
cure and prevention of Alzheimer's disease. Also gives funding to
scientists who might not otherwise be funded.
Bruce L. Miller, MD, Chief Medical Officer
Karen Bedrosian Coyne, President

757 National Alzheimer's Disease Institute
7111 Sweetgum Road   nationalalzdiseaseinstitute.org
Fairview, TN 37602-9384
Investigates and presents information on the ways in which natural
or alternative medicine can slow or prevent dementia. Physician
referrals are provided. The institute is overseen by the National
Fund for Alternative Medicine.
P. Anthony Chapdelaine, Jr., Executive Director
Mary Ann Chapdelaine, President

758 National Institute on Aging
31 Center Drive, MSC 2292   800-222-2225
Bethesda, MD 20892   TTY: 800-222-4225
                                      niaic@nia.nih.gov
                                      www.nia.nih.gov

Seeks to understand the nature of aging, and to extend healthy, ac-
tive years of life. Free resources are available on topics such as
Alzheimer's & dimentia, caregiving, cognitive heath, end of life
care, and more.
Richard J. Hodes MD, Director
Marie A. Bernard, MD, Deputy Director

State Agencies & Associations

Alabama

759 Alzheimer's Association: North Alabama Chapter
4747 Bob Wallace Avenue SW   256-880-1575
Huntsville, AL 35805-4872   800-272-3900
                                      Fax: 256-880-8596
                                      cwhite2@alz.org
                                      www.alz.org
Al Wiggins, Chair
Courtney White, Local Contact

760 Alzheimer's Association: Southeast Alabama Chapter
PO Box 609   334-677-6799
Dothan, AL 36302   800-272-3900
                                      Fax: 334-671-3715
                                      www.alz.org
Kay Jones, Executive Director

761 Alzheimer's Association: Southwest Alabama Chapter
PO Box 9272   334-660-5661
Mobile, AL 36691   800-272-3900
                                      Fax: 334-660-5667
                                      www.alz.org
Bunnie Sutton, Executive Director

Alaska

762 Alzheimer's Disease Resource Agency of Alaska
1750 Abbott Road   907-561-3313
Anchorage, AK 99507   800-272-3900
                                      Fax: 907-561-3315
                                      dnobre@alzalaska.org
                                      www.alz.org
Jackie Brunton, President
Debbie Newsham, Vice President

Arizona

763 Alzheimer's Association: Desert Southwest Chapter
1028 E McDowell Road   602-528-0545
Phoenix, AZ 85006-2622   800-272-3900
                                      Fax: 602-528-0546
                                      deborah.schaus@alz.org
                                      www.alz.org
Serving the state of Arizona and Southern Nevada offices in Phoe-
nix, Tucson, Sun City, Prescott and Las Vegas.
Deborah Schaus, Executive Director
Dawn Boeck, Development Assistant

764 Alzheimer's Association: Northern Arizona
225 Grove Avenue   928-771-9257
Prescott, AZ 86301-2911   800-272-3900
                                      Fax: 520-771-9297
                                      pwinkels@alz.org
                                      www.alz.org
Don Connell, Regional Director
Patty Winkels, Local Contact

765 Alzheimer's Association: Northern Nevada
225 Grove Avenue   928-771-9257
Prescott, AZ 86301   800-272-3900
                                      Fax: 520-771-9297
                                      pwinkels@alz.org
                                      www.alz.org
Meg Fenzi, Regional Director
Patty Winkels, Local Contact

766 Alzheimer's Association: Southern Arizona
5132 East Pima Street 520-322-6601
Tucson, AZ 85712 800-272-3900
Fax: 520-322-6739
kraach@alz.org
www.alz.org

Tormay Newman, Director
Kelly Raach, Local Contact

767 Alzheimer's Association: Southern Arizona Region
3003 S Country Club Road 520-322-6601
Tucson, AZ 85713 800-272-3900
Fax: 520-322-6739
kraach@alz.org
www.alz.org

Heriberto Contreras, Regional Director
Kelly Raach, Local Contact

Arkansas

768 Alzheimer's Arkansas Programs and Services
400 President Clinton Ave 501-265-0027
Little Rock, AR 72205 800-272-3900
Fax: 501-227-6303
sdavis@alz.org
www.alz.org

Phyllis Watkins, Executive Director
Susie Davis, Local Contact

769 Alzheimer's Association: Western Arkansas Chapter
121 Riverfront Drive 479-426-5541
Fort Smith, AR 72901-3454 800-272-3900
Fax: 479-782-3185
sdavis@alz.org
www.alz.org

Rebecca Freeman, Executive Director
Susie Davis, Local Contact

California

770 Alzheimer's Association San Diego/Imperial Chapter
6632 Convoy Court 858-966-3319
San Diego, CA 92111 800-272-3900
Fax: 858-492-4406
walksandiego@alz.org
www.alz.org

The leading voluntary health organization in Alzheimer care, support and research. The mission is to eliminate Alzheimer's disease through the advancement of research; to provide and enhance care and support for all affected; to advocate for policy change; and to reduce the risk of dementia through the promotion of brain health.
Lisa Bruner, Executive Director
Shelita Weinfield, Local Contact

771 Alzheimer's Association: California Central Chapter: Ventura County Office
80 North Wood Road 80 - 4 - 60
Camarillo, CA 93010 800-272-3900
Fax: 805-485-4767
www.alz.org

The local chapter of the National Alzheimer's Association. The chapter stands by people with Alzheimer's disease, their families and professional caregivers through the following programs and services: a telephone help line, support groups, respite grants.
Norma Featherston, Area Director
Carol Swinney, Office Manager

772 Alzheimer's Association: Greater Sacramento
11th St. & N St. 916-930-9080
Sacramento, CA 95814 800-272-3900
Fax: 916-930-9085
estone@alz.org
www.alz.org

Mary Gillon MPA, Regional Director
Erin Stone, Local Contact

773 Alzheimer's Association: Greater North Valley Chapter
1000 Woodland Ave 530-895-9661
Chico, CA 95928-3148 800-272-3900
Fax: 530-872-7470
swatroba@alz.org
www.alz.org

Herb Williams, President
Suzanne Watroba, Local Contact

774 Alzheimer's Association: Los Angeles Chapter
133 N Sunol Drive 323-930-6228
Los Angeles, CA 90063-5017 800-272-3900
Fax: 323-938-1036
bwelch@alz.org
www.alz.org

Earl Greinetz, President
Brian Welch, Local Contact

775 Alzheimer's Association: Monterey County Chapter
5 Custom House Plaza 831-647-9890
Monterey, CA 93940-5337 800-272-3900
Fax: 831-655-9241
janderson@alz.org
www.alz.org

Herb Williams, President
Joy Anderson, Local Contact

776 Alzheimer's Association: North Bay Chapter
4340 Redwood Highway 415-472-4340
San Rafael, CA 94903 800-272-3900
Fax: 415-472-4350
info@alznorcal.org
www.alz.org

Provides a continuum of services for Alzheimer's families, education and referral in Marin, Sonoma and Napa counties. To provide leadership and to eliminate Alzheimer's disease through the advancement of research while enhancing care and support services.
Herb Williams, President
Eduardo Salaz, Vice President

777 Alzheimer's Association: Orange County Chapter
17771 Cowan 949-955-9000
Irvine, CA 92614 800-272-3900
Fax: 949-757-3700
helpoc@alz.org
www.alz.org

Dedicated to providing services, education and advocacy for individuals, families and the community affected by Alzheimer's disease and related memory disorders. Services include: 24/7 help line, support groups, family orientation program and care managers.
Norma Castellano, Program Specialist
Bobbie Babbage, Family Services Coordinator

778 Alzheimer's Association: Riverside/San Bernardino Counties Chapter
5900 Wilshire Boulevard 323-930-6228
Los Angeles, CA 90036 800-272-3900
Fax: 323-938-1036
bwelch@alz.org
www.alz.org

Help line, support groups, information and education for caregivers and community.
400 Members
Earl Greinetz, President
Brian Welch, Local Contact

779 Alzheimer's Association: San Francisco Bay Area Chapter
1060 La Avenida 650-962-8111
Mountain View, CA 94043 800-272-3900
Fax: 650-962-9644
info@alznorcal.org
www.alz.org

Herb Williams, President
Eduardo Salaz, Vice President

780 Alzheimer's Association: Santa Barbara Central Coast Chapter
3400 Calle Real   805-892-4259
Santa Barbara, CA 93105-8820   800-272-3900
                                                    Fax: 805-892-4250
                                                    gbolton@alz.org
                                                    www.alz.org
The Alzheimer's Association California Central Coast Chapter
serves families caring for people with Alzheimer's disease and re-
lated dementia throughout San Luis Obispo, Santa Barbara and
Ventura Counties, offering a variety of educational and supportive
programs.
Rhonda Spiegel, Executive Director
Genny Bolton, Local Contact

781 Alzheimer's Association: Santa Cruz County Chapter
1777-A Capitola Road   831-464-9982
Santa Cruz, CA 95062   800-272-3900
                                                    Fax: 831-464-8930
                                                    info@alznorcal.org
                                                    www.alz.org

Herb Williams, President
Eduardo Salaz, Vice President

Colorado

782 Alzheimer's Association: Greater Grand Junction Area Chapter
2232 N 7th Street   970-256-1274
Grand Junction, CO 81501   800-272-3900
                                                    Fax: 970-256-0569
                                                    www.alz.org
Linda Mitchell, President/CEO
Lisa Miller, Local Contact

783 Alzheimer's Association: Rocky Mountain Chapter
455 Sherman Street   303-813-1669
Denver, CO 80203   800-272-3900
                                                    Fax: 303-813-1670
                                                    jlorentz@alz.org
                                                    www.alz.org
Linda Mitchell, President/CEO
Jill Lorentz, Local Contact

784 American Homes for the Aging: Western
5010 Aspen Drive   303-795-5465
Littleton, CO 80123   Fax: 303-794-0487
Part of the national association representing retirement communities, nursing homes and community services for the elderly.

Connecticut

785 Alzheimer's Association: Connecticut Chapter
99 Trinity Street   860-956-9560
Hartford, CT 06106   800-272-3900
                                                    Fax: 860-956-9590
                                                    walkhelpct@alz.org
                                                    www.alz.org
Works with all individuals and family members affected by Alzhei-
mer's disease and related disorders; ensures humane systems of
care and support and promotes research efforts to treat and cure
Alzheimer's disease.
Christopher Rupp, Chairman
Daniel P Finke, Treasurer

786 Alzheimer's Association: South Central Connecticut Chapter
2911 Dixwell Avenue   203-230-1777
Hamden, CT 06518   800-272-3900
                                                    Fax: 203-230-1712
                                                    www.alz.org
Patricia Clark, Executive Director

Delaware

787 Alzheimer's Association: Delaware Chapter
240 N James Street   302-633-4420
Newport, DE 19804   800-272-3900
                                                    Fax: 302-633-4494
                                                    Wendy.Campbell@alz.org
                                                    www.alz.org
Wendy L Campbell, President
Theresa Haenn, Vice President Development

District of Columbia

788 Alzheimer's Association: Greater Washington DC Chapter
2524 Pensylvania Avenue Southeast   703-359-4440
Washington, DC 20020   800-272-3900
                                                    Fax: 202-483-4164
                                                    alzwalknca@alz.org
                                                    www.alz.org
Help line-telephone referral support groups, caregiver education,
respite services. We have three offices serving DC and surrounding Maryland counties.
Abigail Reinecker, Local Contact

Florida

789 Alzheimer's Association: Broward County Chapter
201 E Sample Road   800-861-7826
Deerfield Beach, FL 33407   800-272-3900
                                                    Fax: 954-786-1538
                                                    barbara.grasch@alz.org
                                                    www.alz.org
Barbara Grasch, Director of Program Services
Ellen Brown, CEO

790 Alzheimer's Association: East Central Florida Chapter
Wickham Road   407-951-7992
Melbourne, FL 32935   800-272-3900
                                                    Fax: 407-729-8044
                                                    jgiovanni@alz.org
                                                    www.alz.org
Joan Giovanni, Local Contact

791 Alzheimer's Association: Florida Gulf Coast Chapter
9365 US Highway 19 N   727-578-2558
Pinellas Park, FL 33782   800-272-3900
                                                    Fax: 727-578-2286
                                                    milnel@alzflgulf.org
                                                    www.alz.org
Provides information and services to families and professionals
dealing with memory related disorders.
Gloria JT Smith, President/CEO
Paul Anderson, Vice President Finance

792 Alzheimer's Association: Greater Miami Chapter
501 Marlins Way   305-891-6228
Miami, FL 33125   800-272-3900
                                                    Fax: 305-751-5551
                                                    snewman@alz.org
                                                    www.alz.org
Reni Rizzo, Community Education Coordinator
Sharon Newman, Local Contact

793 Alzheimer's Association: Greater Orlando Area Chapter
Ampitheatre at 300 Robinson St., Do   407-951-7992
Orlando, FL 32801   800-272-3900
                                                    Fax: 407-228-4201
                                                    jgiovanni@alz.org
                                                    www.alz.org
Stu Gaines, Chair
Joan Giovanni, Local Contact

794 Alzheimer's Association: Greater Palm Beach Area Chapter
600 N Congress Avenue   561-478-3120
Delray Beach, FL 33445   800-272-3900
                                                    Fax: 561-278-4910
                                                    www.alz.org

795 Alzheimer's Association: Northeast Florida
4237 Salisbury Rd   904-281-9077
Jacksonville, FL 32216   800-272-3900
                                                    Fax: 866-281-9078
                                                    mdrinks@alz.org
                                                    www.alz.org
Michelle Drinks, Local Contact

796 Alzheimer's Association: Northern Central Florida Chapter
1001 NW 34th St
Gainesville, FL 32605
904-281-9077
800-272-3900
Fax: 352-372-2038
mdrinks@alz.org
www.alz.org

Michelle Drinks, Local Contact
Tish Sheesley, CEO

797 Alzheimer's Association: Northwest Florida Chapter
119 Hollywood Boulevard
Ft. Walton Beach, FL 32548
850-302-0581
800-272-3900
Fax: 850-302-0583
www.alz.org

798 Alzheimer's Association: Southwest Florida Chapter
4075 Tamiami
Port Charlotte, FL 33952
941-235-7470
800-272-3900
Fax: 941-235-7473
www.alz.org

799 Alzheimer's Association: Tampa Bay Chapter
601 N Old Coachman Rd
Clearwater, FL 33765
727-259-2317
800-272-3900
Fax: 941-380-5701
farinasr@alzflgulf.org
www.alz.org

Gloria JT Smith, President/CEO
Rachel Farinas, Local Contact

800 Alzheimer's Association: Volusia/Flagler Branch
111 N Frederick Avenue
Daytona Beach, FL 32114-5126
407-951-7992
800-272-3900
Fax: 386-238-8293
jgiovanni@alz.org
www.alz.org

Joan Giovanni, Local Contact

801 Alzheimer's Association: West Central Florida Chapter
PO Box 2070
New Port Richey, FL 34656-2070
813-848-8888
800-272-3900
Fax: 813-849-6124
www.alz.org

Georgia

802 Alzheimer's Association: Atlanta Chapter
1925 Century Boulevard
Atlanta, GA 30345-4021
404-728-6066
800-272-3900
Fax: 404-636-9768
rrotunda@alz.org
www.alz.org

Bennett Watts, Chair
Robyn Rotunda, Local Contact

803 Alzheimer's Association: Augusta Chapter
1899 Central Avenue
Augusta, GA 30904-5755
706-731-9060
800-272-3900
Fax: 706-731-9099
kim.franklin@alz.org
www.alz.org

Bennett Watts, Chair
Bruce Flechter, Treasurer

804 Alzheimer's Association: Central Georgia Chapter
277 Martin Luther King Jr Boulevard
Macon, GA 31201-3498
478-746-7050
800-272-3900
Fax: 478-746-6679
kim.franklin@alz.org
www.alz.org

Bennett Watts, Chair
Bruce Flechter, Treasurer

805 Alzheimer's Association: Greater Columbus Chapter
5900 River Road
Columbus, GA 31904-0185
706-327-6838
800-272-3900
Fax: 706-494-0533
cvogler@alz.org
www.alz.org

Bennett Watts, Chair
Christina Vogler, Local Contact

806 Alzheimer's Association: Greater Georgia Chapter
1925 Century Boulevard
Atlanta, GA 30345-4021
404-728-6066
800-272-3900
Fax: 404-636-9768
rrotunda@alz.org
www.alz.org

Bennett Watts, Chair
Robyn Rotunda, Local Contact

807 Alzheimer's Association: Southeast Georgia Chapter
201 Television Circle
Savannah, GA 31406
912-920-2231
800-272-3900
Fax: 912-921-7960
dheddendorf@alz.org
www.alz.org

Deborah Heddendorf, Local Contact

808 Alzheimer's Association: Southwest Georgia Chapter
1512-1 Gillionville Road
Albany, GA 31707
229-388-8219
800-272-3900
Fax: 229-888-2620
dphillips@alz.org
www.alz.org

Maggie Keenan, Office Volunteer
Dan Phillips, Local Contact

Hawaii

809 Alzheimer's Association: Honolulu Chapter
1050 Ala Moana Boulevard
Honolulu, HI 96814
808-591-2771
800-272-3900
Fax: 808-591-9071
ebatalon@alz.org
www.alz.org

Eric Batalon, Local Contact
Chris Shirai, Chairman

810 Alzheimer's Association: West Hawaii Chapter
PO Box 390247
Kailua Kona, HI 96739-0247
808-591-2771
800-272-3900
Fax: 808-322-0008
ebatalon@alz.org
www.alz.org

Eric Batalon, Local Contact

Idaho

811 Alzheimer's Association: Greater Idaho Chapter
1111 S Orchard
Boise, ID 83705-2878
208-384-1788
800-272-3900
Fax: 208-385-7191
suzette.albers-tunnell@alz.org
www.alz.org

Suzette Albers-Tunne, Executive Director

812 Alzheimer's Association: Northern Idaho Chapter
2003 Kootenai Health Way
Coeur D Alene, ID 83814
208-666-2996
800-272-3900
Fax: 509-473-3389
pchristo@alz.org
www.alz.org

PJ Christo, Outreach Coordinator
Joel Loiacono, Executive Director

Illinois

813 Alzheimer's Association: Central Illinois Chapter
606 W Glen Avenue
Peoria, IL 61614-4831
309-681-1100
800-272-3900
Fax: 309-681-1101
kgabbert@alz.org
www.alz.org

Nikki Vulgaris, Executive Director
Kari Gabbert, Local Contact

814 Alzheimer's Association: East Central Illinois Chapter
303 N. Hershey
Bloomington, IL 61704-7337
217-351-1726
800-272-3900
Fax: 217-351-2161
www.alz.org

Provides information, support, and referral services to families and individuals facing Alzheimer's disease. Includes newsletter, support groups, and education.

815 Alzheimer's Association: Four Rivers Chapter
401 N Wall Street
Kankakee, IL 60901

815-936-0464
800-272-3900
Fax: 815-936-9363
www.alz.org

816 Alzheimer's Association: Greater Illinois Chapter
4709 Golf Road
Skokie, IL 60076-1260

847-933-2413
800-272-3900
Fax: 847-933-2417
info@alz.org
www.alz.org

817 Alzheimer's Association: Greater Illinois Chapter: Carbondale Office
402 E Plaza Drive
Carterville, IL 62918-1429

618-985-1095
800-272-3900
Fax: 618-457-7830
GI.Chapter@alz.org
www.alz.org

Jill Schoenborn, Coordinator Outreach & Development

818 Alzheimer's Association: Land of Lincoln Chapter
South Second Street & Southwind Roa
Springfield, IL 62703-4833

217-801-9352
800-272-3900
Fax: 217-726-5185
tarnold@alz.org
www.alz.org

Jane Field, Office Manager
Tina Arnold, Local Contact

819 American Homes for the Aging: Midwest Regional Office
911 N Elm Street
Hinsdale, IL 60521-3641

630-323-6755
800-272-3900
Fax: 630-325-0749
www.alz.org

Regional office of the AHA, a national professional association of nonprofit nursing homes, retirement communities and homes for the aging.

Indiana

820 Alzheimer's Association: Central Indiana Chapter
601 W. New York Street
Indianapolis, IN 46202-1816

317-575-9620
800-272-3900
Fax: 317-582-0669
IndianaWalk@alz.org
www.alz.org

Heather Allen Hershberger, Executive Director
Leslie Bush, Local Contact

821 Alzheimer's Association: Northern Indiana Chapter
922 E Colfax Avenue
S Bend, IN 46617-3112

57 - 2 - 41
800-272-3900
Fax: 57 - 2 - 42
www.alz.org

Iowa

822 Alzheimer's Association: Big Sioux Chapter
401 Gordon Drive
Sioux City, IA 51101-3716

712-279-5802
800-272-3900
Fax: 712-277-8076
tschroeder@alz.org
www.alz.org

Kim McCormick, Executive Director
Terri Schroeder, Local Contact

823 Alzheimer's Association: East Central Iowa Chapter
1570 42nd Street NE
Cedar Rapids, IA 52402

319-294-9699
800-272-3900
Fax: 319-294-0068
amiller2@alz.org
www.alz.org

Kelly Hauer, Executive Director
Abbey Miller, Local Contact

824 Alzheimer's Association: Greater Iowa Chapter
1730 28th Street
W Des Moines, IA 50266

515-440-2722
800-272-3900
Fax: 515-440-6385
Carol.Sipfle@alz.org
www.alz.org

Carol Sipfle, Executive Director
Holly Bradford, Finance Director

825 Alzheimer's Association: Heart of Iowa Chapter
3915 Mortensen Road
Ames, IA 50014-7259

515-440-6383
800-272-3900
Fax: 515-292-0125
cmathany@alz.org
www.alz.org

Chantelle Mathany, Local Contact

826 Greater Iowa Chapter Alzheimer's Association Quadcity Office
736 Federal Street
Davenport, IA 52803-5750

563-324-1022
800-272-3900
Fax: 563-324-6267
Jerry.Schroeder@alz.org
www.alz.org

Jerry Schroeder, Program Specialist
Julie Seier, Community Relations Coordinator

Kansas

827 Alzheimer's Association: Heart of America Chapter
3846 W 75th Street
Prairie Village, KS 66208-4126

913-831-3888
800-272-3900
Fax: 913-831-1916
jan.horn@alz.org
www.alz.org

Debra R Brook, Executive Director
Michelle Niedens, Education Director

828 Alzheimer's Association: Sunflower Chapter
347 S Laura
Wichita, KS 67211-4109

316-267-7333
800-272-3900
Fax: 316-267-6369
lbelton@alz.org
www.alz.org

Marsha Hills, Executive Director
Lanette Belton, Local Contact

Kentucky

829 Alzheimer's Association: Lexington/ Bluegrass Chapter
465 E High Street
Lexington, KY 40507

859-266-5283
800-272-3900
Fax: 859-268-4764
amber.lakin@alz.org
www.alz.org

Debbie Lacy Goodman, VP Awareness & Community Relations
Amber Lakin, Local Contact

830 Alzheimer's Association: Louisville Chapter
6100 Dutchmans Lane
Louisville, KY 40205

502-451-4266
800-272-3900
Fax: 502-456-2701
wvogel@alz.org
www.alz.org

Teri Shirk, Chapter President & CEO
Whitney Vogel, Local Contact

Louisiana

831 Alzheimer's Association: Northeast/Central Louisiana Chapter
2300 Sycamore
Monroe, LA 71201

318-861-8680
800-272-3900
Fax: 318-998-7360
dhayes@alz.org
www.alz.org

Debbie Hayes, Local Contact

832 Alzheimer's Association: Greater New Orleans Chapter
DePaul Hospital

1040 Calhoun Street
New Orleans, LA 70118-5999

504-648-4084
800-272-3900
Fax: 504-648-0493
charrell@alz.org
www.alz.org

Chet Harrell, Local Contact

833 Alzheimer's Services of the Capital Area
3772 N Boulevard
Baton Rouge, LA 70806

225-334-7494
800-548-1211
Fax: 225-387-3664
info@alzbr.org
www.alzbr.org

The mission of Alzheimer's Services of the Capital Area is to provide education and support services to memory impaired individuals as well as caregivers and professionals; and to enhance community awareness of Alzheimer's disease and related disorders.
Barbara Auten, Executive Director

Maine

834 Alzheimer's Association: Maine Chapter
383 U.S. Route 1
Scarborough, ME 04074-2419

207-772-0115
800-272-3900
Fax: 207-289-3705
laurie.trenholm@alz.org
www.alz.org

Joy Heptner, Executive Director
Liz Weaver, Program Director

835 Maine Alzheimer's Care Center
154 Dresden Avenue
Gardiner, ME 04345

207-626-1770

Maryland

836 Alzheimer's Association: Central Maryland Chapter
1850 York Road
Timonium, MD 21093-5122

410-561-9099
800-272-3900
Fax: 410-561-3433
info.maryland@alz.org
www.alz.org

Cass Naugle, Executive Director
Teri Bennett, Helpline Coordinator

837 Alzheimer's Association: Eastern Shore Chapter
909 Progress Circle
Salisbury, MD 21804

410-543-1163
800-272-3900
Fax: 410-546-0184
dmagarelli@alz.org
www.alz.org

Cass Naugle, Executive Director
Damian Magarelli, Local Contact

838 Alzheimer's Association: Western Maryland Chapter
101 Clarke Pl.
Frederick, MD 21701

301-696-0315
800-272-3900
Fax: 301-696-9061
kweddle@alz.org
www.alz.org

To eliminate Alzheimer's disease through the advancement of research and to enhance care and support for individuals their families and caregivers.
Cathy Hanson, Program Coordinator
Kristen Weddle, Local Contact

Massachusetts

839 Alzheimer's Association: Massachusetts Chapter
311 Arsenal Street
Watertown, MA 02472

617-868-6718
800-272-3900
Fax: 617-868-6720
www.alz.org

Nonprofit, national, voluntary health organization dedicated to Alzheimer research and care. Provides 24 hour help line, support groups, a wanderers prevention program early stage patient programs, family educators, professional training, and advocacy.
James Wessle MBA, President & CEO
Betsy Fitzgerald-Cam, Vice President Communications

840 Alzheimer's Association: Western Regional Office: Massachusetts Chapter
264 Cottage Street
Springfield, MA 01104

413-787-1113
800-272-3900
Fax: 413-787-1109
www.alz.org

Nonprofit organization serving family and professional caregivers in seven counties in southwest Michigan. Provides information on Alzheimer's and other diseases, educational programs, resource libraries. Train-the-trainer agency referral, autopsy liaison, and other services.
Marcia McKen Med, Manager
Annie Clattenburg, Coordinator Administrative Services

Michigan

841 Alzheimer's Association: East Central Michigan Chapter
G-3287 Beecher Road
Flint, MI 48503

810-720-2791
800-272-3900
Fax: 810-720-3040
www.alz.org

842 Alzheimer's Association: Greater Michigan Chapter
20300 Civic Center Drive
Southfield, MI 48076

248-351-0280
800-272-3900
Fax: 248-351-0417
www.alz.org

A national network of chapters, is the largest national voluntary health organization committed to finding a cure for Alzheimer's and helping those affected by the disease. Provides a wide range of services and programs for Alzheimer's and other dementia patients for their families and for the general public.

843 Alzheimer's Association: Greater Michigan Chapter: Upper Peninsula Region
1420 Pine Street
Marquette, MI 49855-4521

906-228-3910
800-272-3900
Fax: 906-228-2455
TTY: 877-204-6924
ralmen@alz.org
www.alz.org

Pamela Parkkila, Director
Ruth Almen, Local Contact

844 Alzheimer's Association: Michigan Great Lakes Chapter: West Shore Region
1740 Village Drive
Muskegon, MI 49442-5546

734-475-7043
800-272-3900
Fax: 231-780-1494
mglcwalk@alz.org
www.alz.org

Providing caregiver support groups a help line informational materials community education and a quarterly newsletter.
Barb Betts, Program Coordinator
Stephanie Barnhill, Local Contact

845 Alzheimer's Association: Mid-Michigan Chapter
4604 N Saginaw Road
Midland, MI 48640

989-839-9910
800-272-3900
Fax: 989-839-5910
TTY: 877-204-6924
boneill@alz.org
www.alz.org

Dawn Spicer, Director
Betty O'Neill, Local Contact

846 Alzheimer's Association: Northeast Michigan Chapter
526 W Chisholm St
Alpena, MI 49707

989-356-4087
800-272-3900
Fax: 989-354-7879
sruetz@alz.org
www.alz.org

Shawn Ruetz, Local Contact

847 **Alzheimer's Association: Northwest Michigan Chapter**
921 W. 11th. Street — 616-459-4558
Traverse City, MI 49864 — 800-272-3900
Fax: 231-922-1584
sruetz@alz.org
www.alz.org

Shawn Ruetz, Local Contact

Minnesota

848 **Alzheimer's Association: Minnesota/Dakotas**
1 Twins Way — 952-830-0512
Minneapolis, MN 55403 — 800-272-3900
Fax: 952-830-0513
mnnd-walk@alz.org
www.alz.org

Mary Birchard, Executive Director
Libby Wilhelmy, Local Contact

Mississippi

849 **Alzheimer's Association: Mississippi Chapter**
1900 Dunbarton Drive — 601-987-0020
Jackson, MS 39216 — 800-272-3900
Fax: 601-987-9020
rruello@alz.org
www.alz.org

Barb Dobrosky, Program Director
Rachel Ruello, Local Contact

850 **Alzheimer's Foundation of the South: Mississippi Division**
PO Box 2394 — 228-867-6251
Gulfport, MS 39503 — 800-272-3900
Fax: 228-864-8843
alzms@cs.com
www.alz.org

Rosemary Hudgins, Executive Director

Missouri

851 **Alzheimer's Association: Mid-Missouri Chapter**
2400 Bluff Creek Drive — 573-443-8665
Columbia, MO 65201 — 800-272-3900
Fax: 573-499-9701
cbaker@alz.org
www.alz.org

Linda Newkirk, Executive Director
Chris Baker, Local Contact

852 **Alzheimer's Association: Northwest Missouri-Chapter**
10th and Faraon — 816-364-4467
St. Joseph, MO 64502-1241 — 800-272-3900
Fax: 816-364-2553
brenda.gregg@alz.org
www.alz.org

853 **Alzheimer's Association: Southwest Missouri Chapter**
1500 S Glenstone — 417-886-2199
Springfield, MO 65804 — 800-272-3900
Fax: 417-886-0337
nreed@alz.org
www.alz.org

Rebecca Argilagos, President/CEO
Nate Reed, Local Contact

854 **Alzheimer's Association: St. Louis Chapter**
700 Clark Avenue — 314-801-0465
Saint Louis, MO 63102-3214 — 800-272-3900
Fax: 314-432-3824
stlwalksupport@alz.org
www.alz.org

Joan D'Ambrose, President
Alyssa Vorhies, Local Contact

Montana

855 **Alzheimer's Association: Greater Billings Area Chapter**
2100 South Shiloh Road — 406-252-3053
Billings, MT 59101 — 800-272-3900
Fax: 406-252-2933
sshannon@alz.org
www.alz.org

Kelly Donovan, President
Sharon Shannon, Local Contact

Nebraska

856 **Alzheimer's Association: Great Plains Chap ter**
1500 S. 70th St — 402-420-2540
Lincoln, NE 68506 — 800-272-3900
mfeit@alz.org
www.alz.org

The Alzheimer's Association of the Great Plains is dedicated to supporting those with Alzheimer's disease and their families and friends through specialized programs and services, educating families, communities, and health professionals about Alzheimer's disease.
Karen Noel, President/CEO
Mark Feit, Local Contact

857 **Alzheimer's Association: Lincoln/Greater Nebraska Chapter**
1500 S. 70th St. — 402-420-2540
Lincoln, NE 68506 — 800-272-3900
Fax: 402-420-2541
mfeit@alz.org
www.alz.org

Karen Noel, President/CEO
Mark Feit, Local Contact

858 **Alzheimer's Association: Omaha/Eastern Nebraska Chapter**
3220 Farnam St — 402-502-4301
Omaha, NE 68131-2167 — 800-272-3900
Fax: 402-502-7001
cenoviso@alz.org
www.alz.org

Duane Gross, President and CEO
Cathy Enoviso, Local Contact

Nevada

859 **Alzheimer's Association: Northern Nevada Chapter**
1301 Cordone Avenue — 775-786-8061
Reno, NV 89502-6362 — 800-272-3900
Fax: 775-786-1920
info@alznorcal.org
www.alz.org

Herb Williams, President
Eduardo Salaz, Vice President

860 **Alzheimer's Association: Southern Nevada Chapter**
5190 S Valley View Boulevard — 702-248-2770
Las Vegas, NV 89118-6062 — 800-272-3900
Fax: 702-248-2771
achavez@alz.org
www.alz.org

Luis Carrillo, Regional Director
Albert Chavez, Local Contact

New Hampshire

861 **Alzheimer's Association of Vermont and New Hampshire**
10 Ferry Street — 603-226-5868
Concord, NH 03301-5004 — 800-272-3900
Fax: 603-225-8126
www.alz.org

Robbie Nicol, Chair
Robert Dowd, First Vice Chair

862 Alzheimer's Association: Greater New Jersey Chapter
400 Morris Avenue   973-586-4300
Denville, NJ 07834   800-272-3900
                                         Fax: 973-586-4342
                                             www.alz.org
Provides programs and services to individuals with Alzheimer's
disease, their families and caregivers, including education and
training, support groups, a toll free telephone help line and respite
assistance.

863 Alzheimer's Association: South Jersey Chapter
3 Eves Drive   856-797-1212
Marlton, NJ 08053   800-272-3900
                                         Fax: 609-784-8486
                                    Wendy.Campbell@alz.org
                                             www.alz.org
Wendy L Campbell, President & CEO
Theresa Haenn, Vice President Development

New Mexico

864 Alzheimer's Association: New Mexico Chapter
9500 Montgomery Boulevard NE   505-266-4473
Albuquerque, NM 87111   800-272-3900
                                         Fax: 505-266-0108
                                         nlawrie@alz.org
                                             www.alz.org
Agnes Vallejos, Executive Director
Nika Lawrie, Local Contact

New York

865 Alzheimer's Association: Sullivan/Delaware Chapter
PO Box 911   941-794-3774
Monticello, NY 12701   800-272-3900
                                             www.alz.org

866 Alzheimer's Association: Central New York Chapter
441 W Kirkpatrick Street   315-472-4201
Syracuse, NY 13204-1361   800-272-3900
                                         Fax: 315-472-4206
                                         gfletcher@alz.org
                                             www.alz.org
Larry Malfitano, President
Grant Fletcher, Local Contact

**867 Alzheimer's Association: Hudson Valley/ Rockland/Westchester
NY Chapter**
2 Jefferson Plaza   845-471-2655
Poughkeepsie, NY 12601-4027   800-272-3900
                                         Fax: 845-471-8960
                                  info@alzhudsonvalley.org
                                             www.alz.org
Elaine Sproat, President & CEO
Meg Boyce, Director of Programs & Services

868 Alzheimer's Association: Long Island Chapter
3281 Veterans Memorial Highway   631-580-5100
Ronkonkoma, NY 11779-3521   800-272-3900
                                         Fax: 631-580-3100
                                     Info@alzheimersli.org
                                             www.alz.org
Voluntary health agency that provides care and consultation, information and referral, education, national safe return program and
support groups to individuals with Alzheimer's, their families
and/or caregivers.
Mary Ann Malack-Ragona, Executive Director/CEO
Linda Cody, Director of Development

869 Alzheimer's Association: New York City Chapter
360 Lexington Avenue   646-744-2900
New York, NY 10017   800-272-3900
                                         Fax: 212-490-6037
                                      helpline@alznyc.org
                                         www.alz.org/nyc
Lou-Ellen Barkan, President/CEO
Jed A. Levine, Executive Vice President

870 Alzheimer's Association: Northeastern New York Chapter
4 Pine West Plaza   518-867-4999
Albany, NY 12205-2083   800-272-3900
                                         Fax: 518-867-4997
                                         infoneny@alz.org
                                             www.alz.org
Regional affiliate of national association. Works to educate and
support families, while raising funds in support of research.
Paul A Wajda, Chair
Warren E Garling, Vice Chair

871 Alzheimer's Association: Putnam County Chapter
Robin Hill Corporate Park
15 Mount Ebo Road S   845-278-0343
Brewster, NY 10509-2164   800-272-3900
                                  info@alzhudsonvalley.org
                                             www.alz.org
Stuart Greif, Program Development Specialist

872 Alzheimer's Association: Rochester Chapter
85 Adams Street   585-760-5472
Rochester, NY 14608   800-272-3900
                                         Fax: 585-760-5401
                                     rochesterwalk@alz.org
                                             www.alz.org
Chris Lacey, Local Contact
Judy Lemoncelli, Local Contact

873 Alzheimer's Association: Southern Tier Chapter
401 Hayes Avenue   607-785-7852
Endicott, NY 13760-5421   800-272-3900
                                         Fax: 607-785-4004
                                       alzcny@alzcny.org
                                             www.alz.org
L Jane Hudreck, Regional Director

874 Alzheimer's Association: Western New York Chapter
2805 Wehrle Drive   716-626-0600
Williamsville, NY 14421   800-272-3900
                                         Fax: 717-626-2255
                                  Donna.McKenzie@alz.org~
                                             www.alz.org
David Cascio, President
Linda Sabo, Executive Director

875 Alzheimer's Foundation of Staten Island
789 Post Avenue   718-667-7110
Staten Island, NY 10310-6427   877-574-7068
                                         Fax: 718-667-8431
Not-for-profit health and human services organization, serving
people with Alzheimer's disease and related dementias.
Leilani Joven Pelletie, Executive Director
David Cascio, President

North Carolina

876 Alzheimer's Association: Eastern North Carolina Chapter
1305 Navaho Dr.   919-832-3732
Raleigh, NC 27609   800-272-3900
                                         Fax: 919-832-7989
                                       awatkins@alznc.org
                                             www.alz.org
Dedicated to providing program services education for patients,
families and professional caregivers, advocacy and research.
Alice Watkins, Executive Director
Rita Bhan, Developmental Director

877 Alzheimer's Association: Western North Car olina Chapter
3800 Shamrock Drive   704-532-7390
Charlotte, NC 28215   800-272-3900
                                         Fax: 704-532-5421
                                         infonc@alz.org
                                             www.alz.org
A nonprofit voluntary organization dedicated to improving the
quality of life for those with Alzheimer's and their families
through a broad range of programs, including patient and family
services, education, advocacy and support of research through
national programs.
Beth Croom MA, Director of Programs/Education
Teresa Hoover, Program Associate/Helpline Coordinator

North Dakota

878 Alzheimer's Association: Fargo/Moorhead Regional Center
5225 31st Ave South
Fargo, ND 58104

701-277-9757
800-272-3900
Fax: 701-277-9785
traie.dockter@alz.org
www.alz.org

Gretchen Dobervich, Regional Center Director
Traie Dockter, Local Contact

Ohio

879 Alzheimer's Association: Canton Chapter
408 Ninth St. SW
Canton, OH 44707

800-272-3900
Fax: 330-996-7757
geoachl@alz.org
www.alz.org

Pam Schuellerman, Executive Director
Andy Junn, Development Director

880 Alzheimer's Association: Central Ohio Chapter
330 Huntington Park Lane
Columbus, OH 43215-2112

614-442-2014
800-272-3900
Fax: 614-457-6634
jsega@alz.org
www.alz.org

Kenneth Strong, Executive Director
Jennifer Monroe-Sega, Local Contact

881 Alzheimer's Association: Clark/Champaign, Miami Valley Chapter
1700 S. Patterson Blvd.
Dayton, OH 45409-2620

937-291-3332
800-272-3900
Fax: 937-323-9259
walkmiamivalley@alz.org
www.alz.org

Judy Turner, Executive Director
Marie McLaughlin, Local Contact

882 Alzheimer's Association: Cleveland Area Chapter
23215 Commerce Park Drive
Beachwood, OH 44122-1013

216-721-8457
800-272-3900
Fax: 216-831-8585
www.alz.org

Nancy B Udelson, Executive Director
Robert Bazzarelli, President

883 Alzheimer's Association: Greater Cincinnati Chapter
720 E. Pete Rose Way
Cincinnati, OH 45202-1742

513-721-4284
800-272-3900
Fax: 513-345-8446
diana.bosse@alz.org
www.alz.org

Committed to support education, advocacy and research on behalf of those affected by Alzheimer's disease.
Clarissa Rentz, Executive Director
Diana Bosse, Local Contact

884 Alzheimer's Association: Greater East Ohio Chapter: Greater Youngstown Office
3695B Boardman-Canfield Rd
Canfield, OH 44406-0321

330-533-3300
800-272-3900
Fax: 330-533-3307
geoachl@alz.org
www.alz.org

Pam Schuellerman, Executive Director
Andy Junn, Development Director

885 Alzheimer's Association: Miami Valley Chapter
1700 S. Patterson Blvd.
Dayton, OH 45409-3661

937-291-3332
800-272-3900
Fax: 937-291-0463
walkmiamivalley@alz.org
www.alz.org

Judy Turner, Executive Director
Marie McLaughlin, Local Contact

886 Alzheimer's Association: Northwest Ohio Chapter
75 N. Main St.
Mansfield, OH 44902-7906

419-537-1999
800-272-3900
Fax: 419-522-5318
nvargas@alz.org
www.alz.org

Voluntary health organization committed to finding a cure for Alzheimer's and helping those affected by the disease.
Michael Malone, President
Nick Vargas, Local Contact

887 Alzheimer's Association: West Central Ohio Chapter
200 East High Street
Lima, OH 45801-3468

419-537-1999
800-272-3900
Fax: 419-222-6212
tschindler@alz.org
www.alz.org

A voluntary health agency providing information Alzheimer's disease and related dementias, serving 7 counties: Allen, Auglaize, Hancock, Hardin, Mercer, Putnam and Van Wert. Offers support group meetings in each county and provides a toll-free help line.
Salli Bollin, Executive Director
Toni Schindler, Local Contact

Oklahoma

888 Alzheimer's Association: Oklahoma Chapter
2448 E. 81st Street
Tulsa, OK 74137-7804

918-392-5012
800-272-3900
Fax: 918-481-7745
TTY: 800-493-1411
shauptman@alz.org
www.alz.org

Dedicated to serving Alzheimer's patients, their families, and caregivers through education, outreach, programs, support services and public advocacy.
Judi A Ver Hoef, President/CEO
Sarah Hauptam, Local Contact

Oregon

889 Alzheimer's Association: Columbia-Willamet Chapter
1940 North Victory Boulevard
Portland, OR 97217-1610

503-416-0209
800-272-3900
Fax: 503-413-6909
kara.busick@alz.org
www.alz.org

Judy McKellar, Executive Director
Kara Busick, Local Contact

890 Alzheimer's Association: Cascade/Coast Chapter
100 Day Island Road
Eugene, OR 97401

503-416-0209
800-272-3900
Fax: 541-345-5797
kara.busick@alz.org
www.alz.org

Judy Clarke, Vice President
Kara Busick, Local Contact

891 Alzheimer's Association: Mary's Peak Chapter
1925 NW Circle Boulevard
Corvallis, OR 97330-1312

541-752-1012
800-272-3900
Fax: 541-757-1395
www.alz.org

892 Alzheimer's Association: Mid-Willamette Chapter
PO Box 12768
Salem, OR 97309-0768

503-371-7728
800-272-3900
Fax: 503-571-9842
midwillamatte@alz.org
www.alz.org

Pennsylvania

893 Alzheimer's Association: Delaware Valley Chapter
1 Citizens Bank Way
Philadelphia, PA 19148
215-561-2919
800-272-3900
Fax: 215-561-4663
keely.boyle@alz.org
www.alz.org

Wendy L Campbell, President
Keely Boyle, Local Contact

894 Alzheimer's Association: Greater Pennsylvania Chapter: SW Regional Office
Landmarks Building, 100 Station
Pittsburgh, PA 15219
412-261-5040
800-272-3900
Fax: 412-471-2722
mlong@alz.org
www.alz.org

Education training, information, support groups, free newsletter, telephone support, services to caregivers and diagnosed individuals, as well as professionals.
Diane Balcom, President/CEO
Mellisa Long, Local Contact

895 Alzheimer's Association: Greater Mid-Ohio
1100 Liberty Avenue
Pittsburgh, PA 15222
412-261-5040
800-272-3900
Fax: 412-471-2722
mlong@alz.org
www.alz.org

Education training information support groups free newsletter telephone support services to caregivers and diagnosed individuals as well as professionals.
Bob LeRoy, President/CEO
Mellisa Long, Local Contact

896 Alzheimer's Association: Laurel Mountains Chapter
194 Donohoe Road
Greensburg, PA 15601-1095
412-261-5040
800-272-3900
Fax: 724-837-4567
aspreng@alz.org
www.alz.org

Abby Spreng, Local Contact

897 Alzheimer's Association: Northeast Pennsylvania Chapter
63 North Franklin Street
Wilkes Barre, PA 18701
717-822-4278
800-272-3900
Fax: 717-822-9915
www.alz.org

898 Alzheimer's Association: Northwest Pennsylvania Chapter
726 West Bayfront Parkway
Erie, PA 16507
814-456-9200
800-272-3900
Fax: 814-454-0414
ahurd@alz.org
www.alz.org

Bob LeRoy, President/CEO
Amanda Hurd, Local Contact

899 Alzheimer's Association: South Central Pennsylvania Chapter
3544 North Progress Avenue
Harrisburg, PA 17110
717-651-5020
800-272-3900
Fax: 717-651-5066
tchambers@alz.org
www.alz.org

Bob LeRoy, President/CEO
Tiffani Chambers, Local Contact

Rhode Island

900 Alzheimer's Association: Rhode Island Chapter
245 Waterman Avenue
Providence, RI 02906
401-421-0008
800-272-3900
Fax: 401-941-8988
Donna.McGowan@alz.org
www.alz.org

Elizabeth Morancy, Executive Director
Marge Angilly, Program Director

South Carolina

901 Alzheimer's Association: Low Country Chapter
20 Patriots Point Road
Charleston, SC 29464
843-571-2641
800-272-3900
Fax: 843-571-6020
kalmstedt@alz.org
www.alz.org

Ashton Houghton, VP of Development & Communications
Kim Almstedt, Local Contact

902 Alzheimer's Association: Mid-State South Carolina Chapter
3223 Sunset Blvd
W Columbia, SC 29169-7044
803-791-3430
800-272-3900
Fax: 803-791-8388
www.alz.org

Adelle Stanley, Program Director
Lynee Moore, Director of Development

903 Alzheimer's Association: Upstate South Carolina Chapter
3027 MLK Jr. Blvd
Anderson, SC 29625-5528
864-224-3045
800-272-3900
Fax: 864-225-1387
kwilliams@alz.org
www.alz.org

Cindy Alewine, President/CEO
Kimberly Williams, Local Contact

Tennessee

904 Alzheimer's Association: Eastern Tennessee Chapter
1600 World's Fair Park Drive
Knoxville, TN 37916
865-200-6668
800-272-3900
Fax: 865-544-6249
jim.ward@alz.org
www.alz.org

Janice Wade-Whitehea, Executive Director
Jim Ward, Local Contact

905 Alzheimer's Association: Highland Rim Chapter
201 W Lincoln Street
Tullahoma, TN 37388-1004
931-455-3345
800-272-3900
Fax: 931-455-5396
swood@alz.org
www.alz.org

George Jensen, Chair
Sarah Wood, Local Contact

906 Alzheimer's Association: Memphis Area Office
500 North Pine Lake Drive
Memphis, TN 38134
901-565-0011
800-272-3900
Fax: 901-565-9550
sgraham@alz.org
www.alz.org

George Jensen, Chair
Susan Graham, Local Contact

907 Alzheimer's Association: Middle Tennessee Chapter
4205 Hillsboro Pike
Nashville, TN 37215-2859
615-292-4938
800-272-3900
Fax: 615-386-9768
ajackson1@alz.org
www.alz.org

George Jensen, Chair
Andrew Jackson, Local Contact

908 Alzheimer's Association: Northeast Tennessee Chapter
207 North Boone Street
Johnson City, TN 37604
423-928-4080
800-272-3900
Fax: 423-928-1152
tracey.kendall@alz.org
www.alz.org

Provide support, education, advocacy and research to those affected by Alzheimer's disease and their families.
George Jensen, Chair
Bruce Duncan, Vice Chair

909 **Alzheimer's Association: Southeast Tennessee Chapter**
7625 Hamilton Park Drive 423-265-3600
Chattanooga, TN 37421 800-272-3900
Fax: 423-265-3611
clowery@alz.org
www.alz.org

George Jensen, Chair
Cindy Lowery, Local Contact

Texas

910 **Alzheimer's Alliance: Texarkana Area**
104 Cypress 903-223-8021
Texarkana, TX 75503-7812 877-312-8536
Fax: 903-792-1792

Linda Nickerson, Executive Director
Fran Long, Program Director

911 **Alzheimer's Association: Capital of Texas Chapter**
3520 Executive Center Drive 512-241-0420
Austin, TX 78731 800-272-3900
Fax: 512-241-0430
Annie.lagow@alz.org
www.alz.org

The Alzheimer Association Greater Austin Chapter is dedicated to
providing leadership to enhance care and support services for individuals and their families while promoting the advancement of research eliminate Alzheimer's disease.
Daniel Hamilton, Chair
Annie LaGow, Local Contact

912 **Alzheimer's Association: El Paso Chapter**
4687 N Mesa 915-544-1799
El Paso, TX 79912-1147 800-272-3900
Fax: 915-544-8746
susie.gorman@alz.org
www.alz.org

Mitch Moss, Chair
Susie Gorman, Local Contact

913 **Alzheimer's Association: Greater Beaumont Area Chapter**
8750 Phelan Blvd. 409-833-1613
Beaumont, TX 77706 800-272-3900
Fax: 713-314-1315
walk@alztex.org
www.alz.org

Richard Elbein, Chief Executive Officer
Clarissa Urban, Local Contact

914 **Alzheimer's Association: Greater Dallas Chapter**
4144 N Central Expressway 214-540-2413
Dallas, TX 75204-4228 800-272-3900
Fax: 214-827-2064
dhill@alz.org
www.alz.org

Provides support and assistance to persons affected by Alzhei-
mer's disease and related dementias and their families and care-
givers. Serving Collin, Cooke, Dallas, Deaton, Ellis, Fanning,
Grayson, Hunt, Kaufmau, Navarro and Rockwall counties.
John R Gilchrist Jr, Executive Director
Jack Broyles, Chairman

915 **Alzheimer's Association: Greater East Texas Chapter**
2900 Raguet 713-314-1343
Nacogdoches, TX 75962 800-272-3900
Fax: 936-569-0514
walk@alztex.org
www.alz.org

Phil King, Chief Financial Officer
Jessica Abad-Serpas, Local Contact

916 **Alzheimer's Association: Greater Wichita Falls Chapter**
901 Indiana 940-767-8800
Wichita Falls, TX 76301-3206 800-272-3900
Fax: 940-322-6259
patty.taylor@alz.org
www.alz.org

Theresa Hocker, Executive Director
Patty Taylor, Local Contact

917 **Alzheimer's Association: Houston and Southeast Texas Chapter**
400 Hamilton Street 713-314-1340
Houston, TX 77002 800-272-3900
Fax: 713-314-1315
walk@alztex.org
www.alz.org

Richard Elbein, CEO
Rasheeda Daugherty, Local Contact

918 **Alzheimer's Association: Northeast Texas Chapter**
211 Winchester 903-509-8323
Tyler, TX 75701-8732 800-272-3900
Fax: 903-509-8373
www.alz.org

Jana Humphrey, Executive Director
Sherlon Spurling, Client Services Coordinator

919 **Alzheimer's Association: Rio Grande Valley Region**
222 E Van Buren 956-440-0636
Harlingen, TX 78550 800-272-3900
Fax: 956-440-9290
www.alz.org

A nonprofit organization designed to educate and support individuals with Alzheimer's, their families and caregivers.

920 **Alzheimer's Association: STAR Chapter, Midland Region**
4400 N Big Spring 432-570-9191
Midland, TX 79705 800-272-3900
Fax: 432-683-2345
derdwurm@alz.org
www.alz.org

Mitch Moss, Chair
Debbie Erdwurm, Local Contact

921 **Alzheimer's Association: South Central Texas**
7400 Louis Pasteur Drive 210-822-6449
San Antonio, TX 78229 800-272-3900
Fax: 210-824-8069
bbenavidez@alz.org
www.alz.org

Mitch Moss, Chair
Belinda Benavides, Local Contact

922 **Alzheimer's Association: Tarrant County Chapter**
101 Summit Avenue 817-336-4949
Fort Worth, TX 76102 800-272-3900
Fax: 817-336-4966
lyn.downing@alz.org
www.alz.org

Offers support to those afflicted with Alzheimer's disease and
their families through education, support groups, case management, telephone help line and referral to services (i.e. long term
care, adult daycare, medical assistance, legal assistance etc.).
Theresa Hocker, Executive Director
Lyn Downing, Local Contact

Utah

923 **Alzheimer's Association: Utah Chapter**
296 E. Murray Park Ave 801-265-1944
Salt Lake City, UT 84107 800-272-3900
Fax: 801-269-1226
Emartini@alz.org
www.alz.org

Nick Sussman, Program Director
Elaine Martini, Local Contact

Vermont

924 **Alzheimer's Association: Vermont Chapter**
300 Cornerstone Drive 802-316-3839
Williston, VT 05495-1139 800-272-3900
Fax: 802-229-5231
ashley.witzenberger@alz.org
www.alz.org

Randy Brock, President and Chair
Ashley Witzenberg, Director of Development

Virginia

925 Alzheimer's Association: Central Virginia Chapter
1160 Pepsi Place
Charlottesville, VA 22901

434-973-6122
800-272-3900
Fax: 434-973-4224
alzcwva@alz.org
www.alz.org

Sue Friedman, President and CEO
Brian Phelps, Chair

926 Alzheimer's Association: Greater Richmond Chapter
4600 Cox Road
Glen Allen, VA 23060

804-967-2580
800-272-3900
Fax: 804-967-2588
sherry.peterson@alz.org
www.alz.org

Alzheimer's Association provides support and services to those
with Alzheimer's and their families services include: help line,
support groups, educational programs for family and professional
caregivers, monthly newsletter, lending library, and a speakers
Sherry Peterson, CEO
Marry Ann Johnson, Program Director

927 Alzheimer's Association: National Capital Area Chapter
3701 Pender Drive
Fairfax, VA 22030

703-359-4440
800-272-3900
Fax: 703-359-4441
Danielle.Otsuka@alz.org
www.alz.org

Provides support and services to those diagnosed with Alzheimer's disease and related disorders and their families. Services include information on the disease, care options, caregiving
techniques and research, support groups, education and training,
and advocacy.
Matthew B Aaron, Chair
Danielle Otsuka, Director of Development

928 Alzheimer's Association: Piedmont-Valley Area Chapter
1160 Pepsi Place
Charlottesville, VA 22901

434-973-6122
800-272-3900
Fax: 434-973-4224
mhanson@alz.org
www.alz.org

Sue Friedman, President and CEO
Mary Pat Hanson, Local Contact

929 Alzheimer's Association: Roanoke Salem Chapter
3959 Electric Rd
Roanoke, VA 24018

540-345-7600
800-272-3900
Fax: 540-345-7900
mhanson@alz.org
www.alz.org

Sue Friedman, President and CEO
Mary Pat Hanson, Local Contact

930 Alzheimer's Association: Southeastern Virginia Chapter
6350 Center Drive
Norfolk, VA 23502

757-459-2405
800-272-3900
Fax: 757-461-7902
InfoSEVA@alz.org
www.alz.org

Provides support to people with Alzheimer's disease or related dementia and their families; educates professionals and the public
about Alzheimer's disease and related dementia; supports research
into causes, improved diagnosis, therapies and cures.
Gino V Colombara, Executive Director
Patricia Far Lacey, Director of Education & Family Services

931 Alzheimer's Association: Southside Virginia Chapter
120 S Hill Avenue
S Hill, VA 23970-0310

434-447-3963
800-272-3900
Fax: 434-447-9024
gino.colombara@alz.org
www.alz.org

Gino V Colombara, Executive Director
June Rainey, Education & Family Services Coordinator

Washington

932 Alzheimer's Association: Inland Northwest Chapter
800 N. Howard St.
Spokane, WA 99201

509-473-3390
800-272-3900
Fax: 509-473-3389
sdruffel@alz.org
www.alz.org

Joel Loiacono, Executive Director
Sandi Druffel, Local Contact

**933 Alzheimer's Association: Western & Central Washington
Chapter**
100 W. Harrison St
Seattle, WA 98119

206-529-3898
800-272-3900
Fax: 206-363-5700
walk@alzwa.org
www.alz.org

Nancy Dapper, Executive Director
Justine Stevens, Local Contact

West Virginia

934 Alzheimer's Association: Greater Mid-Ohio Valley Chapter
1920 Park Ave.
Parkersburg, WV 26101

304-865-6775
800-272-3900
wendy.hamilton@alz.org
www.alz.org

Jane Marks, Executive Director
Wendy Hamilton, Local Contact

935 Alzheimer's Association: N Central West Virginia Chapter
1299 Pineview Drive
Morgantown, WV 26505-4543

304-599-1159
800-272-3900
Fax: 304-291-2577
wvinfo@alz.org
www.alz.org

Jane Marks, Executive Director
Jane Siers, Development Director

936 Alzheimer's Association: South West Virginia Chapter
601 Morris St.
Charleston, WV 25301

304-343-2717
800-272-3900
Fax: 304-343-2723
kford@alz.org
www.alz.org

Jane Marks, Executive Director
Kaarmin Ford, Local Contact

Wisconsin

937 Alzheimer's Association: Greater Wisconsin Chapter
La Crosse & Second Streets
La Crosse, WI 54601

608-784-5011
800-272-3900
Fax: 608-784-4428
bwilliams@alz.org
www.alz.org

To eliminate Alzheimer's disease through the advancement of research; to provide and enhance care and support for all affected;
and to reduce the risk of dementia through the promotion of brain
health.
Brad Beckman, President
Brett Williams, Local Contact

938 Alzheimer's Association: Indianhead Chapter
Carson Park Dr
Eau Claire, WI 54703-5996

715-345-2969
800-272-3900
Fax: 715-345-2969
kdavies@alz.org
www.alz.org

Mary B Bouche, Executive Director
Kathy Davies, Local Contact

939 Alzheimer's Association: Lake Superior Chapter
US Highway 2 East   715-392-3255
Ashland, WI 54806-1652   800-272-3900
                                           Fax: 715-682-6561
                                                fcarlson@alz.org
                                                www.alz.org

Kim Kinner, Executive Director
Freda Carlson, Local Contact

940 Alzheimer's Association: Midstate Wisconsin Chapter
1800 S Central Ave   715-845-7440
Marshfield, WI 54449   800-272-3900
                                           Fax: 715-387-5727
                                                aswatek@alz.org
                                                www.alz.org

941 Alzheimer's Association: North Central Wisconsin Chapter
1205 Lincoln St   715-362-7779
Rhinelander, WI 54501   800-272-3900
                                           Fax: 715-362-1879
                                                jstpierre@alz.org
                                                www.alz.org

Kim Kinner, Executive Director
Julie St. Pierre, Local Contact

942 Alzheimer's Association: Northeast Wisconsin Chapter
1265 Lombardi Ave   920-469-2110
Green Bay, WI 54304   800-272-3900
                                           Fax: 920-498-2203
                                                bbartlett@alz.org
                                                www.alz.org

Kim Kinner, Executive Director
Beverly Bartlett, Local Contact

943 Alzheimer's Association: South Central Wisconsin Chapter
1 John Nolen Drive   608-203-8502
Madison, WI 53703   800-272-3900
                                           Fax: 608-232-3407
                                                ehilker@alz.org
                                                www.alz.org

Provides support and assistance to the families of those impacted
by Alzheimer's and related dementias, including educational programs, support groups, information and referral and advocacy.
150 Members
Paul Rusk, Executive Director
Emily Hilker, Local Contact

944 Alzheimer's Association: Southeast Wisconsin Chapter
2900 North Menomonee River Parkway   414-479-8800
Milwaukee, WI 53222   800-272-3900
                                           Fax: 414-479-8819
                                           TTY: 414-479-8466
                                                slatona@alz.org
                                                www.alz.org

To eliminate Alzheimer's disease through advancement of research and to enhance care and support for individuals, their families and caregivers. Individual consultation over the phone or in
person. Extensive library of educational materials for loan or
purchase.
Kendra Albers, Special Events Manager
Shelby LaTona, Development Coordinato

Wyoming

945 Alzheimer's Wyoming
900 Werner Court   307-265-7960
Casper, WY 82602   Fax: 307-265-7960
Alzheimer's Affiliation of Wyoming is an independent organization that makes presentations about Alzheimer's Disease; assists
Alzheimer support groups; provides funds for respite care; maintains a lending library; refers patients and their families to
services.
Mary Hein, Executive Director

Foundations

946 Long Island Alzheimers Foundation
5 Channel Drive   516-767-6856
Port Washington, NY 11050   Fax: 516-767-6864
                                                info@liaf.org
                                                www.liaf.org
To help lighten the burden and improve the quality of life for those
suffering with Alzheimer's disease and related dementias, their
caregivers and their families.
Fred Jenny, Executive Director
Sean Phillips, Director of Development

Libraries & Resource Centers

947 Green-Field Library-Alzheimer's Association
225 N. Michigan Avenue   847-324-0356
Chicago, IL 60601-7633   800-272-3900
                                           Fax: 866-699-1238
                                           TTY: 312-335-5886
                                           TDD: 312-335-8700
                                                greenfield@alz.org
                                                www.alz.org
Located at the national Alzheimer's Association in Chicago this library offers a sizable collection of videos on a variety of subjects
that may interest the Alzheimer's patient family members and
caregivers.
Richard Hovland, COO

Research Centers

**948 Aging and Alzheimer's Disease Center Oregon Health Sciences
University**
Oregon Health Sciences University
3181 SW Sam Jackson Park Road   503-494-8311
Portland, OR 97239-3098   Fax: 503-494-6695
                                                kaye@ohsu.edu
                                                www.ohsu.edu/research/alzheimers
Researches causes and consequences of Alzheimer's disease and
ways of clinical services. Publishes a newsletter twice a year.
Jeffrey Kaye, Director
Joan Benedict, Administrative Coordinator

949 Alzheimer's Disease Center Emory University/VA Medical Center
201 Dowman Drive   404-727-6069
Atlanta, GA 30322   Fax: 404-286-55
                                                emoryadrc@emory.edu
                                                www.med.emory.edu/ADRC
Researchers work to translate advances into improved care and di-
agnosis for Alzheimer's patients.
Allan Levey, Director
Stuart Zola, Co-Director

950 Alzheimer's Disease Center Kentucky University
Sanders-Brown Center on Aging
1030 South Broadway   859-257-1412
Lexington, KY 40504-0230   Fax: 859-323-2866
                                                rdavi3@email.uky.edu
                                                /www.mc.uky.edu/coa
Researchers work to translate advances into improved care and di-
agnosis for Alzheimer's patients.
Linda J. Van Eldik, Ph.D., Director
Vince J Kellen, Chief Information Officer

951 Alzheimer's Disease Center Mayo Clinic Mayo Medical School
Mayo Medical School
200 First Street SW   507-284-2511
Rochester, MN 55905   Fax: 507-538-0161
                                           TDD: 507-2849786
                                                mayoADC@mayo.edu
                                                www.mayoclinic.com
Researchers work to translate advances into improved care and di-
agnosis for Alzheimer's patients.
John H Noseworhty MD, President
William C Rupp MD, Vice President, CEO

952 Alzheimer's Disease Center Pennsylvania University School of Medicine
Ralston House
3615 Chestnut Street   215-662-7810
Philadelphia, PA 19104   Fax: 215-662-7812
jason.karlawish@uphs.upenn.edu
www.pennadc.org
Researchers work to translate advances into improved care and diagnosis for Alzheimer's patients.
John Q Trojanowski, Director

953 Alzheimer's Disease Center: Boston University
Boston University School of Medicine
72 E Concord Street   617-638-5426
Boston, MA 02118   888-458-2823
Fax: 617-414-1197
buad@bu.edu
www.bu.edu/alzresearch
Researchers work to translate advances into improved care and diagnosis for Alzheimer's patients.
Neil W Kowall, Director
Richard Fine, Associate Director

954 Alzheimer's Disease Center: Johns Hopkins University School of Medicine
Johns Hopkins University Department of Pathology
720 Rutland Avenue   410-502-5164
Baltimore, MD 21205   Fax: 410-955-9777
edelman1@jhmi.edu
www.alzresearch.org
Researchers work to translate advances into improved care and diagnosis for Alzheimer's patients.
Marilyn Albert, Director
Philip Wong, Associate Director

955 Alzheimer's Disease Center: University of California, Davis
4860 Y Street   916-734-5496
Sacramento, CA 95817   wjjagust@lbl.gov
alzheimer.ucdavis.edu/
Researchers work to translate advances into improved care and diagnosis for Alzheimer's patients.
Charles DeCarli MD, Clinical Core Director

956 Alzheimer's Disease Center: University of Alabama at Birmingham
1720 7th Avenue S   205-934-3847
Birmingham, AL 35294-0017   Fax: 205-975-7365
adbrain@uab.edu
Researchers work to translate advances into improved care and diagnosis for Alzheimer's patients.
Daniel C Marson, Director
J Michael Wyss, Associate Director

957 Alzheimer's Disease Center: Washington University
1660 S Columbian Way   206-764-2069
Seattle, WA 98108-1597   800-317-5382
Fax: 206-768-5456
wamble@u.washington.edu
www.depts.washington.edu/adrcweb
Researchers work to translate advances into improved care and diagnosis for Alzheimer's patients.
Sydney Lewis, Education and Outreach Coordinator
Nancy Brown, Lead Psychometrist and Autopsy Coordinat

958 Alzheimer's Disease Research Center Washington University School of Medicine
Washington University School of Medicine
4488 Forest Park Avenue   314-286-2683
St Louis, MO 63108   Fax: 314-286-2763
morrisj@abraxas.wustl.edu
www.adrc.wustl.edu
Researchers work to translate advances into improved care diagnosis and treatment for Alzheimer's patients.
John Morris, Director
Virginia D Buckles, Executive Director

959 Alzheimer's Disease Research Center Duke University
Bryan ADRC

2200 W Main Street Suite A200   919-668-0820
Durham, NC 27705   866-444-2372
kwe@duke.edu
adrc.mc.duke.edu
Researchers work to translate advances into improved care and diagnosis for Alzheimer's patients.
Kathleen A Welsh-Bohmer, Director
James Robert Burke, Associate Director

960 Cognitive Neurology and Alzheimer's Disease Center
CNADC
320 E Superior Street   312-908-9339
Chicago, IL 60611   Fax: 312-908-8789
CNADC-Admin@northwestern.edu
www.brain.northwestern.edu
Researchers work to translate advances into improved care and diagnosis for Alzheimer's patients.
Megan Atchu, MA, Research Administrator
Kevin Connolly, Business Administrator

961 Cornell University: Winifred Masterson Burke Medical Research-Dementia
1300 York Avenue   212-746-5454
New York, NY 10065   Fax: 212-821-0576
publicaffairs@med.cornell.edu
www.med.cornell.edu
Clinical and basic studies in metabolic aspects of the nervous system especially Alzheimer's disease.
David J Skorton MD, President
Thomas H Blair lll, Senior Director Administrator

962 Duke University Center for the Study of Aging and Human Development
Duke University
Box 3003   919-660-7500
Durham, NC 27710   Fax: 919-668-0453
webmaster@geri.duke.edu
Basic and clinical research into geriatrics and gerontology focusing on a number of chronic diseases in the elderly including osteoporosis cancer heart disease infectious diseases Alzheimer's disease and other disorders leading to dysmobility.
Harvey Jay Cohen MD, Director
Linda K George, Associate Director

963 Duke University Clinical Research Institute
Headquarters
2400 Pratt Street   919-668-8700
Durham, NC 27705   www.dcri.duke.edu
Multidisciplinary clinical research into the cause and prevention of human diseases such as Alzheimer's.
Robert A Harrington, Director
Elizabeth Be Reed, Chief Operating Officer

964 Indiana University Center for Aging Research
The Center for Aging Research
1050 Wishard Blvd   317-630-6083
Indianapolis, IN 46202-2872   Fax: 317-423-5695
www.medicine.iupui.edu/iucar/?
Researchers work to translate advances into improved care and diagnosis for Alzheimer's patients.
Christopher Callahan, Director
Douglas K Miller, Associate Director

965 Indiana University: Human Genetics Center of Medical & Molecular Genetics
School of Medicine
340 West 10th Street   317-274-8157
Indianapolis, IN 46202-3082   kcornett@iupui.edu
www.medicine.iu.edu
Comprised of a core group of scientists with primary appointments in the Department and a group of molecular biologists from other departments who hold joint appointments in Medical and Molecular Genetics.
D Craig Brater MD, Dean
John F. Fitzgerald, MD, MBA, Executive Associate Dean

966 Institute for Basic Research in Developmental Disabilities
1050 Forest Hill Road   718-494-0600
Staten Island, NY 10314-0001   866- 94- 973
                                          TTY: 866- 933-488
                                          ibr@opwdd.ny.gov
               www.opwdd.ny.gov/institute-for-basic-res
James F Moran, Acting Commissioner

967 Long Island Alzheimers Foundation
5 Channel Drive   516-767-6856
Port Washington, NY 11050   Fax: 516-767-6856
                                          info@liaf.org
                                          www.liaf.org
Researchers work to translate advances into improved care and diagnosis for Alzheimer's patients.
Fred Jenny, Executive Director
Anna Maria Warmuz, Executive Assistant

968 Massachusetts Alzheimers Disease Research Center
Massachusetts ADRC
16th Street   617-726-3987
Charlestown, MA 02129   Fax: 617-724-1480
                                          www.madrc.org
Multi-institutional consortium of Harvard affiliated facilities encompasses five Core units: an Administrative Core a Clinical Core a Database Management and Statistics Core a Neuropathology Core and an Education and Information Transfer Core. The ADRC also supports four specific research projects funded for 3-5 years and annually designates three or four pilot research projects that are funded for 1 year.
John H Growdon, Clinic Director
Bradley T Hyman, Center Director

969 Medical College of Georgia Alzheimers Research Center
1120 15th Street   706-721-0211
Augusta, GA 30912   Fax: 706-721-7063
Clinical and basic research of Alzheimer's disease.
Jerry Buccaf MD, Director
J Warren Beach, Member

970 Michigan Alzheimer's Disease Research Center
University of Michigan
2101 Commonwealth Blvd.,   734-936-4000
Ann Arbor, MI 48105-0316   www.med.umich.edu/alzheimers
Researchers work to translate advances into improved care and diagnosis for Alzheimer's patients.
Sid Gilman MD, Director
Bruno Giordani Ph.D., Core Director

971 Mount Sinai School of Medicine: Alzheimers Disease Research Center
Alzheimer's Disease Research Center
One Gustave L Levy Place   212-241-6696
New York, NY 10029-6574   Fax: 212-369-2344
                                          mary.sano@mssm.edu
                                          www.mssm.edu
Focuses on Alzheimer's disease research.
Mary Sano, Director
Samuel Gandy, Associate Director

972 Neurosciences Institute of the Neurosciences Research Program
The Neurosciences Institute
10640 John Jay Hopkins Drive   858-626-2000
San Diego, CA 92121   Fax: 858-626-2099
                                          info@nsi.edu
                                          www.nsi.edu
Nonprofit organization focusing on Alzheimer's and related disorders.
Gerald M Edelman, President

973 Ohio State University Neuroscience Program
1835 Neil Avenue   614-292-8185
Columbus, OH 43210   Fax: 614-921-44
                                          www.psy.ohio-state.edu
Specializes in brain disorders such as Alzheimer's disease.
Richard Petty, Chair
Scott Burch, Behavioral Neurosciences Area Assistant

974 Taub Institute for Research on Alzheimers Disease and the Aging Brain
630 West 168th Street   212-305-1818
New York, NY 10032   Fax: 212-342-2849
                                          taubinstitute@columbia.edu
                                          www.alzheimercenter.org
Researchers work to translate advances into improved care and diagnosis for Alzheimer's patients.
Michael L Shelanski, Co-Director
Richard Mayeux MD, Co-Director

975 The Alzheimer's Disease & Memory Disorders Center
ADMDC
One Baylor Plaza   713-798-5971
Houston, TX 77030   Fax: 713-798-7434
                                          neurons@bcm.edu
                                          www.bcm.edu/neurology/admdc
Researchers work to translate advances into improved care and diagnosis for Alzheimer's Disease and other memory disorders.
Eli M Mizrahi, Chair, Department of Neurology
Keith Davis, Department Administrator

976 The Sam and Rose Stein Institute for Research on the Aging
University of California San Diego
9500 Gilman Drive   858-534-6299
La Jolla, CA 92093-0664   Fax: 858-534-5475
                                          steininstitute@ucsd.edu
Research on aging and Alzheimer's disease.
Debra Kaine, Director
Maureen Halp MS, Executive Director

977 University Alzheimer Center University of Alabama at Birmingham
University of Alabama at Birmingham
1530 3rd Avenue S   205-934-4011
Birmingham, AL 35294-1150   800-333-6543
                                          Fax: 205-975-7365
                                          TTY: 205-934-4642
                                          adbrain@uab.edu
Researchers work to translate advances into improved care and diagnosis for Alzheimer's patients.
Dr. Carol Garrison, President
Kristen N Burdick, Director of Executive Affairs

978 University Alzheimer Center UHC: Case Western Reserve University
12200 Fairhill Road   216-844-6400
Cleveland, OH 44120   Fax: 216-844-6446
                                          Kathy.Shaw@Case.Edu
                                          www.ohioalzcenter.org
Researchers work to translate advances into improved care and diagnosis for Alzheimer's patients.
Alan Lerner, Co-Director
Kathleen A Smyth, Administrator

979 University of Chicago Dept of Neurology University of Chicago Hospital
University of Chicago Hospital
5841 S Maryland Avenue   773-702-6390
Chicago, IL 60637-1470   Fax: 773-702-9076
                                          cgomez@neurology.bsd.uchicago.edu
                                          neurology.uchicago.edu
Covers Translational Neuroscience Research and research programs in neuroimmunology neuromuscular disease and neurovirology provided the initial foundation and brought national recognition.
Kenneth Goodell, Senior Executive Administrator
Judith Maratea, Administrative Assistant

980 University of Illinois Health Services Research
University of Illinois College of Medicine
1601 Parkview Avenue   815-395-0600
Rockford, IL 61107   Fax: 815-395-5887
                                          prrockford@uic.edu
A unit of the University of Illinois College of Medicine at Rockford serves faculty students health care providers human services agencies and other community organizations throughout Illinois with demographic health social and economic data. The skills data and resources available to faculty and students at the college

are also available to individuals and organizations needing assistance.
Joann Glacken, Research Support Services

981   University of Maryland: Division of Infectious Diseases
UM Baltimore Department of Medicine
655 West Baltimore Street   410-706-7410
Baltimore, MD 21201   Fax: 410-706-0235
rredfield@ihv.umaryland.edu
www.medschool.umaryland.edu
Focuses research on elderly studies including drug use treatments and infectious diseases of the aged.
E. Albert Reece, Vice President
Richard Pierson III MD, Senior Associate Dean for Academic Affai

982   University of Miami: Center on Aging Center on Aging
Center on Aging
1695 NW 9th Avenue   305-355-9080
Miami, FL 33136   Fax: 305-355-9076
ajaret@med.miami.edu
Focuses on aged disorders such as Alzheimer's research.
Sara J Czaja, Co-Director
Charles B. Nemeroff, M.D., Ph.D, Director

983   Yeshiva University: Resnick Gerontology Center
Albert Einstein College of Medicine
Jack and Pearl Resnick Campus   718-920-6722
Bronx, NY 10467   866-633-8255
Fax: 718-655-9672
ljacobs@aecom.yu.edu
www.aecom.yu.edu
Alzheimer's disease and other dementia studies.
Allen M Spiegel MD, Dean
Amy R Ehrlich, Geriatrics Fellowship Program Director

Support Groups & Hotlines

984   Alzheimer's Association Autopsy Assistance Network
Alzheimer s Association
Western/Central Washington Chapter   206-363-5500
Seattle, WA 98125   800-848-7097
Fax: 206-363-5700
rowena.rye@alz.org
http://alzwa.org/resources6.htm
The primary purposes of the Autopsy Assistance Network are: to provide families with information regarding autopsy; to assist in obtaining a confirmed diagnosis; provide tissue for Alzheimer's disease research; and establish diagnosis for purpose of clinical and epidemiological studies.
Nancy Dapper, Executive Director
Rowena Rye, Community Resources

985   Alzheimer's Support Group
Columbus Health Rehabilitation Center
2100 Midway Street   812-372-8447
Columbus, IN 47201   Fax: 812-375-5117
www.columbushrc.com/
The skilled Nursing Center includes a separate unit dedicated to the care of residents with Alzheimer's disease and other forms of dementia. The Alzheimer's program is designed to celebrate the spirit of their residents, striving to offer a comfortable and compassionate environment that emphasizes positive life experiences and active involvement in a daily routine.
Mike Spencer, Executive Director

986   National Health Information Center
Office of Disease Prevention & Health Promotion
1101 Wootton Pkwy   Fax: 240-453-8281
Rockville, MD 20852   odphinfo@hhs.gov
www.health.gov/nhic
Supports public health education by maintaining a calendar of National Health Observances; helps connect consumers and health professionals to organizations that can best answer questions and provide up-to-date contact information from reliable sources; updates on a yearly basis toll-free numbers for health information, Federal health clearinghouses and info centers.
Don Wright, MD, MPH, Director

Books

987   36-Hour Day
Hachette Book Group USA
3 Center Plaza   800-759-0190
Boston, MA 02108   Fax: 800-331-1664
webmaster@hbgusa.com
www.hachettebookgroup.com
A family guide to caring for persons with Alzheimer's disease, related dementing illnesses, and memory loss later in life.
1999
ISBN: 0-446618-76-2
Nancy L. Mace M.A., Author
Peter V. Rabins M.D., M.P.H., Author

988   Alzheimer Early Stages
Daniel Kuhn MSW, author
Hunter House Publishers
424 Church Street   615-255-2665
Nashville, TN 37219   800-266-5592
Fax: 615-255-5081
ordering@hunterhouse.com
www.turnerpublishing.com
First steps in caring and treatments. This book is for family members and friends of those recently diagnosed with Alzheimer's Disase.
288 pages Paperback
ISBN: 0-897933-97-4

989   Alzheimer's Disease
Springer Publishing Company
11 West 42nd Street   212-431-4370
New York, NY 10036-3955   877-687-7476
Fax: 212-941-7842
cs@springerpub.com
www.springerpub.com
This volume presents the latest research and findings on Alzheimer's disease.
1996 224 pages Softcover
ISBN: 0-826196-22-5
Annette Imperati, Marketing Director

990   Alzheimer's Disease Orientation Kit
Alzheimer's Association
225 North Michigan Avenue   312-335-8700
Chicago, IL 60601-1696   800-272-3900
Fax: 866-699-1246
TDD: 312-335-5886
info@alz.org
www.alz.org
A collection of materials developed to familiarize the audience with Alzheimer's disease and its effects on the patient and family. Includes the Orientation to Alzheimer's Disease videotape, Learning Guide and Caregiver Packet.

991   Alzheimer's Disease: A Guide to Federal Programs
Alzheimer's Disease Education & Referral Center
31 Center Drive   800-438-4380
Bethesda, MD 20892-8250   Fax: 301-495-3334
niaic@nia.nih.gov
www.nia.nih.gov/alzheimers
Directory of Alzheimer's disease programs sponsored by federal agencies. Lists agency by agency, it provides locations and telephone numbers for multisite activities and demonstration programs and lists information resources.

992   Alzheimer's Disease: Activity-Focused Care
Butterworth-Heinemann
3255 Bell Helicopter   817-280-2011
Fort Worth, TX 76118   800-366-2665
Fax: 817-280-2321
www.bh.com
Information for professional and family caregivers on activity-focused care for Alzheimer's patients.
436 pages
ISBN: 0-750699-08-6

993   Alzheimer's Disease: Advances in Neurology
Raven Press

1185 Ave of the Americas
New York, NY 10036-2601
304 pages
ISBN: 0-781700-81-7

212-930-9500
800-777-2295

994 Alzheimer's Disease: Questions and Answers
Merit Publishing International
5840 Corporate Way
West Palm Beach, FL 33407

561-697-1116
Fax: 561-477-4961
meritpi@aol.com

Answers questions about Alzheimer's, explains what it is, how it is diagnosed, causes, and how if affects functions of the brain.
1999
ISBN: 1-873413-52-1
Gene Evans, President
Martin Garrido, VP

995 Alzheimer's Disease: Thesaurus
Alzheimer's Disease Education & Referral Center
31 Center Drive
Bethesda, MD 20892-8250

800-438-4380
Fax: 301-495-3334
niaic@nia.nih.gov
www.nia.nih.gov/alzheimers

To help librarians and others to save time and money when searing online for books, journal articles, videos and other materials related to Alzheimer's disease.
140 pages

996 Alzheimer's Disease: Treatment and Family Stress: Directions for Research
Superintendent of Documents
PO Box 371954
Pittsburgh, PA 15250-7954

202-512-2250

Presents a collection of papers giving current information on research investigations that increase the understanding of the nature and consequences of family caregiving.
486 pages

997 Alzheimer's, Stroke and 29 Other Neurological Disorders Sourcebook
Omnigraphics
PO Box 8002
Aston, PA 19014-3993

610-461-3548
800-234-1340
Fax: 610-532-9001
customerservice@omnigraphics.com
www.omnigraphics.com

Provides vital information for the nontechnical reader focusing on Alzheimer's disease, stroke and various neurological disorders. Answers thousands of questions related to afflications of the central nervous system with each chapter reviwing a particular disorder and offers in-depth discussions.
ISBN: 0-780806-66-2
Georgiann Lauginiger, Customer Service Manager

998 Care That Works: A Relationship Approach to Persons with Dementia
John's Hopkins University Press
2715 N Charles Street
Baltimore, MD 21218-4319

410-516-6900
800-537-5487
Fax: 410-516-6998
www.press.jhu.edu

Focuses on building and improving the relationship between the caregiver and the person with Alzheimer's.
272 pages
ISBN: 0-801860-26-1
Jitka M. Zgola, Author

999 Care of Alzheimer's Patients: A Manual for Nursing Home Staff
Lisa P Gwyther, author

Alzheimer's Association
225 North Michigan Avenue
Chicago, IL 60601-1696

312-335-8700
800-272-3900
Fax: 866-699-1246
TDD: 312-335-5886
info@alz.org
www.alz.org

A care guide for nursing home staff. A useful resource for any caregiver or professional.
122 pages
Lisa P. Gwyther, Author

1000 Caregiver Helpbook
Legacy Health System
1015 NW 22nd Avenue
Portland, OR 97210

503-413-6778
Fax: 503-413-6911
www.legacyhealth.org

A helpful guide with useful self care tools for family caregivers of frail or ill older adults.
300 pages Paperback
ISBN: 0-937915-54-6
Kathy Shannon, Manager/Caregiver

1001 Caring for Alzheimer's Patients: A Guide for Family & Healthcare Providers
Plenum Publishing Corporation
233 Spring Street
New York, NY 10013-1522

212-620-8460
800-221-9369
Fax: 212-463-0742
books@plenum.com

Consists of five organizations that furnish information and resources concerning Alzheimer's Disease support groups and hospitals.
308 pages
ISBN: 0-306431-99-8

1002 Complete Guide to Alzheimer's Proofing Your Home
Purdue University Press
509 Harrison Street
West Lafayette, IN 47907-2025

765-494-2038
800-247-6553
Fax: 765-496-2442
pupress@purdue.edu
www.thepress.purdue.edu

Guide on how to modify homes of Alzheimer's patients to facilitate caregiving.
496 pages Paperback
ISBN: 1-557532-02-8
Mark Warner, Author

1003 Confronting Alzheimer's Disease
American Assoc. of Homes and Services for Aging
2519 Connecticut Ave NW
Washington, DC 20008-2008

202-783-2242
Fax: 202-783-2255

A resource for administrators, professional caregivers and families dealing with Alzheimer's disease and related disorders.
225 pages

1004 Court-Related Needs of the Elderly and Persons with Disabilities
Commission on the Mentally Disabled
1800 M Street NW
Washington, DC 20036

202-331-2240

Report of the National Conference, examines the barriers of the judicial system impeding access for the elderly and persons with disabilities.

1005 Developing Support Groups for Individuals with Early-Stage Alzheimer's Disease
Robyn Yale, author

Health Professions Press
PO Box 10624
Baltimore, MD 21285-0624

410-337-9585
888-337-8808
Fax: 410-337-8539
www.healthpropress.com

This one-of-a-kind, step-by-step guidebook has been used as a national and international model to meet the needs of people just diagnosed with Alzheimer's disease. Clinical and administrative issues include selecting group participants, training facilitators and managing unique group topics, interactions and dynamics.
256 pages Paperback
ISBN: 1-878812-62-2
Robyn Yale, Author

1006 Directory of Alzheimer's Disease Treatment Facilities & Home Health Care
Oryx Press
4041 N Central Avenue
Phoenix, AZ 85012-3397

602-265-2651
800-279-4663

A compilation of 1,500 specialized facilities with day care, residential care, diagnosis and treatment facilities.

1007 Ginny: A Love Remembered
Iowa State Press

2121 State Street
Ames, IA 50014

515-292-0155
800-862-6657
Fax: 515-292-3348
iowastatepress.com

This book tells the story of midwest cartoonist Bob Artley's life with his beloved wife and their 10 year battle together against Alzheimer's disease, which finally claimed her.
278 pages Hardcover
ISBN: 0-813821-04-5
Brad Nobiling, Credit Manager

1008 Hospice Alternative
Harper Collins Publishers/Basic Books
10 E 53rd Street
New York, NY 10022-5299

212-207-7057
800-242-7737
Fax: 212-207-7203

An account of the hospice experience. An innovative and humane way of caring for the terminally ill.
256 pages
ISBN: 0-465030-61-0

1009 Hospice Care for Patients with Advanced Progressive Dementia
Springer Publishing Company
536 Broadway
New York, NY 10012

212-431-4370
877-687-7476
Fax: 212-941-7842
marketing@springerpub.com
www.springerpub.com

Discusses adpating hospice care for terminally ill patients with dementia. Topics include infections, eating difficulties, and providing palliative care.
320 pages Hardcover
ISBN: 0-826111-62-9
Annette Imperati, Marketing Director

1010 I'm Just Not Myself Anymore: A Family Guide to Alzheimer's Disease
Northwestern University Press
633 Clark Street
Evanston, IL 60208-4210

312-503-8649
Fax: 847-491-8150
www.northwestern.edu

1993 283 pages Paperback
ISBN: 1-880416-72-7

1011 Interventions for Alzheimer's Disease: A Caregiver's Complete Reference
Ruth M Tappen, author
Health Professions Press
PO Box 10624
Baltimore, MD 21285-0624

410-337-9585
888-337-8808
Fax: 410-337-8539
www.healthpropress.com

For professionals who plan, administer or provide services to Alzheimer's patients.
256 pages Paperback
ISBN: 1-878812-39-4

1012 Key Elements of Dementia Care
Alzheimer's Association
225 North Michigan Avenue
Chicago, IL 60601-1696

312-335-8700
800-272-3900
Fax: 866-699-1246
TDD: 312-335-5886
info@alz.org
www.alz.org

Defines, describes, and illustrates dementia-capable care throughout the range of residential care settings.
1997 90 pages

1013 Nursing Home and You: Partners in Caring for a Relative with Alzheimer's Disease
American Assn. of Homes & Services for the Aging
901 E Street NW
Washington, DC 20004-2037

202-783-2242
800-508-9442
Fax: 202-783-2255

Offers suggestions for families of nursing home residents on how to work with staff to foster smooth transitions.
32 pages

1014 Occupational Therapy Practice Guidelines for Adults with Alzheimer's Disease
American Occupational Therapy Association
4720 Montgomery Lane
Bethesda, MD 20814-1220

301-652-2682
Fax: 240-762-5150
TDD: 800-377-8555
www.aota.org

21 pages
ISBN: 1-569001-46-4

1015 Positive Interactions Program of Activities for People with Alzheimer's
Sylvia Nissenboim, author
Health Professions Press
PO Box 10624
Baltimore, MD 21285-0624

410-337-9585
888-337-8808
Fax: 410-337-8539
www.healthpropress.com

All interactions focus on preventing individual dignity and providing opportunities to experience meaningful involvement and satisfaction. Works in a variety of settings and promotes the OBRA quality of care guidelines.
176 pages 1997
ISBN: 1-878812-40-8
Christine Vroman, Editor
Sylvia Nissenboim, Author/Editor

1016 Rethinking Alzheimer's Care
Sam Fazio, Dorothy Seman, author
Health Professions Press
PO Box 10624
Baltimore, MD 21285-0624

410-337-9585
888-337-8808
Fax: 410-337-8539
www.healthpropress.com

Appropriate for all settings providing long-term care, adult day services, or assisted living, this fresh and humanistic approach to Alzheimer's care will encourage caregivers to rethink the disease experience and explore its possibilities, instead of its limitations.
200 pages Paperback
ISBN: 1-878812-62-9
Jane Stansell, Editor
Sam Fazio, Author/Editor

1017 Speaking Our Minds: Personal Reflections from Individuals with Alzheimer's
WH Freeman and Company
41 Madison Avenue
New York, NY 10010

212-576-9400
888-330-8477
Fax: 212-689-2383
www.macmillanhighered.com/

Personal reflections of people with Alzheimer's disease.
161 pages Hardcover
ISBN: 0-716732-24-6

1018 The Comfort of Home for Alheimer's Disease A Guide for Caregivers
M. Meyer, M. Mittelman, P. Derr, C. Epstein, author
CareTrust Publications LLC
PO Box 10283
Portland, OR 97296-0283

800-565-1533
Fax: 415-673-2005
sales@comfortofhome.com
www.comfortofhome.com

Walks readers through all Alzheimer's stages and cover the basics from undertanding the difference between AD and normal aging, to coping with the behavioral symptoms that come with the diminishing reasoning skills. Additionally, Comfort talks about how to provide safe physical care around other medical conditions the Alzheimer's sufferer may have, due to normal aging. Not the least of all, Comfort provides self-care tips for the caregivers to remain emotionally and mentally healthy.
2008 288 pages
ISBN: 0-978790-30-8

1019 Therapeutic Interventions in Alzheimer's
Aspen Publishers
7201 McKinney Circle
Frederick, MD 21705-0990

301-698-7100
800-638-8437
Fax: 301-695-7931
customerservice@aspenpub.com

A program of functional skills for activities of daily living.
197 pages

1020 **Time for Alzheimer's: A True Story**
Emerald Ink Publishing
7141 Office City Drive   800-324-5663
Houston, TX 77087-3722   www.emeraldink.com
Based on the author's personal experience in caring for her mother.
139 pages
ISBN: 1-885373-13-3

1021 **Understanding Alzheimer's Disease**
University Press of Mississippi
3825 Ridgewood Road   601-432-6205
Jackson, MS 39211-6492   800-737-7788
                                          Fax: 601-432-6217
                                       press@ihl.state.ms.us
                                       www.upress.state.ms.us
Aimed at people with Alzheimer's, family members, caregivers,
health care and human service professionals. Describes Alzheimer's from early to advanced stages. Discusses the care of AD patients, ideas to help families care for the AD patient at home,
reviews treatments for the psychiatric, behavioral and cognitive
effects of AD and describes research efforts to better understand
AD and develop effective therapies. Price $28 Hardcover, $12
Paperback.
1996 150 pages
ISBN: 0-878059-11-3
Neal R. Cutler, M.D., Author
John J. Sramek,Pharm.D., Author

1022 **When We Become the Parent to Our Parents**
MEA Productions
55 Binks Hill Road   603-536-2641
Plymouth, NH 03264   Fax: 603-536-4851
                                          me.allen@juno.com
                                  www.maryemmallen.blogspot.com
Experiences of a woman who cared for her mother and aunt, both
Alzheimer's patients.
62 pages
ISBN: 0-965167-51-8
Mary Emma Allen, Author

Children's Books

1023 **Grandpa Doesn't Know It's Me**
Donna Guthrie, author
Alzheimer's Association
225 North Michigan Avenue   312-335-8700
Chicago, IL 60601-1696   800-272-3900
                                          Fax: 866-699-1246
                                          TDD: 312-335-5886
                                               info@alz.org
                                               www.alz.org
Geared to the concerns of a young child who has a relative with
Alzheimer's disease.
26 pages
Donna Guthrie, Author

1024 **Grandpa's Music: A Story About Alzheimer's**
Alison Acheson, author
Albert Whitman & Company
250 S. Northwest Highway   847-232-2800
Park Ridge, IL 60068-2723   800-255-7675
                                          Fax: 847-581-0039
                                          www.albertwhitman.com
Children's book using text and illustrations to show the effects of
Alzheimer's disease.
ISBN: 0-807530-52-8
Alison Acheson, Author
Joe Campbell, Customer Service

1025 **Just for Children: Helping You Understand Alzheimer's Disease**
Alzheimer's Association

225 North Michigan Avenue   312-335-8700
Chicago, IL 60601-1676   800-272-3900
                                          Fax: 866-699-1246
                                          TDD: 312-335-5886
                                               info@alz.org
                                               www.alz.org
Information about Alzheimer's disease written especially for children.
1997 2 pages Pack of 100

1026 **Let's Talk About When Someone You Love Has Alzheimer's
Disease**
Rosen Publishing Group's PowerKids Press
29 E 21st Street   212-777-3017
New York, NY 10010   800-237-9932
                                          Fax: 888-436-4643
                                    customerservice@rosenpub.com
                                    www.rosenpublishing.com
This book sensitively helps children cope with this unsettling disease.
ISBN: 0-823923-06-1
Elizabeth Weitzman, Author

1027 **Through Tara's Eyes: Helping Children Cope with Alzheimer's
Disease**
American Health Assistance Foundation
22512 Gateway Center Dr.   301-948-3244
Clarksburg, MD 20871   800-437-2423
                                          Fax: 301-258-9454
                                          info@brightfocus.org
                                          www.brightfocus.org
Told from the perspective of Tara who has a grandmother with Alzheimer's disease but does not know anything is wrong with her
grandmother.
36 pages

1028 **What's Wrong with Grandma? A Family Experience with
Alzheimer's**
Margaret Shawver, author
Prometheus Books
59 John Glenn Drive   716-691-0133
Amherst, NY 14228-2197   800-421-0351
                                          Fax: 716-691-0137
                                    marketing@prometheusbooks.com
                                    www.prometheusbooks.com
The story of a family's struggle with Alzheimer's disease as told by
the youngest child.
62 pages Paperback
ISBN: 1-159011-74-2
Margaret Shawver, Author

1029 **Window of Time**
Associated Publishers Group
1501 Country Hospital Rd   615-254-2450
Nashville, TN 37218   800-327-5113
                                          Fax: 615-254-2405
                                          vlill@apgbooks.com
Illustrated book about the relationship between a grandfather with
Alzheimer's and his grandson.
28 pages
ISBN: 0-963633-51-1

Magazines

1030 **Alzheimer Disease and Associated Disorders: An International
Journal**
Raven Press
1185 Ave of the Americas   212-930-9500
New York, NY 10036-2601   800-777-2295
                                          journals.lww.com
A leading international forum for reports of new research findings
and new approaches to diagnosis and treatments. Contributions are
offered from all scientific and medical fields.
Quarterly
ISBN: 0-89303H- -
Charles DeCarli, MD, Editor-in-Chief

1031 Mature Health
Haymarket Group, Ltd.
45 W 34th Street   212-239-0855
New York, NY 10001-3073
Magazine featuring articles on health aspects of aging, as well as articles on recreation and leisure.

1032 Research & Practice
Alzheimer's Association
225 North Michigan Avenue   312-335-8700
Chicago, IL 60601-1696   800-272-3900
                                         Fax: 866-699-1246
                                         TDD: 312-335-5886
                                              info@alz.org
                                              www.alz.org
Provides practical information for healthcare professionals on the current status of prominent areas of Alzheimer research.
Quarterly
ISBN: 2-909342-84-0

Newsletters

1033 Advances: Progress in Alzheimer Research and Care
Alzheimer's Association
225 North Michigan Avenue   312-335-8700
Chicago, IL 60601-1696   800-272-3900
                                         Fax: 866-699-1246
                                         TDD: 312-335-5886
                                              info@alz.org
                                              www.alz.org
Provides information related to research and caregiving.
Quarterly

1034 Aging and Alzheimer's Disease Center Newsletter
Oregon Health Sciences University
3181 SW Sam Jackson   503-494-6976
Portland, OR 97201-3098   Fax: 503-494-7499
                                            kaye@ohsu.edu
                                 www.ohsu.edu/som-alzheimers
Researches causes and consequences of Alzheimer's disease and ways of clinical services.
2x Year
Jeffrey Kaye, Director

1035 Alzheimer Disease and Associated Disorders
Charles Decarli, author
Lippincott Williams & Wilkins
16522 Hunters Green Pkwy   301-223-2300
Hagerstown, MD 21740   800-638-3030
                                         Fax: 301-223-2398
                                            orders@lww.com
                                              www.lww.com
A leading international forum for reports of new research findings and new approaches to diagnosis and treatment.
Quarterly Journal
Charles DeCarli MD, Editor

1036 Alzheimer's Association: Tarrant County Chapter
2630 West Freeway   817-336-4949
Fort Worth, TX 76102   800-471-4422
                                         Fax: 817-336-4966
                                              info@alz.org
                                 www.alz.org/northcentraltexas
Newsletter for those afflicted with Alzheimer's disease. Includes education, support groups, case management, telephone helpline and referral to services (i.e. long term care, adult daycare, medical assistance, legal assistance, etc.).
8 pages
Theresa Hocker, Executive Director
Susanna Luk-Jones, Director Services

1037 LIAFLine Newsletter
Long Island Alzheimers Foundation
5 Channel Drive   516-767-6856
Port Washington, NY 11050   Fax: 516-767-6864
                                              info@liaf.org
                                              www.liaf.org

It is intended for caregivers, service providers and anyone interested in Alzheimer's Disease or the Foundation.
Fred Jenny, Executive Director

Pamphlets

1038 10 Warning Signs of Alzheimer's Disease
Alzheimer's Association
225 N Michigan Avenue   312-335-8700
Chicago, IL 60601-7633   800-272-3900
                                         Fax: 866-699-1246
                                         TDD: 866-403-3073
                                              info@alz.org
                                              www.alz.org
Contains a list of symptoms and answers to the most frequently asked questions.
Pack of 100
Harry Johns, President/CEO

1039 Alzheimer's Disease
National Institutes of Health
9000 Rockville Pike   301-496-4000
Bethesda, MD 20892-0001   TTY: 301-402-9612
                                         NIHinfo@od.nih.gov
                                              www.nih.gov
Contains information on the diagnosis and treatment of Alzheimer's and on research that offers hope for the future. Included is a list of sources of help for both the patient and the family.

1040 Alzheimer's Disease: The Basics
Alzheimer's Association
225 N Michigan Avenue   312-335-8700
Chicago, IL 60601-7633   800-272-3900
                                         Fax: 866-699-1246
                                         TDD: 312-335-5886
                                              info@alz.org
                                              www.alz.org
Symptoms, diagnosis, treatments and more
32 pages
Harry Johns, President/CEO

1041 Behaviors
Alzheimer's Association
225 N Michigan Avenue   312-335-8700
Chicago, IL 60601-7633   800-272-3900
                                         Fax: 866-669-1246
                                         TDD: 312-335-5886
                                              info@alz.org
                                              www.alz.org
The most common behaviors and how to manage them.
12 pages
Harry Johns, President/CEO

1042 Caregiver Stress
Alzheimer's Association
225 N Michigan Avenue   312-335-8700
Chicago, IL 60601-7633   800-272-3900
                                         Fax: 866-699-1246
                                         TDD: 312-335-5886
                                              info@alz.org
                                              www.alz.org
Symptoms of caregiver stress and ways you can become a healthy caregiver.
6 pages
Harry Johns, President/CEO

1043 Caring for Alzheimer's Patients
Human Sciences Press
233 Spring Street   212-620-8000
New York, NY 10013-1522   800-221-9369
This handbook is designed for families, friends, and health-care professionals coping with the myriad of problems encountered by those afflicted with Alzheimer's disease.
308 pages Cloth

1044 Dementia Care Practice Recommendations Phases 1 and 2
Alzheimer's Association

225 N Michigan Avenue 312-335-8700
Chicago, IL 60601-7633 800-272-3900
Fax: 866-699-1246
TDD: 312-335-5886
info@alz.org
www.alz.org

Covers fundamentals of dementia care and six key care practice areas: food and fluid consumption, pain management, social engagement, resident wandering, falls and physical restraint-free care.
32 pages
Harry Johns, President/CEO

1045 Early-Onset Alzheimer's: I'M Too Young to Have Alzheimer's Disease
Alzheimer's Association
225 N Michigan Avenue 312-335-8700
Chicago, IL 60601-7633 800-272-3900
Fax: 866-699-1246
TDD: 312-335-5886
info@alz.org
www.alz.org

Addresses unique challenges for diagnosed individuals who are younger than 65
12 pages
Harry Johns, President/CEO

1046 Early-Stage Alzheimer's: If You Have Alzheimer's Disease What You Should Know
Alzheimer's Association
225 N Michigan Avenue 312-335-8700
Chicago, IL 60601-7633 800-272-3900
Fax: 866-669-1246
TDD: 312-335-5886
info@alz.org
www.alz.org

Coping strategies and tips for living with Alzheimer's
16 pages
Harry Johns, President/CEO

1047 Home Safety for People with Alzheimer's Disease
Alzheimer's Disease Education & Referral Center
31 Center Drive 301-495-3311
Bethesda, MD 20892 800-438-4380
Fax: 301-495-3334
adear@nia.nih.gov
www.nia.nih.gov

For those who provide in-home care for people with Alzheimer's disease or related disorders. The goal is to improve home safety by identifying potential problems in the home and offering possible solutions to help prevent accidents.
32 pages

1048 If You Have Alzheimer's Disease: What You Should Know, What You Should Do
Alzheimer's Association
225 North Michigan Avenue 800-272-3900
Chicago, IL 60611-1696 Fax: 866-699-1246
TDD: 312-335-8700
media@alz.org
www.alz.org

Guide for the person with Alzheimer's disease. Includes suggestions of things to do that will help the person cope.
1994 Pack of 100

1049 Just for Teens: Helping You Understand Alzheimer's Disease
Alzheimer's Association
225 North Michigan Avenue 800-272-3900
Chicago, IL 60611-1696 Fax: 866-699-1246
TDD: 312-335-8700
media@alz.org
www.alz.org

Information about Alzheimer's disease aimed at teenagers.
Pack of 100

1050 Late Stage Care
Alzheimer's Association

225 North Michigan Avenue 800-272-3900
Chicago, IL 60611-1696 Fax: 866-699-1246
TDD: 312-335-8700
media@alz.org
www.alz.org

Suggestions for coping with caregiving problems that commonly occur late in the progression of Alzheimer's disease.
Pack of 100

1051 Legal Plans
Alzheimer's Association
225 N Michigan Avenue 312-335-8700
Chicago, IL 60601-7633 800-272-3900
Fax: 866-699-1246
TDD: 312-335-5886
info@alz.org
www.alz.org

Covers legal documents and how to find a lawyer.
16 pages
Harry Johns, President/CEO

1052 MedicAlert & Alzheimer's Association Safe Return
Alzheimer's Association
225 N Michigan Avenue 312-335-8700
Chicago, IL 60601-7633 800-272-3900
Fax: 866-699-1246
TDD: 312-335-5886
info@alz.org
www.alz.org

Enroll in the nationwide emergency response program that provides help when a person with dementia wanders or has a medical emergency.
1 pages
Harry Johns, President/CEO

1053 Money Matters
Alzheimer's Association
225 N Michigan Avenue 312-335-8700
Chicago, IL 60601-7633 800-272-3900
Fax: 866-699-1246
TDD: 312-335-5886
info@alz.org
www.alz.org

Identifies care costs and how to pay for them.
28 pages
Harry Johns, President/CEO

1054 National Public Policy Program to Conquer Alzheimer's Disease
Alzheimer's Association
225 North Michigan Avenue 312-335-8700
Chicago, IL 60611-1676 800-272-3900
Fax: 866-699-1246
TDD: 312-335-5886
info@alz.org
www.alz.org

Summary of the Association's public policy goals, objectives and policies.
1997-Present 12 pages

1055 Nutrition Screening Initiative
Nutrition Screening Initiative
2626 Pennsylvania Ave NW 202-625-1662
Washington, DC 20037-1618 nsi@gmmb.com

Offers information on nutrition pertaining to older Americans and illnesses such as Alzheimer's disease.

1056 Partnering with Your Doctor: A Guide for Persons with Memory Problems
Alzheimer's Association
225 N Michigan Avenue 312-335-8700
Chicago, IL 60601-7633 800-272-3900
Fax: 866-699-1246
TDD: 312-335-5886
info@alz.org
www.alz.org

Tips on working with your doctor to get the best care.
20 pages
Harry Johns, President/CEO

1057 Phase 3: Dementia Care Practice Recommendations
Alzheimer's Association
225 N Michigan Avenue   312-335-8700
Chicago, IL 60601-7633   800-272-3900
                                              Fax: 866-699-1246
                                              TDD: 312-335-5886
                                                   info@alz.org
                                                    www.alz.org

Covers minimizing physical, emotional and spiritual distress;
maximizing well-being; snsuring communication with the resident, family and care team.
28 pages
Harry Johns, President/CEO

1058 Practice Recommendations for Home Care Professionals
Alzheimer's Association
225 N Michigan Avenue   312-335-8700
Chicago, IL 60601-7633   800-272-3900
                                              Fax: 866-699-1246
                                              TDD: 312-335-5886
                                                   info@alz.org
                                                    www.alz.org

Covers concrete, evidence-based practice suggestions for addressing issues unique to people with dementia living in the community.
68 pages
Harry Johns, President/CEO

1059 Report of the Panel on Alzheimer's Disease
National Clearinghouse for Alcohol and Drug Abuse
PO Box 2345   800-729-6686
Rockville, MD 20857   www.health.org
52 pages

1060 Respite Care Guide
Alzheimer's Association
225 N Michigan Avenue   312-335-8700
Chicago, IL 60601-7633   800-272-3900
                                              Fax: 866-699-1246
                                              TDD: 312-335-5886
                                                   info@alz.org
                                                    www.alz.org

Find help when you need a break from caregiving.
19 pages
Harry Johns, President/CEO

1061 Steps to Diagnosis
Alzheimer's Association
225 North Michigan Avenue   800-272-3900
Chicago, IL 60611-1696   Fax: 866-699-1246
                                              TDD: 312-335-8700
                                                  media@alz.org
                                                    www.alz.org

Educates individuals and their families on the importance of seeking a diagnosis, and the various test completed to obtain an accurate diagnosis.

1062 Steps to Enhancing Communication
Alzheimer's Association
225 North Michigan Avenue   800-272-3900
Chicago, IL 60611-1696   Fax: 866-699-1246
                                              TDD: 312-335-8700
                                                  media@alz.org
                                                    www.alz.org

Offers caregivers techniques for improving their approach to listening to and communication with the individual with Alzheimer's
disease.
1996 Pack of 100

1063 Tax Credits and Deductions
Alzheimer's Association
225 N Michigan Avenue   312-335-8700
Chicago, IL 60601-7633   800-272-3900
                                              Fax: 866-669-1246
                                              TDD: 321-335-5886
                                                   info@alz.org
                                                    www.alz.org

Outlines caregiving tax deductions and credits.
3 pages
Harry Johns, President/CEO

1064 Terms & Tips: An Alzheimer Care Handbook
Marjorie Brandenburg, author
Alzheimer's Association
225 North Michigan Avenue   800-272-3900
Chicago, IL 60611-1696   Fax: 866-699-1246
                                              TDD: 312-335-8700
                                                  media@alz.org
                                                    www.alz.org

Offers an explanation for over 250 terms and offers practical caregiver ideas and tips. Primarily for people with dementia and their
caregivers, family members, and all providers of hands-on
assistance.
1995 84 pages

1065 Treatments for Alzheimer's Disease
Alzheimer's Association
225 N Michigan Avenue   312-335-8700
Chicago, IL 60601-7633   800-272-3900
                                              Fax: 866-699-1246
                                              TDD: 312-335-5886
                                                   info@alz.org
                                                    www.alz.org

Information about FDA-approved drugs.
3 pages
Harry Johns, President/CEO

1066 Useful Information on Alzheimer's Disease
National Clearinghouse for Alcohol and Drug Abuse
PO Box 2345   800-729-6686
Rockville, MD 20857-0001   www.health.org
24 pages

**1067 You Are One of Us: Clergy/Church Connections to Alzheimer
Families**
Alzheimer's Disease Education & Referral Center
31 Center Drive   301-495-3311
Bethesda, MD 20892-8250   800-438-4380
                                              Fax: 301-495-3334
                                              adear@nia.nih.gov
                                          www.nia.nih.gov/alzheimers

Describes how clergy and church members can help families by including patients and their relatives in church activities, visiting patients and developing church programs that support family
caregivers.

Audio & Video

1068 Alzheimer's Association Caregiver Resources
Alzheimer's Association
225 N. Michigan Ave.   312-335-8700
Chicago, IL 60601   800-848-7097
                                              Fax: 866-699-1246
                                              TDD: 312-335-5886
                                                   info@alz.org
                                       http://alzwa.org/resources6.htm

A variety of numerous resources, materials and publications providing information for assisting those with Alzheimer's Disease
including a documentation guide, informational fact sheets on topics such as bathing, dressing, eating and dealing with grief, in addition resources on long term care options and a newsletter.
Nancy Dapper, Executive Director
Rowena Rye, Community Resources

1069 Alzheimer's Association Dementia Care Conference
Alzheimer's Association
225 North Michigan Avenue   312-335-5790
Chicago, IL 60601-7633   800-272-3900
                                              Fax: 866-699-1246
                                              TDD: 312-335-8700
                                          careconference@alz.org
                                         www.alz.org/careconference/

Selected sessions from the conference discussing topics such as assisted living preconference, sexuality, intimacy and lifestyle
changes, and activity intensive changing approaches to Alzheimer
care.
Marisol Sukhu, Hotel/Events Information
Sheryl Trotz, Continuing Education & Presentations

1070 Alzheimer's Association Safe Return Police Training Video
Alzheimer's Association Massachusetts Chapter
225 N. Michigan Ave. 617-868-6718
Chicago, IL 60601 800-548-2111
Fax: 617-868-6720
www.alzmass.org/
An educational package designed to help police officers recognize and respond appropriately to Alzheimer patients who may need assistance. Kit includes 1 videotape and 3 print pieces.
James Wessler, President/Chief Executive Officer
Betsy Fitzgerald, Director of Communications

1071 Alzheimer's Association: Waves of Stone Video and Documentary
Alzheimer's Association Rhode Island Chapter
245 Waterman Street 401-421-3900
Providence, RI 02906 800-272-3900
Fax: 401-421-0115
info@alz.org
http://www.alz-ri.org/Videoshtm.htm
PBS documentary on Alzheimer's disease that discusses both scientific research and caregiver issues.
1994 57 minutes
Elizabeth Morancy, Executive Director
Rita St Pierre, Program Director

1072 Another Home for Mom
Lori Hope, author
Fanlight Productions
32 Court Street 718-488-8900
Brooklyn, NY 11201-1731 800-876-1710
Fax: 718-488-8642
info@fanlight.com
www.fanlight.com
A gentle documentary following one couple as they confront the decision of whether to place the husbands mother, who has Alzheimer's disease, in a nursing home.
1989 27 Minutes
ISBN: 1-572950-77-3

1073 Caring...Sharing: The Alzheimer's Caregiver
Fanflight Productions
32 Court Street 718-488-8900
Brooklyn, NY 11201 800-876-1710
Fax: 718-488-8642
info@fanlight.com
www.fanlight.com
Examines what it means to be a caregiver. This program will be invaluable for any person or group involved in the care of the elderly.
38 minutes
ISBN: 1-572951-22-2
Hal Kirn, Producer

1074 For Those Who Take Care: An Alzheimer's Disease Training Program for Nurses
Alzheimer's Disease Education & Referral Center
31 Center Drive 301-495-3311
Bethesda, MD 20892-8250 800-438-4380
Fax: 301-495-3334
adear@nia.nih.gov
www.nia.nih.gov/alzheimers
Guide for training nursing assistants and nurses' aides in long term care facilities, adult day care and private homes. Manual, text and student handouts. Produced by the University of Kentucky.

Web Sites

1075 Alzheimer Research Forum
www.alzforum.org
The web's most dynamic scientific community dedicated to understanding alzheimer's disease and related disorders.

1076 Alzheimer Support
www.alzheimersupport.com
Serves Alzheimer's sufferers and their loved ones by reporting the latest news in research and treatment, making hard-to-find, recommended nutritional supplements available at manufacturer-direct low prices, and, most importantly, donating profits from each purchase to fund Alzheimer's medical research.

1077 Alzheimer's Association
www.alz.org
The leading, global voluntary health organization in Alzheimer care and support, and the largest private, nonprofit funder of Alzheimer research.

1078 Alzheimer's Disease International
www.alz.co.uk/adi
The international federation of 73 Alzheimer associations around the world, in relations with the World Health Organization.

1079 Healing Well
www.healingwell.com
A social network and support community for patients, caregivers, and families coping with the daily struggles of diseases, disorders and chronic illness.

1080 Health Finder
www.healthfinder.gov
A government website where individuals can find information and tools to help you and those you care about stay healthy.

1081 Healthlink USA
www.healthlinkusa.com
Health information concerning treatment, cures, prevention, diagnosis, risk factors, research, support groups, email lists, personal stories and much more. Updated regularly.

1082 MEDLINEplus Health Information
www.nlm.nih.gov/medlineplus
MedlinePlus is the National Institutes of Health's Web site for patients and their families and friends.

1083 MedicineNet
www.medicinenet.com
An online resource for consumers providing easy-to-read, authoritative medical and health information.

1084 Medscape
www.medscape.com
Medscape offers specialists, primary care physicians, and other health professionals the Web's most robust and integrated medical information and educational tools.

1085 Neurology Channel
www.healthcommunities.com
Find clearly explained, medically accurate information regarding conditions, including an overview, symptoms, causes, diagnostic procedures and treatment options. On this site it is possible to ask questions and get information from a neurologist and connect to people who have similar health interests.

1086 WebMD
www.webmd.com
Provides credible information, supportive communities, and in-depth reference material about health subjects. A source for original and timely health information as well as material from well known content providers.

Description

1087 ## Amyotrophic Lateral Sclerosis

Amyotrophic Lateral Sclerosis, ALS, also called Lou Gehrig's disease, is a neurological disorder that affects the motor nerves in the brain and spinal cord. The cause of ALS is unknown. It is marked by progressive muscle weakness. 14,000-15,000 Americans have ALS. There are two types of ALS; sporadic (90 percent of cases) and familial or genetic (5-10 percent of cases). Sporadic ALS results from newly-arising mutations and familial ALS results from inherited mutations in specific genes, such as SOD1, which encodes the enzyme copper-zinc superoxide dismutase 1, or a gene known as "chromosome 9 open reading frame 72," or C9ORF72.

Initial symptoms may be subtle, but early signs of ALS can include twitching and cramping of muscles (particularly in the hands and feet), as well as difficulty in swallowing. As the disorder progresses, use of legs and arms, breathing, speaking, and swallowing become increasingly difficult.

Although the physical symptoms of ALS are most debilitating, the disease does not seem to impair intellectual functioning, although recent research indicates a significant number of people with ALS who have cognitive defects. Voluntary eye movement (blinking) and the senses also remain unaffected.

Currently, there is no cure for ALS. However, two drugs, riluzole and edaravone are FDA-approved to treat ALS. Riluzole does not reduce neural damage caused by the diseased, but it does prolong survival by several months. Edaravone slows the decline of ALS. A regime of physical therapy and psychological support can help patients and their families.

National Agencies & Associations

1088 **ALS Association National Office**
1275 K Street NW
Washington, DC 20005
202-407-8580
800-782-4747
Fax: 202-464-8869
alsinfo@alsa-national.org
www.alsa.org
National nonprofit voluntary health organization dedicated solely to the fight against amyotrophic lateral sclerosis, including finding a cure for and improving living with ALS. The four priorities are: encouraging, identifying, funding, and monitoring.
Calaneet Balas, President & CEO
Kimberly Maginnis, Senior Vice President, Care Services

1089 **American Association of Neuromuscular & Electrodiagnostic Medicine**
2621 Superior Drive NW
Rochester, MN 55901
507-288-0100
Fax: 507-288-1225
aanem@aanem.org
www.aanem.org
The American Association of Neuromuscular & Electrodiagnostic Medicine (AANEM) is a nonprofit membership association dedicated to the advancement of neuromuscular, musculoskeletal, and electrodiagnostic medicine.
Shirlyn A. Adkins, JD, Executive Director
Millie Suk, JD, MPP, Health Policy Director

1090 **The International Alliance of ALS/MND Associations**
c/o The ALS Association

1275 K Street NW
Washington, DC 20005
202-627-0993
alliance@als-mnd.org
www.alsmndalliance.org
The International Alliance of ALS/MND Associations exists to provide an international community for individual ALS/MND associations from around the world.
Catherine Summings, CAE, MBA, Executive Director

State Agencies & Associations

Alabama

1091 **ALS Association: Alabama Chapter**
300 Cahaba Park Circle
Birmingham, AL 35242
205-213-7289
800-664-1242
Fax: 205-449-9330
info@ALSAlabama.org
webal.alsa.org
ALS Association chapters are multifaceted grass roots organizations that carry out ALSA's mission and strategic goals at the community level. The chapter, with supporting services from the national office, actively pursues the association's goals.
Bobbi Grady, Director, Development & Outreach
Melissa Enfinger, Director Care Services

Arizona

1092 **ALS Association: Arizona Chapter**
360 E. Coronado
Phoenix, AZ 85004
602-297-3800
866-350-2572
Fax: 602-297-3804
info@alsaz.org
webaz.alsa.org
ALS Association chapters are multifaceted grass roots organizations that carry out ALSA's mission and strategic goals at the community level. The chapter, with supporting services from the national office, actively pursues the association's goals.
Taryn Norley, Executive Director
Anissa Franklin, Director of Operations

Arkansas

1093 **ALS Association: Arkansas Chapter**
1200 West Walnut
Rogers, AR 72756
479-621-8700
866-540-7411
Fax: 479-621-8701
info@als-arkansas.org
webar.alsa.org
ALS Association chapters are multifaceted grass roots organizations that carry out ALSA's mission and strategic goals at the community level. The chapter, with supporting services from the national office, actively pursues the association's goals.
Jennifer Necessary, Executive Director

California

1094 **ALS Association: Golden West Chapter**
PO Box 565
Agoura Hills, CA 91376
866-750-2572
info@alsagoldenwest.org
www.alsala.org
Serving Hawaii & 31 counties in CA. ALS Association chapters are multifaceted grass-roots organizations that carry out ALSA's mission and strategic goals at the community level. The chapter — with supporting services from the National Office — actively pursues the Association's goals.
Fred Fisher, President & CEO
Asher Garfinkel, VP Community Outreach

1095 **ALS Association: Golden West Chapter - Greater Los Angeles Office**
28720 Roadside Drive
Agoura Hills, CA 91301
818-865-8067
866-750-2572
Fax: 818-865-8066
info@alsagoldenwest.org
www.alsala.org
ALS Association chapters are multifaceted grass-roots organizations that carry out ALSA's mission and strategic goals at the com-

munity level. The chapter — with supporting services from the National Office — actively pursues the Association's goals.
Robin Eller, Regional Care Manager

1096   ALS Association: Golden West-Greater Bay
1330 Broadway, Ste 1830   510-251-2572
Oakland, CA 94612   800-209-0433
                                       Fax: 510-251-2573
                                       fightALS@alsabayarea.org
ALS Association chapters are multifaceted grass roots organizations that carry out ALSA's mission and strategic goals at the community level. The chapter, with supporting services from the national office, actively pursues the association's goals.
Fred Fisher, President & CEO
Daniel Potapshyn, MA, Regional Care Manager

1097   ALS Association: Greater Sacramento Chapte r
2717 Cottage Way   916-979-9265
Sacramento, CA 95825   Fax: 916-979-9271
                                       lou@alssac.org
                                       www.alssac.org
ALS Association chapters are multifaceted grass roots organizations that carry out ALSA's mission and strategic goals at the community level. The chapter, with supporting services from the national office, actively pursues the association's goals.
Amy Sugimoto, Executive Director
Nancy Wakefield, MA, Director of Patient Services

1098   ALS Association: Greater San Diego Chapter
9929 Hibert Street   858-271-5547
San Diego, CA 92131   Fax: 858-271-5687
                                       miller.keith@alsasd.org
ALS Association chapters are multifaceted grass-roots organizations that carry out ALSA's mission and strategic goals at the community level. The chapter — with supporting services from the National Office — actively pursues the Association's goals.
Steve Becvar, Executive Director
Keith D. Miller, Associate Director, Care Services

1099   ALS Association: Orange County Chapter
3002 Dow Avenue, Unit 204   714-285-1088
Santa Ana, CA 92780   Fax: 714-285-0305
                                       information@alsaoc.org
                                       weboc.alsa.org
Provides information to ALS patients families and caregivers; offers support groups, information and referrals, a loan closet and public awareness information.
Natalie Villegas, Director of Care Services
Kristin Schlick, Project Support Coordinator

Colorado

1100   ALS Association: Rocky Mountain Chapter
10855 Dover Street, Ste 500   303-832-2322
Westminster, CO 80021   866-ALS-3211
                                       Fax: 303-832-3365
                                       info@alsaco.org
                                       www.alscolorado.org
Serving: Wyoming, Colorado. The ALS Association chapters are multifaceted grass-roots organizations that carry out ALSA's mission and strategic goals at the community level. The chapter — with supporting services from the National Office — actively pursues the Association's goals.
Pam Rush-Negri, Executive Director
Leslie Ryan, Care Services Director

Connecticut

1101   ALS Association: Connecticut Chapter
4 Oxford Road   203-874-5050
Milford, CT 06460   877-257-2281
                                       Fax: 203-874-7070
                                       webct.alsa.org
The central source in Connecticut for services and education of ALS patients, families and caregivers. Provides ALS patients with information concerning medical care and facilities, support groups, daily living aids and other services.
Jacky Rose, Development Manager
Kim Buda, Operations Manager

District of Columbia

1102   ALS Association: National Capital Area Chapter
7507 Standish Place   301-978-9855
Rockville, MD 20855   866-348-3257
                                       Fax: 301-978-9854
                                       info@ALSinfo.org
                                       webdc.alsa.org
Offers patient referrals, informational newsletters and brochures, patient support groups and meetings and fund raising for research into finding cures and treatments for ALS.
Judy Taylor, Executive Director
Tremetris Harrell, VP, Programs & Operations

Florida

1103   ALS Association: Florida Chapter
3242 Parkside Center Circle   813-637-9000
Tampa, FL 33619   888-257-1717
                                       Fax: 813-637-9010
                                       jniehoff@alsafl.org
                                       webfl.alsa.org
ALS Association chapters are multifaceted grass-roots organizations that carry out ALSA's mission and strategic goals at the community level. The chapter — with supporting services from the National Office — actively pursues the Association's goals.
Kim Hanna, President & CEO
Julie Niehoff, Director, Marketing & Communications

Georgia

1104   ALS Association: Georgia Chapter
5881 Glenridge Drive   404-636-9909
Atlanta, GA 30328   888-636-9940
                                       Fax: 404-636-9949
                                       info@alsaga.org
                                       www.alsaga.org
Offers meetings, local support groups, patient support equipment loan and research for persons suffering from ALS.
Sarah Embro, Executive Director
Juanita Pharr, Care Services Director

Illinois

1105   Lois Insolia ALS Center at Northwestern Memorial Hospital
5550 West Touhyu   847-679-3311
Skokie, IL 60077   888-ALS-1107
                                       Fax: 847-679-9109
                                       info@lesturnerals.org
                                       www.lesturnerals.org
Utilizes a multidisciplinary approach in treating ALS. Trained specialists provide diagnostic, rehabilitative and supportive services that focus on assessment, care planning and education. Patients and loved ones are encouraged to attend the support groups offered. Provides in-home visits by ALS nurse consultants and social worker, support groups, a lending bank of equipment, and grant programs for financial aid.
Teepu Siddique MD, Director

Indiana

1106   ALS Association: Indiana Chapter
7202 E. 87th Street   317-915-9888
Indianapolis, IN 46256   888-508-3232
                                       Fax: 317-573-9889
                                       info@alsaindiana.org
                                       webin.alsa.org
ALS Association chapters are multifaceted grass-roots organizations that carry out ALSA's mission and strategic goals at the community level. The chapter — with supporting services from the National Office — actively pursues the Association's goals.
Tina Kaetzel, Executive Director
Leslie Weaver, Care Services Coordinator

Kansas

1107 ALS Association: Mid America Chapter Kansas City Metro Area
6950 Squibb Rd   913-648-2062
Mission, KS 66202   800-878-2062
                                                         Fax: 913-642-2431
                                                         info@alsa-midamerica.org
                                                         www.alsa-midamerica.org
ALS Association chapters are multifaceted grass-roots organizations that carry out ALSA's mission and strategic goals at the community level. The chapter — with supporting services from the National Office — actively pursues the Association's goals.
Colleen Wachter, Executive Director
Sally Dwyer, Director, Programs & Services

1108 ALS Association: Mid America Chapter Centr al Kansas Office
3450 N. Rock Road   316-612-0188
Wichita, KS 67226   800-878-2062
                                                         Fax: 316-612-8768
                                                         www.alsa-midamerica.org
ALS Association chapters are multifaceted grass-roots organizations that carry out ALSA's mission and strategic goals at the community level. The chapter — with supporting services from the National Office — actively pursues the Association's goals.
Katelynn Powell, Administrative Director
Cheyenne Layton, Development Manager

Kentucky

1109 ALS Association: Kentucky Chapter
8640 Haines Drive   859-331-1384
Florence, KY 41042   800-406-7702
                                                         Fax: 859-331-1902
                                                         webky.alsa.org
ALS Association chapters are multifaceted grass-roots organizations that carry out ALSA's mission and strategic goals at the community level. The chapter — with supporting services from the National Office — actively pursues the Association's goals.
Mari Bacon, Executive Director
Jennifer Houston, Project Manager

Massachusetts

1110 ALS Association: Massachusetts Chapter
315 Norwood Park S., 1st Fl   781-255-8884
Norwood, MA 02062   800-258-3323
                                                         Fax: 781-326-4940
                                                         info@als-ma.org
Offers informational brochures and newsletters to promote public awareness, support groups and meetings for patients and their families, and referral information for members in the Massachusetts area.
Lynn Aaronson, Executive Director
Jan Oberman, Director Care Services

Michigan

1111 ALS Association: East Michigan Chapter
675 E. Big Beaver Rd, Ste 207   248-680-6540
Troy, MI 48083   866-927-2873
                                                         Fax: 248-680-6543
                                                         randy@alsa-michigan.org
                                                         www.alsofmichigan.org
ALS Association chapters are multi-faceted grass-roots organizations that carry out ALSA's mission. and strategic goals at the community level. The chapter — with supporting services from the National Office — actively pursues the Association's goals.
Tyler MacEachran, Executive Director
Randy Berd, Care Services & Education Coordinator

1112 ALS Association: West Michigan Chapter
678 Front Street, NW   616-459-1900
Grand Rapids, MI 49504   866-927-2873
                                                         Fax: 616-459-4522
                                                         randy@alsa-michigan.org
                                                         webmi.alsa.org
ALS Association chapters are multi-faceted grass-roots organizations that carry out ALSA's mission. and strategic goals at the com-

munity level. The chapter — with supporting services from the National Office — actively pursues the Association's goals.
Tyler MacEachran, Executive Director
Randy Berd, Care Services & Education Coordinator

Minnesota

1113 ALS Association: Minnesota, South Dakota, North Dakota Chapter
333 N Washington Avenue   612-672-0484
Minneapolis, MN 55401   888-672-0484
                                                         Fax: 612-672-9110
                                                         info@alsmn.org
                                                         webmn.alsa.org
ALS Association chapters are multifaceted grass-roots organizations that carry out ALSA's mission and strategic goals at the community level. The chapter — with supporting services from the National Office — actively pursues the Association's goals.
Jennifer Hjelle, Executive Director
Marianne Keuhn, VP, Care Services

Missouri

1114 ALS Association: Mid America Chapter- Southern Missouri Office
2209 Petrus Circle   417-886-5003
Ozark, MO 65721   800-878-2062
                                                         Fax: 417-886-5003
                                                         www.alsa-midamerica.org
ALS Association chapters are multifaceted grass-roots organizations that carry out ALSA's mission and strategic goals at the community level. The chapter — with supporting services from the National Office — actively pursues the Association's goals.
Beth Hanslow, Development Manager
Sherri Murray, Care Services Specialist

1115 ALS Association: St. Louis Regional Chapter
2258 Weldon Parkway   314-432-7257
Saint Louis, MO 63146   888-873-8539
                                                         Fax: 314-432-2991
                                                         info@alsastl.org
                                                         webstl.alsa.org
A chapter serving the Eastern Missouri and Southern Illinois regions dedicated solely to finding the cause and cure of ALS through research, patient support, information and referrals and public awareness.
Maureen Barber-Hill, President
Lori Dobbs, Care Services Coordinator

Nebraska

1116 ALS Association: MidAmerica Chapter - Nebr aska Office
900 s. 74 Plaza, Ste 106   402-991-8788
Omaha, NE 68114   866-762-6361
                                                         Fax: 402-991-3690
                                                         info@alsa-midamerica.org
                                                         www.alsa-midamerica.org
ALS Association chapters are multifaceted grass-roots organizations that carry out ALSA's mission and strategic goals at the community level. The chapter — with supporting services from the National Office — actively pursues the Association's goals.
Shannon Todd, Care Services Specialist
Sherrie Hanneman, Director of Communications

New Hampshire

1117 ALS Association: Northern New England Chapter
The Champlain Mill
10 Ferry Street, Ste 438   603-226-8855
Concord, NH 03301   866-257-6663
                                                         Fax: 603-226-8890
                                                         executive.director@alsanne.org
                                                         www.alsanne.org
ALS Association chapters are multifaceted grass-roots organizations that carry out ALSA's mission and strategic goals at the community level. The chapter — with supporting services from the National Office — actively pursues the Association's goals.
Mauret Brinsor, Executive Director
Christine Richards, Patient Services Manager

1118 ALS Association: New Mexico Chapter
2309 Renard Place SE 505-323-6348
Albuquerque, NM 87106 als@alsanm.org
ALS Association chapters are multifaceted grass-roots organizations that carry out ALSA's mission and strategic goals at the community level. The chapter — with supporting services from the National Office — actively pursues the Association's goals.
Joe Cordova, Executive Director
Michelle Waters, Care Services Coordinator

New York

1119 ALS Association: Greater New York Chapter
42 Broadway 212-619-1400
New York, NY 10004 800-672-8857
Fax: 212-619-7409
als@als-ny.org
www.als-ny.org
ALS Association chapters are multifaceted grass-roots organizations that carry out ALSA's mission and strategic goals at the community level. The chapter — with supporting services from the National Office — actively pursues the Association's goals.
Dorine Gordon, President
Rachel Kent, Communications Manager

1120 ALS Association: Upstate New York Chapter
135 Old Cove Rd, Ste 213 315-413-0121
Liverpool, NY 13090 866-499-7257
Fax: 315-413-0508
info@alsaupstateny.org
webuny.alsa.org
ALS Association chapters are multifaceted grass-roots organizations that carry out ALSA's mission and strategic goals at the community level. The chapter — with supporting services from the National Office — actively pursues the Association's goals.
Elisabeth Krisanda, Executive Director
Rebecca Coulter, Care Services Manager

Ohio

1121 ALS Association: Central & Southern Ohio Chapter
1170 Old Henderson Road 614-273-2572
Columbus, OH 43220 866-273-2572
Fax: 614-273-2573
alsohio@alsohio.org
webcsoh.alsa.org
Offers telephone consultation services, support groups, caregivers support groups, equipment loan bank and a 24 hour telephone answering service for persons with ALS.
Marlin Seymour, Executive Director
Yvonne Dressman, Care Coordinator

1122 ALS Association: Northern Ohio Chapter
6155 Rockside Road 216-592-2572
Independence, OH 44131 888-592-2572
Fax: 216-592-2575
alsa@alsaohio.org
webnoh.alsa.org
Offers telephone consultation services, support groups, caregivers support groups, equipment loan bank and a 24 hour telephone answering service for persons with ALS.
Mary Wilson Wheelock, Executive Director
Lisa Bruening, Director, Care Services

Oregon

1123 ALS Association: Oregon & SW Washington Chapter
700 NE Multnomah 503-238-5559
Portland, OR 97232 800-681-9851
Fax: 503-296-5590
info@alsa-or.org
webor.alsa.org
The ALS Association chapters are multifaceted grass-roots organizations that carry out ALSA's mission and strategic goals at the community level. The chapter — with supporting services from the National Office — actively pursues the Association's goals.
Lance Christian, Executive Director
Aubrey McCauley, Development Director

Pennsylvania

1124 ALS Association: Greater Philadelphia Chapter
321 Norristown Road 215-643-5434
Ambler, PA 19002 877-434-7441
Fax: 215-643-9307
alsassoc@alsphiladelphia.org
www.alsphiladelphia.org
To lead the fight to treat and cure ALS through global research and nationwide advocacy while also empowering people with Lou Gehrig's Disease and their families to live fuller lives by providing them with compassionate care and support.
Marta Rubin-Kiesling, Executive Director
Erich Fasnacht, Chief Development Officer

1125 ALS Association: Western Pennsylvania Chapter
416 Lincoln Avenue 412-821-3254
Pittsburgh, PA 15209 800-967-9296
Fax: 412-821-3549
info@cure4als.org
webwpawv.alsa.org
The mission of this chapter is to provide services and education to ALS patients, families and caregivers through medical information, support groups, assisting health care providers and providing communication devices.
Merritt Holland Epier, Executive Director
Marie Folino, Director, Care Services

South Carolina

1126 ALS Association: South Carolina Chapter
7499 Parklane Rd, Ste 144 803-851-3233
Columbia, SC 29223 Fax: 803-851-3403
infosc@scalsa.org
websc.alsa.org
ALS association chapters are multifaceted grass roots organizations that carry out ALSA's mission and strategic goals at the community level. The chapter, with supporting services from the national office, actively pursues the association's goals.
Gerald H. Talley, Jr, Executive Director
Brett Vowles, Care Services Manager

South Dakota

1127 ALS Association: Minnesota, South Dakota, North Dakota Chapter
PO Box 2223 605-274-0230
Sioux Falls, SD 55401 888-672-0484
Fax: 605-274-0231
info@alsmn.org
webmn.alsa.org
ALS Association chapters are multifaceted grass-roots organizations that carry out ALSA's mission and strategic goals at the community level. The chapter — with supporting services from the National Office — actively pursues the Association's goals.
Mike Stephanson, Director, Marketing & Communications

Tennessee

1128 ALS Association: Tennessee Chapter
4825 Trousdale Drive, Ste 107 615-331-5556
Nashville, TN 37220 877-216-5551
Fax: 615-331-5796
steve.wallace@alstn.org
webtn.alsa.org
ALS Association chapters are multifaceted grass-roots organizations that carry out ALSA's mission and strategic goals at the community level. The chapter — with supporting services from the National Office — actively pursues the Association's goals.
Steve Wallace, CEO
Patty Lane, Director, Care Services

Texas

1129 ALS Association: Greater Houston Office
1213 Hermann Drive, Ste 525   713-942-2572
Houston, TX 77004   877-714-0088
                                           Fax: 713-456-2976
ALS Association chapters are multi-faceted grass roots organizations that carry out ALSA's mission and strategic goals at the community level. he chapter — with supporting services from the National Office — actively pursues the Association's goals.
Alexis Hyett, Operations & Database Coordinator
Eniye Elegon, Regional Development Manager

1130 ALS Association: South Texas Chapter
4939 De Zavala, Ste 105   210-775-5720
San Antonio, TX 78249   877-714-0088
                                           Fax: 210-733-5206
                                  Information@alsasotx.org
                                           www.alstexas.org
ALS Association chapters are multi-faceted grass roots organizations that carry out ALSA's mission and strategic goals at the community level. he chapter — with supporting services from the National Office — actively pursues the Association's goals.
Linda Quiroz, Care Services Coordinator
Stephen Morse, Director, Care Services

1131 ALS Association: Texas Chapter - Austin
1315 Sam Bass Circle, Unit B5   972-924-9886
Round Rock, TX 78681   877-714-0088
                                           Fax: 972-714-0066
                                  k.mansfield@alsa-texas.org
                                           www.alstexas.org
ALS Association chapters are multi-faceted grass roots organizations that carry out ALSA's mission and strategic goals at the community level. he chapter — with supporting services from the National Office — actively pursues the Association's goals.
Katie Mansfield, Regional Development Manager
Janette Steinheimer, Care Services Manager

1132 ALS Association: Texas Chapter - Dallas
2251 Chenault   972-893-1567
Carrollton, TX 75006   877-714-0088
                                           Fax: 972-714-0066
                                  g.hill@alsa-texas.org
                                           www.alstexas.org
ALS Association chapters are multi-faceted grass roots organizations that carry out ALSA's mission and strategic goals at the community level. he chapter — with supporting services from the National Office — actively pursues the Association's goals.
Greg Hill, Director, Communications & Operations
Tanner Hockensmith, Executive Director

Washington

1133 ALS Association: Evergreen Chapter
19226 66th Avenue S.   425-656-1650
Kent, WA 98032   866-786-7257
                                           Fax: 425-656-1649
                                           webwa.alsa.org
The ALS Association chapters are multifaceted grass-roots organizations that carry out ALSA's mission and strategic goals at the community level. The chapter — with supporting services from the National Office — actively pursues the Association's goals.
Rebecca Moore, Executive Director
Caryn Wise, Care Services Director

1134 ALS Association: Oregon & SW Washington Chapter
700 NE Multnomah   503-238-5559
Portland, OR 97232   800-681-9851
                                           Fax: 503-296-5590
                                           info@alsa-or.org
                                           webor.alsa.org
The ALS Association chapters are multifaceted grass-roots organizations that carry out ALSA's mission and strategic goals at the community level. The chapter — with supporting services from the National Office — actively pursues the Association's goals.
Lance Christian, Executive Director
Karen Galloway, Care Services Director

Wisconsin

1135 ALS Association: Southeast Wisconsin Chapter
3333 N Mayfair Rd, Ste 104   414-763-2220
Wauwatosa, WI 53222   Fax: 414-231-9100
                                           info@alsawi.org
                                           www.alsawi.org
Begun in 1987 as a support group this chapter is managed by a Board of Directors from all walks of life and disciplines. All members share a dedication to carry out the mission of Hope Through Research and Support Through Caring. The goal is to help ALS
Melanie Roach-Bekos, Executive Director
Lori Banker-Horner, LPN, BA, Care Services Director

Research Centers

1136 ALS Center at UCSF
350 Parnassus Avenue   415-353-2108
San Francisco, CA 94117   Fax: 415-353-2524
                                           alscenter@ucsf.edu
                                           www.neurology2.ucsf.edu
Research serves as a cornerstone for our patient programs allowing us to translate the most recent advancement in therapies drug development and clinical management into care for our patients.
Catherine Lomen-Hoer, Director
Carolyn Rodriguez, Clinical Coordinator

1137 ALS Clinic at Penn Neurological Institute ALS Association Greater Philadelphia Cha
ALS Association Greater Philadelphia Chapter
321 Norristown Road   215-643-5434
Ambler, PA 19002   Fax: 215-643-9307
                                  brenda@alsphiladelphia.org
                                           www.pennhealth.com/als
A multidisciplinary center for the evaluation and treatment of amyotrophic lateral sclerosis (ALS) and related disorders.
Brenda Edelm LCSW BCD, Director of Patient Services
Lauren Elman, Associate Medical Director

1138 ALS Clinical Department of Neurology
College of Medicine of the University of Vermont
89 Beaumont Avenue   802-656-2154
Burlington, VT 05405-3456   Fax: 802-656-8577
                                           Rup.Tandan@uvm.edu
                                           www.med.uvm.edu
Clinical care facility for ALS patients.
Daniel Mark Fogel, President
Robert Cioffi, Chair

1139 Center for ALS and Related Diorders The Cleveland Clinic DepartmentOf Neurol
The Cleveland Clinic DepartmentOf Neurology
9500 Euclid Avenue   216-444-5538
Cleveland, OH 44195-5227   800-223-2273
                                           Fax: 216-445-4653
                                           TTY: 216-444-0261
                                           my.clevelandclinic.org
Clinical care and research facility for ALS patients.
Erik P Pioro, Director
Kathleen M Kelly, ALS Clinical Coordinator

1140 Les Turner Research Laboratory Northwestern University Medical School
Northwestern University Medical School
5550 W Touhy Avenue   847-679-3311
Skokie, IL 60077   888-ALS-1107
                                           Fax: 847-679-9109
                                           info@lesturnerals.org
                                           www.lesturnerals.org
Scientists and researchers dedicate their time to discover what causes ALS and find a cure for the disease. The international team of scientists at the Laboratory are internationally recognized for their accomplishments in the field of ALS research.
Harvey Gaffen, President
Wendy Abrams, Executive Director

1141 Mayo Clinic: Department of Neurology
200 First Street SW
Rochester, MN 55905   507-284-2511
                                           Fax: 507-284-0161
                                           TDD: 507-284-9786
                                               www.mayo.edu
Ongoing research and treatment for ALS.
John H Noseworthy MD, President
William C Rupp, MD, Vice President, CEO

**1142 Motor Neuron Disease Clinic University of Connecticut Health
        Center**
University of Connecticut Health Center
263 Farmington Avenue   860-679-2000
Farmington, CT 06030   Fax: 860-679-1454
                                            TTY: 860-679-2242
                                               www.uchc.edu
Francisco L. Borges, Chairman
Sanford Cloud Jr., Chair

**1143 Motor Neuron Disease Program University of Michigan Health
        System**
University of Michigan Health System
1500 E Medical Center Drive   734-936-6641
Ann Arbor, MI 48109-316   Fax: 734-153-53
                                           www.med.umich.edu
Regional clinic that is dedicated to the diagnosis of Amyotrophic
Lateral Sclerosis and improving the well-being of patients who
have this disease.
Ora Hirsh Pescovitz MD, Vice President
Douglas L Strong, CEO

1144 Neuromuscular and ALS Center The Clinical Academic Building
The Clinical Academic Building
125 Patterson Street   732-235-7331
New Brunswick, NJ 08901   Fax: 732-235-7344
A multidisciplinary program for the diagnosis evaluation and
long-term management of a host of neuromuscular diseases found
in adults.
Jerry Belsh MD, Director
Annmarie Coyne-West, Patient Care Coordinator

1145 New England Medical Center: ALS Laboratory
800 Washington Street   617-636-5000
Boston, MA 02111-1533   Fax: 617-636-8568
                                       www.tuftsmedicalcenter.org
Specializes in Amyotrophic Lateral Sclerosis research.
Ellen Zane, President, CEO
Margret Vosburgh, Chief Operating Officer

1146 Solomon Park Research Institute
12815 NE 124th Street   425-650-2020
Kirkland, WA 98034   800-470-1817
                                            Fax: 425-650-2028
                                               www.solomon.org
Amyotrophic lateral sclerosis research.
Patric Clapshaw, Director
Sheila Dunagan, Office Manager

1147 Stem Cell Research Program University of Wisconsin-Madison
University of Wisconsin-Madison
1500 Highland Avenue   608-890-0173
Madison, WI 53705-2280   Fax: 608- 26- 526
                                       www.waisman.wisc.edu/scrp
The mission of this program is to understand the molecular mecha-
nisms responsible for the proliferation and differentiation of stem
cells and assess their safety and efficacy following transplantation
into various disease models.
Jacalyn McHugh, Research Program Manager
Anita Bhattacharyya, Principal Ivestigator

1148 Virginia Mason Medical Center Neuroscience Institute
Virginia Mason Medical Center
1100 9th Avenue   206-341-1900
Seattle, WA 98101   888-862-2737
                                           www.virginiamason.org
Clinical care and research.
Gary Kaplan, Chairman, CEO

Support Groups & Hotlines

1149 ALS Association Free Standing Support Groups
ALS Association National Office
27001 Agoura Road   818-880-9007
Calabasas Hills, CA 91301-5104   800-782-4747
                                           Fax: 818-880-9006
                                       alsinfo@alsa-national.org
                                               www.alsa.org
We know of support groups in Alabama, California, Florida, Illi-
nois, New York, Oklahoma, Oregon, Puerto Rico, Utah and Vir-
ginia.
Gary Leo, President
Sondi Scheck, VP Operations/Administration

1150 American Society of Human Genetics
9650 Rockville Pike   301-634-7000
Bethesda, MD 20814-3998   Fax: 301-634-7001
                                               www.faseb.org
This society will locate a genetic counselor in various areas across
the United States for persons with ALS.

1151 Amyotrophic Lateral Sclerosis Toll Free Hotline
ALS Association
27001 Agoura Road   818-880-9007
Calabasas Hills, CA 91301-5104   800-782-4747
                                           Fax: 818-880-9006
                                       alsinfo@alsanational.org
                                               www.alsa.org
Informs individuals with ALS and their families of services avail-
able through the ALS Association.
Gary Leo, President
Sondi Scheck, VP Operations/Administration

1152 Les Turner Amyotrophic Lateral Sclerosis Foundation
5550 West Touhy   847-679-3311
Skokie, IL 60077   888-257-1107
                                           Fax: 847-679-9109
                                       info@lesturnerals.org
                                           www.lesturnerals.org
Support groups offer patients and family members a chance to not
feel alone and frustrated in coping with ALS and offers them the
support of professionals as well as others who are experiencing
similar problems.
Claire Owen, Director Patient Services

1153 National Health Information Center
Office of Disease Prevention & Health Promotion
1101 Wootton Pkwy   Fax: 240-453-8281
Rockville, MD 20852   odphpinfo@hhs.gov
                                           www.health.gov/nhic
Supports public health education by maintaining a calendar of National Health Observances; helps connect consumers and health
professionals to organizations that can best answer questions and
provide up-to-date contact information from reliable sources; updates on a yearly basis toll-free numbers for health information,
Federal health clearinghouses and info centers.
Don Wright, MD, MPH, Director

Books

1154 Amyotrophic Lateral Sclerosis: Guide for Patients and Families
Hiroshi Mitsumoto MD, author

Demos Medical Publishing
11 W 42nd Street   212-683-0072
New York, NY 10036   800-532-8663
                                       support@demosmedical.com
                                           www.demosmedpub.com
Covers every aspect of the management of ALS, from clinical features of the disease, to diagnosis, to an overview of symptom management. Major sections deal with medical and rehabilitative
management, living with ALS, managing advanced disease,
end-of-life issues and resources that can provide support and
assistance in this time of need.
450 pages
ISBN: 1-932603-72-7

1155 Complete Bedside Companion: No-Nonsense Advice to Caring for the Seriously Ill
Rodger McFarlane, Philip Bashe, author
Simon & Shuster
1230 Ave of the Americas   212-698-7094
New York, NY 10020   Fax: 212-698-7171
www.simonandschuster.com
Offers warmth, encouragement, and the medical, legal, financial, and emotional advice you need when caring for an ailing loved one.
1999 544 pages
ISBN: 0-684843-19-6

1156 Easy-to-Swallow, Easy-to-Chew Cookbook
Donna L Weihofen, JoAnne Robbins, Paula A Sullivan, author
Wiley Publishers
111 River Street   201-748-6000
Hoboken, NJ 07030-5774   Fax: 201-748-6088
info@wiley.com
www.wiley.com
Presents a collection of more than 150 nutritious recipes that make eating enjoyable and satisfying for anyone who has difficulty chewing or swallowing. Also shares helpful tips and techniques to make eating easier for the elderly and those with such as Parkinson's, AIDS, or head and neck cancers.
256 pages
ISBN: 0-471200-74-1

1157 Journeys with ALS
DLRC Press
PO Box 61661   757-473-1130
Virginia Beach, VA 23466   800-776-0560
mary@davidlawrence.com
Compiled by an ALS patient, this book contains 33 first person journeys with ALS. Some are hopeful, some are sad, a few are angry. All are powerful, real-life examples of people doing their best to cope, often with humor and high spirits.
1998
ISBN: 1-880731-58-4

1158 Learning to Fall: the Blessings of an Imperfect Life
Philip Simmons, author
Random House
1745 Broadway   www.randomhouse.com
New York, NY 10019
Philip Simmons was just thirty-five years old in 1993 when he learned that he had ALS, or Lou Gehrig's disease, and was told he had less than five years to live. As a young husband and father, and at the start of a promising literary career, he suddenly had to learn the art of dying. Nine years later, he has succeeded, against the odds, in learning the art of living.
176 pages
Philip Simmons, Author

1159 Life on Wheels: for the Active Wheelchair User
Gary Karp, author
O'Reilly Media
1005 Gravenstein Hgwy N   707-827-7000
Sebastopol, CA 95472   800-998-9938
Fax: 707-829-0104
orders@oreilly.com
www.oreilly.com
For people who want to take charge of their life experience. Describes medical issues (paralysis, circulation, rehab, cure research); day-to-day living (exercise, skin, bowel and bladder, sexuality, home access, maintaining a wheelchair); and social issues (self-image, adjustement, friends, family, cultural attitudes, activism)
565 pages
ISBN: 1-565922-53-2
Gary Karp, Author

1160 Non Chew Cookbook
Wilson Publishing Company
5708 Nicollet Avenue S   800-843-2409
Minneapolis, MN 55419   nonchew@excite.com
Soft food recipes good for the whole family.

1161 Realities in Coping with Progressive Neuromuscular Diseases
Charles Press Publishers
2037 Chestnut Street   215-561-2786
Philadelphia, PA 19103   Fax: 215-600-1248
mail@charlespresspub.com
www.charlespresspub.com
Focuses on this fundamental question by bringing together the work of 51 eminent authorities on neurology, nursing, psychology, social work, psychiarty, respiratory therapy, pastoral care and other related disciplines.
248 pages Hardcover only
ISBN: 0-914783-20-3

Newsletters

1162 ALS Today
Les Turner ALS Foundation
5550 West Touhy   847-679-3311
Skokie, IL 60077   888-257-1107
Fax: 847-679-9109
info@lesturnerals.org
www.lesturnerals.org
Offers information on clinical trials, medical updates, recipes, resources and support groups available from the foundation.
3 per year

1163 LINK
ALS Association
27001 Agoura Road   818-880-9007
Calabasas Hills, CA 91301-5104   800-782-4747
Fax: 818-880-9006
alsinfo@alsa-national.org
www.alsa.org
Offers information on a national level to all patients and chapter members of the ALS Association. Medical updates, loan equipment, resources, hotlines, support groups and news of charity and fundraising events are included as well.

1164 Massachusetts Chapter of the ALS Association Newsletter
Massachusetts Chapter of the ALS Association
315 Norwood Park S.   781-255-8884
Norwood, MA 02062-3021   800-258-3323
Fax: 781-255-8811
info@als-ma.org
webma.alsa.org
Offers information on activities, events, charity and fundraising activities, resources and more for members.
BiMonthly
Ginny DelVecchio, President

1165 Peach Lines
ALS Association of Georgia
3795 Manor House Drive   770-642-7962
Marietta, GA 30062-5147
Chapter newsletter offering information on support groups, meetings, hotlines, resources and reviews the newest technology and daily living aids for persons with ALS in the Georgia area.
BiMonthly

1166 Reaching Out
Orange County Chapter of the ALS Association
16787 Beach Boulevard   949-587-9700
Huntington Beach, CA 92647-4848
Offers information on support groups, meetings, charity events, fundraising activities and more for ALS members in the Orange County area.
BiMonthly

1167 South Texas Chapter of the ALS Association Newsletter
8600 Wurzbach Road   210-493-1311
San Antonio, TX 78240   877-714-0088
webtx.alsa.org
Offers chapter information on events, charities, memorials, tributes and resources for persons with ALS and their families.
BiMonthly

1168 ALS News & Views
Western Pennsylvania Chapter-ALS Association

1323 Forbes Avenue   412-261-5940
Pittsburgh, PA 15219-4725
Offers information on resources, medical articles, events, charities, fundraising activities and more for patients with ALS, families and caregivers in the western Pennsylvania region.
8 pages BiMonthly
Rita Patchan, Editor

Pamphlets

1169   **Basic Home Care for ALS Patients**
ALS Association
1275 K Street NW   202-407-8580
Washington, DC 20005   800-782-4747
Fax: 202-289-6801
alsinfo@alsa-national.org
www.alsa.org
Provides basic information about home care for people affected by ALS. This booklet is intended as an introductory guide and should be used along with professional medical care from one's physician, nurse and social worker.
Jane H Gilbert, President/CEO

1170   **Maintaining Good Nutrition with ALS**
ALS Association
1275 K Street NW   202-407-8580
Washington, DC 20005   800-782-4747
Fax: 202-289-6801
alsinfo@alsa-national.org
www.alsa.org
Helps people with ALS overcome the obstacles to eating well. Discusses the importance of nutrition to people with ALS and makes suggestions for dealing with various eating problems.
Jane H Gilbert, President/CEO

Audio & Video

1171   **Driving Force: A Story of Life**
Production House
811 St. John's   847-433-3172
Highland Park, IL 60035   Fax: 847-433-9383
Inspiring video featuring Dr. Frank de Leon Jones, a pychiatrist and ALS patient. Despite his disease and the need for continuous medical ventilation, Dr. de Leon Jones continues his challenging medical practice and physical education responsibilities. This is a film of courage, persistence and love of life. It offers poignant messages for ALS patients, family and caregivers as well as healthcare providers. Available in VHS or DVD.
Howie Samuelson, Executive Director

1172   **Living with ALS: Adapting to Breathing Changes/Use of Non Invasive Ventilation**
ALS Association
1275 K Street NW   202-407-8580
Washington, DC 20005   800-782-4747
Fax: 202-289-6801
alsinfo@alsa-national.org
www.alsa.org
Describes how ALS impacts this vital body function and what can be done to help the person with ALS.
Jane H Gilbert, President/CEO

1173   **Living with ALS: Adjusting to Swallowing Difficulties & Good Nutrition**
ALS Association
1275 K Street NW   202-407-8580
Washington, DC 20005   800-782-4747
Fax: 202-289-6801
alsinfo@alsa-national.org
www.alsa.org
In this video we look at the impact of ALS on swallowing and one's ability to maintain good nutrition. Health care professionals provide guidelines and tips for diet changes and for decision-making regarding a feeding tube; patients and their families share their own experiences and demonstrate their ingenuity in adapting to the

changes that weakened swallowing muscles and structures can cause.
2003
Jane H Gilbert, President/CEO

1174   **Living with ALS: Communication Solutions & Symptom Management**
ALS Association
1275 K Street NW   202-407-8580
Washington, DC 20005   800-782-4747
Fax: 202-289-6801
alsinfo@alsa-national.org
www.alsa.org
Companion video to Living with ALS Manual #3 and 5
Jane H Gilbert, President/CEO

1175   **Living with ALS: Mobility, Activities of Daily Living, Home Adaptions**
ALS Association
1275 K Street NW   202-407-8580
Washington, DC 10005   800-782-4747
Fax: 202-289-6801
alsinfo@alsa-national.org
www.alsa.org
This first video, Functioning When Your Mobility is Affected, covers a range of mobility issues that occur with ALS. Our goal is to help you maximize your mobility, independence, safety and comfort. Health care professionals, persons with ALS and their families not only provide information in this video, but also demonstrate equipment and techniques that can help you maximize your function.
Jane H Gilbert, President/CEO

1176   **Ventilation: Decision Making Process**
Les Turner ALS Foundation
5550 West Touhy   847-679-3311
Skokie, IL 60077   888-257-1107
Fax: 847-679-9109
info@lesturnerals.org
www.lesturnerals.org
Designed for ALS patients, their family members and health professionals. Includes interviews with three ventilator dependent ALS patients, family members and the medical staff from Lois Insolia ALS Center at Northwestern University Medical School. Available for loan to ALS patients.
20 Minutes

Web Sites

1177   **Healing Well**
www.healingwell.com
A social network and support community for patients, caregivers, and families coping with the daily struggles of diseases, disorders and chronic illness.

1178   **Health Finder**
www.healthfinder.gov
A government web site where individuals can find information and tools to help you and those you care about stay healthy.

1179   **Healthlink USA**
www.healthlinkusa.com
Health information concerning treatment, cures, prevention, diagnosis, risk factors, research, support groups, email lists, personal stories and much more. Updated regularly.

1180   **MedWebPlus**
www.medwebplus.com
An independently run site related to everything medical and a few things that aren't.

1181   **MedicineNet**
www.medicinenet.com
An online resource for consumers providing easy-to-read, authoritative medical and health information.

1182   **Medscape**
www.medscape.com

Medscape offers specialists, primary care physicians, and other health professionals the Web's most robust and integrated medical information and educational tools.

1183 Neurology Channel

www.healthcommunities.com

Find clearly explained, medically accurate information regarding conditions, including an overview, symptoms, causes, diagnostic procedures and treatment options. On this site it is possible to ask questions and get information from a neurologist and connect to people who have similar health interests.

1184 WebMD

www.webmd.com

Provides credible information, supportive communities, and in-depth reference material about health subjects. A source for original and timely health information as well as material from well known content providers.

Description

1185 Arthritis

Arthritis is a nonspecific term meaning inflammation of one or more joints. There are over 100 kinds of arthritis, many of them associated with illnesses of other body systems, such as the skin, gut, or liver. Most cases of arthritis are chronic and involve multiple joints. The three most common are rheumatoid arthritis (RA), osteoarthritis (OA), sometimes called degenerative joint disease, and gouty arthritis, or gout. Juvenile Rheumatoid Arthritis (JRA) affects children.

Rheumatoid arthritis may strike either sex at any age, but typically affects women in the early adult years. It is caused by the immune system attacking components of the joints and is marked by considerable joint inflammation, commonly of the hands and feet. RA may also involve the knee, elbow, shoulder, ankle and neck, as well as other body systems in addition to the joints. Osteoarthritis tends to occur later in life, and results from repeated wear and tear most commonly on weight-bearing joints, such as the hip and knee. Osteoarthritis often occurs earlier in people who have injured their joints in sports. Gout, which typically affects men in midlife, reflects a disorder in the body's metabolism of uric acid. Its most common feature is excruciating pain in the big toe.

Joints affected by arthritis are typically painful, stiff, and swollen. Nonspecific treatment may be used for arthritis of any sort. This includes the nonsteroidal anti-inflammatory drugs (NSAIDs), such as aspirin, ibuprofen,or naproxen. Steroids can be injected into the knee in OA or into joints afflicted by gouty arthritis. Oral corticosteroids are indicated for RA or gout. Severe cases of rheumatoid arthritis are generally treated with more specific drugs that attempt to downregulate the body's immune system. Gouty arthritis responds to drugs that alter the production and metabolism of uric acid, such as allopurinol or febuxostat, which inhibit the synthesis of uric acid, or medications like probenecid and lesinurad that increase uric acid excretion by the kidney. Gout is also treated with and oral anti-inflammatory drug called colchicine. For any kind of arthritis, local application of heat and cold, as well as physical therapy, are often helpful. In certain cases, joint surgery is recommended.

National Agencies & Associations

1186 American Chronic Pain Association
PO Box 850
Rocklin, CA 95677
800-533-3231
ACPA@theacpa.org
www.theacpa.org

The ACPA facilitates peer support and education for individuals with chronic pain in its many forms, in order to increase quality of life. Also raises awareness among the healthcare community, and with policy makers.
Penney Cowan, Founder & CEO
Daniel Galia, Director, Global Support

1187 American Juvenile Arthritis Organization
Arthritis Foundation
1355 Peachtree Street NE
Atlanta, GA 30309
404-872-7100
800-283-7800
Fax: 404-872-9559
help@arthritis.org
www.arthritis.org

A council established by the Arthritis Foundation which serves the special needs of the 300,000 young people with arthritis and their families. Provides information, inspiration and advocacy by identifying the needs of children with arthritis and speaks out on their behalf.
Ann M. Palmer, President & CEO
Guy S. Eakin, PhD, Sr Vice President, Scientific Strategy

1188 Arthritis & Autoimmunity Research Centre
Canadian Blood Services Building
67 College Street
Toronto, Ontario, M5G-2M1
416-340-3843
Fax: 416-340-3453
tlockett@uhnres.utoronto.ca
www-old.uhnresearch.ca

The AARC is dedicated to researching the 100 chronic illnesses associated with arthritis and other autoimmune diseases.
Theresa Lockett, Contact

1189 Arthritis Society
393 University Avenue
Toronto Ontario, M5G-1E6
416-979-7228
800-321-1433
Fax: 416-979-8366
info@arthritis.ca
www.arthritis.ca

Promotes, evaluates, and funds research in the areas of causes, prevention, treatment, and cures of arthritis.
Janet Yale, President & CEO
Sian Bevan, PhD, Chief Science Officer

1190 Myositis Association of America
1940 Duke Street
Alexandria, VA 22314
703-553-2632
800-821-7356
tma@myositis.org
www.myositis.org

The MMA seeks to improve the lives of individuals affected by myositis, an inflammation of the muscles, through funding research and increasing public awareness.
Mary McGowan, Executive Director
Tricha Shivas, MBe, Director, Development & Partnerships

1191 National Institute of Arthritis & Musculoskeletal & Skin Diseases
National Institutes of Health
Bethesda, MD 20892-3675
301-495-4484
877-226-4267
Fax: 301-718-6366
TTY: 301-565-2966
NIAMSinfo@mail.nih.gov
www.niams.nih.gov

Supports research into the causes, treatment, and prevention of arthritis and musculoskeletal and skin diseases, the training of basic and clinical scientists to carry out this research, and the dissemination of information on research programs.
Robert H. Carter, MD, Director
Gahan Breithaupt, Assoc. Director, Management & Operations

State Agencies & Associations

Alabama

1192 Alabama Chapter of the Arthritis Foundation
2700 Hwy 280 E
Birmingham, AL 35223-3775
205-979-5700
800-879-7896
Fax: 205-979-4172
info.al@arthritis.org
www.arthritis.org

Founded in 1948 this chapter affects thousands of lives through programs services information and referrals public and professional education and more for residents of Alabama. Research is a great priority of the chapter which supports the advancement
Kristin Whitehurst, Regional VP
Lisa Hemphill, Regional Development Director

Arizona

1193 Arthritis Foundation: Central Arizona Chapter
1313 E. Osborn Road
Phoenix, AZ 85014
602-264-7679
800-477-7679
Fax: 602-264-0563
info.caz@arthritis.org
www.arthritis.org
A nonprofit health agency serving the needs of Arizona residents with arthritis. This chapter provides arthritis self-help courses, aquatic programs, foundation clubs, a juvenile arthritis parent group, exercise programs and informational brochures.
Warren Rizzo, Chair
Robert Leslie, Vice Chair

Arkansas

1194 Arthritis Foundation: Arkansas Chapter
6213 Father Tribou Street
Little Rock, AR 72205-3002
501-664-7242
800-482-8858
Fax: 501-664-6588
info.ar@arthritis.org
www.arthritis.org
Carla Davis, Secretary
Diane Denham, VP Finance/Administration

California

1195 Arthritis Foundation: Northern California Chapter
657 Mission Street
San Francisco, CA 94105-4120
415-356-1230
800-464-6240
Fax: 415-356-1240
info.nca@arthritis.org
www.arthritis.org
Offers research into the causes of arthritis and more effective treatments; serves people in California with arthritis through information and referral services, exercise programs, self-help courses, education and other activities.
PJ Handelhand, President
Deborah Jackson, Senior VP

1196 Arthritis Foundation: San Diego Area Chapter
9089 Clairemont Mesa Boulevard
San Diego, CA 92123-1288
858-492-1090
800-422-8885
Fax: 858-492-9248
info.sd@arthritis.org
www.arthritis.org
Offers various programs and services including professional seminars, a speakers bureau, public forums, exercise classes, patient and family support groups, arthritis self-help courses and medical research to the residents of the San Diego area living with arthritis.
Veronica Braun, President
Sandra Hayhurst, Director Health Promotion

1197 Arthritis Foundation: Southern California Chapter
800 W 6th Street
Los Angeles, CA 90017-3775
323-954-5750
800-954-2873
Fax: 323-954-5790
info.sac@arthritis.org
www.arthritis.org
Cynthia Callihan, Administrative Assistant
Christeen Amloian, Assistant Controller

Colorado

1198 Arthritis Foundation: Rocky Mountain Chapter
2280 S Albion Street
Denver, CO 80222-4906
303-756-8622
800-475-6447
Fax: 303-759-4349
info.rm@arthritis.org
www.arthritis.org
Serves Colorado, Montana, and Wyoming and is dedicated to finding solutions to over 100 forms of arthritis which affect 43 millions of people nationwide.
Kristie Archer, Programs Coordinator
Laura Rosseisen, President

Connecticut

1199 Arthritis Foundation: Southern New England Chapter
35 Cold Spring Road
Rocky Hill, CT 06067
860-563-1177
800-541-8350
Fax: 860-563-6018
info.sne@arthritis.org
www.arthritis.org
A resource center for persons in Southern New England, Connecticut, Maine and Vermont with arthritis. Offers self-help courses, exercise programs, aquatic programs, Dial-A-Doctor help line, and physician referrals.
Stephen Evangelista, CEO
Gail Campbell, CFO

District of Columbia

1200 Arthritis Foundation: Metropolitan Washington Chapter
2011 Pennsylvania Avenue NW
Washington, DC 20006
202-537-6800
Fax: 202-537-6859
info.mwa@arthritis.org
www.arthritis.org
The mission of the Arthritis Foundation is to improve lives through leadership in the prevention control and cure of arthritis and related conditions.
Calaneet Balas, President/CEO
Jacquelyn Hair, Director of Operations

Florida

1201 Arthritis Foundation: Florida Chapter, Gulf Coast Branch
3816 W Linebaugh Avenue
Tampa, FL 33618
813-968-7000
800-850-9455
Fax: 941-795-0348
info.fl.b4@arthritis.org
www.arthritis.org
Dedicated to improving the quality of life for those in the seven county area of Pinellas, Pasco, Citrus, Levy, Hillsborough, Hernando and Polk, who have one or more of over 100 conditions that comprise the disease known as arthritis. Provides patient education and referral services.
Alexa Simpkins, Events Coordinator
Alvi McConahay, Regional Executive Director

Georgia

1202 Arthritis Foundation: Georgia Chapter
2790 Peachtree Road
Atlanta, GA 30305
404-237-8771
800-933-7023
Fax: 404-237-8153
info.ga@arthritis.org
www.arthritis.org
A statewide health organization dedicated to reducing the devastating effects of arthritis by offering programs for people with arthritis and their families, information and educational services for people with arthritis, medical professionals and the general public.
Andrea Collins, Vice President Mission Delivery
Christina Lennon, VP Resource Development

Illinois

1203 Arthritis Foundation: Greater Chicago Chapter
35 E Wacker Drive
Chicago, IL 60601
312-372-2080
800-795-0096
Fax: 312-372-2081
info.gc@arthritis.org
www.arthritis.org
Offers self-help courses, wellness workshops, educational seminars, aquatic programs, brochures and publications for persons with arthritis in the state of Illinois.
Roxanne Bartol, Information Systems Coordinator
Tom Fite, President

1204 Arthritis Foundation: Greater Illinois Chapter
2621 N Knoxville Avenue
Peoria, IL 61604-3623
309-682-6600
Fax: 309-682-6732
greaterillinois@arthritis.org
www.arthritis.org
Craig Rogers, Area Director

Indiana

1205 Arthritis Foundation: Indiana Chapter
615 N Alabama   317-879-0321
Indianapolis, IN 46204   800-783-2342
                                            Fax: 317-876-5608
                                            info.in@arthritis.org
                                            www.arthritis.org
Offers programs and services for the arthritis community of Indiana.
Jenny Conder, Area Vice President
BJ Farrell, Director of Development

Iowa

1206 Arthritis Foundation: Iowa Chapter
2600 72nd Street   515-278-0636
Des Moines, IA 50322-4724   866-378-0636
                                            Fax: 515-278-2603
                                            info.ia@arthritis.org
                                            www.arthritis.org

Julie Dalrymple, Program Coordinator
Doyle Monsma CFRE, President/CEO

Kansas

1207 Arthritis Foundation: Kansas Chapter
1999 N Amidon Avenue   316-263-0116
Wichita, KS 67203-2122   800-362-1108
                                            Fax: 316-263-3260
                                            info.ks@arthritis.org
                                            www.arthritis.org
Serves 103 counties and is governed by the Volunteer Board of Directors elected from throughout the state. Services offered include water exercise classes, arthritis support groups, children's summer camp, loan closet of hospital equipment and self-help programs.
Dennis Bender, Area VP
Valerie Fairchild, Program Director

Kentucky

1208 Arthritis Foundation: Kentucky Chapter
2908 Brownsboro Road   502-585-1866
Louisville, KY 40206   800-633-5335
                                            Fax: 502-585-1657
                                            myoung@arthritis.org
                                            www.arthritis.org
Serves residents of 117 counties in Kentucky and the counties of Floyd and Clark in Indiana. This chapter is a resource center for funding research education programs for health professionals, community education and support services for people with arthritis.
Barbara Perez, President/CEO
Annette Beach, Annual Giving Coordinator

Maryland

1209 Arthritis Foundation: Maryland Chapter
9505 Reisterstown Road   410-654-6570
Owings Mills, MD 21117   800-365-3811
                                            Fax: 410-654-9270
                                            info.md@arthritis.org
                                            www.arthritis.org
This chapter supports research both locally and nationally to help find causes better treatments and ways to prevent the many forms of arthritis. Offers various educational booklets and brochures, a referral service for physician referrals, and other support services.
Barbara Newhouse, CEO
Gail Norman, COO

Massachusetts

1210 Arthritis Foundation: Massachusetts Chapter
29 Crafts Street   617-244-1800
Newton, MA 02458-1287   800-766-9449
                                            Fax: 617-558-7686
                                            info.ma@arthritis.org
                                            www.arthritis.org

Offers essential information research programs and services for the close to one million Massachusetts residents with arthritis.
Suha Bekdash, Administrative Assistant
Carmen Quinonez, Finance Manager

Michigan

1211 Arthritis Foundation: Michigan Chapter Chapter and Metro Detroit
1050 Wilshire Drive   248-649-2891
Troy, MI 48084-1564   800-968-3030
                                            Fax: 248-649-2895
                                            info.mi@arthritis.org
                                            www.arthritis.org
Supports research to prevent, control, and cure arthritis and related diseases. The Foundation also helps improve the lives of people with arthritis and their families by offering self-help classes, exercise programs, support groups, information and referrals.
Mary Sue Langen, Development Manager
Michelle Glazier, President/CEO

Minnesota

1212 Arthritis Foundation: North Central Chapter
1876 Minnehaha Avenue West   651-644-4108
Saint Paul, MN 55104   800-333-1380
                                            Fax: 651-644-4219
                                            info.mn@arthritis.org
                                            www.arthritis.org
A nonprofit organization providing programs and services to anyone affected by arthritis in the Minnesota area. Offers aquatic programs support groups juvenile arthritis support groups, research, grants program and information and referrals.
Chris Davis, Community Development Coordinator
Deb Cassidy, Assistant to the President

Mississippi

1213 Arthritis Foundation: Mississippi Chapter
731 Avignon Drive   601-853-7556
Ridgeland, MS 39157   Fax: 601-853-7516
                                            cbaker@arthritis.org
                                            www.arthritis.org
Many Mississippians volunteer their services to help the chapter with fund raising and program support. Programs include land and water based exercise classes, and support groups, direct assistance to needy individuals to purchase arthritis medications and services.
Cynthia Baker, Development Specialist
Pamela Snow, Programs Director

Missouri

1214 Arthritis Foundation: Eastern Missouri Chapter
9433 Olive Boulevard   314-991-9333
Saint Louis, MO 63132   800-406-2491
                                            Fax: 314-991-4020
                                            info.emo@arthritis.org
                                            www.arthritis.org

Jan Bignall, Director of Development
Karen Shoulders, Director of Programs

1215 Arthritis Foundation: Western Missouri, Greater Kansas City
1900 W 75th Street   913-262-2233
Prairie Village, KS 66208   888-719-5670
                                            Fax: 91 -26 -228
                                            info.wmo@arthritis.org
                                            www.arthritis.org
The only organization in the area representing the National Office in support of its international research program and in providing services throughout the bi-state area. Offers a wide range of services and programs to deal with the needs of persons with arthritis.
Sherri Hayes, Director of Operations
Alyson Watkins, Special Events Coordinator

Nebraska

1216 Arthritis Foundation: Nebraska Chapter
600 N 93rd Street
Omaha, NE 68114
402-330-6130
800-642-5292
Fax: 402-330-6167
mpuccioni@arthritis.org
www.arthritis.org

For close to 40 years the Arthritis Foundation has been the source for help and hope to the 263 000 Nebraskans and residents of Pottawattamie County Iowa with arthritis. Provides a wide variety of services designed to help people better cope with arthritis.
Cindy Doerr, Program Director/Editor
Marzia Pucci Shields, Executive Director

New Jersey

1217 Arthritis Foundation: New Jersey Chapter
555 Route 1 South
Iselin, NJ 08830
732-283-4300
888-467-3112
Fax: 732-283-4633
info.nj@arthritis.org
www.arthritis.org

Offers various programs for the residents of New Jersey including support groups, self-help courses, water exercise and arthritis fitness classes and informational public forums.
Linda Gruskiewicz, President & CEO
Tanya Barbarics, Director

New York

1218 Arthritis Foundation: Central New York Chapter
3300 Monroe Avenue
Rochester, NY 14618
585-264-1480
Fax: 585-264-1517
www.arthritis.org

Melinda Merante, Executive Director
Nicole Mau, Director

1219 Arthritis Foundation: Long Island Chapter
501 Walt Whitman Road
Melville, NY 11747-2189
631-427-8272
Fax: 631-427-3546
into.li@arthritis.org
www.arthritis.org

The mission of the Arthritis Foundation is to fund research to find the cause and cures for arthritis and to improve the quality of life for those affected. There is a wide range of programs available for patients.
Patrick T McAsey, President
Roshane Gillespie, Program Secretary

1220 Arthritis Foundation: New York Chapter
122 E 42nd Street
New York, NY 10168-1898
212-984-8700
Fax: 212-878-5960
nfo.ny@arthritis.org
www.arthritis.org

Offers land exercise programs warm water resources and programs, self-help groups and courses, events and activities video clinics, peer support and a lending library to arthritis sufferers in the New York area.
Suzanne Bliss, President CEO

1221 Arthritis Foundation: Rockland/Orange Unit
Helen Hayes Hospital
Route 9W
W Haverstraw, NY 10993
845-947-3000
Fax: 845-429-9602
ameyerowitz@arthritis.org
www.arthritis.org

Aviva Meyerowitz, Community Outreach Coordinator
Beatrice Jasanya, Community Outreach Coordinator

North Carolina

1222 Arthritis Foundation: Carolinas Chapter
4530 Park Road
Charlotte, NC 28209
704-529-5166
800-365-3811
Fax: 704-529-0626
info.car@arthritis.org
www.arthritis.org

Barbara Newhouse, President CEO
Candy Fuller, Community Development Coordinator

Ohio

1223 Arthritis Foundation: Central Ohio Chapter
3740 Ridge Mill Drive
Hilliard, OH 43026
614-876-8200
Fax: 614-876-8363
info.coh@arthritis.org
www.arthritis.org

Offers information and referral services, self-help courses, aquatics program equipment loans, clinics, home assessment and continuing education to help more than 350,000 people in Central Ohio, including over 5,000 children affected with the 100 types of arthritis
Stephanie Houck, Director of Special Events
David Painter, Director of Outreach

1224 Arthritis Foundation: Northeastern Ohio Chapter
4630 Richmond Road
Cleveland, OH 44128-5525
216-831-7000
800-245-2275
Fax: 216-831-1764
info.neoh@arthritis.org
www.arthritis.org

Barb Cvelbar, Director of Health Promotion
Cheryl Carter, Director of Development

1225 Arthritis Foundation: Northwestern Ohio Chapter
35 E Wacker Drive
Chicago, IL 60601
31 -37 -208
800-735-0096
Fax: 31 -37 -208
info.gc@arthritis.org
www.arthritis.org

Tom Fite, CEO

1226 Arthritis Foundation: Ohio River Valley Chapter
7124 Miami Avenue
Cincinnati, OH 45243
513-271-4545
800-383-6843
Fax: 513-271-4703
info.orv@arthritis.org
www.arthritis.org

Barbara Perez, President/CEO
Edith Nixon, Chair

1227 Arthritis Foundation; Great Lakes Region, Northeastern Ohio
4630 Richmond Road
Cleveland, OH 44128-5525
216-831-7000
800-245-2275
Fax: 216-831-1764
info.neoh@arthritis.org
www.arthritis.org

Mary L Kudasick, Regional VP

Oklahoma

1228 Arthritis Foundation: Oklahoma Chapter
710 W. Wilshire Blvd
Oklahoma City, OK 73116
405-936-3366
800-627-5486
Fax: 405-936-0617
info.ok@arthritis.org
www.arthritis.org

Sherri O'Neil, Executive Director
Sherri Harris, Director Special Events

Pennsylvania

1229 Arthritis Foundation: Central Pennsylvania Chapter
3544 North Progress Avenue
Harrisburg, PA 17110
717-763-0900
800-776-0746
Fax: 717-763-0903
info.cpa@arthritis.org
www.arthritis.org

Serves 28 counties in the central Pennsylvania area. More than 441,233 persons in the chapter area are affected with one of the forms of arthritis seriously enough to require medical care. The chapter offers research services, professional education and training, parent and community services and public health education.
Douglas Knepp, Interim Executive Director

1230 Arthritis Foundation: Southern New England Chapter
35 Cold Spring Road   860-563-1177
Rocky Hill, CT 06067   800-541-8350
                                       Fax: 860-563-6018
                                       info.sne@arthritis.org
                                       www.arthritis.org
Offers programs and services for persons in the Rhode Island area who are living with arthritis.
Stephen Evangelista, CEO
Gail Campbell, CFO

Tennessee

1231 Arthritis Foundation: Southeast Region
421 Great Circle Road   615-254-6795
Nashville, TN 37228   800-454-4662
                                       Fax: 615-254-8316
                                       info.tn@arthritis.org
                                       www.arthritis.org
This chapter serves the residents of Tennessee by offering arthritis support through Life Improvement Series Classes, exercise programs, educational programs, free information, public forums and seminars.
David Popen Esq, CEO

Texas

1232 Arthritis Foundation: North Texas Chapter
4300 Macarthur   214-826-4361
Dallas, TX 75209-6524   800-442-6653
                                       Fax: 214-824-5842
                                       info.ntx@arthritis.org
                                       www.arthritis.org
With over 1.5 million people in the North Texas Chapter area with arthritis, the chapter's mission is to improve lives through leadership in the prevention, control and cure of arthritis and related diseases.
Carla Brandt, CFO/COO
Jane Hynes, Director Administration/Info Systems

Utah

1233 Arthritis Foundation: Utah/Idaho Chapter
448 E 400 S   801-536-0990
Salt Lake City, UT 84111   800-444-4993
                                       Fax: 801-536-0991
                                       info.utid@arthritis.org
                                       www.arthritis.org
A nonprofit organization serving individuals with arthritis and their families in Utah and Idaho by providing invaluable services, programs and activities.
Lisa B Fall, President
Leslie Nelson, Program Director

Vermont

1234 Arthritis Foundation: Northern New England Chapter
6 Chenell Drive   603-224-9322
Concord, NH 03301   800-639-2113
                                       Fax: 603-224-3778
                                       info.sne@arthritis.org
                                       www.arthritis.org
Stephen Evangelista, CEO
Margaret Duffy, Regional Program Director

Virginia

1235 Arthritis Foundation: Virginia Chapter
3805 Cutshaw Avenue   804-359-1700
Richmond, VA 23230   800-456-4687
                                       Fax: 804-359-4900
                                       info.va@arthritis.org
                                       www.arthritis.org
Founded in 1954 this chapter is a nonprofit voluntary health organization dedicated to finding the cause prevention and cure for the entire group of diseases called arthritis. Offered classes books and information to better manage arthritis.
Angela Courtney, Vice President Community Development
C Annie Magnant, President

Washington

1236 Arthritis Foundation: Washington/Alaska Chapter
3876 Bridge Way N   206-547-2707
Seattle, WA 98103   800-746-1821
                                       Fax: 206-547-2707
                                       tzuehl@arthritis.org
                                       www.arthritis.org
Offers arthritis help lines and information lines for residents of Washington state. Provides self-help courses arthritis aquatic programs and resources for persons living with various forms of arthritis.
Barbara Osen, North Puget Sound Branch Director
Kim Mellen, Campaign Coordinator

Wisconsin

1237 Arthritis Foundation: Wisconsin Chapter Foundation
1650 S 108th Street   414-321-3933
W Allis, WI 53214-4021   800-242-9945
                                       Fax: 414-321-0365
                                       www.arthritis.org
Statewide programs offered. Including aquatics exercise programs, support groups, self-help courses, professional education, public education seminars, advocacy counsel, juvenile arthritis support programs and children's camp information and referral help.

Foundations

1238 Arthritis Foundation
1355 Peachtree Street NE   404-872-7100
Atlanta, GA 30309   800-283-7800
                                       Fax: 404-872-0457
                                       help@arthritis.org
                                       www.arthritis.org
A nonprofit organization that depends on volunteers to provide services to help people with arthritis. Supports research to find ways to cure and prevent arthritis and provides services to improve the quality of life for those affected by arthritis. Provides help through information, referrals, speakers bureaus, forums, self-help courses, and various support groups and programs nationwide.
Ann M. Palmer, President & CEO
Guy S. Eakin, PhD, Sr Vice President, Scientific Strategy

Libraries & Resource Centers

1239 New York Chapter of the Arthritis Foundation
122 East 42nd Street   212-984-8700
New York, NY 10168-1898   Fax: 212-878-5960
                                       info.ny@arthritis.org
                                       www.arthritis.org
Offers people with arthritis, their families and all those with an interest in the rheumatic diseases, information on how to live every day to its fullest, even when affected by a chronic disease.

Research Centers

1240 Affiliated Children's Arthritis Centers of New England
New England Medical Center
750 Washington Street   617-636-7285
Boston, MA 02111-1533   Fax: 617-350-8388
Research organization comprised of a network of 15 territory pediatric centers throughout New England and based at the Floating Hospital of New England Medical Center.
Jane G Schaller MD, Coordinator

1241 Arthritis and Musculoskeletal Center: UAB Shelby Interdisciplinary Biomedical Rese
Shelby Interdisciplinary Biomedical Research Bldg

1825 University Boulevard 205-934-0245
Birmingham, AL 35294-2182 Fax: 205-934-1564
rpk@uab.edu
Arthritis and related rheumatic disorders are studied.
Robert Kimbe MD, Director
Jennifer A Croker, Executive Administrator

1242 Boston University Arthritis Center
580 Harrison Avenue 617-638-4590
Boston, MA 02118 Fax: 617-638-5226
mikyork@bu.edu
www.bumc.bu.edu
The research efforts of the Rheumatology Section relate to basic biologic mechanisms in the pathogenesis of scleroderma vasculitis amyloidosis osteoarthritis and systemic lupus erythematosus. There are concordant research efforts in clinical investigation of these disorders including testing of novel therapies.
Karen H Antman, Dean
Paul Monach, Associate Fellowship Program Director

1243 Boston University Medical Campus General Clinical Research Center
72 E Concord Street 617-638-4542
Boston, MA 02118 Fax: 617-638-8890
jkopp@bu.edu
Integral unit of the University Hospital specializing in arthritis and connective tissue studies.
Courtney Alpert, Administrative Coordinator
Janice Kopp, Executive Director

1244 Brigham and Women's Orthopedica and Arthritis Center
Brigham and Women's Hospital
75 Francis Street 617-732-5500
Boston, MA 02115 800-BWH-9999
TTY: 617-732-6458
www.brighamandwomens.org
Research studies into arthritis and rheumatic diseases.
Matthew Lian MD, Director

1245 Central Missouri Regional Arthritis Center Stephen's College Campus
Stephen's College Campus
1205 University Ave 573-882-8097
Columbia, MO 65211 888-702-8818
Fax: 573-884-5509
TDD: 0
Research into arthritis and rheumatic diseases.
Liz Raine, MPH, CHES,, Health Educator
Beth Richards ,BS,TRS, Director

1246 Department of Pediatrics, Division of Rheumatology
Duke University School of Medicine
T909 Children's Health Center 919-684-6575
Durham, NC 27710-1 Fax: 919-684-6616
rheum.pediatrics.duke.edu
Clinical and laboratory pediatric rheumatoid studies.
Laura Schanberg MD, Cochairman
Egla Rabinovich MD, Co-Chairman

1247 Hahnemann University Hospital, Orthopedic Wellness Center
Hahnemann University Hospital
230 N Broad St 215-762-7000
Philadelphia, PA 19102-1511 Fax: 215-762-8109
www.hahnemannhospital.com
Research activity at Hahnemann University into the areas of arthritis.
Dr. Arnold Berman, Director

1248 Medical University of South Carolina
96 Jonathan Lucas Street 843-792-1991
Charleston, SC 29403 800-424-MUSC
Fax: 843-792-7121
www.muschealth.com
Offers basic and clinical research on various types of arthritis.
Richard M Silver, Division Director/Professor
Gary S Gilkeson, Vice Chairman Research

1249 Medical University of South Carolina: Division of Rheumatology & Immunology
96 Jonathan Lucas Street 843-792-1991
Charleston, SC 29403 Fax: 843-792-7121
www.musc.edu
Offers basic and clinical research on various types of arthritis.
Richard M Silver, Division Director/Professor
Gary S Gilkeson, Vice Chairman Research

1250 Multipurpose Arthritis and Musculoskeletal Disease Center
School of Medicine Rheumatology Division
545 Barnhill Drive 317- 27- 843
Indianapolis, IN 46202 Fax: 317-274-1437
medicine.iupui.edu
The mission of this center is to pursue major biomedical research interests relevant to the rheumatic diseases. Current areas of emphasis include articular cartilage biology pathogenesis and treatment of various forms of amyloidosis the pathogenesis of dermatomyositis and immunologic and biochemical markers of cartilage breakdown and repair.
Bernetta Hartman, Executive Assistant to the Chairman
Martin Friedman, VP Medicine Specialties Division, IUHP

1251 National Institute of Arthritis & Musculoskeletal & Skin Diseases
National Institutes of Health
Bethesda, MD 20892-3675 301-495-4484
877-226-4267
Fax: 301-718-6366
TTY: 301-565-2966
NIAMSinfo@mail.nih.gov
www.niams.nih.gov
Supports research into the causes, treatment, and prevention of arthritis and musculoskeletal and skin diseases, the training of basic and clinical scientists to carry out this research, and the dissemination of information on research programs.
Robert H. Carter, MD, Director
Gahan Breithaupt, Assoc. Director, Management & Operations

1252 Oklahoma Medical Research Foundation
825 NE 13th Street 405-271-6673
Oklahoma City, OK 73104-5005 800-522-0211
Fax: 405-271-OMRF
contact@omrf.org
www.omrf.ouhsc.edu
Focuses on arthritis and muscoloskeletal disease research.
Dr Paul Kincade, Head of OMRF's Immunobiology
Philip M Silverman PhD, Member

1253 Rehabilitation Institute of Chicago
345 E Superior Street 312-238-1000
Chicago, IL 60611 800-354-7342
TTY: 312-238-1059
www.ric.org
Expertise in treating a range of conditions from the most complex conditions including cerebral palsy spinal cord injury stroke and traumatic brain injury to the more common such as arthritis chronic pain and sports injuries.
Edward B Case, Executive Vice President and Chief Finan
Joanne C Smith, President and Chief Executive Officer

1254 Rosalind Russell Medical Research Center for Arthritis at UCSF
350 Parnassus Avenue 415-476-1141
San Francisco, CA 94117 Fax: 415-476-3526
rrac@medicine.ucsf.edu
Arthritis research and its probable causes.
Ephraim P Engelman MD, Director
David Wofsy, Associate Director

1255 University of Michigan: Orthopaedic Research Laboratories
University of Michigan Mott Hospital
109 Zina Pitcher Place 734-936-7417
Ann Arbor, MI 48109-2200 Fax: 734-647-0003
Develops and studies the causes and treatments for arthritis including new devices and assistive aids.
Dr SA Goldstein, Director

1256 Warren Grant Magnuson Clinical Center
National Institute of Health

9000 Rockville Pike
Bethesda, MD 20892

301-496-2563
800-411-1222
Fax: 301-480-9793
TTY: 866-411-1010
prpl@mail.cc.nih.gov
www.clinicalcenter.nih.gov

Established in 1953 as the research hospital of the National Institutes of Health. Designed so that patient care facilities are close to research laboratories so new findings of basic and clinical scientists can be quickly applied to the treatment of patients. Upon referral by physicians, patients are admitted to NIH clinical studies.
John Gallin, Director
David Henderson, Deputy Director for Clinical Care

Support Groups & Hotlines

1257   Arthritis Foundation Information Helpline
1355 Peachtree Street NE
Atlanta, GA 30309-0669

844-571-4357
help@arthritis.org
www.arthritis.org

Offers information and referrals, counseling, physicians information and more to persons living with arthritis.
Ann M. Palmer, President & CEO

1258   Kids on the Block Arthritis Programs
Arthritis Foundation
PO Box 19000
Atlanta, GA 31126-1000

404-872-7100
800-283-7800
Fax: 404-872-0457

State and local programs that use puppetry to help children understand what it is like for children and adults who have arthritis.

1259   National Health Information Center
Office of Disease Prevention & Health Promotion
1101 Wootton Pkwy
Rockville, MD 20852

Fax: 240-453-8281
odphpinfo@hhs.gov
www.health.gov/nhic

Supports public health education by maintaining a calendar of National Health Observances; helps connect consumers and health professionals to organizations that can best answer questions and provide up-to-date contact information from reliable sources; updates on a yearly basis toll-free numbers for health information, Federal health clearinghouses and info centers.
Don Wright, MD, MPH, Director

Books

1260   250 Tips for Making Life with Arthritis Easier
Arthritis Foundation Distribution Center
PO Box 6996
Alpharetta, GA 30023-6996

800-207-8633
Fax: 770-442-9742
www.arthritis.com

Learn about helpful services you didn't know were available through you bank, post office, phone company, grocery store, and other businesses you frequent.
88 pages

1261   Arthritis 101: Questions You Have, Answers You Need
Arthritis Foundation Distribution Center
PO Box 6996
Alpharetta, GA 30009-6996

800-207-8633
Fax: 770-442-9742
www.arthritis.com

Expert reviewers answer questions about basic arthritis facts, treatments, research, surgery and more. Also, specific information about six common conditions: rheumatoid arthritis, osteoarthritis, osteoporosis, fibromyalgia, lupus and gout.
144 pages

1262   Arthritis Helpbook: A Tested Self-Management Program for Coping
Kate Lorig and James Fries, author
Da Capo Press
Order Department
Jackson, TN 38301

800-343-4499
Fax: 800-351-5073
www.perseusbooksgroup.com/dacapo

This book teaches people proven techniques to reduce pain and increase dexterity, build a calcium-rich diet and maintain a healthy

weight, design an exercise program that matches their needs, find tips and gadgets that solve common problems, overcome fatigue, depression, and other troubling feelings associated with these health issues, and learn about all available arthritis medications and surgeries.
2006 288 pages 6th Edition
ISBN: 0-201409-63-1

1263   Arthritis Self-Help Products
Aids for Arthritis
35 Wakefield Drive
Medford, NJ 08055-3204

609-654-6918
Fax: 609-654-8631
aidsforarthritis@gmail.com
www.aidsforarthritis.com

Offers lists of arthritis self-help devices.

1264   Arthritis Self-Management
RA Rapaport Publishing
150 W 22nd Street
New York, NY 10011-2421

212-989-0200
800-234-0923
Fax: 212-989-4786
editor@arthritis-self-mgmt.com
www.arthritisselfmanagement.com

Publishes practical, how to information, focusing on the day-to-day and long term aspects of arthritis in a positive and upbeat style. Gives subscribers up-to-date news, facts and advice to help them maintain their wellness and make informed decisions regarding their health.
48+ pages Bi-Monthly
Christine Martin Grove, Editor
Ingrid Strauch, Editor

1265   Arthritis: What Exercises Work
Dava Sobel, Arthur C Klein, author
MacMillan
175 5th Avenue
New York, NY 10010

212-674-5151
800-221-7945
Fax: 212-420-9314
customerservice@mpsvirginia.com
us.macmillan.com

The right exercises for your kind of arthritis, pain-level, age, occupation, and hobbies. The most effective exercises for arthritis available anywhere, supported by medical doctors and backed by the latest research.
200 pages
ISBN: 0-312130-25-1

1266   Arthritis: Your Complete Exercise Guide
Human Kinetics Press
1607 N Market Street
Champaign, IL 61820-5076

217-351-1549
800-873-6759
Fax: 217-351-2674
ce@hkusa.com
www.humankinetics.com

1993 152 pages Paperback
ISBN: 0-873223-92-6
Steve Ruhlig, Marketing Director

1267   Bone Up on Arthritis
Arthritis Foundation
PO Box 6996
Alpharetta, GA 30009-6996

800-207-8633
Fax: 770-442-9742
www.arthritis.com

A self-help education packet designed for home-study use, this program can improve your pain and function levels by teaching proven self-help techniques.
w/Audio Tapes

1268   Clinical Care in the Rheumatic Disease
Arthritis Foundation Distribution Center
PO Box 6996
Alpharetta, GA 30023-6996

800-207-8633
Fax: 770-442-9742
www.arthritis.com

This book was written for all health professionals caring for people with rheumatic diseases and for students in these disciplines.
224 pages

1269   Educational Rights for Children with Arthritis: A Parents Manual
AJAO

1314 Spring Street NW   404-872-7100
Atlanta, GA 30309-2810   www.arthritis.org/
A self-instructional manual helping parents to identify and obtain school services needed by their child with arthritis. Covers laws and special services, explores strategies for working with school personnel and stresses good communication and advocacy techniques.

1270   Exercise Beats Arthritis
Bull Publishing Company
PO Box 1377   303-545-6350
Boulder, CO 80306   800-676-2855
    Fax: 303-545-6354
    www.bullpub.com
Easy-to-follow program will help arthritis sufferers of all ages manage the problems of living with this condition. In depth look at minimizing the pain and limitations of arthritis, keep their joints mobile, increase muscle strength, strengthen bones and ligaments, perform daily tasks more easily.
1998 144 pages
ISBN: 0-923521-45-3
Valerie Sayce, Author
Ian Fraser, Author

1271   Help Yourself Cookbook
Arthritis Foundation
PO Box 6996   800-207-8633
Alpharetta, GA 30023-6996   Fax: 770-442-9742
    www.arthritis.com

158 pages

1272   Living With Rheumatoid Arthritis
John's Hopkins University Press
2715 N Charles Street   410-516-6900
Baltimore, MD 21218-4319   800-537-5487
    Fax: 410-516-6968
    www.press.jhu.edu
This book offers practical and usable answers to the questions of everyday life. The authors provide clear explanations of the causes, diagnosis and treatment of the disease and why medication, joint protection, physical activity and good nutrition are essential components of care.
1993 312 pages Paperback
ISBN: 0-801871-47-6
Tammi L. Shlotzhauer, M.D, Author

1273   Personal Guide to Living Well with Fibromyalgia
Arthritis Foundation Distribution Center
PO Box 6996   800-207-8633
Alpharetta, GA 30023-6996   Fax: 770-442-9742
    www.arthritis.com
With this guide you'll learn the latest information about fibromyalgia, what researchers have uncovered about its causes, and an overview of the best treatment options available. Helpful worksheets and tables allow you to manage your condition and document your progress.
224 pages

1274   Primer on the Rheumatic Diseases
John H Klippel, author
Springer Publishing
233 Spring Street   212-460-1500
New York, NY 0013   Fax: 212-460-1575
    service-ny@springer.com
    www.springer.com
Designed to provide up-to-date information about the major clinical syndromes. One of the most prestigious and comprehensive texts on arthritis and related diseases, including osteoarthritis, rheumatoid arthritis, osteoporosis, lupus, and more than one hundred others.
724 pages
ISBN: 0-387356-64-8
J.H. Klippel, Author
J.H. Stone, Author

1275   Toward Healthy Living: A Wellness Journal
Arthritis Foundation Distribution Center
PO Box 6996   800-207-8633
Alpharetta, GA 30023-6996   Fax: 770-442-9742
    www.arthritis.com

This spiral-bound journal has ample pages where you can record your thoughts, plus scales to monitor your mood and pain. Throughout the book you will also find wisdom from a variety of famous and ordinary people - those who live with chronic ilness, and those whose life lessons can help you gain a more positive outlook on daily living.
144 pages

1276   Understanding Juvenile Rheumatoid Arthritis
American Juvenile Arthritis Organization
PO Box 19000   800-283-7800
Atlanta, GA 31126-1000
A manual for health professionals to use in teaching children with JRA and their families about disease management and self-care.
372 pages

1277   We Can: A Guide for Parents of Children with Arthritis
AJAO
1330 W Peachtree Strt NW   404-872-7100
Atlanta, GA 30309-2904   www.arthritis.org/
Offers parents tips for daily living and practical points for helping their child toward independent adulthood.

Children's Books

1278   Arthritis
Franklin Watts Grolier
90 Old Sherman Turnpike   203-797-3500
Danbury, CT 06816-0001   800-621-1115
    Fax: 203-797-3197
    www.grolier.com
This book offers a clear explanation of the various forms and effects of the disease of arthritis and what treatments are available.
96 pages Grades 7-12
ISBN: 0-531108-01-5

1279   JRA and Me
American Juvenile Arthritis Organization
PO Box 19000   800-283-7800
Atlanta, GA 31126-1000
A workbook for school-aged children who have juvenile arthritis. This book offers a variety of educational games, puzzles and worksheets to teach children about their illness and how to take care of themselves.
57 pages

1280   Living with Arthritis
Franklin Watts Grolier
90 Old Sherman Turnpike   203-797-3500
Danbury, CT 06816-0001   800-621-1115
    Fax: 203-797-3197
    www.grolier.com

Shows how people with arthritis can overcome their pain and lead productive, full lives.
32 pages Grades 5-7

1281   Yard Sale Coloring Book
American Juvenile Arthritis Organization
PO Box 19000   800-283-7800
Atlanta, GA 31126-1000
A coloring/activity book based on a Kids on the Block script, written for third and fourth grade students. It can be used with Kids on the Block performances, as a stand-alone piece or with a free lesson plan packet.

Magazines

1282   Arthritis Today
Arthritis Foundation
1330 W Peachtree Strt NW   404-872-7100
Atlanta, GA 30309-2922   800-933-0032
    Fax: 404-872-9559
    www.arthritis.org
The authoritative and respected source of information for persons with arthritis, their families and health professionals who manage their care. As the official magazine of the Arthritis Foundation, it is backed by the Foundation's experience of 44 years and leadership in the fight against arthritis. This magazine gives its readers

the advice, information and inspiration they need to live better with arthritis.
Monthly

Newsletters

1283 AJAO Newsletter
American Juvenile Arthritis Organization
1330 W Peachtree Strt NW   404-872-7100
Atlanta, GA 31126-2904
Offers information and updates about the organization's activities and events. Legislative information, medical updates, camp information and more for children living with arthritis.
Quarterly
Janet Austin MEd, Editor

1284 Arthritis Accent
Arthritis Foundation Southern N.E. Chapter
35 Cold Spring Road   860-563-1177
Rocky Hill, CT 06067-3166   800-541-8350
Fax: 860-563-6018
sevangel@arthritis.org
www.arthritis.org
Information on chapter events and activities.
Quarterly

1285 Arthritis Foundation: Newsletter of Nebraska Chapter
600 North 93rd Street   402-330-6130
Omaha, NE 68114   800-642-5292
Fax: 402-330-6167
mpuccioni@arthritis.org
www.arthritis.org
Contains information on research, medication, different types of arthritis and features on oustanding volunteers.
3x Year
Cindy Doerr, Program Director/Editor

1286 Arthritis Foundation: Southern Arizona Chapter
6464 E Grant Road   520-290-9090
Tucson, AZ 85715   800-444-5426
Offers updated information and news on chapter activities and events for persons with arthritis.
Monthly
Richard M Brown EdD, CFRE, President

1287 Arthritis News
Arthritis Foundation - WI Chapter
10427 W Lincoln Avenue   414-321-3933
West Allis, WI 53227   800-333-1380
Fax: 414-321-0365
info.wi@arthritis.org
www.arthritis.org
Offers information on activities, events, medical research, information and referrals to persons living in the Wisconsin area that are afflicted with arthritis.
Quarterly
Judy Haugsland, CEO

1288 Arthritis Observer
Rocky Mountain Chapter of the Arthritis Foundation
2280 S Albion Street   303-756-8622
Denver, CO 80222-4906   888-391-9389
Fax: 303-759-4349
www.arthritis.org
Offers chapter information and educational programs to the community as well as updates on fund-raising events, resources, publications and medical updates for the arthritis community.
Quarterly

1289 Arthritis Reporter
New York Chapter of the Arthritis Foundation
122 E 42nd Street   212-984-8700
New York, NY 10168-0002   Fax: 212-878-5960
IMontecino@arthritis.org
www.arthritis.org
Chapter newsletter offering information on upcoming events, activities and groups for the arthritis community.
Quarterly
Ingrid Montecino, President and CEO

1290 Arthritis Update of Rhode Island
Arthritis Foundation Rhode Island Office
Airport Office Park   401-739-3773
Warwick, RI 02886   Fax: 401-739-8990
sevangel@arthritis.org
www.arthritis.org
Offers information, activities, events and updates on the chapter.
Quarterly
Stephen Evangelista, Chief Executive Officer
Gail Campbell, Chief Financial Officer

1291 Arthritis Volunteer
Tennessee Chapter of the Arthritis Foundation
1719 W End Avenue   615-320-7626
Nashville, TN 37203-5123   Fax: 615-329-3982
Keeps members up-to-date on arthritis developments and on programs, services and special events in Tennessee.
Quarterly

1292 Factor Fax
Arthritis Foundation: Northeast California Chapter
3040 Explorer Drive   916-368-5599
Sacramento, CA 95827   800-571-3456
Fax: 916-368-5596
info.neca@arthritis.org
www.arthritis.org
Offers information on all of the chapter's activites, events and resources for the arthritis community of central California.
Patrick Dunlap, VP Events/Programs/Services
Edward Kelley, Motion Coordinator

1293 Focus
Arthritis Foundation: Central Ohio Chapter
3740 Ridge Mill Drive   614-876-8200
Hilliard, OH 43026-9231   Fax: 614-876-8363
www.arthritis.org
Offers updated information on arthritis as well as news of the services and activities of the chapter.
Quarterly
Irene Baird, President

1294 Health Points
TyH Publications
12005 Saguaro Blvd   480-837-7590
Fountain Hills, AZ 85268   800-801-1406
customerservice@e-tyh.com
www.e-tyh.com
National newsletter with articles on complementary therapy, latest nutrition news, disability issues and much more. Focus is on fibromyalgia, chronic fatigue, arthritis and chronic pain.
Quarterly

1295 News Across Our Horizons
Northern & Southern New England Chapter
35 Cold Spring Road   860-563-1177
Rocky Hill, CT 06060   800-541-8350
Fax: 860-563-6018
info.sne@arthritis.org
www.arthritis.org
Chapter newsletter offering information on programs, activities and events of the foundation, medical and research articles and resources for persons with arthritis.

1296 Newsletter of the Central Pennsylvania Chapter
Central Pennsylvania Chapter/Arthritis Foundation
Foster Plaza #11   412-566-1645
Pittsburgh, PA 15220-5459   800-776-0746
Fax: 412-539-1182
info.cpa@arthritis.org
www.arthritis.org
Offers information on activities and events of the Chapter.
Quarterly

1297 Spectrum
Michigan Chapter of the Arthritis Foundation
1050 Wilshire Drive   248-649-2891
Troy, MI 48084-1564   800-968-3030
Fax: 248-649-2895
info.mi@arthritis.org
www.arthritis.org

Arthritis / **Pamphlets**

Promotes various activities and programs and provides current information about arthritis.

1298 Volunteer Voice
Kentucky Chapter of the Arthritis Foundation
410 W Chestnut Street   502-893-9771
Louisville, KY 40202-2368   800-633-5335
Newsletter offering information and updates on chapter activities, events, camps, juvenile programs and government/legislative information.

Pamphlets

1299 Americans with Disabilities Act Resource Manual
Arthritis Foundation
PO Box 7669   404-872-7100
Atlanta, GA 30357-0669   800-283-7800
                                     Fax: 404-872-0457

1300 Ankylosing Spondylitis
Arthritis Foundation
PO Box 7669   404-872-7100
Atlanta, GA 30357-0669   800-283-7800
                                     Fax: 404-872-0457

1301 Arthritis Answers: Basic Information About Arthritis
Arthritis Foundation
PO Box 7669   404-872-7100
Atlanta, GA 30357-0669   800-283-7800
                                     Fax: 404-872-0457

1302 Arthritis Information: Advocacy and Government Affairs
Arthritis Foundation
PO Box 7669   404-872-7100
Atlanta, GA 30357-0669   800-283-7800
                                     Fax: 404-872-0457

1303 Arthritis Information: Children
Arthritis Foundation
PO Box 7669   404-872-7100
Atlanta, GA 30357-0669   800-283-7800
                                     Fax: 404-872-0457
List of materials for children with arthritis, their families and the health professionals who care for them.

1304 Arthritis and Diet Information Package
NAMSIC/National Institutes of Health
1 AMS Circle   301-495-4484
Bethesda, MD 20892-0001   877-226-4267
                                     Fax: 301-718-6366
                                     TTY: 301-565-2966
                                     niamsinfo@mail.nih.gov
                                     www.nih.gov/niams/
Offers information on nutrition and diet pertaining to the arthritis community.
16 pages

1305 Arthritis and Employment: You Can Get the Job You Want
Arthritis Foundation
1330 W Peachtree Strt NW   404-872-7100
Atlanta, GA 30309-0669   800-283-7800
                                     Fax: 404-872-0457
                                     www.arthritis.org
Free brochures offered by Arthiritis Foundation.

1306 Arthritis and Inflammatory Bowel Disease
Arthritis Foundation
PO Box 7669   404-872-7100
Atlanta, GA 30357-0669   800-283-7800
                                     Fax: 404-872-0457

1307 Arthritis and Pregnancy
Arthritis Foundation
1330 W Peachtree Strt NW   404-872-7100
Atlanta, GA 30309-0669   800-283-7800
                                     Fax: 404-872-0457
                                     www.arthritis.org
How arthritis affects pregnancy, managing pregnancy and a new baby.
Mary Anne Dunkin, Writer

1308 Arthritis and Vocational Rehabilitation
Arthritis Foundation
2970 Peachtree Road NW   404-237-8771
Atlanta, GA 30305   800-933-7023
                                     Fax: 404-237-8153
                                     info.ga@arthritis.org
                                     www.arthritis.org

1309 Arthritis in Children Information Package
NAMSIC/National Institutes of Health
1 AMS Circle   301-495-4484
Bethesda, MD 20892-0001   877-226-4267
                                     Fax: 301-718-6366
                                     TTY: 301-565-2966
                                     niamsinfo@mail.nih.gov
                                     www.nih.gov/niams/

1310 Arthritis in Children and La Artritis Infantojuvenil
American Juvenile Arthritis Organization
PO Box 19000   800-283-7800
Atlanta, GA 31126-1000
A medical information booklet about juvenile rheumatoid arthritis. This booklet is written for parents or other adults and includes details about different forms of JRA, medications, therapies and coping issues.

1311 Arthritis on the Job: You Can Work With It
Arthritis Foundation
PO Box 7669   404-872-7100
Atlanta, GA 30357-0669   800-283-7800
                                     Fax: 404-872-0457

1312 Arthritis: Do You Know?
Arthritis Foundation
PO Box 7669   404-872-7100
Atlanta, GA 30357-0669   800-283-7800
                                     Fax: 404-872-0457
A brief overview of arthritis and the services of the Arthritis Foundation.

1313 Aspirin and Other Nonsteroidal Anti-Inflamatory Drugs
Arthritis Foundation
8600 Rockville Pike   404-872-7100
Bethesda, MD 20894-0669   888-346-3656
                                     Fax: 404-872-0457
                                     info@ncbi.nlm.nih.gov
                                     www.ncbi.nlm.nih.gov
A book on hypersensitivity to aspirin and other non steroidal anti-inflammatory drugs (NSAIDs) manifestation.
AL1 de Weck, Author
PM Gamboa, Author

1314 Back Pain
Arthritis Foundation
PO Box 7669   404-872-7100
Atlanta, GA 30357-0669   800-283-7800
                                     Fax: 404-872-0457

1315 Behcet's Disease
Arthritis Foundation
1330 W Peachtree Strt NW   404-872-7100
Atlanta, GA 30309-0669   800-283-7800
                                     Fax: 404-872-0457
                                     www.arthritis.org
Beh‡et's disease, also called Beh‡et's syndrome, is a rare disorder that causes seemingly unrelated symptoms in different parts of the body, including mouth sores, genital sores, eye inflammation, and skin rashes and lesions.

1316 Bursitis, Tendionitis and Other Soft Tissue Rheumatic Syndromes
Arthritis Foundation
PO Box 7669   404-872-7100
Atlanta, GA 30357-0669   800-283-7800
                                     Fax: 404-872-0457

1317 CPPD Crystal Deposition Disease
Arthritis Foundation
1330 W Peachtree Strt NW   404-872-7100
Atlanta, GA 30309-0669   800-283-7800
                                     Fax: 404-872-0457
                                     www.arthritis.org

Calcium pyrophosphate dihydrate crystal deposition disease (CPPD) occurs when these crystals form deposits in the joint and surrounding tissues.

1318   Corticosteriod Medications
Arthritis Foundation
1330 W Peachtree Strt NW   404-872-7100
Atlanta, GA 30309-0669   800-283-7800
                                        Fax: 404-872-0457
                                         www.arthritis.org

Corticosteroids (glucocorticoids) are medications that mimic the effects of the hormone cortisol, which helps reduce inflammation in the body.

1319   Diet and Arthritis
Arthritis Foundation
PO Box 7669   404-872-7100
Atlanta, GA 30357-0669   800-283-7800
                                        Fax: 404-872-0457

1320   Ehlers-Danlos Syndrome
Arthritis Foundation
1330 W Peachtree Strt NW   404-872-7100
Atlanta, GA 30309-0669   800-283-7800
                                        Fax: 404-872-0457
                                         www.arthritis.org

Ehlers-Danlos syndrome (EDS) is a collection of genetic disorders that affect connective tissue.

1321   Exercise and Your Arthritis
Arthritis Foundation
PO Box 7669   404-872-7100
Atlanta, GA 30357-0669   800-283-7800
                                        Fax: 404-872-0457

Types of exercise for people with arthritis and how to do them.

1322   Family
Arthritis Foundation
PO Box 7669   404-872-7100
Atlanta, GA 30357-0669   800-283-7800
                                        Fax: 404-872-0457

Effects of arthritis on family life and ways to cope.

1323   Family: Making the Difference
Arthritis Foundation
PO Box 7669   404-872-7100
Atlanta, GA 30357-0669   800-283-7800
                                        Fax: 404-872-0457

1324   Gold Treatment
Arthritis Foundation
PO Box 7669   404-872-7100
Atlanta, GA 30357-0669   800-283-7800
                                        Fax: 404-872-0457

1325   Gout
Arthritis Foundation
1330 W Peachtree Strt NW   404-872-7100
Atlanta, GA 30309-0669   800-283-7800
                                        Fax: 404-872-0457
                                         www.arthritis.org

Gout is a form of inflammatory arthritis that develops in some people who have high levels of uric acid in the blood.

1326   Guide to Effective Volunteer Lobbying
Arthritis Foundation
PO Box 7669   404-872-7100
Atlanta, GA 30357-0669   800-283-7800
                                        Fax: 404-872-0457

1327   Health, Life and Disability Insurance for People with Arthritis
Arthritis Foundation
PO Box 7669   404-872-7100
Atlanta, GA 30357-0669   800-283-7800
                                        Fax: 404-872-0457

Information about these three types of insurance.

1328   Hydroxychloroquine
Arthritis Foundation
PO Box 7669   404-872-7100
Atlanta, GA 30357-0669   800-283-7800
                                        Fax: 404-872-0457

1329   Individuals with Arthritis
Mainstream
1030 5th Street NW   202-898-1400
Washington, DC 20001-2504
Mainstreaming individuals with arthritis into the workplace.
12 pages

1330   Juvenile Dermatomyositis
Arthritis Foundation
1330 W Peachtree Strt NW   404-872-7100
Atlanta, GA 30309-0669   800-283-7800
                                        Fax: 404-872-0457
                                         www.arthritis.org

Juvenile dermatomyositis (JDM) is an inflammatory disease that causes muscle weakness and a skin rash on the eyelids and knuckles.

1331   Living and Loving: Information About Sexuality and Intimacy
Arthritis Foundation
PO Box 7669   404-872-7100
Atlanta, GA 30357-0669   800-283-7800
                                        Fax: 404-872-0457

1332   Managing Your Activities
Arthritis Foundation
PO Box 7669   404-872-7100
Atlanta, GA 30357-0669   800-283-7800
                                        Fax: 404-872-0457

1333   Managing Your Fatigue
Arthritis Foundation
PO Box 7669   404-872-7100
Atlanta, GA 30357-0669   800-283-7800
                                        Fax: 404-872-0457

1334   Managing Your Health Care
Arthritis Foundation
PO Box 7669   404-872-7100
Atlanta, GA 30357-0669   800-283-7800
                                        Fax: 404-872-0457

1335   Managing Your Pain
Arthritis Foundation
1330 W Peachtree Strt NW   404-872-7100
Atlanta, GA 30309-0669   800-283-7800
                                        Fax: 404-872-0457
                                         www.arthritis.org

Complimentary health lecture by Arthritis Foundation.

1336   Managing Your Stress
Arthritis Foundation
1330 W Peachtree Strt NW   404-872-7100
Atlanta, GA 30309-0669   800-283-7800
                                        Fax: 404-872-0457
                                         www.arthritis.org

Complimentary health lecture by Arthiritis Foundation.

1337   Methotrexate
Arthritis Foundation
1330 W Peachtree Strt NW   404-872-7100
Atlanta, GA 30309-0669   800-283-7800
                                        Fax: 404-872-0457
                                         www.arthritis.org

Methotrexate is one of the most effective and widely used medications for treating rheumatoid arthritis (RA).

1338   Myositis
Arthritis Foundation
1330 W Peachtree Strt NW   404-872-7100
Atlanta, GA 30309-0669   800-283-7800
                                        Fax: 404-872-0457
                                         www.arthritis.org

Myositis is a term meaning inflammation in the muscles. There are several types of myositis, the most common being polymyositis and dermatomyositis.

1339   Osteoarthritis
Arthritis Foundation

1330 W Peachtree Strt NW
Atlanta, GA 30309-0669

404-872-7100
800-283-7800
Fax: 404-872-0457
www.arthritis.org

Osteoarthritis (OA) is the most common chronic condition of the joints.

1340 Osteonecrosis
Arthritis Foundation
1330 W Peachtree Strt NW
Atlanta, GA 30309-0669

404-872-7100
800-283-7800
Fax: 404-872-0457
www.arthritis.org

Osteoporosis drugs called bisphosphonates have been linked with the development of osteonecrosis (bone death) in the jaw.

1341 Overcoming Rheumatoid Arthritis
Michigan Chapter of the Arthritis Foundation
1050 Wilshire Drive
Troy, MI 48084-1564

248-649-2891
800-968-3030
Fax: 248-649-2895
info.mi@arthritis.org
www.arthritis.org

Provides extensive information about the disease and treatment, with an emphasis on what you can do for yourself.

1342 Penicillamine
Arthritis Foundation
PO Box 7669
Atlanta, GA 30357-0669

404-872-7100
800-283-7800
Fax: 404-872-0457

1343 Polyarteritis Nodosa and Wegener's Granulomatosis
Arthritis Foundation
PO Box 7669
Atlanta, GA 30357-0669

404-872-7100
800-283-7800
Fax: 404-872-0457

1344 Polymyalgia Rheumatica and Giant Cell Arthritis
Arthritis Foundation
PO Box 7669
Atlanta, GA 30357-0669

404-872-7100
800-283-7800
Fax: 404-872-0457

1345 Pseudoxanthoma Elasticum Fact Sheet
Arthritis Foundation
PO Box 7669
Atlanta, GA 30357-0669

404-872-7100
800-283-7800
Fax: 404-872-0457

1346 Psoriatic Arthritis Information Package
NAMSIC/National Institutes of Health
1 AMS Circle
Bethesda, MD 20892-0001

301-495-4484
877-226-4267
Fax: 301-718-6366
TTY: 301-565-2966
niamsinfo@mail.nih.gov
www.nih.gov/niams/

1347 Q&A's About Arthritis and Rheumatic Disease
NIH/National Institutes of Health
1 AMS Circle
Bethesda, MD 20892-0001

301-495-4484
877-226-4267
Fax: 301-718-6366
TTY: 301-565-2969
niamsinfo@mail.nih.gov
www.nih.gov/niams

This pamphlet offers information, technical articles and research on arthritis and related disorders. Also included are referral organizations to help patients uncover more information.

1348 Reflex Sympathetic Dystrophy Syndrome Fact Sheet
Arthritis Foundation
PO Box 7669
Atlanta, GA 30357-0669

404-872-7100
800-283-7800
Fax: 404-872-0457
www.arthritis.org

Reactive arthritis is an inflammatory type of arthritis which affects the joints, and may affect the eyes, skin and urinary tract (bladder, vagina, urethra).

1349 Reiter's Syndrome
Arthritis Foundation
1330 W Peachtree Strt NW
Atlanta, GA 30309-0669

404-872-7100
800-283-7800
Fax: 404-872-0457

1350 Rheumatoid Arthritis Information Package
NAMSIC/National Institutes of Health
1 AMS Circle
Bethesda, MD 20892-0001

301-495-4484
877-226-4267
Fax: 301-718-6366
TTY: 301-565-2966
niamsinfo@mail.nih.gov
www.nih.gov/niams

Offers an introduction and definition of rheumatoid arthritis, treatments, causes, objectives, daily living, resources and medical information.

1351 Surgery: Information to Consider
Arthritis Foundation
PO Box 7669
Atlanta, GA 30357-0669

404-872-7100
800-283-7800
Fax: 404-872-0457

1352 Thinking About Tomorrow: A Career Guide for Teens with Arthritis
Arthritis Foundation
PO Box 7669
Atlanta, GA 30357-0669

404-872-7100
800-283-7800
Fax: 404-872-0457

1353 When Your Student Has Arthritis: A Guide for Teachers
Arthritis Foundation
PO Box 7669
Atlanta, GA 30357-0669

404-872-7100
800-283-7800
Fax: 404-872-0457

A medical information booklet written for teachers or other adults who have arthritis. The booklet describes different forms of juvenile arthritis, how arthritis might affect the child at school, and how to help the child work around these problems.

Audio & Video

1354 FIT Video
Arthritis Foundation
550 Pharr Road
Altlanta, GA 30023-6996

404-237-8771
800-933-7023
Fax: 404-237-8153
info.ga@arthritis.org
www.arthritis.org

1355 In Control
Arthritis Foundation
1330 W Peachtree Strt NW
Atlanta, GA 30309-2922

404-872-7100
800-283-7800
Fax: 404-872-0457

An excellent at-home program which includes video, audio cassettes and the Arthritis Helpbook. Provides tools to help meet the challenges of arthritis.

1356 PACE I
Arthritis Foundation
PO Box 6996
Alpharetta, GA 30023-6996

800-207-8633

1357 PACE II
Arthritis Foundation
PO Box 6996
Alpharetta, GA 30023-6996

800-207-8633
Fax: 770-442-9742
www.arthritis.com

1358 Pathways to Better Living
Arthritis Foundation
PO Box 6996
Alpharetta, GA 30023-6996

800-207-8633
Fax: 770-442-9742
www.arthritis.com

1359 Pool Exercise Program
Arthritis Foundation Distribution Center

PO Box 6996
Alpharetta, GA 30023-6996

800-207-8633
Fax: 770-442-9742
www.arthritis.com

This video features water exercises that will help you increase and maintain joint flexibility, strengthen and tone muscles, and increase endurance. All exercises are performed in water at chest level. No swimming skills are necessary.

Web Sites

1360 American Juvenile Arthritis Organization

www.arthritis.com

Serves the special needs of young people with arthritis and their families. Provides information, inspiration and advocacy.

1361 Arthritis Foundation

www.arthritis.org

Provides services to help through information, referrals, speakers bureaus, forums, self-help courses, and various support groups and programs nationwide.

1362 Healing Well

www.healingwell.com

An online health resource guide to medical news, chat, information and articles, newsgroups and message boards, books, disease-related web sites, medical directories, and more for patients, friends, and family coping with disabling diseases, disorders, or chronic illnesses.

1363 Health Finder

www.healthfinder.gov

Searchable, carefully developed web site offering information on over 1000 topics. Developed by the US Department of Health and Human Services, the site can be used in both English and Spanish.

1364 Healthlink USA

www.healthlinkusa.com

Health information concerning treatment, cures, prevention, diagnosis, risk factors, research, support groups, email lists, personal stories and much more. Updated regularly.

1365 MedicineNet

www.medicinenet.com

An online resource for consumers providing easy-to-read, authoritative medical and health information.

1366 Medscape

www.medscape.com

Medscape offers specialists, primary care physicians, and other health professionals the Web's most robust and integrated medical information and educational tools.

1367 National Arthritis & Musculoskeletal & Skin Diseases Information Clearinghouse

www.niams.nih.gov

The mission of the National Institute of Arthritis and Musculoskeletal and Skin Diseases is to support research into the causes, treatment, and prevention of arthritis and musculoskeletal and skin diseases; the training of basic and clinical scientists to carry out this research; and the dissemination of information on research progress in these diseases.

1368 WebMD

www.webmd.com

Provides credible information, supportive communities, and in-depth reference material about health subjects. A source for original and timely health information as well as material from well known content providers.

Description

1369 Asthma

Asthma is a reversible, obstructive respiratory disorder that causes shortness of breath, wheezing, coughing and chest tightness. About 19 million adults and 6.2 million children in the U.S. have asthma, and its incidence is increasing. It is the leading cause of hospitalization for children; however, some children with asthma will outgrow the disorder by the time they are teenagers or adults. Asthma is a compilation of different types of obstructive respiratory diseases that have distinct disease mechanisms and range from mild illness to life-threatening asthmatic attacks.

Numerous environmental factors trigger an asthma attack including allergies, infections, exercise, cold weather and stress. Treatment consists of avoiding or minimizing factors that cause an asthma attack, for example pet dander and pollen.

In addition, several medications, known as bronchodilators, are used to relieve asthma symptoms by opening lung airways. Many of these drugs can be inhaled so that they work directly on the lungs. Inhaled steroids may be used for long-term control. For more recalcitrant forms of asthma, oral corticosteroids may be required. Biological medications, such as omalizumab, benralizumab, reslizumab, mepolizumab, and dipilumab, can also provide excellent long-term relief from particular types of treatment-resistant forms of asthma. Research and new therapies are being directed at trying to find medications that will prevent asthma from occurring. See also *Lung Disease.*

National Agencies & Associations

1370 Administration for Children and Families
330 C Street SW
Washington, DC 20201
202-205-8347
Fax: 202-205-9721
www.acf.hhs.gov
The Administration for Children & Families (ACF) is a division of the U.S. Department of Health & Human Services (HHS). ACF promotes the economic and social well-being of families, children, individuals and communities.
Lynn Johnson, Assistant Secretary
Jerry Milner, Acitng Commissioner, Children & Families

1371 Agency for Healthcare Research and Quality
5600 Fishers Lane
Rockville, MD 20857
301-427-1104
www.ahrq.gov
The Agency for Healthcare Research and Quality's (AHRQ) mission is to produce evidence to make health care safer, higher quality, more accessible, equitable, and affordable, and to work within the U.S. Department of Health and Human Services and with other partners to make sure that the evidence is understood and used.
Gopal Khanna, MBA, Director
Howard E. Holland, Director, Communications

1372 Agency for Toxic Substances and Disease Registry
4770 Buford Hwy NE
Atlanta, GA 30341-3717
770-488-0736
800-232-4636
Fax: 770-488-1547
TTY: 888-232-6348
jah8@cdc.gov
www.atsdr.cdc.gov
The Agency for Toxic Substances and Disease Registry (ATSDR), based in Atlanta, Georgia, is a federal public health agency of the U.S. Department of Health and Human Services. ATSDR serves the public by using the best science, taking responsive public health actions, and providing trusted health information to prevent harmful exposures and diseases related to toxic substances.
Patrick Breysse, PhD, CIH, Director
Jack Hanley, Acting Branch Chief, Central Branch

1373 Allergy & Asthma Network
8229 Boone Boulevard
Vienna, VA 22182
800-878-4403
Fax: 703-288-5271
info@aanma.org
www.allergyasthmanetwork.org
Non-profit membership organization dedicated to eliminating suffering and death due to asthma, allergies and related conditions through education, advocacy, community outreach, and research.
Tonya Winders, President & CEO
Marcela Gieminiani, Director, Outreach

1374 American Academy of Allergy, Asthma & Immunology
555 East Wells Street
Milwaukee, WI 53202-3823
414-272-6071
Fax: 414-272-6070
info@aaaai.org
www.aaaai.org
Strives to serve the public through information on asthma and allergies, as well as referrals to allergists.
Mary-Beth Fasano, President
Giselle S. Mosnaim, Secretary-Treasurer

1375 American College of Allergy, Asthma & Immunology
85 West Algonquin Road
Arlington Heights, IL 60005
847-427-1200
Fax: 847-427-9656
mail@acaai.org
www.acaai.org
Focuses on research and public awareness of allergies, asthma, and immunology. Distributes informational brochures and pamphlets, offers referrals and counseling services, as well as patient care.
Rick Slawny, Executive Diector
Nancy Ryan, Associate Executive Director

1376 American Lung Association
55 W. Wacker Drive
Chicago, IL 60601
800-586-4872
info@lung.org
www.lung.org
The mission of the American Lung Association is to prevent lung disease and promote lung health by fighting disease in all its forms, with special emphasis on asthma, tobacco control and environmental health.
Harold P. Wimmer, National President & CEO
Albert Rizzo, MD, FACP, Chief Medical Officer

1377 Asthma Canada
124 Merton Street
Toronto, Ontario, M4S-2Z2
416-787-4050
866-787-4050
Fax: 416-787-5807
info@asthma.ca
www.asthma.ca
National, volunteer-led organization devoted to enhancing the quality of life for individuals with athsma and respiratory allergies.
Vanessa Foran, President & CEO
Jenna Reynolds, Director, Programs & Services

1378 Birth Defect Research for Children, Inc.
976 Lake Baldwin Lane
Celebration, FL 32814
407-895-0802
staff@birthdefects.org
www.birthdefects.org/allergies
A non-profit organization providing parents and soon-to-be parents with information resources about birth defects, and support services for their children. Offers fact sheets on allergies.
Betty Mekdeci, Executive Director

1379 Canadian Society of Allergy and Clinical Immunology
PO Box 51045
Orleans, K1E-3W4
613-986-5869
Fax: 866-839-7501
info@csaci.ca
www.csaci.ca
Promotes the advancement of the knowledge and practice of allergy, clinical immunology, and asthma for optimal patient care.
Harold Kim, President
Louise Tremblay, Executive Director

1380 **Centers for Disease Control & Prevention: Division of Adolescent & School Health**
1600 Clifton Road   800-232-4636
Atlanta, GA 30329-4027   TTY: 888-232-6348
                                                     www.cdc.gov/HealthyYouth
CDC promotes the health and well-being of children and adolescents to enable them to become healthy and productive adults.

1381 **Centers for Medicare & Medicaid Services**
7500 Security Boulevard   410-786-3000
Baltimore, MD 21244   877-267-2323
                                                     TTY: 866-226-1819
                                                     www.cms.gov
U.S. federal agency which administers Medicare, Medicaid, and the State Children's Health Insurance Program.
Seema Verma, Administrator
Tom Corry, Director

1382 **National Center for Complementary and Integrative Health**
9000 Rockville Pike   888-644-6226
Bethesda, MD 20892   TTY: 866-464-3615
                                                     info@nccih.nih.gov
                                                     nccih.nih.gov
The National Center for Complementary and Integrative Health (NCCIH) is the Federal Government's lead agency for scientific research on the diverse medical and health care systems, practices, and products that are not generally considered part of conventional medicine.
Helene M. Langevin, MD, Director
David Shurtleff, Ph.D., Deputy Director

1383 **National Human Genome Research Institute**
Building 31, Room 4B09   301-402-0911
Bethesda, MD 20892-2152   Fax: 301-402-2218
                                                     www.genome.gov
The National Human Genome Research Institute began as the National Center for Human Genome Research (NCHGR), which was established in 1989 to carry out the role of the National Institutes of Health (NIH) in the International Human Genome Project (HGP).
Eric D. Green, M.D., Ph.D., Director
Lawrence Brody, Ph.D., Director, Division of Genomics & Society

1384 **National Institute for Occupational Safety and Health**
Patriots Plaza 1
395 E Street SW   202-245-0625
Washington, DC 20201   800-232-4636
                                                     Fax: 513-533-8347
                                                     TTY: 888-232-6348
                                                     www.cdc.gov/niosh
The National Institute for Occupational Safety and Health (NIOSH) is the U.S. federal agency that conducts research and makes recommendations to prevent worker injury and illness.
John Howard, MD, Director
Frank Hearl, PE, Chief of Staff

1385 **National Institute of Allergy and Infectious Diseases**
NIAID Office of Communications & Govt Relations
5601 Fishers Lane   301-496-5717
Bethesda, MD 20892-9806   866-284-4107
                                                     Fax: 301-402-3573
                                                     TDD: 800-877-8339
                                                     ocpostoffice@niaid.nih.gov
                                                     www.niaid.nih.gov
Conducts and supports research on allergies; focused on understanding what happens to the body during the allergic process. Educates patients and health care workers in controlling allergic disease; offers various research centers that conduct and evaluate educational programs focused on methods to control allergic diseases.
Anthony S. Fauci, MD, Director

1386 **National Institute of Biomedical Imaging and Bioengineering**
9000 Rockville Pike   301-496-8859
Bethesda, MD 20892   info@nibib.nih.gov
                                                     www.nibib.nih.gov
The mission of the National Institute of Biomedical Imaging and Bioengineering (NIBIB) is to improve health by leading the development and accelerating the application of biomedical technologies.
Bruce J. Tromberg, PhD, Director
Jill Heemskerk, PhD, Deputy Director

1387 **National Institute of Environmental Health Sciences**
105 T.W. Alexander Drive   919-541-3345
Research Triangle Park, NC 27709   webcenter@niehs.nih.gov
                                                     www.niehs.nih.gov
The mission of the NIEHS is to discover how the environment affects people in order to promote healthier lives.
Linda S. Birnbaum, PhD, Director
Richard Woychik, PhD, Deputy Director

1388 **National Institute of General Medical Sciences**
45 Center Drive MSC 6200   301-496-7301
Bethesda, MD 20892-6200   info@nigms.nih.gov
                                                     www.nigms.nih.gov
The National Institute of General Medical Sciences (NIGMS) supports basic research that increases understanding of biological processes and lays the foundation for advances in disease diagnosis, treatment and prevention.
Jon R. Lorsch, PhD, Director
Judith H. Greenberg, PhD, Deputy Director

1389 **U.S. Food and Drug Administration**
10903 New Hampshire Avenue   301-796-8240
Silver Spring, MD 20993-0002   888-463-6332
                                                     www.fda.gov
FDA is responsible for protecting the public health by assuring the safety, efficacy and security of human and veterinary drugs, biological products, medical devices, the nation's food supply, cosmetics, and products that emit radiation.
Norman E. Sharpless, MD, Commissioner
Denise Hinton, Chief Scientist

State Agencies & Associations

Alaska

1390 **Asthma and Allergy Foundation of America: Alaska Chapter**
PO Box 201927   907-349-0637
Anchorage, AK 99520-1927   800-651-4914
                                                     Fax: 907-349-0637
                                                     aafaalaska@gci.net
                                                     www.aafaalaska.com
Serves patients of all ages in Alaska who are affected by asthma and allergies, and also provides resources to healthcare professionals, caregivers and childcare providers.
Dale Knutsen, Executive Director

Maryland

1391 **National Institute of Nursing Research**
31 Center Drive   301-496-0207
Bethesda, MD 20892   Fax: 301-496-8845
                                                     info@ninr.nih.gov
                                                     www.ninr.nih.gov
The mission of the National Institute of Nursing Research (NINR) is to promote and improve the health of individuals, families, communities, and populations.
Patricia A. Grady, Institute Director
Dr. Ann R. Knebel, Deputy Director

Massachusetts

1392 **Asthma and Allergy Foundation of America: New England Chapter**
25 Braintree Hill Office Park   781-444-7778
Braintree, MA 02184   david@aafane.org
                                                     www.asthmaandallergies.org
Serves patients of all ages in Connecticut, Maine, Massachusetts, New Hampshire, Rhode Island and Vermont, who are affected by asthma and allergies, and also provides resources to healthcare professionals, caregivers and childcare providers.
David Guydan, Executive Director

Michigan

1393 Asthma and Allergy Foundation of America: Michigan Chapter
26111 West 14 Mile   248-406-4254
Franklin, MI 48025   888-444-0333
aafamich@sbcglobal.net
www.aafamich.org
Serves patients of all ages in Michigan who are affected by asthma and allergies, and also provides resources to healthcare professionals, caregivers and childcare providers.
Kathleen Felice Slonager, Executive Director

Missouri

1394 Asthma and Allergy Foundation of America: St. Louis Chapter
1500 S Big Bend   314-645-2422
St. Louis, MO 63117   Fax: 314-692-2022
aafa@aafastl.org
www.aafastl.org
Serves patients of all ages in St. Louis and surrounding counties who are affected by asthma and allergies, and also provides resources to healthcare professionals, caregivers and childcare providers. Offers the BREATH asthma and allergy management program for children.
Marjorie Moore, Executive Director

Virginia

1395 National Science Foundation
4201 Wilson Blvd   703-292-5111
Arlington, VA 22230   TDD: 703-292-5090
info@nsf.gov
www.nsf.gov
NSF is the only federal agency whose mission includes support for all fields of fundamental science and engineering, except for medical sciences.
France A. Cordova, Director
Joan Ferrini-Mundy, Chief Operating Officer

Foundations

1396 American Academy of Allergy, Asthma & Immunology Foundation
555 East Wells Street   414-272-6071
Milwaukee, WI 53202-3823   Fax: 414-272-6070
lwiensch@aaaai.org
www.aaaaifoundation.org
Funds research in an effort to prevent and cure asthma and allergic/immunologic diseases.
Lee Wiensch, Executive Director
Anne Koenings, Development Manager

1397 American College of Allergy, Asthma & Immunology Foundation
85 West Algonquin Road   847-427-1200
Arlington Heights, IL 60005   Fax: 847-427-9656
mail@acaai.org
college.acaai.org/acaai-foundation
Funds faculty research grants and travel scholarships.
Richard Weber, President
Stanley Fineman, Vice President

1398 Asthma and Allergy Foundation of America
8201 Corporate Drive   202-466-7643
Landover, MD 20785   800-727-8462
Fax: 202-466-8940
info@aafa.org
www.aafa.org
The AAFA is a non-profit patient organization dedicated to improving the quality of life for people with asthma and allergies and their caregivers, through education, advocacy, funding, and research.
Richard Murray, Chair
Kenneth Mendez, Chief Executive Officer

Research Centers

1399 Brigham and Women's Hospital: Rheumatology Immunology, and Allergy Division
75 Francis Street   61 -73 -550
Boston, MA 02115   Fax: 617-525-1001
TTY: 617-732-6458
www.brighamandwomens.org
Internationally renowned for excellence in clinical care clinical investigation and basic research. A faculty of 36 board certified rheumatologists and allergists provide eldtive urgent and emergency consultations as necessary.
Michael B Brenner MD, Division Chief
Jonathan S Coblyn, Clinical Director Rheumatology

1400 Childrens Hospital Immunology Division Children's Hospital
Children's Hospital
300 Longwood Avenue   61 -35 -600
Boston, MA 02115   www.childrenshospital.org
Organizational research unit of the Children's Hospital that focuses on the causes prevention and treatments of asthma infections and allergies.
Dr. James Mandell, CEO
Sandra Fenwick, President & COO

1401 Clinical Immunology, Allergy, and Rheumatology
Tulane Medical School
1700 Perdido Street   504-988-5187
New Orleans, LA 70112-1210   Fax: 504-988-3686
medsch@tulane.edu
www.som.tulane.edu/medciar
Mauel Lopez MD, Director

1402 Duke Asthma, Allergy and Airway Center
4309 Medical Park Drive   919-620-7300
Durham, NC 27704   www.aaac.duhs.duke.edu/
Raffeal Rau, President
Dr Monica Kraft, Director

1403 Johns Hopkins University: Asthma and Allergy Center
5501 Hopkins Bayview Circle   410-550-2101
Baltimore, MD 21224-6801   Fax: 410-550-3256
jhuallergy@jhmi.edu
www.hopkinsmedicine.org/allergy
Studies of allergic diseases and individuals with allergic disease pulmonary diseases and diseases involving inflammation and immunological processes.
Bruce S Bochner, Director
Peter S Creticos, Clinical Director

1404 National Jewish Division of Immunology
National Jewish Medical and Research Center
1400 Jackson Street   303-398-1337
Denver, CO 80206-2762   80 -42 -889
Fax: 303-270-2125
harbeckr@njc.org
The only medical center in the country whose research and patient care resources are dedicated to respiratory and immunologic diseases.
John Cambier, Chairman
Ronald J Harbeck, Medical Director

1405 Northwestern University: Division of Allergy and Immunology
The Feinberg School of Medicine
251 East Huron Street   312-926-6895
Chicago, IL 60611   Fax: 312-926-6905
rpschleimer@northwestern.edu
www.medicine.northwestern.edu
A referral center of local regional and national stature. Areas of clinical excellence include asthma allergic bronchopulmonary aspergillosis idiopathic anaphylaxis drug allergy occupational immunologic lung disease and allergen immunotherapy.
Douglas E Vaughan MD, Chair
James Foody MD, Vice Chair Clinical Affairs

1406 University of Virginia: General Clinical Research Center
University of Virginia Health System
2515 Lee Street   434-924-2394
Charlottesville, VA 22908-0787   Fax: 434-924-9960
www.healthsystem.virginia.edu/

Focuses on asthmatic disorders.
Arthur Garso Jr MD MPH, Principal Investigator
Eugene J Barrett, Program Director

1407   University of Wisconsin: Asthma, Allergy and Pulmonary
Research Center
600 Highland Avenue   608-263-6400
Madison, WI 53792-2454   Fax: 608-263-6401
                                              www.medicine.wisc.edu
Sheri L Lawrence, MBA, Administrator
Sharon Gehl, MBA, Associate Administrator

Support Groups & Hotlines

1408   National Health Information Center
Office of Disease Prevention & Health Promotion
1101 Wootton Pkwy   Fax: 240-453-8281
Rockville, MD 20852   odphpinfo@hhs.gov
                                              www.health.gov/nhic
Supports public health education by maintaining a calendar of National Health Observances; helps connect consumers and health
professionals to organizations that can best answer questions and
provide up-to-date contact information from reliable sources; updates on a yearly basis toll-free numbers for health information,
Federal health clearinghouses and info centers.
Don Wright, MD, MPH, Director

1409   Physician Referral and Information Line
American Academy of Allergy Asthma and Immunology
555 East Wells Street   414-272-6071
Milwaukee, WI 53202-3889   800-822-2762
                                           Fax: 414-272-6070
                                                  www.aaaai.org
Referral line offering information on allergy and asthma, referral
to an allergy/immunology specialist.

1410   Support for Asthmatic Youth
Asthma and Allergy Foundation of America
1080 Glen Cove Avenue   516-625-5735
Glen Head, NY 11545-1565   Fax: 516-625-2976
A network of educational/support groups for adolescents between
the ages of 9 and 17. All meetings are free and feature guest speak-
ers, informational programs, games and other fun activities.
Renee Theodorakis MA, Director Adolescent Services

Books

1411   Asthma Care Training for Kids
Asthma and Allergy Foundation of America
8201 Corporate Drive   202-466-7643
Landover, MD 20785   Fax: 202-466-8940
                                                  info@aafa.org
                                                  www.aafa.org
Designed to help children ages 7-12 and their parents take charge
of their asthma. In a series of three action filled sessions, children
and their parents meet separately with their peers to learn about
asthma management.

1412   Asthma Organizer
Allergy and Asthma Network/Mothers of Asthmatics
2751 Prosperity Avenue   703-641-9595
Fairfax, VA 22031-4397   800-878-4403
                                           Fax: 703-573-7794
                                       www.mothersofasthmatics.org
Includes daily symptom diary and forms to track medications, office visits and updates to your personal management plan. Information on peak flow monitoring, managing asthma at school,
understanding asthma activators, and allergy-proofing also included. Available in Spanish.
Loose Leaf
Mary McGowan, Executive Director

1413   Asthma Resources Directory
Allergy and Asthma Network/Mothers of Asthmatics
2751 Prosperity Avenue   703-641-9595
Fairfax, VA 22031-4397   800-878-4403
                                           Fax: 703-573-7794
                                       www.mothersofasthmatics.org

Comprehensive listings of thousands of products, services, and resources for allergy and asthma questions.
Mary McGowan, Executive Director

1414   Asthma Self-Help Book
Asthma and Allergy Foundation of America
8201 Corporate Drive   202-466-7643
Landover, MD 20785   Fax: 202-466-8940
                                                  info@aafa.org
                                                  www.aafa.org
A thorough, practical look at asthma that includes information
from the National Heart, Lung and Blood Institute's 1991 Asthma
Guidelines.

1415   Asthma in the School: Improving Control with Peak Flow
Monitoring
Asthma and Allergy Foundation of America
8201 Corporate Drive   202-466-7643
Landover, MD 20785   Fax: 202-466-8940
                                                  info@aafa.org
                                                  www.aafa.org
Comprehensive and practical guide to help the school nurse moni-
tor and assist students with asthma.

1416   Asthma in the Workplace
John H Dekker & Sons
2941 Clydon Street SW   616-538-5160
Grand Rapids, MI 49509   Fax: 616-538-0720
1993 664 pages
ISBN: 0-824787-99-4

1417   Asthma: The Complete Guide
Asthma and Allergy Foundation of America
8201 Corporate Drive   202-466-7643
Landover, MD 20785-2330   800-727-8462
                                           Fax: 202-466-8940
                                                  info@aafa.org
                                                  www.aafa.org
An excellent self-management guide for asthma and allergy patients and their families.
357 pages Paperback

1418   Breathing Disorders: Your Complete Exercise Guide
Human Kinetics
1607 N Market Street   217-351-1549
Champaign, IL 61820-5076   800-873-6759
                                           Fax: 217-351-2674
                                                  ce@hkusa.com
                                              www.humankinetics.com
1993 144 pages Paperback
ISBN: 0-873224-26-4
Steve Ruhlig, Marketing Director

1419   Bronchial Asthma: Principles of Diagnosis and Treatment
Humana Press
999 Riverview Drive   973-256-1699
Totowa, NJ 07512   Fax: 973-256-8341
                                                  www.springer.com
2001 496 pages
ISBN: 0-896038-61-0

1420   Children with Asthma: A Manual for Parents
Allergy Control Products
1620-D Satellite Blvd   203-438-9580
Duluth, GA 30097-0793   800-422-3878
                                           Fax: 203-431-8963
                                              www.allergycontrol.com
Known as the asthma bible, this second edition is sprinkled with
anecdotes by patients and their parents.
296 pages Paperback

1421   Conquering Asthma
Michael Newhouse, MD, author
B.C Decker, Inc.
50 King Street E, Floor 2   905-522-7017
Ontario, Canada L8N 3K7,   800-568-7281
                                           Fax: 905-522-7839
                                              info@bcdecker.com
                                              www.bcdecker.com

This text shows asthmatics how to live a healthier and happier life hardly aware that they have asthma.
1998 107 pages Paperback
ISBN: 1-896998-01-1

1422 Coping with Asthma
Rosen Publishing Group
29 E 21st Street
New York, NY 10010

212-777-3017
800-237-9932
Fax: 888-436-4643
customerservice@rosenpub.com
www.rosenpublishing.com

This book prepares students by explaining to them the dangers of asthma, a condition which, when properly treated, is completely manageable.
ISBN: 0-823929-69-8
Carolyn Simpson, Author

1423 Understanding Asthma
Phil Lieberman, MD, author
University Press of Mississippi
3825 Ridgewood Road
Jackson, MS 39211-6492

601-432-6205
800-737-7788
Fax: 601-432-6217
kburgess@ihl.state.ms.us
www.upress.state.ms.us

A guide to how the disease behaves and how the latest therapies work.
1999 120 pages Paperback
ISBN: 1-578061-42-3
Phil Lieberman, M.D., Author

Children's Books

1424 All About Asthma
Asthma and Allergy Foundation of America
8201 Corporate Drive
Landover, MD 20785-2330

202-466-7643
800-727-8462
Fax: 202-466-8940
info@aafa.org
www.aafa.org

Written by a 10-year-old with asthma, this cleverly illustrated book explains causes and symptoms, and ways to control asthma to lead a normal life.
39 pages Paperback

1425 Asthma
Franklin Watts Grolier
90 Old Sherman Turnpike
Danbury, CT 06816-0001

203-797-3500
800-621-1115
Fax: 203-797-3197
www.grolier.com

This book offers vital information on causes and treatments, plus advice on how to prevent flare-ups.
96 pages Grades 7-12
ISBN: 0-531106-97-7

1426 Asthma Challenge
Asthma and Allergy Foundation of America
8201 Corporate Drive
Landover, MD 20785

202-466-7643
Fax: 202-466-8940
info@aafa.org
www.aafa.org

An exciting new team game for large or small groups. Custom designed, full color, stand up board and two sets of pretested question cards. Teens and adults win AAFA Bucks as they test their knowledge in categories like Sneezes and Wheezes and Asthma Nuts and Bolts.

1427 Best of Superstuff Activity Booklet
American Lung Association
1740 Broadway
New York, NY 10019-4315

212-315-8700

For young children with asthma featuring a series of activities designed to help youngsters cope with asthma.
32 pages Ages 6-8

1428 Bronkie the Bronchiasaurus
Asthma and Allergy Foundation of America

8201 Corporate Drive
Landover, MD 20785-2330

202-466-7643
800-727-8462
Fax: 202-466-8940
info@aafa.org
www.aafa.org

A Super Nintendo role-playing adventure in which players manage the asthma of two dinosaurs. They must avoid triggers, maintain their peak-flow and take daily medications. Only then can they use their strongest defense - the powerful breath blast. Designed for ages 7 to 15.

1429 Childhood Asthma: Learning to Manage
Asthma and Allergy Foundation of America
8201 Corporate Drive
Landover, MD 20785-2330

202-466-7643
800-727-8462
Fax: 202-466-8940
info@aafa.org
www.aafa.org

Self-paced, entertaining activity books for home use featuring practical guidelines for managing childhood asthma with a focus on using peak flow meters.

1430 Clubhouse Kids Learn About Asthma
Asthma and Allergy Foundation of America
8201 Corporate Drive
Landover, MD 20785-2330

202-466-7643
800-727-8462
Fax: 202-466-8940
info@aafa.org
www.aafa.org

Interactive CD-ROM helps children ages 4-12 learn about asthma at their own pace. Sound, animation and game-like features draw players into the life of Janie, who has just been diagnosed with asthma.

1431 I'm a Meter Reader
Allergy and Asthma Network/Mothers of Asthmatics
2751 Prosperity Avenue
Fairfax, VA 22031-4397

703-641-9595
800-878-4403
Fax: 703-573-7794
www.mothersofasthmatics.org

Provides expert advice on how a peak flow meter can help detect when an asthma attack can occur in an easy to understand format with colorful illustrations. Available in Spanish. Companion video, I'm a Meter Reader, available as part of a set for $12.00.
Ages 4-9
Mary McGowan, Executive Director
Nancy Sander, Editor-in-Chief

1432 Let's Talk About Having Asthma
Rosen Publishing Group's PowerKids Press
29 E 21st Street
New York, NY 10010

212-777-3017
800-237-9932
Fax: 888-436-4643
customerservice@rosenpub.com
www.rosenpublishing.com

This book talks about the cause and treatments for asthma as well as the precautions sufferers should take. Recommended for grades K-4.
ISBN: 0-823950-32-8

1433 Lion Who Had Asthma
Asthma and Allergy Foundation of America
8201 Corporate Drive
Landover, MD 20785-2330

202-466-7643
800-727-8462
Fax: 202-466-8940
Info@aafa.org
www.aafa.org

A beautifully illustrated book that encourages preschoolers to use their imaginations and take their asthma medications.
24 pages Hardcover

1434 Luke Has Asthma Too!
Allergy Control Products
PO Box 793
Ridgefield, CT 06877-0793

800-422-3878
Fax: 203-431-8963

This gentle book will make for good reading with children, whether they have asthma or not.

1435 Scorpions
Harper & Row

10 E 53rd Street — 212-207-7000
New York, NY 10022-5299 — www.harpercollins.com
This novel, while not wholly dedicated to examining the ramifications of asthma on a child's life, does incorporate the theme into a compelling narrative.
Grades 6-9
Walter Dean Myers, Author

1436 So You Have Asthma Too!
Allergy and Asthma Network/Mothers of Asthmatics
2751 Prosperity Avenue — 703-641-9595
Fairfax, VA 22031-4397 — 800-878-4403
Fax: 703-573-7794
www.mothersofasthmatics.org
A children's illustrated book, offering a clear description and understanding of childhood asthma. Available in Spanish. Also see companion video, SO YOU HAVE ASTHMA TOO!, available as part of a set for $12.00.
Mary McGowan, Executive Director
Nancy Sander, Editor-in-Chief

1437 Winning Over Asthma
Asthma and Allergy Foundation of America
8201 Corporate Drive — 202-466-7643
Landover, MD 20785-2330 — 800-727-8462
Fax: 202-466-8940
Info@aafa.org
www.aafa.org
Simple coloring book explains asthma through a story about five-year-old Graham.
30 pages Paperback

Magazines

1438 Allergy & Asthma Today
Allergy & Asthma Network
8229 Boone Boulevard — 800-878-4403
Vienna, VA 22182 — Fax: 703-288-5271
info@aanma.org
www.allergyasthmanetwork.org
Medically reviewed magazine for people living with asthma, allergies and other respiratory conditions. Free with Allergy & Asthma Network membership.
40 pages
Gary Fitzgerald, Managing Editor

1439 Controlling Asthma
American Lung Association
1740 Broadway — 212-315-8700
New York, NY 10019-4315
For parents of children with asthma, this newsmagazine tells how parents can help their child deal with the many problems presented by asthma.
16 pages

1440 Starting Strong-Staying Strong: A Resource Guide for Educational Support Groups
Asthma and Allergy Foundation of America
8201 Corporate Drive — 202-466-7643
Landover, MD 20785 — 800-727-8462
Fax: 202-466-8940
info@aafa.org
www.aafa.org
A resource guide to help educational support groups get organized, publicize and remain successful. Great for people who want to start an asthma or allergy support group and for existing group leaders who want to strengthen their programs. Filled with stories of success and struggle from other group leaders, medical advisors and group members across the country. A companion CD-ROM provides additional tips.
Guide + CD-ROM
William McLin, Executive Director
Mike Tringale, Director Marketing/Communications

Newsletters

1441 Advance
Asthma and Allergy Foundation of America
8201 Corporate Drive — 202-466-7643
Landover, MD 20785-2330 — 800-727-8462
Fax: 202-466-8940
Info@aafa.org
www.aafa.org
A bi-monthly, 8 page newsletter for patients and their families filled with timely and useful information about managing asthma and allergies.
BiMonthly

1442 Allergy & Asthma ADVOCATE Newsletter
American Academy of Allergy, Asthma and Immunology
555 East Wells Street — 414-272-6071
Milwaukee, WI 53202 — 800-822-2762
Fax: 414-272-6070
www.aaaai.org
Offers tips and medical information on allergies and asthma via articles written by allied health and physician AAAAI members.
6 pages Quarterly

1443 BReATHE
Asthma and Allergy Foundation of America
8201 Corporate Drive — 800-727-8462
Landover, MD 20785 — info@aafa.org
www.aafa.org
E-newsletter filled with information on how to control asthma and allergies, with stories from patients who are living life without limits.
Bi-Monthly
William McLin, President/CEO
Angel Waldron, Sr Manager Marketing/Communications

1444 FreshAAIR
Asthma and Allergy Foundation of America
8201 Corporate Drive — 202-466-7643
Landover, MD 20785 — 800-727-8462
Fax: 202-466-8940
info@aafa.org
www.aafa.org
Filled with information about asthma, seasonal allergies, food allergies, back-to-school tips for parents, educational materials and more.
Bi-Monthly
William McLin, President/CEO
Angel Waldron, Sr Manager Marketing/Communications

1445 Leaders Link
Asthma and Allergy Foundation of America
8201 Corporate Drive — 800-727-8462
Landover, MD 20785 — info@aafa.org
www.aafa.org
Provides useful and timely insights on how to plan and lead asthma and allergy support group meetings, how to keep your support group active and strong, and useful ideas from other support groups.
Bi-Monthly
William McLin, President/CEO
Angel Waldron, Sr Manager Marketing/Communications

1446 MA Report
Allergy and Asthma Network/Mothers of Asthmatics
2751 Prosperity Avenue — 703-641-9595
Fairfax, VA 22031-4397 — 800-878-4403
Fax: 703-573-7794
www.mothersofasthmatics.org
Offers information on medical breakthroughs, patient care, public awareness, activities and events focusing on the allergy and asthma patient. This newsletter keeps a patient fully informed with medical articles written by experts in the field.
Monthly
Mary McGowan, Executive Director
Nancy Sander, Editor-in-Chief

Pamphlets

1447 About Asthma
American Lung Association
1740 Broadway   212-315-8700
New York, NY 10019-4315
A popular style pamphlet explaining symptoms, treatment and more for persons with asthma.
16 pages

1448 Allergies and You
American Lung Association
1740 Broadway   212-315-8700
New York, NY 10019-4315
Answers basic questions about allergy, particularly as it relates to asthma.

1449 Allergy & Asthma
American Academy of Allergy, Asthma and Immunology
555 East Wells Street   414-272-6071
Milwaukee, WI 53202-3889   800-822-2762
                                       Fax: 414-272-6070
                                       www.aaaai.org
An informational brochure discussing major topics of allerges and asthma.

1450 Asthma Alert
American Lung Association
1740 Broadway   212-315-8700
New York, NY 10019-4315
Quick reference folders with information on asthma, the symptoms and what to do in an emergency.

1451 Asthma Handbook
American Lung Association
1740 Broadway   212-315-8700
New York, NY 10019-4315
Explains asthma, gives self-care methods for handling it and helps patients work more effectively with their doctor.
28 pages

1452 Asthma Lifelines
American Lung Association
1740 Broadway   212-315-8700
New York, NY 10019-4315
Promotional brochure providing descriptions of ALA asthma education materials.
12 pages

1453 Asthma and Allergies in Seniors
American Academy of Allergy, Asthma and Immunology
555 East Wells Street   414-272-6071
Milwaukee, WI 53202   800-822-2762
                                       Fax: 414-272-6070
                                       www.aaaai.org

1454 Asthma and Pregnancy
American Academy of Allergy, Asthma and Immunology
555 East Wells Street   414-272-6071
Milwaukee, WI 53202-3889   800-822-2762
                                       Fax: 414-272-6070
                                       www.aaaai.org

1455 Asthma and the School Child
American Academy of Allergy, Asthma and Immunology
555 East Wells Street   414-272-6071
Milwaukee, WI 53202-3889   800-822-2762
                                       Fax: 414-272-6070
                                       www.aaaai.org

1456 Atopic Dermatitis
American Academy of Allergy, Asthma and Immunology
555 East Wells Street   414-272-6071
Milwaukee, WI 53202-3889   800-822-2762
                                       Fax: 414-272-6070
                                       www.aaaai.org
This brochure offers information on symptoms, diagnosi, treatment, and prognosis.

1457 Being Close
National Jewish Center for Immunology
1400 Jackson Street   303-388-4461
Denver, CO 80206-2762
A booklet offering information to patients suffering from a respiratory disorder such as emphysema, asthma or tuberculosis, that discusses sexual problems and feelings.

1458 Childhood Asthma
American Academy of Allergy, Asthma and Immunology
555 East Wells Street   414-272-6071
Milwaukee, WI 53202-3889   800-822-2762
                                       Fax: 414-272-6070
                                       www.aaaai.org

1459 Childhood Asthma: A Guide for Parents
Asthma and Allergy Foundation of America
8201 Corporate Drive   202-466-7643
Landover, MD 20785-2330   800-727-8462
                                       Fax: 202-466-8940
                                       Info@aafa.org
                                       www.aafa.org
This colorful booklet helps parents learn all about asthma in children.
32 pages

1460 Childhood Asthma: A Matter of Control
American Lung Association
1740 Broadway   212-315-8700
New York, NY 10019-4315
A guide for parents of children with asthma, this booklet covers topics such as identifying asthma signs and symptoms as well as controlling the condition.
28 pages

1461 Consumer Guide to Health Care Plans
American Academy of Allergy, Asthma and Immunology
555 East Wells Street   414-272-6071
Milwaukee, WI 53202-3889   800-822-2762
                                       Fax: 414-272-6070
                                       www.aaaai.org
Gives answers to some commonly asked questions on health care.

1462 Efficacy of Asthma Education, Selected Abstracts
American Lung Association
1740 Broadway   212-315-8700
New York, NY 10019-4315
Abstracts documenting the efficacy of asthma education programs for physicians and other health professionals.

1463 Exercise-Induced Asthma & Bronchospasm
American Academy of Allergy, Asthma and Immunology
555 East Wells Street   414-272-6071
Milwaukee, WI 53202-3889   800-822-2762
                                       Fax: 414-272-6070
                                       www.aaaai.org
This brochure covers testing, treatment, and other advice on how to deal with exercise-induced asthma.

1464 Facts About Asthma
American Lung Association
1740 Broadway   212-315-8700
New York, NY 10019-4315
Primary public information leaflet on asthma.
12 pages

1465 Facts About Peak Flow Meters
American Lung Association
1740 Broadway   212-315-8700
New York, NY 10019-4315
Discusses the use of a peak flow meter for adults and children with asthma.
8 pages

1466 Healthy Breathing
National Jewish Center for Immunology
1400 Jackson Street   303-388-4461
Denver, CO 80206-2762
Offers patients with lung or respiratory disorders information on exercise and healthy breathing.

1467 Helping Others Breathe Easier
Allergy and Asthma Network/Mothers of Asthmatics

2751 Prosperity Avenue   703-641-9595
Fairfax, VA 22031-4397   800-878-4403
     Fax: 703-573-7794
     www.mothersofasthmatics.org
Offers information on educational resources, support groups and the Network for persons afflicted with asthma or allergic disorders.
Mary McGowan, Executive Director
Nancy Sander, Editor-in-Chief

1468   Home Control of Allergies and Asthma
American Lung Association
1740 Broadway   212-315-8700
New York, NY 10019-4315
Discusses substances in the home that may trigger asthma and allergy problems and offers suggestions for controlling them.
12 pages

1469   Inhaled Medications for Asthma
American Academy of Allergy, Asthma and Immunology
555 East Wells Street   414-272-6071
Milwaukee, WI 53202-3889   800-822-2762
     Fax: 414-272-6070
     www.aaaai.org
This brochure gives helpful information on classes of inhaled medication, types of inhalation devices, spacers and holding chambers, how proper training is necessary.

1470   Making the Most of Your Next Doctor Visit
American Academy of Allergy, Asthma and Immunology
555 East Wells Street   414-272-6071
Milwaukee, WI 53202-3889   800-822-2762
     Fax: 414-272-6070
     www.aaaai.org
A personal asthma management monitor. Includes personal tracking charts to help you along.
10 pages

1471   Many Faces of Asthma
American Lung Association
1740 Broadway   212-315-8700
New York, NY 10019-4315
Provides an overview of asthma as a major public health problem, describes what happens during asthma attacks and explains how asthma is treated and managed.
12 pages

1472   Nocturnal Asthma
National Jewish Center for Immunology
1400 Jackson Street   303-388-4461
Denver, CO 80206-2762
Offers information to patients about how to understand and manage asthma at night.

1473   Occupational Asthma
American Academy of Allergy, Asthma and Immunology
555 East Wells Street   414-272-6071
Milwaukee, WI 53202-3889   800-822-2762
     Fax: 414-272-6070
     www.aaaai.org
This brochure also contains a list of most common agents theat cause occupational asthma and who is at risk.

1474   Occupational Asthma: Lung Hazards on the Job
American Lung Association
1740 Broadway   212-315-8700
New York, NY 10019-4315
Discusses occupational asthma, a form of asthma in which airways overreact to various irritants in the workplace.

1475   Outpatient Treatment of Asthma
American Academy of Allergy, Asthma and Immunology
555 East Wells Street   414-272-6071
Milwaukee, WI 53202-3889   800-822-2762
     Fax: 414-272-6070
     www.aaaai.org

1476   Peak Flow Meter: A Thermometer for Asthma
American Academy of Allergy, Asthma and Immunology

555 East Wells Street   414-272-6071
Milwaukee, WI 53202-3889   800-822-2762
     Fax: 414-272-6070
     www.aaaai.org

1477   School Information Packet
Allergy and Asthma Network/Mothers of Asthmatics
2751 Prosperity Avenue   703-641-9595
Fairfax, VA 22031-4397   800-878-4403
     Fax: 703-573-7794
     www.mothersofasthmatics.org
Practical, medical, and legal information for school administrators and parents of students with asthma.
Mary McGowan, Executive Director
Nancy Sander, Editor-in-Chief

1478   Standards for the Diagnosis and Care of Patients with Asthma
American Lung Association
1740 Broadway   212-315-8700
New York, NY 10019-4315
Standards developed by the American Thoracic Society, the medical section of the ALA. For physicians.
24 pages

1479   Student Asthma Action Card
Asthma and Allergy Foundation of America
8201 Corporate Drive   202-466-7643
Landover, MD 20785-2330   800-727-8462
     Fax: 202-466-8940
     Info@aafa.org
     www.aafa.org
Indispensable tool for familiarizing school personnel with asthma triggers, daily medications and emergency directions for each of their students with asthma.

1480   Superstuff
American Lung Association
1740 Broadway   212-315-8700
New York, NY 10019-4315
Kit specifically designed to help the elementary schoolchild with asthma to learn how to manage the condition. The kit contains teaching tools, puzzles, riddles, stories and games.

1481   Teens Talk to Teens About Asthma
Asthma and Allergy Foundation of America
8201 Corporate Drive   202-466-7643
Landover, MD 20785-2330   800-727-8462
     Fax: 202-466-8940
     Info@aafa.org
     www.aafa.org
Quotes and thoughts from teens capture the essence of what it feels like to have asthma.

1482   There are Solutions for the Student with Asthma
American Lung Association
1740 Broadway   212-315-8700
New York, NY 10017
Leaflet telling how parents and school personnel can work together to make life easier for children with asthma.
4 pages

1483   Tips to Remember
American Academy of Allergy, Asthma and Immunology
611 E Wells Street   414-272-6071
Milwaukee, WI 53202-3889
A set of 23 tip sheets offering information on various topics including allergy and asthma treatments, pregnancy and asthma, animal allergies, sinusitis and more.

1484   Tips to Remember Brochures
American Academy of Allergy, Asthma and Immunology
555 East Wells Street   414-272-6071
Milwaukee, WI 53202-3889   800-822-2762
     Fax: 414-272-6070
     www.aaaai.org
Thirty three colorful brochures offered on numerous topics in allergy, asthma, and immunology.

1485   Triggers of Asthma
American Academy of Allergy, Asthma and Immunology

555 East Wells Street
Milwaukee, WI 53202-3889

414-272-6071
800-822-2762
Fax: 414-272-6070
www.aaaai.org

This brochure gives helpful information on what will cause an asthma attack.

1486 Understanding Asthma
National Jewish Center for Immunology
1400 Jackson Street   303-388-4461
Denver, CO 80206
Offers a brief introduction to asthma and then goes into the physiology of asthma, the triggers of asthma, and diagnosis and monitoring of asthma.
27 pages

1487 Understanding Immunology
National Jewish Center for Immunology
1400 Jackson Street   303-388-4461
Denver, CO 80206-2762
Offers information to patients and the public on the body's defenses. Explains how immunity develops, the basics of immunologic medicine and coping with respiratory disorders.

1488 Understanding Your Child with Asthma
National Jewish Center for Immunology
1400 Jackson Street   303-388-4461
Denver, CO 80206-2762   800-222-5264
Offers information on patient care, research, education and adult programs offered by the Association.

1489 Unproven Methods in Diagnosing and Treating Allergies
Asthma and Allergy Foundation of America
8201 Corporate Drive   202-466-7643
Landover, MD 20785-2330   800-727-8462
Fax: 202-466-8940
Info@aafa.org
www.aafa.org

1490 Use of Steroids for Asthma and Allergies
American Academy of Allergy, Asthma and Immunology
555 East Wells Street   414-272-6071
Milwaukee, WI 53202-3889   800-822-2762
Fax: 414-272-6070
www.aaaai.org

1491 What Every Patient Should Know About Asthma & Allergy Medications
American Academy of Allergy, Asthma and Immunology
555 East Wells Street   414-272-6071
Milwaukee, WI 53202-3889   800-822-2762
Fax: 414-272-6070
www.aaaai.org

1492 Your Child and Asthma
National Jewish Center for Immunology
1400 Jackson Street   303-388-4461
Denver, CO 80206-2762
A booklet offering information to parents and family about their child with asthma. Offers information on diagnosis, treatments, triggers and family concerns.

Audio & Video

1493 Asthma Handbook Slides
American Lung Association
1740 Broadway   212-315-8700
New York, NY 10019-4315
Slides and script based on The Asthma Handbook for asthma patients and others.
Film

1494 Asthma Management
American Academy of Allergy, Asthma and Immunology
555 East Wells Street   414-272-6071
Milwaukee, WI 53202-3889   800-822-2762
Fax: 414-272-6070
www.aaaai.org
Although there is currently no cure for asthma, attacks can be controlled by appropriate asthma management. This video describes

what happens during an asthma attack, how your allergists diagnoses asthma, and ways your allergist can help you to manage your condition.
10-13 minutes

1495 Asthma and the Athlete
American Academy of Allergy, Asthma and Immunology
555 East Wells Street   414-272-6071
Milwaukee, WI 53202   800-822-2762
Fax: 414-272-6070
www.aaaai.org

In the past, people with asthma were sometimes discouraged from exercising. Today we know that everyone, including asthmatics, can benefit from physical actilvity. This video details which exercises are best for those with asthma, and how an allergist can help asthmatic athletes to properly manage and treat their disease.
10-13 minutes

1496 Environmental Control Measures
American Academy of Allergy, Asthma and Immunology
555 East Wells Street   414-272-6071
Milwaukee, WI 53202-3889   800-822-2762
Fax: 414-272-6070
www.aaaai.org

By conrtolling your environment, you can reduce your exposure to substances called allergens that trigger your allergic symptoms. This program depicts common outdoor and indoor allergens, methods an allergist uses to diagnose which substances you're allergic to, and how to reduce your exposure to allergic triggers.
10-13 minutes

1497 I'm a Meter Reader
Allergy and Asthma Network/Mothers of Asthmatics
2751 Prosperity Avenue   703-641-9595
Fairfax, VA 22031-4397   800-878-4403
Fax: 703-573-7794
www.mothersofasthmatics.org
Provides expert advice on how a peak flow meter can help detect when an asthma attack can occur in an easy to understand format. Companion book, I'm a Meter Reader, available as part of a set for $12.00.
Video
Mary McGowan, Executive Director
Nancy Sander, Editor-in-Chief

1498 Managing Asthma in School: An Action Plan
Asthma and Allergy Foundation of America
8201 Corporate Drive   202-466-7643
Landover, MD 20785-2330   800-727-8462
Fax: 202-466-8940
Info@aafa.org
www.aafa.org
Gives the basics of asthma and a plan for school nurses, parents and physicians to work together.
14 minutes

1499 Managing Childhood Asthma
American Lung Association
Box 596-COL   212-245-8000
New York, NY 10001   800-586-4872
Fax: 312-440-9374
webmaster@ala.org
www.ala.org
What parents need to know to manage asthma. 22 minutes.
Video

1500 Pharmacologic Therapy of Pediatric Asthma
American Lung Association
1740 Broadway   212-315-8700
New York, NY 10019-4315
A Learning Resource Program developed by a joint committee of the American Thoracic Society and the ALA.
Film

1501 Regular Kid
American Lung Association
1740 Broadway   212-315-8700
New York, NY 10019-4315
This film shows how families and children cope with asthma problems. Proven asthma management strategies are presented through

the experiences of four children with asthma, ranging in age from toddler to teenager.
Film

1502 So You Have Asthma Too!
Allergy and Asthma Network/Mothers of Asthmatics
2751 Prosperity Avenue   703-641-9595
Fairfax, VA 22031-4397   800-878-4403
Fax: 703-573-7794
Offers a clear description and understanding of childhood asthma.
Video
Mary McGowan, Executive Director
Nancy Sander, Editor-in-Chief

1503 What School Personnel Should Know About Asthma
American Lung Association
1740 Broadway   212-315-8700
New York, NY 10019-4315
Professionally produced videotape discussing the triggers, symptoms and management of childhood asthma.
Videotape

1504 You're in Charge: Teens with Asthma
Asthma and Allergy Foundation of America
8201 Corporate Drive   202-466-7643
Landover, MD 20785-2330   800-727-8462
Fax: 202-466-8940
Info@aafa.org
www.aafa.org
Designed for young adults dealing with the daily challenges of asthma management. Teens share their experiences and use of peak flow meters and prescribed medications.
10 minutes

Web Sites

1505 Allergy & Asthma Network
www.allergyasthmanetwork.org
Non-profit membership organization dedicated to eliminating suffering and death due to asthma, allergies and related conditions through education, advocacy, community outreach, and research.

1506 American Academy of Allergy, Asthma & Immunology
www.aaaai.org
Strives to serve the public through information on asthma and allergies, as well as referrals to allergists.

1507 American College of Allergy, Asthma & Immunology
www.acaai.org
Focuses on research and public awareness of allergies, asthma, and immunology. Distributes informational brochures and pamphlets, offers referrals and counseling services, as well as patient care.

1508 American Lung Association
www.lung.org
Offers research, medical updates, fund-raising, educational materials and public awareness campaigns relating to lung disease causes.

1509 Asthma and Allergy Foundation of America
www.aafa.org
The AAFA is a non-profit patient organization dedicated to improving the quality of life for people with asthma and allergies and their caregivers, through education, advocacy, funding, and research.

1510 Gazoontite
www.gazoontite.com
Provides links to websites involving asthma and also asthma-related products, such as books and guides.

1511 Healingwell
www.healingwell.com
A social network and support community for patients, caregivers, and families coping with the daily struggles of diseases, disorders and chronic illness.

1512 Health Finder
www.healthfinder.gov
A government web site where individuals can find information and tools to help you and those you care about stay healthy.

1513 Healthlink USA
www.healthlinkusa.com
Health information concerning treatment, cures, prevention, diagnosis, risk factors, research, support groups, email lists, personal stories and much more. Updated regularly.

1514 MedicineNet
www.medicinenet.com
An online resource for consumers providing easy-to-read, authoritative medical and health information.

1515 Medscape
www.medscape.com
Medscape offers specialists, primary care physicians, and other health professionals the Web's most robust and integrated medical information and educational tools.

1516 WebMD
www.webmd.com
Provides credible information, supportive communities, and in-depth reference material about health subjects. A source for original and timely health information as well as material from well known content providers.

Description

1517 Ataxia

Ataxia refers to a group of diseases characterized by abnormal, uncoordinated movements. Ataxia disrupts muscular coordination, resulting in a staggered gait, the inability to stand or sit straight, and the inability to make smooth, voluntary movements. Other symptoms will vary depending on the type of ataxia but may include deterioration of fine motor skills (which prevents the execution of everyday tasks such a buttoning clothes, opening jars, or handwriting), speech and swallowing difficulties, vision abnormalities, increased fatigue, and cognitive and mood problems. All ataxias involve deterioration of the cerebellum and/or the brain and spinal structures that communicate with it. Conditions that are associated with ataxia may be hereditary or sporadic.

The most common hereditary ataxia is Friedreich's ataxia, which typically begins between 5 and 15 years of age. At first there is gait unsteadiness and slurred speech which progresses to weakness of the extremities. Some patients develop spinal deformity or cardiac problems. Other, less common hereditary ataxias generally begin during adult life. Sporadic cases also begin in adulthood and may be due to toxins, such as alcohol, infections, tumors, or autoimmune conditions, or may be of unknown cause. Sporadic cases are often a symptom of some other disease, such as multiple sclerosis, stroke, or vitamin deficiencies. Although essentially all patients will become wheelchair-dependent at some point, the outlook for long-term survival is good.

Treatment for any of the ataxias is aimed at the underlying cause, but often supportive, with physical therapy, assistive devices, psychological support, career counseling and treatment of complications. Some ataxias are treated with vitamin E or coenzyme Q10, but one type of ataxia, Episodic Ataxia Type 2 (EA2), is treated with acetazolamide. Leg spasticity is relieved by the muscle relaxant baclofen. In some cases, the ataxia progression is delayed by amantadine. And ataxia-associated tremors are treated with primidone, beta-blockers, or benzodiazepams. Genetic counseling is appropriate for those with the hereditary forms and their families.

National Agencies & Associations

1518 American Chronic Pain Association
PO Box 850
Rocklin, CA 95677
800-533-3231
ACPA@theacpa.org
www.theacpa.org

The ACPA facilitates peer support and education for individuals with chronic pain in its many forms, in order to increase quality of life. Also raises awareness among the healthcare community, and with policy makers.
Penney Cowan, Founder & CEO
Daniel Galia, Director, Global Support

1519 International Parkinson and Movement Disorder Society
555 East Wells Street
Milwaukee, WI 53202-3823
414-276-2145
Fax: 414-276-3349
info@movementdisorders.org
www.movementdisorders.org

The MDS is comprised of clinicians, scientists, and other healthcare professionals interested in Parkinson's disease, as well as related neurodegenerative and neurodevelopmental disorders, hyperkinetic movement disorders, and abnormalities in muscle tone and motor control.
Jennie Socha, Executive Director
Erin Weileder, Director, Membership & Communications

Foundations

1520 Ataxia Canada - Claude St-Jean Foundation
1751 Richardson Street
Montreal, Quebec, H3K-1G6
514-321-8684
855-321-8684
ataxie@lacaf.org
lacaf.org

Ataxia Canada seeks to improve the lives of individuals with familial ataxia, and to support research.
Jean Luk Pellerin, President
Francois Theberge, General Manager

1521 National Ataxia Foundation
600 Highway 169 S
Minneapolis, MN 55426
763-553-0020
Fax: 763-553-0167
naf@ataxia.org
www.ataxia.org

The NAF seeks to improve the lives of individuals affected by ataxia through support, education, and research.
Andrew Rosen, Executive Director
Susan Hagen, Patient Services Director

Support Groups & Hotlines

1522 National Health Information Center
Office of Disease Prevention & Health Promotion
1101 Wootton Pkwy
Rockville, MD 20852
Fax: 240-453-8281
odphpinfo@hhs.gov
www.health.gov/nhic

Supports public health education by maintaining a calendar of National Health Observances; helps connect consumers and health professionals to organizations that can best answer questions and provide up-to-date contact information from reliable sources; updates on a yearly basis toll-free numbers for health information, Federal health clearinghouses and info centers.
Don Wright, MD, MPH, Director

Alabama

1523 Alabama Ambassador: National Ataxia Foundation
123 Leigh Ann Road
Hazel Green, AL 35750
256-828-4858
diannebw@aol.com
www.ataxia.org

Ambassadors are often in areas not served by a support group or chapter.
Dianne Blaine-Williamson, NAF Ambassador

1524 Birmingham Support Group: National Ataxia Foundation
16 Oaks Circle
Hoover, AL 35244
205-987-2883
donnellyB6132@aol.com
www.ataxia.org

Becky Donnelly, Group Contact

Arizona

1525 Phoenix Area Support Group: National Ataxi a Foundation
2322 W Sagebrush Drive
Chandler, AZ 85224-2155
480-726-3579
rtg22@cox.net
www.ataxia.org

Rita Garcia, Director

1526 **Tucson Support Group: National Ataxia Foundation**
7665 E Placita Luna Preciosa   520-885-8326
Tucson, AZ 85710   bbeck15@cox.net
    www.ataxia.org

Bart Beck, Director

California

1527 **California Ambassador: National Ataxia Foundation**
315 W Alamos   559-281-9188
Clovis, CA 93612   www.ataxia.org
Mike Betchel, NAF Ambassador

1528 **Los Angeles Support Group: National Ataxia Foundation**
339 W Palmer   818-246-5758
Glendale, CA 91204   www.ataxia.org
Sid Luther, President

1529 **Northern California Support Group: National Ataxia Foundation**
26840 Eldridge Avenue   510-783-3190
Hayward, CA 94544   rsisbig@aol.com
    www.ataxia.com

Deborah Ominctin, Leader

1530 **Orange County Support Group: National Ataxia Foundation**
829 W Gary Ave   323-788-7751
Montebello, CA 90640   dnavar@ucla.edu
    www.ataxia.org

Daniel Navar, Group Leader

1531 **San Diego Support Group: National Ataxia Foundation**
2087 Granite Hills Drive   619-447-3753
El Cajon, CA 92019   sdasg@cox.net
    www.ataxia.org

Earl McLaughlin, Group Leader

Colorado

1532 **Denver Support Group: National Ataxia Foundation**
5902 W Maplewood Drive   303-973-8035
Littleton, CO 80123   tom_sathre@acm.org
    www.ataxia.org

Tom Sathre, Group Leader

Florida

1533 **Florida Ambassador: National Ataxia Foundation**
302 Beach Drive   850-654-2817
Destin, FL 30541   csugars@cox.net
    www.ataxia.org
Ambassadors are often in areas not served by a support group or chapter.
Christina Sugars, NAF Ambassador

1534 **Northwest Florida Support Group: National Ataxia Foundation**
54 Troon Terrace   904-273-4644
Ponte Vedra, FL 32082-3321   jmcgranepvb@bellsouth.net
    www.ataxia.org

June McGrane, Group Leader

1535 **West Central FL Support Group: National Ataxia Foundation**
9753 Elm Way   813-453-1084
Tampa, FL 33635   flataxia@yahoo.com
    www.ataxia.org

Crystal Frohna, Group Leader

Georgia

1536 **Georgia Support Group: National Ataxia Foundation**
320 Peters Street   404-822-7451
Savannah, GA 30313   rookssgj@yahoo.com
    www.ataxia.org

Greg Rooks, Group Leader

Illinois

1537 **Chicago Area Support Group: National Ataxia Foundation**
410 W Mahogany Ct   847-496-7544
Palatine, IL 60067   caasg2@aol.com
    www.ataxia.org

Craig Lisack, Group Leader

1538 **Chicago Metro Support Group: National Ataxia Foundation**
5633 N Kenmore   773-334-1667
Chicago, IL 60660   cmarsh34@ameritech.net
    www.ataxia.org

Chris Marsh, Group Leader

Indiana

1539 **Southern Indiana Support Group: National Ataxia Foundation**
1102 Ridgewood Drive   812-630-4783
Huntingburg, IN 47542   www.ataxia.org
Monica Smith, Group Leader

Louisiana

1540 **Louisiana Support Group: National Ataxia Foundation**
2250 Gause Blvd   985-643-0783
Slidell, LA 70431   ataxia1@earthlink.net
    www.ataxia.org

Charlene Danielson, President
Camille Daglio, Vice-President

Maine

1541 **Maine Support Group: National Ataxia Foundation**
PO Box 113   rollins@gwi.net
Bowdoinham, ME 04008   www.ataxia.org
Kelly Rollins, Group Leader

Maryland

1542 **Chesapeake Area Support Group: National Ataxia Foundation**
3200 Baker Circle   301-644-1836
Adamstown, MD 21710-9666   www.ataxia.org
Carl J Lauter, Group Leader

Massachusetts

1543 **New England Area Support Group: National Ataxia Foundation**
45 Juliette Street   978-475-8072
Andover, MA 01810   www.ataxia.org
Donna Gorzela, Group Leader

Michigan

1544 **Detroit Support Group: National Ataxia Foundation**
20217 Wyoming   313-736-2827
Detroit, MI 48221   www.ataxia.org
Tanya Tunstul, Group Leader

Minnesota

1545 **Minnesota Ambassador: National Ataxia Foundation**
5179 Meadow Drive SE   504-282-7127
Rochester, MN 55904   logoetz@gmail.com
    www.ataxia.org

Lori Goetzman, NAF Ambassador

1546 **Twin Cities Area Support Group: National Ataxia Foundation**
2549 32nd Avenue S   612-724-3487
Minneapolis, MN 55406   lschultz@bitstream.net
    www.ataxia.org

Lenore Healy Schultz, Group Leader

Mississippi

1547 **Mississippi Area Support Group: National Ataxia Foundation**
PO Box 17005   daglio1@bellsouth.net
Hattisburg, MS 39404   www.ataxia.org
Camille Daglio, Group Leader

1548 **Kansas City Support Group: National Ataxia Foundation**
17700 E 17th Terrace Court S   816-257-2428
Independence, MO 64057   www.ataxia.org
Lois Goodman, Group Leader

1549 **Mid Missouri Support Group: National Ataxia Foundation**
1609 Cocoa Court   573-474-7232
Columbia, MO 65202   rogercooley@localnet.com
                                          www.ataxia.org
Roger Cooley, Contact

1550 **Central NY Area Support Group: National Ataxia Foundation**
2849 Bingley Road   johnsons@summitsolutions.net
Cazenovia, NY 13035   www.ataxia.org
Linda Johnson, President

1551 **New York Ambassador National Ataxia Foundation**
36 W Redoubt Rd   763-553-0020
Fishkill, NY 12524   vrabsolutely@aol.com
                                          www.ataxia.org
Valerie Ruggiero, NAF Ambassador

1552 **Tri-State Area Support Group: National Ataxia Foundation**
Northgate 6C   212-844-8711
Bronxville, NY 10708   markmeghan@aol.com
                                          www.ataxia.org
Mark Mitchell, Group Leader

1553 **Central Ohio Support Group: National Ataxia Foundation**
7852 Country Court   440-255-8284
Mentor, OH 44060   wurbanski@oh.rr.com
                                          www.ataxia.org
Cecilia Urbanski, Group Leader

1554 **North East Ohio Support Group National Ataxia Foundation**
PO Box 148   440-693-4454
Mesopotamia, OH 44439   kakah@windstream.net
                                          www.ataxia.org
Joe Miller, President

1555 **Ohio Ambassador: National Ataxia Foundation**
1283 Westfield SW   330-499-4060
North Canton, OH 44720   www.ataxia.org
James Kardos, NAF Ambassador

1556 **Oklahoma Ambassador: National Ataxia Foundation**
5700 SE Hazel Road   918-331-9530
Bartlesville, OK 74006   droopydog36@hotmail.com
                                          www.ataxia.org
Darrell Owens, NAF Ambassador

1557 **Willamette Valley Support Group: National Ataxia Foundation**
Albany General Hospital   541-812-4162
Albany, OR 97321   Fax: 541-812-4614
                                          malindam@samhealth.org
                                          www.ataxia.org
Malinda Moore, President

1558 **Carolinas Support Group: National Ataxia National Ataxia Foundation**
1305 Cely Road   864-220-3395
Easley, SC 29642   cecerussell@hotmail.com
                                          www.ataxia.org
Cece Russell, Group Leader

1559 **Houston Support Group: National Ataxia Foundation**
9405 Highway 6 S   281-693-1826
Houston, TX 77083   angelahcloud@aol.com
                                          www.ataxia.org
Angela Cloud, Group Leader

1560 **North Texas Support Group: National Ataxia Foundation**
7 Wentworth Court   cheve11e@sbcglobal.net
Trophy Club, TX 76262   www.ataxia.org
David Henry Jr, Group Leader

1561 **Texas Ambassador: National Ataxia Foundation**
356 Las Brisas Blvd   830-557-6050
Seguin, TX 78155-0193   acemom@peoplepc.com
                                          www.ataxia.org
Charlene Danielson, President
Camilie Daglio, Vice-President

1562 **Utah Support Group: National Ataxia Foundation**
Moran Eye Clinic   801-585-2213
Salt Lake City, UT 84132   julia.kleinschmidt@hsc.utah.edu
                                          www.ataxia.org
Dr Julia Kleinschmidt, Group Leader

1563 **Washington Ambassador National Ataxia Foundation**
PO Box 19045   509-482-8501
Spokane, WA 99219   www.ataxia.org
Linda Jacoy, Ambassador

1564 **Western WA Support Group: National Ataxia Foundation**
14104 107th Avenue   425-823-6239
Kirkland, WA 98034   www.ataxia.org/chapters/Seattle/default.
Milly Lewendon, Group Leader

Books

1565 **Directory of National Genetic Voluntary Organizations**
Genetic Alliance
4301 Connecticut Ave NW   202-966-5557
Washington, DC 20008-2369   800-336-4363
                                          Fax: 202-966-8553
                                          info@geneticalliance.org
Lists hundreds of organizations and associations dealing with genetic conditions.

1566 **Hereditary Ataxia: Guidebook for Managing Speech & Swallowing**
National Ataxia Foundation
2600 Fernbrook Lane N   763-553-0020
Minneapolis, MN 55447-4752   Fax: 763-553-0167
                                          naf@ataxia.org
                                          www.ataxia.org

1567 **Living with Ataxia**
National Ataxia Foundation
2600 Fernbrook Lane N   763-553-0020
Minneapolis, MN 55447-4752   Fax: 763-553-0167
                                          naf@ataxia.org
                                          www.ataxia.org

Compassionate resource for people who have or may be at risk of having ataxia, and for their families. This book explains the nature and causes of ataxia, the basic genetics that underlie many kinds of ataxia, discusses medical management of ataxia, provides practical advice for everyday living, points the way to many useful resources and assures that living a good life is an entirely reasonable aspiration, even with ataxia.
112 pages

1568 **Ten Years to Live**
National Ataxia Foundation

2600 Fernbrook Lane N 763-553-0020
Minneapolis, MN 55447-4752 Fax: 763-553-0167
naf@ataxia.org
www.ataxia.org
Struggles of the Schut family with hereditary ataxia.
ISBN: 0-962716-63-1

Newsletters

1569 Alert
Alliance of Genetic Support Groups
4301 Connecticut Ave NW 301-652-5553
Washington, DC 20008-2304 800-336-4363
Functions as a vehicle of communication between the Alliance and its constituency. Provides timely and useful information on genetics research.
Monthly

1570 GENES Information Services
Genetic Network of the Empire State
Empire State Plaza 518-474-7148
Albany, NY 12201 Fax: 518-474-8590

1571 Generations
National Ataxia Foundation
2600 Fernbrook Lane N 763-553-0020
Minneapolis, MN 55447-4752 Fax: 763-553-0167
naf@ataxia.org
www.ataxia.org
Provides the latest in ataxia research, information on coping, reference material, updates on chapters and support groups and personal stories on living with ataxia. With a readership of more than 25,000, this publication is distributed throughout the US and the world. This publication is for ataxia families, the medical community, ataxia researchers and interested individuals. This publication is free to NAF members.
Quarterly

1572 Genexus
Great Plains Genetic Service Network
The University of Iowa 319-356-2674
Iowa City, IA 52242 Fax: 319-356-3347

1573 Great Lakes Genetic News
Great Lakes Regional Genetics Group
1500 Highland Avenue 608-266-2907
Madison, WI 53705-2274 Fax: 608-263-3496

1574 MARGIN
Mid-Atlantic Regional Human Genetics Network
260 S Broad Street 215-456-7910
Philadelphia, PA 19102-5021 Fax: 215-456-7911

1575 MSRGSN Newsletter
Mountain States Regional Genetics Service Network
4300 Cherry Creek Drive S 303-692-2423
Denver, CO 80246 Fax: 303-782-5576
joyce.hooker@state.co.us
www.mostgene.org

8-12 pages
Joyce Hooker, Coordinator

1576 NERG News
New England Regional Genetics Group
PO Box 670 207-839-5324
Mount Desert, ME 04660-0670 Fax: 207-839-8637

1577 SERGG
Southeast Regional Genetics Group
PO Box 1642 404-778-8551
Decatur, GA 30031-1642 Fax: 404-778-8562
mlane@sergginc.org
sergginc.org

Pamphlets

1578 Alliance Brochure
Genetic Alliance

4301 Connecticut Ave NW 202-966-5557
Washington, DC 20008-2304 Fax: 202-966-8553
info@geneticalliance.org
www.geneticalliance.org
Explains the services and programs offered by the alliance.

1579 Ataxia Fact Sheet
National Ataxia Foundation
2600 Fernbrook Lane N 763-553-0020
Minneapolis, MN 55447-4752 Fax: 763-553-0167
naf@ataxia.org
www.ataxia.org
Describes ataxia as a symptom and its association with other medical problems as well as the hereditary types.

1580 Familial Spastic Paraplegia
National Ataxia Foundation
2600 Fernbrook Lane N 763-553-0020
Minneapolis, MN 55447-4752 Fax: 763-553-0167
naf@ataxia.org
www.ataxia.org
Defines this disorder and notes symptoms, causes and treatments.

1581 Frenkel's Exercises
National Ataxia Foundation
2600 Fernbrook Lane N 763-553-0020
Minneapolis, MN 55447-4752 Fax: 763-553-0167
naf@ataxia.org
www.ataxia.org
Describes an exercise program designed for those with ataxia.

1582 Friedrich's Ataxia
National Ataxia Foundation
2600 Fernbrook Lane N 763-553-0020
Minneapolis, MN 55447-4752 Fax: 763-553-0167
naf@ataxia.org
www.ataxia.org
Describes symptoms, diagnosis, genetics and hints on coping.

1583 Gene Testing for Ataxia
National Ataxia Foundation
2600 Fernbrook Lane N 763-553-0020
Minneapolis, MN 55447-4752 Fax: 763-553-0167
naf@ataxia.org
www.ataxia.org
Describes the latest information about who should consider it and where to have it done.

1584 Health Insurance
National Ataxia Foundation
2600 Fernbrook Lane N 763-553-0020
Minneapolis, MN 55447-4752 Fax: 763-553-0167
naf@ataxia.org
www.ataxia.org
Offers health insurance advice for persons with ataxia.

1585 Hereditary Ataxia: Brochure
National Ataxia Foundation
2600 Fernbrook Lane N 763-553-0020
Minneapolis, MN 55447-4752 Fax: 763-553-0167
naf@ataxia.org
www.ataxia.org
Describes recessive and dominant ataxias, information on how hereditary ataxia is transmitted and explanations of the NAF's role in education, service and prevention.

1586 Hereditary Ataxia: Fact Sheets
National Ataxia Foundation
2600 Fernbrook Lane N 763-553-0020
Minneapolis, MN 55447-4752 Fax: 763-553-0167
naf@ataxia.org
www.ataxia.org
Various ataxia fact sheets relating to specific forms of hereditary ataxia. Individual ataxia fact sheets include Friederich's ataxia and specific forms of spinocerebellar ataxias (SCAs).

1587 Incorporating Consumers into Regional Genetics Networks
Genetic Alliance

4301 Connecticut Ave NW   202-966-5557
Washington, DC 20008-2304   Fax: 202-966-8553
info@geneticalliance.org
www.geneticalliance.org

1588   **Informed Consent: Participation In Genetic Research Studies**
Genetic Alliance
4301 Connecticut Ave NW   202-966-5557
Washington, DC 20008-2304   Fax: 202-966-8553
www.geneticalliance.org
This booklet explains the nature of genetic research with its benefits and risks.

1589   **Pen-Pal Directory**
National Ataxia Foundation
2600 Fernbrook Lane N   763-553-0020
Minneapolis, MN 55447-4752   Fax: 763-553-0167
naf@ataxia.org
www.ataxia.org
National, state and international directory of others who are affected by ataxia. Available to NAF Pen-Pal members only. Application available.

1590   **Students with Friedreich's Ataxia**
National Ataxia Foundation
2600 Fernbrook Lane N   763-553-0020
Minneapolis, MN 55447-4752   Fax: 763-553-0167
naf@ataxia.org
www.ataxia.org
Worksheet for teachers, parents and others who need to understand the physical constraints of ataxia.

Audio & Video

1591   **Together...There Is Hope**
National Ataxia Foundation
2600 Fernbrook Lane N   763-553-0020
Minneapolis, MN 55447-4752   Fax: 763-553-0167
naf@ataxia.org
www.ataxia.org
Video discussing ataxias genetic patterns of inheritance and the National Ataxia Foundation and its research efforts.

Web Sites

1592   **Healing Well**
www.healingwell.com

An online health resource guide to medical news, chat, information and articles, newsgroups and message boards, books, disease-related web sites, medical directories, and more for patients, friends, and family coping with disabling diseases, disorders, or chronic illnesses.

1593   **Health Finder**
www.healthfinder.gov
Searchable, carefully developed web site offering information on over 1000 topics. Developed by the US Department of Health and Human Services, the site can be used in both English and Spanish.

1594   **Healthlink USA**
www.healthlinkusa.com
Health information concerning treatment, cures, prevention, diagnosis, risk factors, research, support groups, email lists, personal stories and much more. Updated regularly.

1595   **MedicineNet**
www.medicinenet.com
An online resource for consumers providing easy-to-read, authoritative medical and health information.

1596   **Medscape**
www.medscape.com
Medscape offers specialists, primary care physicians, and other health professionals the Web's most robust and integrated medical information and educational tools.

1597   **National Ataxia Foundation**
naf@ataxia.org
www.ataxia.org
Information on ataxia, ataxia research, listing of chapters and support groups and related links. Researchers may download NAF's ataxia reserch application guidelines and forms. Exerpts of articles in NAF's quarterly news publication, Generations. Online registration for NAF's annual membership meetings. Caladar of events on NAF activities. This site is for ataxia familes, the medical community, ataxia reserachers and interested individuals.

1598   **WebMD**
www.webmd.com
Provides credible information, supportive communities, and in-depth reference material about health subjects. A source for original and timely health information as well as material from well known content providers.

Description

1599 **Attention Deficit Hyperactivity Disorder**

Attention Deficit-Hyperactivity Disorder, ADHD, and Attention Deficit Disorder, ADD, are neurologically based disorders. ADHD primarily affects children, with 15.7 percent of the school-age population in the United States having been diagnosed. Approximately one-third of children diagnosed with ADHD retain the diagnosis into adulthood. In about 25 percent of attention deficit cases, hyperactivity is not present, and it is thus labeled ADD. ADHD's three major symptoms are distractibility, impulsivity and hyperactivity. The dominant symptom of ADD is day dreaming or tuning out. ADHD is diagnosed roughly twice as much in boys than girls, and ADHD affects three times as many adolescent males (13 percent) as females (4.2 percent). Studies show that 90 percent have academic problems or are underachievers, although these difficulties may not begin until the middle school years.

While studies suggest that about 50 percent of children with these disorders will improve at puberty, both ADHD and ADD can exist throughout a lifetime and, in fact, may first be diagnosed in teen or adult years.

Often, an affected individual experiences difficulties that can impact learning, peer relations, family life, and self-esteem. These difficulties may manifest themselves through angry outbursts, self-imposed social isolation, blaming others, a quickness to fight, and a high sensitivity to criticism.

Treatment of ADHD and ADD include: education programs with resource or tutorial help;psychological programs to improve self-esteem and help families and individuals deal with associated stress; and medical therapy. Treatment must be individualized to address both intrinsic characteristics of the child and relevant environmental factors and be coordinated with a variety of interventions within the school, home and community.

Many professionals agree that medication, when appropriate, combined with counseling, best controls symptoms. Stimulant medications, such as short-acting, intermediate-acting, long-acting, and transdermal methylphenidate, and short-, intermediate-, and long-acting amphetamine derivatives, are the drugs of choice. Non-stimulants, for children who cannot tolerate stimulants, includes guanfacine, clonidine, and atomoxetine. To identify children with this disorder and to develop the most appropriate treatment plan, parents will need to consult with a psychiatrist, pediatric neurologist, or pediatrician.

National Agencies & Associations

1600 **Attention Deficit Disorder Association**
800-939-1019
add.org

International non-profit organization dedicated to adult Attention Deficit Disorder. ADDA is entirely volunteer-run, and does not maintain a physical office.
Duane Gordon, President
Michelle Frank, PsyD, Vice President

1601 **Canadian ADHD Resource Alliance**
366 Adelaide Street E
416-637-8582
Toronto, Ontario, M5A-3X9
niamh.mcgarry@caddra.ca
www.caddra.ca
Non-profit organization for healthcare and research professionals with interests in the study of ADHD.
Niamh McGarry, Executive Director
Stacey D. Espinet, Education Project Manager

1602 **Center for Parent Information & Resources**
SPAN
35 Halsey Street
973-642-8100
Newark, NJ 07102
malizo@spannj.org
www.parentcenterhub.org
Serves as a central hub of information and products for Parent Centers that serve children with disabilities. Coordinates training, provides an e-newsletter twice a month, and produces specially designed databases.
Debra A. Jennings, Director
Jessica Wilson, Communications Director

1603 **Children & Adults with Attention Deficit /Hyperactivity Disorder**
4221 Forbes Blvd
301-306-7070
Lanham, MD 20706
800-233-4050
Fax: 301-306-7090
www.chadd.org
CHADD's primary objectives are: to provide a support network for parents and caregivers; to provide a forum for continuing education; to be a community resource and disseminate accurate evidence-based information about AD/HD to parents, educators and adults.
Robert Cattoi, Chief Executive Officer
April Gower, Chief Operating Officer

1604 **Council for Exceptional Children**
2900 Crystal Drive
888-232-7733
Arlington, VA 22202-3557
TTY: 866-915-5000
service@cec.sped.org
www.cec.sped.org
Advocates appropriate policies, standards and development for individuals with special needs. Provides professional development for special educators.
Alexander T. Graham, Executive Director
Craig Evans, Director, Operations

1605 **Feingold Association of the US**
11849 Suncatcher Drive
631-369-9340
Fishers, IN 46037
feingold.org
Helps families of children with learning and behavior problems, including attention deficit disorder. Also helps chemically-sensitive and salicylate-sensitive adults. Program is based upon a diet which primarily eliminates certain synthetic food additives.

1606 **Goodwill Industries International, Inc.**
15810 Indianola Drive
800-466-3945
Rockville, MD 20855
contactus@goodwill.org
www.goodwill.org
A nonprofit, community-based organization whose mission is to help people achieve self-sufficiency through the dignity and power of work, serving people who are disadvantaged, disabled or elderly. The mission is accomplished through providing independent living skills, affordable housing, and training and placement in community employment. The GoodWill Network includes 160 independent, local locations across the U.S. and Canada.
S. Dale Jenkins, Chair
Steven C. Preston, President & CEO

1607 **Learning Disabilities Association of America**
PO Box 10369
412-341-1515
Pittsburgh, PA 15234-1349
Fax: 412-344-0224
info@LDAAmerica.org
www.ldaamerica.org

An information and referral center for parents and professionals dealing with learning disabilities.
Stephanie Fedro-Byrom, Operations Manager
Maureen Swanson, Director, Healthy Children Project

1608 National Center for Learning Disabilities
1 Thomas Circle NW   212-545-7510
Washington, DC 20005   www.ncld.org
Nonprofit organization committed to improving the lives of the estimated one in ten children with learning disabilities, and raising public awareness and understanding.
Lindsay E. Jones, Chief Executive Officer
Ace Parsi, Director, Innovation

State Agencies & Associations

Florida

1609 Goodwill Industries-Suncoast
10596 Gandy Boulevard   727-523-1512
St. Petersburg, FL 33702   888-279-1988
                                                      TTY: 727-579-1068
                                                      www.goodwill-suncoast.org
A nonprofit, community-based organization whose mission is to help people achieve self-sufficiency through the dignity and power of work, serving people who are disadvantaged, disabled or elderly. The mission is accomplished through providing independent living skills, affordable housing, and training and placement in community employment.
Heather Ceresoli, CPA, Chair
Deborah A. Passerini, President & CEO

Libraries & Resource Centers

1610 HEATH Resource Center
George Washington University
2134 G Street NW   202-973-0904
Washington, DC 20052-0001   800-544-3284
                                                      Fax: 202-994-3365
                                                      askheath@gwu.edu
                                                      http://www.heath.gwu.edu/
The HEATH Resource Center of The George Washington University, Graduate School of Education and Human Development, is the national clearinghouse on postsecondary education for individuals with disabilities.
Dr Joan Kester, Principal Investigator
Christopher Nace, Research

Support Groups & Hotlines

1611 Attention Deficit Information Network
475 Hillside Ave   617-455-9895
Needham, MA 02194
Offers support and information to families of children with attention deficit disorder, adults with ADD and professionals through an international network of 60 parent and adult chapters.

1612 National Federation of Families for Children's Mental Health
12320 Parklawn Drive   240-403-1901
Rockville, MD 20852   Fax: 240-403-1909
                                                      ffcmh@ffcmh.org
                                                      www.ffcmh.org
Provides advocacy at the national level for the rights of children and youth with emotional, behavioral and mental health challenges and their families; provides leadership and technical assistance to a nation-wide network of family run organizations; and collaborates with family run and other child serving organizations to transform mental health care in America.
Lynda Gargan, PhD, Executive Director
Leann Sherman, Project Coordinator

1613 National Health Information Center
Office of Disease Prevention & Health Promotion
1101 Wootton Pkwy   Fax: 240-453-8281
Rockville, MD 20852   odphpinfo@hhs.gov
                                                      www.health.gov/nhic

Supports public health education by maintaining a calendar of National Health Observances; helps connect consumers and health professionals to organizations that can best answer questions and provide up-to-date contact information from reliable sources; updates on a yearly basis toll-free numbers for health information, Federal health clearinghouses and info centers.
Don Wright, MD, MPH, Director

Books

1614 ADHD Parenting Handbook: Practical Advice for Parents from Parents
Colleen Alexander-Roberts, author
Taylor Trade Publishing
4501 Forbes Boulevard   301-459-3366
Lanham, MD 20706   Fax: 301-429-5743
                                                      custserv@nbnbooks.com
                                                      www.rlpgtrade.com
A compilation of practical advice and tips for handling day-to-day activities that routinely become problematic for ADHD children, such as getting dressed for school, going to bed, performing chores, completing homework, and playing with other children.
Paperback
ISBN: 0-878338-62-4

1615 ADHD in Schools: Assessment and Intervention Strategies
George J DuPaul, Gary Stoner, author
Guilford Publications
370 Seventh Avenue   800-365-7006
New York, NY 10001   Fax: 212-966-6708
                                                      info@guilford.com
                                                      www.guilford.com
Provides essential guidance for school-based professionals meeting the challenges of ADHD at any grade level. Comprehensive and practical, includes several reproducible assessment tools and handouts.
330 pages Paperback
ISBN: 1-593850-89-0

1616 ADHD: Handbook for Diagnosis & Treatment
Western Psychological Services
12031 Wilshire Boulevard   310-478-2061
Los Angeles, CA 90025-1201   800-648-8857
                                                      Fax: 310-478-7838
                                                      www.wpspublish.com
This second edition helps clinicians diagnose and treat Attention Deficit Hyperactivity Disorder. Written by an internationally recognized authority in the field, it covers the history of ADHD, its primary symptoms, associated conditions, developmental course and outcome, and family context. A workbook companion manual is also available.
700 pages

1617 Attention Deficit Disorder: A Different Perception
Underwood-Miller
708 Westover Drive   717-285-2255
Lancaster, PA 17601-1242
1993 180 pages Paperback
ISBN: 0-887331-56-4

1618 Attention Deficit Disorder: Learning Disabilities
Random House
25 Van Zant Street   410-848-1900
East Norwalk, CT 06855-1726   800-726-0600
                                                      Fax: 800-214-1438
                                                      www.randomhouse.com
Realities, myths, and controversial treatments. Section I tries to dispel the myths and discusses proven treatments for ADHD and LD. Section II explains how the scientific community evaluates new treatment methods, and Section III summarizes alternative treatments and discusses scientific evidence pertaining to its usefulness.
256 pages
ISBN: 0-385469-31-4

1619 Attention Deficit Hyperactivity Disorder: What Every Parent Wants to Know
Paul H Brookes Publishing Company

PO Box 10624
Baltimore, MD 21285-0624

301-337-9580
800-638-3775
Fax: 410-337-8539
www.brookespublishing.com

1993 320 pages Paperback
ISBN: 1-557661-41-3
Dante Washington, Customer Service Representative

1620 Coping with ADD/ADHD
Rosen Publishing Group
29 E 21st Street
New York, NY 10010-6209

212-777-3017
800-237-9932
Fax: 888-436-4643
customerservice@rosenpub.com
www.rosenpublishing.com

At least 3.5 million American youngsters suffer from ADD. This book defines the syndrome and provides specific information about treatment and counseling.
150 pages Hardcover
ISBN: 0-823931-96-X

1621 Helping Your ADD Child With or Without Hyperactivity
John F Taylor PhD, author
Random House Inc.
Dep of Library Marketing
New York, NY 10017

800-733-3000
800-726-0600
Fax: 212-940-7381
crownpublicity@randomhouse.com
www.randomhouse.com

Inside this book you will find step-by-step tools for helping your ADD or ADHD child. From extensive screening for spotting the initial signs to the pros and cons of nutritional, psychological, and drug treatments.
2001
ISBN: 0-761527-56-7

1622 Hyperactive Children Grown Up
Gabrielle Weiss, Lily Trokenberg Hechtman, author
Guilford Publications
370 Seventh Avenue
New York, NY 10001

800-365-7006
Fax: 212-966-6708
info@guilford.com
www.guilford.com

Reports findings on the etiology, treatment, and outcome of attention deficits and hyperactivity at all stages of development.
473 pages Paperback
ISBN: 0-898625-96-7

1623 LD Child and the ADHD Child
Suzanne H Stevens, author
John F Blair Publishing
1406 Plaza Drive
Winston-Salem, NC 27103

336-768-1374
800-222-9796
Fax: 336-768-9194
blairpub@aol.com
www.blairpub.com

Helps parents raise their LD and/or ADHD children so that they, too, can grow up to be okay-so that they will be happy, well-adjusted, and successful adults despite the learning and behavior patterns that make them different.
Paperback
ISBN: 0-895871-42-8

1624 Managing Attention Deficit Hyperactivity Disorder in Children:
Sam Goldstein, Michael Goldstein, author
Wiley Publishing
111 River Street
Hoboken, NJ 07030-5774

201-748-6000
Fax: 201-748-6088
info@wiley.com
www.wiley.com

A proven approach to the diagnosis and management of one of the most challenging childhood disorders. In this book the authors describe a proven multidisciplinary approach to the diagnosis and treatment of childhood ADHD, developed at the prestigous Neurology, Learning and Behavior Center in Salt Lake City.
1998 896 pages
ISBN: 0-471121-58-9

1625 Maybe You Know My Kid: A Parent's Guide to Identifying ADHD
Birch Lane Press
120 Enterprise Avenue S
Secaucus, NJ 07094-1902

800-447-2665

The author writes about her family experiences with their son, David, who has attention deficit disorder. Contains a comprehensive review of important issues plus descriptions of some helpful management techniques.
222 pages

1626 Medications for Attention Disorders and Related Medical Problems
Specialty Press
300 NW 70th Avenue
Plantation, FL 33317

954-792-8100
800-233-9273
Fax: 954-792-8545
sales@addwarehouse.com
www.addwarehouse.com

A comprehensive handbook covering the history, characteristics, and causes of ADHD. The equal importance of appropriate academic programming, counseling, and medication are stressed throughout.
415 pages Hardcover

1627 Parents Helping Parents: A Directory of Support Groups for ADD
CibaGelgy, Pharmaceuticals Division
1400 Parkmoor Avenue
San Jose, CA 95126

408-727-5775
855-727-5775
Fax: 408-286-1116
www.php.com

1628 Parents' Hyperactivity Handbook: Helping the Fidgety Child
Plenum Press
233 Spring Street
New York, NY 10013-1578

212-460-1550
800-777-4643
Fax: 212-460-1575
support@apress.com
www.springer.com

1993 306 pages
ISBN: 0-306444-65-8

1629 Rethinking Attention Deficit Disorders
Miriam Cherkes-Julkowski, author
Brookline Books
8 Trumbull Rd
Northampton, MA 01060

413-584-0184
800-666-2665
Fax: 413-584-6184
brooklinebks.com

Gives the classroom teacher useful information that provides ideas and strategies for working with children suffering from ADD.
1997 Paperback
ISBN: 1-571290-37-0

1630 The New ADD in Adults Workbook
Lynn Weiss, PhD, author
Taylor Trade Publishing
4501 Forbes Boulevard
Lanham, MD 20706

301-459-3366
Fax: 301-429-5743
custserv@nbnbooks.com

Not only touches on and dispels the most recent clinical findings, but also emphasizes the bigger perspective, focusing on the empowerment and diversity issues facing all of us on the A.D.D. continuum today. Persuades readers to work through their challenges with practical, prescriptive exercises and insights.
Paperback
ISBN: 0-878338-50-0

1631 You Mean I'm Not Lazy, Stupid or Crazy?
Tyrell & Jerem Press
PO Box 20089
Cincinnati, OH 45220-0089

800-622-6611

A new self-help book is the first written by ADD adults for ADD adults. This comprehensive guide provides accurate information, practical how-tos and moral support.

1632 Attention Deficit/Hyperactivity Disorder
Guilford Publications

370 Seventh Avenue
New York, NY 10012-4068
212-431-9800
800-365-7006
Fax: 212-966-6708
www.guilford.com

A second edition that is the handbook on the diagnosis and treatment of ADHD in the 1990s. A companion workbook is also available with forms that may be photocopied.
747 pages Hardcover
ISBN: 0-898624-43-6

Children's Books

1633 Self-Control Games & Workbook
Western Psychological Services
12031 Wilshire Boulevard
Los Angeles, CA 90025-1201
310-478-2061
800-648-8857
Fax: 310-478-7838

This game is designed to teach self-control in academic and social situations. Addresses a total of 24 impulsive, inattentive and hyperactive behaviors. The companion workbook reinforces the use of positive self-statements, and problem-solving techniques, instead of expressing anger.
Game

1634 Shelley, the Hyperactive Turtle
Deborah Moss, author
Woodbine House
6510 Bells Mill Road
Bethesda, MD 20817
800-843-7323
Fax: 301-897-5838
info@woodbinehouse.com
www.woodbinehouse.com

Reassures young children who are going through the diagnostic process or who are having problems behaving at school or making friends because of AD/HD.
20 pages
ISBN: 1-890627-75-1

Magazines

1635 Attention
Children & Adults with Attention Deficit Disorder
8181 Professional Place
Landover, MD 20785-7221
301-306-7070
800-233-4050
Fax: 301-306-7090
TTY: 301-429-0641
Quarterly

Newsletters

1636 ADHD Report
Guilford Publications
370 Seventh Avenue
New York, NY 10001
800-365-7006
Fax: 212-966-6708
info@guilford.com
www.guilford.com

Examines the nature, diagnosis, and outcomes associated with the disorder, and provides a single reliable guide to the latest developments in the fields of clinical management and education. Includes research findings, as well as ongoing coverage of ADHD in the news.
16 pages BiMonthly

1637 Chadder
Children & Adults with Attention Deficit Disorder
8181 Professional Place
Landover, MD 20785-7221
301-306-7070
800-233-4050
Fax: 301-306-7090
TTY: 301-429-0641
Quarterly

1638 Challenge
Challenge
PO Box 488
West Newbury, MA 01985-0688
978-462-0495
800-233-2322

National newsletter on ADD/ADHD that carries interviews with nationally-known scientists, as well as physicians, psychologists,

social workers, educators, and other practitioners in the field of ADHD.
12 pages BiMonthly
Jean C Harrison, Executive Director

1639 Pure Facts
Feingold Association of the US
PO Box 6550
Alexandria, VA 22306-0550
703-768-3287

Monthly newsletter with articles on nutrition and behavior and lists of approved brand-name foods.

Pamphlets

1640 ADHD
Learning Disabilities Association of America
4156 Library Road
Pittsburgh, PA 15234-1349
412-341-1515
888-300-6710
Fax: 412-344-0224
info@ldaamerica.org
www.ldaamerica.org

A booklet for parents offering information on Attention Deficit Hyperactivity Disorders and learning disabilities.

1641 Attention Deficit Disorders and Hyperactivity
Council for Exceptional Children
2900 Crystal Drive
Arlington, VA 22202
703-620-3660
888-232-7733
Fax: 703-264-9494
TTY: 866-915-5000
service@cec.sped.org
www.cec.sped.org

Published by the Council for Exceptional Children.

1642 COGREHAB
Life Science Associates
1 Fennimore Road
Bayport, NY 11705-2115
631-472-2111
Fax: 631-472-8146
lifesciassoc@pipeline.com

Divided into six groups for diagnosis and treatment of attention, memory and perceptual disorders to be used by and under the guidance of a professional.
$95 - $1,950

1643 Fact Sheet: Attention Deficit Hyperactivity Disorder
Learning Disabilities Association of America
4156 Library Road
Pittsburgh, PA 15234-1349
412-341-1515
888-300-6710
Fax: 412-344-0224
info@ldaamerica.org
www.ldaamerica.org

A pamphlet offering factual information on ADHD.

1644 Helping Adolescents with ADHD and Learning Disabilities
Learning Disabilities Association of America
4156 Library Road
Pittsburgh, PA 15234-1349
412-341-1515
888-300-6710
Fax: 412-344-0224
info@ldaamerica.org
www.ldaamerica.org

Audio & Video

1645 ADD Stepping Out of the Dark
ADD Videos
PO Box 622
New Paltz, NY 12561-0622
845-255-3612
Fax: 845-883-6452

A powerful, effective video, ideal for health professionals, educators and parents providing a visual montage designed to promote an understanding and awareness of attention deficit disorder. Based on actual accounts of those who have ADD, including a neurologist, an office worker, and parents of children with ADD. The video allows the viewer to feel the frustration and lack of attention that ADD brings to many.
Video
Lenae Madonna, Producer
Sheila Buckley, Executive Director

1646 ADHD in Adults
Guilford Publications
370 Seventh Avenue
New York, NY 10001-4068
212-431-9800
800-365-7006
Fax: 212-966-6708
info@guilford.com
www.guilford.com

This program integrates information on ADHD with the actual experiences of four adults who suffer from the disorder. Representing a range of professions, from a lawyer to a mother working at home, each candidly discusses the impact of ADHD on his or her daily life. These interviews are augmented by comments from family members and other clinicians who treat adults with ADHD.
Video

1647 ADHD in the Classroom: Strategies for Teachers
Rusell A Barkley, author
Guilford Publications
370 Seventh Avenue
New York, NY 10001
800-365-7006
Fax: 212-966-6708
info@guilford.com
www.guilford.com

Designed to help teachers create a learning environment that is responsive to the needs of all students, including those with ADHD.

1648 ADHD: What Do We Know?
Guilford Publications
370 Seventh Avenue
New York, NY 10001-4068
212-431-9800
800-365-7006
Fax: 212-966-6708
info@guilford.com
www.guilford.com

An introduction for teachers and special education practitioners, school psychologists and parents of ADHD children. Topics outlined in this video include the causes and prevalence of ADHD, ways children with ADHD behave, other conditions that may accompany ADHD and long-term prospects for children with ADHD.
Video

1649 Around the Clock
Guilford Publications
370 Seventh Avenue
New York, NY 10001-4068
212-431-9800
800-365-7006
Fax: 212-966-6708
info@guilford.com
www.guilford.com

This videotape provides both professionals and parents a helpful look at how the difficulties facing parents of ADHD children can be handled.

1650 Attention Deficit Disorder
Pro-Ed, Inc.
8700 Shoal Creek Blvd
Austin, TX 78757-6897
512-451-3246
800-897-3202
Fax: 800-397-7633
info@proedinc.com
www.proedinc.com/

A video and book providing helpful suggestions for both home and classroom management of students with attention deficit disorder.
216 pages Paperback
ISBN: 0-890797-42-0
Krista Anderson, Technical Advisor
Matt Synatschk, Books & Materials Permissions Editor

1651 Educating Inattentive Children
Western Psychological Services
12031 Wilshire Boulevard
Los Angeles, CA 90025-1201
800-648-8857
Fax: 310-478-7838
An excellent resource for teachers who encounter inattention and hyperactivity in the classroom. It helps teachers distinguish deliberate misbehavior from the incompetent, nonpurposeful behavior of the inattentive child.
Video

1652 It's Just Attention Disorder
Western Psychological Services
12031 Wilshire Boulevard
Los Angeles, CA 90025-1201
310-478-2061
800-648-8857
Fax: 310-478-7838
This ground-breaking videotape takes the critical first steps in treating attention-deficit disorder: it enlists the inattentive or hyperactive child as an active participant in his or her treatment.
Video

1653 Why Won't My Child Pay Attention?
Western Psychological Services
12031 Wilshire Boulevard
Los Angeles, CA 90025-1201
310-478-2061
800-648-8857
Fax: 310-478-7838
Practical and reassuring videotape, noted child psychologist tells parents about two of the most common and complex problems of childhood: inattention and hyperactivity.
Video

Web Sites

1654 Healing Well
www.healingwell.com
A social network and support community for patients, caregivers, and families coping with the daily struggles of diseases, disorders and chronic illness.

1655 Health Finder
www.healthfinder.gov
A government web site, where individuals can find information and tools to help you and those you care about stay healthy.

1656 Healthlink USA
www.healthlinkusa.com
Health information concerning treatment, cures, prevention, diagnosis, risk factors, research, support groups, email lists, personal stories and much more. Updated regularly.

1657 MedicineNet
www.medicinenet.com
An online resource for consumers providing easy-to-read, authoritative medical and health information.

1658 Medscape
www.medscape.com
Medscape offers specialists, primary care physicians, and other health professionals the Web's most robust and integrated medical information and educational tools.

1659 WebMD
www.webmd.com
Provides credible information, supportive communities, and in-depth reference material about health subjects. A source for original and timely health information as well as material from well known content providers.

Description

1660 Autistic Spectrum Disorders

Autistic Spectrum Disorders, ASD, includes (from most to least severe) autism, high-functioning autism (HFA), Asperger's syndrome, and PDD-NOS (pervasive development disorder — not otherwise specified). ASD typically appear during the first three years of life. Autism involves severe impairment of social and communication development. HFA symptoms are less severe, but include delayed language development. Asperger's is similar to HFA, but with no speech delay. PPD-NOS describes autistic categories that do not fit into any of the above. ASD affects behavior, communication, social interaction and other neurological functions.

ASD has numerous symptoms, all of which reduce the child's ability to communicate and interact. Many autistic children have abnormal social relationships, impaired understanding, and uneven intellectual development with mental disability in most cases. They may exhibit repetitive movement (i.e., rocking, spinning, and hand twisting), avoid making eye contact, and have impaired verbal skills. Occasionally, children with ASD will have decreased sensitivity to pain, and have abnormal responses to light, touch and sound. The disorder can include self-injury and bizarre behavior.

ASD is two to four times more common in boys than in girls. It is found in people of all ethnic backgrounds, and throughout the world. In 2009, nine in 1000 children were diagnosed with ASD, up from one in 500 just six years ago.

In some cases, ASD may be linked to damage to the brain or nervous system. Studies of twins with autism point to a possible genetic link. ASD has been associated with the following risk factors: pre- and perinatal birth complications; prenatal infections with certain viruses; abnormalities of the brain detected with a CT scan or MRI (although no specific defects in the brain structure have been consistently identified), and very low birth weight. Childhood vaccines, after extensive epidemiological and laboratory examinations, have been shown to not be a cause for the sharp rise in ASD cases in recent decades.

Although there are no known cures for ASD, experts advocate early and intense behavioral, developmental and speech therapy. Medications may alleviate some of the accompanying behavior problems but provide minimal help for the disorder itself and are generally not used. Antidepressant and anti-anxiety medicines can mitigate some of the persistent anxiety and obsessive behaviors, such as running away from new situations, compulsive checking or washing, or anxiety from strict black-and-white thinking. Selective serotonin reuptake inhibitors (SSRIs) such as sertraline or fluoxetine can sometimes help with mood, anxiety, obsessive thoughts, and compulsive behaviors. They are used off-label. Another class of medicines, atypical antipsychotics, which include aripiprazole, quetiapine, and risperidone, can effectively treat the constant movement, repetitive behaviors, and sleep disturbance in children with autismThere is strong emphasis on early diagnosis, early intervention, and individualized educational programs to provide the opportunity for maximum development for the child with Autistic Spectrum Disorder.

National Agencies & Associations

1661 Autism Research Institute

833-281-7165
info@autism.org
www.autism.com

A clearinghouse for research on autism and related disorders of learning and behavior. Conducts and compiles research findings to provide people with the latest research available.
Stephen M. Edelson, PhD, Executive Director
Denise Fulton, Administrative Director

1662 Autism Services Center
10 - 6th Avenue W
Huntington, WV 25701-0507

304-525-8014
Fax: 304-525-8026
www.autismservicescenter.org

Provides educational information to the public and professional communities on autism; provides case management activities and referrals for persons afflicted with autism and their families.
Jimmie Beirne, Chief Executive Officer
David Finley, Chief Operations Officer

1663 Autism Society of America
4340 East-West Hwy
Bethesda, MD 20814

800-328-8476
info@autism-society.org
www.autism-society.org

A national charitable organization with the mission of providing as much information as possible about autism and the various options, approaches, methods and systems available to parents of children with autism, family members and professionals.
Scott Badesch, President & CEO
John Dabrowski, COO/CFO

1664 Autism Treatment Center of America
2080 S Undermountain Road
Sheffield, MA 01257

413-229-2100
877-766-7473
www.autismtreatmentcenter.org

Provides training programs for parents and professionals caring for children challenged by Autism, Autism Spectrum Disorders, Pervasive Developmental Disorder (PDD), and other developmental disorders.
Barry Neil Kaufman, Co-Founder/Co-Originator
Samahria Lyte Kaufman, Co-Founder/Co-Orginator

1665 Community Services for Autistic Adults & Children
Jane Salzano Center for Autism
8615 E Village Avenue
Montgomery Village, MD 20886

240-912-2220
Fax: 301-926-9384
csaac@csaac.org
csaac.org

Non-profit dedicated to providing support services for children and adults with autism.
Eric Salzano, Executive Director
Paul Martineau, Director, Special Projects & Operations

1666 Council for Exceptional Children
2900 Crystal Drive
Arlington, VA 22202-3557

888-232-7733
TTY: 866-915-5000
service@cec.sped.org
www.cec.sped.org

Advocates appropriate policies, standards and development for individuals with special needs. Provides professional development for special educators.
Alexander T. Graham, Executive Director
Craig Evans, Director, Operations

1667 Dogs for Better Lives
10175 Wheeler Road
Central Point, OR 97502

541-826-9220
800-990-3647
info@dogsforbetterlives.org
dogsforbetterlives.org

Trains ear dogs to alert deaf persons to certain sounds. Dogs are chosen from pet adoption shelters and assigned on the basis of a prioritized waiting list. Four to five months of training teaches them to alert their masters to a number of sounds. Dogs are also available for autistic children.
Lake Matray, President/CEO
Annette Vitello, Operations Director

1668 Goodwill Industries International, Inc.
15810 Indianola Drive
Rockville, MD 20855

800-466-3945
contactus@goodwill.org
www.goodwill.org

A nonprofit, community-based organization whose mission is to help people achieve self-sufficiency through the dignity and power of work, serving people who are disadvantaged, disabled or elderly. The mission is accomplished through providing independent living skills, affordable housing, and training and placement in community employment. The GoodWill Network includes 160 independent, local locations across the U.S. and Canada.
S. Dale Jenkins, Chair
Steven C. Preston, President & CEO

1669 National Institute of Neurological Disorders and Stroke
NIH Neurological Institute
Bethesda, MD 20824

301-496-5751
800-352-9424
www.ninds.nih.gov

Seeks to reduce the burden of neurological disease affecting individuals from all walks of life.
Walter J. Koroshetz, MD, Director
Amy B. Adams, Director, Office of Scientific Liaison

State Agencies & Associations

Alabama

1670 Autism Society of Alabama
4217 Dolly Ridge Rd
Birmingham, AL 35243

205-951-1364
877-4AU-TISM
Fax: 205-967-8244
info@autism-alabama.org
www.autism-alabama.org

Michelle MacDaniel, Program & Community Outreach Coordinator
Melanie Jones, Executive Director

Arizona

1671 Autism Society of Southern Arizona
2600 Wyatt Drive
Tucson, AZ 85712

520-770-1541
Fax: 520-319-5979
info@as-az.org
www.as-az.org

Hailey Thoman, Executive Director

California

1672 Autism Society of California
PO Box 1355
Glendora, CA 91740

562-943-3335
800-869-7069
brubin698@earthlink.net
www.autismsocietyca.org

Beth Burt, President
Sandra Shove, Vice President

Colorado

1673 Autism Society of Colorado
550 S Wadsworth Boulevard
Lakewood, CO 80226-4169

720-214-0794
Fax: 720-274-2744
info@autismcolorado.org
www.autismcolorado.org

District of Columbia

1674 Autism Society of District Columbia
PO Box 31245
Washington, DC 20030

202-561-5300
Fax: 202-561-8634
dcautismsociety@gmail.com
www.autism-society.org/chapter130

Ronald Hampton, President

Florida

1675 Autism Society of Florida
PO Box 677055
Orlando, FL 32867

407-207-3388
www.autismfl.com

Ven Sequenzia, President
Stacy Hoaglund, Vice President/President-Elect

1676 Goodwill Industries-Suncoast
10596 Gandy Boulevard
St. Petersburg, FL 33702

727-523-1512
888-279-1988
TTY: 727-579-1068
www.goodwill-suncoast.org

A nonprofit, community-based organization whose mission is to help people achieve self-sufficiency through the dignity and power of work, serving people who are disadvantaged, disabled or elderly. The mission is accomplished through providing independent living skills, affordable housing, and training and placement in community employment.
Heather Ceresoli, CPA, Chair
Deborah A. Passerini, President & CEO

Georgia

1677 Autism Society of Greater Georgia
8343 Roswell Road
Atlanta, GA 30350

844-404-2742

Jonathan Basinger, Chair
Jere Pittner, Director of Programs

Hawaii

1678 Autism Society of Hawaii
PO Box 178411
Honolulu, HI 96817

808-368-1191
autismhi@gmail.com
www.autismhi.org

Ryan Lee, President
Jessica Wong-Sumida, M.A., J.D., Executive Director

Idaho

1679 Autism Society of Treasure Valley
PO Box 44831
Boise, ID 83711-9404

208-336-5676
Fax: 202-884-5582
Autism.asatvc@yahoo.com
www.asatvc.org

Allison Walters, President

Illinois

1680 Autism Society of Illinois
2200 S Main Street
Lombard, IL 60148-5366

630-691-1270
888-691-1270
Fax: 630-932-5620
www.autismillinois.org

Karen McDonough, Executive Director
Kym Bills, President

Indiana

1681 Autism Society of Indiana
4740 Kingsway Drive
Indianapolis, IN 46205-0252

317-695-0252
Fax: 317-815-0859
info@inautism.org
www.autismsocietyofindiana.org

Joshua Carr, President
Kylee Hope, Vice-President

Iowa

1682 Autism Society of Iowa
4549 Waterford Drive
W Des Moines, IA 50265-2059

515-327-9075
888-722-4799
Fax: 319-557-1169
autism50ia@aol.com
www.autismia.org

James Ball, Ed.D., BCBA-D, Executive Chair
Ron E. Simmons, Vice Chair

Kansas

1683 Autism Society of Kansas Autism Society of America
Autism Society of America
PO Box 860984
Shawnee, KS 66286-2325

913-706-0042
Fax: 316-943-3292

Bill Robinso, President
DeeDee Velasquez-Per, Board Member

Kentucky

1684 Autism Chapter of Bluegrass Chapter
243 Shady Lane
Lexington, KY 40503-2034

859-299-9000
www.asbg.org

Sara Spragens, President

1685 Autism Society of Western Kentucky
230 Second Street Suite 206
Henderson, KY 42419-1647

270-826-0510
nboyett1956@yahoo.com
www.autism.org

Nancy Boyett, President

Louisiana

1686 Autism Society of Louisiana
5430 S Woodchase Court
Baton Rouge, LA 70808

800-955-3760

Pat Giamanco, President

Maine

1687 Autism Society of Maine
72B Main Street
Winthrop, ME 04364-1406

800-273-5200
Fax: 207-377-9434
www.asmonline.org

Kim Humphrey, President
Lynda Mazzola, Vice President

Maryland

1688 Autism Society of Baltimore-Chesapeake
PO Box 10822
Parkville, MD 21234

410-655-7933
info@baltimoreautismsociety.org
www.baltimoreautismsociety.org

Debbie Page, Co-President:
Kay Holman, Vice-President:

Massachusetts

1689 Autism Society of Massachusetts
20 Alice Agnew Drive
Attleboro Falls, MA 2763-2108

877-622-2884
Fax: 774-643-6331
asamasschapter@hotmail.com
www.nationalautismassociation.org

Jo Pike, Co-Founder President/Executive Director
Laura Bono, Founding Board Member

Michigan

1690 Autism Society of Michigan
1213 Center Street
Lansing, MI 48906-5338

517-882-2800
800-223-6722
Fax: 517-862-2816
www.autism-mi.org

Kathy Johnson, President
Penny Bearden, Vice President

Minnesota

1691 Autism Society of Minnesota
2380 Wycliff Street
St Paul, MN 55114-1257

651-647-1083
Fax: 651-642-1230
info@ausm.org
www.ausm.org

Pam Erickson, Executive Director
Laurie Dixon, Associate Director

Missouri

1692 Autism Society of Gateway Chapter
7777 Bonhomme Avenue
St Louis, MO 63105

314-863-0077
Fax: 314-863-7494
PegiSues@aol.com
www.autism-society.org

Pegi Price, President
James Ball, Ed.D., BCBA-D, Executive Chair

Nebraska

1693 Autism Society of Nebraska
1672 Van Dorn Street
Lincoln, NE 68502

402-472-4346
877-375-0120
autismsociety@autismnebraska.org
www.autismnebraska.org

Shawn Neff, President
Georgann Albin, Executive Director

Nevada

1694 Autism Society of Northern Nevada
3490 Southampton Drive
Reno, NV 89509-8911

775-786-9315
Fax: 775-786-0984

Paul Deane, Vice President
Dinah Deane, President

New Hampshire

1695 Autism Society of New Hampshire
PO Box 68
Concord, NH 03302-0068

603-679-2424
Fax: 301-657-0869
www.nhautism.com

Stacey Shannon, President

New Jersey

1696 Autism Society of Southwest New Jersey
10 Shadow Oak Court
Mount Laurel, NJ 08054-2113

856-722-8518
CMedo@aol.com
www.autism-society.org

New Mexico

1697 **Autism Society of New Mexico**
PO Box 30955
Albuquerque, NM 87190
505-332-0306
nmautism@nmautismsociety.org
www.nmautismsociety.org

Sarah Baca, Executive Director
Sharon Esch, President

New York

1698 **Autism Society of Albany**
PO Box 3487
Schenectady, NY 12303
518-355-2191
Fax: 518-355-2191
www.albanyautism.org

Gordon Zuckerman, President
Jenny DeBellis, Treasurer

North Carolina

1699 **Autism Society of North Carolina**
505 Oberlin Road
Raleigh, NC 27605-1345
919-743-0204
800-442-2762
Fax: 919-743-0208
info@autismsociety-nc.org
www.autismsociety-nc.org

Scott Badesch, Chief Executive Officer
David Laxton, Director Communications

North Dakota

1700 **Autism Society of North Dakota**
628 6th Avenue
Alice, ND 58031
701-281-8254
Jocelyn@AutismND.org
www.AutismND.org

Kris Wallman, President
Renie Chadwell, Vice President

Ohio

1701 **Autism Society of Greater Cincinnati**
PO Box 58385
Cincinnati, OH 45258
513-561-2300
Fax: 513-561-4748
www.autismcincy.org

Kay Brown, President
Sue Radabaugh, Vice President

1702 **Autism Society of Ohio Tri-County Chapter**
1749 S Raccoon Road
Austintown, OH 44515
330-720-2066
Terry Chapin, President
Jack Campbell, Vice President

Oklahoma

1703 **Autism Society of Central Oklahoma**
PO Box 720103
Norman, OK 73070
405-370-3220
ASOCO-owner@yahoogroups.com
Jeremy Rand, Contact

Oregon

1704 **Autism Society of Oregon**
PO Box 396
Marylhurst, OR 97036-0396
503-636-1676
888-288-4761
Fax: 503-636-1696
info@oregonautism.com
www.oregonautism.com

Jenny Schoonbee, President
Genevieve Athens, Executive Director

Pennsylvania

1705 **Autism Society of Greater Harrisburg**
PO Box 101
Enola, PA 17025-0856
717-732-8400
800-277-2425
georgia.rackley@verizon.net
www.autismharrisburg.com

Georgia Rackley, President
Sherry Christian, Vice President

Rhode Island

1706 **Autism Society of Rhode Island**
PO Box 16603
Rumford, RI 02916
401-595-3241
www.asa-ri.org
Lisa Rego, President
Claudia Swiader, Vice President

South Carolina

1707 **Autism Society of South Carolina**
806 Twelfth Street
W Columbia, SC 29169
803-750-6988
800-438-4790
Fax: 703-750-8121
scas@scautism.org
www.scautism.org

Craig Stoxen, President & CEO
Tim Conroy, Chief Operating Officer & Vice President

South Dakota

1708 **Autism Society of Black Hills**
521 7th Street
Rapid City, SD 57701-4347
605-737-0377
sheritony@rap.midco.net
www.autismsd.com

Sandy Burns, President
Sheri Perkins

Tennessee

1709 **Autism Society of East Tennessee**
PO Box 30015
Knoxville, TN 37930
865-824-2897
Fax: 865-824-2896
asaetc@gmail.com
www.asaetc.org

Mike Manfredo, President
Roddey M. Coe, Vice President

Texas

1710 **Autism Society of Dallas**
10503 Metric Drive
Dallas, TX 75243
214-208-0792
autismsociety_dallas@yahoo.com
www.autism-society.org

Carolyn Garver, Contact
Pamela Lane, President

Vermont

1711 **Autism Society of Vermont Autism Society of America**
Autism Society of America
PO Box 978
White River Junction, VT 05001-0978
800-559-7398

Virginia

1712 **Autism Society of Northern Virginia**
PO Box 1334
Vienna, VA 22183-1334
703-495-8444
Fax: 703-571-8138
info@asanv.org
www.asanv.org

Kymberly S DeLoatche, Executive Director
Christopher Waddell, President

1713   Autism Society of Washington
P. O. Box 503
Olympia, WA 98507   888-279-4968
      Fax: 253-503-1157
      info@autismsocietyofwa.org
      www.autismsocietyofwa.org

Jeffrey Foster, President
Teresa McCann, Vice-President

1714   Autism Socity of West Virginia
PO Box 1024
Wayne, WV 25570   304-272-9834
Kim Farley, President
Ginny Gattlieb, 1st VP

1715   Autism Society of Wisconsin
1477 Kenwood Drive
Menasha, WI 54952   920-558-4602
      888-428-8476
      Fax: 920-553-0034
      asw@asw4autism.org
      www.asw4autism.org

Robert Johnston, President
Kendra Mateni, Secretary

Libraries & Resource Centers

1716   Emory Autism Resource Center
Emory University School of Medicine
Justin Tyler Traux Building   404-727-8350
Atlanta, GA 30322-0001   Fax: 404-727-3969
      michael.j.morrier@emory.edu
      www.psychiatry.emory.edu/PROGRAMS/autism
The Emory Autism Resource Center is a component of the Department of Psychiatry and Behavioral Sciences of Emory University's School of Medicine. It is the only Georgia resource that provides a comprehensive continuum of services specially designed to meet the needs of children and adults with autism and their families.
Gail G McGee, PhD, Director
Michael J Morrier, MA, Asst Director Research Manager

1717   Indiana Resource Center for Autism (IRCA)
Indiana Institute on Disability & Community
Indiana University-Bloomington   812-855-6508
Bloomington, IN 47408-2696   800-825-4733
      Fax: 812-855-9630
      TTY: 812-855-9396
      prattc@indiana.edu
      www.iidc.indiana.edu/irca
The Indiana Resource Center for Autism staff conduct outreach training and consultations, engage in research, and develop and disseminate information focused on building the capacity of local communities, organizations, agencies, and families to support children and adults across the autism spectrum in typical work, school, home, and community settings.
Dr Cathy Pratt PhD, Director

Research Centers

1718   Center for Neurodevelopmental Studies
5430 W Glenn Drive   623-915-0345
Glendale, AZ 85301   800-352-3792
      Fax: 623-937-5425
      admin@ccnsaz.org
      www.thechildrenscenteraz.org
Effective treatment methods for autism and developmental disabilities are subjects researched and studied at the Center.
Lorna Jean King, Founder
Kent Rideout, Executive Director

1719   Division TEACCH University of North Carolina at Chapel H
University of North Carolina at Chapel Hill

100 Renee Lynne Court   919-966-5156
Carrboro, NC 27510-6305   Fax: 919-966-4003
      teacch@unc.edu
      www.teacch.com
This organization is the division for the treatment and education of Autistic and related communication handicapped children.
Catherine Jones, Office Manager/Parent Intake Coordinator
Elaine Coonrod, Clinical Director

1720   Institute for Basic Research in Developmental Disabilities
1050 Forest Hill Road   718-494-0600
Staten Island, NY 10314-6356   Fax: 718-494-0833
      www.health.gov/NHIC/
Conducts research into neurodegenerative diseases, Alzheimer's disease, developmental disabilities, fragile X syndrome, Down's syndrome, autism, epilepsy and basic science issues underlying all developmental disabilities.

1721   Institute on Communication and Inclusion at Syracuse University
University of Syracuse
370 Huntington Hall   315-443-9379
Syracuse, NY 13244-2340   Fax: 315-443-2274
      icistaff@syr.edu
      http://ici.syr.edu
College offering facilitated learning research into communication with persons who have autism or severe disabilities. Offers books videos and public awareness information on the research projects.
Douglas Biklen, Dean

1722   National Alliance for Autism Research
1 East 33rd Street   212-252-8584
New York, NY 10016   Fax: 212-252-8676
      www.autismspeaks.org
The National Alliance for Autism Research has merged with Autism Speaks to further reach for the goal of finding the causes the best prevention and treatments and a cure for autism.
Peter H Bell, Executive Vice President
Mark Roithmayr, President

1723   State University of New York Health Sciences Center
SUNY Downstate Medical Center
450 Clarkson Avenue   718-270-1000
Brooklyn, NY 11203-2098   Fax: 718-270-1271
      health@downstate.edu
      www.downstate.edu/
Child psychiatry research programs.
John C Larosa, President

1724   The West Virginia Autism Training Center Marshall University
Marshall University
1 John Marshall Drive   304-696-2332
Huntington, WV 25755   800-344-5115
      wvatc@marshall.edu
      www.marshall.edu/coe/atc
The Autism Training Center was established through the efforts of parents of children with autism throughout West Virginia to provide education training and treatment programs for West Virginians who have Autism Pervasive Developmental Disorder (NOS) or Asperger's Disorder and have been formally registered with the Center.

Support Groups & Hotlines

1725   Autism Society of America
4340 East-West Hwy   800-328-8476
Bethesda, MD 20814   info@autism-society.org
      www.autism-society.org
A national charitable organization with the mission of providing as much information as possible about autism and the various options, approaches, methods and systems available to parents of children with autism, family members and professionals.
Scott Badesch, President & CEO
John Dabrowski, COO/CFO

1726 Genetic Alliance
4301 Connecticut Avenue NW
Washington, DC 20008-2369
202-966-5557
800-336-4363
Fax: 202-668-8533
info@geneticalliance.org
www.geneticalliance.org
A nonprofit health advocacy organization committed to transforming through genetics and promoting an environment of openness centered on the health of individuals, families and communities.
Sharon Terry, President/CEO

1727 National Autism Hotline Autism Services Center
Keith Albee Building
929 4th Avenue
Huntington, WV 25710
304-525-8014
Fax: 304-525-8026
www.autismservicescenter.org
Serving people with autism, other developmental disabilities anf those who care for and about them.
Mike Grady, CEO, Autism Services Center
Derek Hyman, President & Treasurer

1728 National Health Information Center
Office of Disease Prevention & Health Promotion
1101 Wootton Pkwy
Rockville, MD 20852
Fax: 240-453-8281
odphpinfo@hhs.gov
www.health.gov/nhic
Supports public health education by maintaining a calendar of National Health Observances; helps connect consumers and health professionals to organizations that can best answer questions and provide up-to-date contact information from reliable sources; updates on a yearly basis toll-free numbers for health information, Federal health clearinghouses and info centers.
Don Wright, MD, MPH, Director

Books

1729 A Miracle to Believe In
Option Indigo Press
2080 S Undermountain Road
Sheffield, MA 01257
413-229-2100
800-714-2779
Fax: 413-229-8931
optioninstitutestore.org/?
A group of people from all walks of life come together and are transformed as they reach out, under the direction of the Kaufmans, to help a little boy the medical world had given up as hopeless.
379 pages
ISBN: 0-440201-08-2
Bears Kaufman, Founder
Samahria Kaufman, Founder

1730 A Parent's Guide to Asperger's Syndrome & High-Functioning Autism
Guilford Press
370 Seventh Avenue
New York, NY 10001
800-365-7006
Fax: 212-966-6708
info@guilford.com
www.guilford.com
For parents of children on the higher end of the autistic spectrum. All educators, the authors provide the basic on diagnosis, causes, and treatment.
2002 278 pages
ISBN: 1-572307-67-6

1731 Activities for Developing Pre-Skill Concepts In Children with Autism
Toni Flowers, author
Autism Society of North Carolina Bookstore
505 Oberlin Road
Raleigh, NC 27605-1345
919-743-0204
800-442-2762
Fax: 919-743-0208
info@autismsociety-nc.org
www.autismsociety-nc.org
Chapters include auditory development, concept development, social development and visual-motor integration.

1732 Asperger Syndrome or High-Functioning Autism?
Eric Schopler, Gary B Mesibov, Linda J Kunce, author
Springer Publishing
233 Spring Street
New York, NY 10013
212-460-1550
800-777-4643
Fax: 212-460-1575
support@apress.com
www.springer.com
The precise relationship between high-functioning autism and Asperger Syndrome is still a subject of debate. Leaders in the field provide a general overview of the disorder and present diverse opinions on diagnosis and assessment-neuropsychological issues-treatment, and related conditions.
428 pages Hardcover
ISBN: 0-306457-45-3

1733 Asperger's Syndrome: A Guide for Parents and Professionals
Taylor & Francis
325 Chestnut Street
Philadelphia, PA 19106
215-625-8900
www.tonyattwood.com
Offers insight into the identification and treatment of children on the higher functioning end of ASD.
201 pages
ISBN: 1-853025-77-1

1734 Autism Society of North Carolina Bookstore
505 Oberlin Road
Raleigh, NC 27605-1345
919-743-0204
800-442-2762
Fax: 919-743-0208
www.autismsociety-nc.org
Offers one of the largest selections of books about autism.

1735 Autism Through the Lifespan: The Eden Model
Woodbine House
6510 Bells Mill Road
Bethesda, MD 20817-1636
301-897-3570
800-843-7323
Fax: 301-897-5838
Presents Eden's comprehensive model for helping children and adults with autism, offering services that extend over their entire lifespan. An overview of what is known about autism today, discussions about Eden's approach to behavior modification, placement and treatment, curriculum from early childhood to adulthood, staffing issues, integration, decision making, and parental roles. Also contains dozens of examples and case histories that illustrate the program's successes.
1998 383 pages Paperback
ISBN: 0-933149-28-x

1736 Autism Treatment Guide
Elizabeth King Gerlach, author
Autism Society of North Carolina Bookstore
505 Oberlin Road
Raleigh, NC 27605-1345
919-743-0204
800-442-2762
Fax: 919-743-0208
info@autismsociety-nc.org
www.autismsociety-nc.org
This 3rd edition offers many of the most current findings in treatments fo autism spectrum disorder. First published in 1993 and updated regularly, this concise handbook provides hundres of resource listings and suggested readings pertaining to ASD. This is a must-have reference book for parents and professionals
2003 157 pages Softcover

1737 Autism and Asperger Syndrome Preparing for Adulthood
Autism Society of North Carolina Bookstore
505 Oberlin Road
Raleigh, NC 27605-1345
919-743-0204
800-442-2762
Fax: 919-743-0208
info@autismsociety-nc.org
www.autismsociety-nc.org
Chapters include topics such as what becomes of adults with ASD, interventions for ASD, problems af communication, social functioning in adulthood, steretyped, ritualistic, and obsessional behaviors, secondary education, post-secondary education, finding and coping with employment, pyschiatric disturbances in adulthood, leagal issues, sexual relationships and marriage, and enhancing independence.
2004 388 pages Softcover

1738 Autism in Adolescents and Adults
Eric Schopler, Gary B Mesibov, author
Springer Publishing
233 Spring Street
New York, NY 10013

121-460-1500
800-777-4643
Fax: 212-460-1575
support@apress.com
www.springer.com

456 pages Hardcover
ISBN: 0-306410-57-4

1739 Autism...Nature, Diagnosis and Treatment
Guilford Press
370 Seventh Avenue
New York, NY 10001

800-365-7006
Fax: 212-966-6708
info@guilford.com
www.guilford.com

Covers perspectives, issues, neurobiological issues and new directions in diagnosis and treatment.
417 pages
ISBN: 0-898627-24-9

1740 Autism: Explaining the Enigma
Uta Frith, author
Wiley Publishing
111 River Street
Hoboken, NJ 07030-5774

201-748-6000
Fax: 201-748-6088
info@wiley.com
www.wiley.com

Includes a new chapter outlining recent developments in neuropsycgological research, and overviews one of the most important theoretical and practical consequences of Frith's original insights into this puzzling condition.
264 pages
ISBN: 0-631229-01-8

1741 Autism: Identification, Education and Treatment
Dianne Zager, author
Lawrence Earlbaum Associates
198 Madison Avenue
New York, NY 10016

201-258-2200
800-926-6579
Fax: 201-236-0072
global.oup.com/academic

Chapters include medical treatments, early intervention and communication development in autism.
2005 608 pages
ISBN: 0-805845-79-8

1742 Autism: The Facts
Simon Baron-Cohen, Patrick Bolton, author
Oxford University Press
2001 Evans Road
Cary, NC 27513

800-445-9714
Fax: 919-677-1303
custserv.us@oup.com
www.oup-usa.org

Explains in a clear, straightforward manner what is known about the condition. Written first and foremost as a guide for parents, but required reading for interested professionals, it covers the recognition and diagnosis of autism, its biological and physiological causes, and the various treatments and educational techniques available.
128 pages
ISBN: 0-192623-27-3

1743 Autistic Adults at Bittersweet Farms
Haworth Press
10 Alice Street
Binghamton, NY 13904-1580

607-722-5857
800-429-6784
Fax: 607-722-0012
www.haworthpress.com

A touching view of an inspirational residential care program for autistic adolescents and adults.
205 pages Paperback
ISBN: 1-560240-57-0

1744 Beyond Gentle Teaching
J.J McGee and F.J Menolascino, author
Springer

233 Spring Street
New York, NY 10013

212-460-1500
800-777-4643
Fax: 212-460-1575
support@apress.com
www.springer.com

252 pages Hardcover
ISBN: 0-306438-56-1

1745 Biology of the Autistic Syndromes
Christopher Gillberg and Mary Coleman, author
Blackwell Publishing, Inc.
Commerce Place
Malden, MA 02148

317-572-3994
800-862-6657
Fax: 781-388-8210
www.blackwellpublishing.com

Autism is not a disease but a syndrome of different diseases. In this completely reworked and updated 3rd edition, the authors adress the difficulties this presents for clinical diagnosis with diagnostic aids and clear guidlines for medical evaluation. This is an essential text text for clinicians and will also be of interest to parents of autistic children.
2000 340 pages
ISBN: 1-898683-22-0

1746 Children with Autism
Woodbine House
6510 Bells Mill Road
Bethesda, MD 20817

800-843-7323
info@woodbinehouse.com
www.woodbinehouse.com

A must-have reference if for the both the new parent coping with a child's recent diagnosis and one who's an experienced advocate. Available online only.
368 pages Paperback

1747 Communication Unbound: How Facilitated Communication Is Challenging Views
Teachers College Press
1234 Amsterdam Avenue
New York, NY 10027

212-678-3929
Fax: 212-678-4149
tcpress@tc.columbia.edu
www.teacherscollegepress.com

Addresses the ways in which we receive persons with autism in our society, our community and our lives.
1993 221 pages

1748 Diagnosis Autism: Now What? 10 Steps to Improve Treatment Outcomes
Lawrence P Kaplan, PhD, author
Autism Society of North Carolina Bookstore
505 Oberlin Road
Raleigh, NC 27605-1345

919-743-0204
800-442-2762
Fax: 919-743-0208
info@autismsociety-nc.org
www.autismsociety-nc.org

This practical guide was written to help parents of children with autism spectrum disorder form successful pediatric partnerships with physicians and other healthcare practitioners involved in their child's diagnosis and treatment. Containing chrts and worksheets, sample questions, research resources, and numerous planning strategies, this guide will aid parents and caregivers as they strive to build collaborative relationships with their child's case management team.
2005

1749 Effective Teaching Methods for Autistic Children
Rosalind C Oppenheim, author
Charles C Thomas Publisher
2600 S 1st Street
Springfield, IL 62704-4730

217-789-8980
800-258-8980
Fax: 217-789-9130
books@ccthomas.com
www.ccthomas.com

The Rimland School for Autistic Children in Evanston, Illinois, with a Foreward by Bernard Rimland. This enlightening monograph is seven chapters detailing the specific problems encountered in teaching autistic children. Anecdotal reports of seven such children bring to light the need for special training and provide an

insight into their handling. Related research is reviewed and discussed.
1974 116 pages Paperback
ISBN: 0-398028-58-3

1750 Encounters with Autistic States
Jason Aronson
P.O.Box 15556
York, PA 17405-7100
646-415-2561
800-782-0015
Fax: 201-840-7242
mail@aronson.com
www.aronson.com
Dr. Victor examines the myths that cloud an understanding of this disorder and describes the meanings of its specific behavioral symptoms.
Hardcover
ISBN: 0-765700-62-

1751 Handbook of Autism and Pervasive Developmental Disorders
Autism Society of North Carolina Bookstore
4340 East-West Hwy
Bethesda, MD 20814-1345
301-657-0881
800-328-8476
Fax: 919-743-0208
info@autism-society.org
www.autism-society.org
A list of contributors address such topics as characteristics of autistic syndromes and interventions.
2005 1317 pages 2 volumes

1752 Helping Children with Autism Learn: Treatment Approaches for Parents
Bryna Siegel, author
Oxford University Press
2001 Evans Road
Cary, NC 27513
800-445-9714
Fax: 919-677-1303
custserv.us@oup.com
www.oup.com
512 pages
ISBN: 0-195325-06-0

1753 Hidden Child: The Linwood Method for Reaching the Autistic Child
Woodbine House
6510 Bells Mill Road
Bethesda, MD 20817-1636
301-897-3570
800-537-3394
Fax: 301-897-5838
info@woodbinehouse.com
www.woodbinehouse.com
Chronicle of the Linwood Children's Center's successful treatment program for autistic children.
286 pages Paperback
ISBN: 0-933149-06-9

1754 I'm Not Autistic on the Typewriter
TASH
11201 Greenwood Avenue N
Seattle, WA 98133-8612
206-361-8870
An introduction to the facilitated communication training method.

1755 Keys to Parenting the Child with Autism
Marlene Targ Brill, M.Ed, author
Barrons Educational Series, Inc.
250 Wireless Boulevard
Hauppauge, NY 11788
800-645-3476
Fax: 631-434-3723
barrons@barronseduc.com
www.barronseduc.com
This book explains what autism is and how it is diagnosed.
2001 224 pages
ISBN: 0-764112-92-9

1756 Let Community Employment Be the Goal for Individuals with Autism
Autism Society of North Carolina Bookstore
505 Oberlin Road
Raleigh, NC 27605-1345
919-743-0204
800-442-2762
Fax: 919-743-0208
www.autismsociety-nc.org
A guide designed for people who are responsible for preparing individuals with autism to enter the work force.
1993 66 pages Booklet

1757 Let Me Hear Your Voice A Family's Triumph Over Autism
Catherine Maurice, author
Autism Society of North Carolina Bookstore
505 Oberlin Road
Raleigh, NC 27605-1345
919-743-0204
800-442-2762
Fax: 919-743-0208
info@autismsociety-nc.org
www.autismsociety-nc.org
The Maurice family's second and third children were diagnosed with autism. This book recounts their experience with a home program using behavior therapy.
1993 371 pages Softcover
ISBN: 0-679408-63-0

1758 Management of Autistic Behavior
Pro-Ed, Inc.
8700 Shoal Creek Blvd
Austin, TX 78757-6897
512-451-3246
800-897-3202
Fax: 800-397-7633
info@proedinc.com
www.proedinc.com
Comprehensive and practical book that tells what works best with specific problems.
450 pages Paperback
ISBN: 0-890791-96-1
Lindy Jordaan, Marketing Coordinator

1759 Navigating the Social World: A Curriculum for Individuals with Asperger's Syndrome
Jeanette McAfee, author
Future Horizons
721 W Abram Street
Arlington, TX 76013
800-489-0727
Fax: 817-277-2270
www.fhautism.com
Addresses the most urgent problems facing those with Asperger's Syndrome, high-functioning autism, and related disorders.
387 pages
ISBN: 1-885477-82-1
Ellen Notbohm, Author
Jed Baker, Author

1760 Neurobiology of Autism
Johns Hopkins University Press
2715 N Charles Street
Baltimore, MD 21218-4319
410-516-6936
Fax: 410-516-6998
This book discusses recent advances in scientific research that point to a neurobiological basis for autism and examines the clinical implications of this research.
272 pages
ISBN: 0-801856-80-9

1761 News from the Border: A Mother's Memoir of Her Autistic Son
Houghton Mifflin Company/Order Processing
222 Berkeley Street
Boston, MA 02116
617-351-5000
800-225-3362
www.hmco.com
A searingly honest account of the author's family experiences with autism. Raising an autistic child is the central, ongoing drama of her married life and this riveting account of acceptance and coping.
1993 384 pages Cloth

1762 Pervasive Developmental Disorders: Finding a Diagnosis and Getting Help
O'Reilly & Associates
1005 Gravenstein Hgwy N
Sebastopol, CA 95472-3858
707-827-7019
800-889-8969
Fax: 707-824-8268
orders@oreilly.com
www.oreilly.com
Published for parents and patients with PDD-NOS and atypical PDD.
Paperback
ISBN: 1-565925-30-0

1763 Please Don't Say Hello
Human Sciences Press
233 Spring Street
New York, NY 10013-1522
212-620-8000

Paul and his family moved into a new neighborhood. Paul's brother was autistic. The children thought that Eddie was retarded until they learned that there were skills that he could do better than they could.
1976 47 pages Paperback
ISBN: 0-898851-99-8

1764 Psychoeducational Profile (PEP-3): TEACCH Individualized Psychoeducational Assessm
Autism Society of North Carolina Bookstore
505 Oberlin Road   919-743-0204
Raleigh, NC 27605-1345   800-442-2762
                                                         Fax: 919-743-0208
                                             info@autismsociety-nc.org
                                             www.autismsociety-nc.org
This is the revised edition of Psychoeducational Profile, a widely recognized assessment tool used to identify the learning strengths and weaknesses of children with autism spectrum disorder (ASD). Developed by Division TEACCH clinicians, this instrument has been updated in several ways, including improved psychometric properties, revised function domains, new items and sub-tests, within-group comparison data, and the addition of key documentation.
2005

1765 Raising a Child with Autism: A Guide to Applied Behavior Analysis for Parents
Taylor & Francis
325 Chestnut Street   215-625-8900
Philadelphia, PA 19106   Fax: 215-625-2940
Applied behavior analysis activities that parents can use with ASD children. Inlcuded is helpful guidance for toilet training, daily living, and increasing communication and sibling interaction.
173 pages
ISBN: 1-853029-10-6

1766 Reaching the Autistic Child: A Parent Training Program
Martin Kozloff, author
Brookline Books/Lumen Editions
8 Trumbull Rd   413-584-0184
Northampton, MA 01060   800-666-2665
                                                         Fax: 413-584-6184
                                             www.brooklinebooks.com
Detailed case studies of social and behavioral change in autistic children and their families show parents how to implement the principles for improved socialization and behavior.
1998 Softcover
ISBN: 1-571290-56-7

1767 Record Book for Individuals with Autism Spectrum Disorders
Marci Wheeler and Cathy Pratt, PhD, author
Autism Society of North Carolina Bookstore
505 Oberlin Road   919-743-0204
Raleigh, NC 27605-1345   800-442-2762
                                                         Fax: 919-743-0208
                                             info@autismsociety-nc.org
                                             www.autismsociety-nc.org
This valuable resource provides a method for organizing and documenting information that will help parents track their child's development. This record book is divided into several categories, including: developmental and family history, sleeping and eating patterns, medical history, education history, behavior problems, skill development, and vital information. The book contains reproducible pages that will help parents keep important information up to date.
2000 44 pages Spiral Bound

1768 Riddle of Autism: A Psychological Analysis
Jason Aronson
P.O.Box 15556   646-415-2561
York, PA 17405-7100   800-782-0015
                                                         Fax: 201-840-7242
                                             mail@aronson.com
                                             www.aronson.com
Dr. Victor examines the myths that cloud an understanding of this disorder and describes the meanings of its specific behavioral symptoms.
356 pages Softcover
ISBN: 1-568215-73-8

1769 Siblings of Children with Autism: A Guide for Families
Woodbine House
6510 Bells Mill Road   301-897-3570
Bethesda, MD 20817   800-537-3394
                                                         Fax: 301-897-5838
                                             info@woodbinehouse.com
                                             www.woodbinehouse.com
Resource for families with autistic children and nonautistic siblings examines the perceptions, needs, compromises, and inevitable stresses that brothers and sisters face.
160 pages
ISBN: 1-890627-29-1

1770 TEACCH Transition Assessment Profile
Autism Society of North Carolina Bookstore
505 Oberlin Road   919-743-0204
Raleigh, NC 27605-1345   800-442-2762
                                                         Fax: 919-743-0208
                                             info@autismsociety-nc.org
                                             www.autismsociety-nc.org
This new assessment profile is a major revision of the AAPEP. This comprehensive test was developed for older children and adolescents with autism spectrum disorder, particularly those who have transition needs. This assessment tool is structured to satisfy those provisions in the 2004 Individuals with Disabilities Education Act, which requires that adolescents be evaluated and also provided with a transition plan.
2007 Kit

1771 Targeting Autism: What We Know, Don't Know and Can Do to Help Young Children
University of California Press
1445 Lower Ferry Road   205-978-5000
Ewing, NJ 08618   800-777-4726
                                                         Fax: 800-999-1958
                                             www.ucpress.com
Provides strong overviews of current work being done with autism and addresses the diferent life cycles of children with the condition through preschool, elementary school, and adolescence.
240 pages
ISBN: 0-520234-80-4

1772 Tasks Galore for the Real World
Laurie Eckenrode, Pat Fennell, and Kathy Hearsey, author
Autism Society of North Carolina Bookstore
505 Oberlin Road   919-743-0204
Raleigh, NC 27605-1345   800-442-2762
                                                         Fax: 919-743-0208
                                             info@autismsociety-nc.org
                                             www.autismsociety-nc.org
These visually structured tasks are strategies that translate complex, everyday life skills into simpler, meaningful learning situations. The myriad of ideas in this guide will be valuable to anyone developing functional, daily living goals for a child or client.
2004

1773 Teach Me Language: A Language Manual for Children with Autism
Sabrina Freeman, PhD and Lorelei Dake, BA, author
Autism Society of North Carolina Bookstore
505 Oberlin Road   919-743-0204
Raleigh, NC 27605-1345   800-442-2762
                                                         Fax: 919-743-0208
                                             info@autismsociety-nc.org
                                             www.autismsociety-nc.org
This book contains behaviorally based exercises and drills that adress common language weaknesses in children and incorporate professional speech pathology methods. These exercises were designed for children who are attentive, able to follow simple directions, have learned the basics of low-level language, and are visual learners. The activities and exercises are appropriate for children and young adults ages 5-18.
1997 410 pages Spiral Bound

1774 Teaching Children with Autism: Strategies to Enhance Communication and Socializing
Kathleen Ann Quill, author
Thomson Delmar Learning

Attn: Order Fullfillment 800-347-7707
Florence, KY 41022 Fax: 800-487-8488
www.delmarlearning.com

This book describes teaching strategies and instructional adaptations which promote communication and socialization in children with autism. It offers specific strategies that capitalize on the individual strengths and learning styles of the autistic child.
1996
ISBN: 0-827362-69-2

1775 Teaching Community Skills and Behaviors to Students with Autism or Related Problems
Indiana Resource Center for Autism
1905 North Range Rd 812-855-6508
Bloomington, IN 47408-2696 Fax: 812-855-9630
TTY: 812-855-9396
iidc@indiana.edu
www.iidc.indiana.edu/irca/fmain1.html

Emphasizing the needs of the person with autism and the philosophy of community integration, this book cover the process of successful community-based teaching.
1988 117 pages

1776 The Autism Sourcebook
Karen Siff Exkorn, author
Autism Society of North Carolina Bookstore
505 Oberlin Road 919-743-0204
Raleigh, NC 27605-1345 800-442-2762
Fax: 919-743-0208
www.autismsociety-nc.org

This comprehensive handbook is for parents of newly diagnosed children who are looking for information about ASD, its diagnosis, treatment options, and practical strategies in one in-depth text.
2005

1777 The Everything Parent's Guide to Children with Autism
Adelle Jameson Tilton, author
Autism Society of North Carolina Bookstore
505 Oberlin Road 919-743-0204
Raleigh, NC 27605-1345 800-442-2762
Fax: 919-743-0208
info@autismsociety-nc.org
www.autismsociety-nc.org

This book offers a wealth of information and reassuring advice for parents of newly diagnosed children. It is filled with hundreds of helpful tips, unique insights, and real-life situations, this is an essential guide for parents and family members.
2004 285 pages Softcover

1778 Understanding the Nature of Autism A Guide to the Autism Spectrum Disorders
Janice E Janzen, author
Autism Society of North Carolina Bookstore
505 Oberlin Road 919-743-0204
Raleigh, NC 27605-1345 800-442-2762
Fax: 919-743-0208
info@autismsociety-nc.org
www.autismsociety-nc.org

Straightforward and comprehensive information that can be used by parents and professionals to develop curricula and programs for children with autism spectrum disorder. This important resource is a standard text used by educators, parents, and caregivers.
2003 508 pages Softcover

1779 When Snow Turns to Rain
Woodbine House
6510 Bells Mill Road 301-897-3570
Bethesda, MD 20817-1636 800-537-3394
Fax: 301-897-5838
info@woodbinehouse.com
www.woodbinehouse.com

A gripping personal account of one family's experiences with autism. Chronicles a family's journey from parental bliss to devastation, as they learn that their son has autism. This book delves into diagnosis, treatments and attitudes toward persons with autism.
1993 250 pages Paperback
ISBN: 0-933149-63-8

1780 Autism Spectrum Disorders: The Complete Guide
Chantal Sicile-Kira, author
Autism Society of North Carolina Bookstore
505 Oberlin Road 919-743-0204
Raleigh, NC 27605-1345 800-442-2762
Fax: 919-743-0208
info@autismsociety-nc.org
www.autismsociety-nc.org

This reference guide was written to help parents, professionals, and other members of the community learn more about autism spectrum disorder, and it presents a thorough overview of the disorder, from diagnosis through adulthood.
2004 360 pages Softcover

Children's Books

1781 Joey and Sam
Illana Katz and Edward Ritvo, MD, author
Autism Society of North Carolina Bookstore
505 Oberlin Road 919-743-0204
Raleigh, NC 27605-1345 800-442-2762
Fax: 919-743-0208
ASNC@aol.com

A unique and invaluable tool for teaching children about others who are different. This awrd-winning and heartwarming sibling storybook examines the similarities and differences in behavior and educational experiences of two brothers, one of whom has autism.
1993 Softcover
ISBN: 1-882388-00-3

1782 Russell is Extra Special
Charles A Amenta III. MD, author
Autism Society of North Carolina Bookstore
505 Oberlin Road 919-743-0204
Raleigh, NC 27605-1345 800-442-2762
Fax: 919-743-0208
info@autismsociety-nc.org
www.autismsociety-nc.org

A sensitive portrayal of an autistic boy written by his father.
Hardcover

1783 Wild Boy of Aveyron
Harlan Lane, author
Harvard University Press
79 Garden Street 617-495-2600
Cambridge, MA 02138 800-405-1619
Fax: 617-495-5898
contact_HUP@harvard.edu
www.hup.harvard.edu

A dramatic account of a wild boy of nature and a young French doctor who shaped the modern education of retarded, deaf, and preschool children.
368 pages
ISBN: 0-674953-00-2

Newsletters

1784 Autism Research Review International
Autism Research Institute
4182 Adams Avenue 619-281-7165
San Diego, CA 92116-2536 Fax: 619-563-6840

A quarterly newsletter published by the Autism Research Institute.
8 pages Quarterly
Dr. Bernard Rimland, Director

Pamphlets

1785 Avoiding Unfortunate Situations
Autism Society of North Carolina Bookstore
505 Oberlin Road 919-743-0204
Raleigh, NC 27605-1345 800-442-2762
Fax: 919-743-0208
info@autismsociety-nc.org
www.autismsociety-nc.org

A collection of tips and information from and about people with autism and other developmental disabilities and their encounters with law enforcement agencies.

1786 Developing a Functional and Longitudinal Individual Plan
Nancy Dalrymple, author

Autism Society of North Carolina Bookstore
1905 North Range Rd   812-855-6508
Bloomington, IN 47408-1345   800-442-2762
                                       Fax: 812-855-9630
                                       iidc@indiana.edu
                                       www.iidc.indiana.edu

It is the author's view that a functional, longitudinal approach should be taken when educating persons with autism spectrum disorder, and that the development of an individualized plan should incorporate school, home, and community. This guide discusses the importance of defining strengths, striving for independent functioning, and determining which activities should recieve priority in the areas of self-care, social and leisure activities, and employment.
1989 11 pages Booklet

1787 Enabling Communication in Children with Autism

Autism Society of North Carolina Bookstore
505 Oberlin Road   919-743-0204
Raleigh, NC 27605-1345   800-442-2762
                                       Fax: 919-743-0208
                                       info@autismsociety-nc.org
                                       www.autismsociety-nc.org

Based on a 2 year research project, the goal of this book is to help teachers develop more communication-enabling enviroments for children with atuism spectrum disorder who use little or no speech. The authors illustrate many communication-enabling strategies, including the minimal speech approach, proximal communication, prompting, and multipointing.
2001 207 pages Softcover

1788 Job Seeker Involvment in Securing Employment
Nancy Kalina, author

Indiana Resource Center for Autism
1905 North Range Rd   812-855-6508
Bloomington, IN 47408-2696   Fax: 812-855-9630
                                       TTY: 812-855-9396
                                       iidc@indiana.edu
                                       www.iidc.indiana.edu/irca/fmain1.html

A walk through the job development process, from identifying job options and writing a resume to negotiating workplace supports with a potential employer. Each step provides opportunities for the peronal with autism, or another disability, to become actively involved in their job search process.
1997 22 pages

1789 Learning to be Independent and Responsible
Nancy Dalrymple, author

Indiana Resource Center for Autism
1905 North Range Rd   812-855-6508
Bloomington, IN 47408-2696   Fax: 812-855-9630
                                       TTY: 812-855-9396
                                       iidc@indiana.edu
                                       www.iidc.indiana.edu/irca/fmain1.html

People with autism build trust in people and environments through successful interactions. Individualized, supportive programs, utilizing positive instructional and environmental supports that lead to increased opportunities, chouse, and motivation are described in this booklet.
1989 11 pages

1790 Parents as Trainers of Legislators, Other Parents and Researchers

Autism Services Center
101 Richmond Street   304-525-8014
Huntington, WV 25702-1513   Fax: 304-525-8026

Reprint offering information on parents of autistic children that learn early in their child's life how little professionals know about autism.

1791 Sex, Sexuality, and the Autism Specrtum
Wendy Lawson, author

Autism Society of North Carolina Bookstore

505 Oberlin Road   919-743-0204
Raleigh, NC 27605-1345   800-442-2762
                                       Fax: 919-743-0208
                                       info@autismsociety-nc.org
                                       www.autismsociety-nc.org

The author, a psychologist, who has Aspergers Syndrome, presents her unique perspective on sexuality and interpersonal relationships. Filled with honest insights and positive advice, this is a valuable guide for persons with ASD and the people who live and work with them.
2005 175 pages Softcover

1792 Son-Rise Method

Option Institute
2080 S Undermountain Road   413-229-2100
Sheffield, MA 01257-9643   Fax: 413-229-8931
                                       information@son-rise.org
                                       www.autismtreatmentcenter.org

Describes a program Barry and Samahria Kaufman developed to help heal their once-autistic son.

1793 What Is Autism

Autism Society of America
4340 East-West Hwy   301-657-0881
Bethesda, MD 20814-3065   800-328-8476
                                       Fax: 301-657-0869
                                       info@autism-society.org
                                       www.autism-society.org

Offers a definition and introduction to autism, produces a wide range of autism information written for various audiences. Offers a quarterly magazine, national conference, nationwide chapter network and many other resources.

Audio & Video

1794 A Sense of Belonging: Including Students with Autism in their School Community

Indiana Resource Center for Autism
1905 North Range Rd   812-855-6508
Bloomington, IN 47408-2696   Fax: 812-855-9630
                                       TTY: 812-855-9396
                                       iidc@indiana.edu
                                       www.iidc.indiana.edu/irca/fmain1.html

Highlights the efforts of two elementary and one middle school in Indiana in teaching students with autism in general education settings. Comments from parents, school administrators, classmates, and educators illustrate the role they each played in supporting students with autism in becoming active learners in their school community. Includes practical strategies for teaching the student with autism.
1997 20 minutes

1795 Autism: A Strange, Silent World

Filmakers Library
3212 Duke Street   212-808-4980
Alexandria, VA 22314   Fax: 212-808-4983
                                       sales@alexanderstreet.com
                                       www.academicvideostore.com

A comprehensive view of autism by focusing on three children of different ages, with very different behaviors. Also introduces us to a remarkable group of parents, teachers and therapists who strive to maximize
VHS/DVD
Sue Oscar, Co-President
Linda Gottesman, Co-President

1796 Autism: A World Apart
Karen Cunninghame, author

Fanlight Productions
32 Court Street   718-488-8900
Brooklyn, NY 11201-1731   800-876-1710
                                       Fax: 718-488-8642
                                       info@fanlight.com
                                       www.fanlight.com

In this documentary, three families show us what the textbooks and studies cannot, what it's like to live with autism day after day, raise

and love children who may be withdrawn and violent and unable to make personal connections with their families.
DVD
ISBN: 1-572959-50-9

1797 Developing IEPs Under the New Idea Regulations
LRP Publications
360 Hiatt Drive   800-341-7874
Palm Beach Gardens, FL 33418-2247   Fax: 215-784-9639
custserve@lrp.com
www.lrp.com
A practical, step-by-step approach makes it easy to understand the legal and educational issues surrounding IEPs.
26 minutes

1798 Discipline Under the New Idea: Practical Methods and Procedures
LRP Publications
360 Hiatt Drive   800-341-7874
Palm Beach Gardens, FL 33418-2247   Fax: 215-784-9639
custserve@lrp.com
www.lrp.com
Provides practical explanation of the discipline methods and procedures school officials are permitted to use for students with disabilities.
26 minutes

1799 Embracing Play: Teaching Your Child with Autism
Woodbine House
6510 Bells Mill Road   301-897-3570
Bethesda, MD 20817   800-537-3394
Fax: 301-897-5838
info@woodbinehouse.com
www.woodbinehouse.com
Guide for parents who incorporate applied behavior analysis with their child.
1993 47 minutes

1800 Functional Behavioral Assessments: How to Do Them Right!
LRP Publications
360 Hiatt Drive   800-341-7874
Palm Beach Gardens, FL 33418-2247   Fax: 215-784-9639
custserve@lrp.com
www.lrp.com
Assist you in understanding why a behavior problem has occured, so you can maximize the effectiveness of a planned intervention.
18 minutes

1801 Getting Started with Facilitated Communication
Syracuse University, Facilitated Communication Ins
370 Huntington Hall   315-443-9379
Syracuse, NY 13244-2340   Fax: 315-443-9218
fcstaff@syr.edu
soeweb.syr.edu/thefci/
Describes in detail how to help individuals with autism and/or severe communication difficulties to get started with facilitated communication.
Videotape

1802 Going to School with Facilitated Communication
Syracuse University, School of Education
805 S Krouse   315-443-2693
Syracuse, NY 13244-0001
A video in which students with autism and/or severe disabilities illustrate the use of facilitated communication focusing on basic principles fostering facilitated communication.
Videotape

1803 I Want My Little Boy Back
Autism Treatment Center of America
2080 S Undermountain Road   413-229-2100
Sheffield, MA 01257   800-714-2779
Fax: 413-229-8931
www.autismtreatmentcenter.org
This BBC documentary follows an English family with a child with autism before, during, and after their time at the Son-Rise Program. It uniquely captures the heart of the Son-Rise Program and is extremely useful in understanding the program's techniques.
Lauren Astor, Public Relations Manager

1804 I'm Not Autistic on the Typewriter
Syracuse University, School of Education
805 S Krouse   315-443-2693
Syracuse, NY 13244-0001
A video introducing facilitated communication, a method by which persons with autism express themselves.
Videotape

1805 Invisible Wall: Autism
PRIMEDIA/Films Media Group
Films for Hum. & Science   800-257-5126
Princeton, NJ 08543   Fax: 609-671-0266
custserv@filmsmediagroup.com
www.films.com/
It features interviews with Ivar Lovaas, the creator of applied behavior analysis therapy.
2001 52 minutes
Dean B Nelson, Chairman & President
Kevin Neary, Chief Financial Officer

1806 Public Schools and Students with Autism: Components of a Defensible Program
LRP Publications
360 Hiatt Drive   800-341-7874
Palm Beach Gardens, FL 33418-2247   Fax: 215-784-9639
custserve@lrp.com
www.lrp.com
This video assists you in understanding transition planning, documentation of student progress and proven strategies you can implement in your program.
13 minutes

1807 Standards and Inclusion: Can We Have Both?
LRP Publications
360 Hiatt Drive   800-341-7874
Palm Beach Gardens, FL 33418-2247   Fax: 215-784-9639
custserve@lrp.com
www.lrp.com
Addresses the critical issues educators face when supporting students with disabilities in inclusive settings. Through dynamic, powerful presentations by two inclusion experts.
40 minutes

1808 Understanding Autism
Suzanne Newman, author
Fanlight Productions
32 Court Street   718-488-8900
Brooklyn, NY 11201-1731   800-876-1710
Fax: 718-488-8642
info@fanlight.com
www.fanlight.com
Parents of children with autism discuss the nature and symptoms of this lifelong disability and outlines a treatment program based on behavior modification principles.
1993 19 Minutes
ISBN: 1-572951-00-1

Web Sites

1809 Autism Research Institute
www.autism.com
A clearinghouse for research on autism and related disorders of learning and behavior. Conducts and compiles research findings to provide people with the latest research available.

1810 Autism Resources
www.autism-resources.com
Provides information and links regarding the developmental disabilities autism and Asperger's Syndrome.

1811 Autism Society of America
www.autism-society.org
A national charitable organization with the mission of providing as much information as possible about autism and the various options, approaches, methods and systems available to parents of children with autism, family members and professionals.

1812 Autism Treatment Center of America
www.autismtreatmentcenter.org

Provides training programs for parents and professionals caring for children challenged by Autism, Autism Spectrum Disorders, Pervasive Developmental Disorder (PDD), and other developmental disorders.

1813 Community Services for Autistic Adults & Children

csaac.org

Non-profit dedicated to providing support services for children and adults with autism.

1814 Healing Well

www.healingwell.com

A social network and support community for patients, caregivers, and families coping with the daily struggles of diseases, disorders and chronic illness.

1815 Health Finder

www.healthfinder.gov

A government web site there individuals can find information and tools to help you and those you care about stay healthy.

1816 Healthlink USA

www.healthlinkusa.com

Health information concerning treatment, cures, prevention, diagnosis, risk factors, research, support groups, email lists, personal stories and much more. Updated regularly.

1817 MedicineNet

www.medicinenet.com

An online resource for consumers providing easy-to-read, authoritative medical and health information.

1818 Medscape

www.medscape.com

Medscape offers specialists, primary care physicians, and other health professionals the Web's most robust and integrated medical information and educational tools.

1819 National Alliance for Autism Research

www.naar.org

The first organization in the United States dedicated to funding and accelerating biomedical research focusing on autism spectrum disorders.

1820 National Institute of Mental Health

www.nimh.nih.gov

Mission is to transform the understanding and treatment of mental illnesses through basic and clinical research, paving the way for prevention, recovery, and cure.

1821 Son Rise Program

www.autismtreatmentcenter.org

A powerful and effective treatment for children and adults challenged by Autism, Autism Spectrum Disorders, Pervasive Developmental Disorder (PDD), Asperger's Syndrome, and other developmental difficulties.

1822 WebMD

www.webmd.com

Provides credible information, supportive communities, and in-depth reference material about health subjects. A source for original and timely health information as well as material from well known content providers.

Description

1823 Birth Defects

Birth defects, or congenital abnormalities, occur in 3 to 4 percent of newborns and can include structural defects of the heart, major blood vessels, kidneys, urinary tract, gastrointestinal tract, skeleton and nervous system. The incidence of specific abnormalities varies with the type of defect. These defects may consist of single abnormalities, or several defects may occur together, often known as a syndrome. Birth defects account for about 21 percent of infant deaths in the United States.

Although in many instances the cause of the defect is unknown, genetic factors may cause many single malformations and syndromes. Some syndromes, such as Down syndrome, result from chromosomal abnormalities. Factors during the pregnancy can sometimes result in defects, such as taking certain drugs (Coumadin, Dilantin), maternal illness (diabetes mellitus), and various infections (toxoplasmosis, syphilis, Rubella).

Prior to birth, ultrasound evaluation of the fetus and testing of the amniotic fluid surrounding it can identify some defects. If a defect is identified and is serious, parents can decide how or if they wish the pregnancy to proceed. Other abnormalities may not be identified until birth. Treatment and outcome vary greatly, depending on the type and severity of the defect. Parents and other family members need honest information and emotional support when caring for a child born with congenital defects. If genetic factors are suspected, the parents should receive genetic counseling. See also *Spina Bifida and Congenital Heart Disease.*

National Agencies & Associations

1824 American Cleft Palate - Craniofacial Association
1504 E Franklin Street
Chapel Hill, NC 27514-2820
919-933-9044
800-242-5338
Fax: 919-933-9604
info@acpa-cpf.org
acpa-cpf.org
Non-profit association of healthcare professionals and other interested individuals in the area of cleft and craniofacial conditions.
Wendy-Jo Toyama, Executive Director
Catherine Choi, Family Services Coordinator

1825 Birth Defect Research for Children, Inc.
976 Lake Baldwin Lane
Celebration, FL 32814
407-895-0802
staff@birthdefects.org
www.birthdefects.org/allergies
A non-profit organization providing parents and soon-to-be parents with information resources about birth defects, and support services for their children. Offers fact sheets on allergies.
Betty Mekdeci, Executive Director

1826 Council for Exceptional Children
2900 Crystal Drive
Arlington, VA 22202-3557
888-232-7733
TTY: 866-915-5000
service@cec.sped.org
www.cec.sped.org
Advocates appropriate policies, standards and development for individuals with special needs. Provides professional development for special educators.
Alexander T. Graham, Executive Director
Craig Evans, Director, Operations

1827 Early Childhood Technical Assistance Center
Campus Box 8040 UNC-CH
Chapel Hill, NC 27599-8040
919-962-2001
Fax: 919-966-7463
TTY: 919-843-3269
ectacenter.org
Assists states and other designated governing jurisdictions as they develop multidisciplinary, coordinated and comprehensive services for children with special needs.
Christina Kasprzak, Co-Director
Megan Vinh, Co-Director

1828 Easterseals
141 W Jackson Blvd
Chicago, IL 60604
312-726-6200
800-221-6827
Fax: 312-726-1494
info@easterseals.com
www.easterseals.com
Provides services to children and adults with disabilities as well as support to their families.
Angela F. Williams, President & CEO
Sharon Watson, Vice President, Communications/Marketing

1829 Federation for Children with Special Needs
529 Main Street
Boston, MA 02129
617-236-7210
800-331-0688
Fax: 617-241-0330
fcsninfo@fcsn.org
www.fcsn.org
A center for parents and parent organizations to work together on behalf of children with special needs.
Pam Nourse, Executive Director
Marilyn Favreau, Director, Statewide Family Engagement

1830 Goodwill Industries International, Inc.
15810 Indianola Drive
Rockville, MD 20855
800-466-3945
contactus@goodwill.org
www.goodwill.org
A nonprofit, community-based organization whose mission is to help people achieve self-sufficiency through the dignity and power of work, serving people who are disadvantaged, disabled or elderly. The mission is accomplished through providing independent living skills, affordable housing, and training and placement in community employment. The GoodWill Network includes 160 independent, local locations across the U.S. and Canada.
S. Dale Jenkins, Chair
Steven C. Preston, President & CEO

1831 Parent Professional Advocacy League
15 Court Square
Boston, MA 02108
866-815-8122
Fax: 617-542-7832
info@ppal.net
www.ppal.net
An organization of families of children with mental, emotional or behavioral needs and concerned professionals. PPAL support groups are run in many areas across the country.
Lisa Lambert, Executive Director
Meri Viano, Associate Director

1832 myFace
333 East 30th Street
New York, NY 10016
917-720-4701
Fax: 917-512-7611
info@myface.org
www.myface.org
Formerly The National Foundation for Facial Reconstruction. It addresses the plight of children with a facial disfigurement by supporting treatment, research, psychosocial support, and medical training.
Priscilla Ma, Executive Director
Dina Zuckerman, Director, Family Programs

State Agencies & Associations

Florida

1833 Goodwill Industries-Suncoast
10596 Gandy Boulevard
St. Petersburg, FL 33702
727-523-1512
888-279-1988
TTY: 727-579-1068
www.goodwill-suncoast.org

A nonprofit, community-based organization whose mission is to help people achieve self-sufficiency through the dignity and power of work, serving people who are disadvantaged, disabled or elderly. The mission is accomplished through providing independent living skills, affordable housing, and training and placement in community employment.

Heather Ceresoli, CPA, Chair
Deborah A. Passerini, President & CEO

Foundations

1834 Cornelia de Lange Syndrome Foundation, Inc
302 W Main Street 860-676-8166
Avon, CT 06001 800-223-8355
Fax: 860-676-8337
info@cdlsusa.org
www.cdlsusa.org
Provides information about birth defects caused by Cornelia de Lange Syndrome, and services for those affected.
Bonnie Royster, Executive Director
Antonie Kline, MD, Medical Director

1835 March of Dimes Foundation
1550 Crystal Drive 888-663-4637
Arlington, VA 22202 www.marchofdimes.org
Seeks to improve the health of babies by preventing birth defects, premature birth, and infant mortality through programs of research, community services, education, and advocacy.
Stacey D. Stewart, President

Research Centers

1836 Boston University Center for Human Genetics
715 Albany Street 617-638-4640
Boston, MA 02118-2394 Fax: 617-638-7092
amilunski@bu.edu
www.bumc.bu.edu
Offers research into genetic disorders and growth disorders.
Dr Karen H Antman, Dean
Jeff Milunsky, Co-Director

1837 California Teratogen Information Service UC San Diego School of Medicine Dept of
UC San Diego School of Medicine Dept of Pediatrics
9500 Gilman Drive 619-294-6291
La Jolla, CA 92093-828 800-532-3749
Fax: 619-220-0228
ctispregnancy@ucsd.edu
www.ctispregnancy.org
Statewide service operated by the California Teratogen Information Service (CTIS) and Clinical Research Program. Our goal is to promote healthy pregnancies through education and research.
Kenneth Lyon Jones MD, Medical Director
Christina D Chambers, Program Director

1838 Department of Reproductive Genetics: Magee Women's Hospital
200 Lothrop Street 412-647-8748
Pittsburgh, PA 15213-2582 800-533-8762
Fax: 412-641-1032
dbrucha@mail.magee.edu
www.upmc.com
Obstetrical and gynecological teaching unit of the University of Pittsburgh School of Medicine. A full-service women's hospital and now has expanded to include a range of services for women and men.
W Allen Hogge, Clinical Investigator
Jie Hu, Assistant Investigator

1839 Division Of Developmental and Behavioral Pediatrics
Children's Hospital Medical Center of Cincinnati
3333 Burnet Avenue 513-636-4200
Cincinnati, OH 45229-3039 800-344-2462
TTY: 513-636-4900
www.cincinnatichildrens.org
The Division of Developmental and Behavioral Pediatrics provides services for infants children and adolescents from birth to age 21 who are experiencing developmental or behavioral problems.
David J Schonfeld, Director
Matthew W Zurad, Business Director

1840 Georgetown University Child Development Center
Box 571485 202-687-5000
Washington, DC 20057-1485 Fax: 202-687-8899
gucdc@georgetown.edu
The mission of the GUCCHD is to bring together policy, research and clinical practice for the betterment of individuals and families, especially children youth and those with special needs including: development disabilities and special health care needs, mental health needs, young children and those in the child welfare system.
John De Gioia, President
Neal Horen, Co-Director Training and Technical Assis

1841 Louisiana State University Genetics Section of Pediatrics
200 Clay Avenue 504-896-9524
New Orleans, LA 70118 Fax: 504-894-3997
ylacas@lsuhsc.edu
www.medschool.lsuhsc.edu

Yves Lacassie, Section Head
Mary Camille Fournet, Research Associate

1842 New England Regional Genetics Group
PO Box 920288 781-444-0126
Needham, MA 02492 Fax: 781-444-0127
mfgnergg@verizon.net
www.nergg.org
Human genetic services and educational planning pertaining to birth defects.
Mary-Frances Garber, Executive Director
Cindy Ingham, Co-Director

1843 Teratology OTIS
1295 N Martin 520-626-3547
Tucson, AZ 85721-202 866-626-6847
contactus@otispregnancy.org
www.otispregnancy.org
Teratology Information Services are comprehensive and multidisciplinary resources for medical consultation on prenatal exposures. TIS interpret information regarding known and potential reproductive risks into risk assessments that are communicated to individuals of reproductive age and health care providers.
Dee Quinn, Executive Director
Lori Wolfe, President

1844 Thomas Jefferson University: Daniel Baugh Institute
329 Jefferson Alumni Hall
1020 Locust Street 215-503-7823
Philadelphia, PA 19107 Fax: 215-503-2636
James.Schwaber@mail.dbi.tju.edu
Cares for both out and in-patients with complex problems involving a wide variety of infectious diseases. The Division has an active clinical research program bringing state-of-the-art treatments to patients.
James Schwaber, Director
Boris N Kholodenko, Director Computational Cell Biology

1845 University of Illinois at Chicago Craniofacial Center
College of Medicine
180 DENT M/C 588 312-996-7546
Chicago, IL 60612 Fax: 312-413-1157
dreisber@uic.edu
www.uic.edu

David J Reisberg, Director

1846 University of Iowa Birth Defects and Genetic Disorders Unit
Iowa Registry for Congenital/Inherited Disorders
100 Oakdale Campus 319-335-3500
Iowa City, IA 52242-5000 866-274-4237
Fax: 319-335-4030
ircid@uiowa.edu
www.uiowa.edu
Established through the joint efforts of the University of Iowa the Iowa Department of Public Health and the Iowa Department of Human Services to monitor birth defects in the state.
Paul A Romitti, Director
Kim Keppler-Noreuil, Clinical Director for Birth Defects

1847 University of Miami: Mailman Center for Child Development
1601 NW 12th Avenue 305-243-6801
Miami, FL 33136-6820 Fax: 305-243-5978
TTY: 305-243-5937
TDD: 305-243-5937
www.pediatrics.med.miami.edu
Focuses on birth defects and children's illnesses.
Dr Robert Stempfel Jr, Director

1848 Wayne State University: CS Mott Center for Human Growth and Development
275 E Hancock Street 313-577-1485
Detroit, MI 48201 Fax: 313-577-8554
home.med.wayne.edu
Human growth and development disorders.
Dr Robert Sokol, Director
Valerie M Parisi, Dean

1849 Wichita Medical Research & Education Foundation
3306 E Central Avenue 316-686-7172
Wichita, KS 67208-3104 Fax: 316-687-0033
www.wichitamedicalresearch.org
The Wichita Medical Research Foundation promotes research for the development of new medical skills and knowledge which serve patients from Wichita and throughout Kansas.
Peggy L Johnson, Executive Director/COO
William Hendry PhD, President

Support Groups & Hotlines

1850 ACPA Family Services
American Cleft Palate-Craniofacial Association
1504 E Franklin Street 919-933-9044
Chapel Hill, NC 27514-2820 800-242-5338
Fax: 919-933-9604
info@acpa-cpf.org
cleftline.org
Provides education, personalized support, and resources for familieis of children with cleft or craniofacial conditions.
Wendy-Jo Toyama, Executive Director
Catherine Choi, Family Services Coordinator

1851 CUNY: Teratogen Information Service
People
1219 N Forest Road 716-634-8132
Williamsville, NY 14221-3292 888-773-0753
Fax: 716-634-3889
www.people-inc.org
Mary Ann Kedron, Ph.D., Chairperson
Joseph J. Abdallah, Vice Chairperson

1852 Connecticut Pregnancy Exposure Information Service
UConn Health Partners
Division of Human Genetics 860-523-6419
West Hartford, CT 06119 800-325-5391
humangenetics.uchc.edu
Provides up-to-date information on all types of exposures during pregnancy or breastfeeding for Connecticut residents or women who have Connecticut physicians.
Philip E Austin, President
James F Abromaitis, Commissioner

1853 Illinois Teratogen Information Service (IT IS)
680 N Lake Shore Drive 312-981-4354
Chicago, IL 60611 800-252-4847
A free statewide service that is financially supported by the Illinois Department of Public Health. Provides information regarding all types of exposures during pregnancy, and is available to women who are pregnant or planning a pregnancy, fathers, physicians, and other health care providers in the State of Illinois
Kristen L Dieter MS/CGC, Genetic Counselor/Coordinator ITIS
Eugene Pergament MD/Ph.D, Medical Geneticist

1854 Indiana Teratogen Information Service
Indiana University Medical Center
975 W Walnut Street 317-274-2241
Indianapolis, IN 46202

A telephone inquiry service that provides central, up-to-date, information from computersized sources, professional articles and expert consultants
David D Weaver MD, Director

1855 Missouri Teratogen Information Service
University of Missouri Health Care
1 Hospital Drive 573-882-7299
Columbia, MO 65212-1 Fax: 573-882-1593
umhs-muhealth@missouri.edu
www.muhealth.org/
The Missouri Teratogen Information Services (MOTIS) helps promote healthy pregnancies by providing, counseling, education and information.
James Ross, Chief Executive Officer
James C Poehling, Chief Operating Officer

1856 National Health Information Center
Office of Disease Prevention & Health Promotion
1101 Wootton Pkwy Fax: 240-453-8281
Rockville, MD 20852 odphpinfo@hhs.gov
www.health.gov/nhic
Supports public health education by maintaining a calendar of National Health Observances; helps connect consumers and health professionals to organizations that can best answer questions and provide up-to-date contact information from reliable sources; updates on a yearly basis toll-free numbers for health information, Federal health clearinghouses and info centers.
Don Wright, MD, MPH, Director

1857 Nebraska Information Service
University of Nebraska Medical Center
985440 Nebraska Medical Center 402-559-5071
Omaha, NE 68198-5440 Fax: 402-559-7248
Teratogen Information Project
Beth Conover APRN, MS, Genetic Counselor
Kathleen Caldwell, Project Assistant

1858 New Jersey Pregnancy Risk Information Service
254 Easton Avenue 732-745-6659
New Brunswick, NJ 8901-1766
DebraLynn Day Salvatore, Medical Director

1859 PALS Support Groups
Parent/Professional Advocacy League
45 Bromfield Street 617-542-7860
Boston, MA 02108 866-815-8122
Fax: 617-542-7832
info@ppal.net
ppal.net
Promotes a strong voice for families of children and adolescents with mental health needs. Advocates for supports, treatment and policies that enale families to live in their communities in an environment of stability and respect.
Lisa Lambert, Executive Director
Christopher Anselmo, Project Coordinator

1860 Pregnancy Healthline: Pennsylvania Hospital
8th & Spruce Streets 215-829-3601
Philadelphia, PA 19107
Betsy Schick-Boschetto MSN

1861 Pregnancy Risk Line
Utah Department of Health
PO Box 141010 801-328-2229
Salt Lake City, UT 84114-1010 800-822-2229
www.health.utah.gov/prl
Provides vaulable information to women who are pregnant, considering becoming pregnant, or breastfeeding, and to their healthcare providers.

1862 Pregnancy Safety Hotline
Western Pennsylvania Hospital
4800 Friendship Avenue 412-687-7233
Pittsburgh, PA 15224-1722 www.wphs.org
Michael Kerr MS

1863 Teratogen Information Services
University of Florida Health Science Center

PO Box 100296
Gainesville, FL 32610-0296
352-392-3050
www.health.ufl.edu
Donna H Poynor MA

1864 Teratogen and Birth Defects Information Project
University of South Dakota
414 E Clark Street
Vermillion, SD 57069-2307
605-677-5011
877-269-6837
Fax: 605-677-6534
urelations@usd.edu
www.usd.edu

James Abbott, University President
Rod Parry, Dean of the Medical School

1865 University of Iowa Teratogen Information Service
University of Iowa Teratogen
200 Hakins Drive
Iowa City, IA 52242
319-353-7877
800-777-8442
www.uihealthcare.com

Donna Katen Bahensky, Chief Executive Officer
Anne Madenrice, Chief Operations Officer

1866 University of Nebraska Medical Center Tera Togen Project
Genetic Medicine-Munroe-Meyer Institute
985430 Nebraska Medical Center
Omaha, NE 68198-5430
402-559-6800
800-656-3937
Fax: 402-559-6688
gbschaef@unmc.edu
www.unmc.edu/dept/mmi/

The section of Genetic Medicine provides comprehensive services for a variety of patients and their families. Direct services include diagnosis, interpretation of risks, supportive counseling, and suggestions/referrals for further management. The department participates in clinics, inpatient consultation, and the Teratogen Information Project.
G Bradley Schaefer MD/FAAP/FACMG, Director Genetics Department

1867 Vermont Pregnancy Risk Information Service
Vermont Regional Genetics Center
1 Mill Street
Burlington, VT 05401-1530
800-932-4609

Alan E Guttmacher MD

Books

1868 Bendectin Report
976 Lake Baldwin Lane
Orlando, FL 32814
407-895-0802
800-313-2232
staff@birthdefects.org
www.birthdefects.org
Report on research connecting the anti-nausea medication, Bendectin, with birth defects. Includes latest judicial opinion confirming $24 million judgment in a Bendectin case.
90 pages

1869 Dursban Report
976 Lake Baldwin Lane
Orlando, FL 32814
407-895-0802
800-313-2232
staff@birthdefects.org
www.birthdefects.org
Report on research and latest EPA findings on Dursban and health problems, including MCS and birth defects.
90 pages

1870 Environmental Birth Defect Digest
976 Lake Baldwin Lane
Orlando, FL 32814
407-895-0802
800-313-2232
staff@birthdefects.org
www.birthdefects.org
Compendium of research briefs from the world medical literature, plus original articles covering birth defects associated with medications, radiation, chemicals, toxic sites, dioxin, pesticides, lead, mercury, Bendectin, aspartame and more.
42 pages

1871 Understanding Birth Defects
Franklin Watts Grolier

90 Old Sherman Turnpike
Danbury, CT 06816-0001
203-797-3500
800-621-1115
Fax: 203-797-3197
www.grolier.com
What birth defects are, their genetic and environmental origins and what can be done to help, plus the problems of low birth weight are discussed.
128 pages
ISBN: 0-531109-55-0

Children's Books

1872 Don't Feel Sorry for Paul
JB Lippincott
530 Walnut Street
Philadelphia, PA 19105
215-521-8300
Fax: 215-521-8902
www.ilkins.com
Paul is seven and was born with deformities of both hands and feet. Paul must wear a prosthesis on both feet so that he can walk. He has a third prosthesis for his right hand. The third prosthesis has a pair of hooks Paul uses as fingers.
94 pages Hardcover
ISBN: 0-397315-88-0

1873 God, the Universe and Hot Fudge Sundaes
Houghton, Mifflin & Company
222 Berkeley Street
Boston, MA 02116-3107
617-351-5000
www.hmco.com

Newsletters

1874 Birth Defect News
Birth Defect Research for Children
976 Lake Baldwin Lane
Celebration, FL 32814
407-895-0802
staff@birthdefects.org
www.birthdefects.org
8 pages Quarterly
Betty Mekdeci, Executive Director

1875 NewsLine
Federation for Children with Special Needs
95 Berkeley Street
Boston, MA 02116-6230
617-482-2915
800-331-0688
Offers information for parents and families on resources, medical updates, activities, fund-raising events and association news for their disabled children.
Quarterly

1876 PAL News
Parent Professional Advocacy League
95 Berkeley Street
Boston, MA 02116-6264
617-482-2915
800-331-0688
Offers information on medical and technological updates in the area of research on birth defects, support groups and family resources for persons with disabled children.
Quarterly

Pamphlets

1877 After School...Then What? The Transition to Adulthood
Federation for Children with Special Needs
95 Berkeley Street
Boston, MA 02116-6230
617-482-2915
800-331-0688
Preparing for the transition after high school for children with special needs.

1878 Agent Orange and Birth Defects
976 Lake Baldwin Lane
Orlando, FL 32814
407-895-0802
800-313-2232
staff@birthdefects.org
www.birthdefects.org
Research booklet, including the latest findings from the National Birth Defect Registry and government research connecting Agent Orange to birth defects.
42 pages

1879 Birth Defects & Genetics: The Genetics Revolution
March of Dimes Birth
1275 Mamaroneck Avenue   914-997-4488
White Plains, NY 10605   Fax: 212-254-3518
                                NY639@marchofdimes.com
                                www.marchofdimes.com
Offers information on genetic testing and what it means to the patient and family members.

1880 Childhood Illnesses in Pregnancy: Chicken Pox & Fifth Disease
March of Dimes
1275 Mamaroneck Avenue   914-997-4488
White Plains, NY 10605   Fax: 212-254-3518
                                NY639@marchofdimes.com
                                www.marchofdimes.com
Located on the March of Dimes website.

1881 Cleft Lip & Palate
March of Dimes
1275 Mamaroneck Avenue   914-997-4488
White Plains, NY 10605   Fax: 212-254-3518
                                NY639@marchofdimes.com
                                www.marchofdimes.com
Located on March of Dimes website.

1882 Club Foot and Other Foot Deformities
March of Dimes
1275 Mamaroneck Avenue   914-997-4488
White Plains, NY 10605   Fax: 212-254-3518
                                NY639@marchofdimes.com
                                www.marchofdimes.com
Located on the March of Dimes website.

1883 Genetic Counseling
March of Dimes
1275 Mamaroneck Avenue   914-997-4488
White Plains, NY 10605   Fax: 212-254-3518
                                NY639@marchofdimes.com
                                www.marchofdimes.com
Located on the March of Dimes website.

1884 Gulf War and Birth Defects
930 Woodcock Road   407-225-7035
Orlando, FL 32812   800-313-2232
                                www.birthdefects.org
Information booklet on recent data from the National Birth Defect Registry and other research related to Gulf War exposures and birth defects.
30 pages

1885 How to Find More About Your Child's Birth Defect or Disability
Association for Birth Defect Children
5400 Diplomat Circle   800-922-9234
Orlando, FL 32810-5603   www.birthdefects.org
An informational fact sheet that encourages parents who have a child with a birth defect or disability to become the expert on the child's disability with some suggestions on how to educate themselves.

1886 Low Birthweight
March of Dimes
1275 Mamaroneck Avenue   914-997-4488
White Plains, NY 10605   Fax: 212-254-3518
                    NY639@marchofdimes.com, www.marchofdimes.com
Fact Sheets: one or two page review written for the general public.

1887 PKU Quick Reference and Fact Sheet
March of Dimes
1275 Mamaroneck Avenue   914-997-4488
White Plains, NY 10605   Fax: 212-254-3518
                                NY639@marchofdimes.com
                                www.marchofdimes.com
Phenylketonuria (PKU) is an inherited disorder that affects the way the body is able to process food. If left untreated, it causes mental retardation. How PKU is passed on and how it is treated are outlined.

1888 Teaching Social Skills to Youngsters with Disabilities
Federation for Children with Special Needs
95 Berkeley Street   617-482-2915
Boston, MA 02116-6230   800-331-0688

Explains the importance of instruction and training to learn appropriate social behavior.

1889 Toxoplasmosis
March of Dimes
1275 Mamaroneck Avenue   914-997-4488
White Plains, NY 10605   Fax: 212-254-3518
                                NY639@marchofdimes.com
                                www.marchofdimes.com
Fact Sheets: one or two page review written for the general public.

Audio & Video

1890 Genetics and Inherited Traits
March of Dimes
1275 Mamaroneck Avenue   914-997-4488
White Plains, NY 10605   Fax: 212-254-3518
                                NY639@marchofdimes.com
                                www.marchofdimes.com
Fact Sheets: one or two page review written for the general public.

1891 Why My Child
5400 Diplomat Circle   407-629-1466
Orlando, FL 32810-5603   800-313-2232
                                www.birthdefects.org
A 9 1/2 minute video that explores the feelings every parent has when their child is born with a birth defect. Emmy-award-winning producer, Karen Dorsett, has created a compelling video that begins with the parents' question, Why my child? and follows through to concerns about links between birth defects and environmental exposures to drugs, pesticides, dioxin, radiation, hazardous wastes, etc.

Web Sites

1892 Birth Defect Research for Children, Inc.
                                www.birthdefects.org
Provides parents and expectant parents with information about birth defects and support services for their children.

1893 Healing Well
                                www.healingwell.com
A social network and support community for patients, caregivers, and families coping with the daily struggles of diseases, disorders and chronic illness.

1894 Health Finder
                                www.healthfinder.gov
A government web site where individuals can find information and tools to help you and those you care about stay healthy.

1895 Healthlink USA
                                www.healthlinkusa.com
Health information concerning treatment, cures, prevention, diagnosis, risk factors, research, support groups, email lists, personal stories and much more. Updated regularly.

1896 March of Dimes Foundation
                                www.marchofdimes.org
Online resources on birth defects.

1897 MedicineNet
                                www.medicinenet.com
An online resource for consumers providing easy-to-read, authoritative medical and health information.

1898 Medscape
                                www.medscape.com
Medscape offers specialists, primary care physicians, and other health professionals the Web's most robust and integrated medical information and educational tools.

1899 WebMD
                                www.webmd.com
Provides credible information, supportive communities, and in-depth reference material about health subjects. A source for original and timely health information as well as material from well known content providers.

Description

1900 Brain Tumors

Brain tumors are either primary (originate in the brain) or metastatic (travel from other cancer sites). About 87,000 people in the United States are diagnosed with primary brain tumors each year; approximately 70 percent of those are benign (noncancerous). Cancerous brain tumors originating in the brain make up roughly 2 percent of all cancers, but they constitute 20 percent of all childhood cancers. They may occur at any age but are most common in early adult and middle life. Metastatic brain tumors (those that spread from other cancers) occur in 20-40 percent of all cancers.

There are many different types of brain tumors, each with a distinctive appearance under the microscope and a characteristic pattern of onset, progression, genetic abnormalities, location and response to treatment. Depending on the exact site and rate of growth of the tumor, symptoms may include change in personality, moodiness, impaired vision and hearing, headaches, nausea, vomiting, seizures, lethargy and a varying degree of weakness. The most common group of primary brain tumors are gliomas, which arise from glial cells, which are the support cells in the central nervous system. Neuronal tumors, or tumors that arise from neurons (those cells that conduct nerve impulses within the nervous system) are far less common than gliomas and tend to occur in younger adults and cause seizures. About 5- 10 percent of brain tumors result from genetic factors that are inherited. In most cases, the cause of an individual's brain tumor is not known.

The treatment of brain tumors, as in many other cancers, consists of a combination of surgical removal, chemotherapy and radiation therapy. The types of chemotherapeutic agents available to treat brain tumors is limited, since most anti-cancer agents do not penetrate the blood-brain barrier. This limitation can be circumvented by injecting agents directly into the brain. Steroids reduce swelling, and antiseizure medications are commonly given. If the disease or its treatment has caused damage to the brain's functioning, the patient may also need physical therapy, speech therapy, or general supportive care. The prognosis depends on the patient's age and on the location, extent and precise type of the tumor. See also *Head Injuries*.

National Agencies & Associations

1901 American Brain Tumor Association

8550 W Bryn Mawr Avenue
Chicago, IL 60631
773-577-8750
800-886-2282
Fax: 773-577-8738
info@abta.org
www.abta.org

Services includes over 40 publications which address brain tumors, their treatment and coping with the disease. Materials address brain tumors in all age groups. Provides free social service consultations and a mentorship program for new brain tumor support groups.
Ralph DeVitto, President & CEO
Nicole Willmarth, PhD, Chief Mission Officer

1902 National Brain Tumor Society

55 Chapel Street
Newton, MA 02458
617-924-9997
Fax: 617-924-9998
development@braintumor.org
www.braintumor.org

Exists to find a cure for brain tumors and strives to improve the quality of life of brain tumor patients and their families. Disseminates educational information and provides access to psycho-social support and raises funds.
David F. Arons, JD, Chief Executive Officer
Kirk Tanner, PhD, Chief Scientific Officer

1903 National Institute of Neurological Disorders and Stroke

NIH Neurological Institute
Bethesda, MD 20824
301-496-5751
800-352-9424
www.ninds.nih.gov

Seeks to reduce the burden of neurological disease affecting individuals from all walks of life.
Walter J. Koroshetz, MD, Director
Amy B. Adams, Director, Office of Scientific Liaison

Foundations

1904 Brain Tumor Foundation of Canada

205 Horton Street E
London, Ontario, N6B-1K7
519-642-7755
800-265-5106
www.braintumour.ca

Seeks to find the cause of, and a cure for, brain tumors while also assisting affected individuals.
Susan Marshall, Chief Executive Officer
Suzanne Fratschko Elliott, Manager, Fundraising & Engagement

1905 Children's Brain Tumor Foundation

1460 Broadway
New York, NY 10036
212-448-9494
866-228-4673
Fax: 212-448-1022
info@cbtf.org
www.cbtf.org

Children's Brain Tumor Foundation (CBTF) is a national organization whose mission is to improve the treatment, quality of life and long-term outlook for children with brain and spinal cord tumors through research, support, education, and advocacy to families and survivors. CBTF provides research and quality of life grants, offers information and support via our toll free line, written educational material, meet the unique needs of childhood brain tumor survivors.
Robert Budlow, Chair
Wade Iwata, Director, Quality of Life Programs

1906 Pediatric Brain Tumor Foundation

302 Ridgefield Court
Asheville, NC 28806
828-665-6891
800-253-6530
Fax: 828-655-6894
info@curethekids.org
www.curethekids.org

Dedicated to finding the cause and cure of childhood brain tumors through the support of medical research. Increases public awareness, aids in early detection and treatment, supports a national database on all primary brain tumors. Helps to provide hope and emotional support for the thousands of children and families affected by this life threatening disease.
Robin Boettcher, President/CEO
Shelley Pressley, National Manager of Family Support

California

1907 Pediatric Brain Tumor Foundation: California Chapter

16911 San Fernando Mission Blvd
Granada Hills, CA 91344
310-650-4782
www.curethekids.org

Provides information and emotional support for families of children with brain tumors. They also raise funds for brain tumor re-

search and provide a telephone network system of parents who offer emotional support.
Tammy Bates, Managing Director
Katie Sheridan, Manager, Family Support Programs

Georgia

1908 Pediatric Brain Tumor Foundation: Georgia Chapter
6065 Roswell Road NE   404-252-4107
Atlanta, GA 30328   Fax: 404-252-4108
                                     www.curethekids.org
Provides information and emotional support for families of children with brain tumors. They also raise funds for brain tumor research and provide a telephone network system of parents who offer emotional support.
Tammy Bates, Managing Director
Katie Sheridan, Manager, Family Support Programs

Research Centers

1909 Brain Research Center Children s Hospital National Medical Cen
Children s Hospital National Medical Center
111 Michigan Avenue NW   202-476-3000
Washington, DC 20010   800-884-5433
                                     Fax: 202-884-5226
                                          tbear@cnmc.org
                                    www.dcchildrens.com

Edwin K Zechman Jr, President
Mark L Batshaw, Chief Medical Officer

1910 Brain Research Foundation
111 W Washington Street   312-759-5150
Chicago, IL 60602   Fax: 312-759-5151
                                         info@theBRF.org
                                           www.thebrf.org
Supports cutting-edge neuroscience research that will lead to novel treatments and prevention of neurological disease and disorders in children and adults. Deliver this commitment through seed grants, which provide early stage fundinf for innovative research projects, as well as educational programs for researchers and the general public.
Nathan Hansom, President
Terre A Constantine PhD, Executive Director

1911 Brain Tissue Resource Center McLean Hospital
McLean Hospital
115 Mill Street   617-855-2000
Belmont, MA 02478   800-272-4622
                                     Fax: 617-855-3199
                            mcleaninfo@mclean.harvard.edu
A centralized resource for the collection and distribution of human brain specimens for brain research.
Francine M Benes, Director
Edward D Bird, Director Emeritus

1912 Central Brain Tumor Registry of the US
244 E Ogden avenue   630-655-4786
Hinsdale, IL 60521   Fax: 630-655-1756
                                          cbtrus@aol.com
                                           www.cbtrus.org
Nonprofit resource for gathering and distributing current statistics on all primary brain tumors for the entire US. Includes data on benign borderline and malignant primary brain tumors.
Carol Kruchko, President /Administrator
Jeri Dolan, Executive Administrator

1913 University of California, San Francisco Brain Tumor Research Center
Department of Neurological Surgery
505 Parnassus Avenue   415-353-7500
San Francisco, CA 94143-0112   Fax: 415-353-2889
                                  garritye@neurosurg.ucsf.edu
Continuously funded by grants from the National Institutes of Health Since 1072, the Brain Tumor Research Center at UCSF is internationally recognized as a major research and treatment center for adults and children with tumors of the brain and spinal cord. This center emphasizes translational research into the biology and behavior of brain tumors - research in which scientists and health care clinicians work in partnership to translate laboratory findings of new or improved forms of therapy.
Charles B Wilson, Director
Michael Gillis, Administrative Director

Support Groups & Hotlines

1914 National Health Information Center
Office of Disease Prevention & Health Promotion
1101 Wootton Pkwy   Fax: 240-453-8281
Rockville, MD 20852   odphpinfo@hhs.gov
                                   www.health.gov/nhic
Supports public health education by maintaining a calendar of National Health Observances; helps connect consumers and health professionals to organizations that can best answer questions and provide up-to-date contact information from reliable sources; updates on a yearly basis toll-free numbers for health information, Federal health clearinghouses and info centers.
Don Wright, MD, MPH, Director

Alabama

1915 Pediatric Brain Tumor Support Group
Children's Hospital
1600 7th Avenue S   205-939-9090
Birmingham, AL 35233-1785
Groups for parents and siblings of brain tumor patients. Related to Children's Hospital of Alabama. Babysitting available.
Paula Teague

Arizona

1916 Arizona Brain Tumor Support Group
Barrow Neurological Ins of St. Joe's Hospital
350 W Thomas Road   623-205-6446
Phoenix, AZ 85013   www.braintumorfoundation.org
Lanette Veres, Director

1917 Southern Arizona Brain Tumor Support Group
Arizona Cancer Cetner
1515 N Campbell Avenue   520-694-4605
Tucson, AZ   www.braintumorfoundation.org
Marsha Drozdoff, Contact

California

1918 Bereavement Group for Children
The Center for Attitudinal Healing
33 Buchanan Drive   415-331-6161
Sausalito, CA 94965   www.braintumor.org
Jimmy Pete, Contact

1919 Brain Tumor Society
National Brain Tumor Society
22 Battery Street   415-834-9970
San Francisco, CA 94111-5520   800-770-8287
                                     Fax: 415-834-9980
                                       info@braintumor.org
                                        www.braintumor.org

N Paul TonThat, Executive Director

1920 Brain Tumor Support Group: Duarte
City of Hope National Medical Center
55 Chapel Street   617-924-9997
Newton, MA 02458   Fax: 617-924-9998
                                        www.braintumor.org
Help you learn more about brain tumors including symptoms, treatment options, and considerations for caregivers.
Heather Ducksworth, Contact

1921 Brain Tumor Support Group: Fresno
Cancer Center at St. Agnes
7130 N Millbrook Avenue   559-450-5528
Fresno, CA 93720   karen.kennedy@samc.com
                                        www.braintumor.org

Karen Kennedy, Contact

1922 Brain Tumor Support Group: Fullerton
St. Jude Medical Plaza

2151 N Harbor Blvd
Fullerton, CA 92835
714-446-7182
kathy.pearson@stjoe.org
www.braintumor.org

Kathy Pearson RN, Contact

1923 Brain Tumor Support Group: Newport Beach
Hoag Hospital
Advanced Technology Pavilion
Newport Beach, CA 92663
949-764-6036
lberberet@hoaghospital.org
www.braintumor.org

Lori Berberet RN, Contact

1924 Brain Tumor Support Group: Orange
UC Irvine-Chao Family Comprehensive Cancer Center
101 The City Drive
Orange, CA 92868
714-456-8609
bakerd@uci.edu
www.braintumor.org

N. Paul TonThat, Chief Executive Officer
Michele Rhee, Director of Program Initiatives

1925 Brain Tumor Support Group: Redding
American Cancer Society
3290 Bechelli Lane
Redding, CA 96002
530-222-1058
www.braintumor.org

1926 Brain Tumor Support Group: Sacramento
UC Davis Ambulatory Care Center
4860 Y Street
Sacramento, CA 95817
916-734-5613
kksmith@ucdavis.edu
www.braintumor.org

Karen Smith RN, Contact
Carolyn Guadagnolo LCSW, Contact

1927 Brain Tumor Support Group: San Diego
Kaiser's Pt Loma Medical Facility
3250 Fordham
San Diego, CA 92117
619-515-9908
www.braintumor.org
Connie Campbell, Contact

1928 Brain Tumor Support Group: San Francisco
UCSF
521 Parnassus Avenue
San Francisco, CA 94143
415-990-4461
mlovely@braintumor.org
www.braintumor.org

Sharon Lamb RN, Contact
Mary Lovely RN, Contact

1929 Brain Tumor Support Group: Santa Barbara
Cancer Center of Santa Barbara
300 W Pueblo Street
Santa Barbara, CA 93105
805-563-5852
www.braintumor.org
Rosario Campuzano, Contact

1930 Brain Tumor Support Group: Stanford
Stanford Cancer Center
875 Blake Wilbur Drive
Stanford, CA 94305
415-990-4461
mlovely@braintumor.org
www.braintumor.org

Joanie Taylor RN, Contact
Sharon Lamb RN, Contact

1931 Brain Tumor Support Group: Westlake Village
The Wellness Community
530 Hampshire Road
Westlake Village, CA 91361
805-379-4777
www.braintumor.org

Rebecca Dekker MFT, Contact

1932 Brain Tumor/Pituitary Patient Support Group
John Wayne Cancer Institute
2200 Santa Monica Blvd
Santa Monica, CA 90404
949-515-9595
pituitarybuddy@hotmail.com
www.braintumor.org

Sharmyn McGraw, Contact

1933 Children Living with Illness
The Center for Attitudinal Healing
33 Buchanan Drive
Sausalito, CA 94965
415-331-6161
Fax: 415-331-4545
www.healingcenter.org

Don Goewey, Executive Director

1934 Glendale Adventist Medical Center Brain Tumor Support Group
Cancer Services
381 Merrill Avenue
Glendale, CA 91026
818-409-3530
www.braintumor.org
Connie Munoz LCSW, Contact

1935 Heads Up!
Northridge Hospital Medical Center
18300 Roscoe Blvd
Northridge, CA 91325
818-885-8500
www.braintumor.org
Wanda Martin, Contact
Robert Salazar, Additional Contact

1936 Neuro-Oncology Information and Support Group
Sister Mary Pia Regional Cancer Center
1800 N California Street
Stockton, CA 95204-6019
209-467-6550
www.stjosephscares.org
For patients and family members living with primary and metastatic brain tumors as well as spinal cord tumors. Free child care and refreshments are provided.
Jim Linderman

1937 Neuroscience Institute Brain Tumor Hotline
Hospital of the Good Samaritan
637 Lucas Avenue
Los Angeles, CA 90017-1912
800-762-1692
info@goodsam.org
www.goodsam.org

Diana Selover, LCSW

1938 Patient Services
22 Battery Street
San Francisco, CA 94111-5520
415-834-9970
800-934-2873
Fax: 415-834-9980
info@braintumor.org
www.braintumor.org

Quickly access brain tumor information and resources.
12 pages
George Gellert, Chief Medical Officer
N. Paul TonThat, Executive Director

1939 Peninsula Support & Education Group for Parents of Children with Brain Tumors
Parents Helping Parents
1400 Parkmoor Avenue
San Jose, CA 95126-3222
408-727-5775
855-727-5775
Fax: 408- 28- 111
info@php.com
www.php.com

A comprehensive family resource center providing information, training, guidance and support to families of children with special needs and the professionals who serve them.
Suzanne Cistulli, Chair
Robert Badagliacco, Treasurer

1940 Support Group for Caregivers of Brain Tumor Patients
UCLA Medical Center
200 UCLA Medical Plaza
Los Angeles, CA 90095
310-206-6731
cabe@mednet.ucla.edu
Cheryl Abe LCSW, Clinical Social Worker
Pamela Hoff LCSW, Clinical Social Worker

1941 Vital Options International
4419 Coldwater Canyon Avenue
Studio City, CA 91604-1479
818-508-5657
Fax: 818-788-5260
info@vitaloptions.org
www.vitaloptions.org

A not-for-profit cancer communications, support, and advocacy organization with a mission, to facilitate a global cancer dialogue.
Selma R Schimmel, CEO/Founder
Juliana Lee, Production Manager

1942 Wellness Community Cancer Support Groups
San Francisco/East Bay
3276 Mc Nutt Avenue
Walnut Creek, CA 94597
925-933-0107
emaslan@yahoo.com
www.braintumor.org

Erika Maslan MFCC, Contact

1943 Wellness Community: South Bay Cities
109 W Torrance Blvd
Redondo Beach, CA 90277   www.braintumor.org
Tom May, Contact

1944 Wellness Community: West Los Angeles
2716 Ocean Park Blvd
Santa Monica, CA 90405   www.braintumor.org

1945 Support Group for Parents of Children with Brain Tumors
Oakland Children's Hospital
747 52nd Street   510-428-3885
Oakland, CA   800-400-PEDS
    www.kidsfirst.org
Trish Murphy

Colorado

1946 Brain Tumor Resource and Vital Encouragement
Childrens Hospital
1056 19th Avenue   303-861-8888
Denver, CO
Pediatric focus. Education and support. Retreats for parents of brain tumor patients.
Jim Shmerling, DHA, FACHE, President & CEO

1947 Colorado Brain Tumor Support Group
Swedish Medical Center   303-806-7420
Englewood, CO 80113   lgibson@thecni.org
    www.braintumorfoundation.org
Lorre Gibson, Contact

Connecticut

1948 Connecticut Brain Tumor Support Group
20 York Street   203-785-7528
New Haven, CT 06510   Fax: 203-688-2395
    www.braintumorfoundation.org
Angela Thomas LCSW, Contact

Delaware

1949 Pediatric Brain Tumor Support Group
Ronald McDonald House
PO Box 269   302-661-4077
Wilmington, DE 19899-3629   izienberg@kidshealth.org
    www.kidshealth.org
Niel Izienberg MD, Chief Executive Officer and Founder

District of Columbia

1950 Washington DC Metropolitan Area Support Group
George Washington University
2150 Pennsylvania Aveneu NW   202-994-4035
Washington, DC 20037-3201
Margaret Fiore, RN

Florida

1951 Angels in the Sun Brain Tumor Support Group
Wellness Community
3900 Clark Road   941-921-5539
Sarasota, FL 34233   www.braintumorfoundation.org
John Kleinbaum, Program Director

1952 Brain Tumor Support Group
Miami Children's Hospital Foundation
3000 SW 62nd Avenue   305-662-8386
Miami, FL 33155   maria.penate@mch.com
Maria Penate RN, Facilitator
Raquel Pasaron, Facilitator

1953 Florida Brain Tumor Association
PO Box 770182   954-755-4307
Coral Springs, FL 33077-0182   sshetsky@fbta.info
    www.fbta.info
Provides hope, support and education to brain tumor survivors, their families and friends; conquers brain tumors by funding re-

search into their causes and cures; and enriches the quality of life of those touched by brain tumors
Sheryl Shetsky, President
Gary L Kornfeld, VP

1954 Florida Brain Tumor Support Group
Healthpark Medical Ctr, Meeting Rm   239-433-4396
Ft Meyers, FL 33919   www.braintumorfoundation.org
Dona Ross, Contact

1955 Florida Brain Tumor Support Group: Deerfield Beach
North Broward Medical Center   954-755-4307
Deerfield Beach, FL 33441   www.fbta.info
Sheryl Shetsky, President
Gary L Kornfeld, VP

1956 Hollywood Area Brain Tumor Support Group
Memorial Regional Hospital   954-265-4725
Hollywood, FL 33021   csurloff@mhs.net
    www.floridabraintumor.com
Sheryl Shetsky, Founder & President
Gary L. Kornfeld, Vice President

1957 Sarasota Area Brain Tumor Support Group
Institute of Advanced Medicine
5880 Rand Avenue   www.fbta.info
Sarasota, FL
Sheryl R Shetsky, President
Gary L Kornfeld, VP

1958 West Palm Beach Area Brain Tumor Support Group
Good Samaritan Medical Center   561-655-5511
West Palm Beach, FL 33401
Sheryl R Shetsky, President
Gary L Kornfeld, VP

Georgia

1959 All Ages Support Group
Brain Tumor Foundation for Children
6065 Roswell Road NE   404-252-4107
Atlanta, GA 30328-4015   Fax: 404-252-4108
    info@braintumorkids.org
    www.braintumorkids.org/
Patient Support Group Activities includes bowling, fishing, craft parties, picnics, sporting events, holiday parties, etc. These activities, social events and more are provided for children of all ages and their families.
Mary Campbell, Executive Director
R Hal Meeks Jr, President

1960 Emory Brain Tumor Support Group
Emory Clinic
Department of Neurosurgery   404-778-3091
Atlanta, GA 30322
Meets the first Thursday of each month with the purpose of providing an opportunity for information-sharing and suport for brain tumor patients, as well as their family, friends and caregivers.
Maxine Brown, Contact

1961 Hearts and Minds
Piedmont Hospital
1968 Peachtree Road NW   404-373-5202
Atlanta, GA   Fax: 404-605-5000
    www.piedmonthospital.org
H.M McFarling, M.D, Chairman
Leslie A. Donahue, President & CEO

1962 SBTF Brain Tumor Support Group
PO Box 422471   404-843-3700
Atlanta, GA 30342   info@sbtf.org
    www.sbtf.org
To improve the quality of life for brain tumor patients and their families.
Costas Hadjipanayis, President
Jennifer Kee Giliberto, Vice President

Illinois

1963 American Brain Tumor Association
8550 W Bryn Mawr Avenue
Chicago, IL 60631

800-886-2282
info@abta.org
www.abta.org

CareLine offered for newly diagnosed patients with brain tumors.
Ralph DeVitto, President & CEO
Nicole Willmarth, PhD, Chief Mission Officer

1964 Brain Tumor Support Group
Northwestern Memorial Hospital
675 N St. Clair
Chicago, IL 60611

312-695-8143
312-695-0990
mmaher@nmff.org
www.cancer.northwestern.edu

Steven Rosen, Director
Leonidas Platanias, MD, PhD, Deputy Director

1965 Parents of Children with Brain Tumors PCBT
Children's Memorial Hospital
2300 Children's Plaza
Chicago, IL 60614

773-880-4316

Meets quarterly and publishes a monthly newsletter. Library available at meetings (at CMH). Educational speakers and family functions.
Gina Baldacci LCSW, Contact

Indiana

1966 Brain Tumor Support Group
Community Hospital East
1500 North Ritter Avenue
Indianapolis, IN 46219

317-355-1411
www.ecommunity.com/east

Michael Kemf, Facilitator
Marsha Cline, Facilitator

1967 Primary Brain Cancer Support Group
Women's Cancer Center at Lutheran Hospital
7950 W Jefferson Boulevard
Fort Wayne, IN 46804

260-435-7959

Linda Jordan RN, Contact

Iowa

1968 Iowa Brain Tumor Support Group
University of Iowa Hospitals
Iowa City, IA 52242

319-356-2557

Lori Roetlin, Contact
Sue May, Additional Contact

1969 Neurological Center of Iowa
Iowa Clinic
5950 University Avenue
Des Moines, IA 50266-1418

515-875-9100
Fax: 515-241-6090
www.iowaclinic.com/

Networks people in similar situations.
Mark A. Reece, Chairman of the Board
Steven A. Keller, Chair Patient Care Committee

1970 Quad Cities Brain Tumor Support Group
Genesis Medical Center
1401 W Central Park
Davenport, IA 52804

563-421-1907

Deb Ide, Contact

Kansas

1971 Gray Matters Support: Kansas City
24050 W 57th Street
Shawnee, KS 66226

graymatters2007@yahoo.com

Debbie Stephenson, Contact

1972 Headstrong Brain Tumor Support Group
Victory in the Valley
3755 E Douglas
Wichita, KS 67218

316-682-7400
info@victoryinthevalley.com
www.victoryinthevalley.org

Cary Cozby, Golf Pro & CEO
Tim Farrell, President, RST Ventures, Inc

Kentucky

1973 Meningioma/Benign Brain Tumor Support Group
Michael Quinlan Brain Tumor Foundation
4012 Dupont Circle
Louisville, KY 40207

502-896-1701

Kathy Quinlan-Thompson, Contact

1974 Wellness Community: Kentucky
1717 Dixie Highway
Fort Wright, KY 41011

859-331-5568
www.cancersupportcincinnati.org

Rick Bryan, Executive Director
Gail Laule, Office Manager

Louisiana

1975 Brain Tumor Support Group
3939 Houma Boulevard, Doctor's Row
Metairie, LA 70005

504-835-5715
gmom224@cox.net
www.braintumor.org

Meets on the third Sunday of each month at 1:30 p.m., call to confirm.
Gayle Johnson, Contact Person

Maine

1976 Brain Tumor Support Group of Maine
Maine Medical Center
22 Bramhall Street
Portland, ME 04102

207-871-4527

Meets on the second Tuesday of each month from 7:00 to 9:00 p.m.
Nancy Fortier LCSW, Contact

Maryland

1977 Brain Tumor Networking Group
10628 Falls Road
Lutherville, MD 21022

410-832-2719
www.loyolamedicine.org

Ronald Petrocelli, Chair
Michael Cathey, Vice Chair

1978 Brain Tumor Support Group: Maryland
NIH Clinical Research Center
9000 Rockville Pike
Bethesda, MD 20892

301-496-6380
garrenn@mail.nih.gov
www.braintumor.org

Nancy Garren, Contact

1979 Brainiacs
Perryville Library
Perryville, MD 21903

410-459-8157

Liz Carrino, Contact

1980 Johns Hopkins Brain Tumor Education Group
Weinberg Building
Baltimore, MD 21231

410-502-2789

Liz Carrino, Contact

1981 Washington DC Metropolitan Area Brain Tumor Support Group
George Washington Ambulatory Center
I & 22nd Street
Middletown, MD 21769

301-371-8660

Lionel Chaiken, Contact
Jeff Schanz, Contact

Massachusetts

1982 Brain Tumor Patient and Caregiver Support Group
Dana Farber Cancer Institute
Boston, MA 02115

617-632-3634

Nancy Tharler LICSW, Contact

1983 Brain Tumor Support Group: Lahey
Lahey Clinic Medical Center
41 Mall Road
Burlington, MA 01805

617-726-1061
www.lahey.org

Michele Lucas MSW LICSW, Contact

1984 Brain Tumor Support Group: Worcester
UMass Memorial Medical Center-University Campus

55 Lake Avenue N
Worcester, MA 01655

508-334-7595
Fax: 800-697-2593
ellen.sharenow@umassmemorial.org
www.braintumor.org

Ellen Sharenow PhD, Contact

1985 Neurological Support Group of St. Luke's Hospital
101 Page Street   508-997-1515
New Bedford, MA 02740-3464
Diane Robinson RN

1986 Parent Education/Support Group
Dana Farber Cancer Institute
44 Binney Street   617-632-3301
Boston, MA 2115   800-525-5068
www.dfci.harvard.edu
For parents of children with brain tumors. Please call for schedule.
Beverly Lavalley Run, Facilitator
Edward Benz Jr, President

Michigan

1987 Brain Tumor Networking Club
Gilda's Club Metro Detroit
3517 Rochester Road   248-577-0800
Royal Oak, MI 48073   Fax: 248-577-0898
Kristen Bernat, Contact

1988 Brain Tumor Support Group for Patients & Families
University of Michigan Medical Center
1500 E Medical Center Drive   734-936-9071
Ann Arbor, MI 48109-0316
Christina Crandall, Contact
Kathy Wilson, Contact

1989 Brain Tumor Support Group: Ann Arbor
St Joseph Mercy Hospital, Cancer Care Center
5301 E Huron River Drive   734-712-3658
Ann Arbor, MI 48106   www.sjmh.com
Paula Nedela RN, Contact

1990 Brain Tumor Support Group: West Bloomfield
Henry Ford Hospital
6777 W Maple   313-916-1796
West Bloomfield, MI 48322
Sandy Remer RN, Contact

Missouri

1991 Brain Cancer Support Group
St John's Hospital
Main Hospital   417-820-3157
Springfield, MO 65804   laura.flowers@mercy.net
Laura Flowers, Contact

1992 Brain Tumor Support Group: Kansas City
St Luke's Hospital of Kansas City
4321 Washington Suite 4000   816-932-6015
Kansas City, MO 64111
Michelle Martin, Contact

1993 Brain Tumor Support and Networking Group
Wellness Community of Greater St. Louis
1058 Old Des Peres Road   314-238-2000
Saint Louis, MO 63131   www.wellnesscommunitystl.org/
Mitchell L Baris, Chair of the Board
Mary Jane Pieroni, CPA, Treasurer

Montana

1994 Cancer Patient/Caregiver Support Group
Wellness Community
1820 W Lincoln Street   406-582-1600
Bozeman, MT 59715   twcmontana@qwest.net
Becky Robideaux, Contact

New Hampshire

1995 Brain Injury/Brain Tumor Support Group
Frisbie Memorial Hospital

Carroll Room
Rochester, NH 03867
Wendy Mitchell LMSW, Contact

New Jersey

1996 Brain Tumor Support Group: New Jersey
90 Bergen Street   973-972-1164
Newark, NJ 07103
LaDawn McClamb, Contact

1997 Brain Tumor Support Group: Toms River
Community Medical Center
99 Highway 37 W   732-557-8270
Toms River, NJ 08755
Sherry Laniado LCSW, Contact

1998 Central New Jersey Brain Tumor Support Group
St. Luke's Roman Catholic Church
300 Clinton Avenue   732-321-7000
North Plainfield, NJ 07063
Patty Anthony RN, Contact
Virginia Shrodo, Contact

New Mexico

1999 People Living Through Cancer Support Groups
3411 Candelaria NE   505-242-3263
Albuquerque, NM 87107   888-441-4439
Fax: 505-242-6756
info@pltc.org
www.pltc.org
A not for profit organization that connects and supports cancer survivors and caregivers by transforming shared individual experiences into enduring hope.
Beth Brown, Executive Director
Mary Ellen Kurucz, Program Director

New York

2000 Brain Tumor Support Group for Patients and Families
Albany Medical Center
Office of NY Oncology/Hematology   845-338-4820
Albany, NY 12208-3412   eehauser@gmail.com
www.braintumor.org/patients-family-frien
Emilie Hauser, Contact

2001 Brain Tumor Support Group: Long Island
230 Main St. Emma Clark Library   516-747-8749
Setauket, NY
Billie Wilczek

2002 Long Island Brain Tumor Support Group
Old Bethpage Public Library
999 Old Country Road   516-996-3705
Plainview, NY 11803
Bob Crescenzo, Contact

2003 Mount Sinai Medical Center Brain Tumor Support Group
Ruttenberg Care Center-Guggenheim Pavilion
1190 Fifth Ave   212-717-3527
New York, NY 10029
Kathleen Maloney-Lutz RN, Contact

2004 New York Brain Tumor Support Group
525 E 68th Street   212-746-3986
New York, NY 10021   wem9011@nyp.org
www.braintumor.org
Wendy Mitchell LMSW, Contact

North Carolina

2005 Brain Tumor Support Group: Raleigh Area
Raleigh Community Hospital
3400 Wake Forest Road   919-846-0923
Raleigh, NC 27609-7373   www.raleighcommunity.com
Lectures, educational materials, and newsletter. Home and hospi-
tal visitation.
Louise Clark, Director

2006 Duke Pediatric Brain Tumor Family Support Program
Preston Robert Tisch Brain Tumor Center
Duke University Medical Center   919-684-5301
Durham, NC 27710   Fax: 919-684-6674
korpi001@mc.duke.edu
www.cancer.duke.edu/btc/

Darell D. Binger, MD, PhD, Director
Allan H Friedman MD, Deputy Director

2007 Preston Robert Tisch Brain Tumor Center at Duke
Cornucopia Cancer Support Center
5517 Durham Chapel Hill Blvd   919-668-6178
Durham, NC 27707   stephanie.english@duke.edu
www.cancer.duke.edu

Stephanie English MSW LCSW, Contact

Ohio

2008 Brain Tumor Support Group: Cincinnati
Wellness Community
4918 Cooper Road   513-791-4060
Cincinnati, OH 45242   Fax: 513-791-8239

2009 Southwest Ohio Brain Tumor Support Group
Kettering Medical Center
3535 Southern Boulevard   937-298-3399
Kettering, OH 45429-1221
Ronald Petrocelli, M.D., Chair
Michael Cathey, Vice Chair

2010 Support Group for Parents of Children with Brain Tumors
Cincinnati Childrens Hospital Medical Center
Childrens Hospital Medical Center   513-636-4200
Cincinnati, OH 45229-3039   800-344-2462
www.cincinnatichildrens.org/default.htm

Thomas Boat, Director
Stephen Daniels, Associate Chair

Oregon

2011 Brain Tumor Education & Support Group
Legacy Good Samaritan Hospital Cancer Center
1130 NW 22nd Ave   503-413-7921
Portland, OR 97210
Wendy Talbot MSW LCSW, Contact
Selma Annala RT CLC, Contact

2012 Central Oregon Brain Tumor Support Group
900 SW 23rd Place   541-350-7243
Redmond, OR 97756   rgklug@crestviewcable.com
Rubyanne Klug, Contact

Pennsylvania

2013 Brain Tumor Community Group
Lancaster General Health Campus
Wellness Conference Room   800-860-9949
Lancaster, PA 17601
Christine Burfete RN, Contact

2014 Brain Tumor Support Group: Johnstown
John P Murtha Neuroscience and Pain Institute
1450 Scalp Avenue   814-534-3797
Johnstown, PA 15904   dlehew@conemaugh.org
www.braintumor.org

N. Paul TonThat, Chief Executive Officer
Michele Rhee, Director of Program Initiatives

2015 Brain Tumor Support Group: Philadelphia
University of PA Hospital-Neurological Institute
3400 Spruce Street   215-615-5240
Philadelphia, PA 19104
Alisha Amendt MSN CRNP, Contact
Arbena Merolli MSW, Contact

2016 Brain Tumor Support Group: Pittsburgh
Cancer Caring Center
4117 Liberty Avenue   412-622-1212
Pittsburgh, PA 15224

2017 Delware Valley Brain Tumor Support Group at Jefferson
Jefferson Health System
Bluemle Life Sciences Building   215-955-4429
Philadelphia, PA 19107
Ann Marie DiBona RN, Contact
Janis Haaf RN, Contact

2018 Pediatric Cancer Foundation of the Lehigh Valley
Camelot for Children
2354 W Emmaus Avenue   610-393-9215
Allentown, PA 18103
Nicole Ronco, Contact

Rhode Island

2019 Brain Tumor Support Group: Providence
Brown University Campus
BioMedical Center   401-789-0126
Providence, RI 02912
Judy Allenson, Contact
Betty Bentley, Contact

2020 Rhode Island Brain & Spine Tumor Foundation
Bethany Home
229 Medway Street   401-272-4177
Providence, RI 02906   ribstf@gmail.com
Colin Shaw, Contact

South Carolina

2021 Brain Tumor Support Group: Charleston
Hollings Cancer Center
86 Jonathon Lucas Street   843-792-8257
Charleston, SC 29445   lizzic@musc.edu
www.braintumor.org

Christa Lizzi RN, Contact

2022 Brain Tumor Support Group: Florence
Florence Neurosurgery and Spine
1204 E Cheves Street   843-206-1910
Florence, SC 29506   info@florenceneurosurgery.com
www.braintumor.org

South Dakota

2023 Cancer Support Group
Sanford Cancer Cetner Oncology Clinic
1020 W 18th Street   605-328-8000
Sioux Falls, SD 57104   www.lls.org/aboutlls/chapters/mn/patient
Sue Halbritter RN NP, Contact

Tennessee

2024 Cancer Support Group: Knoxville
Wellness Community of East Tennessee
2230 Sutherland Avenue   865-546-4661
Knoxville, TN 37919   Fax: 865-522-0938
www.cancersupportet.org

Christi Branscom, President
Beth Lee, Secretary

2025 Cancer Support Group: Nashville
Gilda's Club Nashville
1707 Division Street   615-329-1124
Nashville, TN 37203

2026 Memphis Regional Brain Tumor Survivors Group
Methodist University Hospital
1265 Union Ave   904-757-0806
Memphis, TN 38104
Cherry Welborn, Contact

Texas

2027 Brain Tumor Support Group: El Paso
Rio Grande Cancer Foundation
10460 Vista Del Sol Drive   915-562-7660
El Paso, TX 79925
Jutta Ramirez, Contact
Robert Lefferts, Contact

2028 Central Texas Brain Tumor Support Group
Brain and Spine Center at Brackenridge Hospital
274 Madison Avenue 512-636-1578
New York, NY 10016 866-228-4673
info@cbtf.org
www.cbtf.org
Contains practical information to sort out the complexities of medical procedures, interruptions in school and social life, and uncertainty about the future.
Thomas Lewman, Contact

2029 Houston Area Brain Tumor Network
MD Anderson Cancer Center Brain & Spine Center
1515 Holcombe Blvd 713-794-1777
Houston, TX 77030 spanju@mdanderson.org
Mark Anderson, Contact
Suki Panju, Contact

2030 South Texas Brain Tumor Foundation Support Group
San Antonio Employees Federal Credit Union
6000 NW Loop 410 210-670-9323
San Antonio, TX 78201
Susie Soriano, Contact

Utah

2031 Cancer Wellness House
59 S 1100 E 801-236-2294
Salt Lake City, UT 84102
Karen Elliott

Virginia

2032 Brain Tumor Support Group: Richmond
St Mary's Hospital
Education Center 877-284-3905
Richmond, VA 23226 curebt@hotmail.com
www.abta.org
Ronald Petrocelli, M.D., Chair
Michael Cathey, Vice Chair

2033 Valley Brain Tumor Support Group
Rehab2Health
Shenandoah Memorial Hospital 540-984-4921
Woodstock, VA 22664 vbtsg@shentel.net
Valorie Hockman, Contact

Washington

2034 Brain Cancer Support Group: Port Orchard
2186 Yukon Harbor Rd SE 360-536-5042
Port Orchard, WA 98366 ideas56@msn.com
Victoria Tierney MA RC, Contact

2035 Brain Cancer Support Group: Seattle
Northwest Hospital
Professional Building 206-297-2500
Seattle, WA 98133

2036 Virginia Mason Brain Tumor Support Group
1201 Terry Avenue 206-223-7552
Seattle, WA 98111
Michelle Handler RN, Contact

2037 Wenatchee Valley Brain Tumor Support Group
Wellness Place
1610 Fifth Street 509-679-9574
Wenatchee, WA 98801
Jeff Hastings, Contact
Mary Lowe, Contact

West Virginia

2038 Brain Tumor Support Group: Southern West Virginia
First Presbyterian Church
16 Broad Street 304-744-0393
Charleston, WV 25301-2487
Jeri McDonald

Wisconsin

2039 Brain Tumor Support Group: John Sierzant Lutheran Hospital, Gunderson Clinic
1836 S Avenue 608-791-9862
LaCrosse, WI
Esther Lindeman RN

2040 LODAT: Brain Tumor Support Group
Children's Hospital of Wisconsin
Room 888 414-962-8984
Milwaukee, WI www.braintumor.org
Living One Day At a Time is a parent support group for families of chidren with cancer. Monthly newsletter, informational meetings, social activities for families, and bereavement support.
Frances Swigart

Books

2041 Brain Tumor Resource Directory
National Brain Tumor Foundation
1517 North Point Street 617-924-9997
San Francisco, CA 94123-5520 800-934-2873
Fax: 617-924-9998
nbtf@braintumor.org
www.braintumor.org
Help you learn more about brain tumors including symptoms, treatment options, and considerations for caregivers.
Rob Tufel, Director Patient Services

2042 Death Be Not Proud: A Memoir
Harper Collins
10 E 53rd Street 212-207-7000
New York, NY 10022 www.harpercollins.com
The father of a young man diagnosed with glioblastoma multiforme wrote this 50-year-old classic.
ISBN: 0-060929-89-8

2043 Resource Guide for Parents of Children with Brain and Spinal Cord Tumors
Children's Brain Tumor Foundation
274 Madison Avenue 212-448-9494
New York, NY 10016 866-228-4673
Fax: 212-448-1022
info@cbtf.org
www.cbtf.org
Contains practical information to sort out the complexities of medical procedures, interruptions in school and social life, and uncertainty about the future.
Robert Budlow, President
Joseph B Fay, Executive Director

2044 Support Group Directory
National Brain Tumor Foundation
1517 North Point Street 617-924-9997
San Francisco, CA 94123-5520 800-934-2873
Fax: 617-924-9998
nbtf@braintumor.org
www.braintumor.org
Help you learn more about brain tumors including symptoms, treatment options, and considerations for caregivers.
Rob Tufel, Director Patient Services

2045 That's Unacceptable: Surviving a Brain Tumor: My Personal Story
Rebecca L Libutti, author
Krystal Publishing
PO Box 221 908-889-6038
Martinsville, NJ 08836 800-833-9327
Fax: 908-889-6038
RLibutti@aol.com
Written by a ten-year survivor of glioblastoma multiforme, the book's title was the author's first response to the initial discouragement she received about pursuing aggressive treatment.
198 pages Paperback
RL Libutti

2046 The Essential Guide to Brain Tumors
National Brain Tumor Foundation

1517 North Point Street
San Francisco, CA 94123-5520

617-924-9997
800-934-2873
Fax: 617-924-9998
nbtf@braintumor.org
www.braintumor.org

Help you learn more about brain tumors including symptoms, treatment options, and considerations for caregivers.
80 pages
Rob Tufel, Director Patient Services

2047 Understanding and Coping with Your Child's Brain Tumor
National Brain Tumor Foundation
1517 North Point Street
San Francisco, CA 94123-5520

617-924-9997
800-934-2873
Fax: 617-924-9998
nbtf@braintumor.org
www.braintumor.org

Help you learn more about brain tumors including symptoms, treatment options, and considerations for caregivers.
52 pages
Rob Tufel, Director Patient Services

Children's Books

2048 My Name is Buddy
Dave Bauer, author
National Brain Tumor Foundation
1517 North Point Street
San Francisco, CA 94123-5520

617-924-9997
800-934-2873
Fax: 617-924-9998
nbtf@braintumor.org
www.braintumor.org

Help you learn more about brain tumors including symptoms, treatment options, and considerations for caregivers.
Rob Tufel, Director Patient Services

Newsletters

2049 Butterfly Bulletin
Brain Tumor Foundation for Children
6065 Roswell Road NE
Atlanta, GA 30328-4015

404-252-4107
Fax: 404-252-4108
www.braintumorkids.org

Reporting on news and events of the Brain Tumor Foundation for Children.
Quarterly
Rick Sauers, Chairman/Co-Founder
R Hal Meeks, Jr, President

2050 Caring Hand
Pediatric Brain Tumor Foundation
302 Ridgefield Court
Asheville, NC 28806

828-665-6891
800-253-6530
Fax: 828-655-6894
pbtfus@pbtfus.org
www.curethekids.org

The Pediatric Brain Tumor Foundation works to eliminate the challenges of childhood brain tumors. As the world's largest nonprofit source of funding for pediatric brain tumor research, our mission is to cure the kids.
Michael Traynor, President
Glenn Wilcox, Vice President

2051 Childhood Brain Tumor Foundation Newsletter
Childhood Brain Tumor Foundation
20312 Watkins Meadow Dr
Germantown, MD 20876-4259

310-515-2900
877-217-4166
Fax: 301-515-2900
cbtf@childhoodbraintumor.org
www.childhoodbraintumor.org

It is a volunteer-run organization driven to help educate families whose children have been diagnosed with brain tumors. Our mission is to provide grant funding for researchers to further the cause to find a cure

2052 Helping Hand
Pediatric Brain Tumor Foundation

302 Ridgefield Court
Asheville, NC 28806

828-665-6891
800-253-6530
Fax: 828-655-6894
www.curethekids.org

The Pediatric Brain Tumor Foundation works to eliminate the challenges of childhood brain tumors. As the world's largest nonprofit source of funding for pediatric brain tumor research, our mission is to cure the kids.
Michael Traynor, President
Glenn Wilcox, Vice President

2053 Message Line Newsletter
American Brain Tumor Association
8550 W. Bryn Mawr Ave.
Chicago, IL 60631-4117

773-577-8750
800-886-2282
Fax: 773-577-8738
info@abta.org
www.abta.org

Describes research advances and announces updates to publications.
TriAnnual
Elizabeth Wilson, Executive Director
Geri Jo Duda, RN, Patient Services

2054 SEARCH
National Brain Tumor Foundation
1517 North Point Street
San Francisco, CA 94123-5520

617-924-9997
800-934-2873
Fax: 617-924-9998
nbtf@braintumor.org
www.braintumor.org

Help you learn more about brain tumors including symptoms, treatment options, and considerations for caregivers.
Quarterly
Rob Tufel, Director Patient Services

2055 TLC (Tips for Living And Coping)
American Brain Tumor Association
8550 W. Bryn Mawr Ave.
Chicago, IL 60018-4117

773-577-8750
800-886-2282
Fax: 773-577-8738
info@abta.org
www.abta.org

E-bulletin of news, research and development finds, support and treatment information.
ISBN: 0-944093-37-X
Elizabeth Wilson, Executive Director
Geri Jo Duda, RN, Patient Services

Pamphlets

2056 Clinical Trial Fact Sheet
National Brain Tumor Foundation
1517 North Point Street
San Francisco, CA 94123-5520

617-924-9997
800-934-2873
Fax: 617-924-9998
nbtf@braintumor.org
www.braintumor.org

Help you learn more about brain tumors including symptoms, treatment options, and considerations for caregivers.

2057 Coping with Your Loved One's Brain Tumor
National Brain Tumor Foundation
1517 North Point Street
San Francisco, CA 94123-5520

617-924-9997
800-934-2873
Fax: 617-924-9998
nbtf@braintumor.org
www.braintumor.org

Help you learn more about brain tumors including symptoms, treatment options, and considerations for caregivers.
12 pages Booklet

2058 Dictionary for Brain Tumor Patients
American Brain Tumor Association
8550 W. Bryn Mawr Ave.
Chicago, IL 60631-4117

773-577-8750
800-886-2282
Fax: 773-577-8738
info@abta.org
www.abta.org

Offers a dictionary of terms used in the diagnosis and everday living with brain tumors.
Paperback
ISBN: 0-944093-27-2
Elizabeth Wilson, Executive Director
Geri Jo Duda, RN, Patient Services

2059 Ependymoma
American Brain Tumor Association
8550 W. Bryn Mawr Ave.   773-577-8750
Chicago, IL 60631-4117   800-886-2282
                                     Fax: 773-577-8738
                                          info@abta.org
                                          www.abta.org
ISBN: 0-944093-40-X
Elizabeth Wilson, Executive Director
Geri Jo Duda, RN, Patient Services

2060 Glioblastoma Multiforme and Anaplastic Astrocytoma
American Brain Tumor Association
8550 W. Bryn Mawr Ave.   773-577-8750
Chicago, IL 60631-4117   800-886-2282
                                     Fax: 773-577-8738
                                          info@abta.org
                                          www.abta.org
ISBN: 0-944093-36-1
Elizabeth Wilson, Executive Director
Geri Jo Duda, RN, Patient Services

2061 Living with A Brain Tumor
American Brain Tumor Association
8550 W. Bryn Mawr Ave.   773-577-8750
Chicago, IL 60631-4117   800-886-2282
                                     Fax: 773-577-8738
                                          info@abta.org
                                          www.abta.org
A guide for brain tumor patients.
2004
ISBN: 0-944093-54-X
Elizabeth Wilson, Executive Director
Geri Jo Duda, RN, Patient Services

2062 Medulloblastoma
American Brain Tumor Association
8550 W. Bryn Mawr Ave.   773-577-8750
Chicago, IL 60631-4117   800-886-2282
                                     Fax: 773-577-8738
                                          info@abta.org
                                          www.abta.org
Paperback
ISBN: 0-944093-33-7
Elizabeth Wilson, Executive Director
Geri Jo Duda, RN, Patient Services

2063 Meningioma
American Brain Tumor Association
8550 W. Bryn Mawr Ave.   773-577-8750
Chicago, IL 60631-4117   800-886-2282
                                     Fax: 773-577-8738
                                          info@abta.org
                                          www.abta.org
ISBN: 0-944093-23-X
Elizabeth Wilson, Executive Director
Geri Jo Duda, RN, Patient Services

2064 Metastatic Brain Tumors
American Brain Tumor Association
8550 W. Bryn Mawr Ave.   773-577-8750
Chicago, IL 60631-4117   800-886-2282
                                     Fax: 773-577-8738
                                          info@abta.org
                                          www.abta.org
ISBN: 0-944093-26-4
Elizabeth Wilson, Executive Director
Geri Jo Duda, RN, Patient Services

2065 Oligodendroglioma and Mixed Glioma
American Brain Tumor Association

8550 W. Bryn Mawr Ave.   773-577-8750
Chicago, IL 60631-4117   800-886-2282
                                     Fax: 773-577-8738
                                          info@abta.org
                                          www.abta.org
Pamphlet
ISBN: 0-944093-43-4
Elizabeth Wilson, Executive Director
Geri Jo Duda, RN, Patient Services

2066 Organizing a Support Group
American Brain Tumor Association
8550 W. Bryn Mawr Ave.   773-577-8750
Chicago, IL 60631-4117   800-886-2282
                                     Fax: 773-577-8738
                                          info@abta.org
                                          www.abta.org
Elizabeth Wilson, Executive Director
Geri Jo Duda, RN, Patient Services

2067 Pituitary Tumors
American Brain Tumor Association
8550 W. Bryn Mawr Ave.   773-577-8750
Chicago, IL 60631-4117   800-886-2282
                                     Fax: 773-577-8738
                                          info@abta.org
                                          www.abta.org
Pamphlet
ISBN: 0-944093-44-2
Elizabeth Wilson, Executive Director
Geri Jo Duda, RN, Patient Services

2068 Primer of Brain Tumors
American Brain Tumor Association
8550 W. Bryn Mawr Ave.   773-577-8750
Chicago, IL 60631-4117   800-886-2282
                                     Fax: 773-577-8738
                                          info@abta.org
                                          www.abta.org
A patient's reference manual offering information on brain tumors.
ISBN: 0-944093-35-3
Elizabeth Wilson, Executive Director
Geri Jo Duda, RN, Patient Services

2069 Radiation Therapy of Brain Tumors: A Basic Guide
American Brain Tumor Association
8550 W. Bryn Mawr Ave.   773-577-8750
Chicago, IL 60631-4117   800-886-2282
                                     Fax: 773-577-8738
                                          info@abta.org
                                          www.abta.org
ISBN: 0-944093-28-0
Elizabeth Wilson, Executive Director
Geri Jo Duda, RN, Patient Services

2070 Returning to Work: Strategies for Brain Tumor Patients
National Brain Tumor Foundation
1517 North Point Street   617-924-9997
San Francisco, CA 94123-5520   800-934-2873
                                     Fax: 617-924-9998
                                       nbtf@braintumor.org
                                       www.braintumor.org
Help you learn more about brain tumors including symptoms, treatment options, and considerations for caregivers.
16 pages Brochure
Rob Tufel, Director Patient Services

2071 Stereotactic Radiosurgery
American Brain Tumor Association
8550 W. Bryn Mawr Ave.   773-577-8750
Chicago, IL 60631-4117   800-886-2282
                                     Fax: 773-577-8738
                                          info@abta.org
                                          www.abta.org
ISBN: 0-944093-42-6
Elizabeth Wilson, Executive Director
Geri Jo Duda, RN, Patient Services

2072 Understanding Brain Tumors: Glioblastoma Multiforme
National Brain Tumor Foundation

1517 North Point Street
San Francisco, CA 94123-5520

617-924-9997
800-934-2873
Fax: 617-924-9998
nbtf@braintumor.org
www.braintumor.org

Help you learn more about brain tumors including symptoms, treatment options, and considerations for caregivers.
16 pages
Rob Tufel, Director Patient Services

2073 Using A Medical Library
American Brain Tumor Association
8550 W. Bryn Mawr Ave.
Chicago, IL 60631-4117

773-577-8750
800-886-2282
Fax: 773-577-8738
info@abta.org
www.abta.org

Elizabeth Wilson, Executive Director
Geri Jo Duda, RN, Patient Services

2074 What You Need to Know About Brain Tumors
National Cancer Institute
9609 Medical Center Drive
Bethesda, MD 20892-0001

301-435-3848
800-422-6237
www.cancer.gov

Offers factual information about brain tumors, possible causes, primary and secondary tumors, symptoms, diagnosis, treatment, side effects, followup care, support and medical terms.

2075 When Your Child Returns to School
American Brain Tumor Association
8550 W. Bryn Mawr Ave.
Chicago, IL 60631-4117

773-577-8750
800-886-2282
Fax: 773-577-8738
info@abta.org
www.abta.org

Guides parents and teachers through a successful return to school when a child has had a brain tumor.
Paperback
ISBN: 0-944093-21-3
Elizabeth Wilson, Executive Director
Geri Jo Duda, RN, Patient Services

Audio & Video

2076 Conference Audiotapes
National Brain Tumor Foundation
1517 North Point Street
San Francisco, CA 94123-5520

617-924-9997
800-934-2873
Fax: 617-924-9998
nbtf@braintumor.org
www.braintumor.org

Help you learn more about brain tumors including symptoms, treatment options, and considerations for caregivers.
Rob Tufel, Director Patient Services

2077 Strategies for Healing
National Brain Tumor Foundation
1517 North Point Street
San Francisco, CA 94123

617-924-9997
800-934-2873
Fax: 617-924-9998
nbtf@braintumor.org
www.braintumor.org

Help you learn more about brain tumors including symptoms, treatment options, and considerations for caregivers.
Rob Tufel, Director Patient Services

Web Sites

2078 American Brain Tumor Association
www.abta.org
Provide free social service consultations; a mentorship program for new brain tumor support group leaders; a nationwide database of established support groups; the Connections pen-pal program; networking with organizations that provide services to patients and families; a resource listing of physicians offering investgative treatments.

2079 Brain Tumor Society
braintumor.org
Disseminates educational information and provides access to psycho-social support and raises funds to advance carefully selected scientific research projects, improve clinical care and find a cure.

2080 Healing Well
www.healingwell.com
An online health resource guide to medical news, chat, information and articles, newsgroups and message boards, books, disease-related web sites, medical directories, and more for patients, friends, and family coping with disabling diseases, disorders, or chronic illnesses.

2081 Health Finder
www.healthfinder.gov
Searchable, carefully developed web site offering information on over 1000 topics. Developed by the US Department of Health and Human Services, the site can be used in both English and Spanish.

2082 Healthlink USA
www.healthlinkusa.com
Health information concerning treatment, cures, prevention, diagnosis, risk factors, research, support groups, email lists, personal stories and much more. Updated regularly.

2083 MedicineNet
www.medicinenet.com
An online resource for consumers providing easy-to-read, authoritative medical and health information.

2084 Medscape
www.medscape.com
Medscape offers specialists, primary care physicians, and other health professionals the Web's most robust and integrated medical information and educational tools.

2085 National Brain Tumor Foundation
braintumor.org
Disseminates educational information and provides access to psycho-social support and raises funds to advance carefully selected scientific research projects, improve clinical care and find a cure.

2086 Pediatric Brain Tumor Foundation of the US
www.curethekids.org
Goal is to create an awareness about this growing disease among children and adults so that fundraising programs may continue to expand in increased laboratory research.

2087 WebMD
www.webmd.com
Provides credible information, supportive communities, and in-depth reference material about health subjects. A source for original and timely health information as well as material from well known content providers.

Description

Cancer is a general term for more than 100 diseases characterized by abnormal or uncontrolled growth of cells. The resulting mass, or disease, can invade and destroy surrounding normal tissue. Cancer cells from the tumor can also spread (metastasize) through the blood or lymph (plasmatic fluid) to start new cancers in other parts of the body. In 2018, about 1,735,350 new cancer cases were diagnosed, and about 609,640 Americans died from their disease. Cancer is the second leading cause of death in the U.S., exceeded only by heart disease. Although these figures seem bleak, most cancers are potentially curable if detected at an early stage. Cancer, also called a malignancy (from Latin, meaning bad), can be either a solid tumor (carcinoma), such as lung cancer, or a disorder of blood cell formation, such as leukemia.

Cancer is caused by an interplay of internal and external factors, individually or in combination. Abnormal genes can cause multiple changes that affect cell growth. Environmental factors, such as cigarette smoke, (also called a carcinogen – causing cancer) and exposure to radiation, play a role. Many cancers can be prevented by health awareness. For example, 90 percent of the over one million skin cancers that will be diagnosed this year could be drastically reduced by protection from solar rays.

Lung cancer, one of the most prevalent and hazardous cancers could be drastically reduced by eliminating tobacco use. The American Cancer Society estimates that 30 percent of all cancer deaths are related to cigarette smoking.

Cancer treatment may be curative – removes the tumor in the hope that it will not reoccur, or palliative – prolongs life and minimize discomfort when a cure is not possible. A treatment program typically includes a combination of surgery, radiation therapy, and chemotherapy. Immunotherapy is the newest form of treatment and uses agents known as biologic-response modifiers (BRM), to alter the immune system in its response to malignant growth. Brief descriptions of the more common cancers follow.

Brain Cancer Brain cancer occurs at varying rates but overall it comprises approximately 5.6 cases per 100,000 populations each year. They are most common in early or middle adult life and incidence in the elderly population is increasing. Overall incidence is about equal in males and females.

The seriousness of brain tumors is determined by their size, location, and rate of growth. While brain cancer does not normally spread to others areas, many other cancers have the propensity of spreading throughout the nervous system and producing metastatic tumors in the brain. In adults, these tumors are most commonly from cancer of the lung, breast, or skin (melanoma). Symptoms include headaches, seizures, behavior problems, changes in eating or sleeping habits, lethargy and clumsiness. See also *Brain Tumors*.

Breast Cancer Breast cancer is the most common malignant tumor in women in the western hemisphere. Approximately 268,600 new cases of breast cancer in women are expected to be diagnosed in 2019, in the United States. As many as one in nine women will develop breast cancer during her lifetime. Incidence of breast cancer increases under the following conditions: age; (two-thirds of cases develop after age 55); a close relative (mother, sister) with breast cancer; a previous history of breast cancer; a previous history of breast cancer; exposure to radiation. Other risk factors include not having children, early onset of menstruation, and estrogen replacement therapy.

Early detection can be lifesaving. Many breast cancers are self-diagnosed. More than 80 percent of breast cancers occur as a painless mass. Monthly breast self-examination for women of all ages is crucial. The American Cancer Society recommends that women aged 20-39 have a clinical breast examination performed every three years. Depending on the presence of known risk factors, patients should undergo mammography either yearly or every other year between 40 and 50 years, and yearly after age 50.

Warning signs that can aid women in detecting breast cancer include lumps, swelling, skin irritation, tenderness of the nipple, and dimpling of the skin. Treatments vary, depending on when the cancer is discovered and whether it has spread. Research has shown that the traditional radical mastectomy (removal of the entire breast) can often be replaced by lumpectomy (removal of just the tumor), coupled with radiation therapy. Chemotherapy or hormonal manipulation is also prescribed in some cases. The five year survival rate for localized (not spread) breast cancer has improved in recent years from 78 percent to 97 percent.

Colon and Rectal Cancer In western countries, colon and rectal (colorectal) cancer account for more new cases of cancer per year than any other anatomic site except the lung. The incidence begins to rise at age 40 and peaks at age 60 to 75. Incidence of colorectal cancer increases in people who eat low-fiber diets that are high in animal protein, fat, and refined carbohydrates.

Symptoms vary, depending on the location and size of the tumor. Vague signs include weight loss, reduced appetite, and general malaise. More specific signs include rectal bleeding, blood in the stool, or a change in bowel habits.

A digital rectal examination and testing the stool for the presence of blood are important screening tests. Flexible sigmoidoscopy in which the doctor inserts a thin, flexible tube into the rectum shows tumors in 60 percent of cases. A colonoscopy is performed when a tumor is believed to be higher up the colon. These procedures are used to visualize abnormalities and take tissue samples (biopsy).

Treatment consists of surgical removal of the tumor, followed by radiotherapy and/or chemotherapy.

Leukemia Leukemia is a disorder characterized by uncontrolled growth of abnormal and immature white or red blood cells, and is divided into acute and chronic forms. Although leukemia is often thought of as a childhood disease, it strikes 10 times as many adults as children. New treatment, especially for acute leukemia in children has resulted in dramatic improvements in the 5-year survival rates. Today, the likelihood of disease remission is greater than 95 percent, with 30 percent chance of the disease reappearing.

Warning signs of leukemia are related to the disruption of the different cells in the blood: weakness and fatigue are caused by anemia (decreased red blood cells); easy bruising and hemorrhages (e.g. nosebleeds) from reduced clotting cells (platelets); and repeated infections from abnormal white cells. Generalized symptoms include weight loss and malaise.

Treatment for leukemia includes chemotherapy with a wide variety of anticancer drugs. Transfusions restore red cells and platelets, and frequent infections are treated with antibiotics. Bone marrow transplants, in which new blood cells are provided, are one of the most recent and successful advances in the treatment of this disease.

Liver Cancer Liver cancer incidence has more than tripled since 1980, according to the American Cancer Society, with approximately 42,030 new cases expected in the United States in 2019. Men are three times more likely to develop liver cancer than women. Risk include hepatitis B infection, hepatitis C infection, and exposure to any agent that causes liver damage, including alcohol. The remaining patients have no underlying liver disorder.

Symptoms include abdominal pain, weight loss, and a mass on the upper right side of the abdomen. The outlook for patients with liver cancer is usually grim. Surgery provides the best hope, but is suitable in only a few cases. Most experts remain wary of the benefit of liver transplantation. See also *Liver Disease*.

Lung Cancer Lung cancer is one of the most prevalent cancers with over 150,000 new cases each year. The frequency is increasing rapidly. Originally a disease that primarily affected men older than 60, lung cancer has become the second most common cause of cancer in women.

Cigarette smoking and exposure to industrial substances, such as asbestos, are strongly linked to lung cancer. Recent research has shown that exposure to secondhand smoke increases the risk for this disease.

Warning signs of lung cancer are persistent coughing, shortness of breath, sputum streaked with blood, chest pain, and reoccurring pneumonia or bronchitis. Early detection is difficult, as symptoms do not appear until the disease is in advanced stages. Treatment includes surgical removal of the lung if the cancer has not spread (metastasized) and/or chemotherapy and radiation therapy.

Survival rates depend on tumor size, location, and whether or not the disease has spread. Because lung cancer is so difficult to treat, public health efforts are focused on prevention. See also *Lung Disease*.

Oral Cancer Oral cancer represents approximately 2 percent of all newly diagnosed cancers, and 1.5 percent of cancer deaths. Incidence is more than twice as high in men as in women, and is most frequently found in men over age 40. Risk factors include cigarette, pipe, and cigar smoking, as well as the use of chewing tobacco and excessive intake of alcohol.

Oral cancer symptoms include a sore that bleeds easily, or a lump, thickening, or persistent red or white patch in the mouth. Difficulties in chewing and swallowing are symptoms of progressive disease.

Oral cancer can affect any part of the mouth, and primary care physicians and dentists often detect the disease during routine check-ups. Treatment consists of surgical removal (frequently disfiguring), radiation therapy, or a combination of both.

Ovarian Cancer Ovarian cancer develops in 1 in 78 women and accounts for 4 percent of cancers in women. Despite its low incidence, it is the cause of more deaths in women than any other female reproductive cancer. Incidence rates are highest in the industrialized nations. Risk factors include prior history of breast cancer and not having had children. Women who become pregnant at an early age, who have early menopause, and who use oral contraceptives are at less risk.

Ovarian cancer symptoms usually do not appear until the disease is well developed. The most common sign is an enlarging abdomen from accumulated fluid; digestive disturbance such as discomfort, gas and distention, may also occur.

Often an abdominal mass is discovered during a routine pelvic examination in women who are symptom free. Therefore, women age 18 or older, or earlier if they are sexually active should have annual check-ups. (The Pap smear detects cervical cancer, not ovarian cancer.) Once diagnosed, 78 percent of ovarian cancer patients survive longer than one year and more than 52 percent survive longer than five years. If the disease is diagnosed before it has spread to the other parts of the body, the five-year survival rate is 95 percent.

Treatment includes surgical removal, followed by varying combinations of chemotherapy. As in all cancers, early detection is the key to effective therapy.

Pancreatic Cancer is one of the most dangerous cancers because it is difficult to detect and responds poorly to anticancer therapy. The incidence of this tumor has been increasing during the 21st century with 56,770 people expected to be diagnosed in 2019. Men are affected more commonly than women, and the average age of diagnosis is from 55 to 65 years.

There is an increased incidence in those who smoke, consume a fatty diet and, to a lesser extent, who are diabetics. Chronic inflammation of the pancreas, especially among alcoholics, is also a predisposing cause.

Pancreatic cancer runs a particularly silent course, with no symptoms until it has significant advanced. The overall 5- year survival rate for patients with pancreatic cancer is less than 5 percent. Surgery is the mainstay of therapy, but only is appropriate for 15 percent of patients; radiation and/or chemotherapy are often part of treatment.

Prostate Cancer Approximately 1 in 9 men will develop prostate cancer by 85. Incidence rates are higher among African-Americans and increases with age.

Early prostate cancer is symptom free. Pain and difficulty urinating, are late signs of prostate cancer. More than 50 percent of patients have a nodule that can be felt by a digital examination.

The American Cancer Society recommends that beginning at age 50, the digital rectal examination and PSA (prostatespecific antigen) blood test should be performed annually to men with a life expectancy of at least 10 years, due to the slow growth of prostate cancer. African-American males, who are at a greater risk of developing prostate cancer, should start screening at age 45, as should men with a close relative (father, brother) was diagnosed with prostate cancer at a young age. Surgery, radiation and hormones are all used to treat prostate cancer, depending on age and health of the patient and how far the disease has progressed.

Skin Cancer There are over one million cases of skin cancer that are diagnosed each year. The vast majority of these cases, called basal cell or squamous cell cancers, appear on areas that are most exposed to the sun and are highly curable. Melanoma is the most serious skin cancer and accounts for 4 percent of cases. Diagnosis of melanomas has more than doubled since the mid-70s and is estimated now to develop in 1 of 50 Americans. Similar to the more benign skin cancers, melanoma develops as the result of excessive exposure to the sun and has a higher incidence among those who work outdoors. Persons with fair complexions are at particular risk. The warning signs of skin cancer include a persistent skin lesion, especially those that change in the size, color or shape. Other signs include scaliness, oozing, bleeding, pain or spread of pigmentation.

Prevention plays a key role in the development of melanoma, especially avoiding the sun's ultraviolet rays between 10 a.m. and 3 p.m. Sunscreens and protective clothing should be worn by those who spend the majority of their time outside, those who easily sunburn, and all children. In addition, early detection is critical because, despite advances in treatment, including the use of biologic response modifiers, melanoma is difficult to cure.

Stomach Cancer Stomach (or gastric) cancer is most common among those living in northern areas of the U.S., and poor African-American populations. Its incidence increases with age; more than 75 percent of patients are over 50 years of age.

Diet and infection are believed to play a role in the development of stomach cancer. It is also more common in persons with vitamin B12 deficiency (pernicious anemia). Other causes are under investigation.

Symptoms of stomach cancer are usually vague, and include indigestion, abdominal discomfort, bloating, heartburn, and weight loss.

Removal of the tumor when possible offers the only hope of cure. The prognosis is good if the tumor is limited, but most patients are not diagnosed until their disease has spread.

Testicular Cancer Cancer of the testes accounts for approximately 1 percent of all male cancers. However, unlike most cancers, testicular cancer usually occurs in the 15 to 40 age group; with the average age at diagnosis is 32 years.

The cause of testicular cancer is uncertain, but the incidence is increased in men with cogenital crytorchidism (a failure of one or both testes to descend). Some researchers believe that getting an infection with a virus, such as mumps, may play a role.

Fortunately, testicular cancer is one of the most curable of all cancers, In order to discover it early, men must perform self examination at regular intervals to feel for local abnormal growths such as lumps or nodules. Pain in the scrotal sac can also occur, although more than 90 percent of patients have a painless, solid testicular swelling.

Treatment of testicular cancer may include surgical removal, radiation, and chemotherapy.

Urinary Tract Cancer Urinary tract cancers comprise about 9 percent of new cancer cases each year in men and 4 percent in women. The two most common urinary tract cancers are of the bladder and kidney. Overall, the incidence rate is three times greater among men than women, and usually occurs in patients who are 40-70 years of age. Smoking is the greatest risk factor, with smokers having twice the incidence of nonsmokers.

African-Americans, those living in urban areas, and workers exposed to dye, rubber, or leather are also at higher risk.

Common symptoms of bladder cancer include microscopic or observable blood in the urine and painful, increased, and urgent urination. Pain the lower back may also be present. Bladder cancer may be treated by surgical removal of the tumor combined with chemotherapy. Risk factors for kidney (renal) cancer are cigarette smoking (most important) and obesity in women. Symptoms are similar to those in bladder cancer and may also include weight loss, nausea, and vomiting.

Total removal of the cancerous kidney is the treatment of choice and is used in nearly 90 percent of cases; radiation therapy and chemotherapy are relatively ineffective. Biologic response modifiers are promising but must responses are limited in duration.

Uterine and Cervical Cancer The overall incidence of cervical cancer has decreased over the past 40 years, due mainly to regular checkups and the use of the Pap smear test for early detection. Risk factors include intercourse at an early age, cigarette smoking, multiple sex partners, and history of a sexually transmitted disease. Infection with the virus that causes genital warts (HPV), is the number one cause of cervical cancer.

Warning signs include bleeding outside the normal menstrual cycle or after menopause. Cervical cancer in most patients is treated with surgery, radiation, or a combination of both. Due to a recently developed vaccine that is 100 percent effective against HPV, the rates of cervical cancer have sharply decreased.

The American Cancer Society recommends that all women who are, or have been, sexually active get an annual Pap test and pelvic examination. After three or more consecutive satisfactory examinations with normal findings, the Pap test may be performed less frequently, after being discussed with your health care provider.

Uterine cancer has been increasing since the 1970s. Risk factors include obesity, diabetes, high blood pressure, late onset of menopause, and estrogen-only hormone replacement therapy. Symptoms for most women include some form of abnormal bleeding from the uterus. Treatment for uterine and cervical cancers include surgery, radiation therapy, hormone therapy and, occasionally, chemotherapy.

National Agencies & Associations

2088 ABCD: After Breast Cancer Diagnosis
5775 N Glen Park Road
Glendale, WI 53209
414-977-1780
800-977-4121
Fax: 414-977-1781
abcdinc@abcdmentor.org
www.abcdbreastcancersupport.org
Provides free, personal support and resources to those affected by breast cancer.
Ellen Friebert Schupper, Executive Director
Judy Mindin, Director, Program Services

2089 American Cancer Society
250 Williams Street NW
Atlanta, GA 30303
800-227-2345
www.cancer.org
A nationwide community based voluntary health organization dedicated to eliminating cancer as a major health problem, by preventing, saving lives, and diminishing suffering through research, education, advocacy, and services. Provides free printed materials.
Gary M. Reedy, Chief Executive Officer
Richard C. Wender, MD, Chief Cancer Control Officer

2090 American Childhood Cancer Organization
6868 Distribution Drive
Beltsville, MD 20705
staff@acco.org
www.acco.org
Founded by parents of children with cancer. The ACCO helps families of pediatric and adolescent cancer patients cope with the educational and emotional needs of the disease. The organization is the largest distributor of free childhood cancer books and other materials.
Ruth I. Hoffman, MPH, Chief Executive Director
Angelique Byrd, Coordinator, Operations & International

2091 American Chronic Pain Association
PO Box 850
Rocklin, CA 95677
800-533-3231
ACPA@theacpa.org
www.theacpa.org
The ACPA facilitates peer support and education for individuals with chronic pain in its many forms, in order to increase quality of life. Also raises awareness among the healthcare community, and with policy makers.
Penney Cowan, Founder & CEO
Daniel Galia, Director, Global Support

2092 American Society of Colon and Rectal Surgeons
One Parkview Plaza
Oakbrook Terrace, IL 60181
847-686-2236
www.fascrs.org
ASCRS Represents more than 3,800 board certified colon and rectal surgeons, as well as other surgeons dedicated to advancing and promoting the science and practice of the treatment of patients with cancer, and other diseases affecting the colon and related areas.
David Westman, Executive Director
Susan Tibbitts, Associate Executive Director

2093 Americas Association for the Care of the Children
PO Box 2154
Boulder, CO 80306
303-527-2742
aaccchildren.org
Carries out a variety of programs to promote the health of children. Publishes educational materials on child health of interest to parents, educators and health professionals.
Deborah Young, Executive Director & Founder
Judi Jackson, President

2094 Breast Cancer Action
275 Fifth Street
San Francisco, CA 94103
415-243-9301
Fax: 415-243-3996
info@bcaction.org
www.bcaction.org
Seeks health justice for women at risk of and living with breast cancer.
Karuna Jaggar, Executive Director
Rebecca Saltzman, Deputy Director

2095 Breast Cancer Society of Canada
420 East Street North
Sarnia, N7T-6Y5
519-336-0746
800-567-8767
Fax: 519-336-5725
bcsc@bcsc.ca
www.bcsc.ca
Funds Canadian research into improving detection, prevention, and treatment of breast cancer, as well as to find a cure, and creates awareness through education.
Antoine Abugaber, Chair
Kimberly Carson, Chief Executive Officer

2096 Canadian Breast Cancer Network (CBCN)
331 Cooper Street
Ottawa, Ontario, K2P-0G5
613-230-3044
800-685-8820
Fax: 613-230-4424
cbcn@cbcn.ca
www.cbcn.ca
Survivor-directed, national network of organizations and individuals concerned about breast cancer, representing the concerns of all Canadians affected by breast cancer, and those at risk.
Jenn Gordon, Director, Operations
Niya Chari, Director, Public Affairs & Health Policy

2097 Canadian Cancer Society
55 St. Clair Avenue W
Toronto, Ontario, M4V-2Y7
416-961-7223
888-939-3333
TTY: 866-786-3934
www.cancer.ca
A national community-based organization of volunteers whose mission is the eradication of cancer and the enhancement of the quality of life of people living with cancer.
Andrea Seale, Interim Chief Executive Officer
Sandra Krueckl, Vice President, Cancer Control

2098 Cancer Caring Center
4117 Liberty Avenue
Pittsburgh, PA 15224
412-622-1212
Fax: 412-622-1216
info@cancercaring.org
www.cancercaring.org
Provides a wide variety of support services to cancer patients, their families and friends including support groups, education classes, personal counseling and telephone help line.
Rebecca Whitlinger, Executive Director
Stephanie Scoletti, Director, Support Services

2099 CancerCare
275 7th Avenue
New York, NY 10001
212-712-8400
800-813-4673
Fax: 212-712-8495
info@cancercare.org
www.cancercare.org
National non-profit organization that provides free, professional support services for anyone affected by a cancer diagnosis.
Patricia J. Goldsmith, Chief Executive Officer
Christine Verini, RPh, Chief Operating Officer

2100 Childhood Cancer Canada
21 St. Clair Avenue E
Toronto, Ontario, M4T-1L9
416-489-6440
800-363-1062
Fax: 416-489-9812
info@childhoodcancer.ca
www.childhoodcancer.ca
Invests in national, collaborative research into childhood cancer, as well as supporting education and community programs.
Elizabeth R. Gill, President & CEO
Sandi Hancox, Vice President, Fundraising

2101 Coalition for Advanced Cancer Treatment and Prevention
7111 Sweetgum Road
Fairview, TN 37602-9384
nationalalzdiseaseinstitute.org
Investigates and presents information on the ways in which natural or alternative medicine can prevent and potentially cure cancer. Physician referrals are provided. The institute is overseen by the National Fund for Alternative Medicine.
P. Anthony Chapdelaine, Jr., Executive Director
Mary Ann Chapdelaine, President

2102 Colorectal Cancer Canada
1350 Sherbrooke Street W
Montreal, Quebec, H3G-1J1
877-502-6566
Fax: 514-875-7746
www.coloncancercanada.ca
Seeks to raise public awareness of colorectal cancer, while supporting and advocating for patients. The Colorectal Cancer Association of Canada and Colon Cancer Canada amalgamated in 2017.
Barry D. Stein, President
Bunnie Schwartz, Co-Founder

2103 International Association of Laryngectomees
925B Peachtree Street NE
Atlanta, GA 30309
866-425-3678
theialoffice@gmail.com
www.theial.com
Consists of local clubs worldwide that provide services and information to patients who have undergone laryngectomies, and their families. Members are given information on first aid, postoperative care, rehabilitation, esophageal speech and other speech alternatives. Directories of speech instructors and self-care supplies for the surgical site are distributed.
Helen Grathwohl, President
Susan Reeves, Administrative Manager

2104 Leukemia and Lymphoma Society
3 International Drive
Rye Brook, NY 10573
800-955-4572
www.lls.org
Dedicated to funding blood cancer research, education, and patient services.
Louis J. DeGennaro, PhD, President & CEO
Rob Beck, Chief Operating Officer

2105 National Cancer Institute
9609 Medical Center Drive
Bethesda, MD 20892-9760
800-422-6237
nciinfo@nih.gov
www.cancer.gov
Offers educational information, public awareness, research grants, and more for patients, their families, and health care professionals. Information specialists answer cancer-related questions by phone, LiveHelp instant messaging, and e-mail.
Douglas R. Lowy, MD, Acting Director
James Doroshow, MD, Deputy Director, Clinical Research

2106 National Coalition for Cancer Survivorship
8455 Colesville Road
Silver Spring, MD 20910
301-650-9127
877-622-7937
Fax: 301-565-9670
info@canceradvocacy.org
www.canceradvocacy.org
Survivor-led advocacy organization working exclusively on behalf of people with all types of cancer and their families. Dedicated to assuring quality and care for all Americans.
Shelley Fuld Nasso, Chief Executive Officer
Dan Weber, Director, Communications

2107 National Hospice & Palliative Care Organization (NHPCO)
1731 King Street
Alexandria, VA 22314
703-837-1500
800-646-6460
Fax: 703-837-1233
www.nhpco.org
The organization seeks to improve end-of-life care, widen access to hospice care, and improve quality of life for the dying and their loved ones.
Edo Banach, JD, President & CEO
Hannah Yang Moore, MPH, Chief Advocacy Officer

2108 National Institute on Aging
31 Center Drive, MSC 2292
Bethesda, MD 20892
800-222-2225
TTY: 800-222-4225
niaic@nia.nih.gov
www.nia.nih.gov

Seeks to understand the nature of aging, and to extend healthy, active years of life. Free resources are available on topics such as Alzheimer's & dimentia, caregiving, cognitive heath, end of life care, and more.
Richard J. Hodes MD, Director
Marie A. Bernard, MD, Deputy Director

2109   National Kidney and Urologic Diseases Information Clearinghouse
3 Information Way   800-860-8747
Bethesda, MD 20892-3580   TTY: 866-569-1162
                                            healthinfo@niddk.nih.gov
                                            www.niddk.nih.gov
A service of the Federal Government's National Institute for Diabetes and Digestive and Kidney Diseases. Offers free information about benign prostate enlargement and other non-cancerous urinary tract problems.
Griffin P. Rodgers, Director
Gregory Germino, Deputy Director

2110   National Marrow Donor Program
500 N 5th Street   612-627-5800
Minneapolis, MN 55401-1206   800-627-7692
                                            patientinfo@nmdp.org
                                            bethematch.org
Created to improve the effectiveness of the search for bone marrow donors so that a greater number of bone marrow transplants can be carried out. Operates the Be The Match marrow registry.
C. Randal Mills, PhD, Chief Executive Officer
Dennis L. Confer, MD, Chief Medical Officer

2111   National Ovarian Cancer Coalition
12221 Merit Drive   214-273-4200
Dallas, TX 75251   888-682-7426
                                            Fax: 214-273-4201
                                            nocc@ovarian.org
                                            www.ovarian.org
Aims to raise awareness about ovarian cancer and to promote education about the disease, while dispelling myths and misunderstandings. The coalition is committed to improving the overall survival rate and quality of life for women with ovarian cancer.
Melissa Aucoin, Chief Executive Officer
Megan Murphy, Director, Business Development

2112   Rethink Breast Cancer
50 Carroll Street   416-220-0700
Toronto, Ontario, M4M-3G3   Fax: 416-920-5798
                                            hello@rethinkbreastcancer.com
                                            www.rethinkbreastcancer.com
Is a charity helping young people who are concerned about and affected by breast cancer through innovative breast cancer education, research and support programs.
M.J. DeCoteau, MA, Founder & Executive Director
Tania Kwong, Director, Marketing & Communications

2113   Support for People with Oral and Head and Neck Cancer (SPOHNC)
PO Box 53   800-377-0928
Locust Valley, NY 11560-0053   Fax: 516-671-8794
                                            info@spohnc.org
                                            www.spohnc.org
Non-profit organization addressing the broad emotional, physical, and humanistic needs of oral and head and neck cancer patients.
James Sciubba, DMD, PhD, President
Mary Ann Caputo, Executive Director

State Agencies & Associations

Alabama

2114   American Cancer Society: Alabama
1100 Ireland Way   205-879-2242
Birmingham, AL 35205   Fax: 205-930-8895
                                            www.cancer.org/docroot/com/com_0.asp
The American Cancer Society is the nationwide community-based voluntary health organization dedicated to eliminating cancer as a major health problem by preventing cancer, saving lives and diminishing suffering from cancer, through research and education.
Scarlet Thom (205-930-8889), Media/Public Relations Alabama

2115   Leukemia and Lymphoma Society: Alabama Chapter
Leukemia Society of America
100 Chase Park S   205-989-0098
Birmingham, AL 35244   888-560-9700
                                            Fax: 205-989-0099
                                            www.lls.org/aboutlls/chapters/al/
Dedicated to finding cures for leukemia and related cancers and to improving the quality of life for patients and their families.
Melanie Mooney, Executive Director
Kate McLean, Campaign Coordinator, Special Events

Alaska

2116   American Cancer Society: Alaska
3851 Piper Street   907-277-8696
Anchorage, AK 99508   Fax: 907-263-2073
                                            leslie.jones@cancer.org
                                            www.cancer.org
The American Cancer Society is the nationwide community-based voluntary health organization dedicated to eliminating cancer as a major health problem by preventing cancer saving lives and diminishing suffering from cancer through research and education.
Leslie Jones, Media/Public Relations Alaska

Arizona

2117   American Cancer Society: Arizona
4212 N 16th Street   602-224-0524
Phoenix, AZ 85016   800-227-2345
                                            Fax: 602-778-7699
                                            www.cancer.org
The American Cancer Society is the nationwide community-based voluntary health organization dedicated to eliminating cancer as a major health problem by preventing cancer saving lives, and diminishing suffering from cancer through research and education.
Meg Kondrich, Media/Public Relations Arizona

2118   International Holistic Center
PO Box 15103   928-771-2826
Phoenix, AZ 85060-5103   ihcinc@cox.net
                                            www.holisticresources.org
Provides information and referrals concerning holistic health care in Arizona and beyond.
Stan Kalson, President

2119   Leukemia and Lymphoma Society: Mountain States Chapter
Leukemia Society of America
3877 N 7th Street   602-567-7600
Phoenix, AZ 85014   800-568-1372
                                            Fax: 602-567-7601
                                            www.leukemia-lymphoma.org
Dedicated to finding cures for leukemia and related cancers and to improving the quality of life for patients and their families. Serves New Mexico and the Greater El Paso, TX area.
Tim Metzer, Executive Director

Arkansas

2120   American Cancer Society: Arkansas
901 N University   501-664-3480
Little Rock, AR 72207   Fax: 501-603-5223
                                            jodie.spears@cancer.org
                                            www.cancer.org
The American Cancer Society is the nationwide community-based voluntary health organization dedicated to eliminating cancer as a major health problem by preventing cancer, saving lives, and diminishing suffering from cancer, through research and education.
Jodie Spears, Media/Public Relations Arkansas

2121   Health Resource
933 Faulkner Street   501-329-5272
Conway, AR 72034   800-949-0090
                                            Fax: 501-329-9489
                                            www.thehealthresource.com
A medical information service which provides clients with an individualized, in depth research report on his or her specific health

problem. Reports include latest treatment options, mainstream, experimental and alternative and top specialists.
Janice Guthrie, Director/Researcher
Shirley Effinger, Researcher

California

2122 American Cancer Society Santa Clara County / Silicon Valley / Central Coast Region
747 Camden Avenue
Campbell, CA 95008
408-871-1062
Fax: 408-871-2993
angie.carrillo@cancer.org
www.cancer.org
The American Cancer Society is the nationwide community-based voluntary health organization dedicated to eliminating cancer as a major health problem by preventing cancer, saving lives and diminishing suffering from cancer, through research and education.
Angie Carillo, Media/Public Relations Silicon Valley

2123 American Cancer Society: Central Los Angeles
3333 Wilshire Boulevard
Los Angeles, CA 90010
213-386-6102
Fax: 213-480-0806
katherine.spangle@cancer.org
www.cancer.org
The American Cancer Society is the nationwide community-based voluntary health organization dedicated to eliminating cancer as a major health problem by preventing cancer, saving lives, and diminishing suffering from cancer, through research and education.
Katie Spangle, Media/Public Relations Los Angeles Area

2124 American Cancer Society: East Bay/Metro Region
1700 Webster Street
Oakland, CA 94612
510-832-7012
Fax: 510-763-8826
patty.guinto@cancer.org
www.cancer.org
The American Cancer Society is the nationwide community-based voluntary health organization dedicated to eliminating cancer as a major health problem by preventing cancer, saving lives, and diminishing suffering from cancer, through research and education.
Patty Guinto, Media/Public Relations East Bay Area

2125 American Cancer Society: Fresno/Madera Counties
2222 W Shaw Avenue
Fresno, CA 93711
559-451-0722
Fax: 559-451-0744
www.cancer.org
The American Cancer Society is the nationwide community-based voluntary health organization dedicated to eliminating cancer as a major health problem by preventing cancer, saving lives, and diminishing suffering from cancer, through research and education.
Erica Jones, Media/Public Relations Fresno CA

2126 American Cancer Society: Inland Empire
6355 Riverside Ave
Riverside, CA 92506
951-683-6415
Fax: 951-682-6804
beckie.mooreflati@cancer.org
www.cancer.org
The American Cancer Society is the nationwide community-based voluntary health organization dedicated to eliminating cancer as a major health problem by preventing cancer, saving lives, and diminishing suffering from cancer, through research and education.
Beckie Moore, Media/Public Relations Riverside Region

2127 American Cancer Society: Orange County
1940 E Deere Avenue
Santa Ana, CA 92705-5718
949-261-9446
Fax: 949-261-9419
jennifer.horspool@cancer.org
www.cancer.org
The American Cancer Society is the nationwide community-based voluntary health organization dedicated to eliminating cancer as a major health problem by preventing cancer, saving lives, and diminishing suffering from cancer, through research and education.
Jennifer Horton, Media/Public Relations Orange County

2128 American Cancer Society: Sacramento County
1765 Challenge Way
Sacramento, CA 95815
916-446-7933
Fax: 916-64 -977
www.cancer.org
The American Cancer Society is the nationwide community-based voluntary health organization dedicated to eliminating cancer as a

major health problem by preventing cancer, saving lives, and diminishing suffering from cancer, through research and education.
Maria Robinson, Media/Public Relations Sacramento County

2129 American Cancer Society: San Diego County
2655 Camino Del Rio N
San Diego, CA 92108
619-299-4200
800-227-2345
Fax: 619-296-0928
robin.brown@cancer.org
www.cancer.org
The American Cancer Society is the nationwide community-based voluntary health organization dedicated to eliminating cancer as a major health problem by preventing cancer, saving lives, and diminishing suffering from cancer, through research and education.
Robin Brown, Media/Public Relations San Diego CA

2130 American Cancer Society: San Francisco County
201 Mission Street
San Francisco, CA 94105
415-394-7100
Fax: 415-495-1877
www.cancer.org
The American Cancer Society is the nationwide community-based voluntary health organization dedicated to eliminating cancer as a major health problem by preventing cancer, saving lives and diminishing suffering from cancer, through research and education.
Patty Guinto, Media/Public Relations San Francisco

2131 American Cancer Society: Santa Maria Valley
426 E Barcellus
Santa Maria, CA 93454
805-922-2354
Fax: 805-925-1424
jeb.baird@cancer.org
www.cancer.org
The American Cancer Society is the nationwide community-based voluntary health organization dedicated to eliminating cancer as a major health problem by preventing cancer, saving lives, and diminishing suffering from cancer, through research and education.
Jeb Baird, Media/Public Relations Santa Maria

2132 American Cancer Society: Sonoma County
1451 Guerneville Road
Santa Rosa, CA 95403
707-545-6720
Fax: 707-545-3179
www.cancer.org
The American Cancer Society is the nationwide community-based voluntary health organization dedicated to eliminating cancer as a major health problem by preventing cancer, saving lives, and diminishing suffering from cancer, through research and education.
Angie Carillo, Media/Public Relations Central Coast

2133 Cancer Control Society and Cancer Book House
2043 N Berendo Street
Los Angeles, CA 90027
213-663-7801
Fax: 323-663-7757
www.cancercontrolsociety.com
An informational organization offering books, films, videos, clinic tours and lists of patients with cancer.
Lorraine Rosenthal, Co-Founder
Frank Cousineau, President

2134 City of Hope National Medical Center Beckman Research Institute
Beckman Research Institute
1500 E Duarte Road
Duarte, CA 91010
626-256-4673
800-826-4673
tpogue@coh.org
www.cityofhope.org
City of Hope is an innovative biomedical research, treatment and educational institution dedicated to the prevention and cure of cancer and other life-threatening illness.
Stephen J Foreman, Chair

2135 Leukemia & Lymphoma Society: Orange, Riverside, And San Bernadino Counties
2020 E 1st Street
Santa Ana, CA 92705
714-881-0610
888-535-9300
Fax: 714-881-0616
www.leukemia-lymphoma.org
Dedicated to finding cures for leukemia and related cancers and to improving the quality of life for patients and their families.

2136 Leukemia and Lymphoma Society: San Diego/Hawaii Chapter
Leukemia Society of America

9150 Chesapeake Dr 858-277-1800
San Diego, CA 92123 888-535-9300
Fax: 858-277-1748
www.leukemia.org
Dedicated to finding cures for leukemia and related cancers and to improving the quality of life for patients and their families.
Keith Turner, Executive Director

2137 Leukemia and Lymphoma Society: Greater Sacramento Area Chapter
Leukemia Society of America
4604 Roseville Road 916-348-1793
North Highlands, CA 95660 Fax: 916-348-7864
www.leukemia.org
Dedicated to finding cures for leukemia and related cancers and to improving the quality of life for patients and their families.
Tracy Latino, Executive Director

2138 Leukemia and Lymphoma Society: Greater Los Angeles Chapter
Leukemia Society of America
6033 W Century Boulevard 310-342-5800
Los Angeles, CA 90045 Fax: 310-342-5801
www.leukemia-lymphoma.org
Dedicated to finding cures for leukemia and related cancers and to improving the quality of life for patients and their families.
Donna Lynch, Executive Director

2139 Leukemia and Lymphoma Society: Northern California Chapter
Leukemia Society of America
1390 Market Street 415-625-1100
San Francisco, CA 94102 Fax: 415-625-1155
supportservices@lls.org
www.lls.org
Dedicated to finding cures for leukemia and related cancers and to improving the quality of life for patients and their families.

2140 Leukemia and Lymphoma Society: Orange, Riverside, And San Bernadino Counties
2020 E 1st Street 714-881-0610
Santa Ana, CA 92705 888-535-9300
Fax: 714-881-0616
www.lls.org
Dedicated to finding cures for leukemia and related cancers and to improving the quality of life for patients and their families.

2141 Leukemia and Lymphoma Society: Tri-County Chapter
Leukemia Society of America
2020 E 1st Street 714-881-0610
Santa Ana, CA 92705 888-535-9300
Fax: 714-881-0616
www.leukemia-lymphoma.org
Dedicated to finding cures for leukemia and related cancers and to improving the quality of life for patients and their families.
John Walter, President & CEO
Louis J DeGennaro, Chief Mission Officer

2142 National Health Federation
PO Box 688 626-357-2181
Monrovia, CA 91017 Fax: 626-303-0642
www.thenhf.com
A nonprofit consumer-oriented organization devoted to health matters. Dedicated to preserving freedom of choice in health care issues, prevention of diseases and the promotion of wellness.
Scott Tips, President
Sylvia Provenza, Vice-President

2143 Regional Cancer Foundation
1200 Gough Street 415-775-9956
San Francisco, CA 94109 Fax: 415-346-8652
This foundation offers, at no charge, a second opinion consultation to individuals diagnosed with cancer. The patient and a family member or friend meet with an interdisciplinary panel of local cancer specialists with expertise in radiation therapy, chemotherapy, and cancer treatment plans.
William Gillis, CEO
Arhur J Inerfield, Chairman

2144 Rose Kushner Breast Cancer Advisory Center
PO Box 757 301-897-3445
Malaga Cove, CA 90274 Fax: 301-897-3444
lkkushner@yahoo.com

Provides a mail service offering referrals to health professionals as well as information about detection, diagnosis, treatment and physical and psychological rehabilitation for patients with breast cancer.

Colorado

2145 American Cancer Society: Colorado
2255 S Oneida Street 303-758-2030
Denver, CO 80224 Fax: 303-759-1615
www.cancer.org
The American Cancer Society is the nationwide community-based voluntary health organization dedicated to eliminating cancer as a major health problem by preventing cancer, saving lives and diminishing suffering from cancer, through research and education.
Lynda Solomo, Media/Public Relations Colorado
Joel Quevill, Media/Public Relations Colorado

Connecticut

2146 American Cancer Society: Connecticut
Meriden Executive Park 203-379-4700
Meriden, CT 06450 Fax: 203-379-5060
www.cancer.org
The American Cancer Society is the nationwide community-based voluntary health organization dedicated to eliminating cancer as a major health problem by preventing cancer, saving lives and diminishing suffering from cancer, through research and education.
Simone Upsey, Media/Public Relations NH/MS/NL Counties
Christian Me, Media/Public Relations LF/FF Counties

2147 Leukemia and Lymphoma Society: Connecticut Chapter
Leukemia Society of America
321 Research Parkway 203-379-0445
Meriden, CT 06450 888-282-9465
Fax: 203-379-0451
www.lls.org/aboutlls/chapters/ct/
Founded in 1949 to help serve and educate the communities and residents who have been touched by leukemia, lymphoma, multiple myeloma and Hodgkin's disease.
Jean Montano, Executive Director
Dina Mariani, Deputy Executive Director

2148 Leukemia and Lymphoma Society: Fairfield County Chapter
Leukemia Society of America
25 Third Street 203-967-8326
Stamford, CT 06905 Fax: 203-325-8559
www.lls.org
Dedicated to finding cures for leukemia and related cancers and to improving the quality of life for patients and their families.

Delaware

2149 American Cancer Society: Delaware
92 Reads Way 302-324-4427
New Castle, DE 19720 Fax: 302-324-4233
dawn.ward@cancer.org
www.cancer.org
The American Cancer Society is the nationwide community-based voluntary health organization dedicated to eliminating cancer as a major health problem by preventing cancer, saving lives, and diminishing suffering from cancer, through research and education.
Dawn Ward, Media/Public Relations Delaware

2150 Leukemia and Lymphoma Society: Delaware Chapter
Leukemia Society of America
100 W 10th Street 302-661-7300
Wilmington, DE 19801 800-220-1617
Fax: 302-661-0363
www.leukemia-lymphoma.org
Our mission is to cure leukemia, lymphoma, Hodgkin's disease and myeloma and to improve the quality of life of patients and their families.
Timothy S Durst, Chairman
James Davis, Vice-Chair

District of Columbia

2151 American Cancer Society: District of Columbia
1875 Connecticut Avenue NW 202-483-2600
Washington, DC 20009 Fax: 202-483-1174
www.cancer.org
The American Cancer Society is the nationwide community-based voluntary health organization dedicated to eliminating cancer as a major health problem by preventing cancer, saving lives, and diminishing suffering from cancer, through research and education.
Angela Colli, Media/Public Relations Washington DC

2152 American Institute for Cancer Research
1759 R Street NW 202-328-7744
Washington, DC 20009 800-843-8114
Fax: 202-328-7226
aicrweb@aicr.org
www.aicr.org
Not-for-profit research and educational organization. Provides grants for research into the causes, development, prevention and treatment of cancer through diet and nutrition. Offers publications, research results, conferences and various public services.

2153 Center for Science in the Public Interest
1220 L Street N.W. 202-332-9110
Washington, DC 20005 Fax: 202-265-4954
cspi@cspinet.org
www.cspinet.org
The nation's leading consumer group concerned with food and nutrition issues. Focuses on diseases that result from consuming too many calories, too much fat, sodium and sugar such as cancer and heart disease.
Don Allen, Director of Finance
Tom Gegax, Board of Directors

Florida

2154 American Cancer Society: Florida
2006 W Kennedy Boulevard 813-254-3630
Tampa, FL 33606 Fax: 813-349-4431
www.cancer.org
The American Cancer Society is the nationwide community-based voluntary health organization dedicated to eliminating cancer as a major health problem by preventing cancer, saving lives, and diminishing suffering from cancer, through research and education.
C. Dunlap, Media/Public Relations Tampa Region
Kristen Redd, Media/Public Relations Tampa Region

2155 Leukemia & Lymphoma Society: Suncoast Chapter
3507 E Frontage Road 813-963-6461
Tampa, FL 33607 800-436-6889
Fax: 813-963-1306
www.lls.org
Serves patients with leukemia, lymphoma, multiple myeloma and Hodgkin's disease in Charlotte, Citrus, Collier, DeSoto, Hardee, Hernando, Hillsborough, Lee, Manatee, Pasco, Pinellas and Sarasota counties.

2156 Leukemia and Lymphoma Society: Southern Florida Chapter
Leukemia Society of America
3325 Hollywood Boulevard 954-961-3234
Hallandale, FL 33021 Fax: 954-961-7376
www.lls.org
Dedicated to finding cures for leukemia and related cancers and to improving the quality of life for patients and their families.

2157 Leukemia and Lymphoma Society: Central Florida Chapter
Leukemia Society of America
3319 Maguire Boulevard 407-898-0733
Orlando, FL 32803-3720 Fax: 407-896-8645
www.lls.org
Dedicated to finding cures for leukemia and related cancers and to improving the quality of life for patients and their families.

2158 Leukemia and Lymphoma Society: Northern Florida Chapter
Leukemia Society of America
9143 Phillips Highway 904-538-0721
Jacksonville, FL 32256 800-868-0072
Fax: 904-538-9245
www.lls.org

Dedicated to finding cures for leukemia and related cancers and to improving the quality of life for patients and their families.

2159 Leukemia and Lymphoma Society: Palm Beach Area Chapter
Leukemia Society of America
4360 Northlake Boulevard 561-775-9954
Palm Beach Gardens, FL 33410 888-478-8550
Fax: 561-775-0930
www.lls.org
Dedicated to finding cures for leukemia and related cancers and to improving the quality of life for patients and their families.

Georgia

2160 American Cancer Society: Georgia
50 Williams Street 404-315-1123
Atlanta, GA 30303 Fax: 404-315-9348
elissa.mccrary@cancer.org
www.cancer.org
The American Cancer Society is the nationwide community-based voluntary health organization dedicated to eliminating cancer as a major health problem by preventing cancer, saving lives, and diminishing suffering from cancer, through research and education.
E. McCrary, Media/Public Relations Georgia

2161 Kidscope
2045 Peachtree Road 404-892-1437
Atlanta, GA 30309 www.kidscope.org
A nonprofit organization formed to help families and children better understand the effects from cancer in a parent. The name can also be read as Kids Cope - one of the goals being to improve the chances that a child will successfully cope with the diagnosis.
H Elizabeth King PhD, Board Member
Carol Webb PhD, Board Member

2162 Leukemia and Lymphoma Society: Georgia Chapter
Leukemia Society of America
3715 Northside Parkway 404-720-7900
Atlanta, GA 30327 800-399-7312
Fax: 404-720-7878
dick.brown@lls.org
www.leukemia-lymphoma.org
Dedicated to finding cures for leukemia and related cancers and to improving the quality of life for patients and their families.
Dick Brown, Executive Director
Maureen Quin Davidson, Director TNT

Hawaii

2163 American Cancer Society: Hawaii
2370 Nuuanu Avenue 808-595-7544
Honolulu, HI 96817 800-ACS-2345
Fax: 808-595-7545
TTY: 866-228-4327
www.cancer.org
The American Cancer Society is the nationwide community-based voluntary health organization dedicated to eliminating cancer as a major health problem by preventing cancer, saving lives, and diminishing suffering from cancer, through research and education.
Milton Hirata, Media Relations Contact - Hawaii

Idaho

2164 American Cancer Society: Idaho
2676 Vista Avenue 208-345-2184
Boise, ID 83705 800-ACS-2345
Fax: 208-343-9922
TTY: 866-228-4327
jim.ryan@cancer.org
www.cancer.org
The American Cancer Society is the nationwide community-based voluntary health organization dedicated to eliminating cancer as a major health problem by preventing cancer, saving lives, and diminishing suffering from cancer, through research and education.
Jim Ryan, Media Relations Contact - Idaho

2165 American Cancer Society: Illinois
225 N Michigan Avenue   312-372-0471
Chicago, IL 60601   800-ACS-2345
                                         Fax: 312-372-0910
                                         TTY: 866-228-4327
                                         www.cancer.org
The American Cancer Society is the nationwide community-based voluntary health organization dedicated to eliminating cancer as a major health problem by preventing cancer, saving lives, and diminishing suffering from cancer, through research and education.
Melissa Leeb, Media Relations Contact - Illinois

2166 Leukemia and Lymphoma Society: Illinois Chapter
Leukemia Society of America
651 W Washington Boulevard   312-651-7350
Chicago, IL 60661   800-742-6595
                                         Fax: 312-463-0980
                                         pam.swenk@lls.org
                                         www.lls.org
Dedicated to finding cures for leukemia and related cancers and to improving the quality of life for patients and their families.
Pam Swenk, Executive Director
Jennifer Hufnagel, Director Donor Development

2167 American Cancer Society: Indiana
5635 W 96th Street   317-344-7800
Indianapolis, IN 46278   800-ACS-2345
                                         Fax: 317-344-7810
                                         TTY: 866-228-4327
                                         leslie.smith@cancer.org
                                         www.cancer.org
The American Cancer Society is the nationwide community-based voluntary health organization dedicated to eliminating cancer as a major health problem by preventing cancer, saving lives, and diminishing suffering from cancer, through research and education.
Leslie Smith Babione, Media Relations Contact - Indianapolis
Katie Burton, Media/Public Relations Indiana

2168 Leukemia and Lymphoma Society: Indiana Chapter
Leukemia Society of America
941 E 86th Street   317-726-2270
Indianapolis, IN 46240   800-846-7764
                                         Fax: 317-726-2280
                                         amy.kwas@lls.org
                                         www.lls.org
Dedicated to finding cures for leukemia and related cancers and to improving the quality of life for patients and their families.
Amy Kwas, Executive Director
Sarah Moore, Deputy Executive Director

2169 American Cancer Society: Iowa
8364 Hickman Road   515-253-0147
Des Moines, IA 50325   800-ACS-2345
                                         Fax: 515-253-0806
                                         TTY: 866-228-4327
                                         www.cancer.org
The American Cancer Society is the nationwide community-based voluntary health organization dedicated to eliminating cancer as a major health problem by preventing cancer, saving lives, and diminishing suffering from cancer, through research and education.
Chuck Reed, Media Relations Contact - Iowa

2170 People Against Cancer
604 E Street   515-972-4444
Otho, IA 50569-0010   800-662-2326
                                         Fax: 515-972-4415
                                         info@PeopleAgainstCancer.net
                                         www.peopleagainstcancer.com
A nonprofit grassroots organization whose mission is to find the best cancer therapy for people with cancer worldwide.
Frank Wiewel, Executive Director

2171 American Cancer Society: Kansas City
6700 Antioch   913-432-3277
Merriam, KS 66024   800-ACS-2345
                                         Fax: 913-432-1732
                                         TTY: 866-228-4327
                                         christine.winter@cancer.org
                                         www.cancer.org
The American Cancer Society is the nationwide community-based voluntary health organization dedicated to eliminating cancer as a major health problem by preventing cancer, saving lives, and diminishing suffering from cancer, through research and education.
Christine Winter, Media Relations Contact

2172 Leukemia and Lymphoma Society: Mid-America Chapter
Leukemia Society of America
6811 W 63rd Street   913-262-1515
Shawnee Mission, KS 66202   800-256-1075
                                         Fax: 913-262-2167
                                         janna.lacock@lls.org
                                         www.lls.org
Dedicated to finding cures for leukemia and related cancers and to improving the quality of life for patients and their families.
Janna LaCock, Executive Director
Jill Ring, Development Director

2173 Leukemia and Lymphona Society: Kansas Chapter
Leukemia Society of America
300 N Main   316-266-4050
Wichita, KS 67202   800-779-2417
                                         Fax: 316-266-4960
                                         kelly.gerstenkorn@lls.org
                                         www.lls.org/ks
Cure leukemia, lymphoma, Hodgkin's disease and myeloma and improve the quality of life for patients and their families.
Timothy S Durst, Chairman
James Davis, Vice-Chair

2174 American Cancer Society: Kentucky
701 W Muhammad Ali Boulevard   502-584-6782
Louisville, KY 40203   800-ACS-2345
                                         Fax: 502-584-6767
                                         TTY: 866-228-4327
                                         www.cancer.org
The American Cancer Society is the nationwide community-based voluntary health organization dedicated to eliminating cancer as a major health problem by preventing cancer, saving lives, and diminishing suffering from cancer, through research and education.
Doug Dressman, Executive Director-Louisville

2175 Leukemia and Lymphoma Society: Kentucky Chapter
Leukemia Society of America
600 E Main Street   502-584-8490
Louisville, KY 40202-2661   800-955-2566
                                         Fax: 502-589-5316
                                         karyl.ferman@lls.org
                                         www.lls.org
Founded in 1975 to serve Kentucky and Southern Indiana residents touched by leukemia and its related cancers. Goal is to find a cure for leukemia and its related cancers and to improve the quality of life for patients and their families.
Karyl D Ferman, Executive Director
Katie Anderson, Director Team in Training

2176 American Cancer Society: Louisiana
2605 River Road   504-469-0021
New Orleans, LA 70121   800-ACS-2345
                                         Fax: 504-219-2290
                                         TTY: 866-228-4327
                                         jewel.m.bush@cancer.org
                                         www.cancer.org
The American Cancer Society is the nationwide community-based voluntary health organization dedicated to eliminating cancer as a

major health problem by preventing cancer, saving lives, and diminishing suffering from cancer, through research and education.
Jewel M Bush, Media Relations Contact

Maine

2177 American Cancer Society: Maine
1 Bowdoin Mill Island   207-373-3700
Topsham, ME 04086   800-ACS-2345
                                         Fax: 207-725-6680
                                         TTY: 866-228-4327
                                         www.cancer.org
The American Cancer Society is the nationwide community-based voluntary health organization dedicated to eliminating cancer as a major health problem by preventing cancer, saving lives, and diminishing suffering from cancer, through research and education.
Susan Clifford, Media Relations Contact - Maine

Maryland

2178 American Cancer Society: Maryland
8219 Town Center Drive   410-931-6850
Baltimore, MD 21236   800-ACS-2345
                                         Fax: 410-931-6875
                                         TTY: 866-228-4327
                                         dawn.ward@cancer.org
                                         www.cancer.org
The American Cancer Society is the nationwide community-based voluntary health organization dedicated to eliminating cancer as a major health problem by preventing cancer, saving lives, and diminishing suffering from cancer, through research and education.
Dawn Ward, Media Relations Contact - Baltimore Area

2179 Leukemia and Lymphoma Society: Maryland Chapter
Leukemia Society of America
11350 McCormick Road   410-527-0220
Hunt Valley, MD 21031-2001   800-242-4572
                                         Fax: 410-527-0510
                                         sharon.yateman@lls.org
                                         www.lls.org
Dedicated to finding cures for leukemia and related cancers and to improving the quality of life for patients and their families.
Sharon E Yateman, Executive Director
Allyson Yospe, Deputy Executive Director

Massachusetts

2180 American Cancer Society: Boston
18 Tremont Street   617-556-7400
Boston, MA 02108   800-ACS-2345
                                         Fax: 617-263-6825
                                         TTY: 866-228-4327
                                         kate.langstone@cancer.org
                                         www.cancer.org
The American Cancer Society is the nationwide community-based voluntary health organization dedicated to eliminating cancer as a major health problem by preventing cancer, saving lives, and diminishing suffering from cancer, through research and education.
Kate Langstone, Media Relations Contact - Boston Area

2181 American Cancer Society: Central New England Region-Weston MA
9 Riverside Road   781-894-6633
Weston, MA 02493   800-ACS-2345
                                         Fax: 781-314-2699
                                         TTY: 866-228-4327
                                         jessica.saporetti@cancer.org
                                         www.cancer.org
The American Cancer Society is the nationwide community-based voluntary health organization dedicated to eliminating cancer as a major health problem by preventing cancer, saving lives, and diminishing suffering from cancer, through research and education.
Jessica Saporetti, Media Relations Contact

Michigan

2182 Leukemia and Lymphoma Society: Michigan Chapter
1421 E 12 Mile Road   248-581-3900
Madison Heights, MI 48071   800-456-5413
                                         Fax: 248-581-3901
                                         peggy.shriver@lls.org
                                         www.lls.org
Peggy Shriver, Executive Director
Robin R Rhea, Director Operations

Minnesota

2183 American Cancer Society: Duluth
130 W Superior Street   218-727-7439
Duluth, MN 55802   800-ACS-2345
                                         Fax: 218-727-8069
                                         TTY: 866-228-4327
                                         janis.rannow@cancer.org
                                         www.cancer.org
The American Cancer Society is the nationwide community-based voluntary health organization dedicated to eliminating cancer as a major health problem by preventing cancer, saving lives, and diminishing suffering from cancer, through research and education.
Janis Rannow, Media Relations Contact

2184 American Cancer Society: Mendota Heights Mendota Heights
Mendota Heights
2520 Pilot Knob Road   651-255-8100
Mendota Heights, MN 55120   800-ACS-2345
                                         Fax: 651-255-8133
                                         TTY: 866-228-4327
                                         lou.harvin@cancer.org
                                         www.cancer.org
The American Cancer Society is the nationwide community-based voluntary health organization dedicated to eliminating cancer as a major health problem by preventing cancer, saving lives, and diminishing suffering from cancer, through research and education.
Lou Harvin, Media Relations Contact
Janis Rannow, Media Relations Contact

2185 American Cancer Society: Rochester
2900 43 Street NW   507-287-2044
Rochester, MN 55901   800-ACS-2345
                                         Fax: 507-287-2178
                                         TTY: 866-228-4327
                                         janis.rannow@cancer.org
                                         www.cancer.org
The American Cancer Society is the nationwide community-based voluntary health organization dedicated to eliminating cancer as a major health problem by preventing cancer, saving lives, and diminishing suffering from cancer, through research and education.
Janis Rannow, Media Relations Contact

2186 American Cancer Society: Saint Cloud
3721 23rd Street S   320-255-0220
Saint Cloud, MN 56301   800-239-7028
                                         Fax: 320-255-5517
                                         TTY: 866-228-4327
                                         www.cancer.org
The American Cancer Society is the nationwide community-based voluntary health organization dedicated to eliminating cancer as a major health problem by preventing cancer, saving lives, and diminishing suffering from cancer, through research and education.
Janis Rannow, Media Relations Contact

2187 Leukemia and Lymphoma Society: Minnesota Chapter
5217 Wayzata Boulevard   763-852-3000
Golden Valley, MN 55426   888-220-4440
                                         Fax: 763-852-3001
                                         Murray.Schmidt@lls.org
                                         www.lls.org
Murray Schmidt, Executive Director
Vickie Shaw, Deputy Executive Director

Mississippi

2188 American Cancer Society: Jackson
1380 Livingston Lane   601-362-8874
Jackson, MS 39213   800-ACS-2345
                                                   Fax: 601-362-8876
                                                   TTY: 866-228-4327
                                            kelly.lindsay@cancer.org
                                                     www.cancer.org
The American Cancer Society is the nationwide community-based
voluntary health organization dedicated to eliminating cancer as a
major health problem by preventing cancer, saving lives, and diminishing suffering from cancer, through research and education.
Kelly Lindsay, Media Relations Contact

2189 Leukemia and Lymphoma Society: Mississippi Chapter
408 Fontaine Place   601-956-7447
Ridgeland, MS 39157   877-538-5364
                                                   Fax: 601-956-6957
                                                  Travis.Lee@lls.org
                                                        www.lls.org

Travis Lee, Campaign Director Team in Training
Natalie Michael, Campaign Director Team in Training

Missouri

2190 American Cancer Society: Saint Louis
4207 Lindell Boulevard   314-286-8100
Saint Louis, MO 63108   800-ACS-2345
                                                   Fax: 314-286-8160
                                                   TTY: 866-228-4327
                                         christine.winter@cancer.org
                                                     www.cancer.org
The American Cancer Society is the nationwide community-based
voluntary health organization dedicated to eliminating cancer as a
major health problem by preventing cancer, saving lives, and diminishing suffering from cancer, through research and education.
Christine Winter, Media Relations Contact

Montana

2191 American Cancer Society: Montana
3550 Mullan Road   406-542-2191
Missoula, MT 59808   800-ACS-2345
                                                   Fax: 406-327-0146
                                                   TTY: 866-228-4327
                                               jim.ryan@cancer.org
                                                     www.cancer.org
The American Cancer Society is the nationwide community-based
voluntary health organization dedicated to eliminating cancer as a
major health problem by preventing cancer, saving lives, and diminishing suffering from cancer, through research and education.
Jim Ryan, Media Relations Contact

Nebraska

2192 American Cancer Society: Nebraska
9850 Nicholas Street   402-393-5800
Omaha, NE 68114   800-ACS-2345
                                                   Fax: 402-393-7790
                                                   TTY: 866-228-4327
                                                     www.cancer.org
The American Cancer Society is the nationwide community-based
voluntary health organization dedicated to eliminating cancer as a
major health problem by preventing cancer, saving lives, and diminishing suffering from cancer, through research and education.
Mike Lefler, Media Relations Contact

2193 Leukemia and Lymphoma Society: Nebraska Chapter
10832 Old Mill Road   402-344-2242
Omaha, NE 68154   888-847-4974
                                                   Fax: 402-344-2422
                                               pattie.gorham@lls.org
                                                        www.lls.org

Pattie Gorham, Executive Director
Tonya Schroeder, Patient Services Manager - Portland Area

Nevada

2194 American Cancer Society: Nevada
6165 S Rainbow Boulevard   702-798-6877
Las Vegas, NV 89118   800-ACS-2345
                                                   Fax: 702-798-0530
                                                   TTY: 866-228-4327
                                                     www.cancer.org
The American Cancer Society is the nationwide community-based
voluntary health organization dedicated to eliminating cancer as a
major health problem by preventing cancer, saving lives, and diminishing suffering from cancer, through research and education.
Paulette Anderson, Media Relations Contact

New Hampshire

2195 American Cancer Society: New Hampshire Gail Singer Memorial Building
Gail Singer Memorial Building
2 Commerce Drive   603-472-8899
Bedford, NH 03110   800-ACS-2345
                                                   Fax: 603-472-7093
                                                   TTY: 866-228-4327
                                             peter.davies@cancer.org
                                                     www.cancer.org
The American Cancer Society is the nationwide community-based
voluntary health organization dedicated to eliminating cancer as a
major health problem by preventing cancer, saving lives, and diminishing suffering from cancer, through research and education.
Peter Davies, Media Relations Contact

2196 New Hampshire Cancer Pain Initiative
125 Airport Road   603-225-0900
Concord, NH 03301
Made up of concerned people who have joined together to promote
the alleviation of cancer pain through education, research and advisory activities.

New Jersey

2197 American Cancer Society: New Jersey
2600 US Highway 1   732-297-8000
N Brunswick, NJ 08902   800-ACS-2345
                                                   Fax: 732-297-9043
                                                   TTY: 866-228-4327
                                          marjorie.kaplan@cancer.org
                                                     www.cancer.org
The American Cancer Society is the nationwide community-based
voluntary health organization dedicated to eliminating cancer as a
major health problem by preventing cancer, saving lives, and diminishing suffering from cancer, through research and education.
Marjorie Kaplan, Media Relations Contact

2198 CanHelp
PO Box 1678   800-364-2341
Livingston, NJ 07039   Fax: 888-800-0201
                                                   joan@canhelp.com
                                                     www.canhelp.com
Offers reports for cancer patients on orthodox and alternative ther-
apies and coaching/counseling to help with treatment deci-
sion-making and coping.
Patrick M McGrady, Founder
Joan Runfola LCSW, Director

2199 Leukemia and Lymphoma Society: Northern New Jersey Chapter
Leukemia Society of America
116 South Euclid Avenue   908-654-9445
Westfield, NJ 07090   Fax: 908-654-9496
                                                  gina.panas@lls.org
                                                        www.lls.org
Dedicated to finding cures for leukemia and related cancers and to
improving the quality of life for patients and their families.

2200 Leukemia and Lymphoma Society: Southern New Jersey Chapter
Leukemia Society of America
216 Haddon Avenue   856-869-0200
Westmont, NJ 08108-2811   888-920-8557
                                                   Fax: 856-869-7383
                                                  gina.panas@lls.org
                                                        www.lls.org

Dedicated to finding cures for leukemia and related cancers and to improving the quality of life for patients and their families.

New Mexico

2201 American Cancer Society: New Mexico
10501 Montgomery Boulevard NE
Albuquerque, NM 87111

505-260-2105
800-ACS-2345
Fax: 505-266-9513
TTY: 866-228-4327
john.weisgerber@cancer.org
www.cancer.org

The American Cancer Society is the nationwide community-based voluntary health organization dedicated to eliminating cancer as a major health problem by preventing cancer, saving lives, and diminishing suffering from cancer, through research and education.
John Weisgerber, Media Relations Contact

2202 Leukemia and Lymphoma Society: Mountain States Chapter
Leukemia Society of America
3411 Candelaria NE
Albuquerque, NM 87107

505-872-0141
888-286-7846
Fax: 505-872-2480
gina.panas@lls.org
www.lls.org

Dedicated to finding cures for leukemia and related cancers and to improving the quality of life for patients and their families. Serves New Mexico and the Greater El Paso, TX area.
Deborah Hoffman, Executive Director
Mikki Aronoff, Patient Services Manager - Portland Area

New York

2203 American Cancer Society: Central New York Region/East Syracuse
6725 Lyons Street
E Syracuse, NY 13057

315-437-7025
800-ACS-2345
Fax: 315-437-8233
TTY: 866-228-4327
kim.mcmahon@cancer.org
www.cancer.org

The American Cancer Society is the nationwide community-based voluntary health organization dedicated to eliminating cancer as a major health problem by preventing cancer, saving lives, and diminishing suffering from cancer, through research and education.
Kim McMahon, Media Relations Contact

2204 American Cancer Society: Long Island
75 Davids Drive
Hauppauge, NY 11788

631-436-7070
800-ACS-2345
Fax: 631-436-5380
TTY: 866-228-4327
jennifer.cucurullo@cancer.org
www.cancer.org

The American Cancer Society is the nationwide community-based voluntary health organization dedicated to eliminating cancer as a major health problem by preventing cancer, saving lives, and diminishing suffering from cancer, through research and education.
Jennifer Cucurullo, Media Relations Contact

2205 American Cancer Society: New York City
132 W 32nd Street
New York, NY 10001-3983

212-586-8700
800-ACS-2345
Fax: 212-237-3855
TTY: 866-228-4327
jennifer.cucurullo@cancer.org
www.cancer.org

The American Cancer Society is the nationwide community-based voluntary health organization dedicated to eliminating cancer as a major health problem by preventing cancer, saving lives, and diminishing suffering from cancer, through research and education.
Jennifer Cucurullo, Media Relations Contact

2206 American Cancer Society: Queens Region / Rego Park
97-99 Queens Boulevard
Rego Park, NY 11374

718-263-2224
800-ACS-2345
Fax: 718-261-0758
TTY: 866-228-4327
jennifer.cucurullo@cancer.org
www.cancer.org

The American Cancer Society is the nationwide community-based voluntary health organization dedicated to eliminating cancer as a major health problem by preventing cancer, saving lives, and diminishing suffering from cancer, through research and education.
Jennifer Cucurullo, Media Relations Contact

2207 American Cancer Society: Westchester Region/White Plains
2 Lyon Place
White Plains, NY 10601

914-949-4800
800-ACS-2345
Fax: 914-397-8851
TTY: 866-228-4327
jennifer.cucurullo@cancer.org
www.cancer.org

The American Cancer Society is the nationwide community-based voluntary health organization dedicated to eliminating cancer as a major health problem by preventing cancer, saving lives, and diminishing suffering from cancer, through research and education.
Jennifer Cucurullo, Media Relations Contact

2208 Foundation for Advancement in Cancer Therapy
Old Chelsea Station
New York, NY 10113

212-741-2790
www.fact-ltd.org

Distributes information on cancer prevention and nontoxic therapies for cancer.
Ruth Sackman, President/Co-founder
James H Davis, Vice Chair

2209 Leukemia & Lymphoma Society Chapter: New York City
475 Park Avenue S
New York, NY 10016

212-376-7100
800-955-4572
Fax: 212-448-9214
ossom@lls.org
www.leukemia-lymphoma.org

Dedicated to finding cures for leukemia and related cancers and to improving the quality of life for patients and their families. Educational materials, support services and financial aid available. Volunteer opportunities.
Michael Osso, Executive Director
Sara Lipsky, Deputy Executive Director

2210 Leukemia & Lymphoma Society: Westchester/ Hudson Valley Chapter
1311 Mamaroneck Avenue
White Plains, NY 10605

914-949-0084
Fax: 914-949-0391
www.lls.org/wch

Mission is to cure leukemia, lymphoma, Hodgkin's disease and myeloma, and to improve the quality of life of patients and their families.
Dennis P Chillemi, Executive Director
Diandra Kodl, Deputy Executive Director

2211 Leukemia and Lymphoma Society Chapter: New York City
475 Park Avenue S
New York, NY 10016

212-376-7100
800-955-4572
Fax: 212-448-9214
ossom@lls.org
www.leukemia-lymphoma.org

Dedicated to finding cures for leukemia and related cancers and to improving the quality of life for patients and their families. Educational materials, support services and financial aid available. Volunteer opportunities.
Michael Osso, Executive Director
Sara Lipsky, Deputy Executive Director

2212 Leukemia and Lymphoma Society: Central New York Chapter
Leukemia Society of America
401 N Salina Street
Syracuse, NY 13203

315-471-1050
800-690-8944
Fax: 315-471-6434
chip.lockwood@lls.org
www.lls.org

Dedicated to finding cures for leukemia and related cancers and to improving the quality of life for patients and their families.
Chip Lockwood, Executive Director
Kristen Duggleby, Campaign Director Donor Relations

2213 Leukemia and Lymphoma Society: Long Island Chapter
Leukemia Society of America

555 Broadhollow Road
Melville, NY 11747
631-752-8500
Fax: 631-752-9066
tammy.philie@lls.org
www.lls.org

Established to serve Long Islanders with leukemia, lymphoma, Hodgkin's disease and myeloma, their families and friends.
Tammy Philie, Executive Director
Nicole Kowaleski, Deputy Executive Director

2214 Leukemia and Lymphoma Society: Upstate New York Chapter
Leukemia Society of America
5 Computer Drive W
Albany, NY 12205
518-438-3583
866-255-3583
Fax: 518-438-6431
Maureen.Thornton@lls.org
www.lls.org

Dedicated to finding cures for leukemia and related cancers and to improving the quality of life for patients and their families.
Maureen O'Brien-Thor, Executive Director
Raechel Hunt, Patient Services Manager - Portland Area

2215 Leukemia and Lymphoma Society: Western New York & Finger Lakes Chapter
Leukemia Society of America
4053 Maple Road
Amherst, NY 14226
716-834-2578
800-784-2368
Fax: 716-837-0335
nancy.hails@lls.org
www.lls.org

Dedicated to finding cures for leukemia and related cancers and to improving the quality of life for patients and their families.
Nancy Hails, Executive Director
Luann Burgio, Deputy Executive Director

North Carolina

2216 American Cancer Society: North Carolina
8300 Health Park
Raleigh, NC 27615
919-334-5218
800-ACS-2345
Fax: 919-841-1422
TTY: 866-228-4327
www.cancer.org

The American Cancer Society is the nationwide community-based voluntary health organization dedicated to eliminating cancer as a major health problem by preventing cancer, saving lives, and diminishing suffering from cancer, through research and education.
Jeff Bright, Media Relations Contact

2217 Leukemia and Lymphoma Society: Eastern North Carolina Chapter
Flagship Building
401 Harrison Oaks Boulevard
Cary, NC 27513
919-677-3993
800-936-9337
Fax: 919-677-3992
tiffany.armstrong@lls.org
www.lls.org

Tiffany Armstrong, Executive Director
Loreal Massiah, Patient Services Manager - Portland Area

2218 Leukemia and Lymphoma Society: North Carolina Chapter
Leukemia Society of America
5950 Fairview Road
Charlotte, NC 28210
704-998-5012
800-888-9934
Fax: 704-998-5010
www.lls.org

Dedicated to finding cures for leukemia and related cancers and to improving the quality of life for patients and their families.
Tiffany Armstrong, Executive Director
Loreal Massiah, Patient Services Manager - Portland Area

North Dakota

2219 American Cancer Society: North Dakota
4646 Amber Valley Parkway
Fargo, ND 58104
701-232-1385
800-ACS-2345
Fax: 701-232-1109
TTY: 866-228-4327
jim.ryan@cancer.org
www.cancer.org

The American Cancer Society is the nationwide community-based voluntary health organization dedicated to eliminating cancer as a major health problem by preventing cancer, saving lives, and diminishing suffering from cancer, through research and education.
Jim Ryan, Media Relations Contact

Ohio

2220 American Cancer Society: Ohio
870 Michigan Avenue
Columbus, OH 43215
888-227-6446
Fax: 877-227-2838
TTY: 866-228-4327
www.cancer.org

The American Cancer Society is the nationwide community-based voluntary health organization dedicated to eliminating cancer as a major health problem by preventing cancer, saving lives, and diminishing suffering from cancer, through research and education.
Robert Paschen, Media Relations Contact

2221 Leukemia and Lymphoma Society: Central Ohio Chapter
Leukemia Society of America
2225 City Gate Drive
Columbus, OH 43219
614-476-7194
800-686-CURE
Fax: 614-476-7189
phil.tanner@lls.org
www.lls.org

Dedicated to finding cures for leukemia and related cancers and to improving the quality of life for patients and their families.
Phil Tanner, Executive Director
Dan Swisher, Office Manager

2222 Leukemia and Lymphoma Society: Northern Ohio Chapter
Leukemia Society of America
23297 Commerce Park
Cleveland, OH 44122
216-910-1200
800-589-5721
Fax: 216-910-1201
frank.canning@lls.org
www.lls.org

Dedicated to finding cures for leukemia and related cancers and to improving the quality of life for patients and their families.
Frank Canning, Field Director
Nancy Toghill, Office Manager

2223 Leukemia and Lymphoma Society: Southern Ohio Chapter
Leukemia Society of America
4370 Glendale Milford Rd
Cincinnati, OH 45242
513-698-2828
Fax: 513-361-2109
michelle.steed@lls.org
www.lls.org

Dedicated to finding cures for leukemia and related cancers and to improving the quality of life for patients and their families. This chapter serves a 22-county geographic area.
Michelle Steed, Executive Director
Gene Fisher, Operations Director

Oklahoma

2224 American Cancer Society: Oklahoma
6525 N Meridian
Oklahoma City, OK 73116
405-843-9888
800-ACS-2345
Fax: 405-848-0795
TTY: 866-228-4327
www.cancer.org

The American Cancer Society is the nationwide community-based voluntary health organization dedicated to eliminating cancer as a major health problem by preventing cancer, saving lives, and diminishing suffering from cancer, through research and education.
Christina Li, Media/Public Relations

2225 Leukemia and Lymphoma Society: Oklahoma Chapter
Leukemia Society of America
500 N Broadway
Oklahoma City, OK 73102
405-943-8888
888-828-4572
Fax: 405-943-8355
sherry.martin@lls.org
www.lls.org

Dedicated to finding cures for leukemia and related cancers and to improving the quality of life for patients and their families.
Sherry Marti MSW LCSW, Patient Services Manager - Portland Area
Jill Hull, Campaign Director Team in Training

Oregon

2226 American Cancer Society: Oregon
330 SW Curry Street
Portland, OR 97239

503-295-6422
800-ACS-2345
Fax: 503-228-1062
TTY: 866-228-4327
www.cancer.org

The American Cancer Society is the nationwide community-based voluntary health organization dedicated to eliminating cancer as a major health problem by preventing cancer, saving lives, and diminishing suffering from cancer, through research and education.
Gretchen Rosenberger, Media Relations Contact

2227 Leukemia and Lymphoma Society: Oregon Chapter
Leukemia Society of America
9320 SWBarbur Boulevard
Portland, OR 97219

503-245-9866
800-466-6572
Fax: 503-245-9865
Sarah.Varner@lls.org
www.lls.org

Dedicated to finding cures for leukemia and related cancers and to improving the quality of life for patients and their families.
Sarah Varner, Executive Director
Sue Sumpter, Patient Services Manager - Portland Area

Pennsylvania

2228 American Cancer Society: Harrisburg Capital Area Unit
Capital Area Unit
3211 N Front Street
Harrisburg, PA 17110

215-985-5336
888-227-5445
Fax: 717-231-5784
TTY: 866-228-4327
john.held@cancer.org
www.cancer.org

The American Cancer Society is the nationwide community-based voluntary health organization dedicated to eliminating cancer as a major health problem by preventing cancer, saving lives, and diminishing suffering from cancer, through research and education.
Colleen Fitz, Media Relations Contact
John Held, Media Relations Contact

2229 American Cancer Society: Philadelphia
1626 Locust Street
Philadelphia, PA 19103

215-985-5336
888-227-5445
Fax: 215-985-5406
TTY: 866-228-4327
john.held@cancer.org
www.cancer.org

The American Cancer Society is the nationwide community-based voluntary health organization dedicated to eliminating cancer as a major health problem by preventing cancer, saving lives, and diminishing suffering from cancer, through research and education.
John Held, Media Relations Contact
Colleen Fitz, Media/Public Relations

2230 American Cancer Society: Pittsburgh
320 Bilmar Drive
Pittsburgh, PA 15205

215-985-5336
888-227-5445
Fax: 412-919-1101
TTY: 866-228-4327
www.cancer.org

The American Cancer Society is the nationwide community-based voluntary health organization dedicated to eliminating cancer as a major health problem by preventing cancer, saving lives, and diminishing suffering from cancer, through research and education.
Dan Catena, Media Relations Contact

2231 Leukemia and Lymphoma Society: Central Pennsylvania Chapter
800 Corporate Circle
Harrisburg, PA 17110

717-652-6520
800-822-2873
Fax: 717-652-8614
beth.mihmet@lls.org
www.lls.org

Elizabeth Mihmet, Executive Director
Danielle Bubnis, Patient Services Manager

2232 Leukemia and Lymphoma Society: Eastern Pennsylvania Chapter
555 N Lane
Conshohocken, PA 19428

610-238-0360
800-482-CURE
Fax: 484-530-0833
ursula.raczak@lls.org
www.lls.org

Lydia Hernandez-Vele, Executive Director
Ursula Raczak, Deputy Executive Director

2233 Leukemia and Lymphoma Society: Western Pennsylvania/West Virginia Chapter
Leukemia Society of America
333 E Carson Street
Pittsburgh, PA 15219-1439

412-395-2873
800-726-2873
Fax: 412-395-2888
massaric@lls.org
www.lls.org

Tina Massari, Executive Director
Jeanne Caliguiri, Development Director

Rhode Island

2234 American Cancer Society: Rhode Island
931 Jefferson Boulevard
Warwick, RI 02886

401-722-8480
800-ACS-2345
Fax: 401-421-0535
TTY: 866-228-4327
jim.beardsworth@cancer.org
www.cancer.org

The American Cancer Society is the nationwide community-based voluntary health organization dedicated to eliminating cancer as a major health problem by preventing cancer, saving lives, and diminishing suffering from cancer, through research and education.
Jim Beardsworth, Media Relations Contact

2235 Leukemia and Lymphoma Society: Rhode Island Chapter
1210 Pontiac Avenue
Cranston, RI 02920

401-943-8888
Fax: 401-943-1377
koconisb@lls.org
www.lls.org

Bill Koconis, Executive Director
Gloria Hincapie, Patient Services Manager

South Carolina

2236 American Cancer Society: South Carolina
128 Stonemark Lane
Columbia, SC 29210

803-750-1693
800-ACS-2345
Fax: 803-750-4000
TTY: 866-228-4327
www.cancer.org

The American Cancer Society is the nationwide community-based voluntary health organization dedicated to eliminating cancer as a major health problem by preventing cancer, saving lives, and diminishing suffering from cancer, through research and education.
Mary Jane Wardle, Media Relations Contact

2237 Leukemia and Lymphoma Society: South Carolina Chapter
1247 Lake Murray Boulevard
Irmo, SC 29063

803-749-4299
Fax: 803-749-4088
www.lls.org

2238 Leukemia and Lymphoma Society: South/West
107 Westpark Boulevard
Columbia, SC 29210

803-731-4060
Fax: 803-731-4066
paul.jeter@lls.org
www.lls.org

Paul Jeter, Executive Director
Cassandra Wineglass, Patient Services Manager

South Dakota

2239 American Cancer Society: South Dakota
4904 S Technopolis Drive
Sioux Falls, SD 57106

605-361-8277
800-ACS-2345
Fax: 605-361-8537
TTY: 866-228-4327
www.cancer.org

The American Cancer Society is the nationwide community-based voluntary health organization dedicated to eliminating cancer as a major health problem by preventing cancer, saving lives, and diminishing suffering from cancer, through research and education.
Charlotte Ho, Media Relations Contact

Tennessee

2240 American Cancer Society: Tennessee
2000 Charlotte Avenue   615-327-0991
Nashville, TN 37203   800-ACS-2345
                                            Fax: 615-341-7335
                                             TTY: 866-228-4327
                                              www.cancer.org
The American Cancer Society is the nationwide community-based voluntary health organization dedicated to eliminating cancer as a major health problem by preventing cancer, saving lives, and diminishing suffering from cancer, through research and education.
Brian Gillespie, Media Relations Contact

2241 Leukemia & Lymphoma Society: Tennessee Chapter
404 BNA Drive   615-331-2980
Nashville, TN 37217   800-332-2980
                                            Fax: 615-331-2941
                            winslowm@tn.leukemia-lymphoma.org
                                 www.leukemia-lymphoma.org
Founded in 1982 to better serve the needs of Tennesseans. Offers contribution funded community services, family support groups, free educational materials and financial assistance for those affected by leukemia, Hodgkin's disease, myeloma and lymphomas.
Colleen Grady, Executive Director
Mary Winslow, Patient Services Manager

Texas

2242 American Cancer Society: Texas
2433 Ridgepoint Drive   512-919-1800
Austin, TX 78754   800-ACS-2345
                                            Fax: 512-919-1846
                                             TTY: 866-228-4327
                                      justine.hall@cancer.org
                                              www.cancer.org
The American Cancer Society is the nationwide community-based voluntary health organization dedicated to eliminating cancer as a major health problem by preventing cancer, saving lives, and diminishing suffering from cancer, through research and education.
Justin Hall, Media Relations Contact

2243 Leukemia and Lymphoma Society: North Texas Chapter
Leukemia Society of America
8111 LBJ Freeway   972-239-0959
Dallas, TX 75251   800-800-6702
                                            Fax: 972-239-0892
                                        Tina.Garcia@lls.org
                                                 www.lls.org
Dedicated to finding cures for leukemia and related cancers and to improving the quality of life for patients and their families.
Tina Garcia, Executive Director
Sarah Bayley, Donor Development Director

2244 Leukemia and Lymphoma Society: South/West Texas Chapter
Leukemia Society of America
431 Isom Road   210-377-1775
San Antonio, TX 78216-4170   800-683-2458
                                            Fax: 210-344-3717
                                                 www.lls.org
Dedicated to finding cures for leukemia and related cancers and to improving the quality of life for patients and their families.
Jon Walter, President/CEO
Jimmy Nangle, CFO

2245 Leukemia and Lymphoma Society: Texas Gulf Coast Chapter
Leukemia Society of America
5005 Mitchelldale   713-680-8088
Houston, TX 77092   Fax: 713-683-9504
                                      BillieSue.Parris@lls.org
                                                 www.lls.org
Dedicated to finding cures for leukemia and related cancers and to improving the quality of life for patients and their families.
Billie Sue Parris, Executive Director
Jane Thompson, Office Manager

Utah

2246 American Cancer Society: Utah
941 E 3300 S   801-483-1500
Salt Lake City, UT 84106   800-ACS-2345
                                            Fax: 801-483-1558
                                             TTY: 866-228-4327
                                              www.cancer.org
The American Cancer Society is the nationwide community-based voluntary health organization dedicated to eliminating cancer as a major health problem by preventing cancer, saving lives, and diminishing suffering from cancer, through research and education.
Patricia Monsoor, Media Relations Contact

Vermont

2247 American Cancer Society: Vermont
121 Connor Way   802-872-6300
Williston, VT 05495   800-ACS-2345
                                            Fax: 802-872-6399
                                             TTY: 866-228-4327
                                              www.cancer.org
The American Cancer Society is the nationwide community-based voluntary health organization dedicated to eliminating cancer as a major health problem by preventing cancer, saving lives, and diminishing suffering from cancer, through research and education.
Chris Falk, Media Relations Contact

Virginia

2248 American Cancer Society: Virginia
4240 Park Place Court   804-527-3700
Glen Allen, VA 23060   800-ACS-2345
                                            Fax: 804-527-3797
                                             TTY: 866-228-4327
                                   domenick.casuccio@cancer.org
                                              www.cancer.org
The American Cancer Society is the nationwide community-based voluntary health organization dedicated to eliminating cancer as a major health problem by preventing cancer, saving lives, and diminishing suffering from cancer, through research and education.
Domenick Casuccio, Media Relations Contact

2249 Arlin J Brown Information Center
PO Box 251   540-752-9511
Fort Belvoir, VA 22060-0251
An information clearinghouse on types of cancer health methods and nontoxic cancer therapies.

2250 Leukemia and Lymophoma Society: National Capital Area Chapter
Leukemia Society of America
5845 Richmond Highway   703-399-2900
Alexandria, VA 22303   Fax: 703-399-2901
                                     donna.mckelvey@lls.org
                                                 www.lls.org
Serves the greater Washington DC metropolitan area including Northern Virginia Prince George's and Montgomery counties.
Gabrielle Urquhart, Executive Director
Beth Gorman, Deputy Director

Washington

2251 American Cancer Society: Washington
728 134th Street SW   425-741-8949
Everett, WA 98204   Fax: 425-741-9638
                                      liz.lamb-ferro@cancer.org
                                              www.cancer.org
The American Cancer Society is the nationwide community-based voluntary health organization dedicated to eliminating cancer as a major health problem by preventing cancer, saving lives, and diminishing suffering from cancer, through research and education.
Liz Lamb-Ferro, Media Relations Contact

2252 Washington Leukemia and Lymphoma Society: Alaska Chapter
Leukemia Society of America
530 Dexter Avenue N 206-628-0777
Seattle, WA 98109 888-345-4572
Fax: 206-292-9791
wachapter@lls.org
www.leukemia-lymphoma.org
Dedicated to finding cures for leukemia and related cancers and to improving the quality of life for patients and their families.
Anne Gillingham, Executive Director
Kimberly Conn, Deputy Executive Director

West Virginia

2253 American Cancer Society: West Virginia
301 RHL Boulevard 304-746-9950
Charleston, WV 25309 800-ACS-2345
Fax: 304-746-9962
TTY: 866-228-4327
www.cancer.org
The American Cancer Society is the nationwide community-based voluntary health organization dedicated to eliminating cancer as a major health problem by preventing cancer, saving lives, and diminishing suffering from cancer, through research and education.
Amy Wentz Berner, Media Relations Contact

Wisconsin

2254 American Cancer Society: Wisconsin
N19 W24350 Riverwood Drive 262-523-5500
Waukesha, WI 53188 800-ACS-2345
Fax: 262-523-5533
TTY: 866-228-4327
www.acscan.org/action/wi
The American Cancer Society is the nationwide community-based voluntary health organization dedicated to eliminating cancer as a major health problem by preventing cancer, saving lives, and diminishing suffering from cancer, through research and education.
Peter Balistrieri, Media Relations Contact
Christopher Hansen, President, ACS CAN

2255 Leukemia and Lymphoma Society: Wisconsin Chapter
Leukemia Society of America
200 S Executive Drive 262-790-4701
Brookfield, WI 53005 800-261-7399
Fax: 262-790-4706
bede.barthpotter@lls.org
www.lls.org
Founded in 1963 to serve Wisconsites touched by leukemia, lymphoma, Hodgkin's disease and myeloma.
Bede Barth Potter, Executive Director
Karen Ropel, Deputy Executive Director

Wyoming

2256 American Cancer Society: Wyoming
333 S Beech Street 307-577-4892
Casper, WY 82601 800-ACS-2345
Fax: 307-234-0926
TTY: 866-228-4327
joel.quevillon@cancer.org
www.acscan.org
The American Cancer Society is the nationwide community-based voluntary health organization dedicated to eliminating cancer as a major health problem by preventing cancer, saving lives, and diminishing suffering from cancer, through research and education.
John R Seffrin, CEO,ACS
Christopher Hansen, President, ACS CAN

Foundations

2257 Bone Marrow & Cancer Foundation
515 Madison Avenue 212-838-3029
New York, NY 10022 800-365-1336
Fax: 212-223-0081
thebmf@bonemarrow.org
bonemarrow.org
Goal is to improve the quality of life for bone marrow and stem cell transplant patients and their families by providing financial aid, education, and emotional support.
Christina Merrill, President & CEO
Robert Fishman, Chair

2258 Chemotherapy Foundation
183 Madison Avenue 212-213-9292
New York, NY 10016 Fax: 212-133-31
www.chemotherapyfoundation.com
The Chemotherapy Foundation is dedicated to developing more effective methods of treatment for the control and cure of cancer. They provide educational materials and provide funds for innovative chemotherapy research, and sponsor professional and public educational symposia.
Shirley Cox, Executive Director
Franco Muggia, Chairman & Medical Director

2259 Dermatology Foundation
1560 Sherman Avenue 847-328-2256
Evanston, IL 60201-4808 Fax: 847-328-0509
dfgen@dermatologyfoundation.org
www.dermfnd.org
The Foundation focuses on funding research that will advance patient care, and help develop and retain tomorrow's teachers and clinical leaders in the specialty.
Sandra Rahn Benz, Executive Director
James H Davis, Vice Chair

2260 National Children's Cancer Society
One South Memorial Drive 314-241-1600
Saint Louis, MO 63102 800-882-6227
Fax: 314-241-1996
krudd@children-cancer.org
www.children-cancer.org
Our mission is to improve the quality of life for children with cancer and their families worldwide. We serve as a financial, emotional, educational, and medical resource for those in need, at every stage of their illness and recovery. The NCCS provides direct financial assistance to families for expenses not covered by insurance during their treatment; including transportation, lodging, gas money, medical assistance, health insurance premiums, and phone cards.
Mark Slocomb, Chairman
Mark Stolze, President/CEO

2261 National Foundation for Cancer Research
5515 Security Lane 800-321-2873
Rockville, MD 20852 info@nfcr.org
www.nfcr.org
Contracts with major universities for basic science cancer research in the fields of biophysics, theoretical physics, and biochemistry.
Sujuan Ba, PhD, President & CEO
Brian Wachtel, Executive Director

2262 Prostate Cancer Foundation
1250 Fourth Street 310-570-4700
Santa Monica, CA 90401 800-757-2873
Fax: 310-570-4701
info@pcf.org
www.pcf.org
Seeks to find better treatments and a cure for recurrent prostate cancer by reaching out to individuals, corporations, and others, to harness financial and human resources.
Michael Milken, Founder & Chair
Jonathan W. Simons, MD, President & CEO

2263 Skin Cancer Foundation
205 Lexington Avenue 212-725-5176
New York, NY 10016 Fax: 212-725-5751
info@skincancer.org
www.skincancer.org
Conducts public and medical education programs to help reduce skin cancer. Major goals are to increase public awareness of the importance of taking protective measures against the damaging rays of the sun and to teach people how to recognize the early signs.
Deborah S. Sarnoff, MD, President
Dan Latore, Executive Director

Libraries & Resource Centers

2264 Cancer Federation
PO Box 1298
Banning, CA 92220
951-849-4325
Fax: 951-849-0156
info@cancerfed.org
The Federation is a not-for-profit organization that provides information, counseling, educational materials and meetings for the cancer patients, their families and friends. Also, they fund research and scholarships.
John Steinbacher, Executive Director

2265 Cancer Information Service
National Cancer Institute
6116 Executive Boulevard
Bethesda, MD 20892-8322
301-435-3848
800-422-6237
TTY: 800-332-8615
http://cis.nci.nih.gov/
Kramer Barnett, Director
Adamson Kristin, Administrative Resource Center

2266 Patient Advocates for Advanced Cancer Treatments (PAACT)
PO Box 141695
Grand Rapids, MI 49514-1695
616-453-1477
Fax: 616-453-1846
paact@paactusa.org
Provides support and advocacy for prostate cancer patients, their families, and the general public at risk. Information relative to the advancements in the detection, diagnosis, evaluation, and treatment of prostate cancer. Information, referrals, phone help, conferences, newsletter.
Richard H. Profit, President
Saleem Durvesh, Executive Marketing Director

Research Centers

2267 Purdue Cancer Center Purdue University
Purdue University
201 S University Street
W Lafayette, IN 47907-2064
765-494-9129
Fax: 765-494-9193
cancerresearch@purdue.edu
www.cancer.purdue.edu
Provide a forum for 75 of Purdue's best and brightest scientists to collaborate across campus and nationwide to prevent cancer to ease its detection and to cure it.
Timothy Ratliff, Director
Andrea Gregory-Kreps, Operations Manager

Alabama

2268 Birmingham VA Medical Center: Research and Development
700 S 19th Street
Birmingham, AL 35233
205-933-8101
866-487-4243
Fax: 205-933-4484
www.birmingham.va.gov
An acute tertiary care facility with particularly strong programs in both medicine and surgery and serves as the primary referral center for the state. We provide health care services to eligible veterans in the VA Southeast Network .
Steven L Keller, Acting Chairman
Rica Lewis-Payton, Medical Center Director

2269 Breast Cancer Resource Foundation of Alabama
PO Box 531225
Birmingham, AL 35253
205-996-5463
Fax: 205-975-2432
jgalbrea@uab.edu
www.bcrfa.org
Dedicated to finding a cure for breast cancer.
Dianne Mooney, President
Jennifer Galbreath, Program Director

2270 University of Alabama At Birmingham Comprehensive Cancer Center
UAB Comprehensive Cancer Center
1802 6th Avenue S
Birmingham, AL 35294-3300
205-934-5077
800-UAB-0933
info@ccc.uab.edu
www3.ccc.uab.edu
The Center provides advanced cancer care research and education based on stringent peer-reviewed data.
Edward E Partridge, Director and Associate Director for Comm
Kirby I Bland, Deputy Director

Arizona

2271 Southwest Association for Education in Biomedical Research
PO Box 210101
Tucson, AZ 85721-0101
520-621-3931
Fax: 520-621-3355
swaebr@ahsc.arizona.edu
www.swaebr.org
The mission of the Southwest Association for Education in Biomedical Research is to develop and implement a strong proactive campaign to educate school children as well as the general public in the vital role biomedical research plays in their everyday lives.
Charles Atkinson, President

2272 University of Arizona Cancer Center
1515 N Campbell Avenue
Tucson, AZ 85724-1454
520-626-5279
800-327-2873
www.azcc.arizona.edu
Comprehensive cancer center for diagnosis treatment and prevention.
David S Alberts, Director
Paola Villar Werstler, Director Of Development

California

2273 Burnham Institute Cancer Center The Burnham Institute for Medical Resear
The Burnham Institute for Medical Research
10901 N Torrey Pines Road
La Jolla, CA 92037
858-646-3100
Fax: 858-646-3199
info@sanfordburnham.org
www.sanfordburnham.org
Known for world-class capabilities in stem cell research and drug discovery technologies. Dedicated to revealing the fundamental molecular causes of disease and devising the innovative therapies of tomorrow.
Kristiina Vuori, President & CEO
Gary Raisl, Executive VP,CFO,Treasurer

2274 Cancer Prevention Institute of California
2201 Walnut Avenue
Fremont, CA 94538-2334
510-608-5000
800-511-2300
Fax: 510-608-5095
www.cpic.org
The North California Cancer Center is dedicated to understanding the causes prevention and detection of cancer and to improving the quality of life for individuals living with cancer.
Reed Goertler, Chief Operations Officer
Sally Glaser PhD, CEO

2275 City of Hope Comprehensive Cancer Research Center
1500 E Duarte Road
Duarte, CA 91010
626-256-4673
800-256-4673
Fax: 626-930-5394
tkronitis@coh.org
www.cityofhope.org
Excellence in biomedical research patient-centered medical care and community outreach.
Theodore G Krontiris MD, Director
Richard Jove, Deputy Director

2276 Geraldine Brush Cancer Research Institute California Pacific Medical Center
California Pacific Medical Center
2333 Clay Street #201
San Francisco, CA 94115
415-600-6000
cpmcadmin@sutterhealth.org
www.cpmc.org
Martin Brotman, President
Robert Tomasello, Chairman

2277 Ida and Joseph Friend Cancer Resource Center
1600 Divisadero St.
San Francisco, CA 94143-981
415-885-3693
800-444-2559
Fax: 415-885-3701
cancerresource@ucsfmedctr.org
www.cancer.ucsf.edu/crc/

The Cancer Resource Center supports wellness and the healing process by providing patients and their loved ones with information emotional support and community resources. The CRC maintains a multimedia library provides access to specialized health databases and offers research assistance. We host diverse support groups and classes and direct people to other community resources. All CRC programs are free.
Frank Mccorm PhD, Director

2278 Jonsson Comprehensive Cancer Center University of California At Los Angeles
University of California At Los Angeles
8-684 Factor Building
Los Angeles, CA 90095-1781
310-825-5268
888-662-8252
Fax: 310-206-5553
jcccinfo@mednet.ucla.edu
www.cancer.ucla.edu
UCLA's Jonsson Comprehensive Cancer Center (JCCC) has established an international reputation for developing new cancer therapies providing the best in experimental treatments and expertly guiding and training the next generation of medical researchers.
Judith Gasson, Director
James Economou, Executive Director

2279 Pediatric Cancer Research Laboratory Children's Hospital of Orange County
Children's Hospital of Orange County
1201 W.LA Veta Ave
Orange, CA 92868-3874
714-997-3000
Fax: 714-532-8380
www.choc.org
CHOC is the first hospital devoted exclusively to caring for children in Orange County.
Dr Mitchell Cairo, Director

2280 Rebecca and John Moores UCSD Cancer Center
3855 Health Sciences Drive
La Jolla, CA 92093-0658
585-534-7600
Fax: 858-534-7628
dedavis@ucsd.edu
One of the just 39 centers in the US to hold a National Cancer Institute designation as a Comprehensive Cancer Center. As such it ranks among the top centers in the nation conducting basic and clinical cancer research providing advanced patient care and serving the community through outreach and education programs.
John Alksne, Professor Surgery
Michael Andre, Adjunct Professor Radiology

2281 Salk Institute Cancer Center
Salk Institute for Biological Studies
PO Box 85800
San Diego, CA 92186-5800
858-453-4100
Fax: 858-453-8534
communications@salk.edu
www.salk.edu
The Cancer Center was established in 1970. It is one of only eight basic research cancer centers in the country designated by the National Cancer Institute. The center includes 22 faculty members 150 postdoctoral researchers 45 graduate students and 80 research assistants. It comprises about half of the research at the Salk Institute.
Walter Eckhart, Professor and Laboratory Head
William R Brody, President

2282 Santa Barbara Breast Cancer Institute
5333 Hollister Avenue
Santa Barbara, CA 93111-2341
805-964-8883
Otto Sartorius, Director

2283 Stanford University: Beckman Center for Molecular and Genetic Medicine
School of Medicine, Department of Biochemistry
291 Campus Drive Rm LK3C02
Stanford, CA 94305-5101
650-723-3622
Fax: 650-724-9733
cmgm.stanford.edu
Dr Paul Berg, Emeritus Professor Biochemistry
Philip A Pizzo MD, Dean

2284 USC/Norris Comprehensive Cancer Center
1441 Eastlake Avenue
Los Angeles, CA 90033-1048
323-865-3000
uscnorriscancer.usc.edu

Major regional and national resource for cancer research treatment prevention and education.
Peter A Jones, Director
Nikias C.L Max, President

2285 University of California Berkeley Cancer Research Laboratory
449 Life Science Addition
Berkeley, CA 94720-2751
510-642-4711
Fax: 510-642-5741
crl@berkeley.edu
Basic research with a special emphasis on mammary cancer and tumor immunotherapy.
Astar Winoto, Director
Judith Yee, Manager

2286 University of California: Los Angeles Bone Marrow Transplantation Program
200 UCLA Medical Plaza
Los Angeles, CA 90024
310-206-6889
Treatment of leukemia and anemia.
David W Golde MD, Director
Gabriel Danovitch, M.D., Medical Director, Proffessor of Medicine

Colorado

2287 AMC Cancer Research Center
1600 Pierce Street
Denver, CO 80214
303-233-6501
800-321-1557
Fax: 303-239-3400
contactus@amc.org
www.amc.org
Offers research activities publications meetings educational activities public services testing services community-based cancer control programs and knowledge of cancer mortality rates.
Alice Norton, Executive Director
Gail Eckhardt, Clinical Science

2288 Colorado Cancer Research Program
2253 S Oneida Street
Denver, CO 80224
303-777-2663
888-785-6789
Fax: 303-777-2642
ccrp@co-cancerresearch.org
www.co-cancerresearch.org
A nonprofit community-based cancer program established to provide community hospitals and physicians access to a wide range of cancer research trials in order to provide their patients with greater options for the treatment control and prevention.
Jane Hajovsky, Executive Director
Eduardo Pajon, Principal Investigator

2289 University of Colorado Cancer Center
13001 E 17th Place
Aurora, CO 80045
303-724-3155
800-473-2288
Fax: 303-724-3162
www.uccc.info
UCCC consortium is the hub for cancer research in Colorado. With eight programs 17 shared core resources and nearly 400 members from three universities and six institutions UCCC is responsible for the majority of cancer research in the Rocky Mountain region.
Dan Theodorescu MD PhD, Director
Laurie Gasper MD, Associate Director for Clinical Research

Connecticut

2290 Yale University Comprehensive Cancer Center
333 Cedar Street
New Haven, CT 06520-8028
203-785-4095
866-925-3226
Fax: 203-785-4116
www.yalecancercenter.org
A National Cancer Institute designated comprehensive cancer center for over 30 years Yale Cancer Center is one of only 40 Centers in the nation and the only comprehensive center in Southern New England.
Thomas Lynch, Director
Kevin Vest, PT, MBA, FACHE, Deputy Director

District of Columbia

2291 Georgetown University: Vincent T Lombardi Cancer Research Center
3800 Reservoir Road NW 202-444-4000
Washington, DC 20057
Established in 1970 the Lombardi Comprehensive Cancer Center is named for the legendary Green Bay Packers and Washington Redskins coach Vince Lombardi who was treated for cancer at Georgetown University Hospital.
Louis M Weiner, Director
Peter G Shields, Deputy Director

2292 Howard University Cancer Center
2041 Georgia Avenue NW 202-806-7697
Washington, DC 20060-0001 Fax: 202-462-8928
ladams-campbell@howard.edu
www.cancer.howard.edu
Reduce the burden of cancer through research education and service with emphasis on the unique ethnic and cultural aspects of minority and underserved populations.
Lucile Adams-Campbel, Director
Wayne A I Frederick, Interim Director

2293 Melanoma Research Foundation
1411 K Street NW 202-347-9675
Washington, DC 20005 800-673-1290
Fax: 202-347-9678
info@melanoma.org
www.melanoma.org
Founded in October 1996 by melanoma patients and their families to support research which will lead to cure for melanoma. Strictly a volunteer organization - not one person will receive compensation for his or her efforts.
Steve Silverstein, President & CEO
william G Reilly, President/Owner

Florida

2294 Rambaugh-Goodwin Institute for Cancer Research
1850 NW 69th Avenue 954-587-9020
Plantation, FL 33313 Fax: 954-587-6378
www.rgicr.org
RGI is committed to rapidly developing anti-cancer therapies in conjunction with industrial and academic partners using efficient models of cancer growth and metastasis with the aim of moving novel compounds to market in the shortest time possible.
Claire Thuning-Robin, Director

2295 UM/Sylvester Comprehensive Cancer Center
1475 NW 12th Avenue 305-243-1000
Miami, FL 33136 800-545-2292
www.sylvester.org
UMHC offers an outpatient clinic a 40-bed inpatient unit a comprehensive treatment unit the Mohs surgery center/dermatology clinic the Rosenfield GI Center a cardiology lab and clinic a radiology/imaging suite an interventional radiology clinic the Spine Institute clinics on-site laboratory and pharmacy the Courtelis Center for Psychosocial Oncology the Jill Selevan Chapel a cafeteria as well as administrative offices.
Joan Scheiner, Chair
Jayne S. Malfitano, Vice Chair

Georgia

2296 Emory University: Georgia Center for Cancer Statistics
Rollins School of Public Health
201 Dowman Drive 404-727-6123
Atlanta, GA 30322 Fax: 404-727-7261
gccs@sph.emory.edu
Serves as a cancer registry for five counties of metropolitan Atlanta and ten rural counties of central Georgia.
James W Wagner, President

2297 Emory University: Winship Cancer Institute
1365-C Clifton Road NE 404-778-1900
Atlanta, GA 30322 888-946-7447
www.winshipcancer.emory.edu

A clinical cancer center coordinating basic and clinical cancer research.
Walter Currans, Executive Director
Fadlo Khuri MD, Deputy Directory for Basic Research

Hawaii

2298 Pacific Health Research Institute
3375 Koapaka Street 808-524-4411
Honolulu, HI 96819 Fax: 808-524-5559
info@phrei.org
www.phrihawaii.org
Located in Honolulu Hawaii Pacific Health Research Institute (PHRI) is the largest independent biomedical research institute in the state. Since its founding on 1960 as an independent not for profit 501(c)(3) research institute PHRI today has become a leader in biomedical research in the Pacific. Indeed its researchers are performing complex investigations aimed at conquering some of the most debilitating and lethal diseases that afflict humankind.
Vicki L Shambaugh, MA, MPH, Director
Helen Petrovitch, Executive Director

2299 University of Hawaii: Cancer Research Center
1236 Lauhala Street 808-586-2985
Honolulu, HI 96813 Fax: 808-586-2982
cvogel@crch.hawaii.edu
The mission of the Cancer Research Center of Hawaii is to reduce the burden of cancer through research education and service with an emphasis on the unique ethnic culture and environmental characteristics of Hawaii and the Pacific.
Carl-Wilhelm Vogel, Professor (Researcher)
Michele Carbone, Interim Cancer Center Director

Illinois

2300 Cancer and Leukemia Group B
230 W Monroe 773-702-9171
Chicago, IL 60606 Fax: 312-345-0117
marciak@uchicago.edu
www.calgb.org
Integral unit of the Institute specializing in leukemia research and prevention.
Marcia Kelly, Administrative Coordinator
Michael Kelly, Director Protocol Operations

2301 Kellogg Cancer Care Center Evanston Hospital
Evanston Hospital
2650 Ridge Avenue 847-570-2000
Evanston, IL 60201 888-364-6400
www.enh.org
Integral unit of the Evanston Hospital this center researches treatment and diagnosis of cancer including phase 1 and phase 2 studies.
Mark R Neaman, President, CEO
Jeffery H Hillebrand, COO

2302 Leukemia Research Foundation
3520 Lake Avenue 847-424-0600
Wilmette, IL 60091-1064 888-558-5385
Fax: 847-424-0606
info@lrfmail.org
www.leukemia-research.org
To conquer leukemia lymphoma and myelodysplastic syndromes by funding research into their causes and cures and to enrich the quality of life of those touched by these diseases.
Kevin Radelet, Executive Director
Cindy Kane, Senior Director of Development

2303 Oncology Hematology Associates of Central Illinois
8940 N Wood Sage Road 309-243-3000
Peoria, IL 61615-7828 866-662-6564
www.illinoiscancercare.com

Research into cancer treatments.
Robert Cooper, Director
Paul A S Fishkin, Hematology Internal Medicine Medical O

2304 **Robert H Lurie Comprehensive Cancer Center of Northwestern University**
Galter Pavilion 675 N Street Clair   312-695-0990
Chicago, IL 60611   866-587-4322
    Fax: 312-695-1352
    cancer@northwestern.edu
    www.lurie.northwestern.edu
Lurie Cancer Center is a founding member of the National Comprehensive Cancer Network an exclusive alliance of 21 of the nation's leading cancer centers.
Steven T Rosen, Director
Leonidas Platanias, Deputy Director

2305 **University of Chicago Cancer Research Center**
5841 S Maryland Avenue   773-702-6180
Chicago, IL 60637   877-824-0600
    cancerresources@uccrc.org
The University of Chicago Cancer Research Center (UCCRC) employs a wealth of intellectual technological and financial resources to pursue a comprehensive collaborative research program involving more than 200 renowned scientists and clinicians.
Mary Ellen Connellan, Executive Director
Justin Ullman, President

2306 **University of Chicago: Clinical Nutrition Research Unit**
5841 S Maryland Avenue   773-702-6180
Chicago, IL 60637-1463   877-824-0600
    feedback@bsd.uchicago.edu
    www.uchicago.edu
Provide superior healthcare in a compassionate manner ever mindful of each patient's dignity and individuality.
Michael M Le Beau PhD, Director
James L Madara, CEO

Indiana

2307 **Mary Margaret Walther Program Walther Cancer Institute**
Walther Cancer Institute
9292 N Meridian Street   317-708-6101
Indianapolis, IN 46260   Fax: 317-708-6102
    info@walther.org
    www.walther.org
Focuses research on all types of cancer studies.
Leonard J Betley, Chairman
James E Ruckle, President/CEO

Iowa

2308 **Iowa Oncology Research Association**
300 E Locust   515-244-7586
Des Moines, IA 50309   888-244-6061
    Fax: 515-244-3037
    sherrijr@iora.org
    www.iora.org
Clinical cancer studies and research.
Sherri Rickabaugh, Administrator
Becky Berrett, Research Assistants

2309 **University of Iowa: Holden Comprehensive Cancer Center**
UI Hospitals and Clinics
University of Iowa   319-353-8620
Iowa City, IA 52242-1002   800-777-8442
    Fax: 319-353-8988
    cancer-center@uiowa.edu
    www.uihealthcare.com/depts/cancercenter
The Holden Cancer Center promotes interactive high-quality cancer research high-quality health care related to the prevention detection and treatment of cancer and educates cancer professionals and the citizens of Iowa about cancer.
Jean E Robillard, Vice President for Medical Affairs
Kenneth P Kates, CEO

Kansas

2310 **Kansas State University: Terry C Johnson Center for Basic Cancer Research**
Center for Basic Cancer Research

1 Chalmers Hall   785-532-6705
Manhattan, KS 66506   Fax: 785-532-6707
    marcia@k-state.edu
    www.k-state.edu/cancer.center
The mission of the Terry C. Johnson Center for Basic Cancer Research is to further the understanding of cancers by funding basic cancer research and supporting higher education training and public outreach.
Rob Denell, Director
S Keith Chapes, Associate Director

Kentucky

2311 **Henry Vogt Cancer Research Institute James Graham Brown Cancer Center**
James Graham Brown Cancer Center
2301 S 3rd Street   502-852-5555
Louisville, KY 40208   800-334-8635
    www.louisville.edu/hsc/centers
The overall goal of the scientists in the Henry Vogt Cancer Research Institute is to study mechanisms relevant to tumor cell biology at the basic and translational level in order to provide insights that will contribute to the ultimate prevention and cure of malignant diseases.
Donald M Miller, Director
John W Eaton, Deputy Director

2312 **Kentucky Cancer Program**
2365 Harrodsburg Road   859-219-0772
Lexington, KY 40504-3381   Fax: 859-219-0548
    dka@kcp.uky.edu
    www.kcp.uky.edu
The KCP provides a variety of cancer programs and services to health professionals the public patients and survivors.
Debra Armstong, Director
Diane Frasure, Administrative Associate

2313 **University of Kentucky: Children Cancer Study Group**
Markey Cancer Center
800 Rose Street   859-257-4500
Lexington, KY 40536-93   800-333-8874
    Fax: 859-323-2074
    www.ukhealthcare.uky.edu/markey/
Kentucky Children's Hospital is the only children's hospital in the region. Patients range in age from infants through adolescents and have a variety of illness and injuries.
Michael Karpf, Executive Vice President for Health Affa
Frank Butler, VP for Medical Center Operations

2314 **University of Kentucky: Lucille Parker Markey Cancer Center**
800 Rose Street   859-247-4500
Lexington, KY 40536   800-333-8874
    Fax: 859-323-2074
    www.ukhealthcare.uky.edu/markey/
The Markey Cancer Center mission is to eliminate the morbidity and mortality of cancer through a comprehensive program of research education clinical care and community outreach.
Alfred M Cohen MD FACS, Director
Michael Karpf, Executive Vice President for Health Affa

Louisiana

2315 **Baton Rouge Regional Tumor Registry Mary Bird Perkins Cancer Center**
Mary Bird Perkins Cancer Center
4950 Essen Lane   225-767-0847
Baton Rouge, LA 70809   Fax: 225-215-1215
    www.marybird.org
The Louisiana Tumor Registry is composed of a central office and regional registries that collect and process cancer incidence data from the state's eight established geographic regions. These eight geographic areas are based on Louisiana's historic health districts.
Todd D Stevens, President, CEO
J Gerald Jolly, Chairman

2316 **Tulane University Pulmonary Diseases Critical Care and Enviromental Medicine**
School of Medicine

1430 Tulane Avenue
New Orleans, LA 70112

504-988-5187
800-588-5300
medsch@tulane.edu
www.som.tulane.edu/pulmdis/facilities

Provides state-of-the-art care to patients and teaching to trainees through several areas of academic excellence that include: Interstitial Lung Diseases; Asthma; Cystic Fibrosis; Sleep Disorders; Interventional Pulmonology; Lung Cancer; Smoking Cessation; Critical Care; and Environmental Medicine.
Lee Hamm, MD, Senior Vice President and Dean
Roy Weiner, Associate Dean for Clinical Research

Maryland

2317   Frederick Cancer Research Center
PO Box B
Frederick, MD 21702-1201

301-846-1000
Fax: 301-846-1108
web.ncifcrf.gov

Direct research into the causes treatment and prevention of cancer AIDS and related diseases.
Craig W Reynolds, Associate Director
Jo Anne Barb, Secretary

2318   Johns Hopkins University: Sydney Kimmel Comprehensive Cancer Center
The Harry and Jeanette Weinberg Buidling
401 N Broadway
Baltimore, MD 21231-0005

410-955-5222
www.hopkinskimmelcancercenter.org

Johns Hopkins Kimmel Cancer Center has active programs in clinical research laboratory research education community outreach and prevention and control.
Ronald J Danielles, President
Edward Miller MD, Dean of Medical Faculty, CEO

2319   National Foundation for Cancer Research
5515 Security Lane
Rockville, MD 20852

800-321-2873
info@nfcr.org
www.nfcr.org

Contracts with major universities for basic science cancer research in the fields of biophysics, theoretical physics, and biochemistry.
Sujuan Ba, PhD, President & CEO
Brian Wachtel, Executive Director

2320   Warren Grant Magnuson Clinical Center
National Institute of Health
9000 Rockville Pike
Bethesda, MD 20892

301-496-4000
800-411-1222
Fax: 301-480-9793
TTY: 866-411-1010
prpl@mail.cc.nih.gov

Established in 1953 as the research hospital of the National Institutes of Health. Designed so that patient care facilities are close to research laboratories so new findings of basic and clinical scientists can be quickly applied to the treatment of patients. Upon referral by physicians, patients are admitted to NIH clinical studies.
John Gallin, Clinical Center Director
David Henderson, Deputy Director for Clinical Care

Massachusetts

2321   Boston University Cancer Research Center
820 Harrison Avenue
Boston, MA 02118

617-638-8265
Fax: 617-638-6518
sfenness@bu.edu
www.bumc.bu.edu/clinicaltrials

The Office of Clinical Research (OCR) was established on July 1 1998 to serve as the central focus for clinical research support conduct and training at Boston University Medical Center.
Douglas V Faller, Director
Salli Fennessey, Manager

2322   Dana-Farber Institute: Department of Biostatistics and Computational Biology
450 Brookline Avenue
Boston, MA 02115-5450

617-632-3000
Fax: 617-632-2444
biostatistics@jimmy.harvard.edu
www.dana-farber.org

Integral unit of the Institute organized into laboratories of biostatistics computing and epidemiology.
Marvin Zelen, Researcher
Edward J Benz, President, CEO

2323   David H. Koch Institute for Integrative Ca ncer Research
MIT Center for Cancer
Koch Institute at MIT 76-158
Cambridge, MA 02142

617-253-6403
Fax: 617-324-2238
cancer@mit.edu

The mission of MIT Cancer Center is to apply tools of basic science and technology to determine how cancer is caused progresses and responds to treatment. Through this effort they have developed an increasingly complete understanding of the nature of cancer cells which has led directly to improved treatments for the disease.
Dr Tyler Jacks, Director
Dr Jaqueline Lees, Associate Director

Michigan

2324   Gershenson Radiation Oncology Center Barbara Ann Karmanos Cancer Institute
Barbara Ann Karmanos Cancer Institute
4100 John Road
Detroit, MI 48201

313-745-9191
800-527-6266
Fax: 313-745-2314
info@karmanos.org
www.karmanos.org

Radiation therapy and cancer treatment and research.
Gerold Bepler, President

2325   Meyer L Prentis Comprehensive Cancer Center of Metropolitan Detroit
Barbara Ann Karmanos Cancer Institute
4100 John Road
Detroit, MI 48201

313-745-9191
800-527-6266
Fax: 313-745-2314
info@karmanos.org
www.karmanos.org

Gerald Bepler, President

2326   Meyer L Prentis Comprehensive Cancer Cente Barbara Ann Karmanos Cancer Institute
4100 John Road
Detroit, MI 48201

313-745-9191
800-527-6266
Fax: 313-745-2314
info@karmanos.org
www.karmanos.org

Gerald Bepler, President

2327   University of Michigan: Cancer Center Cancer Research Committee
Cancer Research Committee
1500 E Medical Center Drive
Ann Arbor, MI 48109-094

734-764-0039
800-865-1125
Fax: 734-936-9582
www.cancer.med.umich.edu

The U-M Comprehensive Cancer Center provides its patients diagnostic treatment and support services in a collaborative environment focused on excellence in patient care.
Eric R Fearon, Associate Director for Science
Max S Wicha, Director

2328   Wayne State University Center for Molecular Medicine and Genetics
Wayne State University School of Medicine
3127 Scott Hall
Detroit, MI 48201

313-577-5323
Fax: 313-577-5218
sshaw@wayne.edu
www.genetics.wayne.edu

Research focusing on human conditions such as cancer and neuromuscular disorders.
Lawrence I Grossman, Professor/Director
Jeffrey A Loeb, Associate Director

Minnesota

2329 Mayo Comprehensive Cancer Center
200 First Street SW 507-284-2511
Rochester, MN 55905-0001 Fax: 507-284-0161
TTY: 507-284-9786
www.mayo.edu
Scientists and physician investigators conduct wide-ranging research to improve patient care while training the next generation of medical scholars.
Denis Cortese, President/Chief Executive Officer
Robert A Rizza, Director

2330 University of Minnesota Masonic Cancer Center
Division of Oncology
420 Delaware Street SE 612-624-8484
Minneapolis, MN 55455 800-226-2376
Fax: 612-626-3069
ccinfo@umn.edu
www.cancer.umn.edu
The Masonic Cancer Center fosters this mission by creating a collaborative research environment focused on the causes prevention detection and treatment of cancer; applying that knowledge to improve quality of life for patients and survivors; and sharing its discoveries with other scientists students professionals and the community.
Brian Steeves, Deputy Director
Ann D Cieslak, Executive Director

Missouri

2331 Cancer Research Center
3501 Berrywood Drive 573-875-2255
Columbia, MO 65201 Fax: 873-443-1202
www.cancerresearchcenter.org
Not only does the Cancer Research Center offer research they also offer community outreach programs to educate church groups civic clubs and other organizations about their research and cancer prevention.
Dr. Abe Eisenstark, Research Director
Jack Bozarth, Director

Nebraska

2332 Lincoln Cancer Center
4600 Valley Road 402-483-2827
Lincoln, NE 68510-4844 Fax: 402-483-4184
Barb Morton, Director

2333 University of Nebraska at Omaha Eppley Institute for Research in Cancer
University of Nebraska
985950 Nebraska Medical Center 402-559-4090
Omaha, NE 68198-5950 hmmaurer@unmc.edu
www.unmc.edu/eppley
To improve the health of Nebraska through premier educational programs innovative research the highest quality patient care and outreach to underserved populations.
Harold M Maurer, Chancellor
Thomas H Rosenquist, Vice Chancellor

New Hampshire

2334 Norris Cotton Cancer Center Dartmouth-Hitchcock Medical Center
Dartmouth-Hitchcock Medical Center
One Medical Center Drive 603-653-9000
Lebanon, NH 03756 800-639-6918
Fax: 603-653-9003
cancercenter@dartmouth.edu
www.cancer.dartmouth.edu
The Cancer Center provides a positive environment for treatment cure and recovery for patients with all forms of cancer.
Mark Israel MD, Director
Burton L Eisenberg, Deputy Director

New Mexico

2335 University of New Mexico: Cancer Research and Treatment Center
1201 Camino de Salud NE 505-272-4946
Albuquerque, NM 87131-5001 800-432-6806
Fax: 505-925-0100
One of the nation's 60 premier National Cancer Institute (NCI)-Designated Cancer Centers and we have been named one of America's Best Cancer Hospitals by U.S. News & World Report. UNM Cancer Center provides cancer diagnosis and treatment to over 40% of the adults and virtually all of the children diagnosed with cancer each year in New Mexico.
Cheryl Willman, Director/CEO
John A Trotter, Deputy EVP for Health Sciences

2336 University of New Mexico: Center for Non-Invasive Diagnosis
Mind Imaging Center/University of New Mexico
1101 Yale Boulevard NE 505-277-0111
Albuquerque, NM 87131-0001 Fax: 505-272-4056
Cardiology and cancer research.
David Lepre, Executive Director

New York

2337 Ackerman Institute for the Family
149 E 78th Street 212-879-4900
New York, NY 10075 Fax: 212-744-0206
ackerman@ackerman.org
www.ackerman.org
Independent nonprofit research organization specializing in family therapy teaching and clinical services.
Lois Braverman, President/CEO
Evan Imber-B PhD, Director

2338 Albany Medical College Joint Center for Cancer and Blood Disorders
43 New Scotland Avenue 518-262-3125
Albany, NY 12208 877-AMC-8008
Fax: 518-262-3165
TTY: 518-262-1180
www.amc.edu
Offers research in the fields of cancer and blood disorders focusing on radiotherapy pathology and surgery.
Herbert Abbott, General Pediatric
Kevin Costello, Internal Medicine

2339 Albert Einstein Cancer Center Albert Einstein College of Medicine
Albert Einstein College of Medicine
1300 Morris Park Avenue 718-430-2302
Bronx, NY 10461 Fax: 718-430-2000
aecc@aecom.yu.edu
www.einstein.yu.edu/centers/cancer/
The goal of AECC is to foster basic clinical population-based and translational research that addresses all aspects of the cancer problem.
Allen M Spiegel MD, Dean
David Goldman, Director

2340 Association for Research of Childhood Cancer
PO Box 251 716-681-4433
Buffalo, NY 14225-0251
The Association was chartered by New York State in that year as a not-for-profit corporation whose primary purpose was to fund the major pediatric research centers in Western New York.
Larry Lorenz, Vice President
Anne O'Donnel, President

2341 Bassett Research Institute
One Atwell Road 607-547-3456
Cooperstown, NY 13326 800-227-7388
research.institute@bassett.org
www.bassett.org
Research institute committed to seeking new information and new strategies for preventing detecting and treating disease.
Wiliiam F Streck MD, President/CEO

2342 Cancer Institute of Brooklyn
927 49th Street
Brooklyn, NY 11219-2923
Jo-Ann Hertz, Executive Director

718-972-5816
Fax: 718-972-8693

2343 Cancer Research Institute: New York
One Exchange Plaza 55 Broadway
New York, NY 10006

212-688-7515
800-992-2623
Fax: 212-832-9376
info@cancerresearch.org
www.cancerresearch.org

The Cancer Research Institute is the world's only non-profit organization dedicated exclusively to the support and coordination of laboratory and clinical efforts that will lead to the immunological treatment control and prevention of cancer.
Jill O'Donnel-Tormey, Executive Director
Leslie Anson, Assistant to the Executive Director

2344 Columbia University Comprehensive Cancer Center
630 W 168th Street
New York, NY 10032

212-305-4186
Fax: 212-305-6889
www.cumc.columbia.edu/

Lee Goldman, President
Anne L Taylor, Vice Dean

2345 Medical Foundation of Buffalo Hauptman-Woodward Medical Research Insti
Hauptman-Woodward Medical Research Institute
700 Ellicott Street
Buffalo, NY 14203-1102

716-898-8600
Fax: 716-898-8660
www.hwi.buffalo.edu

Nonprofit organization devoted to cancer research.
Herbert A Hauptman PhD, President/Nobel Laureate
Eaton E Lattman, Executive Director & CEO

2346 Memorial Sloan-Kettering Cancer Center
1275 York Avenue
New York, NY 10065

212-639-2000
888-675-7722
publicaffairs@mskcc.org
www.mskcc.org

Sloan-Kettering Institute has endeavored to lead the way in basic science research oftentimes translating those advances into clinical treatments.
Harold Varmus, President, CEO
Paul A Marks, President Emeritus

2347 New York University Cancer Institute New York University Medical Center
New York University Medical Center
530 First Avenue
New York, NY 10016

212-263-7300
888-769-8633
Fax: 212-263-0715
www.nyucancerinstitute.org

The mission of the NYU Cancer Institute is to decrease and eliminate cancer as a significant health problem throughout New York the national and the world by developing and maintaining excellent programs in patient care research education and prevention.
William Carroll, Director
Lauren E Hackett, Executive Director of Administration

2348 Roswell Park Cancer Institute National Cancer Institute
Elm & Carlton Streets
Buffalo, NY 14263

716-845-2300
877-275-7724
askrpci@roswellpark.org
www.roswellpark.org

Roswell Park Cancer Institute has made fundamental contributions to reducing the cancer burden and has successfully maintained an exemplary leadership role in setting the national standards for cancer care research and education.
Donald L Trump MD, Director
Ann Gioia, Director

2349 State University of New York Health Science Center At Brooklyn
450 Clarkson Avenue
Brooklyn, NY 11203

718-270-1000
www.downstate.edu

Downstate includes Colleges of Medicine Nursing and Health Related Professions and a School of Graduate Studies as well as its own teaching hospital an M.P.H. Program and extensive research facilities.
John C LaRosa, President
John B Clark, Interim Chancellor

2350 University of Rochester: James P Wilmot Cancer Center
601 Elmwood Avenue
Rochester, NY 14642

585-275-5823
866-494-5668
Fax: 585-276-0158
www.urmc.rochester.edu

To use education science and technology to improve health transforming the patient experience with fresh ideas and approaches steeped in disciplined science and delivered by health care professionals who innovate take intelligent risks and care about the lives they touch.
Jonathan W. Friedberg M.D., Director
Gregory Connolly, M.D., Hematology Oncology

North Carolina

2351 Cancer Center of Wake Forest University at Bowman Gray School of Medicine
Wake Forest University School Of Medicine
Medical Center Boulevard
Winston-Salem, NC 27157

336-716-2011
800-446-2255
Fax: 336-716-9593
medadmit@wfubmc.edu
www1.wfubmc.edu/cancer

Provide a superb education as well as personal support. Beyond the academic experiences offered at our medical school we encourage the development of our students as caring physicians dedicated to providing the very best care professionally and personally to all patients.
William B Applegate M D M P, Dean
John D McConnell, CEO

2352 Duke Comprehensive Cancer Center
2424 Erwin Road
Durham, NC 27705

919-684-3377
888-ASK-DUKE
Fax: 919-684-5653
www.cancer.duke.edu

One of only 39 centers in the country designated by the National Cancer Institute (NCI) as a 'comprehensive cancer center ' Duke combines cutting-edge research with compassionate care. Our team of nationally recognized physicians and staff treat nearly 6 000 new patients per year giving them the extensive experience that yields better results. In fact U.S. News & World Report rates Duke #7 in the nation for cancer care and best in the Southeast.
H Kim Lyerly, Director
Anthony Means, Deputy Director

2353 University of North Carolina UNC Lineberger Comprehensive Cancer Center
School of Medicine
450 est Dr
Chapel Hill, NC 27514

919-966-3036
866-869-1856
Fax: 919-966-3015
lccc@med.unc.edu
www.unclineberger.org

The Center provides multidisciplinary programs for most cancers giving patients the benefit of many medical specialists in one place often in one visit.
H Shelton Earp, Director
Michael O'Malley, Associate Director

Ohio

2354 Case Western Reserve University: Ireland Cancer Center
University Hospitals of Cleveland
11100 Euclid Avenue
Cleveland, OH 44106

216-844-1529
888-844-8447
www.uhhospitals.org/irelandcancer

Thomas F Senty, CEO

2355 Children's Hospital Research Foundation
700 Childrens Drive
Columbus, OH 43205-2696

614-722-2000
800-792-8401
Fax: 61 -35 -079
www.nationwidechildrens.org

Offers research activities into Reye's Syndrome genetics and children's cancer chemotherapy.
Richard McClead, Medical Director
Richard J Brilli, Chief Medical Officer

2356 Medical College of Toledo: Cancer Research Division
Department of Pathology
3000 Arlington Avenue   419-383-4000
Toledo, OH 43614-2595   800-321-8383
                                     Fax: 419-383-6130
                                     utmc.webmaster@utoledo.edu
Researches into all aspects of cancer.
Jill Zyrek-Betts, Assistant Professor

2357 Ohio State University Comprehensive Cancer Center
Arthur G James Cancer Hospital
300 W 10th Avenue   614-293-7521
Columbus, OH 43210-1240   michael.caligiuri@osumc.edu
A national and international leader in research, which translates to high-quality patient care and educational programs for residents of Ohio and beyond.
Michael A Caligiuri M D, Director
John C Byrd, Associate Director

2358 Ohio State University General Clinical Research Center
The Ohio State University   614-293-8750
Columbus, OH 43210   Fax: 614-293-3796
                                william.malarkey@osumc.edu
Provides facilities and financial support for inpatient and outpatient cancer research.
William Malaykey, Program Director
David Phillips, Administrative Director

2359 The Cancer Prevention Institute
23 Jasper St   937-227-9400
Dayton, OH 45409   877-274-4543
                                     Fax: 937-297-6970
                                     info@pch-dayton.org
                                www.premiercommunityhealth.org
Nonprofit organization focusing research activities primarily on cancer prevention anti-cancer drugs early diagnosis of cancer and bone marrow toxicity. previously known as the Hipple Cancer Research Center.
Stephen McHugh, Treasurer
Diane Ewing, Chair

Oklahoma

2360 Natalie Warren Bryant Cancer Center St. Francis Hospital
St. Francis Hospital
6600 S Yale Avenue   918-488-6688
Tulsa, OK 74136   webadministrator@saintfrancis.com
Jake Henry Jr, President/Chief Executive Officer
Barry Steichen, Executive Vice President/Chief Administr

2361 Oklahoma Medical Research Foundation Immunobiolgy & Cancer Research
Oklahoma Medical Research Foundation
825 North East 13th Street   405-271-6673
Oklahoma City, OK 73104-5005   800-522-0211
                                     Fax: 405-271-7016
                                     OMRF-President@omrf.org
                                     www.omrf.org
Dr. Stephen Prescott, President

2362 Samuel Roberts Noble Foundation Biomedical Division
Samuel Roberts Noble Foundation
2510 Sam Noble Parkway   580-223-5810
Ardmore, OK 73401   Fax: 580-224-6217
                                     www.noble.org
One of the largest international offshore drilling contractors in the world.
Michael A Cawley, CEO/President
Bill Goddard, Trustee

Pennsylvania

2363 Abramson Cancer Center of the University of Pennsylvania
3535 Market Street   800-789-PENN
Philadelphia, PA 19104-3309   Fax: 215-349-5445
                                craig@mail.med.upenn.edu
                                     www.penncancer.com
National leader in cancer research patient care and education.
Douglas L Fraker MD, Deputy Director
Caryn Lerman, Interim Director

2364 Allegheny Singer Research Institute West Penn Allegheny Health System
West Penn Allegheny Health System
4800 Friendship Avenue   412-362-8677
Pittsburgh, PA 15224   877-284-2000
                                     Fax: 412-359-8610
                                     tchakurd@wpahs.org
                                     www.wpahs.org
Christopher Olivia MD, President, CEO

2365 Eastern Cooperative Oncology Group
1818 Market Street   215-789-3645
Philadelphia, PA 19103   800-4CA-NCER
                                     Fax: 267-256-5291
Studies into cancer including biological response modifiers and cancer studies.

2366 Fox Chase Cancer Center
333 Cottman Avenue   215-728-6900
Philadelphia, PA 19111-2497   888-369-2427
                                     www.fccc.edu
Linda Fliescher MPH PhD, Assistant Vice President for Communicati
Theresa Berger MBE, Project Manager

2367 Temple University FELS Institute for Cancer Research
School of Medicine
3500 N Broad Street   215-707-7000
Philadelphia, PA 19140   Fax: 215-707-7000
                                www.temple.edu/medicine
Policies and programs are oriented toward research and training in cancer-related basic biological and biochemical sciences with progressive extension into the areas of molecular developmental and chemical biology to advance knowledge of the etiology and pathogenesis of cancer. A major goal of the Institute is to utilize the advances made in basic science programs to develop novel targeted therapies for the treatment of cancer.
John M Daly MD, Dean
Diane Omdal, Director, Research Administration

2368 University of Pittsburgh Cancer Institute
5150 Centre Avenue   412-647-2811
Pittsburgh, PA 15232   PCI-INFO@upmc.edu
                                     www.upci.upmc.edu
Since 1985 the UPCI has been committed to improving the understanding of how cancer develops; to characterizing new lifesaving approaches for cancer prevention detection diagnosis and treatment; and to educating future generations of scientists and clinicians.
Nancy E Davidson MD, Committee Chair
Adam Brufsky MD PhD, Associate Director

Rhode Island

2369 Brown University Division of Biology and Medicine
BioMed Research Admin, Brown Medical School
The Warren Alpert Medical School of 401-863-3330
Providence, RI 02912-0001   Fax: 401-863-2660
Interdisciplinary studies in biological and medical sciences including studies in health care problems and fields of research such as cancer and diabetes.
John Perry, Senior Associate Dean
Edward J Wing, Medicine / Biological Sciences

2370 Roger Williams Clinical Cancer Research Center
Roger Williams General Hospital

825 Chalkstone Avenue
Providence, RI 02908
401-456-2000
www.rwmc.com
Kenneth Belcher, President
Sheri L. Smith, Ph.D., Chair

South Carolina

2371 Children's Center for Cancer and Blood Disorders
University of South Carolina School of Medicine
7 Richland Medical Park
Columbia, SC 29203
803-434-7000
www.palmettohealth.org
Joint clinical and basic research of juvenile cancer and blood disorders.
Charles D Beaman Jr, CEO

Tennessee

2372 St. Jude Children's Research Hospital
262 Danny Thomas Place
Memphis, TN 38105
901-495-3300
Fax: 901-495-4011
www.stjude.org
One of the world's premier pediatric cancer research centers.
Harvey J Cohen, Chair
William Evan PharmD, Director/CEO

2373 University of Tennessee Memphis: Cancer Center
66 N. Pauline St
Memphis, TN 38163-0001
901-448-5150
Fax: 901-528-5033
Alvin M Mauer MD, Director

Texas

2374 Baylor University Bone Marrow Transplantation Research Center
Baylor Research Institute
3500 Gaston Avenue
Dallas, TX 75246
214-820-2687
800-422-9567
www.baylorhealth.com
Offers bone marrow transplantation research in leukemia studies.
John B McWhorter, President
Irving D Prengler, VP Medical Staff Affairs

2375 Cancer Therapy and Research Center
7979 Wurzbach Road
San Antonio, TX 78229
210-450-1000
800-340-2872
www.ctrc.net
The mission of the Cancer Therapy & Research Center is to conquer cancer through research prevention and treatment.
Ian M Thompson MD, Director

2376 San Antonio Cancer Institute
7703 Floyd Curl Drive
San Antonio, TX 78229-3900
210-567-7000
Fax: 210-567-2709
www.uthscsa.edu/
Dr Tyler J Curiel, Director
William L Henrich MD MACP, President

2377 Southwest Foundation for Biomedical Research
PO Box 760549
San Antonio, TX 78245-0549
210-258-9400
Advancing the health of our global community through innovative biomedical research.
John R Hurd, Chairman
Lewis J Moorman III, Vice-Chairman

2378 University of Texas: MD Anderson Cancer Center
1515 Holcombe Boulevard
Houston, TX 77030-4009
713-792-2121
800-392-1611
www.mdanderson.org
To eliminate cancer in Texas the nation and the world through outstanding programs that integrate patient care research and prevention and through education for undergraduate and graduate students trainees professionals employees and the public.
John Mendelsohn, President -Executive Committee
Raymond DuBois, Executive Vice President

2379 University of Texas: Medical Branch at Galveston Cancer Center
301 University Boulevard
Galveston, TX 77555
409-772-1011
Fax: 409-747-1938
TTY: 409-772-4200
public.affairs@utmb.edu
www.utmb.edu
The mission of The University of Texas Medical Branch at Galveston is to provide scholarly teaching innovative scientific investigation and state-of-the-art patient care in a learning environment to better the health of society.
B Mark Evers, Director
David L Calender, President

Utah

2380 Brigham Young University Cancer Research Center
181 Benson Science Building
Provo, UT 84602
801-422-3913
cancer_research@byu.edu
Provide a rigorous research training program for students.
Daniel L Simmons, Director
Cecil O. Samuelson, President

2381 Huntsman Cancer Institute University of Utah School of Medicine
University of Utah School of Medicine
2000 Circle of Hope
Salt Lake City, UT 84112
801-585-0303
877-585-0303
Fax: 801-585-5886
public.affairs@hci.utah.edu
www.huntsmancancer.org
Understand cancer from its beginnings to use that knowledge in the creation and improvement of cancer treatments to relieve the suffering of cancer patients and to provide education about cancer risk prevention and care.
Mary C Beckerle, Executive Director
Wallace Akerley, Senior Director of Clinical Research

Vermont

2382 University of Vermont Cancer Center University of Vermont
University of Vermont
E-213 Given Buildinge
Burlington, VT 05405
802-656-4414
877-540-4673
Fax: 802-656-8788
info@vermontcancer.org
www.vermontcancer.org
Richard Branda, Interim Director
Marianne Baggs, Assistant to the Director

Virginia

2383 Cancer Research Foundation of America
1600 Duke Street
Alexandria, VA 22314-3421
703-836-4412
800-227-2732
Fax: 703-836-4413
www.preventcancer.org
Prevention and early detection of cancer through research education and community outreach to all populations including children and the underserved.
Carolyn R Aldige, President and Founder
Marcia Myers Carlucci, Chairman

2384 Virginia Commonwealth University: Massey Cancer Center
401 College Street
Richmond, VA 23298-5017
804-828-0450
877-4MA-SSEY
Fax: 804-828-8453
massey@vcu.edu
www.massey.vcu.edu
The mission of the University of Central Arkansas is to maintain the highest academic quality and to ensure that its programs remain current and responsive to the diverse needs of those it serves.
Gordon D Ginder MD, Director
Steven Grant MD, Associate Director

Washington

2385 Fred Hutchinson Cancer Research Center
1100 Fairview Avenue N   206-288-7222
Seattle, WA 98109-1024   800-804-8824
                              Fax: 206-288-1025
                              hutchdoc@fhcrc.org
                              www.fhcrc.org
At Fred Hutchinson Cancer Research Center our interdisciplinary teams of world-renowned scientists and humanitarians work together to prevent diagnose and treat cancer HIV/AIDS and other diseases.
Lee Hartwell, Director/President
Mark Groudine, Executive Vice President and Deputy Dire

West Virginia

2386 West Virginia University: Mary Babb Randolph Cancer Center
Mary Babb Randolph Cancer Center Clinic
One Medical Center Drive   304-293-4500
Morgantown, WV 26506   877-427-2894
                              Fax: 304-598-4553
                              www.wvucancer.org/pages/
Premier cancer facility with a national reputation of excellence in cancer treatment prevention and research.
Augusto Ochoa, Director
Lori K Acciavatti, Professional Technologists

Wisconsin

2387 University of Wisconsin Paul P Carbone Comprehensive Cancer Center
600 Highland Avenue   608-263-6400
Madison, WI 53792-6164   800-622-8942
                              Fax: 608-263-8613
                              www.cancer.wisc.edu
The University of Wisconsin Paul P. Carbone Comprehensive Cancer Center is the only comprehensive cancer center in Wisconsin as designated by the National Cancer Institute. An integral part of the UW School of Medicine and public Health this cancer center unites more than 250 physicians and scientists who work together in translating discoveries from research laboratories into new treatments that benefit cancer patients.
George Wildi MD, Director
Kelly Sitkin, Development Director

Support Groups & Hotlines

2388 American Cancer Society: San Jose Prostate Cancer Support Group
3369 Union Avenue   408-559-8553
San Jose, CA 95124-2033   www.cancer.org

2389 American Foundation for Urologic Disease: Us Too Line
1128 N Charles Street   301-727-2908
Baltimore, MD 21201-5506   800-828-7866
Provides information and referrals for family members, victims and other individuals concerned with prostate cancer.

2390 American Institute for Cancer Research
1759 R Street NW   202-328-7744
Washington, DC 20009   800-843-8114
                              Fax: 202-328-7226
                              aicrweb@aicr.org
                              www.aicr.org

Melvin Huston, Chairman
Lawrence Pratt, Vice-Chairman

2391 Cancer Information Service
National Cancer Institute
1100 Fairview Avenue North   206-667-4675
Seattle, WA 98109-1024   800-422-6237
                              Fax: 206-667-7792
                              TTY: 800-332-8615
                              www.cancer.gov
Provides the latest and most accurate cancer information to patients, their families, the public, and health professionals. Also provides personalized responses to specific questions about cancer and assistance to smokers who want to quit.
Nancy Zbaren, Program Director

2392 Cancer Support Community
3276 Mc Nutt Avenue   925-933-0107
San Francisco, CA 94597-1909   Fax: 925-933-0249
                              www.cancersupportcommunity.net
Offers understanding, support and guidance to people with cancer and those who care about them.
James Bouquin, President & Executive Director
Margaret Stauffer, Vice President & Program Director

2393 Cancervive
11636 Chayote Street   310-203-9232
Los Angeles, CA 90049   800-486-2873
                              Fax: 310-471-4618
                              cancervivr@aol.com
Dedicated to providing support, public education and advocacy to those who have experienced this disease. The mission of Cancervive is to assist survivors to reclaim their lives after cancer.
Susan Nessim Keeney, Founder/President

2394 Center for Cancer Survival
104 W Anapamu Street   805-962-6221
Santa Barbara, CA 93101-3126
Nonprofit, nonmedical outreach education program teaching specific emotional, mental and spiritual skills for survival on their journey of recovery from cancer.
Richard Sheldon, Founder

2395 Collaborative Medicine Center
10 Willow Street   415-383-3197
Mill Valley, CA 94941-2895
Not specifically a cancer treatment center but works with cancer patients by using a variety of supportive modalities. The emphasis at the center is on helping people learn to support and activate their own healing processes.
Martin L Rossman MD

2396 Commonwealth Cancer Help Program
451 Mesa Road   415-868-0970
Bolinas, CA 94924   Fax: 415-868-2230
                              commonweal@commonweal.org
                              www.commonweal.org/programs/cancer-help/
An educational program designed to help participants reduce the stress of cancer, explore health habits, be with others experiencing the same difficulties and consider information on established and complementary therapeutic options.
Michael Lerner, President
Susan Braun, Executive Director

2397 Corporate Angel Network
Westchester County Airport
One Loop Road   914-328-1313
White Plains, NY 10604-1215   866-328-1313
                              Fax: 914-328-3938
                              info@corpangelnetwork.org
                              www.corpangelnetwork.org
To ease the emotional stress, physical discomfort and financial burden of travel for cancer patients by arranging free flights to treatment cetners, using the empty seats on corporate aircraft flying on routine business.
Peter H. Fleiss, Executive Director
Randall Greene, President & CEO

2398 Exceptional Cancer Patients/ECaP
532 Jackson Park Drive   814-337-8192
Meadville, CT 16335   Fax: 814-337-0699
                              info@ecap-online.org, info@mind-body.org
                              www.ecap-online.org/home.htm
The mission of EcaP/Exceptional Cancer Patients is to provide exceptional resources, comprehensive professional training programs and extraordinary interdisciplinary retreats that help people facing the challenges of cancer and other chronic illnesses discover their inner healing resources.
Bernie Siegal MD, Founder
Barry Bittman MD, Chief Executive Officer

2399 Gilda's Club: Grand Rapids
1806 Bridge Street NW
Grand Rapids, MI 49504   616-453-8300
Fax: 616-453-8355
info@gildasclubgr.org
www.gildasclubgr.org
A free cancer support community of children, adults, families and friends.
Leann Arkema, President/CEO
Davis Sesbastian, Chair

2400 Gilda's Club: New York City
502 Eigth Avenue   718-788-1600
Brooklyn, NY 11215   Fax: 718-788-0322
info@gildasclubnyc.org
www.gildasclubnyc.org
Creates welcoming communities of free support for everyone living with cancer - men, women, teens and children - along with their families and friends. The innovative program is an essential complement to medical care, providing networking and support groups, workshops, lectures and social activities, all free of charge.
Robert Easton, Chairman of the Board
Lily Safani, CEO

2401 Gilda's Club: Quad Cities
1234 E River Drive   319-326-7504
Davenport, IA 52803   877-926-7504
Fax: 563-323-1658
www.gildasclubqc.org
A cancer support community providing people living with cancer, and all who touch their lives, access to other people going through the same experience.
Claudia Robinson, CEO
Melissa Wright, Program Director

2402 Gilda's Club: South Florida
119 Rose Drive   954-763-6776
Fort Lauderdale, FL 33316   Fax: 954-763-6761
info@gildasclubsouthflorida.org
www.gildasclubsouthflorida.org
A free cancer support community for women, men, children, and teens with all types of cancer and their families and friends. Offer networking groups, lectures, workshops, specialized children's and teen programs, and social events in a nonresidential, non-medical, home-like setting.
Shelley Goren, CEO
Sara Howley Callari, Chair

2403 I Can Cope
American Cancer Society
1599 Clifton Road NE   404-320-3333
Atlanta, GA 30329-4250   800-227-2345
www.cancer.org
An educational program for people facing cancer, either personally, or as a friend or family caregiver. Helps dispel cancer myths by presenting straightforward facts and answers to your cancer-related questions

2404 International Association of Cancer Victors and Friends
7740 W Manchester Avenue   310-822-5032
Playa del Rey, CA 90293-8449   Fax: 310-822-4193
Offers reports and information on alternative therapies and recent cancer studies.
Ann Cinquina

2405 JamesCare For Life Support Groups & Services
James Cancer Hospital & Solove Research Institute
300 W 10th Avenue   614-293-5066
Columbus, OH 43210   800-293-5066
Fax: 614-293-2565
jamesline@osumc.edu
www.cancer.osu.edu
JamesCare for Life Cancer Support Groups and Services provides a wide range of resources and services to assist patients and families on their journey. This group offers support for patients and families to share experiences, express concerns, and learn more about the impact of cancer and available treatments.
Michael A Caligiuri, CEO
Jeff Walker, Senior Executive Director

2406 Look Good... Feel Better
American Cancer Society
1599 Clifton Road NE   404-320-3333
Atlanta, GA 30329-4250   800-227-2345
www.lookgoodfeelbetter.org
A community-based, free, national service. Teaches female cancer patients beauty tips to look better and feel good about how they look during chemotherapy and radiation treatments

2407 Lung Cancer Alliance Support Group
888 16th Street NW   202-463-2080
Washington, DC 20006   800-298-2436
kay@lungcanceralliance.org
www.lungcanceralliance.org
Dedicated solely to support and advocacy for all those living with or at risk for lung cancer.
T.Joseph Lopez, Chairman
Cheryl Healton, President & CEO

2408 National Cancer Institute
9609 Medical Center Drive   800-422-6237
Bethesda, MD 20892-9760   nciinfo@nih.gov
www.cancer.gov
Offers educational information, public awareness, research grants, and more for patients, their families, and health care professionals. Information specialists answer cancer-related questions by phone, LiveHelp instant messaging, and e-mail.
Douglas R. Lowy, MD, Acting Director
James Doroshow, MD, Deputy Director, Clinical Research

2409 National Foundation for Cancer Research Hotline
5515 Security Lane   800-321-2873
Rockville, MD 20852   info@nfcr.org
www.nfcr.org
Contracts with major universities for basic science cancer research in the fields of biophysics, theoretical physics, and biochemistry.
Sujuan Ba, PhD, President & CEO
Brian Wachtel, Executive Director

2410 National Health Information Center
Office of Disease Prevention & Health Promotion
1101 Wootton Pkwy   Fax: 240-453-8281
Rockville, MD 20852   odphpinfo@hhs.gov
www.health.gov/nhic
Supports public health education by maintaining a calendar of National Health Observances; helps connect consumers and health professionals to organizations that can best answer questions and provide up-to-date contact information from reliable sources; updates on a yearly basis toll-free numbers for health information, Federal health clearinghouses and info centers.
Don Wright, MD, MPH, Director

2411 National Hospice Helpline
1731 King Street   703-837-1500
Alexandria, VA 22314   800-646-6460
Fax: 703-837-1233
www.nhpco.org
Offers information on hospice in general and offers referrals to local hospice programs.
Edo Branch, JD, President & CEO
Hannah Yang Moore, MPH, Chief Advocacy Officer

2412 PDQ
National Cancer Institute
6116 Executive Boulevard   301-402-5874
Bethesda, MD 20892-8322   800-422-6237
www.cancer.gov
An NCI database that contains the latest information about cancer treatment, screening, prevention, genetics, supportive care, and complementary and alternative medicine, plus clinical trials.
Mark Greene MD, Editor-in-Chief

2413 Reach to Recovery
American Cancer Society
1599 Clifton Road NE   404-320-3333
Atlanta, GA 30329-4250   800-227-2345
www.cancer.org
Provides support for people recentlry diagnosed with breast cancer; people facing a possible diagnosis of breast cancer; those interested in or who have undergone a lumpectomy or mastectomy;

those considering breast reconstruction; those who have lymphedema; those who are undergoing or who have completed treatment such as chemotherapy and radiation therapy; people facing breast cancer recurrence or metastasis

2414 United Ostomy Associations of America Advocacy Hotline
PO Box 512   800-826-0826
Northfield, MN 55057-0512   info@uoaa.org
www.ostomy.org
A national network for bowel and urinary diversion support groups in the United States. The goal is to provide a nonprofit association that will serve to unify and strengthen its member support groups, which are organized for the benefit of people who have, or will have intestinal or urinary diversions and their caregivers.
Dave Rudzin, President

2415 Wainwright House Cancer Support Programs
260 Stuyvesant Avenue   914-967-6080
Rye, NY 10580-3115
Weeklong residential retreats offered four times a year to cancer patients. Retreats are devoted to cancer patient education, health promotion and stress management.
Richard Grossman, Program Director

2416 Women's Suffrage for Prostate Cancer Awareness
743 Caribou Court   800-776-2262
Sunnyvale, CA 94087-4229
Women have banded together here to help people cope with the effects of prostate cancer on their lives and educate others about it. Members understand problems of patients and families and are here to support and educate.
Judith P. Barnhard, CPA, Chairman
May Barnhard, PC, Chairman

Books

2417 3rd Opinion: International Directory to Complementary Therapy Centers
Avery Publishing Group
120 Old Broadway   516-741-2155
New Hyde Park, NY 11040-5000
Discusses over 300 alternative treatment cancer centers, educational centers, support groups and other research services.

2418 A Breast Cancer Journey: Your Personal Guidebook
American Cancer Society
1599 Clifton Road NE   404-320-3333
Atlanta, GA 30329-4250   800-227-2345
Helps women steer through the maze of information, empowering them to take control of their disease, treatment choices, health care team and life. Guidebook format encourages the reader to organize her information in a logical, easily accessible manner, record personal feelings and concerns and understand the details of practical matters such as paperwork and insurance, legal and sexual issues, side effects of treatment, and helping the entire family with support.
440 pages paperback
ISBN: 0-944235-20-4

2419 American Cancer Society Cancer Book
Doubleday & Company
666 5th Avenue   212-765-6500
New York, NY 10103-0001   www.penguinrandomhouse.com
Publishes 135 cancer organizations, centers, support services and various programs.

2420 American Cancer Society's Guide to Complementary/Alternative Cancer Methods
American Cancer Society
1599 Clifton Road NE   404-320-3333
Atlanta, GA 30329-4250   800-227-2345
Helps the public, the consumer and patients and their families understand what works, what's dangerous, and how best to evaluate the hundreds of claims that can be found on the internet and in the popular press. Each entry is researched and based on scientific evidence. Possible problems or complications are identified and clearly highlighted for easy reference. Covers a broad range, in-

cluding herbs, vitamins, minerals, diet, manual healing and biological methods. Clear, understandable language.
464 pages hardcover
ISBN: 0-944235-20-4

2421 American Cancer Society's Guide to Pain Control
American Cancer Society
1599 Clifton Road NE   404-320-3333
Atlanta, GA 30329-4250   800-227-2345
Provides a wealth of information, including talking to your health care team about pain, understanding what pain is and where it comes from, current drug and non-drug treatments and dealing with the financial burden of pain treatment. Includes information on how to record, chart and rate pain, guidelines for pain management, a comprehensive list of medications and other methods of pain relief and an informative resource guide.
400 pages paperback
ISBN: 0-944235-20-4

2422 American Cancer Society's Healthy Eating Cookbook: A Celebration of Food...
American Cancer Society
1599 Clifton Road NE   404-320-3333
Atlanta, GA 30329-4250   800-227-2345
More than 200 pages of irresistable recipes that turn healthy eating into a celebration of good food. Features photos and recipes from a host of the American Cancer Society's celebrity friends and fans. Includes hundreds of recipes, celebrity photos and essays, a handy Smart Substitution reference section and numerous tips for healthy cooking, including smart shopping, using leftovers and eating out.
216 pages hardcover
ISBN: 0-944235-20-4

2423 Bowel Cancer
Oxford University Press
2001 Evans Road   800-445-9714
Cary, NC 27513-2010   800-451-7556
Fax: 919-677-1303
custserv.us@oup.com
Offers information and public awareness on the disease of bowel cancer.
152 pages

2424 Breast Cancer
Branden Publishing Company
Branden Books   617-734-2045
Wellesley, MA 02482   Fax: 617-734-2046
www.branden.com
Paperback
ISBN: 0-828319-49-9

2425 Cancer Dictionary
Facts on File
11 Penn Plaza   212-967-8800
New York, NY 10001   800-322-8755
Fax: 800-678-3633
352 pages Paperback

2426 Cancer Facts and Figures
American Cancer Society
1599 Clifton Road NE   404-320-3333
Atlanta, GA 30329-4250   800-227-2345
Publishes over 57 treatment centers.

2427 Cancer Rates and Risks
National Cancer Institute
Building 31   800-422-6237
Bethesda, MD 20892-0001
This book is a compact guide to statistics, risk factors, and risks for major cancer sites.
136 pages

2428 Cancer Sourcebook
Karen Bellenir, author
Omnigraphics
155 W. Congress   313-961-1340
Detroit, MI 48226-4105   313-961-1383
Fax: 800-875-1340
contact@omnigraphics.com
www.omnigraphics.com

Offers basic information on cancer types, symptoms, diagnostic methods, and treatments. Includes statistics on cancer occurrences worldwide and the risks associated with known carcinogens and activities.
2003 1119 pages
ISBN: 0-780806-33-6

2429 Cancer Therapy: Ind. Consumer's Guide to Non-Toxic Treatment & Prevention
Ralph W. Moss, author
Equinox Press
Cancer Decisions   814-238-3367
Lemont, PA 16851   800-980-1234
    Fax: 814-238-3367
    www.cancerdecisions.com
A must for cancer patients and their families who want: Practical information on the most promising non-toxic treatments; Scientific evidence in readable language; Well-documented resource lists and medical references.
523 pages
ISBN: 1-881025-06-3
Ralph Moss, Medical Writer

2430 Cancer in the Family: Helping Children Cope with a Parent's Illness
American Cancer Society
1599 Clifton Road NE   404-320-3333
Atlanta, GA 30329-4250   800-227-2345
A diagnosis of cancer changes a family forever. Ordinary responsibilities become more demanding, and parents sometimes need assistance in balancing all of their children's needs. This book outlines steps to take to help children understand what happens when a parent has been diagnosed with cancer. Offers suggestions for talking to children, helping them cope, answering difficult questions, managing role changes and disruptions in routines, recognizing signs that your child needs help.
272 pages paperback
ISBN: 0-944235-20-4

2431 Caregiving: A Step-By-Step Resource for Caring for the Person w/Cancer at Home
American Cancer Society
1599 Clifton Road NE   404-320-3333
Atlanta, GA 30329-4250   800-227-2345
This practical guide offers manageable solutions to the myriad conditions and situations the caregiver may face, from physical to emotional conditions and dealing with health care providers and insurance carriers, to taking care of his or her own needs as well as those of the patient. East to use, this handy reference offers thorough, concise check-lists, questions to ask, signs and symptoms to note, and where to turn for more help.
336 pages paperback
ISBN: 0-944235-20-4

2432 Celebrate! Healthy Entertaining for Any Occasion
American Cancer Society
1599 Clifton Road NE   404-320-3333
Atlanta, GA 30329-4250   800-227-2345
You can celebrate in style without taking a break from healthy eating or delicious food. This book combines 20 festive, fun theme menus with easy recipes that don't sacrifice taste. Each menu offers a combination of approximately 8 manageable recipes, including appetizers, main dishes, side dishes, desserts and even beverages. Activities and decorating ideas in each section help make entertaining a breeze.
272 pages paperback
ISBN: 0-944235-20-4

2433 Choices: Realistic Alternatives in Cancer Treatment
Harper Collins
Avenue of the Americas   800-331-3761
New York, NY 10019   Fax: 800-822-4090
    www.naturalpedia.com
Covers a wide gamut of information that includes treatment centers, associations, research groups, and other facilities that are equipped to assist cancer patients and their families.

2434 Colorectal Cancer: A Compassionate Resource for Patients and Their Families
American Cancer Society

5900 Wilshire Boulevard   323-634-0080
Los Angles, CA 90036-4250   800-227-2345
    www.oreilly.com
The information in this article is meant to educate and should not be used as an alternative for professional medical care.
290 pages paperback
ISBN: 0-944235-20-4

2435 Consumer's Guide to Cancer Drugs
American Cancer Society
1599 Clifton Road NE   404-320-3333
Atlanta, GA 30329-4250   800-227-2345
Created for patients, cancer survivors and caregivers. Provides detailed information for the more than 200 medicines used to treat cancer or the symptoms of cancer. Drugs are listed alphabetically by generic name and described in depth. Detailed descriptions include common side effects, precautions and other important facts. All generic and trade names are listed in the index for easy cross-reference. Easy-to-understand language.
448 pages paperback
ISBN: 0-944235-20-4

2436 Coping: A Young Woman's Guide to Breast Cancer Prevention
Rosen Publishing Group
29 E 21st Street   212-777-3017
New York, NY 10010   800-237-9932
    Fax: 888-436-4643
    customerservice@rosenpub.com
    www.rosenpublishing.com
Breast cancer research has revealed the genetic predisposition of some cancers. This guide explains the nature of cancer, the risk of cancer and the ways to reduce that risk, especially for young women with a family history of breast cancer.
ISBN: 0-825929-67-1

2437 Everyone's Guide to Cancer Therapy
Andrews McMeel Publishing, LLC
c/o Simon & Schuster   800-851-8923
Riverside, NJ 08075   Fax: 816-581-7486
    www.andrewsmcmeel.com
How cancer is diagnosed, treated, and managed day to day.
2002 960 pages Paperback
ISBN: 0-740718-56-8

2438 Health Consequences of Smoking: Cancer & Chronic Lung Disease in the Workplace
DIANE Publishing Company
330 Pusey Ave   610-461-6200
Darby, PA 19023   800-782-3833
    Fax: 610-461-6130
    dianepublishing@gmail.com
    www.dianepublishing.net
Examines the relationship between cigarette smoking and occupational exposures. Establishes that in order to protect the workers fully, forces of labor, management, insurers and government must become as engaged in attempts to reduce the prevalence of cigarette smoking as they are in occupational exposure. Tables and figure. Extensive bibliography, index.
542 pages Paperback
ISBN: 0-788123-11-4
Herman Baron, Publisher

2439 Healthy and Hearty Diabetic Cooking
Diabetes Self-Management Books
PO Box 11477   800-664-9269
Des Moines, IA 50381-0001
James Hazlett, Editor

2440 Home Care Guide for Cancer
John's Hopkins University Press
2715 N Charles Street   410-516-6900
Baltimore, MD 21218-4319   800-537-5487
    Fax: 410-516-6998
    www.press.jhu.edu
This easy to use workbook was designed for home caregivers, patients, support groups and education programs; it features easy to

read type and index for quick reference and advice on twenty common cancer caregiving problems.
1996 260 pages Paperback
ISBN: 0-943126-30-4
Peter Houts, Editor

2441 I Choose to Fight: Tom Harper's Courageous Victory Over Cancer
Prentice Hall
15 Columbus Circle 212-373-8000
New York, NY 10023-7707 www.prenhall.com
A semi, auto-biographical account of Tom Harper's ordeal with testicular cancer, an affliction in young men.

2442 Informed Decisions: The Complete Book of Cancer Diagnosis, Treatment and Recovery
American Cancer Society
1599 Clifton Road NE 404-320-3333
Atlanta, GA 30329-4250 800-227-2345
Offers the latest information on every aspect of cancer, from detection to recovery. Covers everything from cancer causes and risk, screening and diagnostic tests, and treatment strategies to coping tips and questions to ask your doctor. Includes tips on how to effectively deal with the system and get the most advanced care in the country. Helps cancer patients and families make the right kinds of decisions- decisions that suit your particular needs and desires, and help you feel in control.
690 pages hardcover
ISBN: 0-944235-20-4

2443 Love Knot
Jones & Bartlett Publishers
40 Tall Pine Drive 978-443-5000
Sudbury, MA 01776 800-832-0034
Fax: 978-443-8000
info@jblearning.com
www.jblearning.com
It is a world-leading provider of instructional, assessment, and learning-performance management solutions for the secondary, post-secondary, and professional markets
232 pages Paperback
ISBN: 0-763714-12-7
Joy Stark, Associate Marketing Manager

2444 My Prostate and Me: Dealing with Prostate Cancer
Addison Books
2719 Houston Avenue 800-829-9653
Houston, TX 77009-7607

2445 National Cancer Institute Fact Book
National Cancer Institute
Building 31 800-422-6237
Bethesda, MD 20892-0001
This book presents general information about the National Cancer Institute including budget data, grants and contracts and historical information.

2446 No Less a Woman
Firestone Touchstone Paperbacks/Simon & Schuster
200 Old Tappan Road 800-999-5479
Old Tappan, NJ 07675-7005
Offers intimate interviews that explore the major issues of coping and surviving breast cancer, from diagnosis and treatment to physical and psychological recovery. In their own words, ten women describe how they successfully adjusted to the changes in their bodies and their feelings about themselves.
288 pages
ISBN: 0-671868-99-3

2447 Organizing and Maintaining Support Groups for Parents
Candlelighters' Childhood Cancer Foundation
7910 Woodmont Avenue 301-657-8401
Bethesda, MD 20814-3015 800-366-2223
Benefits of self-help support groups, activities, referral systems and parent/professional relations.

2448 Prostate Cancer: A Survivor's Guide
Don Kaltenbach and Tim Richards, author
Dattoli Cancer Foundation

2803 Fruitville Road 941-365-5599
Sarasota, FL 24237 800-915-1001
Fax: 941-366-3786
info@dattolifoundation.org
www.dattolifoundation.org
Written with the aid of leading prostate cancer specialists, this book clearly explains tests, the latest statistics and how to interpret them.
updated 2003 256 pages
ISBN: 0-964008-89-0

2449 Prostate Cancer: What Every Man and His Family Needs to Know
American Cancer Society
1599 Clifton Road NE 404-320-3333
Atlanta, GA 30329-4250 800-227-2345
Written by a team of internationally known and respected medical experts, this newly revised edition explains everything a man needs to know about prostate cancer, the most common form of cancer (excluding skin cancer) among American men.
322 pages paperback
ISBN: 0-944235-20-4

2450 Prostate Health Workbook
Newton Malerman, author
Hunter House Publishing
424 Church Street 615-255-2665
Nashville, TE 37219 800-266-5592
Fax: 615-255-5081
ordering@hunterhouse.com
www.turnerpublishing.com
A practical guide for the prostate cancer patients.
2002 160 pages Paperback
Newton Malerman, Author

2451 Singing from the Soul
Bone Marrow Foundation
515 Madison Avenue 212-838-3029
New York, NY 10022-5102 800-365-1336
Fax: 212-223-0081
THEBMF@BoneMarrow.org
www.bonemarrow.org
Jose Carreras' autobiography describes in eloquent detail his bone marrow transplant experience.

2452 Teratologies: A Cultural Study of Cancer
Routledge
8th Floor, 711 3rd Avenue 212-216-7800
New York, NY 10017 Fax: 212-564-7854
orders@taylorandfrancis.com
www.routledge.com
A distinctively feminist look at how cancer is perceived, experienced and theorized in contemporary society. Beginning with powerful personal accounts of her own illness, as well as self-help manuals and patients' personal stories, Jackie Stacey explores changing beliefs about the causes and treatments of cancer in both biomedecine and its increasingly popular alternative counterparts.
304 pages
Jackie Stacey, Author

2453 The Mountain You've Climbed: A Parent's Guide to Childhood Cancer Survivorship
500 North Broadway 314-241-1600
Saint Louis, MO 63101 Fax: 314-241-1996
krudd@children-cancer.org
This guide is designed to answer parent's questions regarding childhood cancer, address issues related to diagnosis and offer suggestions on how to integrate the cancer experience into all areas of the family's life. It addresses issues beginning from the time of diagnosis through the completion of treatment and beyond.
Mark Slocomb, Chairman
Mark Stolze, President/CEO

2454 Understanding Breast Cancer Genetics
Barbara T Zimmerman, PhD, author
University Press of Mississippi
3825 Ridgewood Road 601-432-6205
Jackson, MS 39211-6492 Fax: 601-432-6217
kburgess@ihl.state.ms.us
www.upress.state.ms.us

Clinical explanations for the genetic causes of the disease women most greatly fear.
2004 128 pages Paperback
ISBN: 1-578065-79-8
Barbara T. Zimmerman, Ph.D., Author

2455 Understanding Cancer Therapies
Helen S L Chan, MD, author
University Press of Mississippi
3825 Ridgewood Road   601-432-6205
Jackson, MS 39211-6492   Fax: 601-432-6217
                                    kburgess@ihl.state.ms.us
                                    www.upress.state.ms.us
A practical and hopeful guide to the many treatments available.
2006 144 pages Paperback
ISBN: 1-578066-89-1
Helen S. L. Chan, M.D., Author

2456 Understanding Colon Cancer
A Richard Adrouny, MD; FACP, author
University Press of Mississippi
3825 Ridgewood Road   601-432-6205
Jackson, MS 39211-6492   Fax: 601-432-6217
                                    kburgess@ihl.state.ms.us
                                    www.upress.state.ms.us
For the general reader a concise manual of facts, warnings, prevention, treatments, and forecasts.
2002 168 pages Paperback
ISBN: 1-578062-03-9
A. Richard Adrouny, M.D., F.A.C.P., Author

2457 When a Parent Has Cancer: A Guide to Caring for Your Children
Harper Collins
10 E 53rd Street   212-207-7000
New York, NY 10022   www.harpercollins.com
ISBN: 0-060187-09-3
Wendy S. Harpham M.D., Author

2458 Women and Cancer: A Compassionate Reource for Patients and Their Families
American Cancer Society
1599 Clifton Road NE   404-320-3333
Atlanta, GA 30329-4250   800-227-2345
Concise, thorough and up-to-date, this book provides women who have been diagnosed with cancer information about the four most common cancers of the reproductive system- breast, cervical, endometrial and ovarian cancer. Each chapter describes how each organ is structured and how it functions, and the risks and benefits of new drug therapies, radiation and chemotherapy, and surgical procedures. Includes patient stories and addresses the full range of issues faced by patients and their families.
290 pages paperback
ISBN: 0-944235-20-4

2459 Young People with Cancer: A Handbook for Parents
Barry Leonard, author
DIANE Publishing Company
330 Pusey Avenue   610-461-6200
Darby, PA 19023   800-782-3833
                                    Fax: 610-461-6130
                                    dianepublishing@gmail.com
                                    www.dianepublishing.net
Gives you information on all stages of your child's cancer. It tells you what to expect and suggests ways to prepare for different situations.
109 pages Paperback
ISBN: 0-756736-59-5
Herman Baron, Publisher

Children's Books

2460 Cancer
Franklin Watts Grolier
90 Old Sherman Turnpike   203-797-3500
Danbury, CT 06816-0001   800-621-1115
                                    Fax: 203-797-3197
                                    www.auth.grolier.com

Discusses causes such as chemicals, viruses, radiation and oncogenes, as well as diagnosis, types of cancers, immune defenses and common treatments.
96 pages Grades 7-12
ISBN: 0-531108-03-1

2461 Cancer: Overview Series
Lucent Books
Thomson Gale   800-877-4253
Farmington Hills, MI 48331-9187   Fax: 800-363-4253
                            gale.customerservice@thomson.com
                                    www.gale.com/lucent
Questions are answered for young adults on the issues of cancer prevention and treatment.
1999 112 pages
ISBN: 1-560063-63-7

2462 Help Yourself: Tips for Teenagers with Cancer
National Cancer Institute
Building 31   800-422-6237
Bethesda, MD 20892-0001
This magazine-style booklet is designed to provide information and support adolescents with cancer.
37 pages

2463 Hospital Days: Treatment Ways
National Cancer Institute
Building 31   800-422-6237
Bethesda, MD 20892-0001
Coloring book helping to orient children with cancer to hospital and treatment procedures.
26 pages

2464 Kathy's Hats: A Story of Hope
Trudy Krisher, author
Albert Whitman & Company
250 South Northwest Hgwy   847-232-2800
Suite 320, IL 60068-2723   800-255-7675
                                    Fax: 847-581-0039
                                    mail@awhitmanco.com
                                    www.albertwhitman.com
When Kathy turns nine she learns she has cancer. When she loses her hair due to the chemotherapy, she feels ugly and awkward. This is a matter-of-fact book about a tough time and subject, and its calm and respectable treatment well serves a story that is indeed one of hope.
32 pages Hardcover
ISBN: 0-807541-16-6

2465 Kemo Shark
Kidscope
2045 Peachtree Road   404-233-0001
Atlanta, GA 30309-1107   www.kidscope.org
Color comic book designed to help children with the psychological and physiological changes in a family where a parent has cancer and chemotherapy.

2466 Kid's 1st Cookbook: Delicious-Nutritious Treats to Make Yourself
American Cancer Society
1599 Clifton Road NE   404-320-3333
Atlanta, GA 30329-4250   800-227-2345
Do creepy spiders, sloppy dogs and tornado swirls sound edible to you? They will to kids. Inside this beautifully illustrated hardcover edition are activities, colorful recipes and cooking tips that will turn meal preparation into exciting family fun. Kids of all ages can take charge, don a chef's hat and create delicious and nutricious snacks and dishes for every meal.
96 pages hardcover
ISBN: 0-944235-20-4

2467 Living with Cancer
Franklin Watts Grolier
90 Old Sherman Turnpike   203-797-3500
Danbury, CT 06816-0001   800-621-1115
                                    Fax: 203-797-3197
                                    www.auth.grolier.com

Shows how persons with cancer can overcome their illness and lead productive lives.
32 pages Grades 5-7
ISBN: 0-531108-59-7

2468 My Book for Kids with Cancer
Waterfront Books
98 Brookes Avenue   800-639-6063
Burlington, VT 05401-3326   www.waterfrontbooks.com/
Frustrated because he couldn't find any books about kids who survived cancer, Jason decided to write his own.
32 pages

2469 Our Mom Has Cancer
American Cancer Society
1599 Clifton Road NE   404-320-3333
Atlanta, GA 30329-4250   800-227-2345
When Abigail and Adrienne's mom told them she had cancer, they were afraid. But when the girls couldn't find any books that explained what might happen to their mother and what they might expect, they wrote one themselves. The girls, ages 9 and 11, tell readers that when their mother was tired during treatment, friends and family pitched in to help cook and to push her in her wheelchair. When chemotherapy made their mom's hair fall out, they threw a hat party for her.
32 pages hardcover
ISBN: 0-944235-20-4

2470 Sammie's New Mask: A Coloring Book for Friends of Children with Cancer
500 North Broadway   314-241-1600
Saint Louis, MO 63101   Fax: 314-241-1996
krudd@children-cancer.org
www.thenccs.org
Sammie's New Mask is about a young girl named Sammie and her friend, Jack, who has cancer. This story addresses Sammie's concerns and common misconceptions about cancer. This coloring book is designed for children in kindergarten through third grade.
K-3rd Grade
Mark Slocomb, Chairman
Mark Stolze, President/CEO

2471 Sammy's Mommy Has Cancer: For Children Who Have a Loved One with Cancer
Sherry Kohlenberg, author

Magination Press (American Psychological Assoc.)
750 First Street NE   202-336-5510
Washington, DC 20002-4242   800-374-2721
Fax: 202-336-5502
TDD: 202-336-6123
magination@apa.org
Sherry Kohlenberg wrote this book after she was diagnosed with breast cancer for her son. It is a warm, sensitive, straightforward story that will help young children understand and accept the changes in their lives when a parent is diagnosed with a life threatening illness. Parents will welcome this valuable aid in explaining the illness to their children. Both the story and the introduction offer useful suggestions for involving children in the jiys and sorrows of good and bad days.
1993 32 pages Softcover
ISBN: 0-945354-55-X

2472 Silver Kiss
Delacorte
568 Broadway   212-354-6500
New York, NY 10012-4039   www.foursquare.com
This moving tale describes the feelings of Zoe as her mother dies of cancer and her family attempts to shield her from seeing the slow decline in her mother.
Grades 8-12

2473 Silver Linings: Living with Cancer
Vantage Press
516 W 34th Street   212-736-1767
New York, NY 10001-1395   Fax: 212-736-2273
Highly personal journey of one woman's battle with breast cancer for over thirty-five years. From operations, radiation treatments, and hormone therapy and her faith and hope while induring them.
ISBN: 0-533113-52-0

2474 The Mountain You've Climbed: A Young Adult Guide to Childhood Cancer Survivorship
500 North Broadway   314-241-1600
Saint Louis, MO 63101   Fax: 314-241-1996
krudd@children-cancer.org
www.thenccs.org
This guide is designed to answer questions and address issues related to cancer survivorship for people ages 15 to 24. As survivorship rates continue to increase, the knowledge regarding late-effects also continues to increase. This survivorship guide will answer questions as well as address healthy living styles for your future.
Ages 15-24
Mark Slocomb, Chairman
Mark Stolze, President/CEO

2475 They Never Want to Tell You: Children Talk About Cancer
Harvard University Press
79 Garden Street   617-495-2600
Cambridge, MA 02138   800-448-2242
Fax: 617-495-5898
www.hup.harvard.edu
A comprehensive book that focuses on eight children who share their various experiences with cancer.
Grades 7-12
ISBN: 0-674883-70-5

2476 Waiting for Johnny Miracle
Harper & Row
10 E 53rd Street   212-207-7000
New York, NY 10022-5299
This powerful book focuses on Becky, a 17-year-old girl who must face the fear of cancer after being diagnosed with a malignant tumor. This book brings up the painful issues that come with the pain, treatment and death of cancer.
Grades 8-12

2477 Why God Gave Me Pain
Loyola University Press
3441 N Ashland Avenue   773-281-1818
Chicago, IL 60657-1355
Using a girl's diary entries, this book expounds on the side effects of cancer as well as the psychological ramifications of the debilitating disease.

Magazines

2478 American Journal of Clinical Oncology: Cancer Clinical Trials
Raven Press
1185 Ave of the Americas   212-930-9500
New York, NY 10036-2601   800-777-2295
www.lib.stu.edu.cn
Offers outstanding coverage of ongoing research in cancer treatment. This journal is the primary source for timely updates covering all aspects of cancer management.
BiMonthly
ISBN: 0-277373-2
Luther W Brady, Editor

2479 Cancer Detection and Prevention Journal
Elsevier
Journals Cust Ser Dept.   877-839-7126
Orlando, FL 32887-4800   Fax: 407-363-1354
usjcs@elsevier.com
www.elsevier.com
A peer-refereed journal devoted to cancer prevention by predictive and preventitive oncology. It is uniquely focused on advances in genetics, molecular medicine and biotechnologies that have an impact on clinical oncology modalities.
2002-present

2480 Cancer Nursing: An International Journal for Cancer Care
Lippincott Williams & Wilkins
Wolters Kluwer Health   847-580-5000
Riverwoods, IL 60015-1600   800-638-3030
Fax: 301-223-2400
orders@lww.com
www.lww.com

Addresses the whole spectrum of problems arising in the care and support of cancer patients- prevention and early detection, geriatric and pediatric cancer nursing, medical and surgical oncology, ambulatory care, nutritional support, psychosocial aspects of cancer, patient responces to all treatment modalities, and specific nursing interventions.
BiMonthly
ISBN: 0-162220-X -

2481   Diseases of the Colon and Rectum
American Society of Colon and Rectal Surgeons
85 W Algonquin Road   847-290-9184
Arlington Heights, IL 60005   Fax: 847-290-9203
                                          ascrs@fascrs.org
                                          www.fascrs.org
Diseases of the Colon and Rectum (DCR) is the official journal of the American Society of Colon and Rectal Surgeons and is mailed to all members on a mothly basis as a member benefit. Non-member subscribers have access to the online version of DCR.
journal

2482   Pancreas
Raven Press
1185 Ave of the Americas   212-930-9500
New York, NY 10036-2601   800-777-2295
Provides a central forum for communication of original works involving both basic and clinical research on the exocrine and endocrine pancreas and their consequences in the disease state.
8x Year
ISBN: 0-885317-7 -
Vay Liang W Go, Editor

2483   Practice Parameters
American Society of Colon and Rectal Surgeons
85 W Algonquin Road   847-290-9184
Arlington Heights, IL 60005   Fax: 847-290-9203
                                          ascrs@fascrs.org
                                          www.fascrs.org
Parameters that have been published in the scientific journal Diseases of the Colon and Rectum, along with other scientific journals. They can be found on the website under Professionals.

2484   Roswellness Magazine
Roswell Park Cancer Institute
Elm & Carlton Streets   716-845-2300
Buffalo, NY 14263   877-275-7724
                                          askrpci@roswellpark.org
                                          www.roswellpark.org
A consumer magazine promoting good health habits, cancer prevention and early detection, and the services of Roswell Park Cancer Institute.
2x/year
Donald L Trump MD, FACP, President/CEO
Candace Johnson PhD, Deputy Director

2485   Skin Cancer Foundation Journal
Skin Cancer Foundation
205 Lexington Avenue   212-725-5176
New York, NY 10016   Fax: 212-725-5751
                                          info@skincancer.org
                                          www.skincancer.org
A collection of articles by physicians, scientists and lay writers on the subject.

Newsletters

2486   Candlelighters' Quarterly
Childhood Cancer Foundation
7910 Woodmont Avenue   301-657-8401
Bethesda, MD 20814   800-366-2223
Artlices on living with and treating pediatric/adolescent cancer, written by and for parents and professionals in the field. Includes reviews, resources, pen pal column, and more.

2487   Candlelighters' Youth Newsletter
Childhood Cancer Foundation
7910 Woodmont Avenue   301-657-8401
Bethesda, MD 20814-3015   800-366-2223

Offers information to teenagers and young adults on cancer issues, medical information, camps and programs.
Quarterly

2488   Exceptional Cancer Patients/ECaP Newsletter
Exceptional Cancer Patients/ECaP
532 Jackson Park Drive   814-337-8192
Meadville, CT 16335   Fax: 814-337-0699
E-newsletter with inspirational articles
2x/year
Bernie Siegal MD, Founder
Barry Bittman MD, Chief Executive Officer

2489   Melanoma Newsletter
Skin Cancer Foundation
149 Madison Avenue   212-725-5176
New York, NY 10016-8728   800-754-6490
                                       Fax: 212-725-5751
                                          info@skincancer.org
                                          www.skincancer.org
For medical investigators and practitioners.

2490   Nutrition Action Healthletter
Center for Science in the Public Interest
One Rideau St   613-244-7337
Ottawa, OT 20009-5736   Fax: 613-244-1559
                                          cspi@cspinet.org
                                          www.cspinet.org
The nation's leading consumer group concerned with food and nutrition issues. Focuses on diseases that result from consuming too many calories, too much fat, sodium and sugar such as cancer and heart disease.
16 pages 10 per year
Stephen Schmidt, Editor

2491   Oncology Times: The News Center for the Cancer Care Team
Lippincott Williams & Wilkins
Wolters Kluwer Health   847-580-5000
Riverwoods, IL 60015-1600   800-638-3030
                                       Fax: 301-223-2400
                                          orders@lww.com
                                          www.lww.com
Reports on breaking clinical news in oncology, radiology, surgery, chemotherapy, and biological and gene therapy, as well as the professional, political, reimbursement, and practice management issues that affect those treating cancer patients.
2x Monthly

2492   Options: New Directions in the War on Cancer
People Against Cancer
604 E Street   515-972-4444
Otho, IA 50569-0010   Fax: 515-972-4415
                                    info@peopleagainstcancer.com
                                    www.peopleagainstcancer.com
Published by People Against Cancer.
8 pages
Frank Wiewel, Executive Director

2493   Phoenix: Newsletter
Candlelighters' Childhood Cancer Foundation
7910 Woodmont Avenue   301-657-8401
Bethesda, MD 20814-3015   800-366-2223
For adult survivors of childhood cancer.

2494   Sun and Skin News
Skin Cancer Foundation
149 Madison Avenue   212-725-5176
New York, NY 10016-8728   800-754-6490
                                       Fax: 212-725-5751
                                          info@skincancer.org
                                          www.skincancer.org
Deals with skin cancer and related subjects in nontechnical terms.

2495   Support for People with Oral and Head and Neck Cancer (SPOHNC)
PO Box 53   800-377-0928
Locust Valley, NY 11560-0053   Fax: 516-671-8794
                                          info@spohnc.org
                                          www.spohnc.org

Services include patient networking oportunities, a national news-letter, a resource library, and insurance information and assistance.
James Sciubba, DMD, PhD, President
Mary Ann Caputo, Executive Director

2496 The Phoenix
United Ostomy Associations of America, Inc.
The Phoenix Magazine   949-600-7296
Mission Viejo, CA 92690   800-826-0826
                                                   publisher@uoaa.org
                                                   www.ostomy.org
The Phoenix magazine is the official publication of the United Ostomy Associations of America, Inc. and is published four times a year- December, March, June, and September.
Quarterly

2497 Voice of Hope
National Children's Cancer Society
500 North Broadway   314-241-1600
Saint Louis, MO 63101   Fax: 314-241-1996
                                                   krudd@children-cancer.org
                                                   www.thenccs.org
It educates donors on how their support is furthering the N.C.C.S. mission, and acknowledges supporters. Distributed to donors of the N.C.C.S.
3x/year
Mark Slocomb, Chairman
Mark Stolze, President/CEO

Pamphlets

2498 Advanced Cancer: Living Each Day
National Cancer Institute
Building 31   800-422-6237
Bethesda, MD 20892-0001
Booklet delving into all aspects of everyday living with cancer. Offers information on coping, how children react, facing the unknown, living wills, additional resources and making treatment decisions.
30 pages

2499 After Breast Cancer: A Guide to Followup Care
National Cancer Institute
Building 31   800-422-6237
Bethesda, MD 20892-0001
Explains the importance of checking for possible signs of recurring cancer by receiving regular mammograms, getting breast exams from a doctor, and continuing monthly breast self-exams.
15 pages

2500 Basic Family Library
Candlelighters' Childhood Cancer Foundation
7910 Woodmont Avenue   301-657-8401
Bethesda, MD 20814-3015   800-366-2223
A bibliography of materials on childhood cancers, medical support, death and bereavement and materials for children.

2501 Brachytherapy and IMRT
Michael Dattoli, Jennifer Cash, and Don Kaltenbach, author
Dattoli Cancer Foundation
2803 Fruitville Road   941-365-5599
Sarasota, FL 34237   800-915-1001
                                              Fax: 941-366-3786
                                                   info@dattolifoundation.org
                                                   www.dattolifoundation.org
A primer on seed implants and Intensity Modulated Radiation Therapy (IMRT). This booklet provides a comprehensive overview of prostate cancer treatment protocols that utilize brachytherapy and IMRT either with or without hormonal therapy.
50 pages Booklet

2502 Breast Biopsy: What You Should Know
National Cancer Institute
Building 31   301-496-4000
Bethesda, MD 20892-0001
Offers information on what happens before, during and after a breast biopsy.

2503 Breast Cancer: Understanding Treatment Options
National Cancer Institute
Building 31   800-422-6237
Bethesda, MD 20892-0001
Summarizes the biopsy procedure and examines the pros and cons of various types of breast surgery. It discusses lumpectomy and radiation therapy as primary treatment.
19 pages

2504 Breast Exams: What You Should Know
National Cancer Institute
Building 31   800-422-6237
Bethesda, MD 20892-0001
Provides answers to questions about breast cancer and breast screening methods.
10 pages

2505 Camps for Children with Cancer and their Siblings
Candlelighters' Childhood Cancer Foundation
7910 Woodmont Avenue   301-657-8401
Bethesda, MD 20814-3015   800-366-2223
A listing by state of day and overnight camp programs, children served and programs.

2506 Cancer Tests You Should Know About: A Guide for People 65 and Over
National Cancer Institute
Building 31   800-422-6237
Bethesda, MD 20892-0001
Describes the cancer tests important for people age 65 and older. Informs men and women of the exams they should be requesting when they schedule checkups with their doctors.
14 pages

2507 Cancer of the Bladder: Research Report
National Cancer Institute
Building 31   800-422-6237
Bethesda, MD 20892-0001
Offers information on the types of bladder cancer, mortality rates, diagnosis, symptoms, therapies, rehabilitation, clinical trials, and selected references.

2508 Cancer of the Colon and Rectum: Research Report
National Cancer Institute
Building 31   800-422-6237
Bethesda, MD 20892-0001
Informative pamphlet offering factual statistics on causes and prevention, detection, diagnosis, staging, treatment, followup, clinical trials and selected references.

2509 Cancer of the Ovary: Research Report
National Cancer Institute
Building 31   800-422-6237
Bethesda, MD 20892-0001

2510 Cancer of the Pancreas: Research Report
National Cancer Institute
Building 31   800-422-6237
Bethesda, MD 20892-0001
Offers information on the various types of pancreatic cancer, treatments, surgical procedures, chemotherapy, biological therapy, hormone therapy, clinical trials and selected references.

2511 Cancer of the Uterus: Endometrial Cancer
National Cancer Institute
Building 31   800-422-6237
Bethesda, MD 20892-0001
Offers information on the description and function of the uterus, incidence and mortality, possible causes and prevention, detection, diagnosis, staging, treatment, clinical trials and selected references.

2512 Cancer of the Uterus: Research Report
National Cancer Institute
Building 31   800-422-6237
Bethesda, MD 20892-0001

2513 Candlelighters Guide to Bone Marrow Transplants in Children
Candlelighters' Childhood Cancer Foundation
7910 Woodmont Avenue   301-657-8401
Bethesda, MD 20814-3015   800-366-2223

For parents who are contemplating a BMT or harvest for their child or whose child is undergoing the procedure.

2514 Chemotherapy and You: A Guide to Self-Help During Treatment
National Cancer Institute
Building 31   800-422-6237
Bethesda, MD 20892-0001
Explains chemotherapy and addresses problems and concerns of patients undergoing this treatment.

2515 Chew or Snuff is Real Bad Stuff
National Cancer Institute
Building 31   301-435-3848
Bethesda, MD 20892-2580   800-422-6237
                                               www.nci.nih.gov
Designed for young adults, this brochure describes the health and social effects of using smokeless tobacco products.

2516 Clearing the Air: A Guide to Quitting Smoking
National Cancer Institute
Building 31   800-422-6237
Bethesda, MD 20892-0001
Offers hints on quitting smoking and cancer prevention.
24 pages

2517 Cutaneous Melanoma of the Head and Neck
American Academy of Otolaryngology
1650 Diagonal Road   703-836-4444
Alexandria, VA 22314-3357   Fax: 703-683-5100
                                               www.entnet.org
Self-instruction package.
Paperback
ISBN: 1-567720-22-6

2518 Diet, Nutrition and Cancer Prevention: The Good News
National Cancer Institute
Building 31   800-422-6237
Bethesda, MD 20892-0001
Provides an overview of dietary guidelines that may assist individuals in reducing their risks for some cancers.
16 pages

2519 Diet, Nutrition and Cancer Prevention: A Guide to Food Choices
National Cancer Institute
Building 31   800-422-6237
Bethesda, MD 20892-0001
Describes what is known about diet, nutrition and cancer prevention. Provides information about foods that contain components like fiber, fat and vitamins that may affect a person's risk of getting certain cancers.

2520 Dilemmas of Providing Help in a Crisis: The Role of Friends & Parents
Candlelighters' Childhood Cancer Foundation
7910 Woodmont Avenue   301-657-8401
Bethesda, MD 20814-3015   800-366-2223

2521 Do the Right Thing: Get a Mammogram
National Cancer Institute
Building 31   800-422-6237
Bethesda, MD 20892-0001
Targets black women age 40 and older. Describes the importance of regular mammograms in the early detection of breast cancer.

2522 Eating Hints: Recipes and Tips for Better Nutrition During Cancer Treatment
National Cancer Institute
Building 31   800-422-6237
Bethesda, MD 20892-0001
Provides recipes that help patients meet their needs for good nutrition during treatment.

2523 Facing Forward: A Guide for Cancer Survivors
National Cancer Institute
Building 31   800-422-6237
Bethesda, MD 20892-0001
Presents a concise overview of important survivor issues, including ongoing health needs, psychosocial concerns, insurance and employment.
43 pages

2524 Facts About Lung Cancer
American Lung Association
1740 Broadway   212-315-8700
New York, NY 10019-4315   www.librarylovers.org.au

2525 Facts About Radon
American Lung Association
1740 Broadway   212-315-8700
New York, NY 10019-4315   www.librarylovers.org.au

2526 Help, Hope, Believe
National Children's Cancer Society
500 North Broadway   314-241-1600
Saint Louis, MO 63101   Fax: 314-241-1996
                                               krudd@children-cancer.org
                                               www.thenccs.org

N.C.C.S. Informational Brochure
3x/year
Mark Slocomb, Chairman
Mark Stolze, President/CEO

2527 Helping Children Cope While a Sibling Undergoes Bone Marrow Transplant
Bone Marrow Foundation
515 Madison Avenue   212-838-3029
New York, NY 10022-5102   Fax: 212-223-0081
                                               THEBMF@BoneMarrow.org
                                               www.bonemarrow.org
Discusses the wide array of emotions felt by the entire family as a child receives a bone marrow transplant.

2528 If You've Thought About Breast Cancer
Rose Kushner Breast Cancer Advisory Center
PO Box 224   Fax: 301-897-3444
Kensington, MD 20895-0224

2529 Immune System: How it Works
National Cancer Institute
Building 31   800-422-6237
Bethesda, MD 20892-0001
Written for the high school level, this booklet explains the human immune system for the general public. It describes the sophistication of the body's immune responses, the impact of immune disorders and the relation of the immune system to cancer therapies.
28 pages

2530 Informed Consent: Does the Current Process Reflect Current Treatments
Candlelighters' Childhood Cancer Foundation
7910 Woodmont Avenue   301-657-8401
Bethesda, MD 20814-3015   800-366-2223

2531 Insurance Articles
Candlelighters' Childhood Cancer Foundation
7910 Woodmont Avenue   301-657-8401
Bethesda, MD 20814-3015   800-366-2223
Includes: Tips on securing health insurance for childhood cancer survivors and patients, Stay a step ahead of you insuruer, and others.

2532 Interpreting Your PSA and Related Prostate Cancer Blood Tests
Michael Dattoli, Jennifer Cash, and Don Kaltenbach, author
Dattoli Cancer Foundation
2803 Fruitville Road   941-365-5599
Sarasota, FL 34237   800-915-1001
                                               Fax: 941-366-3786
                                               info@dattolifoundation.org
                                               www.dattolifoundation.org
Provides a comprehensive overview of the PSA (prostate specific antigen) blood test and other related lab tests including the PSA velocity, free and bound PSA, and the PAP (prostatic Acid Phosphatase) blood test.
2006 50 pages Booklet

2533 Leading Self-Help Groups: Report on Workshop for Leaders of Groups
Candlelighters' Childhood Cancer Foundation
7910 Woodmont Avenue   301-657-8401
Bethesda, MD 20814-3015   800-366-2223

2534 Letter to a Friend Whose Child is Newly Diagnosed with Cancer
Candlelighters' Childhood Cancer Foundation
7910 Woodmont Avenue   301-657-8401
Bethesda, MD 20814-3015   800-366-2223

2535 Managing Your Child's Eating Problems During Cancer Treatment
National Cancer Institute
Building 31   800-422-6237
Bethesda, MD 20892-0001
Contains information about the importance of nutrition, side effects of cancer and its treatment.
32 pages

2536 Mastectomy: A Treatment for Breast Cancer
National Cancer Institute
Building 31   800-422-6237
Bethesda, MD 20892-0001
Presents information about the different types of breast surgery, explains what to expect at the hospital and during the recovery period.
25 pages

2537 Melanoma: Research Report
National Cancer Institute
Building 31   800-422-6237
Bethesda, MD 20892-0001
Offers information on types of skin cancer, detection, diagnosis, staging, treatment, clinical trials, selected references and additional information for patients with skin cancer.

2538 Nutrition for Patients Receiving Chemotherapy/Radiation Treatment
National Cancer Institute
Building 31   800-422-6237
Bethesda, MD 20892-0001
Describes the importance of maintaining nutritional intake while receiving chemotherapy and radiation.

2539 Once a Year for a Lifetime
National Cancer Institute
Building 31   800-422-6237
Bethesda, MD 20892-0001
Targets all women age 40 and older describing the importance of regular mammograms in the early detection of breast cancer.

2540 Oral Cancers: Research Report
National Cancer Institute
Building 31   800-422-6237
Bethesda, MD 20892-0001
Describes types of oral cancer, causes and risk factors, symptoms, prevention, detection, diagnosis, treatment, staging, methods of treatments, followup care, clinical trials and selected references for more information.

2541 Pap Test: It Can Save Your Life
National Cancer Institute
Building 31   800-422-6237
Bethesda, MD 20892-0001
Easy-to-read pamphlet tells women of the importance of getting a Pap test, how often to get it done and where to go to get it.

2542 Preparing your Child for a Bone Marrow Transplant
Bone Marrow Foundation
515 Madison Avenue   212-838-3029
New York, NY 10022-5102   Fax: 212-223-0081
THEBMF@BoneMarrow.org
www.bonemarrow.org
Discusses the wide array of emotions felt by the entire family as a child receives a bone marrow transplant.

2543 Questions and Answers About Breast Lumps
National Cancer Institute
Building 31   800-422-6237
Bethesda, MD 20892-0001
Describes some of the most common noncancerous breast lumps and what can be done about them.
22 pages

2544 Questions and Answers About Choosing a Mammography Facility
National Cancer Institute
Building 31   800-422-6237
Bethesda, MD 20892-0001
Lists questions to ask in selecting a quality mammography facility.

2545 Questions and Answers About DES Exposure During Pregnancy and Before Birth
National Cancer Institute
Building 31   800-422-6237
Bethesda, MD 20892-0001

2546 Questions and Answers About Metastatic Cancer
National Cancer Institute
Building 31   800-422-6237
Bethesda, MD 20892-0001
Presents information on detection, treatment methods and common areas of reoccurrence.

2547 Questions and Answers About Pain Control
National Cancer Institute
Building 31   800-422-6237
Bethesda, MD 20892-0001
Discusses pain control using both medical and nonmedical methods.

2548 Radiation Therapy and You: A Guide To Self-Help During Treatment
National Cancer Institute
Building 31   800-422-6237
Bethesda, MD 20892-0001
Explains radiation therapy and addresses concerns of patients receiving radiation treatment.

2549 Recurrence: What Do I Do Now?
Dattoli Cancer Foundation
2803 Fruitville Road   941-365-5599
Sarasota, FL 34237   800-915-1001
Fax: 941-366-3786
info@dattolifoundation.org
www.dattolifoundation.org
This booklet offers comprehensive information on the issues surrounding ruccurence: detection, risk categories, treatment options including radiation, brachytherapy, and hormone therapy.
58 pages Booklet

2550 Research Report: Adult Kidney Cancer and Wilms' Tumor
National Cancer Institute
Building 31   800-422-6237
Bethesda, MD 20892-0001

2551 Skin Cancers, Basal Cell and Squamous Cell Carcinomas: Research Report
National Cancer Institute
Building 31   800-422-6237
Bethesda, MD 20892-0001
Offers information on types of skin cancer, incidence and mortality, risk factors, prevention, symptoms, detection, diagnosis, staging, treatment, followup care and clinical trials.

2552 Students with Cancer: A Resource for the Educator
National Cancer Institute
Building 31   800-422-6237
Bethesda, MD 20892-0001
Designed for teachers who have students with cancer in their classrooms or schools.
22 pages

2553 Sunlight, Ultraviolet Radiation and the Skin
National Cancer Institute
Building 31   800-422-6237
Bethesda, MD 20892-0001

2554 Support Systems for Parents of Children with Cancer
Candlelighters' Childhood Cancer Foundation
7910 Woodmont Avenue   301-657-8401
Bethesda, MD 20814-3015   800-366-2223

2555 Taking Time: Support for People with Cancer & People Who Care for Them
National Cancer Institute

Building 31   800-422-6237
Bethesda, MD 20892-0001
Discusses the emotional sides of cancer. how to deal with the disease and learn to talk with friends, family members and others about cancer.

2556 Talking with Your Child About Cancer
National Cancer Institute
Building 31   800-422-6237
Bethesda, MD 20892-0001
Designed for the parent whose child has been diagnosed with cancer.
16 pages

2557 Testicular Cancer: Research Report
National Cancer Institute
Building 31   800-422-6237
Bethesda, MD 20892-0001

2558 Testicular Self-Examination
National Cancer Institute
Building 31   800-422-6237
Bethesda, MD 20892-0001
Contains information about risks and symptoms of testicular cancer and provides instructions on how to perform testicular self-examination.

2559 What You Need to Know About Bladder Cancer
National Cancer Institute
Building 31   301-496-4000
Bethesda, MD 20892-0001
Offers information on the history, symptoms, diagnosis, treatment, followup care, support groups, medical terms and resources for more information.

2560 What You Need to Know About Cancer
National Cancer Institute
Building 31   800-422-6237
Bethesda, MD 20892-0001
Offers information on signs and symptoms, diagnosis, treatment, early detection and advances in medical technology.

2561 What You Need to Know About Cancer of The Colon and Rectum
National Cancer Institute
Building 31   800-422-6237
Bethesda, MD 20892-0001
Offers information on symptoms, diagnosis, treatments, and support for cancer patients.

2562 What You Need to Know About Cervical Cancer
National Cancer Institute
Building 31   800-422-6237
Bethesda, MD 20892-0001
Areas covered include early detection, symptoms, treatments, diagnosis, followup care, support, medical terms and resources.

2563 What You Need to Know About Esophagal Cancer
National Cancer Institute
Building 31   800-422-6237
Bethesda, MD 20892-0001
Offers information on symptoms, causes, preventions, diagnosis, support, medical terms and available resources.

2564 What You Need to Know About Kidney Cancer
National Cancer Institute
Building 31   800-422-6237
Bethesda, MD 20892-0001
Offers factual information on diagnosis, symptoms, prevention, treatment and referral sources.

2565 What You Need to Know About Larynx Cancer
National Cancer Institute
Building 31   800-422-6237
Bethesda, MD 20892-0001
Offers information on what cancer is, symptoms, diagnosis, treatment options, side effects of medication, rehabilitation, learning to speak again, living with cancer, causes and preventions, medical terms and resources.

2566 What You Need to Know About Lung Cancer
National Cancer Institute
Building 31   800-422-6237
Bethesda, MD 20892-0001
Offers information on types of lung cancer, symptoms, diagnosis, treatments, support, medical terms and resources.

2567 What You Need to Know About Oral Cancers
National Cancer Institute
Building 31   800-422-6237
Bethesda, MD 20892-0001
Offers information on symptoms, diagnosis, treatments, rehabilitation, followup care, support, medical terms and resources for cancer patients.

2568 What You Need to Know About Ovarian Cancer
National Cancer Institute
Building 31   800-422-6237
Bethesda, MD 20892-0001
Early detection, symptoms, diagnosis, treatments, medical terms and resources for further information.

2569 What You Need to Know About Pancreatic Cancer
National Cancer Institute
Building 31   800-422-6237
Bethesda, MD 20892-0001
Offers information on symptoms, diagnosis, treatment, support, medical terms and resources.

2570 What You Need to Know About Prostate Cancer
National Cancer Institute
Building 31   800-422-6237
Bethesda, MD 20892-0001
Offers information on symptoms, diagnosis, treatment options, side effects of medications, followup care, living with cancer and support resources for patients.

2571 What You Need to Know About Skin Cancer
National Cancer Institute
Building 31   800-422-6237
Bethesda, MD 20892-0001
Offers information on types of skin cancer, symptoms, causes, prevention, treatment planning, treating skin cancer, research and medical terms.

2572 What You Need to Know About Testicular Cancer
National Cancer Institute
Building 31   800-422-6237
Bethesda, MD 20892-0001
Offers information on the symptoms, diagnosing of testicular cancer, side effects of treatments, followup care, support for patients, cancer research, medical terms and resources.

2573 What You Need to Know About Uterine Cancer
National Cancer Institute
Building 31   800-422-6237
Bethesda, MD 20892-0001
Offers information on symptoms, diagnosing cancer of the uterus, treatments, followup care, support for patients, medical terms and resources.

2574 What You Need to Know About...
National Cancer Institute
Building 31   800-422-6237
Bethesda, MD 20892-0001
This is a series of booklets, broken down in this directory. Each provides information about a specific type of cancer. These booklets discuss emotional issues, treatment, diagnosis, symptoms and questions to ask the doctor about cancer.

2575 What are Clinical Trials All About?
National Cancer Institute
Building 31   800-422-6237
Bethesda, MD 20892-0001
Explains clinical trials (studies of new cancer treatments) to help patients decide if they want to take part in a trial.

2576 When Cancer Recurs: Meeting the Challenge Again
National Cancer Institute
Building 31   800-422-6237
Bethesda, MD 20892-0001

Offers information on why cancer can recur, where cancers can recur, diagnosing recurrent cancer, treatment methods and resources that offer more help.

2577 When Someone in Your Family Has Cancer
National Cancer Institute
Building 31   800-422-6237
Bethesda, MD 20892-0001
Written for young people whose parent or sibling has cancer.
28 pages

2578 Who is This Person Who Helped Save My Life
Bone Marrow Foundation
515 Madison Avenue   212-838-3029
New York, NY 10022-5102   Fax: 212-223-0081
THEBMF@BoneMarrow.org
www.bonemarrow.org
Discusses the wide range of emotions for a patient in the process of searching for and identifying a donor.

2579 Why Do You Smoke?
National Cancer Institute
Building 31   800-422-6237
Bethesda, MD 20892-0001
Contains a self-test to determine why people smoke and suggest alternatives that can help them stop and prevent cancer.

2580 Wish Fulfillment Organizations
Candlelighters' Childhood Cancer Foundation
7910 Woodmont Avenue   301-657-8401
Bethesda, MD 20814-3015   800-366-2223
A list of groups granting wishes of children with life-threatening, chronic or terminal illnesses, with criteria and contacts.

2581 Young People with Cancer: A Handbook for Parents
National Cancer Institute
Building 31   800-422-6237
Bethesda, MD 20892-0001
Discusses the most common types of childhood cancer, treatments, and side effects and issues that may arise when a child is diagnosed with cancer.
86 pages

Audio & Video

2582 Beyond the Loss of the Breast
Fanlight Productions
4196 Washington Street   617-469-4999
Boston, MA 02131-1731   800-937-4113
Fax: 617-469-3379
fanlight@fanlight.com
www.fanlight.com
This video addresses breast cancer throught the personal narratives and poetry of two women living with recurrent breast cancer and the film maker, whose mother died from metastatic disease.
1994 25 Minutes
ISBN: 1-572951-68-0

2583 Living with Ovarian Cancer
National Ovarian Cancer Coalition
2501 Oak Lawn Avenue   561-393-0005
Dallas, TX 5219   888-682-7426
Fax: 561-393-7275
nocc@ovarian.org
www.ovarian.org
Videotape for women who have been recently diagnosed with ovarian cancer. Created to orient and inform patients and their families; describes the experiences of individuals intimately connected with the disease.
Suzy Lockwood-Rayermann RN, Chair
Julene Fabrizio, President

2584 Not Just a Cancer Patient
Fanlight Productions
4196 Washington Street   617-469-4999
Boston, MA 02131-1731   800-937-4113
Fax: 617-469-3379
fanlight@fanlight.com
www.fanlight.com

Focuses on several articulate teenagers who are undergoing cancer treatment to help caregivers understand the needs and feelings of this population.
1991 23 Minutes
ISBN: 1-572950-86-2

2585 Skin Cancer: Preventable and Curable
Skin Cancer Foundation
149 Madison Avenue   212-725-5176
New York, NY 10016-8728   800-754-6490
Fax: 212-725-5751
info@skincancer.org
www.skincancer.org

Web Sites

2586 American Academy of Dermatology
www.aad.org
An organization of doctors who specialize in diagnosing and treating skin problems.

2587 American Cancer Society
www.cancer.org
Provides free printed materials, offers a range of services to patients and their families.

2588 American Society of Colon and Rectal Surgeons
www.fascrs.org
ASCRS Represents more than 3,800 board certified colon and rectal surgeons, as well as other surgeons dedicated to advancing and promoting the science and practice of the treatment of patients with cancer, and other diseases affecting the colon and related areas.

2589 Association for the Cure of Cancer of the Prostate
www.capcure.org

2590 Bone Marrow & Cancer Foundation
bonemarrow.org
Goal is to improve the quality of life for bone marrow and stem cell transplant patients and their families by providing financial aid, education, and emotional support.
Christina Merrill, President & CEO
Robert Fishman, Chair

2591 Healing Well
www.healingwell.com
An online health resource guide to medical news, chat, information and articles, newsgroups and message boards, books, disease-related web sites, medical directories, and more for patients, friends, and family coping with disabling diseases, disorders, or chronic illnesses.

2592 Health Finder
www.healthfinder.gov
Searchable, carefully developed web site offering information on over 1000 topics. Developed by the US Department of Health and Human Services, the site can be used in both English and Spanish.

2593 Healthlink USA
www.healthlinkusa.com
Health information concerning treatment, cures, prevention, diagnosis, risk factors, research, support groups, email lists, personal stories and much more. Updated regularly.

2594 International Association of Eating Disorders Professionals Foundation
www.iaedp.com
Supplies printed information and sponsors meetings and other activities. Publishes a directory of speech instructors and maintains a list of sources for supplies for laryngectomee.

2595 Leukemia and Lymphoma Society
www.leukemia.org
A national voluntary health agency dedicated to curing leukemia, lymphoma, Hodgkin's disease and myeloma and to improving the quality of life of patients and their families.

2596 MedicineNet
www.medicinenet.com

An online resource for consumers providing easy-to-read, authoritative medical and health information.

2597 Medscape

www.medscape.com

Medscape offers specialists, primary care physicians, and other health professionals the Web's most robust and integrated medical information and educational tools.

2598 National Hospice & Palliative Care Organization (NHPCO)

www.nhpco.org

The organization seeks to improve end-of-life care, widen access to hospice care, and improve quality of life for the dying and their loved ones. NHPCO's website offers information on regulations, advocacy, quality and performance, education, and a variety of other resources.

2599 National Ovarian Cancer Coalition

www.ovarian.org

Aims to raise awareness about ovarian cancer and to promote education about the disease, while dispelling myths and misunderstandings. The coalition is committed to improving the overall survival rate and quality of life for women with ovarian cancer.

2600 Support for People with Oral and Head and Neck Cancer (SPOHNC)

www.spohnc.org

Non-profit organization addressing the broad emotional, physical, and humanistic needs of oral and head and neck cancer patients.

2601 WebMD

www.webmd.com

Provides credible information, supportive communities, and in-depth reference material about health subjects. A source for original and timely health information as well as material from well known content providers.

2602 Webhelp

www.webhelp.com

Provides links to information, including research, treatment, prevention, support, and more.

Description

2603 ## Carpal Tunnel Syndrome

Carpal Tunnel Syndrome, CTS, is a painful, often debilitating condition caused by compression of the median nerve as it passes through the wrist (carpal tunnel) to the hand. CTS most commonly occurs in women aged 30 to 50 years. The incidence is highest among keyboard users, secretaries, musicians, assembly-line workers, and others who engage in repetitive handwork. There are about 3 million cases per year in the U.S.

An initial indication of CTS is a feeling that the hand is asleep. Typically, the patient wakes at night with numbness and tingling of the affected hand. The most serious functional problem occurs when it becomes difficult or impossible to move the thumb into a grasping position with the other fingers. In advanced cases, pain associated with CTS may radiate up the arm to the shoulder. While job-related movement is the most common cause of CTS, people with underlying conditions, such as diabetes, gout, rheumatoid arthritis, obesity and pregnancy, are more prone to experience symptoms. Although less common, the onset of CTS can stem from trauma, such as a blow to the hand or wrist.

Diagnosis involves the Phalen Test, in which the hands are placed together, back to back and the wrist is flexed. This maneuver generally produces tingling of the hand in a patient with CTS, and the Tinel's test, in which the physician presses or taps along the median nerve at inside of the wrist to see if it causes any numbness or tingling in the fingers. Diagnosis is confirmed by testing how quickly an impulse is transmitted along the median nerve.

The condition can most often be successfully treated based on an understanding of workplace movement issues — ergonomics. keyboard users, and those engaged in similar activities, should adjust their seats and backrests to assure that their arms are positioned comfortably during work sessions. For mild cases of CTS, a lightweight brace, especially worn at night, can decrease symptoms by holding the wrist stable. Marked improvement may arise from wearing a brace for a week or two. However, in many cases, it is recommended that the sufferer cease working until symptoms have improved. Exercises and deep-tissue massage can strengthen the wrist and hand.

Over-the-counter anti-inflammatory medications, such as ibuprofen and aspirin, can also reduce symptoms of mild Carpal Tunnel Syndrome. In more acute conditions, cortisone injections may be administered. When symptoms are severe and persistent, surgery may be required to reduce pressure on the nerves. The most common surgery is an open incision technique called open carpal tunnel release, which usually improves the condition dramatically. A newer and less invasive procedure is endoscopic carpal tunnel release, which uses a smaller incision and visualizes the operative field using a fiber optic camera.

National Agencies & Associations

2604 **American Academy of Orthopaedic Surgeons**
9400 West Higgins Road   847-823-7186
Rosemont, IL 60018-4262   800-626-6726
Fax: 847-823-8125
customerservice@aaos.org
www.aaos.org
Provides education and practice management services for orthopaedic surgeons and allied health professionals. Also serves as an advocate for improved patient care, and to inform the public.
Thomas E. Arend, Jr., Chief Executive Officer
Will Shaffer, MD, Medical Director

2605 **American Chronic Pain Association**
PO Box 850   800-533-3231
Rocklin, CA 95677   ACPA@theacpa.org
www.theacpa.org
The ACPA facilitates peer support and education for individuals with chronic pain in its many forms, in order to increase quality of life. Also raises awareness among the healthcare community, and with policy makers.
Penney Cowan, Founder & CEO
Daniel Galia, Director, Global Support

2606 **American Society for Surgery of the Hand**
822 W. Washington Boulevard   312-880-1900
Chicago, IL 60607   Fax: 847-384-1435
info@assh.org
www.assh.org
The mission of the ASSH is to advance the science and practice of hand and upper extremity surgery through education, research, and advocacy on behalf of patients and practitioners.
Mark C. Anderson, CAE, Executive VP & CEO
Pamela Schroeder, Deputy Executive VP

2607 **Arthritis Trust of America**
7111 Sweetgum Road   admin@arthritistrust.org
Fairview, TN 37602-9384   www.arthritistrust.org
The Arthritis Trust of America provides information about auto-immune or collagen tissue diseases such as Rheumatoid Arthritis and related diseases, and the search for a cure. Publications, research, and physician referrals are provided. The trust is overseen by the National Fund for Alternative Medicine.
P. Anthony Chapdelaine, Jr., Executive Director
Mary Ann Chapdelaine, President

2608 **National Institute of Arthritis & Musculoskeletal & Skin Diseases**
National Institutes of Health
Bethesda, MD 20892-3675   301-495-4484
877-226-4267
Fax: 301-718-6366
TTY: 301-565-2966
NIAMSinfo@mail.nih.gov
www.niams.nih.gov
Supports research into the causes, treatment, and prevention of arthritis and musculoskeletal and skin diseases, the training of basic and clinical scientists to carry out this research, and the dissemination of information on research programs.
Robert H. Carter, MD, Director
Gahan Breithaupt, Assoc. Director, Management & Operations

Foundations

2609 American Foundation for Surgery of the Hand
822 W. Washington Boulevard
Chicago, IL 60607

312-880-1900
Fax: 847-384-1435
afsh@assh.org
www.afsh.org

Founded by the Council of the American Society for Surgery of the Hand, the AFSH funds educational services, research, and assists in Society outreach.
Mark C. Anderson, CAE, Executive VP & CEO
Bill Chandler, Chief Financial Officer

Research Centers

2610 National Institute of Arthritis & Musculoskeletal & Skin Diseases
National Institutes of Health
Bethesda, MD 20892-3675

301-495-4484
877-226-4267
Fax: 301-718-6366
TTY: 301-565-2966
NIAMSinfo@mail.nih.gov
www.niams.nih.gov

Supports research into the causes, treatment, and prevention of arthritis and musculoskeletal and skin diseases, the training of basic and clinical scientists to carry out this research, and the dissemination of information on research programs.
Robert H. Carter, MD, Director
Gahan Breithaupt, Assoc. Director, Management & Operations

2611 Orthopaedic Associates of Michigan
1111 Leffingwell Avenue NE
Grand Rapids, MI 49525

616-459-7101
800-582-7244
Fax: 616-957-0444
www.oamichigan.com

Support Groups & Hotlines

2612 National Health Information Center
Office of Disease Prevention & Health Promotion
1101 Wootton Pkwy
Rockville, MD 20852

Fax: 240-453-8281
odphpinfo@hhs.gov
www.health.gov/nhic

Supports public health education by maintaining a calendar of National Health Observances; helps connect consumers and health professionals to organizations that can best answer questions and provide up-to-date contact information from reliable sources; updates on a yearly basis toll-free numbers for health information, Federal health clearinghouses and info centers.
Don Wright, MD, MPH, Director

Books

2613 Occupational Therapy Practice Guidelines for Adults with Carpal Tunnel Syndrome
American Occupational Therapy Association
4720 Montgomery Lane
Bethesda, MD 20814-1220

301-652-6611
Fax: 240-762-5150
TDD: 800-377-8555
www.aota.org

13 pages Paperback
ISBN: 1-569001-47-2

2614 Pain Free Typing Techniques: Simple Solutions to Prevent Strain Injury
Howard Richman, author
Sound Feelings Publishing
18375 Ventura Boulevard
Tarzana, CA 91356

818-757-0600
information@soundfeelings.com
www.soundfeelings.com

This 12 page booklet provides drug-free treatments and suggestions for repetitive motion disorder and cumulative trauma disorders. Unconventional concepts for increasing human performance are revealed, which help prevent computer-related illnesses including hand pain, wrist pain, and other keyboard ergonomics.

Most repetitive motion disorders and overuse injuries can be improved by correcting certain angles and positions.
1999 12 pages Booklet
ISBN: 1-882060-80-6

Pamphlets

2615 Carpal Tunnel Syndrome
Arthritis Foundation
535 Connecticut Avenue
Norwalk, CT 06854-0669

203-828-0349
800-283-7800
Fax: 404-872-0457
jmitchell@belvoir.com

Offers an introduction to Carpal Tunnel, causes, symptoms, diagnosis and resources.

Web Sites

2616 Avoiding Carpal Tunnel Syndrome
www.indiana.edu/~ucsstaff/cts.html
A guide for computer keyboard users, by Mark Sheehan, reprinted from the University Computing Times.

2617 CTD Resource Network
www.ctdrn.org
This is an organization providing educational material and charitable assistance related to the prevention and treatment of cumulative trauma disorders, also known as repetitive strain injuries.

2618 Carpal Tunnel Syndrome Home Page
www.ctsplace.com
Information about carpal tunnel syndrome (CTS) and how to prevent it.

2619 Computer-Related Repetitive Strain Injury
rsi.unl.edu
Contains advice on proper posture and equipment from Paul Marxhausen, an engineering electronics technician.

2620 Health Finder
www.healthfinder.gov
Searchable, carefully developed web site offering information on over 1000 topics. Developed by the US Department of Health and Human Services, the site can be used in both English and Spanish.

2621 MedicineNet
www.medicinenet.com
An online resource for consumers providing easy-to-read, authoritative medical and health information.

2622 Neurology Channel
www.healthcommunities.com
Find clearly explained, medically accurate information regarding conditions, including an overview, symptoms, causes, diagnostic procedures and treatment options. On this site it is possible to ask questions and get information from a neurologist and connect to people who have similar health interests.

2623 RSI Resources
Information on carpal tunnel and other repetitive strain injuries.

Description

2624 Celiac Disease

Celiac disease, also called celiac sprue, is a chronic disease in which the small bowel cannot absorb most nutrients. This inability, called malabsorption, is caused by inflammation of the bowel triggered by a sensitivity to gluten, a cereal protein found in wheat and rye, and less so in barley and oats. In particular, patients with celiac disease react to a protein component of gluten called gliadin.

The disease may appear when a child is first given wheat products, generally in the second year of life. Some cases, however, do not appear until a person is in their twenties, or later, with women showing symptoms 10-15 years earlier than men. Affected children will fail to grow normally. Adults may lose weight despite a voracious appetite. There is no typical presentation of celiac disease. However, painful abdominal distention and passage of large, loose stools are common; iron deficiency anemia and vitamin deficiencies may appear. Other conditions known as non-celiac gluten-related disorders have been proposed, since some patients do not have celiac disease, but seem to improve when gluten is removed from the diet. Unfortunately, many rigorous studies have failed to demonstrate the existence of such a condition.

Family incidence is a valuable clue. Celiac disease is more common in people with Type I diabetes and certain forms of thyroid and skin disease. Blood tests that detect antibodies against transglutaminase, an enzyme that interacts with gliadin peptides, are highly sensitive and specific for diagnosing celiac disease, but the most definitive test is endoscopic examination of a small sample of the inflamed bowel.

Withdrawal of dietary gluten is the treatment for celiac disease; eating even small amounts of gluten-containing foods can prevent remission and cause relapse. Vitamins and minerals may also have to be supplemented. Long-term celiac disease may increase the risk for small bowel cancer and T-cell lymphoma. See also *Gastrointestinal Disorders* and *Crohn's Disease*.

National Agencies & Associations

2625 Academy of Nutrition & Dietetics
120 South Riverside Plaza
Chicago, IL 60606-6995
312-899-0040
800-877-1600
media@eatright.org
www.eatright.org
Offers information and support to those with celiac disease. Serves the public through the promotion of optimal nutrition, health, and well-being. Formerly the American Dietetic Association.
Mary Russell, President
Patricia M. Babjak, Chief Executive Officer

2626 American Celiac Society
266 Midway Drive
New Orleans, LA 70123
504-305-2968
www.americanceliacsociety.org

Promotes education, research, and mutual support for people with dietary disorders.
Annette Bentley, President
James Bentley, Vice President

2627 Canadian Celiac Association
1450 Meyerside Drive
Mississauga, Ontario, L5T-2N5
905-507-6208
800-363-7296
Fax: 905-507-4673
info@celiac.ca
www.celiac.ca
A national organization dedicated to providing services and support to persons with celiac disease and dermatitis herpetiformis through programs of awareness, advocacy, education, and research.
Melissa Secord, Executive Director
Helen Matteer, Manager, Grants & Special Projects

2628 Celiac Society
www.celiacsociety.com
Volunteer organization seeking to raise awareness about and provide information on celiac disease and other gluten-related disorders.

2629 Gluten Intolerance Group
31214 124th Avenue SE
Auburn, WA 98092
253-833-6655
Fax: 253-833-6675
CustomerService@gluten.org
gluten.org
Provides instructional and general information materials, as well as counseling and access to gluten-free products and ingredients to persons with celiac sprue and their families; operates telephone information and referral service, and conducts educational seminars.
Cynthia Kupper, RD, CD, Chief Executive Officer
Channon Quinn, Chief Operating Officer

2630 National Celiac Association
20 Pickering Street
Needham, MA 02492
617-262-5422
888-423-5422
info@nationalceliac.org
nationalceliac.org
Dedicated to helping individuals with celiac disease and gluten sensitivities through education, advocacy, and awareness.
Lee Graham, Executive Director
Kimberly Buckton, Managing Director

2631 Society for the Study of Celiac Disease
3300 Woodcreek Drive
Downers Grove, IL 60515
630-522-7886
info@nasscd.org
www.theceliacsociety.org
Professional organization of physicians, nurses, dietitians, and other healthcare workers in North America, with specialties in treating celiac disease and gluten-related disorders.
Ciaran P. Kelly, MD, President
Kristy Radcliffe, Director, Client Services

Foundations

2632 Celiac Disease Foundation
20350 Ventura Boulevard
Woodlands Hills, CA 91364
818-716-1513
Fax: 818-267-5577
www.celiac.org
Provides services and support to persons with celiac disease and dermatitis herpetiformis, through programs of awareness, education, advocacy and research; telephone information and referral services; medical advisory board annual educational conference and quarterly newsletters.
Marilyn Grunzweig Geller, Chief Executive Officer
Deborah J. Ceizler, Chief Development Officer

Support Groups & Hotlines

2633 Celiac Disease Foundation
20350 Ventura Boulevard
Woodlands Hills, CA 91364
818-716-1513
Fax: 818-267-5577
www.celiac.org
Provides services and support to persons with celiac disease and dermatitis herpetiformis, through programs of awareness, educa-

tion, advocacy and research; telephone information and referral services; medical advisory board annual educational conference and quarterly newsletters.
Marilyn Grunzweig Geller, Chief Executive Officer
Deborah J. Ceizler, Chief Development Officer

2634 National Health Information Center
Office of Disease Prevention & Health Promotion
1101 Wootton Pkwy   Fax: 240-453-8281
Rockville, MD 20852   odphpinfo@hhs.gov
                                      www.health.gov/nhic
Supports public health education by maintaining a calendar of National Health Observances; helps connect consumers and health professionals to organizations that can best answer questions and provide up-to-date contact information from reliable sources; updates on a yearly basis toll-free numbers for health information, Federal health clearinghouses and info centers.
Don Wright, MD, MPH, Director

Books

2635 CSA/USA Cookbook Series
Celiac Sprue Association/USA
PO Box 31700
Omaha, NE 68131   402-558-0600
                                      877-272-4272
                                      Fax: 402-643-4108
                                      celiacs@csaceliacs.org
                                      www.csaceliacs.org
Three cookbooks compiled from CSA members' contributions. Each contains a section of cooking hints, information on adapting recipes and a variety of special topics related to cooking gluten-free.
34 pages Annual
Mary Schluckebier, Executive Director

2636 Cooperative Gluten-Free Commercial Products Listing
Celiac Sprue Association/USA
PO Box 31700
Omaha, NE 68131   402-558-0600
                                      877-272-4272
                                      Fax: 402-643-4108
                                      celiacs@csaceliacs.org
                                      www.csaceliacs.org
Listing of gluten-free products compiled from written documentation recieved by the Celiac Sprue Association from manufacturers and distributors. Also includes vendor information for companies specializing in gluten-free products and phone numbers of companies.
2006 Annual
Mary Schluckebier, Executive Director

2637 Diets to Help Gluten and Wheat Allergy
HarperCollins Canada Limited/Order Department
1995 Markham Road   800-387-0117
Scarborough, M1B-5M8   Fax: 800-668-5788
This book offers sound and practical advice on gluten allergy wheat sensitivity and Celiac disease.
96 pages
ISBN: 0-722529-10-4

2638 The Gluten-Free Gourmet
Bette Hagman, author
Gluten Intolerance Group: GIG
31214 124th Avenue SE
Auburn, WA 98092-3667   253-833-6655
                                      Fax: 253-833-6675
                                      customerservice@gluten.org
                                      www.gluten.net
225 recipes.
272 pages
ISBN: 0-805064-84-2
Cynthia Kupper RDCD, Executive Director

Magazines

2639 Food & Nutrition
120 South Riverside Plaza   312-899-0040
Chicago, IL 60606-6995   800-877-1600
                                     foodandnutrition@eatright.org
                                     www.eatright.org
Formerly the ADA Times, Food & Nutrition is the member and professional magazine of the Academy of Nutrition & Dietetics.

2640 Journal of the Academy of Nutrition and Dietetics
120 South Riverside Plaza   312-899-4831
Chicago, IL 60606-6995   journal@eatright.org
                                     www.eatright.org
Official research publication of the Academy of Nutrition and Dietetics.
Joe Skey, Advertising Contact

Newsletters

2641 GIG Quarterly Magazine
Gluten Intolerance Group: GIG
31214 124th Avenue SE
Auburn, WA 98092-3667   253-833-6655
                                     Fax: 253-833-6675
                                     customerservice@gluten.org
                                     www.gluten.net
Member magazine. Offers updated medical and technological information for patients with celiac disease, their families and healthcare professionals.
Quarterly
Cynthia Kupper RDCD, Executive Director

2642 Lifeline
Celiac Sprue Association/USA
PO Box 31700
Omaha, NE 68131   402-558-0600
                                     877-272-4272
                                     Fax: 402-643-4108
                                     celiacs@csaceliacs.org
                                     www.csaceliacs.org
Quarterly newsletter for members; contains up-to-date research information, personal stories from celiacs, cooking tips, recipes and contact information for support chapters and resource units.
Mary Schluckebier, Executive Director

2643 Whooo's Report
American Celiac Society
PO Box 23455   504-737-3293
New Orleans, LA 70183   amerceliacsoc@netscape.net
Provides practical assistance to members and individuals with celiac disease and information about the disease to the public.

Pamphlets

2644 Celiac Disease
Gluten Intolerance Group: GIG
31214 124th Avenue SE
Auburn, WA 98092-3667   253-833-6655
                                     Fax: 253-833-6675
                                     customerservice@gluten.org
                                     www.gluten.net
Offers facts and statistics on celiac disease.
Cynthia Kupper RDCD, Executive Director

2645 Celiac Disease: A Hidden Epidemic
Peter Greene, MD, author
Harper Collins Publishers
10 East 53rd Street   212-207-7000
New York, NY 10022   www.harpercollins.com
An inside-out examination and explanation of Celiac Disease.
2006 352 pages
ISBN: 0-060766-93-X
Peter H.R. Green M.D., Author
Rory Jones, Author

2646 Dermatitis Herpetiformis
Gluten Intolerance Group: GIG

31214 124th Avenue SE
Auburn, WA 98092-3667
253-833-6655
Fax: 253-833-6675
customerservice@gluten.org
www.gluten.net
Offers facts and statistics on dermatitis herpetformis.
Cynthia Kupper RDCD, Executive Director

2647 Grains and Flours
Celiac Sprue Association/USA
PO Box 31700
Omaha, NE 68131
402-558-0600
877-272-4272
Fax: 402-643-4108
celiacs@csaceliacs.org
www.csaceliacs.org
A variety of different gluten-free flour mixtures, to experiment with and discover your favorite!
Mary Schluckebier, Executive Director

2648 Guide to Gluten-Free Diets
American Allergy Association
PO Box 7273
Menlo Park, CA 94026-7273
650-322-1663
Offers information on safe substitutes for baking and cooking. Differentiates celiac disease from wheat allergy. Sources of gluten in diet with warnings on when to check with the manufacturer.

2649 Patient Packet
Celiac Sprue Association/USA
PO Box 31700
Omaha, NE 68131
402-558-0600
877-272-4272
Fax: 402-643-4108
celiacs@csaceliacs.org
www.csaceliacs.org
A basic information packet for the newly-diagnosed celiac. Provided free of charge to individuals, physicians, dietitians, and family members.
Mary Schluckebier, Executive Director

2650 Quick Start Diet Guide
Gluten Intolerance Group: GIG
31214 124th Avenue SE
Auburn, WA 98092-3667
253-833-6655
Fax: 253-833-6675
customerservice@gluten.org
www.gluten.net
Packet available to download on website.
Cynthia Kupper RDCD, Executive Director

Audio & Video

2651 CD-A NIH Consensus Conference
Celiac Sprue Association/USA
PO Box 31700
Omaha, NE 68131
402-558-0600
877-272-4272
Fax: 402-643-4108
www.csaceliacs.org
Celiac Disease - A NIH Consensus Conference - Reaching Out to Improve the Health of Millions.
Mary Schluckebier, Executive Director

Web Sites

2652 Academy of Nutrition & Dietetics
www.eatright.org
Offers information and support to allergy sufferers. Serves the public through the promotion of optimal nutrition, health, and well-being. Formerly the American Dietetic Association.

2653 American Celiac Society
www.americanceliacsociety.org
Promotes education, research, and mutual support for people with dietary disorders.

2654 Celiac Disease & Gluten-Free Diet Online Resource Center
www.celiac.com
Internet based support organization that provides important resources and information for people on gluten-free diets due to celiac disease, gluten intolerance or wheat allergy.

2655 Celiac Disease Foundation
www.celiac.org
Provides services and support to persons with celiac disease and dermatitis herpetiformis, through programs of awareness, education, advocacy and research; telephone information and referral services; medical advisory board annual educational conference and quarterly newsletters.

2656 Gluten Intolerance Group
gluten.org
Provides instructional and general information materials, as well as counseling and access to gluten-free products and ingredients to persons with celiac sprue and their families; operates telephone information and referral service, and conducts educational seminars.

2657 Healing Well
www.healingwell.com
An online health resource guide to medical news, chat, information and articles, newsgroups and message boards, books, disease-related web sites, medical directories, and more for patients, friends, and family coping with disabling diseases, disorders, or chronic illnesses.

2658 Health Finder
www.healthfinder.gov
Searchable, carefully developed web site offering information on over 1000 topics. Developed by the US Department of Health and Human Services, the site can be used in both English and Spanish.

2659 Healthlink USA
www.healthlinkusa.com
Health information concerning treatment, cures, prevention, diagnosis, risk factors, research, support groups, email lists, personal stories and much more. Updated regularly.

2660 MedicineNet
www.medicinenet.com
An online resource for consumers providing easy-to-read, authoritative medical and health information.

2661 Medscape
www.medscape.com
Medscape offers specialists, primary care physicians, and other health professionals the Web's most robust and integrated medical information and educational tools.

2662 National Celiac Association
nationalceliac.org
Dedicated to helping individuals with celiac disease and gluten sensitivities through education, advocacy, and awareness.
Lee Graham, Executive Director
Kimberly Buckton, Managing Director

2663 WebMD
www.webmd.com
Provides credible information, supportive communities, and in-depth reference material about health subjects. A source for original and timely health information as well as material from well known content providers.

195

Description

2664 ## Cerebral Palsy Syndromes

Cerebral palsy syndromes are nonprogressive syndromes distinguished by impaired posture or voluntary movement that result from prenatal developmental malformations or perinatal or postnatal damage to the central nervous system. The symptoms of these syndromes usually present before two years of age. CP can be caused by birth trauma, insufficient oxygen supplied to the infant at or before birth, excessively high blood levels of bilirubin (kernicterus), premature birth or a severe systemic disease, such as meningitis, during early infancy. However, the exact cause is often difficult to establish.

Children with cerebral palsy may not be identified until they reach 1-2 years of age and may show only lagging motor development. Therefore, children known to be at risk should be followed closely. Increased spastic movements are the most common symptoms, but children may also show weakness, poor sense of balance, involuntary movements and abnormal walking. In more severe cases, difficulty in speaking and mental disability may also be present.

Since there is no known cure for cerebral palsy, the goal of treatment is to develop maximal independence. Therapy may include physical and occupational rehabilitation, the use of leg braces, speech training and special orthopedic surgery. Some children benefit from botulinum toxin injections, benzodiazepines, or other muscle relaxants (e.g., baclofen, tinzidine, or dantrolene) to decrease spasticity. Surgical treatments, such as muscle tendon release or transfer, or in severe cases, re-routing of overactive nerves (dorsal rhizotomy) can benefit patients. Parents need assistance and guidance in understanding their child's status and potential.

National Agencies & Associations

2665 **American Academy for Cerebral Palsy and Developmental Medicine**
555 E Wells St.
Milwaukee, WI 53202
414-918-3014
Fax: 414-276-2146
info@aacpdm.org
www.aacpdm.org
A multidisciplinary scientific society devoted to the study of cerebral palsy and other childhood onset disabilities, promoting professional education for the treatment and management of these conditions and to improving the quality of life for people with the condition.
1550 members
Anniekay Erby, MBA, CAE, Executive Director
Kay Whalen, MBA, CAE, Managing Partner

2666 **American Chronic Pain Association**
PO Box 850
Rocklin, CA 95677
800-533-3231
ACPA@theacpa.org
www.theacpa.org
The ACPA facilitates peer support and education for individuals with chronic pain in its many forms, in order to increase quality of

life. Also raises awareness among the healthcare community, and with policy makers.
Penney Cowan, Founder & CEO
Daniel Galia, Director, Global Support

2667 **Canadian Cerebral Palsy Sports Association**
c/o House of Sport, RA Centre
2451 Riverside Drive
Ottawa, Ontario, K1H-7X7
613-748-1430
888-752-2772
info@ccpsa.ca
www.ccpsa.ca
Athelete-focused national organization administering and governing sport opportunities targeted to athletes with CP and related disabilities.
Jennifer Larson, Program Manager
Peter Leyser, Executive Director

2668 **Easterseals**
141 W Jackson Blvd
Chicago, IL 60604
312-726-6200
800-221-6827
Fax: 312-726-1494
info@easterseals.com
www.easterseals.com
Provides services to children and adults with disabilities as well as support to their families.
Angela F. Williams, President & CEO
Sharon Watson, Vice President, Communications/Marketing

2669 **Independent Living Research Utilization Project**
1333 Moursund
Houston, TX 77030
713-520-0232
Fax: 713-520-5785
TTY: 713-520-0232
ilru@ilru.org
www.ilru.org
A national center for information, training, research, and technical assistance in independent living. Goal is to expand the body of knowledge in independent living and to improve utilization of results of research programs and demonstration projects.
Lex Frieden, Director
Richard Petty, Co-Director

2670 **National Institute of Neurological Disorders and Stroke**
NIH Neurological Institute
Bethesda, MD 20824
301-496-5751
800-352-9424
www.ninds.nih.gov
Seeks to reduce the burden of neurological disease affecting individuals from all walks of life.
Walter J. Koroshetz, MD, Director
Amy B. Adams, Director, Office of Scientific Liaison

2671 **National Rehabilitation Information Center**
8400 Corporate Drive
Landover, MD 20785
800-346-2742
Fax: 301-459-4263
TTY: 301-459-5984
www.naric.com
One of the three components of the office of Special Education and Rehabilitative Services. Operates in concert with the Rehabilitation Services Administration and the Office of Special Education Programs.
Mark X. Odum, Project Director
Jessica H. Chaiken, Media and Information Services Manager

2672 **United Cerebral Palsy Associations**
1825 K Street NW
Washington, DC 20006
202-776-0406
ucp.org
A network of approximately 64 state and local voluntary agencies which provide services, conduct public and professional education programs, and support research in cerebral palsy.
Armando Contreras, President & CEO
Anita Porco, Vice President, Affiliate Network

State Agencies & Associations

Alabama

2673 United Cerebral Palsy of Alabama
301 EA Darden Drive   256-237-8203
Anniston, AL 36202   Fax: 256-235-2388
executivedirector@ecaucp.org
www.ecaucp.org
United Cerebral Palsy provides information, advocacy, referral services for persons with disabilities and/or their families. UCP also operates an equipment loan program, conducts parent workshops, disseminates written literature on topics of interest.
Linda Johns, Executive Director
Shannon Priddy, Development Director

2674 United Cerebral Palsy of East Central Alabama
301 EA Darden Drive   256-237-8203
Anniston, AL 36202   Fax: 256-235-2388
www.ecaucp.org
United Cerebral Palsy provides information, advocacy, referral services for persons with disabilities and/or their families. UCP also operates an equipment loan program, conducts parent workshops, disseminates written literature on topics of interest to people with disabilities.
Donald Turner, Chairman of the Board
John Rogers, Treasurer

2675 United Cerebral Palsy of Greater Birmingha m
120 Oslo Circle   205-944-3900
Birmingham, AL 35211   800-654-4483
Fax: 205-944-3990
gedwards@ucpbham.com
www.ucpbham.com
United Cerebral Palsy provides information, advocacy, referral services for persons with disabilities and/or their families. UCP also operates an equipment loan program, conducts parent workshops, disseminates written literature on topics of interest to people with disabilities.
Gary Edwards, Executive Director
Jennifer H Ellison, Chief Development Officer

2676 United Cerebral Palsy of Huntsville & Tennessee Valley
2075 Max Luther Drive   256-852-5600
Huntsville, AL 35810   Fax: 256-852-6722
tracyc@ucphuntsville.org
www.ucp.org
United Cerebral Palsy provides information, advocacy, referral services for persons with disabilities and/or their families. UCP also operates an equipment loan program, conducts parent workshops, disseminates written literature on topics of interest.
Cheryl Smith, Executive Director
Tim Reeves, President

2677 United Cerebral Palsy of Mobile
3058 Dauphin Square Connector   251-479-4900
Mobile, AL 36607   Fax: 251-479-4998
info@ucpmobile.org
www.ucp.org
United Cerebral Palsy provides information, advocacy, referral services for persons with disabilities and/or their families. UCP also operates an equipment loan program, conducts parent workshops, disseminates written literature on topics of interest.
Glenn Harger, President/CEO
Susan Watson, VP/COO

2678 United Cerebral Palsy of Northwest Alabama
4212 Jackson Highway   256-381-4310
Sheffield, AL 35660   Fax: 256-381-4378
alison@ucpshoals.org
www.ucpshoals.org
United Cerebral Palsy provides information, advocacy, referral services for persons with disabilities and/or their families. UCP also operates an equipment loan program, conducts parent workshops, disseminates written literature on topics of interest.
Alison Isbell, Director
Linda Williamson, Development Director/WEE-CARE Director

2679 United Cerebral Palsy of West Alabama
1100 UCP Parkway   205-345-3031
Northport, AL 35476   Fax: 205-345-3035
www.ucpa.org
United Cerebral Palsy provides information, advocacy, referral services for persons with disabilities and/or their families. UCP also operates an equipment loan program, conducts parent workshops, disseminates written literature on topics of interest.
Lisa D Skelton, Executive Director
Brenda Ewart, Development Director

Alaska

2680 United Cerebral Palsy of Alaska/PARENTS
4743 E Northern Lights Boulevard   907-337-7678
Anchorage, AK 99508   800-478-7678
Fax: 907-337-7671
TTY: 907-337-7629
www.ucpa.org
Provides information, advocacy, referral services for persons with disabilities and/or their families. UCP also operates an equipment loan program, conducts parent workshops, disseminates written literature on topics of interest to people with disabilities.

Arizona

2681 United Cerebral Palsy of Central Arizona
1802 Parkside Lane   602-943-5472
Phoenix, AZ 85027   Fax: 602-943-4936
www.ucpa.org
United Cerebral Palsy provides information, advocacy, referral services for persons with disabilities and/or their families. UCP also operates an equipment loan program, conducts parent workshops, disseminates written literature on topics of interest.
Dan Rossi, Executive Director
Perry Bramlett, Chief Human Resources Officer

2682 United Cerebral Palsy of Southern Arizona
635 N Craycroft Road   520-795-3108
Tucson, AZ 85711   Fax: 520-795-3196
staff@ucpsa.org
www.ucpsa.org
United Cerebral Palsy provides information, advocacy, referral services for persons with disabilities and/or their families. UCP also operates an equipment loan program, conducts parent workshops, disseminates written literature on topics of interest.
Cindy Mars, Executive Director
Gary Bahman, Finance Director

Arkansas

2683 United Cerebral Palsy of Central Arkansas
9720 N Rodney Parham Road   501-224-6067
Little Rock, AR 72227   Fax: 501-227-5591
general@ucpcark.org
www.ucpark.org
United Cerebral Palsy provides information, advocacy, referral services for persons with disabilities and/or their families. UCP also operates an equipment loan program, conducts parent workshops, disseminates written literature on topics of interest.
Woody Connette, Chair
Ian Ridlon, Vice-Chairman

California

2684 United Cerebral Palsy of Central California
4224 North Cedar Avenue   559-221-8272
Fresno, CA 93726-3700   Fax: 559-221-9347
info@ccucp.org
www.ccucp.org/
United Cerebral Palsy provides information, advocacy, referral services for persons with disabilities and/or their families. UCP also operates an equipment loan program, conducts parent workshops, disseminates written literature on topics of interest to people with disabilities.
Mark Lanier, Presdient
Carol Klonnger, Vice-President

2685 United Cerebral Palsy of Greater Sacrament o
191 Lathrop Way   916-565-7700
Sacramento, CA 95815   Fax: 916-565-7773
ucp@ucpsacto.org
www.ucpsacto.org
UCP provides programs and services for people with all types of developmental disabilities. These services include: day programs for adults, an in-home respite service, transportation, independent living services, information and referral services.
Doug Bergman, President/CEO
Tanya Hartle, COO

2686 United Cerebral Palsy of Los Angeles & Ventura Counties
6430 Independence Avenue   818-782-2211
Woodland Hills, CA 91367   Fax: 818-909-9106
mail@ucpla.com
www.ucpla.org
United Cerebral Palsy provides information, advocacy, referral services for persons with disabilities and/or their families. UCP also operates an equipment loan program, conducts parent workshops, disseminates written literature on topics of interest to people with disabilities.
Ronald S Cohen, Chief Executive Officer
Clark Jensen, Chief Operating Officer

2687 United Cerebral Palsy of Orange County
980 Roosevelt   949-333-6400
Irvine, CA 92602   Fax: 949-333-6400
info@ucp-oc.org
United Cerebral Palsy provides information, advocacy, referral services for persons with disabilities and/or their families. UCP also operates an equipment loan program, conducts parent workshops, disseminates written literature on topics of interest.
Paul Pulver, Executive Director~
Lauren Mille Beeler, Director of Therapy Services

2688 United Cerebral Palsy of San Diego County
8525 Gibbs Drive   858-571-7803
San Diego, CA 92123   Fax: 858-571-0919
ucp@ucpsd.org
www.ucpa.org
United Cerebral Palsy provides information, advocacy, referral services for persons with disabilities and/or their families. UCP also operates an equipment loan program, conducts parent workshops, disseminates written literature on topics of interest.
David Carucci, Executive Director
Mary Krieger, Associate Executive Director

2689 United Cerebral Palsy of San Joaquin, Calaveras & Amador Counties
333 W Benjamin Holt Drive   209-956-0290
Stockton, CA 95207   Fax: 209-956-0294
slarson@ucpsj.org
www.ucp.org
United Cerebral Palsy provides information, advocacy, referral services for persons with disabilities and/or their families. UCP also operates an equipment loan program, conducts parent workshops, disseminates written literature on topics of interest to people with disabilities.
Leslie Heier, Interim Executive Director
Theresa Galano-Burke, Executive Assistant

2690 United Cerebral Palsy of San Luis Obispo
3620 Sacramento Drive   805-543-2039
San Luis Obispo, CA 93401   877-UCP-CAR1
Fax: 805-543-2045
shaftmt@aol.com
www.ucp-slo.org
United Cerebral Palsy provides information, advocacy, referral services for persons with disabilities and/or their families. UCP also operates an equipment loan program, conducts parent workshops, disseminates written literature on topics of interest to people with disabilities.
Mark Shaffer, UCP Executive Director
Karl Winkler, UCP Administrative Assistant

2691 United Cerebral Palsy of Santa Barbara County
6430 Independence Avenue   818-782-2211
Woodland Hills, CA 91367   888-733-4227
Fax: 818-909-9106
mail@ucpla.org
www.ucpla.org
United Cerebral Palsy provides information, advocacy, referral services for persons with disabilities and/or their families. UCP also operates an equipment loan program, conducts parent workshops, disseminates written literature on topics of interest.
Ellen Kessler, Chairperson
Nick Roxborough, President

2692 United Cerebral Palsy of Santa Clara & San Mateo Counties
512 E Maude Avenue   650-917-6900
Sunnyvale, CA 94085-4431   Fax: 650-948-8503
www.ucpscsm.org/
United Cerebral Palsy provides information, advocacy, referral services for persons with disabilities and/or their families. UCP also operates an equipment loan program, conducts parent workshops, disseminates written literature on topics of interest.
Stephen Bennett, President/CEO National Office (DC)
Armetta Parker, Marketing/Communications Director (DC)

2693 United Cerebral Palsy of Stanislaus County
1213 13th Street   209-577-2122
Modesto, CA 95353   Fax: 209-577-2392
rlonczak@ucpstan.org
www.ucpstan.org
United Cerebral Palsy provides information, advocacy, referral services for persons with disabilities and/or their families. UCP also operates an equipment loan program, conducts parent workshops, disseminates written literature on topics of interest to people with disabilities.
Robert S Lonczak, Executive Director
Jeanette Jones, Program~Coordinator

2694 United Cerebral Palsy of the Golden Gate
1970 Broadway   510-832-7430
Oakland, CA 94612   Fax: 510-839-1329
info@ucpgg.org
www.ucp.org
United Cerebral Palsy provides information, advocacy, referral services for persons with disabilities and/or their families. UCP also operates an equipment loan program, conducts parent workshops, disseminates written literature on topics of interest.
Karen Glatze, Administrator
Dori Maxon, SNAP Program Director

2695 United Cerebral Palsy of the Inland Empire
35-325 Date Palm Drive   760-321-8184
Cathedral City, CA 92234   877-512-2224
Fax: 760-321-8284
info@ucpie.org
www.ucpie.org
United Cerebral Palsy provides information, advocacy, referral services for persons with disabilities and/or their families. UCP conducts parent workshops, disseminates written literature on topics of interest to people with disabilities.
Roger M Alexander, Chair
Micki James, Vice Chair

2696 United Cerebral Palsy of the North Bay
3835 Cypress Drive   707-766-9990
Petaluma, CA 94954   800-872-5827
Fax: 202-776-0414
info@ucpnb.org
www.ucp.org
United Cerebral Palsy's mission is to advance the independence, productivity and full citizenship of people with disabilities through an affiliate network.
Margaret Farman, Executive Director
Ron Hamilton, Chief of Operations

Colorado

2697 United Cerebral Palsy of Colorado
801 Yosemite Street
Denver, CO 80230-5708
303-691-9339
866-701-2277
Fax: 303-691-0846
www.cpco.org
United Cerebral Palsy provides information, advocacy, referral services for persons with disabilities and/or their families. UCP also operates an equipment loan program, conducts parent workshops, disseminates written literature on topics of interest.
Jim Reuter, Chairman of the Board
Judith I Ham, President/CEO

Connecticut

2698 United Cerebral Palsy of Eastern Connecticut
42 Norwich Road
Quaker Hill, CT 06375
860-447-3800
Fax: 860-443-8272
www.ucp.org
United Cerebral Palsy provides information, advocacy, referral services for persons with disabilities and/or their families. UCP also operates an equipment loan program, conducts parent workshops, disseminates written literature on topics of interest to people with disabilities.
Margaret Morrison, Executive Director
Patricia Mansfield, Executive Director

2699 United Cerebral Palsy of Greater Hartford
80 Whitney Street
Hartford, CT 06105
860-236-6201
Fax: 860-218-2454
www.ucphartford.org
United Cerebral Palsy provides information, advocacy, referral services for persons with disabilities and/or their families. UCP also operates an equipment loan program, conducts parent workshops, disseminates written literature on topics of interest to people with disabilities.
Pam Reid, Regional Administrator
Sean Thompson, In-Home Support Coordinator

2700 United Cerebral Palsy of Southern Connecticut
94-96 South Turnpike Road
Wallingford, CT 06492
203-269-3511
Fax: 203-269-7411
ucpasouthernct@yahoo.com
www.ucpa.org
United Cerebral Palsy provides information, advocacy, referral services for persons with disabilities and/or their families. UCP also operates an equipment loan program, conducts parent workshops, disseminates written literature on topics of interest to people with disabilities.

Delaware

2701 United Cerebral Palsy of Delaware
700 A River Road
Wilmington, DE 19809-2746
302-764-2400
Fax: 302-764-8713
wmccool@ucpde.org
www.ucp.org/ucp_local.cfm/52
United Cerebral Palsy provides information, advocacy, referral services for persons with disabilities and/or their families. UCP also operates an equipment loan program, conducts parent workshops, disseminates written literature on topics of interest.
Michelle Welch, President
D Bruce McClenathan, Vice President

District of Columbia

2702 United Cerebral Palsy of Washington DC
1818 New York Avenue
Washington, DC 20002
202-526-0146
Fax: 202-526-0519
dcarter@ucpdc.org
www.ucpdc.org
United Cerebral Palsy provides information, advocacy, referral services for persons with disabilities and/or their families. UCP also operates an equipment loan program, conducts parent workshops, disseminates written literature on topics of interest.
Mark A Simione, Board President
Roderick Johnson, Board Secretary

2703 United Cerebral Palsy of Washington DC & Northern Virginia
1818 New York Avenue NE
Washington, DC 20002
202-526-0146
Fax: 202-526-0519
www.ucpdc.org
United Cerebral Palsy provides information, advocacy, referral services for persons with disabilities and/or their families. UCP also operates an equipment loan program, conducts parent workshops, disseminates written literature on topics of interest to people with disabilities.
Mark Simione, President
George Connors, 1st Vice President

Florida

2704 United Cerebral Palsy of Central Florida
3305 S Orange Avenue
Orlando, FL 32806
407-852-3300
Fax: 407-852-3301
www.ucpcfl.org
United Cerebral Palsy provides information, advocacy, referral services for persons with disabilities and/or their families. UCP also operates an equipment loan program, conducts parent workshops, disseminates written literature on topics of interest.
Ilene E Wilkins, President & Chief Executive Officer
Jill Wisth, Chief Financial Officer

2705 United Cerebral Palsy of East Central Florida
1100 Jimmy Ann Drive
Daytona Beach, FL 32117
386-274-6474
Fax: 386-274-6532
www.ucp.org
Barry Pollack, President/CEO
Kelly Johanessen, VP of Operations

2706 United Cerebral Palsy of Florida
1830 Buford Court
Tallahassee, FL 32308
850-922-5630
Fax: 850-922-1258
gloriawe@earthlink.net
www.ucp.org
United Cerebral Palsy provides information, advocacy, referral services for persons with disabilities and/or their families. UCP also operates an equipment loan program, conducts parent workshops, disseminates written literature on topics of interest.

2707 United Cerebral Palsy of North Florida: Tender Loving Care
1241 NE Avenue
Panama City, FL 32401
850-769-7960
Fax: 850-769-1060
www.ucp.org
United Cerebral Palsy provides information, advocacy, referral services for persons with disabilities and/or their families. UCP also operates an equipment loan program, conducts parent workshops, disseminates written literature on topics of interest to people with disabilities.

2708 United Cerebral Palsy of Northeast Florida
3311 Beach Boulevard
Jacksonville, FL 32207
904-396-1462
Fax: 904-396-1199
cpnefagency@hotmail.com

2709 United Cerebral Palsy of Northwest Florida
2912 North East Street
Pensacola, FL 32501-1324
850-432-1596
Fax: 850-432-1930
www.ucpnwfl.org/
The number one service provider in Northwest Florida for individuals with cerebral palsy and other developmental disabilities, UCP provides information ,advocacy and referral services for persons with disabilities and/or their families. Additionally, UCP offers individuals assistance with daily living skills training, computer training, basic education, speech, physical and occupational therapy, residential, supported living and finding long-term employment.
Brain Bell, Chair
Michelle Fielder, Vice-Chairman

2710 United Cerebral Palsy of Sarasota-Manatee
1090 S Tamiami Trail
Sarasota, FL 34236
941-957-3599
Fax: 947-957-3499
ucpwendy@aol.com
www.ucpsarasota.org
United Cerebral Palsy provides information, advocacy, referral services for persons with disabilities and/or their families. UCP

also operates an equipment loan program, conducts parent workshops, disseminates written literature on topics of interest.
Barnett A Greenberg, Chairperson
Mark Famiglio, President

2711   United Cerebral Palsy of South Florida
2700 W 81st Street
Hialeah, FL 33016

305-325-1080
Fax: 305-325-1313
info@ucpsouthflorida.org
www.ucp.org

United Cerebral Palsy provides information, advocacy, referral services for persons with disabilities and/or their families. UCP also operates an equipment loan program, conducts parent workshops, disseminates written literature on topics of interest.
Joseph Aniello, President & CEO
Linda Gluck, Vice President & CFO

2712   United Cerebral Palsy of Tallahassee
1830 Buford Court
Tallahassee, FL 32308

850-878-2141
Fax: 850-922-1258
gloriawe@earthlink.net
www.ucp.org

United Cerebral Palsy provides information, advocacy, referral services for persons with disabilities and/or their families. UCP also operates an equipment loan program, conducts parent workshops, disseminates written literature on topics of interest.

2713   United Cerebral Palsy of Tampa Bay
2215 E Henry Avenue
Tampa, FL 33610

813-239-1179
800-749-5155
Fax: 813-237-3091
www.ucptampa.org

United Cerebral Palsy provides information, advocacy, referral services for persons with disabilities and/or their families. UCP also operates an equipment loan program, conducts parent workshops, disseminates written literature on topics of interest to people with disabilities.
Jim King, Executive Director
Dawn Gosselin, Executive Development Assistant / Events

Georgia

2714   United Cerebral Palsy of Georgia
3300 NE Expressway
Atlanta, GA 30341

770-676-2000
Fax: 770-455-8040
info@ucpga.org
www.ucp.org

United Cerebral Palsy provides information, advocacy, referral services for persons with disabilities and/or their families. UCP also operates an equipment loan program, conducts parent workshops, disseminates written literature on topics of interest to people with disabilities.
Diane Wilush, Executive Director
Kevin Walton, Associate Executive Director

Hawaii

2715   United Cerebral Palsy of Hawaii
414 Kuwili Street
Honolulu, HI 96817-5050

808-532-6744
800-606-5654
Fax: 808-532-6747
www.ucpahi.org

United Cerebral Palsy provides information, advocacy, referral services for persons with disabilities and/or their families. UCP also operates an equipment loan program, conducts parent workshops, disseminates written literature on topics of interest.
Jerry Pupillo, President
Stephen Hink, 1st Vice President

Idaho

2716   United Cerebral Palsy of Idaho
5420 W Franklin Road
Boise, ID 83705

208-377-8070
888-289-3281
Fax: 208-322-7133
www.ucp.org

United Cerebral Palsy provides information, advocacy and referral services for persons with disabilities and/or their families.
Kim Kane, Executive Director
Kathy Griffin, Program Director

Illinois

2717   United Cerebral Palsy Land of Lincoln
101 N 16th Street
Springfield, IL 67203

217-525-6522
Fax: 217-525-9017
info@ucpll.org
www.ucp.org

United Cerebral Palsy provides information, advocacy, referral services for persons with disabilities and/or their families. UCP also operates an equipment loan program, conducts parent workshops, disseminates written literature on topics of interest.
Brenda L Yarnell, President/CEO
Kathy Leuelling, Chief Operating Officer

2718   United Cerebral Palsy of East Central Illinois
1023 N Water
Decatur, IL 62523

217-428-5033
Fax: 217-428-5094
ww.ucpa.org

United Cerebral Palsy provides information, advocacy, referral services for persons with disabilities and/or their families. UCP also operates an equipment loan program, conducts parent workshops, disseminates written literature on topics of interest.
Woody Connette, Chair

2719   United Cerebral Palsy of Greater Chicago
547 W Jackson
Chicago, IL 60661

312-765-0419
Fax: 312-765-0503
TTY: 312-368-0179
pdulle@ucpnet.org
www.ucpnet.org

United Cerebral Palsy provides information, advocacy, referral services for persons with disabilities and/or their families. UCP also operates an equipment loan program, conducts parent workshops, disseminates written literature on topics of interest to people with disabilities.
Paul J Dulle, President/CEO
Peggy Childs, Executive Vice President

2720   United Cerebral Palsy of Illinois
310 E Adams
Springfield, IL 62701

877-550-8274
877-550-8274
Fax: 217-528-9739
TTY: 877-550-8274

United Cerebral Palsy provides information, advocacy, referral services for persons with disabilities and/or their families. UCP also operates an equipment loan program, conducts parent workshops, disseminates written literature on topics of interest to people with disabilities.
Don Moss, Executive Director
Alice Foss, Associate Director

2721   United Cerebral Palsy of Southern Illinois
9 Cusumano Professional Plaza Drive
Mount Vernon, IL 62864

618-244-2505
Fax: 618-244-3568
ucpsi@onemain.com
www.ucpa.org

United Cerebral Palsy provides information, advocacy, referral services for persons with disabilities and/or their families. UCP also operates an equipment loan program, conducts parent workshops, disseminates written literature on topics of interest to people with disabilities.

2722   United Cerebral Palsy of Will County
311 S Reed Street
Joliet, IL 60436

815-744-3500
Fax: 815-744-3504
www.ucp.org

United Cerebral Palsy provides information, advocacy, referral services for persons with disabilities and/or their families. UCP also operates an equipment loan program, conducts parent workshops, disseminates written literature on topics of interest to people with disabilities.
Samuel Mancuso, President & Chief Executive Officer
Stephanie Bergner, Family Support/Respite Administrator

2723   United Cerebral Palsy of the Blackhawk Region
7399 Forest Hills Road
Rockford, IL 61111

815-636-7132
Fax: 815-282-8835
ucpbr@aol.com
www.ucpa.org

United Cerebral Palsy provides information, advocacy, referral services for persons with disabilities and/or their families. UCP also operates an equipment loan program, conducts parent workshops, disseminates written literature on topics of interest to people with disabilities.

2724 United Cerebral Palsy: Eastern Seals
230 W Monroe Street 312-726-6200
Chicago, IL 60606 800-221-6827
Fax: 312-726-1494

United Cerebral Palsy provides information, advocacy, referral services for persons with disabilities and/or their families. UCP also operates an equipment loan program, conducts parent workshops, disseminates written literature on topics of interest.
John Rogers, IT consultant
Tyler Howe, Project Manager

Indiana

2725 United Cerebral Palsy Association of Indiana
1915 West 18th Street 317-632-3561
Indianapolis, IN 46202-1016 Fax: 317-632-3338
donnar@ucpaindy.org
www.ucpa.org

United Cerebral Palsy provides information, advocacy, referral services for persons with Cerebral Palsy and/or their families. UCP also provides funding for equipment and operates an equipment loan program, disseminates written literature on topics of interest to people with disabilities.
Donna L Roberts, Executive Director

2726 United Cerebral Palsy Associations
6100 N Keystone Avenue 317-632-3561
Indianapolis, IN 46220 Fax: 317-632-3338
www.ucpaindy.org

United Cerebral Palsy provides information, advocacy, referral services for persons with Cerebral Palsy and/or their families. UCP also provides funding for equipment and operates an equipment loan program, disseminates written literature on topics of interest.
Donna L Roberts, Executive Director
Beth Allison, Case Manager

2727 United Cerebral Palsy of the Wabash Valley
621 Poplar Street 812-232-6305
Terre Haute, IN 47807 Fax: 812-234-3683
ucp.wv@verizon.net

United Cerebral Palsy provides information, advocacy, referral services for persons with disabilities and/or their families. UCP also operates an equipment loan program, conducts parent workshops, disseminates written literature on topics of interest to people with disabilities.
Jacquie Denehie, Executive Director
Brain Garcia, President

Kansas

2728 United Cerebral Palsy of Kansas
5111 E 21st Street 316-688-1888
Wichita, KS 67208 Fax: 316-688-5687
davej@cprf.org
www.ucp.org

United Cerebral Palsy provides information, advocacy, referral services for persons with disabilities and/or their families. UCP also operates an equipment loan program, conducts parent workshops, disseminates written literature on topics of interest.
Dave Jones, Executive Director
Amelia Ornelas, Office Manager

Louisiana

2729 United Cerebral Palsy of Baton Rouge McMains Children's Developmental Center
1805 College Drive 225-923-3420
Baton Rouge, LA 70808 Fax: 225-922-9316
jketcham@mcmainscdc.org
www.mcmainscdc.org

United Cerebral Palsy provides information, advocacy, referral services for persons with disabilities and/or their families. UCP

also operates an equipment loan program, conducts parent workshops, disseminates written literature on topics of interest.
Janet Ketcham, Director
Norman Landry, President

2730 United Cerebral Palsy of Greater New Orleans
1000 Leonidas St & Leake Avenue 504-865-0003
New Orleans, LA 70118 Fax: 504-865-0300
www.ucpgno.org

United Cerebral Palsy provides information, advocacy, referral services for persons with disabilities and/or their families. UCP also operates an equipment loan program, conducts parent workshops, disseminates written literature on topics of interest to people with disabilities.
Tommy Freel, Chair
Joanne Rinardo, Treasurer

Maine

2731 United Cerebral Palsy of Northeastern Maine
700 Mount Hope Avenue 207-941-2952
Bangor, ME 04401 877-603-0030
Fax: 207-941-2955
office@ucpofmaine.org
www.ucp.org

United Cerebral Palsy provides information, advocacy, referral services for persons with disabilities and/or their families. UCP also operates an equipment loan program, conducts parent workshops, disseminates written literature on topics of interest to people with disabilities.
Bobbi-Jo Yeager, Executive Director
Tricia Kail, Director of Services

Maryland

2732 United Cerebral Palsy of Central Maryland
1700 Reistertown Road 410-484-4540
Baltimore, MD 21208-2935 Fax: 410-484-1807
TTY: 800-451-2452
info@ucp-cm.org
www.ucp.org

United Cerebral Palsy provides information, advocacy, referral services for persons with disabilities and/or their families. UCP also operates an equipment loan program, conducts parent workshops, disseminates written literature on topics of interest.
Diane Coughlin, President and CEO
Judy Cox, Assistant to the President

2733 United Cerebral Palsy of Prince Georges & Montgomery Counties
4409 Forbes Boulevard 301-459-0566
Lanham, MD 20706 Fax: 301-459-7691
TTY: 301-459-7691
TDD: 301-262-4982
ucppgmc@aol.com

Provides information, advocacy, referral services for persons with disabilities and/or their families. UCP also operates an equipment loan program, conducts parent workshops, disseminates written literature on topics of interest to people with disabilities.
Charles McNelly, Executive Director
Diane Dekoladenu, Program Director

2734 United Cerebral Palsy of Southern Maryland
221 Chinquapin Round Road 410-280-2003
Annapolis, MD 21401 Fax: 410-269-5757

United Cerebral Palsy provides information, advocacy, referral services for persons with disabilities and/or their families. UCP also operates an equipment loan program, conducts parent workshops, disseminates written literature on topics of interest to people with disabilities.

Massachusetts

2735 United Cerebral Palsy of Berkshire County
208 W Street 413-442-1562
Pittsfield, MA 01201 Fax: 413-499-4077
info@ucpberkshire.org
www.ucp.org

United Cerebral Palsy provides information, advocacy, referral services for persons with disabilities and/or their families. UCP

also operates an equipment loan program, conducts parent workshops, disseminates written literature on topics of interest to people with disabilities.
Christine Singer, Executive Director
Joni Thomas, Director of Development

2736 United Cerebral Palsy of MetroBoston
71 Arsenal Street   617-926-5480
Watertown, MA 02472   Fax: 617-926-3059
                                                           www.ucp.org
United Cerebral Palsy provides information, advocacy, referral services for persons with disabilities and/or their families. UCP also operates an equipment loan program, conducts parent workshops, disseminates written literature on topics of interest.
Todd Kates, Executive Director
Roberta Jaro, Associate Executive Director

Michigan

2737 United Cerebral Palsy of Metropolitan Detroit
23077 Greenfield   248-557-5070
Southfield, MI 48075   Fax: 248-557-0224
                                                       main@ucpdetroit.org
                                                           www.ucp.org
United Cerebral Palsy provides information, advocacy, referral services for persons with disabilities and/or their families. UCP also operates an equipment loan program, conducts parent workshops, disseminates written literature on topics of interest.
Leslynn Angel, President & CEO
Latoya Jones, Chief Financial Officer

2738 United Cerebral Palsy of Michigan
4970 Northwind Drive   517-203-1200
E Lansing, MI 48823   800-828-2714
                                                           Fax: 517-203-1203
                                                     ucp@ucpmichigan.org
                                                           www.ucp.org
United Cerebral Palsy provides information, advocacy, referral services for persons with disabilities and/or their families. UCP also operates an equipment loan program, conducts parent workshops, disseminates written literature on topics of interest.
Linda Potter, Executive Director
Linda Carey, Office Manager

Minnesota

2739 United Cerebral Palsy of Central Minnesota
510 25th Avenue North   320-253-0765
St. Cloud, MN 56303-3255   Fax: 320-253-6753
                                                       info@ucpcentralmn.org
                                                       www.ucpcentralmn.org
Provides information, advocacy, referral services for persons with disabilities and/or their families. UCP conducts parent workshops, disseminates free newsletter. Computers go round recycles quality used computers to persons with disabilities. UCP awards scholarship for post secondary education.
Shelly Gaetz, President
Sue Schlosser, Vice-President

2740 United Cerebral Palsy of Minnesota
1821 University Avenue W   651-646-7588
St Paul, MN 55104-2892   877-528-5678
                                                           Fax: 651-646-3045
                                                     ucpmnStacey@hotmail.com
                                                           www.ucp.org
United Cerebral Palsy provides information, advocacy, referral services for persons with disabilities and/or their families. UCP also operates an equipment loan program, conducts parent workshops, disseminates written literature on topics of interest.
Stacey Vogele, Executive Director
Ramsey Lee, Events Coordinator

Missouri

2741 United Cerebral Palsy of Greater Kansas City
1044 Main Street   816-531-4454
Kansas City, MO 64105   Fax: 816-531-3383
                                                           www.ucp.org

Provides information, advocacy, referral services for persons with disabilities and/or their families. UCP also operates residential programs and care management for seniors.
Bruce A Scott, President & CEO
Sam T Switzer, Senior Vice President & CFO

2742 United Cerebral Palsy of Greater St. Louis
13975 Mancester Rd   636-227-6030
Manchester, MO 63011-3999   Fax: 636-779-2270
                                                       forkoshr@ucpstl.org
                                                       www.ucpheartland.org/
United Cerebral Palsy provides information, advocacy, referral services for persons with disabilities and/or their families. UCP also operates an equipment loan program, conducts parent workshops, disseminates written literature on topics of interest to people with disabilities.
Woody Connette, Chair
Lan Ridlon, Vice Chair

2743 United Cerebral Palsy of Northwest Missouri
3303 Frederick Avenue   816-364-3836
St. Joseph, MO 64506   Fax: 816-390-8546
                                                       ucp@ucpnwmo.org
                                                           www.ucpa.org
United Cerebral Palsy provides information, advocacy, referral services for persons with disabilities and/or their families. UCP also operates an equipment loan program, conducts parent workshops, disseminates written literature on topics of interest to people with disabilities.
Jared Bronner, President
Shawn Drew, Vice-President

Nebraska

2744 United Cerebral Palsy of Nebraska
920 S 107th Avenue   402-502-3572
Omaha, NE 68114   800-729-2556
                                                           Fax: 402-502-6791
                                                           www.ucp.org
United Cerebral Palsy provides information, advocacy, referral services for persons with disabilities and/or their families. UCP also operates an equipment loan program, conducts parent workshops, disseminates written literature on topics of interest.
Carol Hahn, Executive Director
Anne Brodin, Financial & Services Director

Nevada

2745 United Cerebral Palsy of Northern Nevada
4068 S McCarran Boulevard   775-331-3323
Reno, NV 89502-7532   Fax: 775-331-7913
                                                           www.ucpnv.org
United Cerebral Palsy provides information, advocacy, referral services for persons with disabilities and/or their families. UCP also provides employment and supported living services and disseminates written literature on topics of interest.
E. Sue Saunders, Chairperson
Julie Ann Utley, Vice Chairperson

New Jersey

2746 United Cerebral Palsy of Hudson County
721 Broadway   201-436-2200
Bayonne, NJ 07002   Fax: 201-436-6642
                                                     kkearney@ucpofhudsoncounty.org
                                                           www.ucp.org
United Cerebral Palsy provides information, advocacy, referral services for persons with disabilities and/or their families. UCP also operates an equipment loan program, conducts parent workshops, disseminates written literature on topics of interest to people with disabilities.
Nick Starita, Executive Director
Keith J Kearney, Associate Executive Director

2747 United Cerebral Palsy of Morris-Somerset
245 Main Street   908-879-2243
Chester, NJ 07930   Fax: 908-879-8363
                                                           www.ucpa.org
United Cerebral Palsy provides information, advocacy, referral services for persons with disabilities and/or their families. UCP

also operates an equipment loan program, conducts parent workshops, disseminates written literature on topics of interest.

2748 United Cerebral Palsy of New Jersey
1005 Whitehead Road Extension
Ewing, NJ 08638

609-392-4004
888-322-1918
Fax: 609-882-4054
TTY: 609-882-0620
info@cpofnj.org
www.cpofnj.org

United Cerebral Palsy provides information, advocacy, referral services for persons with disabilities and/or their families. UCP also operates an equipment loan program, conducts parent workshops, disseminates written literature on topics of interest.
Mathew Jacobs, President
Warren Kelemen, Vice-President

New York

2749 Center for the Disabled
314 S Manning Boulevard
Albany, NY 12208

518-437-5700
bulgaro@cftd.org
www.cfdsny.org

United Cerebral Palsy provides information, advocacy, referral services for persons with disabilities and/or their families. UCP also operates an equipment loan program, conducts parent workshops, disseminates written literature on topics of interest to people with disabilities.
Alan Krafchin, CEO/President
Patrick J Rielly, Chief Operating Officer

2750 Cerebral Palsy Associations of New York State
90 State Street
Albany, NY 12207

518-436-0178
Fax: 518-436-8619
AffiliateServices@cpofnys.org
www.cpofnys.org

Provides information, advocacy, referral services for persons with disabilities and/or their families. CP also operates an equipment loan program, conducts parent workshops and disseminates written literature on topics of interest to people with disabilities.
Michael Alvaro, Executive Vice President
Susan Constantino, President & CEO

2751 Niagara Cerebral Palsy
9812 Lockport Road
Niagara Falls, NY 14304

716-297-0798
Fax: 716-297-0998
www.ucpaofniagara.com

Provides educational, residential, vocational and recreational programs.

2752 Prospect Child And Family Center
133 Aviation Road
Queensbury, NY 12804

518-798-0170
Fax: 518-798-0533
www.prospectcenter.com

Gary Edie, President
Eli Socolof, Vice-President

2753 United Cerebral Palsy of Chemung County
1118 Charles Street
Elmira, NY 14901

607-734-7107
Fax: 607-734-7334
www.chemungcp.com

United Cerebral Palsy provides information, advocacy, referral services for persons with disabilities and/or their families. UCP also operates an equipment loan program, conducts parent workshops, disseminates written literature on topics of interest to people with disabilities.
Mark Peters, Executive Director
Leisa Alger, Associate Executive Director

2754 United Cerebral Palsy of Fulton & Montgomery Counties
67 Division Street
Amsterdam, NY 12010

518-842-3511
Fax: 518-843-6042
www.ucpa.org

United Cerebral Palsy provides information, advocacy, referral services for persons with disabilities and/or their families. UCP also operates an equipment loan program, conducts parent workshops, disseminates written literature on topics of interest to people with disabilities.

2755 United Cerebral Palsy of Greater Suffolk
250 Marcus Boulevard
Hauppauge, NY 11788

631-232-0011
Fax: 631-232-4422
www.ucp-suffolk.org

United Cerebral Palsy provides information, advocacy, referral services for persons with disabilities and/or their families. UCP also operates an equipment loan program, conducts parent workshops, disseminates written literature on topics of interest.
Stephen H Friedman, President & CEO
James Monnier, Board of Directors

2756 United Cerebral Palsy of Nassau County
380 Washington Avenue
Roosevelt, NY 11575

516-378-2000
Fax: 516-868-4089
info@ucpn.org
www.ucpn.org

United Cerebral Palsy provides information, advocacy, referral services for persons with disabilities and/or their families. UCP also operates an equipment loan program, conducts parent workshops, disseminates written literature on topics of interest to people with disabilities.
Robert Masterson, President
Thomas Connolly, Executive Vice President

2757 United Cerebral Palsy of New York City
80 Maiden Lane
New York, NY 10038-4811

212-683-6700
800-GIV-EUCP
Fax: 212-685-8394
info@ucpnyc.org
www.ucpnyc.org

United Cerebral Palsy provides information, advocacy, referral services for persons with disabilities and/or their families. UCP also operates an equipment loan program, conducts parent workshops, disseminates written literature on topics of interest.
Edward R. Matthews, Chief Executive Officer
Gary Geresi, President

2758 United Cerebral Palsy of Putnam & Southern Dutchess Counties
40 John Barrett Road
Patterson, NY 12563

845-878-9078
Fax: 845-878-3203
hvcs@aol.com
www.ucpa.org

United Cerebral Palsy provides information, advocacy, referral services for persons with disabilities and/or their families. UCP also operates an equipment loan program, conducts parent workshops, disseminates written literature on topics of interest to people with disabilities.

2759 United Cerebral Palsy of Queens: Queens Centers for Progress
81-15 164th Street
Jamaica, NY 11432

718-380-3000
Fax: 718-380-0483
TTY: 718-969-0270
info@queenscp.org
www.queenscp.org

Provides information advocacy and referral services for persons with disabilities and/or their families. Offers an equipment loan program parent workshops and written literature on topics of interest to people with disabilities.
George Wildi Berger, President
Joseph A Cristiano, Vice-President

2760 United Cerebral Palsy of Westchester County
1186 King Street
Rye Brook, NY 10573

914-937-3800
Fax: 914-937-0967
www.cpwestchester.org

United Cerebral Palsy provides information advocacy referral services for persons with disabilities and/or their families. UCP also operates an equipment loan program conducts parent workshops disseminates written literature on topics of interest to people with disabilities.
Richard Osterer, President
Richard Eising, Executive Vice President

2761 United Cerebral Palsy of Western New York
7 Community Drive
Buffalo, NY 14225

716-894-0130
Fax: 716-894-8257
ucpawny1@aol.com
www.ucpa.org

United Cerebral Palsy provides information advocacy referral services for persons with disabilities and/or their families. UCP also operates an equipment loan program conducts parent workshops disseminates written literature on topics of interest to people with disabilities.

2762 United Cerebral Palsy of the North Country
4 Commerce Lane
Canton, NY 13617
315-379-9667
Fax: 315-379-9388
www.cpnorthcountry.org/
United Cerebral Palsy provides information advocacy referral services for persons with disabilities and/or their families. UCP also operates an equipment loan program conducts parent workshops disseminates written literature on topics of interest to people with disabilities.

North Carolina

2763 Easterseals UCP North Carolina & Virginia
5171 Glenwood Ave
Raleigh, NC 27612
919-783-8898
800-662-7119
Fax: 919-782-5486
www.easterseals.com/NCVA
A lifelong partner to families managing disabilities and mental health challenges. Serves more than 20,000 individuals and their families annually through an array of services. Enhances the quality of life for individuals and maximizes their potential for engaging in their communities.
Luanne Welch, President/CEO

Ohio

2764 United Cerebral Palsy of Central Ohio
440 Industrial Mile Road
Columbus, OH 43228-2411
614-279-0109
Fax: 914-279-2527
www.ucpofcentralohio.org
United Cerebral Palsy provides information advocacy referral services for persons with disabilities and/or their families. UCP also operates an equipment loan program conducts parent workshops disseminates written literature on topics of interest to people with disabilities.
Charles Dyas, President/Executive Committee Chair
Diane Dierna, Vice-President

2765 United Cerebral Palsy of Cincinnati
3601 Victory Parkway
Cincinnati, OH 45229
513-221-4606
Fax: 513-872-5262
sschiller@ucp-cincinnati.org
www.ucp-cincinnati.org
United Cerebral Palsy provides information advocacy referral services for persons with disabilities and/or their families. UCP also operates an equipment loan program conducts parent workshops disseminates written literature on topics of interest to people with disabilities.
Susan Schiller, Executive Director, Development Director

2766 United Cerebral Palsy of Greater Cleveland
10011 Euclid Avenue
Cleveland, OH 44106
216-791-8363
Fax: 216-721-3372
sdean@ucpcleveland.org
www.ucpcleveland.org/
United Cerebral Palsy provides information, advocacy, referral services for persons with disabilities and/or their families. UCP also operates an equipment loan program, conducts parent workshops, disseminates written literature on topics of interest to people with disabilities.
Mathew Cox, Chair
Sean Wenger, Vice-Chairman

2767 United Cerebral Palsy of Greater Dane
10011 Euclid Avenue
Cleveland, OH 44106
216-791-8363
Fax: 216-721-3372
sdean@ucpcleveland.org
www.ucpcleveland.org
United Cerebral Palsy provides information advocacy referral services for persons with disabilities and/or their families. UCP also operates an equipment loan program conducts parent workshops disseminates written literature on topics of interest to people with disabilities.
Robert J Darden, President
Douglas A Neary, Vice President

Oklahoma

2768 United Cerebral Palsy of Oklahoma
10400 Greenbriar Place
Oklahoma City, OK 73159
405-759-3562
Fax: 405-917-7082
info@ucpok.org
www.ucpok.org
United Cerebral Palsy provides information advocacy referral services for persons with disabilities and/or their families. UCP also operates an equipment loan program conducts parent workshops disseminates written literature on topics of interest to people with disabilities.

Oregon

2769 United Cerebral Palsy of Oregon & SW Washington
11731 NE Glenn Widing Drive
Portland, OR 97220
503-777-4166
800-473-4581
Fax: 503-771-8048
ucpa@ucpaorwa.org
www.ucp.org
United Cerebral Palsy provides information advocacy referral services for persons with disabilities and/or their families. UCP also operates an equipment loan program conducts parent workshops disseminates written literature on topics of interest to people with disabilities.
Bud Thoune, Executive Director
Doug Taylor, Development and Marketing Director

Pennsylvania

2770 United Cerebral Palsy Central PA
44 S 38th Street
Camp Hill, PA 17011
717-975-0611
Fax: 717-975-0839
kidscenter@ucpcentralpa.org
www.ucp.org
United Cerebral Palsy provides information advocacy referral services for persons with disabilities and/or their families. UCP also operates an equipment loan program conducts parent workshops disseminates written literature on topics of interest to people with disabilities.
Jeffrey W Cooper, President/CEO
Jennifer Brubaker~, Director of Administrative Services

2771 United Cerebral Palsy of Beaver, Butler & Lawrence Counties
101 Hindman Lane
Butler, PA 16001
724-482-4765
Fax: 724-283-5945
www.ucpa.org
United Cerebral Palsy provides information, advocacy, referral services for persons with disabilities and/or their families. UCP also operates an equipment loan program, conducts parent workshops, disseminates written literature on topics of interest to people with disabilities.

2772 United Cerebral Palsy of Northwestern Pennsylvania
3745 W 12th Street
Erie, PA 16505
814-836-9113
Fax: 814-833-3919
www.ucpa.org
United Cerebral Palsy provides information advocacy referral services for persons with disabilities and/or their families. UCP also operates a wheelchair ramp building program, conducts parent workshops and offers adaptive recreation activities.
Laura Eaton, Executive Director

2773 United Cerebral Palsy of Pennsylvania
908 N Second Street
Harrisburg, PA 17102
717-441-6044
866-761-6129
Fax: 717-236-2046
www.ucp.org
United Cerebral Palsy provides information advocacy referral services for persons with disabilities and/or their families. UCP also operates an equipment loan program conducts parent workshops disseminates written literature on topics of interest to people with disabilities.
Joan Martin, Executive Director
Vini Portzline, Policy Information Exchange

2774 United Cerebral Palsy of Philadelphia Vicinity
102 E Mermaid Lane   215-242-4200
Philadelphia, PA 19118   Fax: 215-247-4229
                                      TTY: 215-248-7620
                                      ucpkravitz@aol.com
United Cerebral Palsy provides information advocacy referral services for persons with disabilities and/or their families. UCP also operates an equipment loan program conducts parent workshops disseminates written literature on topics of interest to people with disabilities.
Gary J Weyhmuller, President
David J Barnhart, Vice President

2775 United Cerebral Palsy of Pittsburgh
4638 Centre Avenue   412-683-7100
Pittsburgh, PA 15213   Fax: 412-683-4160
                                      info@ucppittsburgh.org
                                      www.ucp.org
United Cerebral Palsy provides information advocacy referral services for persons with disabilities and/or their families. UCP also operates an equipment loan program conducts parent workshops disseminates written literature on topics of interest to people with disabilities
Al Condeluci, CEO
Joyce Redmerski, Chief Financial Officer

2776 United Cerebral Palsy of South Central Pennsylvania
788 Cherry Tree Court   717-632-5552
Hanover, PA 17331   800-333-3873
                                      Fax: 717-632-2315
                                      phoughton@ucpsouthcentral.org
                                      www.ucp.org
Provides early intervention, in home personal care and community integration services for children and adults with disabilities in York, Adams and Franklin counties.
Paulette Houghton, Executive Director
William Long, Director of Operations

2777 United Cerebral Palsy of Southern Alleghenies Region
119 Jari Drive   814-262-9600
Johnstown, PA 15904   877-371-1110
                                      Fax: 814-262-9650
                                      www.alucp.org
United Cerebral Palsy provides information, advocacy, referral services for persons with disabilities and/or their families. UCP also operates an equipment loan program, conducts parent workshops, disseminates written literature on topics of interest.
Marie Polinsky, CEO
Mark Malzi, CFO

2778 United Cerebral Palsy of Southwestern Pennsylvania
190 N Main Street   724-229-0851
Washington, PA 15301   Fax: 724-229-9252
                                      www.ucp.org
United Cerebral Palsy provides information, advocacy, referral services for persons with disabilities and/or their families. UCP also operates an equipment loan program, conducts parent workshops, disseminates written literature on topics of interest.

2779 United Cerebral Palsy of Western Pennsylvania
2904 Seminary Drive   724-832-8272
Greensburg, PA 15601   Fax: 724-837-8278
                                      www.ucpa.org
United Cerebral Palsy provides information, advocacy, referral services for persons with disabilities and/or their families. UCP also operates an equipment loan program, conducts parent workshops, disseminates written literature on topics of interest.

Rhode Island

2780 United Cerebral Palsy of Rhode Island
200 Main Street   401-728-1800
Pawtucket, RI 02860   Fax: 401-728-0182
                                      info@ucpri.org
                                      www.ucpri.org
United Cerebral Palsy provides information, advocacy, referral services for persons with disabilities and/or their families. UCP also operates an equipment loan program, conducts parent work-

shops, disseminates written literature on topics of interest to people with disabilities.
Peter Quattromani, Executive Director & CEO
Karl Provost, CFO

Tennessee

2781 United Cerebral Palsy of Middle Tennessee
1200 9th Avenue N   615-242-4091
Nashville, TN 37208   Fax: 615-242-3582
                                      request@ucpnashville.org
                                      www.ucpmidtn.org/
United Cerebral Palsy provides information, advocacy, referral services for persons with disabilities and/or their families. UCP also operates an equipment loan program, conducts parent workshops, disseminates written literature on topics of interest to people with disabilities.
Deana Claiborne, Executive Director
Diane Dietrich, Director of Development

2782 United Cerebral Palsy of the Mid-South
3239 players club Parkway   901-761-4277
Memphis, TN 38125   Fax: 901-761-7876
United Cerebral Palsy provides information, advocacy, referral services for persons with disabilities and/or their families. UCP also operates an equipment loan program, conducts parent workshops, disseminates written literature on topics of interest to people with disabilities.
Michael Nolen, Chief Executive Officer
Kelly Burrow, Executive Vice-President of Development

Texas

2783 United Cerebral Palsy of Greater Houston
4500 Bissonet   713-838-9050
Bellaire, TX 77401   Fax: 713-838-9098
                                      www.ucpa.org
United Cerebral Palsy provides information, advocacy, referral services for persons with disabilities and/or their families. UCP also operates an equipment loan program, conducts parent workshops, disseminates written literature on topics of interest to people with disabilities.

2784 United Cerebral Palsy of Metropolitan Dallas
8802 Harry Hines Boulevard   214-247-4505
Dallas, TX 75235   800-999-1898
                                      Fax: 214-351-2610
                                      www.ucpdallas.org
United Cerebral Palsy provides information, advocacy, referral services for persons with disabilities and/or their families. UCP also operates an equipment loan program, conducts parent workshops, disseminates written literature on topics of interest to people with disabilities.
Bill Knudsen, President / Chief Executive Officer
Becky Adams, Chief Operations Officer

2785 United Cerebral Palsy of Tarrant County
1555 Merrimac Circle   817-332-7171
Fort Worth, TX 76107   Fax: 817-332-7601
                                      www.ucp.org
United Cerebral Palsy provides information, advocacy, referral services for persons with disabilities and/or their families. UCP also operates an equipment loan program, conducts parent workshops, disseminates written literature on topics of interest to people with disabilities.

2786 United Cerebral Palsy of Texas
1016 La Posada Drive   512-472-8696
Austin, TX 78752   800-798-1492
                                      Fax: 512-472-8026
                                      www.ucpa.org
United Cerebral Palsy provides information, advocacy, referral services for persons with disabilities and/or their families. UCP also operates an equipment loan program, conducts parent workshops, disseminates written literature on topics of interest.

Utah

2787 United Cerebral Palsy of Utah
PO Box 65219
S Salt Lake, UT 84165
801-266-1805
Fax: 801-266-2404
www.ucpa.org
United Cerebral Palsy provides information, advocacy, referral services for persons with disabilities and/or their families. UCP also operates an equipment loan program, conducts parent workshops, disseminates written literature on topics of interest.

Virginia

2788 Cerebral Palsy of Virginia
5825 Arrowhead Drive
Virginia Beach, VA 23462
757-497-7474
Fax: 757-497-0868
www.cerebralpalsyofvirginia.org
Cerebral Palsy provides information, advocacy, referral services for persons with disabilities and/or their families. Cerebral Palsy also operates an equipment loan program, summer computer camp, art works job training program and much more.
Kathy Prendergast, Executive Director
Michelle Majority, Associate Executive Director

Washington

2789 United Cerebral Palsy of Pierce County
6315 S 19th Street
Tacoma, WA 98466-6217
253-565-1463
Fax: 253-565-1463
www.ucpa.org
United Cerebral Palsy provides information, advocacy, referral services for persons with disabilities and/or their families. UCP also operates an equipment loan program, conducts parent workshops, disseminates written literature on topics of interest to people with disabilities.

Wisconsin

2790 United Cerebral Palsy of Greater Dane County
2801 Coho Street
Madison, WI 53713
608-273-4434
Fax: 608-273-3426
ucpgdc@ucpdane.org
www.ucpdane.org
Provides information, advocacy, referral services for persons with disabilities and/or their families. UCP also conducts parent workshops and disseminates written literature on topics of interest to people with disabilities.
Wade Harrison, President
Rich Cooper, Vice-President

2791 United Cerebral Palsy of North Central Wisconsin
108 Scott Street
Wausau, WI 54401
715-842-8700
800-472-4408
www.ucpa.org
United Cerebral Palsy provides information, advocacy, referral services for persons with disabilities and/or their families. UCP also operates an equipment loan program, conducts parent workshops, disseminates written literature on topics of interest to people with disabilities.

2792 United Cerebral Palsy of Southeastern Wisconsin
7519 W Oklahoma Avenue
Milwaukee, WI 53219
414-329-4500
888-482-7739
Fax: 414-329-4510
TTY: 414-329-4511
info@ucpsew.org
www.ucpsew.org/
United Cerebral Palsy provides information, advocacy, referral services for persons with disabilities and/or their families. UCP also operates an equipment loan program, conducts parent workshops, disseminates written literature on topics of interest to people with disabilities.
Scott Andreson, Presdient
Emmett Prosser, Secretary

2793 United Cerebral Palsy of Wisconsin
206 Water Street
Eau Claire, WI 54703
715-832-1782
Fax: 715-832-8203
www.ucpwcw.org/

United Cerebral Palsy provides information, advocacy, referral services for persons with disabilities and/or their families. UCP also operates an equipment loan program, conducts parent workshops, disseminates written literature on topics of interest to people with disabilities.
Connie Werlein, President
Randi Johnson, Vice-President

Research Centers

2794 Orthopaedic Biomechanics Laboratory Shriners Hospital for Crippled Children
Shriners Hospital for Crippled Children
2181 Westlawn Building
Iowa City, IA 52242-1100
319-335-7529
Fax: 319-335-7530
Offers research and studies into cerebral palsy.
Stephen R Skinner, Clinical Director

Support Groups & Hotlines

2795 Family Support Network
215 Centennial Mall S
Lincoln, NE 68508-1813
402-477-2992
800-245-6081

2796 National Health Information Center
Office of Disease Prevention & Health Promotion
1101 Wootton Pkwy
Rockville, MD 20852
Fax: 240-453-8281
odphpinfo@hhs.gov
www.health.gov/nhic
Supports public health education by maintaining a calendar of National Health Observances; helps connect consumers and health professionals to organizations that can best answer questions and provide up-to-date contact information from reliable sources; updates on a yearly basis toll-free numbers for health information, Federal health clearinghouses and info centers.
Don Wright, MD, MPH, Director

Books

2797 An Introduction to Your Child Who Has Cerebral Palsy
Medic Publishing Company
PO Box 89
Redmond, WA 98073-0089
425-881-2883
Information and answers to questions for parents of children with cerebral palsy.

2798 Children with Cerebral Palsy
Woodbine House
6510 Bells Mill Road
Bethesda, MD 20817-1636
301-897-3570
800-843-7323
Fax: 301-897-5838
info@woodbinehouse.com
www.woodbinehouse.com
Explains what Cerebral Palsy is, and discusses its diagnosis and treatment. Also offers information and advice concerning daily care, early intervention, therapy, educational options and family life.
432 pages Paperback
ISBN: 0-933149-15-8

2799 Discovery Book
United Cerebral Palsy Association
1660 L Street NW
Washington, DC 20036-5602
202-776-0406
800-872-5827
Fax: 202-776-0414
ucpnatl@ucpa.org

2800 Individuals with Cerebral Palsy
Mainstream
1030 5th Street NW
Washington, DC 20001-2504
202-898-1400
Mainstreaming individuals with cerebral palsy into the workplace.
12 pages

2801 Occupational Therapy Practice Guidelines for Adults with Cerebral Palsy
American Occupational Therapy Association

4720 Montgomery Lane
Bethesda, MD 20814-1220

301-652-6611
Fax: 240-762-5150
TDD: 800-377-8555
www.aota.org

15 pages
ISBN: 1-569001-59-6

Children's Books

2802 Can't You Be Still?
Gemma B Publishing
776 Corydon Avenue
Winnipeg, MB, R3M 0Y1,

204-452-7566
Fax: 204-475-9903
gempub@mts.net
www.gemmab.mb.ca

On Ann's first day at school, the other students are both fascinated and horrified by her cerebral palsy. She wins them over by helping them jump into the water and swim. Available in Braille.
24 pages Paperback
ISBN: 0-969647-70-0
Sarah Yates, President

2803 Cerebral Palsy
Franklin Watts Grolier
90 Old Sherman Tpke
Danbury, CT 06816-0001

203-797-3500
800-621-1115
Fax: 203-797-3197
www.auth.grolier.com

A look at the causes, detection, prevention, effects and treatment of Cerebral Palsy.
112 pages Grades 7-12
ISBN: 0-531125-29-7

2804 Here's What I Mean To Say
Gemma B Publishing
776 Corydon Avenue
Winnipeg, MB, R3M 0Y1,

204-452-7566
Fax: 204-475-9903
gempub@mts.net
www.gemmab.mb.ca

In this books Ann's battle to read is assisted by an angel, who helps her read the directions in Jay's computer game. Is the angel read or is this the magic of reading? Available in Braille.
32 pages Paperback
ISBN: 0-969647-72-7
Sarah Yates, President

2805 Mine for Keeps
Little, Brown & Company
34 Beacon Street
Boston, MA 02108-1415

617-227-0730
800-343-9204

Sarah Jean Copeland was born with cerebral palsy. At four years of age she was placed in a school for handicapped children but made such good progress that she could return home. Coming home for Sarah meant a new school, and new adjustments to her parents, two sisters, and her brother. At first Sarah was scared and didn't think she could do all the things she needed to do, but she soon learned her fears were not well-founded.
186 pages Hardcover

2806 My Brother Matthew
Woodbine House
6510 Bells Mill Road
Bethesda, MD 20817-1636

800-843-7323
www.woodbinehouse.com

A book written from the point of view of the brother of Matthew, a boy with multiple disabilities, David describes the incidents characterizing how life in his family changes.
28 pages Grades K-5

2807 Nobody Knows!
Gemma B Publishing
776 Corydon Avenue
Winnipeg, MB, R3M 0Y1,

204-452-7566
Fax: 204-475-9903

An adventure during which a frustrated Ann goes out to find someone who understand what she wants. She meets a turtle and an alligator, who like her don't use words to communicate. Available in Braille.
24 pages Paperback
ISBN: 0-969647-71-9
Sarah Yates, President

Newsletters

2808 Family Support Bulletin
United Cerebral Palsy Associations
1660 L Street NW
Washington, DC 20036-1202

202-842-1266
800-872-5827

Pamphlets

2809 Cerebral Palsy: Facts & Figures
United Cerebral Palsy Associations
1825 K Street NW
Washington, DC 20006

202-776-0406
800-872-5827
Fax: 202-776-0414
www.ucp.org

Offers information on what cerebral palsy is, the effects, causes, types, and prevention.

Audio & Video

2810 A Day At A Time
Filmakers Library
3212 Duke Street
Alexandria, VA 22314-1798

212-808-4980
Fax: 212-808-4983
sales@alexanderstreet.com
www.academicvideostore.com

The story of twin girls with Cerebral Palsy, whose family is determined that they have every opportunity to participate in and lead normal lives. Winner of a number of awards. DVD or VHS $195, Classroom Rental $75
VHS or DVD
Sue Oscar, Co-President

Web Sites

2811 American Academy for Cerebral Palsy and Developmental Medicine

www.aacpdm.org

A multidisciplinary scientific society devoted to the study of cerebral palsy and other childhood onset disabilities, promoting professional education for the treatment and management of these conditions and to improving the quality / life for people with the condition.

2812 Healing Well

www.healingwell.com

An online health resource guide to medical news, chat, information and articles, newsgroups and message boards, books, disease-related web sites, medical directories, and more for patients, friends, and family coping with disabling diseases, disorders, or chronic illnesses.

2813 Health Finder

www.healthfinder.gov

Searchable, carefully developed web site offering information on over 1000 topics. Developed by the US Department of Health and Human Services, the site can be used in both English and Spanish.

2814 Healthlink USA

www.healthlinkusa.com

Health information concerning treatment, cures, prevention, diagnosis, risk factors, research, support groups, email lists, personal stories and much more. Updated regularly.

2815 MedicineNet

www.medicinenet.com

An online resource for consumers providing easy-to-read, authoritative medical and health information.

2816 Medscape

www.medscape.com

Medscape offers specialists, primary care physicians, and other health professionals the Web's most robust and integrated medical information and educational tools.

2817 National Rehabilitation Information Center

www.naric.com

The National Rehabilitation Information Center (NARIC) is the library of the National Institute on Disability, Independent Living, and Rehabilitation Research (NIDILRR.).

2818 Neurology Channel

www.healthcommunities.com

Find clearly explained, medically accurate information regarding conditions, including an overview, symptoms, causes, diagnostic procedures and treatment options. On this site it is possible to ask questions and get information from a neurologist and connect to people who have similar health interests.

2819 United Cerebral Palsy Associations

ucp.org

United Cerebral Palsy (UCP) educates, advocates and provides support services to ensure a life without limits for people with a spectrum of disabilities.

2820 WebMD

www.webmd.com

Provides credible information, supportive communities, and in-depth reference material about health subjects. A source for original and timely health information as well as material from well known content providers.

Description

2821 Chronic Fatigue Syndrome

Chronic Fatigue Syndrome, CFS, is an illness characterized by longstanding fatigue that impairs daily functioning. It may be accompanied by sore throat, swollen glands, muscle and joint pain, headaches, sleeplessness, and impaired memory or concentration. Profound or life-altering fatigue—the disease's hallmark—usually comes on suddenly and persists for at least six months, and often for years.

The cause of CFS is controversial. One theory is that a chronic viral infection is involved. Allergic reactions have also been proposed, and various immunologic abnormalities have been reported. Another theory involves proposed disturbances in the hormonal (endocrine) system. Psychological factors may be the cause, although CFS is distinct from typical depression or anxiety. Because the cause is unknown, there is no single test or group of tests that can diagnose CFS. Therefore, the goal in evaluating an individual with presumed CFS is to exclude other treatable illnesses.

Given the difficulty in proving a diagnosis or understanding the cause of CFS, it is not surprising that many treatments have been offered for it. Antidepressants appear to be the most successful treatment studied so far; as many as 80 percent of patients report benefit. Other therapies, including nutritional supplements, hormones, antiviral drugs and steroids have been mostly disappointing.

Patients with CFS need emotional support from physicians and family, due to the debilitating nature of the disease. Individual and group therapy may help some individuals. The nagging pain and fatigue can be addressed with certain drugs such as pregabalin, duloxetine, amitriptyline, or gabapentin. Physical therapy has also been shown to help, and other patients benefit from stimulants. Alternative treatments, such as antivirals, immunosuppressants, elimination diets, and amalgam extractions have not been shown to provide any definitive improvement in chronic fatigue syndrome patients and should be avoided. See also *Fibromyalgia*.

National Agencies & Associations

2822 American Academy of Sleep Medicine
2510 North Frontage Road
Darien, IL 60561
630-737-9700
Fax: 630-737-9790
contact@aasm.org
www.aasmnet.org
A unique multi-disciplinary organization for both individual members and center members. The individual member branch includes clinicians involved in the diagnosis and treatment of patients with disorders of sleep and alertness.
Kelly A. Carden, MD, President
Steve Van Hout, Executive Director

2823 American Chronic Pain Association
PO Box 850
Rocklin, CA 95677
800-533-3231
ACPA@theacpa.org
www.theacpa.org

The ACPA facilitates peer support and education for individuals with chronic pain in its many forms, in order to increase quality of life. Also raises awareness among the healthcare community, and with policy makers.
Penney Cowan, Founder & CEO
Daniel Galia, Director, Global Support

2824 American Fibromyalgia Syndrome Association
PO Box 32698
Tucson, AZ 85751
520-733-1570
Fax: 520-290-5550
kthorson@afsafund.org
www.afsafund.org
AFSA is a non-profit organization whose primary mission is to seed research in fibromyalgia syndrome and chronic fatigue syndrome.
Kristen Thorson, President
Steve Thorson, Vice President

2825 American Myalgic Encephalomyelitis and Chronic Fatigue Syndrome Society
admin@ammes.org
ammes.org
Serves patients and caregivers via support, advocacy, and education.
Erica Verrillo, Founder

2826 International Association for Chronic Fatigue Syndrome/Myalgic Encephalomyelitis
9650 Rockville Pike
Bethesda, MD 20814
301-634-7701
Fax: 301-634-7099
membership@iacfsme.org
www.iacfsme.org
IACFS/MEA is a non-profit organization of research scientists, physicians, licensed medical healthcare professionals and other individuals and institutions interested in promoting the stimulation, coordination and exchange of ideas for CFS and ME research and patient care.
Newsletter
Staci R. Stevens, MA, Co-President
Lily Chu, MD, MS, Co-President

2827 National Institute of Allergy and Infectious Diseases
Office of Communications & Government Relations
5601 Fishers Lane
Bethesda, MD 20892
301-402-1663
866-284-4107
Fax: 301-402-1020
TDD: 800-877-8339
ocpostoffice@niaid.nih.gov
www.niaid.nih.gov
Offers information and educational materials on Chronic Fatigue Syndrome and other disorders.
Anthony S. Fauci, MD, Director

2828 National ME/FM Action Network
33 Banner Road
Nepean, Ontario, K2H-8V7
613-829-6667
Fax: 613-829-8518
mefminfo@mefmaction.com
www.mefmaction.com
Works to support people with Myalgic Encephalomyelitis, Chronic Fatigue Syndrome, and Fibromyalgia in North America.
Lydia E. Neilson, MSM, Founder & CEO
Margaret Parlor, President

2829 Option Institute
2080 South Undermountain Road
Sheffield, MA 01257
413-229-2100
800-714-2779
Fax: 413-229-8931
participantsupport@option.org
www.option.org
Self-defeating beliefs, along with attitudes and judgments, can lead to a host of physical and psychological challenges, including Chronic Fatigue Syndrome. The Option Institute offers programs designed to help people gain new perspectives on the attitudes and judgments that may be affecting their lives, especially those regarding and surrounding Chronic Fatigue Syndrome.
Barry Kaufman, Co-Founder
Samahria Lyte Kaufman, Co-Founder

2830 Solve ME/CFS Initiative
5455 Wilshire Blvd.   704-364-0016
Los Angeles, CA 90036-0007   solvecfs@solvecfs.org
                                                        solvecfs.org
SMCI works to make Myalgic Encephalomyelitis/Chronic Fatigue
Syndrome better understood, diagnosable, and treatable.
Carol Head, President
Sadie Whittaker, PhD, Chief Scientific Officer

Foundations

2831 National CFIDS Foundation
103 Aletha Road   781-449-3535
Needham, MA 02492   Fax: 781-449-8606
                                                     info@ncf-net.org
                                                     www.ncf-net.org
The goals of the Foundation are to help fund medical research to
find a cause, expedite treatments and eventually a cure for this dev-
astating disease. The NCF also strives to provide information, edu-
cation, and support to those people who have CFIDS (also known
as chronic fatigue syndrome (CFS), myalgic encephalomyelitis
(ME) and many other names)— as well as related illnesses such as
Gulf War Illness (GWI) and Multiple Chemical Sensitivities
(MCS). Provides guides, articles, and newsletters.
Gail Kansky, President
Alan Cocchetto, Medical Director

Support Groups & Hotlines

2832 Centers for Disease Control and Prevention
1600 Clifton Road   800-232-4636
Atlanta, GA 30333   TTY: 888-232-6348
                                                     cdcinfo@cdc.gov
                                                     www.cdc.gov
Collaborating to create the expertise, information, and tools that
people and their communities need to protect their health - through
health promotion, prevention of disease, injury and disability, and
preparedness for new health threats.
Thomas R Frieden MD MPH, Director

2833 Chronic Fatigue Syndrome & Fibromyalgia Support
7250 Clearvista Dr   317-252-9223
Indianapolis, IN 46256
Offers emotional support, education and information about CFS
and FMS through statewide monthly meetings and a quarterly
newsletter. Provides 24-hour hotline and physician/attorney referrals. Financial assistance for members. Support group meets twice
a month at Community Hospital North Professional Building and
at other locations throughout Indiana.

2834 National Health Information Center
Office of Disease Prevention & Health Promotion
1101 Wootton Pkwy   Fax: 240-453-8281
Rockville, MD 20852   odphpinfo@hhs.gov
                                                     www.health.gov/nhic
Supports public health education by maintaining a calendar of National Health Observances; helps connect consumers and health
professionals to organizations that can best answer questions and
provide up-to-date contact information from reliable sources; updates on a yearly basis toll-free numbers for health information,
Federal health clearinghouses and info centers.
Don Wright, MD, MPH, Director

Books

2835 CFIDS in Children Packet
CFIDS Association of America
PO Box 220398   800-442-3437
Charlotte, NC 28222-0398
This packet contains articles about CFIDS and children.
60 pages

2836 CFS Cookbook
CFIDS Association of America
PO Box 220398   800-442-3437
Charlotte, NC 28222-0398

Gourmet recipes designed to combat the monotony associated with
CFIDS, allergy and immune-compromised diets.
218 pages

2837 Chronic Fatigue Syndrome Cookbook: Delicious &
Wellness-Enhancing Recipes
DIANE Publishing Company
330 Pusey Avenue   610-461-6200
Darby, PA 19023   800-782-3833
                                                     Fax: 610-461-6130
                                        dianepublishing@gmail.com
                                             www.dianepublishing.net
These recipes help combat the boredom of the CFS diet usually rec-
ommended and still satisfy all of your nutritional requirements as a
CFS sufferer. In addition, the book includes a comprehensive look
at the do's and don't's of a CFS diet, quick recipes for those days
when you are too tired to cook and an insightful medical
introduction.
218 pages Hardcover
ISBN: 0-756753-28-7
Herman Baron, Publisher

2838 Chronic Fatigue Syndrome and the Yeast Connection
CFIDS Association of America
PO Box 220398   800-442-3437
Charlotte, NC 28222-0398
Dr. Crook explains the possible role of multiple entities, including
yeast overgrowth, allergies and chemical sensitivities, in CFS and
how each contributes to immune dysregulation.
386 pages

2839 Chronic Fatigue Syndrome: Information for Physicians
Barry Leonard, author
DIANE Publishing Company
330 Pusey Avenue   610-461-6200
Darby, PA 19023   800-782-3833
                                                     Fax: 610-461-6130
                                        dianepublishing@gmail.com
                                             www.dianepublishing.net
Includes a historical perspective on chronic fatigue syndrome; epidemiology; clinical picture; evaluation of patients; patient management; etiologic theories; public health service resources; fact
sheet; resources for patients, overview of the CFS research program; NIAID and NIAID/Johns Hopkins hospital study, which
seeks volunteers, management strategies for CFS; the relationship
between nuerally mediatec hypotension and CFS and fibromyalgia
and CFS; solving diagnostic and therapeutic dilemmas.
60 pages Paperback
ISBN: 0-788143-78-6
Herman Baron, Publisher

2840 Chronic Fatigue Syndrome: The Limbic Hypothesis
CFIDS Association of America
PO Box 220398   800-442-3437
Charlotte, NC 28222-0398
A detailed thesis proposing CFS as a limbic system
encephalopathy in the context of a dysregulated neuroimmune sys-
tem.
259 pages

2841 Chronic Fatigue: Your Complete Exercise Guide
Human Kinetics Press
1607 N Market Street   217-351-5076
Champaign, IL 61820-5076   800-747-4457
                                                     Fax: 217-351-1549
                                                     info@hkusa.com
                                             www.humankinetics.com
1993 144 pages Paperback
ISBN: 0-873223-93-4
Steve Ruhlig, Marketing Director

2842 Coping With CFS
CFIDS Association of America
PO Box 220398   704-365-2343
Charlotte, NC 28222-0398   800-442-3437
                                                     Fax: 704-365-9755
                                                     info@cfids.org
                                                     www.cfids.org

Offers practical, established coping strategies for living better with CFIDS. Based on Dr. Friedberg's experiences as a person with CFIDS and a counselor to PWCs.
176 pages
Jon Sterling, Chairman
Kim Kenny, President/CEO

2843 Disability and Chronic Fatigue Syndrome
The Haworth Press
10 Alice Street
Binghamton, NY 13904-1580
607-722-5857
800-429-6784
Fax: 800-895-0582
www.impresaitalia.info
Discusses the difficult subject of how to diagnose disability in chronic fatigue syndrome patients, how to determine the severity of a patient's disability, and how new disability guidelines would make more chronic fatigue patients eligible to apply for disability benefits.
121 pages Paperback
ISBN: 0-789005-01-8
Bill Cohen, Publisher
Sandy Jones, VP Marketing

2844 Doctor's Guide to Chronic Fatigue Syndrome
CFIDS Association of America
PO Box 220398
Charlotte, NC 28222-0398
800-442-3437
Written by one of the world's leading experts on CFIDS.
275 pages

2845 Fifty Things You Should Know About the Chronic Fatigue Syndrome Epidemic
St. Martin's Press
175 5th Avenue
New York, NY 10010-7848
212-674-5151
800-221-7945
Fax: 212-420-9314
1993
ISBN: 0-312950-43-8

2846 Hope and Help for Chronic Fatigue Syndrome
CFIDS Association of America
PO Box 220398
Charlotte, NC 28222-0398
704-365-2343
800-442-3437
Fax: 704-365-9755
info@cfids.org
www.cfids.org
Insight into the experience of having CFIDS, the physical and emotional impact, difficulty in obtaining a diagnosis, available methods of treatment and key strategies for regaining control over your life.
216 pages
Jon Sterling, Chairman
Kim Kenny, President/CEO

2847 International Classification of Sleep Disorders
American Academy of Sleep Medicine
2510 North Frontage Road
Darien, IL 60561
630-737-9700
Fax: 630-737-9790
cme@aasmnet.org
www.aasmnet.org
A comprehensive manual for physicians and other healthcare professionals containing information on 84 sleep disorders. The extensive text describes the diagnostic features of each disorder and includes specific diagnostic and severity criteria for each disorder.
396 pages Paperback

2848 Living with CFS: A Personal Story of the Struggle for Recovery
CFIDS Association of America
PO Box 220398
Charlotte, NC 28222-0398
800-442-3437
Describes the pain associated with the author's loss of livelihood, impaired physical and mental functioning and the strain on his marriage and friendships, while maintaining hope for recovery.
224 pages
ISBN: 1-560250-75-5

2849 Living with ME
CFIDS Association of America
PO Box 220398
Charlotte, NC 28222-0398
800-442-3437
Fax: 704-365-9755

The author describes M.E. (mylagic encephalomyelitis - the British term for chronic fatigue syndrome), and discusses practical methods for coping and comments on various treatments.

2850 Music Appreciation
CFIDS Association of America
PO Box 220398
Charlotte, NC 28222-0398
800-442-3437
A full-length collection of poems by Skloot who has been disabled by CFIDS since 1988.
105 pages

2851 Night-Side: CFS and the Illness Experience
CFIDS Association of America
PO Box 220398
Charlotte, NC 28222-0398
704-365-2343
800-442-3437
Fax: 704-365-9755
info@cfids.org
www.cfids.org
An honest and ultimately hopeful exploration of what it means to have your life shattered by disease.
190 pages
Jon Sterling, Chairman
Kim Kenny, President/CEO

2852 Recovering From the Chronic Fatigue Syndrome: A Guide to Self-Empowerment
Berkley Books
200 Madison Avenue
New York, NY 10016-3903
212-951-8800
This book teaches persons with CFIDS to take control of their illness and to help themselves find the road to recovery.
1993 224 pages Paperback
ISBN: 0-399518-07-0

2853 Running on Empty
CFIDS Association of America
PO Box 220398
Charlotte, NC 28222-0398
704-365-2343
800-442-3437
Fax: 704-365-9755
info@cfids.org
www.cfids.org
Landmark guide to CFIDS has just been revised and re-released. A must read for the newly disgnosed.
315 pages
Jon Sterling, Chairman
Kim Kenny, President/CEO

2854 Self-Caring Fatigue
Rodale Press
604 East Stree
Otho, IA 50569-0099
715-191-0217
515-972-4444
Fax: 515-972-4415
info@peopleagainstcancer.com
A step-by-step plan to uncover and eliminate the causes of chronic fatigue.
1993 320 pages
ISBN: 0-875961-61-4

2855 Solving the Puzzle of CFS
2730 Wilshire Boulevard
Santa Monica, CA 90403-4724
310-453-4424
Fax: 310-966-9196

Magazines

2856 CFIDS Chronicle
CFIDS Association of America
PO Box 220398
Charlotte, NC 28222-0398
704-362-2343
800-442-3437
Fax: 704-365-9755
The largest and most comprehensive periodical specifically pertaining to chronic fatigue syndrome information in the world.

2857 Feel Good Catalog
2895 W Oxford Avenue
Englewood, CO 80110-4370
303-790-1045
800-997-6789
Variety of items to ease pain.

2858 Journal SLEEP
American Academy of Sleep Medicine
One Westbrook Corp Center   708-492-0930
Westchester, IL 60154   Fax: 708-492-0943
Publishes articles ranging from clinical investigations of sleep/wake disorders and medical problems during sleep, to investigations of the basic physiological and biochemical events and anatomical structures involved in normal and abnormal sleep. Includes psychological and psycho-physiological research, as well as research in relevant areas of circadian and biological rhythms.
10x Year
ISBN: 0-161810-5 -

2859 Journal of the Chronic Fatigue Syndrome
Haworth Medical Press
10 Alice Street   607-722-5857
Binghamton, NY 13904-1503   800-429-6784
                                         Fax: 607-722-0012
                                         www.impresaitalia.info
Peer reviewed medical journal containing CFIDS scientific abstract information. Appropriate for patients as well as medical professionals.
Quarterly
Nancy Klimas MD, Founding Co-Editor

Newsletters

2860 Health Points
TyH Publications
17007 E Colony Drive   800-801-1406
Fountain Hills, AZ 85268   editor@e-tyh.com
National newsletter with articles on complementary therapy, latest nutrition news, disability issues and much more. Focus is on fibromyalgia, chronic fatigue, arthritis and chronic pain.
Quarterly

2861 Heart of America News
National Chronic Fatigue Syndrome & Fibromyalgia
PO Box 18426   660-313-2000
Kansas City, MO 64133-8426
Offers scientifically accurate information, medical updates, informational references, articles on coping and living with Chronic Fatigue Syndrome and more, based on peer-reviewed materials.
Quarterly

2862 National Forum
103 Aletha Road   781-449-3535
Needham, MA 02492   Fax: 781-449-8606
                                         info@ncf-net.org
                                         www.ncf-net.org
The Forum's focus: CFIDS/ME, FMS, GWI, MCS and related illnesses.
Gail Kansky, President

2863 Syndrome Sentinel
Massachusetts CFIDS Association
808 Main Street   781-893-4415
Waltham, MA 02451-8533
This quarterly newsletter contains articles written by health-care professionals working with these conditions. Contributors include traditional and alternative experts, as well as personal stories from people with these chronic syndromes and their significant others.

2864 The National Forum
The National CFIDS Foundation
103 Aletha Road   781-449-3535
Needham, MA 02492   Fax: 781-449-8606
                                         info@ncf-net.org
                                         www.ncf-net.org
Offers the latest information on CFIDS treatments being tried throughout the United States.

Pamphlets

2865 Americans with Disabilities Act: CFS and Employment
National Chronic Fatigue Syndrome & Fibromyalgia

PO Box 18426   660-313-2000
Kansas City, MO 64133-8426

2866 CFIDS Membership Packet
CFIDS Association of America
PO Box 220398   800-442-3437
Charlotte, NC 28222-0398   Fax: 704-365-9755
Offers pamphlets, brochures, information on local support groups for members.

2867 CFIDS in Children
CFIDS Association of America
PO Box 220398   800-442-3437
Charlotte, NC 28222-0398
Describes the special difficulties faced by children with CFIDS.

2868 CFS in the Workplace
National Chronic Fatigue Syndrome & Fibromyalgia
PO Box 18426   660-313-2000
Kansas City, MO 64133

2869 Chronic Fatigue Syndrome & School Success
National Chronic Fatigue Syndrome & Fibromyalgia
PO Box 18426   660-313-2000
Kansas City, MO 64133-8426

2870 Chronic Fatigue Syndrome in Children
National Chronic Fatigue Syndrome & Fibromyalgia
PO Box 18426   660-313-2000
Kansas City, MO 64133

2871 Chronic Fatigue Syndrome in Men
National Chronic Fatigue Syndrome & Fibromyalgia
PO Box 18426   660-313-2000
Kansas City, MO 64133-8426

2872 Chronic Fatigue Syndrome: A Pamphlet for Physicians
National Institute of Allergy & Infectious Disease
5601 Fishers Lane   301-402-1663
Bethesda, MD 20892-2520   Fax: 301-402-0120
                                         niaidnews@niaid.nih.gov
                                         www.niaid.nih.gov
Offers information on epidemiology, clinical procedures, evaluations, patient management, neuropsychologic features and etiologic theories.

2873 Chronic Fatigue Syndrome: The Thief of Vitality
National Chronic Fatigue Syndrome & Fibromyalgia
PO Box 18426   660-313-2000
Kansas City, MO 64133-8426

2874 Coping Skills
National Chronic Fatigue Syndrome & Fibromyalgia
PO Box 18426   660-313-2000
Kansas City, MO 64133-8426

2875 Disability Packet
CFIDS Association of America
PO Box 220398   800-442-3437
Charlotte, NC 28222-0398
Includes nine Chronicle articles about disability benefits and how persons with CFIDS can secure Social Security Disability Insurance benefits.
42 pages

2876 Facts About Chronic Fatigue Syndrome
Centers for Disease Control & Prevention
Division of Viral Dis   404-639-3311
Atlanta, GA 30333

2877 Fibromyalgia
National Chronic Fatigue Syndrome & Fibromyalgia
PO Box 18426   660-313-2000
Kansas City, MO 64133-8426

2878 March is Chronic Fatigue Syndrome Awareness Month Tips
National Chronic Fatigue Syndrome & Fibromyalgia
PO Box 18426   660-313-2000
Kansas City, MO 64133

2879 Neuropsychological Rehabilitation Suggestions/Techniques
National Chronic Fatigue Syndrome & Fibromyalgia

PO Box 18426
Kansas City, MO 64133-8426 660-313-2000

2880 School's Guide for Students with CFS
National Chronic Fatigue Syndrome & Fibromyalgia
PO Box 18426
Kansas City, MO 64133-8426 660-313-2000

2881 Social Security Disability Benefits Information
National Chronic Fatigue Syndrome & Fibromyalgia
PO Box 18426
Kansas City, MO 64133-8426 660-313-2000

2882 Suicide is Not an Option
National Chronic Fatigue Syndrome
PO Box 18426
Kansas City, MO 64133-8426 660-313-2000

2883 Understanding CFIDS
CFIDS Association of America
PO Box 220398 800-442-3437
Charlotte, NC 28222-0398
Provides an extensive overview of CFIDS and answers the most commonly asked questions about the disease.

2884 Understanding the Emotions Surrounding CFS
National Chronic Fatigue Syndrome & Fibromyalgia
PO Box 18426
Kansas City, MO 64133-8426 660-313-2000

Audio & Video

2885 Behavioral and Circadian Sleep Problems of Infancy and Childhood
American Academy of Sleep Medicine
2510 North Frontage Road 630-737-9700
Darien, IL 60561 Fax: 708-492-0943
cme@aasmnet.org
www.aasmnet.org
Addresses the problems of sleep disorders in children and outlines the types of disturbances, both of a medical and behavioral nature, that are commonly identified.
66 slides

2886 CFS and Self-Esteem
CFIDS Association of America
PO Box 220398 800-442-3437
Charlotte, NC 28222-0398
Addresses the sources of low self-esteem in persons with CFIDS and offers reassurance and practical techniques for increasing self-confidence.
Audiotape

2887 CFS: Addressing the Realities of a Chronic Illness
National Chronic Fatigue Syndrome & Fibromyalgia
PO Box 18426
Kansas City, MO 64133-8426 660-313-2000
This video offers reliable information featuring patients and a medical professional.

2888 CFS: Unraveling the Mystery
CFIDS Association of America
PO Box 220398 800-442-3437
Charlotte, NC 28222-0398
An excellent videotape for convincing skeptics that CFIDS is a real disease.
Videotape

2889 Chronic Fatigue Syndrome: For Those Who Care
CFIDS Association of America
PO Box 220398 800-442-3437
Charlotte, NC 28222-0398
An audiotape designed for friends and family of persons with CFIDS.
Audiotape

2890 Chronic Fatigue Syndrome: Information, Relaxation/Healing Exercise
CFIDS Association of America

PO Box 220398 800-442-3437
Charlotte, NC 28222-0398
Includes a comprehensive overview of CFS and relaxation/healing and imagery/stress reduction exercises for persons with CFIDS.
Audiotape

2891 Fibromyalgia
National Chronic Fatigue Syndrome & Fibromyalgia
PO Box 18426 660-313-2000
Kansas City, MO 64133
Videotape

2892 HHS Satelite Video on Chronic Fatigue Syndrome and Fibromyalgia Association
National Chronic Fatigue Syndrome and Fibromyalgia
PO Box 18426 660-313-2000
Kansas City, MO 64133-8426

2893 Living Hell: The Real World of Chronic Fatigue Syndrome
CFIDS Association of America
PO Box 220398 800-442-3437
Charlotte, NC 28222-0398
An emotional exposure of the tragedy of CFIDS.
Videotape

2894 Neurocognitive Aspects of CFS
CFIDS Association of America
PO Box 220398 800-442-3437
Charlotte, NC 28222-0398
A description of CFIDS-associated neurocognitive deficits and strategies for coping with them and the embarrassment and frustration they cause.
Audiotape

Web Sites

2895 American Association for Chronic Fatigue Syndrome
www.aacfs.org
A non profit organization of research scientists, physicians, licensed medical healthcare professionals, and other indviduals and institutions interested in promoting the stimulation, coordination, and exchange of ideas for CFS research and patient care.

2896 CFIDS Association of America
solvecfs.org
An organization focused on myalgic encephalomyelitis (ME) and Chronic Fatigue Syndrome (CFS) since being founded in 1987.

2897 Centers for Disease Control and Prevention
www.cdc.gov
CDC works 24/7 to protect America from health, safety and security threats, both foreign and in the U.S. Whether diseases start at home or abroad, are chronic or acute, curable or preventable, human error or deliberate attack, CDC fights disease and supports communities and citizens to do the same.

2898 Healing Well
www.healingwell.com
An online health resource guide to medical news, chat, information and articles, newsgroups and message boards, books, disease-related web sites, medical directories, and more for patients, friends, and family coping with disabling diseases, disorders, or chronic illnesses.

2899 Health Finder
www.healthfinder.gov
Searchable, carefully developed web site offering information on over 1000 topics. Developed by the US Department of Health and Human Services, the site can be used in both English and Spanish.

2900 Healthlink USA
www.healthlinkusa.com
Health information concerning treatment, cures, prevention, diagnosis, risk factors, research, support groups, email lists, personal stories and much more. Updated regularly.

2901 Journal of Chronic Fatigue Syndrome
www.cfs-news.org/jcfs.htm

Offers multidisciplinary original research, practical clinical management, case reports, and literature reviews to keep the entire health care delivery team well informed.

2902 MedicineNet

www.medicinenet.com

An online resource for consumers providing easy-to-read, authoritative medical and health information.

2903 Medscape

www.medscape.com

Medscape offers specialists, primary care physicians, and other health professionals the Web's most robust and integrated medical information and educational tools.

2904 Option Institute

www.option.org

Self-defeating beliefs, along with attitudes and judgments, can lead to a host of physical and psychological challenges, including Chronic Fatigue Syndrome. The Option Institute offers programs designed to help people gain new perspectives on the attitudes and judgments that may be affecting their lives, especially those regarding and surrounding Chronic Fatigue Syndrome. Website features lists of programs, audio and visual resources, and more.

2905 Sleepnet

www.sleepnet.com

Links all the sleep information located on the internet. Provides a place for everyone to read and post questions, or responses.

2906 WebMD

www.webmd.com

Provides credible information, supportive communities, and in-depth reference material about health subjects. A source for original and timely health information as well as material from well known content providers.

Description

2907 Chronic Pain

Chronic pain is defined as pain persisting for more than one month after resolution of an acute injury or pain that persists or recurs for more than three months. The pain may begin for unknown reasons, or may begin with some injury or illness but persist long after the triggering event is gone. There are about three million cases of chronic pain in the U.S. diagnosed each year. Human pain has physiological causes but also has psychological components differing for each person. Many Americans suffer from chronic pain. The annual cost, including treatment and lost work days, now hovers around $635 billion in the US.

Doctors and patients have tried almost every conceivable type of therapy for chronic pain. Drug treatments include narcotics (codeine and morphine), non-narcotic painkillers such as acetaminophen, and nonsteroidal anti-inflammatory drugs such as aspirin, ibuprofen, and naproxen. Use of antidepressants, either alone or in conjunction with pain medications, can be beneficial. Doctors may inject drugs to block the nerves that carry the pain signal, or may even cut the nerve. Physical measures include heat or cold application, application of electrical stimuli (TENS), stretching, acupuncture, local electrical stimulation, brain stimulation, and general conditioning exercises. Psychological treatment includes psychotherapy, meditation, hypnosis and biofeedback-relaxation. Because of the complexity of chronic pain and its treatment, some doctors have begun to specialize in management of pain and have organized multidisciplinary pain clinics which offer expertise from anesthesiology, rheumatology, neurosurgery, psychology and physical therapy.

A realistic goal of therapy is to improve one's daily functioning; for instance, being able to return to work or pleasurable activities. Those able to achieve this status will often state that the pain is still there but that it does not bother them like it once did. Whatever the stage of one's condition, peer support is important, and is available from local in-person support groups or from Internet chat rooms and bulletin boards.

National Agencies & Associations

2908 American Chronic Pain Association
PO Box 850
Rocklin, CA 95677
800-533-3231
ACPA@theacpa.org
www.theacpa.org
The ACPA facilitates peer support and education for individuals with chronic pain in its many forms, in order to increase quality of life. Also raises awareness among the healthcare community, and with policy makers.
Penney Cowan, Founder & CEO
Daniel Galia, Director, Global Support

2909 American Osteopathic Association
142 E. Ontario St.
Chicago, IL 60611-2864
888-626-9262
info@osteopathic.org
www.osteopathic.org

Serving as the professional family for more than 145,000 osteopathic physicians (DOs) and osteopathic medical students, the American Osteopathic Association (AOA) promotes public health and encourages scientific research.
Ronald Burns, President
Adrienne White-Faines, Chief Executive Officer

2910 American Pain Society
8735 W. Higgins Road
Chicago, IL 60631
847-375-4715
info@americanpainsociety.org
www.americanpainsociety.org
A multidisciplinary organization of basic and clinical scientists, practicing clinicians, policy analysts, and others. Mission is to advance pain-related research, education, treatment, and professional practice.
Carly Reisner, Chief Executive Officer
Emily Panci, Manager, Operations

2911 American Physical Therapy Association
1111 North Fairfax Street
Alexandria, VA 22314-1488
703-684-2782
800-999-2782
Fax: 703-684-7343
memberservices@apta.org
www.apta.org
The American Physical Therapy Association (APTA) is an individual membership professional organization representing more than 100,000 member physical therapists (PTs), physical therapist assistants (PTAs), and students of physical therapy.
Justin Moore, Chief Executive Officer
Mandy Frohlich, COO & EVP, Strategic Affairs

2912 Canadian Pain Society
250 Consumers Road
Toronto, ON M2J-4V6
416-642-6379
Fax: 416-495-8723
office@canadianpainsociety.ca
www.canadianpainsociety.ca
Dedicated to healthcare professionals and lay persons with an interest in the field of pain.
Hilary Robinson, Manager

2913 Chronic Pain Association of Canada
PO Box 66017
Edmonton, AB T6J-6T4
780-482-6727
Fax: 780-433-3128
chronicpaincanada.com
Seeks to prevent and alleviate chronic pain, and to improve patients' quality of life.
Barry Ulmer, Executive Director

2914 International Association for the Study of Pain
1510 H Street NW
Washington, DC 20005
202-856-7400
Fax: 202-856-7401
iaspdesk@iasp-pain.org
www.iasp-pain.org
The International Association for the Study of Pain is the leading professional forum for science, practice, and education in the field of pain.
Matthew D'Uva, Executive Director
Colleen Eubanks, Chief Operating Officer

2915 International Pelvic Pain Society
1510 H Street NW
Washington, DC 20005-1020
202-856-7422
Fax: 202-856-7401
info@pelvicpain.org
www.pelvicpain.org
Seeks to recruit, organize, and educate health care professionals actively involved with the treatment of patients who have chronic pelvic pain.
Colleen Eubanks, Executive Director

2916 National Association of Myofascial Trigger Point Therapists
Namtpt.president@gmail.com
www.myofascialtherapy.org
The NAMTPT is a professional organization dedicated to increasing public awareness of and access to myofascial pain treatment.
Kate Simmons, President
Heather Brown, Vice President

2917 National Fibromyalgia & Chronic Pain Association
25 Federal Avenue
Logan, UT 84321
801-200-3627
info@fmcpaware.org
www.fmcpaware.org

Seeks to unite patients, policy makers, and health and science communities to research fibromyalgia and chronic pain illnesses; also provides advocacy, support, and education.
Janet Favero Chambers, President

2918 Reflex Sympathetic Dystrophy Syndrome Association (RSDSA)
99 Cherry Street, PO Box 502   203-877-3790
Milford, CT 06460   877-662-7737
          Fax: 203-882-8362
          info@rsds.org
          www.rsds.org
Non-profit professional and consumer organization founded to support research into the cause, treatment, and cure of reflex sympathetic dystrophy syndrome. RSDSA also organizes support groups, promote awareness among health professionals and develop educational programs.
Jim Broatch, Executive VP & Director
Jeri Krassner, Special Events Coordinator

Support Groups & Hotlines

2919 National Health Information Center
Office of Disease Prevention & Health Promotion
1101 Wootton Pkwy   Fax: 240-453-8281
Rockville, MD 20852   odphpinfo@hhs.gov
          www.health.gov/nhic
Supports public health education by maintaining a calendar of National Health Observances; helps connect consumers and health professionals to organizations that can best answer questions and provide up-to-date contact information from reliable sources; updates on a yearly basis toll-free numbers for health information, Federal health clearinghouses and info centers.
Don Wright, MD, MPH, Director

Books

2920 ACPA Facilitator Guide & Materials
American Chronic Pain Association
PO Box 850   916-632-0922
Rocklin, CA 95677   800-533-3231
          Fax: 916-632-3208
          acpa@theacpa.org
          www.theacpa.org
This guide will help you and others in your community organize an ACPA chapter. The manual contains how-to information on organizing an ACPA chapter, sharing responsibility for the group with others, finding a meeting place, conducting the first meeting, and generating public interest in your area. You must be an ACPA member to purchase this manual.
Penny Cowan, Executive Director

2921 ACPA Family Manual
Penny Cowan, author
American Chronic Pain Association
PO Box 850   916-632-0922
Rocklin, CA 95677   800-533-3231
          Fax: 916-632-3208
          acpa@theacpa.org
          www.theacpa.org
A manual designed with the needs of those who live with a person who has chronic pain.
149 pages
ISBN: 0-967387-82-5
Penny Cowan, Executive Director

2922 ACPA Journal Reflections of You
American Chronic Pain Association
PO Box 850   916-632-0922
Rocklin, CA 95677   800-533-3231
          Fax: 916-632-3208
          acpa@theacpa.org
          www.theacpa.org
A daily meditation and personal journal book which provides positive and motivating thoughts to stimulate your thinking and challenge you to personal growth. Your daily entries in the journal will

help track your progress and show when you have reached your personal goal.
Penny Cowan, Executive Director

2923 ACSM's Exercise Management for Persons with Chronic Disease & Disabilities
Human Kinetics Press
1607 N Market Street   800-747-4457
Champaign, IL 61820-5076   800-747-4457
          Fax: 217-351-1549
          info@hkusa.com
          www.humankinetics.com
1993 384 pages Hardcover
ISBN: 0-736038-72-8
Steve Ruhlig, Marketing Director

2924 Essential Guide to Chronic Illness: The Active Patient's Handbook
James W Long, author
DIANE Publishing Company
330 Pusey Avenue   610-461-6200
Darby, PA 19023   800-782-3833
          Fax: 610-461-6130
          dianepublishing@gmail.com
          www.dianepublishing.net
A comprehensive guide to dealing with nearly 50 chronic illness and conditions from acne to Zollinger-Ellison syndrome, including diabetes, menopause, migraines, rheumatoid arthritis and psoriasis.
625 pages Paperback
ISBN: 0-788169-03-3
Herman Baron, Publisher

2925 From Patient to Person: First Steps
American Chronic Pain Association
PO Box 850   916-632-0922
Rocklin, CA 95677   800-533-3231
          Fax: 916-632-3208
          acpa@theacpa.org
          www.theacpa.org
A workbook designed to help anyone who has a chronic pain problem to gain a better understanding of how one can begin to cope with all the problems that their pain creates.
ISBN: 0-967387-80-9
Penny Cowan, Executive Director

2926 Occupational Therapy Practice Guidelines for Adults with Low Back Pain
American Occupational Therapy Association
4720 Montgomery Lane   301-652-6611
Bethesda, MD 20814-1220   Fax: 240-762-5150
          TDD: 800-377-8555
          www.aota.org
15 pages
ISBN: 1-569001-49-9

2927 Occupational Therapy Practice Guidelines for Adults with Hip Fracture/Replacement
American Occupational Therapy Association
4720 Montgomery Lane   301-652-6611
Bethesda, MD 20814-1220   Fax: 240-762-5150
          TDD: 800-377-8555
          www.aota.org
10 pages
ISBN: 1-569001-48-0

2928 Staying Well: Advanced Pain Management for ACPA Members
American Chronic Pain Association
PO Box 850   916-632-0922
Rocklin, CA 95677   800-533-3231
          Fax: 916-632-3208
          acpa@theacpa.org
          www.theacpa.org
This workbook is designed for those who have a working knowledge of the basics of pain management. This workbook provides additional skills necessary to continue to move forward in the journey to wellness.
ISBN: 0-969387-81-7
Penny Cowan, Executive Director

2929 Understanding Chronic Pain
Angela Koestler, PhD; Ann Myers, MD, author
University Press of Mississippi
3825 Ridgewood Road
Jackson, MS 39211-6492
601-432-6205
Fax: 601-432-6217
kburgess@ihl.state.ms.us
www.upress.state.ms.us
A handbook for people coping with chronic pain and suffering and for those who seek to understand and support them.
2002 184 pages Paperback
ISBN: 1-578064-40-6
Kathy Burgess, Advertising/Marketing Services Manager

2930 Your Pain is Real: Free Yourself from Chronic Pain, Breakthrough Med. Trtmnt.
DIANE Publishing Company
330 Pusey Avenue
Darby, PA 19023
610-461-6200
800-782-3833
Fax: 610-461-6130
dianepublishing@gmail.com
www.dianepublishing.net
A complete, authoritative and hopeful book on the subject of chronic pain relief. Offers revolutionary ways to relieve all types and degrees of painful conditions. Also offers breakthrough medical treatments, clear guidelines for seeking expert care and the latest scientific findings on pain management.
252 pages Hardcover
ISBN: 0-756753-70-8
Herman Baron, Publisher

Newsletters

2931 Health Points
TyH Publications
17007 E Colony Drive
Fountain Hills, AZ 85268
800-801-1406
editor@e-tyh.com
National newsletter with articles on complementary therapy, latest nutrition news, disability issues and much more. Focus is on fibromyalgia, chronic fatigue, arthritis and chronic pain.
Quarterly

Audio & Video

2932 ACPA Relaxation Tapes
American Chronic Pain Association
PO Box 850
Rocklin, CA 95677
916-632-0922
800-533-3231
Fax: 916-632-3208
acpa@theacpa.org
www.theacpa.org
Audio tapes offering information on pain relief, breath relaxation and autogenic relaxation. These tapes are designed to help persons regain control of their bodies through exercises in relaxation techniques. $10.00-$25.00.
Audio Tapes
Penny Cowan, Executive Director

2933 ACPA Video: 10 Steps from Patient to Person
American Chronic Pain Association
PO Box 850
Rocklin, CA 95677
916-632-0922
800-533-3231
Fax: 916-632-3208
acpa@theacpa.org
www.theacpa.org
The video, featuring Penny Cowan, founder of the ACPA, discussed the value of a multidisiplinary pain management program and what is necessary to maintain wellness long term.
Penny Cowan, Executive Director

2934 Affirmation Tape
American Chronic Pain Association
PO Box 850
Rocklin, CA 95677
916-632-0922
800-533-3231
Fax: 916-632-3208
acpa@theacpa.org
www.theacpa.org
Designed to help you focus on positive things about yourself and builds self-esteem.
Penny Cowan, Executive Director

2935 Relaxation Tape
American Chronic Pain Association
PO Box 850
Rocklin, CA 95677
916-632-0922
800-533-3231
Fax: 916-632-3208
acpa@theacpa.org
www.theacpa.org
Tape one includes pain relief and breath relaxation. Tape two includes general relaxation and autogenic relaxation.
Penny Cowan, Executive Director

Web Sites

2936 American Pain Society
americanpainsociety.org
Multidisciplinary organization of basic and clinical scientists, practicing clinicians, policy analysts, and others.

2937 Discovery Health
www.discoverylife.com
A source of information on various health topics, including chronic pain and its symptoms and treatments.

2938 Healing Well
www.healingwell.com
An online health resource guide to medical news, chat, information and articles, newsgroups and message boards, books, disease-related web sites, medical directories, and more for patients, friends, and family coping with disabling diseases, disorders, or chronic illnesses.

2939 Health Finder
www.healthfinder.gov
Searchable, carefully developed web site offering information on over 1000 topics. Developed by the US Department of Health and Human Services, the site can be used in both English and Spanish.

2940 Healthlink USA
www.healthlinkusa.com
Health information concerning treatment, cures, prevention, diagnosis, risk factors, research, support groups, email lists, personal stories and much more. Updated regularly.

2941 International Pelvic Pain Society
www.pelvicpain.org
Seeks to recruit, organize, and educate health care professionals actively involved with the treatment of patients who have chronic pelvic pain.

2942 MedicineNet
www.medicinenet.com
An online resource for consumers providing easy-to-read, authoritative medical and health information.

2943 Medscape
www.medscape.com
Medscape offers specialists, primary care physicians, and other health professionals the Web's most robust and integrated medical information and educational tools.

2944 WebMD
www.webmd.com
Provides credible information, supportive communities, and in-depth reference material about health subjects. A source for original and timely health information as well as material from well known content providers.

Description

2945 Congenital Heart Defects

Congenital heart defects (CHDs) occur in almost 1 percent of all live births, and among birth defects are the leading cause of infant mortality. CHDs result from abnormal heart formation during embryonic development. The heart develops between the 2nd and 6th week of development, and may be affected by genetic mutations, maternal illness (e.g., rubella, diabetes mellitus, systemic lupus erythematosus), maternal systemic medications or toxins (e.g. alcohol abuse), and possibly maternal age. The incidence of CHDs in the population is about eight cases in 1,000 live births. About half of these cardiac defects are minor and can be followed clinically while the other half fall into the categories of major CHDs. This latter group often requires surgery early in life to either completely repair the heart defect or in some cases, to redirect blood through the cardiovascular system to palliate the structural abnormality.

Fetal blood circulation differs from adult circulation in that the umbilical arteries branch from the internal iliac arteries and carry deoxygenated blood to the placenta. The placenta is drained by the umbilical veins, which enter the fetus and conduct blood to the inferior vena cava through the ductus venosus, and, to a lesser extent, to the liver. Most of the highly oxygenated blood that reaches the right side of the heart moves through an opening in the wall of the right atrium, called the foramen ovale, to the left atrium, where it is pumped from the left ventricle into the aorta to supply the head and body.

Deoxygenated blood from the head comes to the heart through the superior vena cava, and moves through the right atrium, into the right ventricle, and is then pumped into the pulmonary artery. From the pulmonary artery, the blood moves, mostly, through a shunt called the ductus arteriosus to the descending aorta. Most of the blood moves through the ductus arteriosus because of high vascular resistance through the fetal pulmonary artery and local prostaglandin synthesis that keeps the ductus arteriosus open. When the baby takes her first breath, vascular resistance precipitously decreases, which raises pressure in the left atrium. Increased left atrial pressure closes the foramen ovale. Increased oxygen concentrations in the lung decrease local prostaglandin synthesis, which closes the ductus arteriosus. Detachment of the placenta causes the umbilical vessels and their shunts to wither and close.

CHDs can be divided into two major categories: acyanotic and cyanotic. Acyanotic CHDs include left-to-right shunting lesions and obstructive lesions. The left to right shunting lesions are the most common of the CHDs and include ventricular septal defects (VSDs) and atrial septal defects (ASDs), which have a total prevalence of 48.4 per 10,000 live births, atrioventricular septal defects (1 in 2,120 live births), and patent ductus arteriosus. In left to right shunting lesions, because of progressive blood flow through openings in the septum causes excess pulmonary blood flow and volumetric overload of the left ventricle. This can cause feeding and breathing problems for infants in the first few months of life, and may lead to heart failure and failure to thrive.

Obstructive lesions prevent normal blood flow, usually as a result of stenosis or narrowing of major blood vessels. Obstruction causes volume overload in the ventricles, which induces ventricular enlargement and may lead to heart failure. The more common left heart obstructive diseases include aortic stenosis (3-6 percent of CHDs), pulmonic stenosis (8-12 percent of CHDs), coarctation of the aorta (1 of 1,500 births) and the hypoplastic left heart syndrome (1 of 4,344 births).

Cyanotic CHDs reduce oxygenation of arterial blood by shunting deoxygenated venous blood from the right side of the heart to the left side.. Infants with cyanotic CHDs may have episodes of turning blue during crying or feeding (known as tet spells).The more common disorders in this group are tetralogy of Fallot (1 in 2,518 births), and transposition of the great arteries (1 in 3,300 births).

With the remarkable advances in neonatal cardiac surgery and interventional cardiac catheterization, almost all of the cardiac malformations can be aggressively addressed with excellent results, even in the youngest and smallest of patients. Overall, survival from all cardiac surgeries in children with CHD is greater than 95 percent, and even for the most complex of CHDs it is approaching 90 percent. These children often require long-term follow-up from a pediatric cardiologist, but the vast majority lead healthy active lives. See also *Birth Defects*.

National Agencies & Associations

2946 Adult Congenital Heart Association
280 N Provindence Road
Media, PA 19063

215-849-1260
888-921-2242
Fax: 215-849-1261
Info@achaheart.org
www.achaheart.org

The Adult Congenital Heart Association (ACHA) is a non-profit organization which seeks to improve the quality of life and extend the lives of adults with congenital heart defects through education, outreach, advocacy,and promotion of research.
Mark Roeder, President & CEO
Danielle M. Hile, Director, Programs

2947 International Society for Adult Congenital Heart Disease (ISACHD)
1500 Sunday Drive
Raleigh, NC 27607
919-861-5578
Fax: 919-787-4916
info@isachd.org
www.isachd.org
To pursue and maintain excellent care for those with congenital heart disease worldwide.
Adrienne Kovacs, PhD, President
Calre P. O'Donnell, Global Affairs/Communications

2948 Kids with Heart National Association for Children's Heart Disorders
michelle@kidswithheart.org
www.kidswithheart.org
Kids with Heart is a non-profit organization dedicated to providing support for families affected by congenital heart defects through surgical care packages.
Michelle Rintamaki, President
Dean Rintamaki, Vice President

2949 Schneeweiss Adult Congenital Heart Disease Center
New York Presbyterian Hospital
161 Fort Washington Avenue
New York, NY 10032
212-305-6936
Fax: 212-305-0490
www.congenitalheart.cuimc.columbia.edu
We provide such diagnostic services such as echocardiography cardiac MRI and cardiac catheterization. Highly specialized care is provided by a team of physicians specifically interested in the problems of adults with congenital heart disease.
Rebecca Ubiera, Office Administrator
Jenny Wang, RDCS, Chief Cardiac Sonographer

Support Groups & Hotlines

2950 National Health Information Center
Office of Disease Prevention & Health Promotion
1101 Wootton Pkwy
Rockville, MD 20852
Fax: 240-453-8281
odphpinfo@hhs.gov
www.health.gov/nhic
Supports public health education by maintaining a calendar of National Health Observances; helps connect consumers and health professionals to organizations that can best answer questions and provide up-to-date contact information from reliable sources; updates on a yearly basis toll-free numbers for health information, Federal health clearinghouses and info centers.
Don Wright, MD, MPH, Director

Web Sites

2951 Heartpoint
www.heartpoint.com
Heartpoint provides information about specific heart defects.

2952 MedicineNet
www.medicinenet.com
An online resource for consumers providing easy-to-read, authoritative medical and health information.

2953 Medline Plus
www.nlm.nih.gov/medlineplus
This website includes information about congenital heart disease and includes links regarding support and treatment.

2954 Yale: Congenital Heart Disease
This web site provides in-depth information regarding various types of heart conditions.

Description

2955 Cooley's Anemia (Thalassemia)

Cooley's anemia, or beta-Thalassemia major, is an inherited disorder characterized by abnormal production of hemoglobin in the red blood cells. There are two forms of beta-Thalassemia: beta-Thalassemia minor, in which the person has no symptoms, and beta-Thalassemia major, or Cooley's anemia, which is a severe, debilitating disease. Although a baby who has Cooley's anemia appears normal at birth, growth rates are impaired, and puberty may be significantly delayed or absent. The patient will develop severe anemia and hyperactivity of the bone marrow. By 1-2 years, patients will present with severe anemia, excessive iron levels (transfusional and absorptive iron overload), jaundice, leg ulcers, and gallstones. The spleen will also be greatly enlarged. Without therapy, there is a general decline. Because of the hyperactivity of the bone marrow the bones of the skull, particularly those of the face, will thicken and become more prominent and pronounced. The long bones are predisposed to fractures and growth delays.

While there is no cure for Cooley's anemia, there are treatments such as blood transfusions, which can reduce some symptoms of the disease. However, children with Cooley's anemia should receive as few transfusions as possible because of the danger of iron overload from the "heme" portion of hemoglobin. Chelation, or binding, of the excess iron associated with multiple, repetitive transfusions is important, and is accomplished with deferoxamine. Removal of the splleen may reduce transfusion requirements. Bone marrow transplants can cure Cooley's Anemia.

Genetic screening of at-risk populations is very important, notably for persons of Mediterranean, African and Southeast Asian ancestry. Prenatal diagnosis can also be performed.

National Agencies & Associations

2956 American Hellenic Educational Progressive Association
1909 Q Street NW
Washington, DC 20009
202-232-6300
Fax: 202-232-2140
ahepa@ahepa.org
www.ahepa.org
Promote Hellenism, education, philanthropy, civic responsibility, and family and individual excellence.
Basil N. Mossaidis, Executive Director
Rosalind Ofuokwu, Director, Membership

2957 American Society of Hematology
2021 L Street NW
Washington, DC 20036
202-776-0544
866-828-1231
Fax: 202-776-0545
www.hematology.org
A professional society serving both clinicians and scientists around the world who are working to conquer blood diseases.
Martha Liggett, Esq., Executive Director
LaFaundra Neville-Ingram, CAP, Executive Assistant

2958 National Association of Special Education Teachers
1250 Connecticut Ave, NW
Washington, DC 20036
800-754-4421
Fax: 800-754-4421
contactus@naset.org
www.naset.org
NASET is a national membership organization dedicated to rendering support and assistance to those preparing for or teaching in the field of special education.
Dr. Roger Pierangelo, Co-Executive Director
Dr. George Giuliani, Co-Executive Director

State Agencies & Associations

California

2959 Cooley's Anemia Foundation (CAF): California
2629 Foothill Boulevard
La Crescenta, CA 91214
800-601-2821
Fax: 212-279-5999
info@cooleysanemia.org
www.cooleysanemia.org
The Cooley's Anemia Foundation (CAF) is dedicated to serving people afflicted with various forms of thalassemia, most notably the major form of this genetic blood disease, Cooley's anemia/thalassemia major. CAF's mission is advancing the treatment and curing the disease.
Christine Giannamore, Coordinator
Gina Cioffi Esq, National Office Executive Director

Illinois

2960 Cooley's Anemia Foundation (CAF): Illinois Oakbrook Towers
Oakbrook Towers
40 N Tower Road
Altbrook, IL 62503
847-602-2616
800-522-7222
Fax: 212-279-5999
info@cooleysanemia.org
www.cooleysanemia.org
The Cooley's Anemia Foundation (CAF) is dedicated to serving people afflicted with various forms of thalassemia most notably the major form of this genetic blood disease Cooley's anemia/thalassemia major. CAF's mission is advancing the treatment and curing the disease.
Bruce Rod, President Illinois Office
Gina Cioffi, National Office Executive Director

Maryland

2961 Cooley's Anemia Foundation (CAF): Capital Area
15321 Peach Orchard Avenue
Silver Spring, MD 20905
301-989-8947
800-522-7222
Fax: 212-279-5999
info@cooleysanemia.org
www.cooleysanemia.org
The Cooley's Anemia Foundation (CAF) is dedicated to serving people afflicted with various forms of thalassemia most notably the major form of this genetic blood disease Cooley's anemia/thalassemia major. CAF's mission is advancing the treatment and curing the disease.
Carl C Vitaliti, President Capital Area Office
Gina Cioffi Esq, National Office Executive Director

Massachusetts

2962 Cooley's Anemia Foundation (CAF): Massachusetts Chapter
44 Joseph Road
Newton, MA 02460-1122
617-332-5952
800-522-7222
Fax: 212-279-5999
info@cooleysanemia.org
www.cooleysanemia.org
The Cooley's Anemia Foundation (CAF) is dedicated to serving people afflicted with various forms of thalassemia most notably the major form of this genetic blood disease Cooley's anemia/thalassemia major. CAF's mission is advancing the treatment and curing the disease.
Rudi Viscomi, President Massachusetts Office
Gina Cioffi, National Office Executive Director

2963 Cooley's Anemia Foundation (CAF): New Jersey Chapter
29 Alyson Place   732-688-2279
Bloomfield, NJ 07003   800-522-7222
                                      Fax: 212-279-5999
                                      info@cooleysanemia.org
                                      www.cooleysanemia.org
The Cooley's Anemia Foundation (CAF) is dedicated to serving people afflicted with various forms of thalassemia most notably the major form of this genetic blood disease Cooley's anemia/thalassemia major. CAF's mission is advancing the treatment and curing the disease.
Christine Somma, President New Jersey Office
Gina Cioffi, National Office Executive Director

New York

2964 Cooley's Anemia Foundation (CAF): Rochester
                                      585-482-5587
                                      800-522-7222
                                      Fax: 212-279-5999
                                      info@cooleysanemia.org
                                      www.cooleysanemia.org
The Cooley's Anemia Foundation (CAF) is dedicated to serving people afflicted with various forms of thalassemia most notably the major form of this genetic blood disease Cooley's anemia/thalassemia major. CAF's mission is advancing the treatment and curing the disease.
Shirley Cammilleri, President Rochester Office
Gina Cioffi Esq, National Office Executive Director

2965 Cooley's Anemia Foundation (CAF): Buffalo
135 Wellington Road   716-834-8903
Buffalo, NY 14216   800-522-7222
                                      Fax: 212-279-5999
                                      info@cooleysanemia.org
                                      www.cooleysanemia.org
The Cooley's Anemia Foundation (CAF) is dedicated to serving people afflicted with various forms of thalassemia most notably the major form of this genetic blood disease Cooley's anemia/thalassemia major. CAF's mission is advancing the treatment and curing the disease.
Dennis Locurto, President Buffalo Office
Gina Cioffi Esq, National Office Executive Director

2966 Cooley's Anemia Foundation (CAF): Long Island
111 Cherry Valley Avenue   516-358-9100
Garden City, NY 11530   800-522-7222
                                      Fax: 516-358-9101
                                      info@cooleysanemia.org
                                      www.cooleysanemia.org
The Cooley's Anemia Foundation (CAF) is dedicated to serving people afflicted with various forms of thalassemia most notably the major form of this genetic blood disease Cooley's anemia/thalassemia major. CAF's mission is advancing the treatment and curing the disease.
Thomas Rotolo, President Long Island Office
Janice Cenzoprano, Vice President Long Island Office

2967 Cooley's Anemia Foundation (CAF): Queens
157-26 9th Avenue   718-746-7677
Beachurst, NY 11357   800-522-7222
                                      Fax: 718-746-7678
                                      info@cooleysanemia.org
                                      www.cooleysanemia.org
The Cooley's Anemia Foundation (CAF) is dedicated to serving people afflicted with various forms of thalassemia most notably the major form of this genetic blood disease Cooley's anemia/thalassemia major. CAF's mission is advancing the treatment and curing the disease.
Paul Tucci, President Queen Office
Abbey Chakalis, Events Manager

2968 Cooley's Anemia Foundation (CAF): Staten Island
16B Dreyer Avenue   718-761-5380
Staten Island, NY 10314   800-522-7222
                                      Fax: 718-761-5381
                                      info@cooleysanemia.org
                                      www.cooleysanemia.org

The Cooley's Anemia Foundation (CAF) is dedicated to serving people afflicted with various forms of thalassemia most notably the major form of this genetic blood disease Cooley's anemia/thalassemia major. CAF's mission is advancing the treatment and curing the disease.
Gina Cioffi Esq, National Office Executive Director
Craig Butler, National Office Communications Director

2969 Cooley's Anemia Foundation (CAF): Suffolk Chapter Office
740 Smithtown Bypass   631-863-0532
Smithtown, NY 11787   800-522-7222
                                      Fax: 631-863-0535
                                      info@cooleysanemia.org
                                      www.cooleysanemia.org
The Cooley's Anemia Foundation (CAF) is dedicated to serving people afflicted with various forms of thalassemia most notably the major form of this genetic blood disease Cooley's anemia/thalassemia major. CAF's mission is advancing the treatment and curing the disease.
Gina Cioffi Esq, National Office Executive Director
Craig Butler, National Office Communications Director

2970 Cooley's Anemia Foundation (CAF): Westches ter/Rockland Chapter
3 Samuel Purdy Lane   914-232-1808
Katonah, NY 10536   800-522-7222
                                      Fax: 212-279-5999
                                      info@cooleysanemia.org
                                      www.cooleysanemia.org
The Cooley's Anemia Foundation (CAF) is dedicated to serving people afflicted with various forms of thalassemia most notably the major form of this genetic blood disease Cooley's anemia/thalassemia major. CAF's mission is advancing the treatment and curing the disease.
Peter Chieco, President Westchester/Rockland Office
Janet Manning, Executive Director

Texas

2971 Cooley's Anemia Foundation (CAF): Texas
4504 Astor Road   214-324-6147
Mesquite, TX 75150-2320   800-522-7222
                                      Fax: 214-324-0612
                                      info@cooleysanemia.org
                                      www.cooleysanemia.org
The Cooley's Anemia Foundation (CAF) is dedicated to serving people afflicted with various forms of thalassemia most notably the major form of this genetic blood disease Cooley's anemia/thalassemia major.
Mateen Shah, President
Gina Cioffi Esq, National Office Executive Director

Foundations

2972 Cooley's Anemia Foundation
330 Seventh Avenue   800-522-7222
New York, NY 10001   Fax: 212-279-5999
                                      info@cooleysanemia.org
                                      www.cooleysanemia.org
Serves individuals affected by the various forms of thalassemia by making advances in treatment, enhancing quality of life, and educating medical professionals.
Peter Chieco, National President
Craig Butler, National Executive Director

2973 Fanconi Anemia Research Fund
1801 Willamette Street   541-687-4658
Eugene, OR 97401   888-326-2664
                                      Fax: 541-687-0548
                                      info@fanconi.org
                                      www.fanconi.org
Funds research and provides education and support services worldwide to families affected with Fanconi anemia: a rare genetic aplastic anemia that leads to bone marrow failure, acute myelogenous leukemia, and squamous cell carcinomas.
Mark Quinlan, Executive Director
Marie Sweeten, Family Services Director

Support Groups & Hotlines

2974 National Health Information Center
Office of Disease Prevention & Health Promotion
1101 Wootton Pkwy
Rockville, MD 20852
Fax: 240-453-8281
odphpinfo@hhs.gov
www.health.gov/nhic
Supports public health education by maintaining a calendar of National Health Observances; helps connect consumers and health professionals to organizations that can best answer questions and provide up-to-date contact information from reliable sources; updates on a yearly basis toll-free numbers for health information, Federal health clearinghouses and info centers.
Don Wright, MD, MPH, Director

Books

2975 Genes, Blood & Courage
129-09 26th Avenue
Flushing, NY 11354
212-598-0911
800-522-7222
www.cooleysanemia.org

2976 What is Cooley's Anemia
330 Seventh Ave
New York, NY 10001
212-279-8090
800-522-7222
Fax: 718-321-3340
info@cooleysanemia.org
www.cooleysanemia.org
Patient and family handbook.
Jayne Restivo, National Executive Director

2977 What is Thalassemia?
Cooley's Anemia Foundation
330 Seventh Ave
New York, NY 10001
212-279-8090
800-522-7222
Fax: 718-321-3340
info@cooleysanemia.org
www.cooleysanemia.org
A guide to help thalassemics and their parents understand thalassemia, the reasons for treatment and the hope for the future.
Jayne Restivo, National Executive Director

Children's Books

2978 Coloring Book on Thalassemia
330 Seventh Ave
New York, NY 10001
212-279-8090
800-522-7222
Fax: 718-321-3340
info@cooleysanemia.org
www.cooleysanemia.org
Available in English, Italian, Greek and Chinese.
Jayne Restivo, National Executive Director

Magazines

2979 AHEPAN Magazine
American Hellenic Educational Progressive Assn
1909 Q Street NW
Washington, DC 20009
202-232-6300
Fax: 202-232-2140
ahepa@ahepa.org
www.ahepa.org
This magazine includes all of the AHEPA organizations.
Quarterly
Basil N Mossaidis, Executive Director

Newsletters

2980 Lifeline
Cooley's Anemia Foundation
330 Seventh Ave
New York, NY 10001
212-279-8090
800-522-7222
Fax: 718-321-3340
info@cooleysanemia.org
www.cooleysanemia.org

A newsletter published by Cooley's Anemia Foundation.
Jayne Restivo, National Executive Director

Pamphlets

2981 Desferal Q&A
330 Seventh Ave
New York, NY 10001
212-279-8090
800-522-7222
Fax: 718-321-3340
info@cooleysanemia.org
www.cooleysanemia.org
Guideline for home infusion.
Jayne Restivo, National Executive Director

2982 What is Thalassemia Trait?
Cooley's Anemia Foundation
330 Seventh Ave
New York, NY 10001
212-279-8090
800-522-7222
Fax: 718-321-3340
info@cooleysanemia.org
www.cooleysanemia.org
This booklet offers information on the thalassemia trait.
1995
Jayne Restivo, National Executive Director

Audio & Video

2983 TAG Annual Patient/Family Conference Video
Cooley's Anemia Foundation
Thalassemia Action Group
New York, NY 10001
800-522-7222
Fax: 212-279-5999
TAG@cooleysanemia.org
www.cooleysanemia.org/
Video from the Thalassemia Action Group/TAG Annual Patient/Family Conference held in March of each year.
Gina Cioffi Esq, National Executive Director
Craig Butler, Communications Director

2984 To Live
Cooley's Anemia Foundation
330 Seventh Avenue
New York, NY 10001
800-522-7222
Fax: 212-279-5999
info@cooleysanemia.org
www.cooleysanemia.org/
An informative and educational video from Cooley's Anemia Foundation.
Gina Cioffi Esq, National Executive Director
Craig Butler, Communications Director

2985 You're Not Alone
Cooley's Anemia Foundation
330 Seventh Avenue
New York, NY 10001
212-279-8090
800-522-7222
Fax: 718-321-3340
info@cooleysanemia.org
www.cooleysanemia.org
An informative and educational video from Cooley's Anemia Foundation.
Gina Cioffi Esq, National Executive Director
Craig Butler, Communications Director

Web Sites

2986 Healing Well
www.healingwell.com
An online health resource guide to medical news, chat, information and articles, newsgroups and message boards, books, disease-related web sites, medical directories, and more for patients, friends, and family coping with disabling diseases, disorders, or chronic illnesses.

2987 Health Finder
www.healthfinder.gov
Searchable, carefully developed web site offering information on over 1000 topics. Developed by the US Department of Health and Human Services, the site can be used in both English and Spanish.

2988 Healthlink USA

www.healthlinkusa.com

Health information concerning treatment, cures, prevention, diagnosis, risk factors, research, support groups, email lists, personal stories and much more. Updated regularly.

2989 MedicineNet

www.medicinenet.com

An online resource for consumers providing easy-to-read, authoritative medical and health information.

2990 Medscape

www.medscape.com

Medscape offers specialists, primary care physicians, and other health professionals the Web's most robust and integrated medical information and educational tools.

2991 WebMD

www.webmd.com

Provides credible information, supportive communities, and in-depth reference material about health subjects. A source for original and timely health information as well as material from well known content providers.

Description

2992 Crohn Disease

Crohn disease is a chronic inflammation in the lining of the digestive tract, and although it can affect any portion of the gastrointestinal tract, from the mouth to the anus, it generally affects the small bowel or part of the colon. The cause is unknown, although certain genetic factors can increase the risk for Crohn disease, and Crohn disease is more common in some families and racial groups. Stress and eating certain foods are not causes of Crohn disease, but I patients with Crohn disease, stress and eating certain foods may cause flare-ups of the disease. Onset is typically before age 30, with the peak incidence between 14 and 24 years.

Common symptoms include diarrhea (which may be bloody), weight loss, fever, abdominal pain and loss of appetite. If the disease is extensive it may cause deficiencies of essential vitamins and other nutrients. Sometimes inflammation occurs outside the gut, attacking the eyes, joints or skin. Local complications include bowel perforation with formation of abscesses or fistulas that drain out to the skin and may become infected. Established chronic Crohn disease is characterized by lifelong exacerbations. These patients carry an increased risk of cancer of the small bowel and colon/rectum.

Therapy depends on the location of the disease and on its severity. To drive active disease to remission and to maintain remission, aminosalicylates are the drugs of choice in cases of mild to modern colonic Crohn disease. Corticosteroids are effective for short-term induction of remission of disease flare-ups. For moderate to severe Crohn disease, thiopurines (azathioprine and mercaptopurine) can maintain remission. An alternative drug is methotrexate. For refractory cases, biological agents can effectively induce and maintain remission. Such agents include tumor necrosis factor inhibitors (infliximab, adalimumab, and certolizumab pegol), interleukin-12 and -23 antagonists (ustekinumab), and integrin receptor antagonists (vendolizumab and natalizumab). Some gastroenterologists also recommend antibiotics in specific cases and probiotics. Surgery may be necessary to treat complications. In all cases, careful attention should be paid to the patient's nutritional status and psychological well-being. See also *Gastrointestinal Disorders* and *Celiac Disease.*

National Agencies & Associations

2993 American Chronic Pain Association
PO Box 850
Rocklin, CA 95677

800-533-3231
ACPA@theacpa.org
www.theacpa.org

The ACPA facilitates peer support and education for individuals with chronic pain in its many forms, in order to increase quality of life. Also raises awareness among the healthcare community, and with policy makers.
Penney Cowan, Founder & CEO
Daniel Galia, Director, Global Support

2994 Inflammatory Bowel Disease Program
Digestive Health Center
Winfield, IL 60190

630-933-1600
Fax: 630-933-1300
TTY: 630-933-4833
www.nm.org

A fully integrated clinical GI program that is part of the Northwestern Medicine Digestive Health Center.

2995 National Digestive Diseases Information Clearinghouse
2 Information Way
Bethesda, MD 20892-3570

800-891-5389
Fax: 703-738-4929
TTY: 866-569-1162
nddic@info.niddk.nih.gov
www.digestive.niddk.nih.gov

Established to increase knowledge and understanding about digestive diseases among people with these conditions and their families, health care professionals, and the general public. To carry out this mission, NDDIC works closely with a coordinating panel of representatives from Federal agencies, voluntary organizations on the national level, and professional groups to identify and respond to informational needs about digestive diseases.

2996 National Institute of Diabetes & Digestive & Kidney Diseases
Office Of Communications and Public Liaison, NIH
31 Center Drive
Bethesda, MD 20892-2560

800-860-8747
TTY: 866-569-1162
healthinfo@niddk.nih.gov
www.niddk.nih.gov

Research areas include diabetes, digestive diseases, endocrine and metabolic diseases, hematologic diseases, kidney disease, liver disease, urologic diseases, as well as matters relating to nutrition and obesity.
Griffin P. Rodgers, MD, MACP, Director
Gregory Germino, MD, Deputy Director

2997 Pediatric Network Initiative - Crohn's & Colitis Foundation
773 Third Avenue
New York, NY 10017

917-476-6511
www.crohnscolitisfoundation.org

Also known as Pediatric Resource Organization for Kids with Inflammatory Intestinal Diseases (PRO-KIIDS), the organization focuses on all aspects of pediatric and adolescent Crohn's disease and ulcerative colitis, including medical, nutritional, psychological and social factors. Activities include information sharing, educational forums, newsletters and hospital outreach programs.
S. Alandra Weaver, Director
Allison Coffrey, Contact

2998 Reach Out for Youth with Ileitis and Colitis, Inc.
1250 Union Turnpike
New Hyde Park, NY 11040

631-293-3102
info@reachoutforyouth.org

Provides educational seminars, and individual and group support to patients and their families. Fundraising efforts support the Center's programs, and clinical and laboratory research.

2999 United Ostomy Associations of America, Inc
PO Box 525
Kennebunk, ME 04043

800-826-0826
www.ostomy.org

A national network for bowel and urinary diversion support groups in the United States. Its goal is to provide a non-profit association that will serve to unify and strengthen its member support groups, which are organized for the benefit of people who have, or will have intestinal or urinary diversions and their caregivers.
Christine Ryan, Executive Director
Jeanine Gleba, Advocacy Manager

3000 Wound Ostomy and Continence Nurses Society
1120 Route 73
Mt Laurel, NJ 08054

888-224-9626
Fax: 856-439-0525
wocn_info@wocn.org
www.wocn.org

Membership comprises nurses that specialize in enterostomal therapy.
Nicolette Zuecca, Chief Executive Officer
Anna Shnayder, Chief Operations Officer

State Agencies & Associations

Alabama

3001 CCFA Alabama Chapter
244 Goodwin Crest Drive
Birmingham, AL 35259
205-941-9900
800-249-1993
Fax: 205-941-1411
www.ccfa.org/chapters/alabama/
Crohn's and Colitis Foundation of America is a non-profit, volunteer-driven organization dedicated to finding the cure for Crohn's disease and ulcerative colitis.
Pat Talty, Executive Director

Arizona

3002 CCFA Southwest Chapter: Arizona
8098 Via de Negocio
Scottsdale, AZ 85258
480-246-3676
877-259-2104
Fax: 480-246-3679
southwest@ccfa.org
www.ccfa.org/chapters/southwest/
Crohn's and Colitis Foundation of America is a non-profit volunteer-driven organization dedicated to finding the cure for Crohn's disease and ulcerative colitis.
Kathie Gadberry, Executive Director
Bernadette Sewer, Development Coordinator

California

3003 CCFA California: Greater Los Angeles Chapter
1640 S Sepulveda Boulevard
Los Angeles, CA 90025
310-478-4500
866-831-9157
Fax: 310-478-4546
losangeles@ccfa.org
www.ccfa.org/chapters/losangeles/
Crohn's and Colitis Foundation of America is a non-profit volunteer-driven organization dedicated to finding the cure for Crohn's disease and ulcerative colitis.
Iyad Zabaneh, Development Coordinator
Kerri Yoder, Education Manager

Colorado

3004 CCFA Rocky Mountain Chapter
1777 S Bellaire Street
Denver, CO 80222
303-639-9163
866-768-2232
Fax: 303-568-0424
rockymountain@ccfa.org
www.ccfa.org/chapters/rockymountain/
Crohn's and Colitis Foundation of America is a non-profit volunteer-driven organization dedicated to finding the cure for Crohn's disease and ulcerative colitis.
Nancy Freimuth, Walk Manager
Mackenzie Lyle, Interim Executive Director

Connecticut

3005 CCFA Central Connecticut Chapter
P O Box 275
Branford, CT 06405
203-208-3130
www.ccfa.org/chapters/centralct/
Crohn's and Colitis Foundation of America is a non-profit volunteer-driven organization dedicated to finding the cure for Crohn's disease and ulcerative colitis.
Sally Connolly, Board President

3006 CCFA Northern Connecticut Affiliate Chapter
PO Box 370614
W Hartford, CT 06137-0614
212-679-1570
800-932-2423
Fax: 212-679-3567
info@ccfa.org
www.ccfa.org/chapters/northernct/
Crohn's and Colitis Foundation of America is a non-profit volunteer-driven organization dedicated to finding the cure for Crohn's disease and ulcerative colitis.
Marilyn Hagg Blohm, Executive Director National Headquarters
Jeff Neale, Public Relations National Headquarters

Florida

3007 CCFA Florida Chapter
2250 N Druid Hills Road
Boca Raton, FL 30329-2391
404-982-0616
877-664-2929
Fax: 404-982-0656
kkeohane@ccfa.org
www.ccfa.org/chapters/florida/
Crohn's and Colitis Foundation of America is a non-profit volunteer-driven organization dedicated to finding the cure for Crohn's disease and ulcerative colitis.
Deborah Barnard, Development Manager
Lacy Woods, Administrator

Georgia

3008 CCFA Georgia Chapter
2250 N Druid Hills Road
Atlanta, GA 30329
404-982-0616
800-472-6795
Fax: 404-982-0656
georgia@ccfa.org
www.ccfa.org/chapters/georgia/
Crohn's and Colitis Foundation of America is a non-profit volunteer-driven organization dedicated to finding the cure for Crohn's disease and ulcerative colitis.
Marcia Greenburg, Executive Director
Karen Rittenbaum, Development Director

Illinois

3009 CCFA Illinois: Carol Fisher Chapter
2250 E Devon Avenue
Des Plaines, IL 60018
847-827-0404
800-886-6664
Fax: 847-827-6563
Illinois@ccfa.org
www.ccfa.org/chapters/illinois/
Crohn's and Colitis Foundation of America is a non-profit volunteer-driven organization dedicated to finding the cure for Crohn's disease and ulcerative colitis.
Marianne Floriano, Executive Director
Kristina Sickles, Development Coordinator

Indiana

3010 CCFA Indiana Chapter
931 E 86th Street
Indianapolis, IN 46240
317-259-8071
800-332-6029
Fax: 317-259-8091
indiana@ccfa.org
www.ccfa.org/chapters/indiana/
Crohn's and Colitis Foundation of America is a non-profit volunteer-driven organization dedicated to finding the cure for Crohn's disease and ulcerative colitis.
Scott Baumruck, Development Director
Dawn Drinkut, Development Assistant

Iowa

3011 CCFA Iowa Chapter
PO Box 1184
Johnston, IA 50131-0016
515-664-8961
Fax: 319-277-6293
iowa@ccfa.org
www.ccfa.org/chapters/iowa/
Crohn's and Colitis Foundation of America is a non-profit volunteer-driven organization dedicated to finding the cure for Crohn's disease and ulcerative colitis.
Tony Kline, Chapter President
Abbie Hansen, Vice President Communications

Kansas

3012 CCFA Mid-America Chapter: Kansas
1034 S Brentwood
St Louis, MO 63117
314-863-4747
800-783-8006
Fax: 314-863-4749
www.ccfa.org/chapters/midamerica/

Crohn's and Colitis Foundation of America is a non-profit volunteer-driven organization dedicated to finding the cure for Crohn's disease and ulcerative colitis.
Steve Skodak, Executive Director
Andi Harrington, Development Manager

Louisiana

3013 CCFA Louisiana Chapter
7611 Maple Street 504-861-3433
New Orleans, LA 70118 866-382-2232
Fax: 504-861-3466
lams@ccfa.org
www.ccfa.org/chapters/louisiana
Crohn's and Colitis Foundation of America is a non-profit volunteer-driven organization dedicated to finding the cure for Crohn's disease and ulcerative colitis.
David Lee Thomas, Development Director
Gail C Smith, Development Assistant

Maryland

3014 CCFA Maryland Chapter
10400 Little Patuxent Parkway 443-276-0861
Columbia, MD 21044 800-618-5583
Fax: 443-276-0865
maryland@ccfa.org
www.ccfa.org/chapters/md-southde
Crohn's and Colitis Foundation of America is a non-profit volunteer-driven organization dedicated to finding the cure for Crohn's disease and ulcerative colitis.
Robert J Milanchus, Regional Executive Director
Mary Glagola, President

Massachusetts

3015 CCFA New England Chapter: Massachusetts
280 Hillside Avenue 781-449-0324
Needham, MA 02494 800-314-3459
Fax: 781-449-0325
ne@ccfa.org
www.ccfa.org/chapters/ne
Crohn's and Colitis Foundation of America is a non-profit volunteer-driven organization dedicated to finding the cure for Crohn's disease and ulcerative colitis.
Jess Adani, Development Manager
Kristin Patmos, Education Manager

Michigan

3016 CCFA Michigan Chapter: Farmington Hills
31313 N Western Highway 248-737-0900
Farmington Hills, MI 78334 Fax: 248-737-0904
michigan@ccfa.org
www.ccfa.org/chapters/michigan
Crohn's and Colitis Foundation of America is a non-profit volunteer-driven organization dedicated to finding the cure for Crohn's disease and ulcerative colitis.
Bernard L Riker, Executive Director
Gilda Hauser, Development Manager

Minnesota

3017 CCFA Minnesota Chapter
1885 University Avenue W 651-917-2424
Saint Paul, MN 55104 888-422-3266
Fax: 651-917-2425
Minnesota@ccfa.org
www.ccfa.org/chapters/minnesota
Crohn's and Colitis Foundation of America is a non-profit volunteer-driven organization dedicated to finding the cure for Crohn's disease and ulcerative colitis.
Maggie Brown, Take Steps Manager
Ruby Lanoux, Development Manager

Missouri

3018 CCFA Mid-America Chapter: Missouri
1034 S Brentwood 314-863-4747
Saint Louis, MO 63117 800-783-8006
Fax: 314-863-4749
info@ccfa.org
www.ccfa.org/chapters/midamerica
Crohn's and Colitis Foundation of America is a non-profit volunteer-driven organization dedicated to finding the cure for Crohn's disease and ulcerative colitis.
Steve Skodak, Executive Director
Andi Harrington, Development Manager

New Jersey

3019 CCFA New Jersey Chapter
45 Wilson Avenue 732-786-9960
Manalapan, NJ 07726 Fax: 732-786-9964
newjersey@ccfa.org
www.ccfa.org/chapters/newjersey
Crohn's and Colitis Foundation of America is a non-profit volunteer-driven organization dedicated to finding the cure for Crohn's disease and ulcerative colitis.
Rosemarie Golombos, Executive Director
Barbara Fedorchak, Chapter Development Manager

New York

3020 CCFA Greater New York Chapter: National Headquarters
386 Park Avenue S 800-932-2423
New York, NY 10016-8804 800-932-2423
Fax: 212-679-3567
info@ccfa.org
www.ccfa.org
Crohn's and Colitis Foundation of America is a non-profit volunteer-driven organization dedicated to finding the cure for Crohn's disease and ulcerative colitis.
Marilyn Hagg Blohm, Executive Director
Jeff Neale, Public Relations/Media Director

3021 CCFA Long Island Chapter
585 Stewart Avenue 516-222-5530
Garden City, NY 11530 Fax: 516-222-5535
longisland@ccfa.org
www.ccfa.org/chapters/longisland
Crohn's and Colitis Foundation of America is a non-profit volunteer-driven organization dedicated to finding the cure for Crohn's disease and ulcerative colitis.
Marilyn Hagg Blohm, Executive Director National Office
Jeff Neale, Public Relations/Media National Office

3022 CCFA Rochester/Southern Tier Chapter
2117 Buffalo Road 585-617-4771
Rochester, NY 14624 800-932-2423
rochester@ccfa.org
www.ccfa.org/chapters/rochester
Crohn's and Colitis Foundation of America is a non-profit volunteer-driven organization dedicated to finding the cure for Crohn's disease and ulcerative colitis.
Marilyn Hagg Blohm, Executive Director National Headquarters
Jeff Neale, Public Relations

3023 CCFA Upstate/Northeastern New York Chapter
4 Normanskill Boulevard 518-439-0252
Delmar, NY 12054 upstateny@ccfa.org
www.ccfa.org/chapters/upstateny
Crohn's and Colitis Foundation of America is a non-profit volunteer-driven organization dedicated to finding the cure for Crohn's disease and ulcerative colitis.
Linda Winston, Chapter President
Peter Purcel MD, Medical Advisory Chair

3024 CCFA Western New York Chapter
2714 Sheridan Drive 716-833-2870
Tonawanda, NY 14150-0224 800-932-2423
www.ccfa.org/chapters/westernny

Crohn's and Colitis Foundation of America is a non-profit volunteer-driven organization dedicated to finding the cure for Crohn's disease and ulcerative colitis.
Marilyn Hagg Blohm, Executive Director National Headquarters
Jeff Neale, Public Relations

North Carolina

3025 CCFA Carolinas Chapter
2901 N Davidson Street 704-332-1611
Charlotte, NC 28205 877-332-1611
Fax: 704-332-1612
carolinas@ccfa.org
www.ccfa.org/chapters/carolinas
Crohn's and Colitis Foundation of America is a non-profit volunteer-driven organization dedicated to finding the cure for Crohn's disease and ulcerative colitis.
Angela Parks, Development Director
Julie Perkins, Special Events/Development Manager

3026 CCFA South Carolina Chapter
2901 N Davidson Street 704-332-1611
Charlotte, NC 28205 877-632-1611
Fax: 704-332-1612
carolinas@ccfa.org
www.ccfa.org/chapters/carolinas
Crohn's and Colitis Foundation of America is a non-profit volunteer-driven organization dedicated to finding the cure for Crohn's disease and ulcerative colitis.
Angela Parks, Development Manager
Tewanna Sanders, Education & Support Manager

Ohio

3027 CCFA Central Ohio Chapter
5008 Pine Creek Drive 614-865-1933
Westerville, OH 43081 800-625-5977
Fax: 614-865-1934
centralohio@ccfa.org
www.ccfa.org/chapters/centralohio
Crohn's and Colitis Foundation of America is a non-profit volunteer-driven organization dedicated to finding the cure for Crohn's disease and ulcerative colitis.
Janelle Gasaway, Take Steps Manager
Kelly Bush, Development Coordinator

3028 CCFA Northeast Ohio Chapter
23775 Commerce Park Road 216-831-2692
Beachwood, OH 44122 866-345-2232
Fax: 216-831-2792
neohio@ccfa.org
www.ccfa.org/chapters/neohio
Crohn's and Colitis Foundation of America is a non-profit volunteer-driven organization dedicated to finding the cure for Crohn's disease and ulcerative colitis.
Kristin Knipp, Development Coordinator
Patty Kaplan, Development Manager NE Ohio Chapter

3029 CCFA Southwest Ohio Chapter
8 Triangle Park Drive 513-772-3550
Cincinnati, OH 45246 877-283-7513
Fax: 513-772-7599
SWOhio@ccfa.org
www.ccfa.org/chapters/swohio
Crohn's and Colitis Foundation of America is a non-profit volunteer-driven organization dedicated to finding the cure for Crohn's disease and ulcerative colitis.
Rachel Spradlin, Take Steps Manager
Jenny Southers, Development Manager SE Ohio Chapter

Oklahoma

3030 CCFA Oklahoma Chapter
4504 E 67th Street 918-523-8540
Tulsa, OK 74136 800-658-1533
Fax: 918-523-8560
www.ccfa.org/chapters/oklahoma

Crohn's and Colitis Foundation of America is a non-profit volunteer-driven organization dedicated to finding the cure for Crohn's disease and ulcerative colitis.
Judy Summers, Regional Executive Director
Christopher Woods, President

Pennsylvania

3031 CCFA Philadelphia/Delaware Valley Chapter
367 E Street Road 215-396-9100
Trevose, PA 19053 888-340-4744
Fax: 215-396-1170
Philadelphia@ccfa.org
www.ccfa.org/chapters/philadelphia
Crohn's and Colitis Foundation of America is a non-profit volunteer-driven organization dedicated to finding the cure for Crohn's disease and ulcerative colitis.
Barbara Berman, Executive Director
Suzanne Rhodeside, Development Director

3032 CCFA Western Pennsylvania/West Virginia Chapter
300 Penn Center Boulevard 412-823-8272
Pittsburgh, PA 15235 877-823-8272
Fax: 412-823-8276
wpawv@ccfa.org
www.ccfa.org/chapters/wpawv
Crohn's and Colitis Foundation of America is a non-profit volunteer-driven organization dedicated to finding the cure for Crohn's disease and ulcerative colitis.
10-12 pages
Jamie Rhoades, Development Manager
Susan Kukic, Executive Director

Tennessee

3033 CCFA Tennessee Chapter
95 White Bridge Road 615-356-0444
Nashville, TN 37205 866-814-2232
Fax: 615-356-0445
tennessee@ccfa.org
www.ccfa.org/chapters/tennessee
Crohn's and Colitis Foundation of America is a non-profit volunteer-driven organization dedicated to finding the cure for Crohn's disease and ulcerative colitis.
Michelle J Chianese, Education & Support Manager
Nicole Boisvert, Walk Manager

Texas

3034 CCFA Houston Gulf Coast/South Texas Chapter
5120 Woodway 713-572-2232
Houston, TX 77056 800-785-2232
Fax: 713-572-2433
infohouston@ccfa.org
www.ccfa.org/chapters/houston
Crohn's and Colitis Foundation of America is a non-profit volunteer-driven organization dedicated to finding the cure for Crohn's disease and ulcerative colitis.
Brandy Bendele, Walk Manager
Erin Fagan, Development Manager

3035 CCFA North Texas Chapter
12801 N Central Expressway 972-386-0607
Dallas, TX 75243 Fax: 972-386-0509
ntexas@ccfa.org
www.ccfa.org/chapters/ntexas
Crohn's and Colitis Foundation of America is a non-profit volunteer-driven organization dedicated to finding the cure for Crohn's disease and ulcerative colitis.
Rachel Wallace, Development Manager
Sharon Seagraves, Executive Director

Virginia

3036 CCFA Greater Washington DC/Virginia Chapter
4085 Chain Bridge Road   703-865-6130
Fairfax, VA 22314   877-807-5271
                                     Fax: 703-865-8873
                              washingtondc@ccfa.org
                       www.ccfa.org/chapters/washingtondc
Crohn's and Colitis Foundation of America is a non-profit volunteer-driven organization dedicated to finding the cure for Crohn's disease and ulcerative colitis.
Eileen Pugh, Executive Director
Stephanie Campbell, Development Coordinator

Washington

3037 CCFA Washington State Chapter
9 Lake Bellevue Drive   425-451-8455
Bellevue, WA 98005   877-703-6900
                                     Fax: 425-451-1708
                                  northwest@ccfa.org
                        www.ccfa.org/chapters/northwest
Crohn's and Colitis Foundation of America is a non-profit volunteer-driven organization dedicated to finding the cure for Crohn's disease and ulcerative colitis.
Linda Huse, Executive Director
Jennifer Simmons, Development Manager

Wisconsin

3038 CCFA Wisconsin Chapter
1126 S 70th Street   414-475-5520
W Allis, WI 53214   877-586-5588
                                     Fax: 414-475-5502
                                  wisconsin@ccfa.org
                        www.ccfa.org/chapters/wisconsin
Crohn's and Colitis Foundation of America is a non-profit volunteer-driven organization dedicated to finding the cure for Crohn's disease and ulcerative colitis.
Jan Lenz, Executive Director
Nadine Davis, Development Coordinator

Foundations

3039 Crohn's & Colitis Foundation
733 Third Avenue   800-932-2423
New York, NY 10017   info@crohnscolitisfoundation.org
                             www.crohnscolitisfoundation.org
CCF's mission is to cure and prevent Crohn's disease and ulcerative colitis through research, and to improve the quality of life of children and adults affected by the disease through education and support. The foundation offers patient and professional support.
Michael Osso, President & CEO
Caren Heller, MD, MBA, Chief Scientific Officer

3040 International Foundation for Functional Gastrointestinal Disorders (IFFGD)
PO Box 170864   414-964-1799
Milwaukee, WI 53217   888-964-2001
                                      iffgd@iffgd.org
                                      www.iffgd.org
Non-profit education, support, and research organization devoted to increasing awareness and understanding of functional gastrointestinal disorders, including irritable bowel syndrome (IBS), constipation, diarrhea, pain, and incontinence. Mission is to inform, assist and support people affected by these disorders.
Nancy J. Norton, Founder
Ceciel T. Rooker, President

Research Centers

3041 Hahnemann University, Krancer Center for Inflammatory Bowel Disease Research
230 N Broad St   215-762-7000
Philadelphia, PA 19102   Fax: 215-762-8109
                              www.hahnemannhospital.com

Research into the causes and treatments of ulcerative colitis and Crohn's disease.
Dr. Harris Clearfield, Director

Support Groups & Hotlines

3042 National Health Information Center
Office of Disease Prevention & Health Promotion
1101 Wootton Pkwy   Fax: 240-453-8281
Rockville, MD 20852   odphpinfo@hhs.gov
                                 www.health.gov/nhic
Supports public health education by maintaining a calendar of National Health Observances; helps connect consumers and health professionals to organizations that can best answer questions and provide up-to-date contact information from reliable sources; updates on a yearly basis toll-free numbers for health information, Federal health clearinghouses and info centers.
Don Wright, MD, MPH, Director

Books

3043 Crohn's Disease and Ulcerative Colitis Fact Book
Crohn's & Colitis Foundation of America
386 Park Avenue S   212-685-3440
New York, NY 10016-8804   800-932-2423
                                     Fax: 212-779-4098
                                      info@ccfa.org
                                      www.ccfa.org
Written in layman's language, this first complete guide is helpful in understanding and coping with inflammatory bowel diseases.

3044 Managing Your Child's Crohn's Disease or Ulcerative Colitis
Crohn's & Colitis Foundation of America
386 Park Avenue S   212-685-3440
New York, NY 10016-8804   800-932-2423
                                     Fax: 212-779-4098
                                      info@ccfa.org
                                      www.ccfa.org
Full-length book on Crohn's disease and ulcerative colitis, specifically targeted for parents of children and teenagers; includes topics on cause and diagnosis, treatment, surgery, hospitalization, diet and nutrition, school and social issues and resources for the patient.
$16.95 Members

3045 Ostomy Book: Living Comfortably with Colostomies, Ileostomies and Urostomies
Barbara Dorr Mullen and Kerry Anne McGinn, author

Bull Publishing Company
PO Box 1377thur Boulevard   800-676-2855
Boulder, CO 80306   Fax: 303-545-6354
                                     www.bullpub.com
This book provides complete information on everything from details of surgery to the management of the appliances. Just as importantly, it is a beautifully told story of the entire expereince from diagnosis through rehabilitation to looking forward to a full and happy life.
ISBN: 0-923521-12-7

3046 People...Not Patients: Source Book for Living with Bowel Disease
Chron's & Colitis Foundation of America
386 Park Avenue S   212-685-3440
New York, NY 10016-8804   800-932-2423
                                     Fax: 212-779-4098
                                      info@ccfa.org
                                      www.ccfa.org
Contains the essential information you need to help you cope with Chron's disease and ulcerative colitis after you leave the doctor's office.

3047 Treating IBD
Crohn's & Colitis Foundation of America
386 Park Avenue S   212-685-3440
New York, NY 10016-8804   800-932-2423
                                     Fax: 212-779-4098
                                      info@ccfa.org
                                      www.ccfa.org

Patient's guide to the medical and surgical management of Inflammatory Bowel Disease, this book gives information on treating crohn's disease and ulcerative colitis, including drug therapies, advances in nutritional care, and recently developed surgical alternatives.

3048 Understanding Crohn Disease and Ulcerative Colitis
Jon Zonderman, Ronald S Vender, MD, author
University Press of Mississippi
3825 Ridgewood Road
Jackson, MS 39211-6492
601-432-6205
Fax: 601-432-6217
kburgess@ihl.state.ms.us
www.upress.state.ms.us
For patients and caregivers an overview of the nature and treatments of inflammatory bowel disease.
2000 128 pages Paperback
ISBN: 1-578062-03-9
Kathy Burgess, Advertising/Marketing Services Manager

Magazines

3049 Colon and Rectal Surgery
International Academy of Proctology
PO Box 1716
Martinsville, IN 46151
765-342-3686
Fax: 765-342-4173
Information for professionals involved with colon and rectal surgery.
George Donnally MD

3050 Digestive Health Matters
Intl. Foundation for Gastrointestinal Disorders
PO Box 170864
Milwaukee, WI 53217-0864
414-964-1799
888-964-2001
Fax: 414-964-7176
iffgd@iffgd.org
www.iffgd.org
Quarterly journal focuses on upper and lower gastrointestinal disorders in adults and children. Educational pamphlets and factsheets are available. Patient and professional membership.

3051 Foundation Focus
Crohn's & Colitis Foundation of America
386 Park Avenue S
New York, NY 10016-8804
212-685-3440
800-932-2423
Fax: 212-779-4098
info@ccfa.org
www.ccfa.org
Magazine for CCFA supporters.

3052 Phoenix Magazine
United Ostomy Association of America
PO Box 512
Northfield, MN 55057
800-826-0826
Fax: 507-645-5168
info@uoaa.org
www.ostomy.org
America's leading ostomy patient magazine providing colostomy, ileostomy, urostomy and continent diversion information, management techniques, new products and much more.
Quarterly
David Rudzin, President

Newsletters

3053 Crohn's Disease, Ulcerative Colitis, and School
Pediatric Crohn's & Colitis Association
PO Box 188
Newton, MA 02468
617-489-5854
questions@pcca.hypermart.net
pcca.hypermart.net
Information on Crohn's Disease and Ulcerative Colitis, including medical, nutritional, psychological and social factors.

3054 IBD File
Crohn's & Colitis Foundation of America
386 Park Avenue S
New York, NY 10016-8804
212-685-3440
800-932-2423
Fax: 212-779-4098
info@ccfa.org
www.ccfa.org

Offers updated information and the latest medical news about Crohn's Disease and Colitis.

3055 Inflammatory Bowel Disease
Gastro-Intestinal Research Foundation
70 E Lake Street
Chicago, IL 60601
312-332-1350
Fax: 312-332-4757
info@girf.org
www.giresearchfoundation.org
Newsletter and patient pamphlet.

3056 Inner Circle
Reach Out for Youth with Ileitis and Colitis
84 Northgate Circle
Melville, NY 11747
516-293-3102
Fax: 516-293-3103
www.rightdiagnosis.com
Provides information to patients with ileitis and colitis and their families.

3057 Inside Story
Reach Out for Youth with Ileitis and Colitis
84 Northgate Circle
Melville, NY 11747
516-293-3102
Fax: 516-293-3103
www.rightdiagnosis.com
Provides information to patients with ileitis and colitis and their families.

Pamphlets

3058 ABC's of Pediatric Inflammatory Bowel Disease
Pediatric Crohn's & Colitis Association
PO Box 188
Newton, MA 02468
617-489-5854
pcca.hypermart.net
Information on Pediatric Inflammatory Disease, including medical, nutritional, psychological and social factors.

3059 CCFA: A Case for Support
Crohn's & Colitis Foundation of America
386 Park Avenue S
New York, NY 10016-8804
212-685-3440
800-932-2423
Fax: 212-779-4098
info@ccfa.org
www.ccfa.org
Reviews the work of the Crohn's and Colitis Foundation of America, sponsors a nationally recognized research program, which seeks to improve treatment and ultimately find the cure for inflammatory bowel disease.

3060 Coping with Crohn's and Colitis is Tough
Crohn's & Colitis Foundation of America
386 Park Avenue S
New York, NY 10016-8804
212-685-3440
800-932-2423
Fax: 212-779-4098
info@ccfa.org
www.ccfa.org
Offers information on the Crohn's and Colitis Association. Also offers factual information and statistics on the diseases.

3061 Crohn's Disease
NDDIC
2 Information Way
Bethesda, MD 20892-0001
301-496-3583
800-891-5389
Fax: 301-907-8906
www.niddk.nih.gov
October 1992

3062 Guide for Children and Teenagers to Crohn's Disease/Ulcerative Colitis
Crohn's & Colitis Foundation of America
386 Park Avenue S
New York, NY 10016-8804
212-685-3440
800-932-2423
Fax: 212-779-4098
info@ccfa.org
www.ccfa.org
Offers important information on these illnesses to children and teens.

3063 Ileostomy Guide
United Ostomy Associations of America, Inc.

PO Box 66
Fairview, TN 37062-0066
800-826-0826
info@uoaa.org
www.ostomy.org

Written for persons who have recently had an ileostomy, this guidebook covers a spectrum of topics including basic facts about ileostomies, information for patients, helpful ideas and practical tips.
28 pages

3064 Questions & Answers About Diet and Nutrition
Crohn's & Colitis Foundation of America
386 Park Avenue S
New York, NY 10016-8804
212-685-3440
800-932-2423
Fax: 212-779-4098
info@ccfa.org
www.ccfa.org

Raises important facts about how diet and nutrition affect persons with Crohn's Disease.

3065 Questions and Answers About Complications
Crohn's & Colitis Foundation of America
386 Park Avenue S
New York, NY 10016-8804
212-685-3440
800-932-2423
Fax: 212-779-4098
info@ccfa.org
www.ccfa.org

Medical facts and complications from surgery.

3066 Questions and Answers About Crohn's Disease & Ulcerative Colitis
Crohn's & Colitis Foundation of America
386 Park Avenue S
New York, NY 10016-8804
212-685-3440
800-932-2423
Fax: 212-779-4098
info@ccfa.org
www.ccfa.org

Offers information on the illness and answers the most frequently asked questions about Crohn's Disease. Also includes a glossary of IBD terms.

3067 Questions and Answers About Emotional Factors in Ileitis and Colitis
Crohn's & Colitis Foundation of America
386 Park Avenue S
New York, NY 10016-8804
212-685-3440
800-932-2423
Fax: 212-779-4098
info@ccfa.org
www.ccfa.org

Answers some of the most commonly asked questions about ileitis and colitis and the role of emotional factors in their cause and course.

3068 Questions and Answers About Pregnancy in Ileitis and Colitis
Crohn's & Colitis Foundation of America
386 Park Avenue S
New York, NY 10016-8804
212-685-3440
800-932-2423
Fax: 212-779-4098
info@ccfa.org
www.ccfa.org

Answers questions about inflammatory bowel disease concerning conception, pregnancy, delivery and nursing.

3069 Questions and Answers About Surgery
Crohn's & Colitis Foundation of America
386 Park Avenue S
New York, NY 10016-8804
212-685-3440
800-343-3637
Fax: 212-779-4098
info@ccfa.org
www.ccfa.org

Answers questions and offers basic facts about surgery for persons suffering from Crohn's Disease and Ulcerative Colitis.

3070 Teacher's Guide to Crohn's Disease and Ulcerative Colitis
Crohn's & Colitis Foundation of America
386 Park Avenue S
New York, NY 10016-8804
212-685-3440
800-932-2423
Fax: 212-779-4098
info@ccfa.org
www.ccfa.org

The purpose of this brochure is to increase the support and encouragement given to young people with Crohn's disease and ulcerative colitis by teachers who understand their illness.

3071 Crohn's Disease, Ulcerative Colitis and Your Child
Crohn's & Colitis Foundation of America
386 Park Avenue S
New York, NY 10016-8804
212-685-3440
800-932-2423
Fax: 212-779-4098
info@ccfa.org; www.ccfa.org

Answers questions about IBD in children, providing information on early signs, growth and developments, treatments and special problems in school.

Web Sites

3072 Crohn's & Colitis Foundation
www.crohnscolitisfoundation.org
CCF's mission is to cure and prevent Crohn's disease and ulcerative colitis through research, and to improve the quality of life of children and adults affected by the disease through education and support. The foundation offers patient and professional support.

3073 Healing Well
www.healingwell.com
An online health resource guide to medical news, chat, information and articles, newsgroups and message boards, books, disease-related web sites, medical directories, and more for patients, friends, and family coping with disabling diseases, disorders, or chronic illnesses.

3074 Health Finder
www.healthfinder.gov
Searchable, carefully developed web site offering information on over 1000 topics. Developed by the US Department of Health and Human Services, the site can be used in both English and Spanish.

3075 Healthlink USA
www.healthlinkusa.com
Health information concerning treatment, cures, prevention, diagnosis, risk factors, research, support groups, email lists, personal stories and much more. Updated regularly.

3076 MedicineNet
www.medicinenet.com
An online resource for consumers providing easy-to-read, authoritative medical and health information.

3077 Medscape
www.medscape.com
Medscape offers specialists, primary care physicians, and other health professionals the Web's most robust and integrated medical information and educational tools.

3078 National Digestive Diseases Information Clearinghouse
www.digestive.niddk.nih.gov
Offers various educational information, resources and reprints focusing on Colitis, Ulcerative Colitis and Crohn's disease.

3079 Pediatric Crohn's and Colitis Association
Focuses on all aspects of pediatric and adolescent Crohn's disease and ulcerative colitis, including medical, nutritional, psychological and social factors. Activities include information sharing, educational forums, newsletters and hospital outreach programs, as well as support of research.

3080 United Ostomy Associations of America, Inc
www.ostomy.org
A national network for bowel and urinary diversion support groups in the United States. Its goal is to provide a non-profit association that will serve to unify and strengthen its member support groups, which are organized for the benefit of people who have, or will have intestinal or urinary diversions and their caregivers.

3081 WebMD
www.webmd.com
Provides credible information, supportive communities, and in-depth reference material about health subjects. A source for original and timely health information as well as material from well known content providers.

Description

3082 Cystic Fibrosis

Cystic fibrosis, CF, is an inherited disease of the exocrine (mucus-producing) glands, primarily affecting the gastrointestinal and respiratory tracts. Cystic fibrosis results from mutations in the CFTR gene, which encodes the cystic fibrosis transmembrane conductance regulator (CFTR). The CFTR protein is a regulator chloride channel and mutations in CFTR lead to the production of suboptimal amounts of functional CFTR or poorly functional CFTR. Without functional CFTR, the cells that line the respiratory airways lack the ability to secrete salt, which further prevents them from secreting water. Poorly hydrated, desiccated secretions become viscous and rubbery and are poorly cleared from the airways and pancreatic ducts. The mucus that should be lubricating the passageways in the lungs and digestive tract instead obstructs them. CF is the most common life-shortening genetic disease in the white population, occurring in 1 in 3,000 white newborns in the United States. Although CF occurs in other ethnic groups, it is far less common (1 in 17,00 African-Americans and 1 in 31,000 Asian Americans).

In the newborn with CF, thick fecal material may cause partial obstruction of the intestine, which then may contort and rupture. Later in life, blockage of secretions from the pancreas results in frequent, foul-smelling, fatty stools, distention of the abdomen and slowed growth. Damage to the lung occurs as thick mucus secretions plug airways. Fifty percent of all patients develop breathing problems marked by a chronic cough, wheezing and repeated lung infections. Blockage of the reproductive tract of males in some cases may render them infertile.

The course of CF is usually determined by the degree to which the lungs are affected and varies greatly from patient to patient. The prognosis is poor, but advances in therapy have helped many survive well into adulthood. New drugs that help the defective CFTR protein properly fold and function have shown remarkable success in some patients (e.g., tezacaftor/ivacaftor and lumacaftor/ivacaftor). Treatment usually includes aggressive use of antibiotics and other drugs to prevent lung complications, physical therapy, adequate nutrition and psychosocial support. Inhaled forms of two antibiotics (tobramycin—Bethkis, and aztreonam—Cayston) have proven quite effective at treating CF-specific respiratory infections.

The first CF gene therapy research began in 1993, and scientists have identified mutations in a CF regulator gene that cause cells to produce abnormally thick mucus. Gene therapy to replace the defective gene with a functional copy is currently under study. Genetic screening is now available.

National Agencies & Associations

3083 Childhood Liver Disease Research Network
340 E. Huron Street   Children-Project-Team@arborresearch.org
Ann Arbor, MI 48104   childrennetwork.org
ChiLDReN works to improve the lives of children and families with rare cholestatic liver diseases, though a network of doctors, nurses, researchers, medical facilities, and support organizations.
Joan M. Hines, MPH, Research Administrator

3084 Cystic Fibrosis Canada
2323 Yonge Street   800-378-2233
Toronto, Ontario, M4P-2C9   www.cysticfibrosis.ca
Non-profit corporation committed to finding a cure for cystic fibrosis through investment in research.
Kelly Grover, President & CEO
John Wallenburg, Chief Scientific Officer

3085 Cystic Fibrosis Worldwide
c/o Cystic Fibrosis Foundation
6931 Arlington Road   301-951-4422
Bethesda, MA 20814   Fax: 301-951-6378
www.cfww.org
CFW is a non-profit organization headquartered in Zurich Switzerland. The purpose and direction of the organization is to assist in improving the quality of life by identifying common problems and attempting to define possible solutions.
Terry Stewart, Board President & CEO
Harry Heijerman, Chief Medical Advisor

Foundations

3086 Cystic Fibrosis Foundation
4550 Montgomery Avenue   301-951-4422
Bethesda, MD 20814   800-344-4823
Fax: 301-951-6378
info@cff.org
www.cff.org
The mission of the Cystic Fibrosis Foundation is to assure the development of the means to cure and control cystic fibrosis and to improve the quality of life for those with the disease.
Preston W. Campbell, III, MD, President & CEO
Marc S. Ginsky, EVP & COO

Libraries & Resource Centers

3087 Children's Hospital of Orange County
455 S Main Street   714-997-3000
Orange, CA 92868-3874   mail@choc.org
www.choc.org
Our mission is to nuture, advance and protect the health and well-being of children.
Kimberly C Cripe, President/CEO

Research Centers

Arizona

3088 Cystic Fibrosis Center: Phoenix Childrens Hospital
1919 E Thomas Road   602-546-1000
Phoenix, AZ 85016   888-908-5437
Fax: 602-460-23
www.phoenixchildrens.com
Robert Meyer, President and Chief Executive Officer
Bruce Morgenstern, Medical Staff President

Arkansas

3089 Arkansas Cystic Fibrosis Center Arkansas Children's Hospital
Arkansas Children's Hospital
1 Children's Way   501-364-1100
Little Rock, AR 72202   Fax: 501-364-3930
TTY: 501-364-1184
pedspulmonary@uams.edu
www.arpediatrics.org

Provide high-quality specialized care to patients from comprehensive diagnosis to ongoing treatment.
John L Carroll, Division Chief
Dennis E Schellhase, Director

California

3090 Children's Hospital of Los Angeles
4650 Sunset Boulevard
Los Angeles, CA 90027
323-660-2450
webmaster@chla.usc.edu
www.childrenshospitalla.org
Provides the highest quality healthcare for children who are the sickest and most seriously injured in our region and beyond.
Richard D Cordova, President/CEO
Rodney B Hanners, Senior Vice President & Chief Operating

3091 Childrens Hospital at Oakland
747 52nd Street
Oakland, CA 94609
510-428-3000
www.childrenshospitaloakland.org
The mission of Children's Hospital Oakland is to ensure the delivery of the highest quality pediatric care for all children through regional primary and subspecialty networks; a strong education and teaching program a diverse workforce state of the art research programs and facilities; and nationally recognized child advocacy efforts.
Bertram Lubin, President and Chief Executive Officer
Kathleen Hogue Gonzalez, Vice President, Research Administration

3092 Cystic Fibrosis Center: Cedars-Sinai Medical Center
Cedars-Sinai Medical Center
8700 Beverly Boulevard
Los Angeles, CA 90048
310-423-3277
800-233-2771
Fax: 310-423-4131
www.cedars-sinai.edu

3093 Cystic Fibrosis Center: University of California at San Francisco
400 Parnassus Avenue
San Francisco, CA 94122-0106
415-353-2961
Fax: 415-476-9278
pulmonary.ucsf.edu
Provides comprehensive evaluation as well as inpatient and outpatient care for patients with cystic fibrosis.
Mary Ellen Kleinhenz, Adult CF Director
Dennis Niels MD, Pediatric CF Director

3094 Cystic Fibrosis Research
2672 Bayshore Parkway
Mountain View, CA 94043
650-404-9975
Fax: 650-404-9981
cfri@cfri.org
www.cfri.org
Cystic Fibrosis Research exists to fund research to provide educational and personal support and spread awareness of Cystic Fibrosis a life threatening genetic disease.
Carroll Jenkins, Executive Director
David Soohoo, Director of Programs

3095 Memorial Miller Children's Hospital Cystic Fibrosis Center
2801 Atlantic Avenue
Long Beach, CA 90806
562-933-2000
Fax: 562-933-8501
enussbaum@memorialcare.org
www.memorialcare.org/miller
provides a multidisciplinary approach to asthma cystic fibrosis sleep disorders and the entire spectrum of chronic and acute lung and airway disorders in children.
Eliezer Nuss, Medical Director
Barry Arbuckle, President

3096 Stanford CF Center Packard Children's Hospital At Stanford
Packard Children's Hospital At Stanford
725 Welch Road
Palo Alto, CA 94304-1601
650-497-8000
cfcenter.stanford.edu
Colleen Dunn, Administrator
Cassie Everson, Research Coordinator

Colorado

3097 Denver Childrens Hospital
1830 Franklin Street
Denver, CO 80218
72-77-136
800-624-6553
Fax: 303-832-9245
TTY: 720-777-9390
www.thechildrenshospital.org
Frank Accurs, Director
Jim Schmerling, President, CEO

Connecticut

3098 University of Connecticut Health Center
263 Farmington Avenue
Farmington, CT 06030-0001
860-679-2000
TTY: 860-679-2242
TDD: 860-679-2242
president@uconn.edu
www.uchc.edu
Philip E Austin, President
Cato T Laurencin, Vice President for Health Affairs

3099 Yale University Cystic Fibrosis Research Center
Yale Pediatrics
333 Cedar Street
New Haven, CT 06510
203-432-4771
sheila.rivera@yale.edu
www.yalepediatrics.org
One of only two in the state of Connecticut the CF Center in the Children's Hospital at the Yale-New Haven Hospital offers a multidisciplinary team approach to provide the most comprehensive state of the art care of CF patients.
Marie Egan, Director
Richard C Levin, President

District of Columbia

3100 Metropolitan DC Cystic Fibrosis Center Children s Hospital National Medical Cen
Children s Hospital National Medical Center
111 Michigan Avenue NW
Washington, DC 20010-2970
202-476-5000
TTY: 800-855-1155
tbear@cnmc.org
www.childrensnational.org
An active clinical and basic science research program that exists within the center.
Roberta Alessi, Senior Vice President
Mark Batshaw, Executive Vice President and Chief Acade

Florida

3101 Cystic Fibrosis Center: All Children's Hospital
Department of Pulmonology
501 6th Street S
Saint Petersburg, FL 33701
727-898-7451
800-456-4543
Fax: 727-767-4218
www.allkids.org
Anthony D Kriseman, Pulmonology
Joseph (Jay) Fleece III, Chair

3102 Miami Childrens Hospital Division of Pulmonology
3100 SW 62nd Avenue
Miami, FL 33155-3309
305-666-6511
800-432-6837
Fax: 305-663-8417
info@mch.com
www.mch.com
Division evaluates and treats many respiratory disorders including asthma chronic lung disease cystic fibrosis pneumonia and tuberculosis. The Division is strongly committed to a multidisciplinary medical approach to these complex disorders.
Moises Simps, Director
M Narendra Kini, President, CEO

3103 Nemours Childrens Clinic
807 Childrens Way
Jacksonville, FL 32207
904-390-3600
Fax: 904-390-3699
www.nemours.org

Nemours Children's Clinic is one integrated multispecialty group practice with locations in four states seeing patients from across the US and the world.
David J Bailey, President, CEO
Robert Bridges, Executive Vice-President

Georgia

3104 Department of Pediatrics Medical College of Georgia
1120 15th Street   706-721-3466
Augusta, GA 30912   Fax: 706-721-7311
Dr William Kanto Jr, Chairperson Pediatrics

3105 Emory University: Cystic Fibrosis Center
201 Dowman Drive   404-727-6123
Atlanta, GA 30322-1028   Fax: 404-727-4828
                                lwolfen@emory.edu
                                www.emory.edu

Lindy Wolfen MD, Director
Jim Wagner, President

Illinois

3106 Comer Children's Hospital at the University of Chicago
5841 S Maryland Avenue   773-702-1000
Chicago, IL 60637   888-824-0200
                                www.uchospitals.edu

3107 Comer Children's Hospital at the Universit
5721 S Maryland Avenue   773-702-1000
Chicago, IL 60637   888-824-0200
                                www.uchicagokidshospital.org
To provide superior healthcare in a compassionate manner ever mindful of each patient's dignity and individuality.

3108 Cystic Fibrosis Center: Childrens Memorial Hospital
2300 Childrens Plaza   773-880-4000
Chicago, IL 60614-3363   800-543-7362
                                www.childrensmemorial.org
The Cystic Fibrosis Center at Children's Memorial Hospital has been a CFF-accredited CF care center since 1963. It is committed to providing exemplary care to each patient and family focused on individualized preventative care active management of lung health and nutrition and patient family education.
Susanna McCo, Director
Patrick M Magoon, President, CEO

3109 Cystic Fibrosis Center: Park Ridge Lutheran General Children's Hospital
Lutheran General Children's Hospital
1775 Dempster Street   847-723-154
Park Ridge, IL 60068   Fax: 847-696-3041
James H Skogsbergh, President, CEO

3110 Loyola University Medical Center: Department of Pediatrics
2160 S 1st Avenue   708-327-9120
Maywood, IL 60153   888-584-7888
                                www.loyolamedicine.org
Vicki Keough, Dean and Professor

3111 Saint Francis Medical Center Peoria Pulmonary Association
530 NE Glen Oak Avenue   309-655-2000
Peoria, IL 61637   www.osfsaintfrancis.org
Dr. Denise Mammolito, President

Indiana

3112 The Riley Cystic Fibrosis Center
1701 North Senate Boulevard   317-962-2000
Indianapolis, IN 46202   800-248-1199
The Riley Cystic Fibrosis Center is the only Cystic Fibrosis Foundation accredited Cystic Fibrosis Center in the state. The Center provides state-of-the-art CF care at Riley and across the state.
Daniel Fink, President, CEO

Iowa

3113 Blank Childrens Hospital Pediatric Pulmonology Clinic
Children's Health Center

1212 Pleasant Street   515-241-6548
Des Moines, IA 50309   www.blankchildrens.org
David Starke, President, CEO
Ken Cheyne, Medical Director

3114 Pediatric Allergy & Pulmonary Division University of Iowa Healthcare
University of Iowa Healthcare
200 Hawkins Drive   319-356-2296
Iowa City, IA 52242   allerpulm@uiowa.edu
                                www.uihealthcare.com/depts/med/pediatric
The Division of Allergy and Pulmonology offers evaluation and management of allergic disorders in children with too many infections and acute and chronic breathing disorders of childhood and adolescence.
Jody Kurtt RN, Director

Kansas

3115 Kansas University Medical Center: Cystic Fibrosis Center
3901 Rainbow Boulevard   913-588-5000
Kansas City, KS 66160   800-332-4199
                                TDD: 913-588-7963
                                gperry@kumc.edu
                                www2.kumc.edu
Barbara F Atkinson, Executive Vice Chancellor

3116 St. Joseph Medical Center Cystic Fibrosis Care and Teaching Center
929 N. St. Francis   316-268-5000
Wichita, KS 67214   Fax: 316-583-90
                                contact@viachristi.org
                                www.viachristi.org
Kay Glasner, Director
Maria Loving, Public Relations Specialist

Kentucky

3117 Kentucky University: Cystic Fibrosis Center
800 Rose Street   859-257-1000
Lexington, KY 40536-0298   800-333-8874
                                Fax: 859-257-7706
                                www.ukhealthcare.uky.edu
The cystic fibrosis team works with more than 175 patients and is dedicated to working with the most advanced therapies to improve the life of every patient.
Jamshed F Kanga, Director
Dr. Michael Karpf, Executive Vice President

3118 Kosair Childrens Cystic Fibrosis Center
Suite 201   502-629-6000
Louisville, KY 40202-2021   www.nortonhealthcare.com
The Cystic Fibrosis Center is one of 120 centers in the United States accredited by the National Cystic Fibrosis Foundation. Specialists provide diagnosis and multidisciplinary care for cystic fibrosis patients of all ages. Professional education and training is also provided.
Nemie Eid, Medical Director
Stephen A Williams, President, CEO

Louisiana

3119 Ernest N Morial Asthma, Allergy & Respiratory Disease Center
Louisiana State University School of Medicine
1901 Perdido Street   504-568-4634
New Orleans, LA 70112-3932   888-695-8647
                                Fax: 504-568-4295
                                www.lsuhsc.edu
Warren R Summer, Director
Larry H. Hollier, President and Chief Operating Officer

Maine

3120 Central Maine Cystic Fibrosis Center
300 Main Street   207-795-0111
Lewiston, ME 04240-7027   Fax: 207-795-2303
                                www.cmhc.org
Ralph V Harder, Director
Peter Chkale, Chief Executive Officer

3121 Maine Medical Center: Cystic Fibrosis Clinical Center
22 Bramhall Street
Portland, ME 04102-3175
207-662-0111
877-339-3107
Fax: 207-775-6024
TTY: 207-662-4900
www.mmc.org
Richard W Peterson, President, CEO

3122 Maine Medical Center: Cystic Fibrosis Clin
22 Bramhall Street
Portland, ME 04102-3175
207-662-0111
877-339-3107
Fax: 207-775-6024
TTY: 207-662-4900
www.mmc.org
Richard W Peterson, President, CEO

Maryland

3123 Cystic Fibrosis Center: National Institute of Health NIDDK
Building 31 Room 9A06
Bethesda, MD 20892-2560
301-496-3583
www2.niddk.nih.gov
Dr Griffin Rodgers, Acting Director

3124 Cystic Fibrosis Foundation
4550 Montgomery Avenue
Bethesda, MD 20814
301-951-4422
800-344-4823
Fax: 301-951-6378
info@cff.org
www.cff.org
The mission of the Cystic Fibrosis Foundation is to assure the development of the means to cure and control cystic fibrosis and to improve the quality of life for those with the disease.
Preston W. Campbell, III, MD, President & CEO
Marc S. Ginsky, EVP & COO

Massachusetts

3125 Baystate Medical Center Wesson Memorial Unit
Wesson Memorial Unit
759 Chestnut Street
Springfield, MA 01199
413-794-0000
Marian.Panto@bhs.org
www.baystatehealth.com
BMC serves as a regional resource for specialty medical care and research while providing comprehensive primary medical services to the community.
Mark R Tolosky, President & Chief Executive Officer
Paula S Dennison, Senior Vice President Human Resources

3126 Childrens Hospital Medical Center Cystic Fibrosis Center
300 Longwood Avenue
Boston, MA 02115
617-355-6000
Fax: 617-730-0373
TTY: 617-730-0152
www.childrenshospital.org
The Cystic Fibrosis Center at Children's Hospital Boston is one of the oldest and largest cystic fibrosis centers in the United States and was founded by Dr. Harry Schwachman one of the earliest physician investigators to help characterize the disorder.
Terry Spence, Director
Sandra Fenwick, President, CEO

3127 Cystic Firbrosis Center: Tufts New England Medical Center
Pediatric Pulmonology and Allergy Department
800 Washington Street
Boston, MA 02111
617-636-5000
www.nemc.org
We strive to heal to comfort to teach to learn and to seek the knowledge to promote health and prevent disease.
Ellen Zane, President and Chief Executive Officer
Margaret Vosburgh, Chief Operating Officer

3128 Massachusetts General Hospital
55 Fruit Street
Boston, MA 02114-2622
617-726-2000
Fax: 617-726-6989
TTY: 617-724-8800
TDD: 617-724-8800
www.massgeneral.org
Peter L Slavin, President
David Torchi, Chairman and Chief Executive Officer

3129 University of Massachusetts Memorial Medical Center
55 Lake Avenue N
Worcester, MA 01655
508-334-1000
www.umassmemorial.org
UMass Memorial Medical Center is the region's trusted academic medical center committed to improving the health of the people of Central New England through excellence in clinical care service teaching and research.
Walter Ettinger, President
George Brenckle, Senior Vice President and Chief Informat

Michigan

3130 East Lansing Cystic Fibrosis Center Michigan State University
Michigan State University
1200 E Michigan Avenue
Lansing, MI 48912
517-364-5440
Fax: 517-364-5413
phd.msu.edu
Eliane F Eakin, Director
H Dele Davies, Department Chair

3131 Kalamazoo Center for Medical Studies Michigan State University
Michigan State University
1000 Oakland Drive
Kalamazoo, MI 49008-1202
269-337-4400
800-275-5267
Fax: 269-337-4234
www.med.wmich.edu
John M. Dunn, Chairman of the Board
Paul A. Spaude, President & CEO

3132 University of Michigan: Cystic Fibrosis Center
A Alfred Taubman Health Care Center
1500 E Medical Center Drive
Ann Arbor, MI 48109-0318
734-936-4000
Fax: 734-936-7635
TTY: 800-649-3777
TDD: 800-649-3777
www.med.umich.edu
Samya Z Nasr, Director
Douglas L Strong, CEO

Minnesota

3133 University of Minnesota: Cystic Fibrosis Center
University of Minnesota Hospital
420 Delaware Street SE
Minneapolis, MN 55455
612-624-0962
800-688-5252
Fax: 612-624-0696
cfcenter@umn.edu
The mission was to develop approaches to understanding and treating the complications of CF.
Warren E Regelmann, Co-Director
Jordan M Dunitz, Co-Director

Mississippi

3134 University of Mississippi Medical Center
2500 N State Street
Jackson, MS 39216-4500
601-984-5046
Fax: 601-984-1973
www.umc.edu
Suzanne Mill, Director
Daniel W Jones, Chancellor

Missouri

3135 Children's Mercy Hospital Children's Mercy Hospitals & Clinics
Children's Mercy Hospitals & Clinics
2401 Gilham Road
Kansas City, MO 64108
816-234-3000
866-512-2168
Fax: 816-842-6107
TTY: 816-234-3816
webmaster@cmh.edu
www.childrensmercy.org
Children's Mercy Hospital provides the highest level of medical care technology services equipment and facilities in promoting the health and well-being of children in the region from birth through adolescence.
Randall L O'Donnell PhD, President/CEO
V Fred Burry, Executive Medical Director/Executive Vic

3136 University of Missouri Columbia Cystic Fibrosis Center
University of Missouri/Dept of Child Health

One Hospital Drive N712
Columbia, MO 65212-1
573-882-6882
Fax: 573-821-54
clarksonb@health.missouri.edu
www.ch.missouri.edu/cysticfibrosis.htm
Peter Konig, Director
Melissa Lawson, Division Director

3137 Washington University: Cystic Fibrosis Center
St. Louis Children's Hospital
660 S Euclid Avenue
Saint Louis, MO 63110
314-454-2694
888-678-4357
Fax: 314-454-2515
www.medschool.wustl.edu/
Dedicated to the treatment of patients with cystic fibrosis (CF) for more than 4 decades. The Cystic Fibrosis Clinical Center and affiliated programs has developed into a premier clinical and research program.
Thomas Ferko, Director

Nebraska

3138 University of Nebraska Medical Center Cystic Fibrosis Center
The Nebraska Medical Center
Omaha, NE 68198-5190
402-552-2000
800-922-0000
Fax: 402-559-7062
necfcntr@unmc.edu
www.unmc.edu
Harold M Maurer, Chancellor
Hari Bandla, Associate Professor

Nevada

3139 Children's Lung Specialists
3838 Meadow Lane
Las Vegas, NV 89107
702-598-4411
Fax: 702-598-1988
The certified Cystic Fibrosis Center of Southern Nevada.
Ruben MD, Director/President/Owner
Craig Nakamu, Assistant Director

New Hampshire

3140 New Hampshire Cystic Fibrosis Care Teaching and Research Center
DarthmouthHitchcock Medical Center
One Medical Center Drive
Lebanon, NH 03756
603-650-5000
Fax: 603-500-07
TTY: 603-650-8034
www.dhmc.org
William Boyl, Director
Dennis Stoke, Director

New Jersey

3141 Monmouth Medical Center: Cystic Fibrosis & Pediatric Pulmonary Center
Monmouth Medical Center
95 Old Short Hills Road
West Orange, NJ 7052
732-222-5200
888-724-7123
Fax: 908-222-4472
info@sbhcs.com
www.sbhcs.com
Peri Kamalakar, Director of Pediatric Hematology/Oncolog

3142 Monmouth Medical Center: Cystic Fibrosis & Monmouth Medical Center
368 Lakehurst Road
Toms River, NJ 08755
732-222-5200
888-724-7123
Fax: 908-222-4472
www.sbhcs.com
Peri Kamalakar, Director of Pediatric Hematology/Oncolog

3143 New Jersey Medical School
185 S Orange Avenue
Newark, NJ 07101-1709
973-972-4595
Fax: 973-972-5965
The mission of New Jersey Medical School is to educate students physicians and scientists to meet society's current and future healthcare needs through patient-centered education; pioneering

research; innovative clinical rehabilitative and preventive care; and collaborative community outreach.
Maria L. Soto-Greene, MD, Vice Dean
Robert L Johnson MD, Dean

New York

3144 Albany Medical College Pediatric Pulmonary & Cystic Fibrosis Center
Department of Pediatrics
43 New Scotland Avenue
Albany, NY 12208
518-262-3125
877-262-8008
Fax: 518-262-6884
www.amc.edu
Scott Scroed, Division Chief

3145 Armond V Mascia Cystic Fibrosis Center NY Medical College
Division of Pediatrics Pulmonology
New York Medical College
Valhalla, NY 10595
914-594-4000
Fax: 914-594-4336
pedpulm@nymc.edu
Provides comprehensive inpatient and outpatient consultation and management for children suffering from a broad variety of respiratory problems. They are the only accredited Cystic Fibrosis center in the Hudson Valley. The center is dedicated to teaching research and patient care.
Allen Dozer, Chief
Karl P Alder MD, President, CEO

3146 CF & Pediatric Pulmonary Care Center
Mount Sinai Hospital
One Gustave L Levy Place
New York, NY 10029-6574
212-241-6500
800-637-4624
Fax: 212-876-3255
www.mountsinai.org
Center staff perform outpatient and inpatient consultations with an integrated multidisciplinary team of professionals who are dedicated specifically to the practice of Pediatric Pulmonary Medicine.
Dennis S Charney, Dean, Executive Vice President

3147 Childrens Lung and Cystic Fibrosis Center
Women and Children's Hospital of Buffalo
140 Hodge Avenue
Buffalo, NY 14222-2099
716-878-7000
Fax: 716-888-3945
www.wchob.org
Services for infants children and teenagers with cystic fibrosis and other chronic respiratory conditions.
Annise Taylor, Manager
Cheryl Klass, President

3148 Cystic Fibrosis Center St. Vincent's Hospital & Medical Center
St. Vincent's Hospital & Medical Center of NY
36 7th Avenue
New York, NY 10011-6600
212-604-8895
Fax: 212-604-3899
www.svcmc.org
Maria Berdel, Co-Director
Patricia Wal MD, Co-Director

3149 Pulomonolgy Morgan Stanley Children's Hospital
Morgan Stanley Children's Hospital
3959 Broadway
New York, NY 10032-3702
212-305-5437
877-NYP-WELL
www.childrensnyp.org
Meyer Kattan, Director

3150 State University of NY Hospital: Upstate Medical Center
750 E Adams Street
Syracuse, NY 13210-1834
315-464-5540
877-464-5540
TDD: 315-464-5769
www.upstate.edu/uh
Stephen R Goodman, Vice President
David R. Smith, President

North Carolina

3151 UNC Cystic Fibrosis Center Department of Pediatrics
Department of Pediatrics
7011 Thurston-Bowles Building
Chapel Hill, NC 27599-7248
919-966-1077
Fax: 919-966-7524

A large multidisciplinary group focused on the pathogenesis and other lung diseases.
Richard C Boucher, Director
Margaret Lei, Director

3152 Western Michigan University School of Medi cine
350 Hanes House
Durham, NC 27710
919-684-3364
888-275-3853
Fax: 919-684-2292
Provides primary and consultative care for patients with various lung diseases on an inpatient and outpatient basis.
Monica Kraft, Division Chief
Gina Brewer, Administrative Assistant

North Dakota

3153 St. Alexius Medical Heart and Lung Clinic
900 E Broadway Avenue
Bismarck, ND 58501
701-530-7000
877-530-5550
Fax: 701-530-8984
TTY: 701-530-5555
TDD: 701-530-5555
www.st.alexius.org
Specializes in services such as cardiac consultation cardiac surgery cardiac catheterization electrophysiology angioplasty intracoronary stents rotoblade asthma emphysema cystic fibrosis chronic lung disease. lung cancer allergy and anesthesia.
John Castleberry, Chair
Sr. Nancy Miller, OSB, President

Ohio

3154 Case Western Reserve University: Cystic Fibrosis Center
10900 Euclid Avenue
Cleveland, OH 44106-2624
216-368-2000
Fax: 216-844-5916
Mds11@case.edu
www.case.edu
Barbara Snyder, President

3155 Columbus Children's Hospital: Cystic Fibrosis Center
700 Childrens Drive
Columbus, OH 43205-0296
614-722-2000
Fax: 614-722-4755
www.nationwidechildrens.org
Dr Steve Allen, CEO
Elizabeth D Allen, Physician

3156 Lewis H Walker MD: Cystic Fibrosis Center
Children's Hospital Medical Center of Akron
One Perkins Square
Akron, OH 44308-1062
330-543-1000
800-262-0333
TTY: 330-543-8080
www.akronchildrens.org/respiratory
One of six CF centers in the state of Ohio providing comprehensive care for patients who suffer from this disease. The center which is part of the Robert T. Stone Respiratory Center actively participates in clinical trials to research new drug therapies to manage cystic fibrosis.
Nathan Krayn, Director Cystic Fibrosis Center
William H Considine, President, CEO

3157 Pediatric Pulmonary Center The Children's Medical Center of Dayton
The Children's Medical Center of Dayton
1 Children's Plaza
Dayton, OH 45404-1815
937-641-3000
800-228-4055
Fax: 937-641-4500
www.childrensdayton.org
David Kinsaul, President, CEO
Robert Fink, Medical Director

3158 University of Cincinnati College of Medicine Division of Pediatrics
Children s Hospital Medical Center
3333 Burnet Avenue
Cincinnati, OH 45229-3039
513-636-4200
800-344-2462
Fax: 513-636-0345
TTY: 513-636-4900
thomas.boat@cchmc.org
www.cincinnatichildrens.org

The University of Cincinnati Department of Pediatrics consists entirely of staff members from Cincinnati Children's Hospital Medical Center one of the nation's leading pediatric research and teaching institutions.
Michael Fisher, President, CEO
Thomas F Boat, Professor of Pediatrics

Oklahoma

3159 University of Oklahoma: Cystic Fibrosis Center
Department of Pediatrics
940 NE 13th Street
Oklahoma City, OK 73104
405-271-4401
Fax: 405-271-8710
brenda-freese@ouhsc.edu
www.oumedicine.com
James A Royall, Professor/Chief Pediatric Pulmonology
Terrence L Stull MD, Chairman

Oregon

3160 Oregon Health & Science University
3181 SW Sam Jackson Park Road
Portland, OR 97239-3098
503-494-8311
www.ohsuhealth.com
Oregon Health & Science University is a leading health and research university that strives for excellence in patient care education research and community service.
Joseph Rober, President
Steven D Stadum, Executive Vice President

Pennsylvania

3161 Cystic Fibrosis Center: Polyclinic Medical Center
Polyclinic Medical Center
PO Box 8700
Harrisburg, PA 17105-8700
717-231-8900
800-334-1007
Fax: 717-782-4679
www.pinnaclehealth.org
Muttiah Gane, Director
Michael A Young, FACHE, President/CEO

3162 Pediatric Pulmonary and Cystic Fibrosis Center
St. Christopher's Hospital for Children
3601 A Street
Philadelphia, PA 19134
215-427-5000
888-STC-RIS
Fax: 215-427-5555
www.stchristophershospital.com
A team of pediatric pulmonary medicine experts treats children with a wide range of acute and chronic lung diseases such as cystic fibrosis bronchopulmonary dysplasia apnea respiratory infections bronchiolitis congenital malformations including chest wall deformities and pneumonia.
Laurie Varlo, Director

3163 University of Pennsylvania: Penn Lung Center
Hospital of The University of Pennsylvania
3 Ravdin Suite F
Philadelphia, PA 19104
215-662-4000
800-789-7366
www.pennhealth.com
Penn Lung Center of the University of Pennsylvania Health System is a multidisciplinary resource for consultation second opinion diagnosis and ongoing treatment of patients with lung disease.
Leslie A Litzky, Associate Professor of Pathology and Lab
Maryl Kreide, Assistant Professor of Medicine

3164 University of Pittsburgh Cystic Fibrosis Center: Children's Hospital
Department of Cell Biology And Physiology
S362 BST
Pittsburgh, PA 15261
412-648-9362
Fax: 412-648-8330
cdpweb@pitt.edu
The primary goal of the Center is to focus the attention of new and established investigators on multidisciplinary approaches designed to improve the understanding and treatment of cystic fibrosis (CF).
Raymond A Frizzell, Director
Carol A Bertrand, Research Assistant Professor

3165 Rhode Island Hospital: Cystic Fibrosis Center
Department of Pediatrics
593 Eddy Street   401-444-4000
Providence, RI 02903   Fax: 401-444-2168
                                                         www.lifespan.org

Michael S Schechter, Director
George A Vecchione, President, CEO

South Carolina

3166 Medical University of South Carolina: Cystic Fibrosis Center
171 Ashley Avenue   803-792-1414
Charleston, SC 29403   800-424-6872
                                                         Fax: 843-876-1435
                                                  www.musc.edu/cfcenter
The objectives of the Cystic Fibrosis Center at MUSC are to offer unsurpassed care to patients with cystic fibrosis to teach medical students house staff medical care providers and general public about cystic fibrosis and to learn about cystic fibrosis through clinical and laboratory research.
Isabel Virella-Lowell, MD, Director
W Stuart Smith, Vice President, Executive Director

Tennessee

3167 Memphis Cystic Fibrosis Center LeBonheur Children's Medical Center
LeBonheur Children's Medical Center
848 Adams Ave   901-287-5437
Memphis, TN 38103   info@lebonheur.org
                                                      www.lebonheur.org

Meri Armour, President, CEO

3168 Vanderbilt Children's Hospital
2200 Childrens Way   615-936-1000
Nashville, TN 37232   866-936-7811
                                              www.vanderbiltchildrens.com
Children's Hospital provides top-level care while including the family as an essential element of a child's treatment plan.
Luke Gregory, Chief Executive Officer
Jonathan Gitlin, Vice Chancellor

Texas

3169 Cook Children's Medical Center: Cystic Fibrosis Clinic
4214 Andrews Highway   432-570-5693
Midland, TX 79701   www.cookchildrens.org
James C Cunningham MD, Director
Paula Webb, Vice President of Nursing Services

3170 Cystic Fibrosis Care and Teaching Center Children's Medical Center
Children's Medical Center
1935 Medical District Dr   214-456-7000
Dallas, TX 75235   Fax: 214-456-2563
                                                      www.childrens.com
The Dallas Cystic Fibrosis Care and Teaching Center manages the outpatient and inpatient care of approximately 400 infants children adolescents and adults.
Claude Prest MD, Director
Brenda Urbanczyk, Practice Administrator

3171 Cystic Fibrosis-Lung Disease Center: Santa Rosa Children's Hospital
CHRISTUS Center for Children and Families
333 N Santa Rosa   210-704-2011
San Antonio, TX 78207   Fax: 210-704-2651
                                                    www.santarosahealth.org
Serving more than 150 000 children each year CSRCH is a 200-plus bed facility and is the only academic Children's hospital in San Antonio partnering with The University of Texas Health Science Center at San Antonio while collaborating with private pediatricians to provide comprehensive pediatric services at one location since 1959.
Donna Beth Willey-Courand MD, Director
Patrick Carrier, President, CEO

3172 Texas Childrens Cystic Fibrosis Care Center
Texas Children's Clinical Care Center
6701 Fannin Street   832-824-1000
Houston, TX 77030   800-364-5437
                                                      Fax: 832-825-3072
                                              www.texaschildrenshospital.org
Provides comprehensive clinical services to help patients families and referring physicians deal with the many problems cystic fibrosis causes.
Mark A. Wallace, President and Chief Executive Officer
Dr. Mark Kline, Physician-in-Chief

3173 Tri-Services Military Cystic Fibrosis Center
Brooke Army Medical Center/Pediatrics Department
3851 Roger Brooke Drive   210-916-3400
Fort Sam Houston, TX 78234-6320   Fax: 210-916-3076
COL Ted Cieslak, Chief of Pediatrics
Joseph Caravalho, Commanding Officer

Utah

3174 University of Utah Intermountain Cystic Fibrosis Center
University Hospital & Clinics
50 N. Medical Drive   801-581-2121
Salt Lake City, UT 84132   800-824-2073
                                                      Fax: 801-585-5350
                                                      www.med.utah.edu
Barbara A Chatfield MD, Director Pediatric Program
Loris Betz, Senior VP, Executive Dean

Vermont

3175 Medical Center Hospital of Vermont Cystic Fibrosis Center
Cystic Fibrosis Center
111 Colchester Avenue   802-847-0000
Burlington, VT 05401-7152   800-358-1144
                                                      Fax: 802-555-2323

Tom Lahiri MD, Director
Melinda L Estes, President, CEO

Virginia

3176 Eastern Virginia Medical School Children's Hospital of The King's Daught
Children's Hospital of The King's Daughters
601 Children's Lane   757-668-7000
Norfolk, VA 23507   healthinfo@chkd.org
                                                         www.chkd.org

Provider of quality children's health services
James D. Dahling, President and Chief Executive Officer
Kathy Abshire, Vice President, Finance

3177 University of Virginia School of Medicine Cystic Fibrosis Center
Department of Pediatrics
PO Box 800793   434-924-2250
Charlottesville, VA 22908   800-251-3627
                                                      Fax: 434-243-6618
                                              www.healthsystem.virginia.edu
Comprehensive care for children and adults with cystic fibrosis.
Steven T DeKosky MD, Vice President, Dean
Sharon L Hostler, Senior Associate Dean

Washington

3178 University of Washington: Cystic Fibrosis Center
University of Washington Medical Center/Adult Prog
1959 NE Pacific Street   206-598-6116
Seattle, WA 98195   Fax: 206-598-4610
                                                      www.washington.edu
UW Medicine works to improve the health of the public by advancing medical knowledge
Ronald Gibson, Center Director
Ronald Gibson, Professor and Center Director

West Virginia

3179 West Virginia University Cystic Fibrosis Center
Pediatrics Department

PO Box 9214
Morgantown, WV 26506-9214
304-293-1201
Fax: 304-293-1216
kmoffett@hsc.wvu.edu
www.hsc.wvu.edu

The Hospital providing the full range of services including allergy/immunology cardiology child development critical care cystic fibrosis endocrinology adolescent medicine gastroenterology genetics and metabolic disease hematology/oncology neonatology nephrology neurology and apnea evaluation. Services provided by faculty with joint appointments include ophthalmology urology orthopedics psychiatry surgery and cardiothoracic surgery.

Kathryn S Moffett MD, Director
Giovanni Piedimonte, Chair

Wisconsin

3180   Medical College of Wisconsin: Cystic Fibrosis Clinic
Children's Hospital of Wisconsin
PO Box 1997
Milwaukee, WI 53201-1997
414-266-2000
877-266-8989
www.chw.org

Children's Hospital and Health System is an independent health care system dedicated solely to the health and well-being of children.

Robert Kliegman MD, Executive VP
Peter J Bartz, Cardiology Pediatric

3181   University of Wisconsin-Madison: Cystic Fibrosis/Pulmonary Center
Clinical Science Center
600 Highland Avenue
Madison, WI 53792
608-263-6400
800-323-8942
www.uwhealth.org

UW Health represents the academic medical care providers of the University of Wisconsin-Madison and its affiliated organizations.

Michael J Rock, Faculty
Prasad S Dalvie, Radiology

Support Groups & Hotlines

3182   National Health Information Center
Office of Disease Prevention & Health Promotion
1101 Wootton Pkwy
Rockville, MD 20852
Fax: 240-453-8281
odphpinfo@hhs.gov
www.health.gov/nhic

Supports public health education by maintaining a calendar of National Health Observances; helps connect consumers and health professionals to organizations that can best answer questions and provide up-to-date contact information from reliable sources; updates on a yearly basis toll-free numbers for health information, Federal health clearinghouses and info centers.

Don Wright, MD, MPH, Director

Books

3183   Cystic Fibrosis: A Guide for Patient and Family
Raven Press
1185 Ave of the Americas
New York, NY 10036-2601
212-930-9500
800-777-2295
253 pages Softcover
ISBN: 0-397516-53-3

3184   Understanding Cystic Fibrosis
Karen Hopkin, PhD, author
University Press of Mississippi
3825 Ridgewood Road
Jackson, MS 39211-6492
601-432-6205
Fax: 601-432-6217
kburgess@ihl.state.ms.us
www.upress.state.ms.us

A useful guide for families and patients.
1998 128 pages Paperback
ISBN: 0-878059-67-9
Kathy Burgess, Advertising/Marketing Services Manager

Children's Books

3185   Give Me One Wish
Norton Publishers
500 5th Avenue
New York, NY 10110-0002
212-354-5500
800-233-4830
www.scholastic.com/

This book reads like a novel because it re-enacts the author's daughter's bout with cystic fibrosis.
Grades 10-12

3186   Robyn's Book: A True Diary
Scholastic
730 Broadway
New York, NY 10003-9511
212-505-3000
800-325-6149

This book chronicles the life of the author and her battle with cystic fibrosis.
Grades 7-12

3187   Toothpick
Holiday
40 E 49th Street
New York, NY 10017-1105
212-688-0085

This book uses relationships between two different teenagers to parallel the life of a person with cystic fibrosis.
Grades 6-9

Newsletters

3188   Better Breathing Bulletin
American Lung Association of Connecticut
45 Ash Street
East Hartford, CT 06108-3294
860-289-5401
800-586-4872
Fax: 860-289-5405
www.alact.org

This newsletter is aimed at persons with chronic lung problems.
John E Zinn, President/CEO

3189   Commitment
Cystic Fibrosis Foundation
6931 Arlington Road
Bethesda, MD 20814-5231
301-951-4422
800-344-4823
Fax: 301-951-6378
info@cff.org
www.cff.org

Offers general information on cystic fibrosis, fund-raising features, public policy and news from across the nation on cystic fibrosis.

Pamphlets

3190   Consumer Fact Sheet
Cystic Fibrosis Foundation
6931 Arlington Road
Bethesda, MD 20814-5231
301-951-4422
800-344-4823
Fax: 301-951-6378
info@cff.org
www.cff.org

Offers a brief introduction to cystic fibrosis, symptoms, causes, treatments and offers illustrations pertaining to drainage positions.

3191   Cystic Fibrosis: A Guide for Parents
American Lung Association
1740 Broadway
New York, NY 10019-4315
212-315-8700

Comprehensive booklet covering topics such as treatment, social aspects, inheritance, genetics and outlook for the future.
24 pages

3192   For Adults with Cystic Fibrosis: Facts on Reproduction
National Maternal and Child Health Clearinghouse
2070 Chain Bridge Road
Vienna, VA 22182-2588
703-442-9051
888-275-4772
Fax: 703-821-2098
ask@hrsa.gov
www.ask.hrsa.gov

The purpose of this booklet is to review the reproductive issues that are unique to individuals with cystic fibrosis.

3193 Foundation Facts
Cystic Fibrosis Foundation
6931 Arlington Road   301-951-4422
Bethesda, MD 20814-5231   800-344-4823
Fax: 301-951-6378
info@cff.org
www.cff.org

Offers information on the fund-raising and grants offered and supported by the foundation.

3194 Here's Everything You'll Need to Save Money with the CFF Health Services
CFF Home Health & Pharmacy Services
6931 Arlington Road   800-342-6967
Bethesda, MD 20814-5223   Fax: 800-233-3504

Offers information on the Cystic Fibrosis Foundation's home health services.

3195 Home Line
Cystic Fibrosis Foundation
6931 Arlington Road   301-951-4422
Bethesda, MD 20814-5231   800-344-4823
Fax: 301-951-6378
info@cff.org
www.cff.org

Offers information on services and programs offered by the foundation.

Audio & Video

3196 Alex: The Life of a Child
Cystic Fibrosis Foundation
6931 Arlington Road   301-951-4422
Bethesda, MD 20814   800-344-4823
Fax: 301-951-6378
info@cff.org
www.cff.org

The story of Alexandra Deford, a young girl who lost her battle with CF at the age of 8, has touched the hearts of millions and has helped to put a face to this disease. Alex's courage and strength is a true inspiration, and in the decades since her death, much progress has been made in the fight against CF. VHS only.
1986 1 Hr 35 Minutes
Robert J Beall, PhD, President/CEO

3197 Embers of the Fire
Mary Kondrat, author
Fanlight Productions
4196 Washington Street   617-469-4999
Boston, MA 02131-1731   800-937-4113
Fax: 617-469-3379
fanlight@fanlight.com
www.fanlight.com

Offers a straight forward explanation of the disease with a primary focus on the stories of several courageous young people with cystic fibrosis during a week at summer camp. Addresses their fears of rejection, isolation and death while demonstrating the ways they have learned to lead fulfilling lives.
1992 28 Minutes
ISBN: 1-572950-98-6

3198 Expanding the Horizon of Hope: 50 Years of Progress
Cystic Fibrosis Foundation
6931 Arlington Road   301-951-4422
Bethesda, MD 20814   800-344-4823
Fax: 301-951-6378
info@cff.org
www.cff.org

This film highlights the progress that has been made in CF research and care over the past 50 years, as well as the challenges that still lie ahead. It pays tribute to all who are involved in the CF effort—from researchers and clinicians, to patients and their families, to volunteers, donors and staff. DVD only.
2005 60 Minutes
Robert J Beall, PhD, President/CEO

3199 Faces of Cystic Fibrosis
Cystic Fibrosis Foundation
6931 Arlington Road   301-951-4422
Bethesda, MD 20814   800-344-4823
Fax: 301-951-6378
info@cff.org
www.cff.org

Through the words of people with CF and their family members, hear the story of how the fight against CF has evolved into a story of hope and optimism that was never possible before...and how none of this would be possible without the dedication and efforts of volunteers. Available in VHS/DVD.
2001 11 Minutes
Robert J Beall, PhD, President/CEO

3200 Information About the Sweat Test
Cystic Fibrosis Foundation
6931 Arlington Road   301-951-4422
Bethesda, MD 20814   800-344-4823
Fax: 301-951-6378
info@cff.org
www.cff.org

See and hear some basic information about the sweat test, the standard diagnostic test for CF. It is intended to help families better understand the sweat testing procedure and what to expect when the test is conducted. VHS only.
3.47 Minutes
Robert J Beall, PhD, President/CEO

Web Sites

3201 Healing Well
www.healingwell.com
An online health resource guide to medical news, chat, information and articles, newsgroups and message boards, books, disease-related web sites, medical directories, and more for patients, friends, and family coping with disabling diseases, disorders, or chronic illnesses.

3202 Health Finder
www.healthfinder.gov
Searchable, carefully developed web site offering information on over 1000 topics. Developed by the US Department of Health and Human Services, the site can be used in both English and Spanish.

3203 Healthlink USA
www.healthlinkusa.com
Health information concerning treatment, cures, prevention, diagnosis, risk factors, research, support groups, email lists, personal stories and much more. Updated regularly.

3204 MedicineNet
www.medicinenet.com
An online resource for consumers providing easy-to-read, authoritative medical and health information.

3205 Medscape
www.medscape.com
Medscape offers specialists, primary care physicians, and other health professionals the Web's most robust and integrated medical information and educational tools.

3206 WebMD
www.webmd.com
Provides credible information, supportive communities, and in-depth reference material about health subjects. A source for original and timely health information as well as material from well known content providers.

Description

3207 Diabetes Mellitus

Diabetes mellitus is a condition in which the body fails to produce sufficient quantities of insulin to control its own blood glucose (sugar) level (type 1 diabetes mellitus) or fails to properly respond to the insulin it makes (type 2 diabetes mellitus). Ordinarily, the pancreas releases enough of insulin to induce the body's cells to absorb and metabolize glucose. In Type I diabetes (formerly called juvenile-onset diabetes, which affects about 10 percent of diabetic patients), damage to the pancreas and destruction of the insulin-producing beta cells causes cessation of insulin production. In Type II, commonly affecting obese individuals older than 40, the pancreas might release normal, reduced, or even elevated levels of insulin, but the body's cells are resistant to the insulin's action. In either case, blood glucose levels rise (hyperglycemia) until sugar begins to appear in the urine. The patient may experience excessive thirst and urination, hunger, weakness and weight loss. In extreme cases, particularly in type 1 diabetics, when their blood sugar is extremely high and they have insufficient levels of insulin to metabolize it, the patient will begin to degrade stored fat and form B-keto acids known as "ketone bodies." Excessive production of ketone bodies can acidify the blood, cause excessive dehydration, and electrolyte imbalances. This condition, known as diabetic ketoacidosis, can cause coma, and, if it remains untreated, death. Long-term complications include anincreased risk of coronary heart disease and other vascular diseases, such as stroke, vision loss and kidney failure, and peripheral neuropathy.

Type I diabetes mellitus appears to be caused by a genetic predisposition that may express itself after an acute insult to the pancreas, often a viral infection. Genetic factors are also important in Type II diabetes which runs strongly in families. It is much more common in obese people, as well as among African-Americans, Hispanics and Native Americans.

Prevention of acute and long-term complications requires careful management including maintaining the proper diet and exercise, blood glucose monitoring and medications. Thorough education of the patient and relevant family members is absolutely critical.

Some individuals with Type II diabetes can control their disease through diet, exercise and weight loss alone. Some will have to take oral medications that help the pancreas make more insulin, sensitizes the body to insulin, or improves the response of the pancreas to blood sugar. Some Type II diabetics, and all Type I diabetics, need to inject themselves with insulin. Research has shown that tight control of diabetes through frequent blood testing and proper adjustment of the dosage of insulin is most beneficial. Insulin is generally given in multiple injections throughout the day, with preparations varying by length of effectiveness. Insulins are either rapid-acting (peak effect at 0.5-1.5 hr peak), regular insulin (peak effect at 2-4 hrs), intermediate insulin (peak at 6-10 hrs) and peakless, long-acting insulins (24-42 hours). Tightest control of glucose levels is achieved by giving insulin through a continuously-connected insulin pump that disperses rapid-acting insulin. With the advent of constant glucose monitors and the software to display such read-outs on personal electronic devices like cell phones (e.g., Dexcom), patients can integrate their insulin delivery through an insulin pump with their blood sugar readings. Such technology can provide very tight blood sugar control. Pancreas transplantation is considered only for patients who also need some other organ, generally a kidney.

National Agencies & Associations

3208 American Association of Diabetes Educators

200 W Madison Street
Chicago, IL 60606

800-338-3633
media@aadenet.org
www.diabeteseducator.org

An independent, multidisciplinary organization of health professionals involved in teaching persons with diabetes. The mission is to enhance the competence of health professionals who teach persons with diabetes and advance the specialty practice of diabetes.
Charles Macfarlane, Chief Executive Officer
Crystal Broj, Chief Technology and Innovation Officer

3209 American Diabetes Association

2451 Crystal Drive
Arlington, VA 22202

888-342-2383
askada@diabetes.org
www.diabetes.org

Voluntary organization concerned with diabetes and its complications. The mission of the organization is to prevent and cure diabetes and to improve the lives of persons with diabetes. Offers a network of offices nationwide.
Tracey D. Brown, MBA, BChE, Chief Executive Officer
Eloise Scavella, MA, Chief Operating & Strategy Officer

3210 Diabetes Action Network for the Blind

1501 Langford Road
Gwynn Oak, MD 21207

410-215-8587
Fax: 410-685-5653
bernienfb75@gmail.com
www.nfb.org

DAN is a division of the National Federation of the Blind. It is a support and information organization of persons losing vision due to diabetes. Provides personal contact and resource information with other blind diabetics about non-visual techniques of independently managing diabetes and monitoring glucose levels.
Bernadette M Jacobs, President

3211 National Certification Board for Diabetes Educators

330 E Algonquin Road
Arlington Heights, IL 60005

847-228-9795
877-239-3233
Fax: 847-228-8469
info@ncbde.org
www.ncbde.org

The Board for Diabetes Educators is dedicated to promoting excellence in the field of diabetes education through the development, maintenance, and protection of the certified Diabetes Educator credential and the certification process.
Leonard Sanders, Chair
Sheryl Traficano, Chief Executive Officer

3212 **National Institute of Diabetes & Digestive & Kidney Diseases**
Office Of Communications and Public Liaison, NIH
31 Center Drive 800-860-8747
Bethesda, MD 20892-2560 TTY: 866-569-1162
healthinfo@niddk.nih.gov
www.niddk.nih.gov
Research areas include diabetes, digestive diseases, endocrine and metabolic diseases, hematologic diseases, kidney disease, liver disease, urologic diseases, as well as matters relating to nutrition and obesity.
Griffin P. Rodgers, MD, MACP, Director
Gregory Germino, MD, Deputy Director

State Agencies & Associations

Alabama

3213 **American Diabetes Association: Alabama**
3918 Montclair Road 205-870-5172
Birmingham, AL 35213 888-DIA-BETE
Fax: 205-879-2903
acasey@diabetes.org
www.diabetes.org
Aimee Casey, Executive Director
Stephanie Willis, Director

3214 **Juvenile Diabetes Research Foundation: Birmingham**
14 Office Park Circle 205-871-0333
Birmingham, AL 35223 Fax: 205-871-0355
www.jdrf.org/alabama
Karin Scott, Executive Director
Sarah Hendren, Special Events Manager

Alaska

3215 **American Diabetes Association: Alaska**
801 W Fireweed Lane 907-272-1424
Anchorage, AK 99503 888-DIA-BETE
Fax: 907-272-1428
mcassano@diabetes.org
www.diabetes.org
Michelle Cassano, Executive Director
Phoebe O'Connell, Manager

Arizona

3216 **American Diabetes Association: Arizona**
8125 N 23rd Avenue 602-861-4731
Phoenix, AZ 85021 Fax: 602-995-1344
www.diabetes.org
Edyth Haro, Manager
Lynda Brown, Special Events Manager

3217 **American Diabetes Association: Arizona, Border Area**
333 W Ft Lowell Rd 520-795-3711
Tucson, AZ 85705 888-DIA-BETE
Fax: 520-795-1179
fgomez@diabetes.org
www.diabetes.org
Fred Gomez, Executive Director
Heidi Goldsmith, Manager

3218 **American Diabetes Association: Atlanta Met**
8125 N 23rd Avenue 602-861-4731
Phoenix, AZ 85021 Fax: 602-995-1344
kbisko@diabetes.org
www.diabetes.org
Karen Bisko, Executive Director
Suzanne Miller, Director

3219 **American Diabetes Association: Northern Arizona**
5333 N 7th Street 602-861-4731
Phoenix, AZ 85014 Fax: 602-995-1344
llandon@diabetes.org
www.diabetes.org
Laura Landon, Executive Director
Suzanne Miller, Programs Director

3220 **Juvenile Diabetes Research Foundation: Phoenix Chapter**
4343 E Camelback Road 602-224-1800
Phoenix, AZ 85018 Fax: 602-224-1801
desertsouthwest@jdrf.org
www.jdrf.org/arizona
Marci Zimmerman, Executive Director
Valerie Jones, Associate Executive Director

Arkansas

3221 **American Diabetes Association: Arkansas**
320 Executive Court 501-221-7444
Little Rock, AR 72205 888-DIA-BETE
Fax: 501-221-3138
rselig@diabetes.org
www.diabetes.org
Rick Selig, Director
Charlotte Williams, Associate Manager

3222 **Juvenile Diabetes Research Foundation: Northwest Arkansas Branch**
4241 Gabel Dr 479-443-9190
Fayetteville, AR 72703 Fax: 479-443-2692
nwarkansas@jdrf.org
www.nwark.jdrf.org
Deb Euculano, Special Events Manager

California

3223 **American Diabetes Association: California**
2720 Gateway Oaks Drive 916-924-3232
Sacramento, CA 95833 888-DIA-BETE
Fax: 916-924-0529
AskADA@diabetes.org
www.diabetes.org/
The American Diabetes Association is a nonprofit health organization providing diabetes research, information and advocacy. Founded in 1940, the American Diabetes Association conducts programs in all 50 states and the District of Columbia.
Michael D Farley CFRE, Chief Community Relations Officer
Richard Kahn PhD, Chief Scientific/Medical Officer

3224 **Diabetes Society of Santa Clara Valley**
4040 Moorpark Avenue 408-241-1922
San Jose, CA 95117 888-DIA-BETE
Fax: 408-241-1972
www.diabetes.org
The Diabetes Society is dedicated to providing education and information to those who have diabetes educating the general public about the seriousness of this disease, and supporting research aimed at preventing complications and finding a cure.
Douglas Metz DPM/MPH, Executive Director
Thomas Smith, Program/Camp Director

3225 **Juvenile Diabetes Research Foundation: Bakersfield Chapter**
712 19th Street 661-636-1305
Bakersfield, CA 93301 Fax: 661-636-1307
Bakersfield@jdrf.org
The Juvenile Diabetes Research Foundation International (JDRF) is a charitable funder and advocate of type 1 (juvenile) diabetes research worldwide. The mission of JDRF is to find a cure for diabetes and its complications through the support of research.
Allison Perkins Thomas, Bakersfield Branch Manager
Arnold Donald, President/CEO Corporate Office (NY)

3226 **Juvenile Diabetes Research Foundation: Inl and Empire Chapter**
1001 East Cooley Drive 909-424-0100
Colton, CA 92324 Fax: 909-424-0044
inlandempire@jdrf.org
www.inlandempire.jdrf.org
The Juvenile Diabetes Research Foundation International (JDRF) is a charitable funder and advocate of type 1 (juvenile) diabetes re-

search worldwide. The mission of JDRF is to find a cure for diabetes and its complications through the support of research.
Jamie Brunelle, Board of Directors
Evelyn Edinin, Board of Directors

3227 Juvenile Diabetes Research Foundation: Los Angeles Chapter
800 West Sixth Street   213-233-9901
Los Angeles, CA 90017   Fax: 213-622-6276
                                                     losangeles@jdrf.org
The Juvenile Diabetes Research Foundation International (JDRF) is a charitable funder and advocate of type 1 (juvenile) diabetes research worldwide. The mission of JDRF is to find a cure for diabetes and its complications through the support of research.
Mark Rieck, Executive Director
Dennis Ellman Esq, Board of Directors President

3228 Juvenile Diabetes Research Foundation: Nor thern California Inland Chapter
1329 Howe Avenue   916-920-0790
Sacramento, CA 95825   Fax: 916-920-0367
                                                     northernca@jdrf.org
                                                     www.jdrf.org/norcal
The Juvenile Diabetes Research Foundation International (JDRF) is a charitable funder and advocate of type 1 (juvenile) diabetes research worldwide. The mission of JDRF is to find a cure for diabetes and its complications through the support of research.
Victoria Webster, Executive Director
Molly Atkinson, Special Events Coordinator

3229 Juvenile Diabetes Research Foundation: Ora nge County Chapter
17992 Mitchell South   949-553-0363
Irvine, CA 92614   Fax: 949-553-8813
                                                     orangecounty@jdrf.org
                                                     www.jdrfoc.org
The Juvenile Diabetes Research Foundation International (JDRF) is a charitable funder and advocate of type 1 (juvenile) diabetes research worldwide. The mission of JDRF is to find a cure for diabetes and its complications through the support of research.
Louise Cummings, Executive Director
John Giovannone, President

3230 Juvenile Diabetes Research Foundation: San Diego Chapter
5677 Oberlin Drive   858-597-0240
San Diego, CA 92121   Fax: 858-597-2072
                                                     sandiego@jdrf.org
The Juvenile Diabetes Research Foundation International (JDRF) is a charitable funder and advocate of type 1 (juvenile) diabetes research worldwide. The mission of JDRF is to find a cure for diabetes and its complications through the support of research.
Linda Riley, Executive Director
Katherine Griswold, Special Events Manager

Colorado

3231 American Diabetes Association: Denver
2480 W 26th Avenue   720-855-1102
Denver, CO 80211   Fax: 720-855-1302
                                                     AskADA@diabetes.org
                                                     www.diabetes.org/
The American Diabetes Association is a nonprofit health organization providing diabetes research, information and advocacy. Founded in 1940 the American Diabetes Association conducts programs in all 50 states and the District of Columbia.
Michael D Farley CFRE, Chief Community Relations Officer
Richard Kahn, Chief Scientific/Medical Officer

3232 Juvenile Diabetes Research Foundation: Colorado Springs Chapter
3710 Sinton Road   719-633-8110
Colorado Springs, CO 80907   Fax: 719-633-8155
                                                     www.jdrfcoloradosprings.org
The Juvenile Diabetes Research Foundation International (JDRF) is a charitable funder and advocate of type 1 (juvenile) diabetes research worldwide. The mission of JDRF is to find a cure for diabetes and its complications through the support of research.
Lynn Page, Branch Manager
Andi Chernushin, President

3233 Juvenile Diabetes Research Foundation: Roc ky Mountain Chapter
5613 DTC Parkway   303-779-0525
Greenwood Village, CO 80111   Fax: 303-720-1630
                                                     RockyMountain@jdrf.org
                                                     www.jdrf.org/rockymountain
The Juvenile Diabetes Research Foundation International (JDRF) is a charitable funder and advocate of type 1 (juvenile) diabetes research worldwide. The mission of JDRF is to find a cure for diabetes and its complications through the support of research.
James Buckles, Executive Director
Nancy L Walters, Special Events Director

Connecticut

3234 American Diabetes Association: Connecticut
306 Industrial Park Road   203-639-0385
Middletown, CT 06457   888-DIA-BETE
                                                     Fax: 860-632-5098
                                                     AskADA@diabetes.org
                                                     www.diabetes.org
The American Diabetes Association is a nonprofit health organization providing diabetes research, information and advocacy. Founded in 1940 the American Diabetes Association conducts programs in all 50 states and the District of Columbia.
Michael D Farley CRFE, Chief Community Relations Officer
Richard Kahn, Chief Scientific/Medical Officer

3235 Juvenile Diabetes Research Foundation: Greater New Haven Chapter
2969 Whitney Avenue   203-248-1880
Hamden, CT 06518   Fax: 203-248-1820
The Juvenile Diabetes Research Foundation International (JDRF) is a charitable funder and advocate of type 1 (juvenile) diabetes research worldwide. The mission of JDRF is to find a cure for diabetes and its complications through the support of research.
Mary K Kessler, Executive Director
Will Martinez, Board of Directors President

3236 Juvenile Diabetes Research Foundation: Fai rfield County Chapter
200 Connecticut Avenue   203-854-0658
Norwalk, CT 06854   Fax: 203-854-0798
                                                     fairfield@jdrf.org
The Juvenile Diabetes Research Foundation International (JDRF) is a charitable funder and advocate of type 1 (juvenile) diabetes research worldwide. The mission of JDRF is to find a cure for diabetes and its complications through the support of research.
Barbara Rose, Executive Director
Michelle Tighe, Special Events Coordinator

3237 Juvenile Diabetes Research Foundation: Nor th Central CT and Western MA
18 North Main Street   860-561-1153
West Hartford, CT 06107   Fax: 860-561-3440
                                                     northcentralct@jdrf.org
The Juvenile Diabetes Research Foundation International (JDRF) is a charitable funder and advocate of type 1 (juvenile) diabetes research worldwide. The mission of JDRF is to find a cure for diabetes and its complications through the support of research.
Mary Ann Slomski, Executive Director
Ellen Kellie, Special Events Coordinator

Delaware

3238 American Diabetes Association: Delaware
100 W 10th Street   302-656-0030
Wilmington, DE 19801   888-342-2383
                                                     Fax: 302-656-7331
                                                     AskADA@diabetes.org
                                                     www.diabetes.org
The American Diabetes Association is a nonprofit health organization providing diabetes research, information and advocacy. Founded in 1940 the American Diabetes Association conducts programs in all 50 states and the District of Columbia.
Michael D Farley CFRE, Chief Community Relations Officer
Richard Kahn, Chief Scientific/Medical Officer

3239 Juvenile Diabetes Research Foundation: Del aware
100 West 10th Street   302-888-1117
Wilmington, DE 19801   Fax: 302-888-1878
                                                    delaware@jdrf.org
                                                www.jdrf.org/delaware
The Juvenile Diabetes Research Foundation International (JDRF) is a charitable funder and advocate of type 1 (juvenile) diabetes research worldwide. The mission of JDRF is to find a cure for diabetes and its complications through the support of research.
Ellen Rubesin, Executive Director
Stephanie Bucksner, Special Events Coordinator

District of Columbia

3240 American Diabetes Association: District of Columbia
1025 Connecticut Avenue NW   202-331-8303
Washington, DC 20036   888-342-2383
                                                Fax: 202-331-1402
                                                  AskADA@diabetes.org
                                                    www.diabetes.org
The American Diabetes Association is a nonprofit health organization providing diabetes research, information and advocacy. Founded in 1940 the American Diabetes Association conducts programs in all 50 states and the District of Columbia.
Michael D Farley CFRE, Chief Community Relations Officer
Richard Kahn, Chief Scientific/Medical Officer

3241 Juvenile Diabetes Research Foundation: Cap itol Chapter
1400 K Street NW   202-371-0044
Washington, DC 20005   Fax: 202-371-0046
                                                    capitol@jdrf.org
The Juvenile Diabetes Research Foundation International (JDRF) is a charitable funder and advocate of type 1 (juvenile) diabetes research worldwide. The mission of JDRF is to find a cure for diabetes and its complications through the support of research.
Pam Gatz, Executive Director
Carrie Hamilton, Special Events Director

Florida

3242 American Diabetes Association: Northeast F lorida/Southeast Georgia
8384 Baymeadows Road   904-730-7200
Jacksonville, FL 32256   888-342-2383
                                                Fax: 940-730-7933
                                                  AskADA@diabetes.org
                                                    www.diabetes.org
The American Diabetes Association is a nonprofit health organization providing diabetes research, information and advocacy. Founded in 1940 the American Diabetes Association conducts programs in all 50 states and the District of Columbia.
Sheri Criswell, Executive Director
Richard Kahn, Chief Scientific/Medical Officer

3243 American Diabetes Association: Seattle
1101 N Lake Destiny Road   407-660-1926
Maitland, FL 32751   Fax: 407-660-1080
                                                  AskADA@diabetes.org
                                                    www.diabetes.org
The American Diabetes Association is a nonprofit health organization providing diabetes research, information and advocacy. Founded in 1940 the American Diabetes Association conducts programs in all 50 states and the District of Columbia.
Pauline Lowe, Executive Director
Richard Kahn, Chief Scientific/Medical Officer

3244 American Diabetes Association: South Coast Regional/Central Florida
1101 North Lake Destiny Road   407-660-1926
Maitland, FL 32751   888-342-2383
                                                Fax: 407-660-1080
                                                  AskADA@diabetes.org
                                                    www.diabetes.org
The American Diabetes Association is a nonprofit health organization providing diabetes research, information and advocacy. Founded in 1940, the American Diabetes Association conducts

programs in all 50 states and the District of Columbia, reaching hundreds of communities.
Michael D Farley CFRE, Chief Community Relations Officer
Richard Kahn, Chief Scientific/Medical Officer

3245 Juvenile Diabetes Research Foundation: Cen tral Florida Chapter
279 Douglas Avenue   407-774-2166
Altamonte Springs, FL 32714   Fax: 407-774-2168
                                                centralflorida@jdrf.org
                                            www.jdrf.org/centralflorida
The Juvenile Diabetes Research Foundation International (JDRF) is a charitable funder and advocate of type 1 (juvenile) diabetes research worldwide. The mission of JDRF is to find a cure for diabetes and its complications through the support of research.
Kendra Presley, Special Events Manager
Gwen Bell, Office Manager

3246 Juvenile Diabetes Research Foundation: Flo rida Sun Coast Chapter
3333 Clark Road   941-929-0621
Sarasota, FL 34231   Fax: 941-929-0602
                                                floridasuncoast@jdrf.org
                                                www.jdrf.org/index.cfm
The Juvenile Diabetes Research Foundation International (JDRF) is a charitable funder and advocate of type 1 (juvenile) diabetes research worldwide. The mission of JDRF is to find a cure for diabetes and its complications through the support of research.
Sara Rankin, Executive Director
Jeannie Kawcak, Special Events Coordinator

3247 Juvenile Diabetes Research Foundation: Gre ater Palm Beach County Chapter
1450 Centrepark Boulevard   561-686-7701
West Palm Beach, FL 33401   Fax: 561-686-7702
                                            greaterpalmbeach@jdrf.org
                                        www.jdrf.org/greaterpalmbeach
The Juvenile Diabetes Research Foundation International (JDRF) is a charitable funder and advocate of type 1 (juvenile) diabetes research worldwide. The mission of JDRF is to find a cure for diabetes and its complications through the support of research.
Lora Hazelwood, Executive Director
Esther Swann, Special Events Coordinator

3248 Juvenile Diabetes Research Foundation: Nor th Florida Chapter
8400 Baymeadows Way   904-739-2101
Jacksonville, FL 32256   Fax: 904-739-2693
                                                  northflorida@jdrf.org
                                            www.jdrf.org/northflorida
The Juvenile Diabetes Research Foundation International (JDRF) is a charitable funder and advocate of type 1 (juvenile) diabetes research worldwide. The mission of JDRF is to find a cure for diabetes and its complications through the support of research.
Brooks Biagini, Executive Director
Wendy Smit, Special Events Assistant

3249 Juvenile Diabetes Research Foundation: Sou th Florida Chapter
3411 NW 9th Avenue   954-565-4775
Fort Lauderdale, FL 33309   Fax: 954-565-4767
                                                  southflorida@jdrf.org
The Juvenile Diabetes Research Foundation International (JDRF) is a charitable funder and advocate of type 1 (juvenile) diabetes research worldwide. The mission of JDRF is to find a cure for diabetes and its complications through the support of research.
Ingrid Velarde, Special Events Coordinator
Katelyn Tolzien, Special Events Coordinator

3250 Juvenile Diabetes Research Foundation: Tam pa Bay Chapter
5959 Central Avenue   727-344-2873
Saint Petersburg, FL 33710   Fax: 727-384-9009
                                                  tampabay@jdrf.org
                                                        www.jdf.org
The Juvenile Diabetes Research Foundation International (JDRF) is a charitable funder and advocate of type 1 (juvenile) diabetes research worldwide. The mission of JDRF is to find a cure for diabetes and its complications through the support of research.
Arnold Donald, President/CEO Corporate Office
Robin Harding, EVP Development & COO

Georgia

3251 American Diabetes Association: Atlanta Met ro
17 Executive Park   404-320-7100
Atlanta, GA 30329   888-342-2383
                                        Fax: 404-320-0025
                                      AskADA@diabetes.org
                                         www.diabetes.org
The American Diabetes Association is a nonprofit health organization providing diabetes research, information and advocacy. Founded in 1940 the American Diabetes Association conducts programs in all 50 states and the District of Columbia, reaching hundreds of communities
Michael Gault, Senior Executive Director
Richard Kahn, Chief Scientific/Medical Officer

3252 American Diabetes Association: Savannah
5105 Paulsen Street   912-353-8110
Savannah, GA 31405   888-343-2383
                                        Fax: 912-353-9114
                                      AskADA@diabetes.org
                                         www.diabetes.org
The American Diabetes Association is a nonprofit health organization providing diabetes research, information and advocacy. Founded in 1940 the American Diabetes Association conducts programs in all 50 states and the District of Columbia.
Maria Center, Director
Richard Kahn, Chief Scientific/Medical Officer

3253 Juvenile Diabetes Research Foundation: Geo rgia Chapter
400 Perimeter Center Terrace   404-420-5990
Atlanta, GA 30346   Fax: 404-420-5995
                                          georgia@jdrf.org
                                     www.jdrfgeorgia.org/
The Juvenile Diabetes Research Foundation International (JDRF) is a charitable funder and advocate of type 1 (juvenile) diabetes research worldwide. The mission of JDRF is to find a cure for diabetes and its complications through the support of research.
Rob Shaw, Executive Director
Scott Whiteside, EVP/General Manager

Hawaii

3254 American Diabetes Association: Hawaii
1500 S Beretania Street   808-947-5979
Honolulu, HI 96826   888-342-2383
                                        Fax: 808-947-5978
                                      AskADA@diabetes.org
                                         www.diabetes.org
The American Diabetes Association is a nonprofit health organization providing diabetes research, information and advocacy. Founded in 1940 the American Diabetes Association conducts programs in all 50 states and the District of Columbia.
Majken Mechling, Executive Director
Richard Kahn, Chief Scientific/Medical Officer

3255 Juvenile Diabetes Research Foundation: Haw aii Chapter
1019 Waimanu Street   808-988-1000
Honolulu, HI 96814   Fax: 808-597-8758
                                           hawaii@jdrf.org
                                              www.jdf.org
The Juvenile Diabetes Research Foundation International (JDRF) is a charitable funder and advocate of type 1 (juvenile) diabetes research worldwide. The mission of JDRF is to find a cure for diabetes and its complications through the support of research.
Arnold Donald, President/CEO Corporate
Robin Harding, EVP/Develpment & COO Corporate

Illinois

3256 American Diabetes Association: Greater Ill inois
2580 Federal Drive   217-875-9011
Decatur, IL 62526   888-342-2383
                                        Fax: 217-875-6849
                                      AskADA@diabetes.org
                                         www.diabetes.org
The American Diabetes Association is a nonprofit health organization providing diabetes research, information and advocacy. Founded in 1940 the American Diabetes Association conducts

programs in all 50 states and the District of Columbia, reaching hundreds of communities.
Donna Scott, Executive Director
Richard Kahn, Chief Scientific/Medical Officer

3257 American Diabetes Association: Northern Il linois
30 North Michigan Avenue   312-346-1805
Chicago, IL 60602   888-343-2383
                                        Fax: 312-346-5342
                                      AskADA@diabetes.org
                                         www.diabetes.org
The American Diabetes Association is a nonprofit health organization providing diabetes research, information and advocacy. Founded in 1940, the American Diabetes Association conducts programs in all 50 states and the District of Columbia, reaching hundreds of communities.
Michael D Farley CFRE (Corporate), Chief Community Relations Officer
Richard Kahn, Chief Scientific/Medical Officer

3258 Juvenile Diabetes Research Foundation: Gre ater Chicago Chapter
500 North Dearborn Street   312-670-0313
Chicago, IL 60610   Fax: 312-670-0250
                                          illinois@jdrf.org
The Juvenile Diabetes Research Foundation International (JDRF) is a charitable funder and advocate of type 1 (juvenile) diabetes research worldwide. The mission of JDRF is to find a cure for diabetes and its complications through the support of research.
Amy Franze, Executive Director
Janine Tobola, Director Office Operations

Indiana

3259 American Diabetes Association: Northern In diana/Northern Ohio
6415 Castleway W Drive   317-352-9226
Indianapolis, IN 46250   888-342-2383
                                        Fax: 317-594-0748
                                      AskADA@diabetes.org
                                         www.diabetes.org
The American Diabetes Association is a nonprofit health organization providing diabetes research, information and advocacy. Founded in 1940 the American Diabetes Association conducts programs in all 50 states and the District of Columbia.
Jennifer Pferrer, Executive Director
Richard Kahn, Chief Scientific/Medical Officer

3260 Diabetes Youth Foundation of Indiana
7311 Tousley Drive   317-750-9310
Indianapolis, IN 46256-9212   Fax: 317-243-4418
                                         dyfjulie@yahoo.com
                                       www.dyfofindiana.org
This nonprofit group whose mission is to improve the lives of children with diabetes and their families.
Julie Shutt, Executive Director
Rick Crosslin, Camp Director

3261 Juvenile Diabetes Research Foundation: Ind iana State Chapter
8465 Keystone Crossing   317-202-0352
Indianapolis, IN 46240   Fax: 317-202-0357
                                       indianastate@jdrf.org
                                      www.jdrf.org/indiana
The Juvenile Diabetes Research Foundation International (JDRF) is a charitable funder and advocate of type 1 (juvenile) diabetes research worldwide. The mission of JDRF is to find a cure for diabetes and its complications through the support of research.
Henry Rodriguez MD, Chapter President

3262 Juvenile Diabetes Research Foundation: Nor thern Indiana Chapter
2004 Ironwood Circle   574-273-1810
South Bend, IN 46635   Fax: 574-273-1870
                                     northernindiana@jdrf.org
                                              www.jdrf.org
The Juvenile Diabetes Research Foundation International (JDRF) is a charitable funder and advocate of type 1 (juvenile) diabetes re-

search worldwide. The mission of JDRF is to find a cure for diabetes and its complications through the support of research.
Arnold Donald, President/CEO Corporate
Robin Harding, EVP/Development & COO Corporate

Iowa

3263 American Diabetes Association: Cedar Rapid s District
St Luke's Resource Center   319-247-5124
Cedar Rapids, IA 52406   888-342-2383
Fax: 319-247-5125
AskADA@diabetes.org
www.diabetes.org
The American Diabetes Association is a nonprofit health organization providing diabetes research, information and advocacy. Founded in 1940 the American Diabetes Association conducts programs in all 50 states and the District of Columbia.
Jennifer Petsche, Manager
Richard Kahn, Chief Scientific/Medical Officer

3264 Juvenile Diabetes Research Foundation: Eas tern Iowa Chapter
701 10th Street SE   319-393-3850
Cedar Rapids, IA 52403   Fax: 319-393-3852
easterniowa@jdrf.org
www.jdrf.org/easterniowa
The Juvenile Diabetes Research Foundation International (JDRF) is a charitable funder and advocate of type 1 (juvenile) diabetes research worldwide. The mission of JDRF is to find a cure for diabetes and its complications through the support of research.
Ann Elise Walsh, Special Events Manager
Mary Henry, Special Events Coordinator

3265 Juvenile Diabetes Research Foundation: Gre ater Iowa Chapter
5444 NW 96th Street   515-986-1512
Johnston, IA 50131   Fax: 515-986-1513
www.jdrf.org/greateriowa
The Juvenile Diabetes Research Foundation International (JDRF) is a charitable funder and advocate of type 1 (juvenile) diabetes research worldwide. The mission of JDRF is to find a cure for diabetes and its complications through the support of research.
Jean Howieson, Special Events Director
Judy Greaves, Office Administrator

Kansas

3266 American Diabetes Association: Kansas
837 S Hillside   316-684-6091
Wichita, KS 67211   888-342-2383
Fax: 316-684-5675
AskADA@diabetes.org
www.diabetes.org
The American Diabetes Association is a nonprofit health organization providing diabetes research, information and advocacy. Founded in 1940 the American Diabetes Association conducts programs in all 50 states and the District of Columbia.
Sarah Beth Webb, Director
Richard Kahn, Chief Scientific/Medical Officer

Kentucky

3267 American Diabetes Association: Kentucky
161 St Matthews Avenue   502-452-6072
Louisville, KY 40207   888-342-2383
Fax: 502-893-2698
AskADA@diabetes.org
www.diabetes.org
The American Diabetes Association is a nonprofit health organization providing diabetes research, information and advocacy. Founded in 1940 the American Diabetes Association conducts programs in all 50 states and the District of Columbia.
Samantha Carroll, Associate Director
Richard Kahn, Chief Scientific/Medical Officer

3268 Juvenile Diabetes Research Foundation: Kentuckiana Chapter
133 Evergreen Road   502-485-9397
Louisville, KY 40243   866-485-9397
Fax: 502-485-9591
kentuckiana@jdrf.org
The Juvenile Diabetes Research Foundation International (JDRF) is a charitable funder and advocate of type 1 (juvenile) diabetes re-

search worldwide. The mission of JDRF is to find a cure for diabetes and its complications through the support of research.
Twynette S Davidson, Executive Director
Joe Salvagne, Chapter President

Louisiana

3269 American Diabetes Association: Louisiana
2644 S Sherwood Forest Boulevard   225-216-3980
Baton Rouge, LA 70816   888-342-2383
Fax: 225-295-7005
AskADA@diabetes.org
www.diabetes.org
Paige Grogan, Associate Manager
Lori Koonce, Associate Manager

3270 Juvenile Diabetes Research Foundation: Bat on Rouge Chapter
9457 Brookline Avenue   225-932-9511
Baton Rouge, LA 70809   Fax: 225-932-9514
batonrouge@jdrf.org
Kristy Andries, President/Development Chair
Danielle Graham, Special Events Assistant

3271 Juvenile Diabetes Research Foundation: Lou isiana Chapter
2201 Veterans Memorial Bouelvard   504-828-2873
Metairie, LA 70002   Fax: 504-828-4922
louisiana@jdrf.org
www.jdrf.org/louisiana
Sam Robinson, President Board of Directors
Becky Spinnato, Vice President Fundraising

3272 Juvenile Diabetes Research Foundation: Shr eveport Chapter
2001 East 70th Street   318-798-1195
Shreveport, LA 71105   Fax: 318-798-1194
Jeff Knutson, President Board of Directors
Craig Floyd, Vice President Fundraising

Maine

3273 American Diabetes Association: Maine
80 Elm Street   207-774-7717
Portland, ME 04101   888-342-2383
Fax: 207-774-7714
AskADA@diabetes.org
www.diabetes.org
Emily Silevinac, Associate Manager
Ryan Williams, Associate Manager

3274 Juvenile Diabetes Research Foundation: New England/Maine Chapter
33 Silver Street   207-761-0133
Portland, ME 04101   Fax: 207-761-1687
Heidi Daniels, New England Chapter Executive Director
Emily Hampton Burgo, Branch Manager

Maryland

3275 American Diabetes Association: Maryland
800 Wyman Park Drive   410-265-0075
Baltimore, MD 21211   888-342-2383
Fax: 410-235-4048
AskADA@diabetes.org
www.diabetes.org
Kathy Rogers, Executive Director
Dotty Raynor, Director

3276 Juvenile Diabetes Research Foundation: Mar yland Chapter
200 East Joppa Road   410-823-0073
Towson, MD 21286   Fax: 410-823-0416
www.jdrf.org/maryland/
Rebecca Maude, Executive Director
Dotty Raynor, Outreach Manager

Massachusetts

3277 American Diabetes Association: Boston
330 Congress Street
Boston, MA 02210
617-482-4580
888-342-2383
Fax: 617-482-1824
AskADA@diabetes.org
www.diabetes.org

Christopher Boynton, Executive Director
Lori Glowacki, Director of Special Events

3278 Juvenile Diabetes Research Foundation: New England/Bay State Chapter
20 Walnut Street
Wellesley, MA 02481
781-431-0700
Fax: 781-431-8836
baystate@jdrf.org

Heidi Daniels, New England Chapter Executive Director
Virginia Irving, Associate Executive Director

Michigan

3279 American Diabetes Association: Michigan
3940 Broadmoor Avenue SE
Grand Rapids, MI 49512
616-458-9341
888-342-2383
Fax: 616-575-9930
AskADA@diabetes.org
www.diabetes.org

Darla Hill, Coordinator
Sharice Purman, Director

3280 Juvenile Diabetes Research Foundation: Metropolitan Detroit/SE Michigan
24359 Northwestern Highway
Southfield, MI 48075-2020
248-355-1133
Fax: 248-355-1188
metrodetroit@jdrf.org
www.jdrfdetroit.org

Rita L Combest, Development Director
Susan Kossik, Development Manager

3281 Juvenile Diabetes Research Foundation: Wes t Michigan Chapter
5075 Cascade Road SE
Grand Rapids, MI 49546
616-957-1838
Fax: 616-957-1169

Annette Guilfoyle, Executive Director
Maxine Gray, Special Events Coordinator

Minnesota

3282 American Diabetes Association: Minnesota
Parkdale Center
Saint Louis Park, MN 55416
763-593-5333
888-342-2383
Fax: 952-582-9000
AskADA@diabetes.org
www.diabetes.org

Jenni Hargraves, Executive Director
Becky Barnett, Associate Manager

3283 Juvenile Diabetes Research Foundation: Min nesota Chapter
2626 East 82nd Street
Bloomington, MN 55425
952-851-0770
800-663-1860
Fax: 952-851-0766
minnesota@jdrf.org
www.jdrf.org/minnesota

Jackie Casey, Executive Director
Angie McCarthy, Special Events Manager

Mississippi

3284 American Diabetes Association: Mississippi
16 Northtown Drive
Jackson, MS 39211
601-932-1118
888-342-2383
Fax: 601-932-1988
AskADA@diabetes.org
www.diabetes.org

The nation's leading voluntary health organization providing diabetes research, information and advocacy. Our mission is to prevent and cure diabetes and to improve the lives of all people affected by diabetes.

Mary D Fortune, Executive Vice President
Stephanie J Coghlan MBA, Senior Regional Director

Missouri

3285 American Diabetes Association: Missouri
1944-A Sunshine
Springfield, MO 65804
417-890-8400
888-342-2383
Fax: 417-890-8484
AskADA@diabetes.org
www.diabetes.org

Renee Paulsell, Executive Director
Jennifer Cotner-Jone, Associate Director

3286 Juvenile Diabetes Research Foundation: St. Louis Chapter
225 S Meramec Avenue
Clayton, MO 63105
314-726-6778
Fax: 314-726-6778
metrostlouis@jdrf.org

M Marie Davis, Executive Director
William Schmitt, Corporate Development

Montana

3287 American Diabetes Association: Montana
3203 3rd Avenue N
Billings, MT 59101
406-256-0616
888-342-2383
Fax: 406-896-0289
AskADA@diabetes.org
www.diabetes.org

Karen Talmadge, Chair
Laurelean Gaines, President

Nebraska

3288 American Diabetes Association: Nebraska
14216 Dayton Circle
Omaha, NE 68137
402-571-1101
888-342-2383
Fax: 402-572-8141
AskADA@diabetes.org
www.diabetes.org

Shawn Murphy, Executive Director
Kortney Krill, Associate Manager

3289 Juvenile Diabetes Research Foundation: Lin coln Chapter
1540 S 70th Street
Lincoln, NE 68506
402-484-8300
Fax: 402-484-8302
lincoln@jdrf.org
www.jdrf.org/lincoln

Deb Gokie, Executive Director
Maggie Pavelka, Special Events Assistant

3290 Juvenile Diabetes Research Foundation: Oma ha Council Bluffs Chapter
9202 W Dodge Road
Omaha, NE 68114
402-397-2873
Fax: 402-572-3343
omaha@jdrf.org
www.jdrf.org/omaha

Shawn Reynolds, Executive Director
Melissa Shapiro, Special Events Coordinator

Nevada

3291 American Diabetes Association: Nevada
2785 E Desert Inn Road
Las Vegas, NV 89121
702-369-9995
888-342-2383
Fax: 702-369-3717
AskADA@diabetes.org
www.diabetes.org

Mary Stokes, Manager
Carly Rohrer, Associate Manager

3292 Juvenile Diabetes Research Foundation: Nevada Chapter
5542 S Fort Apache Road
Las Vegas, NV 89148
702-732-4795
Fax: 702-732-1635
www.jdrf.org/nevada

Stuart Mason, Nevada Chapter Co-Founder
Flora Mason, Nevada Chapter Co-Founder

3293 Juvenile Diabetes Research Foundation: Nor thern Nevada Branch
5335 Kietzke Lane
Reno, NV 89511
775-786-1881
Fax: 775-827-0131
northernnevada@jdrf.org
www.jdrf.org/northernnevada
Molly Dillon, Branch Manager
Arnie Pitts, Board of Directors President

New Hampshire

3294 American Diabetes Association: New Hampshire
249 Canal Street
Manchester, NH 03101
603-627-9579
888-342-2383
Fax: 603-669-1477
www.diabetes.org

3295 Juvenile Diabetes Research Foundation: New England/New Hampshire Chapter
2 Wellman Avenue
Nashua, NH 03064
603-595-2595
Fax: 603-595-2073
newhampshire@jdrf.org
Brooke Edwards, Special Events Coordinator
Heidi Daniels, New England Chapter Executive Director

New Jersey

3296 American Diabetes Association: New Jersey
CentrePoint II Suite 103
Bridgewater, NJ 08807
732-469-7979
888-342-2383
Fax: 732-469-4887
AskADA@diabetes.org
www.diabetes.org
James Roberts, Executive Director
Pamela Hooper, Director

3297 Juvenile Diabetes Research Foundation: South Jersey Chapter
1415 Route 70 E
Cherry Hill, NJ 08034
856-429-1101
Fax: 856-429-1105
southjersey@jdrf.org
www.jdrf.org/southjersey
Stephen Blocher, Executive Director
Robin Berger, Special Events Coordinator

3298 Juvenile Diabetes Research Foundation: Cen tral Jersey Chapter
740 Broad Street
Shrewsbury, NJ 07702
732-219-6654
Fax: 732-219-8722
centraljersey@jdrf.org
Lori McLane, Executive Director
Beckie Burlew, Special Events Coordinator

3299 Juvenile Diabetes Research Foundation: Mid -Jersey Chapter
28 Kennedy Boulevard
East Brunswick, NJ 08816
732-296-7171
Fax: 732-296-1433
midjersey@jdrf.org
www.jdrf.org/NJ/Mid-Jersey
Elizabeth Giardina Preston, Chapter Executive Director
Sandra Hilsenrath, Special Events Coordinator

3300 Juvenile Diabetes Research Foundation: Roc kland County/Northern New Jersey
560 Sylvan Avenue
Englewood Cliffs, NJ 07632
201-568-4838
Fax: 201-568-5360
rockland@jdrf.org
www.jdrf.org/northernnj
Douglas Rouse, Executive Director
Allison Hartstone, Special Events Coordinator

New Mexico

3301 American Diabetes Association: New Mexico
2625 Pennsylvania NE
Albuquerque, NM 87110
505-266-5716
888-342-2383
Fax: 505-268-4533
AskADA@diabetes.org
www.diabetes.org
Betsey Robinson, Associate Director
Lisa Johnson, Manager

3302 Juvenile Diabetes Research Foundation: Albuquerque
2501 San Pedro NE
Albuquerque, NM 87110
505-255-4005
Fax: 505-260-1430
newmexico@jdrf.org
www.jdrf.org/newmexico
Joann Perrine, Branch Manager
Elizabeth Romero, Fundraising Assistant

New York

3303 American Diabetes Association: New York
Pine W Plaza Building 2
Albany, NY 12205
518-218-1755
888-342-2383
Fax: 518-218-0114
AskADA@diabetes.org
www.diabetes.org
Amy R Young, District Director
Karen Dooley, Associate Manager

3304 Juvenile Diabetes Research Foundation
Executive Office/Corporate Headquarters
120 Wall Street
New York, NY 10005-4001
212-725-4925
800-533-2873
Fax: 212-785-9595
info@jdrf.org
www.jdrf.org/
Allan J Lewis, President/Chief Executive Officer
Amy C Franze, EVP Development

3305 Juvenile Diabetes Research Foundation: Long Island/South Shore Chapter
532 Broadhollow Road
Melville, NY 11747
631-414-1126
Fax: 631-414-1133
www.jdrf.org/longisland
Barbara Rogus, Executive Director
Christina Colandro, Special Events Manager

3306 Juvenile Diabetes Research Foundation: Buf falo/Western New York Chapter
331 Alberta Drive
Buffalo, NY 14226
716-833-2873
Fax: 716-833-0199
westernny@jdrf.org
www.jdrf.org/westernny
Karen Swierski, Executive Director
Jennifer Hickok, Special Events Manager

3307 Juvenile Diabetes Research Foundation: Hud son Valley Chapter
Hollowbrook Office Park
Wappinger Falls, NY 12590
845-297-8600
Fax: 845-297-7887
hudsonvalley@jdrf.org
www.letscurediabetes.com
Charlie Lawrence, Branch Manager
Linda Delia, Events Assistant

3308 Juvenile Diabetes Research Foundation: New York Chapter
432 Park Avenue S
New York, NY 10016
212-689-2860
Fax: 212-689-4038
newyorkchapter@jdrf.org
www.nyc.jdrf.org
Mania Boyder, New York City Chapter Executive Director

3309 Juvenile Diabetes Research Foundation: Nor theastern New York
6 Greenwood Drive
East Greenbush, NY 12061
518-477-2873
Fax: 518-477-7004
northeastny@jdrf.org
Bev Kennedy, Executive Director
Darlene Robbiano, Special Events Manager

3310 Juvenile Diabetes Research Foundation: Roc hester Branch/Western New York Chapter
1200-A Scottsville Road
Rochester, NY 14624
585-546-1390
Fax: 585-546-1404
rochester@jdrf.org
www.jdrf.org/rochester
Mary Anne Fox, Executive Director
Lisa Swindon, Senior Development Coordinator

3311 Juvenile Diabetes Research Foundation: Wes tchester County Chapter
30 Glenn Street
White Plains, NY 10603
914-686-7700
Fax: 914-686-7701
westchester@jdrf.org
www.jdrf.org/westchester

Katherine Cintron, Executive Director
Dejan Popovich, Special Events Coordinator

North Carolina

3312 American Diabetes Association: North Carolina
222 South Church Street
Charlotte, NC 28202
704-373-9111
888-342-2383
Fax: 704-373-9113
www.diabetes.org

Dianne Roth, Executive Director

3313 Juvenile Diabetes Research Foundation: Triangle/Eastern North Carolina Chapter
2210 Millbrook Road
Raleigh, NC 27604
919-431-8330
Fax: 919-431-8373
triangle@jdrf.org

Jim Burson, Chapter President
Courtney Davies, Executive Director

3314 Juvenile Diabetes Research Foundation: Cha rlotte Chapter
205 Regency Executive Park Drive
Charlotte, NC 28217
704-561-0828
Fax: 704-561-9920
charlotte@jdrf.org
www.gwc.jdrf.org

Brenning Johnston, Volunteer Coordinator

3315 Juvenile Diabetes Research Foundation: Pie dmont Triad Chapter
1401-B Old Mill Circle
Winston-Salem, NC 27103
336-768-1027
Fax: 336-768-1029
piedmont@jdrf.org
www.jdrf.org/triad

Brad Calloway, President Board of Directors
Tom Brinkley, VP Fundraising & Development

North Dakota

3316 American Diabetes Association: Nashville
1323 23rd Street S
Fargo, ND 58103
701-234-0123
Fax: 701-235-3080
AskADA@diabetes.org
www.diabetes.org

Stephanie Chimeziri, Associate Director

3317 American Diabetes Association: North Dakota
1323 23rd Street South
Fargo, ND 58103
701-234-0123
888-342-2383
Fax: 701-235-3080
www.diabetes.org

Ohio

3318 American Diabetes Association: Ohio
4500 Rockside Road
Independence, OH 44131
216-328-9989
888-342-2383
Fax: 216-328-0007
AskADA@diabetes.org
www.diabetes.org

Jill Pupa, Executive Director
Patti Clair, Associate Director

3319 Juvenile Diabetes Research Foundation/JDRF
1293-H Lyons Road
Dayton, OH 45458
937-439-2873
Fax: 937-439-4086
dayton@jdrf.org
www.jdrf.org/dayton

Karen Myers, Executive Director
Vicky Williams, Office Manager

3320 Juvenile Diabetes Research Foundation: Mid-Ohio Chapter
1550 Old Henderson Rd
Columbus, OH 43220
614-464-2873
Fax: 614-464-2877
midohio@jdrf.org

Staci Perkins, Executive Director
Roberta Smedes, Office Manager

3321 Juvenile Diabetes Research Foundation: Akr on/Canton Chapter
5000 Rockside Road
Canton, OH 44131
888-718-3061
Fax: 216-328-8340

Laura E Maciag, Executive Director
Danielle Thompson, Special Events Manager

3322 Juvenile Diabetes Research Foundation: Gre ater Cincinnati Chapter
8041 Hosbrook Road
Cincinnati, OH 45236-3830
513-793-3223
Fax: 513-936-5333
cincinnati@jdrf.org

Bill Rice, Executive Director
Bethe Ferguson, Special Events Coordinator

3323 Juvenile Diabetes Research Foundation: Tol edo/Northwest Ohio Chapter
3450 W Central Avenue
Toledo, OH 43606
419-873-1377
800-533-2873
Fax: 419-720-6339
www.jdrf.org/northwestohio

Megan Meyer, Executive Director
Marna Cousino, Special Events Coordinator

Oklahoma

3324 American Diabetes Association: Oklahoma
3000 United Founders Boulevard
Oklahoma City, OK 73112
405-840-3881
888-342-2383
Fax: 405-840-3899
AskADA@diabetes.org
www.diabetes.org

Diane Sarantakos, Executive Director
Andrea Barnett, Associate Manager

3325 Juvenile Diabetes Research Foundation: Cen tral Oklahoma Chapter
2601 NW Expressway
Oklahoma City, OK 73112
405-810-0070
888-533-9255
Fax: 405-810-0078
oklahoma@jdrf.org

Renee MacDonald, Executive Director
Shannon Scott, Special Events Coordinator

3326 Juvenile Diabetes Research Foundation: Tul sa Green County Chapter
4606 E 67th Street
Tulsa, OK 74136
918-481-5807
Fax: 918-481-5823
tulsa@jdrf.org
www.jdrf.org/tulsa-green

Brandi Sullivan, Executive Director
Angela Peterson, Special Events Coordinator

Oregon

3327 American Diabetes Association: Oregon
2350 Oakmont Way
Eugene, OR 97401
541-343-0735
888-342-2383
Fax: 541-342-1491
AskADA@diabetes.org
www.diabetes.org

Cynthia Benton, Associate Director

3328 Juvenile Diabetes Research Foundation: Ore gon/SW Washington Chapter
7460 SW Hunziker Street
Portland, OR 97223
503-643-1995
866-598-9074
Fax: 503-598-9087
oregon-washington@jdrf.org
www.jdrf.org/oregon

Ashleigh Farleigh, Special Events Manager
Debbie Secor, Special Events Assistant

Pennsylvania

3329 American Diabetes Association: Pennsylvania
3544 Progress Avenue
Harrisburg, PA 17110
717-657-4310
888-342-2383
Fax: 717-657-4320
www.diabetes.org

3330 American Diabetes Association: Western Pennsylvania
300 Penn Center Boulevard
Pittsburgh, PA 15235
412-824-1181
888-342-2383
Fax: 412-824-2191
AskADA@diabetes.org
www.diabetes.org

Terri Seidman, Area Manager
Steven Shivak, Executive Director

3331 Juvenile Diabetes Research Foundation: Central Pennsylvania Chapter
119 Aster Drive
Harrisburg, PA 17112
717-901-6489
Fax: 717-901-6573
centralpa@jdrf.org
www.jdrf.org/centralpa

Susan Harral, Executive Director
Kate Severs, Special Events Assistant

3332 Juvenile Diabetes Research Foundation: Berks County Chapter
619 Wellington Avenue
West Lawn, PA 19609
610-775-4169
Tammy A. Edwards, Contact

3333 Juvenile Diabetes Research Foundation: Northwestern Pennsylvania Chapter
1700 Peach St
Erie, PA 16501
814-452-0635
Fax: 814-452-0645
northwestpa@jdrf.org
www.jdrf.org/northwestpa

Douglas K White, Executive Director
Amy Bement, Special Events Assistant

3334 Juvenile Diabetes Research Foundation: Philadelphia Chapter
225 City Line Avenue
Bala Cynwyd, PA 19004
610-664-9255
Fax: 610-664-9585
philadelphia@jdrf.org

Ellen Rubesin, Executive Director
Kathy Farren, Special Events Director

3335 Juvenile Diabetes Research Foundation: Western Pennsylvania
960 Penn Avenue
Pittsburgh, PA 15222
412-471-1414
888-528-8788
Fax: 412-471-1417
westernpa@jdrf.org
www.jdrf.org/westernpa

David R Donahue, Executive Director
Kimberly A McElroy, Office Manager

Rhode Island

3336 American Diabetes Association: Rhode Island
146 Clifford St
Providence, RI 02903
401-351-0498
888-342-2383
Fax: 401-351-1674
www.jdf.org

South Carolina

3337 American Diabetes Association: South Carolina
2711 Middleburg Drive
Columbia, SC 29204
803-799-4246
888-342-2383
Fax: 803-799-5792
www.diabetes.org

3338 Juvenile Diabetes Research Foundation: Palmetto Chapter
810 Dutch Square Blvd
Columbia, SC 29210
803-782-1477
Fax: 803-782-8975
palmetto@jdrf.org
www.jdrfpalmetto.org/about.aspx

Michael Slapnik, President
Dana Bruce, Executive Director

3339 Juvenile Diabetes Research Foundation: Low Country Chapter
520 Folly Road
Charleston, SC 29412
843-345-0369
Fax: 843-406-7957
Pam Nestor McAdams, Events/Walk Director South Coastal Chptr

South Dakota

3340 Juvenile Diabetes Research Foundation: Sioux Falls Chapter
PO Box 88540
Sioux Falls, SD 57109-8540
605-338-2295

Tennessee

3341 American Diabetes Association: Nashville
4205 Hillsboro Road
Nashville, TN 37215
615-298-3066
888-342-2383
Fax: 615-292-5357
AskADA@diabetes.org
www.diabetes.org

Glenda Berry, Executive Director
Harlyn Hardin, Director of Programs

3342 American Diabetes Association: Tennessee
5583 Murray Road
Memphis, TN 38119
901-682-8232
888-342-2383
Fax: 901-682-8170
AskADA@diabetes.org
www.diabetes.org

John Carroll, Director
Daniele Cain, Coordinator

3343 Juvenile Diabetes Research Foundation: East Tennessee Chapter
355 Trane Lane
Knoxville, TN 37919
865-544-0768
Fax: 865-544-4312
EastTennessee@jdrf.org

3344 Juvenile Diabetes Research Foundation: Middle Tennessee Chapter
105 Westpark Drive
Nashville, TN 37027
615-383-6781
Fax: 615-383-4284
www.midtennessee.jdrf.org

Joe Bide, Vice President

Texas

3345 American Diabetes Association: Texas
4150 International Plaza
Fort Worth, TX 76109
817-332-7110
888-342-2383
Fax: 817-732-6244
www.diabetes.org

3346 Juvenile Diabetes Research Foundation: South Central Texas Chapter
8700 Crownhill Boulevrad
San Antonio, TX 78209
210-822-5336
Fax: 210-822-1443
scentraltexas@jdrf.org

Doug Koskie, President
Brigitte West, Secretary

3347 Juvenile Diabetes Research Foundation: Dallas Chapter
9400 North Central Expressway
Dallas, TX 75231-5063
214-373-9808
Fax: 214-373-6337
Dave Johnson, President
Michael Keith, Treasurer

3348 Juvenile Diabetes Research Foundation: Greater Fort Worth/Arlington Chapter
3840 Hulen Street
Fort Worth, TX 76107-2127
817-332-2601
Fax: 817-332-5641
grfortworth@jdrf.org
www.jdf.org

3349 Juvenile Diabetes Research Foundation: Houston/Gulf Coast Chapter
2425 Fountain View
Houston, TX 77057
713-334-4400
Fax: 713-334-4040
houston@jdrf.org
www.jdf.org

3350 Juvenile Diabetes Research Foundation: Wes t Texas Chapter
Clay Desta Towers, 10 Desta Drive   432-570-5643
Midland, TX 79705   Fax: 432-682-0765
                                           www.jdf.org

Utah

3351 American Diabetes Association: Utah
1245 E Brickyard Road   801-363-3024
Salt Lake City, UT 84106   888-342-2383
                                           Fax: 801-363-3031
                                           www.diabetes.org

Vermont

3352 American Diabetes Association: Vermont
1 Kennedy Drive   802-654-7716
S Burlington, VT 05403   888-342-2383
                                           Fax: 802-658-9145
                                           www.diabetes.org

Virginia

3353 American Diabetes Association: Richmond
4335 Cox Road   804-225-8038
Glen Allen, VA 23060   888-342-2383
                                           Fax: 804-270-4742
                                           www.diabetes.org

3354 American Diabetes Association: Virginia
870 Greenbrier Circle   757-424-6662
Chesapeake, VA 23320   888-342-2383
                                           Fax: 757-420-0490
                                           www.diabetes.org

3355 Juvenile Diabetes Research Foundation: Gre ater Blue Ridge Chapter
3959 Electric Road   540-772-1975
Roanoke, VA 24018   888-849-0510
                                           Fax: 540-772-6672

Mary Lou Bruce, Board President
Annette Kirby, Secretary

Washington

3356 American Diabetes Association: Seattle
Metropolitan Park E   206-282-4616
Seattle, WA 98101   888-342-2383
                                           Fax: 206-903-8107
                                           www.diabetes.org

Linda Henderson, Executive Director
Sarah Popelka, Director

3357 American Diabetes Association: Washington
1200 Sixth Avenue   509-624-7478
Spokane, WA 99204   888-342-2383
                                           Fax: 509-624-7212
                                           www.diabetes.org

3358 Juvenile Diabetes Research Foundation: Seattle Guild
1215 Fourth Avenue   206-343-0873
Seattle, WA 98161-1101   Fax: 206-343-7015
Nadie Heichel, Executive Director
Becky Baumgardner, Office Manager

3359 Juvenile Diabetes Research Foundation: Sea ttle Chapter
1333 N Northlake Way   206-545-1510
Seattle, WA 98103-8900   Fax: 206-545-1511

3360 Juvenile Diabetes Research Foundation: Spo kane County Area Chapter
9 South Washington   509-459-6307
Spokane, WA 99201   Fax: 509-459-6392
                                           inlandnw@jdrf.org
                                           http://www.jdrf.org/index.cfm

Kay C Dightman, Contact

West Virginia

3361 American Diabetes Association: West Virginia
PO Box 238   304-768-2596
Hurricane, WV 25526   888-342-2383
                                           Fax: 304-562-1887
                                           rahearn@diabetes.org
                                           diabetes.org

Karen Talmadge, Chair
Lurelean Gaines, President

3362 Juvenile Diabetes Research Foundation: Hun tington Chapter
PO Box 2903   304-525-4533
Huntington, WV 25728

Wisconsin

3363 American Diabetes Association: Wisconsin
1701 North Beauregard Street Alexan   608-222-7785
Monona, WI 53713   888-342-2383
                                           Fax: 608-222-7795
                                           bfolco@diabetes.org
                                           www.diabetes.org

Barb Folco, Manager
Jay Kemp, Coordinator

3364 Juvenile Diabetes Research Foundation: Southeastern Chapter
3333 North Mayfair Road   414-453-4673
Wauwatosa, WI 53222   Fax: 414-453-4919
                                           southeastwi@jdrf.org
                                           www.sewi.jdrf.org/

3365 Juvenile Diabetes Research Foundation: Gre ater Madison Chapter
434 S. Yellowstone Drive   608-833-2873
Madison, WI 53719   Fax: 608-833-9214
                                           westernwi@jdrf.org
                                           www.jdrfwesternwisconsin.org/

Douglas Berry, President
Aaron Weinbe Swenson, Treasurer

3366 Juvenile Diabetes Research Foundation: Nor theast Wisconsin Chapter
1800 Appleton Road   920-997-0038
Menasha, WI 54952-0101   Fax: 920-997-0039
                                           northeastwi@jdrf.org
                                           www.jdrf.org

Julie Kersten, Executive Director
Dana Paschen, Special Events Coordinator

Foundations

3367 Juvenile Diabetes Research Foundation International
26 Broadway   800-533-2873
New York, NY 10004   Fax: 212-785-9595
                                           info@jdrf.org
                                           www.jdrf.org

Focuses energies on fund-raising, referrals, educational materials and information pertaining to juvenile diabetes.
Aaron J. Kowalski, PhD, President & CEO
Sandra Hijikata, Chief Development Officer

3368 Juvenile Diabetes Research Foundation Cana da
235 Yorkland Blvd.   647-789-2000
Toronto, Ontario, M2J-4Y8   877-287-3533
                                           Fax: 416-491-2111
                                           general@jdrf.ca
                                           www.jdrf.ca

JDRF concentrates on research projects in three areas: Cure, Treat, and Prevent.
Dave Prowten, President & CEO
Susan Delisle, VP, Philanthropy & Corporate Partnership

Libraries & Resource Centers

3369 Diabetes Control Program
California Department of Health Services

PO Box 997413
Sacramento, CA 95899-7413
916-552-9888
Fax: 916-552-9988
http://www.caldiabetes.org/
Our mission is to prevent diabetes and its complications in California's diverse communities.
Susan Lopez-Payan, Interim Chief

3370 Division of Diabetes Translation
National Center for Chronic Disease Prevention
1600 Clifton Rd
Atlantia, GA 30333-3717
800-232-4636
Fax: 770-488-5966
TTY: 888-232-6348
cdcinfo@cdc.gov
www.cdc.gov/diabetes
The Division of Diabetes Translation's (DDT) goal is to reduce the burden of diabetes in the United States. The division works to achieve this goal by combining support for public health-oriented diabetes prevention and control programs (DPCPs) and translating diabetes research findings into widespread clinical and public health practice.

3371 Health Science Library
Marshall University
1600 Medical Center Drive
Huntington, WV 25701
304-691-1700
www.musom.marshall.edu/library
The Health Sciences Library's primary mission is serving the informational needs of the students, faculty, and staff at Marshall University and the Cabell-Huntington Hospital. The Library also plays an important role in providing information services to hospitals and healthcare professionals in the Huntington and the Tri-State area.
Edward Dzierzak, Director

3372 Joslin Center at University of Maryland Medicine
22 S Greene Street
Baltimore, MD 21201
800-492-5538
TDD: 800735225800
www.umm.edu/joslindiabetes
The Joslin Center at University of Maryland Medicine meets the highest standards of care for people with diabetes. Its programs reflect a philosophy which have been the hallmark of Joslin's care — a comprehensive team approach to diabetes treatment with programs designed to help children and adults with diabetes take charge of their own health and well-being.
Thomas W Donner, MD, Director

3373 Naomi Berrie Diabetes Center at Columbia University Medical Center
Russ Berrie Medical Science Pavillion
1150 St. Nicholas Avenue
New York, NY 10032
212-851-5494
Fax: 212-851-5459
diabetes@columbia.edu
nbdiabetes.org
The special focus of the Naomi Berrie Diabetes Center is on families — a concept that differentiates it from almost every other diabetes treatment facility in America. People with diabetes are strongly encouraged to involve their entire families in the treatment process.
Robin Goland, MD, Co-Director
Rudolph Liebel, Co-Director

3374 National Diabetes Information Clearinghous e
One Information Way
Bethesda, MD 20892-3560
800-860-8747
Fax: 703-738-4929
TTY: 866-8569-116
ndic@info.niddk.nih.gov
diabetes.niddk.nih.gov
To serve as a diabetes informational, educational, and referral resource for health professionals and the public. NDIC is a service of the NIDDK.

3375 Schulze Diabetes Institute
University of Minnesota
420 Delaware Street SE
Minneapolis, MN 55455
612-626-3016
diitinfo@umn.edu
www.med.umn.edu
Formerly the Diabetes Institute for Immunology and Transplantation
David Sutherland MD, PhD, Director
Bernard Hering, Director

3376 Tallahassee Memorial Diabetes Center
Tallahassee Memorial Health Care
1300 Miccosukee Road
Tallahassee, FL 32308
850-431-5404
800-662-4278
Fax: 850-431-6325
www.tmh.org/diabetes
TMH provides comprehensive, patient-centered services to both children and adults. The Diabetes Center uses a team approach that involves the patient, physicians, nurse educators, registered dietitians with access to a diabetes counselor and registered pharmacists and social worker.
Richard M Bergenstal, MD, Medical Director

Research Centers

3377 Barbara Davis Center for Childhood Diabetes
13001 E 17th Place
Aurora, CO 80045-6511
303-724-2323
Fax: 303-724-6839
Research and educational organization.
Marian Rewers, Clinical Director
George S Eisenbarth, Executive Director

3378 Baylor College of Medicine: Children's General Clinical Research Center
One Baylor Plaza
Houston, TX 77030
713-798-4780
Fax: 713-790-1345
pedi-webmaster@bcm.edu
www.bcm.edu/pediatrics
Offers research into juvenile aspects of immunology and infectious diseases including diabetes research activities.
Lisa Bomgaars, Medical Director
Mark A Ward, Director

3379 Benaroya Research Institute Virginia Mason Medical Center
Virginia Mason Medical Center
1201 9th Avenue
Seattle, WA 98101-2795
206-583-6525
Fax: 206-223-7543
info@benaroyaresearch.org
www.benaroyaresearch.org
Immunology and diabetes research.
Robert B Lemon, Chair
Gerald Nepom, Director

3380 Diabetes Education and Research Center The Franklin House
The Franklin House
PO Box 897
Philadelphia, PA 19105
215-829-3426
Fax: 215-829-5807
Is a non-profit organization serving the needs of people living in Philadelphia PA and surrounding communities. The goal of the Foundation is to improve the health of people with diabetes.

3381 Diabetes Research and Training Center: University of Alabama at Birmingham
Department of Medicine
1530 3rd Avenue S
Birmingham, AL 35294-1150
205-934-4011
Fax: 205-934-4389
TTY: 205-934-4642
The DRTC works to develop and evaluate new models of diabetes care and to facilitate translational diabetes research.
Dr Carol Garrison, President
William Ferniany, CEO

3382 Division on Endocrinology Northwestern University Feinberg School
Northwestern University Feinberg School of Medicin
251 East Huron Street
Chicago, IL 60611
312-926-6895
Fax: 312-503-7757
help@medicine.northwestern.edu
www.medicine.northwestern.edu
Nonprofit organization focusing research activities on endocrinology metabolism nutrition and specializing in diabetes.
Joe Bass, MD, PhD, Chief of the Division of Endocrinology
Grazia Aleppo, MD, Director, Endocrinology Clinical Practic

3383 Endocrinology Research Laboratory Cabrini Medical Center
Cabrini Medical Center
227 E 19th Street
New York, NY 10003-7457
212-222-7464
www.cabrininy.org

Focuses on the effects of insulin and insulin-like growth factors on human body functions.
Dr Leonid Poretsky, Director

3384   Indiana University: Area Health Education Center
714 N Senate Avenue   317-278-8893
Indianapolis, IN 46202   Fax: 317-278-0392
                                    ahec@iupui.edu
                                    www.ahec.iupui.edu
A collaborative statewide system for community-based primary health care professions education that fosters the continuing improvement of health care services for all citizens in Indiana.
Richard D Kiovsky, MD, Director
Jonathan C Barclay, Associate Director

3385   Indiana University: Center for Diabetes Research
340 West 10th Street   317-274-8157
Indianapolis, IN 46202-3082   Fax: 317-274-1437
                                     rconsidi@iupui.edu
                                     www.medicine.iu.edu
Our goal is to promote the training of scientists whose research will develop new understandings of the basis of the disease and its complications and to cultivate basic science research that can speed the discovery of more effective therapies.
Robert Considine, Associate Professor of Medicine
D Craig Brater MD, Dean

3386   Indiana University: Pharmacology Research Laboratory
Division of Clinical Pharmacology
1001 W 10th Street   317-630-8795
Indianapolis, IN 46202   Fax: 317-630-8185
                                     www.medicine.iupui.edu/clinpharm
We will train highly skilled compassionate and altruistic professionals both generalists and specialists to be future leaders in medical practice academia and industry.
David A Flockhart, Division Director
John T Callaghan, Associate Professor of Medicine

3387   International Diabetes Center at Nicollet
3800 Park Nicollet Boulevard   952-993-3393
Saint Louis Park, MN 55416-2533   888-825-6315
                                     Fax: 952-993-1302
                                     idcdiabetes@parknicollet.com
                                     www.parknicollet.com/diabetes
Research center which improves the quality of life of individuals with diabetes and those at risk of developing diabetes by undertaking clinical care education research and outreach activities that stimulate and support health.
Richard Berg MD, Executive Director

3388   Joslin Diabetes Center
One Joslin Place   617-732-2400
Boston, MA 02215-5306   800-567-5461
                                     Fax: 617-322-40
                                     diabetes@joslin.harvard.edu
                                     www.joslin.org
An internationally recognized leader in diabetes and endocrine disease treatment research and patient and professional education affiliated with Harvard Medical School. In addition to its headquarters in Boston's Longwood Medical area Joslin has affiliated treatment centers across the nation. Established in 1898.
John L Brooks, Chairman of the Board
Martin J Abrahamson, Senior VP, Medical Director

3389   Metabolic Research Institute
1515 N Flagler Drive   561-802-3060
West Palm Beach, FL 33401   Fax: 561-802-3260
                                     www.metabolic-institute.com
The Metabolic Research Institute specializes in clinical studies involving endocrinology disorders complications of endocrinology disorders metabolic problems and selected renal disease.
William A Kaye, Co-Director
Barry Horowitz, Co-Director

3390   Sansum Diabetes Research Institute
2219 Bath Street   805-682-7638
Santa Barbara, CA 93105-4321   Fax: 805-682-3332
                                     info@sansum.org
                                     www.sansum.org

A research institute devoted to the prevention treatment and cure of diabetes.
Lois Jovanovich, CEO & Chief Scientific Officer
Wendy Bevier, Associate Investigator

3391   University of Chicago: Comprehensive Diabetes Center
5841 S Maryland Avenue   773-702-2371
Chicago, IL 60637   800-989-6740
                                     diabetes@uchospitals.edu
                                     www.kovlerdiabetescenter.org
The University of Chicago Kovler Diabetes Center offers a unique fully comprehensive approach to diagnosing and treating diabetes. Focuses on children adolescents and adults with diabetes as well as individuals at the highest risk for serious complications.
Louis H Philipson, Medical Director
Christopher Rhodes, Kovler Diabetes Center Pediatric Program

3392   University of Colorado: General Clinical Research Center, Pediatric
13001 E 17th Place   720-777-2957
Aurora, CO 80045   Fax: 72 -77 -727
Focuses on developmental studies and diabetes research.
Ronald J Sokol, Program Director
Philip S Zeitler, Associate Program Director

3393   University of Iowa: Diabetes Research Center
Department of Internal Medicine
200 Hawkins Drive   319-353-7842
Iowa City, IA 52242   www.int-med.uiowa.edu
The Diabetes Research Center combines the talents of experienced clinical investigators molecular biologists and vascular physiologists in an integrated multidisciplinary approach toward the study and treatment of abnormalities of vascular reactivity which characterize diabetes mellitus.
Ken Kates, Chief Executive Officer
John Swenning, Associate Director

3394   University of Kansas Cray Diabtetes Center
3901 Rainbow Boulevard   913-588-5000
Kansas City, KS 66160-7376   Fax: 913-588-4023
                                     TTY: 913-588-7963
                                     geaks@kumc.edu
                                     www.kumc.edu
The KU Medical Center is a complex institution whose basic functions include research education patient care and community service involving multiple constituencies at state and national levels.
Barbara Atkinson, Executive Vice Chancellor

3395   University of Massachusetts: Diabetes and Endocrinology Research Center
55 Lake Avenue N   508-856-8989
Worcester, MA 01655   evelyn.vignola@umassmed.edu
                                     www.umassmed.edu
UMMS has exploded onto the national scene as a major center for research, and in the past four decades, UMMS researchers have made pivotal advances in HIV, cancer, diabetes, infectious disease and in understanding the molecular basis of disease.
Micheal F Collins MD, Senior VP
Michael P Czech, Professor and Chair

3396   University of Miami: Diabetes Research Institute
200 S Park Road   954-964-4040
Hollywood, FL 33021   800-321-3437
                                     Fax: 954-964-7036
                                     info@drif.org
                                     www.diabetesresearch.org
The Diabetes Research Institute (DRI) is an innovator in many fields of diabetes research but one of its primary strengths lies in islet cell transplantation, a cellular therapy that restores insulin production to normalize blood sugar control.
Thomas D Stern, Chairman
Camillo Ricordi, DRI Scientific Director

3397   University of New Mexico General Clinical Research Center
University of New Mexico Hospital
The University of New Mexico   505-277-0111
Albuquerque, NM 87131-2240   Fax: 505-272-0266
                                        mburge@salud.unm.edu

Diabetes research.
Steve McKernan, CEO
Richard Larson, Vice President for Research

3398 University of Pennsylvania Diabetes and Endocrinology Research Center
700 Clinical Research Building (CRB   215-898-4365
Philadelphia, PA 19104   Fax: 215-898-5408
                                gburgese@mail.med.upenn.edu
                                www.med.upenn.edu/idom/derc
The Penn Diabetes and Endocrinology Research Center (DERC) participates in the nationwide inter-disciplinary program established over two decades ago by the NIDDK to foster research and training in the areas of diabetes and related endocrine and metabolic disorders.
Mitchell A Lazar, Director
Morris J Birnbaum, Co Director

3399 University of Pittsburgh: Department of Molecular Genetics and Biochemistry
200 Lothrop Street   412-648-9570
Pittsburgh, PA 15261   Fax: 412-624-8997
                                info@mmg.pitt.edu
MMG students and fellows routinely publish their research in outstanding journals, present their science at international conferences and go on to achieve positions at prestigious laboratories and institutions.
J Richard Chaillet, Associate Professor
Bruce A McClane, Professor

3400 University of Tennessee: General Clinical Research Center
1265 Union Avenue   901-516-2212
Memphis, TN 38104   Fax: 901-516-7013
Congress directed the National Institutes of Health to establish clinical research centers throughout the United States to launch an all-out attack on human diseases.
Bruce S Alpert MD, Program Director
Teresa Carr, Research Nurses

3401 University of Texas General Clinical Research Center
7400 Merton Minter Boulevard   409-772-1950
San Antonio, TX 78229   Fax: 409-772-8097
                                public.affairs@utmb.edu
Focuses on diabetes and infectious disease research.
Michael Lich MD, Program Director
Garland D Anderson, Principal Investigator

3402 University of Washington Diabetes: Endocrinology Research Center
DVA Puget Sound Health Care System
1660 S Columbian Way   206-616-4860
Seattle, WA 98108   Fax: 206-764-2693
                                derc@u.washington.edu
                                www.depts.washington.edu/diabetes
The primary purpose of the DERC is to facilitate and enhance the diabetes-related research of approximately 100 Affiliate Investigators at the University of Washington
Jerry P Palmer MD, Director
David E Cummings, Deputy Director

3403 Vanderbilt University Diabetes Center
1211 Medical Center Drive   615-322-5000
Nashville, TN 37232   Fax: 615-936-1667
                                dc.brown@vanderbilt.edu
                                www.mc.vanderbilt.edu/diabetes/vdc
The Vanderbilt Diabetes Center provides complete care for children and adults with diabetes under one roof
Joe C Davis, Chair in Biomedical Sciences
Alvin C Powers, Director Vanderbilt Diabetes Center

3404 Veterans Affairs Medical Center: Research Service
500 Foothill Drive   801-582-1565
Salt Lake City, UT 84148   Fax: 801-584-1289
                                www.va.gov
Diabetes and cancer research.
James Floyd, Director
Byron Bair, Director

3405 Warren Grant Magnuson Clinical Center
National Institute of Health

9000 Rockville Pike   301-496-4000
Bethesda, MD 20892   800-411-1222
                                Fax: 301-480-9793
                                TTY: 866-411-1010
                                prpl@mail.cc.nih.gov
                                clinicalcenter.nih.gov
Established in 1953 as the research hospital of the National Institutes of Health. Designed so that patient care facilities are close to research laboratories so new findings of basic and clinical scientists can be quickly applied to the treatment of patients. Upon referral by physicians, patients are admitted to NIH clinical studies.
John Gallin, Director
David Henderson, Deputy Director for Clinical Care

3406 Washington University: Diabetes Research and Training Center
School of Medicine
660 S Euclid Avenue   314-362-0558
Saint Louis, MO 63110   Fax: 314-747-2692
                                drtc.im.wustl.edu
DRTC investigators were involved in conducting 60 investigator-initiated diabetes-related clinical research protocols on the WU GCRC
Jean Schaffer MD, Professor of Medicine
Kristin E Mondy, Medicine/Infectious Diseases

Support Groups & Hotlines

3407 American Diabetes Association
2451 Crystal Drive   888-342-2383
Arlington, VA 22202   askada@diabetes.org
                                www.diabetes.org
Voluntary organization concerned with diabetes and its complications. The mission of the organization is to prevent and cure diabetes and to improve the lives of persons with diabetes. Offers a network of offices nationwide.
Tracey D. Brown, MBA, BChE, Chief Executive Officer
Eloise Scavella, MA, Chief Operating & Strategy Officer

3408 Diabetes Society
1165 Lincoln Avenue   408-287-3785
San Jose, CA 95125   Fax: 408-287-2701
                                ckassouf@diabetessociety.org
The Diabetes Society was organized in 1963 as the result of efforts by a group of mothers of children with diabetes. Today, the Diabetes Society offers its services to the estimated 140,000 people with diabetes in the Santa Clara Valley.
Greg Price, Board President
Carol Kassouf, CEO

3409 National Health Information Center
Office of Disease Prevention & Health Promotion
1101 Wootton Pkwy   Fax: 240-453-8281
Rockville, MD 20852   odphpinfo@hhs.gov
                                www.health.gov/nhic
Supports public health education by maintaining a calendar of National Health Observances; helps connect consumers and health professionals to organizations that can best answer questions and provide up-to-date contact information from reliable sources; updates on a yearly basis toll-free numbers for health information, Federal health clearinghouses and info centers.
Don Wright, MD, MPH, Director

Books

3410 101 Tips for Improving Your Blood Sugar
American Diabetes Association
2451 Crystal Drive   800-342-2383
Arlington, VA 22202   Fax: 703-549-6995
                                www.diabetes.org
Tips for 101 common situations and questions to reduce the risk of complications from blood sugar at the wrong level.
122 pages
Brenda Montgomery, President, Health Care & Education

3411 Balance Your Act: A Book for Adults with Diabetes
Pritchett & Hull

3440 Oakcliff Road
Atlanta, GA 30340-3079
800-774-1124
1993 96 pages Paperback
ISBN: 0-939838-14-1

3412 Buyer's Guide
American Diabetes Association
2451 Crystal Drive
Arlington, VA 22202
800-342-2383
Fax: 703-549-6995
www.diabetes.org

A catalog listing all manufacturers of insulin, syringes, pumps, test strips, monitors and more.
Brenda Montgomery, President, Health Care & Education

3413 Caring for the Diabetic Soul
American Diabetes Association
2451 Crystal Drive
Arlington, VA 22202
800-342-2383
Fax: 703-549-6995
www.diabetes.org

Restoring emotional balance for yourself and your family.
213 pages
Brenda Montgomery, President, Health Care & Education

3414 Clinical Practice Recommendations
American Diabetes Association
2451 Crystal Drive
Arlington, VA 22202
800-342-2383
Fax: 703-549-6995
www.diabetes.org

Features all current position and consensus statements of the American Diabetes Association.
Brenda Montgomery, President, Health Care & Education

3415 Complete Weight Loss Workbook
American Diabetes Association
2451 Crystal Drive
Arlington, VA 22202
800-342-2383
Fax: 703-549-6995
www.diabetes.org

A unique, brisk, practical workbook that offers a series of fresh, memorable tests, checklists, worksheets, mini-cases, calculation exercises, mental reminders, and other practical aids to losing weight and staying fit for good.
252 pages
Brenda Montgomery, President, Health Care & Education

3416 Computer Planned Menus for Health Professionals
American Diabetes Association
2451 Crystal Drive
Arlington, VA 22202
800-342-2383
Fax: 703-549-6995
www.diabetes.org

Input a patient's dietary prescription, food preferences, and budget, and the program produces individualized menus. Professional version includes license to distribute these customized menus.
Brenda Montgomery, President, Health Care & Education

3417 Control Diabetes the Easy Way
Random House Trade Books
400 Hahn Road
Westminster, MD 21157-4663
800-733-3000
Fax: 800-659-2436
ISBN: 0-679778-03-9

3418 Convenience Food Facts
American Diabetes Association
2451 Crystal Drive
Arlington, VA 22202
800-342-2383
Fax: 703-549-6995
www.diabetes.org

Helps to serve appetizing convenience foods low in sodium, cholesterol, and fat.
459 pages Softcover
Brenda Montgomery, President, Health Care & Education

3419 Cooking a la Heart
American Diabetes Association
2451 Crystal Drive
Arlington, VA 22202
800-342-2383
Fax: 703-549-6995
www.diabetes.org

Recipes that include a complete nutrient profile with diabetic exchanges.
Brenda Montgomery, President, Health Care & Education

3420 Diabetes & Pregnancy: What to Expect
American Diabetes Association

2451 Crystal Drive
Arlington, VA 22202
800-342-2383
Fax: 703-549-6995
www.diabetes.org

Information concerning an unborn baby's development, tests to expect, labor and delivery, birth control, and more.
Brenda Montgomery, President, Health Care & Education

3421 Diabetes A to Z
American Diabetes Association
2451 Crystal Drive
Arlington, VA 22202
800-342-2383
Fax: 703-549-6995
www.diabetes.org

Dictionary-style guidebook discussing basic terms and issues concerning diabetes. Third edition.
202 pages
Brenda Montgomery, President, Health Care & Education

3422 Diabetes Care Made Easy
Chronimed Publishing
PO Box 59032
Minneapolis, MN 55459-0032
612-513-6475
800-848-2793
Fax: 612-443-2806

Written and designed for both adults and for children with limited reading skills, this easy-to-read book explains how to exercise and eat for better health, prevent foot problems, test blood sugar, cope with emotions, take insulin, and more. Also available in Spanish.
180 pages Paperback
ISBN: 1-885115-31-8

3423 Diabetes Education Goals
American Diabetes Association
2451 Crystal Drive
Arlington, VA 22202
800-342-2383
Fax: 703-549-6995
www.diabetes.org

Features advice on how to assess, plan, and evaluate patient education and counseling programs. Covers both short-term and in-depth goals. Focuses on the education process and assessing the unique needs of each patient.
64 pages Softcover
Brenda Montgomery, President, Health Care & Education

3424 Diabetes Low-Fat & No-Fat Meals in Minutes
John Wiley and Sons, Inc.
Cust Ser-Consumer Accts
Indianapolis, IN 46256
877-762-2974
Fax: 800-597-3299
consumers@wiley.com
www.wiley.com

Includes more than 250 recipes, 60 days of diabetic menus, and 16 pages of full-color photographs. Each recipe features a complete nutrition analysis, including diabetic exchanges.
1998 352 pages
ISBN: 1-565610-84-9

3425 Diabetes Medical Nutrition Therapy
American Diabetes Association
2451 Crystal Drive
Arlington, VA 22202
800-342-2383
Fax: 703-549-6995
www.diabetes.org

A professional guide to management and nutrition education resources. Provides in-depth coverage of nutrition assessment, goal setting, intervention, and outcome evaluation. Information is provided on specific resources and case studies are cited for practical examples.
Softcover
Brenda Montgomery, President, Health Care & Education

3426 Diabetes Mellitus: A Practical Handbook
Bull Publishing Company
PO Box 1377
Boulder, CO 80306
800-676-2855
Fax: 303-545-6354
www.bullpub.com

This helpful and user friendly practical guide addresses the everyday concerns of all diabetics.
2002 Paperback
ISBN: 0-923521-72-0

3427 Diabetes Self-Management
RA Rapaport Publishing

150 W 22nd Street
New York, NY 10011-2421
212-989-0200
800-234-0923
Fax: 212-989-4786
www.diabetesselfmanagement.com

Publishes practical, how to information, focusing on the day-to-day and long term aspects of diabetes in a positive and up-beat style. Gives subscribers up-to-date news, facts and advice to help them maintain their wellness and make informed decisions regarding their health.
Ingird Strauch, Executive
Richard A. Rapaport, Publisher

3428 Diabetes Sourcebook
Dawn D Matthews, author
Omnigraphics
155 W. Congress
Detroit, MI 48226-4105
313-961-1340
313-961-1383
Fax: 800-875-1340
contact@omnigraphics.com
www.omnigraphics.com

This Sourcebook contains information for people seeking to understand the risk factors, complications, and management of the different types of diabetes. It includes information about testing, diagnosis, medications, and other topics related to living with diabetes.
2003 622 pages
ISBN: 0-780806-29-8

3429 Diabetes Teaching Guide for People Who Use Insulin
Joslin Diabetes Center
1 Joslin Place
Boston, MA 02215-5306
617-732-2400
Fax: 617-732-2562
diabetes@joslin.harvard.edu
www.joslin.org

Discusses the causes of diabetes, the role of diet and exercise, meal planning and complications. Also provide information on drawing blood, mixing and injecting insulin.

3430 Diabetes Youth Curriculum: A Toolbox for Educators
Chronimed Publishing
PO Box 59032
Minneapolis, MN 55459-0032
612-513-6475
800-848-2793
Fax: 612-443-2806

Program consisting of two volumes: the Curriculum and the Resource and Activities Guide (listed separately). Divided into sections dealing with general development concepts and specific guidelines for ages 6 to 8, 9 to 11, and 12 to 16.
136 pages Paperback
ISBN: 0-937721-49-2

3431 Diabetes: A Guide to Living Well
American Diabetes Association
2451 Crystal Drive
Arlington, VA 22202
800-342-2383
Fax: 703-549-6995
www.diabetes.org

Offers a guide to helping the person with diabetes design a program of individualized self-care and gain the willingness to follow it. Also tells how to deal with diet, exercise, stress, emotions, negative beliefs, and self-image.
242 pages Paperback
ISBN: 1-580402-09-7
Brenda Montgomery, President, Health Care & Education

3432 Diabetes: Your Complete Exercise Guide
Human Kinetics Publishers
PO Box 5076
Champaign, IL 61825-5076
217-351-1549
800-747-4457
Fax: 217-351-5076

Part of the Cooper Clinic and Research Institute Fitness Series providing exercise rehabilitation for persons with diabetes.
144 pages Paperback
ISBN: 0-873224-27-2

3433 Diabetes: Your Questions Answered
Paul Drury and Wendy Gatling, author
Elsevier
Book Cust Ser Dept
St. Louis, MO 63146
800-545-2522
Fax: 800-535-9935
usbkinfo@elsevier.com
www.elsevier.com

This new volume in the popular Your Questions Answered series uses a question-and-answer format to provide easy access to hands-on guidance on the management of diabetes. Its succinct, practical coverage explores the latest evidence-based practice guilines and their interpretation. Case vignettes illustrate the clinical relevance of the material.
2004 380 pages Softcover
ISBN: 0-443073-89-9

3434 Diabetic Gourmet
Diabetes Self-Management Books
PO Box 10676
Des Moines, IA 50336-0676
800-664-9269

3435 Diabetic's Guide to Health and Fitness
Human Kinetics Publishers
PO Box 5076
Champaign, IL 61825-5076
217-351-1549
800-747-4457
Fax: 217-351-5076
272 pages Paperback
ISBN: 0-880113-47-2

3436 Direct and Indirect Costs of Diabetes in the US
American Diabetes Association
2451 Crystal Drive
Arlington, VA 22202
800-342-2383
Fax: 703-549-6995
www.diabetes.org

Examines the specific costs of diabetes, as well as all the costs of health care for people with diabetes and compares those costs with the total cost of health care for the US population without diabetes.
32 pages Softcover
Brenda Montgomery, President, Health Care & Education

3437 Dr. Bernstein's Diabetes Solution
Richard K Bernstein, MD, author
Little, Brown and Company
Haworth Public School
New York, NY 07641
201-384-5526
800-759-0190
Fax: 201-384-8619
publicity@littlebrown.com

A complete guide to achieving normal blood sugars with strong emphasis on diet and up-to-date information on products, insulins, and oral agents.
512 pages Hardcover
ISBN: 0-316099-06-6

3438 Easy & Elegant Entrees
American Diabetes Association
2451 Crystal Drive
Arlington, VA 22202
800-342-2383
Fax: 703-549-6995
www.diabetes.org

Recipes that are low in fat and calories.
Brenda Montgomery, President, Health Care & Education

3439 Exchanges for All Occasions
American Diabetes Association
2451 Crystal Drive
Arlington, VA 22202
800-342-2383
Fax: 703-549-6995
www.diabetes.org

Meal planning suggestions for traveling, entertaining, camping, dining out, and more.
Brenda Montgomery, President, Health Care & Education

3440 Family Cookbook: Volumes I-IV
American Diabetes Association
2451 Crystal Drive
Arlington, VA 22202
800-342-2383
Fax: 703-549-6995
www.diabetes.org

Unforgettable recipes for the whole family. Great for diabetics.
Brenda Montgomery, President, Health Care & Education

3441 Fitness Book: For People with Diabetes
American Diabetes Association
2451 Crystal Drive
Arlington, VA 22202
800-342-2383
Fax: 703-549-6995
www.diabetes.org

Advice on learning to exercise to lose weight, exercise safely, increase your competitive edge, get your mind and body ready to exercise, and more.
149 pages
Brenda Montgomery, President, Health Care & Education

3442 Great Starts & Fine Finishes
American Diabetes Association
2451 Crystal Drive   800-342-2383
Arlington, VA 22202   Fax: 703-549-6995
                                        www.diabetes.org
Healthy select cookbook offering great meals in minutes.
Brenda Montgomery, President, Health Care & Education

3443 Healthy Eater's Guide to Family & Chain Restaurants
American Diabetes Association
2451 Crystal Drive   800-342-2383
Arlington, VA 22202   Fax: 703-549-6995
                                        www.diabetes.org
Advice on safe choices from fast-food menus, complete with nutrition values and exchanges.
Brenda Montgomery, President, Health Care & Education

3444 Healthy Homestyle Cookbook
American Diabetes Association
2451 Crystal Drive   800-342-2383
Arlington, VA 22202   Fax: 703-549-6995
                                        www.diabetes.org
Lay-flat binding for hands-free reference.
181 pages
Brenda Montgomery, President, Health Care & Education

3445 How to Cook for People with Diabetes
American Diabetes Association
2451 Crystal Drive   800-342-2383
Arlington, VA 22202   Fax: 703-549-6995
                                        www.diabetes.org
One hundred and fifty recipes featuring unusual techniques.
205 pages
Brenda Montgomery, President, Health Care & Education

3446 If Your Child Has Diabetes: An Answer Book for Parents
Putnam Publishing Group
200 Madison Avenue   212-951-8400
New York, NY 10016-3903
Provides information and recommendations for parents of children with diabetes on subjects such as school, recreation, medical and life insurance and employment as well as general information about diabetes.

3447 Intensified Insulin Management for You
Chronimed Publishing
PO Box 59032   612-513-6475
Minneapolis, MN 55459-0032   800-848-2793
                                        Fax: 612-443-2806
Manual helping those with diabetes to understand and use an intensified insulin regimen under the guidance of their health care provider. A personalized program for advanced diabetes self-care that focuses on emotional and intellectual goals as well as on how diet and exercise fit into an intensified regimen.
85 pages Paperback
ISBN: 0-937721-84-0

3448 Intensive Diabetes Management
American Diabetes Association
2451 Crystal Drive   800-342-2383
Arlington, VA 22202   Fax: 703-549-6995
                                        www.diabetes.org
Delivers practical advice on how to help your patients achieve better glucose control through intensified management.
128 pages Softcover
Brenda Montgomery, President, Health Care & Education

3449 Learning to Live Well with Diabetes
Chronimed Publishing
PO Box 59032   612-513-6475
Minneapolis, MN 55459-0032   800-848-2793
                                        Fax: 612-443-2806
Updated and revised edition reflects the latest medical advances, technologies, and research. In straight-forward language, it explains how to take charge of your diabetes and live an active, healthy life.
525 pages Paperback
ISBN: 0-937721-79-4

3450 Life with Diabetes: A Series of Teaching Outlines
American Diabetes Association
2451 Crystal Drive   800-342-2383
Arlington, VA 22202   Fax: 703-549-6995
                                        www.diabetes.org
Presents a comprehensive curriculum for diabetes education. Each outline includes a statement of purpose, prerequisites for attending the session, materials needed for teaching the session, recommended teaching method, a content outline, instructor notes, an evaluation and documentation plan, and suggested readings related to each topic.
Brenda Montgomery, President, Health Care & Education

3451 Managing Type II Diabetes
Chronimed Publishing
PO Box 59032   612-513-6475
Minneapolis, MN 55459-0032   800-848-2793
                                        Fax: 612-443-2806
Revised and updated guide for people with Type II diabetes. Offers the latest medical advances and practical advice. Includes tips on dealing with emotions, finding motivation to manage diabetes, preventing and treating complications, monitoring blood glucose, and more.
192 pages Paperback
ISBN: 1-885115-26-1

3452 Managing Your Gestational Diabetes
Chronimed Publishing
PO Box 59032   612-513-6475
Minneapolis, MN 55459-0032   800-848-2793
                                        Fax: 612-443-2806
Gives answers to questions on weight gain, injecting insulin, and preventing complications.
128 pages Paperback
ISBN: 1-565610-52-0

3453 Manual of Pediatric Nutrition
B.C Decker, Inc.
50 King Street E, Floor 2   905-522-7017
Ontario, Canada L8N 3K7,   800-568-7281
                                        Fax: 905-522-7839
                                        info@bcdecker.com
                                        www.bcdecker.com
A comprehensive guide that provides an overview of nutritional care for both healthy and ill pediatric patients.
2005 500 pages
ISBN: 1-550093-08-8

3454 Maximizing the Role of Nutrition in Diabetes Management
American Diabetes Association
2451 Crystal Drive   800-342-2383
Arlington, VA 22202   Fax: 703-549-6995
                                        www.diabetes.org
Integrates medical, nutritional, and behavioral sciences and recognizes the importance of each in total diabetes care.
64 pages Softcover
Brenda Montgomery, President, Health Care & Education

3455 Medical Management of Pregnancy Complicated by Diabetes
American Diabetes Association
2451 Crystal Drive   800-342-2383
Arlington, VA 22202   Fax: 703-549-6995
                                        www.diabetes.org
Information on every aspect of pregnancy and diabetes, providing precise protocols for treatment. Techniques for managing blood glucose levels from the time of conception through every stage of pregnancy.
136 pages Softcover
Brenda Montgomery, President, Health Care & Education

3456 Medical Management of Type I Diabetes
American Diabetes Association
2451 Crystal Drive   800-342-2383
Arlington, VA 22202   Fax: 703-549-6995
                                        www.diabetes.org

Instruction on all issues impacting patients with Type 1 diabetes, including: blood glucose regulation, nutrition, exercise, blood pressure, blood lipid levels, and other key elements.
176 pages Softcover
Brenda Montgomery, President, Health Care & Education

3457 Medical Management of Type II Diabetes
American Diabetes Association
2451 Crystal Drive   800-342-2383
Arlington, VA 22202   Fax: 703-549-6995
                                                        www.diabetes.org
Complete overview of Type II diabetes, including diagnosis and classification, pathogenesis, and prevention/treatment of complications.
112 pages Softcover
Brenda Montgomery, President, Health Care & Education

3458 Month of Meals Set of 5
American Diabetes Association
2451 Crystal Drive   800-342-2383
Arlington, VA 22202   Fax: 703-549-6995
                                                        www.diabetes.org
Each planner offers twenty-eight day's worth of tasty selections including a holiday planner, ethnic meals, fast foods, meat and potatoes, and vegetarian dishes. Available individually.
5 planners
Brenda Montgomery, President, Health Care & Education

3459 Outsmarting Diabetes
Richard S Beaser, author
John Wiley and Sons, Inc.
Cust Ser-Consumer Accts   877-762-2974
Indianapolis, IN 46256   Fax: 800-597-3299
                                                        consumers@wiley.com
                                                        www.wiley.com
Shows how intensive control can dramatically reduce the effects of insulin-dependent diabetes and the risk of long-term complications.
256 pages Paperback
ISBN: 0-471346-94-4

3460 Pumping Insulin
John Walsh PA, CDE and Ruth Roberts, MA, author
Torrey Pines Publishing
The Diabetes Mall   619-497-0900
San Diego, CA 92103   800-988-4772
                                               Fax: 619-497-0900
                                                        www.diabetesnet.com
Features information for achieving excellent blood sugar control, correcting pump problems quickly, and lowering risks for complications.
322 pages Paperback
John Walsh,PA,CDE, Author
Ruth Roberts MA, Author

3461 Quick and Easy Meals and Menus
Diabetes Self-Management Books
PO Box 11066   800-664-9269
Des Moines, IA 50380-0001

3462 Quick and Healthy Recipes & Ideas
American Diabetes Association
2451 Crystal Drive   800-342-2383
Arlington, VA 22202   Fax: 703-549-6995
                                                        www.diabetes.org
More than 190 recipes with complete nutrition information for each.
Brenda Montgomery, President, Health Care & Education

3463 Quick and Hearty Main Dishes
American Diabetes Association
2451 Crystal Drive   800-342-2383
Arlington, VA 22202   Fax: 703-549-6995
                                                        www.diabetes.org
Offers recipes for main courses.
Brenda Montgomery, President, Health Care & Education

3464 Raising a Child with Diabetes: A Guide for Parents
American Diabetes Association

2451 Crystal Drive   800-342-2383
Arlington, VA 22202   Fax: 703-549-6995
                                                        www.diabetes.org
You'll learn how to help your child adjust to insulin to allow for favorite foods, have a busy schedule and still feel healthy and strong, negotiate the twists and turns of being different, and much more.
Brenda Montgomery, President, Health Care & Education

3465 Real Life Parenting of Kids with Diabetes
Virginia Nasmyth Loy, author
McGraw-Hill Companies
Returns Department   877-833-5524
Dubuque, IA 52002   Fax: 609-308-4484
                        pbg.ecommerce_custserv@mcgraw-hill.com
                                                        www.mcgraw-hill.com
Virginia Loy had engineered successful management of her two sons' diabetes for 12 years at the time of publication. She is offering her organized, experienced, and practical advice to parents, for helping children to cope with and manage their diabetes from elementary school through college.
2001 188 pages Paperback
ISBN: 1-580400-83-3

3466 Resource and Activities Guide
Chronimed Publishing
PO Box 59032   612-513-6475
Minneapolis, MN 55459-0032   800-848-2793
                                               Fax: 612-443-2806
For use with the Diabetes Youth Curriculum. Contains 300 educational activities that correspond with the text in the Curriculum and can easily be removed for photocopying.
260 pages Loose Leaf
ISBN: 0-937721-50-6

3467 Right from the Start
American Diabetes Association
2451 Crystal Drive   800-342-2383
Arlington, VA 22202   Fax: 703-549-6995
                                                        www.diabetes.org
Addresses issues such as: learning to take charge, coping, changing one's eating habits, getting fit, self-testing, family issues, preventive care, finances, as well as resources to turn to for further information and support. Available for both Type 1 and Type 2.
Pkg. of 25
Brenda Montgomery, President, Health Care & Education

3468 Savory Soups and Salads
American Diabetes Association
2451 Crystal Drive   800-342-2383
Arlington, VA 22202   Fax: 703-549-6995
                                                        www.diabetes.org
Offers exciting recipes for quick and healthy side dishes.
Brenda Montgomery, President, Health Care & Education

3469 Simple and Tasty Side Dishes
American Diabetes Association
2451 Crystal Drive   800-342-2383
Arlington, VA 22202   Fax: 703-549-6995
                                                        www.diabetes.org
Healthy recipes for the diabetic.
Brenda Montgomery, President, Health Care & Education

3470 Special Celebrations and Parties Cookbook
American Diabetes Association
2451 Crystal Drive   800-342-2383
Arlington, VA 22202   Fax: 703-549-6995
                                                        www.diabetes.org
Offers a list of more than 150 holiday recipes.
Brenda Montgomery, President, Health Care & Education

3471 Take-Charge Guide to Type I Diabetes
American Diabetes Association
2451 Crystal Drive   800-342-2383
Arlington, VA 22202   Fax: 703-549-6995
                                                        www.diabetes.org
Offers answers to the most important questions regarding Type 1 diabetes.
Brenda Montgomery, President, Health Care & Education

3472 Therapy for Diabetes Mellitus and Related Disorders
American Diabetes Association
2451 Crystal Drive
Arlington, VA 22202
800-342-2383
Fax: 703-549-6995
www.diabetes.org
Guides through the treatment of specific problems of persons with diabetes. Represents the views and experience of leading clinicians in a concise, practical approach to treatment.
384 pages
Brenda Montgomery, President, Health Care & Education

3473 Type 2 Diabetes: Your Healthy Living Guide
American Diabetes Association
2451 Crystal Drive
Arlington, VA 22202
800-342-2383
Fax: 703-549-6995
www.diabetes.org
A thorough guide to staying healthy with Type 2. Includes everything from choosing a health care team and eating and exercising properly to self-monitoring, insulin, dealing with complications, and keep mentally fit.
180 pages
Brenda Montgomery, President, Health Care & Education

3474 Using Insulin
Torrey Pines Press
The Diabetes Mall
San Diego, CA 92103
619-497-0900
800-988-4772
Fax: 619-497-0900
www.diabetesnet.com
How to take charge of your blood sugars in diabetes. Information on feeling better, improving your health, and achieving peace of mind.
316 pages Paperback
John Walsh,PA,CDE, Author
Ruth Roberts MA, Author

3475 Voice of the Diabetic
200 East Wells Street
Columbia, MO 65201
573-875-8911
epc@roudley.com
www.nfb.org
Personal stories and practical guidelines by blind diabetics and medical professionals, medical news, resource column and a recipe corner.

3476 Weight Management for Type II Diabetes
John Wiley and Sons, Inc.
Cust Ser-Consumer Accts
Indianapolis, IN 46256
877-762-2974
Fax: 800-597-3299
consumers@wiley.com
www.wiley.com
An interactive, personalized guide that helps you manage your weight and your diabetes by making gradual lifestyle changes. Details how to set reasonable goals, keep pace with an exercise program, design your own meal plan, manage stress, and more.
1997 224 pages Paperback
ISBN: 0-471347-50-7

3477 When Diabetes Complicates Your Life
Chronimed Publishing
PO Box 59032
Minneapolis, MN 55459-0032
612-513-6475
800-848-2793
Fax: 612-443-2806
Directly addresses the subject of diabetic complications. This revised edition includes chapters on nerves and circulation, kidneys, and eyes. Enhancements to the new edition include a chapter on vitamins, herbs, and supplements, and reference to the latest research.
Feb 1998 208 pages Paperback
ISBN: 1-565611-27-6

Children's Books

3478 Diabetes
Franklin Watts Grolier
90 Old Sherman Turnpike
Danbury, CT 06816-0001
203-797-3500
800-621-1115
Fax: 203-797-3197
www.auth.grolier.com

Looks at the differences between juvenile and adult-onset diabetes, discusses the history of the disease, causes, complications and treatments.
128 pages Grades 7-12
ISBN: 0-531108-82-1

3479 Dinosaur Tamer
American Diabetes Association
2451 Crystal Drive
Arlington, VA 22202
800-342-2383
Fax: 703-549-6995
www.diabetes.org
Twenty-five fictional stories that will entertain, enlighten, and ease your child's frustrations about having diabetes. Each tale evaporates the fear of insulin shots, blood tests, going to diabetes camp, and more.
Ages 8-12
Brenda Montgomery, President, Health Care & Education

3480 Even Little Kids Get Diabetes
Connie Pirner, author
Albert Whitman & Company
250 South Northwest Hgwy
Suite 320, IL 60068-2723
847-232-2800
800-255-7675
Fax: 847-581-0039
mail@awhitmanco.com
www.albertwhitman.com
A preschooler tells how it was discovered when she was only two, that she has this common disease and describes her daily treatment and the precautions her family must observe.
24 pages Hardcover
ISBN: 0-807521-58-8
Alison Acheson, Author
Mike Allegra, Author

3481 Everyone Likes to Eat
John Wiley and Sons, Inc.
Customer Service-Consumer Accounts
Indianapolis, IN 46256
877-762-2974
Fax: 800-597-3299
consumers@wiley.com
www.wiley.com
Revised and up-to-date second edition. How children can eat most of the foods they enjoy and still take care of their diabetes. Intended for elementary-school-age children, this guide is filled with activities, puzzles, and problem-solving exercises.
128 pages Paperback
ISBN: 0-471346-82-1

3482 Grilled Cheese
American Diabetes Association
2451 Crystal Drive
Arlington, VA 22202
800-342-2383
Fax: 703-549-6995
www.diabetes.org
Story designed to ease children's fears and frustrations of having diabetes.
Brenda Montgomery, President, Health Care & Education

3483 Kiss the Candy Days Good-bye
Delacorte Press
1540 Broadway
New York, NY 10036-4039
212-354-6500
This book focuses on Jimmy who is surprised to learn he has diabetes after seeming so healthy and fit. The story contains information on symptoms and the dangers of untreated diabetes.
Grades 6-8

3484 Living with Diabetes
Franklin Watts Grolier
90 Old Sherman Turnpike
Danbury, CT 06816-0001
203-797-3500
800-621-1115
Fax: 203-797-3197
Shows how persons with diabetes can control their illness and lead productive lives.
32 pages Grades 5-7
ISBN: 0-531108-44-9

3485 Shira: A Legacy of Courage
Doubleday
666 5th Avenue
New York, NY 10103-0001
212-354-6500

A biographical account of Shira Putter's fight with a rare form of diabetes. Using the victim's diary, this book is both powerful and poignant, as well as an educational resource for all people struggling with diabetes.
Grades 4-9

3486 Sun, the Rain and the Insulin
American Diabetes Association
2451 Crystal Drive
Arlington, VA 22202
800-342-2383
Fax: 703-549-6995
www.diabetes.org
Author chronicles a week at a summer diabetes camp, using her expertise and experience to capture the journey and the fight to cope that all people go through when diabetes hits the family.
Brenda Montgomery, President, Health Care & Education

Magazines

3487 Countdown
Juvenile Diabetes Foundation International
432 Park Avenue S
New York, NY 10016-8013
212-889-7575
Fax: 212-725-7259
Offers the latest news and information in diabetes research and treatment to everyone from an international arena of diabetes investigators to parents of small children with diabetes, from physicians to school teachers, from pharmacists to corporate executives.
Sandy Dylak, Editor

3488 Diabetes
American Diabetes Association
2451 Crystal Drive
Arlington, VA 22202
800-342-2383
Fax: 703-549-6995
www.diabetes.org
A peer-reviewed journal focusing on laboratory research.
Monthly
Brenda Montgomery, President, Health Care & Education

3489 Diabetes Care
American Diabetes Association
2451 Crystal Drive
Arlington, VA 22202
800-342-2383
Fax: 703-549-6995
www.diabetes.org
A peer-reviewed journal emphasizing reviews, commentaries and original research on topics of interest to clinicians.
Monthly
Brenda Montgomery, President, Health Care & Education

3490 Diabetes Forecast
American Diabetes Association
2451 Crystal Drive
Arlington, VA 22202
800-342-2383
Fax: 703-549-6995
www.diabetes.org
The monthly lifestyle magazine for people with diabetes, featuring complete, in-depth coverage of all aspects of living with diabetes.
Monthly
Brenda Montgomery, President, Health Care & Education

3491 Diabetes Spectrum: From Research to Practice
American Diabetes Association
2451 Crystal Drive
Arlington, VA 22202
800-342-2383
Fax: 703-549-6995
www.diabetes.org
A journal translating research into practice and focusing on diabetes education and counseling.
Quarterly
Brenda Montgomery, President, Health Care & Education

3492 Joslin Magazine
Joslin Diabetes Center
1 Joslin Place
Boston, MA 02215-5306
617-732-2400
Fax: 617-732-2562
diabetes@joslin.harvard.edu
www.joslin.org

3493 Voice of the Diabetic
Ed Bryant, author
National Federation of the Blind

200 East Wells Street
Baltimore, MD 21230-4998
410-659-9314
Fax: 410-685-5653
www.nfb.org
The leading publication in the diabetes field. Each issue addresses the problems and concerns of diabetes, with a special emphasis for those who have lost vision due to diabetes. Available in print and on cassette.
28 pages Quarterly
Eileen Ley, Director of Publishing
Elizabeth Lunt, Editor

Newsletters

3494 Clinical Diabetes
American Diabetes Association
2451 Crystal Drive
Arlington, VA 22202
800-342-2383
Fax: 703-549-6995
www.diabetes.org
A bimonthly newsletter providing practical treatment information for primary care physicians.
BiMonthly
Brenda Montgomery, President, Health Care & Education

3495 Diabetes Advisor
American Diabetes Association
2451 Crystal Drive
Arlington, VA 22202
703-549-1500
800-342-2383
Fax: 703-549-6995
askada@diabetes.org
www.diabetes.org
Offers informative articles and research in the area of diabetes for professionals and patients. Offers facts and research on diagnosis, symptoms, technology and the newest devices for persons with diabetes, as well as referral and hotline numbers.
Bi-Monthly
Brenda Montgomery, President, Health Care & Education

3496 Diabetes Dateline
National Diabetes Information Clearinghouse
1 Information Way
Bethesda, MD 20205
301-496-3583
800-860-8747
Fax: 301-907-8906
www.niddk.nih.gov

BiAnnually

3497 Diabetes Educator
American Association of Diabetes Educators
444 N Michigan Avenue
Chicago, IL 60611-3959
312-644-2233
Fax: 312-644-4411
Offers information to health professionals working with persons with diabetes.
James J Balija, Executive Director

3498 Kid's Corner
American Diabetes Association
2451 Crystal Drive
Arlington, VA 22202
800-342-2383
Fax: 703-549-6995
www.diabetes.org
A mini-magazine for kids that offers word searches, puzzles and jokes - plus an encouraging story in each issue about kids with diabetes.
8 pages Quarterly
Brenda Montgomery, President, Health Care & Education

Pamphlets

3499 Dental Tips for Diabetics
National Diabetes Information Clearinghouse
1 Information Way
Bethesda, MD 20892-0001
301-496-3583
800-860-8747
Fax: 301-907-8906
ndic@info.niddk.nih.gov
www.niddk.nih.gov
Discusses the relationship between diabetes and periodontal disease. Describes the symptoms of periodontal problems and preventive measures.

3500   Diabetes Dateline
National Diabetes Information Clearinghouse
1 Information Way   800-860-8747
Bethesda, MD 20892-0001   Fax: 301-634-0716
                                                    TTY: 866-569-1162
                                               ndic@info.niddk.nih.gov
                                               www.diabetes.niddk.nih.gov
This bulletin features news about current issues in diabetes research and control, special events, patient and professional meeting, and new publications available from NDIC and other organizations.
Quarterly

3501   Diabetes and Brief Illness
Chronimed Publishing
PO Box 59032   612-513-6475
Minneapolis, MN 55459-0032   800-848-2793
                                                    Fax: 612-443-2806
This booklet gives self-care instructions and eating suggestions to prevent development of ketoacidosis during brief illness that disrupts normal eating.
12 pages Pack of 10

3502   Diabetes and Exercise
Chronimed Publishing
PO Box 59032   612-513-6475
Minneapolis, MN 55459-0032   800-848-2793
                                                    Fax: 612-443-2806
Exercise and weight loss tips and precautions for those with both insulin and non-insulin-dependent diabetes.
36 pages Pack of 10

3503   Diabetes in Pregnancy
March of Dimes
1275 Mamaroneck Avenue   914-997-4488
White Plains, NY 10605   Fax: 212-254-3518
                                               NY639@marchofdimes.com
                                               www.marchofdimes.com
Fact Sheets: one or two page review written for the general public.

3504   Diabetic Foot Care
American Diabetes Association
2451 Crystal Drive   800-342-2383
Arlington, VA 22202   Fax: 703-549-6995
                                                    www.diabetes.org
Booklet discussing early detection and prompt treatment of diabetic foot problems.
12 pages
Brenda Montgomery, President, Health Care & Education

3505   Gestational Diabetes: What To Expect
American Diabetes Association
2451 Crystal Drive   703-549-1500
Arlington, VA 22202   800-342-2383
                                                    Fax: 703-549-6995
                                                    www.diabetes.org
A complete comprehensive guide for women with gestational diabetes. Explains the stages in your baby's development, the types of prenatal testing you may recieve, and what to expect during labor, delivery, and beyond.
100 pages
ISBN: 1-580402-33-X
Brenda Montgomery, President, Health Care & Education

3506   Healthy Eating
Chronimed Publishing
PO Box 59032   612-513-6475
Minneapolis, MN 55459-0032   800-848-2793
                                                    Fax: 612-443-2806
Offers simple guidelines for choosing healthful foods, lowering fat intake, and timing meals and snacks. Available in Spanish.
Pack of 10

3507   Healthy Food Choices
American Diabetes Association
2451 Crystal Drive   800-342-2383
Arlington, VA 22202   Fax: 703-549-6995
                                                    www.diabetes.org
Pamphlet containing the basics of good nutrition.
Brenda Montgomery, President, Health Care & Education

3508   Hypoglycemia The Other Sugar Disease
Anita Flegg, author
Book Coach Press
3-390 MacKay Street   613-746-3334
Ontario, Canada K1M 2C4,   info@bookcoachpress.com
                                               www4.bookcoachpress.com
This book is filled with dozens of real-life practical tips and will give you the tools to feel better and take control of your life.

3509   Insulin-Dependent Diabetes
National Diabetes Information Clearinghouse
1 Information Way   800-860-8747
Bethesda, MD 20892-0001   Fax: 301-634-0716
                                                    TTY: 866-569-1162
                                               ndic@info.niddk.nih.gov
                                               www.diabetes.niddk.nih.gov
Explains diabetes and how it develops and describes the differences between the two major forms of diabetes, insulin-dependent and noninsulin-dependent.

3510   Low Blood Sugar
Chronimed Publishing
PO Box 59032   612-513-6475
Minneapolis, MN 55459-0032   800-848-2793
                                                    Fax: 612-443-2806
Pack of 10

3511   Noninsulin-Dependent Diabetes
National Diabetes Information Clearinghouse
1 Information Way   800-860-8747
Bethesda, MD 20892-0001   Fax: 301-634-0716
                                                    TTY: 866-569-1162
                                               ndic@info.niddk.nih.gov
                                               www.diabetes.niddk.nih.gov
Describes the symptoms and diagnosis of noninsulin-dependent diabetes; diabetes management, including diet, oral drugs, and insulin; glucose monitoring; and complications.
1992 35 pages

3512   Recognizing and Treating Low Blood Sugar (Hypoglycemia)
Chronimed Publishing
PO Box 59032   612-513-6475
Minneapolis, MN 55459-0032   800-848-2793
                                                    Fax: 612-443-2806
The causes, symptoms, and treatment of low blood sugar are clearly presented in this booklet, including guidelines for using glucagon.
12 pages Pack of 10

3513   Taking Care of Gestational Diabetes
International Diabetes Center at Park Nicollet
3800 Park Nicollet Blvd   952-993-3874
Minneapolis, MN 55416-2699   888-637-2675
                                                    Fax: 952-993-0501
                                               idccustsvc@parknicollet.com
                                               www.idcpublishing.com
Available in Spanish. Empowering women to make healthy choices for a healthy pregnancy, a healthy baby, and a healthy lifestyle. This book covers food planning, testing, targets, medications and more.
242 pages

3514   Understanding Gestational Diabetes
National Diabetes Information Clearinghouse
1 Information Way   800-860-8747
Bethesda, MD 20892-0001   Fax: 301-634-0716
                                                    TTY: 866-569-1162
                                               ndic@info.niddk.nih.gov
                                               www.diabetes.niddk.nih.gov
A guide for women who develop diabetes during pregnancy. It discusses symptoms and diagnosis of gestational diabetes, risk factors, tests during pregnancy and daily management including the use of insulin and blood glucose monitoring.
44 pages

Audio & Video

3515   ADA Clinical Education Series on CD-Rom
American Diabetes Association

2451 Crystal Drive
Arlington, VA 22202

800-342-2383
Fax: 703-549-6995
www.diabetes.org

Features complete texts of Medical Management of Type 1 Diabetes, Medical Management of Type 2 Diabetes, Therapy for Diabetes Mellitus and Related Disorders, 2nd Ed., and Medical Management of Pregnancy Complicated by Diabetes, 2nd Ed.
CD-Rom
Brenda Montgomery, President, Health Care & Education

3516 Black Experience
American Diabetes Association
2451 Crystal Drive
Arlington, VA 22202

703-549-1500
800-342-2383
Fax: 703-549-6995
www.diabetes.org

Designed to increase awareness of diabetes in the black community.
Brenda Montgomery, President, Health Care & Education

3517 Diabetes & Exercise Video
American Diabetes Association
2451 Crystal Drive
Arlington, VA 22202

800-342-2383
Fax: 703-549-6995
www.diabetes.org

A video offering information on how to maintain good health and exercise in controlling diabetes.
Brenda Montgomery, President, Health Care & Education

3518 Label Reading and Shopping
American Diabetes Association
2451 Crystal Drive
Arlington, VA 22202

703-549-1500
800-342-2383
Fax: 703-549-6995
www.diabetes.org

Provides practical information on how to shop and what to look for on labels.
Videotape
Brenda Montgomery, President, Health Care & Education

3519 Living Well with Diabetes
American Diabetes Association
2451 Crystal Drive
Arlington, VA 22202

800-342-2383
Fax: 703-549-6995
www.diabetes.org

Presents two patient role models who are successfully following a treatment plan for noninsulin dependent diabetes.
Videotape
Brenda Montgomery, President, Health Care & Education

3520 On Top of My Game: Living with Diabetes
American Diabetes Association
2451 Crystal Drive
Arlington, VA 22202

800-342-2383
Fax: 703-549-6995
www.diabetes.org

Six patients and their families share their day-to-day frustrations and successes in managing diabetes.
Videotape
Brenda Montgomery, President, Health Care & Education

3521 Physicians Guide to Type I Diabetes
American Diabetes Association
2451 Crystal Drive
Arlington, VA 22202

800-342-2383
Fax: 703-549-6995
www.diabetes.org

Principles of good care in the diagnosis and management of Type I.
Videotape
Brenda Montgomery, President, Health Care & Education

3522 Survival Skills for Diabetic Children
Ajn Company
20 West 44th Street
New York, NY 10036-2961

212-686-7220
800-226-6256
Fax: 212-686-7232
www.chamber.nyc

How to provide insulin-dependent children with education, supervision, and support.
1988 28 minutes

3523 Understanding Diabetes: A User's Guide to Novolin
American Diabetes Association
2451 Crystal Drive
Arlington, VA 22202

800-342-2383
Fax: 703-549-6995
www.diabetes.org

Basic information about diabetes and the role insulin plays in blood glucose control.
Videotape
Brenda Montgomery, President, Health Care & Education

Web Sites

3524 American Association of Diabetes Educators
www.diabeteseducator.org
An independent, multidisciplinary organization of health professionals involved in teaching persons with diabetes. The mission is to enhance the competence of health professionals who teach persons with diabetes and advance the specialty practice of diabetes.

3525 American Diabetes Association
www.diabetes.org
Voluntary organization concerned with diabetes and its complications. The mission of the organization is to prevent and cure diabetes and to improve the lives of persons with diabetes. Offers a network of offices nationwide.
Tracey D. Brown, MBA, BChE, Chief Executive Officer
Eloise Scavella, MA, Chief Operating & Strategy Officer

3526 Diabetes Dictionary
diabetes.niddk.nih.gov
A publication of National Diabetes Information Clearinghouse. The Clearinghouse provides information about diabetes to people with diabetes and to their families, health care professionals, and the public. The NDIC answers inquiries, develops and distributes publications, and works closely with professional and patient organizations and Government agencies to coordinate resources about diabetes.

3527 Diabetes Exercise
www.diabetes-exercise.org
Exists to enhance the quality of life for people with diabetes through exercise and physical fitness.

3528 Healing Well
www.healingwell.com
An online health resource guide to medical news, chat, information and articles, newsgroups and message boards, books, disease-related web sites, medical directories, and more for patients, friends, and family coping with disabling diseases, disorders, or chronic illnesses.

3529 Health Finder
www.healthfinder.gov
Searchable, carefully developed web site offering information on over 1000 topics. Developed by the US Department of Health and Human Services, the site can be used in both English and Spanish.

3530 Healthlink USA
www.healthlinkusa.com
Health information concerning treatment, cures, prevention, diagnosis, risk factors, research, support groups, email lists, personal stories and much more. Updated regularly.

3531 MedicineNet
www.medicinenet.com
An online resource for consumers providing easy-to-read, authoritative medical and health information.

3532 Medscape
www.medscape.com
Medscape offers specialists, primary care physicians, and other health professionals the Web's most robust and integrated medical information and educational tools.

3533 National Diabetes Information Clearinghous e
www.niddk.nih.gov
Offers various materials, resources, books, pamphlets and more for persons and families in the area of diabetes.

3534 WebMD
www.webmd.com

Provides credible information, supportive communities, and in-depth reference material about health subjects. A source for original and timely health information as well as material from well known content providers.

Description

3535 Down Syndrome

Down syndrome is a collection of inherited abnormalities caused by an extra chromosome. Instead of having the normal number of chromosomes (46), children with Down syndrome have an extra copy of chromosome 21 or a smaller portion of chromosome 21. (Because there are three copies of chromosome 21 instead of the normal two, Down syndrome is often called trisomy 21). This chromosomal abnormality results in altered growth and development. Approximately 6,000 children are born with Down syndrome every year in the United States. The overall incidence is about 1 in every 800 live births, but there is a marked variability depending on maternal age. In the early childbearing years, the incidence is about 1/2000 live births; for mothers over 40, it rises to at least 1/100 if not more frequent with advancing age.

Down syndrome is associated with a wide variety of clinical signs, although most individuals do not possess all of them. Common findings include decreased muscle tone, slanting eyes with folds of skin in the inside corners, white spots appearing in the irises of the eyes, and single creases across the palms of one or both hands. Physically, children with Down syndrome have broad feet with short toes, short ears and necks, small heads and small oral cavities. Mental development in the child with Down syndrome is impaired; the mean IQ is approximately 50. Hearing and speech abilities may also be hampered. However, many children with Down syndrome can reach surprisingly highlevels of achievement. Congenital heart disease is found in nearly half of patients, and there is an increased susceptibility to acute leukemia. Down syndrome children show wide symptomatic variation. Today, most patients survive well into adulthood, although problems such as Alzheimer's Disease and psychiatric illness may increase with age.

It is essential that parents enroll their children with Down syndrome in an infant development program. These programs advise parents on how to help a child with Down syndrome in language, cognitive, social and motor skills.

National Agencies & Associations

3536 Administration for Children and Families
330 C Street SW　　　　　　　202-205-8347
Washington, DC 20201　　　　Fax: 202-205-9721
　　　　　　　　　　　　　　www.ACF.HHS.gov
The Administration for Children & Families (ACF) is a division of the U.S. Department of Health & Human Services (HHS). ACF promotes the economic and social well-being of families, children, individuals and communities.
Lynn Johnson, Assistant Secretary
Jerry Milner, Acitng Commissioner, Children & Families

3537 Agency for Healthcare Research and Quality
5600 Fishers Lane　　　　　　301-427-1104
Rockville, MD 20857　　　　　www.ahrq.gov

The Agency for Healthcare Research and Quality's (AHRQ) mission is to produce evidence to make health care safer, higher quality, more accessible, equitable, and affordable, and to work within the U.S. Department of Health and Human Services and with other partners to make sure that the evidence is understood and used.
Gopal Khanna, MBA, Director
Howard E. Holland, Director, Communications

3538 Canadian Down Syndrome Society
2003 14 Street NW　　　　　　403-270-8500
Calgary, Alberta, T2M-3N4　　800-883-5608
　　　　　　　　　　　　Fax: 403-270-8291
　　　　　　　　　　　　　　www.cdss.ca
Resource linking parents and professionals through advocacy, education and providing information.
Laura LaChance, Interim Executive Director

3539 Center for Parent Information & Resources
SPAN
35 Halsey Street　　　　　　　973-642-8100
Newark, NJ 07102　　　　　malizo@spannj.org
　　　　　　　　　　　www.parentcenterhub.org
Serves as a central hub of information and products for Parent Centers that serve children with disabilities. Coordinates training, provides an e-newsletter twice a month, and produces specially designed databases.
Debra A. Jennings, Director
Jessica Wilson, Communications Director

3540 Centers for Disease Control & Prevention: Division of Adolescent & School Health
1600 Clifton Road　　　　　　800-232-4636
Atlanta, GA 30329-4027　　TTY: 888-232-6348
　　　　　　　　　　www.cdc.gov/HealthyYouth
CDC promotes the health and well-being of children and adolescents to enable them to become healthy and productive adults.

3541 Centers for Medicare & Medicaid Services
7500 Security Boulevard　　　410-786-3000
Baltimore, MD 21244　　　　　877-267-2323
　　　　　　　　　　　　TTY: 866-226-1819
　　　　　　　　　　　　　　www.cms.gov
U.S. federal agency which administers Medicare, Medicaid, and the State Children's Health Insurance Program.
Seema Verma, Administrator
Tom Corry, Director

3542 Council for Exceptional Children
2900 Crystal Drive　　　　　　888-232-7733
Arlington, VA 22202-3557　　TTY: 866-915-5000
　　　　　　　　　　　service@cec.sped.org
　　　　　　　　　　　　　www.cec.sped.org
Advocates appropriate policies, standards and development for individuals with special needs. Provides professional development for special educators.
Alexander T. Graham, Executive Director
Craig Evans, Director, Operations

3543 Early Childhood Technical Assistance Center
Campus Box 8040 UNC-CH　　919-962-2001
Chapel Hill, NC 27599-8040　Fax: 919-966-7463
　　　　　　　　　　　　TTY: 919-843-3269
　　　　　　　　　　　　　　ectacenter.org
Assists states and other designated governing jurisdictions as they develop multidisciplinary, coordinated and comprehensive services for children with special needs.
Christina Kasprzak, Co-Director
Megan Vinh, Co-Director

3544 Goodwill Industries International, Inc.
15810 Indianola Drive　　　　800-466-3945
Rockville, MD 20855　　　contactus@goodwill.org
　　　　　　　　　　　　　　www.goodwill.org
A nonprofit, community-based organization whose mission is to help people achieve self-sufficiency through the dignity and power of work, serving people who are disadvantaged, disabled or elderly. The mission is accomplished through providing independent living skills, affordable housing, and training and placement in

community employment. The GoodWill Network includes 160 independent, local locations across the U.S. and Canada.
S. Dale Jenkins, Chair
Steven C. Preston, President & CEO

3545 National Association for Down Syndrome
1460 Renaissance Drive
Park Ridge, IL 60068
630-325-9112
Fax: 847-376-8908
info@nads.org
www.nads.org
A non-for-profit organization founded by parents of children with Down syndrome who felt a need to create a better environment and bring about understanding and acceptance of people with Down syndrome.
Linda Smarto, Director, Programs & Advocacy
Chris Newlon, Coordinator, Family Support & Outreach

3546 National Down Syndrome Congress
30 Mansell Court
Roswell, GA 30076
770-604-9500
800-232-6372
Fax: 770-604-9898
info@ndsccenter.org
www.NDSCcenter.org
The mission of the NDSC is to provide information, advocacy, and support concerning all aspects of life for individuals with Down Syndrome.
David Tolleson, Executive Director
Kathy Edwards, Development Director

3547 National Down Syndrome Society
8 E. 41st Street
New York, NY 10017
800-221-4602
Fax: 646-870-9320
info@ndss.org
www.ndss.org
NDSS supports researchers seeking the causes of and answers to many of the medical, genetic, behavioral and learning problems associated with Down syndrome. Also sponsors symposia and conferences for parents and professionals provides advocacy.
Kandi Pickard, Interim President & CEO
Keisha Landry, Chief of Staff

3548 National Human Genome Research Institute
Building 31, Room 4B09
Bethesda, MD 20892-2152
301-402-0911
Fax: 301-402-2218
www.genome.gov
The National Human Genome Research Institute began as the National Center for Human Genome Research (NCHGR), which was established in 1989 to carry out the role of the National Institutes of Health (NIH) in the International Human Genome Project (HGP).
Eric D. Green, M.D., Ph.D., Director
Lawrence Brody, Ph.D., Director, Division of Genomics & Society

3549 National Institute for Occupational Safety and Health
Patriots Plaza 1
395 E Street SW
Washington, DC 20201
202-245-0625
800-232-4636
Fax: 513-533-8347
TTY: 888-232-6348
www.cdc.gov/niosh
The National Institute for Occupational Safety and Health (NIOSH) is the U.S. federal agency that conducts research and makes recommendations to prevent worker injury and illness.
John Howard, MD, Director
Frank Hearl, PE, Chief of Staff

3550 National Institute of Child Health and Human Development
PO Box 3006
Rockville, MD 20847
800-370-2943
Fax: 866-760-5947
TTY: 888-320-6942
www.nichd.nih.gov
NICHD seeks to better understand disabilities and important events that occur during pregnancy.
Diana W. Bianchi, MD, Director
Constantine Stratakis, Scientific Director

3551 National Institute of Environmental Health Sciences
105 T.W. Alexander Drive
Research Triangle Park, NC 27709
919-541-3345
webcenter@niehs.nih.gov
www.niehs.nih.gov

The mission of the NIEHS is to discover how the environment affects people in order to promote healthier lives.
Linda S. Birnbaum, PhD, Director
Richard Woychik, PhD, Deputy Director

3552 National Institute of General Medical Sciences
45 Center Drive MSC 6200
Bethesda, MD 20892-6200
301-496-7301
info@nigms.nih.gov
www.nigms.nih.gov
The National Institute of General Medical Sciences (NIGMS) supports basic research that increases understanding of biological processes and lays the foundation for advances in disease diagnosis, treatment and prevention.
Jon R. Lorsch, PhD, Director
Judith H. Greenberg, PhD, Deputy Director

3553 The ARC of the United States
The ARC of the United States
1825 K Street NW
Washington, DC 20006
202-534-3700
800-433-5255
Fax: 202-534-3731
info@thearc.org
www.thearc.org
Works to include all children and adults with cognitive, intellectual, and developmental disabilities in every community.
Peter V. Berns, Chief Executive Officer
Trudy Jacobson, Senior Executive Officer, Development

3554 U.S. Food and Drug Administration
10903 New Hampshire Avenue
Silver Spring, MD 20993-0002
301-796-8240
888-463-6332
www.fda.gov
FDA is responsible for protecting the public health by assuring the safety, efficacy and security of human and veterinary drugs, biological products, medical devices, the nation's food supply, cosmetics, and products that emit radiation.
Norman E. Sharpless, MD, Commissioner
Denise Hinton, Chief Scientist

State Agencies & Associations

California

3555 Down Syndrome Association of Los Angeles
16461 Sherman Way
Van Nuys, CA 91406
818-786-0001
Fax: 818-786-0004
info@dsala.org
www.dsala.org
Offers information on Down syndrome, counseling, resources, facts, laws and other forms of information.
Gail Williamson, Executive Director
Sandra Baker, Office Administrator/Spanish Coordinator

Colorado

3556 Mile High Down Syndrome Association
2121 S Oneida Street
Denver, CO 80224
303-797-1699
Fax: 303-756-6144
info@mhdsa.org
www.mhdsa.org

Mac Macsovits, Executive Director
Melissa Davis, Volunteer Coordinator

Connecticut

3557 Connecticut Down Syndrome Congress
263 Farmington Avenue
Farmington, CT 06030-0485
205-351-1157
888-486-8537
manager@ctdownsyndrome.org
www.ctdownsyndrome.org
Sheryl Knapp, Secretary
Walter Glomb, President

Florida

3558 Gold Coast Down Syndrome Organization
2255 Glades Road
Boca Raton, FL 33431
561-912-1231
Fax: 561-912-1232
www.goldcoastdownsyndrome.org

Gold Coast Down syndrome Organization is a private nonprofit corporation dedicated to making the future brighter for people with Down syndrome in Palm Beach County, Florida.
Sue Killan, President
Tina Trujillo, Secretary

3559 Goodwill Industries-Suncoast
10596 Gandy Boulevard   727-523-1512
St. Petersburg, FL 33702   888-279-1988
                                 TTY: 727-579-1068
                             www.goodwill-suncoast.org
A nonprofit, community-based organization whose mission is to help people achieve self-sufficiency through the dignity and power of work, serving people who are disadvantaged, disabled or elderly. The mission is accomplished through providing independent living skills, affordable housing, and training and placement in community employment.
Heather Ceresoli, CPA, Chair
Deborah A. Passerini, President & CEO

Georgia

3560 Down Syndrome Association of Atlanta
2221 Peachtree Rd   404-320-3233
Atlanta, GA 30309   Fax: 404-228-7475
                                    www.dsaatl.org

Hawaii

3561 Hawaii Down Syndrome Congress
419 Keoniana Street   808-949-1999
Honolulu, HI 96815   Conkay@AOL.com
Constance K Smith, President

Indiana

3562 Indiana Down Syndrome Foundation
2625 N. Meridian Street #49   317-925-7617
Indianapolis, IN 46208   888-989-9255
                                Fax: 317-925-7619
                                info@dsindiana.org
Lisa Tokarz-Guiterre, Executive Director
Jeff Huffman, President

Maryland

3563 National Institute on Drug Abuse
6001 Executive Boulevard   301-443-1124
Bethesda, MD 20892   dd279k@nih.gov
                                www.drugabuse.gov
NIDA's mission is to lead the Nation in bringing the power of science to bear on drug abuse and addiction.
Nora D. Volkow, M.D., Director
David Daubert, Acting Associate Director for Management

Massachusetts

3564 Massachusetts Down Syndrome Congress
20 Burlington Mall Road   781-221-0024
Melrose, MA 02176   800-664-MDSC
                                Fax: 781-221-0011
                                mdsc@mdsc.org
                                    www.mdsc.org
Maureen Gallagher, Executive Director
Sarah Cullen, Outreach Coordinator

Minnesota

3565 Down Syndrome Association of Minnesota
656 Transfer Road   651-603-0720
St Paul, MN 55114   800-511-3696
                                Fax: 651-603-0726
                                dsamn@dsamn.org
                                    www.dsamn.org
A non-profit organization dedicated to ensuring that all individuals with Down syndrome and their families receive the support necessary to participate in, contribute to and achieve the fulfillment of life in their community.
Craig Parker, President
Kathleen Forney, Executive Director

New York

3566 Association for Children with Down Syndrome
4 Fern Place   516-933-4700
Plainview, NY 11803   Fax: 516-933-9524
                                msmith@acds.org
                                    www.acds.org
Nonprofit educational program that combines national information and research dissemination with direct services at the local level. Services include early intervention, pre-school, recreation programs and residential homes.
Michael M Smith, Executive Director
Cecilia Barry, Principal

Ohio

3567 Down Syndrome Association of Greater Cinci nnati
644 Linn Street   513-761-5400
Cincinnati, OH 45203-1734   Fax: 513-761-5401
                                dsagc@dsagc.org
                                    www.dsagc.com
The mission of the Down Syndrome Association of Greater Cincinnati is to provide information resources and support to individuals with Down syndrome, their families, and their communities.
Janet Gora, Executive Director
Nora Lindsay Quinn, Event Coordinator

Tennessee

3568 Down Syndrome Association of Middle Tennessee
111 N Wilson Boulevard   615-386-9002
Nashville, TN 37205-2411   Fax: 615-386-9754
                                dsamt@bellsouth.net
                                    www.dsamt.org
A nonprofit organization of families whose mission is to enhance the quality of life for all individuals with Down Syndrome by providing information and support to families professionals and the community.
Sheila Moore, Executive Director
Erin Kice, Program Coordinator

Texas

3569 Down Syndrome Guild of Dallas
701 N Central Expressway   214-267-1374
Richardson, TX 75080-1174   Fax: 972-234-2510
                             www.downsyndromedallas.org
Kelly Drablos, President
Tamara White, Secretary

3570 Texas Association on Mental Retardation
TAMR Headquarters   512-349-7470
Austin, TX 78755   Fax: 512-349-2117
An organization made up of professionals, parents, consumers and advocates. Our goal is to create an accessible system of services and resources which support personal choice and promotes lives of dignity and self-determination.
Pat Holder

Virginia

3571 Down Syndrome Association of Hampton Roads
The Endependence Center   757-466-3696
Norfolk, VA 23502   DSAHR@verizon.net
                                    www.dsahr.org
The Down Syndrome Association of Hampton Roads is a not-for-profit organization serving the needs of individuals with Down Syndrome and their families. The association is supported by a board of directors, an advisory board and dedicated volunteers.
Andrea Anderson, President
Florence Thacker, Secretary

3572 Down Syndrome Association of Wisconsin
3211 South Lake Drive   414-327-3729
Milwaukee, WI 53235   866-327-3729
                                            Fax: 414-327-1329
                                               info@dsaw.org
                                               www.dsaw.org
An organization created by families for families of individuals and
for individuals with Down Syndrome. Our primary mission is to
provide each person with Down Syndrome the support needed to
achieve personal goals and develop self-esteem.
Tom Oday, President
Nicole Cook, Treasurer

Foundations

3573 ALEH Israel Foundation
PO Box 4911   917-936-6305
New York, NY 10185   866-750-2534
                                               www.aleh.org
ALEH is Israel's largest and most advanced network of residential
facilities for children with severe disabilities.
Josh Pruzansky, Director, Development, USA & Canada

3574 ALEH Rehabilitation of Canada
95 Barber Greene Road   416-449-6350
Toronto, Ontario, M3C-3E9   888-824-5477
                                               www.aleh.org
ALEH is Israel's largest and most advanced network of residential
facilities for children with severe disabilities.
Josh Pruzansky, Director, Development, USA & Canada

Libraries & Resource Centers

3575 Adult Down Syndrome Center of Lutheran General Hospital
1999 Dempster Street   847-318-2303
Park Ridge, IL 60068
The Adult Down Syndrome Center is a comprehensive medical resource providing multidisciplinary medical and psychosocial care
for adults with Down syndrome, with an emphasis on health
promotion.
Brian Chicoine MD, Medical Director

3576 Ann Whitehill Down Syndrome Program
Riley Hospital for Children
702 Barnhill Drive   800-248-1199
Indianapolis, IN 46202   www.iuhealth.org
Brings together specialists from many areas to address the medical
and psychosocial needs of children with Down Syndrome. We also
refer the family to local resources for therapy and developmental
programs.
Evans Parker, President
William Cast, CEO

3577 Blick Clinic for Developmental Disabilities
640 W Market Street   330-762-5425
Akron, OH 44303-1465   Fax: 330-762-4019
                                       blickclinic@blickclinic.com
Blick Clinic is a private, non-profit outpatient clinic which began
by a group of parents of children with developmental disabilities
and a few volunteer professionals. Together, they developed the
Clinic into a single, comprehensive source of diagnostic, evaluation, treatment, and support group services to persons with
developmental disabilities.

3578 Center for Disabilities and Development
University of Iowa Hospitals and Clinics
100 Hawkins Drive   319-353-6900
Iowa City, IA 52242-1011   877-686-0031
                                            Fax: 319-356-8284
                                            TTY: 877-686-0032
                                        CDD-Webmaster@uiowa.edu
Provides comprehensive health care and services to people with
disabilities of all ages and their families through a combination of
outpatient, inpatient, and community based programs. UHS provides information, evaluation, treatment recommendations, and
training related to aging and disabilities. UHS provides both

preservice and inservice training programs for service providers
and others who provide services to individuals with disabilities.

3579 Children's Hospital of Philadelphia
34th St & Civic Center Boulevard   215-590-1000
Philadelphia, PA 19104-4399   www.chop.edu
The oldest hospital dedicated exclusively to pediatrics, strives to
be the world leader in the advancement of healthcare for children
by integrating excellent patient care, innovative research and quality professional education into all of its programs.

3580 Children's Neurodevelopment Center
Hasbro Children's Hospital
167 Point Street   401-444-3500
Providence, RI 02903   www.lifespan.org/
The Children's Neurodevelopment Center (CNDC) at Hasbro
Children's Hospital provides evaluation and treatment of children
with neurological, genetic, developmental, metabolic and behav-
ioral disorders.
Timothy J. Babineau, President and Chief Executive Officer
Kenneth E. Arnold, Senior Vice President and General Counse

3581 Dartmouth-Hitchcock Medical Center - Genetics and
Development
One Medical Center Drive   603-653-1400
Lebanon, NH 03756-0001   Fax: 603-653-3585
                                   www.employees.dartmouth-hitchcock.org
Dartmouth-Hitchcock Clinic is committed to a regional, inte-
grated, comprehensive healthcare system, which can evolve under
physician leadership, lay administrative support and public trustee
guidance. DHC and its partnering DHMC organizations are recog-
nized as leaders in using scientific methods to improve health care
delivery.
Carol B Andrew EdD, MS
Mary Beth Dinulos, MD

3582 Developmental Evaluation Clinic
Westchester Institute for Human Development
Cedarwood Hall   914-493-8150
Valhalla, NY 10595-1681   wihd@wihd.org
                                               www.wihd.org
WIHD envisions a future where all people, including children and
adults living with disabilities, fully participate in society, live
healthy and productive lives, and have access to culturally appropriate services and supports, emerging technologies, competent
professionals, caring families, caregivers, and communities.

3583 Developmental Medicine Center (DMC)
Children's Hospital Boston
300 Longwood Avenue   617-355-6000
Boston, MA 02115   Fax: 617-730-0373
                                           TTY: 617-730-0152
                                       www.childrenshospital.org
Provides developmental evaluation and treatment services for
children aged birth to adolescence with a wide range of develop-
mental, behavioral and learning difficulties
Leonard A Rappaport MD, MS, Program Director
Sandra Fenwick, President, CEO

3584 Down Syndrome Center of Western Pennsylvania
One Children's Hospital Drive   412-692-5325
Pittsburgh, PA 15224-2524   Fax: 412-692-5723
                                               www.chp.edu
The Down Syndrome Center of Western Pennsylvania has a lend-
ing library of books, videos, audio cassettes and periodicals; pro-
vides current information about Down syndrome to families and
professionals; maintains a file of articles on issues relating to
Down Syndrome and publishes a quarterly newsletter in conjunction with the Down Syndrome Group of Western Pennsylvania.
Dr William Cohen, MD, Director

3585 Down Syndrome Clinic of Houston
6701 Fannin Street, 16th Floor   832-822-3478
Dallas, TX 75235-7701   Fax: 832-825-3399
                                   downsyndrome@texaschildrenshospital.org
The mission of the Down Syndrome Clinic of Houston is to help in-
dividuals with Down syndrome reach his or her fullest potential.
We accomplish our goal by offering a clinic where children receive

complete evaluations by a multidisciplinary team. Families will obtain needed strategies for management of common concerns.
Nirupama Madduri, MD, Chief of Service
Jennifer Chung, Clinic Coordinator

3586 Dr. Gertrude A Barber National Institute
136 E Avenue
Erie, PA 16507-1899
814-453-7661
Fax: 814-455-1132
BNIerie@barberinstitute.org
www.barberinstitute.org
We believe that all persons have the capacity for growth and fulfillment, and to that end they must be afforded every opportunity to attain the greatest use of thier potential within themselves and their community.
John Barber, JD, President/CEO
Maureen Barber-Carey, EdD, Executive Vice President

3587 Jane and Richard Thomas Center for Down Syndrome
Cincinnati Center for Developmental Disorders
3333 Burnet Avenue
Cincinnati, OH 45229-3039
513-636-4200
800-344-2462
Fax: 513-636-0527
TTY: 513-636-4900
www.cincinnatichildrens.org
The Jane and Richard Thomas Center for Down Syndrome conducts research and offers interdisciplinary evaluations and intervention for infants, children, adolescents and young adults with Down syndrome. By providing a range of comprehensive services within one center, families can now spend less time pursuing services through multiple agencies and professionals.
David J Schonfeld MD, Division Head
Michael Fisher, President and CEO

3588 Kennedy Krieger Institute
707 N Broadway
Baltimore, MD 21205-1888
443-923-9200
800-873-3377
Fax: 410-550-9292
info@kennedykrieger.org
www.kennedykrieger.org
Kennedy Krieger Institute is an internationally recognized facility located in Baltimore, Maryland dedicated to improving the lives of children and adolescents with pediatric developmental disabilities through patient care, special education, research, and professional training. Our clinical programs offer an interdisciplinary approach in treatment tailored to the individual needs of each child.
Gary W Goldstein, President

3589 LaRabida Children's Hospital: Developmental Disabilities & Delays
6501 South Promontory Drive
Chicago, IL 60649
773-363-6700
info@larabida.org
www.larabida.org
La Rabida Children's Hospital is dedicated to excellence in caring for children with chronic illness, disabilities, or who have been abused, allowing them to achieve their fullest potential through expertise and innovation within the health care and academic communities.
Paula Kienberger Jaudes, MD, President/CEO

3590 Marcus Institute for Development and Learning
1920 Briarcliff Road
Atlanta, GA 30329
404-727-9450
Fax: 404-727-9598
Marcus_Info@MarcusInstitute.org
www.marcus.org
Our mission is to provide information, services and programs to people with developmental disabilities and their families, as well as those who live and work with them. We offer integrated state-of-the-art clinical, behavioral, educational and family support services through a single organization to reduce the stress and aggravation for families who may have a child with mild to severe disabilities.
Charles M Shaffer, Jr, President/CEO
Dr Claire Coles, Director Fetal Alcohol Center

3591 MeritCare Children's Hospital Down Syndrome Outpatient Service
Coordinated Treatment Center

736 Broadway
Fargo, ND 58122-4420
701-234-6600
800-828-2901
Fax: 701-234-6965
www.meritcare.com
MeritCare Children's Hospital offers a multidisciplinary outpatient service to help accommodate the special medical developmental, behavioral, family and community needs of patients with Down Syndrome.

3592 Mt. Washington Pediatric Clinic
1708 W Rogers Avenue
Baltimore, MD 21209-4596
410-578-8600
Fax: 410-466-1715
www.mwph.org
The primary purpose of the Mt. Washington Pediatric Hospital and its affiliates is to sponsor and promote the provision of the highest quality pediatric health care services in a nurturing environment.
Sheldon J Stein, President/CEO
Robert H Imhoff, III, VP Development

3593 Santa Rosa Medical Center
PO Box 7330
San Antonio, TX 78207-0330
210-228-2386
www.srmcfl.com
Philip Wright, CEO

3594 UCSF Children's Hospital Health Library
505 Parnassus Avenue
San Francisco, CA 94143
415-476-1000
www.ucsfhealth.org
This Health Library is an online resource to supplement information your doctors, nurses and pharmacists may provide. Our library includes a medical dictionary and an online calendar of our health events. We have news about our research advances and treatments, patient education materials and listings of other helpful Web sites.
Mark Laret, CEO

3595 University of Maryland: Department of Pediatrics
22 South Greene Street
Baltimore, MD 21201
410-328-8667
Fax: 410-328-3981
http://www.umm.edu/pediatrics/
Recognized throughout Maryland and the mid-Atlantic region as a valuable resource for critically and chronically ill children, the University of Maryland Hospital for Children combines state-of-the-art medicine with family-centered care.

3596 University of Washington: Experimental Education Unit
Box 357925
Seattle, WA 98195-7925
206-543-4011
Fax: 206-543-8480
The Experimental Education Unit (EEU) is a state-certified special education school that serves children from birth to age 7 with diverse abilities. Faculty at the EEU conduct research projects, and provide training opportunities to undergraduate and graduate students, educators, and other professionals.
Rick Neel, Director

Research Centers

3597 Institute for Basic Research in Developmental Disabilities
44 Holland Avenue
Albany, NY 12229-0001
718-494-0600
866-946-9733
Fax: 718-494-0833
TTY: 866-933-4889
Conducts research into neurodegenerative diseases Alzheimer's disease developmental disabilities fragile X syndrome Down's Syndrome autism epilepsy and basic science issues underlying all developmental disabilities.
W Ted Brown, Director
Raju K Pullarkat, Chair Developmental Biochemistry

3598 Kennedy Krieger Institute - Down Syndrome
10 Center Drive
Bethesda, MD 20892
301-496-4000
888-554-2080
Fax: 443-923-9138
TTY: 443-923-2645
webmaster@kennedykrieger.org
clinicalcenter.nih.gov
Dedicated to improving the lives of children and adolescents with pediatric developmental disabilities through patient care special education research and professional training.
John Gallin, Director
Char Koller, Research

Support Groups & Hotlines

3599 Down Syndrome Association of Greater Cinci nnati
644 Linn Street   513-761-5400
Cincinnati, OH 45203-1734   Fax: 513-761-5401
www.dsagc.com

Janet Gora, Executive Director
Collette Maddy, Office Coordinator

3600 National Down Syndrome Congress
30 Mansell Court   770-604-9500
Roswell, GA 30076   800-232-6372
Fax: 770-604-9898
info@ndsccenter.org
www.NDSCcenter.org
The mission of the NDSC is to provide information, advocacy, and support concerning all aspects of life for individuals with Down Syndrome.
David Tolleson, Executive Director
Kathy Edwards, Development Director

3601 National Down Syndrome Society Hotline
8 E. 41st Street   800-221-4602
New York, NY 10017   Fax: 646-870-9320
info@ndss.org
www.ndss.org
NDSS supports researchers seeking the causes of and answers to many of the medical, genetic, behavioral and learning problems associated with Down syndrome; sponsors symposia and conferences for parents and professionals; performs advocacy; provides information and refferal through a toll-free number; and develops and disseminates educational materials.
Kandi Pickard, Interim President & CEO
Keisha Landry, Chief of Staff

3602 National Health Information Center
Office of Disease Prevention & Health Promotion
1101 Wootton Pkwy   Fax: 240-453-8281
Rockville, MD 20852   odphpinfo@hhs.gov
www.health.gov/nhic
Supports public health education by maintaining a calendar of National Health Observances; helps connect consumers and health professionals to organizations that can best answer questions and provide up-to-date contact information from reliable sources; updates on a yearly basis toll-free numbers for health information, Federal health clearinghouses and info centers.
Don Wright, MD, MPH, Director

3603 Parents of Children with Down Syndrome
Arc of Montgomery County
11600 Nebel Street   301-984-5777
Rockville, MD 20852-2538   Fax: 301-816-2429
TTY: 301-881-1548
asachs@arcmontmd.org
www.arcmontmd.org/
Activities include formal and informal meetings, parent-to-parent support, contacting new parents of down syndrome children to offer support and information on community resources, providing information on doctors, hospitals and professionals.
Petere Holden, Executive Director
John Slavcoff, President of the Board

Books

3604 ACDS Infant, Toddler & Pre-school Curriculum for Children
Association for Children with Down Syndrome
4 Fern Place   516-933-4700
Plainview, NY 11803   Fax: 516-933-9524
msmith@acds.org
www.acds.org
This curriculum is user friendly for parents, educators, related service professionals and other caregivers. It provides checklists and teaching strategies to facilitate aquisition of skills in cognition, self-help, socialization, speech and language, gross and fine motor skills plus much more.
Michael M. Smith, Executive Director

3605 Babies with Down Syndrome
Woodbine House
6510 Bells Mill Road   301-897-3570
Bethesda, MD 20817-1636   800-843-7323
www.telebyte.com
Praised as the finest book ever written for new parents, this book covers everything they need to know about rearing these beautiful and special children in a loving environment.
237 pages Paperback
ISBN: 0-933149-02-6

3606 Bethy and the Mouse: God's Gifts in Special Packages
Faith and Life Press
718 Main Street   316-283-5100
Newton, KS 67114-0344
A father's account of his special children, Bethy with Down Syndrome and The Mouse who has been born with microcephaley. A tender story of a father's love.
164 pages Paperback
ISBN: 0-873031-11-3

3607 Breast Feeding the Baby with Down Syndrome
LaLeche League International
35 E. Wacker Drive   312-646-6260
Chicago, IL 60601-4048   Fax: 312-644-8557
llli@llli.org
www.llli.org
16 pages Pamphlet

3608 Cara: Growing with a Retarded Child
Temple University Press
1852 North 10th Street   215-926-2140
Philadelphia, PA 19122   800-621-2736
www.temple.edu/tempress
The author offers information and experiences on raising her daughter, Cara, who has Down syndrome.

3609 Communication Skills in Children with Down Syndrome
Woodbine House
6510 Bells Mill Road   800-843-7323
Bethesda, MD 20817   www.woodbinehouse.com
Offers parents a chance to learn what to expect as communication skills progress from infancy through early teenage years. Discussions are included on speech and language therapy, hearing problems, school performance and intelligibility issues.
150 pages Paperback
ISBN: 0-933149-53-0

3610 Current Approaches to Down's Syndrome
Greenwood Publishing Group, Inc/Praeger Publishers
P.O. Box 1911   805-968-1911
Santa Barbara, CA 93117-6926   800-368-6868
Fax: 866-270-3856
CustomerService@abc-clio.com
www.greenwood.com
An exploration of current initiatives relating to Down syndrome in the medical, educational and social fields.
447 pages
ISBN: 0-275902-12-9
Vince Burns, VP
Brian Stratford, Editor

3611 Differences in Common: Straight Talk on Mental Retardation/Down Syndrome
Woodbine House
22 Corporate Woods Blvd   518-738-0020
Albany, NY 12211   800-843-7323
info@dsahrc.org
www.dsahrc.org
A collection of essays by the mother of an adult son who has Down syndrome. Focuses on mainstreaming, terminology, parent groups and advocacy.
M Trainer, Editor

3612 Down Syndrome: A Review of Current Knowledge
Jean-Adolphe Rondal, Juan Perera, and Lynn Nadek, author
John Wiley and Sons, Inc.

111 River Street
Hoboken, NJ 07030

201-748-6000
877-762-2974
Fax: 201-748-6088
info@wiley.com
www.wiley.com

1999 350 pages Hardcover
Stephen M. Smith, President and CEO
John Kritzmacher, EVP, CFO

3613 Down Syndrome: An Update and Review for Primary Care Physicians
Dartmouth-Hitchcock Medical Center
22 Corporate Woods Blvd
Albany, NY 12211-0001

518-738-0020
info@dsahrc.org
www.dsahrc.org

An excellent medical review of Down syndrome intended for physicians.
WC Cooley, Editor

3614 Down Syndrome: The Facts
Oxford University Press
2001 Evans Road
Cary, NC 27513-2010

212-726-6000
800-451-7556
Fax: 919-677-1303
www.oup-usa.org

A book for parents who have a child with Down syndrome written by a pediatrician who works with Down syndrome children.
M Selikowitz, Editor

3615 From 17 Months to 17 Years...A Look at Down Syndrome
Bonnie Lavender
22 Corporate Woods Blvd
Albany, NY 12211

518-738-0020
info@dsahrc.org
www.dsahrc.org

Includes profiles of six families who have children with Down syndrome. Offers photographs and accompanying text that detail each family's experiences with Down syndrome.
B Lavender, Editor
GJ Lega, Editor

3616 Medical and Surgical Care for Children with Down Syndrome
Woodbine House
6510 Bells Mill Road
Bethesda, MD 20817-1636

800-843-7323
www.woodbinehouse.com

Provides detailed and easy-to-understand information for parents on a wide range of medical conditions and treatments including: heart disease, recurrent infections, thyroid problems, eye problems, skin conditions, ear, nose and throat problems, orthopedic conditions, leukemia, facial and dental concerns and neurological problems.
320 pages Paperback
ISBN: 0-933149-54-9

3617 Parent's Guide to Down Syndrome: Toward a Brighter Future
Siegfried M Pueschel, MD, PhD, JD, MPH, author

Brookes Publishing Company
Cust Ser Department
Baltimore, MD 21285-0624

800-638-3775
Fax: 410-337-8539
custserv@brookespublishing.com
www.brookespublishing.com

A comprehensive reference book especially for new parents but useful and informative to seasoned parents as well. Range of topics include a history of Down syndrome, physical characterisitcs, developmental expectations, early intervention, feeding the young child and the school years.
2001 338 pages Paperback
ISBN: 1-557664-52-8

3618 Parents of Children with Down Syndrome
11600 Nebel Street
Rockville, MD 20852-2538

301-984-5792
Fax: 301-816-2429

Activities include formal and informal meetings, parent-to-parent support, contacting new parents of down syndrome children to offer support and information on community resources, providing information on doctors, hospitals and professionals.

3619 Paul
Miriam Perrone
440 Park Avenue
Saint Simons Island, GA 31522-4357

912-638-8551

How a determined mother carved a semi-independent life for her now-grown Down's syndrome child.

3620 Show Me No Mercy
Cokesbury
PO Box 801
Nashville, TN 37202-0801

A father of a young adult man with Down syndrome relates the experience of his attempt to be reunited with his son after a family tragedy separates them.
R Perske, Editor

3621 Since Owen
Johns Hopkins University Press
2715 N Charles Street
Baltimore, MD 21218-2105

410-516-6900
Fax: 410-516-6968
www.press.jhu.edu

A well written book displaying understanding from a veteran parent communicating with other parents of children with disabilities.
466 pages
Kathleen Keane, Director
Erik A. Smist, Director, Finance and Administration

3622 Teaching the Infant with Down Syndrome: A Guide for Parents & Professionals
Pro-Ed, Inc.
8700 Shoal Creek Blvd
Austin, TX 78757-6897

512-451-3246
800-897-3202
Fax: 512-451-8542
info@proedinc.com
www.proedinc.com

A manual providing teaching ideas and activities that can be used to assist an infant's development.
MJ Hanson, Editor

3623 To Give an Edge: A Guide for New Parents of Children with Down's Syndrome
Viking Press
7000 Washington Avenue S
Eden Prairie, MN 55344-3580

612-941-8780

A guide for new parents designed to provide information about the disorder and how other parents of children with Down syndrome have coped.
JE Rynders, Editor
JM Horrobin, Editor

3624 Understanding Down's Syndrome An Introduction for Parents
Brookline Books
8 Trumbull Rd
Northampton, MA 01060

413-584-0184
Fax: 617-734-3952
brbooks@yahoo.com
www.brooklinebooks.com

The author provides answers and explanations to the countless questions directed to him during his twenty years' involvement with Down syndrome individuals and their families.
Softcover
ISBN: 1-571290-09-5

Children's Books

3625 Our Brother Has Down's Syndrome: An Introduction for Children
Firefly Books
50 Staples Avenue
Richmond Hill,

416-499-8412
416-499-8313
www.fireflybooks.com

Two young sisters tell about their little brother with Down syndrome in this color picture book.
21 pages
S Cairo, Editor

3626 Secret Place of the Stairs
Harper & Row
10 E 53rd Street
New York, NY 10022-5299

212-207-7000

A story that weaves many themes, including the institutionalizing of the protagonist's sister, her parents' divorce and her own expectations.
Grades 7-10

3627 **We Can Do It!**
Macmillan
175 Fifth Avenue
New York, NY 10010-6221   646-307-5151
www.macmillan.com
A colorful book of photographs that show the daily activities of
young children with different developmental delays, including
Down syndrome.
L Dwight, Editor

Magazines

3628 **Down Syndrome, Papers and Abstracts for Professionals**
National Down Syndrome Society
8 E. 41st Street
New York, NY 10017   301-963-1857
800-221-4602
info@ndss.org
www.ndss.org
Quarterly review of research literature pertaining to Down syndrome.
Sara Hart Weir, President
Kandi Pickard, Chief of Staff

3629 **Exceptional Parent Magazine**
6 Pickwick Lane
Woodcliff Lake, NJ 07677-5071   617-730-5800
Fax: 201-746-0179
www.eparent.com
A publication dealing with many issues affecting exceptional chil-
dren and their families.
Monthly
Joseph M. Valenzano, Jr., President, CEO
Rick Rader, Editor-in-Chief

Newsletters

3630 **Down Syndrome News**
National Down Syndrome Congress
30 Mansell Court
Roswell, GA 30076-1655   770-604-9500
800-232-6372
Fax: 770-604-9898
NDSC.center@aol.com
www.ndsccenter.org
Contains book reviews, articles and items of interest to those
touched by Down syndrome.
10x Annually
Marilyn Tolbert, President
Bret Bowerman, 1st Vice President

3631 **Down Syndrome Today**
National Down Syndrome Society
8 E. 41st Street
New York, NY 10017   516-654-3242
800-221-4602
www.ndss.org
Offers information, articles, resources and materials for the parent
and professional working and nurturing patients and persons with
Downs syndrome.
Sara Hart Weir, President
Kandi Pickard, Chief of Staff

3632 **National Down Syndrome Society Update**
National Down Syndrome Society
8 E. 41st Street
New York, NY 10017   800-221-4602
Fax: 646-870-9320
www.ndss.org
Offers information on the activities of the society, new breakthroughs in medical technology, articles offering state of the art information to families and individuals with Down syndrome, and
answers to questions about the illness.
12 pages Quarterly
Kandi Pickard, Interim President & CEO
Keisha Landry, Chief of Staff

3633 **On the Up with Down Syndrome**
Carole Shafer, author
Down Syndrome Association of Wisconsin

9401 West Beloit Road   414-327-3729
Milwaukee, WI 53227   866-327-3729
Fax: 414-327-1329
thomtalent@aol.com
www.dsaw.org
Offers the exchange of ideas and experiences. Free to our mem-
bers. Membership is $20.00/year.
Quarterly
Ron Irwin, Board President
Robbin Lyons, Newsletter Contact

Pamphlets

3634 **Alzheimer's Disease and Down Syndrome**
National Down Syndrome Society
8 E. 41st Street
New York, NY 10017   212-460-9330
800-221-4602
www.ndss.org
1995
Sara Hart Weir, President
Kandi Pickard, Chief of Staff

3635 **Down Syndrome**
March of Dimes
1275 Mamaroneck Avenue   914-997-4488
White Plains, NY 10605   Fax: 212-254-3518
NY639@marchofdimes.com
www.marchofdimes.com

3636 **Heart and Down Syndrome**
National Down Syndrome Society
8 E. 41st Street
New York, NY 10017   212-460-9330
800-221-4602
www.ndss.org
1995
Sara Hart Weir, President
Kandi Pickard, Chief of Staff

3637 **Life Planning and Down Syndrome**
National Down Syndrome Society
8 E. 41st Street
New York, NY 10017   212-460-9330
800-221-4602
www.ndss.org
Sara Hart Weir, President
Kandi Pickard, Chief of Staff

3638 **Neurology of Down Syndrome**
National Down Syndrome Society
8 E. 41st Street
New York, NY 10017   212-460-9330
800-221-4602
www.ndss.org
1995
Sara Hart Weir, President
Kandi Pickard, Chief of Staff

3639 **New Parents**
Association for Children with Down Syndrome
4 Fern Place
Plainview, NY 11803   516-933-4700
Fax: 516-933-9524
msmith@acds.org
www.acds.org
Bibliography compiled for parents who have just given birth to a
child with Down syndrome. Free upon reciept of a stamped,
self-addressed envelope.
Michael Smith, Executive Director

3640 **Sexuality in Down Syndrome**
National Down Syndrome Society
8 E. 41st Street
New York, NY 10017   212-460-9330
800-221-4602
www.ndss.org
1995
Sara Hart Weir, President
Kandi Pickard, Chief of Staff

3641 **Speech and Language in Children and Adolescents with Down
Syndrome**
National Down Syndrome Society

8 E. 41st Street
New York, NY 10017
1995
Sara Hart Weir, President
Kandi Pickard, Chief of Staff

212-460-9330
800-221-4602
www.ndss.org

Audio & Video

3642 Adaptation to the Initial Crisis
Lawren Productions
100 Brook Hill Drive
West Nyack, NY 10994-1556

845-353-7500
800-872-7423
Fax: 845-353-4141
online@cambridge.org
www.cambridge.org/us

A family learns to adapt to the birth of a child with a handicap.

3643 Bernardsville Beginnings
National Down Syndrome Society
8 E. 41st Street
New York, NY 10017

212-460-9330
800-221-4602
Fax: 212-979-2873
www.ndss.org

Follows Alison through her first full year in a first grade inclusion program. Step-by-step account of teaching staff preparation, classroom experiences, a portrayal of one girl's successful adjustment, and a whole class matured by the experience.
23 minutes
Sara Hart Weir, President
Kandi Pickard, Chief of Staff

3644 Bittersweet Waltz
National Down Syndrome Society
8 E. 41st Street
New York, NY 10017

212-460-9330
800-221-4602
Fax: 212-979-2873
info@ndss.org
www.ndss.org

Experience of Alec and his first year included in a regular fifth grade class. From a point of view of a parent, a child, and the school administration.
18 minutes
Sara Hart Weir, President
Kandi Pickard, Chief of Staff

3645 Colin and Ricky
Lawren Productions
930 Pitner Avenue
Evanston, IL 60202-1556

847-328-6700
800-421-2363

A young boy comes to deal with his disappointment surrounding the birth of his baby brother with Down syndrome.

3646 Congratulations: An Introduction to Down Syndrome for Parents/Family/Friends
New Challenges
96 Ogden Avenue
White Plains, NY 10605

914-287-0723

Film for parents which addresses some of the most commonly asked questions about raising a child with Down syndrome.

3647 Daddy's Girl
Carle Media
110 W Main Street
Urbana, IL 61801-2715

217-384-4838

A film starring a twelve-year-old actress with Down syndrome, dealing with her divorced father's inability to accept the fact that his daughter has Down syndrome.
Carolyn Baxley

3648 Down Syndrome: See the Potential
National Down Syndrome Society
8 E. 41st Street
New York, NY 10017

800-221-4602
www.ndss.org

Video highlighting the capability of children with Down syndrome.
Sara Hart Weir, President
Kandi Pickard, Chief of Staff

3649 Gifts of Love
National Down Syndrome Society
8 E. 41st Street
New York, NY 10017

212-460-9330
800-221-4602
Fax: 212-979-2873
www.ndss.org

Four families of children with Down syndrome talk about their feelings and experiences with their children, particularly during the first six years. All the children live at home and attend programs in their communities.
25 minutes
Sara Hart Weir, President
Kandi Pickard, Chief of Staff

3650 Infant Motor Development: A Look at the Phases
Communication Skill Builders/Therapy Skill Builder
3830 E Bellevue
Tucson, AZ 85733

520-323-7500

A video depicting development in and activities for infants birth through 12 months.

3651 New Expectations
Lawren Productions
930 Pitner Avenue
Evanston, IL 60202-1556

800-421-2363

Focuses on the emotional and technical aspects of Down syndrome. Highlights four persons at various life stages from infancy to adulthood in the areas of education and employment.

3652 New Set of Fears, a New Set of Hopes
Meyer Children's Rehabilitation Institute
Resource Center
Omaha, NE 68131

402-559-7467
800-232-6372

Explores the way a family adjusts as they go through the life cycle with their child who has Down syndrome.

3653 Opportunities to Grow
National Down Syndrome Society
8 E. 41st Street
New York, NY 10017

212-460-9330
800-221-4602
Fax: 212-979-2873
info@ndss.org
www.ndss.org

Sequel to Gifts of Love video shows how people with Down syndrome, ages 6 to 26, participate equally in all phases of community life. Vignettes of 15 young men and women illustrate how inclusion, education, computer facilitation, socialization programs, and employment training help them to fulfill their potential.
25 minutes
Sara Hart Weir, President
Kandi Pickard, Chief of Staff

3654 Stepping Stones
AIT
PO Box A
Bloomington, IN 47402-0120

800-457-4509

Series of video programs on teaching basic skills to at-risk, special needs and normally developed children.

3655 Thanks Mom and Dad: Profiles of Patrick
University of Washington
CDMRC Mail Stop WJ-10
Seattle, WA 98195-0001

206-543-4011
800-232-6372

Documentary on the life of Patrick, a young man with Down syndrome from birth through his graduation from high school.

3656 You Don't Outgrow Down Syndrome
National Association for Down Syndrome
1460 Renaissance Drive
Park Ridge, IL 60068-4542

630-325-9112
847-376-8908
info@nads.org
www.nads.org

Winner of the second annual International Rehabilitation Film Festival.
Steve Connors, President
Sarah Alzamora, First Vice President

Web Sites

3657 ALEH Israel Foundation
PO Box 4911   917-936-6305
New York, NY 10185   866-750-2534
www.aleh.org
ALEH is Israel's largest and most advanced network of residential facilities for children with severe disabilities.
Josh Pruzansky, Director, Development, USA & Canada

3658 Down Syndrome
www.downsyn.com
A resource for new paretns of children with Down syndrome. Provides a personnel perspective from parents who also have children with Down syndrome.

3659 Healing Well
www.healingwell.com
An online health resource guide to medical news, chat, information and articles, newsgroups and message boards, books, disease-related web sites, medical directories, and more for patients, friends, and family coping with disabling diseases, disorders, or chronic illnesses.

3660 Health Finder
www.healthfinder.gov
Searchable, carefully developed web site offering information on over 1000 topics. Developed by the US Department of Health and Human Services, the site can be used in both English and Spanish.

3661 Healthlink USA
www.healthlinkusa.com
Health information concerning treatment, cures, prevention, diagnosis, risk factors, research, support groups, email lists, personal stories and much more. Updated regularly.

3662 MedicineNet
www.medicinenet.com
An online resource for consumers providing easy-to-read, authoritative medical and health information.

3663 Medscape
www.medscape.com
Medscape offers specialists, primary care physicians, and other health professionals the Web's most robust and integrated medical information and educational tools.

3664 National Down Syndrome Society
www.ndss.org
NDSS supports researchers seeking the causes of and answers to many of the medical, genetic, behavioral and learning problems associated with Down syndrome. Also sponsors symposia and conferences for parents and professionals provides advocacy.

3665 WebMD
www.webmd.com
Provides credible information, supportive communities, and in-depth reference material about health subjects. A source for original and timely health information as well as material from well known content providers.

Description	National Agencies & Associations

Description

3666 Eating Disorders (Anorexia Nervosa, Bulimia)

Anorexia nervosa and bulimia nervosa are eating disorders characterized by a disturbed sense of body image and an irrational fear of obesity. They are manifested by abnormal patterns relating to food and by self-induced, marked weight loss.

Anorexia is a psychiatric disorder in which a relentless fear of gaining weight drives devastating dieting and other habits to prevent weight gain. Anorexics are often unable to maintain a normal weight and often experience excessive weight loss. About 95 percent of persons with this disorder are female, although males can be affected. The onset usually occurs during adolescence and some sufferers are in their 60s. Anorexia nervosa is characterized by self-starvation, food preoccupation and rituals, compulsive exercising, and often a resulting absence of menstrual cycles. The cause is unknown, although social factors appear to play an important role, including advertisements that equate thinness with desirability. Denial is a prominent feature, and sufferers usually resist treatment.

Bulimia nervosa is characterized by recurring cycles of binge eating followed by efforts to avoid weight gain, such as purging through self-induced vomiting, abuse of laxatives and/or diuretics (water pills) and/or appetite suppressants, fasting or dieting, and excessive, compulsive exercise. Unlike patients with anorexia, those with bulimia usually have normal weight. Binges are often triggered by psychological stress and carried out in secret. Warning signs of bulimia include eating uncontrollably, frequent use of the bathroom, erosion of dental enamel of the front teeth (from vomiting), and painless swollen salivary glands. The pharynx and esophagus may be irritated in those who self-induce vomiting, and calluses may be present on the knuckles or of the dominant hand. Bulimia may coexist with anorexia.

Anorexia nervosa is associated with a 10 percent death rate, generally from a sudden disturbance of heart rhythm. Bulimic patients may suffer from wild swings in electrolyte concentrations that may affect muscle and heart function. Fortunately, most sufferers will eventually return to a normal or near-normal body weight, although many continue to struggle with body image and unhealthy eating patterns. Treatment for both illnesses is similar, beginning with the need to restore body weight. Initial treatment may require hospitalization for physical stabilization. Antidepressants, such as fluoxetine may be helpful for bulimia. Long-term psychological treatment and behavior modification is often necessary and focuses on behavioral and emotional growth for both the individual with the eating disorder and their family. See also *Obesity*.

National Agencies & Associations

3667 Academy for Eating Disorders
11130 Sunrise Valley Drive
Reston, VA 20191
703-234-4079
Fax: 703-435-4390
info@aedweb.org
www.aedweb.org
AED is an association of multidisciplinary professionals promoting effective treatment, developing prevention initiatives, advocating for the field, stimulating research and sponsoring an annual conference.
Elissa Myers, Executive Director
Dawn Gannon, Deputy Executive Director

3668 Academy of Nutrition & Dietetics
120 South Riverside Plaza
Chicago, IL 60606-6995
312-899-0040
800-877-1600
media@eatright.org
www.eatright.org
Serves the public through the promotion of optimal nutrition, health, and well-being. Formerly the American Dietetic Association.
Mary Russell, President
Patricia M. Babjak, Chief Executive Officer

3669 Administration for Children and Families
330 C Street SW
Washington, DC 20201
202-205-8347
Fax: 202-205-9721
www.acf.hhs.gov
The Administration for Children & Families (ACF) is a division of the U.S. Department of Health & Human Services (HHS). ACF promotes the economic and social well-being of families, children, individuals and communities.
Lynn Johnson, Assistant Secretary
Jerry Milner, Acitng Commissioner, Children & Families

3670 Agency for Healthcare Research and Quality
5600 Fishers Lane
Rockville, MD 20857
301-427-1104
www.ahrq.gov
The Agency for Healthcare Research and Quality's (AHRQ) mission is to produce evidence to make health care safer, higher quality, more accessible, equitable, and affordable, and to work within the U.S. Department of Health and Human Services and with other partners to make sure that the evidence is understood and used.
Gopal Khanna, MBA, Director
Howard E. Holland, Director, Communications

3671 Bulimia Anorexia Nervosa Association
1500 Ouellette Avenue
Windsor, Ontario, N8X-1K7
519-969-2112
855-969-5530
Fax: 519-969-0227
www.bana.ca
BANA facilitates, advocates, and coordinates support for any individual directly or indirectly affected by eating disorders, and raises public awareness through improved communication and the provision of education within the community.
Luciana Rosu-Sieza, Executive Director
Patrick Kelly, Communications & Office Administrator

3672 Centers for Disease Control & Prevention: Division of Adolescent & School Health
1600 Clifton Road
Atlanta, GA 30329-4027
800-232-4636
TTY: 888-232-6348
www.cdc.gov/HealthyYouth
CDC promotes the health and well-being of children and adolescents to enable them to become healthy and productive adults.

3673 Centers for Medicare & Medicaid Services
7500 Security Boulevard
Baltimore, MD 21244
410-786-3000
877-267-2323
TTY: 866-226-1819
www.cms.gov
U.S. federal agency which administers Medicare, Medicaid, and the State Children's Health Insurance Program.
Seema Verma, Administrator
Tom Corry, Director

3674 Eating Disorders Anonymous
PO Box 55876
Phoenix, AZ 85078-5876
info@eatingdisordersanonymous.org
www.4eda.org

EDA provides support group services for people recovering from eating disorders.

3675 Eating Disorders Coalition for Research, Policy and Action
PO Box 96503-98807
Washington, DC 20090
202-543-9570
Fax: 202-543-9570
www.eatingdisorderscoalition.org
Advocates at the federal level on behalf of people with eating disorders, their families, and professionals working with these populations. Promotes federal support for improved access to care.
David Jaffe, Executive Director
Emilie LaBonte, Assistant Account Executive

3676 Healthy Weight Network
402 S 14th Street
Hettinger, ND 58639
701-567-2646
Fax: 701-567-2602
www.healthyweight.net
Promotes information and resources pertaining to the Health at Any Size paradigm.
Frances M. Berg, MS, Founder/Editor

3677 Jessie's Legacy
1111 Lonsdale Avenue
North Vancouver, BC, V7M-2H4
jessieslegacy@familyservices.bc.ca
jessieslegacy.com
604-988-5281
A program of Family Services of the North Shore, Jessie's Legacy seeks to support youth, families, and professionals involved in body image and eating disorders in BC.
Joanna Zelichowska, Manager

3678 MindWise Innovations
270 Bridge Street
Dedham, MA 02026
781-239-0071
Fax: 781-320-9136
info@mindwise.org
www.mindwise.org
Formerly known as Screening For Mental Health, MindWise Innovations provides resources to schools, workplaces, and communities to address mental health issues, eating disorders, substance abuse, and suicide.
Bryan Kohl, Senior Vice President
Marjie McDaniel, Vice President

3679 National Association of Anorexia Nervosa and Associated Disorders
220 N. Green Street
Chicago, IL 60607
630-577-1330
hello@anad.org
www.anad.org
Works to prevent eating disorders and provides numerous programs — all free — to help victims and families including hotlines, support groups, referrals, information packets and newsletters. Educational/prevention programs include presentations and early detection.
Lynn Slawsky, MPA, PMP, Executive Director
Kristen Portland, Operations Manager

3680 National Center for Complementary and Integrative Health
9000 Rockville Pike
Bethesda, MD 20892
888-644-6226
TTY: 866-464-3615
info@nccih.nih.gov
nccih.nih.gov
The National Center for Complementary and Integrative Health (NCCIH) is the Federal Government's lead agency for scientific research on the diverse medical and health care systems, practices, and products that are not generally considered part of conventional medicine.
Helene M. Langevin, MD, Director
David Shurtleff, Ph.D., Deputy Director

3681 National Eating Disorder Information Centre
ES 7-421, 200 Elizabeth Street
Toronto, Ontario, M5G-2C4
416-340-4156
866-633-4220
Fax: 416-340-4736
nedic@uhn.ca
www.nedic.ca
NEDIC promotes healthy lifestyles, including both healty eating and appropriate, enjoyable exercise, through outreach and education, direct client support, and other programs.
Suzanne Phillips, Program Manager
Rekha Wijayaratna, Development Officer

3682 National Eating Disorders Association
1500 Boradway
New York, NY 10036
212-575-6200
800-931-2237
Fax: 212-575-1650
info@NationalEatingDisorders.org
www.nationaleatingdisorders.org
NEDA aims to eliminate eating disorders and body dissatisfaction through prevention efforts, education, referral and support services, advocacy training, and research.
Claire Mysko, Chief Executive Officer
Christine Novak Micka, Chief Development Officer

3683 National Human Genome Research Institute
Building 31, Room 4B09
Bethesda, MD 20892-2152
301-402-0911
Fax: 301-402-2218
www.genome.gov
The National Human Genome Research Institute began as the National Center for Human Genome Research (NCHGR), which was established in 1989 to carry out the role of the National Institutes of Health (NIH) in the International Human Genome Project (HGP).
Eric D. Green, M.D., Ph.D., Director
Lawrence Brody, Ph.D., Director, Division of Genomics & Society

3684 National Institute for Occupational Safety and Health
Patriots Plaza 1
395 E Street SW
Washington, DC 20201
202-245-0625
800-232-4636
Fax: 513-533-8347
TTY: 888-232-6348
www.cdc.gov/niosh
The National Institute for Occupational Safety and Health (NIOSH) is the U.S. federal agency that conducts research and makes recommendations to prevent worker injury and illness.
John Howard, MD, Director
Frank Hearl, PE, Chief of Staff

3685 National Institute of Environmental Health Sciences
105 T.W. Alexander Drive
Research Triangle Park, NC 27709
919-541-3345
webcenter@niehs.nih.gov
www.niehs.nih.gov
The mission of the NIEHS is to discover how the environment affects people in order to promote healthier lives.
Linda S. Birnbaum, PhD, Director
Richard Woychik, PhD, Deputy Director

3686 Office of Women's Health
200 Independence Avenue SW
Washington, DC 20201
202-690-7650
800-994-9662
Fax: 202-205-2631
womenshealth@hhs.gov
www.womenshealth.gov
Government agency under the Department of Health & Human Services, with free health information for women.
Dorothy Fink, MD, Deputy Asst. Secretary, Women's Health
Nicole Greene, Deputy Director

3687 U.S. Food and Drug Administration
10903 New Hampshire Avenue
Silver Spring, MD 20993-0002
301-796-8240
888-463-6332
www.fda.gov
FDA is responsible for protecting the public health by assuring the safety, efficacy and security of human and veterinary drugs, biological products, medical devices, the nation's food supply, cosmetics, and products that emit radiation.
Norman E. Sharpless, MD, Commissioner
Denise Hinton, Chief Scientist

3688 Up Against Eating Disorders
upagainsted.com
Provides services to loved ones of people with eating disorders, and training to treatment professionals.
Joe Kelly, Founder

3689 Weight-Control Information Network
National Institutes of Health
31 Center Drive
Bethesda, MD 20892-2560
800-860-8747
TTY: 866-569-1162
healthinfo@niddk.nih.gov
www.win.niddk.nih.gov

WIN provides the general public, health professionals, and the media with up-to-date, science-based information on obesity, weight control, physical activity, and related nutritional issues.

State Agencies & Associations

Connecticut

3690 Renfrew Center of Connecticut
1445 E. Putnam Avenue
Wilton, CT 06897
800-736-3739
Fax: 203-563-9936
foundation@renfrew.org
www.renfrewcenter.com

Florida

3691 Renfrew Center of Miami
151 Majorca Avenue
Coral Gables, FL 33134
800-REN-FREW
Fax: 305-445-2729
info@renfrewcenter.com
www.renfrewcenter.com

3692 Renfrew Center of South Florida
7700 Renfrew Lane
Coconut Creek, FL 33073
800-736-3739
Fax: 954-698-9007
info@renfrewcenter.com
www.renfrewcenter.com

Maryland

3693 St. Joseph's Medical Center
7601 Osler Drive
Towson, MD 21204
410-337-1000
www.stjosephtowson.com
John Tolmie, President/CEO

Massachusetts

3694 Massachusetts Eating Disorder Association
92 Pearl Street
Newton, MA 02458
617-558-1881
866-343-MEDA
Fax: 617-558-1771
www.medainc.org
A nonprofit organization dedicated to the treatment and prevention of eating disorders. MEDA provides help line resource and referral, assessments, client consultations, individual therapy, support groups and an intensive evening treatment program.
100+ Members
Rebecca Manley, Founder
Beth Mayer, CEO

New Jersey

3695 American Anorexia Bulimia Association: New Jersey Chapter
10 Station Place
Metuchen, NJ 08840
609-252-0202
Fax: 609-688-1544

3696 Renfrew Center of Northern New Jersey
174 Union Street
Ridgewood, NJ 07450
800-736-3739
Fax: 201-652-6253
info@renfrewcenter.org
www.renfrewcenter.com

New York

3697 Renfrew Center of New York
11 E 36th Street
New York, NY 10016
800-736-3739
Fax: 212-686-1865
info@renfrewcenter.org
www.renfrewcenter.com

3698 Westchester Task Force on Eating Disorders/American Anorexia Bulimia
3 Mount Joy Avenue
Scarsdale, NY 10583-2632
914-472-3701

Pennsylvania

3699 American Anorexia Bulimia Association of Philadelphia
PO Box 1287
Langhorne, PA 19047
215-221-1864
Fax: 215-702-8944
www.aabaphila.org

3700 Pennsylvania Educational Network for Eating Disorders
4801 McKnight Road
Pittsburgh, PA 15237
412-215-7967
www.pened.org
PENED is a nonprofit organization providing education, support, and referral information to the general and professional public.
Anita Sincro Maier, Therapist
Ralph F. Wilps, Therapist

3701 Renfrew Center of Bryn Mawr
735 Old Lancaster Road
Bryn Mawr, PA 19010
800-736-3739
Fax: 610-527-9361
www.renfrewcenter.com

3702 Renfrew Center of Philadelphia
475 Spring Lane
Philadelphia, PA 19128
800-REN-FREW
Fax: 215-482-7390
info@renfrew.org
www.renfrewcenter.com

Foundations

3703 International Association of Eating Disorders Professionals Foundation
PO Box 1295
Pekin, IL 61555-1295
309-346-3341
800-800-8126
Fax: 309-346-2874
iaedpmembers@earthlink.net
www.iaedp.com
IAEDP Offers professional counseling and assistance to the medical community, courts, law enforcement officials and social welfare agencies.
Bonnie Harken, Managing Director
Blanche Williams, Director, International Development

3704 The Emily Program Foundation (merged with Anna Westin Foundation)
1295 Bandana Boulevard W.
St Paul, MN 55108
952-361-3051
www.emilyprogramfoundation.org
The Anna Westin Foundation is dedicated to the prevention and treatment of eating disorders. They are committed to preventing the tragic loss of life to anorexia nervosa and bulimia and to raising public awareness of those dangerous illnesses.
Lisa Radzak, Executive Director
Emily Monson, Outreach & Program Manager

Libraries & Resource Centers

3705 Weight-Control Information Network
National Institutes of Health
31 Center Drive
Bethesda, MD 20892-2560
800-860-8747
TTY: 866-569-1162
healthinfo@niddk.nih.gov
www.win.niddk.nih.gov
WIN provides the general public, health professionals, and the media with up-to-date, science-based information on obesity, weight control, physical activity, and related nutritional issues. WIN provides tip sheets, fact sheets, and brochures for a range of audiences. Some of WIN's content is available in Spanish.

Research Centers

3706 Academy for Eating Disorders
11130 Sunrise Valley Drive
Reston, VA 20191
703-234-4079
Fax: 703-435-4390
info@aedweb.org
www.aedweb.org
AED is an association of multidisciplinary professionals promoting effective treatment, developing prevention initiatives, advo-

cating for the field, stimulating research and sponsoring an annual conference.
Elissa Myers, Executive Director
Dawn Gannon, Deputy Executive Director

3707 Center for the Study of Anorexia and Bulimia
1841 Broadway at 60th Street   212-333-3444
New York, NY 10023   Fax: 212-333-5444
www.icpnyc.org
The Institute is composed of a group of 150 professionally trained licensed psychotherapists who offer a full range of psychotherapeutic services including individual and group psychotherapy and psychoanalysis in addition to more specialized treatment services.
Jim M Pollack CSW, Executive Director/Director of Treatment
Ron Taffel, Chair

3708 Division of Digestive & Liver Diseases of Cloumbia University
630 W 168th Street   212-305-5960
New York, NY 10032-3784   Fax: 212-305-8466
hjw14@columbia.edu
www.cumc.columbia.edu
The Division's faculty members are devoted to research and the clinical care of patients with gastrointestinal, liver and nutritional disorders. The Division is also responsible for the Gastroenterology Training Program at the medical center and for teaching medical students, interns, residents, fellows and attending physicians aspects of gastrointestinal and liver diseases.
Howard J Worman MD, Division Director
Karen Wisdom, Director

3709 Harris Center for Education and Advocacy in Eating Disorders
2 Longfellow Place   617-726-8470
Boston, MA 02114   Fax: 617-726-1595
Conducts research provides a newsletter and information.
David B Herzog MD, Director
David B Herzog, Director

Support Groups & Hotlines

3710 AABA Support Group
Chippenham Medican Center
7101 Jahnke Rd.   804-320-3911
Richmond, VA 23225
Elliot Spanier, Contact

3711 About Kids GI Disorders
IFFGD
PO Box 170864   414-964-1799
Milwaukee, WI 53217-8076   888-964-2001
Fax: 414-964-7176
iffgd@iffgd.org
www.aboutkidsgi.org
About Kids is the pediatric branch of the International Foundation for Functional Gastrointestinal Disorders (IFFGD), a registered nonprofit education and research organization founded in 1991. Their mission is to inform, assist, and support those affected by gastrointestinal (GI) disorders, addressing issues of digestive health in children through support of education and research. IFFGD promotes awareness among the public, health care providers, researchers, and regulators.
Nancy J Norton, President/Founder

3712 Association of Gastrointestinal Motility D isorders
AGMD International Corporate Headquarters
12 Roberts Drive   781-275-1300
Bedford, MA 01730   Fax: 781-275-1304
digestive.motility@gmail.com
www.agmd-gimotility.org
A non-profit international organization which serves as an integral educational resource concerning digestive motility diseases and disorders. Also functions as an important information base for members of the medical and scientific communities. Also provides a forum for patients suffering from digestive motility diseases and disorders as well as their families and members of the medical, scientific, and nutritional communities.
Mary Angela DeGrazia-DiTucci, President/Patient/Founder

3713 Coconut Creek Eating Disorders Support Group
Renfrew Center
7700 NW 48th Avenue   954-698-9222
Coconut Creek, FL 33073-3508   877-367-3383
Fax: 954-698-9007
www.renfrew.org
Samuel Menagad, Director

3714 Eating Disorder Resource Center
330 W 58th Street   212-989-3987
New York, NY 10019   info@edrcnyc.org
www.edrcnyc.org
A specialized treatment program for women and men who were suffering from bulimia. Now EDRC treats eating disorders of all kinds, offering individual, group, family and couples treatment for those challenged by bulimia, binge eating disorder, anorexia and other kinds of body dysmorphia.
Judith Brisman, Director & Founder
Senna Lauer, Marketing Assistant

3715 Eating Disorders Association of New Jersey
10 Station Place   800-522-2230
Metuchen, NJ 08840   Fax: 732-906-9307
info@edanj.org
www.edanj.org
A non-profit state organization whose mission is to provide supportive services and resources to indivudals affected by eating disorders, including family members and friends.

3716 First Presbyterian Church in the City of New York Support Groups
First Presbyterian Church in the City of New York
12 West 12th Street   212-675-6150
New York, NY 10011   fpcnyc@fpcnyc.org
www.fpcnyc.org
The First Presbyterian Church in the City of New York provides numerous programs and supports groups for both adults and children including an educational program for autistic children.
Jon M Walton, Senior Pastor
Sarah Segal Mccaslin, Associate Pastor

3717 Holliswood Hospital Psychiatric Care, Serv ices and Self-Help/Support Groups
87-37 Palermo Street   718-776-8181
Holliswood, NY 11423   800-486-3005
Fax: 718-776-8572
HolliswoodInfo@libertymgt.com
www.holliswoodhospital.com/
The Holliswood Hospital, a 110-bed private psychiatric hospital located in a quiet residential Queens community, is a leader in providing quality, acute inpatient mental health care for adult, adolescent, geriatric and dually diagnosed patients. Holliswood Hospital treats patients with a broad range of psychiatric disorders. Additionally, specialized services are available for patients with psychiatric diagnoses compounded by chemical dependency, or a history of physical or sexual abuse.
Susan Clayton, Support Group Coordinator
Angela Hurtado, Support Group Coordinator

3718 National Association of Anorexia Nervosa and Associated Disorders Helpline
220 N. Green Street   630-577-1330
Chicago, IL 60607   hello@anad.org
www.anad.org
Works to prevent eating disorders and provides numerous programs — all free — to help victims and families including hotlines, support groups, referrals, information packets, and online content. Educational/prevention programs include presentations and early detection.
Lynn Slawsky, MPA, PMP, Executive Director
Kristen Portland, Operations Manager

3719 National Eating Disorder Information Centr e Helpline
ES 7-421, 200 Elizabeth Street   416-340-4156
Toronto, Ontario, M5G-2C4   866-633-4220
Fax: 416-340-4736
nedic@uhn.ca
www.nedic.ca
NEDIC promotes healthy lifestyles, including both healty eating and appropriate, enjoyable exercise, through outreach and educa-

tion, direct client support, and other programs, including a helpline.
Suzanne Phillips, Program Manager
Rekha Wijayaratna, Development Officer

3720   National Eating Disorders Association Helpline
1500 Boradway   212-575-6200
New York, NY 10036   800-931-2237
                                       Fax: 212-575-1650
                      info@NationalEatingDisorders.org
                           www.nationaleatingdisorders.org
NEDA aims to eliminate eating disorders and body dissatisfaction through prevention efforts, education, referral and support services, advocacy training, and research. Also provides a Helpline.
Claire Mysko, Chief Executive Officer
Christine Novak Micka, Chief Development Officer

3721   National Health Information Center
Office of Disease Prevention & Health Promotion
1101 Wootton Pkwy   Fax: 240-453-8281
Rockville, MD 20852   odphpinfo@hhs.gov
                                       www.health.gov/nhic
Supports public health education by maintaining a calendar of National Health Observances; helps connect consumers and health professionals to organizations that can best answer questions and provide up-to-date contact information from reliable sources; updates on a yearly basis toll-free numbers for health information, Federal health clearinghouses and info centers.
Don Wright, MD, MPH, Director

3722   Richmond Support Group
Warwick Medical & Professional Ctr   804-320-7881
Richmond, VA

Books

3723   Anorexia Nervosa & Recovery: A Hunger for Meaning
The Haworth Press
One Haworth Center   616-393-3000
Holland, MI 49423   800-344-2600
                                       getinfo@haworth.com
                                           www.haworth.com
1993 146 pages Paperback
ISBN: 0-918393-95-7

3724   Bearly Any Fat Cookbook
Obesity Foundation
8757 Georgia Avenue   301-563-6526
Silver Spring, MD 20910-2202   301-563-6595
                                         editor@obesity.org
                                            www.obesity.org
Perfect cookbook to assist anyone in a weight reduction program.
Francesca M. Dea, Executive Director
Kathie Cleary, Senior Director, Finance

3725   Body Betrayed
American Psychiatric Press
1400 K Street NW   202-682-6268
Washington, DC 20005-2403   Fax: 202-789-2648
A book concentrating on women, eating disorders and treatments.
440 pages Hardcover
ISBN: 0-880485-22-1

3726   Bulimia: A Guide to Recovery
Gurze Books
PO Box 2238   800-756-7533
Carlsbad, CA 92018-9883   Fax: 760-434-5476
                                           gzcatl@aol.com
                                            www.bulimia.com
This intimate guidebook offers a complete understanding of bulimia and a plan for recovery. It includes a two-week program to stop bingeing, things-to-do instead of bingeing, a two-week guide for support groups, specific advice for loved ones and Eating Without Fear, Hall's story of self-cure which has inspired thousands of other bulimics.
280 pages Paperback
ISBN: 0-936077-31-X

3727   Conversations with Anorexics
Jason Aronson
P.O. Box 15556   800-782-0015
Amsterdam, NL -7100   Fax: 201-840-7242
                                         mail@aronson.com
                                            www.aronson.com
A Compassionate and Hopeful Journey through the Therapeutic Process.
238 pages
ISBN: 1-568212-61-5
Robert D. Aronson, Director
Lisa Rooimans, Assistant

3728   Coping with Eating Disorders
Rosen Publishing Group
29 E 21st Street   212-777-3017
New York, NY 10010   800-237-9932
                                       Fax: 888-436-4643
                         customerservice@rosenpub.com
                                       www.rosenpublishing.com
This book offers practical suggestions on coping with eating disorders.
ISBN: 0-823929-74-4
Barbara Moe, Author

3729   Cult of Thinness
Oxford University Press
2001 Evans Road   212-726-6000
Cary, NC 27513-2010   800-451-7556
                                       Fax: 919-677-1303
                                           www.oup-usa.org
1996 256 pages
ISBN: 0-195082-41-9

3730   Deadly Diet: Recovering from Anorexia & Bulimia
New Harbinger Publications
5674 Shattuck Avenue   800-748-6273
Oakland, CA 94609-1662   Fax: 510-652-5472
                         customerservice@newharbinger.com
                                       www.newharbinger.com
1993 265 pages Paperback
ISBN: 1-879237-42-3

3731   Eating Diorders Resource Catalogue
Gurze Books
PO Box 2238   800-756-7533
Carlsbad, CA 92018-9883   Fax: 760-434-5476
                                            www.bulimia.com
This catalogue of resources contains over 140 books, videos and audiotapes, lists of national organizations and treatment facilities and basic facts about eating disorders. It is widely distributed by individuals who are suffering, their loved ones, the health care professionals who treat them and educators who are working towards prevention.
24 pages Annual

3732   Eating Disorder Sourcebook
Gurze Books
PO Box 2238   800-756-7533
Carlsbad, CA 92018-2238   Fax: 760-434-5476
                                           gzcatl@aol.com
                                            www.bulimia.com
An ideal book for someone with a loved one who has an eating disorder but who knows little about this subject, this new release presents a clear overview of basic issues.
222 pages Paperback

3733   Eating Disorders Resource Catalogue
Gurze Books
PO Box 2238   800-756-7533
Carlsbad, CA 92018-9883   Fax: 760-434-5476
                                            www.bulimia.com
This catalogue of resources contains over 140 books, videos and audiotapes, lists of national organizations and treatment facilities and basic facts about eating disorders. It is widely distributed by individuals who are suffering, their loved ones, the health care professionals who treat them and educators who are working towards prevention.
28 pages Annual

3734 Eating Disorders-Overview Series
Lucent Books
Thomson Gale   800-877-4253
Farmington Hills, MI 48331-9187   Fax: 800-414-5043
gale.customerservice@thomson.com
www.gale.com/lucent
This book examines how eating disorders can be identified, who is
affected by them, and how they can be treated.
2001
ISBN: 1-560066-59-8

3735 Eating Disorders: When Food Turns Against You
Franklin Watts Grolier
90 Old Sherman Tpke   203-797-3500
Danbury, CT 06816-0001   Fax: 203-797-3197
www.grolier.com

1993 96 pages
ISBN: 0-531111-75-0

3736 Emotional Eating: A Practical Guide to Taking Control
Free Press
1230 Ave of the Americas   800-223-7445
New York, NY 10020   Fax: 800-943-9831
info@simonsays.com
www.simonsays.com

1003 200 pages
ISBN: 0-029002-15-0

3737 Encyclopedia of Obesity and Eating Disorders
Facts on File
132 West 31st Street   212-967-8800
New York, NY 10001   800-322-8755
Fax: 800-678-3633
custserv@factsonfile.com
www.infobasepublishing.com
From abdominoplasty to Zung Rating Scale, this volume defines
and explains these disorders, along with medical and other problems associated with them.
272 pages Hardcover

3738 Endorphins: Eating Disorders & Other Addictive Behavior
WW Norton & Company
500 5th Avenue   212-354-5500
New York, NY 10110-0054   800-233-4830
Fax: 212-869-0856
www.wwnorton.com

1993 320 pages
ISBN: 0-393701-56-5

3739 Etiology and Treatment of Bulimia Nervosa
Jason Aronson
P.O.Box 15556   800-782-0015
Amsterdam, NB 1001-7100   Fax: 201-767-1576
www.aronson.com

352 pages Softcover
ISBN: 1-568213-39-5

3740 Evaluation and Management of Eating Disorders
Human Kinetics Publishers
8600 Rockville Pike   217-351-1549
Bethesda, MD 20894-5076   800-747-4457
Fax: 217-351-5076
www.ncbi.nlm.nih.gov

368 pages Cloth
ISBN: 0-873229-11-8

3741 Fear of Being Fat
Jason Aronson
P.O.Box 15556   800-782-0015
Amsterdam, NB 1001-7100   Fax: 201-840-7242
www.aronson.com

366 pages
ISBN: 0-876688-99-7

3742 Getting Better Bit(e) by Bit(e)
Gurze Books
PO Box 2238   800-756-7533
Carlsbad, CA 92018-2238   Fax: 760-434-5476
gzcatl@aol.com
www.bulimia.com

This practical book on recovery from bulimia and binge eating is
packed with lists, exercises, case studies, discussions, insights and
specific things to do. This book also addresses the day-to-day
problems faced by eating disorder sufferers and concentrates on
key behavior changes necessary for progress.
143 pages Paperback

3743 Going Backwards
Scholastic
730 Broadway   212-505-3000
New York, NY 10003-9511   800-325-6149
www.thesaurus.com
A story that weaves the themes of acceptance, death, mortality and
family loyalty to present a controversial plot.
Grades 7-10
Michele Turner, CEO
Jim Conning, SVP of Engineering

3744 Golden Cage: The Enigma of Anorexia Nervosa
Gurze Books
PO Box 2283   800-756-7533
Carlsbad, CA 92018-2283   Fax: 760-434-5476
gzcatl@aol.com
www.bulimia.com

3745 Group Psychotherapy for Eating Disorders
American Psychiatric Press
PO Box 1295   202-682-6268
Pekin, IL 61555-2403   800-800-8126
Fax: 202-789-2648
info@eatingdisordersreview.com
eatingdisordersreview.com
The first book to fully explore the use of group therapy in the treat-
ment of eating disorders.
353 pages Hardcover
ISBN: 0-880484-19-5

3746 Helping Athletes with Eating Disorders
Human Kinetics Publishers
165 West 46th Street   212-575-6200
New York, NY 10036-5076   800-931-2237
Fax: 212-575-1650
https://www.nationaleatingdisorders.org
Gives readers the information they need to identify and address
major eating disorders such as: anorexia, bulimia nervosa, and eat-
ing disorders not otherwise specified.
208 pages Cloth
ISBN: 0-873223-83-7
Ric Clark, Chair
Mary Curran, Vice-Chair

**3747 Hope and Recovery: A Mother-Daughter Story About Anorexia
Nervosa & Bulimia**
Franklin Watts Grolier
65 West 36th St.   800-621-1115
New York, NY 10018-0001   Fax: 800-374-4329
www.kirkusreviews.com/
Mother and daughter tell a story of a young woman's recovery from
the horror of an eating disorder. This compelling account shows
how anorexia and bulimia can affect an entire family.
192 pages
ISBN: 0-531111-40-7
Herb Simon, Chairman
Marc Winkelman, President and Publisher

3748 Hungry Self: Women, Eating and Identity
Gurze Books
PO Box 2283   800-756-7533
Carlsbad, CA 92018-2283   Fax: 760-434-5476
gzcatl@aol.com
www.bulimia.com

3749 Insights in the Dynamic Psychotherapy of Anorexia and Bulimia
Jason Aronson

P.O.Box 15556
Amsterdam, NB 1001-1523

646-415-2561
800-782-0015
Fax: 201-840-7242
www.aronson.com

320 pages Hardcover
ISBN: 0-876685-68-8
Robert D. Aronson, Director
Lisa Rooimans, Assistant

3750   It's Not Your Fault
Gurze Books
PO Box 2238
Carlsbad, CA 92018-2238

800-756-5476
Fax: 760-434-5476
gzcatl@aol.com
www.bulimia.com

In this comprehensive, medically sound guide to overcoming eating disorders, Dr. Marx defines the warnings signs of eating disorders, explores causes, at risk populations, the role of drug therapy and advises patients and families where and how they can find help.

3751   Making Peace with Food
Gurze Books
PO Box 2238
Carlsbad, CA 92018-2238

800-756-7533
Fax: 760-434-5476
gzcatl@aol.com
www.bulimia.com

This unique, full sized workbook is designed to help anyone who experienced compulsive eating, yo-yo dieting, food and body anxiety, or associated eating disorders. Filled with ideas, workbook pages, exercises and resources, Kano's book is an excellent aid to clarifying and overcoming your personal diet/weight struggle.
224 pages Paperback

3752   Meals Without Squeals Sense
Bull Publishing
PO Box 1377
Boulder, CO 80306

303-545-6350
800-676-2855
Fax: 303-545-6354
www.bullpub.com

Straight forward information on childrens growth accompanies age specific, child tested recipes. Explained is how common feeding problems can be solved and show ways to offer children positive experiences with food.
2006 288 pages
ISBN: 1-933503-00-4
Emily Sewell, CFO
Claire Cameron, Director of Marketing

3753   My Name is Caroline
Doubleday
666 Fifth Avenue
New York, NY 10103

212-354-6500

A poignant tale of one woman's battle with bulimia throughout her life as a successful student, athlete, scholar and musician.
Grades 10-12

3754   Obesity: Theory and Therapy
Raven Press
8600 Rockville Pike
Bethesda, MD 20894-2601

212-930-9500
800-777-2295
www.ncbi.nlm.nih.gov

A classic reference for clinicians dealing with obesity, this volume provides the most up-to-date research, preclinical and clinical information.
500 pages
ISBN: 0-881678-84-8

3755   Practice Guidelines for Eating Disorders
American Psychiatric Press
1000 Wilson Boulevard
Arlington, VA 22209-2403

202-682-6268
Fax: 202-789-2648
psychiatryonline@psych.org
psychiatryonline.org

Designed for health care professionals, this guideline includes information on all aspects of anorexia nervosa and bulimia nervosa, including self-induced vomiting, use of laxatives and vigorous exercise to prevent weight gain.
38 pages Paperback
ISBN: 0-890423-00-8

3756   Psychodynamic Technique in the Treatment of the Eating Disorders
Jason Aronson
P.O.Box 15556
Amsterdam, NB 1001-7100

646-415-2561
800-782-0015
Fax: 201-840-7242
mail@aronson.com
www.aronson.com

440 pages Hardcover
ISBN: 0-876686-22-6
Robert D. Aronson, Director
Lisa Rooimans, Assistant

3757   Self-Starvation
Jason Aronson
P.O.Box 15556
Amsterdam, NB 1001-7100

646-415-2561
800-782-0015
Fax: 201-840-7242
mail@aronson.com
www.aronson.com

312 pages Softcover
ISBN: 1-568218-22-2
Robert D. Aronson, Director
Lisa Rooimans, Assistant

3758   Starving to Death in a Sea of Objects
Jason Aronson
P.O.Box 15556
Amsterdam, NB 1001-7100

646-415-2561
800-782-0015
Fax: 201-840-7242
mail@aronson.com
www.aronson.com

How emancipation becomes security for anorexics.
464 pages Softcover
ISBN: 0-876684-35-5
Robert D. Aronson, Director
Lisa Rooimans, Assistant

3759   Surviving an Eating Disorder: Perspectives & Strategies
Gurze Books
PO Box 2238
Carlsbad, CA 92018-2238

800-756-7533
Fax: 760-434-5476
gzcatl@aol.com
www.bulimia.com

Parents, spouses and friends of individuals with food problems will find practical guidelines in this book for helping themselves and their loved ones.
222 pages Paperback

3760   Treating Bulimia: A Psychoeducational Approach
American Anorexia/Bulimia Association
165 W 46th Street
New York, NY 10036-2501

212-575-6200
amanbu@aol.com
lifestream.aol.com

3761   When Food is Love
Gurze Books
PO Box 2238
Carlsbad, CA 92018-2238

760-434-7533
800-756-7533
Fax: 760-434-5467
gzcatl@aol.com
www.gurze.com

Drawing on her own personal experience, Roth explores similarities between eating and loving such as fantasizing, wanting the forbidden, creating drama, control issues, and the experience of relationship.
205 pages Paperback

3762   Withering Child
University of Georgia Press
320 South Jackson Street
Athens, GA 30602

404-542-2830
800-266-5842
Fax: 706-542-2558
www.uga.edu/ugapress

1993 288 pages
ISBN: 0-820315-60-5
Lisa Bayer, Director
Chantel Dunham, Director of Development

Children's Books

3763 Billy's Story
Metro Intergroup of Overeaters Anonymous
117 W 26th Street
New York, NY 10001
212-206-8621
www.billysstory.com

3764 I Was a Fifteen-Year-Old Blimp
Harper & Row
10 E 53rd Street
New York, NY 10022-5299
212-207-7000
This story focuses on Gabby, a teenage girl who overhears others discuss her weight and takes radical steps to become popular.
Grades 6-9

Magazines

3765 BASH Magazine
Bulimia Anorexia Self-Help/Behavior Adaptation
PO Box 39903
Saint Louis, MO 63139-8903
800-762-3334
A journal of eating and mood disorders.
Monthly

3766 Food & Nutrition
120 South Riverside Plaza
Chicago, IL 60606-6995
312-899-0040
800-877-1600
foodandnutrition@eatright.org
www.eatright.org
Formerly the ADA Times, Food & Nutrition is the member and professional magazine of the Academy of Nutrition & Dietetics.

3767 Journal of the Academy of Nutrition and Dietetics
120 South Riverside Plaza
Chicago, IL 60606-6995
312-899-4831
journal@eatright.org
www.eatright.org
Official research publication of the Academy of Nutrition and Dietetics.
Joe Skey, Advertising Contact

Newsletters

3768 AABA Newsletter
American Anorexic and Bulemic Association
905 S. Fillmore
Amarillo, TX 79105-2501
806-345-6300
Fax: 806-345-6363
firm@bf-law.com
www.bf-law.com
This newsletter is published three times a year and is mailed to the members of the AABA. The AABA is a tax-exempt, nonprofit organization with a membership of professionals, sufferers of eating disorders, and their family and friends.

3769 Eating Disorders Review
Gurze Books
PO Box 2238
Carlsbad, CA 92018-9883
800-756-7533
Fax: 760-434-5476
gzcatl@aol.com
www.bulimia.com
Presents current clinical information for the professional treating eating disorders. Features summeries of relevant research from journals and unpublished studies, abstracts, nutritional notes, questions and answers, book reviews and reproducible client handouts.
8 pages BiMonthly
Joel Yager MD, Editor-in-Chief
Liegh Cohn, Publisher

3770 WIN Notes
Weight-control Information Network
1 WIN Way
Bethesda, MD 20892-3665
202-828-1025
877-946-4627
Fax: 202-828-1028
win@mathewsgroup.com
www.niddk.nih.gov/health/nutrit/win.htm
Addresses the health information needs of individuals with weight-control problems. Available on the WIN web site.
BiAnnual
Griffin P. Rodgers, Director

3771 Working Together
Anorexia Nervosa and Associated Disorders
PO Box 7
Highland Park, IL 60035-0007
847-831-3438
Fax: 847-433-4632
www.thesaurus.com
Designed for individuals, families, group leaders and professionals concerned with eating disorders. Provides updates on treatments, resources, conferences, programs, articles by therapists, recovered victims, group members and leaders.
Quarterly
Michele Turner, CEO
Jim Conning, SVP of Engineering

Pamphlets

3772 Applying New Attitudes & Directions
Anorexia Nervosa and Associated Disorders
PO Box 7
Highland Park, IL 60035-0007
847-831-3438
Fax: 847-433-4632
anad20@aol.com
Self-help booklet offering an eight-step program to recovery with suggestions, information and recovery stories.
Dawn Ries, Administrator

Audio & Video

3773 Bulimia: A Guide to Recovery
Gurze Books
PO Box 2238
Carlsbad, CA 92018-2238
800-756-7533
Fax: 760-434-5476
gzcatl@aol.com
www.bulimia.com
This newly rediscovered tape is an inspirational talk by Lindsey Hall on the relationship between bulimia, self-esteem and love. This was one of Lindsey's last public appearances, where she addressed a 1991 eating disorers conference in Colorado Springs.
Audio tape

Web Sites

3774 Academy of Nutrition & Dietetics
www.eatright.org
Offers information and support to allergy sufferers. Serves the public through the promotion of optimal nutrition, health, and well-being. Formerly the American Dietetic Association.

3775 Anorexia Nervosa & Related Eating Disorders
www.anred.com
A nonprofit organization that provides information about anorexia nervosa, bulimia nervosa, binge eating disorder, and other less-well-known food and weight disorders.

3776 GERD Information Resource Center
www.gerd.com
A resource center with educational resources on Gastroesophageal Reflux Disease (GERD).

3777 Gastroenterology Therapy Online
www.gastrotherapy.com
An informational website with resources for many kinds of diseases.

3778 Healing Well
www.healingwell.com
An online health resource guide to medical news, chat, information and articles, newsgroups and message boards, books, disease-related web sites, medical directories, and more for patients, friends, and family coping with disabling diseases, disorders, or chronic illnesses.

3779 Health Finder
www.healthfinder.gov

Searchable, carefully developed web site offering information on over 1000 topics. Developed by the US Department of Health and Human Services, the site can be used in both English and Spanish.

3780 Healthlink USA

www.healthlinkusa.com

Health information concerning treatment, cures, prevention, diagnosis, risk factors, research, support groups, email lists, personal stories and much more. Updated regularly.

3781 MedicineNet

www.medicinenet.com

An online resource for consumers providing easy-to-read, authoritative medical and health information.

3782 Medscape

www.medscape.com

Medscape offers specialists, primary care physicians, and other health professionals the Web's most robust and integrated medical information and educational tools.

3783 National Association for Anorexia Nervosa and Associated Disorders

www.anad.org

ANAD provides educational/prevention programs include presentations and early detection packets for schools and community groups, sponsoring local and national training conferences for health professionals, and working with electronic and print media. Undertakes and encourages research, fights insurance discrimination.

3784 National Association of Anorexia Nervosa and Associated Disorders

www.anad.org

Works to prevent eating disorders and provides numerous programs — all free — to help victims and families including hotlines, support groups, referrals, information packets, and online content. Educational/prevention programs include presentations and early detection.

3785 National Eating Disorders Association

www.nationaleatingdisorders.org

NEDA aims to eliminate eating disorders and body dissatisfaction through prevention efforts, education, referral and support services, advocacy training, and research.

3786 WebMD

www.webmd.com

Provides credible information, supportive communities, and in-depth reference material about health subjects. A source for original and timely health information as well as material from well known content providers.

3787 Weight-Control Information Network

www.win.niddk.nih.gov

The Weight-control Information Network (WIN) provides the general public, health professionals, and the media with up-to-date, science-based information on obesity, weight control, physical activity, and related nutritional issues. WIN provides tip sheets, fact sheets, and brochures for a range of audiences. Some of WIN's content is available in Spanish.

Description

3788 Endometriosis

Endometriosis is a condition characterized by the abnormal implantation of normal endometrial mucosa in locations other than the uterine cavity. These cells respond to the woman's hormonal cycles, and swell and bleed at the time of menses. This causes pain, generally worse with each period, pelvic masses and alterations of the menstrual cycle. The pain may be aggravated by intercourse or defecation. Although the reported incidence varies, endometriosis is commonly found in 6-10 percent of women between the ages of 25 and 44 years. 30-40 percent of women with endometriosis are subfertile.

Because the symptoms of endometriosis depends upon the cyclic production of hormones during the menstrual cycle, regulating the menstrual cycle can ameliorate symptoms. First-line treatments include combination oral contraceptive pills, progestational agents, gonadotropin-releasing hormone (GnRH) analogues, and gonadotropin-releasing hormone antagonists. Treatment depends on the severity of the symptoms and the age and reproductive wishes of the patient. The pain associated with mild cases may be treated with non-steroidal anti-inflammatory drugs. Laparoscopic surgery may destroy some of the ectopic endometrial tissue, and is often used in hopes of improving fertility. Hysterectomy (removal of the uterus or uterus and ovaries) is used for intractable cases, especially in women who do not desire future pregnancy.

National Agencies & Associations

3789 AAGL - Elevating Gynecologic Surgery
6757 Katella Avenue
Cypress, CA 90630

714-503-6200
800-554-2245
lmichels@aagl.org
www.aagl.com

Founded as the American Association of Gynecologic Laparoscopists, AAGL is devoted to promoting and improving minimally invasive gynecologic surgery.
Linda Michels, Executive Director
Linda Bradley, MD, Medical Director

3790 American Chronic Pain Association
PO Box 850
Rocklin, CA 95677

800-533-3231
ACPA@theacpa.org
www.theacpa.org

The ACPA facilitates peer support and education for individuals with chronic pain in its many forms, in order to increase quality of life. Also raises awareness among the healthcare community, and with policy makers.
Penney Cowan, Founder & CEO
Daniel Galia, Director, Global Support

3791 American Society for Reproductive Medicine
1209 Montgomery Highway
Birmingham, AL 35216-2809

205-978-5000
Fax: 205-978-5005
asrm@asrm.org
www.asrm.org

A private, non-profit medical organization devoted to advancing the knowledge, understanding and expertise in all phases of reproductive medicine and biology. Offers patient education brochures, recommended readings and support. Publishes professional journal and consumer publications.
Richard H. Reindollar, MD, Chief Executive Officer

3792 Endometriosis Association International
8585 N 76th Place
Milwaukee, WI 53223

414-355-2200
support@endometriosisassn.org
www.endometriosisassn.org

Self-help organization of women, families, doctors, scientists, and others engaged in information-sharing about endometriosis, with the ultimate goal of prevention and finding a cure. Offers a crisis call hotline, support groups, online community, and healthcare provider lists.

3793 Endometriosis Research Center
630 Ibis Drive
Delray Beach, FL 33444

800-239-7280
Fax: 561-274-0931
askerc@endocenter.org
www.endocenter.org

Non-profit international organization dedicated to helping women and girls suffering from endometriosis. Services include chapter and support groups, crisis/counseling assistance, education of the public and medical community materials including books and videos.
Michelle E. Marvel, Executive Director

3794 HealthyWomen
1 Harding Road
Red Bank, NJ 07701

732-530-3425
877-986-9472
info@healthywomen.org
www.healthywomen.org

Independent, non-profit organization seeking to educate women in all areas of health, to allow them to make informed choices. The HealthyWomen website features numerous tools and health calculators, plus other media.
Beth Battaglino, RN, Chief Executive Officer
Phyllis E. Greenberger, Sr. VP, Science & Health Policy

3795 International Pelvic Pain Society
1510 H Street NW
Washington, DC 20005-1020

202-856-7422
Fax: 202-856-7401
info@pelvicpain.org
www.pelvicpain.org

Seeks to recruit, organize, and educate health care professionals actively involved with the treatment of patients who have chronic pelvic pain.
Colleen Eubanks, Executive Director

3796 National Women's Health Network
1413 K Street
Washington, DC 20005

202-682-2640
Fax: 202-682-2648
nwhn@nwhn.org
www.nwhn.org

Non-profit organization advocating for national policies that protect and promote all women's health, and providing evidence-based independent information.
Cindy Pearson, Executive Director
Sarah Christopherson, Policy Advocacy Director

3797 World Endometriosis Society
1201 West Pender Street
Vancouver, BC, V6E-2V2

604-681-2153
office@endometriosis.ca
endometriosis.ca

WES seeks to advance education, advocacy, clinical care, and research in endometriosis.
Luk y Rombauts, President
Krina Zondervan, Honorary Secretary

Foundations

3798 Fertility Research Foundation
877 Park Avenue
New York, NY 10021

212-744-5500
888-439-2999
Fax: 212-744-6536
info@frfbaby.com
www.frfbaby.com

Offers information on treatment and the latest research on male and female infertility.
Masood Khatamee MD, Executive Director

3799 Hysterectomy Educational Resources & Services (HERS) Foundation
610-667-7757
888-750-4377
hers@hersfoundation.org
www.hersfoundation.com
A nonprofit foundation which provides information about the alternatives to hysterectomy, the risks of the alternatives, and the consequences of the surgery. HERS provides copies of a medical journals, a quarterly newsletter, and a free lending library of books, videos and audio tapes.

Research Centers

3800 Dartmouth Medical School: Microbiology Department
Department of Microbiology & Immunology
1 Rope Ferry Road
Hanover, NH 03755-1404
603-650-1200
877-DMS-1797
Fax: 603-650-1202
microbiology@dartmouth.edu
www.dms.dartmouth.edu
Dartmouth Medical School is a beacon of discovery and learning stimulating inquiry and harnessing ingenuity for new solutions and better health
Ann Hill, Administrative Assistant
Gregory J MacDonald, Assistant Professor of Medicine

3801 Endometriosis Association Research Program : Vanderbuilt University
1211 Medical Center Drive
Nashville, TN 37232
615-322-5000
Fax: 615-343-8881
www.mc.vanderbilt.edu
Heather Arnold, Senior Secretary

3802 Endometriosis Reseach Center and Women's Hospital
The Endometriosis Research Center
630 Ibis Drive
Delray Beach, FL 33444
561-274-7442
800-239-7280
Fax: 561-274-0931
www.endocenter.org
A nonprofit organization dedicated to establishing a center to conduct research and provide women education and treatment.
Ann Koerner, Operations Manager

3803 Endometriosis Research Center
630 Ibis Drive
Delray Beach, FL 33444
800-239-7280
Fax: 561-274-0931
askerc@endocenter.org
www.endocenter.org
Non-profit international organization dedicated to helping women and girls suffering from endometriosis. Services include chapter and support groups, crisis/counseling assistance, education of the public and medical community materials including books and videos.
Michelle E. Marvel, Executive Director

3804 University of Tennessee: Division of Reproductive Endocrinology
956 Court Avenue
Memphis, TN 38163
901-528-5859
TDD: 901-448-7382
Studies into endometriosis.
Dr. Jon Buster, Chief
Kennard Brown, Executive Vice Chancellor & Chief Operat

Support Groups & Hotlines

3805 Endometriosis Association International
8585 N 76th Place
Milwaukee, WI 53223
414-355-2200
support@endometriosisassn.org
www.endometriosisassn.org
Self-help organization of women, families, doctors, scientists, and others engaged in information-sharing about endometriosis, with the ultimate goal of prevention and finding a cure. Offers a crisis call hotline, support groups, online community, and healthcare provider lists.

3806 National Health Information Center
Office of Disease Prevention & Health Promotion
1101 Wootton Pkwy
Rockville, MD 20852
Fax: 240-453-8281
odphpinfo@hhs.gov
www.health.gov/nhic
Supports public health education by maintaining a calendar of National Health Observances; helps connect consumers and health professionals to organizations that can best answer questions and provide up-to-date contact information from reliable sources; updates on a yearly basis toll-free numbers for health information, Federal health clearinghouses and info centers.
Don Wright, MD, MPH, Director

3807 RESOLVE Helpline
1760 Old Meadow Road
McLean, VA 22102
703-556-7172
Fax: 703-506-3266
www.resolve.org
A nationwide network mandated to promote reproductive health and to ensure equal access to all family building options for men and women experienceing infertility or other reproductive disorders.
Barbara Collura, President/ CEO
Margaret Cha Berardelli, Director

Books

3808 Alternatives for Women with Endometriosis Guide by Women for Women
Third Side Press
3 Marina Road
Yarmouth, MA 04096-1863
773-271-3029
Fax: 773-271-0459
thirdside@aol.com
www.womentowomen.com
174 pages
ISBN: 1-879427-12-5

3809 Coping with Endometriosis
Avery Putnam Penguin
375 Hudson Street
New York, NY 10014
212-366-2000
800-847-5515
Fax: 800-775-4829
online@penguinputnam.com
www.penguinputnam.com
Educates readers about the disease, focusing on the particular psychological and emotional concerns that those suffering from endometriosis may have.
322 pages
ISBN: 1-583330-74-7

3810 Endometriosis Sourcebook
Endometriosis Association
8585 N 76th Place
Milwaukee, WI 53223
414-355-2200
800-992-3636
Fax: 414-355-6065
endo@endometriosisassn.org
www.EndometriosisAssn.org
Comprehensive, authorative and up-to-date resource that includes information about treatment options, strategies for coping with the disease and its effects on you and those around you.
473 pages Paperback
ISBN: 0-809232-63-4
Mary Lou Ballweg, Founder/Executive Director

3811 Endometriosis and Infertility and Traditio nal Chinese Medicine
Blue Poppy Press
1990 57th Court N.
Boulder, CO 80301
303-447-8372
800-487-9296
Fax: 303-245-8362
honora@bluepoppy.com
An easy to understand guide to Chinese medicine as it relates to endometriosis and infertility.
105 pages Paperback
ISBN: 0-936185-14-7
Honora Wolfe, Marketing Director

3812 Endometriosis: A Key to Healing through Nutrition
Endometriosis Association

8585 N 76th Place
Milwaukee, WI 53223

414-355-2200
800-992-3636
Fax: 414-355-6065
endo@endometriosisassn.org
www.endometriosisassn.org

An excellent resource tool to help patients begin making changes in their diets.
Mary Lou Ballweg, Founder/Executive Director

3813   Endometriosis: A Natural Approach
Ulysses Press
PO Box 3440
Berkeley, CA 94703

510-601-8301
800-377-2542
Fax: 510-601-8307
ulysses@ulyssespress.com
www.ulyssespress.com

This is a solid resource, written in a clear, basic tone, for anyone who needs information about the widespread disease known as endometriosis. Chapters cover all aspects of endometriosis, from what it is and what causes it, to diagnosis, natural therapies, and conventional treatments.
120 pages
ISBN: 1-569750-88-2
Ray Riegert, Publisher
Leslie Henriques, Co-Publisher

3814   Endometriosis: Advanced Management and Surgical Techniques
Springer Verlag
175 5th Avenue
New York, NY 10010

212-460-1500
800-777-4643
Fax: 212-473-6272
service@springer-ny.com
www.springer-ny.com

This book provides a practical, clinical, and thorough examination of both the medical and surgical treatment of this disease.
Derk Haank, CEO
Martin Mos, COO

3815   Endometriosis: Complete Reference for Taking Charge of Your Health
Contemporary Books/McGraw-Hill Companies
8585 N. 76th Place
Milwaukee, WI 53223

414-355-2200
Fax: 414-355-6065
www.endometriosisassn.org

An authoritative guide on endometriosis, including its prevention and relationship with other diseases. Special sections are dedicated to endo and menopause, endo and teenagers, endo and nutrition, endo and cancer as well as endo and environmental toxins.

Newsletters

3816   Endometriosis Association Newsletter
Endometriosis Association
8585 N 76th Place
Milwaukee, WI 53223

414-355-2200
800-992-3636
Fax: 414-355-6065
endo@endometriosisassn.org
www.EndometriosisAssn.org

Contains research updates and latest health news that affects women and girls with endometriosis. Regular features such as crisis call helpers, news and announcements, and request for contact provide networking and support assistance.
10 pages Bi-Monthly
Mary Lou Ballweg, Executive Director

Pamphlets

3817   Infertility: Causes and Treatment
American College/Obstetricians and Gynecologists
409 12th Street SW
Washington, DC 20024

202-638-5577
800-673-8444
Fax: 304-728-2171
www.acog.com

To obtain a free copy of this publication, please send a self-addressed stamped #10 envelope and request by title.

Audio & Video

3818   Monroe Institute Surgical Support Tapes
Endometriosis Association
8585 N 76th Place
Milwaukee, WI 53223-2633

414-355-2200
800-992-3636
Fax: 414-355-6065
endo@endometriosisassn.org
www.EndometriosisAssn.org

Anxiety is normal for women before surgery, so women with endometriosis will be happy to hear this wonderful series of audiotapes specifically developed for relaxation.
Audiotape
Mary Lou Ballweg, Founder/Executive Director

Web Sites

3819   American Society for Reproductive Medicine
www.reproductivefacts.org

A private, non-profit medical organization devoted to advancing the knowledge, understanding and expertise in all phases of reproductive medicine and biology. Offers patient education brochures, recommended readings and support. Publishes professional journal and consumer publications, and runs the *Reproductive-Facts.org* website for patients.

3820   Endometriosis Association
www.EndometriosisAssn.org

Nonprofit organization dedicated to helping women and girls suffering from endometriosis. Services include chapter and support groups, crisis/counseling assistance, education of the public and the medical community. Materials, including books, video/audiotapes, CDs, newsletters and articles mostly based on data from the Association's research registries and its extensive research program, including a flagship scientific team at Vanderbuilt University School of Medicine.

3821   Endometriosis Research Center
www.endocenter.org

Maintain and offer a vast database of unbased and fact-based materials on every aspect of Endometriosis to practitioners, researchers, patients and all those interested in the disease.

3822   Endometriosis Support Group
Online support group and question forum for endometriosis.

3823   Healing Well
www.healingwell.com

An online health resource guide to medical news, chat, information and articles, newsgroups and message boards, books, disease-related web sites, medical directories, and more for patients, friends, and family coping with disabling diseases, disorders, or chronic illnesses.

3824   Health Finder
www.healthfinder.gov

Searchable, carefully developed web site offering information on over 1000 topics. Developed by the US Department of Health and Human Services, the site can be used in both English and Spanish.

3825   Healthlink USA
www.healthlinkusa.com

Health information concerning treatment, cures, prevention, diagnosis, risk factors, research, support groups, email lists, personal stories and much more. Updated regularly.

3826   HealthyWomen
www.healthywomen.org

Independent, non-profit organization seeking to educate women in all areas of health, to allow them to make informed choices. The HealthyWomen website features numerous tools and health calculators, plus other media.

3827   International Pelvic Pain Society
Seeks to recruit, organize, and educate health care professionals actively involved with the treatment of patients who have chronic pelvic pain.

3828 MedicineNet

www.medicinenet.com

An online resource for consumers providing easy-to-read, authoritative medical and health information.

3829 Medscape

www.medscape.com

Medscape offers specialists, primary care physicians, and other health professionals the Web's most robust and integrated medical information and educational tools.

3830 Universe of Women's Health

www.obgyn.net

A comprehensive website dedicated to women's health.

3831 WebMD

www.webmd.com

Provides credible information, supportive communities, and in-depth reference material about health subjects. A source for original and timely health information as well as material from well known content providers.

Description

3832 Fabry Disease

The inability to degrade complex molecules is a characteristic shared by a cluster of genetic diseases called lysosomal storage diseases. Cells use small, membrane-bound compartment called lysosomes to fully disassemble complex molecules. Lysosomes depend on a specific group of enzymes called "acid hydrolases" to take apart such molecules, and loss-of-function mutations in those genes that encode acid hydrolases lead to lysosomal storage diseases. Fabry disease results from mutations in the GLA gene, which encodes an acid hydrolase called a-galactosidase A. Non-functional a-galactosidase A causes a buildup of complex glycolipids called globotriaosylceramide (GL-3/GB-3). Accumulation of globotriaosylceramide in the body damages blood vessels in the skin and cells in the nervous system, kidney, and heart and leads to the symptoms of Fabry disease. The frequency of Fabry disease is in 1 in 40,000 to 60,000 males (GLA is an X-linked gene).

Symptoms begin during childhood with episodes of pain, particularly in the hands and feet (acroparesthesias) that worsen during exercise and hot weather. Fabry disease also diminishes the ability of the patient to sweat (hypohidrosis) and collections of small, dark red spots appear on the skin (angiokeratomas), usually around the waist. The corneas of the eyes cloud over (corneal opacity), but this usually does not cause significant visual impairment. There is ringing in the ears (tinnitus) followed by hearing loss. The gastrointestinal system is hyperactive with frequent bowel movements shortly after eating. Life-threatening complications include progressive stroke, heart attack, and kidney damage. As kidneys become more involved, many patients require kidney transplants or dialysis. Patients with Fabry disease usually survive into adulthood but have a reduced life expectancy. Some mutations in GLA do not completely eliminate a-galactosidase A activity and individuals with such mutations have milder forms of Fabry disease in which symptoms appear later in life and the disease only affects the heart or kidneys.

Currently, there is no cure for Fabry disease and treatment typically deals with controlling its symptoms. Pain in hands and feet responds to several medications. Gastrointestinal hyperactivity may be controlled by taking a nutritional supplement. Enzyme replacement therapy was given a dramatic boost in 2003 when the FDA approved a new synthetic enzyme, agalsidase-B (Fabrazyme), which is made by Sanofi Genzyme. It is given intravenously and reduces GL-3 accumulation in many types of cells.

National Agencies & Associations

3833 Association for Neuro-Metabolic Disorders
5223 Brookfield Lane   419-885-1809
Sylvania, OH 43560-1809 www.kumc.edu/gec/support/neuro-me.html

Serves as an advocate organization for families of patients with neuro-methabolic disorders such as phenylketonuria, maple syrup urine disease, galactosemia and biotinidase. Provides educational information for parents and children and provides networking.

3834 Canadian Fabry Association
748 Kelly Street   www.fabrycanada.com
Thunder Bay, Ontario, P7E-2A1
Non-profit organization seeking to raise awareness and educate the public about Fabry disease.
Julia Alton, Executive Director
Donna Strauss, Vice President

3835 Genetic and Rare Diseases Information Center
PO Box 8126   301-251-4925
Gaithesburg, MD 20898-8126   888-205-2311
                                   Fax: 301-251-4911
                                   TTY: 888-205-3223
                                   GARDinfo@nih.gov
                                   rarediseases.info.nih.gov
GARD is a program of the National Center for Advancing Translational Sciences and isalso funded by the National Human Genome Research Institute. Provides free and immediate access to accurate, reliable information about genetic and rare diseases. Also provides assistance to patients and families, health professionals and other interested parties.
Anne Pariser, MD, Director, Rare Disease Research

3836 International Center for Fabry Disease
Icahn School of Medicine at Mount Sinai
Box 1498   866-322-7963
New York, NY 10029   fabry.disease@mssm.edu
                               icahn.mssm.edu/research/fabry
Clinical research center attended by a staff of physicians and nurses specially trained to understand and meet the needs of individuals with Fabry disease. Services offered to both men and women of all ages include diagnosis, evaluation and treatment consultation.
Yonina Loskove, Clinical Research Assistant

3837 National Institute of Neurological Disorders and Stroke
NIH Neurological Institute   301-496-5751
Bethesda, MD 20824   800-352-9424
                                   www.ninds.nih.gov
Seeks to reduce the burden of neurological disease affecting individuals from all walks of life.
Walter J. Koroshetz, MD, Director
Amy B. Adams, Director, Office of Scientific Liaison

3838 National Organization for Rare Disorders
55 Kenosia Avenue   203-744-0100
Danbury, CT 06810-1968   800-999-6673
                                   Fax: 203-263-9938
                                   www.rarediseases.org
NORD is a federation of voluntary health organizations dedicated to helping people with rare orphan diseases and assisting the organizations that serve them. It is committed to the identification, treatment, and cure of rare disorders through programs of education, advocacy, research, and service.
Peter Saltonstall, President & CEO
Pamela Gavin, Chief Strategy Officer

3839 National Tay-Sachs and Allied Diseases Association
2001 Beacon Street   617-277-4463
Brighton, MA 02135   info@ntsad.org
                                   www.ntsad.org
Patient advocacy group funding research, raising awareness to prevent diseases, and supporting families and individuals around the world.
Sue Kahn, Executive Director
Diana Pangonis, Director, Family Svcs & Communications

Foundations

3840 National Fabry Disease Foundation
4301 Connecticut Avenue NW   919-732-2799
Washington, DC 20008   800-651-9131
                                   info@fabrydisease.org
                                   www.fabrydisease.org

The NFDF supports the Fabry disease community through education, disease identification, supporting research, advocacy, and providing assistance to those in need.
Jerry Walter, Founder, President and Chair
Derek Halberg, Vice Chair

Research Centers

3841   International Center for Fabry Disease
Icahn School of Medicine at Mount Sinai
Box 1498   866-322-7963
New York, NY 10029   icahn.mssm.edu/research/fabry
Clinical research center attended by a staff of physicians and nurses specially trained to understand and meet the needs of individuals with Fabry disease. Services offered to both men and women of all ages include diagnosis, evaluation and treatment consultation.
Yonina Loskove, Clinical Research Assistant

3842   Lysosomal Disease Center at the University of Pittsburgh
E1650 Biomedical Science Tower   800-334-7980
Pittsburgh, PA 15261   pitt.edu
Offers diagnosis management treatment and genetic counseling for people with or at risk for lysosomal storage disease and their families.
John A Barrenger MD PhD, Director
Erin O'Rourk, Manager

3843   National Gaucher Disease Foundation
2227 Idlewood Road   770-934-2910
Tucker, GA 30084   800-504-3189
                                        Fax: 770-934-2911
                                  rhonda@gaucherdisease.org
                                      www.gaucherdisease.org
Provides information and assistance for those affected by Gaucher disease.
Rhonda P Buyers, CEO/Executive Director
Barbara Lichtenstein, Programs Director National Gaucher Care

Support Groups & Hotlines

3844   Fabry Support & Information Group
108 NE 2nd Street Suite C   660-463-1355
Concordia, MO 64020   Fax: 660-463-1356
                                              info@fabry.org
                                              www.fabry.org
To raise awareness of Fabry disease and its symptoms. The website provides mutual self-help by linking patients and family members/caregivers. In this way they can support and encourage one another.
J Johnson, Founder

3845   National Health Information Center
Office of Disease Prevention & Health Promotion
1101 Wootton Pkwy
Rockville, MD 20852   Fax: 240-453-8281
                                           odphpinfo@hhs.gov
                                          www.health.gov/nhic
Supports public health education by maintaining a calendar of National Health Observances; helps connect consumers and health professionals to organizations that can best answer questions and provide up-to-date contact information from reliable sources; updates on a yearly basis toll-free numbers for health information, Federal health clearinghouses and info centers.
Don Wright, MD, MPH, Director

Web Sites

3846   A World of Genetic Societies
                                        www.faseb.org/genetics
FASEB's Mission is to advance health and welfare by promoting progress and education in biological and biomedical sciences through service to member societies and collaborative advocacy.

3847   Alliance of Genetic Support Groups
                                        www.geneticalliance.org

Genetic Alliance is a nonprofit health advocacy organizations. Its network includes more than 1,200 disease-specific advocacy organizations, as well as thousands of universities, private companies, government agencies, and public policy organizations. The network is a dynamic and growing open space for shared resources, creative tools, and innovative programs.

3848   Fabry Support & Information Group
                                              www.fabry.org
Fabry Support & Information Group (FSIG) is a 501(c)(3) nonprofit organization. There mission is to raise awareness of Fabry disease and its symptoms. The FSIG website provides mutual self-help by linking patients and family members/caregivers. In this way they can support and encourage one another. An increased understanding of Fabry disease and emotional support may alleviate some of the burden associated with this rare disorder.

3849   Gene Clinics
                                           www.genetests.org
GeneTests is a medical genetics information resource developed for physicians, genetic counselors, other healthcare providers and researchers.

3850   International Storage Disease Collaborative
                                  www.pediatrics.med.umn/edu/isdcsg/
This study group focuses on stem cell and bone marrow transplantation. Has discussion page/general information.

3851   MedicineNet
                                         www.medicinenet.com
An online resource for consumers providing easy-to-read, authoritative medical and health information.

3852   Morbus Fabry
                                             home.t-online.de
Fabry information and links to other sites.

3853   National Organization for Rare Disorders
                                          www.rarediseases.org
NORD is a federation of voluntary health organizations dedicated to helping people with rare orphan diseases and assisting the organizations that serve them. It is committed to the identification, treatment, and cure of rare disorders through programs of education, advocacy, research, and service. Website features resources for patients and families, patient organizations, and clinicians and researchers.

3854   National Society of Genetic Counselors
                                                    nsgc.org
The National Society of Genetic Counselors (NSGC) promotes the professional interests of genetic counselors and provides a network for professional communication. Local and national continuing education opportunities and the discussion of all issues relevant to human genetics and the genetic counseling profession are an integral part of membership in NSGC.

3855   OMIM: Fabry Disease
                                        omim.org/entry/301500
Description of disease and links to research papers written.

3856   Pediatric Database: Fabry Disease
Description of disease.

3857   Support-Group.Com: Fabry Disease
                                        www.support-group.com
Fabry Disease discussion forum.

Description

3858 Fibromyalgia Syndrome

Fibromyalgia syndrome, FMS, also called fibrositis or fibromyositis, is a long-lasting, chronic condition that causes muscle pain and fatigue. It strikes mostly women between the ages of 20 and 50, and may affect as many as one in 20 adult females. The main symptoms are pain and tenderness throughout the entire body. The pain ranges from mild discomfort to complete disability and may vary from day to day. Physical over-exertion, changes in weather, drafty environments, stress, depression, and hormonal changes can all contribute to flare-ups in FMS symptoms.

In addition to widespread pain, FMS also causes a decreased sense of energy, disturbances of sleep, and varying degrees of anxiety and depression. Other medical conditions sometimes associated with fibromyalgia include tension headaches, migraine, irritable bowel syndrome, premenstrual tension syndrome, chronic fatigue syndrome, cold intolerance, and restless leg syndrome.

A physician's diagnosis of FMS is usually based on the following criteria: widespread musculoskeletal pain; tenderness at 11 or more of 18 specific tender points, which are exquisitely more tender than adjacent sites; and scans of the brain. Fibromyalgia may remit spontaneously with decreased stress but can recur at frequent intervals or become chronic.

There is currently no commonly accepted cure for this condition. Nonsteroidal anti-inflammatory drugs (NSAIDs) such as aspirin, ibuprofen, or naproxen can effectively address musculoskeletal pain. For severe pain, opiate pain relievers may be used. Specific antidepressants called selective norepinephrine reuptake inhibitors (SNRIs), in particular duloxetine and milnacipran, can help alleviate both pain and fatigue. Nerve-based pain is effectively treated with a drug called pregabalin. All drug treatments should be accompanied by lifestyle changes. Patients may also benefit from regular aerobic exercises, local applications of heat, gentle massage and reduced stress in their lives. A healthy diet, and regular sleep schedule are also essential elements for fibromyalgia patients. See also *Chronic Fatigue Syndrome.*

National Agencies & Associations

3859 American Chronic Pain Association
PO Box 850   800-533-3231
Rocklin, CA 95677   ACPA@theacpa.org
www.theacpa.org
The ACPA facilitates peer support and education for individuals with chronic pain in its many forms, in order to increase quality of life. Also raises awareness among the healthcare community, and with policy makers.
Penney Cowan, Founder & CEO
Daniel Galia, Director, Global Support

3860 American Fibromyalgia Syndrome Association
PO Box 32698   520-733-1570
Tucson, AZ 85751   Fax: 520-290-5550
kthorson@afsafund.org
www.afsafund.org
AFSA is a non-profit organization whose primary mission is to seed research in fibromyalgia syndrome and chronic fatigue syndrome.
Kristen Thorson, President
Steve Thorson, Vice President

3861 International Myopain Society
PO Box 268   info@myopain.org
Nine Mile Falls, WA 99026   www.myopain.org
Community of healthcare professionals, researchers, educators, and others dedicated to improve care for individuals with soft tissue pain syndromes like myofascial pain syndrome and fibromyalgia syndrome.
Rae Gleason, Executive Director

3862 National Fibromyalgia & Chronic Pain Association
25 Federal Avenue   801-200-3627
Logan, UT 84321   info@fmcpaware.org
www.fmcpaware.org
Seeks to unite patients, policy makers, and health and science communities to research fibromyalgia and chronic pain illnesses; also provides advocacy, support, and education.
Janet Favero Chambers, President

3863 National Fibromyalgia Association
3857 Birch Street   nfa@fmaware.org
Newport Beach, CA 92660   www.fmaware.org
Develops and extends programs dedicated to improving the quality of life for people with Fibromyalgia by increasing the awareness of the public media government and medical communities. Supports an ongoing media presence and assist local support groups.
Lynne Matallana, Founder/President

3864 National Fibromyalgia Partnership (NFP)
PO Box 2355   www.fmpartnership.org
Centreville, VA 20122
Non-profit, membership organization which publishes medically accurate information on Fibromyalgia to patients, health care professionals and the public. It also provides support and start-up information to support groups.
Russell Rothenberg, MD, Chair, Medical Advisory Board

3865 National ME/FM Action Network
33 Banner Road   613-829-6667
Nepean, Ontario, K2H-8V7   Fax: 613-829-8518
mefminfo@mefmaction.com
www.mefmaction.com
Works to support people with Myalgic Encephalomyelitis, Chronic Fatigue Syndrome, and Fibromyalgia in North America.
Lydia E. Neilson, MSM, Founder & CEO
Margaret Parlor, President

3866 Option Institute
2080 South Undermountain Road   413-229-2100
Sheffield, MA 01257   800-714-2779
Fax: 413-229-8931
participantsupport@option.org
www.option.org
Self-defeating beliefs, along with attitudes and judgments, can lead to a host of physical and psychological challenges, including Chronic Fatigue Syndrome. The Option Institute offers programs designed to help people gain new perspectives on the attitudes and judgments that may be affecting their lives, especially those regarding and surrounding Chronic Fatigue Syndrome.
Barry Kaufman, Co-Founder
Samahria Lyte Kaufman, Co-Founder

Libraries & Resource Centers

3867 Fibromyalgia Resources Group
103 Sherwood Hill Road   845-278-5944
Brewster, NY 10509   Fax: 845-278-2641
kindness@fibrobetsy.com

Personalized patient service searches and distributes information on patient recommended, fibromyalgia literate doctors world wide. Information packet is included with each doctor list emailed. Doctor recommendations are welcome.
Betsy Jacobson, President

Support Groups & Hotlines

3868 Fibromyalgia Network
PO Box 31750
Tucson, AZ 85751-1750
520-290-5508
800-853-2929
Fax: 520-290-5550
inquiry@fmnetnews.com
www.fmnetnews.com
Provides individuals with ad-free, patient-focused information that can be use today.

3869 National Health Information Center
Office of Disease Prevention & Health Promotion
1101 Wootton Pkwy
Rockville, MD 20852
Fax: 240-453-8281
odphpinfo@hhs.gov
www.health.gov/nhic
Supports public health education by maintaining a calendar of National Health Observances; helps connect consumers and health professionals to organizations that can best answer questions and provide up-to-date contact information from reliable sources; updates on a yearly basis toll-free numbers for health information, Federal health clearinghouses and info centers.
Don Wright, MD, MPH, Director

3870 Rocky Mountain CFIDS/FMS Association
7020 E Girard Avenue
Denver, CO 80224
303-423-7367
link@rmcfa.org
www.rmcfa.org
An educational resource for patients, medical professionals and those affected by these diseases.
Tim Smith, President
Mike Munoz, Executive Director

Books

3871 All About Fibromyalgia
Oxford University Press
198 Madison Avenue
New York, NY 10016-4314
212-726-6033
800-451-7556
Fax: 212-726-6447
www.oup-usa.org
ISBN: 0-195147-53-7

3872 Delicate Balance: Living Successfully with Chronic Illness
Perseus Books Group
5500 Central Avenue
Boulder, CO 80301
800-386-5656
Fax: 303-449-3356
info@perseuspublishing.com
Up to date and practical advice and inspiration for the millions of Americans who struggle daily against chronic illness. From locating a suitable healthcare provider and making sense of the powerful emotions that accompany chronic illness, to seeking accomodations from the Americans with Disabilities Act, this book is helpful and hopeful.
312 pages
ISBN: 0-738203-23-8

3873 Fibromyalgia
NAMSIC/National Institutes of Health
1 AMS Circle
Bethesda, MD 20892-0001
301-495-4484
877-226-4267
Fax: 301-718-6366
TTY: 301-565-2966
niamsinfo@mail.nih.gov
www.nih.gov/niams

3874 Fibromyalgia & Other Central Pain Syndromes
Daniel Wallace, Daniel Clauw, author
Lippincott Williams & Wilkins

16522 Hunters Green Pkwy
Hagerstown, MD 21740-2116
301-223-2300
800-638-3030
Fax: 301-223-2400
orders@lww.com
www.lww.com
Devoted to fibromyalgia and other centrally mediated chronic pain syndromes. Leading experts examine the latest research findings on these syndromes and present evidence-based reviews of current controversies.
2005
ISBN: 0-781752-61-2

3875 Fibromyalgia Guidelines: The Concensus Diagnosis & Treatment Protocols
FM-CFS Canada
16522 Hunters Green Pkwy
Hagerstown, MD 21740-5P5
301-223-2300
800-638-3030
Fax: 301-223-2400
orders@lww.com
www.lww.com
This entire special issue of the Journal of Musculoskeletal Pain [JMP] is devoted to presentation of what will likely to be called the Canadian Consensus Document on Fibromyalgia Syndrome (FMS). The document encompasses a very broad scope, involving a clinical case definition, diagnosis, and management of FMS.
130 pages

3876 Fibromyalgia Relief Book: 213 Ideas for Improving Your Quality of Life
Walker & Company
435 Hudson Street
New York, NY 10014
212-727-8300
Fax: 212-727-0984
www.walkerbooks.com
208 pages Paperback
ISBN: 0-802775-53-5
Josh Wood, Sales Director

3877 Fibromyalgia Supporter
Anadem Publishing Company
3620 N High Street
Columbus, OH 43214
800-633-0055
Fax: 614-262-6630
anadem@anadem.com
www.anadem.com

3878 Fibromyalgia Survivor
Anadem Publishing Company
3620 N High Street
Columbus, OH 43214
800-633-0055
Fax: 614-262-6630
anadem@anadem.com
www.anadem.com
ISBN: 0-964689-12-X

3879 Fibromyalgia Syndrome and Chronic Fatigue Syndrome in Young People
Fibromyalgia Network
PO Box 31750
Tucson, AZ 85751-1750
800-853-2929
Fax: 520-290-5550
www.fmnetnews.com
Guide for parents.
Kristin Thorson, Editor

3880 Fibromyalgia and Chronic Myofascial Pain Syndrome: a Survivor Manual
New Harbinger Publishers
5674 Shattuck Avenue
Oakland, CA 94609
800-748-6273
Fax: 510-652-5472
customerservice@newharbinger.com
www.newharbinger.com
Written from the perspective of myofacial pain syndrome.
432 pages

3881 Fibromyalgia, Managing the Pain
Anadem Publishing Company
3620 N High Street
Columbus, OH 43214-3611
800-633-0055
Fax: 614-262-6630
anadem@anadem.com
www.anadem.com
Comprehensive guide to the syndrome, including chapters on diagnosis, medication, physical medicine treatments, occupational ad-

justments, advice on flare ups and some medical and legal aspects of FMS.

3882 Inside Fibromyalgia
Anadem Publishing Company
3620 N High Street   614-262-2539
Columbus, OH 43214   800-633-0055
                                                          Fax: 614-262-6630
                                                          anadem@anadem.com
                                                          www.anadem.com
Written by a physician who has fibromyalgia. From the newest medications to alternative therapies and everything in between, Dr. Pellegrino helps you develop a plan for healing today and tomorrow.
Paperback
ISBN: 1-890018-36-8

3883 Laugh at Your Muscles
Anadem Publishing Company
3620 N High Street   800-633-0055
Columbus, OH 43214-3611   Fax: 614-262-6630
                                                          anadem@anadem.com
                                                          www.anadem.com

3884 Taking Charge of Fibromyalgia
FMS Educational Systems
P O Box 500   503-315-7257
Salem, OR 97308   Fax: 503-315-7205
                                                          nfra@firstpac.com
Written by three professionals who have fibromyalgia and who often update the book.

3885 Taking Control of TMJ: Your Total Wellness Program
Robert O Uppgaard, DDS, author
New Harbinger Publications
5674 Shattuck Avenue   800-748-6273
Oakland, CA 94609   Fax: 510-652-5472
                                                          customerservice@newharbinger.com
                                                          www.newharbinger.com
Six-step wellness program helps readers understand what TMJ is and provides exercises to improve jaw functioning, relieve pain and deal with trigger points, eliminate harmful habits, deal with contributing stress, and evaluate and improve your diet and exercise habits. Additional chapters cover the connection between TMJ, whiplash, and fibromyalgia.
2004 200 pages Paperback
ISBN: 1-572241-26-8

3886 Understanding Post-Traumatic Fibromyalgia
Anadem Publishing Company
3620 N High Street   800-633-0055
Columbus, OH 43214-3611   Fax: 614-262-6630
                                                          anadem@anadem.com
                                                          www.anadem.com
Anyone with post-traumatic fibromyalgia will benefit from reading this book focusing exclusively on this condition.

Magazines

3887 FM Monograph
National Fibromyalgia Partnership
140 Zinn Way   866-725-4404
Linden, VA 22642   Fax: 866-666-2727
                                                          mail@fmpartnership.org
                                                          www.fmpartnership.org
Publishes a print quarterly (available online and in booklet form in English, Spanish, and French) which provides information on fibromyalgia symptoms, diagnosis, treatment, and research. Comprehensive resource packets and reprints are also available on a variety of subjects. Technical support is provided to fibromyalgia support organizations worldwide.
Quarterly
Tamara Liller, President

3888 Fibromyalgia AWARE
National Fibromyalgia Association

1000 Bristol Street N.   714-921-0150
Newport Beach, CA 92660   Fax: 714-921-6920
                                                          nfa@FMaware.org
                                                          www.FMaware.org
Official publication of the National Fibromyalgia Association. Available to members and contributors.

3889 Fibromyalgia Frontiers
National Fibromyalgia Partnership (NFP)
PO Box 160   866-725-4404
Linden, VA 22642   Fax: 866-666-2727
                                                          mail@fmpartnership.org
                                                          www.fmpartnership.org
Publishes a print quarterly (available online and in booklet form in English, Spanish, and French) which provides information on fibromyalgia symptoms, diagnosis, treatment, and research. Comprehensive resource packets and reprints are also available on a variety of subjects. Technical support is provided to fibromyalgia support organizations worldwide. Included with membership into NFP.
Quarterly
Tamara Liller, President

3890 Journal of Musculoskeletal Pain
Haworth Medical Press
10 Alice Street   607-722-5857
Binghamton, NY 13904-1503   800-429-6784
                                                          Fax: 607-722-0012
                                                          getinfo@haworthpress.com
                                                          www.haworthpress.com
Peer reviewed medical journal containing FMS scientific abstract information. Appropriate for medical professionals as well as amateur.
Quarterly

Newsletters

3891 Fibromyalgia Clinic Kentfield Rehabilitation Newsletter
Fibromyalgia Clinic
25 Sir Francis Drake Blvd   714-230-3150
Santa Ana, CA 92799   Fax: 714-850-0153
                                                          www.dynamicchiropractic.com

3892 Florida Fibromyalgia News
FMS Association of Florida
P.O. Box 100221   352-265-8901
Gainesville, FL 32610-4848   painresearch@medicine.ufl.edu
                                                          rheum.med.ufl.edu
Quarterly newsletter.

3893 Health Points
TyH Publications
17007 E Colony Drive   800-801-1406
Fountain Hills, AZ 85268   editor@e-tyh.com
                                                          www.healthpts.com
National newsletter with articles on complementary therapy, latest nutrition news, disability issues and much more. Focus is on fibromyalgia, chronic fatigue, arthritis and chronic pain.
Quarterly
J. Mark Lambright, President & CEO
Don Springer, Chief Operating Officer

3894 Healthwatch
CFIDS and Fibromyalgia Health Resource
2040 Alameda Padre Serra   800-366-6056
Santa Barbara, CA 93103   Fax: 805-963-4515
                                                          www.prohealth.com
Healthwatch serves fibromyalgia and chronic fatigue syndrome sufferers by focusing on reporting the latest news in research and treatment, making hard-to-find nutritional supplements available at low prices, and raising needed funds for medical research.

3895 Journal of Musculoskeletal Medicine
Cliggott Publishing Company
27 Warren Street   201-487-9655
Hackensack, NJ 07601-6074   Fax: 201-487-9656
                                                          wspc@wspc.com
                                                          www.worldscientific.com

This journal provides a unique and efficient monthly update on the management of musculoskeletal disorders. Offers articles regarding orthopedics, rheumatology, sports medicine, etc.

3896 To Your Health and Healthpoints
To Your Health
12005 Saguaro Blvd   480-837-7590
Fountain Hills, AZ 85268   800-801-1406
                                      Fax: 480-837-1875
                                      www.e-tyh.com
Resource catalogue and newspaper for FMS, CFIDS, arthritis, and chronic pain. Features vitamins and health products developed specifically for FMS and CFIDS making hard-to-find, recommended nutritional supplements available to fibromyalgia and chronic fatigue syndrome sufferers at a manufacturer-direct low price.

Audio & Video

3897 Audio Cassette Program on Fibromyalgia
Arthritis Foundation/Research Cassettes
111 E Wacker Drive   312-616-3470
Chicago, IL 60601-3713
Covers treatment and research taped during a patient education forum.

3898 Fibromyalgia Interval Training
Arthritis Foundation Distribution Center
235 East 42nd Street   800-879-3477
New York, NY 10017-6996   Fax: 770-442-9742
                                      www.arthritis.com
Designed for people with fibromyalgia, the video features warm water exercises in shallow and deep water, including warmup, stretching, upper and lower body exercises, aerobics, strengthing, cool-down and relaxation. Designed to help you manage the pain, stiffness and fatigue of fibromyalgia.

3899 Fibromyalgia Stretch Video & Strength and Toning Video
Oregon Fibromyalgia Foundation
1221 SW Yamhill   503-228-3217
Portland, OR 97205   www.myalgia.com
These videos offer comprehensive stretching and strength and toning regimens developed by exercise physiologist Sharon Clark PhD, FNP, specifically for people with FMS. Fibromyalgia patients are shown demonstrating these unique stretching and strength and toning programs. Prices are per video and do not include shipping and handling.

3900 Fibromyalgia: Face to Face
Ontario Fibromyalgia Association
250 Cloor Street E   416-979-7228
Toronto, Ontario, M4W
A 14 minute insight into living with FMS from people, including children, who are coping with this syndrome.

3901 Improving Muscle Tone and Strength
Oregon Fibromyalgia Foundation
235 Berry Road   207-224-7471
Hartford, ME 04220   www.atabendintheroad.com
A video developed by exercise physiologist Sharon Clark, PhD, RN, specifically for people with fibromyalgia.

Web Sites

3902 American Fibromyalgia Research Association
                                      www.afsafund.org
Charitable organization whose primary mission is to seed research in FMS and CFS. We acknowledge that patient and physician education, public awareness and advocacy are all important ingredients in aiding the lives of people with FMS and CFS.

3903 Healing Well
                                      www.healingwell.com
An online health resource guide to medical news, chat, information and articles, newsgroups and message boards, books, disease-related web sites, medical directories, and more for patients, friends, and family coping with disabling diseases, disorders, or chronic illnesses.

3904 Health Finder
                                      www.healthfinder.gov
Searchable, carefully developed web site offering information on over 1000 topics. Developed by the US Department of Health and Human Services, the site can be used in both English and Spanish.

3905 Healthlink USA
                                      www.healthlinkusa.com
Health information concerning treatment, cures, prevention, diagnosis, risk factors, research, support groups, email lists, personal stories and much more. Updated regularly.

3906 MedicineNet
                                      www.medicinenet.com
An online resource for consumers providing easy-to-read, authoritative medical and health information.

3907 Medscape
                                      www.medscape.com
Medscape offers specialists, primary care physicians, and other health professionals the Web's most robust and integrated medical information and educational tools.

3908 My Fibromyalgia & Chronic Fatigue Syndrome
                                      www.fms-help.com
A compassionate, Christian-based site for people with Fibromyalgia (FMS), Chronic Fatigue & Immune Dysfunction Syndrome (CFIDS) and Myalgic Encephalomyelitis (M.E.)

3909 National Fibromyalgia Association
                                      www.fmaware.org
Information for fibromyalgia patients and the general public.

3910 National Fibromyalgia Partnership (NFP)
                                      www.fmpartnership.org
Non-profit, membership organization which publishes medically accurate information on Fibromyalgia to patients, health care professionals and the public. It also provides support and start-up information to support groups.

3911 Neurology Channel
                                      www.healthcommunities.com
Find clearly explained, medically accurate information regarding conditions, including an overview, symptoms, causes, diagnostic procedures and treatment options. On this site it is possible to ask questions and get information from a neurologist and connect to people who have similar health interests.

3912 Option Institute
                                      www.option.org
Self-defeating beliefs, along with attitudes and judgments, can lead to a host of physical and psychological challenges, including Fibromyalgia. The Option Institute offers programs designed to help people gain new perspectives on the attitudes and judgments that may be affecting their lives, especially those regarding and surrounding Fibromyalgia. Website features lists of programs, audio and visual resources, and more.

3913 WebMD
                                      www.webmd.com
Provides credible information, supportive communities, and in-depth reference material about health subjects. A source for original and timely health information as well as material from well known content providers.

Description

3914 ## Gastrointestinal Disorders

The gastrointestinal tract is responsible for masticating food brought into the body into smaller particles, digesting that food so that the complex macromolecules in food are degraded into simple precursors, absorbing those precursors into the bloodstream, and then expelling the remainder.

Motility disorders of the gastrointestinal (GI) tract are conditions in which there is a failure of normal top-to-bottom movement of gastric contents. Endocrine disorders, such as hypothyroidism or diabetes mellitus, can cause bowel motility disorders, as can certain medications, such as opioid pain killers, diuretics, heart medicines (i.e., verapamil), or tricyclic antidepressants. In reflux, the food content moves from the stomach back into the esophagus, irritating that organ and causing heartburn, the most common symptom. This is known as GERD, or gastro-esophageal reflux disease, and sometimes causes choking or coughing. Complications include inflammation and even ulceration of the esophagus. It is a problem in infants, but also occurs in adults especially with advancing age. Occasionally, an ulcer may develop in a segment of the GI tract, typically in the stomach or duodenum. Proton-pump inhibitors are the first-line treatment for GERD. An infectious agent, Helicobacter pylori, plays a central role in peptic ulcer disease. H. pylori infections are treated with a combination of antibiotics, proton-pump inhibitors, and bismuth sulfate (Pepto-Bismol). In achalasia, the normal movement of food down the GI tract by peristalsis is disrupted, and contents of the esophagus are unable to move into the stomach. As a result, the person chokes on food or liquid. Chest pain and coughing at night may also occur. Achalasia is treated with surgical stretching of the esophagus or Botox injections into the esophagus.

Other motility disorders reflect the bowel's inability to move its contents forward properly. Children may be born with Hirschsprung's disease in which peristalsis is absent or abnormal in the large bowel, resulting in partial or complete obstruction. The most common motility disorder in adults is called irritable bowel syndrome (IBS); also known as functional bowel or spastic colitis. IBS can cause variable degrees of abdominal pain and bloating, diarrhea and/or constipation, and is treated with medications that either relieve gut spasticity (e.g., dicyclomine), decrease bowel motility (loperamide, eluxadoline, rifaximin, or alosetron), or increase bowel motility (fiber, laxatives, lubiprostone, linaclotide, plecanatide).

Outpouchings in the walls of the lower GI tract, called diverticula, sometimes trap nutrient waste, and may become infected, bleed, and rupture. Finally, the digestive tract may fail in its primary task of absorbing nutrients, known as malabsorption syndromes. Rarely it will absorb too much of something. In hemochromatosis, for instance, the bowel takes in too much iron from the diet, and the excess is stored in and damages the liver, pancreas, heart, and gonads. More commonly, the body absorbs too little nutrient rather than too much. For instance, celiac disease, or sprue, is a disorder caused by intolerance to gluten, a cereal protein in wheat rye, barley, and oats. Lactose intolerance is an inability to digest a carbohydrate (lactose) in dairy products, and, consequently, bacteria in the bowel ferment lactose and produce organic acids and gas. This results in stomach pain, flatulence, and diarrhea. Treatment for malabsorption syndromes includes dietary modifications and, in more serious cases, supplementation with intravenous feedings known as parenteral nutrition.

National Agencies & Associations

3915 **Academy of Nutrition & Dietetics**
120 South Riverside Plaza
Chicago, IL 60606-6995
312-899-0040
800-877-1600
media@eatright.org
www.eatright.org
Serves the public through the promotion of optimal nutrition, health, and well-being. Formerly the American Dietetic Association.
Mary Russell, President
Patricia M. Babjak, Chief Executive Officer

3916 **American College of Gastroenterology**
6400 Goldsboro Road
Bethesda, MD 20817
301-263-9000
www.gi.org
ACG serves clinical and scientific information needs of member physicians and surgeons, who specialize in digestive and related disorders. Emphasis is on scholarly practice, teaching and research.
Mark B. Popchapin, MD, FACG, President
Daniel J. Pambianco, MD, FACG, Secretary

3917 **American Gastroenterological Association National Office**
National Office
4930 Del Ray Avenue
Bethesda, MD 20814
301-654-2055
Fax: 301-654-5920
member@gastro.org
www.gastro.org
AGA fosters the development and application of the science of gastroenterology by providing leadership and aid including patient care, research, teaching, continuing education, scientific communication and matters of national health policy.
Tom Serena, Executive Vice President
Sarah Fitzpatrick, Executive Office Coordinator

3918 **American Hemochromatosis Society**
PO Box 950871
Lake Mary, FL 32795-0871
407-829-4488
888-655-4766
Fax: 407-333-1284
mail@americanhs.org
www.americanhs.org
Educates the public, the medical community and the media by distributing the most current information available on hereditary hemochromatosis (HH) including DNA screening for HH and pediatric HH; also facilitates patient empowerment through an online network.
Sandra Thomas, President/Founder

3919 **American Motility Society**
45685 Harmony Lane
Belleville, MI 48111   734-699-1130
                                   Fax: 734-699-1136
                                 admin@motilitysociety.org
                                 www.motilitysociety.org
Promotes research and sponsors professional education seminars about gastrointestinal motility topics including disorders of esophageal, gastric, small intestinal, and colonic function; and sponsors biennial meetings (even years), syposia and courses.
John Pandolfino, MD, President
Lori Ennis, Executive Director

3920 **American Pancreatic Association**
                   www.american-pancreatic-association.org
Provides forum for presentation of scientific research related to the pancreas.
Anil Rustgi, MD, President
Ashok Saluja, Secretary-Treasurer

3921 **American Society for Gastrointestinal Endoscopy**
3300 Woodcreek Drive   630-573-0600
Downers Grove, IL 60515   800-353-2743
                                   Fax: 630-963-8332
                                       info@asge.org
                                       www.asge.org
ASGE provides information, training, and practice guidelines about gastrointestinal endoscopic techniques.
Barbara Connell, CAE, Chief Executive Officer
Adjournia Jones, Manager, Operations

3922 **American Society for Parenteral and Enteral Nutrition (ASPEN)**
8401 Colesville Road   301-587-6315
Silver Spring, MD 20910   Fax: 301-587-2365
                                 aspen@nutritioncare.org
                                 www.nutritioncare.org
Offers information and continuing medical education to professionals involved in the care of parenterally and enterally fed patients. Membership includes complimentary subscriptions to two peer reviewed journals.
Wanda Johnson, Chief Executive Officer
Peggi Guenter, PhD, RN, Senior Director, Clincal Practice

3923 **Cyclic Vomiting Syndrome Association**
PO Box 270341   414-342-7880
Milwaukee, WI 53227   cvsa@cvsaonline.org
                                   www.cvsaonline.org
CVSA provides opportunities for patients, families and professionals to offer and receive support and share knowledge about cyclic vomiting syndrome; actively promotes and facilitates medical research about nausea and vomiting.
Kathleen Adams, President Emerita & Co-Founder
Kristin Koch, Secretary

3924 **Digestive Disease National Coalition**
507 Capitol Court NE   202-544-7497
Washington, DC 20002   Fax: 202-546-7105
                                     herzog@hmcw.org
                                       www.ddnc.org
Informs the public and the health care community about digestive disorders; seeks Federal funding for research, education, and training; and represents members' interests regarding Federal and State legislation that affects digestive diseases research.
Nancy Ginter, Chair
James DeGerome, MD, Director, Development

3925 **National Digestive Diseases Information Clearinghouse**
2 Information Way   800-891-5389
Bethesda, MD 20892-3570   Fax: 703-738-4929
                                    TTY: 866-569-1162
                                 nddic@info.niddk.nih.gov
                                 www.digestive.niddk.nih.gov
Established to increase knowledge and understanding about digestive diseases among people with these conditions and their families, health care professionals, and the general public. To carry out this mission, NDDIC works closely with a coordinating panel of representatives from Federal agencies, voluntary organizations on the national level, and professional groups to identify and respond to informational needs about digestive diseases.

3926 **North American Society for Pediatric Gastroenterology, Hepatology & Nutrition**
714 N. Bethlehem Pike   215-641-9800
Ambler, PA 19002   Fax: 215-641-1995
                                 naspghan@naspghan.org
                                 www.naspghan.org
Promotes research and provides a forum for professionals in the areas of pediatric GI liver disease, gastroenterology, and nutrition. Associated with fellow organizations in Europe and Australia (ESPGAN, AUSPGAN).
Margaret K. Stallings, Executive Director
Kim Rose, Associate Director

3927 **Northwestern Medicine Digestive Health Center**
Digestive Health Center
Winfield, IL 60190   630-933-1600
                                   Fax: 630-933-1300
                                   TTY: 630-933-4833
                                       www.nm.org
Multifaceted program to meet the needs of people who suffer from gastrointestinal problems; offers literature, videotapes and educational meetings and, if medical care is needed, appropriate referrals are made.

3928 **Society for Surgery of the Alimentary Tract**
500 Cummings Center   978-927-8330
Beverly, MA 01915   Fax: 978-524-0498
                                       www.ssat.com
SSAT provides a forum for exchange of information among physicians specializing in alimentary tract surgery.
Steven C. Stain, MD, Chair

3929 **Society of American Gastrointestinal Endoscopic Surgeons**
11300 W Olympic Boulevard   310-437-0544
Los Angeles, CA 90064   www.sages.org
SAGES encourages study and practice of gastrointestinal endoscopy laparoscopy and minimal access surgery.
Horacio J. Asbun, MD, President
Fredrick J. Brody, MD, Secretary

3930 **Society of Gastroenterology Nurses and Associates**
330 N Wabash Avenue   312-321-5165
Chicago, IL 60611   800-245-7462
                                   Fax: 312-673-6694
                                       info@sgna.org
                                       www.sgna.org
SGNA provides members with continuing education opportunities practice and training guidelines, and information about trends and development in the field of gastroenterology.
Kim Eskew, MBA, CAE, Executive Director
Mollie Corbett, Operations Manager

3931 **United Ostomy Associations of America, Inc**
PO Box 525   800-826-0826
Kennebunk, ME 04043   www.ostomy.org
A national network for bowel and urinary diversion support groups in the United States. Its goal is to provide a non-profit association that will serve to unify and strengthen its member support groups, which are organized for the benefit of people who have, or will have intestinal or urinary diversions and their caregivers.
Christine Ryan, Executive Director
Jeanine Gleba, Advocacy Manager

Foundations

3932 **American Porphyria Foundation**
4900 Woodway   713-266-9617
Houston, TX 77056   866-APF-3635
                                   Fax: 713-840-9552
                                 porphyrus@porphyriafoundation.com
                                 www.porphyriafoundation.com
The APF is dedicated to improving the health and well-being of individuals and families affected by porphyria. Our mission is to enhance public awareness about porphyria, develop educational programs and distributing educational material for patients and physicians and support research to improve treatment and ultimately lead to a cure.
Desiree H Lyon, Executive Director
James Young, Chairman

3933 Gastro-Intestinal Research Foundation
70 East Lake Street   312-332-1350
Chicago, IL 60601-5907   Fax: 312-332-4757
                                                      info@girf.org
                                         www.giresearchfoundation.org
Provides funds for equipment, laboratories and the support of investigators and young physicians in the University of Chicago Gastroenterology Section, a group of full-time dedicated doctors who seek solutions to all kinds of gastrointestinal illnesses, affecting the esophagus, the stomach, the small intestine, the large intestine, the liver, the gallbladder, and the pancreas.
Kimberly Coady, Executive Director
Eric Berlin, President

3934 International Foundation for Functional Gastrointestinal Disorders (IFFGD)
PO Box 170864   414-964-1799
Milwaukee, WI 53217   888-964-2001
                                                      iffgd@iffgd.org
                                                      www.iffgd.org
Non-profit education, support, and research organization devoted to increasing awareness and understanding of functional gastrointestinal disorders, including irritable bowel syndrome (IBS), constipation, diarrhea, pain, and incontinence. Mission is to inform, assist and support people affected by these disorders.
Nancy J. Norton, Founder
Ceciel T. Rooker, President

3935 NASPGHAN Foundation
714 N. Bethlehem Pike   215-641-9800
Ambler, PA 19002   Fax: 215-641-1995
                                                      naspghan@naspghan.org
                                                      www.naspghan.org
The foundation's sole mission is to improve treatment and management of gastrointestinal, hepatobiliary, pancreatic, and nutritional disorders in children.
Menno Verhave, President

3936 North American Society for Pediatric Gastroenterology, Hepatology & Nutrition
714 N. Bethlehem Pike   215-641-9800
Ambler, PA 19002   Fax: 215-641-1995
                                                      naspghan@naspghan.org
                                                      www.naspghan.org
Promotes research and provides a forum for professionals in the areas of pediatric GI liver disease, gastroenterology, and nutrition. Associated with fellow organizations in Europe and Australia (ESPGAN, AUSPGAN).
Margaret K. Stallings, Executive Director
Kim Rose, Associate Director

3937 Oley Foundation
43 New Scotland Ave   518-262-5079
Albany, NY 12208-3478   800-776-6539
                                             Fax: 518-262-5528
                                                      www.oley.org
Promotes and advocates education and research in home parenteral and enteral nutrition; provides support and networking to patients through information clearinghouse and regional volunteer networks; sponsors meetings and conferences, including annual patient/clinician conference; maintains speakers bureau.
Joan Bishop, Executive Director
Roslyn Dahl, Communications & Development

3938 Society for Surgery of the Alimentary Foundation
500 Cummings Center   978-927-8330
Beverly, MA 01915   Fax: 978-524-0498
                                                      ssat.com/foundation
Provides funding for surgeon-scientists.
Jeffrey B. Matthews, MD, Chair

Research Centers

3939 ACG Institute for Clinical Research and Education
6400 Goldsboro Road   301-263-9000
Bethesda, MD 20817   gi.org/acg-institute
Innovation center and source of funding for clinically oriented research and education into gastroenterology.
Nicholas J. Shaheen, MD, MPH, FACG, Director

3940 Baylor College of Medicine: General Clinical Research Center for Adults
One Baylor Plaza   713-798-4951
Houston, TX 77030   dbier@bcm.edu
                                                      www.bcm.edu/pediatrics
Endocrinology, genetics and gastroenterology research.
Dennis M Bier MD, Program Director
Paul Klotman, President

3941 Digestive Disorders Associates Ridgely Oaks Professional Center
Ridgely Oaks Professional Center
621 Ridgely Avenue   41 -22 -488
Annapolis, MD 21401   800-273-0505
                                             Fax: 410-224-6971
                                             TTY: 800-735-2258
                                                      www.dda.net
Specialize in the diagnosis and treatment of diseases of the entire digestive system including esophagus stomach small and large intestine colon liver pancreas and gall bladder.
Michael S Epstein, Founder
Charles E King, Doctor

3942 Gastro-Intestinal Research Foundation
70 E Lake Street   312-332-1350
Chicago, IL 60601-5915   Fax: 312-332-4757
                                                      info@girf.org
                                         www.giresearchfoundation.org
Founded to help combat gastrointestinal diseases. Raises funds to support research at the Center for study of the Digestive Diseases at the University of Chicago Medical Center and to support advanced training for scientists. Sponsors educational activities for the public.
Kimberly Coady, Executive Director
Eric Berlin, President

3943 University of California: Davis Gastroenterology & Nutrition Center
Pediatric GI Medical Center
4900 Broadway   91- 73- 904
Sacramento, CA 95820-2214   www.ucdmc.ucdavis.edu
Research into gastrointestinal mobility and electro-physiology nutrition support and references for the public and patient evaluations.
Bonnie Hyatt, Assistant Director
Jenny Carrick, Senior Director of Communications and Ma

3944 University of California: Los Angeles Center for Ulcer Research
LA Medical Center
Building 115 Room 117   310-312-9284
Los Angeles, CA 90073   Fax: 310-268-4963
                                                      cureadmn@mednet.ucla.edu
                                                      www.cure.med.ucla.edu
Offers basic and clinical research related to peptic ulcer disease including causes checks and balances and stress-ulcer relationships.
Enrique Rozengurt, Director
Emeran Mayer, Co-Director

3945 University of Michigan Michigan Gastrointestinal Peptide Research Ctr.
U-M Health System
1500 E Medical Center Drive   734-936-4000
Ann Arbor, MI 48109   Fax: 734-763-2535
                                                      www.med.umich.edu/mgpc
Research into gastroenterology including chemistry of gut hormones is studied.
Chung Owyang MD, Director
Juanita Merc MD PhD, Associate Director

3946 University of Pennsylvania: Harrison Department of Surgical Research
3400 Spruce Street   215-662-4000
Philadelphia, PA 19104   800-789-PENN
                                             Fax: 215-615-0471
Offers research and studies on surgical transplantations gastrointestinal physiology.
Julie Hagan Koehler MBA, Business Director
Georgina Suarez, Administrative Assistant

Support Groups & Hotlines

3947 National Health Information Center
Office of Disease Prevention & Health Promotion
1101 Wootton Pkwy
Rockville, MD 20852
Fax: 240-453-8281
odphpinfo@hhs.gov
www.health.gov/nhic
Supports public health education by maintaining a calendar of National Health Observances; helps connect consumers and health professionals to organizations that can best answer questions and provide up-to-date contact information from reliable sources; updates on a yearly basis toll-free numbers for health information, Federal health clearinghouses and info centers.
Don Wright, MD, MPH, Director

3948 Pull-thru Network
2312 Savoy Street
Hoover, AL 35226-1528
205-978-2930
www.pullthrough.org
Dedicated to the needs of those born wutith anorectal malformation or colon disease and any of the associated diagnoses.

Magazines

3949 ASAP Forum
ASAP International Corporate Headquarters
19 Carroll Road
Woburn, MA 01801
781-935-9776
Fax: 781-933-4151
asapgi@sprynet.com
Educates the general public and medical community about chronic intestinal pseudo-obstruction (CIP) and other related digestive motility disorders; serves as an integral source of information for patients of all ages with CIP and related disorders, their families, and members of the medical community.

3950 American Journal of Gastroenterology
American College of Gastroenterology
6400 Goldsboro Rd
Bethesda, MD 20817
301-263-9000
gi.org/journals-publications
Serves clinical and scientific information needs of member physicians and surgeons, who specialize in digestive and related disorders. Emphasis is on scholarly practice, teaching, and research.

3951 American Journal of Gastrointestinal Surgery
Society for Surgery of the Alimentary Tract
500 Cummings Center
Beverly, MA 01915
978-927-8330
Fax: 978-524-8890
ssat@prri.com
www.ssat.com
Provides information for physicians specializing in gastrointestinal surgery.
Robin S. McLeod, Chair
Fabrizio Michelassi, President

3952 Clinical Perspectives in Gastroenterology
American Gastroenterological Association
4930 Del Ray Avenue
Bethesda, MD 20814
301-654-2055
Fax: 301-654-5920
member@gastro.org
www.gastro.org
Focuses on research, medical and professional developments in the science of gastroenterology.
John I. Allen, President
Michael Camilleri, President-Elect

3953 Digestive Health Matters
Intl. Foundation for Gastrointestinal Disorders
PO Box 170864
Milwaukee, WI 53217
414-964-1799
888-964-2001
Fax: 414-964-7176
iffgd@iffgd.org
www.iffgd.org
Quarterly journal focuses on upper and lower gastrointestinal disorders in adults and children. Educational pamphlets and factsheets are available. Patient and professional membership.
Nancy Norton, President

3954 Food & Nutrition
120 South Riverside Plaza
Chicago, IL 60606-6995
312-899-0040
800-877-1600
foodandnutrition@eatright.org
www.eatright.org
Formerly the ADA Times, Food & Nutrition is the member and professional magazine of the Academy of Nutrition & Dietetics.

3955 Gastroenterology
American Gastroenterological Association
4930 Del Ray Avenue
Bethesda, MD 20814-3002
301-654-2055
Fax: 301-654-5920
member@gastro.org
www.gastro.org
Focuses on research, medical and professional developments in the science of gastroenterology.
John I. Allen, President
Michael Camilleri, President-Elect

3956 Gastroenterology Nursing
Society of Gastroenterology Nurses and Associates
330 N. Wabash Ave.
Chicago, IL 60611
312-321-5165
800-245-7462
Fax: 312-673-6694
sgna@sba.com
www.sgna.org
Provides members with information about trends and development in the field of gastroenterology nursing.
Colleen Keith, President
Lisa Fonkalsrud, President-Elect

3957 Gastrointestinal Endoscopy
American Society for Gastrointestinal Endoscopy
3300 Woodcreek Dr.
Downers Grove, IL 60515
630-573-0600
866-353-2743
Fax: 630-963-8332
info@asge.org
www.asge.org
Provides information, training, and practice guidelines about gastrointestinal endoscopic techniques.
Adjournia Jones, Manager of Operations
Angela Saylor, Accounting Assistant Manager

3958 Journal of Parenteral and Enteral Nutrition
ASPEN
8630 Fenton Street
Silver Spring, MD 20910-3805
301-587-6315
Fax: 301-587-2365
aspen@nutr.org
www.nutritioncare.org
Offers information to professionals involved in the care of parenterally and enterally fed patients.
100 pages BiMonthly
Adrian Nickel, Director Communications/Marketing

3959 Journal of Pediatric Gastroenterology and Nutrition
N American Society for Pediatric Gastroenterology
6900 Grove Road
Thorofare, NJ 08086
609-848-1000
Fax: 609-848-5274
www.jpgn.org/
Provides information for professionals in the areas of pediatric GI liver disease, gastroenterology, and nutrition.

3960 Journal of the Academy of Nutrition and Dietetics
120 South Riverside Plaza
Chicago, IL 60606-6995
312-899-4831
journal@eatright.org
www.eatright.org
Official research publication of the Academy of Nutrition and Dietetics.
Joe Skey, Advertising Contact

3961 Nutrition in Clinical Practice
ASPEN
8630 Fenton Street
Silver Spring, MD 20910-3805
301-587-6315
Fax: 301-587-2365
aspen@nutr.org
www.nutritioncare.org
Offers information to professionals involved in the care of parenterally and enterally fed patients.
100 pages BiMonthly
Adrian Nickel, Director Communications/Marketing

3962 Pancreas
American Pancreatic Association
3 Bethesda Metro Center
Bethesda, MD 20814-6904
301-961-1508
866-726-2737
Fax: 301-657-9776
info@pancreasfoundation.org
pancreasfoundation.org
Provides information on scientific research related to the pancreas.
Joseph M. Titlebaum, Chair
Jessica Kruse, Secretary

3963 Phoenix Magazine
United Ostomy Association of America
PO Box 512
Northfield, MN 55057
800-826-0826
Fax: 507-645-5168
info@uoaa.org
www.uoa.org
America's leading ostomy patient magazine providing colostomy, ileostomy, urostomy and continent diversion information, management techniques, new products and much more.
Quarterly
David Rudzin, President

Newsletters

3964 APF Newsletter
4900 Woodway
Houston, TX 77056
713-266-9617
Fax: 713-840-9552
porphyrus@aol.com
www.porphyriafoundation.com
Provides updates on treatment and research, as well as informative articles on patients and specialists who treat porphyria. It's mailed to all Sponsors of the APF.
Desiree H Lyon, Executive Director
James V. Young, Chairman

3965 ASAP Capsule
ASAP International Corporate Headquarters
19 Carroll Road
Woburn, MA 01801
781-935-9776
Fax: 781-933-4151
asapgi@sprynet.com
Professional membership newsletter for ASAP, an organization which educates the general public and medical community about chronic intestinal pseudo-obstruction (CIP) and other related digestive motility disorders; serves as an integral source of information for patients of all ages with CIP and related disorders, their families, and members of the medical community.

3966 ASAP Digest
ASAP International Corporate Headquarters
19 Carroll Road
Woburn, MA 01801
781-935-9776
Fax: 781-933-4151
asapgi@sprynet.com
General membership newsletter for ASAP. Educates the general public and medical community about chronic intestinal pseudo-obstruction (CIP) and other related digestive motility disorders; serves as an integral source of information for patients of all ages with CIP and related disorders, their families, and members of the medical community.

3967 Clinical Updates
American Society for Gastrointestinal Endoscopy
3300 Woodcreek Dr.
Downers Grove, IL 60515
630-573-0600
Fax: 630-963-8332
info@asge.org
www.asge.org
Provides information, training, and practice guidelines about gastrointestinal endoscopic techniques.
Quarterly
Colleen M. Schmitt, President
Douglas O. Faigel, President-elect

3968 Code V
Cyclic Vomiting Syndrome Association (CVSA)
13180 Caroline Court
Elm Grove, WI 53122-1732
614-837-2586
Fax: 614-837-6543
drwaites@infinet.com
Newsletter for members of the CVSA.

3969 Hemochromatosis Awareness
Hemochromatosis Foundation
PO Box 8569
Albany, NY 12208
518-489-0972
Fax: 518-489-0227
www.hemochromatosis.org
Provides information to the public, families, professionals and government agencies about hereditary hemochromatosis (HH); conducts and raises funds for research; encourages early screening for HH; holds symposiums and meetings; and offers genetic counseling along with support for patients, families, and professionals.
Margit Krikker MD, Medical Director

3970 Ironic Blood
Iron Overload Diseases Association
433 Westward Drive
Taylors, SC 29687-5123
561-840-8512
Fax: 561-842-9881
info@irondisorders.org
www.irondisorders.org
Information for hemochromatosis patients and families.

3971 Lifeline Letter
Oley Foundation
Albany Medical Center
Albany, NY 12208-3478
518-262-5079
800-776-6539
Fax: 518-262-5528
bishopj@mail.amc.edu
www.oley.org
Information on home parenteral and enteral nutrition for patients and the public.
16 pages Bi-Monthly
Joan Bishop, Executive Director

3972 Ostomy Quarterly
United Ostomy Association
P.O. Box 512
Northfield, MN 55057
800-826-0826
info@uoa.org
www.uoa.org
First person stories, ostomy management advice from an ET and MD, organization news and ostomy product information.
72 pages Quarterly
Susan Burns, President
Jim Murray, 1st Vice President

3973 Pull-thru Network News
Pull-thru Network
4 Woody Lane
Westport, CT 06880
203-221-7530
Pullthrunw@aol.com
members.aol.com/pullthrunw/Pullthru.html
Provides information to patients and families of children who have had or will have pull-through surgery to correct an imperforate anus or associated malformation, Hirschsprung's disease, or other fecal incontinence problems.

3974 SGNA News
Society of Gastroenterology Nurses and Associates
330 N. Wabash Ave.
Chicago, IL 60611
312-321-5165
800-245-7462
Fax: 312-321-5165
sgna@sba.com
www.sgna.org
Provides members with information about trends and development in the field of gastroenterology.

3975 WIN Notes
Weight-control Information Network
1 WIN Way
Bethesda, MD 20892-3665
301-496-3583
877-946-4627
Fax: 202-828-1028
Addresses the health information needs of individuals with weight-control problems. Available on the WIN web site.
BiAnnual

Pamphlets

3976 Acute Intermittent Porphyria
American Prophyria Foundation
PO Box 22712
Houston, TX 77227
713-266-9617
www.enterprise.net

An informational brochure published by the American Porphyria Foundation.

3977 Common Questions About Porphyria
American Prophyria Foundation
PO Box 22712
Houston, TX 77227
713-266-9617
www.enterprise.net
An informational brochure published by the American Porphyria Foundation.

3978 Diet and Nutrition in Porphyria
American Prophyria Foundation
PO Box 22712
Houston, TX 77227
713-266-9617
www.enterprise.net
An informational brochure published by the American Porphyria Foundation.

3979 Drugs and Porphyria
American Prophyria Foundation
PO Box 22712
Houston, TX 77227
713-266-9617
www.enterprise.net
An informational brochure published by the American Porphyria Foundation.

3980 Erythropoietic Protoporphyria
American Prophyria Foundation
PO Box 22712
Houston, TX 77227
713-266-9617
www.enterprise.net
An informational brochure published by the American Porphyria Foundation.

3981 Hematin
American Prophyria Foundation
PO Box 22712
Houston, TX 77227
713-266-9617
www.enterprise.net
An informational brochure published by the American Porphyria Foundation.

3982 Iron Overload Alert
Iron Overload Diseases Association
433 Westward Drive
Taylors, SC 29687-5123
561-840-8512
Fax: 561-842-9881
info@irondisorders.org
www.irondisorders.org
Information for hemochromatosis patients and families.

3983 Issues in Women's Gastrointestinal Health
Gastro-Intestinal Research Foundation
70 E Lake Street
Chicago, IL 60601
312-332-1350
Fax: 312-332-4757
info@girf.org
www.giresearchfoundation.org
Patient education pamphlet.
Howard Grill, President

3984 Porphyria Cutanea Tarda
American Prophyria Foundation
PO Box 22712
Houston, TX 77227
713-266-9617
www.enterprise.net
An informational brochure published by the American Porphyria Foundation.

Audio & Video

3985 A Day in the Life of a Child
Albany Medical Center
Albany, NY 12208-3478
518-262-5079
800-776-6539
Fax: 518-262-5528
www.oley.org
In this video you are welcomed into the household of the Miller family. The Millers have three children, one of whom is tube fed. Jessica has been dependent on tube-feedings since birth, and her family is prepared to show you just what that means. They share tips for keeping a sterile environment in a house with three children, and tips for helping Jessica fit in with her peers.
Joan Bishop, Executive Director

3986 Cleveland Clinic Teaching Conference
Hemochromatosis Foundation

PO Box 8569
Albany, NY 12208
518-489-0972
Fax: 518-489-0227
www.hemochromatosis.org
Provides information to the public, families, and professionals about hereditary hemochromatosis.

3987 Family Teaching Conference
Hemochromatosis Foundation
PO Box 8569
Albany, NY 12208
518-489-0972
Fax: 518-489-0227
www.hemochromatosis.org
Provides information to the public, families, and professionals about hereditary hemochromatosis.

3988 Life with Mic-Key
Albany Medical Center
Albany, NY 12208-3478
518-262-5079
800-776-6539
Fax: 518-262-5528
www.oley.org
Serves as an informative and introductory guide for adapting to life with a Mic-key low profile feeding tube. Low profile means that the Mic-key tube lies very close to the patient's body and does not stick out. It's slim design allows more air to circulate around the stoma site and makes it easy to care for. The Mic-key tube uses a balloon to hold it in place and comes with several important accessories, including two types of extensions sets and an anti-reflux valve.
10 Minutes
Joan Bishop, Executive Director

3989 Mealtime Notions - The 'Get Permission' Approach to Mealtimes and Oral Motor
Marsha Dunn Klein, MED, OTR/L, author
Albany Medical Center
Albany, NY 12208-3478
518-262-5079
800-776-6539
Fax: 518-262-5528
www.oley.org
This video explores the development of trusting feeding relationships, understanding the child's pace, and strategies for increasing permissive behavior. Tools discussed in this video include an introduction to the sensory continuum, a description of the around the bowl technique, and tips for removing the stress from your child's mealtime.
10 Minutes
Joan Bishop, Executive Director

Web Sites

3990 Academy of Nutrition & Dietetics
www.eatright.org
Offers information and support to allergy sufferers. Serves the public through the promotion of optimal nutrition, health, and well-being. Formerly the American Dietetic Association.

3991 American College of Gastroenterology
www.gi.org
ACG serves clinical and scientific information needs of member physicians and surgeons, who specialize in digestive and related disorders. Emphasis is on scholarly practice, teaching, and research.

3992 American Gastroenterological Association
www.gastro.org
AGA fosters the development and application of the science of gastroenterology by providing leadership and aid including patient care, research, teaching, continuing education, scientific communication and matters of national health policy.

3993 American Hemochromatosis Society
www.americanhs.org
Educates the public, the medical community, and the media by distributing the most current information available on hereditary hemochromatosis (HH), including DNA screening for HH and pediatric HH; also facilitates patient empowerment through an online network.

3994 American Porphyria Foundation
www.porphyriafoundation.com

Advances awareness, research, and treatment of the porphyrias; provides self-help services for members; and provides referrals to porphyria treatment specialists.

3995 **American Pseudo-Obstruction and Hirschsprung's Disease Society**

Promotes public awareness of gastrointestinal motility disorders, in particular intestinal pseudo-obstruction and Hirschsprung's Disease; provides education and support to individuals and families of children who have been diagnosed with these disorders through parent-to-parent contact, publications, and educational symposia; and encourages and supports medical research in the area of gastrointestinal motility disorders.

3996 **American Society for Gastrointestinal Endoscopy**

www.asge.org

ASGE provides information, training, and practice guidelines about gastrointestinal endoscopic techniques.

3997 **American Society of Abdominal Surgeons**

www.abdominalsurg.org

ASAS sponsors extensive continuing education program for physicians in the field of abdominal surgery and maintains library.

3998 **Background on Functional Gastrointestinal Disorders**

www.med.unc.edu

Statistical background information on gastrointestinal disorders.

3999 **Children's Motility Disorder Foundation**

www.motility.org

CMDF works to increase awareness of pediatric motility disorders in the general public and among the physicians most likely to encounter children suffering from these conditions, such as pediatricians and family practice doctors. Supports medical research regarding the causes, treatment, and potentially life-threatening disorders.

4000 **Cyclic Vomiting Syndrome Association**

www.cvsaonline.org

CVSA provides opportunities for patients, families and professionals to offer and receive support and share knowledge about cyclic vomiting syndrome; actively promotes and facilitates medical research about nausea and vomiting.

4001 **Gastrointestinal Research Foundation**

www.giresearchfoundation.org

Founded to help combat gastrointestinal diseases. Raises funds to support research at the Center for the study of the Digestive Diseases at the University of Chicago Medical Center and to support advanced training for scientists. Sponsors educational activities for the public.

4002 **Healing Well**

www.healingwell.com

An online health resource guide to medical news, chat, information and articles, newsgroups and message boards, books, disease-related web sites, medical directories, and more for patients, friends, and family coping with disabling diseases, disorders, or chronic illnesses.

4003 **Health Finder**

www.healthfinder.gov

Searchable, carefully developed web site offering information on over 1000 topics. Developed by the US Department of Health and Human Services, the site can be used in both English and Spanish.

4004 **Healthlink USA**

www.healthlinkusa.com

Health information concerning treatment, cures, prevention, diagnosis, risk factors, research, support groups, email lists, personal stories and much more. Updated regularly.

4005 **Hemochromatosis Foundation**

www.hemochromatosis.org

Provides information to the public, families, and professionals about hereditary hemochromatosis (HH); conducts and raises funds for research; encourages early screening for HH; holds symposiums and meetings; and offers genetic counseling along with support for patients, families, and professionals.

4006 **International Foundation for Functional Gastrointestinal Disorders (IFFGD)**

www.iffgd.org

Non-profit education, support, and research organization devoted to increasing awareness and understanding of functional gastrointestinal disorders, including irritable bowel syndrome (IBS), constipation, diarrhea, pain, and incontinence. Mission is to inform, assist and support people affected by these disorders.

4007 **MedicineNet**

www.medicinenet.com

An online resource for consumers providing easy-to-read, authoritative medical and health information.

4008 **Medscape**

www.medscape.com

Medscape offers specialists, primary care physicians, and other health professionals the Web's most robust and integrated medical information and educational tools.

4009 **National Digestive Diseases Information Clearinghouse**

www.digestive.niddk.nih.gov

Offers various educational information, resources and reprints focusing on Colitis, Ulcerative Colitis and Crohn's disease.

4010 **North American Society for Pediatric Gastroenterology, Hepatology & Nutrition**

www.naspghan.org

NASPGHAN strives to improve the care of infants, children and adolescents with digestive disorders by promoting advances in clinical care, research and education.

4011 **Nutrition in Clinical Practice**

www.nutritioncare.org

NCP is indexed by PubMed (MEDLINE), Cumulative Index to Nursing and Allied Health Literature, International Nursing Index, International Pharmaceutical Index, Reference Update, Silver Platter, TOXLINE and UMI.

4012 **Oley Foundation**

www.oley.org

Enriches the lives of those requiring home IV & tube feeding through education, outreach, & networking.

4013 **Pull-thru Network**

www.pullthrunetwork.org

Pull-thru Network (PTN) was founded in 1988 and has grown to be one of the largest organizations in the world dedicated to the needs of those born with an anorectal malformation or colon disease and any of the associated diagnoses

4014 **Society for Surgery of the Alimentary Tract**

www.ssat.com

SSAT provides a forum for exchange of information among physicians specializing in alimentary tract surgery.

4015 **Society of American Gastrointestinal Endoscopic Surgeons**

www.sages.org

SAGES encourages study and practice of gastrointestinal endoscopy, laparoscopy and minimal acces surgery.

4016 **The Inside Tract**

theinsidetract.sgna.org

Content brand of the Society of Gastroenterology Nurses and Associates, with an online portal featuring analysis, editorials, behind the scenes, education, and more.

4017 **United Ostomy Associations of America, Inc**

www.ostomy.org

A national network for bowel and urinary diversion support groups in the United States. Its goal is to provide a non-profit association that will serve to unify and strengthen its member support groups, which are organized for the benefit of people who have, or will have intestinal or urinary diversions and their caregivers.

4018 **WebMD**

www.webmd.com

Provides credible information, supportive communities, and in-depth reference material about health subjects. A source for original and timely health information as well as material from well known content providers.

Description

4019 Gaucher Disease

Gaucher disease is an inherited lysosomal storage disease that results from mutations in the GBA gene, which encodes the enzyme B-glucocerebros. B-glucocerebrosidase degrades a complex lipid called glucocerebroside into glucose and a simpler lipid called ceramide. In the absence of functional B-glucocerebrosidase, glucocerebroside accumulates to toxic levels that causes cells to die. There are several types of Gaucher disease, each with different types of symptoms. Type 1 Gaucher disease is the mildest form and does not affect the central nervous system. The main symptoms are enlargement of the liver and spleen, anemia, easy bruising as a result of low numbers of blood platelets, lung disease, and bone abnormalities such as bone pain, fractures, and arthritis. Types 2 and 3 Gaucher disease affect the nervous system and in addition to the symptoms of Type 1 Gaucher disease, types 2 and 3 can cause abnormal eye movements, seizures, and brain damage. Type 2 Gaucher disease usually causes life-threatening problems that begin in infancy. Type 3 Gaucher disease is milder and worsens slower than type 2. The most severe type of Gaucher disease is called the perinatal lethal form. Most infants with the perinatal lethal form of Gaucher disease survive for only a few days after birth. A cardiovascular type of Gaucher disease causes the heart valves to harden (calcify). People with the cardiovascular form of Gaucher disease may also have eye abnormalities, bone disease, and mild enlargement of the spleen. Diagnosis is based on finding Gaucher typical cells in the bone marrow, and genetic tests.

The treatment for Gaucher disease is enzyme replacement, which is administered intravenously. There are three FDA-approved products for enzyme replacement treatment of Gaucher disease: imiglucerase (Cerezyme), velaglucerase-a ((VPRIV), and taliglucerase (Elelyso). Removal of the spleen and blood transfusions may be necessary. Current research is aimed at gene therapy.

National Agencies & Associations

4020 Jewish Genetics Disaese Center
Icahn School of Medicine at Mt Sinai
1425 Madison Avenue   212-659-6700
New York, NY 10029   Fax: 212-360-1809
                        icahn.mssm.edu/research/jewish-genetics
Created to raise funds for and to inform the public about genetic diseases which afflict descendants of eastern and central European Jews. It sponsors medical symposia from time to time.
Robert J. Desnick, PhD, MD, Center Director

4021 National Organization for Rare Disorders
55 Kenosia Avenue   203-744-0100
Danbury, CT 06810-1968   800-999-6673
                        Fax: 203-263-9938
                        www.rarediseases.org
NORD is a federation of voluntary health organizations dedicated to helping people with rare orphan diseases and assisting the organizations that serve them. It is committed to the identification, treatment, and cure of rare disorders through programs of education, advocacy, research, and service.
Peter Saltonstall, President & CEO
Pamela Gavin, Chief Strategy Officer

Foundations

4022 National Gaucher Foundation
5410 Edson Lane   800-504-3189
Rockville, MD 20852   ngf@gaucherdisease.org
                        www.gaucherdisease.org
National foundation providing information and assistance for those affected by Gaucher disease, as well as education and outreach to increase public awareness.
Brian Berman, President & CEO
Amy Blum, Chief Operating Officer

4023 National Gaucher Foundation of Canada
83 Winnegreen Court   613-867-6344
Ottawa, Ontario, K1G-5S3   info@gauchercanada.ca
                        gauchercanada.ca
Group of volunteers, comprised of individuals, families, health professionals, and organizations interested in improving the health and well-being of anyone affected with Gaucher disease.
Christine White, President

Research Centers

4024 Children's Gaucher Research Fund
8110 Warren Court   916-797-3700
Granite Bay, CA 95746   Fax: 916-797-3707
                        research@childrensgaucher.org
                        www.childrensgaucher.org
A nonprofit organization that raises funds to coordinate support research to find a cure for Type 2 and Type 3 Gaucher Disease.
Roscoe Brady, MD, Scientific Advisory Board
Gregory Grabowski, MD, Scientific Advisory Board

4025 Comprehensive Gaucher Treatment Center at Tower Hermatology Oncology
9090 Wilshire Boulevard   310-888-8680
Beverly Hills, CA 90211   888-248-4456
                        Fax: 310-285-7298
                        info@gaucherwest.com
                        www.gaucherwest.com
The Comprehensive Gaucher Treatment Center at Tower Hermatology Oncology under the direction of Dr. Barry Rosenbloom provides clinical evaluations for the diagnosis and treatment of patient's with Gaucher disease. We provide a multi-disciplinary program that includes Hermatology Genetics Orthopedics and Radiology. To ensure continuity of care we provide assistance to other physicians regarding testing diagnosis evaluation and management of the Gaucher patient.
Barry Rosenbloom, Director
Cheryl Elzinga, Gaucher Coordinator

4026 LAC/USC Imaging Science Center
1975 Zonal Avenue   323-442-1900
Los Angeles, CA 90089-9034   Fax: 323-442-2722
Provides a Gaucher Disease radiology consultant: Michael R Terk MD.and Muskuloskeletal Imaging.
Coreen Rodgers, COO
Sherri Sammon, Associate Director

Support Groups & Hotlines

4027 Brave Kids
151 Sawgrass Corners Drive   904-280-1895
Ponte Vedra Beach, FL 32082   800-568-1008
                        Fax: 904-280-1897
                        www.bravekids.org
An organization that offers support for parents and children suffering from serious health problems.
Kristen Fitzgerald, Founder

4028 **National Health Information Center**
Office of Disease Prevention & Health Promotion
1101 Wootton Pkwy   Fax: 240-453-8281
Rockville, MD 20852   odphpinfo@hhs.gov
                                       www.health.gov/nhic
Supports public health education by maintaining a calendar of National Health Observances; helps connect consumers and health professionals to organizations that can best answer questions and provide up-to-date contact information from reliable sources; updates on a yearly basis toll-free numbers for health information, Federal health clearinghouses and info centers.
Don Wright, MD, MPH, Director

Newsletters

4029 **Gaucher Disease Newsletter**
National Gaucher Foundation
61 General Early Drive   301-816-1515
Harpers Ferry, WV 25425-3151   800-504-3189
                                       Fax: 770-934-2911
                                       rhonda@gaucherdisease.org
                                       www.gaucherdisease.org
Offers information on the latest research, treatments and technology for persons affected by Gaucher Disease. Also includes legislative and medical information.
Quarterly
Brian E. Berman, President
Michael David Epstein, Chairman/Secretary

Pamphlets

4030 **Gaucher Disease Fact Sheet**
National Gaucher Foundation
61 General Early Drive   301-816-1515
Harpers Ferry, WV 25425-3151   800-504-3189
                                       Fax: 770-934-2911
                                       rhonda@gaucherdisease.org
                                       www.gaucherdisease.org
Offers information on what Gaucher Disease is, the symptoms, risks, treatments and the workings of the National Gaucher Foundation.
Brian E. Berman, President
Michael David Epstein, Chairman/Secretary

4031 **Living with Gaucher Disease**
National Gaucher Foundation
61 General Early Drive   301-816-1515
Harpers Ferry, WV 25425-3151   800-504-3189
                                       Fax: 770-934-2911
                                       rhonda@gaucherdisease.org
                                       www.gaucherdisease.org
A guide for parents, families and relatives that teach them how to deal with and cope with a diagnosis of Gaucher Disease.
24 pages
Brian E. Berman, President
Michael David Epstein, Chairman/Secretary

Audio & Video

4032 **Pain & Hope**
National Gaucher Foundation
61 General Early Drive   301-816-1515
Harpers Ferry, WV 25425-3151   800-504-3189
                                       Fax: 770-934-2911
                                       rhonda@gaucherdisease.org
                                       www.gaucherdisease.org
A patient and family perspective on Gaucher Disease.
Brian E. Berman, President
Michael David Epstein, Chairman/Secretary

Web Sites

4033 **Gaucher Disease Homepage**
                                       www.gaucherdisease.org

Information on Gaucher disease, including symptoms, treatment, prevalence, resources, support, and news.

4034 **Healing Well**
                                       www.healingwell.com
An online health resource guide to medical news, chat, information and articles, newsgroups and message boards, books, disease-related web sites, medical directories, and more for patients, friends, and family coping with disabling diseases, disorders, or chronic illnesses.

4035 **Health Finder**
                                       www.healthfinder.gov
Searchable, carefully developed web site offering information on over 1000 topics. Developed by the US Department of Health and Human Services, the site can be used in both English and Spanish.

4036 **Healthlink USA**
                                       www.healthlinkusa.com
Health information concerning treatment, cures, prevention, diagnosis, risk factors, research, support groups, email lists, personal stories and much more. Updated regularly.

4037 **MedicineNet**
                                       www.medicinenet.com
An online resource for consumers providing easy-to-read, authoritative medical and health information.

4038 **Medscape**
                                       www.medscape.com
Medscape offers specialists, primary care physicians, and other health professionals the Web's most robust and integrated medical information and educational tools.

4039 **National Organization for Rare Disorders**
                                       www.rarediseases.org
NORD is a federation of voluntary health organizations dedicated to helping people with rare orphan diseases and assisting the organizations that serve them. It is committed to the identification, treatment, and cure of rare disorders through programs of education, advocacy, research, and service. Website features resources for patients and families, patient organizations, and clinicians and researchers.

4040 **WebMD**
                                       www.webmd.com
Provides credible information, supportive communities, and in-depth reference material about health subjects. A source for original and timely health information as well as material from well known content providers.

Description

4041 Growth Disorders

There are many conditions that make a child grow more slowly than average. Any sort of severe chronic illness, especially one involving the digestive system, may cause this. Certain genetic conditions such as Turner syndrome, a sex chromosome abnormality or achondroplasia (skeletal maldevelopment) will predictably limit growth and eventual adult height. Endocrine, or hormonal, causes of short stature include underactivity of the thyroid gland (hypothyroidism) or hypopituitary dwarfism, in which the anterior lobe of the pituitary gland fails to secrete sufficient quantities of growth hormone (GH). Poor nutrition, especially insufficient dietary protein intake (kwashiorkor), can also stunt growth. Finally, there are many cases where the child's height is significantly below that of peers, yet none of these conditions is present. This may reflect two parents who are themselves quite short, or may be completely unexplained.

If slow growth is related to low levels of GH, therapy with synthetic GH is extremely effective. Regular injections will be necessary for a prolonged period until an acceptable height is reached.

Regardless of the underlying cause, a child whose disorder is recognized at birth or who is not growing as quickly as the rest of his or her peers should receive a complete evaluation by a pediatric endocrinologist or other growth specialist.

National Agencies & Associations

4042 Dwarf Athletic Association of America

www.daaa.org

Develops, promotes and provides quality amateur level athletic opportunities for dwarf athletes in the US, including the annual U.S. National Dwarf Games.

4043 Genetic Alliance

4301 Connecticut Avenue NW
Washington, DC 20008-2369
202-966-5557
Fax: 202-966-8553
info@geneticalliance.org
www.geneticalliance.org

Non-profit organization seeks to transform healthcare for the better for individuals, families, and communities.

Sharon Terry, MA, President & CEO
Natasha Bonhomme, Chief Strategy Officer

4044 Goodwill Industries International, Inc.

15810 Indianola Drive
Rockville, MD 20855
800-466-3945
contactus@goodwill.org
www.goodwill.org

A nonprofit, community-based organization whose mission is to help people achieve self-sufficiency through the dignity and power of work, serving people who are disadvantaged, disabled or elderly. The mission is accomplished through providing independent living skills, affordable housing, and training and placement in community employment. The GoodWill Network includes 160 independent, local locations across the U.S. and Canada.

S. Dale Jenkins, Chair
Steven C. Preston, President & CEO

4045 Little People of America

617 Broadway
Sonoma, CA 95476
714-368-3689
888-572-2001
Fax: 714-721-1896
info@lpaonline.org
www.lpaonline.org

Focuses research, support and information on persons who are short in stature.

Mark Povinelli, President
Deb Himsel, Executive Director

4046 National Institute of Child Health and Human Development

PO Box 3006
Rockville, MD 20847
800-370-2943
Fax: 866-760-5947
TTY: 888-320-6942
www.nichd.nih.gov

NICHD seeks to better understand disabilities and important events that occur during pregnancy.

Diana W. Bianchi, MD, Director
Constantine Stratakis, Scientific Director

State Agencies & Associations

Florida

4047 Goodwill Industries-Suncoast

10596 Gandy Boulevard
St. Petersburg, FL 33702
727-523-1512
888-279-1988
TTY: 727-579-1068
www.goodwill-suncoast.org

A nonprofit, community-based organization whose mission is to help people achieve self-sufficiency through the dignity and power of work, serving people who are disadvantaged, disabled or elderly. The mission is accomplished through providing independent living skills, affordable housing, and training and placement in community employment.

Heather Ceresoli, CPA, Chair
Deborah A. Passerini, President & CEO

Foundations

4048 Human Growth Foundation

997 Glen Cove Avenue
Glen Head, NY 11545
516-671-4041
800-451-6434
Fax: 516-671-4055
hgf1@hgfound.org
www.hgfound.org

Our mission is to help children, and adults with disorders of growth and growth hormone through research, education, support, and advocacy. The Foundation is dedicated to helping medical science to better understand the process of growth. It is composed of concerned parents and friends of children, and adults, with growth problems; and, interested health professionals.

Patricia D Costa, Executive Director
Pisit Pitukcheewanont, President

4049 MAGIC Foundation for Children's Growth

6645 West North Avenue
Oak Park, IL 60302
708-383-0808
800-362-4423
Fax: 708-383-0899
dianne@magicfoundation.org
www.magicfoundation.org

Provides support services for the families of children afflicted with a wide variety of chronic and/or critical disorders, syndromes and that affect a child's growth.

Dianne Tamburrino, Executive Director
Susan Smith, Director Medical Education

4050 March of Dimes Foundation

1550 Crystal Drive
Arlington, VA 22202
888-663-4637
www.marchofdimes.org

Seeks to improve the health of babies by preventing birth defects, premature birth, and infant mortality through programs of research, community services, education, and advocacy.

Stacey D. Stewart, President

Research Centers

4051 Case Western Reserve University: Bolton Brush Growth Study Center
2123 Abington Road   216-368-4649
Cleveland, OH 44106-4905   Fax: 216-368-3204
mgh4@po.cwru.edu
dental.cwru.edu/bolton-brush
Investigations and research into the growth and development of the human body. Extensive collection of longitudinal human growth data.
Mark G Hans, Director
Aaron Weinbe, Associate Professor and Chairman

4052 International Skeletal Dysplasia Registry Medical Genetics Institute
Medical Genetics Institute
8700 Beverly Boulevard   310-423-3277
Los Angeles, CA 90048   800-233-2771
Fax: 310-423-0462
www.csmc.edu
Provides patient services for skeletal dysplasia patients particularly research in dwarfism.
David L Rimoin MD PhD, Director
Xiao-Ning Chen, Research Scientist

4053 New Jersey Institute of Technology Center for Biomedical Engineering
University Heights   973-596-8449
Newark, NJ 07102-1982   Fax: 973-596-6056
william.c.hunter@njit.edu
www.njit.edu
Offers research into facial and bone disorders.
Robert A Altenkirch, President
Joel Bloom, Vice President

4054 WM Krogman Center for Research in Child Growth and Development
3101 Walnut Street   215-898-1470
Philadelphia, PA 19104-6003   mannj@upenn.edu
www.upenn.edu
Focuses research and studies on growth disorders and birth defects.
Amy Gutmann, President

Support Groups & Hotlines

4055 National Health Information Center
Office of Disease Prevention & Health Promotion
1101 Wootton Pkwy   Fax: 240-453-8281
Rockville, MD 20852   odphpinfo@hhs.gov
www.health.gov/nhic
Supports public health education by maintaining a calendar of National Health Observances; helps connect consumers and health professionals to organizations that can best answer questions and provide up-to-date contact information from reliable sources; updates on a yearly basis toll-free numbers for health information, Federal health clearinghouses and info centers.
Don Wright, MD, MPH, Director

Books

4056 Growing Children: A Parent's Guide
Human Growth Foundation
997 Glen Cove Avenue   516-671-4041
Glen Head, NY 11545   800-451-6434
Fax: 516-671-4055
hgf1@hgfound.org
www.hgfound.org
Offers parents information on the normal pattern of their child's growth, growth charts, recognition of growth problems, evaluation of growth problems and resources for more information.
Pisit Pitukcheewanont, President
Emily L. Germain-Lee, Vice President

4057 Short and OK
Human Growth Foundation
997 Glen Cove Avenue   516-671-4041
Glen Head, NY 11545   800-451-6434
Fax: 516-671-4055
hgf1@hgfound.org
www.hgfound.org
Guide for parents of short children offering information on behavior issues, medical issues and psychological warning signs.
54 pages
Pisit Pitukcheewanont, President
Emily L. Germain-Lee, Vice President

Pamphlets

4058 Achondroplasia
Human Growth Foundation
997 Glen Cove Avenue   516-671-4041
Glen Head, NY 11545   800-451-6434
Fax: 516-671-4055
hgf1@hgfound.org
www.hgfound.org
Signs, causes and prevention of achondroplasia.
Pisit Pitukcheewanont, President
Emily L. Germain-Lee, Vice President

4059 Growth Hormone Testing
Human Growth Foundation
997 Glen Cove Avenue   516-671-4041
Glen Head, NY 11545   800-451-6434
Fax: 516-671-4055
hgf1@hgfound.org
www.hgfound.org
What to expect during the testing period.
Pisit Pitukcheewanont, President
Emily L. Germain-Lee, Vice President

4060 Intrauterine Growth Retardation
Human Growth Foundation
997 Glen Cove Avenue   516-671-4041
Glen Head, NY 11545   800-451-6434
Fax: 516-671-4055
hgf1@hgfound.org
www.hgfound.org
Explains some of the reasons for an infant's failure to grow normally in intrauterine life.
Pisit Pitukcheewanont, President
Emily L. Germain-Lee, Vice President

4061 Most Frequently Asked Questions with Growth Hormone Deficiency
Human Growth Foundation
997 Glen Cove Avenue   516-671-4041
Glen Head, NY 11545   800-451-6434
Fax: 516-671-4055
hgf1@hgfound.org
www.hgfound.org
Provides a brief overview for parents about Growth Hormone Deficiency.
Pisit Pitukcheewanont, President
Emily L. Germain-Lee, Vice President

4062 Septo-Optic Dysplasia
Human Growth Foundation
997 Glen Cove Avenue   516-671-4041
Glen Head, NY 11545   800-451-6434
Fax: 516-671-4055
hgf1@hgfound.org
www.hgfound.org
Also known as DeMorsier Syndrome. Describes the disease and the different treatments that can lead to the significant improvement in the quality of life.
Pisit Pitukcheewanont, President
Emily L. Germain-Lee, Vice President

Web Sites

4063   Alliance of Genetic Support Groups

www.geneticalliance.org

Genetic Alliance is a nonprofit health advocacy organization. Its network includes more than 1,200 disease-specific advocacy organizations, as well as thousands of universities, private companies, government agencies, and public policy organizations. The network is a dynamic and growing open space for shared resources, creative tools, and innovative programs.

4064   Atomz

www.pediatricservices.com

Provides resources to help all families obtain the information they need for the development of their children. Pediatric Services offers bilingual services - English and Espanol.

4065   Healing Well

www.healingwell.com

An online health resource guide to medical news, chat, information and articles, newsgroups and message boards, books, disease-related web sites, medical directories, and more for patients, friends, and family coping with disabling diseases, disorders, or chronic illnesses.

4066   Health Finder

www.healthfinder.gov

Searchable, carefully developed web site offering information on over 1000 topics. Developed by the US Department of Health and Human Services, the site can be used in both English and Spanish.

4067   Healthlink USA

www.healthlinkusa.com

Health information concerning treatment, cures, prevention, diagnosis, risk factors, research, support groups, email lists, personal stories and much more. Updated regularly.

4068   Human Growth Foundation

www.HGFound.org

Organization committed to expanding and accelerating research into growth hormone deficiency. Provides education and support to those affected by growth disorders and their families and fosters the exchange of information with the medical community.

4069   March of Dimes Foundation

www.marchofdimes.org

Online resources on birth defects.

4070   MedicineNet

www.medicinenet.com

An online resource for consumers providing easy-to-read, authoritative medical and health information.

4071   Medscape

www.medscape.com

Medscape offers specialists, primary care physicians, and other health professionals the Web's most robust and integrated medical information and educational tools.

4072   OHSU Homepage Search

www.ohsu.edu

A search which provides several links for information on growth disorders.

4073   WebMD

www.webmd.com

Provides credible information, supportive communities, and in-depth reference material about health subjects. A source for original and timely health information as well as material from well known content providers.

Description

4074 Head Injuries

Head Injuries, or Traumatic Brain Injuries, cover a range of severity. There are 1.7 million traumatic brain injuries each year, and presently, there are 5.3 million Americans living with a disability because of a head or brain injury. Concussion, the most common injury, is the momentary loss of consciousness. It usually resolves without any major complications. Damage can result from penetration of the skull or from acceleration/deceleration of the brain that occurs in severe automobile accidents. Injuries can include brain bruising and bleeding into the brain, resulting in swelling that can be life threatening because the skull, as a rigid structure, cannot expand.

Postconcussion syndrome commonly follows a mild injury and can include temporary headaches, dizziness, mild mental slowing and sleepiness. A moderate head or brain injury results in loss of consciousness usually lasting from minutes to a few hours, followed by a few days or weeks of confusion. Loss of consciousness for greater than two minutes implies a worse outcome. Cognitive and psychological impairments lasting many months or even permanently are usual consequences of moderate injury. A severe injury almost always results in prolonged unconsciousness or coma lasting days to weeks or longer. People who sustain a severe head or brain injury often have brain contusions, hematomas (a collection of blood) and/or damage to the nerve fibers or axons. Many people who sustain a severe brain injury make significant improvements in the first year or two. After that improvement tends to diminish down but may continue for years. Some physical and/or cognitive impairments are permanent. See also *Brain Tumors*.

National Agencies & Associations

4075 American Brain Tumor Association
8550 W Bryn Mawr Avenue
Chicago, IL 60631
773-577-8750
800-886-2282
Fax: 773-577-8738
info@abta.org
www.abta.org

Services includes over 40 publications which address brain tumors, their treatment and coping with the disease. Materials address brain tumors in all age groups. Provides free social service consultations and a mentorship program for new brain tumor support groups.
Ralph DeVitto, President & CEO
Nicole Willmarth, PhD, Chief Mission Officer

4076 American Chronic Pain Association
PO Box 850
Rocklin, CA 95677
800-533-3231
ACPA@theacpa.org
www.theacpa.org

The ACPA facilitates peer support and education for individuals with chronic pain in its many forms, in order to increase quality of life. Also raises awareness among the healthcare community, and with policy makers.
Penney Cowan, Founder & CEO
Daniel Galia, Director, Global Support

4077 American Head and Neck Society
11300 W Olympic Blvd.
Los Angeles, CA 90064
310-437-0559
310-437-0585
admin@ahns.info
www.ahns.info

The society seeks to advance education, research, and quality of care for hed and neck oncology patients.
Christina Kasendorf, Executive Director
J.J. Jackman, Associate Executive Director

4078 Brain Injury Association of America
1608 Spring Hill Road
Vienna, VA 22182
703-761-0750
Fax: 703-761-0755
info@biausa.org
www.biausa.org

The BIA's mission is to create a better future through brain injury prevention, research, education, and advocacy. Offers information on state and national offices, treatment and rehabilitation, conferences, prevention, financial development and more.
Susan H. Connors, President & CEO
Mary S. Reitter, Executive Vice-President & COO

4079 Family Caregiver Alliance/National Center on Caregiving
101 Montgomery Street
San Francisco, CA 94104
415-434-3388
800-445-8106
www.caregiver.org

Caregiver information and assistance via phone or e-mail; fact sheets and publications describing and documenting caregiver needs and services.
Jacquelyn Kung, PhD, Chief Executive Officer
Wyatt Ritchie, MBA, Managing Director

4080 International Brain Injury Association
5909 Ashby Manor Place
Alexandria, VA 22313
703-960-0027
Fax: 703-960-6603
congress@internationalbrain.org
www.internationalbrain.org

Provides scientific and medical leadership worldwide in the field of brain injury.
David Arciniegas, Chairman & CEO
Nathan Zasler, Vice Chairman & Vice CEO

4081 TBI: Traumatic Brian Injury
www.tbi.org

The Perspective Network was changed to TBI in 2015; it provides forums and resources for persons with families, caregivers, friends and the professionals who serve them. Their goals are to promote a sense of community and to increase public awareness of brain injury.
Elaine Jones, Contact

State Agencies & Associations

Alabama

4082 Alabama Head Injury Foundation
3100 Lorna Road
Hoover, AL 35216
205-823-3818
800-433-8002
Fax: 205-823-4544
ahif1@bellsouth.net
http://www.ahif.org

Services provided to Alabamians with traumatic brain injury or spinal cord injury include information, housing, respite care, recreation programs, resource coordination.
Keith Belt, President
Charles D Priest, Executive Director

Arizona

4083 Brain Injury Association of Arizona
5025 E Washington Street
Phoenix, AZ 85034
602-508-8024
888-500-9165
Fax: 602-508-8285
info@biaaz.org
www.biaaz.org

Information and resources for brain injury survivors and their families. Support group listings available. Educational training, con-

ference for families and survivors, neuro-specific resources and helpline.
Lisa Counters, President
Rebecca Armendariz, VicePresident

Arkansas

4084 Brain Injury Association of Arkansas
PO Box 26236   501-374-3585
Little Rock, AR 72221-6236   800-444-6443
                                      Fax: 501-918-6595
                                      info@brainassociation.org

Dana Austen, President
Kortney Coats, Vice President

Colorado

4085 Brain Injury Association of Colorado
4200 W Conejos Place   303-355-9969
Denver, CO 80204   800-955-2443
                                      Fax: 303-355-9968
                                      www.biacolorado.org

William Levis, President
Gavin Attwood, Executive Director

Connecticut

4086 Brain Injury Association of Connecticut
200 Day Hill Road   86 - 2 - 02
Windsor, CT 06095   800-278-8242
                                      Fax: 86 - 2 - 05
                                      general@biact.org
                                      www.biact.org

500 Members
Paul A Slager, President
Julie Peters, Executive Director

Delaware

4087 Brain Injury Association of Delaware
840 Walker Road   302-346-2083
Dover, DE 19904   800-411-0505
                                      Fax: 888-258-3694

Devon Dorman, President
Esther Curtis, Executive Director

Florida

4088 Brain Injury Association of Florida
1637 Metropolitan Boulevard   850-410-0103
Tallahassee, FL 32308   800-992-3442
                                      Fax: 850-410-0105
                                      biaftalla@biaf.org
                                      www.biaf.org

Valerie E Breen, President/CEO

4089 Choices for Work Program Goodwill Industries-Suncoast
Goodwill Industries-Suncoast
10596 Gandy Boulevard   727-523-1512
St Petersburg, FL 33702   888-279-1988
                                      Fax: 727-563-9300
                                      TTY: 727-579-1068
                                      gw.marketing@goodwill-suncoast.com
                                      www.goodwill-suncoast.org
A nonprofit community based organization whose purpose is to improve the quality of life for people who are disabled, disadvantaged and/or aged. This mission is accomplished through a staff of over 1,200 employees providing independent living skills, affordable housing, career assessment and job skills training and opportunities.
Deborah A. Passerini, President
Oscar J. Horton, Chair

4090 Pensacola Brain Injury TBI/ABI Support Group
TBI/ABI Support Group
2001 N E Street   850-457-2870
Pensacola, FL 32507   hens8250@bellsouth.net

Survivors and caregivers oriented association. Publishes monthly magazine.
Peggy Henshall, Support Group Coordinator

Hawaii

4091 Brain Injury Association of Hawaii
420 Kuwili Street   808-791-6942
Honolulu, HI 96817-1474   Fax: 808-454-1975
                                      biahi@hawaiiantel.net
                                      www.biausa.org/Hawaii

Ian Mattoch, President
Mary Wilson, Executive Director

Idaho

4092 Brain Injury Association of Idaho
PO Box 414   208-342-0999
Boise, ID 83701-0414   888-374-3447
                                      Fax: 208-333-0026
                                      info@biaid.org
                                      www.biaid.org

Michelle Featherston, President

Illinois

4093 Brain Injury Association of Illinois
PO Box 64420   312-726-5699
Chicago, IL 60664-0420   800-699-6443
                                      Fax: 312-630-4011
                                      info@biail.org
                                      www.biail.org

Philicia L Deckard, Executive Director
Irene Pedersen, Founder

Indiana

4094 Brain Injury Association of Indiana
9531 Valparaiso Court   317-356-7722
Indianapolis, IN 46268   866-854-4246
                                      Fax: 31 - 8 - 17
                                      info@biai.org

Anna Garrett, Executive Director
Laura C Trexler, TBI Grant Program Director

Iowa

4095 Brain Injury Association of Iowa
7025 Hickman Road   319-466-7455
Urbandale, IA 50322   800-444-6443
                                      Fax: 800-381-0812
                                      info@biaia.org
                                      www.biaia.org

Geoffrey Lauer, Executive Director

Kansas

4096 Brain Injury Association of Kansas and Greater Kansas City
6405 Metcalf Avenue   913-754-8883
Overland Park, KS 66202   800-444-6443
                                      Fax: 816-842-1531
                                      info@biaks.org
                                      www.biaks.org

Rob Flores, President
Betsy Johnson, Executive Director

Kentucky

4097 Brain Injury Association of Kentucky
7410 New Lagrange Roadd   502-493-0609
Louisville, KY 40222   800-592-1117
                                      Fax: 502-426-2993
                                      www.biak.us

Chell Austin, Executive Director
Wes Wilkinson, Development Director

Maine

4098 Brain Injury Association of Maine
13 Washington Street
Waterville, ME 04901
207-861-9900
800-275-1233
Fax: 207-861-4617
info@biame.org
www.biame.org

Mary Lombardo, President
Leslie DuVall, Director of Operations

Maryland

4099 Brain Injury Association of Maryland
2200 Kernan Drive
Baltimore, MD 21207
410-448-2924
800-221-6443
Fax: 410-448-3541
info@biamd.org
www.biamd.org

Patricia Janus, President
Diane Tripplet, Executive Director

Massachusetts

4100 Brain Injury Association of Massachusetts
30 Lyman Street
Westborough, MA 01581
508-475-0032
800-242-0030
Fax: 508-475-0400
biama@biama.org
www.biama.org

Shahriar Khaksari, President
Arlene Korab, Executive Director

Michigan

4101 Brain Injury Association of Michigan
7305 Grand River
Brighton, MI 48114-2334
810-229-5880
800-444-6443
Fax: 810-229-8947
info@biami.org
www.biami.org
Our mission is to enhance the lives of those affected by brain injury through education, advocacy, research and local support groups and to reduce the incidence of brain injury through prevention.
Katie Knight, Program Coordinator
Michael F Dabbs, President

Minnesota

4102 Brain Injury Association of Minnesota
34 13th Avenue NE
Minneapolis, MN 55413
612-378-2742
800-669-6442
Fax: 612-378-2789
info@braininjurymn.org
www.braininjurymn.org

20-24 pages
Andrew Kiragu, Board Chairman

Mississippi

4103 Brain Injury Association of Mississippi
2727 Old Canton
Jackson, MS 39296-5912
601-981-1021
800-444-6443
Fax: 601-981-1039
info@msbia.org
www.msbia.org

Howard T Katz, Chairman
Lee Jenkins, Executive Director

Missouri

4104 Brain Injury Association of Missouri
10270 Page Avenue
Saint Louis, MO 63132-1322
314-426-4024
800-444-6443
Fax: 314-426-3290
info@biamo.org
www.biamo.org

Information and referral services and support groups through the state of Missouri.
John Bennett, President of the Board
Terrie Price, VP

Montana

4105 Brain Injury Association of Montana
1280 S 3rd W
Missoula, MT 59801
406-541-6442
800-241-6442
Fax: 406-541-4360
biam@biamt.org
www.biamt.org

Bobbi Perkins, President
Kristen Morgan, Program Director

New Hampshire

4106 Brain Injury Association of New Hampshire
109 N State Street
Concord, NH 03301
603-225-8400
800-773-8400
Fax: 603-228-6749
mail@bianh.org
www.bianh.org

Brant Elkind, President
Steven Wade, Executive Director

New Jersey

4107 Brain Injury Association of New Jersey
825 Georges Road
N Brunswick, NJ 08902
732-745-0200
800-669-4323
Fax: 732-745-0211
info@bianj.org
www.bianj.org

Barbara Parker, President

New Mexico

4108 Brain Injury Association of New Mexico
3234 Candelaria NE
Albuquerque, NM 87107
505-292-7414
88 - 2 - 74
Fax: 505-271-8983
info@braininjurynm.org
www.braininjurynm.org

John Tiwald, Board President
Mark Pedrotty, VP

New York

4109 Brain Injury Association of New York State
10 Colvin Avenue
Albany, NY 12206-1242
518-459-7911
800-228-8201
Fax: 518-482-5285
info@bianys.org
www.bianys.org

Marie Cavallo, President
Judith Avner, Executive Director

4110 RRTC on Community Integration of Persons with TBI
2323 S Shepherd
Houston, TX 77019
713-630-0526
800-732-8124
Fax: 713-630-0529
terri.hudler-hull@memorialhermann.org
www.tbicommunity.org
Karen A Hart PhD, Director Of Training
Sunil Kothari, Medical Director

North Carolina

4111 Brain Injury Association of North Carolina
2113 Cameron Street
Raleigh, NC 27605
919-833-9634
800-377-1464
Fax: 919-833-5415
bianc@bianc.net
www.tbicommunity.org

Cindy Boyd, Board Chairman
Sandra Farmer, President

Ohio

4112 Brain Injury Association of Ohio
855 Grand View Avenue
Columbus, OH 43215-1123
614-481-7100
866-644-6242
Fax: 614-481-7103
help@biaoh.org
www.biaoh.org

Jon Fishpaw, President
Suzanne Minnich, Executive Director

Oklahoma

4113 Brain Injury Association of Oklahoma
PO Box 88
Hillsdale, OK 73743-0088
580-233-4363
800-444-6443
Fax: 580-233-4546
brainhelp@braininjuryoklahoma.org˜
www.braininjuryoklahoma.org

Tracy Grammer, President
Gary Clarke, Chairman

Oregon

4114 Brain Injury Association of Oregon
PO Box 549
Molalla, OR 97038
503-740-3155
800-544-5243
Fax: 503-961-8730
info@biaoregon.org
www.biaoregon.org

Tootie Smith, President
Sherry Stock, Executive Director

Pennsylvania

4115 Brain Injury Association of Pennsylvania
950 Walnut Bottom Road
Carlisle, PA 17015
717-657-3601
866-635-7097
Fax: 717-692-5567
info@biapa.org
www.biapa.org

Drew Nagele, Chairman of Board Development Committee
Stewart L Cohen, Chairman

Rhode Island

4116 Brain Injury Association of Rhode Island
935 Park Avenue
Cranston, RI 02910-2743
401-461-6599
Fax: 401-461-6561
braininjuryctr@biaofri.org

Michael Baker, Co-President
Colleen McCarthy, Co-President

South Carolina

4117 Brain Injury Association of South Carolina
800 Dutch Square Boulevard
Columbia, SC 29210
803-731-9823
877-TBI-FACT
Fax: 803-731-4804
scbraininjury@bellsouth.net
www.biausa.org/sc

Elaine Phillips, President
Joyce Davis, Executive Director

Tennessee

4118 Brain Injury Association of Tennessee
955 Woodland St
Nashville, TN 37206
615-248-5878
877-757-2428
Fax: 615-383-1176
biaoftn@yahoo.com
www.biaoftn.org

Guynn Edwards, President
Pam Bryan, Executive Director

Texas

4119 Brain Injury Association of Texas
316 W 12th Street
Austin, TX 78701
512-326-1212
800-392-0040
Fax: 512-478-3370
www.biatx.org

Jane Boutte, President

Utah

4120 Brain Injury Association of Utah
1800 S W Temple
Salt Lake City, UT 84115
801-484-2240
800-281-8442
Fax: 801-484-5932
biau@sisna.com
www.biau.org

Teresa Such-Niebar, President
Ron S Roskos, Executive Director

Vermont

4121 Brain Injury Association of Vermont
92 S Main Street
Waterbury, VT 05676
802-244-6850
877-856-1772
Fax: 802-244-4005
support1@biavt.org
www.biavt.org

Marsha Bancroft, President
Trevor Squirrell, Executive Director

Virginia

4122 Brain Injury Association of America's National Family Helpline
1608 Spring Hill Road
Vienna, VA 22182
703-761-0750
800-444-6443
Fax: 703-761-0755
FamilyHelpline@biausa.org
www.biausa.org

Greg Oshanick, Chairman
Susan Conners, President and CEO

4123 Brain Injury Association of Virginia
1506 Willow Lawn Drive
Richmond, VA 23230
804-355-5748
800-444-6443
Fax: 804-355-6381
info@biav.net
www.biav.net

Anne McDonnell, Executive Director
Lynette Scott, Program Director

Washington

4124 Brain Injury Association of Washington
800 Jefferson Street
Seattle, WA 98104
206-388-0900
800-523-5438
Fax: 206-388-0901
info@biawa.org
www.biawa.org

Richard Adler, President
Gene van den Bosch, Executive Director

West Virginia

4125 Brain Injury Association of West Virginia
PO Box 574
Institute, WV 25112-0574
304-766-4892
800-356-6443
Fax: 304-766-4940
mdavis@brainman.com

Michael W Davis, Board of Director
Linda Arthur, Board of Director

Wisconsin

4126 Brain Injury Association of Wisconsin
21100 W Capitol Drive
Pewaukee, WI 53072
262-790-9660
800-882-9282
Fax: 262-790-9670
admin@execpc.com
www.biaw.org

Advocacy, education, prevention, information, resources, and support groups in regards to traumatic brain injury.
David Voss, President
Mark Warhus, Executive Director

Wyoming

4127 Brain Injury Association of Wyoming
111 W 2nd Street   307-473-1767
Casper, WY 82601   800-643-6457
                                                       Fax: 307-237-5222

Larry Plemmons, President
Jack Nokes, Director

Foundations

4128 Brain Trauma Foundation
708 Third Avenue   212-772-0608
New York, NY 10017-4201   Fax: 212-772-2035
                                                       info@braintrauma.org
                                                       www.braintrauma.org
Our goal at the Brain Trauma Foundation is to improve the outcome of TBI patients through Guideline development, clinical research, professional education, and quality improvement programs.
Quarterly
Jamshid Ghajar, MD, President
Pamela Drexel, Executive Director

Research Centers

4129 Brady Institute Jamaica Hospital Medical Center
Jamaica Hospital Medical Center
8900 Van Wyck Expressway   718-206-6000
Jamaica, NY 11418-2897   Fax: 718-206-6559
                                                       www.jamaicahospital.org
The James and Sarah Brady Institute for Traumatic Brain Injury.
David P Rosen, President & CEO
Neil Foster Phillips, Chairman

4130 Dana Alliance for Brain Initiatives
745 Fifth Avenue   212-223-4040
New York, NY 10151   Fax: 212-317-8721
                                                       danainfo@dana.org
                                                       www.dana.org
A non-profit organization of more than 250 neuroscientists which was formed to help provide information about the personal and public benefits of brain research.
Jane Nevins, Vice President
Edward F Rover, President

4131 Institute for Rehabilitation and Research
1333 Moursund Street   713-799-5000
Houston, TX 77030   800-447-3422
                                                       Fax: 713-874-1798
                                                       tirr.referrals@memorialhermann.org
                                                       www.tirr.org
Carl Josehart, CEO
Gerard F. Francisco, Chief Medical Officer

4132 New York University Medical Center Head Trauma Program
Reet   212-998-9819
New York, NY 10010-4020   Fax: 212-340-7158
Research pertaining to young adults suffering from head injuries.
Dr Yehuda Ben-Yishay, Coordinator

4133 Ohio State University Laboratory of Psychobiology
1835 Neil Avenue   614-292-8185
Columbus, OH 43210-1222   Fax: 614-292-4537
                                                       www.psy.ohio-state.edu/labs
Studies done on recovery of function after brain damage.
Laura Peterson, Lab Coordinator
James Walton, Research Associate

4134 Rehabilitation Institute of Michigan
261 Mack Avenue   313-745-1203
Detroit, MI 48201   Fax: 313-745-2376
                                                       www.rimrehab.org

Physical medicine and rehabilitation medicine.
William H Restum PhD, President
Horacio Varg Jr, Interim Executive Director

4135 Thomas Jefferson University Ischemia-Shock Research Center
1020 Locust Street   215-503-4400
Philadelphia, PA 19107-6731   Fax: 215-503-9920
                                                       jgsbs-info@jefferson.edu
                                                       www.jefferson.edu
Promotes research into head injuries and clinical studies.

4136 Thomas Jefferson University Ischemia-Shock
1020 Walnut Street   215-955-6000
Philadelphia, PA 19107   Fax: 215-923-7932
                                                       www.jefferson.edu
Promotes research into head injuries and clinical studies.

4137 Tulane University: US-Japan Biomedical Research Laboratories
1430 Tulane Avenue   504-988-5187
New Orleans, LA 70112   Fax: 504-394-7169
                                                       medsch@tulane.edu
                                                       www.tulane.edu/som/
Focuses research efforts on neuroendocrinology and neurosciences.
Benjamin P Sachs, MB, BS, Senior Vice President, Dean
Mary Brown, MBA, Vice President

4138 UCLA Neuropsychiatric Institute
760 Westwood Plaza   310-825-2631
Los Angeles, CA 90095   800-825-9989
                                                       Fax: 310-825-9179
                                                       pwhybrow@mednet.ucla.edu
                                                       www.semel.ucla.edu
Devote to teach research and patient care in psychiatry neuroscience and related fields.
Peter Whybrow, Director

4139 University of California: Irvine Brain Imaging Center
101 The City Drive S   949-824-7872
Irvine, CA 92697-3960   Fax: 949-824-7873
                                                       BIC@msx.hsis.uci.edu
Offers PET scan analysis of brain functions focusing on brain damage brain tumors and head injuries.
Steven L Small, PhD, MD, Director
David B Keator, MCS, Technical Director

4140 University of California: San Francisco Laboratory for Neurotrauma
1001 Potrero Avenue   415-206-8313
San Francisco, CA 94110-3518   www.ucsf.edu
Research done into traumatic brain and head injuries.
Lawrence H Pitts MD

4141 University of Memphis: Department of Psych ology
Memphis State University
202 Psychology Building   901-678-2000
Memphis, TN 38152   Fax: 901-678-2579
                                                       psycadvise@memphis.edu
                                                       www.memphis.edu/psychology/
Evaluation and development of assessment and treatment procedures for neurologically impaired persons.
Guy Mittleman, Professor Director of CAPR
Frank Andrasik, Professor, Chair

4142 Virginia Commonwealth University: Rehab Research and Training Center
1314 W Main Street   804-828-1851
Richmond, VA 23284-2011   Fax: 804-828-2193
                                                       TTY: 804-828-2494
                                                       www.vcu.edu/rrtcweb/
Focuses research on traumatic brain and head injuries.
Paul Wehman, Director
Jeanne Dalton, Public Relations Assistant Specialist

4143 Wayne State University: Gurdjian-Lissner Biomechanics Laboratory
Department of Neurological Surgery
4160 John R Street   313-831-0777
Detroit, MI 48201   877-486-7978
                                                       Fax: 313-966-0368
                                                       www.neurosurgery.med.wayne.edu

Head and neck injury research.
Murali Guthikonda, MD, FACS, Professor (Clinician-Educator) and Chair
Patti Bekowies, MBA, Chief Administrative Officer

Support Groups & Hotlines

4144 National Health Information Center
Office of Disease Prevention & Health Promotion
1101 Wootton Pkwy
Rockville, MD 20852

Fax: 240-453-8281
odphpinfo@hhs.gov
www.health.gov/nhic

Supports public health education by maintaining a calendar of National Health Observances; helps connect consumers and health professionals to organizations that can best answer questions and provide up-to-date contact information from reliable sources; updates on a yearly basis toll-free numbers for health information, Federal health clearinghouses and info centers.
Don Wright, MD, MPH, Director

Alabama

4145 Alabama Head Injury Foundation Helpline
3100 Lorna Road
Hoover, AL 35216-5451

205-823-3818
800-433-8002
Fax: 205-823-4544
ahifl@bellsouth.net
www.ahif.org/

The Alabama Head Injury Foundation (AHIF) was founded by professionals and families in 1983 to increase public awareness of Traumatic Brain Injury (TBI) and to stimulate the development of supportive services. AHIF provides accessible resources, services and programs that meet the unique needs of individuals with traumatic brain injury (TBI) as well as spinal cord injury (SCI) in certain programs.
Charles D Priest, Executive Director
Janet Massey, Executive Assistant

Arizona

4146 Brain Injury Association of Arizona
5025 E Washington Street
Phoenix, AZ 85034

602-508-8024
888-500-9165
Fax: 602-508-8285
info@biaaz.org
www.biaaz.org

Information and resources for brain injury survivors and their families. Support group listings available. Educational training, conference for families and survivors, neuro-specific resources and helpline.
Kim Halloran, Executive Director
Jeanne Andersen, Information & Referral Manager

Arkansas

4147 Brain Injury Association of Arkansas Helpl ine
PO Box 26236
Little Rock, AR 72221-6236

501-374-3585
866-610-4841
Fax: 501-918-6595
info@brainassociation.org

Founded in 1980, the Brain Injury Association of America (BIAA) is a national organization serving and representing individuals, families and professionals who are touched by a life-altering, often devastating, traumatic brain injury (TBI). BIAA provides information, education and support through its network of chartered state affiliates, local chapters and support groups across the country to assist the 5.3 million Americans currently living with traumatic brain injury and their families.
Dana Austen, President Arkansas State Office
Kortney E Gold, Vice President

California

4148 Brain Injury Association of California Hel pline
3501 Mall View Road
Bakersfield, CA 93306

661-872-4903
Fax: 661-873-2508
calbiainfo@yahoo.com
www.biacal.org/

Founded in 1980, the Brain Injury Association of America (BIAA) is a national organization serving and representing individuals, families and professionals who are touched by a life-altering, often devastating, traumatic brain injury (TBI). BIAA provides information, education and support through its network of chartered state affiliates, local chapters and support groups across the country to assist the 5.3 million Americans currently living with traumatic brain injury and their families.
Paula Daoutis, Administrative Director
Ursula Pesta, Project Coordinator

4149 Jodi House
625 Chapala St.
Santa Barbara, CA 93101

805-563-2882
Fax: 805-563-3982
info@jodihouse.org
www.jodihouse.org

Jodi House is a community-based, post-rehabilitation day program that provides opportunities for social interaction, life skill training, recreation, and support for adults living with acquired brain injury (i.e. from head trauma, tumor, and stroke) and their families.
Gayle Cummings, Co-President
Timothy Morton-Smith, Co-President/Vice President of Finance

Colorado

4150 Brain Injury Association of Colorado Helpline
1385 South Colorado Boulevard
Denver, CO 80222

303-355-9969
800-955-2443
Fax: 303-355-9968
biacolo@aol.com
www.BIAColorado.org

Dannis Schanel, LCSW, CBIST, President
Gavin Attwood, Exececutive Director

Connecticut

4151 Brain Injury Association of Connecticut Helpline
200 Day Hill Road
Windsor, CT 06095-1304

860-219-0291
800-278-8242
Fax: 860-219-0568
general@biact.org
www.biact.homestead.com/

Supports persons with brain injuries and their families by promoting services to facilitate full inclusion within their local community and to increase awareness and understanding of brain injury and its prevention through community education.
500 Members
Paul A. Slager, Esq., President
Dr. Johnny Magwood, BSME, MBA, DBA, Vice President

Delaware

4152 Brain Injury Association of Delaware Helpl ine
32 West Loockerman Street
Dover, DE 19904

302-346-2083
800-411-0505
Fax: 302-678-3183
www.biaofde.org//

Founded in 1980, the Brain Injury Association of America (BIAA) is a national organization serving and representing individuals, families and professionals who are touched by a life-altering, often devastating, traumatic brain injury (TBI). BIAA provides information, education and support through its network of chartered state affiliates, local chapters and support groups across the country to assist the 5.3 million Americans currently living with traumatic brain injury and their families.
Elizabeth Furber, President Delaware State Office
Timothy J Walker, Vice President

Florida

4153 Brain Injury Association of Florida
1637 Metropolitan Blvd
Tallahassee, FL 32308

850-410-0103
800-992-3442
Fax: 850-410-0105
admin@biaf.org
www.biaf.org

Gary Clarke, Chairman
Valerie Breen, President/CEO

Hawaii

4154 Brain Injury Association of Hawaii
420 Kuwili Street 808-436-8977
Honolulu, HI 96817 biahi@hawaiiantel.net
Dedicated to serving those affected by brain injury throughgh advocacy, prevention, and support
Mary Wilson, Executive Director
Ian Mattoch, President

Illinois

4155 American Brain Tumor Association
8550 W Bryn Mawr Avenue 800-886-2282
Chicago, IL 60631 info@abta.org
www.abta.org
CareLine offered for newly diagnosed patients with brain tumors.
Ralph DeVitto, President & CEO
Nicole Willmarth, PhD, Chief Mission Officer

4156 Brain Injury Association of Illinois Helpline
PO Box 64420 312-726-5699
Chicago, IL 60664-420 800-699-6443
Fax: 312-630-4011
info@biail.org
www.biail.org
Works with all people with brain inquiries and their families with professionals who serve them. Provides camp oppurtunities, support groups, educational seminars, information and referrals and a quarterly newsletter.
Irene Pedersen, Founder
Philicia L Deckard, Executive Director

Indiana

4157 Brain Injury Association of Indiana Helpli ne
9531 Valparaiso Court 317-356-7722
Indianapolis, IN 46268 866-854-4246
Fax: 317-802-1768
info@biai.org
www.biai.org
Founded in 1980, the Brain Injury Association of America (BIAA) is a national organization serving and representing individuals, families and professionals who are touched by a life-altering, often devastating, traumatic brain injury (TBI). BIAA provides information, education and support through its network of chartered state affiliates, local chapters and support groups across the country to assist the 5.3 million Americans currently living with traumatic brain injury and their families.
Nancy Ritter, Chairperson
Anna Garrett, Executive Director

Iowa

4158 Brain Injury Alliance of Iowa Helpline
Brain Injury Association of America
7025 Hickman Road 319-272-2312
Urbandale, IA 50322 855-444-6443
Fax: 319-272-2109
info@biaia.org
www.biaia.org
Geoffrey Lauer, Executive Director
Natasha Retz, Director of Programs and Services

Kansas

4159 Brain Injury Association of Kansas and Greater Kansas City Helpline
6701 W. 64th Street 913-754-8883
Overland Park, KS 66202 800-783-1356
Fax: 816-842-1531
rabramowitz@biaks.org
www.biaks.org
Whitney Sunderland, President
Robin Abramowitz, Executive Director

Kentucky

4160 Brain Injury Alliance of Kentucky
7321 New LaGrange Road 502-493-0609
Louisville, KY 40222 800-592-1117
Fax: 502-426-2993
www.biak.us
Founded in 1980, the Brain Injury Association of America (BIAA) is a national organization serving and representing individuals, families and professionals who are touched by a life-altering, often devastating, traumatic brain injury (TBI). BIAA provides information, education and support through its network of chartered state affiliates, local chapters and support groups across the country to assist the 5.3 million Americans currently living with traumatic brain injury and their families.
Andrew Horne, President Kentucky State Office
Chell Austin, Executive Director

Louisiana

4161 Brain Injury Association of Louisiana Help line
c/o National Headquarters Office
8325 Oak Street 504-982-0685
New Orleans, LA 70118 800-444-6443
Fax: 703-761-0755
info@biala.org
www.biala.org/
Founded in 1980, the Brain Injury Association of America (BIAA) is a national organization serving and representing individuals, families and professionals who are touched by a life-altering, often devastating, traumatic brain injury (TBI). BIAA provides information, education and support through its network of chartered state affiliates, local chapters and support groups across the country to assist the 5.3 million Americans currently living with traumatic brain injury and their families.
Janet Clark, Chairman
Tommy Lotz, Executive Director

Maryland

4162 Brain Injury Association of Maryland Helpl ine
Kernan Hospital
2200 Kernan Drive 410-448-2924
Baltimore, MD 21207 800-221-6443
Fax: 410-448-3541
info@biamd.org
www.biamd.org
Founded in 1980, the Brain Injury Association of America (BIAA) is a national organization serving and representing individuals, families and professionals who are touched by a life-altering, often devastating, traumatic brain injury (TBI). BIAA provides information, education and support through its network of chartered state affiliates, local chapters and support groups across the country to assist the 5.3 million Americans currently living with traumatic brain injury and their families.
Mark Huslage, President Maryland State Office
Bryan Thomas Pugh, Executive Director

Massachusetts

4163 Brain Injury Association of Massachusetts Helpline
30 Lyman Street 508-475-0032
Westborough, MA 01581 800-242-0030
Fax: 508-475-0400
TTY: 508-948-0593
biama@biama.org
www.biama.org
Founded in 1980, the Brain Injury Association of America (BIAA) is a national organization serving and representing individuals, families and professionals who are touched by a life-altering, often devastating, traumatic brain injury (TBI). BIAA provides information, education and support through its network of chartered state affiliates, local chapters and support groups across the country to assist the 5.3 million Americans currently living with traumatic brain injury and their families.
Teresa Hayes, President Massachusetts State Office
Mathew Martino, Executive Board

4164 VALT Support Group (Vital Active Life After Trauma)
53 Linden Street 617-277-6327
Brookline, MA 02149

Michigan

4165 Brain Injury Association of Michigan Helpline
7305 Grand River 810-229-5880
Brighton, MI 48114-2334 800-444-6443
Fax: 810-229-8947
info@biami.org
www.biami.org

Deborah Newton, Chair
Michael F Dabbs, President

Minnesota

4166 Brain Injury Alliance of Minnesota
34 13th Avenue North East 612-378-2742
Minneapolis, MN 55413 800-669-6442
Fax: 612-378-2789
info@braininjurymn.org
www.braininjurymn.org

Tom Gode, Executive Director

Mississippi

4167 Brain Injury Association of Mississippi Helpline
2727 Old Canton Road 601-981-1021
Jackson, MS 39216-5912 800-444-6443
Fax: 601-981-1039
ljenkins@msbia.org
www.msbia.org/

Howard T Katz, MD, Chair
Lee Jenkins, Executive Director

Missouri

4168 Brain Injury Association of Missouri Helpline
2265 Schuetz Road 314-426-4024
St Louis, MO 63146-1322 800-444-6443
Fax: 314-426-3290
info@biamo.org
www.biamo.org
Information and referral services and support groups throughout
the state of Missouri.
Eric Hart, Psy.D, Board President
Stephanie Cooper, Executive Director

Montana

4169 Brain Injury Alliance of Montana
1280 South 3rd Street West 406-541-6442
Missoula, MT 59801 800-241-6442
Fax: 406-243-2349
kristen@biamt.org
www.biamt.org

Kristen Morgan, MSW, Program Director
Molly Walsh, Outreach Coordinator

New Hampshire

4170 Brain Injury Association of New Hampshire
Brain Injury Association of America
109 N State Street 603-225-8400
Concord, NH 03301-4447 800-773-8400
Fax: 603-228-6749
mail@bianh.org
www.bianh.org

Laura Flashman, PhD, President
Steven D Wade, Executive Director

New Jersey

4171 Brain Injury Alliance of New Jersey
Brain Injury Association of America

825 Georges Road 732-745-0200
North Brunswick, NJ 08902 800-669-4323
Fax: 732-745-0211
info@bianj.org
www.bianj.org

Edward Kim, MD, MBA, Chairperson
Barbara Geiger-Parker, President/CEO

New Mexico

4172 Brain Injury Alliance of New Mexico
3232 Candelaria NE 505-292-7414
Albuquerque, NM 87107 888-292-7415
Fax: 505-271-8983
www.braininjurynm.org
Founded in 1980, the Brain Injury Association of America (BIAA)
is a national organization serving and representing individuals,
families and professionals who are touched by a life-altering, often
devastating, traumatic brain injury (TBI). BIAA provides information, education and support through its network of chartered state
affiliates, local chapters and support groups across the country to
assist the 5.3 million Americans currently living with traumatic
brain injury and their families.
John Tiwald, Board President New Mexico State Office
Mark Pedrotty, PhD, Vice President

New York

4173 Brain Injury Association of New York State Helpline
10 Colvin Avenue 518-459-7911
Albany, NY 12206-1242 800-228-8201
Fax: 518-482-5285
info@bianys.org
www.bianys.org

Marie Cavallo, Ph.D, President
Judith Avner, Executive Director

4174 Cafe Plus
216 W Manlius Street 315-446-3124
East Syracuse, NY 13057
For people who have survived a head-injury or some type of head
trauma.
David Listowski, Manager

4175 Hy Feinstein Clubhouse
Long Island Head Injury Association
300 Kennedy Drive 631-543-2245
Hauppauge, NY 11788 Fax: 631-543-2261
lgiordano@headinjuryassoc.org
The LIHIA provides a place for people with head injury to participate in meaningful work, to have the opportunity to meet and build
friendships and ultimately seek employment within the
community.
Stuart Gleiber, President
Leonard Feinstein, Vice President

North Carolina

4176 Brain Injury Association of North Carolina Helpline
2113 Cameron Street 919-833-9634
Raleigh, NC 27605 800-377-1464
Fax: 919-833-5415
bianc@bianc.net
www.bianc.net/

Susan Baker, Director of Finance
Cindy Boyd, Fundraising Chair

North Dakota

4177 Brain Injury Association of North Dakota
1225 South 12th Street 877-525-2724
Bismarck, ND 58504 Fax: 701-845-1175
www.braininjurynd.com/
Founded in 1980, the Brain Injury Association of America (BIAA)
is a national organization serving and representing individuals,
families and professionals who are touched by a life-altering, often
devastating, traumatic brain injury (TBI). BIAA provides information, education and support through its network of chartered state
affiliates, local chapters and support groups across the country to

assist the 5.3 million Americans currently living with traumatic brain injury and their families.
April Fairfield, Executive Director
Rebecca Quinn, Eastern Region Contact

Ohio

4178 Brain Injury Association of Ohio
855 Grandview Avenue   614-481-7100
Columbus, OH 43215-1000   800-444-6443
                                         Fax: 614-481-7103
                                              help@biaoh.org
                                              www.biaoh.org

Stephanie Ramsey, President
Jon Fishpaw, First Vice President

Oklahoma

4179 Brain Injury Association of Oklahoma Helpl ine
3015 E. Skelly Dr.   918-789-0406
Tulsa, OK 74105-0088   800-765-6809
                                         Fax: 918-712-9019
                                   braininjuryoklahoma@gmail.com
                                   www.braininjuryoklahoma.org
Founded in 1980, the Brain Injury Association of America (BIAA) is a national organization serving and representing individuals, families and professionals who are touched by a life-altering, often devastating, traumatic brain injury (TBI). BIAA provides information, education and support through its network of chartered state affiliates, local chapters and support groups across the country to assist the 5.3 million Americans currently living with traumatic brain injury and their families.
Adam Sherman, PhD, President Oklahoma State Office
Mary Dobbs, Vice-President

Oregon

4180 Brain Injury Alliance of Oregon
Brain Injury Association of America
2145 NW Overton Street   503-413-7707
Portland, OR 97210   800-544-5243
                                         Fax: 503-413-6849
                                              biaor@biaoregon.org
                                              www.biaoregon.org
Non-profit providing information and referral, support groups, prevention, education, training, and advocacy for those with brain injury, families, and professionals.
Ralph Wiser, President
Chuck McGilvrary, Vice-President

Rhode Island

4181 Brain Injury Association of Rhode Island H elpline
935 Park Avenue   401-461-6599
Cranston, RI 02910-2743   Fax: 401-461-6561
                                              www.biausa.org/RI/
Founded in 1980, the Brain Injury Association of America (BIAA) is a national organization serving and representing individuals, families and professionals who are touched by a life-altering, often devastating, traumatic brain injury (TBI). BIAA provides information, education and support through its network of chartered state affiliates, local chapters and support groups across the country to assist the 5.3 million Americans currently living with traumatic brain injury and their families.
Michael L. Baker, Co-President
Sharon Brinkworth, Executive Director

Tennessee

4182 Brain Injury Association of Tennessee Help line
955 Woodland Street   615-248-2541
Nashville, TN 37206   800-444-6443
                                         Fax: 615-383-1176
                                              biaoftn@yahoo.com
                                              www.braininjurytn.org/
Founded in 1980, the Brain Injury Association of America (BIAA) is a national organization serving and representing individuals, families and professionals who are touched by a life-altering, often devastating, traumatic brain injury (TBI). BIAA provides informa-

tion, education and support through its network of chartered state affiliates, local chapters and support groups across the country to assist the 5.3 million Americans currently living with traumatic brain injury and their families.
Guynn Edwards, President Tennessee State Office
Pam Bryan, Executive Director

Utah

4183 Brain Injury Alliance of Utah
Brain Injury Association of America
5280 Commerce Dr.   801-716-4993
Murray, UT 84107   800-281-8442
                                         Fax: 801-716-4995
                                              info@biau.org
                                              www.biau.org/

Antonietta Anna Russo, Ph.D., President
Ron S Roskos, Executive Director

Vermont

4184 Brain Injury Association of Vermont Helpli ne
92 South Main Street   802-244-6850
Waterbury, VT 05676   877-856-1772
                                         Fax: 802-244-4005
                                              support1@biavt.org
                                              www.biavt.org
Founded in 1980, the Brain Injury Association of America (BIAA) is a national organization serving and representing individuals, families and professionals who are touched by a life-altering, often devastating, traumatic brain injury (TBI). BIAA provides information, education and support through its network of chartered state affiliates, local chapters and support groups across the country to assist the 5.3 million Americans currently living with traumatic brain injury and their families.
Marsha Bancroft, President Vermont State Office
Trevor Squirrell, Executive Director

Virginia

4185 Brain Injury Association of Virginia Helpline
1506 Willow Lawn Dr   804-355-5748
Richmond, VA 23230-5018   800-444-6443
                                         Fax: 804-355-6381
                                              info@biav.net
                                              www.biav.net
Nonprofit organization providing information and resources related to brain injury to individuals with brain injuries, their families and professionals who deal with brain injury.
Kimberly Moore, President
Anne McDonnell, Executive Director

Washington

4186 Brain Injury Association of Washington Hel pline
P.O. Box 3044   206-467-4800
Seattle, WA 98114   877-982-4292
                                         Fax: 206-467-4808
                                              info@braininjurywa.org
                                              www.braininjurywa.org/
Founded in 1980, the Brain Injury Association of America (BIAA) is a national organization serving and representing individuals, families and professionals who are touched by a life-altering, often devastating, traumatic brain injury (TBI). BIAA provides information, education and support through its network of chartered state affiliates, local chapters and support groups across the country to assist the 5.3 million Americans currently living with traumatic brain injury and their families.
Mark T Long, President Washington State Office
Deborah Crawley, Executive Director

4187 Brain Injury Resource Center
Brain Injury Resource Center
PO Box 84151   206-621-8558
Seattle, WA 98124-5451   Fax: 206-329-4355
                                              brain@headinjury.com
                                              www.headinjury.com

Disseminates head injury information and provides referrals to facilitate adjustment to life following head injury. Organizes seminars for professionals, head injury survivors, and their families.
Constance Miller MA, Founder/President
B Parker Lindner MPA, Communications Specialist

West Virginia

4188 Brain Injury Association of West Virginia Helpline
Brain Injury Association of America
PO Box 574   304-400-4506
Institute, WV 25112-574   800-356-6443
                                        Fax: 304-766-4940
                                        mdavis@brainman.com

Michael W Davis, President

Wisconsin

4189 Brain Injury Alliance of Wisconsin
21100 W. Capitol Dr.   262-790-9660
Brookfield, WI 53072   800-882-9282
                                        Fax: 262-790-9670
                                        admin@execpc.com
                                        www.biaw.org
Founded in 1980, the Brain Injury Association of America (BIAA) is a national organization serving and representing individuals, families and professionals who are touched by a life-altering, often devastating, traumatic brain injury (TBI). BIAA provides information, education and support through its network of chartered state affiliates, local chapters and support groups across the country to assist the 5.3 million Americans currently living with traumatic brain injury and their families.
Audrey Nelson, President Wisconsin State Office
Lori Schultz, Executive Director

Wyoming

4190 Brain Injury Alliance of Wyoming
111 West 2nd Street   307-473-1767
Casper, WY 82601   800-643-6457
                                        Fax: 307-237-5222
                                        www.wybia.org/

Dorothy Cronin, Director

Books

4191 An Educational Challenge: Meeting the Needs of Students with Brain Injury
Brain Injury Association
2775 South Quincy Street   703-998-2020
Arlington, VA 22206   800-444-6443
                                        Fax: 703-236-6001
                                        info@brainline.org
                                        www.brainline.org

Noel Gunther, Executive Director
Christian Lindstrom, Director

4192 Brain Injury Glossary
HDI Publishers
5215 Ashe Rd.   661-872-3408
Bakersfield, CA 93313   800-922-4994
                                        Fax: 661-872-5150
                                        spersel@neuroskills.com
                                        www.neuroskills.com
Contains glossary and descriptions of health care providers.
Mark J. Ashley, President and CEO

4193 Brainlash
Demos Medical Publishing
11 West 42nd Street   212-683-0072
New York, NY 10036   Fax: 212-683-0118
                                        support@demosmedical.com
                                        www.demosmedpub.com
Maximize your recovery from mild brain injury.
376 pages
ISBN: 1-888799-37-4
Dr. Diana M Schneider

4194 Coming Home: A Discharge Manual for Families of Persons with a Brain Injury
HDI Publishers
5215 Ashe Rd.   661-872-3408
Bakersfield, CA 93313   800-922-4994
                                        Fax: 661-872-5150
                                        spersel@neuroskills.com
                                        www.neuroskills.com

Mark J. Ashley, President and CEO

4195 Communication Disorders Following Traumatic Brain Injury
Pro-Ed, Inc.
8700 Shoal Creek Blvd   512-451-3246
Austin, TX 78757-6897   800-897-3202
                                        Fax: 800-397-7633
                                        info@proedinc.com
                                        www.proedinc.com
For graduates and professionals, this text takes a holistic approach toward treating the client with traumatic brain injury.
439 pages Paperback
ISBN: 0-890792-95-X
Lindy Jordaan, Marketing Coordinator

4196 Dano Cerebral: Guia Para Familias y Cuidadores
Brain Injury Association/HDI Publishers/Catalogue
PO Box 131401   800-321-7037
Houston, TX 77219   Fax: 713-526-7787
This book, written in Spanish, is a thorough, well-researched guide for people with brain injury, their families and caregivers. Up-to-date information covers such topics as Intensive Care- admittance and discharge; Mechanics of brain injury; Coma; Consequences of brain injury; Mental and Emotional symptoms among many others.
158 pages 1994

4197 From the Ashes
Phoenix Project
PO Box 84151   206-621-8558
Seattle, WA 98124-5451   brain@headinjury.com
                                        www. headinjury.com
A self-help book that addresses the trauma that comes with a head injury and introduces methods of building a fulfilling and productive life.
108 pages

4198 Handbook of Head Truma: Acute Care to Recovery
Plenum Publishing Corporation
233 Spring Street   212-620-8000
New York, NY 10013-1522   800-221-9369
                                        Fax: 212-463-0742
                                        books@plenum.com

466 pages
ISBN: 0-306439-47-6
Nathan R. Selden, President
Zoher Ghogawala, VP

4199 Head Injury and the Family: A Life and Living Perspective
St. Lucie Press
100 E Linton Boulevard   407-274-9906
Delary Beach, FL 33483   Fax: 407-274-9927
One of the best books written in this area. Easy to read, written with family, caregivers and patients in mind. Includes exercises and vignettes.

4200 Integrating Community Resources
HDI Publishers
540 Gaither Road   301-427-1104
Rockville, MD 20850   800-321-7037
                                        Fax: 713-956-2288
                                        www.ahrq.gov

4201 Living with Brain Injury: A Guide for Families
Brain Injury Association/HDI Publishers/Catalogue
PO Box 131401   512-785-4469
Houston, TX 77219   800-321-7037
                                        Fax: 713-526-7787
                                        www.richardsenelick.com
This book will help readers- families, persons with brain injury and professionals alike- through this uncharted territory. topics include: How brain injury is caused and how it can be treated: Physi-

cal, cognitive and behavioral symptoms; Questions family members commonly ask.
145 pages 1998
Richard C. Senelick, Author

4202 National Directory of Brain Injury Rehabilitatiom
Brain Injury Association
2775 South Quincy Street
Arlington, VA 22206
703-998-2020
800-444-6443
Fax: 703-236-6001
info@brainline.org
www.brainline.org
Desk reference for professionals listing brain injury rehabilitation programs and individual service providers nationwide.
Noel Gunther, Executive Director
Christian Lindstrom, Director

4203 National Directory of Head Injury Rehabilitation Services
Brain Injury Association
2775 South Quincy Street
Arlington, VA 22206
703-998-2020
800-444-6443
Fax: 703-236-6001
info@brainline.org
www.brainline.org
Noel Gunther, Executive Director
Christian Lindstrom, Director

4204 Planning for the Future
Brain Injury Association
2775 South Quincy Street
Arlington, VA 22206
703-998-2020
800-444-6443
Fax: 703-236-6001
info@brainline.org
www.brainline.org
This book provides a meaningful life for a child with a disability after your death.
Noel Gunther, Executive Director
Christian Lindstrom, Director

4205 Recovery from Brain Damage in the Elderly
Aspen Publishers
8600 Rockville Pike
Bethesda, MD 20894-0990
800-638-8437
www.ncbi.nlm.nih.gov
Recovery and rehabilitation techniques in the area of brain damage in the elderly.

4206 Sexuality and the Person with Traumatic Brain Injury
Brain Injury Association
1000 Thomas Jefferson
Washington, DC 20007
202-403-5600
800-444-6443
Fax: 703-236-6001
TTY: 877-334-3499
msktc@air.org
www.msktc.org

4207 Stress Management Following Head Injury: Strategies for Families and Caregivers
Brain Injury Association
2775 South Quincy Street
Arlington, VA 22206
703-998-2020
800-444-6443
Fax: 703-236-6001
info@brainline.org
www.brainline.org
Noel Gunther, Executive Director
Christian Lindstrom, Director

4208 TBI Tool Kit
HDI Publishers
2775 South Quincy Street
Arlington, VA 22206
703-998-2020
800-321-7037
Fax: 713-956-2288
info@brainline.org
www.brainline.org
Noel Gunther, Executive Director
Christian Lindstrom, Director

4209 Traumatic Brain Injury Rehabilitation: Brain Injury Consortium Monograph Series
St. Lucie Press

250 Greenwich St.
New York, NY 10007
212-772-0608
Fax: 407-274-9927
www.braintrauma.org
Assistive technology, under the Americans with Disabilities Act, is that designed for and used by individuals with the intent of eliminating, ameliorating, or compensating for functional limitations. Coverage includes impaired functions that limit vocational outcome, behavior concerns in the workplace, maximizing a client's residual knowledge skills, use of computers and adapting work environments.
Jamshid Ghajar, President
Alan Quasha, Chairman

4210 Traumatic Head Injury: Cause, Consequence and Challenge
Brain Injury Association/HDI Publishers/Catalogue
785 Market St.
San Francisco, CA 94103
800-445-8106
Fax: 713-526-7787
A resource book on traumatic brain injury which translates technical medical information on brain injury into simple, easy-to-understand language for persons with brain injury and their families. Covered topics: a general overview of brain injury; similarities and differences among people with brain injury; types and consequences of brain injury; recovery and rehabilitation; accepting and coping with change.
60 pages 1993
Ping Hao, President
Jacquelyn Kung, VP

4211 Why Did it Happen on a School Day: My Family's Experience with Brain Injury
Brain Injury Association
2775 South Quincy Street
Arlington, VA 22206
703-998-2020
800-444-6443
Fax: 703-236-6001
www.brainline.org
Noel Gunther, Executive Director
Christian Lindstrom, Director

4212 Working After Brain Injury
HDI Publishers
2775 South Quincy Street
Arlington, VA 22206
703-998-2020
800-321-7037
Fax: 713-956-2288
www.brainline.org
Noel Gunther, Executive Director
Christian Lindstrom, Director

Magazines

4213 Journal of Head Trauma Rehabilitation
Aspen Publishers
2001 Market Street
Philadelphia, PA 19103-3129
215-521-8300
800-638-8437
www.lww.com
Scholarly journal designed to provide information on clinical management and rehabilitation of the head-injured for the practicing professional.

Jennifer E. Brogan, Vice President
Kivmars Bowling, Senior Publisher

4214 Mouth Magazine
PO Box 558
Topeka, KS 66601-0558
785-272-2578
Fax: 785-272-7348
www.mouthmag.org
Bi-monthly magazine with subscription.
Lucy Gwin, Editor-designer
Cal Grandy, General Officer

Newsletters

4215 BIAW News
Brain Injury Association of Wisconsin

N63 W23583 Main Street
Sussex, WI 53089

262-790-9660
800-882-9282
Fax: 262-790-9670
admin@biaw.org
www.biaw.org

David Voss, President
Mark Warhus, Executive Director

4216 Brain Injury Source
Brain Injury Association
1608 Spring Hill Road
Vienna, VA 22182

703-761-0750
800-444-6443
Fax: 703-761-0755
www.biausa.org

Written for and by professionals in the field. Blends professionally written articles on information and research in brain injury with a user friendly format that incorporates graphics and charts to effectively deliver the messages. Full color.
50+ pages Quarterly

4217 Brain Waves
Brain Injury Association of Florida
1637 Metropolitan Blvd
Tallahassee, FL 32308

850-410-0103
800-992-3442
Fax: 850-410-0105
admin@biaf.org
www.biaf.org

Each issue highlights a topic related to TBI and TBI resources.
Bi-Annually
Valerie E Breen, President/CEO

4218 Brainstorm
Brain Injury Association of Arizona
5025 E. Washington Street
Phoenix, AZ 85034

602-508-8024
888-500-9165
Fax: 602-323-9165
info@biaaz.org
www.biaaz.org

A newsletter serving persons with brain injury, their families and professionals.
8 pages Quarterly
Robert Djergaian, Board President
Tom Nielsen, Vice President

4219 TBI Challenge!
Brain Injury Association of America
1608 Spring Hill Road
Vienna, VA 22182-3010

703-761-0750
800-444-6443
Fax: 703-761-0755
www.biausa.org

Exclusively for and about persons with brain injury. Provides information to individuals with brain injury and their families. Professionals will benefit from the perspectives provided in Kid's Corner, Relatively Speaking, Ask the Lawyer, Information and Resources and Ask the Doctor.
bimonthly

Pamphlets

4220 A Survey of Accredited and Other Rehabilitation Facilities
Brain Injury Association
6951 East Southpoint Road
Tucson, AZ 85756

703-236-6000
800-444-6443
Fax: 520-318-1129
www.carf.org

Education, training and cognitive rehabilitation in barin injury programs.
Herb Zaretsky, Board Chair

4221 About Head Injuries
Channing L Bete Company
P.O.BOX 84151
Seattle, WA 98124

206-621-8558
800-628-7733
www.headinjury.com

Covers basic information including identifying the members of the treatment team and how to take care of yourself as a caregiver.

4222 Adolescents with Closed Head Injuries: A Report of Initial Cognitive Deficits
Brain Injury Association
P.O.BOX 84151
Seattle, WA 98124

206-621-8558
800-444-6443
Fax: 703-236-6001
www.headinjury.com

4223 Basic Questions About Head Injury & Disability
Brain Injury Association
P.O.BOX 84151
Seattle, WA 98124

206-621-8558
800-444-6443
Fax: 703-236-6001
www.headinjury.com

4224 Behavioral and Psychosocial Sequelae of Pediatric Head Injury
Brain Injury Association
P.O.BOX 84151
Seattle, WA 98124

206-621-8558
800-444-6443
Fax: 703-236-6001

4225 Brain Damage is a Family Affair
Brain Injury Association
P.O.BOX 84151
Seattle, WA 98124

206-621-8558
800-444-6443
Fax: 703-236-6001
www.headinjury.com

4226 Brain Injuries: A Guide for Families & Caretakers
Brain Injury Association
P.O.BOX 84151
Seattle, WA 98124

206-621-8558
800-444-6443
Fax: 703-236-6001
www.headinjury.com

4227 Brain Injury: A Home Based Cognitive Rehabilitation Program
HDI Publishers
2775 South Quincy Street
Arlington, VA 22206

703-998-2020
800-321-7037
Fax: 713-956-2288
info@brainline.org
www.brainline.org

4228 Catastrophic Injury Cases: The Relationship of Traumatic Brain Injury
Brain Injury Association
P.O.BOX 84151
Seattle, WA 98124

206-621-8558
800-444-6443
Fax: 703-236-6001
www.headinjury.com

4229 Children with Disabilities: Understanding Sibling Issues
Brain Injury Association
P.O.BOX 84151
Seattle, WA 98124

206-621-8558
800-444-6443
Fax: 703-236-6001
www.headinjury.com

4230 Counseling Head Injured Patients: Guidelines for Community Health Workers
Brain Injury Association
P.O.BOX 84151
Seattle, WA 98124

206-621-8558
800-444-6443
Fax: 703-236-6001
www.headinjury.com

4231 Education Concerns for the Traumatically Head Injured Student
Brain Injury Association
P.O.BOX 84151
Seattle, WA 98124

206-621-8558
800-444-6443
Fax: 703-236-6001
www.headinjury.com

4232 From One Family Member to Another
Brain Injury Association
P.O.BOX 84151
Seattle, WA 98124

206-621-8558
800-444-6443
Fax: 703-236-6001
www.headinjury.com

A mother tells the story of her son's injury and recovery. Gives suggestions for structuring the home environment.

4233 Guide to Selecting and Monitoring Head Injury Rehabilitation Services
Brain Injury Association
P.O.BOX 84151
Seattle, WA 98124
206-621-8558
800-444-6443
Fax: 703-236-6001
www.headinjury.com

4234 Head Injury Survivor on Campus: Issues & Resources
Brain Injury Association
P.O.BOX 84151
Seattle, WA 98124
206-621-8558
800-444-6443
Fax: 703-236-6001
www.headinjury.com

4235 Head Injury: A Booklet for Families
Brain Injury Association
P.O.BOX 84151
Seattle, WA 98124
206-621-8558
800-444-6443
Fax: 703-236-6001
www.headinjury.com

4236 Head Injury: A Guide for Families
HDI Publishers
P.O.BOX 84151
Seattle, WA 98124
206-621-8558
800-321-7037
Fax: 713-956-2288
www.headinjury.com
Structured by problem with examples and practical coping strategies.

4237 Hearing Loss Following Head Injury
Brain Injury Association
P.O.BOX 84151
Seattle, WA 98124
206-621-8558
800-444-6443
Fax: 703-236-6001
www.headinjury.com

4238 Hiring Persons with a Brain Injury: What to Expect
HDI Publishers
P.O.BOX 84151
Seattle, WA 98124
206-621-8558
800-321-7037
Fax: 713-956-2288
www.headinjury.com

4239 Individual Psychotherapy with the Brain Injured Adult
Brain Injury Association
P.O.BOX 84151
Seattle, WA 98124
206-621-8558
800-444-6443
Fax: 703-236-6001
www.headinjury.com
Review of literature on substance abuse and head injury. Includes statistics, and treatment options, strategies and extensive bibliography.

4240 Information General Sobre: Lesion Cerebral
Brain Injury Association
P.O.BOX 84151
Seattle, WA 98124
206-621-8558
800-444-6443
Fax: 703-236-6001
www.headinjury.com

4241 Introductory Information for Families
Brain Injury Association
P.O.BOX 84151
Seattle, WA 98124
206-621-8558
800-444-6443
Fax: 703-236-6001
www.headinjury.com
A collection of readings on basic information about TBI and a guide for selecting rehabilitation facilities.

4242 Know Your Brain
Nat'l Institute of Neurological Disorders & Stroke
PO Box 5801
Bethesda, MD 20824
301-496-5751
800-352-9424
Fax: 301-402-2186
www.ninds.nih.gov
Basic information about the brain, neuroscience research, and disorders of the brain.

4243 Legal and Financial Issues for Families
Brain Injury Association
P.O.BOX 84151
Seattle, WA 98124
206-621-8558
800-444-6443
Fax: 703-236-6001
www.headinjury.com
Packet designed for families that explores some of the legal and financial issues faced after TBI.

4244 Life After Brain Injury: Who am I
HDI Publishers
2775 South Quincy Street
Arlington, VA 22206
703-998-2020
800-321-7037
Fax: 713-956-2288
info@brainline.org
www.brainline.org
A well-structured book. Dicusses specific problems areas. Includes good examples and gives lists of practical coping strategies.

4245 Mild Brain Injury: Damage and Outcome
Brain Injury Association
P.O.BOX 84151
Seattle, WA 98124
206-621-8558
800-444-6443
Fax: 703-236-6001
www.headinjury.com

4246 Neuropsychology of Attention and Memory
Brain Injury Association
P.O.BOX 84151
Seattle, WA 98124
206-621-8558
800-444-6443
Fax: 703-236-6001
www.headinjury.com

4247 Persisting Problems After Mild Head Injury: A Review of the Syndrome
Brain Injury Association
P.O.BOX 84151
Seattle, WA 98124
206-621-8558
800-444-6443
Fax: 703-236-6001
www.headinjury.com

4248 Post-Traumatic Headaches: Subtypes & Behavioral Treatments
Brain Injury Association
P.O.BOX 84151
Seattle, WA 98124
206-621-8558
800-444-6443
Fax: 703-236-6001
www.headinjury.com

4249 Recovery and Cognitive Retraining After Craniocerebral Trauma
Brain Injury Association
P.O.BOX 84151
Seattle, WA 98124
206-621-8558
800-444-6443
Fax: 703-236-6001
www.headinjury.com

4250 Relationships Between Personality Disorders
Brain Injury Association
P.O.BOX 84151
Seattle, WA 98124
206-621-8558
800-444-6443
Fax: 703-236-6001
www.headinjury.com
Social Disturbances and physical disability following TBI.

4251 Resources List of Organizations
Brain Injury Association
P.O.BOX 84151
Seattle, WA 98124
206-621-8558
800-444-6443
Fax: 703-236-6001
www.headinjury.com

4252 Severe Brain Injury
Brain Injury Association
P.O.BOX 84151
Seattle, WA 98124
206-621-8558
800-444-6443
Fax: 703-236-6001
www.headinjury.com
This pamphlet is in hand out format and would be appropriate for use in clinic or hospital setting.

4253 Spouses of Persons Who Are Brain Injured: Overlooked Victims
Brain Injury Association

P.O.BOX 84151
Seattle, WA 98124

206-621-8558
800-444-6443
Fax: 703-236-6001
www.headinjury.com

4254 Stress Management Following Head Injury: Strategies for Families & Caregivers
Brain Injury Association
P.O.BOX 84151
Seattle, WA 98124

206-621-8558
800-444-6443
Fax: 703-236-6001
www.headinjury.com

4255 Subarachnoid Hemorrhage & Aneurysm
University Hospital & Clinics
269 Hanover Street
Hanover, MA 02339

781-826-5556
888-272-4602
Fax: 781-826-5566
debra@bafound.org
www.bafound.org

This pamphlet includes easy to read, general information plus a glossary and schematic diagrams. This pamphlet would be most appropriate for use with recently head injured patients.
Christine Buckley, Executive Director??
Debra Coulter?, Director of Information Technology

4256 Substance Abuse Task Force White Paper
Brain Injury Association
P.O.BOX 84151
Seattle, WA 98124

206-621-8558
800-444-6443
Fax: 703-236-6001
www.headinjury.com

Review of literature on substance abuse and head injury. Includes statistics, and treatment options, strategies and extensive bibliography.

4257 Susan's Dad: A Child's Story of Head Injury
Brain Injury Association
P.O.BOX 84151
Seattle, WA 98124

206-621-8558
800-444-6443
Fax: 703-236-6001
www.headinjury.com

4258 Teaching Persons with A Brain Injury: What to Expect
HDI Publishers
1608 Spring Hill Road
Vienna, VA 22182

703-761-0750
800-444-6443
Fax: 703-761-0755
www.biausa.org

Daniel S. Chamberlain, Chairman
Susan H. Connors, President and CEO

4259 Unseen Injury: Minor Head Injury
Brain Injury Association
P.O.BOX 84151
Seattle, WA 98124

206-621-8558
800-444-6443
Fax: 703-236-6001
www.headinjury.com

4260 What is Anoxic Brain Injury
Brain Injury Association
P.O.BOX 84151
Seattle, WA 98124

206-621-8558
800-444-6443
Fax: 703-236-6001
www.headinjury.com

4261 When Your Child Goes to School After an Injury
Brain Injury Association
P.O.BOX 84151
Seattle, WA 98124

206-621-8558
800-444-6443
Fax: 703-236-6001
www.headinjury.com

4262 When Your Child is Seriously Injured: The Emotional Impact on Families
Brain Injury Association
P.O.BOX 84151
Seattle, WA 98124

206-621-8558
800-444-6443
Fax: 703-236-6001
www.headinjury.com

4263 Working After A Head Injury
HDI Publishers
1608 Spring Hill Road
Vienna, VA 22182

703-761-0750
800-444-6443
Fax: 703-761-0755
www.biausa.org

Daniel S. Chamberlain, Chairman
Susan H. Connors, President and CEO

Audio & Video

4264 A Fate Better than Death
Brain Injury Association
P.O.BOX 84151
Seattle, WA 98124

206-621-8558
800-444-6443
Fax: 703-236-6001
www.headinjury.com

Video features 4 young adults with traumatic brain injury. Focuses on support groups.

4265 Neuropsychological Assessment: What it Does & Does Not Do
Brain Injury Association
P.O.BOX 84151
Seattle, WA 98124

206-621-8558
800-444-6443
Fax: 703-236-6001
www.headinjury.com

This pamphlet is in hand out format and would be appropriate for use in clinic or hospital setting.

4266 Peter Wegner Is Alive and Well and Living in Providence
Filmakers Library
3212 Duke Street
Alexandria, VA 22314-1798

212-808-4980
Fax: 212-808-4983
sales@alexanderstreet.com
www.filmakers.com

Peter Wegner was a professor at Brown University when he recveived an award in London and was hit by a bus there. The film follows the challenges and decisions faced by his family, in dealing with the serious brain injuries sustained. Comatose, brain surgery, how can a person decide the right path for their loved one? Winner of American Psychology Award. DVD or VHS $195, Classroom Rental $55
VHS or DVD
Sue Oscar, Co-President

4267 Unseen Injury: Minor Head Injury
Brain Injury Association
P.O.BOX 84151
Seattle, WA 98124

206-621-8558
800-444-6443
Fax: 703-236-6001
www.headinjury.com

Designed specifically for viewing by family members.

4268 Surviving Coma: The Journey Back
Brain Injury Association
P.O.BOX 84151
Seattle, WA 98124

206-621-8558
800-444-6443
Fax: 703-236-6001
www.headinjury.com

21 minutes

Web Sites

4269 Agency for Healthcare: Research Facility

www.ahcpr.gov

The Agency for Healthcare Research and Quality's (AHRQ) mission is to produce evidence to make health care safer, higher quality, more accessible, equitable, and affordable, and to work within the U.S. Department of Health and Human Services and with other partners to make sure that the evidence is understood and used.

4270 American Brain Tumor Association

www.abta.org

Provide free social service consultations; a mentorship program for new brain tumor support group leaders; a nationwide database of established support groups; the Connections pen-pal program; networking with organizations that provide services to patients and families; a resource listing of physicians offering inv[e]stgative treatments.

4271 Brain Injury Association of America

www.biausa.org

Seeking to improve the quality of life for people with brain injuries and their families through information and resource referral, legislative advocacy, prevention awareness, and professional education. BIA's mission is to create a better future through brain injury prevention, research, education and advocacy.

4272 Brain Research Institute: Medicine School University of California, Los Angeles

www.bri.ucla.edu

The UCLA Brain Research Institute (BRI) is a catalyst for education, outreach, and research collaborations among current and future scientists, engineers and clinicians who seek to understand the healthy and diseased brain.

4273 Headinjury.Com

www.headinjury.com

Maintained by the Head Injury Hotline, a non-profit clearinghouse founded and operated by head injury activist. The primary goal are to empower through education, resources and support. The basic premise is that the medical system is deeply flawed and that the brain injury rehab industry is no exception. The site integrates resources from diverse organizations including support groups, rehabilitation and research sites.

4274 Healing Well

www.healingwell.com

An online health resource guide to medical news, chat, information and articles, newsgroups and message boards, books, disease-related web sites, medical directories, and more for patients, friends, and family coping with disabling diseases, disorders, or chronic illnesses.

4275 Health Finder

www.healthfinder.gov

Searchable, carefully developed web site offering information on over 1000 topics. Developed by the US Department of Health and Human Services, the site can be used in both English and Spanish.

4276 Healthlink USA

www.healthlinkusa.com

Health information concerning treatment, cures, prevention, diagnosis, risk factors, research, support groups, email lists, personal stories and much more. Updated regularly.

4277 MedicineNet

www.medicinenet.com

An online resource for consumers providing easy-to-read, authoritative medical and health information.

4278 Medscape

www.medscape.com

Medscape offers specialists, primary care physicians, and other health professionals the Web's most robust and integrated medical information and educational tools.

4279 Neurology Channel

www.healthcommunities.com

Find clearly explained, medically accurate information regarding conditions, including an overview, symptoms, causes, diagnostic procedures and treatment options. On this site it is possible to ask questions and get information from a neurologist and connect to people who have similar health interests.

4280 Road Less Traveled

Dedicated to survivors and families of victims of Traumatic Brain Injury.

4281 TBI Help

www.tbihelp.com

Information concerning head injury.

4282 TBI: Traumatic Brian Injury

www.tbi.org

The Perspective Network was changed to TBI in 2015; it provides forums and resources for persons with families, caregivers, friends and the professionals who serve them. Their goals are to promote a sense of community and to increase public awareness of brain injury.

4283 Traumatic Brain Injury

www.traumaticbraininjury.com

Internet resource for education, advocacy, research and support for brain injury survivors, their families, and medical and rehabilitation professionals.

Description

4284 Hearing Impairment

Approximately 48 million Americans have some degree of hearing impairment or deafness. This common problem affects people of all ages, and the loss can range from mild to severe.

Hearing loss is divided into four categories: conductive, sensorineural, mixed and central. Conductive hearing loss is caused by a defect in the external ear canal or middle ear, and can be helped by hearing aids, medical treatment or surgery. Sensorineural hearing loss results from damage to the inner ear and to the auditory nerve that transmits sound waves to the brain. Mixed hearing loss is a combination of conductive and sensorineural defects. Central hearing loss results from impairment of the auditory pathways in the brain that process auditory nerve impulses.

Hearing loss may be present at birth or begin later in life. Causes include infections (such as meningitis), injury, prolonged noise exposure, hereditary diseases and side effects of certain drugs (E.g., aminoglycosides, loop diuretics). Amplification of sound with hearing aids helps almost all persons with mild-to-severe conductive or sensorineural hearing loss. Profoundly deaf persons who cannot be helped by hearing aids may benefit from a cochlear implant, a specialized device inserted into the inner ear. Children with hearing impairments may have slow or inaccurate speech development, or problems with concentration. Early diagnosis usually helps children improve their auditory ability, through the use of hearing aids, educational programs and speech therapy. Hearing loss in adults, if moderate or severe, is usually obvious to the patient family members. In young children, however, the problem is easily overlooked and the opportunity for early intervention can be lost.

National Agencies & Associations

4285 AbleData
103 W. Broad Street
Falls Church, VA 22046
800-227-0216
Fax: 703-356-8314
TTY: 703-992-8313
abledata@neweditions.net
abledata.acl.gov
An information and referral service that uses computer listings and a large file system to answer requests related to assistive devices. Houses a large file system library and contacts with other sources which enables them to answer just about any question.

4286 Academy of Doctors of Audiology
446 East High Street
Lexington, KY 40507
866-493-5544
Fax: 859-271-0607
info@audiologist.org
www.audiologist.org
ADA encourages audiology training programs to include pertinent aspects of hearing aid dispensing in their curriculum.
Stephanie Czuhajewski, Executive Director
Adam Haley, Coordinator, Government Affairs

4287 Academy of Rehabilitative Audiology
ara@audrehab.org
www.audrehab.org
Provides professional education, research, and interest in programs for hearing handicapped persons.
Kristin Vasil-Dilaj, PhD, President

4288 Administration for Children and Families
330 C Street SW
Washington, DC 20201
202-205-8347
Fax: 202-205-9721
www.acf.hhs.gov
The Administration for Children & Families (ACF) is a division of the U.S. Department of Health & Human Services (HHS). ACF promotes the economic and social well-being of families, children, individuals and communities.
Lynn Johnson, Assistant Secretary
Jerry Milner, Acitng Commissioner, Children & Families

4289 Agency for Healthcare Research and Quality
5600 Fishers Lane
Rockville, MD 20857
301-427-1104
www.ahrq.gov
The Agency for Healthcare Research and Quality's (AHRQ) mission is to produce evidence to make health care safer, higher quality, more accessible, equitable, and affordable, and to work within the U.S. Department of Health and Human Services and with other partners to make sure that the evidence is understood and used.
Gopal Khanna, MBA, Director
Howard E. Holland, Director, Communications

4290 Agency for Toxic Substances and Disease Registry
4770 Buford Hwy NE
Atlanta, GA 30341-3717
770-488-0736
800-232-4636
Fax: 770-488-1547
TTY: 888-232-6348
jah8@cdc.gov
www.atsdr.cdc.gov
The Agency for Toxic Substances and Disease Registry (ATSDR), based in Atlanta, Georgia, is a federal public health agency of the U.S. Department of Health and Human Services. ATSDR serves the public by using the best science, taking responsive public health actions, and providing trusted health information to prevent harmful exposures and diseases related to toxic substances.
Patrick Breysse, PhD, CIH, Director
Jack Hanley, Acting Branch Chief, Central Branch

4291 American Academy of Audiology
11480 Commerce Park Drive
Reston, VA 20191
703-790-8466
800-222-2336
Fax: 703-790-8631
infoaud@audiology.org
www.audiology.org
A professional organization of individuals dedicated to providing high quality hearing care to the public. Provides professional development education and research and provides increased public awareness of hearing disorders and audiologic services.
Tanya Tolpegin, Executive Director
Dina Santucci, Senior Director, Business Development

4292 American Academy of Otolaryngology - Head and Neck Surgery
1650 Diagonal Road
Alexandria, VA 22314-3357
703-836-4444
memberservices@entnet.org
www.entnet.org
The missions of the AAO-HNS and its foundation are to advance the art and science of otolaryngology-head and neck surgery through state-of-the-art education, research and learning; and to unite, serve and represent the interests of its members and their families.
Duane J. Taylor, MD, President
James C. Denneny III, MD, Executive Vice President & CEO

4293 American Association of the Deaf-Blind
248 Rainbow Drive
Livingston, TX 77399-2048
AADB-Info@aadb.org
www.aadb.org
Promotes better opportunities and services for deaf-blind people. The mission of this organization is to assure that a comprehensive, coordinated system of services is accessible to all deaf-blind people, enabling them to achieve their maximum potential.
600 Members
Rene Pellerin, President
Mindy Dill, Vice President

4294 American Auditory Society
PO Box 779   877-746-8315
Pennsville, NJ 08070   Fax: 650-763-9185
                                          amaudsoc@comcast.net
                                          www.amauditorysoc.org
Publishes Ear & Hearing and The Bulletin of the American Auditory Society.
Sumitrajit Dhar, PhD, President
Darla M. Eastlack, Executive Director

4295 American Deafness and Rehabilitation Association
6522 Calm River Way   office@adara.org
Louisville, KY 40299   www.adara.org
ADARA is a partnership of national organizations, local affiliates, professional sections, and individual members working together to support social services.
John Gournaris, PhD, President
Charles Sterling, Office Manager

4296 American Society for Deaf Children
PO Box 23   800-942-2732
Woodbine, MD 21797   info@deafchildren.org
                                          www.deafchildren.org
A non-profit, parent-helping-parent organization promoting a positive attitude toward signing and deaf culture. Also provides support, encouragement, and current information about deafness to families with deaf and hard of hearing children.
Avonne Brooker-Rutowski, President
Lisalee Egbert, PhD, Vice President

4297 American Speech-Language-Hearing Association
2200 Research Boulevard   301-296-5700
Rockville, MD 20850   800-638-8255
                                          Fax: 301-296-8580
                                          TTY: 301-296-5650
                                          actioncenter@asha.org
                                          www.asha.org
A professional and scientific organization for speech-language pathologists and audiologists concerned with communication disorders. Provides informational materials and a toll-free HELPLINE number for consumers to inquire about speech, language or hearing disorders.
Arlene A. Pietranton, PhD, CAE, Chief Executive Officer
Elena Plante, PhD, CCC-SLP, Vice President, Science and Research

4298 American Tinnitus Association
PO Box 424049   800-634-8978
Washington, DC 20042-4049   www.ata.org
Provides information about tinnitus and referrals to local contacts/support groups nationwide. Also provides a bibliography service, funds scientific research related to tinnitus and offers workshops to professionals. Works to promote public education.
Torryn Brazell, CAE, CMP, Chief Executive Officer
Jodi Asmus, Communications Specialist

4299 Association of Late-Deafened Adults
8038 Macintosh Lane   815-332-1515
Rockford, IL 61107-5336   TTY: 815-332-1515
                                          info@alda.org
                                          www.alda.org
Serves as a resource and information center for late-deafened adults and works to increase public awareness of the special needs of late-deafened adults.
Richard Brown, President
Cynthia Moynihan, Vice President

4300 Canadian Hard of Hearing Association
75 Albert Street   613-526-1584
Ottawa, Ontario, K1P-5E7   800-263-8068
                                          Fax: 613-526-4718
                                          TTY: 613-526-2692
                                          chhanational@chha.ca
                                          www.chha.ca
Acts as Canada's national voice for all people with hearing loss.
Christopher Sutton, National Executive Director
Karla Wilson, Manager, Administration and Finance

4301 Center for Parent Information & Resources
SPAN

35 Halsey Street   973-642-8100
Newark, NJ 07102   malizo@spannj.org
                                          www.parentcenterhub.org
Serves as a central hub of information and products for Parent Centers that serve children with disabilities. Coordinates training, provides an e-newsletter twice a month, and produces specially designed databases.
Debra A. Jennings, Director
Jessica Wilson, Communications Director

4302 Center on Employment: Rochester Institute of Technology
National Technical Institute for the Deaf
52 Lomb Memorial Drive   585-475-6400
Rochester, NY 14623-5604   TTY: 585-475-6400
                                          ntidcoe@rit.edu
                                          www.ntid.rit.edu/nce
Operated by the National Technical Institute for the Deaf at Rochester Institute of Technology, the NTIC Center on employment was established to promote successful employment of RIT's deaf students and graduates.
John Macko, Director
Lorie Fidurko, Office Assistant

4303 Centers for Medicare & Medicaid Services
7500 Security Boulevard   410-786-3000
Baltimore, MD 21244   877-267-2323
                                          TTY: 866-226-1819
                                          www.cms.gov
U.S. federal agency which administers Medicare, Medicaid, and the State Children's Health Insurance Program.
Seema Verma, Administrator
Tom Corry, Director

4304 Convention of American Instructors of the Deaf
PO Box 377   office.manager@caid.org
Bedford, TX 76095-0377   www.caid.org
An organization that promotes professional development, communication and information among educators of deaf individuals and other interested people.
Christina Yuknis, PhD, President
Chong Min Lee, Communications Officer

4305 Dogs for Better Lives
10175 Wheeler Road   541-826-9220
Central Point, OR 97502   800-990-3647
                                          info@dogsforbetterlives.org
                                          dogsforbetterlives.org
Trains ear dogs to alert deaf persons to certain sounds. Dogs are chosen from pet adoption shelters and assigned on the basis of a prioritized waiting list. Four to five months of training teaches them to alert their masters to a number of sounds. Dogs are also available for autistic children.
Lake Matray, President/CEO
Annette Vitello, Operations Director

4306 EAR Foundation
1817 Patterson Street   615-627-2724
Nashville, TN 37203   800-545-4327
                                          Fax: 615-627-2728
                                          TTY: 615-627-2724
                                          TDD: 615-627-2724
                                          info@earfoundation.org
                                          www.earfoundation.org
A national non-profit organization committed to the goal of better hearing and balance through public and professional education programs including The Meniere's Network and the Young Ears program. The Meniere's Network is a national network of patient outreach.
Amy Nielsen, Associate Director

4307 Hands & Voices
PO Box 3093   303-492-6283
Boulder, CO 80307   parentadvocate@handsandvoices.org
                                          www.handsandvoices.org
Non-profit, parent-led organization supporting families of children who are deaf or hard of hearing with online resources, programs, and chapters across the country.
Janet DesGeorges, Executive Director
Lisa Kovacs, Director, Programs

4308 Hands Organization: Advocacy Network for the Deaf and Hearing Impaired
Advocacy Network For The Deaf And Hearing Impaired
PO Box 17755 773-978-8552
Chicago, IL 60617-0755 TTY: 773-978-8552
Advocacy for the deaf and hearing impaired; information and referrals educational events sign language summer youth camps and newsletters.

4309 Hear Now: Starkey Hearin Foundation
The Starkey Hearing Foundation
6700 Washington Avenue S 866-354-3254
Eden Prairie, MN 55344 Fax: 952-828-6900
info@StarkeyFoundation.org
www.sotheworldmayhear.org
Committed to making technology accessible to deaf and hard of hearing individuals throughout the United States. Also raises funds to provide hearing aids, cochlear implants and related services to children and adults who have hearing losses.
Richard Brown, President
Brady Forseth, Executive Director

4310 Hearing Education and Awareness for Rocker s
1405 Lyon Street 415-409-3277
San Francisco, CA 94115 Fax: 415-552-4296
TTY: 415-476-7600
hear@hearnet.com
www.hearnet.com
Educates the public about the real dangers of hearing loss resulting from repeated exposure to excessive noise levels.
Kathy Peck, Executive Director
John Doyle, Secretary

4311 Hearing Health Foundation
363 Seventh Avenue 212-257-6140
New York, NY 10001 TTY: 888-435-6104
info@hhf.org
www.hearinghealthfoundation.org
The nation's largest voluntary health organization entirely committed to public awareness and support for basic and clinical research into deafness and hearing disabilities. Sponsors a broad program of innovative research and education.
Nadine Deghan, CEO
Laura Friedman, Communications & Programs Manager

4312 Hearing Industries Association
777 6th Street NW 202-975-0905
Washington, DC 20001 www.hearing.org
HIA represents hearing aid manufacturers, suppliers, distributors, and hearing health professionals.
Kate Carr, President
Carole Rogin, Strategic Advisor

4313 Hearing Loss Association of America
7910 Woodmont Avenue 301-657-2248
Bethesda, MD 20814-3079 Fax: 301-913-9413
TTY: 301-657-2248
info@hearingloss.org
www.hearingloss.org
Promotes awareness and information about hearing loss communication assistive devices and alternative communication skills through publications exhibits and presentations.
Barbara Kelley, Executive Director

4314 Helen Keller National Center for Deaf/Blind Youth and Adults
141 Middle Neck Road 516-944-8900
Sands Point, NY 11050-1299 Fax: 516-944-7302
TTY: 516-944-8637
hkncinfo@hknc.org
www.hknc.org
The national center and its 10 regional offices providing diagnostic evaluations comprehensive vocational and personal adjustment training and job preparation and placement for people who are deaf/blind from every state and territory.

4315 House Ear Institute
2100 W 3rd Street 213-483-4431
Los Angeles, CA 90057 800-388-8612
Fax: 213-483-8789
TTY: 213-484-2642
TDD: 213-484-2642
info@hei.org
www.hei.org
A national non-profit otologic research and educational institute that provides information on hearing and balance disorders.
John W House MD, President
James D Boswell, CEO

4316 International Hearing Dog
5901 E 89th Avenue 303-287-3277
Henderson, CO 80640 Fax: 303-287-3425
TTY: 303-287-3277
TDD: 303-287-3277
info@hearingdog.org
www.ihdi.org
Trains dogs to hear for deaf persons - telephones, doorbells, babies etc.
Samuel Cheris, Chairman
Valerie Foss-Brugger, President/ Executive Director

4317 International Hearing Society
16880 Middlebelt Road 734-522-7200
Livonia, MI 48154 800-521-5247
Fax: 734-522-0200
tom.higgins8@verizon.net
www.ihsinfo.org
A nonprofit professional association which represents Hearing Instrument Specialists in the United States, Canada and several other countries. The society is recognized for promoting and maintaining the highest possible standards for its members.
Richard Giles, President
Kathleen Mennillo, Executive Director

4318 John Tracy Clinic
806 W Adams Boulevard 213-748-5481
Los Angeles, CA 90007-2505 800-522-4582
Fax: 213-749-1651
TTY: 213-747-2924
www.jtc.org/
An educational facility for preschool age children who have hearing losses and their families. In addition to on-site services worldwide correspondence courses in English and Spanish are offered to parents whose children are of preschool age and are hard of hearing.
Michael D. Barker, Chair
J. Gaston Kent, President and Chief Executive Officer

4319 Listening and Spoken Language Knowledge Ce nter
3417 Volta Place NW 202-337-5220
Washington, DC 20007 Fax: 202-337-8314
TTY: 202-337-5221
info@agbell.org
www.listeningandspokenlanguage.org/
The world's oldest and largest membership organization promoting the use of spoken language by children and adults who are hearing impaired. Members include parents of children with hearing loss, adults who are deaf or hard of hearing and educators.
Lyn Robertson, Ph.D., President
Alexander T Graham, Executive Director/CEO

4320 National Association of the Deaf
8630 Fenton Street 301-587-1788
Silver Spring, MD 20910-4500 Fax: 301-587-1791
nad.info@nad.org
www.nad.org
The nation's largest constituency organization safeguarding the accessibility and civil rights of 28 million deaf and hard of hearing Americans in education, employment, health care and telecommunications. A private, nonprofit organization.
Howard A. Rosenblum, CEO
Lizzie Sorkin, Director, Communications

4321 National Captioning Institute
3725 Concorde Parkway
Chantilly, VA 20151
703-917-7600
Fax: 703-917-9853
TTY: 703-917-7600
jagudelo@ncicap.org
www.ncicap.org

Advocates captioned television for people who want to see, as well as hear, the dialogue of a television program. It not only enables deaf and hard-of-hearing people to understand all of a program's content but it is also beneficial for new Americans learning English.
Gene Chao, President, CEO
Drake Smith, Chief Technology Officer

4322 National Center for Voice and Speech: University of Iowa
The University Of Iowa
250 Hawkins Drive
Iowa City, IA 52242
319-335-6600
Fax: 319-335-6603
ingo-titze@uiowa.edu
www.ncvs.org

This is a consortium of institutions focusing on voice and speech disorders. The members of this consortium are the University of Iowa, the Denver Center for Performing Arts, the University of Wisconsin-Madison and the University of Utah.
Ingo Titze PhD, Executive Director
Lynn Maxfield, PhD, Associate Director

4323 National Consortium on Deaf-Blindness
Teaching Research
345 N Monmouth Avenue
Monmouth, OR 97361
800-438-9376
Fax: 503-838-8150
TTY: 800-854-7013
info@nationaldb.org
www.nationaldb.org

Collects organizes and disseminates information related to children and youth who are deaf-blind and connects consumers of deaf-blind information to sources of information about deaf-blindness assistive technology and deaf-blind people.
John Reiman
Kathy McNulty

4324 National Family Association for Deaf-Blind
141 Middle Neck Road
Sands Point, NY 11050
800-225-0411
Fax: 516-883-9060
NFADB@aol.com
www.nfadb.org

NFADB advocates for all persons who are deaf-blind of any chronological age and cognitive ability, supports national policy to benefit people who are deaf-blind, encourages the founding and strengthening of family organizations in each state and shares information.
Clara Berg, President
Dr Stephanie Smith, VP

4325 National Human Genome Research Institute
Building 31, Room 4B09
Bethesda, MD 20892-2152
301-402-0911
Fax: 301-402-2218
www.genome.gov

The National Human Genome Research Institute began as the National Center for Human Genome Research (NCHGR), which was established in 1989 to carry out the role of the National Institutes of Health (NIH) in the International Human Genome Project (HGP).
Eric D. Green, M.D., Ph.D., Director
Lawrence Brody, Ph.D., Director, Division of Genomics & Society

4326 National Institute of Biomedical Imaging and Bioengineering
9000 Rockville Pike
Bethesda, MD 20892
301-496-8859
info@nibib.nih.gov
www.nibib.nih.gov

The mission of the National Institute of Biomedical Imaging and Bioengineering (NIBIB) is to improve health by leading the development and accelerating the application of biomedical technologies.
Bruce J. Tromberg, PhD, Director
Jill Heemskerk, PhD, Deputy Director

4327 National Institute of Environmental Health Sciences
105 T.W. Alexander Drive
Research Triangle Park, NC 27709
919-541-3345
webcenter@niehs.nih.gov
www.niehs.nih.gov

The mission of the NIEHS is to discover how the environment affects people in order to promote healthier lives.
Linda S. Birnbaum, PhD, Director
Richard Woychik, PhD, Deputy Director

4328 National Institute on Deafness and other Communication Disorders
National Institutes Of Heath
31 Center Drive
Bethesda, MD 20892-2320
301-496-7243
800-241-1044
Fax: 301-402-0018
TTY: 800-241-1055
nidcdinfo@nidcd.nih.gov
www.nidcd.nih.gov

A national resources center for information about hearing, balance, smell, taste, voice, speech and language.
Dr. James F Battey, Jr., M.D., Ph.D, Director
Marin Allen PhD, Chief Office of Health Communication

4329 National Organization for Hearing Research Foundation
P.O. Box 421
Narberth, PA 19072
610-649-6114
Fax: 610-668-1428
TTY: 610-664-3135
info@nohrfoundation.org
www.nohrfoundation.org

This organization is a nonprofit private foundation seeking to fund exceptional researchers with $5 000 seed money grants.

4330 Rainbow Alliance of the Deaf
PO Box 1616
Langley, WA 98260
www.deafrad.org

A national organization serving the deaf gay and lesbian community. Represents approximately 24 chapters throughout the United States Canada and Europe.
Henry Carter, President
Steven Schumacher, Secretary

4331 Registry of Interpreters for the Deaf
333 Commerce Street
Alexandria, VA 22314
703-838-0030
Fax: 703-838-0454
TTY: 703-838-0459
ridinfo@rid.org
www.RID.org

A membership organization with almost 4 000 members including professional interpreters and translators persons with deafness or hearing impairments and professionals in related fields.
Brenda Walker Prudhom, President/Board of Directors
Shane H. Feldman, Executive Director

4332 Society of Hearing Impaired Physicians
1999 Mowry Avenue
Fremont, CA 94538-1622
510-797-2939
Fax: 510-797-0168
fphship@aol.com

This Society aids and assists physicians medical students and prospective medical students whose hearing impairment may necessitate different tools and/or approaches to medical practice and training.

4333 Telecommunications for the Deaf
8630 Fenton Street
Silver Spring, MD 20910
301-589-3786
Fax: 301-589-3797
TTY: 301-589-3006
www.tdi-online.org

A nonprofit consumer advocacy organization promoting full visual and other access to information and telecommunications for people who are deaf, hard of hearing, deaf-blind and speech impaired.
Claude Stout, Executive Director
Scott Recht, Business Manager

4334 Tripod
1727 W Burbank Boulevard
Burbank, CA 91506
818-972-2080
Fax: 818-972-2090
TTY: 818-972-2080
info@tripod.org
www.tripod.org

TRIPOD is a nonprofit organization dedicated to providing support and services for deaf and hard of hearing children and their families. TRIPOD offers model local educational programs, Montessori, bilingual parent, infant, toddler and preschool programs.

4335 U.S. Food and Drug Administration
10903 New Hampshire Avenue   301-796-8240
Silver Spring, MD 20993-0002   888-463-6332
                                      www.fda.gov
FDA is responsible for protecting the public health by assuring the safety, efficacy and security of human and veterinary drugs, biological products, medical devices, the nation's food supply, cosmetics, and products that emit radiation.
Norman E. Sharpless, MD, Commissioner
Denise Hinton, Chief Scientist

4336 USA Deaf Sports Federation
PO Box 22011   HomeOffice@usdeafsports.org
Santa Fe, NM 87502   www.usdeafsports.org
A governing body for all deaf sports and recreation in the United States.
Jeffrey L. Salit, President
Brianne Burger, Secretary

State Agencies & Associations

Alabama

4337 Alabama Institute for Deaf and Blind
205 East South Street   256-761-3200
Talladega, AL 35160   Fax: 256-761-3344
                                 TTY: 256-761-3200
                                 mascia.john@aidb.state.al.us
                                 www.aidb.org
Dr. John Mascia, President
Dr. Frieda Meacham, Vice President, Instructional Programs

Arizona

4338 Arizona Association of the Deaf
5025 N Central Avenue   tposedly@aol.com
Phoenix, AZ 85012   www.azadinc.org
This organization shall be organized and operated exclusively to promote the welfare of deaf and hard of hearing residents of the state of Arizona in education, economic, security, social equality, and just rights and privileges as citizens.
Tom Buell, President
Joy Saunders, Vice President

Arkansas

4339 Arkansas Association of the Deaf
26 Corporate Hill Drive   hdketchum@aol.com
Little Rock, AR 72205   www.arkad.org
The mission of the Arkansas Association of the Deaf is to promote the educational, economic, and social welfare of Arkansans who are deaf or hard of hearing.
Holly Ketchum, President
Billie Jordan, 1st Vice President

District of Columbia

4340 Shiloh Senior Center for the Hearing Impaired
913 P Street NW   202-232-1425
Washington, DC 20001   TTY: 202-667-9779
Senior programs, sponsored by the DC Office on Aging in co-ordination with grantee: Shiloh Baptist Church serving the entire Metro Washington area's deaf and hard-of-hearing senior citizens.

Florida

4341 Florida Association of the Deaf
7852 Mansfield Hollow Rd.   june@fadcentral.org
Delray Beach, FL 33446   www.fadcentral.org

The mission of the Florida Association of the Deaf is to promote, protect, and preserve the rights and quality of life of Deaf and hard of hearing individuals in the state of Florida.
June McMahon, President
Lissette Molina, Vice President

Georgia

4342 Georgia Association of the Deaf
PO Box 615   turqcat9992000@yahoo.com
Hiram, GA 30141-1616   www.gadeaf.org
Julie Burton, President
Russell Fleming, Vice President

Illinois

4343 Illinois Association of the Deaf
PO Box 1275   773-237-1877
Oak Park, IL 60304   Fax: 847-740-2319
                                 TTY: 847-740-2319
                                 botz@iadeaf.org
                                 www.iadeaf.org
The Illinois Association of the Deaf is a non-profit, political, educational, social economic, welfare of the deaf, and cultural organization made up of deaf, hard of hearing, and hearing members.
Angela Botz, President
Crystal Kelley Schwartz, Vice-President

Kansas

4344 Kansas Association of the Deaf
PO Box 10085   785-273-0612
Olathe, KS 66051   Fax: 785-273-9063
                                 president@deafkansas.org
                                 www.deafkansas.org
The mission of the Kansas Association of the Deaf a state-wide, non-profit organization is to assure that an extensive, organized system of services is accessible to all deaf or hard of hearing people in Kansas.
Ann Cooper, President
Pam Siebert, Vice-President

Kentucky

4345 Kentucky Association of the Deaf
1707 Richmond Drive   Fax: 606-272-7747
Louisville, KY 40205-1407   TTY: 606-223-3999
                                 www.kydeaf.org
The mission of the Kentucky Association of the Deaf is to advocate for the deaf and hard of hearing in Kentucky by promoting equality, accessibility, and quality of life through employment, services, education and welfare.
Sharon White, President
Arlen Finke, Vice-President

Louisiana

4346 Louisiana Association of the Deaf
3112 Valley Creek Drive   225-341-6406
Baton Rouge, LA 70808   Fax: 225-923-1235
                                 TTY: 225 923-1266
                                 info@lad1908.org
                                 www.lad1908.org
Lou Cannon, President
Cindy Robillard, VP

Massachusetts

4347 Massachusetts State Association of the Deaf
PO Box 276   781-388-9114
Reading, MA 01867   Fax: 781-388-9015
                                 TTY: 781-388-9115
                                 MSADeaf@aol.com
                                 www.msad.org
The Massachusetts State Association of the Deaf is a statewide nonprofit organization serving the estimated 350 000 deaf and hard of hearing Massachusetts citizens and their families.
Justine Barros, President
Michelle Donatello, Vice President

Michigan

4348 Michigan Deaf Association
6093 133rd Ave
Saugatuck, MI 49453
Fax: 586-775-0906
info@mideaf.org
www.mideaf.org

MDA is a non-profit, tax exempt organization with a mission to help improve the lives of Deaf and Hard of Heating citizens of Michigan. MDA is affiliated with he National Association of the Deaf whose mission is to promote, protect, and preserve the rights of the deaf and hearing impaired communities.
Scot A Pott, President
Kat Vogtmann, 1st Vice-President

New York

4349 Center for Hearing and Communication
50 Broadway
New York, NY 10004
917-305-7700
Fax: 917-305-7888
TTY: 917-305-7999
www.chchearing.org

A private not-for-profit rehabilitation agency for infants, children and adults who are hard of hearing and deaf. The League's mission is to improve the quality of life for people with all degrees of hearing loss.
Laurie Hanin, Executive Director
Ellen Lafargue, Director Audiology

North Carolina

4350 North Carolina Association of the Deaf
1200 Revolution Mill Drive
Greensboro, NC 27405
919-773-2974
Fax: 919-834-0127
NCAD2011@gmail.com

Christina Bryant, Chairperson

North Dakota

4351 North Dakota Association of the Deaf
1115 11th Avenue North
Fargo, ND 58102
www.nddeaf.org

The North Dakota Association of the Deaf is actively involved in issues affecting Deaf citizens in North Dakota.
Michele Rolewitz, President
Cody Duncan, Vice President

Oklahoma

4352 Oklahoma Association of the Deaf
2737 Sunnybrook Lane
Enid, OK 73703
Mlznull@aol.com
www.ok-oad.org

The purpose of Oklahoma Association of the Deaf is to promote the interests of the deaf and to advance the social, educational, cultural and economic well-being of the deaf.
Lynn Null, President
Ka Ann Varner, Vice President

Oregon

4353 Oregon Association of the Deaf
999 Locust Street NE
Salem, OR 97301
www.deaforegon.com

The Oregon Association of the Deaf is a non-profit organization working toward a better life for the deaf. Their mission is to create an opportunity for the Deaf of Oregon to join together in planning, devising, conducting and participating in activities.
Daniel Sloan, Committee
Wendy Stanley, Committee

Rhode Island

4354 Rhode Island Association of the Deaf
PO Box 40853
Providence, RI 02940
riadsec@gmail.com
www.riadeaf.blogspot.in/

Heather Niedbala, Vice-President
Neil Leahey, Treasurer

Texas

4355 Texas Association of the Deaf
PO Box 1982
Manchaca, TX 78652-3570
www.deaftexas.org

Texas Association of the Deaf is an organization for persons who are deaf or hard of hearing. It is a membership organization to provide information and education including surveys and studies to bring the viewpoint on various issues affecting the lives of the deaf and hearing impaired.
Steve C Baldwin, President
Chris Kearney, VP

Virginia

4356 National Science Foundation
4201 Wilson Blvd
Arlington, VA 22230
703-292-5111
TDD: 703-292-5090
info@nsf.gov
www.nsf.gov

NSF is the only federal agency whose mission includes support for all fields of fundamental science and engineering, except for medical sciences.
France A. Cordova, Director
Joan Ferrini-Mundy, Chief Operating Officer

4357 Virginia Association of the Deaf
5251 College Drive
Dublin, VA 24084
757-587-9555
Fax: 757-461-5376
TTY: 757-461-7527
vadpresident007@yahoo.com
www.vad.org

LaDonna Larsen, President
Chuck Kelley, VP

Wisconsin

4358 Wisconsin Association of the Deaf
PO Box 114
Delavan, WI 53115-4230
608-825-9791
TTY: 414-607-3297
wisdeaf@gmail.com
www.wisdeaf.org/

The mission of the Wisconsin Association of the Deaf is to ensure that a comprehensive and coordinated system of resources is accessible to Wisconsin people who are deaf or hard of hearing, enabling them to achieve their maximum potential.
Jenny Buechner-Madison, President
Steph Buell, Vice President

Wyoming

4359 Deaf Association of Wyoming
PO Box 20107
Cheyenne, WY 82003
307-635-1125

The Deaf Association of Wyoming is a state non-profit organizations; which is associated with the Association of the Deaf. Membership is open to all deaf persons, parents of deaf children, interpreters, professionals who work with deaf and all interested parties.
Heather Parsons, President
Bill Bitner, VP

Foundations

4360 AAO-HNS Foundation
1650 Diagonal Road
Alexandria, VA 22314-3357
703-836-4444
memberservices@entnet.org
www.entnet.org

Philanthropic arm of the American Academy of Otolaryngology - Head and Neck Surgery, funding research, humanitarian and international programs.
Lee D. Eisenberg, MD, MPH, Coordinator, Development
Cecelia Schmalbach, MD, Coordinator, Research and Quality

4361 American Academy of Audiology Foundation
11480 Commerce Park Drive 703-790-8466
Reston, VA 20191 800-222-2336
Fax: 703-790-8631
infoaud@audiology.org
www.audiology.org
Promotes philanthropy and supports research, education, and advocacy in audiology and hearing science.
Tanya Tolpegin, Executive Director
Dina Santucci, Senior Director, Business Development

4362 American Hearing Research Foundation
275 N. York Street 630-617-5079
Elmhurst, IL 60126 Fax: 630-563-9181
info@american-hearing.org
www.american-hearing.org
Supports medical research and education into the causes, prevention, and cures of deafness, hearing losses and balance disorders. Also keeps physicians and the public informed of the latest developments in hearing research and education.
Richard G. Muench, Chair
Alan G. Micco, MD, President

Libraries & Resource Centers

4363 Captioned Films/Videos
National Association of the Deaf
8630 Fenton Street 301-587-1788
Silver Spring, MD 20910-4500 Fax: 301-587-1791
TTY: 301-587-1789
www.nad.org
The mission of the National Association of the Deaf is to promote,protect,and preserve the rights and quality of life of eaf and hard of hearing individuals in the United States of America.
Jason Stark, Director-Described and Captioned Media P

4364 Captioned Media Program
National Association of the Deaf
8630 Fenton Street 301-587-1788
Silver Spring, MD 20910-4500 Fax: 301-587-1791
TTY: 301-587-1789
www.nad.org
Free loans of educational and entertainment captioned films and videos for deaf and hard of hearing people.
Jason Stark, Director

4365 Friends of Libraries for Deaf Action USA
2930 Craiglawn Road 202-727-2255
Silver Spring, MD 20904-1816 Fax: 301-572-5168
TTY: 301-572-5168
folda86@aol.com
www.folda.net/
Library services for people with disabilities.
Alice L Hagemeyer, President
Merrie A Davidson, Associate

4366 Library Services to the Deaf Community
District of Columbia Public Library
901 G Street NW 202-727-2145
Washington, DC 20001 TTY: 202-727-2255
library_deaf_dc@yahoo.com
www.dclibrary.org
Assures that the deaf community is aware of existing library and information services by the District of Columbia Public Library; promotes public awareness about the deaf community, deaf history and culture, American Sign Language, and assistive technology for people with hearing loss.
John W Hill Jr, President
Bonnie R Cohen, VP

4367 Listening and Spoken Knowledge Center
3417 Volta Place NW 202-337-5220
Washington, DC 20007-2737 Fax: 202-337-8314
TTY: 202-337-5221
info@agbell.org
www.listeningandspokenlanguage.org/
Contains one of the world's largest historical collections of publications, documents and information on deafness. In addition to the main collection, which includes books, periodicals and indexed

clipping files dating from the turn of the century, the library also houses a significant archival collection dealing with the history of deafness since the 16th century.
Lyn Robertson, Ph.D., President
Alexander T Graham, Executive Director/CEO

4368 Wallace Memorial Library
Rochester Institute of Technology
90 Lomb Memorial Drive 585-475-2562
Rochester, NY 14623
Information on physical disabilities and deafness.
Chandra McKenzie, Assistant Provost/Director

Research Centers

4369 Boys Town National Research Hospital
555 N 30th Street 402-498-6511
Omaha, NE 68131 800-320-1171
Fax: 402-498-6331
TTY: 800 320-1171
www.boystownhospital.org
An internationally recognized center for state-of-the-art research diagnosis treatment of patients with ear diseases hearing and balance disorders cleft lip and palate and speech/language problems. Also includes programs such as Parent/Child Workshops Center for Childhood Deafness Register for Heredity Hearing Loss Center for Hearing research Center for Abused Handicapped and summer programs for gifted deaf teens and college students.
John K Arch, Executive VP
Edward M. Kolb, Medical Director

4370 Center for Hearing Loss in Children Boystown National Research Hospital
Boystown National Research Hospital
555 N 30th Street 402-498-6511
Omaha, NE 68131-2136 800-282-6657
Fax: 402-498-6331
TTY: 800 320-1171
chilic@boystown.org
www.boystownhospital.org
The Center for Hearing Loss in Children unites professionals from a variety of disciplines to focus on research training information dissemination and continuing education in the area of childhood deafness.
John K Arch, Executive VP
Edward M. Kolb, Medical Director

4371 Central Institute for the Deaf
825 S Taylor Avenue 314-977-0132
Saint Louis, MO 63110-1502 877-444-4574
Fax: 314-977-0023
TTY: 314-977-0037
rfeder@cid.edu
www.cid.edu
Central Institute for the Deaf is a private nonprofit auditory-oral school for children who have hearing impairments. We teach children with hearing loss birth-12 to listen talk and succeed in the mainstream.
Ned Lemkemeier, President
Robin M Feder, Executive Director

4372 City University of New York Center for Research in Speech and Hearing
365 Fifth Avenue 212-817-7000
New York, NY 10016-4309 877-428-6942
Fax: 212-817-1537
strangepin@aol.com
www.gc.cuny.edu
Programmable research of digital and auditory hearing aids and sensory aids for the speech and hearing impaired person.
Dr. William Kelly, President
Marilyn Marzolf, Chief of Staff

4373 Civitan International Research Center
1530 3rd Avenue S 205-934-8900
Birmingham, AL 35294-0001 800-UAB-CIRC
Fax: 205-975-6330
www.circ.uab.edu

Studies of deaf children.
Dr Harald Sontheimer, Director
Dr Alan Percy, Medical Director

4374 Cleveland Hearing and Speech Center
11635 Euclid Avenue   216-231-0787
Cleveland, OH 44106-4319   Fax: 216-231-2135
                             TTY: 216-231-5266
                             jkeatley@chsc.org
                             www.chsc.org
Offers research and studies into speech language and hearing disorders.
David J Abood, President
Bernard P Henri PhD, Executive Director

4375 David T Siegel Institute for Communicative Disorders
Humana Hospital-Michael Reese
3033 S Cottage Grove Avenue   773-791-2900
Chicago, IL 60616-3346   Fax: 773-791-4014
Conducts behavioral research on language development and sign language for the deaf.
Edward Applebaum, Chief Service

4376 Eaton-Peabody Laboratory of Auditory Physiology
Massachusetts Eye & Ear Institute
243 Charles Street   617-573-3745
Boston, MA 02114-3002   Fax: 617-720-4408
                             eplweb@mit.edu
                             research.meei.harvard.edu/EPL
Auditory system and auditory information processing including ear-brain interactions in normal and pathologic hearing.
John Fernandez, President, CEO
Thane Benson, Consultant

4377 Gallaudet University: Center for Auditory and Speech Sciences
800 Florida Avenue NE   202-651-5000
Washington, DC 20002-3660   866-637-0102
                             Fax: 202-651-5295
                             TTY: 202-651-5005
                             www.gallaudet.edu
Develops new hearing tests that use speech sounds to measure hearing loss.
Dr T Alan Hurwitz, President
Deborah DeStefano, Special Assistant to the President

4378 Hear Center
301 E Del Mar Boulevard   626-796-2016
Pasadena, CA 91101   Fax: 626-796-2320
                             info@hearcenter.org
                             www.hearcenter.org
Auditory and verbal program designed to help hearing impaired children infants and adults lead normal and productive lives. Seeks to develop auditory techniques to aid people who have communication problems due to deafness.
Ellen Simon, Executive Director
Deborah Lorino, Office Manager

4379 Houston Ear Research Foundation
7737 SW Freeway   713-771-9966
Houston, TX 77074-1867   800-843-0807
                             Fax: 713-771-0546
                             TTY: 800-843-0807
                             www.houstoncochlear.org
Aims to improve health care and education for deaf and hearing-impaired children.
Jan Gilden, Clinical Audiologist
Mary Lynn McDonald

4380 Loyola University of Children: Parmly Hearing Institute
1032 W Sheridan Road   773-274-3000
Chicago, IL 60660   Fax: 773-508-2719
                             webmaster@luc.edu
                             www.luc.edu
Engage in the comparative study of sensory systems including hearing vision speech perception vestibular function and the special senses of the lateral-line organ and electroreception in fish.
Richard Fay, PhD, Director
Dr William Yost, Professor of Psychology

4381 Northern Illinois University Research and Training Center
1425 W Lincoln Highway   815-753-1000
DeKalb, IL 60115-2825   800-892-3050
                             Fax: 815-753-6520
                             helpdesk@niu.edu
                             www.niu.edu
Conducts research resource development and training/technical assistance projects geared toward enhancing the employment independent living and quality of life outcomes for traditionally underserved people who are deaf.
Douglas D Baker, President

4382 Ohio State University Otological Research Laboratories
410 W 10th Avenue   614-293-8103
Columbus, OH 43210   800-293-5123
                             Fax: 614-293-5506
                             OSUCareConnection@osumc.edu
                             www.medicalcenter.osu.edu
Clinical and basic research in otology.
Larry Anstine, CEO
Peter Geier, Chief Operating Officer

4383 Ohio University Therapy Associates: Hearing, Speech and Language Clinic
W218 Grover Center   740-593-1000
Athens, OH 45701   Fax: 740-593-0287
                             webteam@ohio.edu
Focuses on hearing and speech impairments.
Brooke Hallowell, Director
Davida Parsons, Clinical Director

4384 Oregon Health Sciences University Oregon Hearing Research Center Tinnitus Clinic
3181 S W Sam Jackson Park Road   503-494-7954
Portland, OR 97239-3098   Fax: 503-945-5656
                                 TTY: 503-494-0910
                                 ohrc@ohsu.edu
The first medical clinic in the world established exclusively for the treatment of chronic tinnitus. During the last 25 years we have successfully treated more than 7 000 patients with severe tinnitus. The Clinic also treats patients with hyperacusis (hypersensitivity to sounds).
William Martin PhD, Director
Baker Yong-Bing Shi, MD, PhD, Assistant Professor

4385 Regional Resource Center on Deafness Western Oregon State College
Western Oregon State College
345 N Monmouth Avenue   503-838-8444
Monmouth, OR 97361   877-877-1593
                             TTY: 503-838-8000
                             rrcd@wou.edu
                             www.wou.edu/education/sped/rrcd.php
Improve the employment and independent living status of deaf and hard-of-hearing people by increasing the number of rehabilitation professionals and their community partners nationwide who have the necessary knowledge and communication skills to serve this population.
Cheryl Davis, Director
Konnie Sayers, Administrative Assistant

4386 Rehabilitation Engineering on Hearing Enha ncement
Lexington Center
800 Florida Avenue NE   202-651-5335
Washington, DC 20002   Fax: 202-651-5324
                             TTY: 202-651-5335
                             info@hearingresearch.org
                             www.hearingresearch.org
A federally funded center that conducts research into hearing aid technology and alternate technologies.
Matthew H Bakke Ph D, Director
James J Mahshie PhD, Director

4387 Research and Training Center for Persons Who are Deaf or Hard of Hearing
University of Arkansas
26 Corporate Hill Drive   501-686-9691
Little Rock, AR 72205-3822   Fax: 501-686-9698
                             TTY: 501-686-9691
                             dwatson@uark.edu

Rehabilitation of deaf and hearing impaired individuals.
Douglas Watson, Director
Glenn B Anderson, Professor Director of Training

4388 Rochester Institute of Technology: Nationa l Technical Institute for the Deaf
Lyndon Baines Johnson Building
52 Lomb Memorial Drive   585-475-6400
Rochester, NY 14623   Fax: 585-475-5978
                                        TTY: 585-475-6400
                                     gbuckley@ntid.rit.edu
                                          www.ntid.rit.edu
Provides technical and professional education and training for deaf students.
Dr Gerard Buckley, President

4389 Scottish Rite Center for Childhood Language Disorders
2800 - 16th Street NW   202-232-8155
Washington, DC 20009-3602   Fax: 202-483-8169
                                                  dcsr.org
Association offering speech-language evaluations and treatment hearing screening and consultation and referrals to children ages birth to 18 years with hearing or speech disorders.
Dr Tommie L Robinson, Director

4390 Speech Simulation Research Foundation
PO Box 824   757-442-2755
Nassawadox, VA 23413-0824
Focuses on hearing and speech disorders.
Monte Penney, Director

4391 State University College at Fredonia Youngerman Clinic
W123 Thompson Hall   716-673-3203
Fredonia, NY 14063   Fax: 716-673-3332
                                  melissa.sidor@fredonia.edu
                                         www.fredonia.edu
Studies communication disorders including hearing and speech.
Melissa Sidor, Director

4392 State University College at Plattsburgh Auditory Research Laboratory
101 Broad Street   518-564-2000
Plattsburgh, NY 12901-2170   www.plattsburgh.edu
Dr John Ettling, President
Anne Hansen, Vice-President

4393 Syracuse University Institute for Sensory Research
Syracuse University
621 Skytop Road   315-443-4164
Syracuse, NY 13244-1   Fax: 315-443-1184
                                           rlsmith@syr.edu
                                            www.isr.syr.edu
Sensory processing and hearing disorders.
Robert L Smith, Director

4394 Temple University Speech and Hearing Science Laboratories
1801 N Broad Street   215-204-7000
Philadelphia, PA 19122   president@temple.edu
                                            www.temple.edu
Speech and hearing studies.
Neil D Theobald, President
Kevin G Clark, Senior Advisor to the President/Interim

4395 Temple University: Section of Auditory Research
1801 N Broad Street   215-204-7000
Philadelphia, PA 19122   Fax: 215-707-6417
                                       president@temple.edu
                                            www.temple.edu

Neil D Theobald, President
Kevin G Clark, Senior Advisor to the President/Interim

4396 The University of Memphis: School of Communication Sciences and Disorders
Memphis State University
101 Wilder Tower   901-678-2111
Memphis, TN 38152-3520   800-669-2678
                                         Fax: 901-251-82
                                   recruitment@memphis.edu
                                       www.memphis.edu/ausp

Offers research into hearing loss and deafness as well as speech impairments.
Shirley C Raines, President
Walt Manning, Associate Director

4397 Trace Center University of Wisconsin: Madison
University of Wisconsin: Madison
1550 Engineering Drive   608-262-6966
Madison, WI 53706-2274   Fax: 608-262-8848
                                        TTY: 608-263-5408
                                        info@trace.wisc.edu
                                           trace.wisc.edu
Research and development center working with communication control and computer access technologies for people with disabilities.
Gregg C Vanderheiden, Center Director
Julie Gamradt, Communication Director

4398 University of Alabama Speech and Hearing Center
5721 USA Drive N   251-445-9378
Mobile, AL 36688-2   Fax: 251- 44- 937
                                www.southalabama.edu/alliedhealth/speech
Providing undergraduate master's and doctoral programs that challenge the student to achieve the highest standards of academic learning scientific inquiry and clinical excellence.
Robert E Moore, Chair
Elizabeth M Adams, Assistant Professor of Audiology

4399 University of Chicago: Temporal Bone Laboratory for Ear Research
5841 S Maryland Avenue   773-702-1000
Chicago, IL 60637-1463   888-824-0200
                                       Fax: 773-702-6809
                                        www.uchospitals.edu
Focuses on hearing impairments and deafness research.
Dr Raul Hinojasa, Director

4400 University of Maine: Communication Science s & Disorders
5724 Dunn Hall   207-581-2006
Orono, ME 04469-5724   Fax: 207-581-2060
                                 Luanne.Wasson@umit.maine.edu
                                  www.umaine.edu/comscidis
Speech disorders of adults and children including hearing impairments and deafness.
Judy Stickles, Clinic Director
Amy Engler Booth, Audiologist

4401 University of Michigan Communicative Disorders Clinic
412 Maynard Street   734-764-1817
Ann Arbor, MI 48109-2054   Fax: 734-764-7084
Focuses on communicative disorders including hearing impairments and speech disorders.
Mary Sue Coleman, President
Joerg Lahann, Assistant Professor of Biomedical Engine

4402 University of Michigan: Kresge Hearing Research Institute
1150 W Medical Center Drive   734-764-8111
Ann Arbor, MI 48109-0500   Fax: 734-764-0014
                                        TTY: 734-764-8110
                                            josef@umich.edu
                                       www.khri.med.umich.edu
Focuses on hearing and auditory disorders.
Josef M Miller, Director
Sue Kelch, Research Administrator

4403 University of Nebraska: Lincoln
1400 R Street   402-472-7211
Lincoln, NE 68588   Fax: 402-472-7697
                                           jbernthal1@unl.edu
                                               www.unl.edu
Focuses on hearing impairments and deaf research.
Harvey Perlman, Chancellor
Marjorie Kostelnik, Dean Education Human Science

4404 University of North Carolina at Chapel Hill Division of Speech & Hearing
321 S. Columbia Street   919-966-1007
Chapel Hill, NC 27599-1   Fax: 919-966-0100
                                        idiana@med.unc.edu
                                     www.med.unc.edu/ahs/sphs

The Division of Speech and Hearing Sciences prepares clinical practitioners in speech-language pathology and audiology to be scholars teachers and researchers in both the theoretical and applied aspects of human communication sciences and disorders.
Jackson Roush, PhD, Director
Lee McLean, PhD, Professor and Associate Dean

4405   University of Oklahoma: Health Sciences Ce nter
University of Oklahoma
1100 N Lindsey   405-271-4000
Oklahoma City, OK 73104   Fax: 405-713-60
                                        www.ouhsc.edu
Dr. Dewayne Andrews, Senior Vice President and Provost
Kenneth D Rowe, Vice President for Administration and Fi

4406   University of Texas at Dallas Callier Center for Communication Disorders
1966 Inwood Road   214-905-3000
Dallas, TX 75235-7205   Fax: 214-905-3022
                                        TDD: 214-905-3012
                                        roeser@callier.utdallas.edu
Focuses on communication and behavioral disorders including hearing impairments and deafness research.
Tom Campbell, Executive Director
Phillip L Wilson, Head of Audiology

4407   University of Washington Department of Speech & Hearing Sciences
1417 NE 42nd Street   206-685-7400
Seattle, WA 98105-6246   Fax: 206-543-1093
                                        www.depts.washington.edu/sphsc/
Communication sciences and disorders.
Joan Hanson, Clinic Manager
Mary Wood, Assistant to the Chair

4408   Yeshiva University: Institute of Communication Disorders
Montefiore Medical Center
500 West 185th Street   212-960-5400
New York, NY 10033   Fax: 718-515-8235
                                        mfried@montefiore.org
                                        www.yu.edu
Studies on communicative disorders including speech and hearing.
Richard M Joel, President
Josh Joseph, VP, Chief of Staff

Support Groups & Hotlines

4409   Aurora of Central New York
518 James Street   315-422-7263
Syracuse, NY 13203-2282   Fax: 315-422-4792
                                        TTY: 315-422-9746
                                        TDD: 315-422-9746
                                        auroracny@auroraofcny.org
Professional counseling services helps to assist individuals and their families deal with the trauma of hearing or vision loss.
Debra Chaken, Executive Director

4410   Beginnings for Parents of Children Who are Deaf or Hard of Hearing
302 Jefferson Street   919-715-4092
Raleigh, NC 27605   800-541-4327
                                        Fax: 919-715-4093
                                        TTY: 919-715-4092
                                        raleigh@ncbegin.org
                                        www.ncbegin.org/
Beginnings provides support to parents of deaf and hard-of-hearing children in an unbiased, family-centered atmosphere. In addition, Beginnings also offers impartial information on communication options, placement and educational programs, and workshops for professional personnel who work with deaf and hard-of-hearing children. Advocacy and support for young people from birth to age 21 is available.
Jim Johnson, President
Dr Joni Y Alberg, Executive Director

4411   Children of Deaf Adults
PO Box 30715   805-682-0997
Santa Barbara, CA 93130-0715   www.coda-international.org

Promotes family awareness and individual growth in hearing children of deaf parents.
Carmel Batson, President
Millie Brother, Founder

4412   Children's Rights Program
Alexander Graham Bell Association
3417 Volta Place NW   202-337-5220
Washington, DC 20007   866-337-5220
                                        Fax: 202-337-8314
                                        info@agbell.org
                                        www.agbell.org
Actively advocates for the legal rights of children with hearing impairments and for legislation to upgrade the delivery of services to children and adults who are hearing impaired.
Gerri A Hanna, Director Advocacy/Policy

4413   Dial-a-Hearing Screening Test
PO Box 1880   610-544-7700
Media, PA 19063   800-222-3277
                                        Fax: 610-543-2802
                                        dahst@aol.com
Hearing help information center. Provides local phone number for Dial-a-Hearing Screening Test and hearing information.
George Biddle, Executive Director

4414   International Hearing Society
International Hearing Society (IHS)
16880 Middlebelt Road   734-522-7200
Livonia, MI 48154   800-521-5247
                                        Fax: 734-522-0200
                                        chelms@ihsinfo.org
                                        http://ihsinfo.org/IhsV2/Home/Index.cfm
Hearing Aid Helpline, a service of International Hearing Society (IHS), provides a referral service for locating qualified hearing healthcare professionals. IHS is a professional association representing Hearing Instrument Specialists worldwide engaged in the practice of testing human hearing, selecting, fitting and dispensing of hearing instruments. Founded in 1951, the Society conducts programs in competency accreditation, education, training promoting specialty-level certification.
Richard Giles, President
Kathleen Mennillo, Executive Director

4415   John Tracy Clinic on Deafness
806 W Adams Boulevard   213-748-5481
Los Angeles, CA 90007-2599   800-522-4582
                                        Fax: 213-749-1651
                                        www.jtc.org
Hotline.
Michael D Barker, Chair
J.Gaston Kent, President & CEO

4416   National Health Information Center
Office of Disease Prevention & Health Promotion
1101 Wootton Pkwy   Fax: 240-453-8281
Rockville, MD 20852   odphpinfo@hhs.gov
                                        www.health.gov/nhic
Supports public health education by maintaining a calendar of National Health Observances; helps connect consumers and health professionals to organizations that can best answer questions and provide up-to-date contact information from reliable sources; updates on a yearly basis toll-free numbers for health information, Federal health clearinghouses and info centers.
Don Wright, MD, MPH, Director

4417   Project Eyes and Ears
1844 T Street SE   202-889-7045
Washington, DC 20020-4635   Fax: 202-889-6312
Disseminates information about resources to families and service providers, provides transition services for pre-kindergarten children who are deaf-blind and integrates children into normalized settings.
Janice Wellborn

Books

4418   A Child with Hearing Loss in Your Classroom? Don't Panic!
Alexander Graham Bell Association

3417 Volta Place NW 202-337-5220
Washington, DC 20007-2737 Fax: 202-337-8314
TTY: 202-337-5220
info@agbell.org
www.listeningandspokenlanguage.org
Designed for mainstream teachers, this booklet discusses educational needs for students with hearing impairments. It especially focuses on students' language skills and their abilities to follow directions, learn new concepts, and comprehend reading. Candid advice about getting support from professionals, implementing and maintaining an IEP, improving classroom acoustic environments and using the PATERR approach.
1993 25 pages

4419 A New Civil Right: Telecommunications Equality for Deaf and Hard of Hearing
Karen Peltz Strauss, author
Hearing Loss Association of America
7910 Woodmont Avenue 301-657-2248
Bethesda, MD 20814-3079 Fax: 301-913-9413
TTY: 301-657-2249
info@hearingloss.org
www.hearingloss.org
This book provides a compelling picture of the challenges and the realization that FCC regulation is required for people with hearing loss to receive the functional equivalence of what everyone else takes for granted.
2006 Hardcover
Anna Gilmore Hall, Executive Director
Lise Hamlin, Director of Public Policy

4420 A Quiet World: Living with Hearing Loss
David G Myers, author
Hearing Loss Association of America
7910 Woodmont Avenue 301-657-2248
Bethesda, MD 20814-3079 Fax: 301-913-9413
TTY: 301-657-2249
info@hearingloss.org
A social psychologist, teacher, and author. The Author's gradual hearing loss caused serious trouble in his career and in his relationships with loved ones as he approached 50. He tells the story of his journey from denial to acceptance to an exploration of the technologies that offer help.
2000 Hardcover
Anna Gilmore Hall, Executive Director
Lise Hamlin, Director of Public Policy

4421 ASL PAH! Deaf Students' Essays About their Language
Sign Media
4020 Blackburn Lane 301-421-0268
Burtonsville, MD 20866-1167 800-475-4756
Fax: 301-421-0270
TTY: 301-421-4460
info@signmedia.com
www.signmedia.com
Tape/text combination featuring student essays on the role of ASL in their lives. The tape offers additional insights from the student authors. The text is not a transcript of the tape.
1979 Paperback/Video
ISBN: 0-932130-14-3
Barabara Olmert, Director Marketing

4422 ASL in Schools: Policies and Curriculum
Gallaudet University
800 Florida Avenue, NE 773-568-1550
Washington, DC 20002-3819 800-621-2736
Fax: 800-621-8476
TTY: 888-630-9347
gupress@gallaudet.edu
gupress.gallaudet.edu
Conference participants questioned experts on bilingual education for deaf students and discussed policy issues faced by educators across the United States.
139 pages

4423 Academic Acceptance of ASL
Gallaudet University

800 Florida Avenue, NE 773-568-1550
Washington, DC 20002-3819 800-621-2736
Fax: 800-621-8476
TTY: 888-630-9347
gupress@gallaudet.edu
gupress.gallaudet.edu
This monograph presents a dozen articles that demonstrate clearly and convincingly that the study of ASL affords the same educational values and the same intellectual rewards as the study of any other foreign language.
196 pages

4424 Access for All: Integrating Deaf, Hard of Hearing and Hearing Preschoolers
Gallaudet University
800 Florida Avenue, NE 773-568-1550
Washington, DC 20002-3819 800-621-2736
Fax: 800-621-8476
TTY: 888-630-9347
gupress@gallaudet.edu
gupress.gallaudet.edu
Describes a model program for integrating the Deaf and hard of hearing children in early education.
150 pages Book & Video

4425 American Deaf Culture
Gallaudet University
800 Florida Avenue, NE 773-568-1550
Washington, DC 20002-3819 800-621-2736
Fax: 800-621-8476
TTY: 888-630-9347
gupress@gallaudet.edu
gupress.gallaudet.edu
This book presents a collection of classic articles which have been selected to provide a variety of perspectives on language and culture of deaf people in America.
132 pages

4426 American Deaf Culture: An Anthology
Sign Media
4020 Blackburn Lane 301-421-0268
Burtonsville, MD 20866-1167 800-475-4756
Fax: 301-421-0270
TTY: 301-421-4460
info@signmedia.com
www.signmedia.com
Features deaf and hearing authors offering their experience and perspectives on cultural values, ASL, social interaction in the Deaf community, education, folklore and more.
Paperback
ISBN: 0-932130-09-7
Barbara Olmert, Director Marketing
Sherman Wilcox, Editor

4427 American Sign Language: A Beginning Course
National Association of the Deaf
8630 Fenton Street 301-587-1788
Silver Spring, MD 20910-4500 Fax: 301-587-1791
TTY: 301-587-1789
nad.info@nad.org
nad.org
An interactive approach to teaching and learning American Sign Language, with 700 sign illustrations, each accompanied by an object drawing.
199 pages Paperback
ISBN: 0-913072-64-8
Christopher Wagner, President
Melissa S. Draganac-Hawk, Vice-President

4428 An Invisible Condition: The Human Side of Hearing Loss
SHHH Publications
7910 Woodmont Avenue 301-657-2248
Bethesda, MD 20814-3572 Fax: 301-913-9413
www.hearingloss.org
Offers editorials from the SHHH Journal that have shaped the past decade of self help with their focus on the plight and hopes and the aspirations of hard of hearing people everywhere.
Rocky Stone, Author

4429 Angels and Outcasts: An Anthology of Deaf Characters in Literature
Gallaudet University
800 Florida Avenue, NE
Washington, DC 20002-3819

773-568-1550
800-621-2736
Fax: 800-621-8476
TTY: 888-630-9347
gupress@gallaudet.edu
gupress.gallaudet.edu

Collection of writings by and about deaf people revealing attitudes and prejudices common to western cultures.
375 pages
Trent Batson, Co-Editor
Eugene Bergman, Co-Editor

4430 Approaching Equality
TJ Publishers
817 Silver Spring Avenue
Silver Spring, MD 20910-4617

301-585-4440
800-999-1168
Fax: 301-585-5930
TTY: 301-585-4441
tjpubinc@aol.com

Written by the former chair of the Commission on the Education of the deaf, this book reviews the dramatic developments in the education of deaf children.
112 pages Softcover
ISBN: 0-932666-39-6
Angela K Thames, President
Jerald A Murphy, VP

4431 Assessment & Management of Mainstreamed Hearing-Impaired Children
Pro-Ed, Inc.
8700 Shoal Creek Blvd
Austin, TX 78757-6897

512-451-3246
800-897-3202
Fax: 800-397-7633
www.proedinc.com

The theoretical and practical considerations of developing appropriate programming for hearing-impaired children who are being educated in mainstream educational settings are presented in this book.
415 pages Hardcover
ISBN: 0-890794-58-8
Linda Jordan, Marketing Coordinator

4432 Assessment of Hearing Impaired People
Gallaudet University
800 Florida Avenue, NE
Washington, DC 20002-3819

773-568-1550
800-621-2736
Fax: 800-621-8476
TTY: 888-630-9347
gupress@gallaudet.edu
gupress.gallaudet.edu

This is a comprehensive review of 62 tests used by educational institutions, rehabilitation agencies, and mental health centers.
128 pages Softcover

4433 At Home Among Strangers
Gallaudet University
800 Florida Avenue, NE
Washington, DC 20002-3819

773-568-1550
800-621-2736
Fax: 800-621-8476
TTY: 888-630-9347
gupress@gallaudet.edu
gupress.gallaudet.edu

Details the history and culture of the deaf community.
336 pages
Jerome D. Schein, Author

4434 Basic Course in Manual Communication
National Association of the Deaf
8630 Fenton Street
Silver Spring, MD 20910-4500

301-587-1788
Fax: 301-587-1791
TTY: 301-587-1789
nad.info@nad.org
nad.org

Over 700 signs are grouped according to shape, location, and movement. Also includes dialogues for practice.
158 pages Paperback
Christopher Wagner, President
Melissa S. Draganac-Hawk, Vice-President

4435 Basic Sign Communication: Student Materials
National Association of the Deaf
8630 Fenton Street
Silver Spring, MD 20910-4500

301-587-1788
Fax: 301-587-1791
TTY: 301-587-1789
nad.info@nad.org
nad.org

Includes study and reference materials for all three levels of Basic Sign Communication.
232 pages Paperback
ISBN: 0-913072-56-7
Christopher Wagner, President
Melissa S. Draganac-Hawk, Vice-President

4436 Basic Sign Communication: Vocabulary
National Association of the Deaf
8630 Fenton Street
Silver Spring, MD 20910-4500

301-587-1788
Fax: 301-587-1791
TTY: 301-587-1789
nad.info@nad.org
nad.org

Features sections on Sign Vocabulary, Numbers, and Classifiers. Contains 1000 illustrated signs, organized alphabetically by gloss for quick reference.
162 pages Paperback
ISBN: 0-913072-55-9
Christopher Wagner, President
Melissa S. Draganac-Hawk, Vice-President

4437 Basic Vocabulary and Language Thesaurus for Hearing Impaired Children
Alexander Graham Bell Association
3417 Volta Place NW
Washington, DC 20007-2737

202-337-5220
Fax: 202-337-8314
TTY: 202-337-5220
info@agbell.org
www.listeningandspokenlanguage.org

This simple thesaurus lists spontaneous vocabulary used by normally hearing children and lets patients and teachers check so that children with hearing losses have mastered these words.
1977 76 pages

4438 Basic Vocabulary: American Sign Language for Parents and Children
TJ Publishers
817 Silver Spring Avenue
Silver Spring, MD 20910-4617

301-585-4440
800-999-1168
Fax: 301-585-5930
TTY: 301-585-4441
tjpubinc@aol.com

Carefully selected words and signs include those families use every day. Alphabetically organized vocabulary incorporates developmental lists helpful to both deaf and hearing children and over 1,000 clear sign language illustrations.
240 pages Softcover
ISBN: 0-932666-00-0
Angela K Thames, President
Jerald A Murphy, VP

4439 Being in Touch
Gallaudet University
800 Florida Avenue, NE
Washington, DC 20002-3819

773-568-1550
800-621-2736
Fax: 800-621-8476
TTY: 888-630-9347
gupress@gallaudet.edu
gupress.gallaudet.edu

Provides information on hearing and vision loss.
80 pages

4440 Best Practices in Educational Interpreting
Sign Enhancers

4450 La Crosse Ave
San Diego, CA 92117-2941

503-304-4501
800-767-4461
Fax: 503-304-1063
TTY: 503-304-4501
www.signenhancers.com

Specific recommendations of best practices for working in preschool through graduate school. Case studies focus on real-life situations with suggested solutions and questions for further thought.
269 pages
ISBN: 0-205263-11-9

4441 Between Friends
Beltone Electronics Corporation
2601 Patriot Blvd.
Glenview, IL 60026-6772

847-832-3300
800-235-8663
www.beltone.com

For hearing aid wearers: quizzes, jokes, health, recipes and financial items.
6 pages
Renee Rockoff, Editor

4442 Black and Deaf in America
TJ Publishers
817 Silver Spring Avenue
Silver Spring, MD 20910-4617

301-585-4440
800-999-1168
Fax: 301-585-5930
TTY: 301-585-4441
tjpubinc@aol.com

An in depth look at some of the problems of the black deaf community, including undereducation and underemployment. This book
includes an important chapter on signs used in the black community and presents interviews with prominent Black deaf individuals who share their joys, fears and hope for the future.
91 pages Softcover
ISBN: 0-932666-18-3
Angela K Thames, President
Jerald A Murphy, VP

4443 Blueprint for Conversational Competence
Alexander Graham Bell Association
3417 Volta Place NW
Washington, DC 20007-2737

202-337-5220
Fax: 202-337-8314
TTY: 202-337-5220
info@agbell.org
www.listeningandspokenlanguage.org

A book that develops conversational skills in children with hearing
impairments.
175 pages

4444 Book of Name Signs
Gallaudet University
800 Florida Avenue, NE
Washington, DC 20002-3819

773-568-1550
800-621-2736
Fax: 800-621-8476
TTY: 888-630-9347
gupress@gallaudet.edu
gupress.gallaudet.edu

This text discusses the rules for ASL name sign formulation and
their appropriate uses and presents a list of over 400 name signs.
112 pages

4445 Broken Ears: Wounded Hearts
Gallaudet University
800 Florida Avenue, NE
Washington, DC 20002-3819

773-568-1550
800-621-2736
Fax: 800-621-8476
TTY: 888-630-9347
gupress@gallaudet.edu
gupress.gallaudet.edu

An intimate journey into the lives of a deaf, multihandicapped
child and her young hearing parents.
186 pages Hardcover

4446 CUED Speech Resource Book for Parents of Deaf Children
Alexander Graham Bell Association
3417 Volta Place NW
Washington, DC 20007-2737

202-337-5220
Fax: 202-337-8314
TTY: 202-337-5220
info@agbell.org
www.listeningandspokenlanguage.org

A comprehensive book describing cued speech, getting started,
your child's rights in and out of school and families expectations
with special attention on siblings and peer relationships.
832 pages Hardcover

4447 Can't Your Child Hear?
Gallaudet University
800 Florida Avenue, NE
Washington, DC 20002-3819

773-568-1550
800-621-2736
Fax: 800-621-8476
TTY: 888-630-9347
gupress@gallaudet.edu
gupress.gallaudet.edu

Is deafness a difference to be accepted or a defect to be corrected?
This comprehensive reference will help parents, as well as educators and other professionals, recognize their options in understanding and handling a child who is deaf.
340 pages Softcover

4448 Chelsea: The Story of a Signal Dog
Gallaudet University
800 Florida Avenue, NE
Washington, DC 20002-3819

773-568-1550
800-621-2736
Fax: 800-621-8476
TTY: 888-630-9347
gupress@gallaudet.edu
gupress.gallaudet.edu

A story of a young deaf couple and their dog who acts as their ears.
169 pages

4449 Choices in Deafness
Woodbine House
6510 Bells Mill Road
Bethesda, MD 20817-1636

800-843-7323
info@woodbinehouse.com
www.woodbinehouse.com

Serving as an invaluable guide to the world of deaf education, this
expanded edition covers a wide variety of communication options
for children with hearing impairments. By providing medical, audiological, and educational information. It also contains numerous
case studies. This indispensible book is an outstanding resource
for parents.
1996 212 pages
ISBN: 0-933149-09-3
Sue Schwartz, Ph.D., Author/ Editor

4450 Chuck Baird
Gallaudet University
800 Florida Avenue, NE
Washington, DC 20002-3819

773-568-1550
800-621-2736
Fax: 800-621-8476
TTY: 888-630-9347
gupress@gallaudet.edu
gupress.gallaudet.edu

Contains 35 full-color plates of the artwork of the deaf artist.
55 pages

4451 Classroom Notetaker
Alexander Graham Bell Association
3417 Volta Place NW
Washington, DC 20007-2737

202-337-5220
Fax: 202-337-8314
TTY: 202-337-5220
info@agbell.org
www.listeningandspokenlanguage.org

This detailed manual for instructors, administrators and staff note
takers promotes classroom notetaking within long-term educational programs as vital for students who are deaf and hard of hearing from elementary school to college. This book will help readers
to sell a notetaking program to schools and will give a good foundation for designing and implementing a notetaking program in a
school or college.
1996 150 pages

**4452 Closer Look: The English Program at the Model Secondary
School for the Deaf**
Gallaudet University

800 Florida Avenue, NE
Washington, DC 20002

773-568-1550
800-621-2736
Fax: 800-621-8476
TTY: 888-630-9347
gupress@gallaudet.edu
gupress.gallaudet.edu

Program highlighting student-centered activities using carefully selected novels and literature texts to enhance students' reading comprehension and writing abilities through interaction with real literature.
67 pages

4453 Cochlear Implant Auditory Training Guidebook
Alexander Graham Bell Association
3417 Volta Place NW
Washington, DC 20007-2737

202-337-5220
Fax: 202-337-8314
TTY: 202-337-5220
info@agbell.org
www.listeningandspokenlanguage.org

This guidebook full of reproducible masters was designed for parents and professionals working with children ages four and up who have cochlear implants. It includes an easy to follow hierarchy for listening goals and a quick placement test to help you find where to start.
236 pages

4454 Cochlear Implantation for Infants and Children
Alexander Graham Bell Association
3417 Volta Place NW
Washington, DC 20007-2737

202-337-5220
Fax: 202-337-8314
TTY: 202-337-5220
info@agbell.org
www.listeningandspokenlanguage.org

This comprehensive text presents the surgical, medical, audiological speech and language and habilitation aspects of cochlear implants in infants and children.
1997 263 pages

4455 Cognition, Education and Deafness
Gallaudet University
800 Florida Avenue, NE
Washington, DC 20002-3819

773-568-1550
800-621-2736
Fax: 800-621-8476
TTY: 888-630-9347
gupress@gallaudet.edu
gupress.gallaudet.edu

The work of 54 authors is gathered in this definitive collection of current research on deafness and cognition. The articles are grouped into seven sections: cognition, problem solving, thinking processes, language development, reading methodologies, measurement of potential and intervention programs.
260 pages Hardcover

4456 Communicate with Me: Conversation Skills for Deaf Students
Gallaudet University
800 Florida Avenue, NE
Washington, DC 20002-3819

773-568-1550
800-621-2736
Fax: 800-621-8476
TTY: 888-630-9347
gupress@gallaudet.edu
gupress.gallaudet.edu

Students learn how to begin and end conversations, choose appropriate topics and maintain subjects.
160 pages

4457 Communication Access for Persons with Hearing Loss
Mark Ross, author
Hearing Loss Association of America
7910 Woodmont Avenue
Bethesda, MD 20814-3079

301-657-2248
Fax: 301-913-9413
TTY: 301-657-2249
info@hearingloss.org
www.hearingloss.org

Communication access for persons with hearing loss covers both visual and hearing techniques devoted to persons with hearingloss, ranging from mild to profound.
Anna Gilmore Hall, Executive Director
Lise Hamlin, Director of Public Policy

4458 Communication Issues Among Deaf People
Gallaudet University
800 Florida Avenue, NE
Washington, DC 20002-3819

773-568-1550
800-621-2736
Fax: 800-621-8476
TTY: 888-630-9347
gupress@gallaudet.edu
gupress.gallaudet.edu

Monograph discussing important aspects of communication including total communication and the value of ASL.
138 pages

4459 Communication Issues Among Deaf People: Eyes, Hands and Voices
National Association of the Deaf
8630 Fenton Street
Silver Spring, MD 20910-4500

301-587-1788
Fax: 301-587-1791
TTY: 301-587-1789
nad.info@nad.org
nad.org

Includes over thirty relevant articles reflecting a wide range of perceptions and attitutes on communication among deaf people.
145 pages
Christopher Wagner, President
Melissa S. Draganac-Hawk, Vice-President

4460 Communication Rules for Hard of Hearing People
Hearing Loss Association of America
7910 Woodmont Avenue
Bethesda, MD 20814-3079

301-657-2248
Fax: 301-913-9413
TTY: 301-657-2249
info@hearingloss.org
www.hearingloss.org

To open the world of communication to people with hearing loss through education, information, support and advocacy.
Anna Gilmore Hall, Executive Director
Lise Hamlin, Director of Public Policy

4461 Communication and Adult Hearing Loss
Alexander Graham Bell Association
3417 Volta Place NW
Washington, DC 20007-2737

202-337-5220
Fax: 202-337-8314
TTY: 202-337-5220
info@agbell.org
www.listeningandspokenlanguage.org

This informative book was written for anyone who wants to communicate more effectively with a person with adult hearing loss.
1993 136 pages

4462 Comprehensive Signed English Dictionary
Harris Communications
6541 City W Parkway
Eden Prairie, MN 55344-3248

612-906-1180
Fax: 612-946-0924
gupress.gallaudet.edu

Complete dictionary offers 3100 signs, including signs reflecting contemporary vocabulary.
457 pages
Harry Bornstein, Co-Editor
Karen L. Saulnier, Co-Editor

4463 Consumer Handbook on Dizziness and Vertigo
Dennis Poe, MD, author
Hearing Loss Association of Amercia
7910 Woodmont Avenue
Bethesda, MD 20814-3079

301-657-2248
Fax: 301-913-9413
TTY: 301-657-2249
info@hearingloss.org
www.hearingloss.org

Learn the differences between dizziness and vertigo.
Hardcover
ISBN: 0-966182-64-2
Anna Gilmore Hall
Lise Hamlin, Director of Public Policy

4464 Conversational Sign Language II: An Intermdiate Advanced Manual
Harris Communications
6541 City W Parkway
Eden Prairie, MN 55344-3248

612-906-1180
Fax: 612-946-0924
gupress.gallaudet.edu

This book presents English words and their American Sign Language equivalents.
218 pages
William J. Madsen, Author

4465 Dancing Without Music
Gallaudet University
800 Florida Avenue, NE   773-568-1550
Washington, DC 20002-3819   800-621-2736
                                       Fax: 800-621-8476
                                       TTY: 888-630-9347
                                       gupress@gallaudet.edu
                                       gupress.gallaudet.edu
Investigates being deaf and its social ramifications.
320 pages
Beryl Lieff Benderly, Author

4466 Deaf Children in Public Schools Placement, Context, and Consequences
Gallaudet University
800 Florida Avenue, NE   773-568-1550
Washington, DC 20002-3819   800-621-2736
                                       Fax: 800-621-8476
                                       TTY: 888-630-9347
                                       gupress@gallaudet.edu
                                       gupress.gallaudet.edu
Assesses the progress of three second-grade deaf students to demonstrate the importance of placement, context, and language in their development.
August 1997 250 pages
ISBN: 1-563680-62-9
Claire L. Ramsey, Author

4467 Deaf Culture, Our Way
Gallaudet University
800 Florida Avenue, NE   773-568-1550
Washington, DC 20002-3819   800-621-2736
                                       Fax: 800-621-8476
                                       TTY: 888-630-9347
                                       gupress@gallaudet.edu
                                       gupress.gallaudet.edu
A revised edition of Silence is Golden, Sometimes, this new edition contains sections on Classic Humor, Bathroom Tales, Classic Hazards and New Technology.
115 pages

4468 Deaf Empowerment, Emergence, Struggle and Rhetoric
Gallaudet University
800 Florida Avenue, NE   773-568-1550
Washington, DC 20002-3819   800-621-2736
                                       Fax: 800-621-8476
                                       TTY: 888-630-9347
                                       gupress@gallaudet.edu
                                       gupress.gallaudet.edu
Examines the rhetorical foundation that motivated Deaf people to work for social change during the past two centuries. Assesses the goal of a multicultural society and offers suggestions for community building through a new humanitarianism.
July 1997 192 pages Hardcover
ISBN: 1-563680-61-0

4469 Deaf Heritage: A Narrative History of Deaf America
National Association of the Deaf
8630 Fenton Street   301-587-1788
Silver Spring, MD 20910-4500   Fax: 301-587-1791
                                       TTY: 301-587-1789
                                       nad.info@nad.org
                                       nad.org
In-depth history of Deaf America contains pictures, vignettes, and biographical profiles.
483 pages Paperback
Christopher Wagner, President
Melissa S. Draganac-Hawk, Vice-President

4470 Deaf Heritage: Student Text and Workbook
National Association of the Deaf

8630 Fenton Street   301-587-1788
Silver Spring, MD 20910-4500   Fax: 301-587-1791
                                       TTY: 301-587-1789
                                       nad.info@nad.org
                                       nad.org
Each chapter is followed by a vocabulary section and workbook activities including questions and follow-up activities for students.
115 pages Paperback
Christopher Wagner, President
Melissa S. Draganac-Hawk, Vice-President

4471 Deaf History Unveiled: Interpretations from the New Scholarship
Gallaudet University
800 Florida Avenue, NE   773-568-1550
Washington, DC 20002-3819   800-621-2736
                                       Fax: 800-621-8476
                                       TTY: 888-630-9347
                                       gupress@gallaudet.edu
                                       gupress.gallaudet.edu
Essays written by internationally renowned deaf studies scholars.
316 pages
John Vickrey Van Cleve, Editor

4472 Deaf Like Me
Gallaudet University
800 Florida Avenue, NE   773-568-1550
Washington, DC 20002-3819   800-621-2736
                                       Fax: 800-621-8476
                                       TTY: 888-630-9347
                                       gupress@gallaudet.edu
                                       gupress.gallaudet.edu
Written by the uncle and father of a deaf girl, this is an account of parents coming to terms with deafness.
292 pages
Thomas S. Spradley, Co-Author
James P. Spradley, Co-Author

4473 Deaf President Now! The 1988 Revolution at Gallaudet University
Gallaudet University
800 Florida Avenue, NE   773-568-1550
Washington, DC 20002-3819   800-621-2736
                                       Fax: 800-621-8476
                                       TTY: 888-630-9347
                                       gupress@gallaudet.edu
                                       gupress.gallaudet.edu
This book chronicles the events leading up to the revolution in which deaf people won social change for themselves and all disabled people.
240 pages
John B. Christiansen, Co-Author
Sharon N. Barnartt, Co-Author

4474 Deaf Sport: The Impact of Sports Within the Deaf Community
Gallaudet University
800 Florida Avenue, NE   773-568-1550
Washington, DC 20002-3819   800-621-2736
                                       Fax: 800-621-8476
                                       TTY: 888-630-9347
                                       gupress@gallaudet.edu
                                       gupress.gallaudet.edu
Describes the full ramifications of athletics for deaf people.
224 pages
David A. Stewart, Author

4475 Deaf Students and the School-to-Work Transition
Gallaudet University
800 Florida Avenue, NE   773-568-1550
Washington, DC 20002-3819   800-621-2736
                                       Fax: 800-621-8476
                                       TTY: 888-630-9347
                                       gupress@gallaudet.edu
                                       gupress.gallaudet.edu
Studies severely and profoundly hearing impaired students as they leave high school and enter the work force.
278 pages

4476 Deaf Studies Curriculum Guide
Gallaudet University

800 Florida Avenue, NE   773-568-1550
Washington, DC 20002-3819   800-621-2736
Fax: 800-621-8476
TTY: 888-630-9347
gupress@gallaudet.edu
gupress.gallaudet.edu
Designed to help students explore the history, language and culture of deaf people.
250 pages

4477   Deaf Women: A Parade Through the Decades
Gallaudet University
800 Florida Avenue, NE   773-568-1550
Washington, DC 20002-3819   800-621-2736
Fax: 800-621-8476
TTY: 888-630-9347
gupress@gallaudet.edu
gupress.gallaudet.edu
A compilation of information, history, anecdotes and research that showcases many deaf women from all walks of American life.
192 pages

4478   Deaf and Hard of Hearing Individuals
Mainstream
1030 5th Street NW   202-898-1400
Washington, DC 20001-2504
Mainstreaming deaf individuals into the workplace.
12 pages

4479   Deaf in America: Voices from a Culture
Gallaudet University
800 Florida Avenue, NE   773-568-1550
Washington, DC 20002-3819   800-621-2736
Fax: 800-621-8476
TTY: 888-630-9347
gupress@gallaudet.edu
gupress.gallaudet.edu
Written by authors who are themselves deaf.
134 pages

4480   Deafness and Child Development
Gallaudet University
800 Florida Avenue, NE   773-568-1550
Washington, DC 20002-3819   800-621-2736
Fax: 800-621-8476
TTY: 888-630-9347
gupress@gallaudet.edu
gupress.gallaudet.edu
Provides rational, informed and balanced approaches to the effects of deafness in child development.
236 pages

4481   Deafness: 1993-2013
National Association of the Deaf
8630 Fenton Street   301-587-1788
Silver Spring, MD 20910   Fax: 301-587-1791
TTY: 301-587-1789
nad.info@nad.org
nad.org
Over 30 articles cover such topics as magnet schools, deaf identity, technology, multicultural education, communication, leadership, and sign language research.
Paperback
Christopher Wagner, President
Melissa S. Draganac-Hawk, Vice-President

4482   Deafness: A Personal Account
Faber & Faber
19 Union Square W   781-721-1427
New York, NY 10003-3304   www.faber.co.uk
Poet, critic and translator David Wright's enduring memoir (now with a substantial new introduction by the author) describes with humor and insight his early life, his development as a poet, and little-known history of deaf education.
202 pages

4483   Deafness: An Autobiography
Gallaudet University

800 Florida Avenue, NE   773-568-1550
Washington, DC 20002-3819   800-621-2736
Fax: 800-621-8476
TTY: 888-630-9347
gupress@gallaudet.edu
gupress.gallaudet.edu
This book is intended to explore the author's own experiences with deafness, and satisfy the curiosity about the condition of deaf people.
238 pages

4484   Deafness: Historical Perspectives
National Association of the Deaf
8630 Fenton Street   301-587-1788
Silver Spring, MD 20910   Fax: 301-587-1791
TTY: 301-587-1789
nad.info@nad.org
nad.org
Focuses on the history of deaf people. Topics cover a spectrum from a history of deaf theaters, to a genealogy of our first deaf families, to a conversation with a ghost.
Paperback
Christopher Wagner, President
Melissa S. Draganac-Hawk, Vice-President

4485   Deafness: Life and Culture II
National Association of the Deaf
8630 Fenton Street   301-587-1788
Silver Spring, MD 20910   Fax: 301-587-1791
TTY: 301-587-1789
nad.info@nad.org
nad.org
Continues to explore the variety and diversity of the deaf experience.
133 pages Paperback
ISBN: 0-913072-79-6
Christopher Wagner, President
Melissa S. Draganac-Hawk, Vice-President

4486   Directory of Auditory-Oral Programs
Alexander Graham Bell Association
3417 Volta Place NW   202-337-5220
Washington, DC 20007-2737   Fax: 202-337-8314
TTY: 202-337-5220
info@agbell.org
www.listeningandspokenlanguage.org
This directory lists auditory/oral programs in public and private schools, auditory-oral programs in speech and hearing centers and therapists who offer private tutoring and auditory-oral therapy.
67 pages

4487   Discovering Sign Language
Gallaudet University
800 Florida Avenue, NE   773-568-1550
Washington, DC 20002-3819   800-621-2736
Fax: 800-621-8476
TTY: 888-630-9347
gupress@gallaudet.edu
gupress.gallaudet.edu
Here is a book of information about deaf people and sign communication.
104 pages Softcover

4488   Douglas Tilden, the Man and His Legacy
Gallaudet University
800 Florida Avenue, NE   773-568-1550
Washington, DC 20002-3819   800-621-2736
Fax: 800-621-8476
TTY: 888-630-9347
gupress@gallaudet.edu
gupress.gallaudet.edu
A beautiful tribute to the Deaf sculptor, Douglas Tilden.
216 pages

4489   Ear Book
Gallaudet University

800 Florida Avenue, NE
Washington, DC 20002-3819
773-568-1550
800-621-2736
Fax: 800-621-8476
TTY: 888-630-9347
gupress@gallaudet.edu
gupress.gallaudet.edu

A how-to book on obtaining and using an otoscope, recognizing and managing common ear disorders, when to call the doctor and when your child needs ear tubes.
136 pages Softcover

4490 Ear Gear: A Student Workbook on Hearing and Hearing Aids
Gallaudet University
800 Florida Avenue, NE
Washington, DC 20002-3819
773-568-1550
800-621-2736
Fax: 800-621-8476
TTY: 888-630-9347
gupress@gallaudet.edu
gupress.gallaudet.edu

Attractive workbook designed to teach elementary-age children about hearing loss and the use of hearing aids.
75 pages

4491 Educating Deaf Children Bilingually
Gallaudet University
800 Florida Avenue, NE
Washington, DC 20002-3819
773-568-1550
800-621-2736
Fax: 800-621-8476
TTY: 888-630-9347
gupress@gallaudet.edu
gupress.gallaudet.edu

Discusses perspectives and practices of educating deaf children with goals of age-level achievement.
120 pages

4492 Educating the Deaf: Psychology, Principles and Practices
Gallaudet University
800 Florida Avenue, NE
Washington, DC 20002-3819
773-568-1550
800-621-2736
Fax: 800-621-8476
TTY: 888-630-9347
gupress@gallaudet.edu
gupress.gallaudet.edu

Offers extensive coverage of the background and history of the education of the deaf, as well as specific information on working with multihandicapped students.
383 pages

4493 Education and Deafness
Longman Publishing Group
95 Church Street
White Plains, NY 10601-1515
914-993-5000

This comprehensive introduction to educating students with hearing impairments provides extensive coverage of the interrelated issues that affect the teaching of these students. It concentrates on the severely to profoundly hearing impaired but includes an entire chapter devoted to students whose impairments are less severe (hard-of-hearing students).
320 pages Paperback
ISBN: 0-801300-26-6

4494 Educational and Development Aspects of Deafness
Gallaudet University
800 Florida Avenue, NE
Washington, DC 20002-3819
773-568-1550
800-621-2736
Fax: 800-621-8476
TTY: 888-630-9347
gupress@gallaudet.edu
gupress.gallaudet.edu

Book detailing the ongoing revolution in the education of deaf children.
415 pages
Donald F. Moores, Co-Editor
Kathryn P. Meadow-Orlans, Co-Editor

4495 Empowerment and Black Deaf Persons
Gallaudet University

800 Florida Avenue, NE
Washington, DC 20002-3819
773-568-1550
800-621-2736
Fax: 800-621-8476
TTY: 888-630-9347
gupress@gallaudet.edu
gupress.gallaudet.edu

Conference proceedings focusing on the guidance and training of African American deaf individuals.
175 pages

4496 Encyclopedia of Deafness and Hearing Disorders
Facts on File
11 Penn Plaza
New York, NY 10001
212-967-8800
800-322-8755
Fax: 800-678-3633

A comprehensive guide to all aspects of hearing impairments.

4497 Eye-Centered: A Study of Spirituality of Deaf People
NCOD
814 Thayer Avenue
Silver Spring, MD 20910-4500
301-587-7992

The findings of the five-year De Sales Project conducted by The National Catholic Office for the Deaf.

4498 FM Auditory Trainers: A Winning Choice for Students, Teachers and Parents
Alexander Graham Bell Association
3417 Volta Place NW
Washington, DC 20007-2737
202-337-5220
Fax: 202-337-8314
TTY: 202-337-5220
info@agbell.org
www.listeningandspokenlanguage.org

A practical guide to the selection and use of FM trainers in class or at home.
67 pages

4499 For Teachers of the Hearing Impaired
Gallaudet University
800 Florida Avenue, NE
Washington, DC 20002-3819
773-568-1550
800-621-2736
Fax: 800-621-8476
TTY: 888-630-9347
gupress@gallaudet.edu
gupress.gallaudet.edu

Contains practical articles by and for teachers of hearing impaired children.

4500 Foundations of Spoken Language for Hearing Impaired Children
Alexander Graham Bell Association
3417 Volta Place NW
Washington, DC 20007-2737
202-337-5220
Fax: 202-337-8314
TTY: 202-337-5220
info@agbell.org
www.listeningandspokenlanguage.org

This guide traces the individual progress of a child's speech development.
1978 87 pages

4501 Free Hand: Education of the Deaf
TJ Publishers
817 Silver Spring Avenue
Silver Spring, MD 20910-4617
301-585-4440
800-999-1168
Fax: 301-585-5930
TTY: 301-585-4441
tjpubinc@aol.com

Based on the proceedings of a 1990 symposium on the educational uses of ASL, A Free Hand presents papers by prominent educators, researchers and linguists in the changing role of American sign language in the classroom.
204 pages Softcover
ISBN: 0-932666-40-X
Angela K Thames, President
Jerald A Murphy, VP

4502 GA and SK Etiquette
Gallaudet University

800 Florida Avenue, NE
Washington, DC 20002-3819

773-568-1550
800-621-2736
Fax: 800-621-8476
TTY: 888-630-9347
gupress@gallaudet.edu
gupress.gallaudet.edu

This booklet presents guidelines for proper usage of the TDD.
53 pages

4503   Gallaudet Encyclopedia of Deaf People and Deafness
Gallaudet University
800 Florida Avenue, NE
Washington, DC 20002-3819

773-568-1550
800-621-2736
Fax: 800-621-8476
TTY: 888-630-9347
gupress@gallaudet.edu
gupress.gallaudet.edu

Three-volume set of research and information on deaf people and deafness.
1400 pages
John V. Van Cleve, Editor

4504   Growing Together: Information for Parents of Deaf & Hard of Hearing Children
Gallaudet University
800 Florida Avenue, NE
Washington, DC 20002-3819

773-568-1550
800-621-2736
Fax: 800-621-8476
TTY: 888-630-9347
gupress@gallaudet.edu
gupress.gallaudet.edu

This publication answers questions often asked by parents of children with a hearing loss.
92 pages

4505   Handtalk Zoo
Macmillan Publishing Company
6535 Nova Drive
Davie, FL 33317-6221

954-530-8746
800-257-5755
Fax: 954-530-6247
post@mcp.com
www.mcp.com

Wonderful photographs are used to show children at the zoo communicating with sign language.
28 pages Hardcover
ISBN: 0-027008-01-0

4506   Hearing Aid Handbook
Gallaudet University
800 Florida Avenue, NE
Washington, DC 20002-3819

773-568-1550
800-621-2736
Fax: 800-621-8476
TTY: 888-630-9347
gupress@gallaudet.edu
gupress.gallaudet.edu

A complete guide for wearers and clinicians for the use and maintenance of hearing aids.
172 pages Paperback
Donna S. Wayner, Author

4507   Hearing Impaired Children and Youth and Developmental Disabilities
Gallaudet University
800 Florida Avenue, NE
Washington, DC 20002-3819

773-568-1550
800-621-2736
Fax: 800-621-8476
TTY: 888-630-9347
gupress@gallaudet.edu
gupress.gallaudet.edu

Offers insights from 24 experts to help clarify relationships between hearing impairments and developmental difficulties.
416 pages

4508   Hearing Loss Help
Impact Publications
9104 Manassas Drive
Manassas Park, VA 20111-5211

703-361-7300
Fax: 703-335-9469
query2@impactpublications.com
www.impactpublications.com

Self-help guide provides factual information on how we hear, and on the causes and symptoms of hearing loss. Gives practical information on ways to improve everyday communication and create better listening conditions, and covers assistive listening devices.

4509   Hearing Loss and Hearing Aids: A Bridge to Healing
Richard Carmen, author
Hearing Loss Association of America
7910 Woodmont Avenue
Bethesda, MD 20814-3079

301-657-2248
Fax: 301-913-9413
TTY: 301-657-2249
info@hearingloss.org
www.hearingloss.org

The Consumer Handbook on hearing loss and hearing aids.
Softcover
ISBN: 0-966182-61-8
Anna Gilmore Hall, Executive Director
Lise Hamlin, Director of Public Policy

4510   Hispanic Deaf
Gallaudet University
800 Florida Avenue, NE
Washington, DC 20002-3819

773-568-1550
800-621-2736
Fax: 800-621-8476
TTY: 888-630-9347
gupress@gallaudet.edu
gupress.gallaudet.edu

Hispanic students now make up the largest minority in education for deaf students. This timely collection includes articles by many of the professionals most closely involved with the education of this very special population.
213 pages Hardcover

4511   History of Special Education: From Isolation to Integration
Gallaudet University
800 Florida Avenue, NE
Washington, DC 20002-3819

773-568-1550
800-621-2736
Fax: 800-621-8476
TTY: 888-630-9347
gupress@gallaudet.edu
gupress.gallaudet.edu

Comprehensive volume examining the facts and events that shaped this field in Western Europe, United States and Canada.
464 pages
Margret A. Winzer, Author

4512   Hollywood Speaks
Gallaudet University
800 Florida Avenue, NE
Washington, DC 20002-3819

773-568-1550
800-621-2736
Fax: 800-621-8476
TTY: 888-630-9347
gupress@gallaudet.edu
gupress.gallaudet.edu

How deafness has been treated in movies and how it provides yet another window onto social history in addition to a fresh angle from which to view Hollywood.
167 pages Hardcover

4513   Hometown Heroes: Successful Deaf Youth in America
Gallaudet University
800 Florida Avenue, NE
Washington, DC 20002-3819

773-568-1550
800-621-2736
Fax: 800-621-8476
TTY: 888-630-9347
gupress@gallaudet.edu
gupress.gallaudet.edu

A lively book showcasing more than 40 deaf and hard-of-hearing teenagers in the United States.
108 pages

4514   How Hearing Impacts Relationships
Richard Carmen, author
Hearing Loss Association of America
7910 Woodmont Avenue
Bethesda, MD 20814-3079

301-657-2248
Fax: 301-913-9413
TTY: 301-657-2249
info@hearingloss.org
www.hearingloss.org

At last families of loved ones with untreated hearing loss can know they are not alone and what options are available.
Softcover
ISBN: 0-966182-63-4
Anna Gilmore Hall, Executive Director
Lise Hamlin, Director of Public Policy

4515 How the Student with Hearing Loss Can Succeed in College
Alexander Graham Bell Association
3417 Volta Place NW
Washington, DC 20007-2737
202-337-5220
Fax: 202-337-8314
TTY: 202-337-5220
info@agbell.org
www.listeningandspokenlanguage.org
This revised book details how students who are deaf or hard of hearing and professionals must work together for students in college to be successful.
1996 304 pages

4516 How to Survive a Hearing Loss
Gallaudet University
800 Florida Avenue, NE
Washington, DC 20002-3819
773-568-1550
800-621-2736
Fax: 800-621-8476
TTY: 888-630-9347
gupress@gallaudet.edu
gupress.gallaudet.edu
This book presents the results of the author's intensive research about hearing and the ear.
241 pages
Charlotte Himber, Author

4517 Hug Just Isn't Enough
Gallaudet University
800 Florida Avenue, NE
Washington, DC 20002-3819
773-568-1550
800-621-2736
Fax: 800-621-8476
TTY: 888-630-9347
gupress@gallaudet.edu
gupress.gallaudet.edu
Photos of deaf children and excerpts from interviews with parents of deaf youngsters.

4518 I Didn't Hear the Dragon Roar
Gallaudet University
800 Florida Avenue, NE
Washington, DC 20002-3819
773-568-1550
800-621-2736
Fax: 800-621-8476
TTY: 888-630-9347
gupress@gallaudet.edu
gupress.gallaudet.edu
The remarkable true story of a deaf woman's journey from Hong Kong to Katmandu.
251 pages

4519 IDEA Advocacy for Children Who are Deaf or Hard of Hearing
Alexander Graham Bell Association
3417 Volta Place NW
Washington, DC 20007-2737
202-337-5220
Fax: 202-337-8314
TTY: 202-337-5220
info@agbell.org
www.listeningandspokenlanguage.org
This book offers up to date information about the 1997 Individuals with Disabilities Education Act which affects children who are deaf or hard of hearing.
1997 96 pages

4520 Implications and Complications for Deaf Students of Full Inclusion Movement
Gallaudet University
800 Florida Avenue, NE
Washington, DC 20002-3819
773-568-1550
800-621-2736
Fax: 800-621-8476
TTY: 888-630-9347
gupress@gallaudet.edu
gupress.gallaudet.edu
A collection of papers discussing the full inclusion movement.
80 pages

4521 In Silence: Growing Up Hearing in a Deaf World
Gallaudet University
800 Florida Avenue, NE
Washington, DC 20002-3819
773-568-1550
800-621-2736
Fax: 800-621-8476
TTY: 888-630-9347
gupress@gallaudet.edu
gupress.gallaudet.edu
Author's story of growing up as a hearing child of deaf parents.
335 pages
Ruth Sidransky, Author

4522 In This Sign
Gallaudet University
800 Florida Avenue, NE
Washington, DC 20002-3819
773-568-1550
800-621-2736
Fax: 800-621-8476
TTY: 888-630-9347
gupress@gallaudet.edu
gupress.gallaudet.edu
A modern classic following a family of deaf parents and their hearing impaired child through several decades of growth and pain, tragedy and triumph.
275 pages

4523 Inclusion?
Gallaudet University
800 Florida Avenue, NE
Washington, DC 20002-3819
773-568-1550
800-621-2736
Fax: 800-621-8476
TTY: 888-630-9347
gupress@gallaudet.edu
gupress.gallaudet.edu
This book defines quality education for deaf and hard of hearing students.
213 pages

4524 International Directory of Periodicals Related to Deafness
Gallaudet University
800 Florida Avenue, NE
Washington, DC 20002-3819
773-568-1550
800-621-2736
Fax: 800-621-8476
TTY: 888-630-9347
gupress@gallaudet.edu
gupress.gallaudet.edu
Offers information on more than 500 magazines and journals related to deafness.
150 pages

4525 International Telephone Directory for TDD Users
Gallaudet University
800 Florida Avenue, NE
Washington, DC 20002-3819
773-568-1550
800-621-2736
Fax: 800-621-8476
TTY: 888-630-9347
gupress@gallaudet.edu
gupress.gallaudet.edu
Offers 12,000 TDD members and organizations serving deaf people.
190 pages

4526 Introduction to Communication
Gallaudet University
800 Florida Avenue, NE
Washington, DC 20002-3819
773-568-1550
800-621-2736
Fax: 800-621-8476
TTY: 888-630-9347
gupress@gallaudet.edu
gupress.gallaudet.edu
Curriculum materials exploring the areas of sound, hearing and interpersonal communication.
100 pages

4527 Invisible Condition: The Human Side of Hearing Loss
Howard E Stone, author
Hearing Loss Association of America

7910 Woodmont Avenue
Bethesda, MD 20814-3079

301-657-2248
Fax: 301-913-9413
TTY: 301-657-2249
info@hearingloss.org
www.hearingloss.org

A collection of 14 years of editorials by the author from the SHHH Journal. An inspiration book that transcends hearing loss.
1993
Anna Gilmore Hall, Executive Director
Howard E. Stone, Author

4528   Its Your Turn Now: Using Dialogue Journals with Deaf Students
Gallaudet University
800 Florida Avenue, NE
Washington, DC 20002-3819

773-568-1550
800-621-2736
Fax: 800-621-8476
TTY: 888-630-9347
gupress@gallaudet.edu
gupress.gallaudet.edu

Based on years of experience, this book reviews teachers' questions and answers.
130 pages

4529   Journey Into the Deaf World
DawnSignPress
6130 Nancy Ridge Drive
San Diego, CA 92121-3223

858-625-0600
800-549-5350
Fax: 858-625-2336
TTY: 858-625-0600
comments@dawnsign.com
www.dawnsign.com

Provides explanation about the nature and meaning of the deaf world. Comprehensive work discusses latest findings and theories for deaf studies students and professionals working with deaf people.
528 pages Paperback
ISBN: 0-915035-63-4
Harlan Lane, Co-Author
Robert Hoffmeister, Co-Author

4530   Journey Out of Silence
Dora Tinglestad Weber, author

Hearing Loss Association of America
7910 Woodmont Avenue
Bethesda, MD 20814-3079

301-657-2248
Fax: 301-913-9413
TTY: 301-657-2249
info@hearingloss.org
www.hearingloss.org

Dora Weber, who made a long and arduous journey out of silence, shares her experiences in an effort to encourage those who are hearing impaired and to increase the sensitivity of those who are not.
Softcover
ISBN: 1-890676-30-6
Anna Gilmore Hall, Executive Director
Lise Hamlin, Director of Public Policy

4531   Joy of Signing
Gospel Publishing House
1445 N Boonville Avenue
Springfield, MO 65802-1894

417-831-8000
800-641-4310
Fax: 417-862-5881
CustSrvOrders@ag.org
gospelpublishing.com

Illustrated sign language text with descriptions of the origin of selected signs and examples of how each is used. Second edition.
352 pages
Lottie L. Riekehof, Author

4532   Kaleidoscope of Deaf America
Harris Communications
8630 Fenton Street
Silver Spring, MD 20910-3248

301-587-1788
Fax: 301-587-1791
TTY: 301-587-1789
nad.org

Puts you in touch with the trends, the events and the thinking that is shaping your future.
79 pages

4533   Kendall Demonstration Elementary School Curriculum Guides
Gallaudet University
800 Florida Avenue, NE
Washington, DC 20002-3819

773-568-1550
800-621-2736
Fax: 800-621-8476
TTY: 888-630-9347
gupress@gallaudet.edu
gupress.gallaudet.edu

These guides provide detailed information to help teachers organize curriculum, structure classes and develop individualized education programs.
18 months+

4534   Kid-Friendly Parenting with Deaf and Hard of Hearing Children
Gallaudet University
800 Florida Avenue, NE
Washington, DC 20002-3819

773-568-1550
800-621-2736
Fax: 800-621-8476
TTY: 888-630-9347
gupress@gallaudet.edu
gupress.gallaudet.edu

A step-by-step guide offering parents hundreds of ideas and play activities for children ages 3 to 12.
336 pages
Daria Medwid, Co-Author
Denise Chapman Weston, Co-Author

4535   Learning to Hear Again
Alexander Graham Bell Association
3417 Volta Place NW
Washington, DC 20007-2737

202-337-5220
Fax: 202-337-8314
TTY: 202-337-5220
info@agbell.org
www.listeningandspokenlanguage.org

This audiologic rehabilitation curriculum guide is designed to help audiologists and speech language pathologist provide rehabilitation and education for adults with hearing losses. The authors are practicing audiologists and have used these methods successfully in individual and group sessions. This comprehensive manual comprises lesson plans, activities and materials ready to be duplicated and distributed to clients.
1996 224 pages

4536   Learning to See: American Sign Language as a Second Language
Gallaudet University
800 Florida Avenue, NE
Washington, DC 20002-3819

773-568-1550
800-621-2736
Fax: 800-621-8476
TTY: 888-630-9347
gupress@gallaudet.edu
gupress.gallaudet.edu

Provides a comprehensive introduction to the history and structure of ASL to the deaf community.
134 pages

4537   Least Restrictive Environment: The Paradox of Inclusion
LRP Publications
P.O. Box 24668
West Palm Beach, FL 33416-0980

800-341-7874
Fax: 561-622-2423
custserv@lrp.com
www.lrp.com

Analyzes relevant federal law and the inclusion reform movement, and discusses the premise that an effort to force one generic placement on all children will create more problems than thought imaginable.
Paperback

4538   Legal Rights for the Deaf and Hard of Hearing
Hearing Loss Association of America
7910 Woodmont Avenue
Bethesda, MD 20814-3079

301-657-2248
Fax: 301-913-9413
TTY: 301-657-2249
info@hearingloss.org
www.hearingloss.org

A comprehensive analysis of recent laws passed to protect the rights of and guarantee equal access for people with hearing loss.

The book explains in layman's terminology how legislation affects individuals with disabilities in everyday life.
2002 Softcover
Anna Gilmore Hall, Executive Director
Lise Hamlin, Director of Public Policy

4539 Legal Rights of Hearing-Impaired People
Gallaudet University
800 Florida Avenue, NE
Washington, DC 20002-3819
773-568-1550
800-621-2736
Fax: 800-621-8476
TTY: 888-630-9347
gupress@gallaudet.edu
gupress.gallaudet.edu
Includes updated interpretations of legislation affecting hearing-impaired people, including chapters dealing with the ADA.
297 pages

4540 Lessons in Laughter: The Autobiography of a Deaf Actor
Gallaudet University
800 Florida Avenue, NE
Washington, DC 20002-3819
773-568-1550
800-621-2736
Fax: 800-621-8476
TTY: 888-630-9347
gupress@gallaudet.edu
gupress.gallaudet.edu
Born deaf of deaf parents, Bernard Bragg dreamed of using sign language to act. This book recounts how he starred in his own television show.
237 pages

4541 Let's Learn About Deafness
Gallaudet University
800 Florida Avenue, NE
Washington, DC 20002-3819
773-568-1550
800-621-2736
Fax: 800-621-8476
TTY: 888-630-9347
gupress@gallaudet.edu
gupress.gallaudet.edu
Hands-on school classroom activities for the deaf student.
82 pages

4542 Listen to Me: Auditory Exercises for Adults
Alexander Graham Bell Association
3417 Volta Place NW
Washington, DC 20007-2737
202-337-5220
Fax: 202-337-8314
TTY: 202-337-5220
info@agbell.org
www.listeningandspokenlanguage.org
Helps hard of hearing teenagers and adults to listen, lip read, pick up clues from conversations and remember what they have heard.
65 pages

4543 Listen with the Heart: Relationships and Hearing Loss
Hearing Loss Association of America
7910 Woodmont Avenue
Bethesda, MD 20814-3079
301-657-2248
Fax: 301-913-9413
TTY: 301-657-2249
info@hearingloss.org
www.hearingloss.org
Written for family and friends as well as professionals. It is an excellent text for college and graduate level courses in psychology, mental health counseling, speech and hearing, special education, and deaf education.
Anna Gilmore Hall, Executive Director
Michael A. Harvey, Author

4544 Listening
National Catholic Office for the Deaf
7201 Buchnan Street
Landover Hills, MD 20784-4500
301-577-1684
Info@ncod.org
www.ncod.org
Published as a pastoral service for the hearing impaired.

4545 Listening & Talking
Alexander Graham Bell Association

3417 Volta Place NW
Washington, DC 20007-2737
202-337-5220
Fax: 202-337-8314
TTY: 202-337-5220
info@agbell.org
www.listeningandspokenlanguage.org
This guide promotes spoken language in young hearing-impaired children.
191 pages

4546 Listening to Learn: A Handbook for Parents with Hearing-Impaired Children
Alexander Graham Bell Association
3417 Volta Place NW
Washington, DC 20007-2737
202-337-5220
Fax: 202-337-8314
TTY: 202-337-5220
info@agbell.org
www.listeningandspokenlanguage.org
Developed by teachers, this handbook provides parents with the essential steps necessary to develop effective spoken communication with their children.
98 pages

4547 Listening: Ways of Hearing in a Silent World
Hannah Merker, author
Hearing Loss Association of America
7910 Woodmont Avenue
Bethesda, MD 20814-3079
301-657-2248
Fax: 301-913-9413
TTY: 301-657-2249
info@hearingloss.org
www.hearingloss.org
This book is about one woman's evocative account of her perceptions and rememberance of sound.
1999
Anna Gilmore Hall, Executive Director
Lise Hamlin, Director of Public Policy

4548 Literature Journal
Gallaudet University
800 Florida Avenue, NE
Washington, DC 20002-3819
773-568-1550
800-621-2736
Fax: 800-621-8476
TTY: 888-630-9347
gupress@gallaudet.edu
gupress.gallaudet.edu
This book includes extensive examples of student and teacher entries taken from actual journals of deaf high school students.
44 pages

4549 Living with Hearing Loss
Marcia B Dugan, author
Hearing Loss Association of America
7910 Woodmont Avenue
Bethesda, MD 20814-3079
301-657-2248
Fax: 301-913-9413
TTY: 301-657-2249
info@hearingloss.org
www.hearingloss.org
Living with Hearing Loss takes the reader from A to Z on the kinds and causes of hearing loss and its common early signs. Topics Include: Seeking Professional Evaluations, Hearing Aids, Assistive Technology, Speechreading, Communication Tips, Cochlear Implants, Dealing with Tinnitus, and resources.
2003
ISBN: 1-563681-34-0
Anna Gilmore Hall, Executive Director
Lise Hamlin, Director of Public Policy

4550 Looking Back: A Reader on the History of Deaf Communities & Sign Language
Gallaudet University
800 Florida Avenue, NE
Washington, DC 20002-3819
773-568-1550
800-621-2736
Fax: 800-621-8476
TTY: 888-630-9347
gupress@gallaudet.edu
gupress.gallaudet.edu
Renowned researchers from around the world present provocative findings in six areas relating to the deaf culture.
558 pages

4551 Loss for Words
Gallaudet University
800 Florida Avenue, NE
Washington, DC 20002-3819
773-568-1550
800-621-2736
Fax: 800-621-8476
TTY: 888-630-9347
gupress@gallaudet.edu
gupress.gallaudet.edu

The author's touching story of her life as an interpreter for her parents, head of her household by the age of eight and a teacher and helper to both of her deaf parents.
208 pages

4552 Mainstreaming Deaf and Hard of Hearing Students
Gallaudet University
800 Florida Avenue NE
Washington, DC 20002-3695
773-568-1550
800-621-2736
Fax: 800-621-8476
TTY: 888-630-9347
gupress@gallaudet.edu
gupress.gallaudet.edu

Gallaudet University is the world leader in liberal education and career development for deaf and hard-of-hearing undergraduate students.
40 pages

4553 Man Without Words
Gallaudet University
800 Florida Avenue, NE
Washington, DC 20002-3819
773-568-1550
800-621-2736
Fax: 800-621-8476
TTY: 888-630-9347
gupress@gallaudet.edu
gupress.gallaudet.edu

Author relates her experiences teaching sign language to a 27 year old deaf Mexican man who had no education and no language.
203 pages

4554 Martimer
APSEA-RCHI
Box 308
Amherst, NS, B4H 3Z6,
902-667-3808
Fax: 902-667-0893
Periodical describing programs and services provided by the APSEA Resource Center for the Hearing Impaired.
Phyllis Cameron, Editor

4555 Mask of Benevolence: Disabling the Deaf Community
Gallaudet University
800 Florida Avenue, NE
Washington, DC 20002-3819
773-568-1550
800-621-2736
Fax: 800-621-8476
TTY: 888-630-9347
gupress@gallaudet.edu
gupress.gallaudet.edu

Written by a doctor who does not view deafness as a handicap but rather a different state of hearing.
310 pages

4556 Meeting Halfway in ASL
MSM Productions
1095 Meigs Street
Rochester, NY 14620-3380
716-442-6370
Fax: 716-442-6371
TTY: 716-442-6370
Books@deaflife.com
www.deaflife.com

Illustrated photographic sign-language book containing 1,300 photos.
ISBN: 0-963401-67-
Bernard Bragg, Co-Author
Jack R. Olson, Co-Author

4557 Meeting the Challenge: Hearing-Impaired Professionals in the Workplace
Gallaudet University
800 Florida Avenue, NE
Washington, DC 20002-3819
773-568-1550
800-621-2736
Fax: 800-621-8476
TTY: 888-630-9347
gupress@gallaudet.edu
gupress.gallaudet.edu

Provides information on communication methods, educational backgrounds and job search tactics used by more than 1500 participants and their current employment conditions.
236 pages

4558 Mental Health Services for Deaf People
Gallaudet University
800 Florida Avenue, NE
Washington, DC 20002-3819
773-568-1550
800-621-2736
Fax: 800-621-8476
TTY: 888-630-9347
gupress@gallaudet.edu
gupress.gallaudet.edu

Contains information on over 350 mental health programs and services for deaf people across the United States.
210 pages

4559 Missing Words: The Family Handbook on Adult Hearing Loss
Gallaudet University
800 Florida Avenue, NE
Washington, DC 20002-3819
773-568-1550
800-621-2736
Fax: 800-621-8476
TTY: 888-630-9347
gupress@gallaudet.edu
gupress.gallaudet.edu

Written by a mother who lost her hearing and her daughter, learning to cope.
304 pages

4560 Mother Father Deaf: Living Between Sound and Silence
Harvard University Press
79 Garden Street
Cambridge, MA 02138-1423
617-495-2600
800-448-2242
Fax: 617-495-5898
contact_hup@harvard.edu
www.hup.harvard.edu

Based on interviews with 150 adult hearing children of deaf parents who chart the sometimes difficult middle ground between spoken and signed language.
Paul Preston, Author

4561 Moving Toward the Standards
Gallaudet University
800 Florida Avenue, NE
Washington, DC 20002-3819
773-568-1550
800-621-2736
Fax: 800-621-8476
TTY: 888-630-9347
gupress@gallaudet.edu
gupress.gallaudet.edu

A national action plan for mathematics education reform for the deaf.
55 pages

4562 Music in Motion
Modern Signs Press
PO Box 1181
Los Alamitos, CA 90720-1181
562-596-8548
800-572-7332
Fax: 562-795-6614
TTY: 562-493-4168
modsigns@modernsignspress.com
www.modernsignspress.com

Includes guitar notes and glossary of sign descriptions for 325-word vocabulary.
109 pages
ISBN: 0-916708-07-1

4563 NAD Deaf Awareness Kit
National Association of the Deaf
8630 Fenton Street
Silver Spring, MD 20910
301-587-1788
Fax: 301-587-1791
TTY: 301-587-1789
nad.info@nad.org
nad.org

Includes information that can be used both during Deaf Awareness Week and year-round to recognize the accomplishments and heritage of the deaf community.
Christopher Wagner, President
Melissa S. Draganac-Hawk, Vice-President

4564 Never the Twain Shall Meet: The Communications Debate
Gallaudet University
800 Florida Avenue, NE   773-568-1550
Washington, DC 20002-3819   800-621-2736
                                      Fax: 800-621-8476
                                      TTY: 888-630-9347
                                      gupress@gallaudet.edu
                                      gupress.gallaudet.edu
Should sign language be used in the education of Deaf children or
should they be forced to deal with a hearing, speaking world on its
own terms?.
129 pages

4565 Next Step
Gallaudet University
800 Florida Avenue, NE   773-568-1550
Washington, DC 20002-3819   800-621-2736
                                      Fax: 800-621-8476
                                      TTY: 888-630-9347
                                      gupress@gallaudet.edu
                                      gupress.gallaudet.edu
A national conference focusing on issues related to substance
abuse in the deaf and hard of hearing population.
209 pages

4566 No Sound
Harris Communications
6541 City W Parkway   612-906-1180
Eden Prairie, MN 55344-3248   Fax: 612-946-0924
A moving, highly informative autobiography of Julius Wiggins,
founder and president of the newspaper Silent News. Second
edition.
211 pages

4567 No Walls of Stone: An Anthology of Literature by Deaf Writers
Gallaudet University
800 Florida Avenue, NE   773-568-1550
Washington, DC 20002-3819   800-621-2736
                                      Fax: 800-621-8476
                                      TTY: 888-630-9347
                                      gupress@gallaudet.edu
                                      gupress.gallaudet.edu
Short fiction, essays, verse and drama written by the deaf and hard
of hearing writer.
240 pages
Jill Jepson, Editor

4568 None So Deaf
Gallaudet University
800 Florida Avenue, NE   773-568-1550
Washington, DC 20002-3819   800-621-2736
                                      Fax: 800-621-8476
                                      TTY: 888-630-9347
                                      gupress@gallaudet.edu
                                      gupress.gallaudet.edu
A student history of education of deaf people and the development
of sign language.
51 pages Paperback

4569 Odyssey of Hearing Loss: Tales of Triumph
Michael A Harvey, PhD, author
Hearing Loss Association of America
7910 Woodmont Avenue   301-657-2248
Bethesda, MD 20814-3079   Fax: 301-913-9413
                                      TTY: 301-657-2249
                                      info@hearingloss.org
                                      www.hearingloss.org
A glimpse into the lives of 10 people; each showing how sharing
insights about hearing loss helps people on the road to healing and
a life well examined.
Anna Gilmore Hall, Executive Director
Michael A. Harvey, Author

4570 Okada Hearing Ear Guide
RR 1 Box 640F   414-275-5226
Fontana, WI 53125-9714
Trains dogs to aid hearing-impaired persons.

4571 On My Own
Gallaudet University
800 Florida Avenue, NE   773-568-1550
Washington, DC 20002-3819   800-621-2736
                                      Fax: 800-621-8476
                                      TTY: 888-630-9347
                                      gupress@gallaudet.edu
                                      gupress.gallaudet.edu
Book examining doorbell devices, alarm clocks, telephone ampli-
fiers and other assistive devices for the deaf.
50 pages Teacher's Guide

4572 Oral Interpreting Selections from Papers from Kirsten Gonzales
Alexander Graham Bell Association
3417 Volta Place NW   202-337-5220
Washington, DC 20007-2737   Fax: 202-337-8314
                                      TTY: 202-337-5220
                                      info@agbell.org
                                      www.listeningandspokenlanguage.org
These six easy to read articles discuss speech reading and oral interpreting. The articles answer questions that are frequently asked
by professionals and the general public.
30 pages

4573 Other Side of Silence
Gallaudet University
800 Florida Avenue, NE   773-568-1550
Washington, DC 20002-3819   800-621-2736
                                      Fax: 800-621-8476
                                      TTY: 888-630-9347
                                      gupress@gallaudet.edu
                                      gupress.gallaudet.edu
Explores the deaf community through interviews from across the
country.
256 pages

4574 Our Forgotten Children
Alexander Graham Bell Association
3417 Volta Place NW   202-337-5220
Washington, DC 20007-2737   Fax: 202-337-8314
                                      TTY: 202-337-5220
                                      info@agbell.org
                                      www.listeningandspokenlanguage.org
This simple book describes characteristics of hard-of-hearing children in the school and discusses their educational requirements,
psychological and social needs and amplification options.
68 pages

4575 Our Forgotten Children: Hard of Hearing Pupils in the Schools
Julia M Davis, PhD, author
Hearing Loss Association of America
7910 Woodmont Avenue   301-657-2248
Bethesda, MD 20814-3079   Fax: 301-913-9413
                                      TTY: 301-657-2249
                                      info@hearingloss.org
                                      www.hearingloss.org
Important resource about the educational environment.
2001
Anna Gilmore Hall, Executive Director
Lise Hamlin, Director of Public Policy

4576 Outsiders in a Hearing World
Gallaudet University
800 Florida Avenue, NE   773-568-1550
Washington, DC 20002-3819   800-621-2736
                                      Fax: 800-621-8476
                                      TTY: 888-630-9347
                                      gupress@gallaudet.edu
                                      gupress.gallaudet.edu
The author gives a sociologist's view of what it is like to be deaf.
240 pages

4577 Parents and Teachers: Partners in Language Development
Alexander Graham Bell Association
3417 Volta Place NW   202-337-5220
Washington, DC 20007-2737   Fax: 202-337-8314
                                      TTY: 202-337-5220
                                      info@agbell.org
                                      www.listeningandspokenlanguage.org

Outlines the essential role of the teacher and parent in the development of language in the school aged child with hearing impairment.
386 pages

4578 Perigee Visual Dictionary of Signing
Harris Communications
6541 City W Parkway   612-906-1180
Eden Prairie, MN 55344-3248   Fax: 612-946-0924
An A-to-Z guide to American Sign Language vocabulary.
450 pages

4579 Perspectives Folio: Mainstreaming
Gallaudet University
800 Florida Avenue, NE   773-568-1550
Washington, DC 20002-3819   800-621-2736
                                                        Fax: 800-621-8476
                                                        TTY: 888-630-9347
                                                        gupress@gallaudet.edu
                                                        gupress.gallaudet.edu
Presents 14 articles from Perspectives magazine that offer practical, experience-based advice on mainstreaming for parents and students themselves.
39 pages

4580 Perspectives on Deafness
National Association of the Deaf
8630 Fenton Street   301-587-1788
Silver Spring, MD 20910   Fax: 301-587-1791
                                                        TTY: 301-587-1789
                                                        nad.info@nad.org
                                                        nad.org
Focuses on the many perspectives which constitute diversity within the deaf community.
Paperback
Christopher Wagner, President
Melissa S. Draganac-Hawk, Vice-President

4581 Place of Their Own: Creating the Deaf Community in America
Gallaudet University Press
800 Florida Avenue, NE   773-568-1550
Washington, DC 20002-3819   800-621-2736
                                                        Fax: 800-621-8476
                                                        TTY: 888-630-9347
                                                        gupress@gallaudet.edu
                                                        gupress.gallaudet.edu
Traces the history of deaf people and views deafness not from the perspective of a pathology, but of culture, not as a disease or disability to overcome or be cured, but as the distinguishing characteristic of a distinct community of individuals whose history and achievement are worthy of study.

4582 Politics of Deafness
Gallaudet University
800 Florida Avenue, NE   773-568-1550
Washington, DC 20002   800-621-2736
                                                        Fax: 800-621-8476
                                                        TTY: 888-630-9347
                                                        gupress@gallaudet.edu
                                                        gupress.gallaudet.edu
Embarks upon a postmodern examination of the search for identity in deafness and its relationship to the prevalent Hearing culture that has marginalized Deaf people.
June 1997 304 pages Softcover
ISBN: 1-563680-58-0
Owen Wrigley, Author

4583 Possible Dream: Mainstream Experiences of Hearing-Impaired Students
Alexander Graham Bell Association
3417 Volta Place NW   202-337-5220
Washington, DC 20007-2737   Fax: 202-337-8314
                                                        TTY: 202-337-5220
                                                        info@agbell.org
                                         www.listeningandspokenlanguage.org
This collection highlights the experiences of auditory-oral children who are Bell Association financial aid winners and their families.
66 pages
Mildred L Oberkotter, Editor

4584 Post Milan
Gallaudet University
800 Florida Avenue, NE   773-568-1550
Washington, DC 20002-3819   800-621-2736
                                                        Fax: 800-621-8476
                                                        TTY: 888-630-9347
                                                        TDD: 800-621-8476
                                                        gupress@gallaudet.edu
                                                        gupress.gallaudet.edu
Timely issues covering trends in ASL and ASL/English literacy.
323 pages

4585 PreReading Strategies
Gallaudet University
800 Florida Avenue, NE   773-568-1550
Washington, DC 20002-3819   800-621-2736
                                                        Fax: 800-621-8476
                                                        TTY: 888-630-9347
                                                        gupress@gallaudet.edu
                                                        gupress.gallaudet.edu
Here is a wealth of good advice for preparing students to understand what they read, building comprehension and enjoyment.
65 pages

4586 Psychoeducational Assessment of Hearing-Impaired Students
Pro-Ed, Inc.
8700 Shoal Creek Blvd   512-451-3246
Austin, TX 78757-6897   800-897-3202
                                                        Fax: 512-451-8542
                                                        info@proedinc.com
                                                        www.proedinc.com
This book includes a comprehensive presentation of issues and procedures related to the assessment of hearing-impaired students.
251 pages Paperback
ISBN: 0-890794-55-3
Lindy Jordaan, Marketing Coordinator

4587 Reading and Deafness
Pro-Ed, Inc.
8700 Shoal Creek Blvd   512-451-3246
Austin, TX 78757-6897   800-897-3202
                                                        Fax: 800-397-7633
                                                        info@proedinc.com
                                                        www.proedinc.com
Three areas are looked at in this book: deaf children's prereading development of real-world knowledge; cognitive abilities and linguistic skills.
422 pages Hardcover
ISBN: 0-887441-07-6
Lindy Jordaan, Marketing Coordinator

4588 Rebuilt: My Journey Back to the Hearing World
Michael Chorost, author
Hearing Loss Association of America
7910 Woodmont Avenue   301-657-2248
Bethesda, MD 20814-3079   Fax: 301-913-9413
                                                        TTY: 301-657-2249
                                                        info@hearingloss.org
                                                        www.hearingloss.org
Brimming with insight and written with charm and self-deprecating humor, Rebuilt unveils, in personal terms, the astounding possibilities of a new technological age.
240 pages Paperback
ISBN: 0-618717-60-9
Anna Gilmore Hall, Executive Director
Lise Hamlin, Director of Public Policy

4589 Say That Again, Please
Gallaudet University
800 Florida Avenue, NE   773-568-1550
Washington, DC 20002-3819   800-621-2736
                                                        Fax: 800-621-8476
                                                        TTY: 888-630-9347
                                                        gupress@gallaudet.edu
                                                        gupress.gallaudet.edu
This book serves to enlighten those who are interested.
370 pages

4590 **Schedules of Development for Hearing Impaired Infants and their Parents**
Alexander Graham Bell Association
3417 Volta Place NW
Washington, DC 20007-2737
202-337-5220
Fax: 202-337-8314
TTY: 202-337-5220
info@agbell.org
www.listeningandspokenlanguage.org
Written for parents and teachers, this assessment record of verbal learning will help to evaluate each child's language development.
1977 14 pages

4591 **Science of Sound**
Gallaudet University
800 Florida Avenue, NE
Washington, DC 20002-3819
773-568-1550
800-621-2736
Fax: 800-621-8476
TTY: 888-630-9347
gupress@gallaudet.edu
gupress.gallaudet.edu
This exciting book is carefully designed to help hearing-impaired students understand, use and enjoy the principles of sound.
32 pages

4592 **Seeds of Disquiet: One Deaf Woman's Experience**
Gallaudet University
800 Florida Avenue, NE
Washington, DC 20002-3819
773-568-1550
800-621-2736
Fax: 800-621-8476
TTY: 888-630-9347
gupress@gallaudet.edu
gupress.gallaudet.edu
This book relates to the story of how Cheryl Heppner reacted to two severe losses in her hearing.
192 pages

4593 **Seeing Voices: A Journey Into the World of the Deaf**
Gallaudet University
800 Florida Avenue, NE
Washington, DC 20002-3819
773-568-1550
800-621-2736
Fax: 800-621-8476
TTY: 888-630-9347
gupress@gallaudet.edu
gupress.gallaudet.edu
Dr. Sacks takes us into the world of deaf people.
180 pages

4594 **Sign Communication: A Family Affair**
Gallaudet University
800 Florida Avenue, NE
Washington, DC 20002-3819
773-568-1550
800-621-2736
Fax: 800-621-8476
TTY: 888-630-9347
gupress@gallaudet.edu
gupress.gallaudet.edu
Book designed to help hearing parents communicate effectively with their deaf children on issues of good health and personal growth.
132 pages

4595 **Sign Language Feelings**
Gallaudet University
800 Florida Avenue, NE
Washington, DC 20002-3819
773-568-1550
800-621-2736
Fax: 800-621-8476
TTY: 888-630-9347
gupress@gallaudet.edu
gupress.gallaudet.edu
Worksheets teach signs for happy, sad and all of the feelings in between.

4596 **Sign Language Interpreters and Interpreting**
Gallaudet University
800 Florida Avenue, NE
Washington, DC 20002-3819
773-568-1550
800-621-2736
Fax: 800-621-8476
TTY: 888-630-9347
gupress@gallaudet.edu
gupress.gallaudet.edu

This monograph presents articles about personal characteristics and abilities of interpreters, the effects of lag time on interpreter errors, and the interpretation of register.
161 pages

4597 **Sign Language Made Simple**
Gospel Publishing House
1445 N Boonville Avenue
Springfield, MO 65802-1894
417-862-2781
800-641-4310
Fax: 417-862-7566
CustSrvOrders@ag.org
gospelpublishing.com
Illustrated sign language text with descriptions of the origin of selected signs and examples of how each is used. Second edition.
240 pages
Edgar D. Lawrence, Author

4598 **Sign Language Talk**
Franklin Watts Grolier
557 Broadway
New York, NY 10012-0001
573-632-1632
800-724-6527
Fax: 203-797-3197
www.grolier.com
Using 300 easy-to-follow illustrations, this book introduces the structure of sign language, shows how sentences are formed and how signed conversations differ from spoken ones.
96 pages
ISBN: 0-531105-97-0

4599 **Sign Language and the Deaf Community: Essays in Honor of William Stokoe**
National Association of the Deaf
8630 Fenton Street
Silver Spring, MD 20910
301-587-1788
Fax: 301-587-1791
TTY: 301-587-1789
nad.info@nad.org
nad.org
Collection of essays, written by professionals in the field of sign language research and usage, describing how information has dramatically altered society's understanding of deaf people and their culture.
267 pages Paperback
Christopher Wagner, President
Melissa S. Draganac-Hawk, Vice-President

4600 **Signed English Starter**
Harris Communications
6541 City W Parkway
Eden Prairie, MN 55344-3248
612-906-1108
Fax: 612-946-0924
gupress.gallaudet.edu
The first book to use when learning Signed English.
208 pages
Harry Bornstein, Co-Author
Karen L. Saulnier, Co-Author

4601 **Signing Exact English**
Modern Signs Press
PO Box 1181
Los Alamitos, CA 90720-1181
562-596-8548
800-572-7332
Fax: 562-795-6614
TTY: 562-493-4168
modsigns@modernsignspress.com
www.modernsignspress.com
A reference manual containing manual signs representing nearly 4,000 words, plus signs for letters, numbers, prefixes and suffixes.
1993 479 pages Softcover
ISBN: 0-196708-23-3

4602 **Signing Illustrated**
Gallaudet University
800 Florida Avenue, NE
Washington, DC 20002-3819
773-568-1550
800-621-2736
Fax: 800-621-8476
TTY: 888-630-9347
gupress@gallaudet.edu
gupress.gallaudet.edu
A guide presenting illustrations of over 1,350 signs.
85 pages

4603 Signing Naturally: Teacher's Curriculum Guide-Level 1
DawnSignPress
6130 Nancy Ridge Drive 619-625-0600
San Diego, CA 92121-3223 800-549-5350
Fax: 619-625-2336
DawnSign@aol.com
www.dawnsign.com

Guide and video.
336 pages 22 minutes
ISBN: 0-915035-07-3

4604 Signs Everywhere
Modern Signs Press
PO Box 1181 562-596-8548
Los Alamitos, CA 90720-1181 800-572-7332
Fax: 562-795-6614
TTY: 562-493-4168
modsigns@modernsignspress.com
www.modernsignspress.com
Includes signs for cities, towns and states through United States,
Canada and Mexico. Drawings and descriptions of the signs ac-
company maps showing locations of states and cities.
280 pages
ISBN: 0-916708-05-5

4605 Signs for Computing Terminology
National Association of the Deaf
8630 Fenton Street 301-587-1788
Silver Spring, MD 20910-4500 Fax: 301-587-1791
TTY: 301-587-1789
nad.info@nad.org
nad.org
Contains over 600 computer related sign illustrations used by deaf
and hearing computer specialists.
182 pages Paperback
ISBN: 0-913072-63-X
Christopher Wagner, President
Melissa S. Draganac-Hawk, Vice-President

4606 Silent Alarm: On the Edge with a Deaf EMT
Gallaudet University
800 Florida Avenue, NE 773-568-1550
Washington, DC 20002-3819 800-621-2736
Fax: 800-621-8476
TTY: 888-630-9347
gupress@gallaudet.edu
gupress.gallaudet.edu
Silent Alarm tells the gripping story of survival and the good that
the author did as a topnotch EMT.
160 pages
Steven L. Schrader, Author

4607 Silent Garden: Raising Your Deaf Child
Gallaudet University
800 Florida Avenue, NE 773-568-1550
Washington, DC 20002 800-621-2736
Fax: 800-621-8476
TTY: 888-630-9347
gupress@gallaudet.edu
gupress.gallaudet.edu
Provides parents with a firm foundation for making the difficult
decisions necessary for their deaf child's future. Includes information on critical concerns, communication, technological alternative, and reassurance through case studies and interviews.
304 pages Softcover
ISBN: 1-563680-58-0

**4608 Simultaneous Communication, ASL and Other Communication
Modes**
Gallaudet University
800 Florida Avenue, NE 773-568-1550
Washington, DC 20002-3819 800-621-2736
Fax: 800-621-8476
TTY: 888-630-9347
gupress@gallaudet.edu
gupress.gallaudet.edu
This monograph presents four major articles that examine issues
surrounding communications in an educational environment.
236 pages

4609 Sing Praise
Sunday School Board of the Southern Baptists
127 9th Avenue N 800-458-2772
Nashville, TN 37234-0001
For use by interpreters to the deaf.

4610 Sociolinguistics in Deaf Communities
Gallaudet University
800 Florida Avenue, NE 773-568-1550
Washington, DC 20002-3819 800-621-2736
Fax: 800-621-8476
TTY: 888-630-9347
gupress@gallaudet.edu
gupress.gallaudet.edu
The first volume in a series offering assessments and up-to-date in-
formation on sign language linguistics.
280 pages
Ceil Lucas, Editor

4611 Software to Go
Gallaudet University
800 Florida Avenue, NE 773-568-1550
Washington, DC 20002-3819 800-621-2736
Fax: 800-621-8476
TTY: 888-630-9347
gupress@gallaudet.edu
gupress.gallaudet.edu
Lists and describes commercial software that may be borrowed by
educators of hearing impaired students.
100 pages

4612 Sound and Sign, Childhood Deafness and Mental Health
Gallaudet University
800 Florida Avenue, NE 773-568-1550
Washington, DC 20002-3819 800-621-2736
Fax: 800-621-8476
TTY: 888-630-9347
gupress@gallaudet.edu
gupress.gallaudet.edu
Presents research to support beliefs that deaf children should be
educated using a combination manual and oral communication in
residual hearing and speech.
265 pages

4613 Speak to Me
Gallaudet University
800 Florida Avenue, NE 773-568-1550
Washington, DC 20002-3819 800-621-2736
Fax: 800-621-8476
TTY: 888-630-9347
gupress@gallaudet.edu
gupress.gallaudet.edu
A story of a single mother confronted with the deafness of her son.
160 pages
Marcia Calhoun Forecki, Author

4614 Speech and the Hearing-Impaired Child
Alexander Graham Bell Association
3417 Volta Place NW 202-337-5220
Washington, DC 20007-2737 Fax: 202-337-8314
TTY: 202-337-5220
info@agbell.org
www.listeningandspokenlanguage.org
Provides a systematic approach to the teaching of speech and a
challenge to all involved in the development of spoken language
skills in hearing-impaired children.
402 pages

4615 Speechreading in Context
Gallaudet University
800 Florida Avenue, NE 773-568-1550
Washington, DC 20002-3819 800-621-2736
Fax: 800-621-8476
TTY: 888-630-9347
gupress@gallaudet.edu
gupress.gallaudet.edu
This useful guide for teachers and therapists approaches
speechreading instruction with the help of context cues.
32 pages

4616 Speechreading: A Way to Improve Understand ing
Harriet Kaplan, author
Hearing Loss Association of America
7910 Woodmont Avenue
Bethesda, MD 20814
301-657-2248
Fax: 301-913-9413
TTY: 3016572249
info@hearingloss.org
www.hearingloss.org
Discusses the nature and process of speechreading, its benefits, and its limitations. This useful book clarifies commonly-held misconceptions about speechreading. The beginning chapters address difficult communication situations and problems related to the speaker, the speechreader, and the environment It then offers strategies to manage them.
160 pages Paperback
Anna Gilmore Hall, Executive Director
Lise Hamlin, Director of Public Policy

4617 Study of American Deaf Folklore
Gallaudet University
800 Florida Avenue, NE
Washington, DC 20002-3819
773-568-1550
800-621-2736
Fax: 800-621-8476
TTY: 888-630-9347
gupress@gallaudet.edu
gupress.gallaudet.edu
Presents a discussion of the different functions that folklore serves in the community.
156 pages

4618 Substance Abuse and Recovery: Empowerment of Deaf Persons
Gallaudet University
800 Florida Avenue, NE
Washington, DC 20002-3819
773-568-1550
800-621-2736
Fax: 800-621-8476
TTY: 888-630-9347
gupress@gallaudet.edu
gupress.gallaudet.edu
Professionals in the field of substance abuse and deafness present their views on abuse.
217 pages

4619 Talk with Me
Alexander Graham Bell Association
3417 Volta Place NW
Washington, DC 20007-2737
202-337-5220
Fax: 202-337-8314
TTY: 202-337-5220
info@agbell.org
www.listeningandspokenlanguage.org
Written by a clinical psychologist and mother, this book educates parents and professionals about crucial early decisions that affect the speech, language, auditory, social and emotional development of children with hearing impairments.
222 pages

4620 Teaching English to the Deaf as a Second Language
Depart. of English, Gallaudet University
800 Florida Avenue NE
Washington, DC 20002
773-568-1550
800-621-2736
Fax: 800-621-8476
TTY: 888-630-9347
gupress@gallaudet.edu
gupress.gallaudet.edu
Publishes articles of practical interest to classroom teachers of hearing impaired and second language students.

Kendall Green

4621 There's a Hearing Impaired Child in my Class
Gallaudet University
800 Florida Avenue, NE
Washington, DC 20002-3819
773-568-1550
800-621-2736
Fax: 800-621-8476
TTY: 888-630-9347
gupress@gallaudet.edu
gupress.gallaudet.edu
This complete package provides basic facts about deafness, practical strategies for teaching hearing impaired children, and the question-and-answer information for all students.
44 pages

4622 Thirteen Keys to A Successful High School Experience
Alexander Graham Bell Association
3417 Volta Place NW
Washington, DC 20007-2737
202-337-5220
Fax: 202-337-8314
TTY: 202-337-5220
info@agbell.org
www.listeningandspokenlanguage.org
In this booklet, three students who have profound hearing losses share their mainstream education experiences. This booklet is great for teachers of any age child and many of the suggestions to make mainstreaming easier are practical and easy to implement.
1996 28 pages

4623 Toward Effective Public School Programs for Deaf Students
Thomas N. Kluwin, Donald F. Moores, Gonter Gaustad, authors
Teachers College Press
1234 Amsterdam Avenue
New York, NY 10027
212-678-3929
Fax: 212-678-4149
tcpress@tc.columbia.edu
www.teacherscollegepress.com
Examining various options for providing effective education-including the highly controversial practice of mainstreaming-the editors base their study on one of the largest and longest-running studies ever of public school programs for the deaf.
272 pages
ISBN: 0-807731-59-5
Martha Gonter Gaustad, Editors

4624 Understanding Deafness Socially
Gallaudet University
800 Florida Avenue, NE
Washington, DC 20002-3819
773-568-1550
800-621-2736
Fax: 800-621-8476
TTY: 888-630-9347
gupress@gallaudet.edu
gupress.gallaudet.edu
Articles on the social dynamics of deafness.
196 pages

4625 Understanding Ear Infections
Alexander Graham Bell Association
3417 Volta Place NW
Washington, DC 20007-2737
202-337-5220
Fax: 202-337-8314
TTY: 202-337-5220
info@agbell.org
www.listeningandspokenlanguage.org
Based on medical research, this clinical aid for medical and hearing professionals explains ear infections and their complications to patients and their families. Sturdily designed of cardboard and spiral-bound, each page has photos and diagrams that explain each topic and answer commonly asked questions about ear infections.
1993 27 pages

4626 Viewpoints on Deafness
National Association of the Deaf
8630 Fenton Street
Silver Spring, MD 20910
301-587-1788
Fax: 301-587-1791
TTY: 301-587-1789
nad.info@nad.org
nad.org
Monograph presents a collection of viewpoints on deafness.
157 pages Paperback
Christopher Wagner, President
Melissa S. Draganac-Hawk, Vice-President

4627 Visible Speech
SRC Software Research Corporation
Box 4277, Station A
Victoria, BC, V8X 3X8,
250-727-3744
Computerized speech culture, analysis and computer-based speech training.
6 pages
AE Wright, Publisher

4628 Voyage to an Island
Gallaudet University

800 Florida Avenue, NE
Washington, DC 20002-3819
773-568-1550
800-621-2736
Fax: 800-621-8476
TTY: 888-630-9347
gupress@gallaudet.edu
gupress.gallaudet.edu

This book recounts the story of how the author, a deaf woman from Finland, adjusts to moving to the exotic island of St. Lucia.
248 pages
Raija Nieminen, Author

4629 Week the World Heard Gallaudet
Gallaudet University
800 Florida Avenue, NE
Washington, DC 20002-3819
773-568-1550
800-621-2736
Fax: 800-621-8476
TTY: 888-630-9347
gupress@gallaudet.edu
gupress.gallaudet.edu

This book gives the readers a day-by-day description of the Deaf President Now movement as it unfolded from March 6 to 13, 1988.
176 pages Paperback

4630 What is an Audiogram?
Gallaudet University
800 Florida Avenue, NE
Washington, DC 20002-3819
773-568-1550
800-621-2736
Fax: 800-621-8476
TTY: 888-630-9347
gupress@gallaudet.edu
gupress.gallaudet.edu

Here's a cheery friend to solve the mysteries of the audiogram.
16 pages

4631 What's that Pig Outdoors? A Memoir of Deafness
Henry Kisor, author
Penguin Group
1325 South Oak Street
Champaign, IL 61820-3657
217-333-0950
800-526-0275
Fax: 217-244-8082
uipress@uillinois.edu
www.press.uillinois.edu

Life of a journalist who is deaf and lives in a hearing world lipreading. Discusses some of the technical advances which help the deaf.
288 pages Hardcover
ISBN: 0-140148-99-2
Henry Kisor, Author

4632 When Your Child is Deaf: A Guide for Parents
Alexander Graham Bell Association
3417 Volta Place NW
Washington, DC 20007-2737
202-337-5220
Fax: 202-337-8314
TTY: 202-337-5220
info@agbell.org
www.listeningandspokenlanguage.org

This book gives encouragement and advice to parents on their essential roles in teaching speech to their child.
182 pages

4633 When the Mind Hears
Gallaudet University
800 Florida Avenue, NE
Washington, DC 20002-3819
773-568-1550
800-621-2736
Fax: 800-621-8476
TTY: 888-630-9347
gupress@gallaudet.edu
gupress.gallaudet.edu

Told largely from the vantage point of Laurent Clerc.
460 pages

4634 Who Speaks for the Deaf Community?
National Association of the Deaf

8630 Fenton Street
Silver Spring, MD 20910
301-587-1788
Fax: 301-587-1791
TTY: 301-587-1789
nad.info@nad.org
nad.org

Paperback
Christopher Wagner, President
Melissa S. Draganac-Hawk, Vice-President

4635 Wired for Sound
Gallaudet University
800 Florida Avenue, NE
Washington, DC 20002-3819
773-568-1550
800-621-2736
Fax: 800-621-8476
TTY: 888-630-9347
gupress@gallaudet.edu
gupress.gallaudet.edu

Secondary school edition of Ear Gear, this attractive workbook is designed to give older students an in-depth understanding of hearing and hearing aids.
156 pages
Carole Bugosh Simko, Author

4636 Working with Deaf People: Accessibility and Accommodation in the Workplace
2600 S 1st Street
Springfield, IL 62704-4730
217-789-8980
Fax: 217-789-9130
books@ccthomas.com
www.ccthomas.com

Reveals the kinds of patterns of work adjustment problems that can surface among deaf employees, including the points of view of both supervisors an deaf people.
250 pages Paperback
ISBN: 0-398061-26-2
Charles C Thomas, Publisher

4637 Working with Deaf Persons in Sunday School
Sunday School Board of the Southern Baptists
127 9th Avenue N
Nashville, TN 37234-0001
800-458-2772

Provides guidance for organizing and conducting Sunday School classes/departments for deaf children, youth and adults.

4638 Writer's Workshop
Gallaudet University
800 Florida Avenue, NE
Washington, DC 20002-3819
773-568-1550
800-621-2736
Fax: 800-621-8476
TTY: 888-630-9347
gupress@gallaudet.edu
gupress.gallaudet.edu

Offers suggestions to teachers who are interested in turning the classroom into an environment where students learn to express themselves in writing.
95 pages

4639 You Just Don't Understand
Deborah Tannen, author
Hearing Loss Association of America
7910 Woodmont Avenue
Bethesda, MD 20814-3079
301-657-2248
Fax: 301-913-9413
TTY: 301-657-2249
info@hearingloss.org
www.hearingloss.org

Studded with lively and entertaining examples of real conversations, this book gives you the tools to understand what went wrong — and to find a common language in which to strengthen relationships at work and at home. A classic in the field of interpersonal relations, this book will change forever the way you approach conversations.
Softcover
ISBN: 0-060959-62-2
Anna Gilmore Hall, Executive Director
Lise Hamlin, Director of Public Policy

4640 You and Your Deaf Child
Gallaudet University

800 Florida Avenue, NE
Washington, DC 20002-3819

773-568-1550
800-621-2736
Fax: 800-621-8476
TTY: 888-630-9347
gupress@gallaudet.edu
gupress.gallaudet.edu

This guide for parents explores how families interact to deal with the special impact of a child who is hearing impaired.
1997 224 pages 2nd edition
John W. Adams, Author

Children's Books

4641   ABC's of Finger Spelling
Modern Signs Press
PO Box 1181
Los Alamitos, CA 90720-1181

562-596-8548
800-572-7332
Fax: 562-795-6614
TTY: 562-493-4168
modsigns@modernsignspress.com
www.modernsignspress.com

Helps teach upper and lower case letters of the alphabet. Includes printed letters and easy-to-follow drawings of the hand shapes.
60 pages
ISBN: 0-916708-13-6

4642   Alphabet of Animal Signs
Garlic Press
899 South College Mall Rd
Bloomington, IN 47401-5337

541-345-0063
800-789-0554
Fax: 800-789-5576
kadler@ipgbook.com
www.garlicpress.com

Presents animal illustrations and associated signs for each letter of the alphabet.
16 pages Paperback
ISBN: 0-931993-65-2
Stan Collins, Author

4643   Animal Signs: A First Book of Sign Language
Gallaudet University
800 Florida Avenue, NE
Washington, DC 20002-3819

773-568-1550
800-621-2736
Fax: 800-621-8476
TTY: 888-630-9347
gupress@gallaudet.edu
gupress.gallaudet.edu

Full-color photos of animals and their signs.
16 pages Ages 1-4
Debbie Slier, Author

4644   Another Handful of Stories
Gallaudet University
800 Florida Avenue, NE
Washington, DC 20002-3819

773-568-1550
800-621-2736
Fax: 800-621-8476
TTY: 888-630-9347
gupress@gallaudet.edu
gupress.gallaudet.edu

Second book contains a series of 37 stories told by deaf individuals.
124 pages

4645   At Grandma's House
Modern Signs Press
PO Box 1181
Los Alamitos, CA 90720-1181

562-596-8548
800-572-7332
Fax: 562-795-6614
TTY: 562-493-4168
modsigns@modernsignspress.com
www.modernsignspress.com

Pictures, signs and printed words tell the tale of April, a cuddly little rabbit who loves to play with her beloved Grandma.
28 pages

4646   Be Happy, Not Sad
Modern Signs Press

PO Box 1181
Los Alamitos, CA 90720

562-596-8548
800-572-7332
Fax: 562-795-6614
TTY: 562-493-4168
modsigns@modernsignspress.com
www.modernsignspress.com

These books help children understand hard to explain emotions through signing. Includes Be Happy Not Sad coloring workbook.
2 Book Set

4647   Belonging
Gallaudet University
800 Florida Avenue, NE
Washington, DC 20002-3819

773-568-1550
800-621-2736
Fax: 800-621-8476
TTY: 888-630-9347
gupress@gallaudet.edu
gupress.gallaudet.edu

Gustie Blaine loses her hearing after an illness and must now learn to accept her loss and understand the changes it brings.
176 pages
Virginia M. Scott, Author

4648   Chris Gets Ear Tubes
Gallaudet University
800 Florida Avenue, NE
Washington, DC 20002-3819

773-568-1550
800-621-2736
Fax: 800-621-8476
TTY: 888-630-9347
gupress@gallaudet.edu
gupress.gallaudet.edu

A helpful book for parents and children to share concerning ear tubes and hospitals.
44 pages

4649   Clerc: The Story of His Early Years
Gallaudet University
800 Florida Avenue, NE
Washington, DC 20002-3819

773-568-1550
800-621-2736
Fax: 800-621-8476
TTY: 888-630-9347
gupress@gallaudet.edu
gupress.gallaudet.edu

A novel by Laurent Clerc, a deaf teacher who helped Gallaudet establish schools to educate deaf Americans.
208 pages

4650   Come Sign with Us: Sign Language Activities for Children
Gallaudet University
800 Florida Avenue, NE
Washington, DC 20002-3819

773-568-1550
800-621-2736
Fax: 800-621-8476
TTY: 888-630-9347
gupress@gallaudet.edu
gupress.gallaudet.edu

Revised version, offering more follow-up activities, including many in context, to teach children sign language. Features more than 300 line drawings of both adults and children signing familiar words, phrases, and sentences using ASL. Shows how to form each sign exactly and also presents the origins of ASL, facts about deafness, and the deaf community.
160 pages Softcover
ISBN: 1-563680-51-3
Jan C. Hafer, Co-Author
Robert M. Wilson, Co-Author

4651   Day We Met Cindy
Gallaudet University
800 Florida Avenue, NE
Washington, DC 20002-3819

773-568-1550
800-621-2736
Fax: 800-621-8476
TTY: 888-630-9347
gupress@gallaudet.edu
gupress.gallaudet.edu

A picture storybook telling the story of Cindy, the hearing impaired aunt of one of the students of a first grade class.
32 pages
Anne Marie Starowitz, Author

4652 Finger Alphabet
Gallaudet University
800 Florida Avenue, NE
Washington, DC 20002-3819
773-568-1550
800-621-2736
Fax: 800-621-8476
TTY: 888-630-9347
gupress@gallaudet.edu
gupress.gallaudet.edu
Includes activities for improving fingerspelling.
30 pages

4653 Flying Fingers Club
Gallaudet University
800 Florida Avenue, NE
Washington, DC 20002-3819
773-568-1550
800-621-2736
Fax: 800-621-8476
TTY: 888-630-9347
gupress@gallaudet.edu
gupress.gallaudet.edu
Three young friends, one deaf and two hearing find they can communicate secretly in sign language.
104 pages

4654 Gift of the Girl Who Couldn't Hear
Alexander Graham Bell Association
3417 Volta Place NW
Washington, DC 20007-2737
202-337-5220
Fax: 202-337-8314
TTY: 202-337-5220
info@agbell.org
www.listeningandspokenlanguage.org
This fictional novel for middle school readers introduces Eliza, a gifted singer and Lucy, her best friend who has been deaf since birth.
79 pages

4655 Goldilocks and the Three Bears
Gallaudet University
800 Florida Avenue, NE
Washington, DC 20002-3819
773-568-1550
800-621-2736
Fax: 800-621-8476
TTY: 888-630-9347
gupress@gallaudet.edu
gupress.gallaudet.edu
Offers children ages 3-8 the classic story with new words and matching signs in Signed English.
48 pages Casebound
ISBN: 1-563680-57-2
Harry Bornstein, Co-Author
Karen L. Saulnier, Co-Author

4656 Grandfather Moose
Modern Signs Press
PO Box 1181
Los Alamitos, CA 90720-1181
562-596-8548
800-572-7332
Fax: 562-795-6614
TTY: 562-493-4168
modsigns@modernsignspress.com
www.modernsignspress.com
Offers exciting and beautifully illustrated rhymes, games and chants in sign language.
32 pages

4657 Handful of Stories
Gallaudet University
800 Florida Avenue, NE
Washington, DC 20002-3819
773-568-1550
800-621-2736
Fax: 800-621-8476
TTY: 888-630-9347
gupress@gallaudet.edu
gupress.gallaudet.edu
Sometimes incredible, moving and amusing, these stories are based on the personal experiences of deaf storytellers.
118 pages

4658 Handmade Alphabet
Gallaudet University

800 Florida Avenue, NE
Washington, DC 20002-3819
773-568-1550
800-621-2736
Fax: 800-621-8476
TTY: 888-630-9347
gupress@gallaudet.edu
gupress.gallaudet.edu
This book presents 26 beautiful color drawings showing a hand forming a letter of the manual alphabet.
26 pages

4659 Hasta Luego, San Diego
Gallaudet University
800 Florida Avenue, NE
Washington, DC 20002-3819
773-568-1550
800-621-2736
Fax: 800-621-8476
TTY: 888-630-9347
gupress@gallaudet.edu
gupress.gallaudet.edu
A Flying Fingers Club mystery.
104 pages
Jean F. Andrews, Author

4660 Hearing Loss
Franklin Watts Grolier
557 Broadway
New York, NY 10012-0001
203-797-3500
800-724-6527
Fax: 203-797-3197
www.grolier.com
Offers a concise explanation of how and why hearing losses occur, how the ear works and how to protect your hearing.
144 pages Grades 7-12
ISBN: 0-531125-19-0

4661 I Have a Sister, My Sister is Deaf
TJ Publishers
817 Silver Spring Avenue
Silver Spring, MD 20910-4617
301-585-4440
800-999-1168
Fax: 301-585-5930
TTY: 301-585-4441
tjpubinc@aol.com
An emphatic, affirmative look at the relationship between siblings, as a young deaf child is affectionately described by her older sister. This Coretta Scott King honor award winner helps young children develop an understanding that deaf children share the same interests as hearing children.
1977 32 pages Softcover
ISBN: 0-064430-59-6
Angela K Thames, President
Jerald A Murphy, VP

4662 I Was So Mad!
Modern Signs Press
PO Box 1181
Los Alamitos, CA 90720-1181
562-596-8548
800-572-7332
Fax: 562-795-6614
TTY: 562-493-4168
modsigns@modernsignspress.com
www.modernsignspress.com
Includes manual alphabet and glossary of signs.
40 pages
ISBN: 0-916708-16-0

4663 In Our House
Modern Signs Press
PO Box 1181
Los Alamitos, CA 90720-1181
562-596-8548
800-572-7332
Fax: 562-795-6614
TTY: 562-493-4168
modsigns@modernsignspress.com
www.modernsignspress.com
This colorful picturebook tells the story of Joy and Jason helping Mom and Dad around the house. Has a 140-word vocabulary listed in an alphabetical glossary.
32 pages
ISBN: 0-191670-81-1

4664 Invisible Inc #4
Alexander Graham Bell Association

3417 Volta Place NW   202-337-5220
Washington, DC 20007-2737   Fax: 202-337-8314
TTY: 202-337-5220
info@agbell.org
www.listeningandspokenlanguage.org

The intrepid trio accept an invitation to doom as they solve the mystery behind their school's haunted computer.
1996 42 pages

4665   **King Midas With Selected Sentences in ASL**
Gallaudet University
800 Florida Avenue, NE   773-568-1550
Washington, DC 20002-3819   800-621-2736
Fax: 800-621-8476
TTY: 888-630-9347
gupress@gallaudet.edu
gupress.gallaudet.edu

Fairytale retold with full color illustrations and American Sign Language sentences.
72 pages Casebound
ISBN: 0-930323-75-0

4666   **Learning to Sign in my Neighborhood**
Gallaudet University
800 Florida Avenue, NE   773-568-1550
Washington, DC 20002-3819   800-621-2736
Fax: 800-621-8476
TTY: 888-630-9347
gupress@gallaudet.edu
gupress.gallaudet.edu

Here are signs to learn and pictures to color, all in one friendly book.
32 pages

4667   **Little Green Monsters**
Modern Signs Press
PO Box 1181   562-596-8548
Los Alamitos, CA 90720-1181   800-572-7332
Fax: 562-795-6614
TTY: 310-493-4168
modsigns@modernsignspress.com
www.modernsignspress.com

Forty-five word vocabulary in signs and printed words introduces concept of directionality. Includes manual alphabet and glossary of signs.
36 pages

4668   **Little Red Riding Hood**
Gallaudet University
800 Florida Avenue, NE   773-568-1550
Washington, DC 20002-3819   800-621-2736
Fax: 800-621-8476
TTY: 888-630-9347
gupress@gallaudet.edu
gupress.gallaudet.edu

A beloved folktale that is told in American Sign Language format.
48 pages
Harry Bornstein, Co-Author
Karen L. Saulnier, Co-Author

4669   **Living with Deafness**
Franklin Watts Grolier
557 Broadway   203-797-3500
New York, NY 10012-0001   800-724-6527
Fax: 203-797-3197
www.grolier.com

Shows how deaf persons can overcome their disability and live happy, productive lives.
32 pages Grades 5-7
ISBN: 0-531108-42-2

4670   **Mandy**
Gallaudet University
800 Florida Avenue, NE   773-568-1550
Washington, DC 20002-3819   800-621-2736
Fax: 800-621-8476
TTY: 888-630-9347
gupress@gallaudet.edu
gupress.gallaudet.edu

A beautiful story about a young deaf girl's relationship with her grandmother.
32 pages

4671   **Matthew Pinkowski's Special Summer**
Gallaudet University
800 Florida Avenue, NE   773-568-1550
Washington, DC 20002-3819   800-621-2736
Fax: 800-621-8476
TTY: 888-630-9347
gupress@gallaudet.edu
gupress.gallaudet.edu

Matthew begins his special summer by moving to Minnesota, where he meets some special friends.
150 pages

4672   **Messy Monsters, Jungle Joggers and Bubble Baths**
Alexander Graham Bell Association
3417 Volta Place NW   202-337-5220
Washington, DC 20007-2737   Fax: 202-337-8314
TTY: 202-337-5220
info@agbell.org
www.listeningandspokenlanguage.org

This child's work book is filled with poems, stories and delightful drawings that make speaking lip reading and using residual hearing fun for the elementary school aged child.
97 pages

4673   **Mother Goose in Sign**
Garlic Press
899 South College Mall Rd   541-345-0063
Bloomington, IN 47401-5337   800-789-0554
Fax: 800-789-5576
orders@ipgbook.com
www.garlicpress.com

Fully illustrated Mother Goose nursery rhymes in sign language.
16 pages Paperback
ISBN: 0-931993-66-0
SH Collins, Contact

4674   **My ABC Signs of Animal Friends**
DawnSignPress
6130 Nancy Ridge Drive   619-625-0600
San Diego, CA 92121-3223   800-549-5350
Fax: 619-625-2336
DawnSign@aol.com
www.dawnsign.com

Sign language primer for both hearing and deaf children from birth to age five.
32 pages
ISBN: 0-915035-31-6

4675   **My First Book of Sign**
Gallaudet University
800 Florida Avenue, NE   773-568-1550
Washington, DC 20002-3819   800-621-2736
Fax: 800-621-8476
TTY: 888-630-9347
gupress@gallaudet.edu
gupress.gallaudet.edu

This book makes signing fun for children from three to eight.
76 pages

4676   **My Signing Book of Numbers**
Gallaudet University
800 Florida Avenue, NE   773-568-1550
Washington, DC 20002-3819   800-621-2736
Fax: 800-621-8476
TTY: 888-630-9347
gupress@gallaudet.edu
gupress.gallaudet.edu

Picture book helps children learn their numbers in sign language.
56 pages

4677   **Nick's Mission**
Alexander Graham Bell Association

3417 Volta Place NW
Washington, DC 20007-2737

202-337-5220
Fax: 202-337-8314
TTY: 202-337-5220
info@agbell.org
www.listeningandspokenlanguage.org

Twelve-year-old Nick plans to spend his summer vacation at the lake, snorkeling and playing with Wags, his dog, not at speech therapy as his mother has planned. But the summer will embroil Nick and Wags in an exciting mystery that includes kidnapping, smuggling, stolen macaws and maybe even speech therapy.
1996 148 pages

4678 Now I Understand
Gallaudet University
800 Florida Avenue, NE
Washington, DC 20002-3819

773-568-1550
800-621-2736
Fax: 800-621-8476
TTY: 888-630-9347
gupress@gallaudet.edu
gupress.gallaudet.edu

Explores what happens when a hard-of-hearing boy is mainstreamed.
56 pages

4679 Number and Letter Games
Gallaudet University
800 Florida Avenue, NE
Washington, DC 20002-3819

773-568-1550
800-621-2736
Fax: 800-621-8476
TTY: 888-630-9347
gupress@gallaudet.edu
gupress.gallaudet.edu

A fascinating way to learning sign language with games, riddles and map skills for children and adults.
30 pages

4680 Nursery Rhymes from Mother Goose
Gallaudet University
800 Florida Avenue, NE
Washington, DC 20002-3819

773-568-1550
800-621-2736
Fax: 800-621-8476
TTY: 888-630-9347
gupress@gallaudet.edu
gupress.gallaudet.edu

The complete nursery rhyme is presented in Signed English.
64 pages

4681 Popsicles are Cold
Modern Signs Press
PO Box 1181
Los Alamitos, CA 90720-1181

562-596-8548
800-572-7332
Fax: 562-795-6614
TTY: 562-493-4168
modsigns@modernsignspress.com
www.modernsignspress.com

Colorful pictures and rhyming words highlight this storybook with a 33-word vocabulary in signs and printed words.
32 pages

4682 Season of Change
Gallaudet University
800 Florida Avenue, NE
Washington, DC 20002-3819

773-568-1550
800-621-2736
Fax: 800-621-8476
TTY: 888-630-9347
gupress@gallaudet.edu
gupress.gallaudet.edu

A cheerful teenager tired of having people treat her as a problem just because she does not hear very well.
108 pages
Lois L. Hodge, Author

4683 Secret Signing: A Sign Language Activity Book
Gallaudet University
800 Florida Avenue, NE
Washington, DC 20002-3819

773-568-1550
800-621-2736
Fax: 800-621-8476
TTY: 888-630-9347
gupress@gallaudet.edu
gupress.gallaudet.edu

Children will enjoy this activity book with signs.
64 pages Level K-1

4684 Secret in the Dorm Attic
Gallaudet University
800 Florida Avenue, NE
Washington, DC 20002-3819

773-568-1550
800-621-2736
Fax: 800-621-8476
TTY: 888-630-9347
gupress@gallaudet.edu
gupress.gallaudet.edu

Susan, Donald and Matt are back, as the Flying Fingers Club solving yet another mystery.
104 pages

4685 Sesame Street Sign Language ABC
Gallaudet University
800 Florida Avenue, NE
Washington, DC 20002-3819

773-568-1550
800-621-2736
Fax: 800-621-8476
TTY: 888-630-9347
gupress@gallaudet.edu
gupress.gallaudet.edu

Muppets learn words and letters signed by Linda Bove.
30 pages

4686 Sesame Street Sign Language Fun
Gallaudet University
800 Florida Avenue, NE
Washington, DC 20002-3819

773-568-1550
800-621-2736
Fax: 800-621-8476
TTY: 888-630-9347
gupress@gallaudet.edu
gupress.gallaudet.edu

This book uses the Muppets to explain concepts such as opposites, words and feelings.
62 pages

4687 Sign Numbers
Modern Signs Press
PO Box 1181
Los Alamitos, CA 90720-1181

562-596-8548
800-572-7332
Fax: 562-795-6614
TTY: 562-493-4168
modsigns@modernsignspress.com
www.modernsignspress.com

A manual teaching sign language and written numbers that includes printed numbers and easy-to-follow drawings of the number hand shapes.
60 pages

4688 Sign-Me-Fine
Gallaudet University
800 Florida Avenue, NE
Washington, DC 20002-3819

773-568-1550
800-621-2736
Fax: 800-621-8476
TTY: 888-630-9347
gupress@gallaudet.edu
gupress.gallaudet.edu

Written for young adults, this book introduces American Sign Language and how it differs from English.
120 pages
Laura Greene, Co-Author
Eva Barash Dicker, Co-Author

4689 Signed Language Coloring Books
Gallaudet University
800 Florida Avenue, NE
Washington, DC 20002-3819

773-568-1550
800-621-2736
Fax: 800-621-8476
TTY: 888-630-9347
gupress@gallaudet.edu
gupress.gallaudet.edu

Six coloring books made up of easy-to-color pictures that include the printed, signed and fingerspelled words for each image.
16 pages

4690 Signing for Kids
Gallaudet University

800 Florida Avenue, NE   773-568-1550
Washington, DC 20002-3819   800-621-2736
      Fax: 800-621-8476
      TTY: 888-630-9347
      gupress@gallaudet.edu
      gupress.gallaudet.edu

Contains 17 chapters dealing with special areas of interest to children like pets, family, friends and people.
142 pages

4691   **Signs for Me: Basic Vocabulary for Children, Parents and Teachers**
DawnSignPress
6130 Nancy Ridge Drive   619-625-0600
San Diego, CA 92121-3223   800-549-5350
      Fax: 619-625-2336
      DawnSign@aol.com
      www.dawnsign.com

ASL/English vocabulary primer filled with all the basics for pre-schoolers. The focus is on learning ASL signs and English words for better language development. Illustrates the meaning of the sign, the sign itself, and the English word in bold print.
112 pages
ISBN: 0-915035-27-8

4692   **Silent Dances**
Gallaudet University
800 Florida Avenue, NE   773-568-1550
Washington, DC 20002-3819   800-621-2736
      Fax: 800-621-8476
      TTY: 888-630-9347
      gupress@gallaudet.edu
      gupress.gallaudet.edu

Space adventure story featuring a deaf graduate of Gallaudet University.
275 pages

4693   **Silent Garden: Raising Your Deaf Child**
Alexander Graham Bell Association
3417 Volta Place NW   202-337-5220
Washington, DC 20007-2737   Fax: 202-337-8314
      TTY: 202-337-5220
      info@agbell.org
      www.listeningandspokenlanguage.org

This book provides parents of deaf children with crucial information on the possibilities afforded their children. Ogden, deaf since birth and a professor of deaf studies offers parents the foundation for making the difficult decisions necessary to start their children on the road to realizing their full potential.
1996 313 pages

4694   **Silent Observer**
Gallaudet University
800 Florida Avenue, NE   773-568-1550
Washington, DC 20002-3819   800-621-2736
      Fax: 800-621-8476
      TTY: 888-630-9347
      gupress@gallaudet.edu
      gupress.gallaudet.edu

Lovely illustrations tell the story of an affectionate memoir of childhood presented through the eyes of a deaf girl.
48 pages
Christy MacKinnon, Writer and Illustrator

4695   **Simple Signs**
Gallaudet University
800 Florida Avenue, NE   773-568-1550
Washington, DC 20002-3819   800-621-2736
      Fax: 800-621-8476
      TTY: 888-630-9347
      gupress@gallaudet.edu
      gupress.gallaudet.edu

Charming, full-color pictures and hints introducing ASL to children.
32 pages

4696   **Sleeping Beauty**
Gallaudet University

800 Florida Avenue, NE   773-568-1550
Washington, DC 20002-3819   800-621-2736
      Fax: 800-621-8476
      TTY: 888-630-9347
      gupress@gallaudet.edu
      gupress.gallaudet.edu

Classic story with full-color illustrations and line drawings of more than 30 sentences rendered in ASL, offering new dimensions of imagination while also strengthening young readers' language skills.
64 pages
ISBN: 0-930323-97-1

4697   **Songs in Sign**
Gallaudet University
800 Florida Avenue, NE   773-568-1550
Washington, DC 20002-3819   800-621-2736
      Fax: 800-621-8476
      TTY: 888-630-9347
      gupress@gallaudet.edu
      gupress.gallaudet.edu

Fully illustrated sign English.
30 pages

4698   **Very Special Sister**
Gallaudet University
800 Florida Avenue, NE   773-568-1550
Washington, DC 20002-3819   800-621-2736
      Fax: 800-621-8476
      TTY: 888-630-9347
      gupress@gallaudet.edu
      gupress.gallaudet.edu

Tells the story of Laura who is deaf and her delight at the fact that she will soon have a brother.
36 pages
Dorothy Hoffman Levi, Author

4699   **Where Is Spot?**
Gallaudet University
800 Florida Avenue, NE   773-568-1550
Washington, DC 20002-3819   800-621-2736
      Fax: 800-621-8476
      TTY: 888-630-9347
      gupress@gallaudet.edu
      gupress.gallaudet.edu

A Signed English edition of a childhood favorite.
20 pages

4700   **Word Signs: A First Book of Sign Language**
Gallaudet University
800 Florida Avenue, NE   773-568-1550
Washington, DC 20002-3819   800-621-2736
      Fax: 800-621-8476
      TTY: 888-630-9347
      gupress@gallaudet.edu
      gupress.gallaudet.edu

Full-color photos of basic words and their signs.
16 pages Ages 1-4
Debbie Slier, Author

Magazines

4701   **American Annals of the Deaf**
Convention of American Instructors of the Deaf
800 Florida Avenue NE   773-568-1550
Washington, DC 20002-3660   800-621-2736
      Fax: 800-621-8476
      TTY: 888-630-9347
      gupress@gallaudet.edu
      gupress.gallaudet.edu

Scholarly journal at the forefront of research related to the education of deaf people. Annual reference Issue identifies programs and services for deaf people nationwide.
64 pages 5x Year
Donald Moores, Editor
Mary E Carew, Managing Editor

4702   **American Journal of Audiology**
American Speech-Language-Hearing Association

2200 Research Boulevard
Rockville, MD 20850-3226

301-897-5700
800-498-2071
actioncenter@asha.org
www.asha.org

AJA is a twice-yearly journal of clinical practice for audiologists and hearing researchers.
Russell L Malone PhD, Editor

4703 American Journal of Speech-Language Pathology
American Speech-Language-Hearing Association
10801 Rockville Pike
Rockville, MD 20852-3226

301-897-5700
800-638-8255
Fax: 301-296-8580
TTY: 301-296-5650
ajslp.pubs.asha.org

AJSLP reports peer-reviewed, primary research findings (basic and applied) concerning an array of clinically oriented topics transcending all aspects of clinical practice in speech-language pathology.
Russell L Malone PhD, Editor

4704 Audiology Today
11480 Commerce Park Drive
Reston, VA 20191-2019

703-790-8466
800-222-2336
Fax: 703-476-5157
infoaud@audiology.org
www.audiology.org

AT is the American Academy of Audiology's award-winning magazine of, by, and for audiologists.
David Fabry, PhD, Content Editor
Amy Miedema, CAE, Executive Editor

4705 Auricle
Auditory-Verbal International
2121 Eisenhower Avenue
Alexandria, VA 22314-4688

703-739-1049
Fax: 703-739-0395
TTY: 703-739-0874
audiverb@aol.com
www.auditory-verbal.org

To provide the choice of listening and speaking as the way of life for children and adults who are deaf on hard of hearing.
Magazine
Sara Lake, Executive Director/CEO/Publisher
Mary Benson, Executive Assistant

4706 Deaf Life
MSM Productions
1095 Meigs Street
Rochester, NY 14620-3380

716-442-6370
Fax: 585-442-6371
www.deaflife.com

This magazine focuses on profiles, news, controversial issues, cultural topics and more relating to the Deaf community.
50 pages Monthly
Matthew Moore, Publisher

4707 Deaf Sports Review
American Athletic Association of the Deaf
PO Box 910338
Lexington, KY 40591-1737

801-393-8710
Fax: 801-393-2263
TTY: 801-393-7916
HomeOffice@usdeafsports.org
www.usdeafsports.org

A magazine that describes deaf athletes and past and upcoming events.
Quarterly
Shirley Platt, Editor

4708 Deaf USA
Eye Festival Communications
6917B Woodley Avenue
Van Nuys, CA 91406-4844

818-902-9800
Fax: 818-902-9840

Provides news coverage on all activities and issues of interest to deaf and hard of hearing readers as well as professionals and associates within this specialized market.
Monthly
David Rosenbaum, Editor

4709 Deaf-Blind American
American Association of the Deaf-Blind

PO Box 8064
Silver Spring, MD 20907-4500

301-563-9064
800-735-2258
Fax: 301-588-8705
TTY: 301-588-6545
aadb-info@aadb.org
www.aadb.org

A journal of the American Association of the Deaf-Blind with articles on new technology, legislation news affecting deaf-blind Americans, success stories on deaf-blind, conference news, and many other topics of interest to deaf-blind people.
4x Year
Jamie McNamara, Editor

4710 Hearing Health
363 Seventh Avenue
New York, NY 10001

212-257-6140
866-454-3924
info@hhf.org
hearinghealthfoundation.org

A publication for deaf and hard-of-hearing people, as well as hearing health care professionals, libraries, agencies, schools and organizations.
BiMonthly
Paula Bartone-Bonillas, Editor

4711 Journal of AAA
American Academy of Audiology
1735 N Lynn Street
Arlington, VA 22209-2019

703-524-1923
800-222-2336
Fax: 703-524-2303

James Jerger, Editor

4712 Journal of Speech-Language-Hearing Research
American Speech-Language-Hearing Association
10801 Rockville Pike
Rockville, MD 20852-3226

301-897-5700
800-638-8255
Fax: 301-296-8580
TTY: 301-296-5650
ajslp.pubs.asha.org

The bimonthly Journal of Speech, Language, and Hearing Research (JSHLR)-an online-only, international, peer-reviewed scholarly journal-has been published continuously since 1936.
Russell L Malone PhD, Editor

4713 Language, Speech and Hearing Services in the Schools
American Speech-Language-Hearing Association
10801 Rockville Pike
Rockville, MD 20852

301-897-5700
800-638-8255
Fax: 301-296-8580
TTY: 301-296-5650
ajslp.pubs.asha.org

Professional journal for clinicians, audiologists and speech-language pathologists.

Russell L Malone PhD, Editor

4714 NADmag
National Association of the Deaf
8630 Fenton Street
Silver Spring, MD 20910

301-587-1788
Fax: 301-587-1791
TTY: 301-587-1789
nad.info@nad.org
nad.org

Each NADmag focuses on a specific theme, such as technology and telecommunications, human services, deaf culture, education, and interpreting.
32 pages Bi-Monthly
Christopher Wagner, President
Melissa S. Draganac-Hawk, Vice-President

4715 Perspectives in Education and Deafness
Gallaudet University
800 Florida Avenue, NE
Washington, DC 20002-3819

773-568-1550
800-621-2736
Fax: 800-621-8476
TTY: 888-630-9347
gupress@gallaudet.edu
gupress.gallaudet.edu

A practical, reader-friendly magazine, offering help and advice in and beyond the classroom, tuned to the needs of today's students, teachers, and families.
5x Annually
Mary Abrams Perica, Editor

4716 SHHH Journal
Self Help For Hard of Hearing People
7910 Woodmont Avenue   301-657-2248
Bethesda, MD 20814-3079   Fax: 301-913-9413
                              TTY: 301-657-2249
                              www.hearingloss.org
An educational journal about hearing loss for hard-of-hearing people.
BiMonthly
Barbara G Harris, Editor

4717 Silent News
1425 Jefferson Road   716-272-4900
Rochester, NY 14623-3139   Fax: 716-272-4904
                              TTY: 716-272-4900
Covers news and events of interest to deaf and hard-of-hearing people all over the world.
Monthly
Tom Willard, Editor

4718 Silent News Job Bulletin
1425 Jefferson Road   716-272-4900
Rochester, NY 14623-3139   Fax: 716-272-4904
                              TTY: 716-272-4900
Lists current job openings and career opportunities working with deaf and hard-of-hearing people.
BiAnnually

4719 Tinnitus Today
American Tinnitus Association
PO Box 5   503-248-9985
Portland, OR 97207-0005   800-634-8978
                              Fax: 503-248-0024
                              tinnitus@ata.org
                              www.ata.org
A quarterly magazine published by the American Tinnitus Association.
28 pages Quarterly
ISBN: 1-530656-9 -
Cara James, Executive Director
Paul Morris, Development Director

4720 USA Deaf Sports Federation
PO Box 22011   homeoffice@usdeafsports.org
Santa Fe, NM 87502   www.usdeafsports.org
A glossy magazine called Deaf Sports Review featuring articles on all deaf sports and recreation.
Jeffrey L. Salit, President
Brianne Burger, Secretary

4721 Volta Review
Alexander Graham Bell Association
3417 Volta Place NW   202-337-5220
Washington, DC 20007-2737   Fax: 202-337-8314
                              TTY: 202-337-5220
                              info@agbell.org
                              www.listeningandspokenlanguage.org
A professionally reviewed journal highlighting research and studies in the field of deafness.
5x Year
Michelle Vanderhoff, Managing Editor

4722 Volta Voices
Alexander Graham Bell Association
3417 Volta Place NW   202-337-5220
Washington, DC 20007-2737   Fax: 202-337-8314
                              TTY: 202-337-5220
                              info@agbell.org
                              www.listeningandspokenlanguage.org
A magazine highlighting inspirational stories from parents of children who are deaf, legislative news, technology update and stories

pertaining to speech, speech reading, and the use of residual hearing.
BiMonthly
Michelle Vanderhoff, Managing Editor

4723 World Around You
Gallaudet University
800 Florida Avenue, NE   773-568-1550
Washington, DC 20002-3819   800-621-2736
                              Fax: 800-621-8476
                              TTY: 888-630-9347
                              gupress@gallaudet.edu
                              gupress.gallaudet.edu
A current events magazine directed at keeping junior high and high school deaf and hard-of-hearing students informed about deaf people and the deaf community.
5x Year
Cathryn Carroll, Editor

Newsletters

4724 AAAD Bulletin
American Athletic Association of the Deaf
3607 Washington Boulevard   801-393-8710
Ogden, UT 84403-1737   Fax: 801-393-2263
                              TTY: 801-393-7916
A newsletter describing deaf athletes and upcoming events.
Quarterly
Shirley Platt, Editor

4725 ADARA Updated
ADARA
PO Box 251554   501-868-8850
Little Rock, AR 72225-1554   Fax: 501-868-8812
Updates readers on events, resources, legislation, information of national interest, conferences, workshops and employment opportunities. Information from and about local chapters, special interest sections, and national organizations is included in this publication.
Quarterly
Nanncy Long PhD, Editor

4726 ALDA News
Association of Late-Deafened Adults
8038 Macintosh Lane   815-332-1515
Rockford, IL 61107   Fax: 877-907-1738
                              TTY: 815-332-1515
                              info@alda.org
                              www.alda.org
Marilyn Howe, Publisher

4727 Adult Bible Lessons for the Deaf
Sunday School Board of the Southern Baptists
127 9th Avenue N   800-458-2772
Nashville, TN 37234-0001
Bible study quarterly that relates to the needs of deaf and hearing impaired persons.
Quarterly

4728 Audiology Express
American Academy of Audiology
1735 N Lynn Street   703-524-1923
Arlington, VA 22209-2019   800-222-2336
                              Fax: 703-524-2303

4729 Better Hearing News
Better Hearing Institute
5021B Backlick Road   703-642-0580
Annandale, VA 22003-6043   800-327-9355
                              Fax: 703-750-9302
Quarterly
Jerry J Rizzo, Executive Director

4730 Canine Listener
Dogs for the Deaf

10175 Wheeler Road
Central Point, OR 97502

541-826-9220
800-990-3647
Fax: 541-826-6696
TTY: 541-826-9220
TDD: 541-826-9220
info@dogsforthedeaf.org
www.dogsforthedeaf.org

Offers information on various dogs for the deaf that are available, hotlines, support groups and articles on the newest technology for the hard of hearing person.
Quarterly
Robin Dickson, President/CEO

4731 Caption Center News
Caption Center
125 Western Avenue
Boston, MA 02134-1008

617-429-9225
Fax: 617-562-0590

Reports developments in closed captioning for persons with hearing impairments.

4732 Deaf Artists of America
302 Goodman Street N
Rochester, NY 14607-1148

716-244-3460
Fax: 716-244-3690
TTY: 716-244-3460

Tom Willard, Editor

4733 Deaf Episcopalian
Episcopal Conference of the Deaf
PO Box 27459
Philadelphia, PA 19118-0459

215-247-1059
Bmose@aol.com
www.ecdeaf.org

Preston H. Colangelo Dn., Contact

4734 Deaf Work
Baptist Sunday School Board
127 9th Avenue N
Nashville, TN 37234-0002

615-251-2000

Offers information for religious workers and church educators who teach the handicapped.

4735 Deafpride Advocate
Deafpride
1350 Potomac Avenue SE
Washington, DC 20003-4412

202-675-6700

4736 Endeavor
American Society for Deaf Children
800 Florida Avenue, NE
Washington, DC 20002-1373

717-334-7922
800-942-2732
Fax: 410-795-0965
TTY: 717-334-7922
asdc1@aol.com
www.deafchildren.org

Newsletter for parents of deaf children.
36 pages Quarterly
Tami Hossler, Editor

4737 Frat
National Fraternal Society of the Deaf
1300 W NW Highway
Mt Prospect, IL 60056-2217

847-392-9282
Fax: 847-392-9298
TTY: 708-392-1409

Offers fraternal insurance information and news about members.
BiMonthly
Wayne D Shook, Editor

4738 GA-SK Newsletter
Telecommunications for the Deaf
8630 Fenton Street
Silver Spring, MD 20910-3822

301-589-3786
Fax: 301-589-3797
TTY: 301-589-3006

A newsletter focusing on issues for the deaf and hearing impaired person.
Quarterly
Barry Solomon, Editor
Alfred Sonnenstrahl, Manager

4739 Gallaudet Today
Galladet University

800 Florida Avenue, NE
Washington, DC 20002

202-651-5000
Fax: 212-599-0039
president@gallaudet.edu
www.gallaudet.edu

A university publication with both general and special issues on deafness-related topics.
Quarterly
Vickie Walter, Editor

4740 Hear
Deafness Research Foundation
15 W 39th Street
New York, NY 10018-3806

212-768-1181

Offers information on the Foundation's activities and events, technical updates on assistive devices, legislative and medical information on the latest breakthroughs and laws for the hearing impaired, book reviews and resources.
Monte H Jacoby, Executive Director

4741 NTID Focus
National Technical Institute for the Deaf
52 Lomb Memorial Drive
Rochester, NY 14623-5604

716-475-6906
Fax: 716-475-5623
TTY: 716-475-6906
ntidmc@rit.edu
www.rit.edu/ntid

A college publication featuring news and stories about NTID programs and community members.
TriAnnual
Kathryn Shwartz, Editor

4742 Newsletter of American Hearing Research
American Hearing Research Foundation
275 N. York Street
Elmhurst, IL 60126-4539

630-617-5079
Fax: 630-563-9181
blederer@american-hearing.org
www.american-hearing.org

Concerned with hearing research and education.
6-8 pages 3 per year
William L Lederer, Executive Director
Sharon Parmet, Development/Communications Associate

4743 Newsline
Sertoma Foundation
1912 E Meyer Boulevard
Kansas City, MO 64132-1141

816-333-8300
Fax: 816-333-4320
infosertoma@sertomahq.org
www.sertoma.org

Reports on activities of the Sertoma Foundation in the field of speech and hearing impairments.

4744 Otoscope
EAR Foundation
1817 Patterson Street
Nashville, TN 37203

615-329-7807
800-545-4327
Fax: 615-329-7935
TTY: 615-329-7849
ear@earfoundation.org
www.earfoundation.org

8-14 pages Quarterly
Amy Nielsen, Director Educational Programs

4745 Research at Gallaudet
Gallaudet University
800 Florida Avenue, NE
Washington, DC 20002-3819

773-568-1550
800-621-2736
Fax: 800-621-8476
TTY: 888-630-9347
gupress@gallaudet.edu
gupress.gallaudet.edu

Newsletter reporting research and activities of the Institute.

4746 Speech and Deafness Newsletter
Hearing, Speech
1620 18th Avenue
Seattle, WA 98122-2798

206-323-5770

Agency newsletter for membership and community.
8 pages
Patty Tumberg, Editor

4747 Tech Talk
Caption Center
125 Western Avenue 617-492-9225
Boston, MA 02134-1008 Fax: 617-562-0590

4748 USA Deaf Sports Federation
PO Box 22011 HomeOffice@usdeafsports.org
Santa Fe, NM 87502 www.usdeafsports.org
A matte newsletter called USADSF Bulletin featuring articles on all deaf sports and recreation.
Jeffrey L. Salit, President
Brianne Burger, Secretary

Pamphlets

4749 25 Ways to Promote Spoken Language in Your Child with a Hearing Loss
Alexander Graham Bell Association
3417 Volta Place NW 202-337-5220
Washington, DC 20007-2737 Fax: 202-337-8314
TTY: 202-337-5220
info@agbell.org
www.listeningandspokenlanguage.org
This pamphlet teaches twenty-five golden rules about preparing your child to listen and to speak.
1995 62 pages

4750 Aging and Hearing Loss: Some Commonly Asked Questions
National Information Center on Deafness
800 Florida Avenue NE 773-568-1550
Washington, DC 20002-3660 800-621-2736
Fax: 800-621-8476
TTY: 888-630-9347
gupress@gallaudet.edu
gupress.gallaudet.edu
Discusses the hearing evaualtion, tests used to determine type and extent of hearing loss and what an audiogram tells us.

4751 Alerting and Communication Devices for Deaf and Hard of Hearing People
National Information Center on Deafness
800 Florida Avenue NE 773-568-1550
Washington, DC 20002 800-621-2736
Fax: 800-621-8476
TTY: 888-630-9347
gupress@gallaudet.edu
gupress.gallaudet.edu
Describes general communication in everyday life.
Loraine DiPietro, M.A., Co-Author
Pettyt Williams, Ph.D., Co-Author

4752 Alexander Graham Bell's Life
Alexander Graham Bell Association
3417 Volta Place NW 202-337-5220
Washington, DC 20007-2737 Fax: 202-337-8314
TTY: 202-337-5220
info@agbell.org
www.listeningandspokenlanguage.org
This pamphlet highlights Alexander Gram Bell's professional and personal involvement with deafness as a teacher of the deaf; a friend of many notable persons, including Helen Keller; a scientist interested in acoustics; the inventor of the telephone; and the founder of the Bell Association.
1996

4753 All About the New Generation of Hearing Aids
National Information Center on Deafness
800 Florida Avenue NE 773-568-1550
Washington, DC 20002-3660 800-621-2736
Fax: 800-621-8476
TTY: 888-630-9347
gupress@gallaudet.edu
gupress.gallaudet.edu
Explains the terms digital hearing aid, and digitally controlled hearing aid.

4754 Assistive Devices Demonstration Centers
National Information Center on Deafness
800 Florida Avenue NE 773-568-1550
Washington, DC 20002-3660 800-621-2736
Fax: 800-621-8476
TTY: 888-630-9347
gupress@gallaudet.edu
gupress.gallaudet.edu
A resource list identifying demonstration centers across the United States.

4755 Books for Parents of Deaf and Hard of Hearing Children
National Information Center on Deafness
800 Florida Avenue NE 773-568-1550
Washington, DC 20002 800-621-2736
Fax: 800-621-8476
TTY: 888-630-9347
gupress@gallaudet.edu
gupress.gallaudet.edu
Identifies books written for parents and everday experiences of deaf and hard of hearing children.

4756 Care of the Ears and Hearing for Health
American Hearing Research Foundation
275 N. York Street 630-617-5079
Elmhurst, IL 60126-4539 Fax: 630-563-9181
blederer@american-hearing.org
www.american-hearing.org
Offers information on ear infections relating to chronic progressive deafness.
William L Lederer, Executive Director
Sharon Parmet, Development/Communications Associate

4757 Consumer's Guide to Hearing Aids
Hearing Loss Association of America
7910 Woodmont Avenue 301-657-2248
Bethesda, MD 20814-3079 Fax: 301-913-9413
TTY: 301-657-2249
info@hearingloss.org
www.hearingloss.org
Color booklet illustrating the different styles of hearing aids and comparing different models and features. Illustrates the technology pyramid and hearing aid pricing.
2006 24 pages
Anna Gilmore Hall, Executive Director
Lise Hamlin, Director of Public Policy

4758 Deaf Culture Videotapes
National Information Center on Deafness
800 Florida Avenue NE 773-568-1550
Washington, DC 20002-3660 800-621-2736
Fax: 800-621-8476
TTY: 888-630-9347
gupress@gallaudet.edu
gupress.gallaudet.edu
This list identifies deaf culture and deaf history videotapes available from the Historic Film Collection of the National Association of the Deaf.

4759 Deaf Culture: Suggested Readings
National Information Center on Deafness
800 Florida Avenue NE 773-568-1550
Washington, DC 20002-3660 800-621-2736
Fax: 800-621-8476
TTY: 888-630-9347
gupress@gallaudet.edu
gupress.gallaudet.edu
A selected reading list providing annotations for 62 books highlighting the community, and history of deaf people.

4760 Deafness: A Fact Sheet
National Information Center on Deafness
800 Florida Avenue NE 773-568-1550
Washington, DC 20002-3660 800-621-2736
Fax: 800-621-8476
TTY: 888-630-9347
gupress@gallaudet.edu
gupress.gallaudet.edu

4761 Developing Cognition in Young Children Who are Deaf
Hope

343 A Erickson Hall
East Lansing, MI 48824-4648
435-752-9533
Fax: 435-752-9533
catalyst@kent.edu
www.deafed.net

Presents interesting, updated information on the importance of early cognition development in young children who are deaf. Contains many ideas for ways to promote early thinking skills, especially those that promote and enhance early communication and language development.

4762 Ear and Hearing
National Information Center on Deafness
800 Florida Avenue NE
Washington, DC 20002-3660
773-568-1550
800-621-2736
Fax: 800-621-8476
TTY: 888-630-9347
gupress@gallaudet.edu
gupress.gallaudet.edu

An illustrated publication of the ear and what can go wrong with it.

4763 Educating Deaf Children: An Introduction
National Information Center on Deafness
800 Florida Avenue NE
Washington, DC 20002-3660
773-568-1550
800-621-2736
Fax: 800-621-8476
TTY: 888-630-9347
gupress@gallaudet.edu
gupress.gallaudet.edu

Describes the different settings in which deaf children are currently educated.

4764 Facts About Hearing Aids
Alexander Graham Bell Association
3417 Volta Place NW
Washington, DC 20007-2737
202-337-5220
Fax: 202-337-8314
TTY: 202-337-5220
info@agbell.org
www.listeningandspokenlanguage.org

This brochure describes defferent types of hearing aids, factors to consider when choosing a hearing aid, the best way to go about purchasing a hearing aid. It also addresses cost and provides information on hearing conservation.

4765 Facts and Fancies About Hearing Aids
American Hearing Research Foundation
275 N. York Street
Elmhurst, IL 60126-4539
630-617-5079
Fax: 630-563-9181
blederer@american-hearing.org
www.american-hearing.org

Offers information on types of hearing aids and hearing aid evaluations.
William L Lederer, Executive Director
Sharon Parmet, Development/Communications Associate

4766 Genetics and Deafness
National Information Center on Deafness
800 Florida Avenue NE
Washington, DC 20002-3660
773-568-1550
800-621-2736
Fax: 800-621-8476
TTY: 888-630-9347
gupress@gallaudet.edu
gupress.gallaudet.edu

Written for deaf people and their families who wish to learn more about the relationship between heredity and deafness.

4767 Hearing Loss: Information for Professionals in the Aging Network
National Information Center on Deafness
800 Florida Avenue NE
Washington, DC 20002-3660
773-568-1550
800-621-2736
Fax: 800-621-8476
TTY: 888-630-9347
gupress@gallaudet.edu
gupress.gallaudet.edu

Introduces professionals in the aging network to the realities of hearing loss.

4768 How Does Your Child Hear and Talk?
American Speech-Language-Hearing Association

2200 Research Boulevard
Rockville, MD 20850-3226
301-296-5700
800-638-8255
Fax: 301-296-8580
TTY: 301-296-5650
nsslha@asha.org
www.asha.org

Offers a chart to parents on children's growth pertaining to their hearing and speech.

4769 Late-Deafened Adults: A Selected Annotated Bibliography
National Information Center on Deafness
800 Florida Avenue NE
Washington, DC 20002-3660
773-568-1550
800-621-2736
Fax: 800-621-8476
TTY: 888-630-9347
gupress@gallaudet.edu
gupress.gallaudet.edu

A selected reading list of books and articles for late-deafened people and their families.

4770 Leading National Publications of and for Deaf People
National Information Center on Deafness
800 Florida Avenue NE
Washington, DC 20002
773-568-1550
800-621-2736
Fax: 800-621-8476
TTY: 888-630-9347
gupress@gallaudet.edu
gupress.gallaudet.edu

Identifies publications with national circulations to deaf audiences.

4771 Making New Friends
National Information Center on Deafness
800 Florida Avenue NE
Washington, DC 20002-3660
773-568-1550
800-621-2736
Fax: 800-621-8476
TTY: 888-630-9347
gupress@gallaudet.edu
gupress.gallaudet.edu

Identifies resources that offer opportunities for deaf people.

4772 Meniere's Disease: Hearing Loss & Inner Ear Blood Flow
Self Help for Hard of H
7910 Woodmont Avenue
Bethesda, MD 20814-3079
301-657-2248
Fax: 301-913-9413
TTY: 301-657-2249
national@shhh.org
www.hearingloss.org

Includes a personal narrative.

4773 National Information Center on Deafness Brochure
National Information Center on Deafness
800 Florida Avenue NE
Washington, DC 20002
773-568-1550
800-621-2736
Fax: 800-621-8476
TTY: 888-630-9347
gupress@gallaudet.edu
gupress.gallaudet.edu

A description of services offered by NICD.

4774 Noise Can Be Harmful to Your Health
Deafness Research Foundation
15 W 39th Street
New York, NY 10018-3806
212-768-1181

Offers information, including a chart of noise levels, low to harmful, and the effects these noise levels have on your hearing.

4775 Otitis Media
Deafness Research Foundation
15 W 39th Street
New York, NY 10018-3806
212-768-1181

Offers information on Otitis Media, prevention, causes, treatments and symptoms.

4776 Perspectives Folio: Parent-Child
Gallaudet University

800 Florida Avenue, NE
Washington, DC 20002-3819
773-568-1550
800-621-2736
Fax: 800-621-8476
TTY: 888-630-9347
gupress@gallaudet.edu
gupress.gallaudet.edu

Seven articles emphasizing family communication while providing important information for parents about deafness and the deaf culture.
29 pages

4777 Publications from the National Information Center on Deafness
National Information Center on Deafness
800 Florida Avenue NE
Washington, DC 20002-3660
773-568-1550
800-621-2736
Fax: 800-621-8476
TTY: 888-630-9347
gupress@gallaudet.edu
gupress.gallaudet.edu

Order form and explanations of NICD publications.

4778 Questions and Answers About Employment of Deaf People
National Information Center on Deafness
800 Florida Avenue NE
Washington, DC 20002-3660
773-568-1550
800-621-2736
Fax: 800-621-8476
TTY: 888-630-9347
gupress@gallaudet.edu
gupress.gallaudet.edu

4779 Questions and Answers on Hearing Loss
Self Help for Hard of H
7910 Woodmont Avenue
Bethesda, MD 20814-3079
301-657-2248
Fax: 301-913-9413
TTY: 301-657-2249
national@shhh.org
www.hearingloss.org

4780 So You Have Had an Ear Operation...What Next?
American Hearing Research Foundation
275 N. York Street
Elmhurst, IL 60126-4539
630-617-5079
Fax: 630-563-9181
www.american-hearing.org

Offers information on ear infections and surgery.
William L Lederer, Executive Director
Sharon Parmet, Development/Communications Associate

4781 Statewide Services for Deaf and Hard of Hearing People
National Information Center on Deafness
800 Florida Avenue NE
Washington, DC 20002
773-568-1550
800-621-2736
Fax: 800-621-8476
TTY: 888-630-9347
gupress@gallaudet.edu
gupress.gallaudet.edu

A resource list of states that have established commissions and other offices to serve deaf people.

4782 Travel Resources for Deaf and Hard of Hearing People
National Information Center on Deafness
800 Florida Avenue NE
Washington, DC 20002
773-568-1550
800-621-2736
Fax: 800-621-8476
TTY: 888-630-9347
gupress@gallaudet.edu
gupress.gallaudet.edu

A publication list of travel industry resources for deaf and hard of hearing people.

4783 What are TTY's? TDDs? TTs?
National Information Center on Deafness
800 Florida Avenue NE
Washington, DC 20002-3660
773-568-1550
800-621-2736
Fax: 800-621-8476
TTY: 888-630-9347
gupress@gallaudet.edu
gupress.gallaudet.edu

Discusses text telephones used by deaf people.

4784 World of Sound
International Hearing Society

16880 Middlebelt Road
Livonia, MI 48154-3367
313-478-2610
Fax: 313-478-4520

The purpose of this booklet is to provide basic information for those with questions about hearing loss, hearing aids and Hearing Instrument Specialists.

4785 You Don't Have to Hate Meetings: Try Computer-Assisted Notetaking Instead
Self Help for Hard of H
7910 Woodmont Avenue
Bethesda, MD 20814-3079
301-657-2248
Fax: 301-913-9413
TTY: 301-657-2249
national@shhh.org
www.hearingloss.org

Audio & Video

4786 ASL Poetry: Selected Works of Clayton Valli
DawnSignPress
6130 Nancy Ridge Drive
San Diego, CA 92121-3223
858-625-0600
800-549-5350
Fax: 858-625-2336
TTY: 858-625-0600
comments@dawnsign.com
www.dawnsign.com

Twenty one original Valli poems recited by a diversity of native signers. Guided experience through the richness of poetry in another language.
105 minutes
ISBN: 0-915035-23-5
Clayton Valli, Director

4787 Basic Course in American Sign Language Vid eotape Package
TJ Publishers
2544 Tarpley Road
Carrollton, TX 75006
972-416-0800
800-999-1168
Fax: 972-416-0944
customerservice@tjpublishers.com
www.tjpublishers.com/index.html

The A Basic Course in American Sign Language Vocabulary Videotape features four Deaf models signing each vocabulary word contained in all 22 lessons of the text plus the alphabet and numbers. The tape has captions and voice which can be turned off to sharpen visual acuity. It is ideal for classroom reinforcement and independent home study.
Angela K Thames, President
Jerald A Murphy, VP

4788 Beginning Reading and Sign Language Video
TJ Publishers
2544 Tarpley Road
Carrollton, TX 75006
972-416-0800
800-999-1168
Fax: 972-416-0944
customerservice@tjpublishers.com
www.tjpublishers.com/index.html

Learning sign improves reading, motor skills and visual perception and increases language acquisition abilities. For kids from 2 to 12, this video picture book features deaf actress Susan Bressler signing over a hundred words at the zoo, at home and around the community.
Video
Angela K Thames, President
Jerald A Murphy, VP

4789 Come Sign With Us
Gallaudet University
800 Florida Avenue, NE
Washington, DC 20002-3819
773-568-1550
800-621-2736
Fax: 800-621-8476
TTY: 888-630-9347
gupress@gallaudet.edu
gupress.gallaudet.edu

Lessons including fingerspelling and signing are overviewed.
90 minutes
ISBN: 1-563680-50-5
Jan C. Hafer, Co-Author
Robert M. Wilson, Co-Author

4790 Deaf Children Signers
Harris Communications
15155 Technology Drive
Eden Prairie, MN 55344   952-906-1180
                                800-825-6758
                            Fax: 952-906-1099
                            TTY: 800-825-9187
                            info@harriscomm.com
                            www.harriscomm.com
This 5-part collection of children signers is great for children, teachers, parents and interpreters.
Robert Harris Ph.D, Founder/President/CEO

4791 Deaf Culture Autobiographies
Harris Communications
15155 Technology Drive
Eden Prairie, MN 55344   952-906-1180
                                800-825-6758
                            Fax: 952-906-1099
                            TTY: 800-825-9187
                            info@harriscomm.com
                            www.harriscomm.com
Inspiring videotapes offer encouragement and enlightenment to the hearing impaired. Total of eight videotapes.
Robert Harris Ph.D, Founder/President/CEO

4792 Deaf Culture Series
Harris Communications
15155 Technology Drive
Eden Prairie, MN 55344   952-906-1180
                                800-825-6758
                            Fax: 952-906-1099
                            TTY: 800-825-9187
                            info@harriscomm.com
                            www.harriscomm.com
Each video in this 5-part series features a variety of Deaf talent. It is an excellent resource for Deaf studies programs, Interpreter Preparation programs and Sign Language programs.
Robert Harris Ph.D, Founder/President/CEO

4793 Deaf Mosaic Series
Harris Communications
15155 Technology Drive
Eden Prairie, MN 55344   952-906-1180
                                800-825-6758
                            Fax: 952-906-1099
                            TTY: 800-825-9187
                            info@harriscomm.com
                            www.harriscomm.com
A national magazine show produced monthly by Gallaudet University, this show has been awarded nine Emmys. As the only nation-wide program about the Deaf community, these videotapes are the best of the best from the shows programs.
Robert Harris Ph.D, Founder/President/CEO

4794 Diagnosis and Treatment of Unilateral Hearing Loss
American Academy of Otolaryngology
1650 Diagonal Road
Alexandria, VA 22314-3357   703-836-4444
                            Fax: 703-683-5100
                            www.entnet.org
This CD-ROM focuses on evaluation and treatment of unilateral hearing loss arising from skull base lesion.

4795 Do You Hear That?
Alexander Graham Bell Association
3417 Volta Place NW
Washington, DC 20007-2737   202-337-5220
                            Fax: 202-337-8314
                            TTY: 202-337-5220
                            info@agbell.org
                            www.listeningandspokenlanguage.org
This video documents auditory-verbal therapy as it is practiced at North York General Hospital in Toronto, Canada.
1992 35 minutes

4796 Fantastic Series
Gallaudet University Bookstore
800 Florida Avenue NE
Washington, DC 20002-3660   773-568-1550
                                800-621-2736
                            Fax: 800-621-8476
                            TTY: 888-630-9347
                            gupress@gallaudet.edu
                            gupress.gallaudet.edu

Tapes designed to encourage both deaf and hearing children to use their imaginations.
Ages 6-10

4797 Fingers that Tickle and Delight
National Association of the Deaf
8630 Fenton Street
Silver Spring, MD 20910   301-587-1788
                            Fax: 301-587-1791
                            TTY: 301-587-1789
                            nad.info@nad.org
                            nad.org
One woman's experience from childhood, school, marriage, her career as a teacher and interpreter trainer, and her life as an entertainer. Closed captioned.
13+ 32 minutes
Christopher Wagner, President
Melissa S. Draganac-Hawk, Vice-President

4798 Fingerspelling and Numbers Software
American Sign Language (ASL) Productions
c/o Harris Communications
Eden Prairie, MN 55344   952-906-1180
                                800-767-4461
                            Fax: 952-906-1099
                            TTY: 800-767-4461
                            ASLProductions@harriscomm.com
Fingerspelling practice partner that allows you to control the speed and vocabulary level. Requires Windows 3.1 or greater.
Robert Harris Ph.D, Founder/President-Harris Communications
Jenna Cassell, Founder ASL Productions

4799 Getting in Touch
Research Press
2612 N Mattis Avenue
Champaign, IL 61822-1053   217-352-3273
                                800-519-2707
                            Fax: 217-352-1221
                            rp@researchpress.com
                            www.researchpress.com
Shows how to create an individualized communications system based on the abilities and needs of the child. Illustrates seven basic communication procedures that involve the use of touch cues and object cues.

4800 Gospel of Luke
Gallaudet University Bookstore
800 Florida Avenue NE
Washington, DC 20002-3660   773-568-1550
                                800-621-2736
                            Fax: 800-621-8476
                            TTY: 888-630-9347
                            gupress@gallaudet.edu
                            gupress.gallaudet.edu
A set of five videotapes of the Gospel of Luke told in ASL.
Set of five

4801 Granny Good's Sign of Christmas
Gallaudet University Bookstore
800 Florida Avenue NE
Washington, DC 20002-3660   773-568-1550
                                800-621-2736
                            Fax: 800-621-8476
                            TTY: 888-630-9347
                            gupress@gallaudet.edu
                            gupress.gallaudet.edu
Twas The Night Before Christmas told in American Sign Language.

4802 Hearing Loss and Rehabilitation
American Academy of Otolaryngology
1650 Diagonal Road
Alexandria, VA 22314-3357   703-836-4444
                            Fax: 703-683-5100
                            www.entnet.org
Slides

4803 I Can Hear!
Alexander Graham Bell Association
3417 Volta Place NW
Washington, DC 20007-2737   202-337-5220
                            Fax: 202-337-8314
                            TTY: 202-337-5220
                            info@agbell.org
                            www.listeningandspokenlanguage.org

This inspirational video describes the auditory-verbal approach for developing speech and language for hearing impaired children and adults.
1992 23 minutes

4804 I Can Hear!: II
Alexander Graham Bell Association
3417 Volta Place NW
Washington, DC 20007-2737
202-337-5220
Fax: 202-337-8314
TTY: 202-337-5220
info@agbell.org
www.listeningandspokenlanguage.org
An exciting videotape that gives more examples of auditory-verbal therapy and a variety of kids who have been taught to speak using this method.
1996 19 minute video

4805 I See What You Say: Self Help Lip Reading Program
Alexander Graham Bell Association
3417 Volta Place NW
Washington, DC 20007-2737
202-337-5220
Fax: 202-337-8314
TTY: 202-337-5220
info@agbell.org
www.listeningandspokenlanguage.org
Easy to follow videotape and manual for consumers teaches visual recognition of speech sounds in single words and phrases.
1995 54 minutes

4806 Interpreters in Public Schools Kit
Sign Media
4020 Blackburn Lane
Burtonsville, MD 20866-1167
301-421-0268
800-475-4756
Fax: 301-421-0270
TTY: 301-421-4460
info@signmedia.com
www.signmedia.com
Videotapes individually specialized for administrators, classroom teachers and for interpreters. Provides practical insights to some of the most crucial issues and problems facing mainstreamed programs. Contains reproducible printed material.
Three videos
Barbara Olmert, Director Marketing

4807 Interview with Kirsten Gonzales
Alexander Graham Bell Association
3417 Volta Place NW
Washington, DC 20007-2737
202-337-5220
Fax: 202-337-8314
TTY: 202-337-5220
info@agbell.org
www.listeningandspokenlanguage.org
Interviews a longtime user and trainer of oral interpreters who offers techniques in articulation and natural gestures.
20 minutes

4808 It's Not Just Hearing AIDS: Deaf People and the Epidemic
National Association of the Deaf
8630 Fenton Street
Silver Spring, MD 20910
301-587-1788
Fax: 301-587-1791
TTY: 301-587-1789
nad.info@nad.org
nad.org
Straightforward and factual information on how AIDS is transmitted, who gets AIDS, procedures for an HIV test, and an interview with a person who actually has the AIDS virus.
9 - 13+ Video
Christopher Wagner, President
Melissa S. Draganac-Hawk, Vice-President

4809 Joy of Signing
Gallaudet University Bookstore
800 Florida Avenue NE
Washington, DC 20002-3660
773-568-1550
800-621-2736
Fax: 800-621-8476
TTY: 888-630-9347
gupress@gallaudet.edu
gupress.gallaudet.edu
Three tapes full of useful information to help increase skill and comfort with sign.
1 Videotape

4810 King Midas
Gallaudet University
800 Florida Avenue, NE
Washington, DC 20002-3819
773-568-1550
800-621-2736
Fax: 800-621-8476
TTY: 888-630-9347
gupress@gallaudet.edu
gupress.gallaudet.edu
Now the tale of King Midas and his golden touch is charmingly retold with full-color illustrations, and key sentences shown in American Sign Language (ASL).
30 minutes
ISBN: 0-930323-71-8
Robert Newby, Author

4811 King Midas Videotape
Gallaudet University Bookstore
800 Florida Avenue NE
Washington, DC 20002-3660
773-568-1550
800-621-2736
Fax: 800-621-8476
TTY: 888-630-9347
gupress@gallaudet.edu
gupress.gallaudet.edu
Story of King Midas told in American Sign Language.
Robert Newby, Author

4812 Learning to Communicate: The First Three Years Videotape
Alexander Graham Bell Association
3417 Volta Place NW
Washington, DC 20007-2737
202-337-5220
Fax: 202-337-8314
TTY: 202-337-5220
info@agbell.org
www.listeningandspokenlanguage.org
This video shows normal communication development in young children under three years of age. It discusses factors which can affect speech and language development, including anatomy and environment. Closed captioned.
11 minutes

4813 Let's Be Friends
Britannica Film Company
345 4th Street
San Francisco, CA 94107-1206
415-597-5555
The teacher left the room and asked Shelly, a hearing impaired child to be the mother. Margaret, an emotionally disturbed child, became frightened and verbally attacked Shelly. The teacher worked to get them to become friends and understand each other's problems.
Films

4814 Once Upon a Time - Children's Classics Ret old in American Sign Language
Harris Communications
15155 Technology Drive
Eden Prairie, MN 55344
952-906-1180
800-825-6758
Fax: 952-906-1099
TTY: 800-825-9187
info@harriscomm.com
www.harriscomm.com
Children's classics come alive on videotapes.
Robert Harris Ph.D, Founder/President/CEO

4815 Parent Sign Video Series
TJ Publishers
2544 Tarpley Road
Carrollton, TX 75006
972-416-0800
800-999-1168
Fax: 972-416-0944
customerservice@tjpublishers.com
www.tjpublishers.com/index.html
Ten instructional videotapes specifically designed for parents of deaf children, present frequently used vocabulary and phrases. The tapes are perfect for home use and as a compliment to sign language and educational programs. Deaf and hearing parents, each having a deaf and a hearing child, reflect common communication needs of all families.
Video
Angela K Thames, President
Jerald A Murphy, VP

4816 Read My Lips
Alexander Graham Bell Association
3417 Volta Place NW
Washington, DC 20007-2737
202-337-5220
Fax: 202-337-8314
TTY: 202-337-5220
info@agbell.org
www.listeningandspokenlanguage.org
A six videotape series that takes adults from lip reading to basic words to complex phrases and sentences in a variety of real life situations.

4817 See What I'm Saying
Thomas Kaufman, author
Fanlight Productions
32 Court Street
Brooklyn, NY 11201-1731
718-488-8900
800-876-1710
Fax: 718-488-8642
rentals@icarusfilms.com
www.fanlight.com
Follows Patricia, a deaf child from a hearing, Spanish speaking family, through her first year of elementary school. Illustrates how the acquisition of communication skills enhances a child's self-esteem, confidence and family relationships. Open captioned.
1992 31 Minutes
ISBN: 1-572950-90-0

4818 Seeing and Hearing Speech: Lessons in Lipreading and Listening
Hearing Loss Association of America
7910 Woodmont Avenue
Bethesda, MD 20814-3079
301-657-2248
Fax: 301-913-9413
TTY: 301-657-2249
info@hearingloss.org
www.hearingloss.org
This CD-Rom helps people with hearing loss learn to combine what they see with what they hear to understand speech better in difficult situations. This interactive CD-ROM contains carefully planned lessons to improve speech understanding through lipreading.
CD-ROM
Anna Gilmore Hall, Executive Director
Lise Hamlin, Director of Public Policy

4819 Show & Tell: Explaining Hearing Loss to Teachers
Alexander Graham Bell Association
3417 Volta Place NW
Washington, DC 20007-2737
202-337-5220
Fax: 202-337-8314
TTY: 202-337-5220
info@agbell.org
www.listeningandspokenlanguage.org
This video introduces mainstreamed teachers to the challenges that hearing impairments impose on normal communication.
20 minutes

4820 Show 'N' Tell Stories
Modern Signs Press
PO Box 1181
Los Alamitos, CA 90720-1181
562-596-8548
800-572-7332
Fax: 562-795-6614
TTY: 562-493-4168
modsigns@modernsignspress.com
www.modernsignspress.com
A bilingual storytelling series for Deaf children and their families, featuring both Signing Exact English (SEE) and American Sign Language (ASL).
Videotape

4821 Sign-Me-A-Story
DawnSignPress
6130 Nancy Ridge Drive
San Diego, CA 92121-3223
858-768-0428
800-549-5350
Fax: 858-625-2336
TTY: 858-625-0600
info@dawnsign.com
www.dawnsign.com/
Linda Bove, the deaf actress from Sesame Street, introduces children to American Sign Language. Teaches simple signs and then acts out fairy tales. Stories are voiced and closed captioned, accessible to all.
30 minutes
ISBN: 0-394892-32-1
Joe Dannis, Founder/Publisher/President

4822 Sleeping Beauty Videotape
Gallaudet University Bookstore
800 Florida Avenue NE
Washington, DC 20002-3660
773-568-1550
800-621-2736
Fax: 800-621-8476
TTY: 888-630-9347
gupress@gallaudet.edu
gupress.gallaudet.edu
Presents the entire story of Sleeping Beauty told in American Sign Language.

4823 Sleeping Beauty: With Selected Sentences in ASL
Gallaudet University
800 Florida Avenue, NE
Washington, DC 20002-3819
773-568-1550
800-621-2736
Fax: 800-621-8476
TTY: 888-630-9347
gupress@gallaudet.edu
gupress.gallaudet.edu
Features the full story in ASL and includes vocabulary and sentence structure focusing on adjectives, with a voice-over throughout.
30 minutes
ISBN: 0-930323-98-X

4824 Sound Hearing
Hearing Loss Association of America
7910 Woodmont Avenue
Bethesda, MD 20814-3079
301-657-2248
Fax: 301-913-9413
TTY: 301-657-2249
info@hearingloss.org
www.hearingloss.org
Provides listening samples to illustrate sound, hearing, and hearing loss. Listeners will hear as people who have hearing loss might, listening to music, a story, etc.
CD-ROM, 26 mins
Anna Gilmore Hall, Executive Director
Lise Hamlin, Director of Public Policy

4825 Telecoil: Plugging Into Sound
Hearing Loss Association of America
7910 Woodmont Avenue
Bethesda, MD 20814-3079
301-657-2248
Fax: 301-913-9413
TTY: 301-657-2249
info@hearingloss.org
www.hearingloss.org
In The Telecoil: Plugging Into Sound, members of SHHH give accounts of their experiences with using the telecoil, describing how the telecoil makes a noticeable difference in their social and professional lives.
Open Captioned
Anna Gilmore Hall, Executive Director
Lise Hamlin, Director of Public Policy

4826 Telecoil: Plugging into Sound
7910 Woodmont Avenue
Bethesda, MD 20814-3079
301-657-2248
Fax: 301-913-9413
TTY: 301-657-2249
national@shhh.org
www.hearingloss.org
Guide for consumers concerning why they should include a telecoil in their hearing aid. SHHH members are featured, talking about their experiences. Includes 50 brochures. Open-captioned.
1996 10 minutes

4827 Telling Stories
Harris Communications
15155 Technology Drive
Eden Prairie, MN 55344
952-906-1180
800-825-6758
Fax: 952-906-1099
TTY: 800-825-9187
info@harriscomm.com
www.harriscomm.com

This international, award winning play, now on video, uses the symbols and myths drawn from the struggles between the world of the deaf and the world of the hearing.
Robert Harris Ph.D, Founder/President/CEO

4828   Treasure
Gallaudet University Bookstore
800 Florida Avenue NE   773-568-1550
Washington, DC 20002-3660   800-621-2736
                                                              Fax: 800-621-8476
                                                              TTY: 888-630-9347
                                                              gupress@gallaudet.edu
                                                              gupress.gallaudet.edu
Ella Mae Lentz, a well-known deaf poet, signs some of her poems.

4829   Unheard Voices
Hearing Loss Association of America
7910 Woodmont Avenue   301-657-2248
Bethesda, MD 20814-3079   Fax: 301-913-9413
                                                              TTY: 301-657-2249
                                                              info@hearingloss.org
                                                              www.hearingloss.org
Unheard Voices is a candid and compassionate portrayal of people coping with the life-changing impact of hearing loss. Open-captioned.
23 minutes
Anna Gilmore Hall, Executive Director
Barbara Kelley, Deputy Executive Director

Web Sites

4830   AbleData
                                                              abledata.acl.gov
An information and referral service that uses computer listings and a large file system to answer requests related to assistive devices. Houses a large file system library and contacts with other sources which enables them to answer just about any question.

4831   Alexander Graham Bell Association
                              www.listeningandspokenlanguage.org
They helps families, health care providers and education professionals understand childhood hearing loss and the importance of early diagnosis and intervention. Through advocacy, education, research and financial aid, AG Bell helps to ensure that every child and adult with hearing loss has the opportunity to listen, talk and thrive in mainstream society.

4832   American Academy of Audiology
                                                              www.audiology.org
Provides professional development, education and research and provides increased public awareness of hearing disorders and audiologic services.

4833   American Academy of Otolaryngology - Head and Neck Surgery
                                                              www.entnet.org
Advance the art and science of otalaryngology-head and neck surgury through state-of-the-art education, research, and learning; and to unite, serve, and represent the interests of its members and their patients to the public.

4834   American Society for Deaf Children
                                                              www.deafchildren.org
Provides support, encouragement, and current information about deafness to families with deaf and hard of hearing children.

4835   American Tinnitus Association
                                                              www.ata.org
Provides information about tinnitus and referrals to local contacts/support groups nationwide.

4836   DeafEd.net
                                                              www.deafed.net
Educational information and opportunities for deaf/hard of hearing children; run in conjunction with Hands & Voices.

4837   EAR Foundation
                                                              www.earfoundation.org
Provides the general public support services promoting the integration of the hearing and balance impaired into mainstream society and to educate young people and adults about hearing

preservation and early detection of hearing loss, enabling them to prevent at an early age hearing and balance disorders.
Molli C. Conti, Executive Director

4838   Healing Well
                                                              www.healingwell.com
An online health resource guide to medical news, chat, information and articles, newsgroups and message boards, books, disease-related web sites, medical directories, and more for patients, friends, and family coping with disabling diseases, disorders, or chronic illnesses.

4839   Health Finder
                                                              www.healthfinder.gov
Searchable, carefully developed web site offering information on over 1000 topics. Developed by the US Department of Health and Human Services, the site can be used in both English and Spanish.
Rick Smith, President & CEO
Rebecca Frank, Chief Development Officer

4840   Healthlink USA
                                                              www.healthlinkusa.com
Health information concerning treatment, cures, prevention, diagnosis, risk factors, research, support groups, email lists, personal stories and much more. Updated regularly.

4841   Hear Now
                                              www.starkeyhearingfoundation.org
Hear Now is the application-based program of Starkey Hearing Foundation that provides assistance to low-income Americans. Each person they help is fit with new, top-of-the-line digital hearing aids that are customized to their hearing loss.
Molli C. Conti, Executive Director

4842   Hearing Education and Awareness for Rocker
                                                              www.hearnet.com
Educates the public about the real dangers of hearing loss resulting from repeated exposure to excessive noise levels.

4843   Hearing Health Foundation
                                                              hearinghealthfoundation.org

4844   Hearing Industries Association
777 6th Street NW   202-975-0905
Washington, DC 20001   www.hearing.org
HIA represents hearing aid manufacturers, suppliers, distributors, and hearing health professionals. The website features articles on hearing aids and childhood hearing impairment.
Kate Carr, President
Carole Rogin, Strategic Advisor

4845   House Ear Institute
                                                              houseclinic.com
A national non-profit otologic research and educational institute that provides information on hearing and balance disorders.

4846   John Tracy Clinic
                                                              www.jtc.org
An educational facility for preschool age children who have hearing losses and their families. In addition to on-site services, worldwide correspondence courses in English and Spanish are offered to parents whose children are of preschool age and are hard of hearing, deaf, or deaf-blind.

4847   MedicineNet
                                                              www.medicinenet.com
An online resource for consumers providing easy-to-read, authoritative medical and health information.

4848   Medscape
                                                              www.medscape.com
Medscape offers specialists, primary care physicians, and other health professionals the Web's most robust and integrated medical information and educational tools.

4849   National Association of the Deaf
                                                              www.nad.org
Focus on advocacy, captioned media, deafness-related information/publications, legal assistance and more.

4850   National Captioning Institute
                                                              ncicap.org

Advocates captioned television for people who want to see, as well as hear, the dialogue of a television program. It not only enables deaf and hard-of-hearing people to understand all of a program's content, but it is also beneficial for new Americans learning English as a second language, as well as children learning to read.

4851 National Information Center on Deafness

www.gallaudet.edu

Provides information or referrals on questions about deafness, including general information, education, research, legislation, assistive devices and more. Offers a bibliography of readings available on 30 topics relating to deafness.

4852 National Information Clearinghouse on Children Who are Deaf-Blind

nationaldb.org

Collects, organizes and disseminates information related to children and youth who are deaf-blind and connects consumers of deaf-blind information to sources of information about deaf-blindness, assistive technology and deaf-blind people.

4853 National Institute on Deafness and Other Communication Disorders

A national resources center for information about hearing, balance, smell, taste, voice, speech and language.

4854 Registry of Interpreters for the Deaf

www.RID.org

Professional interpreters and translators, persons with deafness or hearing impairments and professionals in related fields.

4855 Self-Help for Hard of Hearing People

www.hearingloss.org

Promotes awareness and information about hearing loss, communication, assistive devices, and alternative communication skills through publications, exhibits and presentations.

4856 USA Deaf Sports Federation

www.usdeafsports.org

Website published by a governing body for all deaf sports and recreation in the United States.

4857 WebMD

www.webmd.com

Provides credible information, supportive communities, and in-depth reference material about health subjects. A source for original and timely health information as well as material from well known content providers.

Description

4858 Heart Disease

There is a wide range of heart (cardiac) diseases that can be divided into several major categories: heart failure; abnormalities of electrical conduction; heart rate and rhythm; and malfunction of the heart valves. Coronary artery disease relates to the arteries that supply oxygen to the heart muscle itself.

Heart failure is the general inability of the heart to function effectively as the pumping mechanism to distribute oxygenated blood and nutrients to the cells and tissues. As the heart's pumping action declines, blood does not get distributed properly and normal circulation gets disrupted. As a result, the fluid accumulates, or backs up, causing swelling (edema) in the body, often noticeable in the ankles, as well as within the lungs (pulmonary edema) causing difficulty in breathing. Numerous mechanisms are responsible for heart failure, so treatment is aimed at the underlying causes, improving heart contractibility (and thus pump efficiency) with drugs like digoxin, reducing the workload on the heart with drugs like beta-blockers and antihypertensive agents like ACE inhibitors and ARBs (angiotensin II receptor antagonists), and removal of excess fluid through the kidneys with diuretics.

Problems in the electrical conduction that makes the heart contract result in irregular heart rate and rhythm, either slower, faster, or, in life-threatening situations, absence of heart beat or ineffective heart contractions. Specific medications and procedures are used in treatment, again depending on the underlying problem.

New diagnostic (angiography) and therapeutic catheter techniques have been developed to accurately identify the rhythm problem, and in some cases, cure it by ablating the tissue responsible for the abnormal activity.

Malfunctions of heart valves are also common, but surgical advances enable successful repair and replacement of defective or diseased valves.

The arteries that directly supply the heart (known as coronary arteries) can also be affected by disease processes. Deposits or fatty plaques may cause narrowing of the arteries (atherosclerosis), or the arteries can become blocked by a clot that originated somewhere else in the body. Either way, the heart may be deprived of oxygenated blood and the particular muscle that is fed by the artery is injured or dies. Angina is chest pain produced when the heart is not receiving enough oxygen but no direct damage occurs. A heart attack (or myocardial infarction) occurs when the heart is deprived of its blood for a significant amount of time because of atherosclerotic blockage of one or more coronary arteries. The outcome of a heart attack depends on the amount of damage sustained by the affected heart muscle and the speed with which treatment is started. Immediate medical intervention has a marked effect on long-term prognosis. Administration of agents that dissolve the clot (blood thinners, antithrombotics) significantly reduce heart attack deaths when given within 6 hours of the onset of chest pain. Catheter interventions (angioplasty) can include balloons and metallic stents that are placed in coronary arteries to push obstructions against the arterial walls thereby re-opening the vessel. The most recent advance is drug-coated stents that prevent reformation of the clot.

The symptoms of heart disease are varied, but may include chest pain, difficulty breathing, fatigue, palpitations, dizziness and fainting. Investigations into stem cell transplantations to heart damaged heart muscle are underway. See also *Congenital Heart Disease.*

National Agencies & Associations

4859 American Autoimmune Related Diseases Association
22100 Gratiot Avenue 586-776-3900
Eastpointe, MI 48021 800-598-4668
Fax: 586-776-3903
aarda@aarda.org
www.aarda.org
Awareness, education, referrals for patients with any type of auto-immune disease.
Virginia T. Ladd, President & Executive Director
Laura Simpson, Assistant Director

4860 American Heart Association
7272 Greenville Avenue 888-478-7653
Dallas, TX 75231 800-242-8721
www.heart.org
The American Heart Association is the nation's oldest, largest volunteer organization devoted to fighting cardiovascular diseases and stroke. Funds research and raises public awareness of heart diseases.
Nancy Brown, CEO
Ivor J. Benjamin, MD, FAHA, President

4861 Canadian Adult Congenital Heart Network
222 Queen Street 877-569-3407
Ottawa, Ontario, K1P-5V9 cachnet@css.ca
www.cachnet.org
Organization founded to share knowledge and skills among congenital heart disease professionals in order to create a community committed to caring for individuals with congenital heart disease.
Ariane Marelli, MD, President
Candice Silversides, MD, Vice President

4862 Children's Heart Society
9920 63 Avenue   780-454-7665
Edmonton, Alberta, T6E-0G9   childrensheart@shaw.ca
                                                  www.childrensheart.ca
Supports families of children with acquired and congenital heart disease.
Gerry Cruz, President
Andrea Luft-Kerr, Vice President

4863 National Heart, Lung & Blood Institute
31 Center Drive   nhlbiinfo@nhlbi.nih.gov
Bethesda, MD 20892   www.nhlbi.nih.gov
Trains, conducts research, and educates in order to promote the prevention and treatment of heart, lung, and blood disorders.
Gary H. Gibbons, MD, Director
Nakela Cook, MD, MPH, FACC, Chief of Staff

4864 Pulmonary Hypertension Association (PHA)
801 Roeder Road   301-565-3004
Silver Spring, MD 20910   800-748-7274
                                         pha@PHAssociation.org
                                           www.PHAssociation.org
A non-profit organization for pulmonary hypertension patients, families, caregivers and PH-treating medical professionals. PHA works to provide support, education, and find a cure for pulmonary hypertension.
Brad A. Wong, President & CEO
Azalea Candelaria, Vice President

Research Centers

4865 Arizona Heart Institute
2632 N 20th Street   602-266-2200
Phoenix, AZ 85006-1300   800-345-4278
                                              Fax: 602-604-5047
                                                   www.azheart.com
Edward Diethrich, Medical Director and Founder

4866 Baylor College of Medicine: Debakey Heart Center
Texas Medical Center
1 Baylor Plaza   713-798-4710
Houston, TX 77030-3411   Fax: 713-798-3692
                                               president@bcm.edu
                                                 www.bcm.tmc.edu
Research activities have an emphasis on therapeutic intervention and prevention of heart disease.
James T Hackett, Chair
Paul Klotman MD, President

4867 Bees-Stealy Research Foundation
2001 4th Avenue   619-235-8744
San Diego, CA 92101-2303   Fax: 619-234-8190
Basic cardiac research.
HD Peabody Jr, Director

4868 Bockus Research Institute Graduate Hospital
Graduate Hospital
415 S 19th Street
Philadelphia, PA 19146-1464   215-893-2000
Offers research in cardiovascular diseases with emphasis on muscle tissue studies.
Dr Robert Cox, Director

4869 Boston University, Whitaker Cardiovascular Institute
715 Albany Street   617-638-4887
Boston, MA 02118   Fax: 617-638-4066
                                                  www.bumc.bu.edu
Offers basic and clinical care research relating to cardiovascular diseases.
Gary J Balady MD, Clinical Investigator

4870 Cardiovascular Research and Training Center University of Alabama
THT Room 311   205-934-3624
Birmingham, AL 35294-6   Fax: 205-345-96
Robert C Bueourge, Director

4871 Children's Heart Institute of Texas
PO Box 3966   512-887-4505
Corpus Christi, TX 78463-3966   Fax: 512-887-0539
Offers research and statistical information on pediatric cardiology.
Laura Berlanga, Director

4872 Cleveland Clinic Lerner Research Institute
9500 Euclid Avenue   216-444-3900
Cleveland, OH 44195   Fax: 216-444-3279
                                                    dicorlp@ccf.org
                                                   www.lerner.ccf.org
Research institute focusing on diseases of the cardiovascular system.
Paul E DiCorleto PhD, Institute Chairman
Guy M Chisolm, III, PhD, Institute Vice-Chair

4873 Columbia University Irving Center for Clinical Research Adult Unit
Presbyterian Hospital
116 Street and Broadway   212-854-1754
New York, NY 10027   Fax: 212-053-13
                                               askcuit@columbia.edu
                                                  www.columbia.edu
Research center focusing on pulmonary diseases.
Lee C Bollinger, President
John H Coatsworth, Provost

4874 Congenital Heart Disease Anomalies Support, Education & Resources CHASER
2112 N Wilkins Road   419-825-5575
Swanton, OH 43558-9445   Fax: 419-825-2880
                                                     www.csun.edu
An organization established to meet the emotional and educational needs of parents and professionals who deal with congenital heart disease in children. Offers resource materials and support for parent to parent networking.

4875 Creighton University Cardiac Center
3006 Webster Street   402-280-4566
Omaha, NE 68131-2137   800-237-7828
                                              Fax: 402-280-4938
                                          thecardiaccenter.creighton.edu
Research into the clinical aspects of cardiology and heart disease.
Tami Ward, Nurse Practitioner
Kimberly Harm, Nurse Practitioner

4876 Duke University Pediatric Cardiac Catheterization Laboratory
T901/Children's Health Center   919-681-4080
Durham, NC 27705-0001   Fax: 919-681-2714
                                               john.rhodes@duke.edu
                                                 pediatrics.duke.edu
Research into pediatric cardiology.
Joseph St Geme, III, MD, Chair
Kay Marshall, Chief Administrator

4877 Florida Heart Research Institute
4770 Biscayne Boulevard   305-674-3020
Miami, FL 33137   Fax: 305-535-3642
                                               pak@floridaheart.org
                                           www.miamiheartresearch.org
General cardiovascular research.
Kathleen T DuCasse, Chief Executive Officer

4878 Framingham Heart Study
73 Mount Wayte Avenue   508-935-3418
Framingham, MA 01702-5828   Fax: 508-626-1262
                                            LLehmann1@partners.org
                                        www.framinghamheartstudy.org
Lisa Soleymani Lehmann, M.D.,, Chair

4879 General Clinical Research Center at Beth Israel Hospital
330 Brookline Avenue   617-667-7000
Boston, MA 02215-5400   800-667-5356
                                              TDD: 800-439-0183
                                                     www.bidmc.org
Studies into cardiology pulmonary disorders and heart disease.
Stephen B Kay, Chair
Kevin Tabb, MD, President & Chief Executive Officer

4880 General Clinical Research Center: University of California at LA
Center for Health Sciences

10833 Le Conte Avenue — 310-825-7177
Los Angeles, CA 90095 — Fax: 310-206-5012
Cardiovascular and heart disease disorders and illness research.
Isidro Salus MD, Program Director
Gerald Levey, Principal Investigator

4881 Hahnemann University Likoff Cardiovascular Institute
Broad & Vine Streets — 215-854-8100
Philadelpia, PA 19102
Diseases of the heart and vessels.
William S Frankl MD, Director

4882 Harvard Throndike Laboratory Harvard Medical Center
Harvard Medical Center
330 Brookline Avenue — 617-735-3020
Boston, MA 02215-5400 — Fax: 617-735-4833
Dr James Morgan, Director

4883 Heart Disease Research Foundation
50 Court Street — 718-649-6210
Brooklyn, NY 11201-4801
Robert A Teters, Director

4884 Heart Research Foundation of Sacramento
1007 39th Street — 916-456-3365
Sacramento, CA 95816-5502
Dr Frink, Founder/Principal Investigator

4885 Hope Heart Institute
1380 112th Ave. NE — 425-456-8700
Bellvue, WA 98004 — Fax: 425-456-8701
info@hopeheart.org
www.hopeheart.org
Heart and blood vessel research.
Dr Lester R Sauvage MD, Founder
Cherie Skager, Interim Executive Director

4886 John L McClellan Memorial Veterans' Hospital Research Office
4300 W 7th Street — 501-257-1000
Little Rock, AR 72205-5446 — Fax: 501-671-2510
Karl David Straub MD, Chief Staff

4887 Krannert Institute of Cardiology
1801 N Senate Boulevard — 317-962-0500
Indianapolis, IN 46202-4832 — 800-843-2786
Fax: 317-962-0501
medicine.iupui.edu/krannert
The cardiovascular program at the Indiana University School of Medicine is recognized throughout the world for its commitment to excellence in patient care research and education. While we're known for our experience and ability to take care of the most complex cardiovascular problems we are equally focused on prevention and early detection.
Peng-Sheng Chen, MD, Division Director
Eric Williams, MD, Associate Dean

4888 Loyola University of Chicago Cardiac Transplant Program
2160 S 1st Avenue — 708-216-9000
Maywood, IL 60153-3304 — 888-584-7888
Fax: 708-216-4918
www.loyolamedicine.org/
Loyola University Health System is committed to excellence in patient care and the education of health professionals. They believe that our Catholic heritage and Jesuit traditions of ethical behavior academic distinction and scientific research lead to new knowledge and advance our healing mission in the communities we serve.
Larry M Goldberg, President & CEO
Wendy S Leutgens, Senior Vice President and COO

4889 Medstar Georgetown University Hospital Facility
3800 Reservoir Road NW — 202-444-2000
Washington, DC 20007-2195 www.georgetownuniversityhospital.org
Studies of medical sciences with particular emphasis on heart disease.
Dr Richard Goldberg, President

4890 Mount Sinai Medical Center
4300 Alton Road — 305-674-2121
Miami Beach, FL 33140-2997 — Fax: 305-743-09
www.msmc.com

General cardiovascular research.
Steven D Sonenreich, President & Chief Executive Officer

4891 Oklahoma Medical Research Foundation: Cardiovascular Research Program
825 NE 13th Street — 405-271-6673
Oklahoma City, OK 73104-5097 — 800-522-0211
Fax: 405-271-3980
contact@omrf.org
www.omrf.ouhsc.edu
The Cardiovascular Biology Research Program investigates fundamental mechanisms involved in blood coagulation inflammation and atherogenesis with special emphasis on the regulation of theses processes.
Dr Stephen M Prescott, President
Mike D Morgan, Executive Vice President & COO

4892 Pennsylvania State University Artificial Heart Research Project
Milton S Hershey Medical Center
500 University Drive — 717-531-8407
Hershey, PA 17033-2391 — Fax: 717-531-5011
www.psu.edu
William S Pierce MD, Director

4893 Preventive Medicine Research Institute
900 Bridgeway — 415-332-2525
Sausalito, CA 94965-2158 — Fax: 415-325-30
Tandis@pmri.org
www.pmri.org
Nonprofit organization focusing on prevention and treatment of heart disease through modification of diet exercise and relaxation techniques.
Dean Ornish, MD, Founder & President
Anne Ornish, Vice President, Director of Program Deve

4894 Purdue University William A Hillenbrand Biomedical Engineering Center
AA Potter Engineering Center
206 S. Martin Jischke Drive — 765-494-2995
W Lafayette, IN 47907-2032 — 877-598-4233
Fax: 765-494-6628
WeldonBME@purdue.edu
engineering.purdue.edu/BME
Cardiology and heart disease research.
Brian J Knoy, Director of Development
Kathryn Copper, Secretary

4895 Rockefeller University Laboratory of Cardiac Physiology
1230 York Avenue — 212-327-8000
New York, NY 10065 — Fax: 212-327-7974
pubinfo@rockefeller.edu
www.rockefeller.edu
Causes of cardiac arrhythmias and prevention of heart disease.
David Rockfeller, Honorary Chair
Russell L Carson, Chair

4896 San Francisco Heart & Vascular Institute
1900 Sullivan Avenue — 650-991-6712
Daly City, CA 94015-2200 — 800-82H-EART
Fax: 650-755-7315
www.sfhi.com
At Seton Medical Center we are committed to providing a full range of high quality services and state-of-the-art cardiovascular treatments for our patients. Our medical nursing and social services staff provide quality care and compassion as a coordinated team focusing on the medical emotional and spiritual needs of patients and their families.
Colman J Ryan, MD, Executive Medical Director
Michael Girolami, MD, Chief of Cardiology

4897 Specialized Center of Research in Ischemic Heart Disease
1802 6th Avenue South — 205-934-4011
Birmingham, AL 35294-0001 — 800-822-8816
Coronary artery disease.
Will Ferniany, CEO
Becky Armstrong, Program Manager

4898 Texas Heart Institute St Lukes Episcopal Hospital
St Lukes Episcopal Hospital

6770 Bertner Avenue
Houston, TX 77030-0345

832-355-4011
800-292-2221
Fax: 713-791-3089
mmattsson@heart.thi.tmc.edu
www.texasheartinstitute.org

Denton A Cooley MD, President Emeritus
James T Willerson MD, President, Medical Director

4899   University of Alabama at Birmingham: Congenital Heart Disease Center
1720 2nd Avenue South
Birmingham, AL 35294

205-934-4011
Fax: 205-934-7514
TDD: 205-934-4642
www.uab.edu

Ray L Watts, MD, President
Linda Lucas, PhD, Provost

4900   University of California San Diego General Clinical Research Center
UCSD Medical Center
200 W Arbor Drive
San Diego, CA 92103-1910

619-543-3102
858-657-7000
Fax: 619-435-36

General clinical research.
Paul Viviano, Chief Executive Officer and Associate Vi
Margarita Baggett, Interim Chief Operating Officer and Chie

4901   University of California: Cardiovascular Research Laboratory
Center for Health Sciences
UCLA Medical Center
Los Angeles, CA 90024

310-825-6824
Fax: 310-206-5777

Cellular and subcellular cardiac conditions.
Dr Glenn Langer, Director

4902   University of Cincinnati Department of Pathology & Laboratory Medicine
234 Goodman Street
Cincinnati, OH 45219-0529

513-584-7284
Fax: 513-584-3892
pathology@uc.edu
pathology.uc.edu

Fred V Lucas, MD, Chair of Pathology
James Hill, Business Manager

4903   University of Iowa: Iowa Cardiovascular Center
College of Medicine
200 Hawkins Drive
Iowa City, IA 52242

319-335-8588
Fax: 319-335-6969
www.int-med.uiowa.edu

The purpose is to coordinate the cardiovascular programs of the College into a more cohesive unit to permit us to 1) utilize our cardiovascular resources optimally 2) intensify expand and integrate basic and clinical research programs in areas related to cardiovascular research and 3) evaluate the role of new measures for prevention diagnosis and treatment of cardiovascular disease.
Barry London, MD, PhD, Director Cardiovascular Medicine

4904   University of Michigan Pulmonary and Critical Care Division
University Hospital
1500 E Medical Center Drive
Ann Arbor, MI 48109

734-647-9342
888-287-1084
Fax: 734-763-4585

Kevin Michael Chan, MD, Division Director

4905   University of Michigan: Cardiovascular Med icine
325 Briarwood Circle
Ann Arbor, MI 48108-0001

734-647-9000
Fax: 734-936-0133

Focuses on the diagnosis, treatment and prevention of cardiovascular and heart diseases.
Kim Allen Eagle, MD, Division Director

4906   University of Missouri Columbia Division of Cardiothoracic Surgery
School of Medicine
Columbia, MO 65212

573-882-2121
Fax: 573-884-0437
AldenM@missouri.edu
www.missouri.edu

Cardiac surgery research.
Mike Alden, Director
Brian Foster, Provost

4907   University of Pennsylvania Muscle Institut e
School of Medicine
700A Clinical Research Building
Philadelphia, PA 19104-2646

215-573-9758
Fax: 215-898-2653
mafoster@mail.med.upenn.edu
www.med.upenn.edu/pmi/

Studies in tissue science.
E. Michael Ostap, PhD, Director

4908   University of Pittsburgh: Human Energy Research Laboratory
4200 Fifth Avenue
Pittsburgh, PA 15260-0001

412-624-4141
www.pitt.edu

Focuses on exercise and cardiac rehabilitation.
Mark A Nordenberg, Chancellor
Patricia E Beeson, Provost and Senior Vice Chancellor

4909   University of Rochester: Clinical Research Center
601 Elmwood Avenue
Rochester, NY 14642-0001

585-275-2907
Fax: 585-256-3805
germaine_reinhardt@urmc.rochester.edu
www.urmc.rochester.edu/crc/

Studies of normal tissue functions pertaining to heart diseases.
Thomas A Pearson, MD, MPH, PhD, Director, Principal Investigator
Giovanni Schifitto , MD, Program Director

4910   University of Southern California: Coronary Care Research
1200 N State Street
Los Angeles, CA 90033-1029

213-226-7242

Dr. L Julian Haywood, Director

4911   University of Tennessee: Division of Cardiovascular Diseases
920 Madison Avenue
Memphis, TN 38163-0001

901-448-5750
Fax: 901-448-8084
www.utmem.edu\cardiology

Cardiovascular system disorders including heart disease prevention and treatment.
Karl T Weber MD, Director

4912   University of Texas Southwestern Medical Center at Dallas
University of Texas
5323 Harry Hines Boulevard
Dallas, TX 75390-7208

214-648-3111
Fax: 214-483-11
www.utsouthwestern.edu

Cardiology department research.
Daniel K Podolsky, MD, President
J. Gregory Fitz, MD, Executive Vice President

4913   University of Utah: Artificial Heart Research Laboratory
50 North Medical Drive
Salt Lake City, UT 84132-1414

801-581-2121
Fax: 801-581-4044
healthsciences.utah.edu

Cardiac and blood vessel research.
Allen Stephens, Associate Director

4914   University of Utah: Cardiovascular Genetic Research Clinic
420 Chipeta Way
Salt Lake City, UT 84132-0001

801-581-3888
Fax: 801-581-6862
www.medicine.utah.edu/internalmedicine/c

Cardiovascular genetics research.
Dr Roger Williams, Founder

4915   Urban Cardiology Research Center
2300 Garrison Boulevard
Baltimore, MD 21216-2308

410-945-8600

Causes diagnosis and treatment of cardiovascular diseases.
Arthur White MD, Director

4916   Warren Grant Magnuson Clinical Center
National Institute of Health
10 Center Drive MSC 1078
Bethesda, MD 20892

301-496-3311
800-411-1222
Fax: 301-496-2390
TTY: 866-411-1010
mmichael@cc.nih.gov
www.dnrc.nih.gov/reports/programs/ncc.as

Established in 1953 as the research hospital of the National Institutes of Health. Designed so that patient care facilities are close to research laboratories so new findings of basic and clinical scien-

tists can be quickly applied to the treatment of patients. Upon referral by physicians, patients are admitted to NIH clinical studies.
Madeline Michael, Chief, Clinical Nutrition Services

4917 Yeshiva University General Clinical Research Center
500 West 185th Street 212-960-5400
New York, NY 10033 www.yu.edu
Cardiovascular research.
Dr Henry Kressel, Chairman
Richard M Joel, President

Support Groups & Hotlines

4918 Mended Hearts
8150 N. Central Expressway 214-206-9259
Dallas, TX 75206 888-432-7899
Fax: 214-295-9552
info@mendedhearts.org
www.mendedhearts.org
Mutual support for persons who have heart disease, their families, friends, and other interested persons.
Gordon Littlefield, President of the Board
Donnette Smith, Executive Vice President

4919 Mitral Valve Prolapse Program of Cincinnati Support Group
10525 Montgomery Road 513-745-9911
Cincinnati, OH 45242 kscordo@wright.edu
Brings together persons frightened by their symptoms in order to learn to better cope with MVP. Fosters use of non-drug therapies. Supervised exercise sessions, diagnostic evaluations and specialized testing. Information and referrals, conferences, literature, group meetings, MVP Hot Line, and assistance in starting groups.

4920 National Health Information Center
Office of Disease Prevention & Health Promotion
1101 Wootton Pkwy Fax: 240-453-8281
Rockville, MD 20852 odphpinfo@hhs.gov
www.health.gov/nhic
Supports public health education by maintaining a calendar of National Health Observances; helps connect consumers and health professionals to organizations that can best answer questions and provide up-to-date contact information from reliable sources; updates on a yearly basis toll-free numbers for health information, Federal health clearinghouses and info centers.
Don Wright, MD, MPH, Director

4921 National Society for MVP and Dysautonomia
880 Montclair Road 205-595-8229
Birmingham, AL 35213 866-595-8229
Fax: 205-595-8222
nancysawyermd@bellsouth.net
Assists individuals suffering from mitral valve prolapse syndrome and dysautonomia to find support and understanding. Education on symptoms and treatment. Other areas of focus are Fibromyalgia and Sjogren's Syndrome.
Nancy Sawyer, MD

4922 Pulmonary Hypertension Association
801 Roeder Road 301-565-3004
Silver Spring, MD 20910 800-748-7274
Fax: 301-565-3994
PHCR@PHAssociation.org
www.phassociation.org
A nonprofit organization funded and for pulmonary hypertension patients. Our mission is to seek a cure, provide hope, support, education and to promote awareness and advocate for the PH community.
Brad Wong, President & CEO
Kelly Williams, VP, Communications & Marketing

4923 Society of Mitral Valve Prolapse Syndrome
PO Box 431 630-250-9327
Itasca, IL 60143-0431 Fax: 630-773-0478
bonnie0107@aol.com
www.mitralvalveprolapse.com/
Provides support and education to patients, families and friends about mitral valve prolapse syndrome.
Jim Durante, Co-Founder
Bonnie Durante, Co-Founder

Books

4924 Advances in Cardiac and Pulmonary Rehabilitation
Haworth Press
10 Alice Street 607-722-5857
Binghamton, NY 13904-1580 800-429-6784
Fax: 607-722-0012
www.haworthpress.com
Enhance your rehabilitation program with this authoritative volume.
74 pages Hardcover
ISBN: 0-866569-86-0

4925 Congenital Heart Disease
Northwestern University Press
625 Colfax Street 847-491-5313
Evanston, IL 60208-4210 800-621-2736
1993 300 pages
ISBN: 1-880416-82-4
Dory Kranz, Executive Director
Pip Marks, Director Outreach Services

4926 Dr. Dean Ornish's Program for Reversing Heart Disease
Random House Trade Books
400 Hahn Road 800-733-3000
Westminster, MD 21157-4663 Fax: 800-659-2436
deanornish.com/books
ISBN: 0-804110-38-7
Andrea Liptak, Founder

4927 Expert Guide to Beating Heart Disease: What You Absolutely Must Know
Dr. Harlan M. Krumholz, author
HarperCollins
195 Broadway 212-207-7000
New York, NY 10007-5299 orders@harpercollins.com
www.harpercollins.com
Translates key medical data into clear guidelines capturing the highest treatment standards for heart disease. Profiles care alternatices from supplements to stress reduction as well as treatments on the horizon.
2005 288 pages
ISBN: 0-060578-34-3
Brian Murray, President and CEO
Michael Morrison, President and Publisher

4928 Heart Disease
Franklin Watts Grolier
90 Old Sherman Turnpike 203-797-3500
Danbury, CT 06816-0001 800-621-1115
Fax: 203-797-3197
www.grolier.com
Using diagrams, this book discusses strokes and other blood vessel disorders, as well as their treatment and prevention.
112 pages Grades 7-12
ISBN: 0-531108-84-8
Debbie Fields, Executive Director

4929 Heart of a Child: What Families Need to Know About Heart Disorders
Johnss Hopkins University Press
2715 N Charles Street 410-935-6900
Baltimore, MD 21218-4319 800-537-5487
Fax: 410-516-6968
www.press.jhu.edu
1993 352 pages Paperback
ISBN: 0-801866-36-7
Doris Farrelly, Contact

4930 Living with Heart Disease
Franklin Watts Grolier
90 Old Sherman Turnpike 203-797-3500
Danbury, CT 06816-0001 800-621-1115
Fax: 203-797-3197
www.grolier.com

Shows how persons with heart disease can overcome their illness and lead productive lives.
32 pages Grades 5-7
ISBN: 0-531108-45-7
Dory Kranz, Executive Director
Pip Marks, Director Outreach Services

4931 Mitral Valve Prolapse Syndrome/Dysautonomia Survival Guide
Society of Mitral Valve Prolapse Syndrome
PO Box 431   630-250-9327
Itasca, IL 60143-0431   Fax: 630-773-0478
                                           bonnie0107@aol.com
                                           www.mitralvalveprolapse.com
Provides support and education to patients, families and friends about mitral valve prolapse syndrome.
175 pages
ISBN: 1-572243-03-1

4932 What Every Woman Must Know About Heart Disease
Warner Books
1271 Ave of the Americas   212-484-2900
New York, NY 10020-1300   Fax: 818-507-5596
                                           www.twbookmark.com

1996
ISBN: 0-446519-86-3

4933 Women Take Heart
Putnam Publishing Group
1380 112th Ave NE   425-456-8700
Bellevue, WA 98004-3903   Fax: 425-456-8701
                                           www.hopeheart.org

1993 224 pages
ISBN: 0-399138-88-9
Cherie Skager, Executive Director
Carol Coughlin, Manager of Development Operations

4934 Women and Heart Disease
Random House Trade Books
400 Hahn Road   301-592-8573
Bethesda, MD 20824-4663   800-733-3000
                                           Fax: 800-659-2436
                                           www.nhlbi.nih.gov

ISBN: 0-345386-20-5
Kathleen B. O'Sullivan, Executive Officer
Ariel Herman, Deputy Executive Officer

Children's Books

4935 Village by the Sea
Franklin Watts Grolier
90 Old Sherman Turnpike   203-797-3500
Danbury, CT 06816-0001   Fax: 203-797-3197
                                           www.grolier.com
This story focuses on the relationship between Emma and her father as he prepares to undergo bypass surgery.
Grades 5-8

Newsletters

4936 American Heart Association News
American Heart Association
7272 Greenville Avenue   214-706-1162
Dallas, TX 75231-5129   800-242-8721
                                           Fax: 214-696-5211
                                           www.heart.org
News reports and journal reports on the latest information concerning heart disease.

4937 And the Beat Goes On
Society of Mitral Valve Prolapse Syndrome
PO Box 431   630-250-9327
Itasca, IL 60143-0431   Fax: 630-773-0478
                                           bonnie0107@aol.com
                                           www.mitralvalveprolapse
Bi-monthly newsletter. Provides support and education to patients, families and friends about mitral valve prolapse syndrome.
6 pages

4938 Heartstyle
American Heart Association
7272 Greenville Avenue   214-706-1162
Dallas, TX 75231-5129   800-242-8721
                                           Fax: 214-696-5211
                                           www.heart.org
Reports on heart and blood vessel diseases and stroke.
Quarterly

4939 MVPS & Anxiety
Society of Mitral Valve Prolapse Syndrome
PO Box 431   630-250-9327
Itasca, IL 60143-0431   Fax: 630-773-0478
                                           bonnie0107@aol.com

6 pages

Pamphlets

4940 About High Blood Pressure
American Heart Association
7272 Greenville Avenue   214-706-1162
Dallas, TX 75231-5129   800-242-8721
                                           Fax: 214-696-5211
                                           www.heart.org
Offers information on what blood pressure is, risk factors and at risk persons.

4941 American Heart Association Diet
American Heart Association
7272 Greenville Avenue   214-706-1162
Dallas, TX 75231-5129   800-242-8721
                                           Fax: 214-696-5211
                                           www.heart.org
An eating plan for healthy americans.

4942 Cholesterol and Your Heart
American Heart Association
7272 Greenville Avenue   214-706-1162
Dallas, TX 75231-5129   800-242-8721
                                           Fax: 214-696-5211
                                           www.heart.org
Offers information on lowering blood cholesterol levels.

4943 Congenital Heart Defects
March of Dimes
1275 Mamaroneck Avenue   914-997-4488
White Plains, NY 10605   Fax: 212-254-3518
                                           NY639@marchofdimes.com
                                           www.marchofdimes.com

4944 E is for Exercise
American Heart Association
7272 Greenville Avenue   214-706-1162
Dallas, TX 75231-5129   800-242-8721
                                           Fax: 214-696-5211
                                           www.heart.org
Offers information on what kinds of exercise are the best and how to exercise properly.

4945 Easy Food Tips for Heart Healthy Eating
American Heart Association
7272 Greenville Avenue   214-706-1162
Dallas, TX 75231-5129   800-242-8721
                                           Fax: 214-696-5211
                                           www.heart.org
Offers food selection hints for fat-controlled meals.

4946 Eat Well, But Wisely
American Heart Association
7272 Greenville Avenue   214-706-1162
Dallas, TX 75231-5129   800-242-8721
                                           Fax: 214-696-5211
                                           www.heart.org
Offers information on good nutrition to reduce the risks of heat attacks.

4947 Exercise and Your Heart
American Heart Association

7272 Greenville Avenue   214-706-1162
Dallas, TX 75231-5129   800-242-8721
Fax: 214-696-5211
www.heart.org

Offers information on how to get enough exercise from daily activities, what the benefits of exercise are and what the risks of exercising are.

4948   Heart Defects
Association of Birth Defect Children
7272 Greenville Avenue   800-242-8721
Dallas, TX 75231-5603   www.heart.org
Informational sheet on the causes, symptoms and statistics of heart defects and heart disease in children.

4949   How to Have Your Cake and Eat It Too
American Heart Association
7272 Greenville Avenue   214-706-1162
Dallas, TX 75231-5129   800-242-8721
Fax: 214-696-5211
www.heart.org

A guide to low-fat, low-cholesterol eating.

Web Sites

4950   American Heart Association
www.heart.org
Supports research, education and community service programs with the objective of reducing premature death and disability from cardiovascular diseases and stroke; coordinates the efforts of health professionals, and other engaged in the fight against heart and circulatory disease.

4951   Healing Well
www.healingwell.com
An online health resource guide to medical news, chat, information and articles, newsgroups and message boards, books, disease-related web sites, medical directories, and more for patients, friends, and family coping with disabling diseases, disorders, or chronic illnesses.

4952   Health Finder
www.healthfinder.gov
Searchable, carefully developed web site offering information on over 1000 topics. Developed by the US Department of Health and Human Services, the site can be used in both English and Spanish.

4953   Healthlink USA
www.healthlinkusa.com
Health information concerning treatment, cures, prevention, diagnosis, risk factors, research, support groups, email lists, personal stories and much more. Updated regularly.

4954   MedicineNet
www.medicinenet.com
An online resource for consumers providing easy-to-read, authoritative medical and health information.

4955   Medscape
www.medscape.com
Medscape offers specialists, primary care physicians, and other health professionals the Web's most robust and integrated medical information and educational tools.

4956   National Heart, Lung and Blood Institute
www.nhlbi.nih.gov
Primary responsibility of this organization is the scientific investigation of heart, blood vessel, lung and blood disorders. Oversees research, demonstration, prevention, education, control and training activities in these fields and emphasizes the prevention and control of heart diseases.

4957   WebMD
www.webmd.com
Provides credible information, supportive communities, and in-depth reference material about health subjects. A source for original and timely health information as well as material from well known content providers.

Description

4958 ## Hemophilia

Hemophilia is an inherited disorder that disrupts the body's normal blood clotting function. There are two main types of hemophilia; hemophilia A, a clotting factor VIII deficiency that accounts for 80 percent of all hemophilia cases, and hemophilia B, a clotting factor IX deficiency and is clinically indistinguishable from hemophilia A. Hemophilia A occurs in about 1 of every 5,000 male births, and about 20,000 Americans are affected with the disorder and, currently, there is no cure.

Hemophilia results from mutations in X chromosome-linked genes. As a result, hemophilia affects males almost exclusively, with females being carriers, whose sons have a 50 percent chance of having the disorder.

Hemophiliacs, like anyone else, will bleed if injured, but they will bleed longer and more profusely. They may also bleed in response to injuries that are inconsequential in other people. For instance, normal daily activities may cause bleeding within a joint, leading to severe pain and swelling, and over time destroying the joint.

The severity of hemophilia varies dramatically depending on the factor VIII and IX levels, thus, affecting a person's prognosis and need for therapy. Treatment is with transfusions of the appropriate clotting factor, and usually has to be repeated frequently. Most hemophiliacs treated with plasma concentrate in the early 1980s are infected with HIV contracted from contaminated blood and transfusions. HIV is now responsible for over half of deaths among hemophiliacs. About 30% of patients with severe hemophilia A who are treated with repeated factor VIII infusions will develop antibodies to factor VIII. In such cases, a recombinant, humanized, bispecific monoclonal antibody called emicizumab is used for hemophilia A patients. Emicizumab binds to clotting factors IX and X and binds them together to form an active complex that allows normal clotting to occur without the need for exogenous factor VIII treatment.

Most hemophiliacs are now treated at comprehensive hemophilia centers, which offer not just factor replacement but multispecialty expertise, sophisticated laboratory testing, physical therapy and psychological support. New techniques allow for identification of carrier females in these families. This is important for genetic counseling and family planning. New gene therapies with adeno-associated virus vectors have been shown to be both safe and effective and may be ready for mass deployment in the near future.

National Agencies & Associations

4959 **American Red Cross Blood Services**
2025 E Street, NW
Washington, DC 20006
202-303-5214
800-733-2767
lkeefe@arlingtonredcross.org
www.redcrossblood.org
Distributes a wide variety of plasma therapeutics to benefit people with hemophilia A and B, immune disorders and hypoalbuminemia.
Bonnie McElveen Hunter, Chairman of the Board
Gail J McGovern, President & CEO

4960 **Baxter Hyland Division**
One Baxter Parkway
Deerfield, IL 60015-1900
224-948-2000
800-422-9837
Fax: 800-568-5020
www.baxter.com
Government affairs office that monitors and selectively lobbies on issues relating to Medicare Medicaid Orphan Drugs and other subjects relating to hemophilia.
Robert L Parkinson, Jr, Chairman of the Board & CEO
David P Scharf, Corporate Vice President and General Cou

4961 **Canadian Hemophilia Society**
301-666 Sherbrooke Street West
Montreal, Quebec, H3A-1E7
514-848-0503
800-668-2686
Fax: 514-848-9661
chs@hemophilia.ca
www.hemophilia.ca
Strives to improve the health and quality of life for all people with inherited bleeding disorders and to find a cure.
Paul Wilton, President
David Page, National Executive Director

4962 **Hemophilia Health Services**
201 Great Circle Road
Nashville, TN 37228
615-352-2500
866-712-5200
Fax: 800-330-0756
www.hemophiliahealth.com
Largest homecare company devoted solely to serving people with bleeding disorders.
Ken Trader, VP of Sales and Marketing

4963 **National Hemophilia Foundation**
7 Penn Plaza
New York, NY 10001
212-328-3700
800-424-2634
Fax: 212-328-3777
info@hemophilia.org
www.hemophilia.org
Dedicated to the treatment and the cure of hemophilia, related bleeding disorders and complications of those disorders or their treatment, including HIV infection, as well as improving the quality of life of all those affected.
Val Bias, CEO
Neil Frick, VP, Research & Medical Information

4964 **National Institute of Diabetes & Digestive & Kidney Diseases**
Office Of Communications and Public Liaison, NIH
31 Center Drive
Bethesda, MD 20892-2560
800-860-8747
TTY: 866-569-1162
healthinfo@niddk.nih.gov
www.niddk.nih.gov
Research areas include diabetes, digestive diseases, endocrine and metabolic diseases, hematologic diseases, kidney disease, liver disease, urologic diseases, as well as matters relating to nutrition and obesity.
Griffin P. Rodgers, MD, MACP, Director
Gregory Germino, MD, Deputy Director

4965 **World Federation of Hemophilia**
1425, boul. Ren,-L,vesque
Montreal, H3G1T-1T7
514-875-7944
Fax: 514-875-8916
wfh@wfh.org
www.wfh.org
An international not-for-profit organization to improving the lives of people with hemophilia and related bleeding disorders.
Alain Baumann, CEO
Antonio Jose Almeida, Director, Programs & Education

State Agencies & Associations

Alabama

4966 Hemophilia and Bleeding Disorders of Alaba ma, Inc.
151 Market Place
Montgomery, AL 36117-1640

334-277-9446
855-469-4232
Fax: 334-272-9167
www.hbda.us/

Brian Ward, Chairman
Vicki Jackson, Executive Director

Arkansas

4967 Hemophilia Foundation of Arkansas
351 Valley Oak Lane
Austin, AR 72007

501-941-3109
888-941-4366
angieclark1315@sbcglobal.net
www.hemophilia.org

Angie Clark, President
John Little, VP

California

4968 Central California Chapter of the National Hemophilia Foundation
PO Box 163689
Sacramento, CA 95816

916-448-0370
Fax: 916-489-1569
cchfsac@yahoo.com
www.cchfsac.org

A very small and family-oriented chapter. Offers an active youth group, an annual summer camp, a men's and women's group and various family activities for persons living in the central California valley from its center in Sacramento to the borders of Nevada.
Sean Hubbert, President
Tracey Huntington, Vice-President

4969 Hemophilia Association of San Diego County
3550 Camino Del Rio North
San Diego, CA 92108

619-325-3570
Fax: 619-325-4350
info@hasdc.org
www.hasdc.org

Provides summer camp programs for young persons with hemophilia, sponsors educational programs for the general public, sponsors support groups for parents to help them deal with hemophilia, monitors legislation pertaining to hemophilia and related conditions.
Mike Brown, Board President
Melissa Pregill, Executive Director

4970 Hemophilia Foundation of Northern California
6400 Hollis Street
Emeryville, CA 94608-3024

510-658-3324
Fax: 510-658-3384
merlin.wedepohl@hemofoundation.org
www.hemofoundation.org

A volunteer, nonprofit organization serving the needs of people with hemophilia and other related bleeding disorders in 35 counties in Northern California. Provides hemophilia literature, scholarships, youth programs and annual summer camps.
Merlin Wedepohl, Executive Director
Nancy Trunzo, Office Manager and Walk Manager

4971 Hemophilia Foundation of Southern California
6720 Melrose Avenue
Hollywood, CA 90038

323-525-0440
800-371-4123
Fax: 323-525-0445
hfsc@hemosocal.org
www.hemosocal.org

Tamara Kato, President
Linda Corrente, Executive Director

Colorado

4972 Colorado Chapter National Hemophilila Foun dation
2465 Sheridan Blvd
Edgewater, CO 80214

720-626-1263
88 - 7 - 02
info@cohemo.org
www.cohemo.org

Amy Board, Executive Director

Florida

4973 Florida Hemophilia Association
915 Middle River Drive
Ft Lauderdale, FL 33304

813-367-0050
888-880-8330
Fax: 813-367-0051
dadamkin@floridahemophilia.org
www.floridahemophilia.org

Barbie Arrebola, President
Debbi Adamkin, Executive Director

Georgia

4974 Hemophilia Foundation of Georgia
8800 Roswelll Road
Atlanta, GA 30350

770-518-8272
Fax: 770-518-3310
mail@hog.org
www.hog.org

Established to help Georgia residents with hemophilia lead normal and productive lives. Because this organization is comprised of patients, their friends and families, it is especially motivated to provide the best in personalized and comprehensive services.
Patricia Dominic, CEO
Andrew Maurer, Chief Governance Officer

Hawaii

4975 Hemophilia Foundation of Hawaii Kapiolani Medical Center
Kapiolani Medical Center
45-1031B. Wailele Road
Kaneohe, HI 96744

808-782-5506
Fax: 808-638-2910
hawaiihemophiliafoundation@hotmail.com
www.hawaiihemo.org/

Cinda Hueu, President
Jennifer Chun, Executive Director

Idaho

4976 Hemophilia Foundation of Idaho
4696 Overland Road
Boise, ID 83705-1622

208-344-4476
866-453-4476
Fax: 208-344-4476
tmagrini@hemophilia.org
www.idahoblood.org/

Shane Bell, President
Taryn Magrini, Executive Director

Illinois

4977 Hemophilia Foundation of Illinois
332 S. Michigan Avenue
Chicago, IL 60604

312-427-1495
Fax: 312-427-1602
brobinson.hfi@mindspring.com

Serves as an information source referral service and advocate for persons with hemophilia and their families. The mission of this chapter is to provide counseling, educational information and support services to persons affected by hemophilia and related disorders.
Mike Toohey, President
Robert P Robinson, Executive Director

Indiana

4978 Hemophilia Foundation of Indiana
5172 E 65th Street
Indianapolis, IN 46220

317-570-0039
800-241-2873
Fax: 317-570-0058
www.hemophiliaofindiana.org

Scott Ehnes, Executive Director
Briana Vieke, Program Director

Kentucky

4979 Kentucky Hemophilia Foundation
1850 Taylor Avenue
Louisville, KY 40213

502-456-3233
800-582-2873
Fax: 502-456-3234
info@kyhemo.org
www.kyhemo.org

Assists individuals with hemophilia and related inherited bleeding disorders through education, advocacy and support services. Services include quarterly newsletter, post secondary education scholarship, summer camp for children, seminars and support functions.
Quarterly
Eric Marcum, President
Ursela Lacer, Executive Director

Louisiana

4980 Louisiana Chapter of the National Hemophilia Foundation
3636 S Sherwood Forest   225-291-1675
Baton Rouge, LA 70816-2285   800-749-1680
                                Fax: 225-291-1679
                                contact@lahemo.org
                                www.lahemo.org/

Lori Keels, Executive Director
Edgar Guedry, President

Maryland

4981 Hemophilia Foundation of Maryland
13 Class Court   410-661-2307
Parkville, MD 21234-2602   800-964-3131
                                Fax: 410-661-2308
                                Miller8043@comcast.net
                                www.hfmonline.org
The Hemophilia foundation of Maryland is a private not for profit organization which devotes its efforts to improving the quality of life for persons affected with bleeding disorders and their complications.
Harvey Gates, President
Emma Miller-Clark, Executive Director

Massachusetts

4982 New England Hemophilia Association
347 Washington Street   781-326-7645
Dedham, MA 02026   Fax: 781-329-5122
                                info@newenglandhemophilia.org
                                www.newenglandhemophilia.org
New England Hemophilia Association is dedicated to improving the quality of life for persons with bleeding disorders (hemophilia, von Willebrands, and other factor deficiencies) and their families through education, support and advocacy.
Patrick Mancini, President
Kevin R Sorge, Executive Director

Michigan

4983 Hemophilia Foundation of Michigan
1921 W Michigan Avenue   734-544-0015
Ypsilanti, MI 48197   800-482-3041
                                Fax: 734-544-0095
                                hfm@hfmich.org
                                www.hfmich.org
Coordinates funding, professional education, and networking, with Hemophilia Treatment Centers in Michigan, Indiana, and Ohio. Provides educational services, including workshops, meetings, symposiums, and numerous publications.
Carrie Reaume, Executive Director
Suzanne Kapica, Regional Coordinator

Minnesota

4984 Hemophilia Foundation of Minnesota and the Dakotas
750 S Plaza Drive   651-406-8655
Mendota Heights, MN 55120   Fax: 651-406-8656
                                hemophiliafound@visi.com
                                www.hfmd.org
A nonprofit organization established to be a leader and a catalyst within the community to enable and inspire members to impact their own lives, with the ultimate aim of cures for both hemophilia and HIV/AIDS.
John Schulte, President/Board of Directors
James Paist, Executive Director

Mississippi

4985 Mississippi Hemophilia Foundation
PO Box 13608   601-957-2706
Jackson, MS 39236   haleyjones80@yahoo.com
                                www.mshemophilia.com/

Haley Jones, President
Leslee Loden, Vice-President

Missouri

4986 Gateway Hemophilia Association
14248 F Manchester Road   314-482-5973
Manchester, MO 63011   877-623-8300
                                Fax: 314-729-7033
                                NicFahey@gatewayhemophilia.org
                                www.gatewayhemophilia.org

Nic Fahey, President
Bridget Tyrey, Executive Director

Nebraska

4987 Nebraska Chapter of the National Hemophilia Foundation
215 Centennial Mall S   402-742-5663
Lincoln, NE 68508   Fax: 402-742-5677
                                office@nebraskanhf.org
The mission of this chapter is to provide support, education, communication and advocacy for men, women and children challenged by Hemophilia. Services provided include a toll free telephone hotline for persons seeking information on HIV and hemophilia.
Jason Everts, President
Kristi Harvey-Simi, Executive Director

Nevada

4988 Hemophilia Foundation of Nevada
7473 W. Lake Mead Blvd.   702-564-4368
Las Vegas, NV 89128   Fax: 702-446-8134
                                www.hfnv.org

Dennis Flynn, President Executive Committee
Kelli Walters, Executive Director

New Mexico

4989 Hemophilia Foundation of New Mexico
PO Box 51494   505-341-9321
Albuquerque, NM 87181   866-341-9321
                                Fax: 505-292-5818
                                www.hemophilia.org

Lori Long, President
Loretta Cordova, Executive Director

New York

4990 Hemophilia Center of Western New York
936 Delaware Ave   716-896-2470
Buffalo, NY 14209   866-434-6551
                                Fax: 716-218-4010
                                info@hemophiliawny.com
                                www.hemophiliawny.com

Robert Long, Chairman
Thomas Long, President

4991 National Hemophilia Foundation: Mary M. Gooley Hemophilia Center
1415 Portland Avenue   585-922-5700
Rochester, NY 14621   Fax: 585-922-5775
                                www.hemocenter.org

Robert Fox, CEO/ President
Linda Magliocco, Senior Vice President

North Carolina

4992 Hemophilia Foundation of North Carolina
260 Town Hall Dr.   919-319-0014
Morrisville, NC 27560   800-990-5557
                                Fax: 919-319-0016
                                info@hemophilia-nc.org
                                www.hemophilia-nc.org

A nonprofit organization that serves as an information source for the hemophilia community of North Carolina. Supply the most up-to-date information concerning hemophilia and hemophilia related HIV/AIDS.
Steven Peretti, PhD, President
Leonard Poe, Vice President & Advocacy Chair

Ohio

4993 Central Ohio Chapter of the National Hemophilia Foundation
200 E. Campus View Blvd
Columbus, OH 43235-0345
614-985-3752
800-847-0345
Fax: 614-985-3601
ralexander@hemophilia.org
www.nhfcentralohio.org
Jeff Stewart, President
Rob Alexander, Executive Director

4994 Northern Ohio Chapter of the National Hemophilia Foundation
One Independence Place
5000 Rockside Road
Independence, OH 44131
216-834-0051
800-554-HEMO
Fax: 216-834-0055
www.nohf.org
Marlene Piatak, President
Janet Tooley, Executive Director

4995 Northwest Ohio Hemophilia Association
2121 Hughes Drive
Toledo, OH 43606
419-291-5882
Fax: 419-479-3269
carla@nwohemophilia.org
www.nwohemophilia.org/
Jim Knepp, President
Carla Wells, Executive Director

4996 Southwestern Ohio Chapter of the National Hemophilia Foundation
3131 S Dixie Drive
Moraine, OH 45439
937-298-8000
Fax: 937-298-8080
info@swohiohemophilia.org
www.swohiohemophilia.org
This chapter serves persons with hemophilia and blood clotting disorders in an 11 county area. It is dedicated to offering people with hemophilia and related blood disorders and their families educational opportunities about the diseases.
Dena Shepard, President
John Gale, Executive Director

Oklahoma

4997 Oklahoma Chapter of the National Hemophilia Foundation
720 W. Wilshire Blvd
Oklahoma City, OK 73116
405-463-6634
800-735-3855
tayers@okhemophilia.org
www.okhemophilia.org
Tom Ayers, President
Bob Goodley, Executive Director

Oregon

4998 Hemophilia Foundation of Oregon
10940 SW Barnes Rd #129
Portland, OR 97225
503-297-7207
Fax: 503-297-0127
info@hemophiliaoregon.org
www.hemophiliaoregon.org/
Jeremy Swanlund, President
Marita Postma, Executive Director

Pennsylvania

4999 Delaware Valley Chapter of the National Hemophilia Foundation
14 E. 6th Street
Lansdale, PA 19446
215-393-3611
Fax: 215-393-9419
hemophilia@navpoint.com
www.hemophiliasupport.org
Thomas Galvin, President
William Widerman, Vice-President

5000 Western Pennsylvania Chapter of the National Hemophilia Foundation
20411 Rt. 19
Cranberry Township, PA 16066
724-741-6160
800-824-0016
Fax: 724-741-6167
info@westpennhemophilia.org
www.westpennhemophilia.org
Brings together and serves as a focal point for those segments of the community most concerned with hemophilia. They include medical and social service providers, people with hemophilia and their families educators and the general public.
Scott E Miller, President
Nathan Rost, Vice-President

Rhode Island

5001 Rhode Island Hemophilia Foundation
347 Washington Street
Dedham, MA 02026
781-326-7645
Fax: 781-329-5122
info@newenglandhemophilia.org
www.newenglandhemophilia.org
Patrick Mancini, President
Kevin R Sorge, Executive Director

South Carolina

5002 Hemophilia Association of South Carolina
PO Box 3874
Sumter, SC 29151
864-350-9941
888-829-4849
www.hemophiliaofsouthcarolina.net/
Sue Martin, President

Tennessee

5003 Tennessee Hemophilia & Bleeding Disorder Foundation
1819 Ward Drive
Murfreesboro, TN 37129-5281
615-900-1486
888-703-3269
Fax: 615-900-1487
mary@thbdf.org
www.thbdf.org
Offers a hemophilia clinic, social workers and consultants, a state hemophilia program, blood donor programs, counseling programs, genetic counseling, literature and resources, summer camp, grants, and more for the hemophilia and HIV/AIDS community.
Kent Russ, President
Mary Hord, Executive Director

Texas

5004 Lone Star Chapter of the National Hemophilia Foundation
10500 NW Freeway
Houston, TX 77092
713-686-6100
888-LSC-NHF1
Fax: 832-383-4601
Debbiedelariva@yahoo.com
www.lonestarhemophilia.org
Nick Zasowski, President

5005 Texas Central Chapter of the National Hemophilia Foundation
12700 Hillcrest Road
Dallas, TX 75230
972-386-3865
Fax: 214-654-9954
mail@texcen.org
www.texcen.org
A group of volunteers seeking solutions to the various aspects of the hemophilia problem. Supports blood drives sponsors a summer camp for hemophiliac children, conducts educational member meetings, arranges for genetic counseling and sponsors group support meetings.
Shannon Brush, President
Brendan Hayes, Executive Director

Utah

5006 Utah Chapter of the National Hemophilia Foundation
772 E 3300 S
Salt Lake City, UT 84106
801-484-0325
877-463-6893
Fax: 801-746-2488
www.hemophiliautah.org

Offers educational information, pamphlets, fundraising events and more for persons and families affected by hemophilia.
Reg Ecker, President
Scott Muir, Executive Director

Virginia

5007 **Hemophilia Association of the Capital Area**
10560 Main Street 703-352-7641
Fairfax, VA 22030-1504 Fax: 540-427-6589
admin@HACAcares.org
www.hacacares.org
A nonprofit organization serving persons with bleeding disorders and their families in northern Virginia Washington DC and Montgomery and Prince George's Counties in Maryland. This chapter's mission is to improve the quality of life for persons with hemophilia.
Miriam Goldstein, President
Karen Krzmarzick, Executive Director

5008 **United Virginia Chapter of the National Hemophilia Foundation**
PO Box 188 804-748-7896
Midlothian, VA 23113-8824 800-266-8438
Fax: 800-266-8438
info@vahemophilia.org
www.vahemophilia.org

Kelly Waters, Executive Director
Heather Conner, Administrative Assistant

Washington

5009 **Bleeding Disorder Foundation of Washington**
9639 Firdale Avenue 206-533-1660
Edmonds, WA 98020 Fax: 206-533-1686
general@bdfwa.org
www.bdfwa.org
Caprice Sauter, President
Stephanie Simpson, Executive Director

5010 **Inland Empire Bleeding Disorders**
1010 Riverside Drive 509-967-7417
W Richland, WA 99353 866-710-4323
iebd4u@verizon.net
www.hemophilia.org
Debbie Campeau, President
Jill McCary, President

Wisconsin

5011 **Great Lakes Hemophilia Foundation**
638 N 18th Street 414-257-0200
Milwaukee, WI 53233 888-797-GLHF
Fax: 414-257-1225
info@glhf.org
www.glhf.org
The only Wisconsin organization that addresses the physical, emotional social and financial needs of individuals affected by hemophilia. This chapter supports high-quality cost-effective programs for patient care, education, research and public awareness.
Bill Finn, President
Danielle Leitner Baxter, Executive Director

Foundations

5012 **National Hemophilia Foundation**
7 Penn Plaza 212-328-3700
New York, NY 10001 800-424-2634
Fax: 212-328-3777
info@hemophilia.org
www.hemophilia.org
The National Hemophilia Foundation is dedicated to finding better treatments and cures for bleeding and clotting disorders and to preventing the complications of these disorders through education, advocacy and research.
Val Bias, CEO
Neil Frick, VP, Research & Medical Information

Research Centers

5013 **Albany Medican Center**
43 New Scotland Avenue 518-262-3125
Albany, NY 12208-3479 800-773-7080
Fax: 518-262-6320
albanyhtc@mail.amc.edu
www.amc.edu
Providing excellence in medical education biomedical research and patient care.
Joanne Faunce, President

5014 **Albert Einstein Medical Center Hemophilia Program**
5501 Old York Road 215-456-7890
Philadelphia, PA 19141 Fax: 215-456-6179
www.einstein.edu
With humanity humility and honor to heal by providing exceptionally intelligent and responsive healthcare and education for as many as we can reach
Barry R Freedman, CEO/ President
John Finger, Chief Administrative Officer

5015 **American Red Cross Hemophilia Center**
2025 E Street, NW 202-303-5214
Washington, DC 20006-0905 800-733-2767
Fax: 608-233-8318
www.redcross.org
Greg Mandell, CEO
Sandra Fenwick, President

5016 **Boston Hemophilia Center Fegan 5 Children's Hospital**
Fegan 5 Children's Hospital
300 Longwood Avenue 617-355-6000
Boston, MA 02115 800-355-7944
Fax: 617-730-0152
TTY: 617-730-0152
www.childrenshospital.org
The program offers comprehensive care to people with hemophilia and their families. Our services range from medical treatment counseling and support to discounts on clotting-factor replacement and other products that people with hemophilia require.
Dr James Mandell, CEO
Sandra Fenwick, President

5017 **Bowman Grey School of Medicine: Hemophilia Diagnostic Center**
Wake Forest University
Department of Pediatrics 919-716-4324
Winston Salem, NC 27157-0001 Fax: 910-716-7100
Christine A MD, Director
Michael Fisher, CEO

5018 **Children's Hospital Hemophilia Treatment Center**
3333 Burnet Avenue 513-636-4200
Cincinnati, OH 45229 800-344-2462
Fax: 513-636-5599
TTY: 513-636-4900
www.cincinnatichildrens.org
Cincinnati Children's will improve child health and transform delivery of care through fully integrated globally recognized research education and innovation.
Ralph Gruppo Cohen MD, Medical Director

5019 **Childrens Hospital of Philadelphia Hemophilia Program**
Division of Hematology
34th Street and Civic Center Boulev 215-590-3437
Philadelphia, PA 19104 800-879-2467
Fax: 215-903-92
www.chop.edu
The Children's Hospital of Philadelphia the oldest hospital in the United States dedicated exclusively to pediatrics strives to be the world leader in the advancement of healthcare for children by integrating excellent patient care innovative research and quality professional education into all of its programs.
Leslie J Raffini, Physician
Char Witmer, Physician

5020 **Christus Santa Rosa Health System**
Children's Hospital

333 N Santa Rosa Street
San Antonio, TX 78207-3108
210-704-2011
877-ALL-KIDZ
Fax: 210-704-2396
www.christussantarosa.org

Patrick Carrier, Presindent, CEO

5021 Comprehensive Hemophilia Diagnostic and Treatment Center
University of North Carolina
101 Manning Drive
Chapel Hill, NC 27514
919-966-4131
Fax: 919-966-3036
lccc@med.unc.edu
www.unchealthcare.org
Multidisciplinary clinics are dedicated to patients with hemophilia (through the Comprehensive Hemophilia Diagnostic and Treatment Center) sickle cell disease brain tumors late effects of anticancer therapy as well as general hematology/oncology.
William RN

5022 Comprehensive Pediatric Hemophilia Center University of South Florida
University of South Florida
450 W Drive
Tampa, FL 33612-4742
813-974-2201
Sara Griggs Kirschke

5023 Eastern Michigan Hemophilia Center St. Joseph Hospital
St. Joseph Hospital
302 Kensington Avenue
Flint, MI 48503-2044
810-762-8656
Leslie RN

5024 Eau Claire Hemophilia Center
900 W Clairemont Avenue
Eau Claire, WI 54701
715-839-4418
Fax: 715-833-4976
Vicky Anders RN, Program Manager

5025 Fairview-University Hemophilia & Thrombosis Center
Harvard Street at E River Road
Minneapolis, MN 55455
612-626-6455
800-688-5252
Fax: 612-625-4955
Serves over 700 adults and children in Minnesota with inherited bleeding disorders. Offers access to current technologies and treatments. Special programs include patient support group family retreats and camps.
Linda Swanso Macfarlane, Director

5026 Great Plains Regional Hemophilia Center University of Iowa Hospitals
University of Iowa Hospitals
200 Howkins Drive
Iowa City, IA 52242
319-384-8442
800-777-8442
Fax: 319-567-59
www.uiowa.edu

Donald E Fahner MD

5027 Greater Grand Rapids Pediatric Hemophilia Program
DeVos at Spectrum Health Systems
100 Michigan NE
Grand Rapids, MI 49503
616-391-2033
James B Trujillo, Financial Administer
W Hoots, Medical Director

5028 Gulf States Hemophilia Diagnostic and Treatment Center
University of Texas Health Science Center Houston
6655 Travis Street
Houston, TX 77030-3005
713-500-8360
800-464-1440
Fax: 713-500-8364
www.livingwithhaemophilia.com
Marisela Thompson, Chief Executive Officer
Joan Curran, Chief Government Relations and External

5029 Gundersen Clinic Comprehensive Hemophilia Treatment Center
Gundersen Clinic
1900 S Avenue
LaCrosse, WI 54601
608-782-7300
800-362-9567
Fax: 608-775-6692
www.gundersenhealth.org/
Jeffrey E Thompson, Chief Executive Officer
Julio Bird, Executive Vice President

5030 Hematology Treatment Center of the Great Lakes Hemophilia Foundation
638 North 18th Street
Milwaukee, WI 53233-2178
414-257-0200
888-797-GLHF
Fax: 414-257-1225
info@glhf.org
www.glhf.org
Bill Finn, President
Danielle Leitner Baxter, Executive Director

5031 Hemophilia Association of the Huntington Area
Marshall University School of Medicine
1600 Medical Center Drive
Huntington, WV 25703-1518
304-691-1384
877-691-1600
Fax: 304-691-1375
McKowen, Dean, Vice President
Andrew Tendleton, Medical Director

5032 Hemophilia Center of Central Pennsylvania Penn State Milton S Hershey Medical Cent
Penn State Milton S Hershey Medical Center
500 University Drive
Hershey, PA 17033
717-531-8521
800-243-1455
Fax: 717-310-4021
TTY: 717-531-4395
www.pennstatehershey.org/
Harold L Paz, Chief Executive Officer
Alan L Brechbill, Executive Director

5033 Hemophilia Center of Rhode Island Rhode Island Hospital
Rhode Island Hospital
593 Eddy Street
Providence, RI 02903
401-444-5184
Fax: 401-444-5017
www.rirad.org
Brian Stainken, President
Terrance Healey, Vice-President

5034 Hemophilia Center of West Virginia University Health Sciences Center
University Health Sciences Center
Medical Center Drive
Morgantown, WV 26506
304-293-4229
Fax: 304-293-3793
John S Holmberg, Executive Director
Thomas Long, President

5035 Hemophilia Center of Western New York Erie County Medical Center
Erie County Medical Center
936 Delaware Ave
Buffalo, NY 14209-3021
716-896-2470
866-434-6551
Fax: 716-218-4010
www.hemophiliawny.com
The center provides a variety of services to the hemophilia and HIV/AIDS community. Included among these services are diagnostics registration outpatient treatment home care programs home visits school visits dental services and counseling services. Offers an adult unit and a pediatric unit.
Robert Long, Chairman
Thomas Long, President

5036 Hemophilia Center of the Huntington Hospital
100 W California Boulevard
Pasadena, CA 91105-3023
626-397-5000
www.huntingtonhospital.com
At Huntington our mission is to excel at the delivery of health care to our community.
Stephen Ralph, President and Chief Executive Officer
Jim Noble, Executive Vice President, COO and CFO

5037 Hemophilia Clinic: Childrens' Rehabilitation Service
1870 Pleasant Avenue
Mobile, AL 36617
334-479-8617
800-879-8163
Fax: 334-450-5037
www.hemophilia.org
Dianna Jackson

5038 Hemophilia Treatment Center at Children's National Medical Center
Department of Hematology/Oncology

111 Michigan Avenue NW
Washington, DC 20010
202-884-3622
Fax: 202-884-2976
www.livingwithhaemophilia.com

Gordon L Cowen, President

5039   Los Angeles Orthopaedic Hospital
2400 S Flower Street
Los Angeles, CA 90007-2629
213-742-1000
Fax: 213-742-1103
www.orthohospital.org

Anthony A Scaduto, M.D, Presindent, CEO

5040   Louisiana Comprehensive Hemophilia Care Center
1430 Tulane Avenue
New Orleans, LA 70112-2699
504-988-5433
Fax: 504-883-08
cleissi@tulane.edu
tulane.edu

Cindy Leissinger, MD, Chief

5041   Maine Hemophilia Treatment Center
19 Bramhall Street
Portland, ME 04102
207-885-7683
Fax: 207-885-7565
Nancy Roy Langstraat, Director

5042   Mayo Comprehensive Hemophilia Center Mayo Clinic
Mayo Clinic
200 1st Street SW
Rochester, MN 55905
507-284-2511
800-660-4582
Fax: 507-284-8286
www.mayoclinic.org/hemophilia/

A World Federation of Hemophilia-designated International Hemophilia Training Center provides multidisciplinary assessment and care of persons with bleeding disorders. Offers consultation with hemotologists specializing in the care of pediatric and adult patients a special consultation laboratory testing center and more.
Harlan ARNP

5043   Miami Comprehensive Hemophilia Center Jackson Medical Towers
Jackson Medical Towers
1500 NW
Miami, FL 33136-3609
305-243-4791
Fax: 305-324-9785
Susan Schmal MD, Head Physician

5044   Michigan State University Hemophilia Comprehensive Care Clinic
Michigan State University
2900 Hannah Boulevard
E Lansing, MI 48823
517-353-9385
800-759-5595
Fax: 517-353-9421

John Penner Gioia RN

5045   Missouri Illinois Regional Hemophilia Comprehensive Treatment Center
3635 Vista Avenue & Grand Boulevard
Saint Louis, MO 63104-1003
314-268-5275
Fax: 314-268-5104
Kathleen P Crist MD, Vice President

5046   Mountain State Regional Hemophilia Center
University of Arizona Health Sciences Center
1501 N Campbell Avenue
Tucson, AZ 85724-0001
520-626-1197
Fax: 520-626-1460
phanthourath@ahsc.arizona.edu
www.ahsc.arizona.edu

Anoma Phanthourath, Deputy & Chief of Staff

5047   Nadeene Brunini Comprehensive Hemophilia Care Center
St Michael s Medical Center
197 Route 18 South
East Brunswick, NJ 08816-2011
732-249-6000
Fax: 732-249-7999
hemnj@comcast.net
www.hanj.org

Hemophilia and other bleeding disorder treatment center.
Louis

5048   North Dakota Comprehensive Hemophilia Center
Roger Maris Cancer Center
820 4th Street N
Fargo, ND 58122-0001
701-234-7544
800-437-4010
Fax: 701-234-7592

A treatment center for diseases of hemotosis and thrombosis which includes a clinical research program in bleeding disorders. Hemotologists are available for consultation 24 hours a day.

5049   North Dakota Hemostasis and Thrombosis Treatment Center
Roger Maris Cancer Center
820 4th Street N
Fargo, ND 58122-0001
701-234-7544
800-437-4010
Fax: 701-234-7577
www.meritcare.com

A treatment center for diseases of hemotosis and thrombosis which includes a clinical research program in bleeding disorders. Hemotologists are available for consultation 24 hours a day.
Dr Nathan Podolsky MD, President

5050   North Texas Comprehensive Pediatric Hemophilia Center
1935 Motor Street
Dallas, TX 75235-7701
214-456-2382
Fax: 214-456-6133
Andrea Johns Steele, President
Ann Gilbert, Director

5051   Northwest Ohio Hemophilia Treatment Center
The Toledo Hospital
2142 N Cove Boulevard
Toledo, OH 43606-3895
419-471-2291
Fax: 412-916-01

5052   Oklahoma Comprehensive Hemophilia Diagnostic Treatment Center
940 NE 13th Street
Oklahoma City, OK 73126-0307
405-271-3661
800-688-5288
Fax: 405-271-3756

Beverly Stev Kasper, Hematology
Richard W Cook, Chairman, CEO

5053   Puget Sound Blood Center
921 Terry Avenue
Seattle, WA 98104-1256
206-292-6500
800-398-7888
schedule@psbc.org
www.psbc.org

Dr. James P AuBuchon, President, CEO
David C Fennell, Chief Operating Officer and Chief Inform

5054   Regional Hemophilia Treatment Center Children's Hospital of Michigan
Children's Hospital of Michigan
1921 W. Michigan Avenue
Ypsilanti, MI 48197-2196
734-544-0015
800-482-3041
Fax: 734-544-0095
www.hfmich.org

Carrie Reaume, Executive Director
Suzanne Kapica, Regional Coordinator

5055   Richland Memorial Comprehensive Pediatric Hemophilia Center
Children's Hospital for Cancer & Blood Disorders
7 Richland Medical Park Drive
Columbia, SC 29203
803-434-3533
Fax: 803-434-4598
Daniel Fink, Chief Executive Officer & President

5056   Riley Hemophilia & Hemophilia Center Riley Hospital for Children
Riley Hospital for Children
705 Riley Hospital Drive
Indianapolis, IN 46202-5200
317-944-5000
800-248-1199
Fax: 317-278-0616

Jeff Sperring, MD, Presindent, CEO
Paul R Haut, MD, Chief Medical Officer

5057   SouthWestern Medical Center
University of Texas Southwestern Medical Center
5323 Harry Hines Boulevard
Dallas, TX 75390-7208
214-648-3111
www.utsouthwestern.edu
Daniel K Podolsky, MD, President
J. Gregory Fitz, MD, Executive Vice-President

5058   Southern Tier Hemophilia Center United Health Services-Wilson Hospital
United Health Services-Wilson Hospital
33-57 Harrison Street
Johnson City, NY 13790
607-763-6436
Fax: 607-763-5514
Doris Michal RN

5059 St. Joseph's Hemophilia Center
2927 N 7th Avenue
Phoenix, AZ 85013-4102   602-406-3770
Rachel Stuar MD, Director

5060 Ted R Montoya Hemophilia Program University of New Mexico
University of New Mexico
Albuquerque, NM 87131-0001   505-277-0111
                                          800-225-5866
                                          Fax: 505-272-6845
                                          www.unm.edu
Prasad Mathe Barchi, President

5061 Tennessee Hemophilia and Bleeding Disorder Foundation
1819 Ward Drive   615-900-1486
Murfreesboro, TN 37129   888-703-3269
                                          Fax: 615-900-1487
                                          mary@thbdf.org
                                          www.thbdf.org
Kent Russ, President
Mary Hord, Executive Director

5062 The Vanderbilt Hemostasis Clinic
2200 Children's Way   615-936-1765
Nashville, TN 37232-9830   866-372-5663
                                          Fax: 615-936-8400
                                          www.mc.vanderbilt.edu/vhtc
The mission of the Vanderbilt Hemostasis-Thrombosis Clinic is to provide the highest quality compassionate care for individuals with inherited disorders of bleeding or clotting. The team emphasizes the empowerment of patients in their own care while also providing opportunities to participate in scientific advances in the diagnosis and treatment of bleeding and clotting disorders.
Anne T Neff, Director of Hemostasis Clinic
Mary G Hudson, Nurse Coordinator

5063 Thomas Jefferson University: Cardenza Foundation for Hematologic Research
1020 Walnut Street   215-955-6000
Philadelphia, PA 19107-5005   Fax: 215-955-2342
                                          www.jefferson.edu
Robert L Abildgaard MD

5064 Tufts Medical Center
Tufts New England Medical Center
800 Washington Street   617-636-5000
Boston, MA 02111-1526   Fax: 617-636-7738
                                          www.tuftsmedicalcenter.org
Comprehensive care for pediatric and young adult individuals with bleeding and prothrombotic disorders.
Eric Beyer, President and Chief Executive Officer
Michael Wagner, Chief Medical Officer

5065 UCD Northern Central California Hemophilia Program
PO Box 163689   916-448-0370
Sacramento, CA 95816-2208   Fax: 916-489-1569
                                          cchfsac@yahoo.com
                                          www.cchfsac.org
An all-volunteer nonprofit organization dedicated to helping people with bleeding disorders.
Sean Hubbert, President
Tracey Huntington, Vice President

5066 UCSD Comprehensive Hemophilia Treatment Center
9500 Gilman Drive   619-471-0336
La Jolla, CA 92093   Fax: 858-822-6444
                                          kdherbst@ucsd.edu
                                          hem-onc.ucsd.edu
Sanford J Shattil, M.D., Professor of Medicine
Edward Ball, MD, Professor of Medicine

5067 University Medical Center Hemophilia Program
1800 W Charleston Boulevard   702-383-2000
Las Vegas, NV 89102-2329   www.umcsn.com
Lawrence Weekly, Chair
Chris Giunchigliani, Vice Chair

5068 University Treatment Center of University Hospitals of Cleveland
11100 Euclid Avenue   216-844-8447
Cleveland, OH 44106   888-844-8447
                                          Fax: 216-844-5431
                                          www.uhhospitals.org
Thomas F Zenty III, CEO

5069 University of Cincinnati Adult Hemophilia Treatment Program
231 Bethesda Avenue   513-558-4233
Cincinnati, OH 45267-0001   Fax: 513-558-3878
Kathleen E Coleman, President

5070 University of Michigan Hemophilia Center
1500 E Medical Center Drive   734-764-1817
Ann Arbor, MI 48109   Fax: 734-635-15
                                          www.umich.edu
Mary Sue Hord, Executive Director

5071 Vermont Regional Hemophilia Center
108 Cherry Street   802-863-7200
Burlington, VT 05402   800-464-4343
                                          Fax: 802-865-7754
                                          vtadap@vdh.state.vt.us
                                          healthvermont.gov
Provides care to persons with types of bleeding disorders. We see people from Vermont and upstate New York.
Miriam Huste Kinsaul, President, CEO
Emmett Broxson, Director Hemothology

5072 West Central Ohio Hemophilia Center Childens Medical Center
Childens Medical Center
1 Childrens Plaza   937-641-3000
Dayton, OH 45404-1815   800-228-4055
                                          Fax: 937-641-5878
                                          www.childrensdayton.org
The center provides complete care for individuals and families with hemophilia and related bleeding disorders. Some of the services offered include a comprehensive clinic emergency treatment network consultations diagnostic coagulation laboratory home infusion programs HIV/AIDS education and counseling and more.
Elizabeth H Ey, Chair
Deborah Feldman, President/ CEO

Support Groups & Hotlines

5073 National Health Information Center
Office of Disease Prevention & Health Promotion
1101 Wootton Pkwy   Fax: 240-453-8281
Rockville, MD 20852   odphpinfo@hhs.gov
                                          www.health.gov/nhic
Supports public health education by maintaining a calendar of National Health Observances; helps connect consumers and health professionals to organizations that can best answer questions and provide up-to-date contact information from reliable sources; updates on a yearly basis toll-free numbers for health information, Federal health clearinghouses and info centers.
Don Wright, MD, MPH, Director

Books

5074 Avoiding Indecision and Hesitation with Hemophilia-Related Emergencies
American Health Consultants
7 Penn Plaza   212-328-3700
New York, NY 10001   800-688-2421
                                          Fax: 212-328-3777
                                          http://www.hemophilia.org
Provides detailed information necessary for physicians, and ED staff to deal effectively and expeditiously with hemophilia emergencies.
12 pages
Neil Frick, VP for Research
John Indence, VP for Marketing & Communications

5075 Federal Medicaid Drug Program
1730 E Street NW   202-628-9292
Washington, DC 20006-5300

Discusses changes in government reimbursement and its effect on plasma derived products distributed by the American Red Cross. Includes law information, individual state billing procedures and Medicaid program coverage for the hemophilia community.

5076   Guide to Insurance Coverage for People with Hemophilia
Armour Pharmaceutical Company
820 First Street NE   202-675-6984
Washington, DC 20002-3930   800-230-9797
                                     Fax: 972-616-6211
                                   www.hemophiliafed.org
An educational guide designed to assist with health insurance concerns.
Tracy Cleghorn, President
Scott Boling, Co-Vice President

5077   Hemophilia Camp Directory
National Hemophilia Foundation
116 W 32nd Street   212-219-8180
New York, NY 10001-3212   800-424-2634
                                     Fax: 212-328-3777
                                     www.hemophilia.org
Lists camps in the United States for children with hemophilia and other coagulation disorders.
16 pages

5078   Procedure Coding for Hemophilia Treatment
Armour Pharmaceutical Company
820 First Street NE   202-675-6984
Washington, DC 20002-3930   800-230-9797
                                     Fax: 972-616-6211
                                   www.hemophiliafed.org
Educational guide designed to facilitate the appropriate use of CPT codes for the hemophilia community.
Tracy Cleghorn, President
Scott Boling, Co-Vice President

Children's Books

5079   Adventures of Maxx
Nova Factor
1620 Century Centery Pkwy   901-348-8129
Memphis, TN 38137   800-424-2634
                                     Fax: 901-385-3778
                                     legendofmaxx.com
An activity book for children with hemophilia, this publication is intended to be both educational and entertaining.
15 pages

5080   Children's Hemophilia Book
Porton Products Limited
37-39 West Main St.   978-352-7657
Georgetown, MA 01833-2006   Fax: 978-352-6254
                                    info@kelleycom.com
                                    www.kelleycom.com
Coloring book that discusses what hemophilia is, bleeding episodes and treatment from a child's point of view.
25 pages

5081   Harold Talks About How He Inherited Hemophilia
Kentucky Hemophilia Foundation
1850 Taylor Avenue   502-456-3233
Louisville, KY 40213-1571   800-582-2873
                                     Fax: 502-634-9995
                                      info@kyhemo.org
                                      www.kyhemo.org
Children's brochure explaining hemophilia causes, symptoms and living a regular life.

5082   Harold's Secret: A Boy with Hemophilia
Bayer
400 Morgan Lane   203-937-2765
West Haven, CT 06516-4175
A comic book for youngsters pertaining to children with hemophilia and understanding of the illness among school friends.
16 pages

5083   Understanding Hemophilia: A Young Person's Guide
Armour Pharmaceuticals Company

820 First Street NE   202-675-6984
Washington, DC 20002-3930   800-230-9797
                                     Fax: 972-616-6211
                                   www.hemophiliafed.org
This publication is designed for young persons with hemophilia. Presented in very basic and accessible language, this text with colored illustrations points out what hemophilia is, how to cope and more.
91 pages

Magazines

5084   HEMALOG
Maleria Medica
101 W 23rd Street   212-725-5151
New York, NY 10011-2490   Fax: 212-725-2794
                                   hemalog@hotmail.com
                                     www.humalog.com
The purpose of Hemalog is to serve as a national forum for the hemophilia community, providing current news, information, opinion and contact with others in the community. The material contained in this journal reflects the experience and opinion of a wide range of people connected with hemophilia and encourages story and art contributions.
36 pages Quarterly

5085   HemAware
National Hemophilia Foundation
7 Penn Plaza   212-328-3700
New York, NY 10001-3212   800-424-2634
                                     Fax: 212-328-3777
                                     www.hemophilia.org
NHF magazine that offers treatment news about bleeding disorders and provides comprehensive articles on the latest developments in treatment and research as well as highlighting new programs and new resources in the field.
Bi-Monthly
Neil Frick, VP for Research
John Indence, VP for Marketing & Communications

5086   Human Factor
Hemophilia Health Services
410 West Lowe   641-472-4480
Fairfield, IA 52556-4206   800-800-6606
                                     Fax: 641-472-5412
                                    hfi@humanfactors.com
                                    www.humanfactors.com
This journal is provided as a free service for the purpose of informing, educating and empowering the hemophilia community.
Quarterly
Eric Schaffer, CEO
Jay More, Global President

Newsletters

5087   Artery
Hemophilia Foundation of Michigan
1921 W. Michigan Avenue   734-544-0015
Ypsilanti, MI 48197-2973   800-482-3041
                                     Fax: 734-544-0095
                                       www.hfmich.org
Offers information on the chapter's activities and events, support groups and hotlines, technical and medical updates pertaining to the hemophilia and HIV/AIDS community.
Quarterly

5088   Big Red Factor
National Hemophilia Foundation: Nebraska
215 Centennial Mall South   402-742-5663
Lincoln, NE 68508   Fax: 402-742-5677
                                 www.nebraskanhf.org/chapter/
Chapter newsletter offering legislative and medical updates, technology, resources, assistive devices and more for persons affected by hemophilia and other blood disorders.

5089   Bloodlines
Hemophilia Association of San Diego County

3550 Camino del Rio North 619-325-3570
San Diego, CA 92108 Fax: 619-325-4350
info@hasdc.org
www.hasdc.org

Updates membership on the newest techniques and technologies on the treatment of hemophilia.
Quarterly

5090 Concentrate
Hemophilia of North Carolina
2 Centerview Drive 919-852-4788
Greensboro, NC 27407-3708

Offers information on summer camps, resources, book reviews, parent information and articles pertaining to hemophilia.
Monthly

5091 Factor Nine News
Coalition for Hemophilia B
225 W 34th Street 212-628-3445
New York, NY 10122 Fax: 212-554-6906
cfb@web-depot.com

Offers information on FDA approvals, annual meetings and the latest in technology and information regarding hemophilia.

5092 Hemophilia NewsBriefs
Great Lakes Hemophilia Foundation
638 North 18th Street 414-257-0200
Milwaukee, WI 53233 Fax: 414-257-1225
info@glhf.org
www.glhf.org

Bill Finn, President
Jeff Koopmeiners, Vice President

5093 Infusion
Kentuckian Hemophilia Foundation
982 Eastern Parkway 510-634-8161
Louisville, KY 40217-1571 800-582-CURE
Fax: 510-568-6111
www.hfnconline.org

Offers information on summer camps, association activities and events, national projects touching on hemophilia and HIV related disorders and articles on the newest breakthroughs and technology for fighting bleeding disorders.
Quarterly

5094 Initiatives
Quantum Health Resources
790 The City Drive S 714-750-1610
Orange, CA 92868-4941

Aimed at keeping patients and other interested individuals informed on important economic trends, legislation and medical issues.
Quarterly

5095 Linking Factor
National Hemophila Foundation: Utah Chapter
340 E 400 S 800-800-6606
Salt Lake City, UT 84111-2909

A newsletter offering chapter association news and information.
BiMonthly

5096 New England Hemophilia Association Newsletter
347 Washington St. 781-326-7645
Dedham, MA 02026-4558 800-228-6342
Fax: 781-329-5122
info@newenglandhemophilia.org
www.newenglandhemophilia.org

New England Hemophilia Association is dedicated to improving the quality of life for persons with bleeding disorders (hemophilia, von Williebrands, and other factor deficiencies) and their families through education, support and advocacy. NEHA is a chapter of the National Hemophilia Foundation.
Quarterly
Patrick Mancini, President
William McCartney, Treasurer

5097 TN Hemo & Bleeding Disorders Foundation Newsletter
TN Hemo & Bleedin Disorders Foundation

1819 Ward Drive 615-220-4868
Murfreesboro, TN 37129-5281 888-703-3269
Fax: 615-220-4889
www.thbdf.org

3x/year
Suzie Harlan, President
Chris Cassada, Vice President

5098 Ways & Means
Quantum Health Resources
790 The City Drive S 714-750-1610
Orange, CA 92868-4941

Features pertinent health care information for hemophilia patients and their families.
Quarterly

5099 Infusion
Northern California Chapter of the NHF
7700 Edgewater Drive 650-568-NCHF
Oakland, CA 94621-3023

Informs members of medical, dental and orthopedic treatment advances and the latest research in the field. Helps to keep people with hemophilia and their families aware of relevant local and national meetings and includes important updates regarding research and treatment.
BiMonthly
Alim Somani, President
John Michell, Chief Operating Officer

Pamphlets

5100 Anyone Can Have a Bleeding Problem
Hemophilia Foundation of Michigan
411 Huronview Boulevard 734-761-2535
Ann Arbor, MI 48103-2973 800-482-3041

Offers information on Hemophilia and Von Willebrand's Disease. How persons can get it, prevention and causes of the illnesses.

5101 Article Reprint Exchange
HANDI-The National Hemophilia Foundation
7 Penn Plaza 212-328-3700
New York, NY 10001-3212 800-424-2634
Fax: 212-328-3777
www.hemophilia.org

Offers various reprinted articles concerning hemophilia and the newest medical technology.
Neil Frick, VP for Research
John Indence, VP for Marketing & Communications

5102 Basics of HIV Disease: Questions and Answers
National Hemophilia Foundation
7 Penn Plaza 212-328-3700
New York, NY 10001-3212 800-424-2634
Fax: 212-328-3777
www.hemophilia.org

This publication contains basic information about hemophilia and HIV disease.
1992 28 pages
Neil Frick, VP for Research
John Indence, VP for Marketing & Communications

5103 Clotting Agents Are Lifesavers
Hemophilia Foundation of Michigan
411 Huronview Boulevard 734-761-2535
Ann Arbor, MI 48103-2973

Offers information on what hemophilia is, treatments, occurances, heredity, Von Willebrand's Disease, patient services and direct services for hemophiliacs and HIV/AIDS patients.

5104 Comprehensive Care
National Hemophilia Foundation
7 Penn Plaza 212-328-3700
New York, NY 10001-3212 800-424-2634
Fax: 212-328-3777
www.hemophilia.org

Discusses the nature of comprehensive care and its functions and defines the care team. Also touches upon essential resources, HIV, and the benefits of comprehensive care.
1991 12 pages
Neil Frick, VP for Research
John Indence, VP for Marketing & Communications

5105 Comprehensive Services for Persons with Hemophilia
Hemophilia Foundation of Minnesota/Dakotas
7 Penn Plaza   212-328-3700
New York, NY 10001-3712   Fax: 212-328-3777
                                                                    www.hemophilia.org
Offers information on what hemophilia is and information and resources for persons with hemophilia and other bleeding disorders.
Neil Frick, VP for Research
John Indence, VP for Marketing & Communications

5106 Consumer Bill of Rights and Responsibilities for Healthcare Service
National Hemophilia Foundation
7 Penn Plaza   212-328-3700
New York, NY 10001-3212   800-424-2634
                                                               Fax: 212-328-3777
                                                                    www.hemophilia.org
Serves as a set of goals for both the provider and consumer in seeking, providing, and receiving high quality health care within a setting of honesty and respect.
1994
Neil Frick, VP for Research
John Indence, VP for Marketing & Communications

5107 Countdown to a Cure
Louisiana Hemophilia Foundation
3636 S Sherwood Forest   225-291-1675
Baton Rouge, LA 70816-2285   Fax: 225-291-1679
                                                          lahemophilia@hipoint.net
                                                     www.louisianahemophilia.org/
Offers information on chapter resources and services for hemophiliacs and their families. Offers information and services to families/patients affected by bleeding disorders.

5108 Fight Hemophilia with Facts Not Fiction
Great Lakes Hemophilia Foundation
638 North 18th Street   414-257-0200
Milwaukee, WI 53233   Fax: 414-257-1225
                                                                    www.glhf.org
Offers information on what hemophilia is, research information and treatments.

5109 Get Real and Be Safe!
National Hemophilia Foundation
7 Penn Plaza   212-328-3700
New York, NY 10001-3212   800-424-2634
                                                               Fax: 212-328-3777
                                                                    www.hemophilia.org
Comic book style, this pamphlet offers information to young adults on the hazards and precautions of sex. Offers an Ask The Doctor question and answer section to books and resources for young adults on safer sex and HIV/AIDS.
1991 14 pages
Neil Frick, VP for Research
John Indence, VP for Marketing & Communications

5110 Guidelines for Finding Childcare
National Hemophilia Foundation
7 Penn Plaza   212-328-3700
New York, NY 10001-3212   800-424-2634
                                                               Fax: 212-328-3777
                                                                    www.hemophilia.org
Information for parents on how to hire a good babysitter, information on daycare centers, how to tell daycare staff about hemophilia, cooperative childcare and suggested reading for parents.
1987 10 pages
Neil Frick, VP for Research
John Indence, VP for Marketing & Communications

5111 HIV Disease in People with Hemophilia: Your Questions Answered
National Hemophilia Foundation

7 Penn Plaza   212-328-3700
New York, NY 10001-3212   800-424-2634
                                                               Fax: 212-328-3777
                                                                    www.hemophilia.org
Discusses hemophilia and HIV disease, AIDS, management of HIV disease, risks to sexual partners, and issues for children with hemophilia.
1991 48 pages
Neil Frick, VP for Research
John Indence, VP for Marketing & Communications

5112 HIV Infection and Hemophilia
Hemophilia Foundation of Illinois
7 Penn Plaza   212-328-3700
New York, NY 10001-4434   800-424-2634
                                                               Fax: 212-328-3777
                                                                    www.hemophilia.org
Offers information on HIV/AIDS relating to persons with hemophilia.
Neil Frick, VP for Research
John Indence, VP for Marketing & Communications

5113 Hemophilia: Current Medical Management
National Hemophilia Foundation
7 Penn Plaza   212-328-3700
New York, NY 10001-3212   800-424-2634
                                                               Fax: 212-328-3777
                                                                    www.hemophilia.org
Provides an overview of all aspects of hemophilia treatment, including prophylaxis, home therapy, inhibitors, orthopedic solutions, surgery, and dental care.
1994 30 pages
Neil Frick, VP for Research
John Indence, VP for Marketing & Communications

5114 How to Control Bleeds: Inspired by Vince, an 8-year-old Boy with Hemophilia
Bayer
400 Morgan Lane   203-937-2765
West Haven, CT 06516-4175
An educational comic book story by Vince about hemophilia and treatment for bleeds.
26 pages

5115 Living with HIV: Talking with Your Child
Bobbie Steinhart, author
National Hemophilia Foundation
7 Penn Plaza   212-328-3700
New York, NY 10001-3212   800-424-2634
                                                               Fax: 212-328-3777
                                                                    www.hemophilia.org
A pamphlet directed at caregivers of young children living with hemophilia and HIV disease.
1990 8 pages
Neil Frick, VP for Research
John Indence, VP for Marketing & Communications

5116 Mild Hemophilia
National Hemophilia Foundation
7 Penn Plaza   212-328-3700
New York, NY 10001-3212   800-424-2634
                                                               Fax: 212-328-3777
                                                                    www.hemophilia.org
Defines mild hemophilia and details its discovery, diagnosis, inheritance, symptoms, treatment, and activity limitations.
1994 25 pages
Neil Frick, VP for Research
John Indence, VP for Marketing & Communications

5117 Participating in a Clinical Trial: Your Life, Your Choice
National Hemophilia Foundation
7 Penn Plaza   212-328-3700
New York, NY 10001-3212   800-424-2634
                                                               Fax: 212-328-3777
                                                                    www.hemophilia.org
This brochure explains what clinical trials are and what they are like for patients, describes what kinds of HIV therapies are being tested in clinical trials, and lists questions to ask before joining a

trial. This publication is ideal for patients, their families, and/or healthcare personnel who counsel HIV-positive patients.
1994 6 pages
Neil Frick, VP for Research
John Indence, VP for Marketing & Communications

5118 Physical Therapy in Hemophilia
Nationa Hemophilia Foundation
7 Penn Plaza   212-328-3700
New York, NY 10001-3832   800-424-2634
                                      Fax: 212-328-3777
                                        www.hemophilia.org
Targeted at physical therapy students or new therapists at comprehensive hemophilia care clinics. Also provides basic treatment care information for persons with hemophilia and their families.
1986 13 pages
Neil Frick, VP for Research
John Indence, VP for Marketing & Communications

5119 Simple & Complex: A Hemophilia Primer
Western Pennsylvania Chapter of the NHF
8326 Naab Rd   412-685-2231
Indianapolis, IN 46260-1531   Fax: 412-683-2568
                                            www.ihtc.org
Offers information on what hemophilia is, explains AIDS and HIV infection, offers information on the treatments for hemophilia and what hemophilia care costs.
Ike G. Batalis, President and CEO
Phillip E. Himelstein, Founder

5120 Student with Hemophilia: A Resource for the Educator
National Hemophilia Foundation
7 Penn Plaza   212-328-3700
New York, NY 10001-3212   800-424-2634
                                      Fax: 212-328-3777
                                        www.hemophilia.org
Written for teachers, nurses, and other school personnel, this booklet aims to dispel the myths and fears surrounding hemophilia.
1995 16 pages
Neil Frick, VP for Research
John Indence, VP for Marketing & Communications

5121 Treatment of Hemophilia: Current Orthopedic Management
Marvin Gilbert, Jerome Wiedel, author
National Hemophilia Foundation
7 Penn Plaza   212-328-3700
New York, NY 10001-3212   800-424-2634
                                      Fax: 212-328-3777
                                        www.hemophilia.org
Covers a wide range of orthopedic treatment issues, including hemophilic arthropathy, clinical considerations, diagnostic imaging, surgical and nonsurgical treatments, hemophilic synovitis, soft-tissue bleeding, the hemophilia pseudotumor, fracture care, other musculoskelatal problems, and HIV infections.
1995 25 pages
Neil Frick, VP for Research
John Indence, VP for Marketing & Communications

5122 Understanding Hepatitis
Leonard Seeff, Maribel Johnson, author
National Hemophilia Foundation
7 Penn Plaza   212-328-3700
New York, NY 10001-3212   800-424-2634
                                      Fax: 212-328-3777
                                        www.hemophilia.org
Provides comprehensive information about viral hepatitis for people with bleeding disorders, their caregivers, and families. Discusses the different hepatitis viruses, viral transmissions, how the liver is affected by hepatitis, blood product concerns, prevention, diagnosis, treatment, and psychosocial issues.
1997 24 pages
Neil Frick, VP for Research
John Indence, VP for Marketing & Communications

5123 Von Willebrand Disease: A Guide for Patients and Families
Hemophilia Health Services
6820 Charlotte Pike   800-800-6606
Nashville, TN 37209-4206

Offers information on this disease, explains the causes, treatments, prevention and offers resources and books.

5124 What Is Hemophilia?
Hemophilia Foundation of Georgia
8800 Roswell Road   770-518-8272
Atlanta, GA 30328-1689   800-866-4366
                                      Fax: 770-518-3310
                                             www.hog.org
Offers information on what hemophilia is, common factors in hemophilia, the cost and treatments offered to hemophiliacs and more.
Dan Maddock, Chief Governance Officer
Amy Greene, Secretary

5125 What Women Should Know About HIV Infection AIDS and Hemophilia
Hemophilia Foundation of Illinois
7 Penn Plaza   212-328-3700
New York, NY 10001-4434   800-424-2634
                                      Fax: 212-328-3777
                                        www.hemophilia.org
For spouses/partners of men with hemophilia and women with bleeding disorders. Provides information about HIV/AIDS and how it affects women in the hemophilia community.
25 pages
Neil Frick, VP for Research
John Indence, VP for Marketing & Communications

5126 What You Should Know About Hemophilia
National Hemophilia Foundation
7 Penn Plaza   212-328-3700
New York, NY 10001-3212   800-424-2634
                                      Fax: 212-328-3777
                                        www.hemophilia.org
Defines hemophilia, explains its effects, and provides a historical overview of treatment and treatment complications.
1991 13 pages
Neil Frick, VP for Research
John Indence, VP for Marketing & Communications

5127 Who Will Tell Them of Your Special Needs?
MedicAlert
2323 Colorado Avenue   800-432-5378
Turlock, CA 95382-2018
Offers information on MedicAlert bracelets, personal identification medical information needed for treatment in case of emergency.

Audio & Video

5128 Song of Superman
National Hemophilia Foundation
7 Penn Plaza   212-328-3700
New York, NY 10001-3212   800-424-2634
                                      Fax: 212-328-3777
                                        www.hemophilia.org
Designed to help young people with bleeding disorders come to terms with their HIV status, sexuality, and living with HIV. The video explores issues of disclosure in relationships and safer sex through dramatic scenes and frank testimonials by young people living with hemophilia and/or HIV. The companion workbook contains group exercises that follow each of the main topics of the video and serve as a bridge to discussion.
1993 49 pages
Neil Frick, VP for Research
John Indence, VP for Marketing & Communications

5129 Treat Yourself to a Brighter Future - It's Time to Hit the Freedom Trail
c/o Hemophilia Association of the Capital Area
10560 Main Street   703-352-7641
Fairfax, VA 22030-7182   Fax: 540-427-6589
                                        admin@HACAcares.org
A booklet and videotape published by the American Red Cross providing a list of required supplies and equipment for self-infusion concentrates for persons with hemophilia A. It is an instructional

piece for home self-infusion and concise text and illustrations depict seven steps for self-infusion.

20 pages Video & Booklet
Steve Long, President
Eboni Morris, Vice President

Web Sites

5130 American Red Cross Blood Services

www.redcross.org/services/biomed

Distributes a wide variety of plasma therapeutics to benefit people with hemophilia A and B, immune disorders and hypoalbuminemia.

5131 Healing Well

www.healingwell.com

An online health resource guide to medical news, chat, information and articles, newsgroups and message boards, books, disease-related web sites, medical directories, and more for patients, friends, and family coping with disabling diseases, disorders, or chronic illnesses.

5132 Health Finder

www.healthfinder.gov

Searchable, carefully developed web site offering information on over 1000 topics. Developed by the US Department of Health and Human Services, the site can be used in both English and Spanish.

5133 Healthlink USA

www.healthlinkusa.com

Health information concerning treatment, cures, prevention, diagnosis, risk factors, research, support groups, email lists, personal stories and much more. Updated regularly.

5134 MedicineNet

www.medicinenet.com

An online resource for consumers providing easy-to-read, authoritative medical and health information.

5135 Medscape

www.medscape.com

Medscape offers specialists, primary care physicians, and other health professionals the Web's most robust and integrated medical information and educational tools.

5136 National Hemophilia Foundation

www.hemophilia.org

Information on the treatment and the cure of hemophilia, related bleeding disorders and complications of those disorders or their treatment, including HIV infection, as well as improving the quality of life of all those affected.

5137 WebMD

www.webmd.com

Provides credible information, supportive communities, and in-depth reference material about health subjects. A source for original and timely health information as well as material from well known content providers.

Description

5138 Hepatitis

Hepatitis, or inflammation of the liver, has multiple causes and several stages. Hepatitis is usually caused by viruses, excess alcohol consumption, or certain drugs. Less common causes include infectious diseases, accidental poisoning, and auto-immune diseases in which the body attacks its own liver. Hepatitis can be acute or, if it lasts longer than six months, chronic.

The severity of the disease is highly variable. Acute viral hepatitis is mainly caused by hepatitis A virus (HAV), hepatitis B virus (HBV), hepatitis C virus (HCV), hepatitis D virus (HDV), and hepatitis E virus (HEV), and to a much lesser extent, Epstein-Barr virus (EBV). In cases of acute hepatitis, there are no symptoms in the early stage. Early symptoms include vague abdominal pain, fever, loss of appetite, vomiting, and nausea. HBV infections may also cause hives and joint pain. After 3-10 days, the patient's urine darkens, and the skin starts to acquire a yellowish tinge (jaundice). The liver is enlarged and tender, and in a minority of cases the spleen also enlarges. Recovery takes 2-4 weeks, and jaundice lasts 4-8 weeks. If the disease becomes chronic, as in the case of HBV and HCV infections, chronic alcoholism, certain autoimmune diseases, and fatty liver disease (nonalcoholic steatohepatitis or NASH), the liver may become irreversibly scarred (cirrhosis). Cirrhosis causes weakness, fatigue and weight loss. Late stage disease includes fluid accumulation in the abdominal cavity (ascites), gastrointestinal bleeding and mental changes. Abdominal pain and liver enlargement are generally present. Advanced cirrhosis is a risk factor for cancer of the liver. Fulminant hepatitis is a rare condition that consists of massive liver cell death as a result of certain infections, exposure to toxic agents or drug-induced liver injury (e.g., acetaminophen, isoniazid, and methyldopa). Patients in these cases become acutely ill with jaundice, rapid changes in mental status, and even unexplained bleeding. If the patient has pre-existing liver disease, they tend to deteriorate quite rapidly.

HAV is a common virus that is spread by contaminated food and water, and generally causes a mild to moderately severe illness that runs its course over several weeks and disappears without further damage. HBV is also very common, and is spread by bodily fluids, generally through blood transfusion, sexual intercourse, sharing of needles or contaminated items like shaving razors and tattoo needles. The disease may resolve without further consequences, but frequently becomes chronic and may lead to cirrhosis as well as chronic infections.

HCV is also spread through blood transfusion and needle sharing. Although it is not usually severe at onset, it can lead to the same serious consequences as type B. HDV is also spread by blood products, and only infects people who already have HBV. HDV/HBV coinfection is associated with a more severe course. HBV is transmitted by either contaminated food or water, and is geographically restricted to particular regions. Most patients recover spontaneously, HEV does not cause chronic disease, except in some patients with compromised immune systems. A vaccine is available in China, but not the U.S.

Prevention of any of these forms of viral hepatitis depends on avoiding the usual routes of transmission. In addition, there is an effective vaccine available for HAV and HBV. Close family contacts of persons with this disease should receive the vaccine if they have not yet received it as part of routine childhood immunization.

Treatment of hepatitis is largely supportive, but antiviral drugs and interferon are used in certain stages of Type B and Type C infection. Combination drug treatments can completely cure patients of HCV. End-stage or overwhelming infection may necessitate liver transplantation. See also *Liver Disease.*

National Agencies & Associations

5139 Centers for Disease Control & Prevention Hepatitis Branch
1600 Clifton Road NE   800-232-4636
Atlanta, GA 30329-4018   TTY: 888-232-6348
www.cdc.gov/hepatitis
Monitors the rates of viral hepatitis in the United States, provides epidemiologic assistance for outbreaks of viral hepatitis and coordinates studies to define the risk factors for acute and chronic viral hepatitis.

5140 HIV/Hepatitis C in Prison (HIP) Committee
California Prison Focus   510-665-1935
San Francisco, CA 94103   contact@prisons.org
www.prisons.org/hivin
The HIV/HCV in Prison Committee of California Prison Focus works on behalf of prisoners to fight for consistent access to quality medical care including access of all new HIV and hepatitis C medications, diagnostic testing and combination therapies.
Michelle Wexler MD, Executive Director
Diane C Peterson, Associate Director for Immunization

5141 Hepatitis Foundation International
8121 Georgia Avenue   301-565-9410
Silver Spring, MD 20910   800-891-0707
Fax: 301-879-6890
info@hepatitisfoundation.org
www.hepatitisfoundation.org
Grassroots support network for persons with viral hepatitis. Provides education about the prevention diagnosis and treatment of viral hepatitis as well as phone network support and various literature.
Ivonne Fuller Cameron, CEO
Jackie Lewis, Operations Director

5142 Immunization Action Coalition
2550 University Avenue West   651-647-9009
Saint Paul, MN 55114   Fax: 651-647-9131
admin@immunize.org
www.immunize.org
The mission of the Immunization Action Coalition is to boost immunization rates and prevent disease. The coalition promotes physician, community and family awareness of and responsibility for

appropriate immunization of all children and adults against all diseases.
Deborah L Wexler, MD, Executive Director
Litjen Tan, MS, PhD, Chief Strategy Officer

5143 Inter-Provincial Roof Consultants, Ltd.
5828 176th Street   604-576-5740
Surrey, V3S 4-6J9   800-616-2437
                                      Fax: 604-576-5790
Through partnerships and collaboration, will work to reduce the incidence of new HIV/AIDS/HEP C and other blood borne pathogens and to improve the quality of life for those infected and affected.
Sean M Lang, President/Owner/Chief Consultant/Spec Wr
Mike Kosman, Consultant/Spec Writer/Roof Observer

5144 National Hepatitis C Coalition
PO Box 5058   951-766-8238
Hemet, CA 92544   www.nationalhepatitis-c.org
The National Hepatitis C Coalition is a 501(c)(3) tax exempt organization that relies on private donations from good folks like you in order to continue helping others with hepatitis C.
Patty Krueger, Co-Founder

Foundations

5145 Hepatitis B Foundation
3805 Old Easton Road
Doylestown, PA 18902   215-489-4900
                                      Fax: 215-489-4313
                                           info@hepb.org
                                           www.hepb.org
We are dedicated to finding a cure and improving the quality of life for those affected by hepatitis B worldwide. Our commitment includes funding focused research, promoting disease awareness, supporting immunization and treatment initiatives, and serving as the primary source of information for patients and their families, the medical and scientific community, and the general public.

Joel Rosen, Chairman, Esq
Timothy M Block, PhD, President

Libraries & Resource Centers

5146 Hepatitis Education Project
911 Western Avenue   206-732-0311
Seattle, WA 98104   Fax: 206-732-0312
                                           hep@scn.org
                                      www.hepeducation.org
The mission of the Hepatitis Education Project is to help raise awareness among patients, medical personnel and the public of the facts concerning hepatitis patients and the resources available to help those who live with the disease.
Steve Graham, President
Michael Ninburg, Executive Director

Support Groups & Hotlines

5147 Christ Hospital Hepatitis C Support Group
Christ Hospital
176 Palisade Avenue   201-795-1230
Jersey City, NJ 07306   dkatz65717@aol.com
For anyone interested in becoming advocates for increasing awareness of this illness.
Graham, President
Michael Ninburg, Executive Director

5148 Hepatitis Education Project
911 Western Avenue   206-732-0311
Seattle, WA 98104   hepinfo@hepeducation.org
                                      www.hepeducation.org
Helps raise awareness among patients, medical personeel and the public of the facts concerning hepatitis patients and the resources available to help those who live with the disease
Steve Graham, President
Michael Ninburg, Executive Director

5149 National Health Information Center
Office of Disease Prevention & Health Promotion
1101 Wootton Pkwy   Fax: 240-453-8281
Rockville, MD 20852   odphpinfo@hhs.gov
                                      www.health.gov/nhic
Supports public health education by maintaining a calendar of National Health Observances; helps connect consumers and health professionals to organizations that can best answer questions and provide up-to-date contact information from reliable sources; updates on a yearly basis toll-free numbers for health information, Federal health clearinghouses and info centers.
Don Wright, MD, MPH, Director

Books

5150 Hepatitis B Prevention: A Resource Guide
National Digestive Diseases Info. Clearinghouse
2 Information Way   301-496-3583
Bethesda, MD 20824   800-891-5389
                                      Fax: 301-907-8906
                                           www.niddk.nih.gov
Designed to assist health care and other professionals who work in planning or administering hepatitis B prevention programs.
252 pages

5151 Understanding Hepatitis
James L Achord, MD, author
University Press of Mississippi
3825 Ridgewood Road   601-432-6205
Jackson, MS 39211-6492   Fax: 601-432-6217
                                      kburgess@ihl.state.ms.us
                                      www.upress.state.ms.us
For general readers a comprehensive discussion of the causes and of the treatments of hepatitis.
2002 152 pages Paperback
ISBN: 1-578064-36-8

5152 Viral Hepatitis: Scientific Basis and Clinical Management
Churchill Livingstone
PO Box 3188   201-319-9800
Secaucus, NJ 07096-3188   800-553-5426
                                      Fax: 201-319-9659
                                      www.harcourt-international.com/cl/
1997 800 pages Hardcover
ISBN: 0-443057-97-4

Magazines

5153 Hepatitis Magazine
Quality Publishing Services
523 N Sam Houston Pkwy E   281-272-2744
Houston, TX 77060   800-310-7047
                                      Fax: 281-847-5440
Magazine for those with hepatitis. Price listed is for a one year subscription.
Quarterly

Newsletters

5154 **American Liver Foundation: Progress Newsletter**
39 Broadway
New York, NY 10006-4826

212-668-1000
800-465-4837
Fax: 212-483-8179
info@liverfoundation.org
www.liverfoundation.org

The American Liver Foundation is the nation's leading nonprofit organization promoting liver health and disease prevention. ALF provides research education and sdvocacy for those affected by liver-related diseases, including hepatitis
8 pages 2 per year

5155 **B Connected**
3805 Old Easton Road
Doylestown, PA 18902

215-489-4900
Fax: 215-489-4313
info@hepb.org
www.hepb.org

Features practical health tips, frequently asked questions, and other useful information for patients and families to live well with chronic hepatitis B. Available in both print and online versions.
3x/year
Joel Rosen, Chairman
Timothy M. Block, President

5156 **B-Informed Newsletter**
Hepatitis B Foundation
3805 Old Easton Road
Doylestown, PA 18902

215-489-4900
Fax: 215-489-4313
info@hepb.org
www.hepb.org

Includes a Drug Watch of approved and experimental therapies for Hepatitis B, reasearch updates, Foundation news and events, and feature articles on special topics. Available in print and online.
Joel Rosen, Chairman
Timothy M. Block, President

5157 **Hepatitis Alert**
Hepatitis Foundation International (HFI)
8121 Georgia Avenue
Silver Spring, MD 20910-1423

301-565-9410
800-891-0707
Fax: 973-875-5044
hfi@intac.com
www.hepfi.org

Provides information for the public, patients, educators, and medical professionals about the diagnosis, treatment, and prevention of viral hepatitis.
Karen Wirth, Chair
Dane R. Christiansen, Vice Chair

5158 **Hepatitis B Coalition News**
Hepatitis B Coalition
2550 University Ave W
Saint Paul, MN 55114-6328

651-647-9009
Fax: 651-647-9131
www.immunize.org

Newsletter with brochures, articles, videotapes, audio-cassette tapes and manuals for different ethnic populations.
Deborah L. Wexler, MD, Executive Director
Litjen Tan, MS, PhD, Chief Strategy Officer

5159 **NEEDLE TIPS & the Hepatitis B Coalition News**
Hepatitis B Coalition
2550 University Ave W
St. Paul, MN 55114-6328

651-647-9009
Fax: 651-647-9131
admin@immunize.org
www.immunize.org

Information on immunization for health professionals.
28 pages 2x Year
Deborah L. Wexler, MD, Executive Director
Litjen Tan, MS, PhD, Chief Strategy Officer

5160 **VACCINATE ADULTS! Coalition News**
Hepatitis B Coalition
2550 University Ave W
St. Paul, MN 55114-6328

651-647-9009
Fax: 651-647-9131
admin@immunize.org
www.immunize.org

Information on immunization: adult medicine specialist.
12 pages 2x Year
Deborah L. Wexler, MD, Executive Director
Litjen Tan, MS, PhD, Chief Strategy Officer

Pamphlets

5161 **Advice to Parents of Children with HBV**
Hepatitis B Foundation
3805 Old Easton Road
Doylestown, PA 18902

215-489-4900
Fax: 215-489-4313
info@hepb.org
www.hepb.org

Provides information to people affected by hepatitis B and their loved ones. Current HBV research, telephone numbers, and a medical glossary.
Joel Rosen, Chairman
Timothy M. Block, President

5162 **Caring for Your Liver**
Hepatitis Foundation International (HFI)
8121 Georgia Avenue
Silver Spring, MD 20910-1423

301-565-9410
800-891-0707
Fax: 973-875-5044
hfi@intac.com
www.hepfi.org

Information for the person with hepatitis.
Karen Wirth, Chair
Dane R. Christiansen, Vice Chair

5163 **Caution! Treating Children with Acetaminophen**
Hepatitis Foundation International (HFI)
8121 Georgia Avenue
Silver Spring, MD 20910-1423

301-565-9410
800-891-0707
Fax: 973-875-5044
hfi@intac.com
www.hepfi.org

Information on hepatitis.
Karen Wirth, Chair
Dane R. Christiansen, Vice Chair

5164 **Chronic Viral Hepatitis Backgrounder**
Schering Corporation
2000 Galloping Hill Road
Kenilworth, NJ 07033

908-298-4000
www.sch-plough.com

Offers information and statistics on viral hepatitis.

5165 **Cirrhosis: Many Causes**
American Liver Foundation
39 Broadway
New York, NY 10066-1000

212-668-1000
800-223-0179
Fax: 212-483-8179
info@liverfoundation.org
www.liverfoundation.org

Gives basic facts about cirrhosis including causes, signs, symptoms and treatments.
David Ticker, Chief Financial Officer
Lynn Seim, Chief Operating Officer

5166 **Diagnosis and Treatment**
Hepatitis Foundation International (HFI)
8121 Georgia Avenue
Silver Spring, MD 20910-1423

301-565-9410
800-891-0707
Fax: 973-875-5044
hfi@intac.com
www.hepfi.org

Information for the person with hepatitis.
Karen Wirth, Chair
Dane R. Christiansen, Vice Chair

5167 **Health Insurance**
Hepatitis Foundation International (HFI)
8121 Georgia Avenue
Silver Spring, MD 20910-1423

301-565-9410
800-891-0707
Fax: 973-875-5044
hfi@intac.com
www.hepfi.org

Information on hepatitis and health insurance.
Karen Wirth, Chair
Dane R. Christiansen, Vice Chair

5168 Helpful Tips for Carriers of HBV
Hepatitis Foundation International (HFI)
8121 Georgia Avenue   301-565-9410
Silver Spring, MD 20910-1423   800-891-0707
                                            Fax: 973-875-5044
                                                 hfi@intac.com
                                                 www.hepfi.org

Information for people with Hepatitis B.
Karen Wirth, Chair
Dane R. Christiansen, Vice Chair

5169 Hepatitis
National Institute of Allergy & Infectious Disease
5601 Fishers Lane   301-402-1663
Bethesda, MD 20892-0001   Fax: 301-402-0120
                                           niaidnews@niaid.nih.gov
A pamphlet discussing the cause, symptoms, transmission, diagnosis, tests, prevention and the latest research on Hepatitis.

5170 Hepatitis A and B Vaccination
Hepatitis Foundation International (HFI)
8121 Georgia Avenue   301-565-9410
Silver Spring, MD 20910-1423   800-891-0707
                                            Fax: 973-875-5044
                                                 hfi@intac.com
                                                 www.hepfi.org

Information on hepatitis vaccination.
Karen Wirth, Chair
Dane R. Christiansen, Vice Chair

5171 Hepatitis A, B & C
Hepatitis Foundation International (HFI)
8121 Georgia Avenue   301-565-9410
Silver Spring, MD 20910-1423   800-891-0707
                                            Fax: 973-875-5044
                                                 hfi@intac.com
                                                 www.hepfi.org

Information for the person with hepatitis.
Karen Wirth, Chair
Dane R. Christiansen, Vice Chair

5172 Hepatitis A, B & C: Liver Disease You Should Know About
American Liver Foundation
1425 Pompton Avenue   800-465-4837
Cedar Grove, NJ 07009   Fax: 973-256-3214
                                           info@liverfoundation.org
                                           www.liverfoundation.org
Explains viral hepatitis, transmission, symptoms, testing and acute chronic hepatitis.

5173 Hepatitis B Prevention
National Center For Infectious Diseases
Hepatitis Branch   404-332-4555
Atlanta, GA 30333
Explains what hepatitis B is, what behaviors are risky and how to protect oneself against it.

5174 Hepatitis Fact Sheet
                          www.cdc.gov/ncidod/diseases/hepatitis/c
Offers information on the causes, symptoms, prevention and treatments for hepatitis.

5175 How Many Times a Day Do You Risk Being Infected with Hepatitis B?
American Liver Foundation
1425 Pompton Avenue   800-465-4837
Cedar Grove, NJ 07009   Fax: 973-256-3214
                                           info@liverfoundation.org
                                           www.liverfoundation.org
A flyer emphasizing the importance of vaccination against hepatitis B.

5176 Is Your Liver Giving You the Silent Treatment?
Hepatitis Foundation International (HFI)

8121 Georgia Avenue   301-565-9410
Silver Spring, MD 20910-1423   800-891-0707
                                            Fax: 973-875-5044
                                                 hfi@intac.com
                                                 www.hepfi.org
Provides information for patients with hepatitis.
Karen Wirth, Chair
Dane R. Christiansen, Vice Chair

5177 Living with Hepatitis C: Self Help Tips
Hepatitis Foundation International (HFI)
8121 Georgia Avenue   301-565-9410
Silver Spring, MD 20910-1423   800-891-0707
                                            Fax: 973-875-5044
                                                 hfi@intac.com
                                                 www.hepfi.org

Information for people with Hepatitis C.
Karen Wirth, Chair
Dane R. Christiansen, Vice Chair

5178 Protect Yourself and Those You Love Against HBV
Hepatitis B Foundation
3805 Old Easton Road   215-489-4900
Doylestown, PA 18902   Fax: 215-489-4313
                                                 info@hepb.org
                                                 www.hepb.org

Provides information to people affected by hepatitis B and their loved ones.
Joel Rosen, Chairman
Timothy M. Block, President

5179 Q and A: Hepatitis B Prevention
SmithKline Beecham Pharmaceuticals
1 Franklin Plaza   215-751-4000
Philadelphia, PA 19102-1282
Informational booklet written for healthcare personnel by the manufacturer of Engerix-B vaccine, reviews hepatitis B prevention.

5180 Someone You Know Has Hepatitis B
Hepatitis B Foundation
3805 Old Easton Road   215-489-4900
Doylestown, PA 18902   Fax: 215-489-4313
                                                 info@hepb.org
                                                 www.hepb.org
Provides information to people affected by hepatitis B and their loved ones.
Joel Rosen, Chairman
Timothy M. Block, President

5181 Tips on Coping with Chronic Hepatitis
Hepatitis Foundation International (HFI)
8121 Georgia Avenue   301-565-9410
Silver Spring, MD 20910-1423   800-891-0707
                                            Fax: 973-875-5044
                                                 www.hepfi.org

Information for people with hepatitis.
Karen Wirth, Chair
Dane R. Christiansen, Vice Chair

5182 Viral Hepatitis: Everybody's Problem?
American Liver Foundation
39 Broadwa   212-668-1000
New York, NY 10006-1000   800-223-0179
                                            Fax: 212-483-8179
                                           info@liverfoundation.org
                                           www.liverfoundation.org
Covering a broad range of topics including: a definition of the disease, descriptions of types of infections, transmission, symptoms, treatment options and prevention of hepatitis.
David Ticker, Chief Financial Officer
Lynn Seim, Chief Operating Officer

5183 What Health Care Workers Should Know About Hepatitis B
Channing L Bete Company
2550 University Ave W   651-647-9009
St. Paul, MN 55114   800-628-7733
                                            Fax: 651-647-9131
                                                 www.immunize.org

Presents information in easy-to-read, simple English for health care workers about hepatitis B.
15 pages
Deborah L. Wexler, MD, Executive Director
Litjen Tan, MS, PhD, Chief Strategy Officer

Audio & Video

5184 Hepatitis B Video
Hepatitis B Foundation
3805 Old Easton Road
Doylestown, PA 18902
215-489-4900
Fax: 215-489-4313
info@hepb.org
www.hepb.org
Provides information to people affected by hepatitis B and their loved ones.
Joel Rosen, Chairman
Timothy M. Block, President

5185 Hepatitis C: A Viral Mystery
Terry Strauss, Stephen Steady, author
Fanlight Productions
4196 Washington Street
Boston, MA 02131-1731
617-469-4999
800-937-4113
Fax: 617-469-3379
fanlight@fanlight.com
www.fanlight.com
This timely video is about living with a serious, chronic illness. In addition to discussing the medical treatments available, the video also explores alternatives which appear to help some people.
2000 30 Minutes
ISBN: 1-572953-08-X

Web Sites

5186 HIV/Hepatitis C in Prison (HIP) Committee
www.prisons.org/hivin.htm
Fighting for consistent access to quality medical care including access to all new HIV and Hepatitis C medications, diagnostic testing and combination therapies.

5187 Healing Well
www.healingwell.com
An online health resource guide to medical news, chat, information and articles, newsgroups and message boards, books, disease-related web sites, medical directories, and more for patients, friends, and family coping with disabling diseases, disorders, or chronic illnesses.

5188 Health Finder
www.healthfinder.gov
Searchable, carefully developed web site offering information on over 1000 topics. Developed by the US Department of Health and Human Services, the site can be used in both English and Spanish.

5189 Healthlink USA
www.healthlinkusa.com
Health information concerning treatment, cures, prevention, diagnosis, risk factors, research, support groups, email lists, personal stories and much more. Updated regularly.

5190 Healthy Lives

5191 Hepatitis B Coalition
www.immunize.org
The Immunization Action Coalition (IAC) works to increase immunization rates and prevent disease by creating and distributing educational materials for health professionals and the public that enhance the delivery of safe and effective immunization services.

5192 Hepatitis Information Network

5193 MedicineNet
www.medicinenet.com
An online resource for consumers providing easy-to-read, authoritative medical and health information.

5194 Medscape
www.medscape.com
Medscape offers specialists, primary care physicians, and other health professionals the Web's most robust and integrated medical information and educational tools.

5195 WebMD
www.webmd.com
Provides credible information, supportive communities, and in-depth reference material about health subjects. A source for original and timely health information as well as material from well known content providers.

Description

5196 Hydrocephalus

The normal brain and spinal cord are surrounded with a water-based substance called cerebrospinal fluid (CSF) that collects within the brain in several larger pools called ventricles, which are connected to one another through tiny channels. The CSF is formed in some of these ventricles by specialized tissues called choroid plexi, and it circulates widely and is eventually reabsorbed. If CFS production exceeds reabsorption, or if the fluid is prevented from circulating because of blockages within the aqueducts that connect the ventricles, it may build up pressure that expands the ventricles and presses on the normal brain tissue, causing hydrocephalus, or water on the brain.

Hydrocephalus can cause change in behavior, headache, visual loss, vomiting and weakness. Hydrocephalus may due to congenital malformations of the brain and present from birth. If it occurs in a child whose skull bones have not yet fused together, it may cause the head to enlarge. There are three main causes of obstructive hydrocephalus in infants. The first is aqueductal stenosis, in which the outflow channels from the third to the fourth ventricles may be excessively narrowed as a result of hemorrhage, tumors, infections, or developmental malformation. The second is Dandy Walker malformation, which results in a cystic enlargement of the 4th ventricle during fetal life that leads to failure of the cerebellum to form properly. The third is Chiari II malformation, which occurs concomitantly with spinal bifida or syringomyelia.

In adults whose brains are encased in the rigid skull, there is no room to expand and pressure builds up in the brain. Excess CSF may be in response to infection such as meningitis or to blockage of CSF movement by tumor. Treatment and outlook depend on the underlying cause. Diuretics can decrease total fluid content in the body and relieve some of the pressure in the brain. Medical therapy may cause limited temporary improvement. Surgical treatment may be able to correct the underlying cause. If it cannot, the surgeon may still give substantial relief by placing a shunt which allows extra CSF to drain from the ventricles to some other part of the body.

National Agencies & Associations

5197 Hydrocephalus Association
4340 East West Highway
Bethesda, MD 20814-4447
301-202-3811
888-598-3789
Fax: 301-202-3813
info@hydroassoc.org
www.hydroassoc.org
Provides support, education and advocacy for families affected by hdrocephalus and professionals.
Brett Weitz, Chair
Susan Fiorella, Vice Chair

5198 National Hydrocephalus Foundation
12413 Centralia Road
Lakewood, CA 90715-1653
562-924-6666
info@nhfonline.org
www.nhfonline.org

A national organization providing information and education, along with peer-to-peer support, physician referrals and more.
Michael Fields, President & Treasurer
Debbi Fields, Executive Director

5199 Spina Bifida & Hydrocephalus Association of Nova Scotia
15 Laura Drive
Nova Scotia, B3G-1K3
902-679-1124
800-304-0450
Fax: 902-679-1433
info@sbhans.ca
www.sbhans.ca
A non-profit, registered charitable organization affiliated with the Spina Bifida and Hydrocephalus Association of Canada.

5200 The Kidney Foundation of Canada
310-5160 Decarie Boulevard
Montreal, Quebec, H3X-2H9
514-369-4806
800-361-7494
Fax: 514-369-2472
info@kidney.ca
www.kidney.ca
A national volunteer organization committed to reducing the burden of kidney disease through funding research, providing education and support, and increasing public awareness and commitment to advancing kidney health and organ donation.
Greg Robbins, President
Terry Tomkins, Treasurer

5201 World Hypertension League
ceo@whleague.org
whleague.org
Devoted to the advancement of hypertension prevention and control through joint efforts of all national leagues and societies.

State Agencies & Associations

Maryland

5202 Hydrocephalus Association
4340 East West Highway
Bethesda, MD 20814
301-202-3811
888-598-3789
Fax: 301-202-3813
info@hydroassoc.org
www.hydroassoc.org
Founded in 1976 this group was formed as a group of concerned families and patients with hydrocephalus to share information and experiences in dealing with this disease locally and nationwide.
Barrett O'Connor, Chair
Dawn Mancuso, Chief Executive Officer

Michigan

5203 Hydrocephalus Support Group of Michigan Children's Hospital of Michigan
Children's Hospital of Michigan
3901 Beaubien
Detroit, MI 48201
313-745-5437
Fax: 313-993-8744
Founded in 1992 this group provides information to families and gives them support.
Mary Smellie

Pennsylvania

5204 Hydrocephalus Association of Philadelphia
PO Box 2099
Boothwyn, PA 19061-8099
610-497-0375
Fax: 610-497-2836
Founded in 1992 the Association provides support information advocacy and telephone support to families in Pennsylvania New Jersey and Delaware.
Halmi, Director

Rhode Island

5205 Hydrocephalus Association of Rhode Island
PO Box 343
Valley Falls, RI 02864-0343
401-723-6065
Founded in 1993 the mission of this Association is to provide information support and advocacy for individuals with hydrocephalus and for friends and family members.
Gabriella Pike, President

Texas

5206 Hydrocephalus Association of North Texas
PO Box 670552   214-528-2877
Dallas, TX 74637-0552   http://nhfonline.org/treatment.php?id=or
Founded in 1987 the mission is to provide information and support
to parents of children with hydrocephalus in the state of Texas and
neighboring states.
Beverly Pozzi

Washington

5207 Children's Hydrocephalus Support Group
PO Box 1611   425-482-0479
Woodinville, WA 98072   lpoliski@hydrosupport.org
                                                    www.hydrosupport.org
Founded in 1993 the group of Seattle provides support to individu-
als with hydrocephalus.
Lori Poliski, Co-Founder
Paul Gross, Co-Founder

Support Groups & Hotlines

5208 Hydrocephalus Parents Support Group
1325 Louis Street   908-722-4691
Manville, NJ 08835
Founded in 1993, the group provides support for parents of chil-
dren with hydrocephalus.
Andrea

5209 National Health Information Center
Office of Disease Prevention & Health Promotion
1101 Wootton Pkwy   Fax: 240-453-8281
Rockville, MD 20852   odphpinfo@hhs.gov
                                                    www.health.gov/nhic
Supports public health education by maintaining a calendar of National Health Observances; helps connect consumers and health
professionals to organizations that can best answer questions and
provide up-to-date contact information from reliable sources; updates on a yearly basis toll-free numbers for health information,
Federal health clearinghouses and info centers.
Don Wright, MD, MPH, Director

Books

5210 Hydrocephalus: A Guide for Patients, Families, and Friends
O'Reilly and Associates
1005 Gravenstein Hwy N   707-827-7019
Sebastopol, CA 95472   800-889-8969
                                               Fax: 707-824-8268
                                               order@oreilly.com
                                               www.oreilly.com
Hydrocephalus: A Guide for Patients, Families, and Friends provides individuals and families with the guidance, information and
support needed to make the right decisions at the right time.
350 pages Paperback
ISBN: 1-565924-10-X

5211 Spina Bifida Association of America: Insights into Spina Bifida
Spina Bifida Association of America
1600 Wilson Blvd.
Arlington, VA 22209-4226   202-944-3285
                                               800-621-3141
                                               Fax: 202-944-3295
                                               sbaa@sbaa.org
                                               www.sbaa.org
News on medical, legislative and education topics relevant to indi-
viduals with spina bifida.
bi-monthly
Megan Sorensen, Chair
Wilson Neyland, Chair-Elect

Children's Books

5212 Loving Ben
Delacorte

1540 Broadway   212-354-6500
New York, NY 10036-4039
This is a moving story of a sister who cares for her baby brother and
tries to help him learn despite his birth defects and deteriorating
health.
Grades 7-10

Newsletters

5213 Alliance of Genetic Support Groups
4301 Connecticut Ave NW   202-966-5557
Washington, DC 20008   800-336-4363
                                               Fax: 202-966-8553
                                               info@geneticalliance.org
                                               www.geneticalliance.org
A coalition of voluntary genetic support groups, consumers and
professionals addressing the needs of individuals and families af-
fected by genetic disorders from a national perspective.
Sharon Terry, President and CEO
Jeffrey Giorgi, Communications & Operations Assistant

5214 Hydrocephalus Association Newsletter
Hydrocephalus Association
4340 East West Highway   301-202-3811
Bethesda, MD 20814-2912   888-598-3789
                                               Fax: 301-202-3813
                                               info@hydroassoc.org
                                               www.hydroassoc.org
Offers information on association news, conference articles, meet-
ings, support and educational groups.
12 pages Quarterly
Aseem Chandra, Chair
Craig Brown, Senior Vice Chair

5215 Hydrocephalus Parents Support Group Newsletter
PO Box 1611   425-482-0479
Woodinville, WA 98072   lpoliski@hydrosupport.org
                                                    www.hydrosupport.org
Founded in 1993, the group provides support for parents of chil-
dren with hydrocephalus.

5216 Hydrocephalus Support Group Newsletter
PO Box 1611   425-482-0479
Woodinville, WA 98072-4236   Fax: 314-995-4108
                                               lpoliski@hydrosupport.org
                                               www.hydrosupport.org
Founded in 1986, this group provides information, education and
support to anyone dealing with hydrocephalus.

5217 National Hydrocephalus Foundation Newsletter
12413 Centrailia Road   562-924-6666
Lakewood, CA 90715-1623   888-857-3434
                                               Fax: 562-924-6666
                                               nhfonline.org
Founded in 1979, the foundation is a national organization whose
purpose is to provide information and education, along with peer
support newsletter quarterly. Group meeting quarterly in Long
Beach, CA. $35 a year.
Quarterly
Debbi Fields, Executive Director

5218 New York University Medical Center Auxiliary of Tisch Hospital
560 1st Avenue   212-263-5040
New York, NY 10016
Conducts national symposiums on hydrocephalus.

Pamphlets

5219 About Hydrocephalus: A Book for Families
Hydrocephalus Association
4340 East West Highway   301-202-3811
Bethesda, MD 20814-2912   888-598-3789
                                               Fax: 301-202-3813
                                               info@hydroassoc.org
                                               www.hydroassoc.org

A booklet in either English or Spanish, detailing all aspects of hydrocephalus from diagnosis and treatment to complications and follow-up care.
36 pages Paperback
Aseem Chandra, Chair
Craig Brown, Senior Vice Chair

5220 About Normal Pressure Hydrocephalus: A Book for Adults & Their Families
Hydrocephalus Association
870 Market Street
San Francisco, CA 94102-2912
415-732-7040
888-598-3789
Fax: 415-732-7044
info@hydroassoc.org
www.hydroassoc.org
Booklet discusses the diagnosis and treatment of adult-onset normal pressure hydrocephalus.
24 pages Paperback
Dory Kranz, Executive Director
Pip Marks, Director Outreach Services

5221 Directory of Neurosurgeons Who Treat Adults
Hydrocephalus Association
870 Market Street
San Francisco, CA 94102-2912
415-732-7040
888-598-3789
Fax: 415-732-7044
info@hydroassoc.org
www.hydroassoc.org
Names and addresses of neurosurgeons who treat adult-onset normal pressure hydrocephalus and adult-acquired hydrocephalus, listed alphabetically and geographically.
Dory Kranz, Executive Director
Pip Marks, Director Outreach Services

5222 Directory of Pediatric Neurosurgeons
Hydrocephalus Association
870 Market Street
San Francisco, CA 94102-2912
415-732-7040
888-598-3789
Fax: 415-732-7044
info@hydroassoc.org
www.hydroassoc.org
Names and addresses of more than 200 neurosurgeons who specialize in pediatrics, listed alphabetically and geographically.
Dory Kranz, Executive Director
Pip Marks, Director Outreach Services

5223 Endoscopic Third Ventriculotomy
Hydrocephalus Association
870 Market Street
San Francisco, CA 94102-2912
415-732-7040
888-598-3789
Fax: 415-732-7044
info@hydroassoc.org
www.hydroassoc.org
Series includes information on primary care, learning disabilities, eye problems, social skills development, headaches, endoscopic third ventriculostomy, shunts and more.
Dory Kranz, Executive Director
Pip Marks, Director Outreach Services

5224 Eye Problems Associated with Hydrocephalus in Children
Hydrocephalus Association
870 Market Street
San Francisco, CA 94102-2912
415-732-7040
888-598-3789
Fax: 415-732-7044
info@hydroassoc.org
www.hydroassoc.org
Series includes information on primary care, learning disabilities, eye problems, social skills development, headaches, endoscopic third ventriculostomy, shunts and more.
Dory Kranz, Executive Director
Pip Marks, Director Outreach Services

5225 Fact Sheet: Hydrocephalus
Hydrocephalus Association
870 Market Street
San Francisco, CA 94102-2912
415-732-7040
888-598-3789
Fax: 415-732-7044
info@hydroassoc.org
www.hydroassoc.org

Available in Spanish.
Dory Kranz, Executive Director
Pip Marks, Director Outreach Services

5226 Headaches and Hydrocephalus
Hydrocephalus Association
870 Market Street
San Francisco, CA 94102-2912
415-732-7040
888-598-3789
Fax: 415-732-7044
info@hydroassoc.org
www.hydroassoc.org
Series includes information on primary care, learning disabilities, eye problems, social skills development, headaches, endoscopic third ventriculostomy, shunts and more.
Dory Kranz, Executive Director
Pip Marks, Director Outreach Services

5227 Hospitalization Tips
Hydrocephalus Association
870 Market Street
San Francisco, CA 94102-2912
415-732-7040
888-598-3789
Fax: 415-732-7044
info@hydroassoc.org
www.hydroassoc.org
1997
Dory Kranz, Executive Director
Pip Marks, Director Outreach Services

5228 How to Be an Assertive Parent on the Treatment Team
Hydrocephalus Association
870 Market Street
San Francisco, CA 94102-2912
415-732-7040
888-598-3789
Fax: 415-732-7044
info@hydroassoc.org
www.hydroassoc.org
Dory Kranz, Executive Director
Pip Marks, Director Outreach Services

5229 ID Card for Third Ventriculostomy Patients
Hydrocephalus Association
870 Market Street
San Francisco, CA 94102-2912
415-732-7040
888-598-3789
Fax: 415-732-7044
info@hydroassoc.org
www.hydroassoc.org
Dory Kranz, Executive Director
Pip Marks, Director Outreach Services

5230 LINK Directory Information
Hydrocephalus Association
870 Market Street
San Francisco, CA 94102-2912
415-732-7040
888-598-3789
Fax: 415-732-7044
info@hydroassoc.org
www.hydroassoc.org
A nationwide network of individuals listed in directory format giving members direct access to others in similar circumstances.
Dory Kranz, Executive Director
Pip Marks, Director Outreach Services

5231 Learning Disabilities in Children with Hydrocephalus
Hydrocephalus Association
870 Market Street
San Francisco, CA 94102-2912
415-732-7040
888-598-3789
Fax: 415-732-7044
info@hydroassoc.org
www.hydroassoc.org
Available in Spanish.
Dory Kranz, Executive Director
Pip Marks, Director Outreach Services

5232 Nonverbal Learning Disorder Syndrome
Hydrocephalus Association

870 Market Street
San Francisco, CA 94102-2912

415-732-7040
888-598-3789
Fax: 415-732-7044
info@hydroassoc.org
www.hydroassoc.org

1998
Dory Kranz, Executive Director
Pip Marks, Director Outreach Services

5233 Prenatal Hydrocephalus: A Book for Parents
Hydrocephalus Association
870 Market Street
San Francisco, CA 94102-2912

415-732-7040
888-598-3789
Fax: 415-732-7044
info@hydroassoc.org
www.hydroassoc.org

Dory Kranz, Executive Director
Pip Marks, Director Outreach Services

5234 Resource Guide
Hydrocephalus Association
870 Market Street
San Francisco, CA 94102-2912

415-732-7040
888-598-3789
Fax: 415-732-7044
info@hydroassoc.org
www.hydroassoc.org

A comprehensive listing of 450 articles on all aspects of hydrocephalus. Articles may be ordered from the association for a small fee.
Dory Kranz, Executive Director
Pip Marks, Director Outreach Services

5235 Resource Guide: Normal Pressure Hydrocephalus/Adult Onset
Hydrocephalus Association
870 Market Street
San Francisco, CA 94102-2912

415-732-7040
888-598-3789
Fax: 415-732-7044
info@hydroassoc.org
www.hydroassoc.org

Dory Kranz, Executive Director
Pip Marks, Director Outreach Services

5236 Social Skills Development in Children with Hydrocephalus
Hydrocephalus Association
870 Market Street
San Francisco, CA 94102-2912

415-732-7040
888-598-3789
Fax: 415-732-7044
info@hydroassoc.org
www.hydroassoc.org

Dory Kranz, Executive Director
Pip Marks, Director Outreach Services

5237 Survival Skills for the Family Unit
Hydrocephalus Association
870 Market Street
San Francisco, CA 94102-2912

415-732-7040
888-598-3789
Fax: 415-732-7044
info@hydroassoc.org
www.hydroassoc.org

Dory Kranz, Executive Director
Pip Marks, Director Outreach Services

5238 Understanding Your Child's Education Needs/Individualized Education Program
Hydrocephalus Association
870 Market Street
San Francisco, CA 94102-2912

415-732-7040
888-598-3789
Fax: 415-732-7044
info@hydroassoc.org
www.hydroassoc.org

Dory Kranz, Executive Director
Pip Marks, Director Outreach Services

Audio & Video

5239 Hydrocephalus: A Neglected Disease
Guardians of Hydrocephalus Research Foundation

2640 East 28 Street
Brooklyn, NY 11235-2023

718-743-9650
Fax: 718-743-9650
GHRF2618@aol.com
www.homestead.com

The Guardians of Hydrocephalus Research Foundation (GHRF) is a non-profit group dedicated to research into the cause and treatment of hydrocephalus
Marie Fischetti, Founder

Web Sites

5240 Healing Well
www.healingwell.com
An online health resource guide to medical news, chat, information and articles, newsgroups and message boards, books, disease-related web sites, medical directories, and more for patients, friends, and family coping with disabling diseases, disorders, or chronic illnesses.

5241 Health Finder
www.healthfinder.gov
Searchable, carefully developed web site offering information on over 1000 topics. Developed by the US Department of Health and Human Services, the site can be used in both English and Spanish.

5242 Healthlink USA
www.healthlinkusa.com
Health information concerning treatment, cures, prevention, diagnosis, risk factors, research, support groups, email lists, personal stories and much more. Updated regularly.

5243 Hydrocephalus Association
www.hydroassoc.org
Provides support, education and advocacy for families and professionals. The goal is to insure that families and individuals dealing with the complexities of hydrocephalus receive personal support, comprehensive educational materials and on-going medical care.

5244 Hydrocephalus Center
www.patientcenters.com/hydrocephalus
An online reference that was created especially as a resource for those with hydrocephalus and their families.

5245 MedicineNet
www.medicinenet.com
An online resource for consumers providing easy-to-read, authoritative medical and health information.

5246 Medscape
www.medscape.com
Medscape offers specialists, primary care physicians, and other health professionals the Web's most robust and integrated medical information and educational tools.

5247 Neurology Channel
www.healthcommunities.com
Find clearly explained, medically accurate information regarding conditions, including an overview, symptoms, causes, diagnostic procedures and treatment options. On this site it is possible to ask questions and get information from a neurologist and connect to people who have similar health interests.

5248 WebMD
www.webmd.com
Provides credible information, supportive communities, and in-depth reference material about health subjects. A source for original and timely health information as well as material from well known content providers.

Description

5249 Hypertension

Hypertension is an abnormal elevation of blood pressure. Blood pressure is noted as a top number (systolic) over a bottom number (diastolic) with a reading of 120/80 being recognized as normal. Hypertension is defined as a systolic pressure greater than 130 and/or a diastolic pressure greater than 90. It is a common disorder that affects about 33 percent of the population. Primary, or essential, hypertension is the most common form, and it has no known cause. It is more prevalent in African-Americans, males, and those with a family history of high blood pressure. Other risk factors include obesity, diabetes, high levels of fat and cholesterol, smoking, sedentary lifestyle and psychological stress. It is a significant risk factor for coronary heart disease, heart failure, stroke, and kidney failure.

Patients with hypertension generally have no symptoms. Diagnosis is made by simple measurement with a blood pressure cuff. Several measurements are necessary at different times to establish the diagnosis.

Treatment of hypertension is done in a step-wise fashion beginning with lifestyle modifications (weight reduction, regular exercise, smoking cessation, a low salt, fat and cholesterol diet and improved stress reduction). If medications are necessary, doctors can choose from a wide variety of effective and usually well-tolerated drugs that include ACE inhibitors, angiotensin II receptor antagonists, beta-blockers, calcium channel blockers, and diuretics. Therapy generally must be lifelong. Home monitoring of blood pressure can also help with blood pressure control.

Occasionally the blood pressure may be refractory, or difficult to control with medicines. In this instance, screening is needed for unusual causes of hypertension, such as renovascular disease (narrowing of the arteries feeding the kidneys), hyperaldosteronism (a tumor or overgrowth of the adrenal gland which secretes hormones that raise the blood pressure), or aortic coarctation (a congenital malformation of the major blood vessels near the heart.) If no specifically treatable cause is identified, the patient will require combination therapy with high doses of drugs. Given a commitment to doing so, it is almost always possible to control the pressure.

National Agencies & Associations

5250 National Heart, Lung & Blood Institute
31 Center Drive
Bethesda, MD 20892
nhlbiinfo@nhlbi.nih.gov
www.nhlbi.nih.gov
Trains, conducts research, and educates in order to promote the prevention and treatment of heart, lung, and blood disorders.
Gary H. Gibbons, MD, Director
Nakela Cook, MD, MPH, FACC, Chief of Staff

5251 National Stroke Association
9707 E Easter Lane
Centennial, CO 80112
info@stroke.org
www.stroke.org
A national organization whose sole purpose is to reduce the incidence and impact of stroke through prevention, treatment, rehabilitation and research and support for stroke survivors and their families.

5252 Pulmonary Hypertension Association (PHA)
801 Roeder Road
Silver Spring, MD 20910
301-565-3004
800-748-7274
pha@PHAssociation.org
www.PHAssociation.org
A non-profit organization for pulmonary hypertension patients, families, caregivers and PH-treating medical professionals. PHA works to provide support, education, and find a cure for pulmonary hypertension.
Brad A. Wong, President & CEO
Azalea Candelaria, Vice President

Research Centers

5253 Creighton University Midwest Hypertension Research Center
601 N 30th Street
Omaha, NE 68131-2137
402-280-4507
Fax: 402-280-4101
Dr William PhD, Director

5254 Hahnemann University: Division of Surgical Research
230 N Broad Street
Philadelphia, PA 19102
215-762-7000
866-884-4HUH
Fax: 215-762-8109
www.hahnemannhospital.com
Studies hypertension and management of stress ulcers.
Teuro Matsum Carretero, Division Head
William H Beierwaltes, Scientist

5255 Henry Ford Hospital: Hypertension and Vascular Research Division
2799 W Grand Boulevard
Detroit, MI 48202-2689
313-972-1693
Fax: 313-876-1479
ocarret1@hfhs.org
www.hypertensionresearch.org
Basic biomedical research seeks to understand: The role of vasoconstrictors and vasodilators (angiotensin II bradykinin nitric oxide natriuretic peptides) in the regulation of blood pressure development of hypertension and development of target organ damage (myocardial infarction heart failure vascular injury and renal disease); The generation of reactive oxygen species by blood vessels and kidney cells and how this contributes to target organ damage; and The mechanisms by which therape
William H Beierwaltes, Ph.D., Faculty
Oscar A Carretero, Faculty

5256 Indiana University: Hypertension Research Center
425 University Boulevard
Indianapolis, IN 46202-0001
317-274-4591
800-274-4862
Fax: 317-278-0673
The mission of the Center is to conduct research in the causes diagnosis treatment and prevention of high blood pressure and its complications.
Dr Myron Rom MPH, Director
Eric Schips, Divisional Administrator

5257 New York University General Clinical Research Center
NYU Medical Center
550 First Avenue
New York, NY 10016
212-263-7300
Fax: 212-263-8501
www.med.nyu.edu
Focuses in the areas of hypertension and studies into endocrinology.
Robert I Grossman, MD, Dean & CEO
Steven B Abramson, MD, Senior Vice President and Vice Dean for

5258 University of Michigan: Division of Hypertension
1500 E Medical Center
Ann Arbor, MI 48109
734-615-0863
855-855-0863
www.med.umich.edu
Excellence in medical education patient care and research.
Douglas L Stoulil, Study Coordinator

5259 University of Minnesota: Hypertensive Research Group
611 Beacon Street SE
Minneapolis, MN 55455   612-624-1438
Research pertaining to hypertension and stress disorders.
Jack Massry, Head

5260 University of Southern California: Division of Nephrology
2025 Zonal Avenue   323-442-5100
Los Angeles, CA 90033-1034   Fax: 213-226-3958
Research into hypertension and sleep disorders.
Gbemisola A Adeseun, MD, MPH, Faculty
Vito M Campese, MD, Faculty

5261 University of Virginia: Hypertension and Atherosclerosis Unit
Medical Center   804-924-8470
Charlottesville, VA 22908-0001   Fax: 804-924-2581
Dr Carlos DVM, Director

5262 Wake Forest University: Arteriosclerosis Research Center
Department of Comparative Medicine
300 S Hawthorne Road   336-764-3600
Winston-Salem, NC 27103-2732   Fax: 336-764-5818
Hypertension research.
Thomas Clark

Support Groups & Hotlines

5263 National Health Information Center
Office of Disease Prevention & Health Promotion
1101 Wootton Pkwy   Fax: 240-453-8281
Rockville, MD 20852   odphpinfo@hhs.gov
                                                        www.health.gov/nhic
Supports public health education by maintaining a calendar of National Health Observances; helps connect consumers and health professionals to organizations that can best answer questions and provide up-to-date contact information from reliable sources; updates on a yearly basis toll-free numbers for health information, Federal health clearinghouses and info centers.
Don Wright, MD, MPH, Director

Books

5264 Courage: Poems & Positive Thoughts for Stroke Survivors
National Stroke Association
9707 E Easter Lane   303-649-9299
Centennial, CO 80112-3747   800-787-6537
                                                        Fax: 303-649-1328
                                                        info@stroke.org
                                                        www.stroke.org
Words of inspiration from survivors and caregivers.
83 pages
Colette Lafosse, Director Rehabilitation/Recovery Program

5265 Discovery Circles
National Stroke Association
9707 E Easter Lane   303-649-9299
Centennial, CO 80112-3747   800-787-6537
                                                        Fax: 303-649-1328
                                                        info@stroke.org
                                                        www.stroke.org
NSA's guide to organizing and facilitating stroke support groups. This detailed manual describes the support group structure and the facilitator's role.
213 pages
Dave Egger, Publisher
Nancy Coulter, Editor

5266 Magic of Humor in Caregiving
National Stroke Association
9707 E Easter Lane   303-649-9299
Centennial, CO 80112-3747   800-787-6537
                                                        Fax: 303-649-1328
                                                        info@stroke.org
                                                        www.stroke.org
A dynamic researching tool focusing on the necessity of humor in daily caregiving interaction.
Colette Lafosse, Director Rehabilitation/Recovery Program
James R. Sherman, Author

5267 Management of Hypertension
EMIS Medical Publishers
Durant, OK 74702-1607   580-924-0643
                                                        800-225-0694
                                                        Fax: 580-924-9414
ISBN: 0-929240-62-6
Kenneth H. Coope, Publisher

5268 November Days
National Stroke Association
9707 E Easter Lane   303-649-9299
Centennial, CO 80112-3747   800-787-6537
                                                        Fax: 303-649-1328
                                                        info@stroke.org
                                                        www.stroke.org
A caregiver's story of her struggle with a loved one's stroke.
225 pages

5269 Ted's Stroke: The Caregiver's Story
National Stroke Association
9707 E Easter Lane   303-649-9299
Centennial, CO 80112-3747   800-787-6537
                                                        Fax: 303-649-1328
                                                        info@stroke.org
                                                        www.stroke.org
Personal experiences, guidance and tips for caregivers.
175 pages
ISBN: 0-962487-61-9
Seven Locks, Publisher

5270 Women in Your Life: Protect Yourself, Protect Your Family
National Stroke Association
9707 E Easter Lane   303-649-9299
Centennial, CO 80112-3747   800-787-6537
                                                        Fax: 303-649-1328
                                                        info@stroke.org
                                                        www.stroke.org
Valuable information about the unique toll stroke takes on women.
Colette Lafosse, Director Rehabilitation/Recovery Program

Magazines

5271 American Journal of Hypertension
American Society of Hypertension
45 Main Street   212-696-9099
New York, NY 11201   Fax: 347-916-0267
                                                        ash@ash-us.org
                                                        www.ash-us.org

5272 Ethnicity & Disease
International Society on Hypertension in Blacks
2045 Manchester Street NE   404-875-6263
Atlanta, GA 30324-4110   Fax: 404-875-6334
                                                        member@ishib.org
                                                        www.ishib.org
International journal on ethnic minority population differences in diease patterns. Provides a comprehensive source of information on the causal relationships in the etiology of common illnesses through the study of ethnic patterns of disease.
Quarterly
John Willey, Publisher
Melanie T Cockfield, Director Administration

5273 Ethnicity Disease
International Society on Hypertension in Blacks
2045 Manchester Street NE   404-875-6263
Atlanta, GA 30324-4110   Fax: 404-875-6334
                                                        member@ishib.org
Determined to accomplish the overall mission to improving the health and life expectancy of ethnic minority populations around

the world. Publishes a quarterly journal and holds an annual conference.
150 pages Quarterly
Christopher T Fitzpatrick, CEO
Melanie T Cockfield, Director Administration

5274 Magazine of the National Institute of Hypertension Studies
13217 Livernois Avenue   313-931-3427
Detroit, MI 48238-3162
Association news.

Newsletters

5275 News Report
National Hypertension Association
324 E 30th Street   212-889-3557
New York, NY 10016-8329   Fax: 212-447-7032
nathypertension@aol.com
www.nathypertension.org
Offers information and medical updates regarding hypertension. Recent book publication: 100 Questions and Answers about Hypertension by WM Manger, MD, PhD, and RW Gifford, Jr, MT available throught National Hypertension Association.
W.M. Manger MD, PhD, Chairman

Pamphlets

5276 African-Americans and Stroke
National Stroke Association
9707 E Easter Lane   303-649-9299
Centennial, CO 80112-3747   800-787-6537
Fax: 303-649-1328
info@stroke.org
www.stroke.org
Colette Lafosse, Director Rehabilitation/Recovery Program

5277 Aneurysm Answers
National Stroke Association
9707 E Easter Lane   303-649-9299
Centennial, CO 80112-3747   800-787-6537
Fax: 303-649-1328
info@stroke.org
www.stroke.org
Colette Lafosse, Director Rehabilitation/Recovery Program

5278 Check Your Pulse, America: Atrial Fibrillation
National Stroke Association
9707 E Easter Lane   303-649-9299
Centennial, CO 80112-3747   800-787-6537
Fax: 303-649-1328
info@stroke.org
www.stroke.org
Colette Lafosse, Director Rehabilitation/Recovery Program

5279 Cholesterol and Stroke
National Stroke Association
9707 E Easter Lane   303-649-9299
Centennial, CO 80112-3747   800-787-6537
Fax: 303-649-1328
info@stroke.org
www.stroke.org
Colette Lafosse, Director Rehabilitation/Recovery Program

5280 High Blood Pressure and Stroke
National Stroke Association
9707 E Easter Lane   303-649-9299
Centennial, CO 80112-3747   800-787-6537
Fax: 303-649-1328
info@stroke.org
www.stroke.org
Colette Lafosse, Director Rehabilitation/Recovery Program

5281 Mobility: Issues Facing Stroke Survivors and Their Families
National Stroke Association

9707 E Easter Lane   303-649-9299
Centennial, CO 80112-3747   800-787-6537
Fax: 303-649-1328
info@stroke.org
www.stroke.org
Colette Lafosse, Director Rehabilitation/Recovery Program

5282 Recurrent Stroke
National Stroke Association
9707 E Easter Lane   303-649-9299
Centennial, CO 80112-3747   800-787-6537
Fax: 303-649-1328
info@stroke.org
www.stroke.org
Colette Lafosse, Director Rehabilitation/Recovery Program

5283 Smoking Cessation: Be Smoke Free in 3 Minutes
National Stroke Association
9707 E Easter Lane   303-649-9299
Centennial, CO 80112-3747   800-787-6537
Fax: 303-649-1328
info@stroke.org
www.stroke.org
Colette Lafosse, Director Rehabilitation/Recovery Program

5284 Transient Ischemic Attack
National Stroke Association
9707 E Easter Lane   303-649-9299
Centennial, CO 80112-3747   800-787-6537
Fax: 303-649-1328
info@stroke.org
www.stroke.org
Seemant Chaturvedi MD, Author
Steven R. Levine MD, Author

Audio & Video

5285 Stroke: Touching the Soul of Your Family
National Stroke Association
9707 E Easter Lane   303-649-9299
Centennial, CO 80112-3747   800-787-6537
Fax: 303-649-1328
info@stroke.org
www.stroke.org
Fifteen minute video chronicling three stroke survivors and their courageous struggle to overcome daily challenges and educate others about stroke.
Colette Lafosse, Director Rehabilitation/Recovery Program

Web Sites

5286 American Society of Hypertension
To organize and conduct educational seminars, materials, and products in all aspects of hypertension and other cardiovascular diseases.

5287 Healing Well
www.healingwell.com
An online health resource guide to medical news, chat, information and articles, newsgroups and message boards, books, disease-related web sites, medical directories, and more for patients, friends, and family coping with disabling diseases, disorders, or chronic illnesses.

5288 Health Finder
www.healthfinder.gov
Searchable, carefully developed web site offering information on over 1000 topics. Developed by the US Department of Health and Human Services, the site can be used in both English and Spanish.

5289 Healthlink USA
www.healthlinkusa.com
Links to websites which may include treatment, cures, diagnosis, prevention, support groups, email lists, messageboards, personal stories, risk factors, statistics, research and more.

5290 Hypertension: Journal of the American Heart Association
hyper.ahajournals.org

Lists current issues of journals about hypertension and the American Heart Association.

5291 Inter-American Society of Hypertension

www.iashonline.org

Website hosted by IASH, a non-profit professional organization devoted to the understanding, prevention and control of hypertension and vascular diseases in the American population. Members from 20 different countries in the Americas as well as Europe, Australia and Asia. Stimulates research and the exchange of ideas in hypertension and vascular diseases among physicians and scientists. Promotes the detection, control and prevention of hypertension and other cardiovascular risk factors.

5292 Lifeclinic.Com

www.lifeclinic.com

Online information about blood pressure, hypertension, diabetes, cholesterol, stroke, heart failure and more. Maintains current, up-to-date and accurate information for patients to help them manage their conditions better and to improve communications between them and their doctors.

5293 Mayo Clinic Health Oasis

www.mayohealth.org

Mission is to empower people to manage their health, by providing useful and up-to-date information and tools that reflect the expertise and standard of excellence of the Mayo Clinic.

5294 MedicineNet

www.medicinenet.com

An online resource for consumers providing easy-to-read, authoritative medical and health information.

5295 Medscape

www.medscape.com

Medscape offers specialists, primary care physicians, and other health professionals the Web's most robust and integrated medical information and educational tools.

5296 National Heart, Lung & Blood Institute

www.nhlbi.nih.gov

Information on the scientific investigation of heart, blood vessel, lung and blood disorders. Oversee research, demonstration, prevention, education and training activities in these fields and emphasizes the control of stroke.

5297 WebMD

www.webmd.com

Provides credible information, supportive communities, and in-depth reference material about health subjects. A source for original and timely health information as well as material from well known content providers.

Description

5298 Impotence

Impotence, also called erectile dysfunction (ED), is defined as the inability of a male to achieve and maintain an erection of sufficient quality to allow sexual intercourse. ED is very common, affecting millions of American males. Although it may occur at any age, it becomes dramatically more common with advancing age. Impotence may be caused by diabetes, circulatory disturbance, genital injury, hormonal disorders, medication side effects, depression, surgery (for instance, prostate removal) and many less well-characterized physical and psychological states. Impotence may be situational, that is, involving place, time, partner and degree of self-esteem.

Few cases of impotence are completely cured, but several kinds of effective treatment exist, including correction, if possible, of underlying causes. Oral medications that increase blood flow to the penis have been effective in many instances (phosphodiesterase-5 inhibitors). Psychological factors that accompany ED should be considered in every case, including behavioral therapy and counseling, as needed.

National Agencies & Associations

5299 Center for Reconstructive Urology
333 City Boulevard W   714-456-2951
Orange, CA 92868   Fax: 714-456-7263
www.centerforreconstructiveurology.org
A regional, national, and internation tertiary referral center committed to the treatment of male urethra disorders.
Joel Gelman, MD, Director

5300 National Institute of Diabetes & Digestive & Kidney Diseases
31 Center Drive   800-860-8747
Bethesda, MD 20892-2560   TTY: 866-569-1162
healthinfo@niddk.nih.gov
www.niddk.nih.gov
Research areas include diabetes, digestive diseases, endocrine and metabolic diseases, hematologic diseases, kidney disease, liver disease, urologic diseases, as well as matters relating to nutrition and obesity.
Griffin P. Rodgers, MD, MACP, Director
Gregory Germino, MD, Deputy Officer

5301 Urology Care Foundation
1000 Corporate Boulevard   410-689-3700
Linthicum, MD 21090   800-828-7866
Fax: 410-689-3998
info@urologycarefoundation.org
www.urologyhealth.org
A charitable organization whose mission is the prevention and cure of urologic diseases through the expansion of research, education, and public awareness.
Harris M. Nagler, MD, FACS, President
Gopal H. Badlani, MD, Secretary

Research Centers

5302 Central New York Male Sexual Dysfunction Center
357 Genesee Street   315-363-8862
Oneida, NY 13421   888-269-6732
Fax: 315-363-5477
www.cnymsdc.com
Burman, Director

5303 Male Sexual Dysfunction Clinic
3401 N Central Avenue   800-788-2873
Chicago, IL 60634   800-788-2873
Fax: 847-231-4130
Helping men overcome male sexual dysfunctions such as impotence since 1981.
Sheldon O MD, Director

5304 New York Male Reproductive Center: Sexual Dysfunction Unit
161 Fort Washington Avenue   212-305-0123
New York, NY 10032   Fax: 212-305-0126
The New York Male Reproductive Center at Columbia-Presbyterian Medical Center offers state-of-the-art diagnosis and treatment for impotence. Treatments include surgical and non-surgical procedures.
Ridwan Shabs

Support Groups & Hotlines

5305 Impotence Information Center
PO Box 9   800-843-4315
Minneapolis, MN 55440
MacKenzie, Founder

5306 Impotents Anonymous
8630 Fenton Street   301-588-5777
Silver Spring, MD 20910-3803
Serves as an educational organization providing concerned individuals with information regarding impotence.
Bruce

5307 National Health Information Center
Office of Disease Prevention & Health Promotion
1101 Wootton Pkwy   Fax: 240-453-8281
Rockville, MD 20852   odphpinfo@hhs.gov
www.health.gov/nhic
Supports public health education by maintaining a calendar of National Health Observances; helps connect consumers and health professionals to organizations that can best answer questions and provide up-to-date contact information from reliable sources; updates on a yearly basis toll-free numbers for health information, Federal health clearinghouses and info centers.
Don Wright, MD, MPH, Director

Books

5308 Impotence: How to Overcome It
HealthProInk Publishing
562 Wind Drift Lane   313-355-3686
Spring Lake, MI 49456-2168
Priyantha Hettiarachchi, Author

5309 It's Not All in Your Head
Impotence Institute of America
8201 Corporate Drive   301-577-0650
Landover, MD 20785-2230
A couple's guide to overcoming impotence.
Gordon J. G. Asmundson PhD, Author
Steven Taylor PhD, Author

Newsletters

5310 Impotence Worldwide
8201 Corporate Drive   301-577-0650
Landover, MD 20785-2230
Provides information from professionals and lay persons concerning impotence plus manufactured product information.
Monthly

5311 Your Sexuality & Health
Impotence Resource Center
333 City Boulevard West,   714-456-2951
Orange, CA 92868-1593   800-433-4215
Fax: 714-456-7263
nfo@centerforreconstructiveurology.org
www.centerforreconstructiveurology.org

Quarterly newsletter that features articles by medical experts and highlights current research and tidbits of healthy living advice.
Quarterly

Pamphlets

5312 Answers to the Most Asked Questions About Impotence
Impotence World Services
8201 Corporate Drive   301-577-0650
Landover, MD 20785-2230

5313 Impotence Causes and Treatments
American Medical Systems
10700 Bren Road E   952-933-4666
Minnetonka, MN 55343   800-843-4315
                                   Fax: 952-930-6157
                                   www.visitams.com
Offers information on what impotence is, physical and emotional causes, treatments, questions and answers.

5314 Male Treatment Guide
Impotence Resource Center
333 City Boulevard West,   714-456-2951
Orange, CA 92868-1593   800-433-4215
                                   Fax: 714-456-7263
                    nfo@centerforreconstructiveurology.org
                    www.centerforreconstructiveurology.org
Explains impotence - what it is, what causes it and how it is treated.
Free

5315 Woman's Perspective
Impotence Resource Center
334 City Boulevard West,   714-456-2952
Orange, CA 92869-1593   800-433-4215
                                   Fax: 714-456-7264
                    nfo@centerforreconstructiveurology.org
                    www.centerforreconstructiveurology.org
Talking with your partner about impotence and choosing a treatment together.
Free

Audio & Video

5316 Impotence Treatment Options
Impotence Resource Center
335 City Boulevard West,   714-456-2953
Orange, CA 92870-1593   800-433-4215
                                   Fax: 714-456-7265
                    nfo@centerforreconstructiveurology.org
                    www.centerforreconstructiveurology.org
Actual taping of a men's sexual health seminar - presented by Gary Leach, MD.

5317 Male Treatment Guide
Impotence Resource Center
336 City Boulevard West,   714-456-2954
Orange, CA 92871-1593   800-433-4215
                                   Fax: 714-456-7266
                    nfo@centerforreconstructiveurology.org
                    www.centerforreconstructiveurology.org
Explains impotence - what it is, what causes it and how it is treated.
Audio Tape

5318 Medical Management of Impotence
Impotence Resource Center
337 City Boulevard West,   714-456-2955
Orange, CA 92872-1593   800-433-4215
                                   Fax: 714-456-7267
                    nfo@centerforreconstructiveurology.org
                    www.centerforreconstructiveurology.org

5319 Woman's Perspective
Impotence Resource Center
338 City Boulevard West,   714-456-2956
Orange, CA 92873-1593   800-433-4215
                                   Fax: 714-456-7268
                    nfo@centerforreconstructiveurology.org
                    www.centerforreconstructiveurology.org

Talking with your partner about impotence and choosing a treatment together.
Audio Tape

Web Sites

5320 American Foundation for Urologic Disease
                                   www.urologyhealth.org
The Urology Care Foundation is committed to promoting urology research and education. They work with researchers, healthcare professionals, patients and caregivers to improve patients' lives.

5321 Family Meds
At Familymeds.com VIPPS certified online pharmacy, they process all of our prescriptions through a fully U.S. and Connecticut licensed and accredited pharmacy based in Farmington, CT.

5322 Healing Well
                                   www.healingwell.com
An online health resource guide to medical news, chat, information and articles, newsgroups and message boards, books, disease-related web sites, medical directories, and more for patients, friends, and family coping with disabling diseases, disorders, or chronic illnesses.

5323 Health Finder
                                   www.healthfinder.gov
Searchable, carefully developed web site offering information on over 1000 topics. Developed by the US Department of Health and Human Services, the site can be used in both English and Spanish.

5324 Healthlink USA
                                   www.healthlinkusa.com
Health information concerning treatment, cures, prevention, diagnosis, risk factors, research, support groups, email lists, personal stories and much more. Updated regularly.

5325 Impotence Resource Center of the Geddings Osbon Sr Foundation
                    www.centerforreconstructiveurology.org
A regional, national, and international tertiary referral center dedicated to the treatment of disorders of the male urethra and external genitalia. In addition to patient care, there mission includes clinical and laboratory research and teaching.

5326 Impotence Specialists.com
Offers information on physicians in your area, treatment options, online resources and more. A guide to the nation's impotence specialists.

5327 Impotence World Association
Informs and educates the public on the subject of impotence and its causes and treatments. Serving the impotence industry since 1983 by bringing total care to the treatment of impotence.

5328 MedicineNet
                                   www.medicinenet.com
An online resource for consumers providing easy-to-read, authoritative medical and health information.

5329 Medscape
                                   www.medscape.com
Medscape offers specialists, primary care physicians, and other health professionals the Web's most robust and integrated medical information and educational tools.

5330 WebMD
                                   www.webmd.com
Provides credible information, supportive communities, and in-depth reference material about health subjects. A source for original and timely health information as well as material from well known content providers.

Description

5331 Incontinence

Urinary incontinence is the involuntary leakage of urine, whether during waking or sleeping hours. One common type is urge incontinence, resulting from involuntary bladder contractions. The person feels a sudden urge to urinate, so intense that it may not be controlled long enough to reach the toilet. Common causes of urge incontinence are urinary tract infections, spinal cord injury, and kidney stones. Stress incontinence is the instantaneous leakage of urine without bladder contractions. It manifests as loss of urine during stress events, such as coughing, sneezing, laughing, or lifting. This may occur in women due to weak bladder tone from multiple pregnancies. In men, stress incontinence can occur after prostate removal or trauma to the bladder. Overflow incontinence, in which the bladder cannot control urine output, can be caused by nerve injury, alcoholism, and some diseases. Symptoms include urgency and having to urinate more often (frequency) and at night (nocturia). Interstitial cystitis or bladder pain syndrome increases urinary frequency and urgency, accompanied by pain as the bladder fills. Interstitial cystitis can result from the immune system attacking the bladder or routine abuse of the drug ketamine.

Treatment of incontinence focuses on therapy for the underlying causes. Infections are treated with the appropriate antibiotics.

Treatment of incontinence focuses on therapy for the underlying causes. Infections are treated with the appropriate antibiotics. Stress incontinence in women can be treated with exercises to strengthen the bladder muscles. Medications have side effects and can provide short-term relief but should not be relied upon for long-term relief. Two main group of medications include antimuscarinic medications (e.g., oxybutynin, solifenacin, darifenacin) and mirabegron (a B3 receptor agonterstitial cystitis is treated with oral pentosan polysulfate and DMSO, which is administered straight into the bladder. Other therapies include biofeedback and electrical stimulation. Severe cases may require surgical repair. Urinary incontinence remains largely a neglected problem, despite the fact that it can often be successfully treated.

National Agencies & Associations

5332 National Association for Continence
PO Box 1019
Charleston, SC 29402-1019
843-377-0900
800-BLA-DDER
Fax: 843-377-0905
memberservices@nafc.org
www.nafc.org
Founded as Help for Incontinent People, NAFC is the foremost consumer advocacy organization dedicated to helping people who struggle with incontinence and related voiding dysfunction. Its mission is focused on public education, awareness and collaboration.
Donna Browdie, Chair
James Firman EdD, President/CEO

5333 National Council on Aging
251 18th Street S.
Arlington, VA 22202
571-527-3900
Fax: 202-479-0735
TTY: 202-479-6674
info@ncoa.org
www.ncoa.org
The nation's first charitable organization dedicated to promoting the dignity, independence, well-being and contributions of older Americans. The council has a goal of improving the health and economic well-being of 10 million older adults by 2020.
James P. Firman, EdD, President & CEO
Howard Bedlin, VP, Public Policy & Advocacy

5334 National Institute of Diabetes & Digestive & Kidney Diseases
Office Of Communications and Public Liaison, NIH
31 Center Drive
Bethesda, MD 20892-2560
800-860-8747
TTY: 866-569-1162
healthinfo@niddk.nih.gov
www.niddk.nih.gov
Research areas include diabetes, digestive diseases, endocrine and metabolic diseases, hematologic diseases, kidney disease, liver disease, urologic diseases, as well as matters relating to nutrition and obesity.
Griffin P. Rodgers, MD, MACP, Director
Gregory Germino, MD, Deputy Director

5335 Simon Foundation for Continence
PO Box 815
Wilmette, IL 60091
847-864-3913
800-237-4666
Fax: 847-864-9758
info@simonfoundation.org
www.simonfoundation.org
Seeks to remove the stigma around incontinence; provides educational materials to patients, their families, and the health care professionals who provide patient care.
Cheryl B. Gartley, Founder & President
Elizabeth A. LaGro, Vice President

5336 Urology Care Foundation
1000 Corporate Boulevard
Linthicum, MD 21090
410-689-3700
800-828-7866
Fax: 410-689-3998
info@urologycarefoundation.org
www.urologyhealth.org
A charitable organization whose mission is the prevention and cure of urologic diseases through the expansion of research, education and public awareness.
Harris M. Nagler, MD, FACS, President
Gopal H. Badlani, MD, Secretary

Foundations

5337 International Foundation for Functional Gastrointestinal Disorders (IFFGD)
PO Box 170864
Milwaukee, WI 53217
414-964-1799
888-964-2001
iffgd@iffgd.org
www.iffgd.org
Non-profit education, support, and research organization devoted to increasing awareness and understanding of functional gastrointestinal disorders, including irritable bowel syndrome (IBS), constipation, diarrhea, pain, and incontinence. Mission is to inform, assist and support people affected by these disorders.
Nancy J. Norton, Founder
Ceciel T. Rooker, President

Support Groups & Hotlines

5338 Greater New York Pull-Thru Network
62 Edgewood Avenue
Wyckoff, NJ 07481
201-891-5977
National support network providing emotional support and information to patients and families of children who have had or will have a pull-thru type surgery to correct an imperforate anus or associated malformation, Hirschsprung's or other fecal incontinence problems. Support group meetings held quarterly.

5339 National Health Information Center
Office of Disease Prevention & Health Promotion
1101 Wootton Pkwy   Fax: 240-453-8281
Rockville, MD 20852   odphpinfo@hhs.gov
                                                  www.health.gov/nhic
Supports public health education by maintaining a calendar of National Health Observances; helps connect consumers and health professionals to organizations that can best answer questions and provide up-to-date contact information from reliable sources; updates on a yearly basis toll-free numbers for health information, Federal health clearinghouses and info centers.
Don Wright, MD, MPH, Director

5340 Simon Foundation Helpline for Incontinence Information
Simon Foundation for Continence
PO Box 815   847-864-3913
Wilmette, IL 60091   800-237-4666
                                                  Fax: 847-864-9758
                                                  info@simonfoundation.org
                                                  www.simonfoundation.org
Offers information and help to persons with incontinence problems and professionals who work with them.
Cheryle Brown MD, Director

5341 University of California at San Francisco Women's Continence Center
2356 Sutter Street   415-885-7788
San Francisco, CA 94115   877-366-8532
                                                  coe.ucsf.edu/wcc
Offers a comprehensive array of clinical services for women with incontinence, urethal or bladder dysfuntion and pelvic support problems.
Jeanette S Vecchiarello, President/Board of Directors
Doni DeBolt, Executive Director

Books

5342 Managing Incontinence: a Guide to Living with Loss of Bladder Control
Simon Foundation for Incontinence
PO Box 815   847-864-3913
Wilmette, IL 60091   800-237-4666
                                                  Fax: 847-864-9768
                                                  simoninfo@simonfoundation.org
                                                  www.simonfoundation.org
Seeks to bring the topic of incontinence out of the closet and remove the associated stigma; provides information to patients, their families and the health care professionals who provide patient care.
Quarterly
Cheryle B Gartley, President
Cheryle Gartley, Author

5343 Pocket Guide for Continence Care
National Association for Continence
PO Box 1019   843-377-0900
Charleston, SC 29402   800-252-3337
                                                  Fax: 843-377-0905
                                                  memberservices@nafc.org
                                                  www.nafc.org
Condensed version of the Blueprint for Continence Care, this guide is designed for a first line supervisor or any health care professional in any eldercare environment to help address any issues related to bladder health. The guide is perfect for a quick referral because it can actually fit in the healthcare professional's pocket.
Nancy Muller, Executive Director
Caryn Antos, Publicity/Publications Associate

5344 Resource Guide: Products and Services for Incontinence
National Association for Continence
PO Box 1019   843-377-0900
Charleston, SC 29402   800-252-3337
                                                  Fax: 843-377-0905
                                                  memberservices@nafc.org
                                                  www.nafc.org
Complete directory of products and services available. Categories include disposable products, reusable products, skin care products, deodorizing products, pelvic organ support devices, medica-

tions to treat incontinence and others. Also includes a listing of distributors and mail/phone order companies.
Nancy Muller, Executive Director
Caryn Antos, Publicity/Publications Associate

5345 Your Personal Guide to Bladder Health
National Association for Continence
PO Box 1019   843-377-0900
Charleston, SC 29402   800-252-3337
                                                  Fax: 843-377-0905
                                                  memberservices@nafc.org
                                                  www.nafc.org
Designed for residents of assisted living environments, other older individuals living independently and their involved family members. It encompasses a wide variety of informative topics, including diet and daily habits, pelvic muscle exercises odor control and more.
48 pages
Nancy Muller, Executive Director
Caryn Antos, Publicity/Publications Associate

Magazines

5346 Digestive Health Matters
Intl. Foundation for Gastrointestinal Disorders
PO Box 170864   414-964-1799
Milwaukee, WI 53217-0864   888-964-2001
                                                  Fax: 414-964-7176
                                                  iffgd@iffgd.org
                                                  www.iffgd.org
Quarterly journal focuses on upper and lower gastrointestinal disorders in adults and children. Educational pamphlets and factsheets are available. Patient and professional membership.

Newsletters

5347 Discoveries
National Association for Continence
PO Box 1019   843-377-0900
Charleston, SC 29402   800-252-3337
                                                  Fax: 843-377-0905
                                                  memberservices@nafc.org
                                                  www.nafc.org
Compendium comprised of the most recently released incontinence products and newly approved protocol. Includes editorial sections, authored by leading clinicians and researchers, describing new product technology and research in other medical advances related to continence care.
32 pages BiAnnual
Nancy Muller, Executive Director
Caryn Antos, Publicity/Publications Associate

5348 Informer
Simon Foundation for Incontinence
PO Box 815   847-864-3913
Wilmette, IL 60091   800-237-4666
                                                  Fax: 847-864-9768
                                                  simoninfo@simonfoundation.org
                                                  www.simonfoundation.org
Seeks to bring the topic of incontinence out of the closet and remove the associated stigma; provides information to patients, their families, and the health care professionals who provide patient care.
Quarterly
Cheryle B Gartley, President
Bret Easton Ellis, Author

5349 Intestinal Fortitude
Intestinal Disease Foundation
One Station Square   412-261-5888
Pittsburgh, PA 15219   Fax: 412-471-2722
Newsletter, brochures and books for Intestinal Disease Foundation members.
Dwight Franklin, Author

5350 Participate
IFFGD

PO Box 17864
Milwaukee, WI 53217-0864

414-964-1799
888-964-2001
Fax: 414-964-7176
iffgd@iffgd.org
www.aboutincontinence.org

Provides information for people affected by the various forms of functional bowel disorders, including irritable bowel syndrome, constipation, diarrhea, pain and incontinence.
Quarterly

5351 Pull-Thru Network News
Greater New York Pull-Thru Network
62 Edgewood Avenue
Wyckoff, NJ 07481-3456

201-891-5977
www.pullthrough.org

Quarterly newsletter for patients and families who have had or will have a pull-thru type surgery to correct an imperforate anus or associated malformation, Hirschsprung's or other fecal incontinence problem.

5352 Quality Care
National Association for Continence
PO Box 1019
Charleston, SC 29402

843-377-0900
800-252-3337
Fax: 843-377-0905
memberservices@nafc.org
www.nafc.org

Quarterly newsletter addressing causes, symptoms, management and treatment options for incontinence and related disorders.
Quarterly
Nancy Muller, Executive Director
Caryn Antos, Publicity/Publications Associate

Pamphlets

5353 Bladder Control for Women
National Kidney and Urologic Diseases Information
3 Information Way
Bethesda, MD 20892-3580

800-891-5390
Fax: 301-907-8906
nkudic@info.nidkk.nih.gov
www.kidney.niddk.nih.gov

Comprehensive introduction to the causes, symptoms, and treatments for bladder control problems in women.

5354 Exercising Your Pelvic Muscles
National Kidney and Urologic Diseases Information
3 Information Way
Bethesda, MD 20892-3580

800-891-5390
Fax: 301-907-8906
nkudic@info.nidkk.nih.gov
www.kidney.niddk.nih.gov

A description of exercises for the pelvic floor muscles, called Kegel exercises, and how they can help to restore or maintain bladder control.

5355 Menopause and Bladder Control
National Kidney and Urologic Diseases Information
3 Information Way
Bethesda, MD 20892-3580

800-891-5390
Fax: 301-907-8906
nkudic@info.nidkk.nih.gov
www.kidney.niddk.nih.gov

An introduction to the changes to your body that occur during menopause, how these changes can result in loss of bladder control, and how your health care team can help you restore or maintain bladder control.

5356 NAFC Fact Sheets
National Association for Continence
PO Box 1019
Charleston, SC 29402

843-377-0900
800-252-3337
Fax: 843-377-0905
memberservices@nafc.org
www.nafc.org

Offering helpful tips and information on a variety of topics, the sheets provide consumers and professionals with the necessary information on managing incontinence. Some titles include medications, diet and daily habits, odor control, prostatectomy and many more.
Nancy Muller, Executive Director
Caryn Antos, Publicity/Publications Associate

5357 Pregnancy, Childbirth, and Bladder Control
National Kidney and Urologic Diseases Information
3 Information Way
Bethesda, MD 20892-3580

800-891-5390
Fax: 301-907-8906
nkudic@info.nidkk.nih.gov
www.kidney.niddk.nih.gov

A look at the effects that pregnancy and childbearing can have on bladder control and ways you can counter those effects.

5358 Talking to Your Health Care Team About Bladder Control
National Kidney and Urologic Diseases Information
3 Information Way
Bethesda, MD 20892-3580

800-891-5390
Fax: 301-907-8906
nkudic@info.nidkk.nih.gov
www.kidney.niddk.nih.gov

Tips for giving your health care provider the information needed to diagnose and treat your bladder control problem. Includes a questionnaire for you to fill out and take to your first appointment.

5359 Urinary Incontinence in Women
National Kidney and Urologic Diseases Information
3 Information Way
Bethesda, MD 20892-3580

800-891-5390
Fax: 301-907-8906
nkudic@info.nidkk.nih.gov
www.kidney.niddk.nih.gov

An overview of the types, diagnosis, and treatment of urinary incontinence in women.

5360 What Your Female Patients Want to Know About Bladder Control
National Kidney and Urologic Diseases Information
3 Information Way
Bethesda, MD 20892-3580

800-891-5390
Fax: 301-907-8906
nkudic@info.nidkk.nih.gov
www.kidney.niddk.nih.gov

Fact sheet with tips for health care providers on raising the issue of incontinence with female patients who may be reluctant to talk about their problem.

5361 Your Body's Design for Bladder Control
National Kidney and Urologic Diseases Information
3 Information Way
Bethesda, MD 20892-3580

800-891-5390
Fax: 301-907-8906
nkudic@info.nidkk.nih.gov
www.kidney.niddk.nih.gov

An introduction to the female urinary system. Includes diagrams of the bladder and pelvic floor muscles.

5362 Your Daily Bladder Diary
National Kidney and Urologic Diseases Information
3 Information Way
Bethesda, MD 20892-3580

800-891-5390
Fax: 301-907-8906
nkudic@info.nidkk.nih.gov
www.kidney.niddk.nih.gov

An easy-to-use form for patients to note liquid intake, trips to the bathroom, urine leaks, and other details that may help explain your incontinence.

5363 Your Medicines and Bladder Control
National Kidney and Urologic Diseases Information
3 Information Way
Bethesda, MD 20892-3580

800-891-5390
Fax: 301-907-8906
www.kidney.niddk.nih.gov

Booklet describing the effects that your medications could have on bladder control, with a recommendation for discussing all your medicines with your doctor.

Audio & Video

5364 Solution Starts with You
Simon Foundation for Continence
PO Box 815
Wilmette, IL 60091

847-864-3913
800-237-4666
Fax: 847-864-9758
cbgartley@simonfoundation.org
www.simonfoundation.org

Seeks to bring the topic of incontinence out of the closet and remove the associated stigma; provides information to patients, their

families, and the health care professionals who provide patient care.
Quarterly
Cheryle Gartley, Founder/President
Jasmine Schmidt, Director of Education

Web Sites

5365 American Foundation for Urologic Disease

www.urologyhealth.org
The Urology Care Foundation is committed to promoting urology research and education. They work with researchers, healthcare professionals, patients and caregivers to improve patients' lives.

5366 Healing Well

www.healingwell.com
An online health resource guide to medical news, chat, information and articles, newsgroups and message boards, books, disease-related web sites, medical directories, and more for patients, friends, and family coping with disabling diseases, disorders, or chronic illnesses.

5367 Health Finder

www.healthfinder.gov
Searchable, carefully developed web site offering information on over 1000 topics. Developed by the US Department of Health and Human Services, the site can be used in both English and Spanish.

5368 Healthlink USA

www.healthlinkusa.com
Health information concerning treatment, cures, prevention, diagnosis, risk factors, research, support groups, email lists, personal stories and much more. Updated regularly.

5369 MedicineNet

www.medicinenet.com
An online resource for consumers providing easy-to-read, authoritative medical and health information.

5370 Medscape

www.medscape.com
Medscape offers specialists, primary care physicians, and other health professionals the Web's most robust and integrated medical information and educational tools.

5371 National Association for Continence

www.nafc.org
Interactive website packed with useful information about diagnosis, treatment options and management solutions for incontinence. The site currently features a specialist search engine of healthcare providers who have recieved specific training in the diagnosis and treatment of incontinence to assist consumers in locating a specialist in their area. Other features include archived Quality Care articles, a message board, online database of active support groups and much more.

5372 Simon Foundation for Continence

www.simonfoundation.org
Seeks to bring the topic of incontinence out of the closet and remove the associated stigma; provides educational materials to patients, their families, and the health care professionals who provide patient care.

5373 WebMD

www.webmd.com
Provides credible information, supportive communities, and in-depth reference material about health subjects. A source for original and timely health information as well as material from well known content providers.

Description

5374 Infertility

Infertility is defined as the failure to achieve conception by couples who have not used contraception for at least one year, and affects 1 in 5 couples in the United States.

Female causes of infertility include dysfunction of the ovaries (20 percent of couples), blockage of the tubes connecting the ovaries to the uterus (30 percent), and abnormal secretions (5 percent). Women older than 35 tend to, on average, have reduced ovarian reserves, especially if they only have one functional ovary. Infertility in males is mostly related to sperm disorders (35 percent of couples), either insufficient production of sperm, ineffective sperm, or defective delivery of sperm. Unidentified factors account for the remaining 10 percent of couples.

A variety of tests are needed to determine the exact cause of infertility and then identify the appropriate treatment options. Failure to conceive can be both an emotional and financial burden on couples. Counseling and psychological support are important parts of treatment. Assisted reproductive technologies are available, to help infertile couples conceive, but such procedures are very expensive and require a substantial commitment for success.

National Agencies & Associations

5375 American Pregnancy Association
3007 Skyway Circle N
Irving, TX 75038
800-672-2296
info@americanpregnancy.org
www.americanpregnancy.org
Provides the public with information about reproductive disease and supports families during struggles with pregnancy, infertility, and adoption. Exists to serve the unique needs of men and women confronting infertility issues.

5376 American Society for Reproductive Medicine
1209 Montgomery Highway
Birmingham, AL 35216-2809
205-978-5000
Fax: 205-978-5005
asrm@asrm.org
www.asrm.org
A private, non-profit medical organization devoted to advancing the knowledge, understanding and expertise in all phases of reproductive medicine and biology. Offers patient education brochures, recommended readings and support. Publishes professional journal and consumer publications.
Richard H. Reindollar, MD, Chief Executive Officer

5377 HealthyWomen
1 Harding Road
Red Bank, NJ 07701
732-530-3425
877-986-9472
info@healthywomen.org
www.healthywomen.org
Independent, non-profit organization seeking to educate women in all areas of health, to allow them to make informed choices. The HealthyWomen website features numerous tools and health calculators, plus other media.
Beth Battaglino, RN, Chief Executive Officer
Phyllis E. Greenberger, Sr. VP, Science & Health Policy

5378 International Council on Infertility Information Dissemination
5765 F Burke Centre Parkway
Burke, VA 22015
INCIIDinfo@inciid.org
www.inciid.org

Provides information on infertility, pregnancy loss, adoption, high risk pregnancy and parenting.
Marla Neufeld, Esq., Board
Geoffrey Sher, MD, Board

5379 Lilliput Families
8391 Auburn Boulevard
Citrus Heights, CA 95610
916-238-3503
855-912-2622
info@lilliput.org
www.lilliput.org
Adoption agency bridging the gap between foster care, public and private sectors.
Karen Alvord, LCSW, CEO
Carol Ramirez, LCSW, Chief Programs Officer

5380 National Women's Health Network
1413 K Street
Washington, DC 20005
202-682-2640
Fax: 202-682-2648
nwhn@nwhn.org
www.nwhn.org
Non-profit organization advocating for national policies that protect and promote all women's health, and providing evidence-based independent information.
Cindy Pearson, Executive Director
Sarah Christopherson, Policy Advocacy Director

5381 RESOLVE: The National Infertility Association
7918 Jones Branch Drive
McLean, VA 22102
703-556-7172
Fax: 703-506-3266
info@resolve.org
www.resolve.org
A nationwide non-profit organization serving the unique needs of those striving to build a family. Provides informed help to people who are experiencing infertility.
Barbara Collura, President & CEO
Marnee Beck, Manager

State Agencies & Associations

Alabama

5382 RESOLVE of Alabama
1760 Old Meadow Road
McLean, VA 22102
703-556-7172
888-473-3062
Fax: 703-506-3266
info@southeast.resolve.org
www.southeast.resolve.org/
Barbara Nelson, President
Denny Ceizyk, VP

Arizona

5383 RESOLVE of Valley of the Sun
PO Box 36252
Phoenix, AZ 85067-6252
602-995-3933
resolveaz@hotmail.com
Tina Collura, President/CEO
Margaret Chandler Berardelli, Director, Development

Arkansas

5384 RESOLVE Affiliate of Northwest Arkansas
2230 Country Way
Fayetteville, AR 72703-4215
501-521-3763
888-895-6055
info@southcentral.resolve.org
www.southcentral.resolve.org/
Barbara Waldron, CA/San Diego Chair

California

5385 RESOLVE of Greater Los Angeles
PO Box 12529
Newport Beach, CA 92658
310-326-2630
877-203-7771
info@southwest.resolve.org
www.southwest.resolve.org
Mari Waldron, CA/San Diego Chair

5386 RESOLVE of Greater San Diego
PO Box 12529
Newport Beach, CA 92658-7385
Mari Munoz, Northern California Coordinator
310-326-2630
877-203-7771

5387 RESOLVE of Northern California
312 Sutter Street
San Francisco, CA 94108
415-788-6772
888-591-6663
Fax: 415-788-6774
www.northpacific.resolve.org/
Volunteer-based organization that provides infertility education
adoption information advocacy and support.
Tracie Fletcher, Local Area Affiliate Chair

Colorado

5388 RESOLVE of Colorado
PO Box 260725
Littleton, CO 80163-0725
303-469-5261
888-592-4449
www.mountain.resolve.org/

Jennifer Malave, Support Services
Maryann Post, Helpline Coordinator

Connecticut

5389 RESOLVE of Fairfield County
PO Box 930
S Norwalk, CT 06856-0930
914-686-1490
888-765-2810
Fax: 203-255-2561
info@northeast.resolve.org

Anne Odeen-Lodato,, Chair
Erin Lasker, Executive Director

5390 RESOLVE of Greater Hartford
PO Box 290964
Wethersfield, CT 06129
781-890-2225
admin@resolvenewengland.org
www.resolvenewengland.org/

Pam Bare, Regional Chair
Cindy Peterson, Volunteer Coordinator

District of Columbia

5391 RESOLVE of the Washington Metro Area
PO Box 3423
Merrifield, VA 22116-3423
202-362-5555
888-583-4441
Cindy Gedaro, Florida, Orlando Coordinator

Florida

5392 RESOLVE Affiliate of Central Florida
1050 W Morse Boulevard
Winter Park, FL 32789
407-637-0142
888-473-3062
resolveofcentralflorida@gmail.com
www.southeast.resolve.org/
Susanna Witt, Florida, Tampa Coordinator
Kathy Fountain, Florida, Tampa Coordinator

5393 RESOLVE of North Florida
1929 Logging Lane
Jacksonville, FL 32221-2071
904-737-0140
888-473-3062
Nicole@theadoptionconsultancy.com
www.southeast.resolve.org/

Nicole Linder, Cooordinator

5394 RESOLVE of South Florida
3342 SW 51 Street
Ft Lauderdale, FL 33312
954-749-9500
888-473-3062
resolvesf@yahoo.com
www.southeast.resolve.org/

Elise Badey, Coordinator
Renee Whitley, Advocacy Chair

Georgia

5395 RESOLVE of Georgia
3904 N Druid Hills Road
Decatur, GA 30333
404-233-8443
888-473-3062
Katie9924@hotmail.com

Kate Collura, President/CEO
Margaret Chandler Berardelli, Director, Development

Hawaii

5396 RESOLVE of Hawaii
PO Box 29193
Honolulu, HI 96820
808-528-8559
888-591-6663
info@resolveofhawaii.org
www.res.pub30.convio.net/Regions/north-p
Barbara Collura, President/CEO
Margaret Chandler Berardelli, Director, Development

Illinois

5397 RESOLVE of Illinois
PO Box 56
Hinsdale, IL 60521
773-743-1623
888-255-1399
info@greatlakes.resolve.org
www.res.pub30.convio.net/Regions/great-l
Barbara Collura, President/CEO
Margaret Chandler Berardelli, Director, Development

Indiana

5398 RESOLVE of Indiana
5155 Sandy Court
Pittsboro, IN 46167-9129
317-329-9519
888-255-1399
info@greatlakes.resolve.org
www.res.pub30.convio.net/Regions/great-l
Barbara Collura, President/CEO
Margaret Chandler Berardelli, Director, Development

Iowa

5399 RESOLVE Affiliate of Iowa
1348 Atlantic
Dunuque, IA 52001
319-557-2763
888-959-0333
info@midwest.resolve.org
www.res.pub30.convio.net/Regions/midwest
Barbara Verhiley, Kentucky State Coordinator

Kentucky

5400 RESOLVE of Kentucky
851 Van Dyke Mill Road
Taylorsville, KY 40071-9502
502-834-7568
888-255-1399
www.res.pub30.convio.net/Regions/great-l
Stephanie Collura, President/CEO
Margaret Chandler Berardelli, Director, Development

Louisiana

5401 RESOLVE of Louisiana
PO Box 55693
Metairie, LA 70055-5693
504-454-6987
888-895-6055
info@southcentral.resolve.org
www.res.pub30.convio.net/Regions/south-c
Barbara Bare, Regional Chair
Cindy Peterson, Volunteer Coordinator

Massachusetts

5402 RESOLVE of the Bay State
395 Totten Pond Road
Waltham, MA 02451-1553
781-890-2225
Fax: 781-890-2249
admin@resolvenewengland.org
www.resolvenewengland.org/
Information on the Massachusetts chapter of a national, nonprofit
consumer based infertility support organization. Information and a
variety of services to answer your questions about infertility, treatments, coping techniquesand insurance issues.
1,000 Homes
Pam Rollinger, Detroit, MI Area Coordinator

Michigan

5403 RESOLVE of Michigan
3601 W Thirteen Mile Road 586-412-8712
Royal Oak, MI 48068-9998 888-255-1399
info@greatlakes.resolve.org
www.res.pub30.convio.net/Regions/great-l
Kathy Collura, President/CEO
Margaret Chandler Berardelli, Director, Development

Minnesota

5404 RESOLVE of Minnesota
1161 E Wayzata Boulevard 651-659-0333
Wayzata, MN 55391 888-959-0333
www.res.pub30.convio.net/Regions/midwest
Barbara Myrick, Missouri Local Area Coordinator

Missouri

5405 RESOLVE of St. Louis, Missouri
PO Box 411072 314-567-8788
Saint Louis, MO 63141-3072 888-959-0333
MMyrickResolveMissouri@Yahoo.com
Melissa Isaacson, Nevada Chair

Nevada

5406 RESOLVE of Nevada
Barbara Greenspun Women's Care Center
8280 W Warm Springs Road 702-616-4900
Las Vegas, NV 89074 877-203-7771
rpbooklover@cox.net
Robyn Odeen-Lodato, Chair
Erin Lasker, Executive Director

New Hampshire

5407 RESOLVE of New Hampshire
131 Daniel Webster Highway 781-890-2225
Nashua, NH 03060-5224 admin@resolvenewengland.org
www.resolvenewengland.org/
Pam Griffiths, New Jersey Coordinator

New Jersey

5408 RESOLVE of New Jersey
1830 Front Street 908-322-9180
Scotch Plains, NJ 07076-0335 888-RNJ-2810
griffithskm@yahoo.com
www.res.pub30.convio.net/Regions/northea
Kim Rodriguez, New Mexico State Coordinator

New Mexico

5409 RESOLVE of New Mexico
PO Box 93386 505-291-5066
Albuquerque, NM 87199 888-895-6055
nmresolve@yahoo.com
www.res.pub30.convio.net/Regions/south-c
Rachel Soto-Lugo, President Advocacy Chair
April R Simanoff, VP Outreach Coordinator

New York

5410 RESOLVE of Long Island
PO Box 303 631-385-5026
Long Island, NY 11714
Arelys Malave, Support Services
Maryann Post, Helpline Coordinator

5411 RESOLVE of New York City
178 Columbus Avenue 212-799-7400
New York, NY 10023 888-765-2810
info@northeast.resolve.org
www.res.pub30.convio.net/Regions/northea
Anne Malave, Support Services
Maryann Post, Helpline Coordinator

5412 RESOLVE of the Capital District
PO Box 14591 518-242-3848
Albany, NY 12212-4591 888-765-2810
www.res.pub30.convio.net/Regions/northea
Anne Pell, North Carolina Coordinator

North Carolina

5413 RESOLVE of North Carolina
101 Gettysburg Drive 919-380-8497
Cary, NC 27513 888-473-3062
resolvenc@gmail.com
www.southeast.resolve.org/
Terry Collura, President/CEO
Margaret Chandler Berardelli, Director, Development

Ohio

5414 RESOLVE of Ohio
3000 NW Boulevard 614-340-0905
Columbus, OH 43221 888-255-1399
Fax: 614-340-0916
info@greatlakes.resolve.org
www.res.pub30.convio.net/Regions/great-l
Barbara Zornes, Oklahoma State Coordinator

Oklahoma

5415 RESOLVE of Oklahoma
PO Box 18151 405-949-8857
Oklahoma City, OK 73154-0151 888-895-6055
christina-zornes@ouhsc.edu
www.res.pub30.convio.net/Regions/south-c
Christy Collura, President/CEO
Margaret Chandler Berardelli, Director, Development

Oregon

5416 RESOLVE of Oregon
PO Box 175 503-762-0449
Scappoose, OR 97056 888-591-6663
resolve_oregon@yahoo.com
Barbara Fries, Philadelphia Coordinator

Pennsylvania

5417 RESOLVE of Philadelphia
PO Box 2456 215-849-3920
Southeastern, PA 19399-2456 888-765-2810
phillyresolve@gmail.com
Katie Collura, President/CEO
Margaret Chandler Berardelli, Director, Development

5418 RESOLVE of Pittsburgh
PO Box 11203 703-861-2910
Pittsburgh, PA 15238-0203 888-255-1399
info@greatlakes.resolve.org
www.res.pub30.convio.net/Regions/great-l
Barbara

5419 RESOLVE of South central Pennsylvania
PO Box 402 717-234-8583
Camp Hill, PA 17001-0402
Odeen-Lodato,, Chair
Erin Lasker, Executive Director

Rhode Island

5420 RESOLVE of the Ocean State
PO Box 28201 781-890-2225
Providence, RI 02908-0201 admin@resolvenewengland.org
www.resolvenewengland.org/
Pam Collura, President/CEO
Margaret Chandler Berardelli, Director, Development

South Carolina

5421   RESOLVE of South Carolina
204 Fernbrook Circle   864-542-9092
Spartanburg, SC 29307-2966   888-473-3062
                                    www.southeast.resolve.org/
Barbara Myers, Tennessee Coordinator

Tennessee

5422   RESOLVE of Tennessee
4770 Riverdale Road   615-244-5582
Memphis, TN 38141-8529   888-473-3062
                                    resolvetn@gmail.com
                                    www.southeast.resolve.org/
Jessica Collura, President/CEO
Margaret Chandler Berardelli, Director, Development

Texas

5423   RESOLVE of Central Texas
PO Box 49783   512-453-2171
Austin, TX 78765   888-895-6055
                        info@southcentral.resolve.org
            www.res.pub30.convio.net/Regions/south-c
Barbara Collura, President/CEO
Margaret Chandler Berardelli, Director, Development

5424   RESOLVE of Dallas/Fort Worth
434 N Manus Drive   888-895-6055
Dallas, TX 77244   info@southcentral.resolve.org
            www.res.pub30.convio.net/Regions/south-c
Barbara Collura, President/CEO
Margaret Chandler Berardelli, Director, Development

5425   RESOLVE of Houston
PO Box 441212   713-975-5324
Houston, TX 77244-1212   888-895-6055
                        info@southcentral.resolve.org
            www.res.pub30.convio.net/Regions/south-c
Barbara Collura, President/CEO
Margaret Chandler Berardelli, Director, Development

5426   RESOLVE of South Texas
PO Box 782061   210-967-6771
San Antonio, TX 78278   888-895-6055
Barbara Barron, Salt Lake City Coordinator

Utah

5427   RESOLVE of Utah
PO Box 57531   801-483-4024
Salt Lake City, UT 84157-0531   888-592-4449
                                    resolveutah@gmail.com
Jennifer Odeen-Lodato,, Chair
Erin Lasker, Executive Director

Vermont

5428   RESOLVE of Vermont
PO Box 1094   781-890-2225
Williston, VT 05495-1094   admin@resolvenewengland.org
                            www.resolvenewengland.org/
Pam Guthrie, Chair
Carol Knoph, Chair

Wisconsin

5429   RESOLVE of Wisconsin
PO Box 13842   262-521-4590
Wauwatosa, WI 53213-0842   888-255-1399
Barbara Jansen, Executive Director
Asgerally T Fazleabas, President

5430   Society for the Study of Reproduction
1619 Monroe Street   608-256-2777
Madison, WI 53711-2063   Fax: 608-256-4610
                                    ssr@ssr.org
                                    www.ssr.org

International scientific society promotes the study of reproductive
biology by fostering interdisciplinary communication within the
science by holding conferences and by publishing meritorious
studies.
2,400 members
Susan S Suarez, President
Judith Jansen, Executive Director

Foundations

5431   Fertility Research Foundation
877 Park Avenue   212-744-5500
New York, NY 10021   888-439-2999
                                Fax: 212-744-6536
                                    www.frfbaby.com
Offers information on treatment and the latest research on male
and female infertility.
Masood Khatamee MD, Executive Director

5432   Hysterectomy Educational Resources & Services (HERS)
Foundation
                                    610-667-7757
                                    888-750-4377
                                hers@hersfoundation.org
                                    www.hersfoundation.com
A nonprofit foundation which provides information about the alternatives to hysterectomy, the risks of the alternatives, and the
consequences of the surgery. HERS provides copies of a medical
journals, a quarterly newsletter, and a free lending library of
books, videos and audio tapes.

Research Centers

5433   California Center for Population Research
759 Chestnut Street   413-784-5252
Springfield, MA 01199-1001   www.tufts.edu
Dr Donald Higby, Director

5434   Fertility Clinic at the Shepherd Spinal Center
Shepherd Spinal Center
2020 Peachtree Road NW   404-352-2020
Atlanta, GA 30309-1465   www.shepherd.org
This clinic makes it possible for paralyzed men to father children.
Gary Ulicny, Chief Executive Officer

5435   Fertility and Women's Health Care Center
130 Maple Street   413-781-8220
Springfield, MA 01103-2202   Fax: 413-732-9088
Conducts basic and clinical studies of male and female infertility.
Ronald K Burke MD, Head

5436   Melpomene Institute for Women's Health Research
550 Rice Street   651-789-0140
Saint Paul, MN 55103   Fax: 651-292-9417
                                shawne@melpomene.org
                                    www.melpomene.org
Focuses on women's health including fertility issues.
Judy Mahle Lutter, President

5437   University of California: UCLA Population Research Center
4284 Public Affairs Building   310-206-7566
Los Angeles, CA 90095-2006   Fax: 310-825-8762
                                stats@ccpr.ucla.edu
                                    www.ccpr.ucla.edu
Clinical investigations of overpopulation and infertility.
Judith A Seltzer, Director
Jennie Brand, Associate Director

5438   University of Michigan Reproductive Sciences Program
1500 East Medical Center Drive   734-764-8123
Ann Arbor, MI 48109   Fax: 734-763-5992
                                juckno@umich.edu
            www.med.umich.edu/OBGYN/research/rsp/
Research done into reproductive medicine and infertility treat-
ments.
Timothy R. B Johnson, Chair
Janet Hall, Clinical Department Administrator

5439 Vanderbilt University: Center for Fertility and Reproductive Research
Nashville, TN 37232-0001   615-322-6576
     Fax: 615-343-4902
Reproductive biology and fertility research.

5440 Wayne State University: University Women's Care
26400 W 12 Mile Road   248-352-8200
Southfield, MI 48034   Fax: 248-356-8224
     wayne.edu
Reproductive endocrine infertility and gynecologic surgery research. The research spans the woman's life cycle. Research projects include: endometriosis polycystic ovary syndrome sexual dysfunction fibroids and menopause. Additional studies pertaining to women's health and male infertility.
Elizabeth Pu MD, Associate Professor
Nancy Angel RN, Research Nurse Coordinator

Support Groups & Hotlines

5441 National Health Information Center
Office of Disease Prevention & Health Promotion
1101 Wootton Pkwy   Fax: 240-453-8281
Rockville, MD 20852   odphpinfo@hhs.gov
     www.health.gov/nhic
Supports public health education by maintaining a calendar of National Health Observances; helps connect consumers and health professionals to organizations that can best answer questions and provide up-to-date contact information from reliable sources; updates on a yearly basis toll-free numbers for health information, Federal health clearinghouses and info centers.
Don Wright, MD, MPH, Director

5442 National Infertility Network Exchange
PO Box 204   516-794-5772
East Meadow, NY 11554   Fax: 516-794-0008
     www.nine-infertility.org/
The National Infertility Network Exchange (NINE) is a national, notfor profit organization for persons and couples with impaired fertility. NINE supportes the decision of legal and medical means to build families as well as the decision to remain childfree.

Books

5443 Adopt the Baby You Want
Simon & Schuster
1230 Ave of the Americas   212-698-7000
New York, NY 10020-1586   800-223-2348
A how-to adoption book written by an attorney specializing in all areas of adoption.
272 pages
Susan Shultz, Author
Michael R. Sullivan, Author

5444 Adopting After Infertility: The Decision, the Commitment, the Experience
American Society for Reproductive Medicine
1209 Montgomery Highway   205-978-5000
Birmingham, AL 35216-2809   Fax: 205-978-5018
     asrm@asrm.com
     www.asrm.com
Emphasizes the importance of communication between partners and offers several guidelines for maintaining a healthy relationship during such a stressful process.
318 pages

5445 Adoption Directory
American Society for Reproductive Medicine
1209 Montgomery Highway   205-978-5000
Birmingham, AL 35216-2809   Fax: 205-978-5018
     asrm@asrm.com
     www.asrm.com
An extensive reference text covering such specifics as state statutes, adoption agencies, exchanges and agencies.
515 pages

5446 Adoption Fact Book
American Society for Reproductive Medicine
1209 Montgomery Highway   205-978-5000
Birmingham, AL 35216-2809   Fax: 205-978-5018
     asrm@asrm.com
     www.asrm.com
A comprehensive source of statistics, regulations and facts on adoption.
277 pages

5447 Adoption Resource Book
Harper Collins
10 E 53rd Street   212-207-7000
New York, NY 10022-5299   800-242-7737
Explores and describes all types and styles of adoption and provides excellent resources for each path taken.
421 pages Third edition
Lois Gilman, Author

5448 Baby of Your Own: New Ways to Overcome Infertility
Taylor Publishing Company
1550 W Mockingbird Lane   214-637-2800
Dallas, TX 75235-5007
Provides current information regarding the psychological aspects of infertility.
244 pages

5449 Conquering Infertility: A Guide for Couples
Prentice Hall Press
15 Columbus Circle   212-373-8000
New York, NY 10023-7707
Covers various aspects of infertility.

5450 Consumer's Guide to Insurance
American Society for Reproductive Medicine
1209 Montgomery Highway   205-978-5000
Birmingham, AL 35216-2809   Fax: 205-978-5018
     asrm@asrm.com
     www.asrm.com
A how-to book for infertile couples who are experiencing difficulty with insurance reimbursement.
106 pages

5451 Consumer's Legal Guide to Today's Health Care
American Society for Reproductive Medicine
1209 Montgomery Highway   205-978-5000
Birmingham, AL 35216-2809   Fax: 205-978-5018
     asrm@asrm.com
     www.asrm.com
Provides accurate and up-to-date information concerning patient rights and medical care.
384 pages
Stephen L. Isaacs, Author

5452 Designs on Life
American Society for Reproductive Medicine
1209 Montgomery Highway   205-978-5000
Birmingham, AL 35216-2809   Fax: 205-978-5018
     asrm@asrm.com
     www.asrm.com
Provides real life stories regarding assisted reproductive technology.
276 pages

5453 Family Bonds: Adoption and the Politics of Parenting
American Society for Reproductive Medicine
1209 Montgomery Highway   205-978-5000
Birmingham, AL 35216-2809   Fax: 205-978-5050
A well organized book is written for people struggling with some of the issues encountered in their journey through infertility and ultimately adoption.
1993 273 pages
Elizabeth Bartholet, Author

5454 Fertility and Pregnancy Guide for DES Daughters and Sons
American Society for Reproductive Medicine
1209 Montgomery Highway   205-978-5000
Birmingham, AL 35216-2809   Fax: 205-978-5018
     asrm@asrm.com
     www.asrm.com

Guide offering information related to the reproductive potential of individuals who have been exposed to DES in utero.
48 pages

5455 For Want of a Child: A Psychologist and His Wife Explore Infertility
Continuum Publishing Corporation
370 Lexington Avenue   212-532-3650
New York, NY 10017-6503
A psychologist and his wife go through the emotional effects and challenges of infertility.

5456 Getting Pregnant When You Thought You Couldn't
Warner Books
1271 Ave of the Americas   www.twbookmark.com
New York, NY 10020
A concise guide to understanding infertility that covers issues from diagnosis to treatment and is useful for couples at any stage of infertility treatment.
1993 512 pages
Helane S. Rosenberg, Author

5457 Guide for the Childless Couple
American Society for Reproductive Medicine
1209 Montgomery Highway   205-978-5000
Birmingham, AL 35216-2809   Fax: 205-978-5018
                                asrm@asrm.com
                                www.asrm.com
A short text which focuses on the emotional aspects of infertility, including its effects on marriage and self-esteem.
201 pages

5458 Guide to In Vitro Fertilization & Other Assisted Reproduction Methods
Pharos Books
200 Park Avenue   212-692-3700
New York, NY 10166-0005   800-221-4816
This book discusses assisted reproductive technologies from a laboratory and a patient's perspective.

5459 Having Your Baby By Donor Insemination
Houghton Mifflin Company
222 Berkeley Street   617-351-5000
Boston, MA 02116   www.hmco.com
A resource guide to donor insemination which discusses the experience, traditions and techniques of donor insemination, sperm freezing, and known vs. anonymous donors.
352 pages

5460 Healing the Infertile Family
University of California Press
1445 Lower Ferry Road   205-978-5000
Ewing, NJ 08618   800-777-4726
                                Fax: 800-999-1958
This well-written book is dedicated to the psychological concerns of the infertile couple.
335 pages
ISBN: 0-520211-80-4

5461 Hormones
American Society for Reproductive Medicine
1209 Montgomery Highway   205-978-5000
Birmingham, AL 35216-2809   Fax: 205-978-5018
                                asrm@asrm.com
                                www.asrm.com
Highly recommended text for patients who are suffering from reproductive disorders.
216 pages

5462 How Can I Help?: A Handbook for Practical Suggestions for Infertility
American Society for Reproductive Medicine
1209 Montgomery Highway   205-978-5000
Birmingham, AL 35216-2809   Fax: 205-978-5018
                                asrm@asrm.com
                                www.asrm.com
Designed to provide greater understanding of the infertility experience.
18 pages

5463 How to Be a Successful Fertility Patient
American Society for Reproductive Medicine
1209 Montgomery Highway   205-978-5000
Birmingham, AL 35216-2809   Fax: 205-978-5018
                                asrm@asrm.com
                                www.asrm.com
Offers extensive interviews with dozens of male and female infertility patients.
1993 447 pages
Peggy Robin, Author

5464 In Pursuit of Fertility
American Society for Reproductive Medicine
1209 Montgomery Highway   205-978-5000
Birmingham, AL 35216-2809   Fax: 205-978-5018
                                asrm@asrm.com
                                www.asrm.com
A comprehensive text which can be used as a tool for couples who want to achieve an understanding of their problem as well as treatment options.
348 pages
Robert R. Franklin, Author

5465 In Vitro Fertilization
Facts on File
11 Penn Plaza   212-967-8800
New York, NY 10001   800-322-8755
                                Fax: 800-678-3633
The A.R.T. of making babies. (Assisted Reproductive Technology) A complete and caring overview of the options available to infertile couples.
208 pages Hardcover
ISBN: 0-816032-69-6

5466 Infertility Book: A Comprehensive Medical & Emotional Guide
American Society for Reproductive Medicine
1209 Montgomery Highway   205-978-5000
Birmingham, AL 35216-2809   Fax: 205-978-5018
                                asrm@asrm.com
                                www.asrm.com
Enables the infertile couple to learn how to take control and educate themselves about the trials and tribulations of infertility treatment.
420 pages Softcover
Robert D. Nachtigall, Author
Carla Harkness, Author

5467 Infertility: A Comprehensive Text
Appleton & Lange
11 W 19th Street   203-838-4400
New York, NY 10011-4209   800-423-1359
A medical reference book.

5468 Issues in Reproductive Management
Thieme Med Publishers
381 Park Avenue S   212-683-5088
New York, NY 10016-8806   Fax: 212-779-9020
1993
ISBN: 0-865775-05-2

5469 Lethal Secrets: The Psychology of Donor Insemination
Warner Books
1271 Ave of the Americas   An interview of a cross-section of people who participated in donor insemination.
New York, NY 10020
1993 277 pages
ISBN: 1-567430-20-1

5470 Lifeline: The Action Guide to Adoption Search
American Society for Reproductive Medicine
1209 Montgomery Highway   205-978-5000
Birmingham, AL 35216-2809   Fax: 205-978-5018
                                asrm@asrm.com
                                www.asrm.com
A very interesting text describing how an adoptee or adoptive parent may track down birth parents.
384 pages
Virgil L. Klunder, Author

5471 Long-Awaited Stork: A Guide to Parenting After Infertility
Jossey-Bass

350 Sansome Street
San Francisco, CA 94104
415-433-1740
Fax: 415-433-0499
webperson@jbp.com
www.josseybass.com

An excellent resource for couples who are moving from being patients to being parents.
300 pages
ISBN: 0-787940-53-4
Ellen Sarasohn Glazer, Author

5472 Love Cycles: The Science of Intimacy
Random House
1540 Broadway
New York, NY 10036
212-782-9000
Fax: 212-302-7985
www.athenainstitute.com

Book providing patients with refreshing, scientific concepts of rhythms and relationships between the sexes.
330 pages
Winifred B. Cutler, Author

5473 Loving Journeys Guide to Adoption
American Society for Reproductive Medicine
1209 Montgomery Highway
Birmingham, AL 35216-2809
205-978-5000
Fax: 205-978-5018
asrm@asrm.com
www.asrm.com

Describes the basic prerequisits agencies and social workers expectations of prospective adoptive parents. Part two offers a directory of state-by-state listings of public and private adoption agencies and adoption attorneys.
394 pages
Elaine L. Walker, Author

5474 Male Body
Firestone Touchstone Paperbacks/Simon & Schuster
200 Old Tappan Road
Old Tappan, NJ 07675-7005
800-999-5479

An informative and reassuring reference written to meet increasing interest in male health issues. This book discusses varied aspects of health such as infections and injuries, vasectomies, the emotional aspects of sexual difficulties and preventive measures that can be taken against AIDS and other sexually transmitted diseases.
208 pages
ISBN: 0-671864-26-2

5475 Men, Women and Infertility
American Society for Reproductive Medicine
1209 Montgomery Highway
Birmingham, AL 35216-2809
205-978-5000
Fax: 205-978-5018
asrm@asrm.com
www.asrm.com

A helpful book offering suggestions for a positive self-image and high self-esteem through the trauma of infertility.
1993 256 pages
Aline P. Zoldbrod, Author

5476 Miscarriage Women: Sharing from the Heart
American Society for Reproductive Medicine
1209 Montgomery Highway
Birmingham, AL 35216-2809
205-978-5000
Fax: 205-978-5018
asrm@asrm.com
www.asrm.com

A well organized book offering help and information to benefit patients who have experienced pregnancy loss as well as professionals working with these couples.
1993 258 pages
Shelly Marks, Author
Marie Allen, Author

5477 Missed Conceptions: Overcoming Infertility
McGraw-Hill
1221 Ave of the Americas
New York, NY 10020
212-512-2000

Book about infertility and the emotional agony that goes along with it. Addresses all aspects surrounding infertility care and offers in-depth discussions of the many fertility options now available.
377 pages

5478 Motherhood: A Feminist Perspective
American Society for Reproductive Medicine
1209 Montgomery Highway
Birmingham, AL 35216-2809
205-978-5000
Fax: 205-978-5018
asrm@asrm.com
www.asrm.com

A compilation of papers from conference proceedings designed to define motherhood. Offers information on infertility, emotional and financial difficulties and daily living.
234 pages

5479 Mothers of Thyme: Customs and Rituals of Infertility and Miscarriage
Lida Rose Press
PO Box 15076
Ann Arbor, MI 48106

An interesting book that offers details on rituals and misconceptions concerning infertility and miscarriage.
128 pages
ISBN: 0-962595-75-6

5480 Never to Be a Mother
Harper Collins Publishers
10 E 53rd Street
New York, NY 10022-5299
212-207-7000
800-242-7737

Offers childless women a plan for confronting their grief, anger and guilt, as well as offering alternative ways to mother and live.

5481 No-Hysterectomy Option
American Society for Reproductive Medicine
1209 Montgomery Highway
Birmingham, AL 35216-2809
205-978-5000
Fax: 205-978-5018
asrm@asrm.com
www.asrm.com

An excellent reference for women faced with decisions regarding hysterectomy.
265 pages
Herbert A. Goldfarb, Author

5482 One Women's Passionate Quest to Complete Her Family
Viking Penguin
375 Hudson Street
New York, NY 10014-3658
212-366-2000

The author presents a highly emotional account of the years of anguish, disappointment, and finally the joy she achieved in trying to complete her family.

5483 Overcoming Infertility
Doubleday
666 5th Avenue
New York, NY 10103-0001
212-765-6500
800-223-6834

Paints a clear picture of the medical and emotional aspects of infertility.

5484 Preventing Miscarriage: The Good News
American Society for Reproductive Medicine
1209 Montgomery Highway
Birmingham, AL 35216-2809
205-978-5000
Fax: 205-978-5018
asrm@asrm.com
www.asrm.com

Provides information on possible causes of miscarriages with information on infections, abnormalities and more.
240 pages Softcover
Jonathan Scher, Author
Carol Dix, Author

5485 Reproductive Hazards in the Workplace: Mending Jobs, Managing Pregnancies
Regina H Kenen, PhD, author
Haworth Press
10 Alice Street
Binghamton, NY 13904-1580
607-722-5857
800-429-6784
Fax: 607-722-0012
www.haworthpress.com

Offers information on the history and present of potential reproductive hazards. Includes pregnancy hazard hotlines, specific contact points where women can get information on working environments and more.
286 pages Hardcover
ISBN: 1-560241-54-3

5486 Resolving Infertility
RESOLVE: National Infertility Association
1310 Broadway 617-623-1156
Somerville, MA 02144-1779 888-623-0744
Fax: 617-623-0252
info@resolve.org
www.resolve.org
Understanding the options and choosing solutions when you want to have a baby is a definitive resource to help you sort out the options and negative through the experience with confidence. This book tells you everything you need to know about infertility treatment and exploring other family building options.
370 pages
ISBN: 0-062735-22-5
Bonny Gilbert, Executive Director
Diane Aronson, Author

5487 Science and Babies: Private Decisions, Public Dilemmas
American Society for Reproductive Medicine
1209 Montgomery Highway 205-978-5000
Birmingham, AL 35216-2809 Fax: 205-978-5018
asrm@asrm.com
www.asrm.com
Offers a superb summary of key reproductive issues ranging from conception to contraception.
250 pages

5488 Silent Sorrow
Delta-Dell Publishers
666 5th Avenue 212-765-6500
New York, NY 10103-0001 800-223-6834
A book dealing with the emotional and psychological aspects of losing a child.

5489 Surrogate Motherhood: The Legal and Human Issues
Harvard University Press
79 Garden Street 617-495-2600
Cambridge, MA 02138-1423
A discussion of the psychological, legal and policy questions raised by surrogacy.

5490 Surviving Infertility
Tapestry Books
PO Box 359 908-806-6695
Ringoes, NJ 08551-0359 800-765-2367
Fax: 732-288-2999
A valuable source of support and practical advice for coping with the many intense feelings associated with being infertile.
389 pages

5491 Surviving Pregnancy Loss: A Complete Sourcebook for Women & Their Families
American Society for Reproductive Medicine
1209 Montgomery Highway 205-978-5000
Birmingham, AL 35216-2809 Fax: 205-978-5018
asrm@asrm.com
www.asrm.com
Contains practical approaches to coping with the emotional and psychological problems associated with pregnancy loss.
298 pages
Bonnie Gradstein, Author
Rochelle Friedman, Author

5492 Sweet Grapes: How to Stop Being Infertile and Living Again
American Society for Reproductive Medicine
1209 Montgomery Highway 205-978-5000
Birmingham, AL 35216-2809 Fax: 205-978-5018
asrm@asrm.com
www.asrm.com
Recommended for couples nearing the end of their options or for those who are unsure if they wish to pursue infertility therapy.
Michael Carter, Author
Jean W. Carter, Author

5493 To Love a Child
Addison Wesley Publishing
PO Box 165 518-859-4424
Clifton Park, MA 12065 800-447-2226
directoratTLC@aol.com
www.toloveachild.net

A thoughtful and informative overview of alternatives to bio/genetic parenting.

5494 Understanding and Infertility
Tapestry Books
PO Box 359 908-806-6695
Ringoes, NJ 08551-0359 800-765-2367
Fax: 732-288-2999
Provides specific advice to the family on how to be supportive of members and/or friends who suffer from infertility.
28 pages

5495 WHO Laboratory Manual
American Society for Reproductive Medicine
1209 Montgomery Highway 205-978-5000
Birmingham, AL 35216-2809 Fax: 205-978-5018
asrm@asrm.com
www.asrm.com

Third edition

5496 Waiting: A Diary of Loss and Hope in Pregnancy
American Society for Reproductive Medicine
1209 Montgomery Highway 205-978-5000
Birmingham, AL 35216-2809 Fax: 205-978-5018
asrm@asrm.com
www.asrm.com
Provides clear insight into coping with the trials and tribulations of infertility.
121 pages

5497 Without Child
American Society for Reproductive Medicine
1209 Montgomery Highway 205-978-5000
Birmingham, AL 35216-2809 Fax: 205-978-5018
asrm@asrm.com
www.asrm.com
Covers topics including the doctor-patient relationship, religion and infertility, living child-free and the adoption process for persons without children investigating their options.
226 pages

5498 Women Without Children
Pharos Books
200 Park Avenue 212-692-3700
New York, NY 10166-0005 800-221-4816
Offers women without children support through their struggle and decision making.

Children's Books

5499 Mommy, Did I Grow in Your Tummy? Where Some Babies Come From
American Society for Reproductive Medicine
1209 Montgomery Highway 205-978-5000
Birmingham, AL 35216-2809 Fax: 205-978-5018
asrm@asrm.com
www.asrm.com
Illustrated book that helps parents explain the different ways children can come into the world, including IVF, surrogacy, game donation and adoption.
28 pages Ages 4-8
Kathy Clo, Author
Elaine R. Gordon, Author

Magazines

5500 American Society for Reproductive Medicine: Clinic Specific Annual Report
1209 Montgomery Highway 205-978-5000
Birmingham, AL 35216-2809 Fax: 205-978-5018
asrm@asrm.org
www.asrm.org
Gives the success rates of treatment for fertility centers around the country.

5501 Biology of Reproduction
1603 Monroe Street
Madison, WI 53711-2021   608-256-2777
                                      Fax: 608-256-4610
                                      bor@ssr.org
                                      www.biolreprod.org

A monthly, peer-reviewed journal.
250 pages Monthly

5502 Family Building Magazine
RESOLVE: National Infertility Association
1310 Broadway   617-623-1156
Somerville, MA 02144-1779   888-623-0744
                                      Fax: 617-623-0252
                                      info@resolve.org
                                      www.resolve.org

Offers various information on the newest technology and advances
in infertility treatments, support groups, helplines, centers and in
depth articles written by professionals in the field.
15-18 pages Quarterly
Bonny Gilbert, Executive Director

5503 Infertility and Adoption
RESOLVE: National Infertility Association
1310 Broadway   617-623-1156
Somerville, MA 02144-1779   888-623-0744
                                      Fax: 617-623-0252
                                      info@resolve.org
                                      www.resolve.org

Published by RESOLVE: The National Infertility Association.
Bonny Gilbert, Executive Director
Roy Sokol, Author

5504 Journal of Occupational & Environmental Medicine
Williams & Wilkins
351 W Camden Street   301-528-4000
Baltimore, MD 21201-7912   800-638-0672

Newsletters

5505 Hers Newsletter
Hysterectomy Educational Resources & Services
422 Bryn Mawr Avenue   610-667-7757
Bala Cynwyd, PA 19004-2708   800-777-4377
                                      Fax: 610-667-8096
                                      hersfdn@aol.com
                                      www.hersfoundation.com

Offers information and support for women who have had or are go-
ing through hysterectomies.
Quarterly
Nora W Coffey, President

5506 RESOLVE of the Bay State
PO Box 541553   781-647-1614
Waltham, MA 02454-1553   Fax: 781-899-7207
                                      www.resolveofthebaystate.org
Information on the Massachusetts chapter of a national, nonprofit,
consumer based infertility support organization. Information on a
variety of services to answer your questions about infertility, treatments, coping techniques, insurance issues and family building
options.

Pamphlets

5507 ART-Assisted Reproductive Technologies
Serono Symposia USA
100 Longwater Circle   800-283-8088
Norwell, MA 02061-1616

5508 Abnormal Uterine Bleeding
American Society for Reproductive Medicine
1209 Montgomery Highway   205-978-5000
Birmingham, AL 35216-2809   Fax: 205-978-5018
                                      asrm@asrm.com
                                      www.asrm.com

1996
Malcolm G. Munro, Author

5509 Adoption
American Society for Reproductive Medicine
1209 Montgomery Highway   205-978-5000
Birmingham, AL 35216-2809   Fax: 205-978-5018
                                      asrm@asrm.com
                                      www.asrm.com

1990

5510 Affording Your Infertility
Serono Symposia USA
100 Longwater Circle   800-283-8088
Norwell, MA 02061-1616

5511 Age and Fertility
American Society for Reproductive Medicine
1209 Montgomery Highway   205-978-5000
Birmingham, AL 35216-2809   Fax: 205-978-5018
                                      asrm@asrm.com
                                      www.asrm.com

1996

5512 Bibliography
RESOLVE: National Infertility Association
1310 Broadway   617-623-1156
Somerville, MA 02144-1779   888-623-0744
                                      Fax: 617-623-0252
                                      info@resolve.org
                                      www.resolve.org

Annotated guide to books and articles on medical and emotional
aspects of infertility.
Bonny Gilbert, Executive Director

5513 Birth Defects of the Female Reproductive System
American Society for Reproductive Medicine
1209 Montgomery Highway   205-978-5000
Birmingham, AL 35216-2809   Fax: 205-978-5018
                                      asrm@asrm.com
                                      www.asrm.com

1993

5514 Coping with the Holidays
RESOLVE
1310 Broadway   781-643-0744
Somerville, MA 02144-1779

5515 Donor Insemination
American Society for Reproductive Medicine
1209 Montgomery Highway   205-978-5000
Birmingham, AL 35216-2809   Fax: 205-978-5018
                                      asrm@asrm.com
                                      www.asrm.com

1995
Christopher L. R. Barratt, Author
Ian Douglas Cooke, Author

5516 Early Menopause (Premature Ovarian Failure)
American Society for Reproductive Medicine
1209 Montgomery Highway   205-978-5000
Birmingham, AL 35216-2809   Fax: 205-978-5018
                                      asrm@asrm.com
                                      www.asrm.com

1996

5517 Ectopic Pregnancy
American Society for Reproductive Medicine
1209 Montgomery Highway   205-978-5000
Birmingham, AL 35216-2809   Fax: 205-978-5018
                                      asrm@asrm.com
                                      www.asrm.com

1996
Isabel Stabile, Author

5518 Emotional Aspects of Infertility
RESOLVE: National Infertility Association
1310 Broadway   617-623-1156
Somerville, MA 02144-1779   888-623-0744
                                      Fax: 617-623-0252
                                      info@resolve.org
                                      www.resolve.org

Published by RESOLVE: The National Infertility Association.
Bonny Gilbert, Executive Director

5519 Ending Infertility Treatment
RESOLVE: National Infertility Association
1310 Broadway   617-623-1156
Somerville, MA 02144-1779   888-623-0744
                                            Fax: 617-623-0252
                                            info@resolve.org
                                            www.resolve.org
Published by RESOLVE: The National Infertility Association.
Bonny Gilbert, Executive Director

5520 Endometriosis
American Society for Reproductive Medicine
1209 Montgomery Highway   205-978-5000
Birmingham, AL 35216-2809   Fax: 205-978-5018
                                            asrm@asrm.com
                                            www.asrm.com
Available in Spanish.
1994
Michael Vernon, Author
Dian Shepperson Mills, Author

5521 Environmental Toxins and Fertility
RESOLVE: National Infertility Association
1310 Broadway   617-623-1156
Somerville, MA 02144-1779   888-623-0744
                                            Fax: 617-623-0252
                                            info@resolve.org
                                            www.resolve.org
Published by the National Infertility Association (RESOLVE).
Bonny Gilbert, Executive Director

5522 Fertility After Cancer Treatment
American Society for Reproductive Medicine
1209 Montgomery Highway   205-978-5000
Birmingham, AL 35216-2809   Fax: 205-978-5018
                                            asrm@asrm.com
                                            www.asrm.com
1995

5523 Getting Started: How Do I Know If I'm Infertile?
RESOLVE
1310 Broadway   781-643-0744
Somerville, MA 02144-1779

5524 Hirsutism and Polycystic Ovarian Syndrome
American Society for Reproductive Medicine
1209 Montgomery Highway   205-978-5000
Birmingham, AL 35216-2809   Fax: 205-978-5018
                                            asrm@asrm.com
                                            www.asrm.com
1995

5525 Husband Insemination
American Society for Reproductive Medicine
1209 Montgomery Highway   205-978-5000
Birmingham, AL 35216-2809   Fax: 205-978-5018
                                            asrm@asrm.com
                                            www.asrm.com
1995

5526 IVF & GIFT: A Guide to Assisted Reproductive Technologies
American Society for Reproductive Medicine
1209 Montgomery Highway   205-978-5000
Birmingham, AL 35216-2809   Fax: 205-978-5018
                                            asrm@asrm.com
                                            www.asrm.com
Available in Spanish.
1995

5527 If You are Having Trouble Conceiving
American Society for Reproductive Medicine
1209 Montgomery Highway   205-978-5000
Birmingham, AL 35216-2809   Fax: 205-978-5018
                                            asrm@asrm.com
                                            www.asrm.com

5528 Infertility Insurance
Serono Symposia USA
100 Longwater Circle   800-283-8088
Norwell, MA 02061-1616

5529 Infertility: An Overview
American Society for Reproductive Medicine
1209 Montgomery Highway   205-978-5000
Birmingham, AL 35216-2809   Fax: 205-978-5018
                                            asrm@asrm.com
                                            www.asrm.com
Available in Spanish.
1994

5530 Infertility: Causes and Treatment
American College/Obstetricians and Gynecologists
409 12th Street SW   www.acog.com
Washington, DC 20024
To obtain a free copy of this publication, please send a self-addressed stamped #10 envelope and request by title. (#AP002)
Nicole Ellisson, Author

5531 Infertility: Coping and Decision Making
American Society for Reproductive Medicine
1209 Montgomery Highway   205-978-5000
Birmingham, AL 35216-2809   Fax: 205-978-5018
                                            asrm@asrm.com
                                            www.asrm.com
1995

5532 Infertility: The Emotional Roller Coaster
Serono Symposia USA
100 Longwater Circle   800-283-8088
Norwell, MA 02061-1616

5533 Insights Into Infertility
Serono Symposia USA
100 Longwater Circle   800-283-8088
Norwell, MA 02061-1616

5534 Introduction to Infertility: The First Steps
RESOLVE: National Infertility Association
1310 Broadway   617-623-1156
Somerville, MA 02144-1779   888-623-0744
                                            Fax: 617-623-0252
                                            info@resolve.org
                                            www.resolve.org
Published by RESOLVE: The National Infertility Association.
Bonny Gilbert, Executive Director

5535 Laparoscopy and Hysteroscopy
American Society for Reproductive Medicine
1209 Montgomery Highway   205-978-5000
Birmingham, AL 35216-2809   Fax: 205-978-5018
                                            asrm@asrm.com
                                            www.asrm.com
1995

5536 Male Infertility
Serono Symposia USA
100 Longwater Circle   800-283-8088
Norwell, MA 02061-1616

5537 Male Infertility and Vasectomy Reversal
American Society for Reproductive Medicine
1209 Montgomery Highway   205-978-5000
Birmingham, AL 35216-2809   Fax: 205-978-5018
                                            asrm@asrm.com
                                            www.asrm.com
1995

5538 Managing Family & Friends
RESOLVE
1310 Broadway   781-643-0744
Somerville, MA 02144-1779

5539 Miscarriage
American Society for Reproductive Medicine
1209 Montgomery Highway   205-978-5000
Birmingham, AL 35216-2809   Fax: 205-978-5018
                                            asrm@asrm.com
                                            www.asrm.com
1995

5540 Myths & Facts
RESOLVE

1310 Broadway
Somerville, MA 02144-1779

781-643-0744

5541 Ovulation Detection
American Society for Reproductive Medicine
1209 Montgomery Highway   205-978-5000
Birmingham, AL 35216-2809   Fax: 205-978-5018
                                         asrm@asrm.com
                                         www.asrm.com

1995

5542 Ovulation Drugs
American Society for Reproductive Medicine
1209 Montgomery Highway   205-978-5000
Birmingham, AL 35216-2809   Fax: 205-978-5018
                                         asrm@asrm.com
                                         www.asrm.com

1995

5543 Patient Information Series Publications
American Society for Reproductive Medicine
1209 Montgomery Highway   205-978-5000
Birmingham, AL 35216-2809   Fax: 205-978-5018
                                         asrm@asrm.com
                                         www.asrm.com

Offers a set of 20 various brochures ranging from artificial insemination to male infertility problems.

5544 Pelvic Pain
American Society for Reproductive Medicine
1209 Montgomery Highway   205-978-5000
Birmingham, AL 35216-2809   Fax: 205-978-5018
                                         asrm@asrm.com
                                         www.asrm.com

1997

5545 Pregnancy After Infertility
American Society for Reproductive Medicine
1209 Montgomery Highway   205-978-5000
Birmingham, AL 35216-2809   Fax: 205-978-5018
                                         asrm@asrm.com
                                         www.asrm.com

1997

5546 Premenstrual Syndrome (PMS)
American Society for Reproductive Medicine
1209 Montgomery Highway   205-978-5000
Birmingham, AL 35216-2809   Fax: 205-978-5018
                                         asrm@asrm.com
                                         www.asrm.com

1997
Syndrome Sullivan, Author
Ronald V. Norris, Author

5547 Third Party Reproduction (Donor Eggs, Donor Sperm, Donor Embryos, & Surrogacy)
American Society for Reproductive Medicine
1209 Montgomery Highway   205-978-5000
Birmingham, AL 35216-2809   Fax: 205-978-5018
                                         asrm@asrm.com
                                         www.asrm.com

1996

5548 Tubal Factor Infertility
American Society for Reproductive Medicine
1209 Montgomery Highway   205-978-5000
Birmingham, AL 35216-2809   Fax: 205-978-5018
                                         asrm@asrm.com
                                         www.asrm.com

1995

5549 Understanding: A Guide to Impaired Fertility for Family and Friends
American Society for Reproductive Medicine
1209 Montgomery Highway   205-978-5000
Birmingham, AL 35216-2809   Fax: 205-978-5018
                                         asrm@asrm.com
                                         www.asrm.com

A pamphlet designed for families of patients with infertility and for distribution to individuals who may want to become involved in the counseling and support of these couples.
28 pages
Patricia I. Johnston, Author

5550 Unexplained Infertility
American Society for Reproductive Medicine
1209 Montgomery Highway   205-978-5000
Birmingham, AL 35216-2809   Fax: 205-978-5018
                                         asrm@asrm.com
                                         www.asrm.com

1997

5551 Uterine Fibroids
American Society for Reproductive Medicine
1209 Montgomery Highway   205-978-5000
Birmingham, AL 35216-2809   Fax: 205-978-5018
                                         asrm@asrm.com
                                         www.asrm.com

1997
Togas Tulandi, Author

Audio & Video

5552 Candid Talk About Loss in Adoption
Mary Martin Mason
4505 York Avenue S   612-922-1136
Minneapolis, MN 55410-1422
Discusses losses incurred by the adopted persons and adoptive persons issues for children adopted into different race families.
Videotape

5553 Coping with Infertility
Distributed By UC Video
425 Ontario Street SE   612-627-4444
Minneapolis, MN 55414-3002
Features five couples talking about their infertility experiences.
Odessa Flores

5554 Infertility: Exploring the Male Factor
American Society for Reproductive Medicine
1209 Montgomery Highway   205-978-5000
Birmingham, AL 35216-2809   Fax: 205-978-5018
                                         asrm@asrm.com
                                         www.asrm.com

A well-orchestrated video discussing male factor infertility, including the infertility workup, physical exam, semen analysis, and surgical options available.
1993 47 minutes

5555 One, Two, Three, Zero: Infertility
Filmmaker's Library
133 E 58th Street   212-355-6545
New York, NY 10022-1236
Videotape

5556 Six Phases of Infertility Treatment: Medical & Emotional Aspects
RESOLVE of Maryland
PO Box 19049   410-243-0235
Baltimore, MD 21284-9049
Gives an overview of infertility treatment, addressing the medical and emotional aspects.
Videotape

5557 So You're Going to Adopt
Mary Martin Mason
4505 York Avenue S   612-922-1136
Minneapolis, MN 55410-1422
This video prepares adoptive parents for pre and post adoption issues.
Videotape

Web Sites

5558 Adopt-A-Special-Kid America

www.adoptaspecialkid.org

Adopt-A-Special-Kid provides information on adoption of children with special needs.

5559 **American Society for Reproductive Medicine**

www.reproductivefacts.org

A private, non-profit medical organization devoted to advancing the knowledge, understanding and expertise in all phases of reproductive medicine and biology. Offers patient education brochures, recommended readings and support. Publishes professional journal and consumer publications, and runs the ReproductiveFacts.org website for patients.

5560 **Center for Disease Control**

www.cdc.gov

Reproductive health information source. Also a resource for the Society of Reproductive Technology. Invitro fertilization data reports and men's reproductive health. Interesting well balanced site.

5561 **Fertilethoughts.com**

www.fertilethoughts.com

A support sytem concerned with helping reach a goal of finding the perfect doctor, the diagnosis, as well as the treatment.

5562 **Healing Well**

www.healingwell.com

An online health resource guide to medical news, chat, information and articles, newsgroups and message boards, books, disease-related web sites, medical directories, and more for patients, friends, and family coping with disabling diseases, disorders, or chronic illnesses.

5563 **Health Finder**

www.healthfinder.gov

Searchable, carefully developed web site offering information on over 1000 topics. Developed by the US Department of Health and Human Services, the site can be used in both English and Spanish.

5564 **Healthlink USA**

www.healthlinkusa.com

Health information concerning treatment, cures, prevention, diagnosis, risk factors, research, support groups, email lists, personal stories and much more. Updated regularly.

5565 **HealthyWomen**

www.healthywomen.org

Independent, non-profit organization seeking to educate women in all areas of health, to allow them to make informed choices. The HealthyWomen website features numerous tools and health calculators, plus other media.

5566 **Infertility Books**

www.infertilitybooks.com

Nonprofit site includes book titles regarding infertility and a short explanation of each book and how to get it.

5567 **International Council on Infertility Information Dissemination**

www.inciid.org

A nonprofit organization that helps individuals and couples explore their family-building options.

5568 **Internet Health Resources**

www.ihr.com/infertility

This web site provides extensive information about IVF, ICSI, infertility clinics, donor egg and surrogacy services, sperm banks, pharmacies, infertility books and videotapes, sperm testing, infertility newsgroups and support organizations, and drugs and medications.

5569 **Ivf.com**

www.ivf.com

Goal is to provide the latest women's healthcare innovations to address infertility, polycystic ovaries, endometriosis, and pelvic pain treatment.

5570 **MedicineNet**

www.medicinenet.com

An online resource for consumers providing easy-to-read, authoritative medical and health information.

5571 **Medscape**

www.medscape.com

Medscape offers specialists, primary care physicians, and other health professionals the Web's most robust and integrated medical information and educational tools.

5572 **National Institutes of Health**

www.medlineplus.gov

Information regarding all aspects of infertility. Some of the topics include: Latest news, overview of anatomy and physiology, clinical trails, diagnoses and symptoms, treatment, genetics, plus lots of links to other sites. Type infertility into the search engine.

5573 **RESOLVE**

www.resolve.org

Provides help to people who are experiencing the infertility crisis and strives to increase the visibility of infertility issues via concerted advocacy and public education.

5574 **Uterine Artery Embolization**

Provides information on Uterine Artery Embolization, or Uterine Fibroid Embolization as an alternative to hysterectomy or myomectomy as a treatment for uterine fibroids.

5575 **WebMD**

www.webmd.com

Provides credible information, supportive communities, and in-depth reference material about health subjects. A source for original and timely health information as well as material from well known content providers.

Description

5576 Kidney Disease

The diseases that affect the kidney can be divided into diseases of the kidney itself, such as nephritis, polycystic kidney disease, hereditary nephropathies, kidney infections and stones, and diseases of other body systems that cause damage to the kidneys, such as diabetes, high blood pressure and lupus. In either instance, disruption of kidney function results in failure to remove excess fluids and wastes from the blood. This may lead to end stage kidney, or renal, failure.

Symptoms of kidney disease and their severity, depend on the underlying cause. If there is damage or disease in the urinary tract, there can be pain when urinating, blood in the urine, or changes in frequency and urgency of urination. If excess fluid cannot be removed, there may be swelling around the eyes and ankles. When the kidney is damaged directly, back or flank tenderness may be present. In many cases, kidney disease causes no symptoms until the advanced stages, although it may be detected much earlier through tests of blood or urine. Because the kidneys regulate the rate of red blood cell production, kidney damage can also cause anemia. Kidney damage will also prevent effective modulation of blood pressure.

Treatment is directed to the cause, and may include antibiotics for infections, removal of kidney stones by surgery or ultrasound waves, management of the systemic disease such as diabetes, dietary modification, especially of salt and protein intake, and close monitoring and correction of fluid and electrolyte imbalances. Treatment may also include control of high blood pressure, which can be caused by kidney disease and further damage the kidney. Immune- or drug-related nephritis can be treated with corticosteroids. The most severe cases of kidney failure require either dialysis, in which the blood's toxins are mechanically filtered and removed, or a kidney transplant.

National Agencies & Associations

5577 American Association of Kidney Patients
14440 Bruce B. Downs Boulevard
Tampa, FL 33613
813-636-8100
800-749-2257
Fax: 813-636-8122
info@aakp.org
www.aakp.org

Offers support and information for kidney patients and their families.
Richard Knight, MBA, President
Daniel Abel, Vice President

5578 American Kidney Fund
11921 Rockville Pike
Rockville, MD 20852
800-638-8299
866-300-2900
helpline@kidneyfund.org
www.kidneyfund.org

A non-profit national health organization providing direct financial assistance to thousands of Americans who suffer from kidney disease.
LaVarne A. Burton, President & CEO
Donald J. Roy, Jr., CPA, Executive Vice President, COO & CFO

5579 National Institute of Diabetes & Digestive & Kidney Diseases
Office Of Communications and Public Liaison, NIH
31 Center Drive
Bethesda, MD 20892-2560
800-860-8747
TTY: 866-569-1162
healthinfo@niddk.nih.gov
www.niddk.nih.gov

Research areas include diabetes, digestive diseases, endocrine and metabolic diseases, hematologic diseases, kidney disease, liver disease, urologic diseases, as well as matters relating to nutrition and obesity.
Griffin P. Rodgers, MD, MACP, Director
Gregory Germino, MD, Deputy Director

5580 National Kidney Foundation
30 E 33rd Street
New York, NY 10016
800-622-9010
855-653-2273
Fax: 212-689-9261
info@kidney.org
www.kidney.org

A health organization dedicated to preventing kidney and urinary tract diseases, improving the health and well-being of individuals and families affected and increasing the availability of all organs for transplantation.
Michael J. Choi, MD, President
Kevin Longino, CEO

State Agencies & Associations

Alabama

5581 Alabama Chapter of the American Association of Kidney Patients
PO BOX 12505
Birmingham, AL 35202-2238
205-934-2111
800-750-3331
Fax: 205-975-6682
jack@alkidney.org
www.alkidney.org

Gwen Deierhoi, President
E.W. Jackson III, Executive Director

Arizona

5582 Arizona Kidney Foundation
4203 E Indian School Road
Phoenix, AZ 85018
602-840-1644
Fax: 602-840-2360
www.azkidney.org

Leonard J McDonald, Chair
Jeffrey D Neff, Chief Executive Officer

5583 Central Arizona Chapter of the American Association of Kidney Patients
4401 W Hatcher Road
Glendale, AZ 85302-3821
602-939-7248
Dale A Ester, President

Arkansas

5584 National Kidney Foundation of Arkansas
1818 N Taylor Street
Little Rock, AR 72207
501-664-4343
800-622-9010
Fax: 816-221-7984
nkfar@kidney.org
www.kidney.org

Nonprofit health organization. Our mission is to prevent kidney and urinary tract disease improve the health and well being of individuals and families affected by these diseases and increase the availability of all organs for transplantation.
R D Todd Baur, Member of the Board of Directors
Derek E Bruce, Member of the Board of Directors

California

5585 Harbor-South Bay Orange County Chapter of the American Assoc. of Kidney Patients
PO Box 8
Seal Beach, CA 90740
714-527-8009
delrita@aol.com
www.aakp.org

Rita McQuire, President

5586 Los Angeles Chapter of the American Association of Kidney Patients
9854 National Boulevard
Los Angeles, CA 90034
310-364-1807
aakpla@yahoo.com
www.aakp.org
Robin Siegal, President

5587 National Kidney Foundation of Northern California
131 Steuart Street
San Francisco, CA 94105
415-543-3303
888-427-5653
Fax: 415-543-3331
infopacific@kidney.org
www.kidney.org/site/503/index.cfm
Work with kidney patients both pre ESRD dialysis and transplant. Financial assistance educational workshops scholarships children's and family camps transplant games information and referral.
Brad J Small, Division President
Connie M Nieri, Division Director of Finance/Operations

5588 National Kidney Foundation of Southern California
15490 Ventura Boulevard
Sherman Oaks, CA 91403
818-783-8153
800-747-5527
Fax: 818-783-8160
nkfsca@kidney.org
www.kidney.org
Pier Merone, Division President
Natalie Kanooni, Division Program Manager

5589 Redding Chapter of the American Association of Kidney Patients
790 Pioneer Drive
Redding, CA 96001-0258
530-241-6451
teamward@c-zone.net
www.aakp.org

5590 Sacramento Valley Chapter of the American Association of Kidney Patients
565 Morrison Avenue
Sacramento, CA 95838
916-924-1996

Colorado

5591 Colorado Chapter of the American Association of Kidney Patients
PO Box 8442
Denver, CO 80201
303-758-8610

5592 National Kidney Foundation of Colorado: Idaho, Montana, and Wyoming
650 South Cherry Street
Denver, CO 80246
720-748-9991
800-596-7943
Fax: 720-748-1273
nkfcmw@kidney.org
www.kidney.org/site/505/
Brandi Krause, State Director
Stacey Lux, Development Director

5593 Western Slope Chapter of the American Association of Kidney Patients
1539 Ptarmigan Ridge
Grand Junction, CO 81056
970-244-9196
Vicki Hathaway, CEO
Donna Sciacca, Director of Patient Programs/Services

Connecticut

5594 National Kidney Foundation of Connecticut
1463 Highland Avenue
Cheshire, CT 06410
203-439-7912
800-441-1280
Fax: 203-439-7934
nkfct@kidney.org
www.kidney.org/site/102/index.cfm
Marcia Hilditch, Program Manager
Deb Ramada, Development Coordinator

District of Columbia

5595 Georgetown University Center for Hypertension and Renal Disease Research
3800 Reservoir Road NW
Washington, DC 20007
202-687-9183
Fax: 202-687-7893

International institute for basic and clinical investigation education and clinical practice in hypertension and renal disease.
Christopher Englert, Jr. CAE, President/CEO

5596 National Kidney Foundation of the National Capital Area
5335 Wisconsin Avenue NW
Washington, DC 20015-2030
202-244-7900
Fax: 202-244-7405
infowdc@kidney.org
www.kidney.org/site/203/index.cfm
Pamela D Gatz, Division President
Sherrita Lancaster, Division Office Manager

Florida

5597 American Association of Kidney Patients
2701 N Rocky Point Drive
Tampa, FL 33607
813-636-8100
800-749-2257
Fax: 813-636-8122
info@aakp.org
www.aakp.org
Sam Pederson, President
Paul T Conway, Vice-President

5598 Kidney Association of South Florida
6801 Lake Worth Road
Lake Worth, FL 33467
561-434-4559
jansym@bellsouth.net
www.aakp.org
Jan Symonette, President

5599 National Kidney Foundation of Florida
1040 Woodcock Road
Orlando, FL 32803
407-894-7325
800-927-9659
Fax: 407-895-0051
nkf@kidneyfla.org
www.kidney.org/site/204/index.cfm
Andrew Helfan, President
Stephanie Hutchinson, CEO

5600 South Florida Chapter of the American Association of Kidney Patients
5217 Northlake Boulevard
Palm Beach Gardens, FL 33418
561-471-2588
diazgray@aol.com
www.aakp.org
Robert Kirby, President

5601 Sunshine Chapter of the American Association of Kidney Patients
PO Box 4716
Hialeah, FL 33014-0716
305-821-4827
Elaine Printup

Georgia

5602 Atlanta Georgia Chapter of the American Association of Kidney Patients
6409 Lakeview Drive
Buford, GA 30518
404-932-1100
Pamela Sachs, Division President
Tracy Jenny, Division Program Director

5603 National Kidney Foundation of Georgia
2951 Flowers Road S
Atlanta, GA 30341
770-452-1539
800-633-2339
Fax: 770-452-7564
nkfga@kidney.org
www.kidney.org
Barbara McDowell, President

5604 Rome Georgia Chapter of the American Association of Kidney Patients
118 Woodcrest Drive
Rome, GA 30161
706-232-8989
Hazel Hayashida, Chief Executive Officer
Diana Pinard, Director of Organization Planning

Hawaii

5605 National Kidney Foundation of Hawaii
1314 S King Street   808-593-1515
Honolulu, HI 96814   800-488-2277
                                Fax: 808-589-5993
                                Glen@kidneyhi.org
                                www.kidneyhi.org
Hawaii's leading voluntary health agency to the education prevention and treatment of kidney and urinary tract diseases and increase the availability of all organs for transplantation in Hawaii.
Aileen Utterdyke, President
Glen Hayashida, CEO

Idaho

5606 National Kidney Foundation of Colorado, Idaho, Montana, and Wyoming
650 South Cherry Street   720-748-9991
Denver, CO 80246   800-596-7943
                                Fax: 720-748-1273
                                nkfcmw@kidney.org
                                www.kidney.org/site/505/
Brandi Krause, State Director
Stacey Lux, Development Director

Illinois

5607 Chicagoland Chapter of the American Association of Kidney Patients
70 Lincoln Oaks Drive   708-325-3475
Chicago, IL 60514
Gloria Lang, Chief Executive Officer
Kate Grubbs O'Connor, Chief Operating Officer

5608 National Kidney Foundation of Illinois
215 W Illinois   312-321-1500
Chicago, IL 60654   Fax: 312-321-1505
                                kidney@nkfi.org
                                www.nkfi.org
Mark L Schwartz, President
Kate Grubbs O'Connor, Chief Executive Officer

Indiana

5609 National Kidney Foundation of Indiana
911 E 86th Street   317-722-5640
Indianapolis, IN 46240-1840   800-382-9971
                                Fax: 317-722-5650
                                nkfi@kidneyindiana.org
                                www.kidney.org/site/303/index.cfm
The mission of the NKFI is to prevent kidney and urinary tract disease improve the health and well-being of individuals and family affected by these disease and increase the availability of all organs for transplantation.
Margie Evans Fort, Chief Executive Officer
Heather Gallagher, Communications Director

Iowa

5610 Iowa Chapter of the Association of Kidney Patients
2203 75th Place   319-391-1194
Davenport, IA 52806-1107
Dave Hagarty, Executive Director
Lori Donald, Accounting Coordinator

Kansas

5611 National Kidney Foundation of Kansas and Western Missouri
6405 Metcalf Avenue   913-262-1551
Overland Park, KS 66202   800-596-7943
                                Fax: 913-722-4841
                                nkfkswmo@kidney.org
                                www.kidney.org/site/305/index.cfm
Sherri Denny, Regional Administrative Assistant
Alexandra Wilson, Special Events Manager

Kentucky

5612 National Kidney Foundation of Kentucky
250 E Liberty Street   502-585-5433
Louisville, KY 40202   800-737-5433
                                Fax: 502-585-1445
                                infonkfk@kidney.org
                                www.nkfk.org
April Enix, Director of Development
Nital Desai, Community Outreach Manager

Louisiana

5613 Bayou Area Chapter of the American Association of Kidney Patients
PO Box 400   504-532-3542
Lockport, LA 70374
Louisiana Kranze, Chief Executive Officer
Tracey Eldridge, Director of Special Events

5614 National Kidney Foundation of Louisiana
8200 Hampson Street   504-861-4500
New Orleans, LA 70118   800-462-3694
                                Fax: 504-861-1976
                                info@kidneyla.org
                                www.kidneyla.org
Shawn Donelon, Chairman
Torie Kranze, Chief Executive Officer

Maine

5615 National Kidney Foundation of Maine
85 Astor Avenue   781-278-0222
Norwood, ME 02062   800-542-4001
                                Fax: 781-278-0333
                                nkfofmrnv@kidneyhealth.org
                                www.kidney.org/site/105/index.cfm
Andrea Savisky RN CNN, Division Program Director
Mark Daley, Division Donor Records Director/User Ser

Maryland

5616 National Kidney Foundation of Maryland
Heaver Plaza, 1301 York Road   410-494-8545
Lutherville, MD 21093-2136   800-671-5369
                                Fax: 410-494-8549
                                www.kidneymd.org
Also covers the Harrisburg area of Pennsylvania and portions of Virginia and West Virginia.
Cassie Shafer, President/CEO
Christie Vera, Vice President of Development and Market

Massachusetts

5617 National Kidney Foundation of MA/RI/NH/VT
85 Astor Avenue   781-278-0222
Norwood, MA 02062   800-542-4001
                                Fax: 781-278-0333
                                nkfofmrnv@kidneyhealth.org
                                www.kidney.org/site/105/index.cfm
Andrea Savisky RN CNN, Division Program Director
Mark Daley, Division Donor Records Director/User Ser

Michigan

5618 Michigan Kidney Foundation
1169 Oak Valley Drive   734-222-9800
Ann Arbor, MI 48108   800-482-1455
                                Fax: 734-222-9801
                                info@nkfm.org
                                www.nkfm.org
Andrew Boschma, Chairman
Daniel M Carney, President/CEO

Minnesota

5619 National Kidney Foundation of Minnesota
1970 Oakcrest Avenue
Saint Paul, MN 55113
651-636-7300
800-596-7943
Fax: 651-636-9700
jille@kidney.org
www.kidney.org/site/313/index.cfm
Also covers North Dakota and South Dakota.
Jill Evenocheck, Division President
Amy Busack, Regional Vice-President

Mississippi

5620 National Kidney Foundation of Mississippi
3000 Old Canton Road
Jackson, MS 39216
601-981-3611
800-232-1592
Fax: 601-981-3612
gail@kidneyms.org
www.kidneyms.org

Paul Howell, President
Lee Parrott, Vice President

Missouri

5621 National Kidney Foundation of Eastern Missouri and Metro East
1001 Craig Road
Creve Coeur, MO 63146
314-961-2828
800-489-9585
Fax: 314-961-0888
nkfemo@kidney.org
www.kidney.org/site/308/index.cfm
Chad Iseman, State Director
Alayna Tatum, Special Events Manager

Montana

5622 National Kidney Foundation of Colorado/Idaho/Montana/Wyoming
650 South Cherry Street
Denver, CO 80246
720-748-9991
800-596-7943
Fax: 720-748-1273
nkfcmw@kidney.org
www.kidney.org/site/505/
Brandi Krause, State Director
Stacey Lux, Development Director

Nebraska

5623 Nebraska Kidney Association
11725 Arbor Street
Omaha, NE 68144-2116
402-932-7200
800-642-1255
Fax: 402-933-0087
www.kidneyne.org
Improve the lives of all Nebraskans through advocacy, education, early disease detection and patient services.

New Hampshire

5624 National Kidney Foundation of MA/RI/NH/VT
85 Astor Avenue
Norwood, MA 02062
781-278-0222
800-542-4001
Fax: 781-278-0333
nkfofmrnv@kidneyhealth.org
www.kidney.org/site/105/index.cfm
Andrea Savisky RN CNN, Division Program Director
Mark Daley, Division Donor Records Director/User Ser

New Jersey

5625 Garrett Mountain Chapter of the American Association of Kidney Patients
PO Box 8496
Haledon, NJ 07538
973-523-3959
Hurwitz, President

5626 Meadowlands Chapter of the American Association of Kidney Patients
PO Box 3032
Clifton, NJ 07012-3032
201-471-5674
Howard

5627 Northern New Jersey Chapter of the American Association of Kidney Patients
1095 Stone Street
Rahway, NJ 07065-1913
732-382-1092
Burnett

New Mexico

5628 National Kidney Foundation of New Mexico
3167 San Mateo Boulevard NE
Albuquerque, NM 87110
505-830-3542
800-282-0190
Fax: 816-221-7984
nkfnm@kidney.org
www.kidney.org

Connie Giarrusso, President
Shirley Baer, Executive Director

New York

5629 Kidney & Urology Foundation of America
2 West 47th Street
New York, NY 10036
212-629-9770
800-633-6628
Fax: 212-629-5652
info@kidneyurology.org
www.kidneyurology.org
Sam Giarrusso, President
Kerri Shapiro, Director of Operations/Administration

5630 Long Island Chapter of the American Association of Kidney Patients
2 Maplewood Avenue
Farmingdale, NY 11735
516-756-9126
Margie Ng Makhuli, Chief Executive Officer
Laura Squadrito, Director of Programs and Services

5631 National Kidney Foundation of Central New York
731 James Street
Syracuse, NY 13203
315-476-0311
877-8KI-DNEY
Fax: 315-476-3707
info@cnykidney.org
www.kidney.org/site/110/index.cfm
Nannette Carbone, Chief Executive Officer
Susan Burns, Director of Administration

5632 National Kidney Foundation of Northeast New York
1971 Western Avenue
Albany, NY 12203
518-458-9697
800-622-9010
Fax: 518-458-9690
www.kidney.org/about/local_info.cfm?sear
Carol MS Ed CFRE, Executive Director
Mary Jones, Division Development Director

5633 National Kidney Foundation of Western New York
310 Packetts Landing
Fairport, NY 14450
585-598-3963
800-724-9421
Fax: 585-598-3966
infoupny@kidney.org
www.kidney.org/site/109/index.cfm
Nonprofit health organization.
Joanne Spink, Division President
Megan Alchowiak, Community Outreach Manager

5634 New York Chapter of the American Association of Kidney Patients
450 Clarkson Avenue
Brooklyn, NY 11203
718-270-1548
linda.cohen@downstate.edu
www.aakp.org
Linda Welch, Kidney Early Evaluation Program Contact

North Carolina

5635 **National Kidney Foundation of North Carolina**
5950 Fairview Road   704-552-1351
Charlotte, NC 28210   800-356-5362
     Fax: 704-552-7870
     www.nkfnc.org
Kenya Welch, Kidney Early Evaluation Program Contact

Ohio

5636 **Miami Valley Ohio Chapter of the American Association of Kidney Patients**
4511 W State Route   513-698-5847
W Milton, OH 45383
Bob B Gold, Division President
Danielle Estep, Division Program Director

5637 **National Kidney Foundation of Ohio**
2800 Corporate Exchange Drive   614-882-6184
Columbus, OH 43231-2804   800-242-2133
     Fax: 614-882-6564
     nkfoh@kidney.org
     www.nkfofohio.org
Patti V.B. Gold, Division President
Danielle Estep, Division Program Director

Oklahoma

5638 **American Association of Kidney Patients: Tulsa Chapter**
911 North Woodland Drive   918-241-3969
Sand Springs, OK 74063   800-749-2257
     jasonmikles@hotmail.com
Jason Tallent, CEO

5639 **National Kidney Foundation of Oklahoma**
10600 S Pennsylvania Avenue   816-221-9559
Oklahoma City, OK 73170   800-622-9010
     Fax: 816-221-7984
     nkfok@kidney.org
     www.kidney.org/about/local_info.cfm?sear
Jeff Baumgardner, CEO
Glenda McClure, Operations Manager

Pennsylvania

5640 **Lehigh Valley Chapter of the American Association of Kidney Patients**
1242 N 19th Street   610-776-1091
Allentown, PA 18104-3058   info@aakp.org
     www.aakp.org
Jill Spink, Division President
Mary Reilly, Development Director

5641 **National Kidney Foundation of Delaware Valley**
111 S Independence Mall E   215-923-8611
Philadelphia, PA 19106   800-697-7007
     Fax: 215-923-2199
     nkfdv@kidney.org
     www.kidney.org/site/112/index.cfm
Also covers Delaware and Southern New Jersey.
Joseph Mullen, Chairman
Joanne Spink, Division President

5642 **National Kidney Foundation of Western Pennsylvania**
3109 Forbes Avenue   412-261-4115
Pittsburgh, PA 15213   800-261-4115
     Fax: 412-261-1405
     info@kidneyall.org
     www.kidney.org/site/113/index.cfm
Also covers Northern West Virginia.
James Sullivan, Chairman
David Vanella, Vice Chairman

Rhode Island

5643 **National Kidney Foundation of MA/RI/NH/VT**
85 Astor Avenue   781-278-0222
Norwood, MA 02062   800-542-4001
     Fax: 781-278-0333
     nkfofmrnv@kidneyhealth.org
     www.kidney.org/site/105/index.cfm
Andrea Savisky RN CNN, Division Program Director
Mark Daley, Division Donor Records Director/User Ser

South Carolina

5644 **National Kidney Foundation of South Carolina**
508 Hampton Street   803-798-3870
Columbia, SC 29201   800-488-2277
     Fax: 803-799-3871
     karen.bailey@kidney.org
     www.kidney.org/site/209/index.cfm
Beth Irick, Division President
Karen Bailey, Division Senior Administrative Assistant

South Dakota

5645 **National Kidney Foundation Serving Minneso ta, Dakotas & Iowa Division Office**
1970 Oakcrest Avenue   651-636-7300
Saint Paul, MN 55113   800-596-7943
     Fax: 651-636-9700
     jille@kidney.org
     www.kidney.org/site/313/index.cfm
Jill Evenocheck, Division President
Amy Busack, Regional Vice President

Tennessee

5646 **National Kidney Foundation of East Tennessee**
5201 Kingston Pike   865-688-5481
Knoxville, TN 37919-1523   800-242-2133
     Fax: 865-688-5495
     nkfetn@kidney.org
     www.kidney.org/about/local_info.cfm?sear
The National Kidney Foundation of East Tennessee works to prevent kidney and urinary tract diseases improve the health and well-being of individuals and family members affected by these diseases and increase the availability of all organs for transplantation.
Helen

5647 **National Kidney Foundation of West Tennessee**
857 Mount Moriah Road   901-683-6185
Memphis, TN 38117   800-273-3869
     Fax: 901-683-6189
     info@nkfwtn.org
     www.kidney.org/about/local_info.cfm?sear
Bruce Skyer, Chief Executive Officer
Joseph Vassalotti, MD, Chief Medical Officer

5648 **National Kidney Foundation of West Texas**
5429 Lyndon B Johnson Fwy   214-351-2393
Dallas, TX 75240   877-543-6397
     Fax: 214-351-3797
     texasinfo@kidney.org
     www.kidney.org/site/406/index.cfm
Marrie Collins, President
Mark Edwards, Division Program Director

5649 **Tennessee Kidney Foundation**
95 White Bridge Road   615-383-3887
Nashville, TN 37205-2613   800-380-3887
     Fax: 615-383-2647
     www.tennesseekidneyfoundation.org
Ron Carter, President
Bob Horton, First Vice President

Texas

5650 American Association of Kidney Patients: Piney Woods Chapter
PO Box 1012 903-537-7031
Mount Vernon, TX 75457 800-749-2257
Edwin Wager, President

5651 Lone Star Chapter of the American Association of Kidney Patients
10042 Sugarloaf Drive 210-523-1605
San Antonio, TX 78245 www.aakp.org
Robert Eaton, CEO
Cameron Hernholm, Director of Development

5652 National Kidney Foundation of North Texas
5429 Lyndon B Johnson Freeway 214-351-2393
Dallas, TX 75240 877-543-6397
Fax: 214-351-3797
texasinfo@kidney.org
www.kidney.org/site/406/index.cfm
Public and professional education about kidney and urinary tract diseases. Peer mentoring medical emergency identification jewelry kidney early evaluation program Camp Reynal transplant games.
Marrie Collins, President
Mark Edwards, Division Program Director

5653 National Kidney Foundation of Southeast Texas
5429 Lyndon B Johnson Freeway 214-351-2393
Dallas, TX 75240 877-543-6397
Fax: 214-351-3797
texasinfo@kidney.org
www.kidney.org/site/406/index.cfm
Provides services for people who suffer with kidney and urinary tract diseases.
Marrie Collins, President
Mark Edwards, Division Program Director

5654 National Kidney Foundation of Texas
5429 Lyndon B Johnson Fwy 214-351-2393
Dallas, TX 75240 877-543-6397
Fax: 214-351-3797
texasinfo@kidney.org
www.kidney.org/site/406/index.cfm
Marie Collins, Division President
Mark Edwards, Divisional Program Director

5655 National Kidney Foundation of the Texas Coastal Bend
PO Box 9172 361-884-5892
Corpus Christi, TX 78469 Fax: 361-884-2332
info@coastalbendkidneyfoundation.org
www.coastalbendkidneyfoundation.org
Bess Stone, President
Becky Gardner, Executive Director

Utah

5656 National Kidney Foundation of Utah
3707 N Canyon Road 801-226-5111
Provo, UT 84604-4585 800-869-5277
Fax: 801-226-8278
NKFU@KidneyUT.org
www.kidneyut.org
Serving kidney dialysis and transplant patients through out Utah providing patient service and support programs medical research and public and patient education regarding kidney disease and its treatment and prevention and the promotion of organ donations.
E.J. Garn, Chairman
Deen Vetterli, Chief Executive Officer

Vermont

5657 National Kidney Foundation of MA/RI/NH/VT
85 Astor Avenue 781-278-0222
Norwood, MA 02062 800-542-4001
Fax: 781-278-0333
nkfofmrnv@kidneyhealth.org
www.kidney.org/site/105/index.cfm
Andrea Savisky RN CNN, Division Program Director
Mark Daley, Division Donor Records Director/User Ser

Virginia

5658 National Kidney Foundation of Virginia
1622 East Parham Road 804-288-8342
Richmond, VA 23228 800-543-6398
Fax: 804-282-7835
www.kidney.org/site/203/index.cfm
An affiliate of the National Kidney Foundation it serves kidney patients and their families in Virginia and portions of West Virginia. Mission includes professional and public education prevention and working to increase the availability of all organs for donation.
Eleanor Myers, Regional Program Director
Liz King, Community Outreach Manager

Wisconsin

5659 National Kidney Foundation of Wisconsin
16655 W Bluemound Road 262-821-0705
Brookfield, WI 53005-5935 800-543-6393
Fax: 262-821-5641
nkfw@kidneywi.org
www.kidneywi.org
Offers prevention detection and education programs for those at risk for kidney disease. The National Kidney Foundation of Wisconsin is making life's better through its programs and services. Brochures are offered at no charge.
Mary Braband, Chair
Cindy Huber, Chief Executive Officer

Wyoming

5660 National Kidney Foundation of Colorado/Idaho/Montana/Wyoming
650 South Cherry Street 720-748-9991
Denver, CO 80246 800-596-7943
Fax: 720-748-1273
nkfcmw@kidney.org
www.kidney.org/site/505/
Brandi Krause, State Director
Stacey Lux, Development Director

Research Centers

5661 Kidney Disease Institute
Wadsworth Center for Laboratories and Research
Empire State Plaza 518-474-7354
Albany, NY 12237 Fax: 518-737-71
dohweb@health.state.ny.us
www.nyhealth.gov
An information and referral organization for polycystic kidney disease autoimmune kidney disease and transplantation.
Andrew M Cuomo, Governor
Nirav R Shah, Commissioner

5662 Lovelace Medical Foundation
2425 Ridgecrest Drive SE 505-348-9400
Albuquerque, NM 87108-5127 Fax: 505-348-8567
info@lrri.org
www.lrri.org
Jackie Lovelace Johnson, Director
Frank Bond, Director

5663 Lovelace Respiratory Research Institute
615 S Preston Street 502-852-7350
Louisville, KY 40202-0001 Fax: 502-852-7643
kdpnet.kdp.louisville.edu
Educates residents and patients regarding kidney diseases and offers a dialysis clinic for people afflicted with kidney disease.
George R Ottensmeyer, President

5664 Nevada Kidney Disease & Hypertension Cente rs
210 S Desplaines Street 312-654-2720
Chicago, IL 60661 Fax: 312-654-0118
charlotte.chapple@ainmd.com
www.ainmd.com/
A medical group practicing nephrology in the Chicago metropolitan area and it suburbs. Includes 21 nephrologists with expertise in many areas in the field of nephrology including hypertension chronic and acute renal failure hemodialysis and peritoneal dialy-

sis glomerulonephritis acid base disturbances fluid and electrolytes management. Provides personal high quality care to patients with kidney diseases.
Eduardo Kantor MD, Founder

5665   PKD Foundation Polycystic Kidney Disease Foundation
Polycystic Kidney Disease Foundation
9221 Ward Parkway   816-931-2600
Kansas City, MO 64114-3367   800-PKD-CURE
                                              Fax: 816-931-8655
                                           pkdcure@pkdcure.org
                                              www.pkdcure.org
The foundation exists to win the war with PKD. Their mission is to promote research into the treatment and cure of polycystic kidney disease by raising financial support for peer approved biomedical research projects and fostering public awareness among medical professionals patients and the general public.
Frank Condella, Jr, Chair
Michelle Davis, Interim CEO and Chief Development Office

5666   University of Kansas Kidney and Urology Research Center
3901 Rainbow Boulevard   913-588-5000
Kansas City, KS 66160   Fax: 913-588-3995
                                           TTY: 913-588-7963
                                              www.kumc.edu

Jared J Brosius, Chief
Joseph Messana, Professor/ Service Chief

5667   University of Michigan Nephrology Division
University of Michigan Health System
1500 E Medical Center Drive   734-936-5645
Ann Arbor, MI 48109   Fax: 734-763-4151
                    www.med.umich.edu/intmed/nephrology
Focuses on kidney research.
Eric Mullen, Division Administrator
Susan Geisser, Financial Consultant

5668   University of Rochester: Nephrology Research Program
601 Elmwood Avenue   585-275-3660
Rochester, NY 14642-0001   Fax: 716-442-9201
                                           www.urmc.rochester.edu
Focuses on kidney disorders.
David A Bushinsky, MD, Division Chief

5669   Warren Grant Magnuson Clinical Center
National Institute of Health
10 Center Drive MSC 1078   301-496-3311
Bethesda, MD 20892   800-411-1222
                                           Fax: 301-496-2390
                                           TTY: 866-411-1010
                                           mmichael@cc.nih.gov
Established in 1953 as the research hospital of the National Institutes of Health. Designed so that patient care facilities are close to research laboratories so new findings of basic and clinical scientists can be quickly applied to the treatment of patients. Upon referral by physicians, patients are admitted to NIH clinical studies.
John Slatopolsky, Director

5670   Washington University Chromalloy American Kidney Center
One Barnes-Jewish Hospital Plaza   314-362-7209
Saint Louis, MO 63110-1036   Fax: 314-747-3743
                                           renal.wustl.edu
Offers a dialysis unit for people afflicted with kidney disease.
Dr Eduardo Lanning RN/JD, President Board of Directors
Sean Tully, Vice President Board of Directors

Support Groups & Hotlines

5671   Kidneeds
Greater Cedar Rapids Community Foundation
200 First Street Southwest   319-366-2862
Cedar Rapids, IA 52404   Fax: 319-386-0431
                                           kidneedsmpgn@yahoo.com
                                           www.medicine.uiowa.edu/kidneeds/
Primary mission of kidneeds is to fund research on membranoproliferative giomerulonephritis type 2 (MPON type 2, aka, dense deposit disease). Phone support and annual newsletter

availiable. No computerized version availiable. No mailing list availble.
Lynne

5672   National Health Information Center
Office of Disease Prevention & Health Promotion
1101 Wootton Pkwy   Fax: 240-453-8281
Rockville, MD 20852   odphpinfo@hhs.gov
                                           www.health.gov/nhic
Supports public health education by maintaining a calendar of National Health Observances; helps connect consumers and health professionals to organizations that can best answer questions and provide up-to-date contact information from reliable sources; updates on a yearly basis toll-free numbers for health information, Federal health clearinghouses and info centers.
Don Wright, MD, MPH, Director

Books

5673   Family and ADPKD: A Guide for Children and Parents
Polycystic Kidney Disease Foundation
9221 Ward Parkway   816-931-2600
Kansas City, MO 64114   800-753-2873
                                           Fax: 816-931-8655
                                           pkdcure@pkdcure.org
                                              www.pkdcure.org
This book focuses on the questions most commonly asked by children and parents about ADPKD. It is divided into two sections: one for children and one for parents.
48 pages
ISBN: 0-961456-75-2
Dave Switzer, National Director, Educational Programs
Arlene B. Chapman, Author

5674   Kidney Beginnings: A Patient's Guide to Li ving with Reduced Kidney Function
American Association of Kidney Patients
3505 E Frantage Road   813-636-8100
Tampa, FL 33607   800-749-2257
                                           Fax: 813-636-8122
                                           info@aakp.org
                                              www.aakp.org
Provides patients with the information they need to take control of their healthcare and do what is necessary to preserve and protect their kidney function. The book addresses concerns of those at risk for kidney disease and their family members; featuring information about the workings of the kidneys, common medications, hypertention, testing, and answers to health, diet and lifestyle questions.
62 pages
Kim Buettner, Executive Director

5675   Kidney Cooking
National Kidney Foundation of Georgia
1639 Tullie Circle NE   404-248-1315
Atlanta, GA 30329-2304
A unique cookbook with over one hundred recipes that have been analyzed for sodium, potassium and protein content.

5676   Nutrition & the Kidney
Little Brown & Company
34 Beacon Street   617-227-0730
Boston, MA 02108-1415   Fax: 617-227-4633
1993 480 pages
ISBN: 0-316575-00-3

5677   PKD Patient's Manual
Polycystic Kidney Disease Foundation
9221 Ward Parkway   816-931-2600
Kansas City, MO 64114   800-753-2873
                                           Fax: 816-931-8655
                                           pkdcure@pkdcure.org
                                              www.pkdcure.org
Covers everything from cysts to how persons can be active if they have ARPKD.
Dave Switzer, National Director, Educational Programs

5678   Q&A on PKD
Polycystic Kidney Disease Foundation

9221 Ward Parkway
Kansas City, MO 64114 816-931-2600
 800-753-2873
Fax: 816-931-8655
pkdcure@pkdcure.org
www.pkdcure.org
A goldmine of information for the PKD patient and physician. Includes 88 pages of PKD questions and answers by the scientific advisers of the PKR Foundation.
88 pages Paperback
ISBN: 0-961456-72-8
Dave Switzer, National Director, Educational Programs

5679 Real Lifestyles Manual
R&D Laboratories
4204 Glencoe Avenue 800-338-9066
Marina Del Rey, CA 90292-5612
A complete renal guide including diets for hemodialysis and CAPD patients. Delicious menus, ADA exchange lists, gourmet recipes with nutritional analysis for renal patients and exercises.

5680 Your Child, Your Family & ARPKD
Polycystic Kidney Disease Foundation
9221 Ward Parkway 816-931-2600
Kansas City, MO 64114 800-753-2873
Fax: 816-931-8655
pkdcure@pkdcure.org
www.pkdcure.org
This second edition book focuses on the questions most commonly asked about ARPKD in order to help families understand more about the disease.
Dave Switzer, National Director, Educational Programs

5681 Your Child, Your Family and Autosomal Recessive Polycystic Kidney Disease
Polycystic Kidney Disease Foundation
9221 Ward Parkway 816-931-2600
Kansas City, MO 64114 800-753-2873
Fax: 816-931-8655
pkdcure@pkdcure.org
www.pkdcure.org
This secong edition book focuses on the questions most commonly asked about autosomal recessive PKD in order to help families understand more about the disease.
26 pages Paperback
Dave Switzer, National Director, Educational Programs

Magazines

5682 Kindey Beginnings: The Magazine
American Association of Kidney Patients
3505 E Frantage Road 813-636-8100
Tampa, FL 33607 800-749-2257
Fax: 813-636-8122
info@aakp.org
www.aakp.org
This quarterly member magazine provides articles, news items and information of interest to those at risk or recently diagnosed with kidney disease, their famliy, and healthcare professionals.
Kmi Buettner, Executive Director

5683 aakpRENALIFE
American Association of Kidney Patients
35052 E Frantage Road 813-636-8100
Tampa, FL 33607 800-749-2257
Fax: 813-636-8122
info@aakp.org
www.aakp.org
The official publication for AAKP members, offering articles, news and health care information for kidney patients,and health care professionals.
BiMonthly
Kim Buettner, Executive Director

Newsletters

5684 Family Focus
National Kidney Foundation

30 E 33rd Street 212-889-2210
New York, NY 10016-5337 800-622-9010
Fax: 212-689-9261
www.kidney.org
A patient and family newspaper targeted toward dialysis populations.
Quarterly

5685 PKD Progress
PKD Foundation
4901 Main Street 816-931-2600
Kansas City, MO 64112-2634 800-753-2873
Fax: 816-931-8655
pkdcure@pkdcure.org
www.pkdcure.org
Offers information and updated medical news for persons and professionals with an interest in kidney disorders.
Monthly
Dave Switzer, Marketing/Public Relations Director

5686 Renal Recipes Quarterly
R&D Laboratories
4204 Glencoe Avenue 800-338-9066
Marina Del Rey, CA 90292-5612
Features timely holiday and ethnic food menus and recipes, shopping and food tips, analysis of nutrients and calculation of food exchanges.
Quarterly

5687 Transplant Chronicles
National Kidney Foundation
30 E 33rd Street 212-889-2210
New York, NY 10016 800-622-9010
Fax: 212-689-9261
www.kidney.org
A patient and family newsletter targeted towards transplant recipients.
Quarterly

Pamphlets

5688 About Kidney Stones
National Kidney Foundation
30 E 33rd Street 212-889-2210
New York, NY 10016 800-622-9010
Fax: 212-689-9261
www.kidney.org
Discusses causes, treatment and prevention of kidney stones.

5689 Advance Directives: A Guide for Patients and Their Families
National Kidney Foundation
30 E 33rd Street 212-889-2210
New York, NY 10016-5337 800-622-9010
Fax: 212-689-9261
www.kidney.org
Everyone has the right to make an advance directive, which is a legal document stating how you want decisions made concerning your medical care when your no longer able to make them yourself. This booklet describes the different types of advance directives and the medical decisions they cover.
12 pages Package

5690 American Kidney Fund Helps When Nobody Else Will
American Kidney Fund
6110 Executive Boulevard 301-881-3052
Rockville, MD 20852-3915 800-638-8299
Fax: 301-881-0898
helpline@AFINC.org
www.kidneyfund.org
Focuses on the services and programs offered by the American Kidney Fund.

5691 At Home with AAKP
American Association of Kidney Patients
3505 E Frantage Road 813-636-8100
Tampa, FL 33607 800-749-2257
Fax: 813-636-8122
info@aakp.org
www.aakp.org

A free publication, this was developed to address the growing need for information about home dialysis treatment options.
Kim Buettner, Executive Director

5692 Children and Kidney Disease
American Kidney Fund
6110 Executive Boulevard
Rockville, MD 20852-3915
301-881-3052
800-638-8299
Fax: 301-881-0898
www.arbon.com/kidney/

5693 Choosing a Treatment for Kidney Failure
National Kidney Foundation
30 E 33rd Street
New York, NY 10016
212-889-2210
800-622-9010
Fax: 212-689-9261
www.kidney.org
Introduces treatment options for kidney failure and explains the pros and cons of each.
16 pages

5694 Diabetes and Kidney Disease
National Kidney Foundation
30 E 33rd Street
New York, NY 10016-5337
212-889-2210
800-622-9010
Fax: 212-689-9261
www.kidney.org
Explains the connection between diabetes and kidney disease covering prevention, recognition and treatments.
12 pages Pkg. of 100
Edgar V. Lerma, Author
Vecihi Batuman, Author

5695 Dialysis Patient: An Informative Guide for the Dentist
American Kidney Fund
6110 Executive Boulevard
Rockville, MD 20852-3915
301-881-3052
800-638-8299
Fax: 301-881-0898
www.arbon.com/kidney/

5696 Diet Guide for the CAPD Patient
American Kidney Fund
6110 Executive Boulevard
Rockville, MD 20852-3915
301-881-3052
800-638-8299
Fax: 301-881-0898
www.arbon.com/kidney/

5697 Diet Guide for the Hemodialysis Patient
American Kidney Fund
6110 Executive Boulevard
Rockville, MD 20852-3915
301-881-3052
800-638-8299
Fax: 301-881-0898
www.arbon.com/kidney/

5698 Facts About Kidney Diseases and Their Treatment
American Kidney Fund
6110 Executive Boulevard
Rockville, MD 20852-3915
301-881-3052
800-638-8299
Fax: 301-881-0898
www.arbon.com/kidney/
Offers information about what kidneys are and their functions, diagnosis and treatment of kidney disease.

5699 Facts About Kidney Stones
American Kidney Fund
6110 Executive Boulevard
Rockville, MD 20852-3915
301-881-3052
800-638-8299
Fax: 301-881-0898
www.arbon.com/kidney/

5700 Glomerulonephritis
National Kidney Foundation
30 E 33rd Street
New York, NY 10016-5337
212-889-2210
800-622-9010
Fax: 212-689-9261
www.kidney.org
Defines the types of Glomerulonephritis, signs, causes and symptoms.
8 pages Pkg. of 100
Graeme Catto, Author

5701 Hemodialysis
National Kidney Foundation
30 E 33rd Street
New York, NY 10016
212-889-2210
800-622-9010
Fax: 212-689-9261
www.kidney.org
Introduces and explains the hemodialysis treatment process.
12 pages Pkg. of 100
C. Ronco, Author
M.H. Rosner, Author

5702 High Blood Pressure and Your Kidneys
National Kidney Foundation
30 E 33rd Street
New York, NY 10016-5337
212-889-2210
800-622-9010
Fax: 212-689-9261
www.kidney.org
Offers a description of hypertension, including symptoms, detection, causes and effects. Also available in Spanish.
8 pages Pkg. of 100
Dr.Randall Hammett, Author

5703 High Blood Pressure and its Effects on the Kidneys
American Kidney Fund
6110 Executive Boulevard
Rockville, MD 20852
301-881-3052
800-638-8299
Fax: 301-881-0898
www.arbon.com/kidney/

5704 Kid
American Kidney Fund
6110 Executive Boulevard
Rockville, MD 20852-3915
301-881-3052
800-638-8299
Fax: 301-881-0898
www.arbon.com/kidney/

5705 Kidney Disease: A Guide for Patients and Their Families
American Kidney Fund
6110 Executive Boulevard
Rockville, MD 20852
301-881-3052
800-638-8299
Fax: 301-881-0898
www.arbon.com/kidney/
Offers information on how the kidneys work, symptoms of kidney disease, kidney failure and treatment alternatives.

5706 Kidney Transplant: A New Lease on Life
National Kidney Foundation
30 E 33rd Street
New York, NY 10016
212-889-2210
800-622-9010
Fax: 212-689-9261
www.kidney.org
A brochure that answers common questions about transplants, such as patient expectations, drug therapy, complications including rejection and recovery.
10 pages Pkg. of 100

5707 Kidneys for Kids
American Kidney Fund
6110 Executive Boulevard
Rockville, MD 20852-3915
301-881-3052
800-638-8299
Fax: 301-881-0898
www.arbon.com/kidney/

5708 Nutrition and Changing Kidney Function
National Kidney Foundation
30 E 33rd Street
New York, NY 10016-5337
212-889-2210
800-622-9010
Fax: 212-689-9261
www.kidney.org
Explains how to slow the progression of kidney disease by controlling the intake of vitamins, minerals, fluids, calories and proteins.
12 pages Pkg. of 100

5709 Organ Donor Program
National Kidney Foundation
30 E 33rd Street
New York, NY 10016-5337
212-889-2210
800-622-9010
Fax: 212-689-9261
www.kidney.org

A comprehensive description of the organ donor program that explains organ and tissue donation, brain death, routine inquiry and becoming an organ donor.
12 pages Pkg. of 100

5710   Peritoneal Dialysis
National Kidney Foundation
30 E 33rd Street   212-889-2210
New York, NY 10016   800-622-9010
                                                    Fax: 212-689-9261
                                                    www.kidney.org

Introduces and explains the peritoneal dialysis treatment process
8 pages
K.D. Nolph, Author

5711   Understanding Nephrotic Syndrome
American Kidney Fund
6110 Executive Boulevard   301-881-3052
Rockville, MD 20852-3915   800-638-8299
                                                    Fax: 301-881-0898
                                                    www.arbon.com/kidney/

5712   Urinary Tract Infections
National Kidney Foundation
30 E 33rd Street   212-889-2210
New York, NY 10016-5337   800-622-9010
                                                    Fax: 212-689-9261
                                                    www.kidney.org

Defines urinary tract infections, its symptoms, causes and treatments.
10 pages Pkg. of 100

5713   Warning Signs of Kidney Disease
National Kidney Foundation
30 E 33rd Street   212-889-2210
New York, NY 10016-5337   800-622-9010
                                                    Fax: 212-689-9261
                                                    www.kidney.org

A one-panel leaflet that numbers and lists the six early warning signs of kidney disease.
Pkg. of 100

5714   Winning the Fight Against Silent Killers
National Kidney Foundation
30 E 33rd Street   212-889-2210
New York, NY 10016-5337   800-622-9010
                                                    Fax: 212-689-9261
                                                    www.kidney.org

Written for the African-American community, this brochure discusses the increased risk of high blood pressure and diabetes in this population.
12 pages Pkg. of 100

5715   Your Kidneys: Master Chemists of the Body
National Kidney Foundation
30 E 33rd Street   212-889-2210
New York, NY 10016-5337   800-622-9010
                                                    Fax: 212-689-9261
                                                    www.kidney.org

Offers an overview of kidneys and urinary system, describing the kidneys' filtering system, hereditary, congenital and acquired kidney diseases.
12 pages Pkg. of 100

Audio & Video

5716   It's Just Part of My Life
National Kidney Foundation
30 E 33rd Street   212-889-2210
New York, NY 10016-5337   800-622-9010
                                                    Fax: 212-689-9261
                                                    www.kidney.org

A 15-minute program for adolescent dialysis patients and their families.

5717   People Like Us
National Kidney Foundation

30 E 33rd Street   212-889-2210
New York, NY 10016-5337   800-622-9010
                                                    Fax: 212-689-9261
                                                    www.kidney.org

A seven-part video series targeted toward the newly-diagnosed chronic kidney disease patient.
Simon Greenall, Author

Web Sites

5718   American Association of Kidney Patients
                                                    www.aakp.org
Serves the needs and interests of kidney patients, for kidney patients, the purpose of this Association is to help patients and their families cope with the emotional, physical and social impact of kidney disease.

5719   American Kidney Fund
                                                    www.akfinc.org/
A nonprofit, national health organization providing direct financial assistance to thousands of Americans who suffer from kidney disease.

5720   Healing Well
                                                    www.healingwell.com
An online health resource guide to medical news, chat, information and articles, newsgroups and message boards, books, disease-related web sites, medical directories, and more for patients, friends, and family coping with disabling diseases, disorders, or chronic illnesses.

5721   Health Finder
                                                    www.healthfinder.gov
Searchable, carefully developed web site offering information on over 1000 topics. Developed by the US Department of Health and Human Services, the site can be used in both English and Spanish.

5722   Healthlink USA
                                                    www.healthlinkusa.com
Links to websites which may include treatment, cures, diagnosis, prevention, support groups, email lists, messageboards, personal stories, risk factors, statistics, research and more.

5723   MedicineNet
                                                    www.medicinenet.com
An online resource for consumers providing easy-to-read, authoritative medical and health information.

5724   Medscape
                                                    www.medscape.com
Medscape offers specialists, primary care physicians, and other health professionals the Web's most robust and integrated medical information and educational tools.

5725   Polycystic Kidney Research Foundation
                                                    www.pkdcure.org
Provide information on research into the cause, treatment, and cure of polycystic kidney disease by raising financial support for peer approved biomedical research projects and fostering public awareness among medical professionals, patients and the general public.

5726   WebMD
                                                    www.webmd.com
Provides credible information, supportive communities, and in-depth reference material about health subjects. A source for original and timely health information as well as material from well known content providers.

Description

5727 Liver Disease

Liver disease covers a wide range of disorders that can result in chronic liver damage, such as scarring (fibrosis) or the development of cirrhosis. An estimated 43,000 Americans die each year from liver disease.

Specific liver diseases that damage the liver include infections (e.g., viral hepatitis), chronic alcoholism or drug abuse, medications, substance abuse, and certain systemic illnesses. Severe disease can permanently damage the liver, causing it to fail totally. The most common causes of liver failure are viruses, drugs, and toxins. Less common causes include vascular (e.g., hepatic vein thrombosis, portal vein thrombosis, and hepatic sinusoidal obstruction syndrome) and metabolic disorders (e.g., Reye Syndrome, Wilson disease, acute fatty liver of pregnancy).

Common signs of liver damage are fatigue, loss of appetite, nausea and tea-colored urine. Yellowing of the skin and the whites of the eye (jaundice) is seen in 50 percent of cases. Other symptoms include liver enlargement and tenderness, and fluid collection in the abdominal cavity. A shriveling liver indicates more chronic and severe damage. The main signs of live failure are jaundice, bleeding disorders (coagulopathy), and brain inflammation (encephalopathy) as a result of increase ammonium production.

Treatment for liver disease depends on the underlying cause. In less severe injury, due to its remarkable capacity to heal itself, the liver can completely recover. In cases of acetaminophen intoxication, N-acetylcysteine is an effective antidote if given in a timely manner. Liver transplantation is accepted as appropriate treatment for end-stage liver dysfunction. See also *Hepatitis*.

National Agencies & Associations

5728 Administration for Children and Families
330 C Street SW
Washington, DC 20201

202-205-8347
Fax: 202-205-9721
www.acf.hhs.gov

The Administration for Children & Families (ACF) is a division of the U.S. Department of Health & Human Services (HHS). ACF promotes the economic and social well-being of families, children, individuals and communities.
Lynn Johnson, Assistant Secretary
Jerry Milner, Acitng Commissioner, Children & Families

5729 Agency for Healthcare Research and Quality
5600 Fishers Lane
Rockville, MD 20857

301-427-1104
www.ahrq.gov

The Agency for Healthcare Research and Quality's (AHRQ) mission is to produce evidence to make health care safer, higher quality, more accessible, equitable, and affordable, and to work within the U.S. Department of Health and Human Services and with other partners to make sure that the evidence is understood and used.
Gopal Khanna, MBA, Director
Howard E. Holland, Director, Communications

5730 Agency for Toxic Substances and Disease Registry
4770 Buford Hwy NE
Atlanta, GA 30341-3717

770-488-0736
800-232-4636
Fax: 770-488-1547
TTY: 888-232-6348
jah8@cdc.gov
www.atsdr.cdc.gov

The Agency for Toxic Substances and Disease Registry (ATSDR), based in Atlanta, Georgia, is a federal public health agency of the U.S. Department of Health and Human Services. ATSDR serves the public by using the best science, taking responsive public health actions, and providing trusted health information to prevent harmful exposures and diseases related to toxic substances.
Patrick Breysse, PhD, CIH, Director
Jack Hanley, Acting Branch Chief, Central Branch

5731 American Association for the Study of Liver Diseases
1001 N Fairfax Street
Alexandria, VA 22314

703-299-9766
Fax: 703-299-9622
aasld@aasld.org
www.aasld.org

Physicians, researchers, and allied hepatology health professionals dedicated to preventing and curing liver disease by fostering research on liver diseases.
Michael W. Fried, MD, FAASLD, President
Meena B. Bansal, MD, FAASLD, Secretary

5732 American Liver Foundation
39 Broadway
New York, NY 10006

212-668-1000
800-465-4837
Fax: 212-483-8179
info@liverfoundation.org
www.liverfoundation.org

ALF raises awareness of liver disease through education, advocacy, and research for the prevention, treatment, and cure of liver disease, and provides support services to those affected.
Tom Nealon, President & CEO
Lynn Gardiner Seim, Executive Vice President & COO

5733 Association for Glycogen Storage Disease
PO Box 896
Durant, IA 52747

563-514-4022
info@agsdus.org
www.agsdus.org

Organization for parents of and individuals with glycogen storage disease (GSD) to communicate, share useful information, provide support, create awareness of GSD, and to foster research on glycogen storage diseases.
Iris Ferrecchia, President
Jessica Knepler, Vice President

5734 Centers for Medicare & Medicaid Services
7500 Security Boulevard
Baltimore, MD 21244

410-786-3000
877-267-2323
TTY: 866-226-1819
www.cms.gov

U.S. federal agency which administers Medicare, Medicaid, and the State Children's Health Insurance Program.
Seema Verma, Administrator
Tom Corry, Director

5735 Children's Liver Association For Support Services (CLASS)
PO Box 186
Monaca, PA 15061

724-581-5527
classkidscaresgmail.com
www.classkids.org

An organization dedicated to addressing the emotional, educational and financial needs of families with children affected by liver disease and transplantation.
William E. Berquist, MD, Chairman
Aimee Seningen, MD, Treasurer

5736 National Center for Complementary and Integrative Health
9000 Rockville Pike
Bethesda, MD 20892

888-644-6226
TTY: 866-464-3615
info@nccih.nih.gov
nccih.nih.gov

The National Center for Complementary and Integrative Health (NCCIH) is the Federal Government's lead agency for scientific research on the diverse medical and health care systems, practices,

and products that are not generally considered part of conventional medicine.
Helene M. Langevin, MD, Director
David Shurtleff, Ph.D., Deputy Director

5737   National Human Genome Research Institute
Building 31, Room 4B09   301-402-0911
Bethesda, MD 20892-2152   Fax: 301-402-2218
www.genome.gov
The National Human Genome Research Institute began as the National Center for Human Genome Research (NCHGR), which was established in 1989 to carry out the role of the National Institutes of Health (NIH) in the International Human Genome Project (HGP).
Eric D. Green, M.D., Ph.D., Director
Lawrence Brody, Ph.D., Director, Division of Genomics & Society

5738   National Institute for Occupational Safety and Health
Patriots Plaza 1
395 E Street SW   202-245-0625
Washington, DC 20201   800-232-4636
Fax: 513-533-8347
TTY: 888-232-6348
www.cdc.gov/niosh
The National Institute for Occupational Safety and Health (NIOSH) is the U.S. federal agency that conducts research and makes recommendations to prevent worker injury and illness.
John Howard, MD, Director
Frank Hearl, PE, Chief of Staff

5739   National Institute of Biomedical Imaging and Bioengineering
9000 Rockville Pike   301-496-8859
Bethesda, MD 20892   info@nibib.nih.gov
www.nibib.nih.gov
The mission of the National Institute of Biomedical Imaging and Bioengineering (NIBIB) is to improve health by leading the development and accelerating the application of biomedical technologies.
Bruce J. Tromberg, PhD, Director
Jill Heemskerk, PhD, Deputy Director

5740   National Institute of Diabetes & Digestive & Kidney Diseases
Office Of Communications and Public Liaison, NIH
31 Center Drive   800-860-8747
Bethesda, MD 20892-2560   TTY: 866-569-1162
healthinfo@niddk.nih.gov
www.niddk.nih.gov
Research areas include diabetes, digestive diseases, endocrine and metabolic diseases, hematologic diseases, kidney disease, liver disease, urologic diseases, as well as matters relating to nutrition and obesity.
Griffin P. Rodgers, MD, MACP, Director
Gregory Germino, MD, Deputy Director

5741   National Institute of Environmental Health Sciences
105 T.W. Alexander Drive   919-541-3345
Research Triangle Park, NC 27709 webcenter@niehs.nih.gov
www.niehs.nih.gov
The mission of the NIEHS is to discover how the environment affects people in order to promote healthier lives.
Linda S. Birnbaum, PhD, Director
Richard Woychik, PhD, Deputy Director

5742   National Institute of General Medical Sciences
45 Center Drive MSC 6200   301-496-7301
Bethesda, MD 20892-6200   info@nigms.nih.gov
www.nigms.nih.gov
The National Institute of General Medical Sciences (NIGMS) supports basic research that increases understanding of biological processes and lays the foundation for advances in disease diagnosis, treatment and prevention.
Jon R. Lorsch, PhD, Director
Judith H. Greenberg, PhD, Deputy Director

5743   U.S. Food and Drug Administration
10903 New Hampshire Avenue   301-796-8240
Silver Spring, MD 20993-0002   888-463-6332
www.fda.gov
FDA is responsible for protecting the public health by assuring the safety, efficacy and security of human and veterinary drugs, biological products, medical devices, the nation's food supply, cosmetics, and products that emit radiation.
Norman E. Sharpless, MD, Commissioner
Denise Hinton, Chief Scientist

State Agencies & Associations

Arizona

5744   American Liver Foundation Arizona Chapter
4545 E Shea Boulevard   602-953-1800
Phoenix, AZ 85028   866-953-1800
Fax: 602-953-1806
mmcracken@liverfoundation.org
www.liverfoundation.org
Melissa McCracken, Executive Director
Ashley Drew, Events Manager

California

5745   American Liver Foundation Greater Los Angeles Chapter
5777 Century Boulevard   310-670-4624
Los Angeles, CA 90045   Fax: 310-670-4672
tfantini@liverfoundation.org
www.liverfoundation.org
Taly Fantini, Executive Director

5746   American Liver Foundation Northern CA Chapter
870 Market Street   415-248-1060
San Francisco, CA 94102   800-292-9099
Fax: 415-248-1066
gmartin@liverfoundation.org
www.liverfoundation.org
Greg Martin, Executive Director

5747   American Liver Foundation San Diego Chapte r
2515 Camino del Rio S   619-291-5483
San Diego, CA 92108   800-749-2630
Fax: 619-295-7181
mdemotto@liverfoundation.org
www.liverfoundation.org
Michele De Motto, Executive Director

Colorado

5748   American Liver Foundation Rocky Mountain Division
1660 S Albion Street   303-988-4388
Denver, CO 80222   Fax: 303-988-4398
jmccormack@liverfoundation.org
www.liverfoundation.org
Joe McCormack, Executive Director

Connecticut

5749   American Liver Foundation: Connecticut Chapter
127 Washington Avenue   203-234-2022
N Haven, CT 06473   Fax: 203-234-1386
jthompson@liverfoundation.org
www.liverfoundation.org
Offers support for patients and families provides educational meetings and conferences raising vital liver research dollars; encouraging the beautifully unselfish gift of organ donation and the medical miracle of organ transplantation.
12 pages Quarterly
JoAnn Thompson, Executive Director

Florida

5750   American Liver Foundation Gulf Coast Chapter
202 S 22nd Street   813-248-3337
Ybor City, FL 33605   Fax: 813-248-3340
jbourgeois@liverfoundation.org
www.liverfoundation.org
Jennifer Nillias, Executive Director

Illinois

5751 American Liver Foundation Illinois Chapter
67 East Madison Street   312-377-9030
Chicago, IL 60603   Fax: 312-377-9035
info@illinois-liver.org
www.illinois-liver.org

Kevin Sutton, Executive Director
Kristin Gray, Development Coordinator

Indiana

5752 American Liver Foundation Indiana Chapter
PO BOX 36085   317-635-5074
Indianapolis, IN 46236   877-548-3730
Fax: 317-635-5075
dsparksunsworth@liverfoundation.org
www.liverfoundation.org

Katrina Marshall, Executive Director

Maryland

5753 National Institute on Alcohol Abuse and Alcoholism
Bethesda, MD   888-69 -4222
niaaaweb-r@exchange.nih.gov
www.niaaa.nih.gov
NIAAA supports and conducts research on the impact of alcohol use on human health and well-being. It is the largest funder of alcohol research in the world.
Dr. George Koob, Director
Kenneth R. Warren, Ph.D., Deputy Director

5754 National Institute on Drug Abuse
6001 Executive Boulevard   301-443-1124
Bethesda, MD 20892   dd279k@nih.gov
www.drugabuse.gov
NIDA's mission is to lead the Nation in bringing the power of science to bear on drug abuse and addiction.
Nora D. Volkow, M.D., Director
David Daubert, Acting Associate Director for Management

Michigan

5755 American Liver Foundation Michigan Chapter
21886 Farmington Road   248-615-5768
Farmington, MI 48336   888-MYL-IVER
Fax: 248-615-5778
michigan@liverfoundation.org
www.liverfoundation.org

Jennifer L Stibbe, Executive Director
Meghan Likes, Community Events Coordinator

Minnesota

5756 American Liver Foundation Minnesota Chapte r
2626 E 82nd Street   952-854-6181
Bloomington, MN 55425   Fax: 952-854-6956
dgirard@liverfoundation.org
www.liverfoundation.org
Dee Girard, Executive Director

Missouri

5757 American Liver Foundation Greater Kansas City Chapter
16 Hampton Village Plaza   314-352-7377
St. Louis, MO 63109   866-455-4837
Fax: 612-892-8442
rmattler@liverfoundation.org
www.liverfoundation.org

Richard Mattler, Executive Director

New York

5758 American Liver Foundation Greater New York Chapter
39 Broadway   212-943-1059
New York, NY 10006   877-307-7507
Fax: 212-943-1314
greaterny@liverfoundation.org
www.liverfoundation.org

Randa Adib, Director, Development
Stephanie Paul, Gala Director

5759 American Liver Foundation Western New York Chapter
25 Canterbury Road   585-271-2859
Rochester, NY 14607   Fax: 585-271-8642
nkoris@liverfoundation.org
www.liverfoundation.org

Nancy Rodwa MNO, Executive Director

Pennsylvania

5760 American Liver Foundation Delaware Valley Chapter
1341 North Delaware Avenue   215-425-8080
Philadelphia, PA 19125   Fax: 215-425-8181
iallison@liverfoundation.org
www.liverfoundation.org
Ivory Allison, Executive Director

5761 American Liver Foundation Western Pennsylv ania
100 W Station Square Drive   412-434-7044
Pittsburgh, PA 15219   Fax: 412-434-7040
samasartis@liverfoundation.org
www.liverfoundation.org

Suzanna Masartis, Executive Director

Tennessee

5762 American Liver Foundation Midsouth Chapter
PO BOX 486   901-766-7668
Ellendale, TN 38029   866-756-7668
Fax: 901-881-3842
midsouth@liverfoundation.org
www.liverfoundation.org

Winn Stephenson, Division Founder
Tina Sandoval, Board Chair

Virginia

5763 National Science Foundation
4201 Wilson Blvd   703-292-5111
Arlington, VA 22230   TDD: 703-292-5090
info@nsf.gov
www.nsf.gov
NSF is the only federal agency whose mission includes support for all fields of fundamental science and engineering, except for medical sciences.
France A. Cordova, Director
Joan Ferrini-Mundy, Chief Operating Officer

Washington

5764 American Liver Foundation Pacific Northwest Chapter
PO BOX 22108   212-668-1000
Seattle, WA 98122   800-465-4837
Fax: 206-443-1511
www.liverfoundation.org

Dr. Stephen Corrigan Rayhill, MD, Director
Dr. Andrew Precht, MD, Director

Wisconsin

5765 American Liver Foundation Wisconsin Chapter
1845 N Farwell Avenue   414-763-3435
Milwaukee, WI 53202   Fax: 414-961-7288
dgirard@liverfoundation.org
www.liverfoundation.org

Dee Girard, Executive Director

Foundations

5766 National Gaucher Foundation
5410 Edson Lane
Rockville, MD 20852
800-504-3189
ngf@gaucherdisease.org
www.gaucherdisease.org
National foundation providing information and assistance for those affected by Gaucher disease, as well as education and outreach to increase public awareness.
Brian Berman, President & CEO
Amy Blum, Chief Operating Officer

Research Centers

5767 Clinical Research Center: Pediatrics Children's Hospital Research Foundation
Children's Hospital Research Foundation
Elland & Bethesda Avenues
Cincinnati, OH 45229
513-559-4412
Fax: 513-559-7431
Studies of pediatric acquired diseases including liver disease and Reye's Syndrome.
Dr James G Redeker, Co-director

5768 University of California Liver Research Unit
7601 E Imperial Highway
Downey, CA 90242
562-940-8961
Fax: 562-940-6628
Dr Allan Lee MD Facp, Professor InteRNal Medicine / Director

5769 University of Texas Southwestern Medical Center
5323 Harry Hines Boulevard
Dallas, TX 75390-9151
214-645-8300
Fax: 214-645-7999
www.utsouthwestern.edu
Daniel K Podolsky, MD, President
J. Gregory Fitz, Executive Vice President

5770 University of Texas Southwestern Medical
5323 Harry Hines Boulevard
Dallas, TX 75390
214-645-8300
Fax: 214-645-7999
news@utsouthwestern.edu
www.utsouthwestern.edu
Daniel K Podolsky, MD, President
J. Gregory Fitz, Executive Vice President

5771 Yeshiva University Marion Bessin Liver Research Center
Albert Einstein College of Medicine
1300 Morris Park Avenue
Bronx, NY 10461-1975
718-430-2000
Fax: 718-918-0857
www.einstein.yu.edu/centers/liver-resear
Liver disease research and therapy.
Allan W Wolkoff, MD, Director
David A Shafritz, MD, Associate Director

Support Groups & Hotlines

5772 Children's Liver Association for Support S ervices
25379 Wayne Mills Place
Valencia, CA 91355
661-263-9099
877-679-8256
Fax: 661-263-9099
admin@classkids.org
www.classkids.org
Dedicated to addressing the emotional, educational, and financial needs of families with children with liver disease or liver transplantation. Telephone hotline, newsletter, parent matching, literature and financial assistance. supports research and educates public about organ donations.
Mark Sumner, Co-Founder
Diane Sumner, Co-Founder

5773 National Health Information Center
Office of Disease Prevention & Health Promotion
1101 Wootton Pkwy
Rockville, MD 20852
Fax: 240-453-8281
odphpinfo@hhs.gov
www.health.gov/nhic
Supports public health education by maintaining a calendar of National Health Observances; helps connect consumers and health professionals to organizations that can best answer questions and provide up-to-date contact information from reliable sources; up-

dates on a yearly basis toll-free numbers for health information, Federal health clearinghouses and info centers.
Don Wright, MD, MPH, Director

5774 National Reye's Syndrome Foundation
426 N Lewis Street
Bryan, OH 43506
419-636-2679
800-233-7393
Fax: 419-636-9897
www.reyessyndrome.org
Devoted to conquering Reye's syndrome, primarily a children's disease affecting the liver and brain, but can affect all ages. Provides support, information and referrals. Encourages research.
John Symonds, Executive Director

5775 Wilson's Disease Association
5572 North Diversey Boulevard
Milwaukee, WI 53217
414-961-0533
866-961-0533
Fax: 330-264-0974
info@wilsonsdisease.org
www.wilsonsdisease.org
Serves as a communications support network for individuals affected by Wilson's disease; distributes information to professionals and the public; makes referrals; and holds meetings.
8 pages
Mary L Graper, President
Stefanie F Kaplan, Vice-President

Books

5776 Liver Cancer
Churchill Livingstone
PO Box 3188
Secaucus, NJ 07096-3188
201-319-9800
800-553-5426
Fax: 201-319-9659
www.churchillmed.com
1997 640 pages Hardcover
ISBN: 0-443054-81-9
Steven A. Curley, Author

5777 Liver Disease in Children
Mosby Year Book
11830 Westline Indus Drv
Saint Louis, MO 63146-3313
314-872-8370
800-325-4177
1993 800 pages
ISBN: 1-556443-77-2
Frederick J. Suchy, Author
Ronald J. Sokol, Author

Magazines

5778 American Association for the Study of Liver Diseases
1729 King Street
Alexandria, VA 22314
703-299-9766
Fax: 703-299-9622
aasld@aasld.org
www.aasld.org
Information for professionals interested in disease of the liver and biliary tract.
Sherrie H Cathcart, Executive Director

5779 Hepatology
American Assoc. for the Study of Liver Disease
1729 King Street
Alexandria, VA 22314
703-299-9766
Fax: 703-299-9622
aasld@aasld.org
www.aasld.org
Information for professionals interested in disease of the liver and biliary tract.
Sherrie H Cathcart, Executive Director

Newsletters

5780 Children's Liver Association for Support S ervices Newsletter
25379 Wayne Mills Place
Valencia, CA 91355

661-263-9099
877-679-8256
Fax: 661-263-9099
SupportSrv@aol.com
www.classkids.org

Dedicated to addressing the emotional, educational, and financial needs of families with children with liver disease or liver transplantation. Telephone hotline, newsletter, parent matching, literature and financial assistance. supports research and educates public about organ donations.
Yearly
Diane Summer, President Board of Directors
Ann Whitehead RN/JD, Vice President Board of Directors

5781 Liver Update
American Liver Foundation
1425 Pompton Avenue
Cedar Grove, NJ 07009-1000

973-256-2550
800-465-4837
Fax: 973-256-3214
info@liverfoundation.org
www.liverfoundation.org

Clinical newsletter for physicians.
BiAnnually
Rick Smith, President & CEO
Rebecca Frank, Chief Development Officer

5782 LiverLink
Alagille Syndrome Alliance
10630 SW Garden Park Plc
Tigard, OR 97223-3832

503-639-6217
www.liverlink.com

Newsletter for Alagille Syndrome.

5783 Progress
American Liver Foundation
1425 Pompton Avenue
Cedar Grove, NJ 07009-1000

973-256-2550
800-465-4837
Fax: 973-256-3214
info@liverfoundation.org
www.liverfoundation.org

Newsletter about liver disease and ALF.
TriAnnually
Rick Smith, President & CEO
Rebecca Frank, Chief Development Officer

Pamphlets

5784 Alcohol and the Liver: Myth vs. Facts
American Liver Foundation
1425 Pompton Avenue
Cedar Grove, NJ 07009-1000

973-256-2550
800-223-0179
www.liverfoundation.org

Rick Smith, President & CEO
Rebecca Frank, Chief Development Officer

5785 Biliary Atresia
American Liver Foundation
1425 Pompton Avenue
Cedar Grove, NJ 07009-1000

973-857-2626
800-223-0179
info@liverfoundation.org
www.liverfoundation.org

Rick Smith, President & CEO
Kazuhiko Bessho, Author

5786 Diet and Your Liver
American Liver Foundation
1425 Pompton Avenue
Cedar Grove, NJ 07009-1000

973-256-2550
800-223-0179
Fax: 973-256-3214
info@liverfoundation.org
www.liverfoundation.org

Rick Smith, President & CEO
Rebecca Frank, Chief Development Officer

5787 Facts on Liver Transplantation
American Liver Foundation

1425 Pompton Avenue
Cedar Grove, NJ 07009-1000

973-256-2550
800-223-0179
Fax: 973-256-3214
info@liverfoundation.org
www.liverfoundation.org

Rick Smith, President & CEO
Rebecca Frank, Chief Development Officer

5788 Fatty Liver
American Liver Foundation
1425 Pompton Avenue
Cedar Grove, NJ 07009-1000

973-256-2550
800-223-0179
Fax: 987-256-3214
info@liverfoundation.org
www.liverfoundation.org

Rick Smith, President & CEO
Sandra Cabot, Author

5789 Gallstones
American Liver Foundation
1425 Pompton Avenue
Cedar Grove, NJ 07009-1000

973-256-2550
800-223-0179
Fax: 973-256-3214
info@liverfoundation.org
www.liverfoundation.org

Rick Smith, President & CEO
M. M. Fisher, Author

5790 Getting Help to Hepatitis
American Liver Foundation
1425 Pompton Avenue
Cedar Grove, NJ 07009-1000

973-256-2550
800-223-0179
Fax: 973-256-3214
info@liverfoundation.org
www.liverfoundation.org

Rick Smith, President & CEO

5791 Hemochromatosis
American Liver Foundation
1425 Pompton Avenue
Cedar Grove, NJ 07009-1000

973-256-2550
800-223-0179
Fax: 973-256-3214
info@liverfoundation.org
www.liverfoundation.org

Rick Smith, President & CEO
James C. Barton, Author

5792 Hepatitis A, B & C
American Liver Foundation
1425 Pompton Avenue
Cedar Grove, NJ 07009-1000

973-256-2550
800-223-0179
Fax: 973-256-3214
info@liverfoundation.org
www.liverfoundation.org

Rick Smith, President & CEO

5793 Hepatitis B: Your Child at Risk
American Liver Foundation
1425 Pompton Avenue
Cedar Grove, NJ 07009-1000

973-256-2550
800-223-0179
Fax: 973-256-3214
info@liverfoundation.org
www.liverfoundation.org

Rick Smith, President & CEO

5794 How Can You Love Me
American Liver Foundation
1425 Pompton Avenue
Cedar Grove, NJ 07009-1000

973-857-2626
800-223-0179
Fax: 973-256-3214
info@liverfoundation.org
www.liverfoundation.org

Rick Smith, President & CEO

5795 Liver Function Tests
American Liver Foundation

1425 Pompton Avenue
Cedar Grove, NJ 07009-1000

973-256-2550
800-223-0179
Fax: 973-256-3214
info@liverfoundation.org
www.liverfoundation.org

Rick Smith, President & CEO

5796   Liver Transplant Fund
American Liver Foundation
1425 Pompton Avenue
Cedar Grove, NJ 07009-1000

973-256-2550
800-223-0179
Fax: 973-256-3214
info@liverfoundation.org
www.liverfoundation.org

Rick Smith, President & CEO

5797   Liver Transplantation
American Liver Foundation
1425 Pompton Avenue
Cedar Grove, NJ 07009-1000

973-857-2626
800-223-0179
Fax: 973-256-3214
info@liverfoundation.org
www.liverfoundation.org

Rick Smith, President & CEO
Dilip Chakravarty, Author

5798   Viral Hepatitis
American Liver Foundation
1425 Pompton Avenue
Cedar Grove, NJ 07009-1000

973-256-2550
800-223-0179
Fax: 973-256-3214
info@liverfoundation.org
www.liverfoundation.org

Rick Smith, President & CEO

5799   Your Liver Lets You Live
American Liver Foundation
1425 Pompton Avenue
Cedar Grove, NJ 07009-1000

973-256-2550
800-223-0179
Fax: 973-256-3214
info@liverfoundation.org
www.liverfoundation.org

Rick Smith, President & CEO

Web Sites

5800   American Association for the Study of Liver Diseases

www.aasld.org/
Conducts symposia and educational courses for professionals interested in disease of the liver and biliary tract. The leading organization for advancing the science and practice of hepatology.

5801   Children's Liver Alliance

www.liverkids.org.au/
Empowering the hearts and minds of children with liver disease, their families and the medical professionals who care for them.

5802   Healing Well

www.healingwell.com
An online health resource guide to medical news, chat, information and articles, newsgroups and message boards, books, disease-related web sites, medical directories, and more for patients, friends, and family coping with disabling diseases, disorders, or chronic illnesses.

5803   Health Finder

www.healthfinder.gov
Searchable, carefully developed web site offering information on over 1000 topics. Developed by the US Department of Health and Human Services, the site can be used in both English and Spanish.

5804   Healthlink USA

www.healthlinkusa.com
Health information concerning treatment, cures, prevention, diagnosis, risk factors, research, support groups, email lists, personal stories and much more. Updated regularly.

5805   Liver Support

www.liversupport.com
Information about the world's safest, most powerful liver-protecting supplement, milk thistle. Specifically facts about the safe, yet highly potent, Phytosome form.

5806   MedicineNet

www.medicinenet.com
An online resource for consumers providing easy-to-read, authoritative medical and health information.

5807   Medscape

www.medscape.com
Medscape offers specialists, primary care physicians, and other health professionals the Web's most robust and integrated medical information and educational tools.

5808   WebMD

www.webmd.com
Provides credible information, supportive communities, and in-depth reference material about health subjects. A source for original and timely health information as well as material from well known content providers.

Description

5809 Lung Disease

Globally, lung diseases are among the most common medical conditions. Since the lungs are in intimate contact with a person's environment, they may be damaged by many different agents, including dust particles, gases and infectious organisms. The majority of lung, or pulmonary, diseases are related to exposure to external irritants, such as cigarette smoke, asbestos, bacteria and viruses. Because the lungs must expand to take in oxygen and contract to expel the metabolic waste product carbon dioxide, lung disease can result from problems with the gas exchange system or the mechanics of breathing.

The most common chronic lung diseases are those that affect the airways, which include emphysema and chronic bronchitis; both are part of the class of diseases called Chronic Obstructive Pulmonary Disease, or COPD. Most cases, though not all, are associated with tobacco usage. High-risk occupations for lung disease include mining, farming, building construction and certain types of manufacturing. Other types of lung disease that affects the airways include asthma, in which the airways are sensitized to allergens (molecules to which to patient is allergic) and experience persistent inflammation that, if untreated, can permanently narrow the airways; acute bronchitis in which an infectious agent causes inflammation in the airways; and cystic fibrosis, a genetic disease that causes the airways to become obstructed with thick, rubbery mucus that encourages respiratory infections and prevents proper air exchange.

Other lung diseases affect the terminal bronchioles and the tiny air sacs (alveoli) into which they terminate. These diseases include pneumonias caused by bacterial infections of the lungs, tuberculosis, which is a slow-progressing pneumonia caused by *Mycobacterium tuberculosis*, pulmonary edema, which is caused by leakage of fluid from blood vessels into the alveoli as a result of lung damage or heart failure, pneumoconiosis or black lung from the inhalation of fine coal dust or asbestos, acute respiratory distress syndrome, which is caused by severe, direct damage to the lungs and requires immediate respiratory support, emphysema, usually as a result of smoking, and lung cancer. Lung cancer may be primary (originating in the lung) or secondary (spread, or metastasized, from another area). Bronchogenic cancer accounts for more than 90 percent of all lung tumors; cigarette smoking is the principal cause. Lung cancer is usually seen in people with COPD, because the two conditions have similar causes.

Lung disease can also affect the tissue that lies between the alveoli (the interstitium), or the pleural membranes that surround the lungs. Pneumonias or pulmonary edemas can adversely affect the lung interstitium, as can a host of other so-called "interstitial lung diseases," which include sarcoidosis, autoimmune diseases, and idiopathic pulmonary fibrosis (IPF). Fluid that leaks into the pleural membranes (pleural effusion) can prevent the lungs from properly expanding and can cause trouble breathing. Likewise, damage to the thoracic body wall cause air to leak into the pleural space (pneumothorax), and the increased air pressure can collapse the lung and prevent it from re-expanding. Cancer of the pleural membranes (mesothelioma) is a consequence of repeated exposure to asbestos.

Other lung disorders are secondary to other diseases, and include clots that originate from other sites in the body (pulmonary embolism) and obstruct pulmonary circulation, systemic illnesses that inhibit breathing mechanics, such as myasthenia gravis or amyotrophic lateral sclerosis, and skeletal abnormalities or obesity that interfere with chest expansion during breathing.

Symptoms of lung disease may include coughing, sputum production, breathlessness, and sometimes fever or chest pain. In advanced cases, breathlessness is constant, and cyanosis (a bluish discoloration of the lips and fingernails) may occur. In the case of severe pneumonias or severe lung cancer, the sputum might be flecked with blood.

Diagnosis of pulmonary disorders depends on a very careful history, physical examination, chest x-ray and pulmonary function testing, or spirometry. These measures are also important in following disease progression and response to treatment. Other chest imaging techniques, such as computed tomography (CT) scans and MRIs, and examination of fluid in the lung and lung tissue help establish a diagnosis. Recent research indicates that PET (positron emission tomography) scans may be helpful in the earlier diagnosis and treatment of lung cancer.

Treatment of lung disease depends on the underlying cause. Management of COPD includes avoiding tobacco or other environmental exposure, antibiotics to control infections and heavy sputum production, and drugs (inhaled B_2-adrenergic agonists and antimuscarinics) to dilate narrowed airways. Inhaled steroids can also decrease inflammation in the airways and increase gas exchange. In advanced cases, breathing oxygen directly by nasal prongs improves quality of life and survival. In older patients, bronchial thermoplasty is an option to widen chronically narrowed airways.

Lung transplantation has occasionally been attempted, usually when COPD is due to a genetic disorder. Early screening for lung cancer has been disappointing; quitting smoking early is the only meaningful way of reducing one's risk of dying of the disease. Treatment may include surgery, radiation, or chemotherapy; success depends on the stage of the tumor and its precise type as determined by tissue biopsy.

Severe Acute Respiratory Syndrome, known as SARS, is an infectious disease that first appeared in China in 2002. SARS is caused by a corona-virus, which is related to the virus behind the common cold. The symptoms of SARS are a fever, greater than 100.4 degrees, fatigue, headache and chills. It is also accompanied by a dry cough and difficulty breathing, owing to the inflamed lungs. Until effective treatment or a vaccine is developed, prevention in SARS-infected areas includes isolating patients, wearing protective surgical masks, and restricting travel. Since 2004, no cases of SARS have been reported. In 2017, Chinese researchers traced the source of the SARS virus to cave-dwelling horseshoe bats in Yunnan province.

National Agencies & Associations

5810 American Association for Respiratory Care
9425 N MacArthur Boulevard
Irving, TX 75063-4706

972-243-2272
Fax: 972-484-2720
info@aarc.org
www.aarc.org

The national and international professional association for respiratory care.
Tom Kallstrom, Executive Director
Shawna Strickland, Associate Executive Director

5811 American Lung Association
55 W. Wacker Drive
Chicago, IL 60601

800-586-4872
info@lung.org
www.lung.org

The mission of the American Lung Association is to prevent lung disease and promote lung health by fighting disease in all its forms, with special emphasis on asthma, tobacco control and environmental health.
Harold P. Wimmer, National President & CEO
Albert Rizzo, MD, FACP, Chief Medical Officer

5812 National Jewish Health
1400 Jackson Street
Denver, CO 80206

800-222-5864
877-225-5654
physicianline@njhealth.org
www.nationaljewish.org

Leading respiratory hospital in the nation offering comprehensive diagnosis, treatment and rehabilitation of people with chronic obstructive pulmonary disease, asthma, allergies and other respiratory and immune diseases.
Richard Baer, Chair
Michael Salem, MD, President & CEO

5813 Pulmonary Fibrosis Foundation
230 E Ohio Street
Chicago, IL 60611

888-733-6741
Fax: 866-587-9158
info@pulmonaryfibrosis.org
www.pulmonaryfibrosis.org

Dedicated to finding a cure for and raising awareness of pulmonary fibrosis.
William T. Schmidt, President & CEO
Scott Staszak, COO

5814 Pulmonary Hypertension Association (PHA)
801 Roeder Road
Silver Spring, MD 20910

301-565-3004
800-748-7274
pha@PHAssociation.org
www.PHAssociation.org

A non-profit organization for pulmonary hypertension patients, families, caregivers and PH-treating medical professionals. PHA works to provide support, education, and find a cure for pulmonary hypertension.
Brad A. Wong, President & CEO
Azalea Candelaria, Vice President

5815 US Environmental Protection Agency: Indoor Environments Division
1200 Pennsylvania Avenue NW
Washington, DC 20460

800-424-8802
www.epa.gov/iaq

Responsible for implementing EPA's Indoor Environments Program, a voluntary program to address indoor air pollution.
Andrew Wheeler, Administrator
Henry Darwin, Acting Deputy Administrator

5816 White Lung Association
PO Box 1483
Baltimore, MD 21203-1483

info@whitelung.org
www.whitelung.org

A national non-profit organization dedicated to the education of the public to the hazards of asbestos exposure. The association developed programs of public education and consults with victims of asbestos exposure, school boards, building owners and government representatives.
Jim Perry, Director of Development

State Agencies & Associations

Alabama

5817 American Lung Association of Alabama
PO BOX 2178
Ridgeland, AL 35244

601-206-5810
Fax: 202-452-1805
inquiries@breathehealthy.org

Robin Robinson, Chair
Sara Dreiling, Chief Executive Officer

Alaska

5818 American Lung Association of Alaska
500 W International Airport Road
Anchorage, AK 99518-1105

907-276-5864
800-LUN-GUSA
Fax: 907-565-5587
mstoneking@aklung.org
www.lung.org/associations/states/alaska/

Marge Pfeifer, President/CEO

Arizona

5819 American Lung Association of Arizona
102 W McDowell Road
Phoenix, AZ 85003-1299

602-258-7505
800-LUN-GUSA
Fax: 602-258-7507
calexander@lungarizona.org

Through research education and advocacy the American Lung Association of Arizona works to prevent lung disease and promote lung health. Our areas of focus are asthma air quality and tobacco control.
Terry Daane, Chair
Stacey Mortenson, Executive Director

Arkansas

5820 American Lung Association of Arkansas
211 Natural Resources Drive
Little Rock, AR 72205-1539

501-224-5864
800-880-5864
Fax: 501-224-5654
www.lungark.org

Karen S Abate, President/CEO
Sylvia Goodin, Secretary

California

5821 American Lung Association of California
424 Pendleton Way
Oakland, CA 94621-2189
510-638-5864
Fax: 510-638-8984
cainfo@lung.org

A.Linda Hinojosa, Chair
Jane Warner, President/CEO

Colorado

5822 American Lung Association of Colorado
5600 Greenwood Plaza Boulevard
Greenwood Village, CO 80111
303-388-4327
800-LUN-GUSA
Fax: 303-377-1102
http://www.lung.org/associations/states/

Curt Huber, Executive Director
Connor Michael, Communications Manager

Connecticut

5823 American Lung Association of Connecticut
45 Ash Street
E Hartford, CT 06108-3272
860-289-5401
800-586-4872
Fax: 860-289-5405
www.alact.org

Part of the American Lung Association the oldest voluntary health agency dedicated to fighting a single disease. Highest priorities are asthma tobacco control and clean air.
Lisa Brown, VP Community Outreach
Susan DeNardo, Development Director

Delaware

5824 American Lung Association of Delaware
630 Churchmans Road
Wilmington, DE 19702-3280
302-737-6414
800-LUN-GUSA
Fax: 888-415-5757
llyons@lunginfo.org
www.lung.org/associations/charters/mid-a

Christopher Carney, Chair
Deborah Brown, CEO

District of Columbia

5825 American Lung Association of the District of Columbia
1301 Pennsylvania Avenue NW
Washington, DC 20004-2617
202-785-3355
lungdc@lung.org

Resource for information and programs in the area of lung health, including asthma, tobacco control, air quality, sarcoidosis, and turberculosis.
Dennis C Alexander, Regional Executive Director
Marc Ittelson, Regional Development Director

Florida

5826 American Lung Association of Florida
6852 Belfort Oaks Place
Jacksonville, FL 32216-5216
904-743-2933
800-940-2933
Fax: 904-743-2916
alaf@lungfla.org
www.lung.org/associations/states/florida

Works for the prevention and control of lung disease through education, advocacy and research.
Marcia Williams, Chairwoman
Martha C Bogdan, President/CEO

Georgia

5827 American Lung Association of Georgia
2452 Spring Road
Smyrna, GA 30080-3862
770-434-5864
Fax: 770-319-0349
Marcia Williams, Chairwoman of the Board
Martha C Bogdan, President/CEO

Hawaii

5828 American Lung Association of Hawaii
650 Iwilei Road
Honolulu, HI 96817
808-537-5966
Fax: 808-537-5971
lleslie@ala-hawaii.org

Lorraine Leslie, Hawaii Director
Debbie Apolo, Tobacco Control Manager

Idaho

5829 American Lung Association of Idaho
1412 W Idaho
Boise, ID 83702
208-345-5864
800-LUN-GUSA
Fax: 208-345-5896
www.lung.org/associations/states/idaho/

Wimmer, CEO
Kim Streib, Vice President Finance

Illinois

5830 American Lung Association of Illinois
55 West Wacker Drive
Chicago, IL 60601
312-781-1100
800-LUN-GUSA
Fax: 318-781-9250
info@lungil.org

Frank Keldermans, Chair
Lewis Bartfield, President/CEO

Indiana

5831 American Lung Association of Indiana
115 W Washington Street
Indianapolis, IN 46204-1470
317-819-1181
800-LUN-GUSA
Fax: 317-819-1187
info@lungin.org

Alan D Rowe, Chair
Lewis Bartfield, President/CEO

Iowa

5832 American Lung Association of Iowa
2530 73rd Street
Des Moines, IA 50322-1800
515-309-9507
800-LUN-GUSA
Fax: 515-334-9564
info@lungia.org
www.lung.org/associations/states/iowa/

Alan D Rowe, Chair
Lewis Bartfield, President/CEO

Kansas

5833 American Lung Association of Kansas
6701 W. 64th Street
Overland Park, KS 66202-2419
913-912- 719
800-LUN-GUSA
Fax: 913-912-7206
inquiries@breathehealthy.org
www.lung.org/associations/charters/plain

Robin Robinson, Chair
Veena B Antony, Director

Kentucky

5834 American Lung Association of Kentucky
4100 Churchman Avenue
Louisville, KY 40215-0067
502-363-2652
800-LUN-GUSA
Fax: 502-363-0222
bgottschalk@midlandlung.org

Barry Gottschalk, President/CEO
Robert Singletary, Vice President - Finance & Administratio

Louisiana

5835 American Lung Association of Louisiana
2325 Severn Avenue
Metairie, LA 70001-6918
504-828-5864
800-586-4872
Fax: 504-828-5867
inquiries@breathehealthy.org
www.lung.org/associations/charters/plain
Robin Robinson, Chair
Veena B Antony, Director

Maine

5836 American Lung Association of Maine
122 State Street
Augusta, ME 04330
207-622-6394
888-241-6566
Fax: 207-626-2919
info@lungne.org
www.lung.org/associations/states/maine/
Ross P Lanzafame, Chairman of the Board
John F Emanuel, Secretary/ Treasurer

Maryland

5837 American Lung Association of Maryland
211 East Lombard Street
Baltimore, MD 21202
443-451-4950
800-LUN-GUSA
Fax: 410-560-0829
lungmd@lungusa.org
Dennis C Alexander, Regional Executive Director
Marc Ittelson, Regional Development Director

Massachusetts

5838 American Lung Association of Massachusetts
5 Mountain Road
Burlington, MA 01903
781-272-2866
Adams, CEO
Nicole Crumpton, Executive Office Manager

Michigan

5839 American Lung Association of Michigan
1475 E 12 Mile Road
Madison Heights, MI 48071
248-784-2000
800-543-LUNG
Fax: 248-784-2008
midland@midlandlung.org
Barry Gottschalk, President/CEO
Robert Singletary, Vice President-Finance & Administration

Minnesota

5840 American Lung Association of Minnesota
490 Concordia Avenue
Saint Paul, MN 55103-2441
651-227-8014
800-LUN-GUSA
Fax: 651-227-5459
info@lungmn.org
Angie Carlson, PhD, Chair
Lewis Bartfield, President/CEO

Mississippi

5841 American Lung Association of Mississippi
PO Box 2178
Ridgeland, MS 39158
601-206-5810
Fax: 601-206-5813
inquiries@breathehealthy.org
www.lung.org/associations/charters/plain
Robin Robinson, Chair
Veena B Antony, Director

5842 American Lung Association of Missouri
6701 W. 64th Street
Overland Park, KS 66202
913-912- 719
Fax: 913-912-7206
inquiries@breathehealthy.org
www.lung.org/associations/charters/plain
Robin Robinson, Chair
Veena B Antony, Director

Missouri

5843 American Lung Association of Eastern Missouri
1118 Hampton Avenue
Saint Louis, MO 63139-3196
314-645-5505
Fax: 314-645-7128
www.lungusa2.org/missouri/index.html

5844 American Lung Association: Kansas City Office
2400 Troost
Kansas City, MO 64108
816-842-5242
Fax: 816-842-5470
National health association dedicated to promoting lung health and preventing lung disease.

Montana

5845 American Lung Association of Northern Rockies
825 Helena Avenue
Helena, MT 59601-3459
406-442-6556
Fax: 406-442-2346
ala-nr@ala-nr.org
www.lungusa.org

Nebraska

5846 American Lung Association of Nebraska
8990 West Dodge
Omaha, NE 68114
402-502-4950
800-LUN-GUSA
Fax: 402-502-3112
inquiries@breathehealthy.org
www.lung.org/associations/charters/plain
Robin Robinson, Chair
Veena B Antony, Director

Nevada

5847 American Lung Association of Nevada
10615 Double R Boulevard
Reno, NV 89521
775-829-LUNG
800-LUN-GUSA
Fax: 775-829-5850
www.lungusa.org
Lisa Genasci, Executive Director
Heather Lunsford, Development & Program Manager

New Hampshire

5848 American Lung Association of New Hampshire
1800 Elm Street
Manchester, NH 03104
603-369-3977
800-83L-UNGS
Fax: 603-369-3978
info@lungne.org
Ross P Lanzafame, Chairman of the Board
John F Emanuel, Secretary/ Treasurer

New Jersey

5849 American Lung Association of New Jersey
1031 Route 22 West
Bridgewater, NJ 08807-3410
908-685-8040
Fax: 888-415-5757
jgrinwald@lunginfo.org
www.lung.org/associations/charters/mid-a
Christopher Carney, Chair
Deborah Brown, CEO

New Mexico

5850 American Lung Association of New Mexico
5911 Jefferson Street NE
Albuquerque, NM 87109
505-265-0732
800-LUN-GUSA
Fax: 505-260-1739
info@lungnewmexico.org
Support group for adults with lung disease. Also offers lung health education.
Deborah Hoffman, Executive Director
JoAnna DeMaria, Director of Programs

Lung Disease / State Agencies & Associations

New York

5851 American Lung Association of New York State
418 Broadway
Albany, NY 12207-2804
518-465-2013
800-499-LUNG
Fax: 781-890-4280
info@lungne.org
www.lung.org/associations/charters/north
Brian Simonds, Chair
Jeff Seyler, President/CEO

North Carolina

5852 American Lung Association of North Carolina
514 Daniels Street
Raleigh, NC 27605
919-424-6069
800-586-4872
Fax: 919-856-8530
lungnc@lungusa.org
www.lungnc.org
Better breathing clubs for chronic lung disease patients.
Dennis C Alexander, Regional Executive Director
Marc Ittelson, Regional Development Director

North Dakota

5853 American Lung Association of North Dakota
212 N. 2nd Street
Bismarck, ND 58501
701-223-5613
800-252-6325
Fax: 701-223-5727
info@lungnd.org
http://www.lung.org/associations/states/
A voluntary health agency whose objective is the conquest of lung disease and the promotion of lung health. We sponsor Super Asthma Saturday and open airways for schools events to educate asthmatics and their families and Dakota Superkids Asthma Camp for kids 8-15 with asthma. Smoking cessation classes for adults and youth.
Alan D Rowe, Chair
Lewis Bartfield, President/CEO

Ohio

5854 American Lung Association of Ohio
1950 Arlingate Lane
Columbus, OH 43228-4102
614-279-1700
800-LUN-GUSA
Fax: 614-279-4940
alao@ohiolung.org
Barry Gottschalk, President/CEO
Robert Singletary, Vice President - Finance & Administratio

Oklahoma

5855 American Lung Association of Oklahoma
11212 N May Avenue
Oklahoma City, OK 73120
405-748-4674
800-LUN-GUSA
Fax: 405-748-6274
inquiries@breathehealthy.org
Robin Robinson, Chair
Veena B Antony, Director

Oregon

5856 American Lung Association of Oregon
7420 SW Bridgeport Road
Tigard, OR 97224-7790
503-924-4094
800-LUN-GUSA
Fax: 503-924-4120
www.lung.org/associations/states/oregon/

Pennsylvania

5857 American Respiratory Alliance of Western Pennsylvania
201 Smith Drive
Cranberry Township, PA 16066
724-772-1750
800-220-1990
Fax: 724-772-1180
info@healthylungs.org
www.healthylungs.org

Dedicated to the prevention and control of lung disease through education training, direct services, research funding and advocacy since 1904.
Christine R Cavan, Director
Robert Petix, Chair/Executive Committee

5858 Breathe Pennsylvania
3001 Old Gettysburg Road
Camp Hill, PA 17011
717-541-5864
800-932-0903
Fax: 888-415-5757
dbrown@lunginfo.org
www.lung.org/associations/charters/mid-a
Provide education, research and information on lung disease and lung health, including asthma, tobacco prevention and cessation, chronic obstructive pulmonary disease, indoor and outdoor air quality, children's summer camps, support groups and specialty programs.
Christopher Carney, Chair
Deborah Brown, CEO

Rhode Island

5859 American Lung Association of Rhode Island
260 W Exchange Street
Providence, RI 02903-3700
401-421-6487
800-586-4872
Fax: 401-331-5266
info@lungne.org
Brian Simonds, Chair
Jeff Seyler, President/CEO

South Carolina

5860 American Lung Association of South Carolina
44-A Markfield Drive
Charleston, SC 29407-2344
843-556-8451
800-849-5864
Fax: 843-766-3294
alasc1@lungsc.org
Marcia Williams, Chairwoman of the Board
William R Cook, Chair-Elect

South Dakota

5861 American Lung Association of South Dakota
401 East 8th Street
Sioux Falls, SD 57103-0233
605-336-7222
800-873-5864
Fax: 605-336-7227
info@lungsd.org
Alan D Rowe, Chair
Lewis Bartfield, President/CEO

Tennessee

5862 American Lung Association of Tennessee
1 Vantage Way
Nashville, TN 37228
615-329-1151
800-LUN-GUSA
Fax: 615-329-1723
gbost@midlandlung.org
A statewide organization the oldest national health agency in the US. Our mission is to prevent lung disease and to promote lung health. Our program priorities include environmental health asthma education tobacco control for children and finding a cure.
Dr Steven Coulter, Chairman
Barry Gottschalk, President/CEO

Texas

5863 American Lung Association of Texas
5926 Balcones Drive
Austin, TX 78731
512-467-6753
800-252-LUNG
Fax: 512-467-7621
inquiries@breathehealthy.org
www.texaslung.org
Robin Robinson, Chair
Veena B Antony, Director

5864 American Lung Association of Utah
1930 S 1100 E   801-484-4456
Salt Lake City, UT 84106-2317   800-548-8252
                                              Fax: 801-484-5461
                                www.lung.org/associations/states/utah/
Troy Neerings, Chair
W. Glenn Lanham, Executive Director

5865 American Lung Association of Virginia
9702 Gayton Road   804-955-4910
Richmond, VA 23238   800-345-5864
                                              Fax: 804-267-5634
                                              lungva@lungusa.org
                                              www.lungva.org
Dennis C Alexander, Regional Executive Director
Marc Ittelson, Regional Development Director

5866 American Lung Association of Washington
822 John Street   206-441-5100
Seattle, WA 98109   800-732-9339
                                              Fax: 206-441-3277
Marina Crickenberger, Executive Director
Chantal Fields, Assistant Executive Director

5867 American Lung Association of West Virginia
2102 Kanawha Blvd   304-342-6600
East Charleston, WV 25311   800-LUN-GUSA
                                              Fax: 888-415-5757
                                              cfields@lunginfo.org
Christopher Carney, Chair
Deborah Brown, CEO

5868 American Lung Association of Wisconsin
13100 W Lisbon Road   262-703-4200
Brookfield, WI 53005-2508   800-LUN-GUSA
                                              Fax: 262-781-5180
                                              info@lungwi.org
Alan D Rowe, Chair
Lewis Bartfield, President/CEO

Research Centers

5869 Enzymology Research Laboratory Dept. of Veterans Affairs Medical Center
Dept. of Veterans Affairs Medical Center
150 Muir Road   925-228-6800
Martinez, CA 94553
Studies affecting emphysema in mankind.
Michael C Gaussig, President

5870 National Jewish Center for Immunology
1400 Jackson Street   303-388-4461
Denver, CO 80206   877-225-5654
                                              www.nationaljewish.org
Offers basic and clinical research into the causes and treatments of various lung diseases and respiratory problems.
Rafeul Alam, Division Chief

5871 University of Utah Rocky Mountain Center for Occupational & Environmental Health
University of Utah
391 Chipeta Way   801-581-4800
Salt Lake City, UT 84108   Fax: 801-817-24
                                              TTY: 801-581-7224
                                              rmoser@rmcoeh.utah.edu
                                              medicine.utah.edu/rmcoeh/
Provides graduate and continuing education programs in occupational medicine occupational health nursing ergonomics and safety industrial hygiene and hazardous materials. Additionally provides clinical evaluations and consultations in the listed areas.
Dennis Lloyd, Chair
Sen Karen Mayne, Advisory Member

5872 Warren Grant Magnuson Clinical Center
National Institute of Health
10 Center Drive MSC 1078   301-496-3311
Bethesda, MD 20892   800-411-1222
                                              Fax: 301-496-2390
                                              TTY: 866-411-1010
                                              mmichael@cc.nih.gov
Established in 1953 as the research hospital of the National Institutes of Health. Designed so that patient care facilities are close to research laboratories so new findings of basic and clinical scientists can be quickly applied to the treatment of patients. Upon referral by physicians, patients are admitted to NIH clinical studies.
John Mark, Lung Help Line Director

Support Groups & Hotlines

5873 American Lung Association HelpLine
55 W. Wacker Drive   800-586-4872
Chicago, IL 60601   www.lung.org
Provides state-by-state association information, and offers support group referrals.

5874 Lung Facts
National Jewish Center for Immunology
1400 Jackson Street   303-388-4461
Denver, CO 80206   877-225-5654
                                              Fax: 303-270-2220
                                              allstetterw@njc.org
                                              www.nationaljewish.org
An automated information service with recorded health messages developed by Lung Line Information Service. The information provided on this system offers help and support, as well as medical updates for persons suffering from lung diseases.
Michael

5875 National Health Information Center
Office of Disease Prevention & Health Promotion
1101 Wootton Pkwy   Fax: 240-453-8281
Rockville, MD 20852   odphpinfo@hhs.gov
                                              www.health.gov/nhic
Supports public health education by maintaining a calendar of National Health Observances; helps connect consumers and health professionals to organizations that can best answer questions and provide up-to-date contact information from reliable sources; updates on a yearly basis toll-free numbers for health information, Federal health clearinghouses and info centers.
Don Wright, MD, MPH, Director

Books

5876 American Lung Association Family Guide to Asthma and Allergies
American Lung Association
55 W. Wacker Drive   800-586-4872
Chicago, IL 60601   info@lung.org
                                              www.lungusa.org
Norman H. Edelman, Author

5877 Health Consequences of Smoking: Cancer & Chronic Lung Disease in the Workplace
DIANE Publishing Company
330 Pusey Avenue   610-461-6200
Darby, PA 19023   800-782-3833
                                              Fax: 610-461-6130
                                              dianepublishing@gmail.com
                                              www.dianepublishing.net
Examines the relationship between cigarette smoking and occupational exposures. Establishes that in order to protect the workers fully, forces of labor, management, insurers and government must become as engaged in attempts to reduce the prevalence of ciga-

rette smoking as they are in occupational exposure. Tables and figure. Extensive bibliography, index.

542 pages Paperback
ISBN: 0-788123-11-4
Herman Baron, Publisher

5878 Management of Acute Exacerbations of Chronic Obstructive Pulmonary Disease
DIANE Publishing Company
330 Pusey Avenue   610-461-6200
Darby, PA 19023   800-782-3833
                                Fax: 610-461-6130
                                dianepublishing@gmail.com
                                www.dianepublishing.net
This report describes evidence about the clinical assessment and management of patients presenting with acute exacerbation of chronic obstructive pulmonary disease, a frequent cause of health care utilization, morality and decreased quality of life.

256 pages Paperback
ISBN: 0-756721-99-7
Herman Baron, Publisher

5879 Seven Steps to a Smoke-Free Life
American Lung Association
1740 Broadway   212-315-8700
New York, NY 10019-4315   800-586-4872
                                info@lungusa.org
                                www.lungusa.org

Pamphlets

5880 Around the Clock with COPD
American Lung Association
1740 Broadway   212-315-8700
New York, NY 10019-4315   800-586-4872
                                info@lungusa.org
                                www.lungusa.org
A booklet with non-medical helpful hints written by persons living with a chronic lung disease for others.

5881 Asbestos in Your Home
American Lung Association
1740 Broadway   212-315-8700
New York, NY 10019-4315   800-586-4872
                                info@lungusa.org
                                www.lungusa.org
Offers information on asbestos.

5882 Black Lung
National Jewish Center for Immunology
1400 Jackson Street   303-388-4461
Denver, CO 80206-2762   800-222-5864
Offers information on black lung and the respiratory system.

5883 Emphysema
American Lung Association of Connecticut
45 Ash Street   860-289-5401
East Hartford, CT 06108-3294   800-586-4872
                                Fax: 860-289-5405
                                www.alact.org
Offers information on who gets emphysema, how it attacks, causes, effects, prevention and treatment.
John E Zinn, President/CEO

5884 Exercise Guidelines for the Person with Lung Disease
American Lung Association of Connecticut
45 Ash Street   860-289-5401
East Hartford, CT 06108-3294   800-586-4872
                                Fax: 860-289-5405
                                www.alact.org
Offers exercise information and illustrations for persons with lung disease.
John E Zinn, President/CEO

5885 Facts About AAT Deficiency-Related Emphysema
American Lung Association

1740 Broadway   212-315-8700
New York, NY 10019-4315   800-586-4872
                                info@lungusa.org
                                www.lungusa.org
Offers information on this type of emphysema, risk factors, development, symptoms and early detection.

5886 Facts About Asbestos
American Lung Association
1740 Broadway   212-315-8700
New York, NY 10019-4315   800-586-4872
                                info@lungusa.org
                                www.lungusa.org
Offers information on lung hazards on the job and what employers can do to protect themselves and the people that work for them.

5887 Facts About Asthma
American Lung Association
1740 Broadway   212-315-8700
New York, NY 10019-4315   800-586-4872
                                info@lungusa.org
                                www.lungusa.org

5888 Steps to a Better Understanding of Lung Cancer: A Patient and Family Guide
American Lung Association
1740 Broadway   212-315-8700
New York, NY 10019-4315   800-586-4872
                                info@lungusa.org
                                www.lungusa.org
A booklet with non-medical helpful hints written by persons living with a chronic lung disease for others.

5889 Understanding Emphysema
National Jewish Center for Immunology
1400 Jackson Street   303-388-4461
Denver, CO 80206-2762   800-222-5864
Offers information on emphysema, causes, treatments, symptoms and prevention.

Audio & Video

5890 Keeping the Balance
Fanlight Productions
4196 Washington Street   617-469-4999
Boston, MA 02131-1731   800-937-4113
                                Fax: 617-469-3379
                                fanlight@fanlight.com
                                www.fanlight.com
Siblings of children with serious lung disease share their experiences of being the normal child, exploring the frequent conflict between their feelings of love and concern and their resentment over the attention denied to them because of the sibling's illness. Offers advice on how parents can keep the balance between the needs of all of their children.

1993 23 Minutes
ISBN: 1-572950-89-7

5891 Sickle Cell Disease: Faces of Our Children
Fanlight Productions
4196 Washington Street   617-469-4999
Boston, MA 02131-1731   800-937-4113
                                Fax: 617-469-3379
                                fanlight@fanlight.com
                                www.fanlight.com
This program examines the devastating impact of sickle cell disease on these young people and their families and caregivers. It will be an important tool for increasing awareness in the community and among healthcare and social service providers in community clinics, hospitals, and other settings.

1999 14 Minutes
ISBN: 1-572953-05-5

Web Sites

5892   American Lung Association

www.lung.org

Offers research, medical updates, fund-raising, educational materials and public awareness campaigns relating to lung disease causes.

5893   Healing Well

www.healingwell.com

An online health resource guide to medical news, chat, information and articles, newsgroups and message boards, books, disease-related web sites, medical directories, and more for patients, friends, and family coping with disabling diseases, disorders, or chronic illnesses.

5894   Health Central

www.healthcenter.com

Provides support group and diagnostic information regarding lung disease.

5895   Health Finder

www.healthfinder.gov

Searchable, carefully developed web site offering information on over 1000 topics. Developed by the US Department of Health and Human Services, the site can be used in both English and Spanish.

5896   Healthlink USA

www.healthlinkusa.com

Health information concerning treatment, cures, prevention, diagnosis, risk factors, research, support groups, email lists, personal stories and much more. Updated regularly.

5897   Lung Disease

www.lungusa.org

The American Lung Association's website, including information on diseases A to Z, living with lung disease, tobacco control, air quality, data, statistics, research, and more.

5898   MedicineNet

www.medicinenet.com

An online resource for consumers providing easy-to-read, authoritative medical and health information.

5899   Medscape

www.medscape.com

Medscape offers specialists, primary care physicians, and other health professionals the Web's most robust and integrated medical information and educational tools.

5900   National Heart, Lung & Blood Institute

www.nhlbi.nih.gov

A website maintained by the National Institute of Health offering general information regarding the heart, lungs, and blood.

5901   WebMD

www.webmd.com

Provides credible information, supportive communities, and in-depth reference material about health subjects. A source for original and timely health information as well as material from well known content providers.

Description

5902 Mental Illness/General

Mental illness includes disorders of mood, thinking and behavior, with psychiatry being the branch of medicine responsible for their study, diagnosis, treatment, and prevention. Mental illness may be determined by genetic, physical, chemical, psychological, and social factors. Mental or emotional illness includes such conditions as major depression, schizophrenia, bipolar disorder (i.e., manic depression), panic and other anxiety disorders, substance abuse and dependence, and dementia and other cognitive disorders.

Psychiatric diagnoses generally are based on criteria outlined in *Diagnostic and Statistical Manual of Mental Disorders* (DSM-V), published by the American Psychiatric Association. Depending on the specific diagnosis, treatment can include medication, counseling, behavior modification, psychotherapy, and modification of the patient's environment. See also *Mental Illness/Depression* and *Mental Illness/Schizophrenia*.

National Agencies & Associations

5903 Action Autonomie
3958 Rue Dandurand 514-525-5060
Montreal, Quebec, H1X-1P7 Fax: 514-525-5580
lecollectif@actionautonomie.qc.ca
www.actionautonomie.qc.ca
Community organization for individuals with mental illness who unite their efforts collectively in order to defend their rights. Action Autonomie educates others on their rights while navigating the mental health care system.

5904 American Academy of Child and Adolescent Psychiatry (AACAP)
3615 Wisconsin Avenue NW 202-966-7300
Washington, DC 20016-3007 Fax: 202-464-0131
clinical@aacap.org
www.aacap.org
Promotes the healthy development of children, adolescents, and families through advocacy, education, and research.
Karen Dineen Wagner, MD, PhD, President
Bennett L. Leventhal, MD, Treasurer

5905 American Association on Intellectual and Developmental Disabilities
8403 Colesville Road 202-387-1968
Silver Spring, MD 20910 Fax: 202-387-2193
mnygren@aaidd.org
www.aamr.org
Promotes progressive policies, scientific research, effective practices and universal human rights for people with intellectual and developmental disabilities.
Margaret A. Nygren, EdD, Executive Director & CEO

5906 American Psychiatric Association
800 Maine Avenue SW 202-559-3900
Washington, DC 20024 apa@psych.org
www.psychiatry.org
A medical specialty society representing a growing membership of psychiatrists. Offers information for psychiatrists, medical students, patients and families.

5907 American Psychological Association
750 First Street NE 202-336-5500
Washington, DC 20002-4242 800-374-2721
TTY: 202-336-6123
www.apa.org
Advancing the creation, communication and application of psychological knowledge to benefit society and improve people's lives.
Rosie Phillips Davis, PhD, President
Jean A. Carter, PhD, Treasurer

5908 Association of Children's Residential Centers
648 N Plankinton Avenue 877-332-2272
Milwaukee, WI 53203 www.togetherthevoice.org
Brings professionals together to advance the frontiers of knowledge regarding therapeutic living environments for adolescents with behavioral health disorders.
Joe Ford, President
Kari Sisson, Executive Director

5909 Canadian Federation of Mental Health Nurses
7270 Woodbine Avenue www.cfmhn.ca
Markham, Ontario, L3R-4B9
A national voice for psychiatric and mental health nurses in Canada, providing resources relevant to the field.
Florence Budden, President
Sherette Currie, Director of Membership

5910 Canadian Mental Health Association (CMHA)
250 Dundas Street W 416-646-5557
Toronto, Ontario, M5T-2Z5 info@cmha.ca
www.cmha.ca
Promotes the mental health of all and supports the recovery of people experiencing mental illness.

5911 Community Access, Inc.
17 Battery Place 212-780-1400
New York, NY 10004 www.communityaccess.org
A non-profit agency providing housing and advocacy for people with disabilities.
Stephen H. Chase, President
Dan Wurtzel, Vice President

5912 Goodwill Industries International, Inc.
15810 Indianola Drive 800-466-3945
Rockville, MD 20855 contactus@goodwill.org
www.goodwill.org
A nonprofit, community-based organization whose mission is to help people achieve self-sufficiency through the dignity and power of work, serving people who are disadvantaged, disabled or elderly. The mission is accomplished through providing independent living skills, affordable housing, and training and placement in community employment. The GoodWill Network includes 160 independent, local locations across the U.S. and Canada.
S. Dale Jenkins, Chair
Steven C. Preston, President & CEO

5913 Mental Health America
500 Montgomery Street 703-684-7722
Alexandria, VA 22314 800-969-6642
Fax: 703-684-5968
www.mentalhealthamerica.net
Formerly known as the National Mental Health Association, Mental Health America is committed to helping all people live mentally healthier lives by promoting awareness of mental health.
340+ Members
Tom Starling, EdD, Chair
Jennifer L. Bright, MPA, Secretary & Treasurer

5914 National Alliance for Hispanic Health
1501 16th Street NW 866-783-2645
Washington, DC 20036-1401 www.healthyamericas.org
Members are Spanish-speaking mental health professionals and patients and those interested in services and decision-making that consider culture and community.
Augustine Chris Baca, MPA, Chairperson
Jane L. Delgado, PhD, MS, President & CEO

5915 National Alliance on Mental Illness (NAMI)
3803 N Fairfax Drive 703-524-7600
Arlington, VA 22203 800-950-6264
info@nami.org
www.nami.org

Committed to building better lives for the millions of Americans affected by mental illness by raising awareness and offering community support.
Adrienne Kennedy, MA, President
Lacey Berumen, PhD, LAC, MNM, First Vice President

5916 National Association of State Mental Health Program Directors
66 Canal Center Plaza   703-739-9333
Alexandria, VA 22314   Fax: 703-548-9517
                                        www.nasmhpd.org
Offers referrals to state mental health programs, services and physicians for persons with mental illness.
Brian Hepburn, MD, Executive Director
Aaron J. Walker, MPA, Senior Policy Associate

5917 National Council for Behavioral Health
1400 K Street NW   202-684-7457
Washington, DC 20005   communications@thenationalcouncil.org
                                    www.thenationalcouncil.org
Represents community mental health centers working on Capitol Hill to ensure funding for community mental health services. Offers technical support and guidance and serves as a liaison with state organizations and other mental health related organizations.
Linda Rosenberg, MSW, President & CEO
Jeannie Campbell, Executive Vice President & COO

5918 National Federation of Families for Children's Mental Health
15800 Crabbs Branch Way   240-403-1901
Rockville, MD 20855   www.ffcmh.org
Provides leadership to develop and sustain a nationwide network of family-run organizations.
Sherrie Luthe, President
Lynda Gargan, PhD, Executive Director

5919 National Institute of Mental Health
6001 Executive Boulevard   866-615-6464
Rockville, MD 20852-9663   Fax: 301-443-4279
                                         TTY: 866-415-8051
                                         nimhinfo@nih.gov
                                         www.nimh.nih.gov
The National Institute of Mental Health works to transform the understanding and treatment of mental illnesses through basic and clinical research, paving the way for prevention, recovery, and cure.
Joshua A. Gordon, MD, PhD, Director

5920 Option Institute
2080 South Undermountain Road   413-229-2100
Sheffield, MA 01257   800-714-2779
                                         Fax: 413-229-8931
                                    participantsupport@option.org
                                         www.option.org
Self-defeating beliefs, along with attitudes and judgments, can lead to a host of physical and psychological challenges. The Option Institute offers programs designed to help people gain new perspectives on the attitudes and judgments that may be affecting their lives.
Barry Kaufman, Co-Founder
Samahria Lyte Kaufman, Co-Founder

5921 Parent Professional Advocacy League
15 Court Square   866-815-8122
Boston, MA 02108   Fax: 617-542-7832
                                         info@ppal.net
                                         www.ppal.net
An organization of families of children with mental, emotional or behavioral needs and concerned professionals. PPAL support groups are run in many areas across the country.
Lisa Lambert, Executive Director
Meri Viano, Associate Director

5922 The Coalition of Behavioral Health
123 William Street   212-742-1600
New York, NY 10038   Fax: 212-742-2080
                                    jalvarez@coalitionny.org
                                         www.coalitionny.org

An advocacy organization of New York's mental health community representing over 100 non-profit community health agencies that serve clients in the five boroughs of New York City.
Amanda Saake, Director
Marlo Pasion, Associate Director

5923 World Federation for Mental Health
PO Box 807   Fax: 703-490-6926
Occoquan, VA 22125   info@wfmh.com
                                         www.wfmh.com
International organization dedicated to improving the care and treatment of individuals with mental disorders, and raising public awareness and understanding of mental health.
Alberto Trimboli, President
Janet Paleo, Treasurer

State Agencies & Associations

Alabama

5924 National Alliance on Mental Illness of Alabama: NAMI Alabama
1401 I-85 Parkway   334-396-4797
Montgomery, AL 36106-1902   800-626-4199
                                         Fax: 334-396-4794
                                    wlaird@namialabama.org
                                         www.namialabama.org
Will O'Rear, President
Sue Guffey, 1st Vice President

Alaska

5925 National Alliance on Mental Illness of Alaska
144 W 15th Avenue   907-277-1300
Anchorage, AK 99501-5106   800-478-4462
                                         Fax: 907-277-1400
                                         trishmcd@nami.org
                                    www.nami.org/sites/alaska
Scott Owens, Co-President
Pat Dobbins, Co-President

Arizona

5926 Mentally Ill Kids In Distress
2642 E Thomas Road   602-253-1240
Phoenix, AZ 85016-2723   800-35M-IKID
                                         Fax: 602-253-1250
                                    Phoenix@MIKID.org
                                         www.mikid.org
Steve Carter, President
Vicki L Johnson, Executive Director

5927 National Alliance on Mental Illness of Arizona
5025 E. Washington Street   602-244-8166
Phoenix, AZ 85034-1604   Fax: 602-252-1349
                                         www.namiaz.org
Provides emotional support education and advocacy to persons of all ages who are affected by serious mental illnesses. Supports research to find a cure.
Robert McCabe

5928 Navaho Nation K'E Project: Tuba City Children & Families Advocacy Corp
PO Box 3937   520-283-5415
Tuba City, AZ 86045   Fax: 520-283-5413
Rueben Clark

5929 Navaho Nation K'E Project: Winslow Children & Families Advocacy Corp
HC 63 Box E   520-657-3234
Winslow, AZ 86047   Fax: 520-657-3207
Jayne

Arkansas

5930 Arkansas FFCMH Jane Burgan
Jane Burgan

PO Box 56667
Little Rock, AR 72115-4023

501-374-7218
Fax: 501-374-2711
pammarshall7218@sbcglobal.net
www.affcmh.org/

Billie Denney, Board Member
James Wilson, Board Member

5931 NAMI Arkansas
1012 Autumn Road
Little Rock, AR 72211-2222

501-661-1548
800-844-0381
Fax: 501-312-7540
nami-ar@namiarkansas.org
www.nami.org

Grassroots organization that focuses on improving mental health services. The mission is three prong: Support, Education, and Advocacy. Support Group meetings are held at 11 locations across the state.
Rick Scott, First Vice President
Karen H Henry, President

California

5932 NAMI California
1851 Heritage Lane
Sacramento, CA 95815-3218

916-567-0163
Fax: 916-567-1757
nami.california@namicalifornia.org
www.namicalifornia.org

Dorothy Hendrickson, President
Jessica Cruz, Executive Director

5933 United Advocates for Children of California
2035 Hurley Way
Sacramento, CA 95825

916-643-1530
866-643-1530
Fax: 916-643-1592
info@uacf4hope.org
www.uacf4hope.org

Carmen Diaz, President
Mary Jane Gross, Treasurer

Colorado

5934 Colorado FFCMH
2950 Tennyson Street
Denver, CO 80212

303-572-0302
888-569-7500
Fax: 303-433-1605
tdillingham@coloradofederation.org
www.coloradofederation.org

5935 FFCMH: Denver/Aurora Chapter
12485 E 13th Avenue
Aurora, CO 80011

303-343-1019
Fax: 720-859-9367

Carmen Mohr, President
Carol Reynolds, Executive Director

5936 National Alliance for the Mentally Ill of Colorado
2280 S Albion Street
Denver, CO 80222-3334

303-321-3104
888-566-6264
Fax: 303-321-0912
admin@namicolorado.org
www.namicolorado.org

The National Alliance for the Mentally Ill Of Colorado is a statewide, grassroots, nonprofit organization whose mission is; To give strength and hope to individuals with mental illness and their families.
Greg C Coleman, President
Scott Glaser, Executive Director

5937 No. Colorado FFCMH
2950 Tennyson Street
Denver, CO 80212

303-572-0302
888-569-7500
Fax: 303-433-1605
www.coloradofederation.org

Meltz

Connecticut

5938 Families United For CMH, Inc.
PO Box 151
New London, CT 06320

860-537-6125
Fax: 860-537-6130
www.familiesunited.org

Morgan Correll, President
Sheila King, Executive Director

5939 National Alliance for the Mentally Ill of Connecticut
576 Farmington Avenue
Hartford, CT 06105

860-882-0236
800-215-3021
Fax: 860-882-0240
membership@namict.org
www.namict.org

Kate Mattias, Executive Director

Delaware

5940 Alliance for the Mentally Ill in Delaware (AMID)
2400 W 4th Street
Wilmington, DE 19805-3306

302-427-0787
888-427-2643
Fax: 302-427-2075
namide@namide.org
www.namide.org

Mary Berger, President
John P Smoots, Treasurer

5941 Delaware FFMCH
19 Baltusrol Court
Dover, DE 19904

302-730-0325
866-994-0000
Fax: 302-730-8952
marags1@aol.com
www.ffcmh.org

Earline McArthur, Director Development/Communications

5942 Mental Health Association of Delaware
100 W 10th Street
Wilmington, DE 19801

302-654-6833
800-287-6423
Fax: 302-654-6838
jlafferty@mhainde.org
www.mhainde.org

Janet M Brown, President
James Lafferty, Executive Director

District of Columbia

5943 DC Threshold Alliance for the Mentally Ill
422 8th Street SE
Washington, DC 20003-2832

202-546-0646
Fax: 202-546-6817
www.nami.org/MSTemplate.cfm?MicrositeID=

Lois Fitzgerald, President
Mary J DiPietro, Secretary

5944 Family Advocacy and Support Association
PO Box 74884
Washington, DC 20056
Lynne M Gladysz, Chair
R Lee Waits, President

202-234-2325
Fax: 202-576-7154

Florida

5945 Florida Alliance for the Mentally Ill
1030 E. Lafayette Street
Tallahassee, FL 32301-2646

850-671-4445
877-626-4352
Fax: 850-671-5272
Info@namiflorida.org
www.namiflorida.org

James Sleeper, President
Judith Evans, Executive Director

5946 Florida FFCMH: Tampa Chapter
13301 Bruce B Downs Boulevard
Tampa, FL 33612

813-974-7930
Fax: 813-974-7712
ffcmh@earthlink.net

Linda M Gladysz, Chair
R Lee Waits, President/CEO

5947 **Goodwill Industries-Suncoast**
10596 Gandy Boulevard
St. Petersburg, FL 33702

727-523-1512
888-279-1988
TTY: 727-579-1068
www.goodwill-suncoast.org

A nonprofit, community-based organization whose mission is to help people achieve self-sufficiency through the dignity and power of work, serving people who are disadvantaged, disabled or elderly. The mission is accomplished through providing independent living skills, affordable housing, and training and placement in community employment.
Heather Ceresoli, CPA, Chair
Deborah A. Passerini, President & CEO

Georgia

5948 **Georgia Alliance for the Mentally Ill**
3050 Presidential Drive
Atlanta, GA 30340-3916

770-234-0855
800-728-1052
Fax: 770-234-0237
namigeorgia@namiga.org
www.namiga.org

Bill Kissel, President
Eric Spencer, Executive Director

Hawaii

5949 **NAMI: The Local Affiliate of the National Alliance for the Mentally Ill**
770 Kapiolani Boulevard
Honolulu, HI 96813-2025

808-591-1297
Fax: 808-591-2058
info@namihawaii.org
namihawaii.org

Members include consumers families health professionals and interested persons/organizations. Programs include advocacy support and education and are free and open to the public. Office has lending library of books and videos. Newsletter is published.
6 pages Quarterly
Carol Kozlovich, President
Kathleen Hasegawa, Executive Director

Idaho

5950 **FFCMH: Idaho Chapter**
704 North 7th Street
Boise, ID 83702

208-433-8845
800-905-3436
Fax: 208-433-8337
info@idahofederation.org
www.idahofederation.org

Stephen Graci, Executive Director
Cindy Shotton, Administrative Assistant

5951 **Idaho Alliance for the Mentally Ill**
4097 Bottle Bay Road
Sagle, ID 83860-0068

208-242-7430
800-572-9940
Fax: 208-673-6685
namiidaho@yahoo.com
www.nami.org/MSTemplate.cfm?MicrositeID=

Douglas McKnight, President
Tom Hanson, Vice President

Illinois

5952 **Illinois Alliance for the Mentally Ill**
218 W Lawrence Avenue
Springfield, IL 62704-2612

217-522-1403
800-346-4572
Fax: 217-522-3598
namiil@sbcglobal.net
il.nami.org

Hugh Brady, President
Brian Allen, Vice President

5953 **Illinois Federation of Families**
PO Box 413
McHenry, IL 60051

847-265-0500
800-871-8400
Fax: 847-265-0501
www.iffcmh.net

Cynthia Hamilton

Indiana

5954 **FFCMH: Indiana Chapter**
2205 Costello Drive
Anderson, IN 46011

765-622-0601
866-247-8547
Fax: 765-622-0643
indianafedfam@comcast.net

Brenda Hamilton

5955 **Family Action Network**
PO Box 322
Winnetka, IN 60093-2206

765-643-4357
info@familyactionnetwork.net
www.familyactionnetwork.net

Susan Rooney, Co-Chair
Lonnie Stonitsch, Co-Chair

5956 **NAMI Indiana**
PO Box 22697
Indianapolis, IN 46222-0697

317-925-9399
800-677-6442
Fax: 317-925-9398
info@namiindiana.org
www.namiindiana.org/

Grass roots advocacy support and educational group for families affected by severe and persistent mental illnesses.
Joshua G Sprunger, Executive Director
Joanne Abbott, Program Director

Iowa

5957 **FFCMH: Iowa Chapter**
106 S Booth
Anamosa, IA 52205

319-462-2187
888-400-6302
Fax: 319-462-6789
help@iffcmh.org
www.iffcmh.org

Lori Reynolds, Executive Director
Heidi Reynolds, Program Director

5958 **NAMI Iowa: National Alliance on Mental Illness**
5911 Meredith Drive
Des Moines, IA 50322-1903

515-254-0417
800-417-0417
Fax: 515-254-1103
www.namiiowa.com

Dawn Adams

Kansas

5959 **Keys for Networking: Kansas FFCMH**
900 South Kansas Avenue
Topeka, KS 66612

785-233-8732
800-499-8732
Fax: 785-235-8732
jadams@keys.org
www.keys.org

Mary Ellen Conlee, President
Greg Whittaker, Treasurer

5960 **NAMI Kansas: Kansas' Voice on Mental Illness**
610 SW 10th Ave
Topeka, KS 66612-0675

785-233-0755
800-539-2660
Fax: 785-233-4804
info@namikansas.org
www.nami.org/MSTemplate.cfm?Site=NAMI_Ka

John Brennan, President
Mr Richard D Cagan, Executive Director

Kentucky

5961 **KY Partnership For Families and Children**
207 Holmes Street
Frankfort, KY 40601

502-875-1320
800-369-0533
Fax: 502-875-1399
kpfc@kypartnership.org
www.kypartnership.org

Carol W Cecil, Executive Director
Joy Varney, Associate Director

5962 Kentucky Alliance for the Mentally Ill
808 Monticello Street
Somerset, KY 42501-1277
606-451-6935
800-257-5081
Fax: 606-677-4052
namiky@nami.org
www.nami.org/MSTemplate.cfm?micrositeID=
Wendy Morris, Chair
Bertha Diaz-Story, 1st Vice Chair

Louisiana

5963 Louisiana Alliance for the Mentally Ill
5534 Galeria Drive
Baton Rouge, LA 70816-2398
225-291-6262
800-437-0303
Fax: 225-926-8773
info@namilouisiana.org
www.namilouisiana.org
Stephanie Boyd, President
Mitch Bergeron, Vice President

Maine

5964 Maine Alliance for the Mentally Ill
1 Bangor Street
Augusta, ME 04330-4701
207-622-5767
800-464-5767
Fax: 207-621-8430
info@namimaine.org
www.namimaine.org
Valerie Gamache, President
Cathy Kidman, Interim Executive Director

5965 United Families for Children's Mental Health
PO Box 2107
Augusta, ME 04338-2107
207-622-3309
Fax: 207-622-1661
Pat Bellack, Executive Director
Dana Lefko

Maryland

5966 National Alliance for the Mentally Ill: Maryland
10630 Little Patuxent Parkway
Columbia, MD 21044-4486
410-884-8691
877-878-2371
Fax: 410-884-8695
amimd@aol.com
md.nami.org
Chris Griffin, President
Kate Farinholt, Executive Director

5967 Parents Supporting Parents of MD
PO Box 30
Kensington, MD 20895-0030
800-498-5551
Marge_Samels@umail.umd.edu
Marge Sagalyn, President
Toby Fisher, Director of Public Policy

Massachusetts

5968 Massachusetts Alliance for the Mentally Ill
400 W Cummings Park
Woburn, MA 01801-6528
781-938-4048
800-370-9085
Fax: 781-938-4069
helpline@namimass.org
www.namimass.org
Lynda Cutrell, President
Laurie Martinelli, Executive Director

Michigan

5969 Association for Children's Mental Health
6017 W Street Joseph Highway
Lansing, MI 48917
517-372-4016
888-226-4543
Fax: 517-372-4032
acmhjane@sbcglobal.net
www.acmh-mi.org
Jane Shank, Interim Executive Director
Mary Porter, Business Manager

5970 JIMHO Affiliated Centers (Justice in Mental Health Organization)
520 Cherry Street
Lansing, MI 48933
517-371-2221
800-831-8035
Fax: 517-371-5770
brwellwood@aol.com
www.jimho.org
JIMHO advocates for the rights and dignity that all people suffering from mental or emotional illness deserve.
Huebl, President
Sharon Solomon, Executive Director

5971 Michigan Alliance for the Mentally Ill
921 N Washington Avenue
Lansing, MI 48906-5137
517-485-4049
800-331-4264
Fax: 517-485-2333
namimichigan@acd.net
mi.nami.org
Hubert Lloyd, President
Sue Abderholden, Executive Director

Minnesota

5972 Minnesota Alliance for the Mentally Ill
800 Transfer Road
Saint Paul, MN 55114-1146
651-645-2948
888-NAM-IHEL
Fax: 651-645-7379
namihelps@namimn.org
www.namihelps.org
Barb Lindberg, President
Sue Abderholden, Executive Director

5973 Minnesota Association for Children's Mental Health
165 Western Avenue
Saint Paul, MN 55102
651-644-7333
800-528-4511
Fax: 651-644-7391
info@macmh.org
www.macmh.org
Joel V Oberstar, MD, President
Deborah Saxhaug, Executive Director

Mississippi

5974 Mississippi Alliance for the Mentally Ill
411 Briarwood Drive
Jackson, MS 39206-3058
601-899-9058
800-357-0388
Fax: 601-956-6380
stateoffice@namims.org
www.namims.org/
Debbie Waller, President
Hank Rainer, Vice President

5975 Mississippi Families as Allies
5166 Keele Street
Jackson, MS 39206
601-355-0915
800-833-9671
Fax: 601-355-0919
info@msfaacmh.org
www.msfaacmh.org
Joy Hogge, PhD, Executive Director
Cynthia Moore-Hardy, MS, Director of Respite Services

Missouri

5976 MO-SPAN
440 Rue Saint Francois
Florissant, MO 63031
314-972-0600
Fax: 314-972-0606
www.mo-span.org
Donna Dittrich, Executive Director
Tina VarVera, Administrative Assistant

5977 Missouri Coalition Alliance for the Mentally Ill
230 W Dunklin Street
Jefferson City, MO 65101-3260
573-634-7727
800-374-2138
Fax: 573-761-5636
Keele@aol.com
Keele, Executive Director
Karren Jones, President

5978 NAMI of Missouri
1001 SW Boulevard
Jefferson City, MO 65109-2501

573-634-7727
800-374-2138
Fax: 573-761-5636
namimosjf@yahoo.com
www.nami.org/MSTemplate.cfm?MicrositeID=

A nonprofit education adudcacy, referal and support organization serving people with mental illness and their families.
12 pages newsletter
Cinda Holloway, President and Chairman
Cindi Keele, Executive Director

Montana

5979 Family Support Network
1002 10th Street W
Billings, MT 59102

406-256-7783
877-376-4850
Fax: 406-256-9879
www.mtfamilysupport.org

Barbara Milhelish, President
Matt Kuntz, Executive Director

5980 Montana Alliance for the Mentally Ill Mihelish's Residence
Mihelish's Residence
616 Helena Avenue
Helena, MT 59601-6946

406-443-7871
888-280-6264
Fax: 406-862-6352
info@namimt.org
www.namimt.org

Matt Kuntz, Executive Director
Carole Denton, President

Nebraska

5981 National Alliance for the Mentally Ill: Nebraska (NAMI)
415 South 25th Avenue
Omaha, NE 68131-2986

402-345-8101
877-463-6264
Fax: 402-346-4070
nami.nebraska@nami.org

NAMI is a nonprofit organization dedicated to providing support, education and advocacy to and for anyone whose life has been touched by a mental illness.
Tim Cuddigan, President
Steve Spelic, Vice President

Nevada

5982 Nevada Alliance for the Mentally Ill
2251 N Rampart Boulevard
Las Vegas, NV 89128

702-310-5764
Fax: 775-329-1618

Joe Abate

New Hampshire

5983 Granite State FFCMH
940 Mammoth Road
Manchester, NH 03104

603-296-0692
gsffcmh@aol.com
www.ffcmh.org

Kathleen Cohen, Executive Director
Win Saltmarsh, Development Director

5984 National Alliance for the Mentally Ill: New Hampshire
85 North State Street
Concord, NH 03301-4020

603-225-5359
800-242-6264
Fax: 603-228-8848
info@naminh.org
www.naminh.org

Family support and advocacy for consumers and family members.
Michele Grennon, President
Ken Norton, Executive Director

New Jersey

5985 All Access Mental Health
Information
819 Alexander Road
Princeton, NJ 08540

609-452-2088
Fax: 609-452-0627
info@aamh.org
www.aamh.org

This organization was founded to create a permanent community support system for mentally ill and developmentally disabled adults and their families living in the Greater Mercer County area of New Jersey.
Cynthia Murphy, President
Lauren Murphy, Vice-President

5986 Community Mental Health Foundation
610 Industrial Avenue
Paramus, NJ 07652

201-986-5070
Fax: 201-265-3543

Perrin, President
Sylvia Axelrod, Executive Director

5987 New Jersey Alliance for the Mentally Ill
1562 Route 130
N Brunswick, NJ 08902-3004

732-940-0991
Fax: 732-940-0355
info@naminj.org
www.naminj.org

Mark Perrin, MD, President
Sylvia Axelrod, Executive Director

New Mexico

5988 Navaho Nation K'E Project Children and Families Advocacy Corp
PO Box 309
Tohatchi, NM 87325

505-733-2474
Fax: 505-733-2444

Vera Balwin

5989 Navajo Nation K'E Project: Shiprock Children & Families Advocacy Corp
PO Box 1240
Shiprock, NM 87420

505-368-4479
Fax: 505-368-5582

Evelyn Beckett, President
Elaine Jones, Executive Director

5990 New Mexico Alliance for the Mentally Ill
8015 Mountain Rd NE
Albuquerque, NM 87110-3086

505-260-0154
Fax: 505-260-0342
naminm@aol.com
www.nami.org/MSTemplate.cfm?MicrositeID=

Patricia D Romero, President

New York

5991 Children's Mental Health Coalition of WNY, Inc.
814 Kenmore Avenue
Buffalo, NY 14216

716-871-8997
Fax: 716-871-8656
mtskorupa@aol.com

Mary Pierce, Executive Director
Joan Cullen, Program Director/Family Specialist

5992 Families Together in New York State
737 Madison Avenue
Albany, NY 12209

518-432-0333
888-326-8644
Fax: 518-434-6478
info@ftnys.org
www.ftnys.org

Vicky McCarthy, President
Paige Pierce, Executive Director

5993 New York Alliance for the Mentally Ill
99 Pine Street
Albany, NY 12207

518-462-2000
800-950-3228
Fax: 518-462-3811
info@naminys.org
www.naminys.org

Thomas Easterly, President
Paul A Capofari, 1st Vice President

5994 Parents United Network: Parsons Child Family Center
60 Academy Road
Albany, NY 12208

518-426-2600
Fax: 518-447-5234
communications@parsonscenter.org
www.parsonscenter.org

Rose Mary Bailly, President
John Henley, Chief Executive Officer

North Dakota

5995 North Dakota Alliance for the Mentally Ill
PO Box 3215
Minot, ND 58702-6016
701-770-8063
Fax: 701-725-4334
l.lund8@hotmail.com
www.namind.org/

Linda Lund, President

5996 North Dakota FFCMH
PO Box 3061
Bismarck, ND 58502-3061
701-222-3310
800-484-2263
Fax: 701-222-3310
carlottamccleary@bis.midco.nrt
www.ndffcmh.org/

Carlotta McCleary, Executive Director
Deb Jendro, Parent Coordinator

Ohio

5997 1st Capital FFCMH
394 Chestnut Street
Chillicothe, OH 45601
740-775-2674
Fax: 740-775-7834
Rosemary Snider, President
Jim Mauro, Executive Director

5998 Ohio Alliance for the Mentally Ill
1225 Dublin Road
Columbus, OH 43215
614-224-2700
800-686-2646
Fax: 614-224-5400
TTY: 866-924-1478
namiohio@namiohio.org
www.namiohio.org

Bob Spada, President
Terry Russell, Executive Director

Oklahoma

5999 Oklahoma Alliance for the Mentally Ill
4200 Perimeter Drive
Oklahoma City, OK 73112-6200
405-230-1900
800-583-1264
Fax: 405-230-1903
namiok@coxinet.net
www.namioklahoma.org/

Paula Walker, President
Traci Cook, Executive Director

6000 Tulsa Unified FFCMH
1022 N Howard
Tulsa, OK 74115
918-838-8033
sherryscoobydoo@aol.com
www.ffcmh.org

Sherry Gorger, Education Program Director
Cora Palazzolo, Communications Coordinator

Oregon

6001 NAMI-Oregon
4701 SE 24th Avenue
Portland, OR 97202-1552
503-230-8009
800-343-6264
Fax: 503-230-2751
namioregon@namior.org
www.nami.org/MSTemplate.cfm?Site=NAMI_Or
Providing support education and advocacy for people with biological mental illness and their families. The in-state 800 phone number is Oregon's NAMI-Line. Callers to this line are provided with information about mental illnesses and referrals to support and treatment services.
Chris Bouneff, Executive Director
Michelle Madison, Events Manager/Outreach Coordinator

6002 Oregon Family Support Network
1300 Broadway Street
Salem, OR 97301
503-363-8068
800-323-8521
Fax: 503-390-3161
www.ofsn.org

David De Fiebre, Board President
Sandy Bumpus, Executive Director

Pennsylvania

6003 Parents Involved Network
1211 Chestnut Street
Philadelphia, PA 19107
215-751-1800
800-688-4226
Janet Jordan Jr, Executive Director
Jyoti Shah, President

6004 Pennsylvania Alliance for the Mentally Ill
2149 N 2nd Street
Harrisburg, PA 17011-1005
717-238-1514
800-223-0500
Fax: 717-238-4390
TTY: 800-890-6093
nami-pa@nami-pa.org
www.nami-pa.org/

Suzanne Vogel-Scibilia, M.D, President
James W Jordan, Jr, Executive Director

Rhode Island

6005 National Alliance for the Mentally Ill of Rhode Island (NAMI)
154 Waterman Street
Providence, RI 02906-4312
401-331-3060
800-749-3197
Fax: 401-274-3020
www.namirhodeisland.org

Marcia Boyd, Esq, President
Chaz J Gross, Executive Director

South Carolina

6006 NAMI-SC: National Alliance on Mental Illness: South Carolina
PO BOX 1267
Columbia, SC 29202-1267
803-733-9592
800-788-5131
Fax: 803-733-9593
namisc@namisc.org
www.namisc.org

Advocacy, Education and Support
Joan Herbert, MS, President
Bill Lindsey, Executive Director

South Dakota

6007 NAMI South Dakota
PO Box 88808
Sioux Falls, SD 57109-1204
605-271-1871
800-551-2531
Fax: 605-271-1871
namisd@midconetwork.com

Shelly Jablonski, President
Sita Diehl, Executive Director

Tennessee

6008 Tennessee Alliance for the Mentally Ill
1101 Kermit Drive
Nashville, TN 37217-2126
615-361-6608
800-467-3589
Fax: 615-361-6698
rpbaxter@comcast.net
www.namitn.org

Dick Baxter, President
Jeff Fladen, Executive Director

Texas

6009 Central Texas FFCMH
6814 Orange Blossom
Austin, TX 78744
512-282-7126
Fax: 512-282-5817
mattie_dixon@hotmail.com
Mattie Owens

6010 North Texas FFCMH
722 E Summitt
Sherman, TX 75090
patoadv@msn.com
Pat Nazaroff

6011 San Antonio Bexar County FFCMH
2516 Bandara
San Antonio, TX 78238
210-523-2351
Fax: 210-523-2352
ideasjn@aol.com

Joseph Peyson, Executive Director
Donna Fisher, President

6012 Texas Alliance for the Mentally Ill
Foundtain Park Plaza III   512-693-2000
Austin, TX 78704   800-633-3760
Fax: 512-693-8000
kjeschke@namitexas.org
www.namitexas.org

Andrea Hazlitt, Board President
Ed Dickey, Vice President

6013 Texas FFCMH
7800 Shoal Creek Road   512-407-8844
Austin, TX 78752   866-893-3264
Fax: 512-407-8266
PattiDerr@txffcmh.org
www.txffcmh.org

Patti Muller, President
Sherri Wittwer, Executive Director

Utah

6014 Utah Alliance for the Mentally Ill
1600 West 2200 South   801-323-9900
West Valley City, UT 84119-1701   877-230-6264
Fax: 801-323-9799
rebecca@namiut.org
www.namiut.org

Zara Juillerat, President
Rebecca Glathar, Executive Director

Vermont

6015 Vermont Alliance for the Mentally Ill
162 S Main Street   802-244-1396
Waterbury, VT 05676-1519   800-639-6480
Fax: 802-244-1405
info@namivt.org
www.nami.org/MSTemplate.cfm?Site=NAMI_Ve
Karen Kelley, Chair
Wendy Beinner, President/CEO

6016 Vermont FFCMH
600 Blair Park Road   802-876-7021
Williston, VT 05495-0607   800-639-6071
Fax: 802-329-2135
vffcmh@vffcmh.org
www.vffcmh.org

Ted Tighe, President
Kathy Holsopple, Executive Director

Virginia

6017 Virginia Alliance for the Mentally Ill
PO Box 8260   804-285-8264
Richmond, VA 23226-1903   888-486-8264
Fax: 804-285-8464
namiva@verizon.net
www.namivirginia.org/

Robert Cluck, President
Mira Signer, Executive Director

Washington

6018 NAMI Washington (National Alliance for the Mentally Ill of Washington)
7500 Greenwood Avenue North   206-783-4288
Seattle, WA 98103-5580   800-782-9264
office@namiwa.org
www.namiwa.org/
Advocacy, support and education for the mentally ill, their families and friends.
Gordon Bopp, President
Jim Bloss, Vice President

6019 Washington FFCMH
801 E 141 Street   253-537-2145
Tacoma, WA 98445-2768   Fax: 253-537-2162
acvmarge@comcast.net
www.ffcmh.org/

Marge Coleman, President
Terrie Isaly, Fast Track Program Director

West Virginia

6020 Mountain State/Parents/Children/ Adolescents Network
1201 Garfield Street   304-233-5399
McMechen, WV 26040   800-CHI-LD35
Fax: 304-233-3847
www.mspcan.org
Joyce Floyd, President
Hope Coleman, Vice President

6021 NAMI West Virginia
PO Box 2706   304-342-0497
Charleston, WV 25330-2706   800-598-5653
Fax: 304-342-0499
namiwv@aol.com
Educational advocacy and support for families consumers and friends of people with mental illnesses.
Randal Rutkowski, Co-President
Terence Schnapp, Interim Executive Director

Wisconsin

6022 Wisconsin Alliance for the Mentally Ill
4233 W Beltline Highway   608-268-6000
Madison, WI 53711-3814   800-236-2988
Fax: 608-268-6004
nami@namiwisconsin.org
www.namiwisconsin.org
Jim Connors, President
Julianne Carbin, Executive Director

6023 Wisconsin Family Ties
16 N Carroll Street   608-267-6888
Madison, WI 53703   800-422-7145
Fax: 608-267-6801
info@wifamilyties.org
www.wifamilyties.org
Hugh Johnson, President
Deion Hagemeister, Vice-President

Wyoming

6024 Wyoming Alliance for the Mentally Ill
133 W 6th Street   307-265-2573
Casper, WY 82601-3124   888-882-4968
Fax: 307-234-0440
www.namiwyoming.org/
Marty Coe, President
Tammy Noel, Executive Director

Foundations

6025 Family Service Foundation, Inc.
5301 76th Avenue   301-459-2121
Landover Hills, MD 20784   Fax: 301-459-0675
www.fsfinc.org
Provides mental health and other support services to clients in the State of Mayland.
Gordon A. Raley, MSW, Chief Executive Officer
Thomas Valayathil, EdD, Director, Behavioral Health Services

Libraries & Resource Centers

6026 Alta Bates Summit Medical Center
2001 Dwight Way   510-204-4444
Berkeley, CA 94704-2608   www.altabatessummit.org/
Alta Bates Summit Medical Center has made community healthcare a priority. We are proud of our many areas of clinical excellence including cardiovascular, behavioral health, women and infants, orthopedics, rehabilitation, and oncology care.
Carolyn McGee, Medical Librarian

6027 Central Louisiana State Hospital Medical and Professional Library
242 West Shamrock Street   318-484-6363
Pineville, LA 71360   Fax: 318-484-6284
bentonmcgee@hotmail.com

The Consortium was established to increase and better utilize the health information resources of Central Louisiana. Information offered on psychiatry, psychology and mental health.
Carol Rogers, Director

6028   National Mental Health Consumer's Self-Help Clearinghouse
1211 Chestnut Street   267-507-3810
Philadelphia, PA 19107   800-553-4539
                                           Fax: 215-636-6312
                                           info@mhselfhelp.org
                                           www.mhselfhelp.org
The National Mental Health Consumers' Self-Help Clearinghouse, the nation's first national consumer technical assistance center, has played a major role in the development of the mental health consumer movement. The consumer movement strives for dignity, respect, and opportunity for those with mental illnesses.
Joseph Rogers, Executive Director
Susan Rogers, Director

6029   National Mental Health Consumers' Self- Help Clearinghouse
1211 Chestnut Street   267-507-3810
Philadelphia, PA 19107   800-553-4539
                                           Fax: 215-636-6312
                                           www.mhselfhelp.org
The National Mental Health Consumers' Self-Help Clearinghouse, the nation's first national consumer technical assistance center, has played a major role in the development of the mental health consumer movement. The consumer movement strives for dignity, respect, and opportunity for those with mental illnesses. Consumers—those who receive or have received mental health services—continue to reject the label of 'those who cannot help themselves.'
Joseph Rogers, Executive Director
Susan Rogers, Director

Research Centers

6030   Anxiety Disorders Center University of Wisconsin
University of Wisconsin
Department of Psychiatry   608-263-6100
Madison, WI 53719-0001
Provides evaluation and treatment for individuals suffering from anxiety disorders as well as training and education for clinicians.
Andy Alexander, PhD, Professor
Ruth Benca, MD, PhD, Professor

6031   Institute of Psychiatry and Human Behavior: University of Maryland
655 West Baltimore Street   410-706-7410
Baltimore, MD 21201-1542   Fax: 410-706-0235
                                           alehman@psych.umaryland.edu
                                           www.medschool.umaryland.edu
Studies in psychiatric disorders.
Anthony Lehm MD, Director
Craig Vantyke, Chief Executive Officer

6032   Jane & Terry Semel Institute for Neuroscie nce & Human Behavior
Neuropsychiatric Institute
760 Westwood Plaza   310-825-2631
Los Angeles, CA 90095   800-825-9989
                                           www.semel.ucla.edu
Studies behavior disorders and psychosocial adaptation and the future.
Peter Whybrow, Director
Fawzy Fawzy, Associate Director

6033   Langley Porter Psychiatric Institute University of California
University of California
401 Parnassus Avenue   415-476-7365
San Francisco, CA 94143-9911   www.universityofcalifornia.edu
Conducts clinical studies of psychiatric disorders.
Samuel Barno Faucher, Director

6034   Medical College of Pennsylvania: Eastern Psychiatric Institute
3200 Henry Avenue   215-842-6990
Philadelphia, PA 19129-1137
Offers research into all aspects of mental illness.
Michael Spohn, Director

6035   Menninger Clinic: Department of Research
12301 S. Main Street   713-275-5140
Houston, TX 77035-0829   800-351-9058
                                           Fax: 785-350-5392
                                           www.menningerclinic.com/
Focuses research on mental illness and mental health issues.
B. Christoph Frueh, PhD, Director of Clinical Research
Chris Fowler, PhD, Associate Director of Clinical Research

6036   Mental Illness Research and Education Institute
Eastern State Hospital
PO Box 800   509-299-3121
Medical Lake, WA 99022-800   Fax: 509-997-15
Governmental organization focusing on mental illness research.
Harold David, Director

6037   NIH Clinical Center
National Institute of Health
9000 Rockville Pike   301-496-4000
Bethesda, MD 20892   800-411-1222
                                           Fax: 301-402-2984
                                           TTY: 866-411-1010
                                           prpl@mail.cc.nih.gov
                                           www.cc.nih.gov
Established in 1953 as the research hospital of the National Institutes of Health. Designed so that patient care facilities are close to research laboratories so new findings of basic and clinical scientists can be quickly applied to the treatment of patients. Upon referral by physicians patients are admitted to NIH clinical studies.
John I Gallin, MD, Clinical Center Director
David Henderson, MD, Deputy Director for Clinical Care

6038   State University of New York At Stony Brook: Mental Health Research
450 Clarkson Avenue   718-270-1270
Brooklyn, NY 11203-2056   www.stonybrook.edu
Benjamin S Hsiao, Phd, Vice President for Research

6039   Thresholds Psychiatric Rehabilitation
2700 N Ravenswood Avenue   773-281-3800
Chicago, IL 60614-1894   Fax: 773-818-90
                                           thresholds@thresholds.org
                                           www.luc.edu
A psychosocial rehabilitation agency serving persons with severe and persistent mental illness.
Tom MD, Director
Peter Whybrow, Director

6040   University of Michigan: Mental Health Research Institute
205 Washtenaw Place   734-763-1817
Ann Arbor, MI 48109   UMresearch@umich.edu
                                           www.umich.edu
Focuses on the diagnosis treatment and prevention of mental illnesses and disorders.
Dr Bernard Schulz, Chair of Psychiatry

6041   University of Minnesota Department of Psychiatry
420 Delaware Street SE   612-624-2430
Minneapolis, MN 55455-374   Fax: 612-265-91
                                           www.umn.edu
Behavior and mental illness research.
S Charles PhD, Director

6042   University of Missouri: Columbia Missouri Institute of Mental Health
5247 Fyler Avenue   573-634-8787
Saint Louis, MO 63139-1300   Fax: 314-644-8834
Mental health policy and ethics studies.
Danny Weddin MD, Director

6043   University of Pittsburgh: Western Psychiatric Institute & Clinic
3811 Ohara Street   412-246-6356
Pittsburgh, PA 15213-2593   Fax: 412-246-6350
                                           reitzpm@msx.upmc.edu
                                           www.pitt.edu
Advancement of basic and clinical knowledge in mental health and psychiatric care.
Thomas Detre Camarata, Acting Director

6044   Vanderbilt Kennedy Center
Vanderbilt University

110 Magnolia Center
Nashville, TN 37203-5701

615-322-8240
Fax: 615-228-36
kc@vanderbilt.edu

Mental health research.
Donna G Eskind, Chair
Cathy S Brown, Past Chair

6045 Veterans Medical Center: Mental Health Clinical Research Center
3801 Miranda Avenue
Palo Alto, CA 94304-1207

650-858-3941
www.va.gov

Jerome Gallin, Director
David Henderson, Deputy Director for Clinical Care

6046 Yeshiva University: Soundview-Throgs Neck Community Mental Health Center
2527 Glebe Avenue
Bronx, NY 10461-3109

718-904-4400
Fax: 718-931-7307

Mental health mental illness and recovery from mental illness research.
Dr Itamar

Support Groups & Hotlines

6047 National Health Information Center
Office of Disease Prevention & Health Promotion
1101 Wootton Pkwy
Rockville, MD 20852

Fax: 240-453-8281
odphpinfo@hhs.gov
www.health.gov/nhic

Supports public health education by maintaining a calendar of National Health Observances; helps connect consumers and health professionals to organizations that can best answer questions and provide up-to-date contact information from reliable sources; updates on a yearly basis toll-free numbers for health information, Federal health clearinghouses and info centers.
Don Wright, MD, MPH, Director

Alabama

6048 Alabama Education of Homeless Children and Youth Program
Alabama State Department of Education
5348 Gordon Persons Building
Montgomery, AL 36130-3901

334-242-8199
Fax: 334-420-9633

The major responsibilities of the Federal Programs Section are to administer all federally funded education programs and to provide technical assistance to local education agencies and schools. These responsibilities include promoting, supervising, and coordinating statewide educational programs with federal programs in addition to assisting schools in developing, revising, and implementing their school wide plans.
Maggie McDonald, Program/Education Director
Augusta Reimer, Leadership Project Coordinator

Alaska

6049 National Alliance for the Mentally Ill (NA MI) Alaska
144 West 15th Avenue
Anchorage, AK 99501-5106

907-227-1300
800-478-4462
Fax: 907-227-1400

NAMI Alaska is a grassroots, 501(c)(3) nonprofit, support, educational and advocacy organization of consumers, families, and friends of people with severe brain disorders such as schizophrenia, schizo-affective disorder, bipolar disorder, major depressive disorder, obsessive-compulsive disorder, panic and anxiety disorders, and attention deficit/hyperactivity disorder. In addition, NAMI provides information and referral services and works with local media on stories about mental illness.
Scott Owens, Co-President
Pat Dobbins, Co-President

Arizona

6050 Navajo Nation Office of Special Education & Rehabilitation Services (OSERS)
PO Box 1420
Window Rock, AZ 86515

928-871-6338
866-341-9918
Fax: 928-871-7865
osers@navajo.org
www.osers.navajo-nsn.gov/

Navajo OSERS is a program within the Division of DINE Education, which offers vocational rehabilitation to people with disabilities. Vocational Rehabilitation includes an array of services, which are funded by a grant to the Navajo Nation from the U.S. Department of Education. The goal of vocational rehabilitation is to assist people with disabilities to obtain or maintain employment.
Treva M Roanhorse, Director
Paula S Seanez, Assistant Director

Colorado

6051 Laradon Services for Children and Adults w ith Developmental Disabilities
5100 Lincoln Street
Denver, CO 80216

303-296-2400
866-381-2163
Fax: 303-296-4012
TDD: 7209746821
www.laradon.org/

Laradon specializes in services to children and adults with developmental disabilities, operating 15 programs that are designed to help each individual develop to his or her fullest potential and maximize self-sufficiency.
John Galvin, Chairman
Frank Lucero, PhD, Executive Director

Florida

6052 Florida Institute for Family Involvement (FIFI)
3927 Spring Creek Highway
Crawfordville, FL 32327

305-293-7626
877-926-3514
Fax: 863-582-9358
HewFLMOM@aol.com

Florida Institute for Family Involvement (FIFI), an affiliate of Federation of Families for Children's Mental Health (FFCMH), enhances, facilitates, and supports family and consumer involvement in the development of responsive, family centered, and community based systems of care. FIFI works in collaboration with state, federal, and private programs to develop a resource and training information center to enable individuals to advocate for appropriate services and make wise service choices.
Connie Hawke, Co-Director
Tara Bremer, Co-Director

6053 Parent Education Network (PEN) Project Health
Family Network on Disabilities of Florida
2735 Whitney Road
Clearwater, FL 33760

727-523-1130
800-825-5736
Fax: 727-523-8687
wilbur@fndfl.org

The PEN Project provides: information on specific disabilities; individual assistance by telephone, email, and in-person; referrals to local, state, and national resources; opportunities for youths with disabilities to be involved in training to parents and students; and, collaboration with Family Network on Disabilities Heart and Hope annual statewide conference for families.
Wilbur Smith, Co-Chief Executive Officer
Anna M McLaughlin, Co-Chief Executive Officer

Georgia

6054 Georgia Parent Support Network (GPSN)
1381 Metropolitan Parkway
Atlanta, GA 30310

404-758-4500
Fax: 404-758-6833
rheba.smith@gpsn.org
www.gpsn.org/

Georgia Parent Support Network (GPNS) provides support, education, and advocacy for children and youth with mental illness,

emotional disturbances, and behavioral differences and their families.
Kathy Dennis, Board President
Sue L Smith, Ed.D, Chief Executive Officer

Hawaii

6055   Hawaii Families As Allies (HFAA)
99-209 Moanalua Road   808-487-8785
Aiea, HI 96701   866-361-8825
                                   Fax: 808-487-0514
                                        hfaa@hfaa.net
                                        www.hfaa.net/
Hawaii Families as Allies (HFAA) is a statewide parent-controlled family network organization that provides support, services and information for families of children and adolescents with emotional and/or behavioral challenges. HFAA is the Hawaii state chapter of the Federation of Families for Children's Mental Health, a national organization that advocates for service system change so that families are valued and treated as true partners.
Linda Machado, Executive Director
Charlene Daraban, Family Resource Specialist

Illinois

6056   CANDU Parent Group
24W 681 Woodcrest Drive   630-983-9027
Naperville, IL 60540
Cathy Dennis

6057   KALEIDOSCOPE
1340 S. Damen Avenue   773-278-7200
Chicago, IL 60608   Fax: 773-278-5663
                                   TTY: 773-292-4086
                                  info@kaleidoscope4kids.org
                                  www.kaleidoscope4kids.org
William J Binder, Chair
Ivy Walker, Vice Chairman-Secretary

6058   Parents Information Network FFCMH
1926 1700th Avenue   217-735-1662
Lincoln, IL 62656
Bridget Van Gogh, President

Indiana

6059   NAMI Indiana - National Alliance on Mental Illness
PO Box 22697   317-925-9399
Indianapolis, IN 46222-0697   800-677-6442
                                   Fax: 317-925-9398
                                        info@namiindiana.org
                                        www.namiindiana.org
NAMI Indiana is a non-profit grassroots organization dedicated to improving the lives of people afflicted by serious and persistent mental illness. NAMI Indiana consists of families, consumers, and professionals that are dedicated to helping families through a network of support, education, advocacy, and promotion of research. NAMI Indiana is affiliated with the National Alliance on Mental Illness (NAMI), which is located in Arlington, Virginia.
Joshua G Sprunger, Executive Director
Joanne Abbott, Program Director

Iowa

6060   Iowa Federaion of Families for Children's Mental Health (FFCMH)
106 South Booth   319-462-2187
Anamosa, IA 52205   888-400-6302
                                   Fax: 319-462-6789
The mission of Iowa Federation of Families for Children's Mental Health is to link families to community, county and state partners for needed supports and services; and to promote systems change that will enable families to live in a safe, stable and respectful environment.
Lori Reynolds, Executive Director
Heidi Reynolds, Program Director

Kentucky

6061   Kentucky IMPACT
275 E Main Street   502-564-7610
Frankfort, KY 40621
Sandra Welles, Executive Director

Minnesota

6062   Emotional Health Anonymous
PO Box 4245   651-647-9712
St Paul, MN 55104-0245   Fax: 651-647-1593
                                        www.emotionsanonymous.org
A twelve-step organization, similar to Alcoholics Anonymous. Compsed of people who come together in weekly meetings for the purpose of working toward recovery from emotional difficulties.
Karen Mead, Executive Director

6063   PACER Center
8161 Normandale Boulevard   952-838-9000
Bloomington, MN 55437-1044   800-537-2237
                                   Fax: 952-838-0199
                                   TTY: 952-838-0190
                                        pacer@pacer.org
                                        www.pacer.org
Paula F Goldberg, Executive Director
Mary Schrock, Chief Operating and Development Officer

Missouri

6064   MO-SPAN Southwest Region
210 W Vine Street   660-679-5767
Butler, MO 64730
Eldonna Dittrich, Executive Director
Tina Vervara, Administrative Assistant

6065   MOSPAN Northwest Region
440 Rue Street Fran‡ois   314-972-0600
Jefferson City, MO 63031   Fax: 314-720-06
Donna Taycher, Executive Director

Nevada

6066   Nevada PEP
2101 S. Jones Boulevard   702-388-8899
Las Vegas, NV 89146   800-216-5188
                                   Fax: 702-388-2966
                                        KTaycher@nvpep.org
                                        www.nvpep.org
A statewide non-profit helping families who have children with disabilities, and the professionals who work with them. Support groups, training, workshops, lending resource library. Services are provided at no cost.
Karen Taycher, Executive Director
Stephanie Vrsnik, Community Development Director

New Hampshire

6067   National Alliance for the Mentally Ill: New Hampshire
85 North State Street   603-225-5359
Concord, NH 03301   800-242-6264
                                   Fax: 603-228-8848
                                        info@naminh.org
                                        www.naminh.org
Family support and advocacy for consumers and family members.
Michele Grennon, President
Ken Norton, Executive Director

New Mexico

6068   Navajo Nation Office Special Education & R ehabilitation Services
IHS PO Box 1337   505-722-1454
Gallup, NM 87301   Fax: 505-722-1554
                                        osers@navajo.org
                                        www.osers.navajo-nsn.gov/
Navajo OSERS is a program within the Division of DINE Education, which offers vocational rehabilitation to people with disabilities. Vocational Rehabilitation includes an array of services, which are funded by a grant to the Navajo Nation from the U.S. Depart-

ment of Education. The goal of vocational rehabilitation is to assist people with disabilities to obtain or maintain employment.
Treva M Roanhorse, Director
Paula S Seanez, Assistant Director

New York

6069   Mental Health Association in Dutchess Coun ty
253 Mansion Street   845-473-2500
Poughkeepsie, NY 12601   Fax: 845-473-4870
                                                           www.mhadc.com/
The Mental Health Association in Dutchess County promotes mental well-being and advances the recovery from mental illness, provides rehabilitation programs and support services for adults with a history of mental illness and their families.
Joseph Ellman, President
Andrew O'Grady, Executive Director

6070   Mental Health Association in Orange County
Mental Health Association of Orange County
73 James P. Kelly Way   845-342-2400
Middletown, NY 10940-1906   800-832-1200
                                                      Fax: 845-343-9665
                                                  mha@mhaorangeny.com
                                              www.mhaorangeny.com/
Mental Health Association of Orange County/MHA is a private, not-for-profit organization seeking to promote the mental health and emotional well being of Orange County residents. Under the leadership of a volunteer Board of Directors, MHA's staff members, consultants and volunteers provide free mental health services to thousands of Orange County residents each year. Several volunteers answer several hotlines, provide companionship, public education, direct services and assist with fundraisers.
David Goggins, President
Nadia Allen, Executive Director

North Dakota

6071   ND FFCMH Region II
PO Box 3061   701-222-1223
Bismarck, ND 58502-3061   Fax: 701-250-8835
                                                            www.ffcmh.org
Carlotta Jendro, Executive Director

6072   ND Region V FFCMH Chapter-Federation of Fa milies for Children's Mental Health
1104 2nd Avenue South   701-235-9923
Fargo, ND 58103   Fax: 701-235-9923
                                                 ndffrgv@nbinternet.com
                                        www.ffcmh.org/who_chapters.php
The FFCMH, a national family-run organization serves to: provide advocacy at the national level for the rights of children and youth with emotional, behavioral and mental health challenges and their families; provide leadership and technical assistance to a nation-wide network of family run organizations; and, collaborate with family run and other child serving organizations to transform mental health care in America.
Deborah Sevart, Executive Director

6073   ND Region VII FFCMH-Federation of Families for Children's Mental Health
2252 La Corte Loop   701-258-1628
Bismarck, ND 58503   Fax: 701-258-1628
                                                       ndffrg7@btinet.net
                                        www.ffcmh.org/who_chapters.php
The FFCMH, a national family-run organization serves to: provide advocacy at the national level for the rights of children and youth with emotional, behavioral and mental health challenges and their families; provide leadership and technical assistance to a nation-wide network of family run organizations; and, collaborate with family run and other child serving organizations to transform mental health care in America.
Becky Beale Psy.D, Group Programs Director
David J Coleman Ph.D, Director of Psychological Services

Ohio

6074   Child & Adolescent Behavioral Health
919 2nd Street NE   330-454-7917
Canton, OH 44704   Fax: 330-452-8860
                                                      bsnyder@casrv.org
                                           www.childandadolescent.org/
The Child and Adolescent Service Center (CASC) was founded and incorporated in 1976 by a standing committee of the Stark County Mental Health Foundation. CASC provides dynamic leadership through innovative service, training and evaluation and is committed to providing culturally-sensitive programs and services throughout the community.
Lisa Warburton-Gregory, President
Michael Johnson, Chief Executive Officer

6075   First Ohio Chapter: FFCMH
4505 Quaker Court   330-726-9570
Canfield, OH 44406-9131   Fax: 330-726-9031
The Federation of Families for Children's Mental Health (FFCMH) is a national organization dedicated exclusively to helping children with mental health needs and their families achieve a better quality of life.
Chrysanne Cianon, Executive Director
Brenda Alego, Assistant Director

Rhode Island

6076   Parent Support Network of Rhode Island
1395 Atwood Avenue   401-467-6855
Johnston, RI 02919   800-483-8844
                                                      Fax: 401-467-6903
                                                    c.ciano@psnri.org
                                                         www.psnri.org
Family-run organization whose mission is to provide support, education and advocacy to parents of children at risk for or who have emotional, behavioral, and/or mental health challenges.
Linda Winfield, Board President
Cathy Ciano, Executive Director

South Carolina

6077   Federation of Families of South Carolina
810 Dutch Square Boulevard   803-772-5210
Columbia, SC 29210-2344   866-779-0402
                                                      Fax: 803-772-5212
                                                FedFamSC@yahoo.com
                                                  www.fedfamsc.org/
Kathleen Scharer, President
Roxann McKinnon, Vice President

Tennessee

6078   Tennessee Voices for Children
701 Bradford Avenue   615-269-7751
Nashville, TN 37204   800-670-9882
                                                      Fax: 615-269-8914
                                                    tvc@tnvoices.org
                                                     www.tnvoices.org
Michele Johnson, President
Paula Sandidge, M.D, Board Secretary

Texas

6079   Harris County FFCMH
431 Breeze Park Drive   713-455-8962
Houston, TX 77015
Elizabeth Cerar, Executive Director
Karen Greenwell, Community Education Coordinator

Utah

6080   Allies with Families
505 East 200 South   801-433-2595
Salt Lake City, UT 84102-2979   877-477-0764
                                                      Fax: 801-521-0872
                                          Allies@AlliesWithFamilies.org
                                             www.allieswithfamilies.org

Allies with Families was created in 1991 to offer practical support and resources for parents and their children and youth who face serious emotional, behavioral and mental health challenges. It was created to support all families in the state of Utah.
Lori Cerar, Executive Director
Karen Greenwell, Project Director and Newsletter Editor

Vermont

6081 Vermont FFCMH
PO Box 1577   802-244-1955
Williston, VT 05495-0507   800-639-6071
                                              Fax: 802-329-2135
                                              vffcmh@vffcmh.org
                                              www.ffcmh.org/find-local-chapter
The Federation of Families for Children's Mental Health (FFCMH) is a national organization dedicated exclusively to helping children with mental health needs and their families achieve a better quality of life,
Kathleen Holsopple

Virginia

6082 PACCT
8032 Mechanicsville Turnpike   804-559-6833
Mechancsville, VA 23111   Fax: 804-559-6835
Joyce Scheibe

6083 PACCT of Roanoke Valley
PO Box 21112   703-989-5042
Roanoke, VA 24018   Fax: 703-989-5675
Sue Critchlow, Director
Sandra Spencer, Executive Director Corporate Office (MD)

Washington

6084 Common Voice for Pierce County Parents
10402 Kline Street   253-537-2145
Lakewood, WA 98445-2768   Fax: 253-537-2162
                                                 nrascon@dadsmove.org
A Common Voice for Pierce County Parents is affiliated with the Federation of Families for Children's Mental Health (FFCMH), a national organization dedicated exclusively to helping children with mental health needs and their families achieve a better quality of life.
Sherry Lyons

Wisconsin

6085 We Are the Children's Hope/Support Group
First Love Outreach Ministries
PO Box 06204   414-263-1323
Milwaukee, WI 53206   Fax: 414-263-1148
                                                 zelodius@aol.com
                                                 www.firstlovelifecoaching.com
Pr Zelodius Gerlosky

Wyoming

6086 Concerned Parent Coalition
1125 Sioux Avenue   307-682-6684
Gillette, WY 82718-6529
Michelle Nikkel, Executive Director
Carla Schroeder, Deputy Director

6087 Uplift
200 W 17th Street   307-778-8686
Cheyenne, WY 82003   888-875-4383
                                                 Fax: 307-778-8681
                                                 uplift@upliftwy.org
                                                 www.upliftwy.org
Peggy Logan, President
Richard Yep, Executive Director

Books

6088 Anatomy of a Psychiatric Illness
American Psychiatric Press

1400 K Street NW   202-682-6268
Washington, DC 20005-2403   Fax: 202-789-2648
Answers questions, provides clinical anecdotes, explains what medical science does and does not know about mental illnesses and discusses compassion and hard scientific facts surrounding the psychiatric profession.
230 pages
ISBN: 0-880485-21-3
Keith Russell Ablow, Author

6089 Assessing Psychopathology and Behavior Problems: Mentally Ill Persons
National Clearinghouse for Alcohol and Drug Abuse
PO Box 2345   800-729-6686
Rockville, MD 20857-0001   www.health.org
239 pages

6090 Caring for People with Severe Mental Disorders: A National Plan
Superintendent of Documents
PO Box 371954   202-512-2250
Pittsburgh, PA 15250-7954
This report offers, from three panels of expert consultants, recommendations for strengthening both services research and research resources that should lead to improvement of the standard and provision of care for persons who have severe mental disorders.
80 pages

6091 Complete Mental Health Directory
Grey House Publishing
4919 Route 22   518-789-8700
Amenia, NY 12501   800-562-2139
                                                 Fax: 518-789-0545
                                                 books@greyhouse.com
                                                 www.greyhouse.com
Offers critical and comprehensive information on disorders, support groups, clinical management, government agencies, professional conferences, research centers and training.
687 pages
ISBN: 1-930956-06-1
Leslie Mackenzie, Publisher

6092 Creating New Options
Bazelon Center for Mental Health Law
1101 15th Street NW   202-467-5730
Washington, DC 20005-5002   Fax: 202-223-0409
                                                 TDD: 202-467-4342
                                                 pubs@bazelon.org
                                                 www.bazelon.org
Training for corrections administrators and staff on access to federal benefits for people with mental illnesses who are leacing jail or prison. Available as a manual ($7.50),a PowerPoint presentation on CD ($5), or both ($11).
2008
Lee Carly, Communications Director

6093 Creating a Circle of Learning: The Church and the Mentally Ill
National Alliance for the Mentally Ill
PO Box 753   301-524-7600
Waldorf, MD 20604-0753   Fax: 301-843-0159
                                                 www.NAMI.org
A curriculum designed to sensitize adults in the church to the plight of people with severe mental illnesses and their families. Leaders can teach the study as 12 one-hour lessons or six two-hour lessons. The teaching sessions build on a Biblical-based theological reflection calling congregations to minister to their brothers and sisters with mental illnesses.
1997

6094 Culture and the Restructuring of Community Mental Health
William A Vega, author
Greenwood Publishing Group, Inc.
PO Box 6926   800-225-5800
Portsmouth, NH 03802-6926   Fax: 877-231-6980
                                                 service@greenwood.com
                                                 www.greenwood.com
Examines treatment, organizational planning and research issues and offers a critique of the theoretical and programmatic aspects of

providing mental health services to traditionally undeserved populations.
168 pages
ISBN: 0-313268-87-8
William Vega, Author
John W. Murphy, Author

6095 Dealing with Mental Incapacity
Center for Public Representation
PO Box 260049   608-251-4008
Madison, WI 53726-0049   800-369-0388
                                        Fax: 608-251-1263
This manual contains a comprehensive introduction to the problem of guardianship as well as chapters of financial and health care planning tools, guardianship under Wisconsin law, protective placement and Watts reviews.
Training Manual

6096 Design of Rehabilitation Services in Psychiatric Hospital Settings
American Occupational Therapy Association
PO Box 1725   301-948-9626
Rockville, MD 20849-1725   800-729-2082
Presents a design for constructing a rehabilitation system that will ensure the delivery of quality services to patients in a psychiatric hospital setting.
130 pages
Jeanette Bair, Executive Director

6097 Dimensions of State Mental Health Policy
Greenwood Publishing Group, Inc/Praeger Publishers
PO Box 6926   800-225-5800
Portsmouth, NH 03802-6926   Fax: 877-231-6980
                                  service@greenwood.com
                                     www.greenwood.com
Introduces students to the emerging field of state mental health policy.
320 pages
ISBN: 0-275932-52-4

6098 Dual Diagnosis of Major Mental Illness and Substance Disorder
National Alliance for the Mentally Ill
PO Box 753   703-524-7600
Waldorf, MD 20604-0753   Fax: 703-524-9094
                                         www.NAMI.org
Written for professionals, readable for families including descriptions of model programs.

6099 Educating Patients and Families About Mental Illness: A Practical Guide
Aspen Publishers
7201 McKinney Circle   800-638-8437
Frederick, MD 21704-8356
Introducing the manual to specifically address educating your patients and their families about mental illness.
496 pages
Cynthia Bisbee, Author

6100 Elderly with Chronic Mental Illness
Springer Publishing Company
536 Broadway   212-431-4370
New York, NY 10012-3955   877-687-7476
                                     Fax: 212-941-7842
                             marketing@springerpub.com
                                     www.springerpub.com
384 pages Hardcover
ISBN: 0-826172-80-6
Annette Imperati, Marketing Director

6101 Elders Assert Their Rights
Bazelon Center for Mental Health Law
1101 15th Street NW   202-467-5730
Washington, DC 20005-5002   Fax: 202-223-0409
                                    TDD: 202-467-4342
                                      pubs@bazelon.org
                                       www.bazelon.org
A guide for residents, family members and advocates to the legal rights of elderly people with mental disabilities in nursing homes.
Paperback
Lee Carly, Communications Director

6102 Encyclopedia of Mental Health
Facts on File
11 Penn Plaza   212-967-8800
New York, NY 10001   800-322-8755
                                     Fax: 800-678-3633
Here, readers will find inciseve definitions of theories, syndromes, symptons, treatments, and contemporary issues in easy-to-understand language.
480 pages Hardcover

6103 Encyclopedia of Phobias, Fears, and Anxieties
Facts on File
11 Penn Plaza   212-967-8800
New York, NY 10001   800-322-8755
                                     Fax: 800-678-3633
500 pages Hardcover

6104 Evaluation and Treatment of the Psychogeriatric Patient
Diane Gibson, MS, author
Haworth Press
10 Alice Street   607-722-5857
Binghamton, NY 13904-1580   800-429-6784
                                     Fax: 607-722-0012
                                     www.haworthpress.com
This pertinent book assists occupational therapists and other health care providers in developing up-to-date psychogeriatric programs.
111 pages Hardcover
ISBN: 1-560240-52-1

6105 Family Caregiving in Mental Illness
National Alliance for the Mentally Ill
PO Box 753   301-524-7600
Waldorf, MD 20604-0753   Fax: 301-843-0159
                                         www.NAMI.org
Examines patients' rights and treatment needs from the point of view of all those involved. Focuses on family burden and research and theoretical perspectives that influence mental health professionals.
1996
Amir Ella, Author

6106 Federal Law of the Mentally Handicapped
William Hein & Company
1285 Main Street   716-882-2600
Buffalo, NY 14209-1987
Chronological compilation of all relevant federal laws dealing with the mentally handicapped along with supporting documentation necessary to create a complete legislative history.
42 volumes/set

6107 Focal Group Psychotherapy for Mental Health Professionals
New Harbinger Publications
5674 Shattuck Avenue   800-748-6273
Oakland, CA 94609-1662   Fax: 510-652-5472
                                   www.newharbinger.com
Definitive guide to leading brief, theme-based groups. This book offers an extensive week-by-week description of the basic concepts and interventions for 14 theme or focal groups.
544 pages

6108 Handbook of Mental Health and Mental Disor der Among Black Americans
Greenwood Publishing Group, Inc.
PO Box 6926   800-225-5800
Portsmouth, NH 03802-6926   Fax: 877-231-6980
                                     www.greenwood.com
In addition to providing a wealth of new data on the mental health status of black communities, this handbook presents analyses of specific social, structural, and cultural conditions that affect the lives of individual black Americans.
352 pages
ISBN: 0-313263-30-2

6109 How to Live with a Mentally Ill Person: A Handbook of Day-to-Day Strategies
National Alliance for the Mentally Ill
PO Box 753   301-524-7600
Waldorf, MD 20604-0753   Fax: 301-843-0159
                                         www.NAMI.org

Offers self-help-styled advice to caregivers. Includes personal experiences, education, stigma, coping, and the mental health system.
1996

6110 Last in Line
Bazelon Center for Mental Health Law
1101 15th Street NW   202-467-5730
Washington, DC 20005-5002   Fax: 202-223-0409
                                                         TDD: 202-467-4342
                                                         pubs@bazelon.org
                                                         www.bazelon.org
discusses barriers to community integration of older adults with mental illnesses, and recommendations for change.
2006 72 pages
Lee Carly, Communications Director
James Stewart Bain, Author

6111 Living with Mental Handicaps
Jessica Kingsley Publishers
118 Pentonville Road   071-833-2307
London, England,   Fax: 071-837-2917
The focus of this book lies in its insistence that mentally handicapped people make transitions like the rest of us from youth to old age.
176 pages

6112 Madness in the Streets
Free Press
866 3rd Avenue   800-323-7445
New York, NY 10022-6221   Fax: 800-943-9831
                                                         www.simonsays.com
How psychiatry and the law abandoned the mentally ill.
436 pages
ISBN: 0-029153-80-8
Virginia C Armat, Author
Rael Jean Isaac, Author

6113 Making Child Welfare Work
Bazelon Center for Mental Health Law
1101 15th Street NW   202-467-5730
Washington, DC 20005-5002   Fax: 202-223-0409
                                                         TDD: 202-467-4342
                                                         pubs@bazelon.org
                                                         www.bazelon.org
How the RC lawsuit forged new partnership to protect children and sustain families. The story of systems reform from the bottom up and the rededication of a burocracy to focus on the children and families it is meant to serve.
1998 126 pages
Lee Carly, Communications Director

6114 Managed Mental Health Care
American Psychiatric Press
1400 K Street NW   202-682-6268
Washington, DC 20005-2403   Fax: 202-789-2648
This text presents the collective wisdom of 40 experts experienced in clinical and managerial issues in managed care.
425 pages Hardcover
ISBN: 0-880483-55-5

6115 Managing Managed Care: A Mental Health Practitioner's Survival Guide
American Psychiatric Press
1400 K Street NW   202-682-6268
Washington, DC 20005-2403   Fax: 202-789-2648
Provides an easy-to-learn system for communicating with external reviewers and documenting quality of care.
200 pages Hardcover
ISBN: 0-880483-69-5

6116 Manic Depressive Illness
National Alliance for the Mentally Ill
PO Box 753   703-524-7600
Waldorf, MD 20604-0753   Fax: 703-524-9094
                                                         www.NAMI.org
A definitive overview of bipolar disorder.

6117 Medicare Rx Consumer Workbook
Mental Health America

2000 N Beauragard Strt   703-684-7722
Alexandria, VA 22311   800-969-6642
                                                         Fax: 703-684-5968
                                                         TTY: 800-433-5959
                                                         www.mentalhealthamerica.net
This workbook is designed to help you as a mental health consumer to get educated about and get enrolled in the new Medicare prescription drug program. Designed as a pocket folder, the workbook includes basic language explanations, tips for enrollment preparation, questions you should ask regarding plan options, worksheets, and definitions.

6118 Membership Directory
Natl. Council for Community Behavioral Healthcare
12300 Twinbrook Parkway   301-984-6200
Rockville, MD 20852   www.icai.org

6119 Mental Disability Law: A Primer
Commission on The Mentally Disabled
1800 M Street NW   202-331-2240
Washington, DC 20036-5802
An updated and expanded version of the 1984 edition. Addresses the considerations involved in representing clients with mental disabilities.

6120 Mental Health Care in Prisons and Jails
Vance Bibliographies
PO Box 229   217-762-3831
Monticello, IL 61856-0229
A bibliography regarding health care in prisons.
30 pages
ISBN: 0-792006-94-1

6121 Mental Health Concepts and Techniques for the Occupational Therapy Assistant
Raven Press
1185 Ave of the Americas   212-930-9500
New York, NY 10036-2601   800-777-2295
This text offers clear and easily understood explanations of the various theoretical and practice health models. Second edition.
344 pages
ISBN: 0-781700-74-4

6122 Mental Health Law Reporter
Business Publishers, Inc.
PO Box 17592   800-274-6737
Baltimore, MD 21297
Brings you the most timely, focused and thorough information on the legal issues that concern you in mental health litigation.
monthly
Leonard Eiserer, Publisher

6123 Mental Health: Counseling Services
Vance Bibliographies
PO Box 229   217-762-3831
Monticello, IL 61856-0229
Selected annotated bibliography on counseling services for the mentally handicapped from a black perspective.
23 pages
ISBN: 1-555903-76-2

6124 Mental Illness-Opposing Viewpoints Series
Greenhaven Press
Thomson Gale   800-877-4253
Farmington Hills, MI 48333-9187   Fax: 800-414-5043
                                                         gale.customerservice@thomson.com
                                                         www.gale.com/greenhaven
In-depth overview of the topic written for upper elementary and junior/senior high school students.
2006
ISBN: 1-560061-68-5

6125 Mental and Physical Disability Law Report
American Bar Association
1800 M Street NW   202-331-2240
Washington, DC 20036-5802
Covers case law, legislative and regulatory developments that affect persons with mental or physical disabilities.

6126 Mentally Ill Individuals
Mainstream
1030 5th Street NW
Washington, DC 20001-2504   202-898-1400
Mainstreaming mentally ill individuals into the workplace.
12 pages

6127 Mood Apart: Depression, Mania, and Other Afflictions of the Self
National Alliance for the Mentally Ill
PO Box 753   301-524-7600
Waldorf, MD 20604-0753   Fax: 301-843-0159
                                    www.NAMI.org
Discussion of depression and mania includes the symptoms, human costs, biological underpinnings, and therapies. Uses case histories, appendices, and historical references.
1997

6128 National Plan for Research on Child and Adolescent Mental Disorders
Superintendent of Documents
PO Box 371954
Pittsburgh, PA 15250-7954   202-512-2250
Summarizes the current knowledge about the prevalence and causes of mental disorders among children, identifies the possible treatments and prevention strategies and notes promising areas of research.
64 pages

6129 Occupational Therapy Practice Guidelines for Adults with Mood Disorders
American Occupational Therapy Association
4720 Montgomery Lane   301-652-2682
Bethesda, MD 20824-1220   Fax: 301-652-7711
                                    TDD: 800-377-8555
                                    www.aota.org
27 pages
ISBN: 1-569001-10-3
Leslie L. Jackson, Author
Arbesman Marian, Ph.D, Author

6130 Playing Cure
Jason Aronson
PO Box 15100   800-782-0015
York, PA 17405-7100   www.aronson.com
400 pages Hardcover
ISBN: 0-765700-21-2
Donna M. Cangelosi, Author
Heidi Kaduson, Author

6131 Protection and Advocacy Program for the Mentally Ill
US Department of Health and Human Services
5600 Fishers Lane   301-443-3667
Rockville, MD 20857-0001   www.uls-dc.org/
Federal formula grant program to protect and advocate the rights of people with mental illnesses who are in residential facilities and to investigate abuse and neglect in such facilities.
Natalie Reatia, Chief

6132 Somatization Disorder in the Medical Setting
Superintendent of Documents
PO Box 371954
Pittsburgh, PA 15250-7954   202-512-2250
Somatization is a process in which psychological distress is expressed in multiple physical symptoms that have no discernible medical cause.
98 pages

6133 Strengthening the Role of Families in States' Early Intervention Systems
CEC, Department K00757   703-471-9543
Herdon, VA 22091
Policy guide for procedural safeguards for infants and toddlers under Part H of the Individuals with Disabilities Education Act.
213 pages Report

6134 Surviving Mental Illness
National Alliance for the Mentally Ill
14738 72nd Avenue   718-261-3772
Flushing, NY 11367-0753   Fax: 703-524-9094
                            www.survivingmentalillness.net

The subjective experiences of people with multiple diagnoses including schizophrenia, bipolar disorder and manic depression.

6135 Teaching Adults with Mental Handicaps
Sunday School Board of the Southern Baptists
127 9th Avenue N   800-458-BSSB
Nashville, TN 37234-0001
Offers guidelines in methods of teaching adults with mental handicaps, their needs, outreach ideas, curriculum resources, adaptation procedures, and ministry suggestions.

6136 Troubled Journey
National Alliance for the Mentally Ill
PO Box 753   301-524-7600
Waldorf, MD 20604-0753   Fax: 301-843-0159
                                    www.NAMI.org
Long associated with NAMI's former Siblings and Adult Children Network, the authors use their years of listening to stories - plus Marsh's professional experience - to provide a book that offers support to siblings and a caring and heartfelt approach to healing.
1997
Faith Cook, Author

6137 Turning Point
American Psychiatric Press
1400 K Street NW   202-682-6268
Washington, DC 20005-2403   Fax: 202-789-2648
                            www.turningpoint.org.in
The first comprehensive chronicle of the contributions made by conscientious objectors who volunteered for service in America's mental hospitals and state institutions for the developmentally disabled.
314 pages Hardcover
ISBN: 0-880485-60-4
Tiffany Snow, Author

6138 Understanding Depression
Patricia Ainsworth, MD, author
University Press of Mississippi
3825 Ridgewood Road   601-432-6205
Jackson, MS 39211-6492   Fax: 601-432-6217
                            kburgess@ihl.state.ms.us
                            www.upress.state.ms.us
A clear explanation for those who know the illness personally and for those who want to understand them.
2000 120 pages Paperback
ISBN: 1-578061-69-5
J. Raymond DePaulo, Author
Leslie Alan Horvitz, Author

6139 Understanding Mental Retardation
Patricia Ainsworth, MD; Pamela C Baker, PhD, author
University Press of Mississippi
3825 Ridgewood Road   601-432-6205
Jackson, MS 39211-6492   Fax: 601-432-6217
                            kburgess@ihl.state.ms.us
                            www.upress.state.ms.us
A resource for parents, caregivers, and counselors.
2004 192 pages Paperback
ISBN: 1-578066-47-6
Edward Zigler, Author
Robert M. Hodapp, Author

6140 Understanding Panic and Other Anxiety Disorders
Benjamin Root, MD, author
University Press of Mississippi
3825 Ridgewood Road   601-432-6205
Jackson, MS 39211-6492   Fax: 601-432-6217
                            kburgess@ihl.state.ms.us
                            www.upress.state.ms.us
A patients guide to panic disorders, panic attacks, and other stress-related maladies.
2000 128 pages Paperback
ISBN: 1-578062-45-4
Kathy Burgess, Advertising/Marketing Services Manager
Root Benjamin, Author

6141 Victims of Dementia
Haworth Press

10 Alice Street
Binghamton, NY 13904-1580

607-722-5857
800-429-6784
Fax: 607-722-0012
www.haworthpress.com

Provides an in-depth look at the concept, construction and operation of Wesley Hall, a special living area at the Chelsea United Methodist retirement home in Michigan.
1993 155 pages Hardcover
ISBN: 1-560242-64-0

6142   Way to Go: School Success for Children wit h Mental Health Care Needs
Bazelon Center for Mental Health Law
1101 15th Street NW
Washington, DC 20005-5002

202-467-5730
Fax: 202-223-0409
TDD: 202-467-4342
pubs@bazelon.org
www.bazelon.org

A report and fact sheets that document how states and school districts have successfully combined school-wide positive behavior support (PBS) with effective mental health services to foster a school environment that is conducive to learning, and improves children's lives. Order book and fact sheets sheets seperately or together. Pricing according to volume begins at $25 per book, $10 per fact sheet, or $29 for the combination.
1998
Lee Carly, Communications Director

6143   What

6144   What Fair Housing Means for People with Disabilities
Bazelon Center for Mental Health Law
1101 15th Street NW
Washington, DC 20005-5002

202-467-5730
Fax: 202-223-0409
TDD: 202-467-4342
pubs@bazelon.org
www.bazelon.org

Explains in plain language how three federal laws protect the housing rights of people with mental or physical disabilities. 2003 edition available as pdf download.
2006 56 pages
Lee Carly, Communications Director
Judge David L. Bazelon, Author

6145   When Madness Comes Home
National Alliance for the Mentally Ill
PO Box 753
Waldorf, MD 20604-0753

301-524-7600
Fax: 301-843-0159
www.NAMI.org

Personal accounts offer first-hand, day-to-day experiences with mental illness of a sibling (mostly) and partner/spouse (briefly) and discuss the effects of growing up in a family whose energies are focused on an ill family member.
1997
Victoria Secunda, Author

6146   When Someone You Love Has a Mental Illness
National Alliance for the Mentally Ill
PO Box 753
Waldorf, MD 20604-0753

703-524-7600
Fax: 703-524-9094
www.NAMI.org

Excellent for families recently stricken with severe mental illness.

Children's Books

6147   Compassion Books, Inc.
7036 State Highway 80 S
Burnsville, NC 28714-7569

828-675-5909
800-970-4220
Fax: 828-675-9687
orders@compassionbooks.com
www.compassionbooks.com

Hand picked resources to help people through loss, grief and changes of all kinds. Carry over 400 books and videos on death and dying, bereavement and change, comfort and healing, hope and much more.
Bruce Greene, VP

Magazines

6148   AJMR
American Association on Mental Retardation
444 N Capitol Street NW
Washington, DC 20001-1508

202-387-1968
800-424-3688
Fax: 202-387-2193
AAMR@access.digex.net
www.aamr.org

Provides information on the latest program advances, current research, and information on products and services in the developmental disabilities field.
BiMonthly

6149   American Journal of Psychiatry
American Psychiatric Association
1000 Wilson Boulevard
Arlington, VA 22209-2492

703-907-7322
800-368-5777
Fax: 703-907-1091
ajp.psychiatryonline.org

Professional papers on topics in psychiatry.
Monthly
Public Affairs, Division

6150   American Psychologist
American Psychological Association
750 First Street NE
Washington, DC 20002-4242

202-336-5510
800-374-2721
Fax: 202-336-5502
TDD: 202-336-6123
www.apa.org

Articles on current issues in psychology as well as empirical, theoretical and practical articles on broad aspects of psychology.
9x a year

6151   Journal of Clinical Psychology
Clinical Psychology Publishing Company
4 Conant Square
Brandon, VT 05733-1018

802-247-6877

Scholarly research reports in the field of psychology.

6152   Mental Retardation
American Association on Mental Retardation
444 N Capitol Street NW
Washington, DC 20001-1508

202-387-1968
800-424-3688
Fax: 202-387-2193
AAMR@access.digex.net
www.aamr.org

Provides information on the latest program advances, current research, and information on products and services in the developmental disabilities field.
BiMonthly
James R. Patton, Author

6153   Psychopharmacology Bulletin
Superintendent of Documents/NIMH Journal
PO Box 371954
Pittsburgh, PA 15250-7954

202-512-2250

Emphasizes rapid, informal dissemination of recent research findings that have not previously appeared in the more formal literature.
Quarterly

6154   Psychosocial Rehabilitation Journal
Int'l Assoc. of Psychosocial Rehab. Services
730 Commonwealth Avenue
Boston, MA 02215-1209

617-353-3549

Discusses issues, programs and research on psychiatric rehabilitation.

Newsletters

6155   ACMH Newsletter
Association for Children's Mental Health
1705 Coolidge Road
East Lansing, MI 48823-1735

517-336-7222
800-782-0883

Offers the latest information, including unmet needs and notices of relevant agency and legislative activities, hearings, public meet-

ings and other opportunities for promoting children's mental health.
Quarterly
Gail Allen, Director
Marla Holle, Parent Advocate

6156 Advocate
National Alliance for the Mentally Ill
200 N Glebe Road   703-524-7600
Arlington, VA 22203-3754   Fax: 703-524-9094
Offers reviews of books, medical information, legislative information and Alliance activities for persons with mental illness, their families and professionals who work with them.
Quarterly

6157 Mental Health Law News
Interwood Publications
PO Box 20241   513-221-3715
Cincinnati, OH 45220-0241
Mental health case law summaries.
6 pages Monthly
ISBN: 0-889017-0 -
Frank J Bardack, Editor

6158 News & Notes
American Association on Mental Retardation
444 N Capitol Street NW   202-387-1968
Washington, DC 20001-1508   800-424-3688
                                          Fax: 202-387-2193
                                             www.aamr.org
Covers legislative, program, and research developments of interest to the field, as well as international news, Association activities, job ads and other classifieds, and upcoming events.
BiMonthly

Pamphlets

6159 14 Worst Myths About Recovered Mental Patients
National Institutes of Health
5600 Fishers Lane   301-496-4000
Rockville, MD 20857-0001   Fax: 301-443-6349
                                           NIHInfo@nih.gov
                                              www.nih.gov
Refutes false beliefs that stigmatize recovered mental patients and suggests ways that the public can help advance the truth.

6160 Bipolar Disorder
National Institutes of Health
5600 Fishers Lane   301-443-3706
Rockville, MD 20857-0001   Fax: 301-443-6349
                                           NIHInfo@nih.gov
                                              www.nih.gov
A short booklet offering a concise description of this disorder, which is also called manic-depressive illness.
Francis Mark Mondimore, Author

6161 Coping with Mental Illness in the Family
National Alliance for the Mentally Ill
PO Box 753   703-524-7600
Waldorf, MD 20604-0753   Fax: 703-524-9094
                                              www.NAMI.org
A handbook for families.

6162 Dual Diagnosis: Substance Abuse and Mental Illness
National Alliance for the Mentally Ill
PO Box 753   703-524-7600
Waldorf, MD 20604-0753   Fax: 703-524-9094
                                              www.NAMI.org
A booklet for families and consumers.

6163 Helping Families Understand PTSD
National Veterans Services Fund
PO Box 2465   203-656-0003
Darien, CT 06820-0465   Fax: 203-656-1957
                                           NatVetSvc@aol.com
                                        www.valdezhousing.com
Pamphlet

6164 Let's Talk Facts About Childhood Disorders
American Psychiatric Association
1400 K Street NW   202-682-6220
Washington, DC 20005-2492
Offers information on depression and depressive disorders including the causes, symptoms, treatments, anxiety, and various other phobias.
Public Affairs, Division

6165 Mental Health Problems of Vietnam Veterans
National Veterans Services Fund
PO Box 2465   203-656-0003
Darien, CT 06820-0465   Fax: 203-656-1957
                                           NatVetSvc@aol.com
                                        www.valdezhousing.com
Pamphlet

6166 Minority Advocacy Notebook
Bazelon Center for Mental Health Law
1101 15th Street NW   202-467-5730
Washington, DC 20005-5002   Fax: 202-223-0409
                                         TDD: 202-467-4342
                                           pubs@bazelon.org
                                             www.bazelon.org
Selected materials and models from our manual on outreach and advocacy for African Americans and Latinos with mental disabilities; includes Impediments to Services and Advocacy for Black and Hispanic People with Mental Illness.
1998
Lee Carly, Communications Director

6167 New Challenge: Responding to Families
Federation for Children with Special Needs
95 Berkeley Street   617-482-2915
Boston, MA 02116-6230   800-331-0688
Addresses the needs of children with emotional, behavioral and mental disorders and their families.

6168 PTSD and the Family: Secondary Traumatization
National Veterans Services Fund
PO Box 2465   203-656-0003
Darien, CT 06820-0465   Fax: 203-656-1957
                                           NatVetSvc@aol.com
                                        www.valdezhousing.com
Pamphlet

6169 Plain Talk About...Dealing with the Angry Child
Superintendent of Documents
PO Box 371954   202-512-2250
Pittsburgh, PA 15250-7954
A flyer that offers suggestions for helping children cope with their anger in a healthy and constructive way.

6170 Plain Talk About...Handling Stress
Superintendent of Documents
PO Box 371954   202-512-2250
Pittsburgh, PA 15250-7954
Information on stress and how you can make it work for you rather than against you.

6171 Psychotherapy with Traumatized Vietnam Combatants
National Veterans Services Fund
PO Box 2465   203-656-0003
Darien, CT 06820-0465   Fax: 203-656-1957
                                           NatVetSvc@aol.com
                                        www.valdezhousing.com
Pamphlet

6172 Triumph Over Fear
National Alliance for the Mentally Ill
PO Box 753   703-524-7600
Waldorf, MD 20604-0753   Fax: 703-524-9094
                                              www.NAMI.org
Step-by-step treatment plans for the many faces of phobias, panic disorder, obsessive-compulsive disorder, and post-traumatic stress. Includes case histories.
1994 Softcover
Rosalynn Carter, Author
Jerilyn Ross, Author

Audio & Video

6173 And After Tomorrow
G. Allan Roeher Institute
4700 Keele Street   416-661-9611
Downsview, ON, M3J 1P3,
A film about lives of people with a mental handicap and their families, in which parents and friends speak candidly about their personal experiences.
Films

6174 With a Little Help from My Friends
L'institut Roeher Institute
York University   416-661-9611
North York, ON, M3J 1P3,   Fax: 416-661-5701
This three-part video provides insight into inclusive education for people with mental handicaps.

Web Sites

6175 American Psychological Association
www.apa.org
Mission is to advance psychology as a science and professional organization that represents psychology in the United States.

6176 Coalition of Voluntary Mental Health Agencies
www.cvmha.org/
An umbrella advocacy organization of New York's mental health community, representing over 100 non-profit community based mental health agencies that serve more than 300,000 clients in the five boroughs of New York City and its environs.

6177 Community Access
www.cairn.org/
A nonprofit agency providing housing and advocacy for people with psychiatric disabilities.

6178 Federation of Families for Children's Mental Health
www.ffcmh.org/
Providing leadership to develop and sustain a nationwide network of family-run organizations.

6179 Healing Well
www.healingwell.com
An online health resource guide to medical news, chat, information and articles, newsgroups and message boards, books, disease-related web sites, medical directories, and more for patients, friends, and family coping with disabling diseases, disorders, or chronic illnesses.

6180 Health Finder
www.healthfinder.gov
Searchable, carefully developed web site offering information on over 1000 topics. Developed by the US Department of Health and Human Services, the site can be used in both English and Spanish.

6181 Healthlink USA
www.healthlinkusa.com
Health information concerning treatment, cures, prevention, diagnosis, risk factors, research, support groups, email lists, personal stories and much more. Updated regularly.

6182 Internet Mental Health
www.mentalhealth.com
A site whose goal is to improve understanding, diagnosis, and treatment of mental illness throughout the world. Includes information on specific disorders, medications, diagnosis, research, news, and other internet links.

6183 MedicineNet
www.medicinenet.com
An online resource for consumers providing easy-to-read, authoritative medical and health information.

6184 Medscape
www.medscape.com
Medscape offers specialists, primary care physicians, and other health professionals the Web's most robust and integrated medical information and educational tools.

6185 Mental Health America (formerly NMHA) Information Center
www.mentalhealthamerica.net
Provides informational materials, lobbies for Federal mental health legislation, stimulates funding of research on the causes and treatment of mental illnesses.

6186 National Alliance for the Mentally Ill
www.nami.org
Over 900 affiliate groups nationwide offer support to members, advocate better lives for their loved ones, support research efforts and educate the public to reduce the stigma attached to serious mental illnesses.

6187 National Mental Health Services Knowledge Exchange Network
www.mentalhealth.org
Leading the national system that delivers mental health services. Provides the treatment and support services neede by adults with mental disorders and children with serious emotional problems.

6188 WebMD
www.webmd.com
Provides credible information, supportive communities, and in-depth reference material about health subjects. A source for original and timely health information as well as material from well known content providers.

6189 World Federation for Mental Health
www.wfmh.com
Mission is to promote, among all people and nations, the highest possible level of mental health in its broadest biological, medical, educational, and social aspects.

Description

6190 ## Mental Illness/Depression

Depression is a mood disorder that can cause marked impairment of physical and social function and work capacity. It differs from normal grief which occurs in response to a significant disappointment, separation, or loss. It affects twice as many women as men and is more common in people with a family history of depression. Depression comes in three forms: disruptive mood dysregulation, which occurs in children and is characterized by persistent irritability and out-of-control behavior, major depressive disorder, which is a discrete depressive episode that lasts two weeks or more, and persistent depressive disorder, which is a persistent depressed or irritable mood that lasts for more than a year.

Research is gathering evidence of the relationship between depression and chemical imbalances in the brain. Clinical depression can also be associated with medication or other physical illnesses.

Common symptoms associated with depression include irritability, sleeping problems, changes in appetite, sadness, apathy, loss of interest in previously enjoyed activities and anxiety. Depression frequently disrupts a person's relationship with friends, family members and colleagues. It is also associated with alcohol and substance abuse. Suicide is the cause of death in approximately 15 percent of untreated patients.

Treatment must be tailored to the individual and can include talk therapy and/or medication. Newer groups of antidepressant medications (SSRIs and SNRIs) havemarkedly improved the success of treatment. Patient and family education can play a crucial role. See also *Mental Illness/General* and *Mental Illness/Schizophrenia*.

National Agencies & Associations

6191 **American Chronic Pain Association**
PO Box 850
Rocklin, CA 95677
800-533-3231
ACPA@theacpa.org
www.theacpa.org
The ACPA facilitates peer support and education for individuals with chronic pain in its many forms, in order to increase quality of life. Also raises awareness among the healthcare community, and with policy makers.
Penney Cowan, Founder & CEO
Daniel Galia, Director, Global Support

6192 **American Counseling Association**
6101 Stevenson Avenue
Alexandria, VA 22304
800-347-6647
Fax: 800-473-2329
www.counseling.org
Non-profit professional and educational organization dedicated to the growth and enhancement of the counseling profession.
Richard Yep, CEO
Brandi McIntyre, Executive Assistant

6193 **American Psychiatric Association**
800 Maine Avenue SW
Washington, DC 20024
202-559-3900
apa@psych.org
www.psychiatry.org

A medical specialty society representing a growing membership of psychiatrists. Offers information for psychiatrists, medical students, patients and families.

6194 **Anxiety Disorders Association of America**
8701 Georgia Avenue
Silver Spring, MD 20910
240-485-1001
Fax: 240-485-1035
information@adaa.org
www.adaa.org
ADAA is a national non-profit organization dedicated to the prevention, treatment, and cure of anxiety, depression, OCD, PTSD, and related disorders and to improving the lives of all people who suffer from them through education, practice, and research.
Mary E. Beth Salcedo, MD, President
Luana Marques, PhD, President-Elect

6195 **Brain & Behavior Research Foundation**
747 Third Avenue
New York, NY 10017
646-681-4888
800-829-8289
info@bbrfoundation.org
www.bbrfoundation.org
Awards funding and grants to scientists around the world in order to advance brain and behavioral science.
Steve Lieber, Chair
Donald M. Boardman, Treasurer

6196 **International Foundation for Research and Education for Depression (iFred)**
PO Box 17598
Baltimore, MD 21297
800-239-1265
Fax: 443-782-0739
info@ifred.org
www.ifred.org
Eliminating mental health stigma through prevention, research, and education.
Tom Dean, Chair
Susan Minamyer, Secretary

6197 **Mental Health America**
500 Montgomery Street
Alexandria, VA 22314
703-684-7722
800-969-6642
Fax: 703-684-5968
www.mentalhealthamerica.net
Formerly known as the National Mental Health Association, Mental Health America is committed to helping all people live mentally healthier lives by promoting awareness of mental health.
Tom Starling, EdD, Chair
Jennifer L. Bright, MPA, Secretary & Treasurer

6198 **MindWise Innovations**
270 Bridge Street
Dedham, MA 02026
781-239-0071
Fax: 781-320-9136
info@mindwise.org
www.mindwise.org
Formerly known as Screening For Mental Health, MindWise Innovations provides resources to schools, workplaces, and communities to address mental health issues, substance abuse, and suicide.
Bryan Kohl, Senior Vice President
Marjie McDaniel, Vice President

6199 **National Alliance on Mental Illness**
3803 N Fairfax Drive
Arlington, VA 22203
703-524-7600
800-950-6264
info@nami.org
www.nami.org
Committed to building better lives for the millions of Americans affected by mental illness by raising awareness and offering community support.
Adrienne Kennedy, MA, President
Lacey Berumen, PhD, LAC, MNM, First Vice President

6200 **National Anxiety Foundation**
3135 Custer Drive
Lexington, KY 40517-4001   www.nationalanxietyfoundation.org
859-272-7166
Offers information and help to persons with panic disorders, manic and depressive disorders and mental illness.
Stephen M. Cox, MD, President & Director
Donald F. Klein, MD, DSc, Senior Scientific Advisor

6201 Option Institute
2080 South Undermountain Road 413-229-2100
Sheffield, MA 01257 800-714-2779
Fax: 413-229-8931
participantsupport@option.org
www.option.org
Self-defeating beliefs, along with attitudes and judgments, can lead to a host of physical and psychological challenges. The Option Institute offers programs designed to help people gain new perspectives on the attitudes and judgments that may be affecting their lives.
Barry Kaufman, Co-Founder
Samahria Lyte Kaufman, Co-Founder

Research Centers

6202 University of Pennsylvania: Depression Research Unit
School of Medicine
Department of Psychiatry 215-662-3462
Philadelphia, PA 19104 Fax: 215-662-6443
Focuses on mental health and depression.
Jay D MD, Chairman
Alex Cabrera, Clinic Manager

6203 University of Texas Mental Health Clinical Research Center
University of Texas
5323 Harry Hines Boulevard 214-645-8300
Dallas, TX 75390 Fax: 214-645-7999
www.utsouthwesteRN.edu
Research activity of major and atypical depression.
Daniel K Podolsky, MD, President
J. Gregory Fitz, Executive Vice President

6204 Yale University: Behavioral Medicine Clinic
Yale School of Medicine
333 Cedar Street 203-432-7960
New Haven, CT 06510 www.medicine.yale.edu
Focuses on mental disorders including schizophrenia and depression.
Peter Salovey, President
Richard Belitsky, Deputy Dean for Education

6205 Yale University: Ribicoff Research Facilities/CT Mental Health Center
34 Park Street 203-789-7300
New Haven, CT 06511 Fax: 203-562-7079
Clinical research in the areas of schizophrenia depression and mental disorders.
George Henin Ashenden, President

Support Groups & Hotlines

6206 Depression and Bipolar Support Alliance
730 N Franklin Street 312-642-0049
Chicago, IL 60654 800-826-3632
Fax: 312-642-7243
adoederlein@dbsalliance.org
www.dbsalliance.org
Consists of approximately 900 patient groups providing support and direct services to persons with clinical depression and/or bipolar disorder.
Lucinda Jewell, Chair
Allen Doederlein, President

6207 National Health Information Center
Office of Disease Prevention & Health Promotion
1101 Wootton Pkwy Fax: 240-453-8281
Rockville, MD 20852 odphpinfo@hhs.gov
www.health.gov/nhic
Supports public health education by maintaining a calendar of National Health Observances; helps connect consumers and health professionals to organizations that can best answer questions and provide up-to-date contact information from reliable sources; updates on a yearly basis toll-free numbers for health information, Federal health clearinghouses and info centers.
Don Wright, MD, MPH, Director

Books

6208 Columbia University Complete Home Guide to Mental Health
Henry Holt & Company
115 W 18th Street 212-886-9200
New York, NY 10011-4113 Fax: 212-633-0748
www.cumc.columbia.edu
A compendium of information on all aspects of mental health; written primarily for the lay reader.
476 pages

6209 Coping with Depression and Mood Disorders
Rosen Publishing Group
29 E 21st Street 212-777-3017
New York, NY 10010 800-237-9932
Fax: 888-436-4643
customerservice@rosenpub.com
www.rosenpublishing.com
With an emphasis on life's myriad difficulties, the authors help teens find practical ways to cope with depression.
ISBN: 0-823929-73-6
Lawrence Clayton PhD, Author
Sharon Carter, Author

6210 Depression Sourcebook
Brian P. Quinn, author
McGraw-Hill Companies
Returns Department 877-833-5524
Dubuque, IA 52002 Fax: 614-759-3749
pbg.ecommerce_custserv@mcgrw-hill.com
www.mcgraw-hill.com
Everything anyone afflicted with a depressive disorder - or the people who care about them - need to know about unipolar and bipolar depression.
2000 288 pages
ISBN: 0-737303-79-4
Amy L. Sutton, Author

6211 Depression and its Treatment
Warner Books
1271 Ave of the Americas 212-522-7200
New York, NY 10020-1300
A layman's guide to help one understand and cope with America's #1 mental health problem.
157 pages

6212 Depressive Illnesses: Treatments Bring New Hope
Superintendent of Documents
PO Box 371954 202-512-2250
Pittsburgh, PA 15250-7954
Offers the general public an overview of the various depressive illnesses. Topics include causes, symptoms and types of depression, clinical evaluation and treatment, helpful suggestions for family and friends, and other sources of information.
28 pages

6213 Encyclopedia of Depression
Facts on File
11 Penn Plaza 212-967-8800
New York, NY 10001 800-322-8755
Fax: 800-678-3633
This volume defines and explains all terms and topics relating to depression.
170 pages Hardcover

6214 Essential Guide to Psychiatric Drugs
St. Martin's Press
175 5th Avenue 212-674-5151
New York, NY 10010-7848 800-221-7945
Fax: 212-420-9314
Basic information on 123 drugs used for depression, anxiety and bipolar illness.

6215 Everything You Need to Know About Depression
Rosen Publishing Group
29 E 21st Street 212-777-3017
New York, NY 10010 800-237-9932
Fax: 888-436-4643
customerservice@rosenpub.com
www.rosenpublishing.com

An important resource for teens who are looking for help with depression.
Grades 7-12
ISBN: 0-823934-39-X
Elanor H Ayer, Author

6216 Inside Manic Depression
Sunnyside Press
PO Box 1717   619-424-3348
San Marcos, CA 92079-1717
The true story of one victim's triumph over despair. A first person account.
176 pages

6217 Medical Management of Depression
EMIS Medical Publishers
PO Box 6100   580-924-0643
Durant, OK 74702-1607   800-225-0694
     Fax: 580-924-9414
ISBN: 0-929240-62-6

6218 Mood Apart
Basic Books
10 E 53rd Street   212-207-7057
New York, NY 10022-5244
An overview of the depression and manic depression and the available treatments for them.
363 pages

6219 Overcoming Depression
Harper & Row
10 E 53rd Street   212-207-7000
New York, NY 10022-5299
318 pages Paperback

6220 Panic Disorder in the Medical Setting
Superintendent of Documents
PO Box 371954   202-512-2250
Pittsburgh, PA 15250-7954
This book serves the primary care physicians as a helpful guide in recognizing and treating panic disorder in patients and in identifying those who need psychiatric consultation or rerferrals.
1993 135 pages

6221 Pastoral Care of Depression
The Haworth Press
10 Alice Street   607-722-5857
Binghamton, NY 13904-1580   800-429-6784
     Fax: 607-895-0582
     getinfo@haworth.com
     www.haworth.com
Helps caregivers by overcoming the simplistic myths about depressive disorders and probing the real issues.
Paperback
ISBN: 0-789002-65-5

6222 Prozac Nation: Young & Depressed in America: A Memoir
Houghton Mifflin Company
Wayside Road   800-225-3362
Burlington, MA 01803
Struck with depression at 11, now 27, Wurtzel chronicles her struggle with the illness. Witty, terrifying and sometimes funny, it tells the story of a young life almost destroyed by depression.
317 pages

6223 Psychotherapy of Severe and Mild Depression
Jason Aronson
PO Box 15100   800-782-0015
York, PA 17405-7100   Fax: 201-840-7242
     www.aronson.com
464 pages Softcover
ISBN: 1-568211-46-5

6224 Questions & Answers About Depression & Its Treatment
Ivan K Goldberg, MD, author
Charles Press Publishers
PO Box 15715   215-561-2786
Philadelphia, PA 19103-0715   Fax: 215-561-0191
     mailbox@charlespresspub.com
     www.charlespresspub.com

All the questions you'd like to ask, asked and answered.
139 pages
ISBN: 0-914783-68-8

6225 Report of the Secretary's Task Force on Youth Suicide, Volume 1
Superintendent of Documents
PO Box 371954   202-512-2250
Pittsburgh, PA 15250-7954
A comprehensive review of information about youth suicide. The task force recommendations are presented in Volume 1.
110 pages

6226 Touched with Fire:- Manic Depressive Illness & the Artistic Temperment
Free Press
866 3rd Avenue   Fax: 800-943-9831
New York, NY 10022-6221   www.simonsays.com
Describing and discussing the markedly increased rates of severe mood disorders and suicides among the artistically creative and the reasons why.
370 pages

6227 Winter Blues
Norman E Rosenthal, author
Guilford Press
72 Spring Street   800-265-7006
New York, NY 10012-4019   Fax: 212-966-6708
     info@guilford.com
     www.guilford.com
Complete information about Seasonal Affective Disorder and its treatment.
2005
ISBN: 1-593852-14-2

6228 Women and Depression
Springer Publishing Company
536 Broadway   212-431-4370
New York, NY 10012-3955   877-687-7476
     Fax: 212-941-7842
     marketing@springerpub.com
     www.springerpub.com
This volume examines depression in women within a developmental context. It ranges from issues in childhood and adolescence through premenstrual syndrome and postpartum depression to issues of menopause and aging.
328 pages Hardcover
ISBN: 0-826151-40-X
Annette Imperati, Marketing Director

6229 Yesterday's Tomorrow
Hazelden
15251 Pleasant Valley Rd   651-257-4010
Center City, MN 55012-9640   800-328-9000
     Fax: 651-213-4426
     www.hazelden.org
A meditation book that shows why and how recovery works, from the author's own experiences.
432 pages Paperback
ISBN: 1-568381-60-3

Children's Books

6230 Compassion Books, Inc.
7036 State Highway 80 S   828-675-5909
Burnsville, NC 28714-7569   800-970-4220
     Fax: 828-675-9687
     orders@compassionbooks.com
     www.compassionbooks.com
Hand picked resources to help people through loss, grief and changes of all kinds. Carry over 400 books and videos on death and dying, bereavement and change, comfort and healing, hope and much more.
Bruce Greene, VP

Newsletters

6231 NFDI Newsletter
National Foundation for Depressive Illness
PO Box 2257   212-268-4260
New York, NY 10116-2257   800-248-4344
                                          Fax: 212-268-4434
                                               pross@att.net
                                            www.depression.org
To correct the myths and misconceptions surrounding the illness
and help reverse the devastating effects depression has on the individual and our society and to inform the public, primary health care
providers, other healthcare professionals and corporations about
depression and manic depression and to provide the information
about correct diagnosis and treatment and the availability of
qualified doctors and support groups.
4 pages Quarterly

Pamphlets

6232 Depression is a Treatable Illness: A Patients Guide
Department of Health & Human Services
2101 E Jefferson Street   301-217-1245
Rockville, MD 20852-4908
Tells about major depressive disorder, which is only one form of
depressive illness. This booklet answers important questions regarding this disorder and gives information on where to go for
more help.

6233 If You're Over 65 and Feeling Depressed...
National Institutes on Mental Health
5600 Fishers Lane   301-443-3706
Rockville, MD 20857-0001   Fax: 301-443-6349
Many older people believe that their age alone is responsible for
feelings of exhaustion, helplessness and worthlessness. This brochure discusses the causes of depression in the older years, symptoms, types of treatment and where to go for help.
12 pages

6234 Let's Talk About Depression
Superintendent of Documents
PO Box 371954   202-512-2250
Pittsburgh, PA 15250-7954
Targeted especially for inner-city youth. The colorful design will
capture attention and focus on depression in a way that young peo-
ple will understand and identify with.

6235 Lithium and Manic Depression
Lithium Info. Center-Dean Foundation for Health
8000 Excelsior Drive   608-836-8070
Madison, WI 53717-1972
A guidebook about lithium and its effects on bipolar affective disorders and manic depression.
1992 32 pages

6236 Living Without Depression & Manic Depression: A Workbook
National Alliance for the Mentally Ill
3803 N. Fairfax Drive   703-524-7600
Arlington, VA 22203-0753   800-950-6264
                                          Fax: 703-524-9094
                                               www.NAMI.org
Workbook offering checklists and helpful advice targeted for indi-
viduals whose depressive illness is stabilized.
1994
Jim Payne, President
Ralph E. Nelson, Jr., First Vice President

6237 Panic Disorder
National Institutes of Health
5600 Fishers Lane   301-443-3706
Rockville, MD 20857-0001   Fax: 301-443-6349
Written for the lay public, this pamphlet contains a description of
panic disorder, gives the symptoms, describes treatment methods,
and encourages the person who has the symptoms to seek
treatment.

6238 Plain Talk About Depression
Superintendent of Documents

PO Box 371954   202-512-2250
Pittsburgh, PA 15250-7954
A flyer discussing types of depression, major depression, symp-
toms and causes.

6239 Understanding Panic Disorder
National Institutes of Health
5600 Fishers Lane   301-443-3706
Rockville, MD 20857-0001   Fax: 301-443-6349
Offers information on what an panic disorder is, symptoms,
causes, treatment, medications and therapy.

6240 Useful Information on Phobias and Panic
Superintendent of Documents
PO Box 371954   202-512-2250
Pittsburgh, PA 15250-7954
This booklet provides information on both phobias and panic.
Symptoms, causes and treatments of these disorders are referred
to. If you know someone who is excessively fearful, this booklet
will be of great help to them in understanding their problem.
40 pages 50 copies

6241 What to Do When a Friend is Depressed: Guide for Students
Superintendent of Documents
PO Box 371954   202-512-2250
Pittsburgh, PA 15250-7954
Offers information on depression and its symptoms and suggests
things a young person can do to guide a depressed friend in finding
help.

6242 What to Do When an Employee is Depressed: A Guide for Supervisors
Superintendent of Documents
PO Box 371954   202-512-2250
Pittsburgh, PA 15250-7954
A D/ART program brochure that will enable an employer to recog-
nize the symptoms of depression in an employee and offers sugges-
tions on what to say to the employee to encourage him or her to seek
help.

Audio & Video

6243 Four Lives: A Portrait of Manic Depression
Fanlight Productions
4196 Washington Street   617-469-4999
Boston, MA 02131-1731   800-937-4113
                                          Fax: 617-469-3379
                                          fanlight@fanlight.com
                                            www.fanlight.com
Four patients, families and psychiatrists share their perspectives
on living with manic depression.
1987 60 Minutes
ISBN: 1-572950-29-3

6244 Taking Control of Depression
                                               800-228-2495
Dramatic program offering new hope in the understanding and
treatment of depression, with actor Ed Asner and Alan Xenakis,
M.D.

6245 When Someone You Love Suffers from Depression
Medcom/Trainex
                                               800-320-1444
Helping family and friends identify depression in a loved one - of-
fers ways to help stop the suffering and get appropriate treatment.

Web Sites

6246 Healing Well
                                            www.healingwell.com
An online health resource guide to medical news, chat, information and articles, newsgroups and message boards, books, disease-related web sites, medical directories, and more for patients,
friends, and family coping with disabling diseases, disorders, or
chronic illnesses.

6247   Health Finder

www.healthfinder.gov

Searchable, carefully developed web site offering information on over 1000 topics. Developed by the US Department of Health and Human Services, the site can be used in both English and Spanish.

6248   Healthlink USA

www.healthlinkusa.com

Health information concerning treatment, cures, prevention, diagnosis, risk factors, research, support groups, email lists, personal stories and much more. Updated regularly.

6249   MedicineNet

www.medicinenet.com

An online resource for consumers providing easy-to-read, authoritative medical and health information.

6250   Medscape

www.medscape.com

Medscape offers specialists, primary care physicians, and other health professionals the Web's most robust and integrated medical information and educational tools.

6251   National Anxiety Foundation

www.lexington-on-line.com/naf.html

Offers information and help to persons with panic disorders, manic and depressive disorders and mental illness.

6252   National Foundation for Depressive Illness

www.ifred.org

iFred engages with individuals and organizations to execute high-impact and effective campaigns that educate the public about support and treatment for depression.

6253   WebMD

www.webmd.com

Provides credible information, supportive communities, and in-depth reference material about health subjects. A source for original and timely health information as well as material from well known content providers.

Description

6254 Mental Illness/Schizophrenia

Schizophrenia is a chronic mental illness that is characterized by disturbances of thinking, feeling, and behavior. Schizophrenia usually begins in late adolescence or early adult life, with a lifetime prevalence between 0.2 to 1 percent. Despite popular perceptions, schizophrenia is not the same as split personality disorder. Although its specific cause is unknown, most cases of schizophrenia are believed to result from a complex interaction between biologic, inherited and environmental factors.

Symptoms of schizophrenia vary in type and severity and may include loss of contact with reality (psychosis), delusions (false beliefs) and auditory hallucinations (hearing voices), incoherent thought patterns, catatonic behavior, and a flat or grossly inappropriate emotional state (flattened affect).

Drug treatment with antipsychotics is the cornerstone of managing schizophrenia. When treated early, patients tend to respond quickly and more fully. Effective drugs have been available for several decades, and have revolutionized treatment of the disease. However, these drug treatments may be limited by side effects (especially movement disorders resembling Parkinson disease) and by the patient's failure or refusal to stay on treatment. Patient non-compliance is sometimes addressed with long-acting injectable medications. A new class of drugs, lacking the Parkinson-like side effects, and sometimes dramatically more effective than previously used drugs known as the second-generation antipsychotics, became available during the 1990s. Their use is limited by high costs and the threat of potentially serious side effects, which differ for each drug. Treatment also includes counseling, social support, rehabilitation, and skills retraining. Poor outcome frequently leads to extensive and long-term disability. Psychological and educational interventions can reduce the rate of relapse. People close to persons with schizophrenia are often very affected by the disease and can be helped by support and advocacy groups. See also *Mental Illness/General* and *Mental Illness/Depression*.

National Agencies & Associations

6255 Brain & Behavior Research Foundation
747 Third Avenue 646-681-4888
New York, NY 10017 800-829-8289
info@bbrfoundation.org
www.bbrfoundation.org
Awards funding and grants to scientists around the world in order to advance brain and behavioral science.
Steve Lieber, Chair
Donald M. Boardman, Treasurer

6256 International Society for the Study of Trauma and Dissociation
1420 New York Avenue 202-803-6332
Washington, DC 20005 Fax: 202-747-2864
info@isst-d.org
www.isst-d.org

The International Society for the Study of Trauma and Dissociation is a non-profit, professional association organized to develop clinically effective and empirically based resources and responses to trauma and dissociation.
Christine Forner, BA, BSW, MSW, President
D. Michael Coy, MA, LICSW, Treasurer

6257 National Alliance on Mental Illness (NAMI)
3803 N Fairfax Drive 703-524-7600
Arlington, VA 22203 800-950-6264
TDD: 703-516-7227
info@nami.org
www.nami.org
Committed to building better lives for the millions of Americans affected by mental illness by raising awareness and offering community support.
Adrienne Kennedy, MA, President
Lacey Berumen, PhD, LAC, MNM, First Vice President

Research Centers

6258 Huxley Insititute-American Schizophrenic Association
The Association Driving effective, low-cost treatment to patients with schizophrenia and help them in a cooperative effort to cope with the disorder.
Abram Carpenter Jr, Director
Vito J Seskunas, Deputy Director for Administration

6259 Maryland Psychiatric Research Center
655 W. Baltimore Street 410-402-7666
Baltimore, MD 21201 Fax: 410-788-3837
www.mprc.umaryland.edu/default.asp
Providing treatment to patients with schizophrenia and related disorders educating professionals and consumers about schizophrenia and conducting basic and translational research into the manifestations causes and treatment of schizophrenia.
Robert Buchanan, MD, Interim Director
Vito J Seskunas, Deputy Director for Administration

6260 National Alliance for Research on Schizophrenia and Depression
Grants Office
60 Cutter Mill Road 516-829-0091
Great Neck, NY 11021 800-829-8289
Fax: 516-487-6930
info@bbrfoundation.org
www.bbrfoundation.org/
Research focusing on varieties of mental illness and mental disorders.
Steve Lieber, Chairman of the Board
Jeffrey Borenstein, M.D., President & CEO

6261 Schizophrenia Research Branch: Division of Clinical and Treatment Research
5600 Fisher Lane, Parklawn Building 301-443-4707
Rockville, MD 20857 Fax: 301-443-6000
Plans, supports, and conducts programs of research, research training, and resource development of schizophrenia and related disorders. Reviews and evaluates research developments in the field and recommends new program directors. Collaborates with organizations in and outside of the National Institue of Mental Health (NIMH) to stimulate work in the field through conferences and workshops.

6262 Tennessee Neuropsychiatric Institute Middle Tennessee Mental Health Institute
Middle Tennessee Mental Health Institute
221 Stewarts Ferry Pike 615-902-7535
Nashville, TN 37217
Michael Eber Andreassen MD, Director

6263 University of Iowa Mental Health Clinical Research Center
University of Iowa Hospitals & Clinics
200 Hawkins Drive 319-356-1553
Iowa City, IA 52242 877-575-2864
Fax: 319-353-8300
Schizophrenia studies and other cognitive disorder research.
Nancy C

Support Groups & Hotlines

6264 National Health Information Center
Office of Disease Prevention & Health Promotion
1101 Wootton Pkwy   Fax: 240-453-8281
Rockville, MD 20852   odphpinfo@hhs.gov
                                       www.health.gov/nhic
Supports public health education by maintaining a calendar of National Health Observances; helps connect consumers and health professionals to organizations that can best answer questions and provide up-to-date contact information from reliable sources; updates on a yearly basis toll-free numbers for health information, Federal health clearinghouses and info centers.
Don Wright, MD, MPH, Director

Books

6265 Encyclopedia of Schizophrenia and the Psychotic Disorders
Facts on File
11 Penn Plaza   212-967-8800
New York, NY 10001   800-322-8755
                                       Fax: 800-678-3633
This volume details recent theories and research findings on schizophrenia and psychotic disorders, together with a complete overview of the field's history.
368 pages Hardcover

6266 Experiences of Schizophrenia
Guilford Press
72 Spring Street   800-365-7006
New York, NY 10012   Fax: 212-966-6708
                                       info@guilford.com
                                       www.guilford.com
This authoritative book presents new information on seasonal affective disorder. It includes remedies such as recent advances in light box therapy, research on the effectiveness of antidepressants, and new recipes to counterbalance unhealthy winter food cravings. This book also helps distinguish various degrees of the disorder ranging from winter blues to full blown SAD, and provides a self test that readers can use to evaluate their own seasonal mood changes.
2005 372 pages
ISBN: 1-593852-14-2

6267 Occupational Therapy Practice Guidelines for Adults with Schizophrenia
American Occupational Therapy Association
4720 Montgomery Lane   301-652-2682
Bethesda, MD 20824-1220   Fax: 301-652-7711
                                       TDD: 800-377-8555
                                       www.aota.org
24 pages
ISBN: 1-569001-53-7

6268 Return from Madness
Jason Aronson
PO Box 15100   800-783-0015
York, PA 17405-7100   www.aronson.com
256 pages Hardcover
ISBN: 1-568216-25-4

6269 Schizophrenia and Primitive Mental States
Jason Aronson
PO Box 15100   800-782-0015
York, PA 17405-7100   Fax: 201-840-7242
                                       www.aronson.com
288 pages Softcover
ISBN: 0-765700-27-1

6270 Schizophrenia: From Mind to Molecule
American Psychiatric Press
1400 K Street NW   202-682-6268
Washington, DC 20005-2403   Fax: 202-789-2648
Presents a change in the scientific understanding and outlook regarding the devastating disorder of schizophrenia. It provides a thorough, up-to-date look at schizophrenia that includes neural behavioral studies, technologies and medical treatments.
274 pages Hardcover
ISBN: 0-880489-50-2

Children's Books

6271 Year it Rained
MacMillan Publishing Company
866 3rd Avenue   212-702-2000
New York, NY 10022-6221
The story of a girl traumatized by an alcoholic father and her desire to commit suicide. Hospitalized for schizophrenia, Elizabeth reaches a catharsis and, with the help of a poet, discovers that her talent and therapy may be in writing.
Grades 7-10

Magazines

6272 Dissociation
ISSMP&D
5700 Old Orchard Road   847-966-4322
Skokie, IL 60077-1036   Fax: 847-966-9418
A professional journal offering the latest information about the issues and research into multiple personalities and related disorders.

6273 Schizophrenia Bulletin
Superintendent of Documents/NIMH Journal
PO Box 371954   202-512-2250
Pittsburgh, PA 15250-7954
Serves as a forum for multidisciplinary exchange of information about schizophrenia and is exclusively devoted to the exploration of this severe disorder.
Quarterly

Newsletters

6274 ISSD News
Int'l Society for the Study of Dissociation
8400 Westpark Drive   703-610-9037
McLean, VA 22102   Fax: 703-610-0234
                                       info@isst-d.org
                                       www.isst-d.org
Includes current news from other onzations of interest to members, information about recent articles and books, news from US and international affiliates and the latest issues concerning multiple personality/dissociative states.
17 pages 6 times a year
Lynette S. Danylchuk, President
Christine Forner, Treasurer

Pamphlets

6275 Schizophrenia
National Alliance for the Mentally Ill
3803 N. Fairfax Drive   703-524-7600
Arlington, VA 22203-3754   800-950-6264
                                       Fax: 703-524-9094
                                       www.NAMI.org
Part of the NAMI medical information series offering information on the causes, symptoms and treatments of Schizophrenia.
Jim Payne, President
Ralph E. Nelson, Jr., First Vice President

Web Sites

6276 Healing Well
                                       www.healingwell.com
An online health resource guide to medical news, chat, information and articles, newsgroups and message boards, books, disease-related web sites, medical directories, and more for patients, friends, and family coping with disabling diseases, disorders, or chronic illnesses.

6277 Health Finder

www.healthfinder.gov

Searchable, carefully developed web site offering information on over 1000 topics. Developed by the US Department of Health and Human Services, the site can be used in both English and Spanish.

6278 Healthlink USA

www.healthlinkusa.com

Health information concerning treatment, cures, prevention, diagnosis, risk factors, research, support groups, email lists, personal stories and much more. Updated regularly.

6279 International Society for the Study of Dissociation

www.issd.org

Association that promotes research and training in the identification of treatment of multiple personality.

6280 MedicineNet

www.medicinenet.com

An online resource for consumers providing easy-to-read, authoritative medical and health information.

6281 Medscape

www.medscape.com

Medscape offers specialists, primary care physicians, and other health professionals the Web's most robust and integrated medical information and educational tools.

6282 National Alliance for the Mentally Ill

www.nami.org

Mental health organization dedicated to building better lives for the millions of Americans affected by mental illness.

6283 Schizophrenia Therapy Online Resource Center

A website which provides effective and lasting alternatives to traditional treatment for individuals suffering with schizophrenia. Offers an effective and full continium of services ranging from psychopharmacology to individual and group psychotherapy to social rehabilitation, supported work experience, assertive community training and supported housing.

6284 WebMD

www.webmd.com

Provides credible information, supportive communities, and in-depth reference material about health subjects. A source for original and timely health information as well as material from well known content providers.

Description

6285 Migraine

Roughly 45 million Americans suffer from chronic headaches, the most disabling of which is migraine. 18 percent of women and about six percent of men suffer from migraines. Classified as a neurovascular headache, migraine headaches are caused by cortical spreading depression (CSD), which is a spontaneous self-propagating wave of neuronal activity that begins at the rear of the brain and spreads across the cerebral cortex. CSD induces the release of neurotransmitters that activate the trigeminal vascular system that subsequently dilates the blood vessels in the dura mater, increases inflammation and sensitization and activation of pain receptors in the brain. This brings on intense pain and nausea, and the focal loss of vision or numbness involving one side of the body. More than 50 percent of patients have a family history of migraine. They also appear to have a hormonal component, being more common in women and often affected by menstrual cycles or pregnancy.

Management of migraine begins with careful observation for triggering agents like foods, alcohol, or irregular sleep patterns. Acute treatment to stop a migraine involves a class of drugs called triptans that antagonize the action of the 5-hydroxytryptamine (5-HT or serotonin) that aggravates the migraine process. They block inflammation and can abort migraine in about 70 percent of patients. Sumatriptan, the prototype, is available in oral, nasal sprays and powders, and subcutaneous injection forms. Ergot drugs (dihydroergotamine mesylate and ergotamine + caffeine), also available in oral, sublingual, nasal, suppository and injectable forms, work by helping the swollen blood vessels constrict down to normal size. If headaches become very frequent, doctors may recommend preventive therapy, which requires daily drug administration. Drugs used in this way include beta-blockers and calcium-channel blockers, which were originally developed for hypertension and heart disease, and certain medicines ordinarily used for depression or seizures. In 2018, the FDA approved erenumab, a once-monthly, subcutaneously-injected monoclonal antibody that inactivates the calcitonin gene-related peptide receptor for preventative treatment for migraines in adults. Calcitonin gene-related peptide (CGRP) is a potent vasodilator that dramatically increases in concentration during migraine attacks.

Pain medications should be used sparingly. Nonsteroidal anti-inflammatory drugs, such as ibuprofen are best for mild to moderate headaches. Narcotic medications should be avoided except under special circumstances and with strict guidelines. Most migraine sufferers can be satisfactorily managed by their primary care physician or a neurologist, but in refractory cases a multi-disciplinary headache center may be of help.

Tension is the other common cause of disabling headaches. They are not migraines and are not considered neurovascular headaches but are mentioned here because they are so common. Some of the resources listed in this section may be helpful for persons with tension headache.

National Agencies & Associations

6286 American Academy of Neurology
201 Chicago Avenue
Minneapolis, MN 55415

612-928-6000
800-879-1960
Fax: 612-454-2746
memberservices@aan.com
www.aan.com

A medical specialty society established to advance knowledge of neurology and promote the best possible care for patients with neurological disorders.
James C. Stevens, MD, FAAN, President
Ann H. Tilton, MD, FAAN, Vice President

6287 American Chronic Pain Association
PO Box 850
Rocklin, CA 95677

800-533-3231
ACPA@theacpa.org
www.theacpa.org

The ACPA facilitates peer support and education for individuals with chronic pain in its many forms, in order to increase quality of life. Also raises awareness among the healthcare community, and with policy makers.
Penney Cowan, Founder & CEO
Daniel Galia, Director, Global Support

6288 American Headache Society
19 Mantua Road
Mount Royal, NJ 08061

856-423-0043
Fax: 856-423-0082
ahshq@talley.com
www.americanheadachesociety.org

Professional society of health care providers who study and treat headache and facial pain. AHS brings physicians from various fields and specialties together to share concepts and developments about headaches and related conditions.
Kathleen B. Digre, MD, FAHS, President
Andrew C. Charles, MD, FAHS, Treasurer

6289 American Migraine Foundation
19 Mantua Road
Mount Royal, NJ 08061

856-423-0043
Fax: 856-423-0082
amf@talley.com
www.americanmigrainefoundation.org

A non-profit alliance of headache sufferers and physicians who are working together to improve the quality of care and the quality of information available to people with chronic or severe headache conditions.
Linda McGillicuddy, CEO
Nim Lalvani, MPH, Director

6290 Help for Headaches
515 Richmond Street
London, Ontario, N6A-5M3

519-434-0008
brent@helpforheadaches.org
www.headache-help.org

A non-profit organization, and a registered Canadian charity that is committed to supporting those suffering from headaches.
G. Brent Lucas, BA, Director

6291 Migraine Awareness Group: A National Understanding for Migraineurs (MAGNUM)
100 N Union Street
Alexandria, VA 22314

www.migraines.org

Works to bring public awareness to the fact that migraine is a true organic neurological disease.
Michael John Coleman, President & Executive Director
Terri Miller Burchfield, Executive VP & Legislative Director

6292 National Headache Foundation
820 N Orleans
Chicago, IL 60610-3131
312-274-2650
888-643-5552
info@headaches.org
www.headaches.org

A non-profit organization committed to serving as an information resource to headache sufferers, their families and the healthcare providers who treat them. Promotes research into potential headache causes and treatments.
Seymour Diamond, MD, Executive Chair & Founder
Arthur Martin, MD, President

Research Centers

6293 Baltimore Headache Institute
11 E Chase Street
Baltimore, MD 21202
410-547-0200
Brian E Goldstein, Director

6294 San Francisco Clinical Research Center
909 Hyde Street
San Francisco, CA 94109
415-673-4600
Fax: 415-673-9352
SFHACLIN@aol.com

This research center also specializes in diagnosis of Alzheimer's related dementia in addition to migraine headaches.
Jerome Goldstein, M.D., Director
Guy Engelmann, M.D., Team Member

Support Groups & Hotlines

6295 National Health Information Center
Office of Disease Prevention & Health Promotion
1101 Wootton Pkwy
Rockville, MD 20852
Fax: 240-453-8281
odphpinfo@hhs.gov
www.health.gov/nhic

Supports public health education by maintaining a calendar of National Health Observances; helps connect consumers and health professionals to organizations that can best answer questions and provide up-to-date contact information from reliable sources; updates on a yearly basis toll-free numbers for health information, Federal health clearinghouses and info centers.
Don Wright, MD, MPH, Director

Books

6296 Conquering Headache
Alan Rapoport, MD, author
B.C Decker, Inc.
50 King Street E, Floor 2
Ontario, Canada L8N 3K7,
905-522-7017
800-568-7281
Fax: 905-522-7839
www.bcdecker.com

Conquering Headache, Fourth Edition provides the information needed to conquer headaches and improve the quality of life.
2003 128 pages Paperback
ISBN: 1-550092-33-2
Alan M. Rapoport, Author
Fred D. Sheftell, Author

6297 Freedom from Headaches
Simon & Schuster Order Department
200 Old Tappan Road
Old Tappan, NJ 07675-7095
800-999-5479
Headache pain is unlike any other pain; when your head throbs, your entire body suffers.
ISBN: 0-671254-04-9
Joel R. Saper, Author

6298 Handbook of Headache Disorders
Essential Medical Information Systems
PO Box 1607
Durant, OK 74702-1607
580-924-0643
800-225-0694
Fax: 580-924-9414

1993 Paperback
ISBN: 0-929240-62-6

6299 Handbook of Headache Management: A Practic al Guide to Diagnosis & Treatment
Williams & Wilkins
351 W Camden Street
Baltimore, MD 21201-7912
301-528-4000
800-638-0672
1993 224 pages
ISBN: 0-683058-01-0
Paolo Martelletti, Editor
Timothy J Steiner, Editor

6300 Migraine and Other Headaches: Vascular Mechanisms
Raven Press
1185 Ave of the Americas
New York, NY 10036-2601
212-930-9500
800-777-2295
www.raven.com

Leading international experts present new concepts on the mechanisms of migraine and other vascular headaches and detail the latest strategies for diagnosis and treatment of migraine with and without aura, tension-type headaches, cluster headaches and other vascular disorders.
368 pages
ISBN: 0-881677-95-7

6301 Migraine: The Complete Guide
American Council for Headache Education
19 Mantua Road
Mount Royal, NJ 08061
856-423-0258
800-255-2243
Fax: 856-423-0082
achehq@talley.com
www.achenet.org

A comprehensive resource book for people with migraine, their families and physicians (updated in 1999) by Lynne M Constantine, Suzanne Scott and ACHE.
Teri Robert, Chair
Dr. Paul Winner, Co-Chair

6302 Overcoming Headaches & Migraines
Longmeadow Press
19 Mantua Road
Mount Royal, NJ 08061-1469
856-423-0258
800-255-2243
Fax: 856-423-0082
achehq@talley.com
www.achenet.org

1993 128 pages Paperback
ISBN: 0-681417-92-7
Teri Robert, Chair
Dr. Paul Winner, Co-Chair

6303 Understanding Migrain and Other Headaches
Stewart J Tepper, MD, author
University Press of Mississippi
3825 Ridgewood Road
Jackson, MS 39211-6492
601-432-6205
Fax: 601-432-6217
press@ihl.state.ms.us
www.upress.state.ms.us

A comprehensive overview of causes, diagnoses, and treatments.
2004 112 pages Paperback
ISBN: 1-578065-92-5
Chip Mercer, Sales Representative
Jim Barkley, Sales Representative

6304 Wolff's Headaches & Other Head Pain
Oxford University Press
2001 Evans Road
Cary, NC 27513-2010
212-726-6000
800-445-9714
Fax: 919-677-1303
custserv.us@oup.com
www.oup-usa.org

1993
ISBN: 0-195082-50-8

Newsletters

6305 Headache
American Council for Headache Education

19 Mantua Road   856-423-0258
Mount Royal, NJ 08061   800-255-2243
       Fax: 856-423-0082
       achehq@talley.com
       www.achenet.org

The ACHE 12 page quarterly newsletter provides valuable and current information on new treatments, as well as time proven headache management strategies. All articles are written or reviewed by headache experts from the American Headache Society (AHS). Recent issues have included articles by headache experts on drug and nondrug treatment options and information on new treatments and research is regularly included.
Quarterly
Teri Robert, Chair
Dr. Paul Winner, Co-Chair

6306   **NHF Head Lines**
National Headache Foundation
820 N Orleans   312-274-2650
Chicago, IL 60610-3132   888-643-5552
       Fax: 312-640-9049
       info@headaches.org
       www.headaches.org

Offers the latest information on headaches, causes and treatments. Contains news on drugs and medical forums, in depth discussions of headaches and preventions and a question and answer section in which physicians respond to reader inquiries and support group information.
16 pages Quarterly
Arthur H. Elkind, President
Vincent Martin, Vice President

Pamphlets

6307   **52 Proven Stress Reducers**
National Headache Foundation
820 N Orleans   312-274-2650
Chicago, IL 60610   888-643-5552
       Fax: 312-640-9049
       info@headaches.org
       www.headaches.org

Members only.
Suzanne Simons, Executive Director

6308   **About Headaches**
National Headache Foundation
820 N Orleans   312-274-2650
Chicago, IL 60610   888-643-5552
       Fax: 312-640-9049
       info@headaches.org
       www.headaches.org

Contains an in depth look at headaches, tips on when to seek medical advice, methods of treatment and more.
16 pages
Suzanne Simons, Executive Director

6309   **Analgesic Rebound Headaches: Fact Sheet**
National Headache Foundation
820 N Orleans   312-274-2650
Chicago, IL 60610   888-643-5552
       Fax: 312-640-9049
       info@headaches.org
       www.headaches.org

Offers information on analgesic agents or drugs used to control pain including migraine and other types of headaches.
Suzanne Simons, Executive Director

6310   **Cluster Headache: Fact Sheet**
National Headache Foundation
820 N Orleans   312-274-2650
Chicago, IL 60610   888-643-5552
       Fax: 312-640-9049
       info@headaches.org
       www.headaches.org

Offers information on cluster headaches and the treatment available for them. This information sheet can be downloaded from the web site.
Suzanne Simons, Executive Director

6311   **Diet and Headache: Fact Sheet**
National Headache Foundation
820 N Orleans   312-274-2650
Chicago, IL 60610   888-643-5552
       Fax: 312-640-9049
       info@headaches.org
       www.headaches.org

Offers information on what foods should be avoided and what foods trigger headaches in all migraine sufferers. This information sheet can be dowloaded from the web site.
Suzanne Simons, Executive Director

6312   **Headache Facts: What Everyone Should Know**
American Council for Headache Education
19 Mantua Road   856-423-0258
Mount Royal, NJ 08061   800-255-2243
       Fax: 856-423-0082
       achehq@talley.com
       www.achenet.org

Teri Robert, Chair
Dr. Paul Winner, Co-Chair

6313   **Headache Handbook**
National Headache Foundation
820 N Orleans   312-274-2650
Chicago, IL 60610   888-643-5552
       Fax: 312-640-9049
       info@headaches.org
       www.headaches.org

Gives information on causes and types of headaches as well as treatments available.
8 pages
Teri Robert, Chair
Dr. Paul Winner, Co-Chair

6314   **Headache in Children: Fact Sheet**
National Headache Foundation
820 N Orleans   312-274-2650
Chicago, IL 60610   888-643-5552
       Fax: 312-640-9049
       info@headaches.org
       www.headaches.org

Offers information on vascular headaches, tension-type headaches, traction and inflammatory headaches and treatment. This information sheet can be downloaded from the web site.
Suzanne Simons, Executive Director

6315   **Hormones and Migraines: Fact Sheet**
National Headache Foundation
820 N Orleans   312-274-2650
Chicago, IL 60610   888-643-5552
       Fax: 312-640-9049
       info@headaches.org
       www.headaches.org

Offers information on the link between hormones and migraines.
Suzanne Simons, Executive Director

6316   **How to Talk to Your Doctor About Headaches**
National Headache Foundation
820 N Orleans   312-274-2650
Chicago, IL 60610   888-643-5552
       Fax: 312-640-9049
       info@headaches.org
       www.headaches.org

Learn how to keep a headache diary to pinpoint symptoms and effective diagnosis.
Suzanne Simons, Executive Director

6317   **Impact of Migraine: A Disabling and Costly Condition**
American Council for Headache Education
19 Mantua Road   856-423-0258
Mount Royal, NJ 08061   800-255-2243
       Fax: 856-423-0082
       achehq@talley.com
       www.achenet.org

Teri Robert, Chair
Dr. Paul Winner, Co-Chair

6318 **Migraine and Coexisting Conditions: Other Illnesses That May Affect Migraine**
American Council for Headache Education
19 Mantua Road
Mount Royal, NJ 08061

856-423-0258
800-255-2243
Fax: 856-423-0082
achehq@talley.com
www.achenet.org

Teri Robert, Chair
Dr. Paul Winner, Co-Chair

6319 **Migraine: Fact Sheet**
National Headache Foundation
820 N Orleans
Chicago, IL 60610

312-274-2650
888-643-5552
Fax: 312-640-9049
info@headaches.org
www.headaches.org

Offers information on migraines and treatments.
Suzanne Simons, Executive Director

6320 **Tap the Best Resource**
National Headache Foundation
820 N Orleans
Chicago, IL 60610

312-274-2650
888-643-5552
Fax: 312-640-9049
info@headaches.org
www.headaches.org

Informational brochure offering facts and statistics on headaches. Everything from muscle contraction, vascular headaches, sinus headaches, TMJ and much more.
Suzanne Simons, Executive Director

6321 **Tension-Type Headache: Fact Sheet**
National Headache Foundation
820 N Orleans
Chicago, IL 60610

312-274-2650
888-643-5552
Fax: 312-640-9049
info@headaches.org
www.headaches.org

Offers information on the least known type of headache, chronic tension-type headaches. This information sheet can be downloaded from the web site.
Teri Robert, Chair
Dr. Paul Winner, Co-Chair

6322 **What's the Best Medicine for My Headaches?**
American Council for Headache Education
19 Mantua Road
Mount Royal, NJ 08061

856-423-0258
800-255-2243
Fax: 856-423-0082
achehq@talley.com
www.achenet.org

Teri Robert, Chair
Dr. Paul Winner, Co-Chair

Audio & Video

6323 **Relaxation Tape**
National Headache Foundation
820 N Orleans
Chicago, IL 60610

312-274-2650
888-643-5552
Fax: 312-640-9049
info@headaches.org
www.headaches.org

Contains techniques to assist the listener in experiencing greater self control and relaxation.
Audio Tape
Suzanne Simons, Executive Director

6324 **Stretch and Relax Tape**
National Headache Foundation
820 N Orleans
Chicago, IL 60610

312-274-2650
888-643-5552
Fax: 312-640-9049
info@headaches.org
www.headaches.org

Based on a series of progressive relaxation techniques which involve the tightening and relaxing of specific muscle groups.
Audio Tape
Suzanne Simons, Executive Director

Web Sites

6325 **American Academy of Neurology**
www.aan.com/
A professional organization representing neurologists worldwide.

6326 **American Council for Headache Education (ACHE)**
www.achenet.org
The ACHE website offers an extensive library of headache information, including a searchable database of past articles from our newsletter, discussion forums that provide virtual contact with leading headache specialists and fellow headache sufferers, a searchable database of physicians to find a specialist in your area and more.

6327 **American Headache Society**
www.americanheadachesociety.org
The American Headache Society (AHS) is a professional society of health care providers dedicated to the study and treatment of headache and face pain. Educating physicians, health professionals and the public and encouraging scientific research are the primary functions of this organization.

6328 **American Medical Association**
Journal of the American Medical Association
www.ama-assn.org/
An organized web site focusing on treatment options, education and support available to those suffering from migraine headaches.

6329 **Cluster Headaches**
www.clusterheadaches.com
A web site devoted completely and exclusively to those that suffer from cluster headaches.

6330 **Healing Well**
www.healingwell.com
An online health resource guide to medical news, chat, information and articles, newsgroups and message boards, books, disease-related web sites, medical directories, and more for patients, friends, and family coping with disabling diseases, disorders, or chronic illnesses.

6331 **Health Finder**
www.healthfinder.gov
Searchable, carefully developed web site offering information on over 1000 topics. Developed by the US Department of Health and Human Services, the site can be used in both English and Spanish.

6332 **Healthlink USA**
www.healthlinkusa.com
Health information concerning treatment, cures, prevention, diagnosis, risk factors, research, support groups, email lists, personal stories and much more. Updated regularly.

6333 **MedicineNet**
www.medicinenet.com
An online resource for consumers providing easy-to-read, authoritative medical and health information.

6334 **Medscape**
www.medscape.com
Medscape offers specialists, primary care physicians, and other health professionals the Web's most robust and integrated medical information and educational tools.

6335 **Medsupport**
michiganheadache.com
The Michigan Headache Clinic has been evolving in Michigan since 1981 and consists of our centrally located headache clinic, our web-based headache information pages and a working relationship we have developed with many skilled colleagues in different parts of Michigan over the years.

6336   Migraine Awareness Group: A National Understanding for Migraineurs

www.migraines.org/

Works to bring public awareness, utilizing the electronic, print, and artistic mediums, to the fact that migraine is a true organic neurological disease.

6337   National Headache Foundation

www.headaches.org

Information for headache sufferers, their families, and the physicians who treat them.

6338   Neurology Channel

www.healthcommunities.com

Find clearly explained, medically accurate information regarding conditions, including an overview, symptoms, causes, diagnostic procedures and treatment options. On this site it is possible to ask questions and get information from a neurologist and connect to people who have similar health interests.

6339   WebMD

www.webmd.com

Provides credible information, supportive communities, and in-depth reference material about health subjects. A source for original and timely health information as well as material from well known content providers.

Description

6340 Multiple Sclerosis

Multiple sclerosis, MS, is a chronic disease that affects the central nervous system and impairs many of its functions. Over 400,000 Americans have MS. Although its cause is unknown, an immunologic abnormality is suspected. There also appear to be both genetic and environmental factors involved. Interestingly, the incidence of MS increases the further one lives from the equator.

Age of onset is typically between 20 and 40 years, and women are affected somewhat more than men. MS destroys the protective myelin sheath that surrounds nerve fibers. This special sheath normally allows passage of electrical signals through the brain, spinal cord, and nerves of the body. The disease is characterized by remissions and recurring exacerbations. The clinical signs vary depending on the area of demyelination and can include: generalized or focal weakness; difficulty walking; clumsiness; slurred speech; easy fatigability; numbness and tingling; visual loss; incontinence (loss of bladder and bowel control); loss of sexual function; and problems with short-term memory, judgment, or reason.

Significant strides are being made in both treating and understanding MS. Currently there is no curative treatment, but corticosteroids, interferon-B the highly effective natalizumab and other more convenient oral medications (dimethyl fumarate, fingolimod, and teriflunomide) shorten or prevent relapses.

Supportive treatment includes medications to control muscle spasticity, fatigue and pain. Maintaining a normal lifestyle is recommended, as are avoiding fatigue and exposure to excessive heat. Physical therapy may also be helpful. Because of the debilitating nature of MS, counseling, psychiatric support, and antidepressant medication may be warranted.

National Agencies & Associations

6341 American Chronic Pain Association
PO Box 850   800-533-3231
Rocklin, CA 95677   ACPA@theacpa.org
www.theacpa.org
The ACPA facilitates peer support and education for individuals with chronic pain in its many forms, in order to increase quality of life. Also raises awareness among the healthcare community, and with policy makers.
Penney Cowan, Founder & CEO
Daniel Galia, Director, Global Support

6342 Multiple Sclerosis Association of America
375 Kings Highway N   800-532-7667
Cherry Hill, NJ 08034   Fax: 856-661-9797
msaa@mymsaa.org
www.mymsaa.org
A national non-profit organization dedicated to enriching the quality of life for everyone affected by multiple sclerosis.
Robert Manley, Chair
Sue Rehmus, Vice Chair

6343 Multiple Sclerosis Foundation
6520 N Andrews Avenue   954-776-6805
Fort Lauderdale, FL 33309-2132   888-673-6287
Fax: 954-938-8708
admin@msfocus.org
www.msfocus.org
The foundation offers free services including educational programs, homecare, support groups, assistive technology for individuals with MS.
Alan R. Segaloff, Executive Director
Eric Schenck, President

6344 National Institute of Neurological Disorders and Stroke
NIH Neurological Institute   301-496-5751
Bethesda, MD 20824   800-352-9424
www.ninds.nih.gov
Seeks to reduce the burden of neurological disease affecting individuals from all walks of life.
Walter J. Koroshetz, MD, Director
Amy B. Adams, Director, Office of Scientific Liaison

6345 National Multiple Sclerosis Society
New York, NY   800-344-4867
nat@nmss.org
www.nationalmssociety.org
Serves persons with MS, their families, health professionals and the interested public. Provides funding for research, public and professional education, advocacy and the design of rehabilitative and psychosocial programs.
Sylvia Lawry, Founder
Cynthia Zagieboylo, President & CEO

State Agencies & Associations

Alabama

6346 National Multiple Sclerosis Society: Alabama Chapter
813 Shades Creek Parkway   205-879-8881
Birmingham, AL 35209   800-FIG-HTMS
Fax: 205-879-8869
alc@nmss.org
www.nationalmssociety.org/alc
Dedicated to serving people with MS and their families by providing programs and services designed to enhance quality of life.
Frank D McPhillips, Chairman
Jan Bell, Chapter President

Alaska

6347 National Multiple Sclerosis Society: Alaska Chapter
511 W 41st Avenue   907-563-1115
Anchorage, AK 99503-6643   800-344-4867
Fax: 907-562-6673
www.nationalmssociety.org/aka
Nonprofit organization providing equipment loan, information and referral, leading library, self-help groups, advocacy, education, training, newsletter, educational programs, volunteer opportunities, exercise/aquatics, newly diagnosed support and educational material.
Gary Wells, Regional Development Manager
Pam McElrath, President, All American Chapter

Arizona

6348 National Multiple Sclerosis Society Desert Southwest Chapter
National Multiple Sclerosis Society
5025 E. Washington Street   480-968-2488
Phoenix, AZ 85034-2343   800-344-4867
Fax: 602-966-4049
info@aza.nmss.org
www.nationalmssociety.org
Serves Central and Northern Arizona.

Arkansas

6349 National Multiple Sclerosis Society: Arkansas Chapter
Evergreen Place

1100 N University Avenue
Little Rock, AR 72207-6367

501-663-8104
800-344-4867
Fax: 501-666-4355
arr@nmss.org
www.nationalmssociety.org/arr

Rick Selig, Division Manager

California

6350 Central California Chapter National Multiple Sclerosis Society
National Multiple Sclerosis Society
334 Shaw Avenue
Clovis, CA 93612-3839

209-325-9293
Fax: 209-325-9295
www.nationalmssociety.org

Dan Dietrich, Development Director
Karen Nunn, Service Director

6351 National Multiple Sclerosis Society: Southern California Chapter
2440 S Sepulveda Boulevard
Los Angeles, CA 90064

310-479-4456
800-344-4867
Fax: 310-479-4436
ms@cal.nmss.org
www.nationalmssociety.org

Leon A LeBuffe, President

6352 National Multiple Sclerosis Society Channel Islands Chapter
14 W Valerio Street
Santa Barbara, CA 93101

805-682-8783
800-344-4867
Fax: 805-563-1489
can_info@nmss.org
www.nationalmssociety.org

Joan Young, Chapter President

6353 National Multiple Sclerosis Society: Silicon Valley Chapter
2589 Scott Boulevard
Santa Clara, CA 95050-2508

408-988-7557
800-344-4867
Fax: 408-988-1816
cau@nmss.org
www.nationalmssociety.org

Funds, researches and supports people with MS and their families
to end the devastating effects of multiple sclerosis.
Carla Hines, Chapter President
Michelle Spam-Allen, Program Director

6354 Northern California Chapter National Multiple Sclerosis Society
National Multiple Sclerosis Society
1700 Owens Street
San Francisco, CA 94158

415-230-6678
800-344-4867
Fax: 415-230-6652
can_info@nmss.org
www.nationalmssociety.org

David Hartman, Chapter President
Denise Casey, Director of Chapter Programs

6355 Orange County Chapter National Multiple Sclerosis Society
National Multiple Sclerosis Society
5950 La Place Court
Carlsbad, CA 92008-5677

760-448-8400
800-344-4867
Fax: 949-833-3104
msinfo@mspacific.org
www.nationalmssociety.org

Richard V Israel, Chapter President
Karen Hooper, Vice President Programs & Services

6356 San Diego Area Chapter National Multiple Sclerosis Society
National Multiple Sclerosis Society
12121 Scripps Summit Dr
San Diego, CA 92131-1498

619-974-8640
800-486-6762
Fax: 760-804-9266
www.nationalmssociety.org

Allan Shaw, Chapter President
Karen Barton, Service Director

Colorado

6357 National MS Society: Colorado Chapter
900 S Broadway
Denver, CO 80209-3442

303-698-7400
800-344-4867
Fax: 303-698-7421
co-wyreceptionist@nmss.org

Carrie Nolan, President
Mary Ann Peters, Executive Assistant

Connecticut

6358 National MS Society: Greater Connecticut Chapter
659 Tower Avenue
Hartford, CT 06112

860-913-2550
800-344-4867
Fax: 860-761-2466
info@ctfightsMS.org

Lisa Gerrol, President and Chief Professional Officer
Cheryl Donati, Executive Vice President

Delaware

6359 National MS Society: Delaware Chapter
2 Mill Road
Wilmington, DE 19806-2175

302-655-5610
800-344-4867
Fax: 302-655-0993
kate.cowperthwait@msdelaware.org
www.nationalmssociety.org/chapters/DED/i

Provides the encouragement, materials and skills needed to
achieve and maintain a productive lifestyle with multiple sclerosis. The organization is a voluntary, nonprofit entity.
1100 members
Kate Cowperthwait, Chapter President
Helen Serbu, Director of Finance

District of Columbia

6360 National MS Society: National Capital Chapter
1800 M Street
Washington, DC 20036-1003

202-296-5363
800-344-4867
Fax: 202-296-3425

J Christophe Broullire, Chapter President
Kevin Dougherty, Vice President Programs and Services

Florida

6361 Central Florida Chapter
2701 Maitland Center Parkway
Orlando, FL 32751-6726

407-478-8880
800-344-4867
Fax: 407-478-8893
www.nationalmssociety.org/chapters/FLC/i

Tami Caesar, President
Ryan Bumgardner, Bike MS Manager

6362 Florida Gulf Coast Chapter National Multiple Sclerosis Society
National Multiple Sclerosis Society
4919 Memorial Highway
Tampa, FL 33634-3540

813-889-8303
800-344-4867
Fax: 813-889-8313

Judy Wilkinson, Service Director
Tim Hanke, Chairman

6363 National Multiple Sclerosis Society: North Florida Chapter
4237 Salisbury Road
Jacksonville, FL 32216-8171

904-332-6810
800-344-4867
Fax: 904-332-0898
TDD: 800-955-8770
www.nationalmssociety.org/fln

Jennifer Lee, Chapter President
Sabrah Witkamp, Client Program Director

6364 South Florida Chapter National Multiple Sclerosis Society
National Multiple Sclerosis Society
3201 W Commercial Boulevard
Fort Lauderdale, FL 33309-6350

954-731-4224
800-344-4867
Fax: 954-739-1398
fls@nmss.org
fls.nationalmssociety.org

Karen Dresbach, Chapter President
Fred Zuckerman, Chairman

Georgia

6365 National MS Society: Georgia Chapter
1117 Perimeter Center W   678-672-1000
Atlanta, GA 30338-3097   800-344-4867
                                                          Fax: 678-672-1015
                                                          gaa.mailbox@nmss.org

Roy A Rangel, Chapter President
Nicole Hill, Director of Finance & Administrative

Hawaii

6366 National MS Society: Hawaii Chapter
418 Kuwili Street   808-532-0806
Honolulu, HI 96817   800-344-4867
                                                          Fax: 808-532-0814

Jeffrey D Peier, Chairman
Pam McElrath, President

Idaho

6367 National MS Society: Idaho Division
6901 W Emerald Street   208-388-4253
Boise, ID 83704   800-344-4867
                                                          Fax: 208-388-1907

Pam McElrath, Chapter President
Suzanne Bland, Executive Vice President

Illinois

6368 National MS Society: Chicago, Greater Illinois Chapter
525 West Monroe Street   312-922-8000
Chicago, IL 60661-3814   800-344-4867
                                                          Fax: 312-922-2752
                                                          www.nationalmssociety.org
The Greater Illnois Chapter is comprised of all the Illinoisans whohave chosen to fight MS and the work that they do through the National Multiple Sclerosis Society Volunteers, staff, healthcare workers, researchers, donors, advocated, and partners together represent the Greater Illinoisans Chapter, and all the many ways it's possible to join the fight against multiple sclerosis.
Steven Pratapous, Chapter President

Indiana

6369 National MS Society: Indiana State Chapter
3500 DePauw Blvd.   317-870-2500
Indianapolis, IN 46268   800-344-4867
                                                          Fax: 317-870-2520
                                                          Indiana@nmss.org

Tiffany Bogard, Chapter President
Lisa Coffman, Director of Chapter Programs

Iowa

6370 National MS Society: Iowa Chapter
8187 University Boulevard   515-270-6337
Clive, IA 50325   800-344-4867
                                                          Fax: 515-270-0337
                                                          mark.davis@nmss.org

Brett Ridge, Chapter President
Mark Davis, Area Director

Kansas

6371 National MS Society: Mid-America Chapter
7611 State Line   913-432-3926
Kansas City, KS 64114-2915   800-344-4867
                                                          Fax: 816-361-2369
                                                          info@nmsskc.org
The National Multiple Sclerosis Society is a not-for-profit organization serving people with MS in every state. The Mid-America Chapter serves the 25,000 people who are affected by MS in eastern Kansas and western Missouri.
Kay Julian, Chapter President
Amy Goldstein, Program Director

6372 National MS Society: South Central & West Kansas Division
9415 E Harry Street   316-264-7043
Wichita, KS 67211-1515   800-344-4867
                                                          Fax: 316-264-5436
Cammy Mathews, Donor Relations Coordinator
Becky Kimbell, Regional Programs and Services Manager

Kentucky

6373 National MS Society: Kentucky Chapter
1201 Story Avenue   502-451-0014
Louisville, KY 40206   800-344-4867
                                                          Fax: 502-581-1010
                                                          KYW@NMSS.ORG
                                                          www.nationalmssociety.org

Jeff Hamilton, Chairman
Stacy Funk, Chapter President

Louisiana

6374 National Multiple Sclerosis Society: Louisiana
4613 Fairfield Street   504-832-4013
Metairie, LA 70006   800-344-4867
                                                          Fax: 504-831-7188

Brian Berrigon, Chapter President
Crystal Smith, Director of Programs and Services

Maine

6375 National MS Society: Maine Chapter
170 US Route One   800-344-4867
Falmouth, ME 04105   800-344-4867
                                                          Fax: 207-781-7961
The National Multiple Sclerosis Societ is dedicated to enind the devastating the devastating effects of multiple sciersis, a chronic, disease of the central nervous system often diagnosed in young adults
Robin Doughty, Director of Finance & Operations
Denise Clavette, Chapter President

Maryland

6376 National MS Society: Maryland Chapter Hunt Valley Business Center
Hunt Valley Business Center
2219 York Road.   443-641-1200
Timonium, MD 21093   800-344-4867
                                                          Fax: 443-641-1201

Mark Roeder, Chapter President
Nicole Weedon, Executive Assistant/Office Manager

Massachusetts

6377 National MS Society: Massachusetts Chapter
101A 1st Avenue   781-890-4990
Waltham, MA 02451-1160   800-344-4867
                                                          Fax: 781-890-2089
                                                          CommunicationsGNE@nmss.org
Linda Guiod, Executive Vice President
Arlyn White, Chapter President & CEO

Michigan

6378 National MS Society: Michigan Chapter
21311 Civic Center Drive   248-351-2190
Southfield, MI 48076   800-344-4867
                                                          Fax: 248-350-0029
                                                          www.nationalmssociety.org/mig
Offer a variety of programs and services benefiting people with multiple sclerosis and their family members. Programs include educational seminars, information and referrals, peer support, advocacy, free legal clinic, financial assistance for medical equipment, medical transportation, home care, technical assistance and much more
Elana Sullivan, Chapter President
Melissa Ryan, Executive Administrative Assistant

Minnesota

6379 National MS Society: Minnesota Chapter
200 12th Avenue S   612-335-7900
Minneapolis, MN 55415   800-344-4867
                                         Fax: 612-335-7997
                                         INFO@MSSOCIETY.ORG

Mississippi

6380 National Multiple Sclerosis Society: Alaba ma-Mississippi Chapter
145 Executive Drive   601-856-5831
Madison, MS 39110-9198   800-344-4867
                                         Fax: 601-856-7173
                                         alc@nmss.org
                                         www.nationalmssociety.org/alc
Angie Jackson, Area Director
Andi Agnew, Programs and Services Coordinator

Missouri

6381 National MS Society: Gateway Area Chapter
1867 Lackland Hill Parkway   314-781-9020
Saint Louis, MO 63146-3545   800-344-4867
                                         Fax: 314-781-1440
Sponsors research and offers educational programs, counseling, lending library, referral services, independent living aids, legislative advocacy and therapeutic recreation for people with MS.
Phyllis Robsham, Chapter President
Kathi Taylor, Executive Assistant

Montana

6382 National MS Society: Montana Division
1629 Avenue D   406-252-5927
Billings, MT 59102   800-344-4867
                                         Fax: 406-252-5956
                                         MTT@NMSS.ORG
Rebecca Wiehe, Regional Programs and Services Manager
Heather Ohs, Regional Development Manager

Nebraska

6383 National MS Society: Midlands Chapter Community Health Plaza
Community Health Plaza
328 S 72nd Street   402-505-4000
Omaha, NE 68114-2153   800-344-4867
                                         Fax: 402-572-3002
                                         NEN@NMSS.ORG
Lisa Brink, Chapter President
Milton Trabal, Director of Finance

Nevada

6384 Natioanl Multiple Sclerosis Society Desert Southwest Chapter
National Multiple Sclerosis Society
6000 S Eastern Avenue   702-736-1478
Las Vegas, NV 89119-3157   800-344-4867
                                         Fax: 702-736-2487
                                         NVL@NMSS.ORG
Serves southern Nevada & northwest Arizona.
Nicole Rainey, Development Coordinator Special Events
Linda Nowell, Programs and Services Coordinator

6385 National MS Society: Great Basin Sierra Chapter
4600 Keitzke Lane   702-329-7180
Reno, NV 89502   800-344-4867
                                         Fax: 775-827-3167
Linda Lott, Regional Development Manager
Danielle Lutzow, Programs and Services Coordinator

New Hampshire

6386 National MS Society: Central New England Chapter
101A First Avenue   781-890-4990
Waltham, MA 02451-1115   800-493-9255
                                         Fax: 781-490-2089
                                         CommunicationsGNE@nmss.org
                                         www.nationalmssociety.org
Serving people with MS in Massachusetts and New Hampshire.
Judy Cotton, Director Chapter Services
Arlyn White, Chapter President & CEO

New Jersey

6387 National MS Society: Greater North Jersey Chapter
1 Kalisa Way   201-967-5599
Paramus, NJ 07652-3550   800-344-4867
                                         Fax: 201-967-7085
                                         Njminfo@nmss.org
                                         www.nationalmssociety.org/chapters/NJM/i
Michael Elkow, Chapter President
Marianne Maddocks, Vice President of Operations

6388 National MS Society: Mid-Jersey Chapter
246 Monmouth Road   732-660-1005
Oakhurst, NJ 07755   800-344-4867
                                         Fax: 732-660-1388
                                         Njminfo@nmss.org
The National Multiple Sclerosis Society is the only voluntary health agency that supports an international program of scientific research designed to cure, prevent and treat MS.
Michael Elkow, Chapter President
Marianne Maddocks, Vice President of Operations

New Mexico

6389 National MS Society: Rio Grande Division
4125-A Carlisle Boulevard NE   505-243-2792
Albuquerque, NM 87107   800-344-4867
                                         Fax: 505-244-0629
                                         NMX@NMSS.ORG
Maggie Schold, Development Coordinator Special Events
Sheri Wharton, Programs and Services Coordinator

New York

6390 National MS Society: Long Island Chapter
40 Marcus Drive   631-864-8337
Melville, NY 11747   800-344-4867
                                         Fax: 631-864-8342
The National Multiple Sclerosis Society, Long Island Chapter, is dedicated to helping people with MS and their families live useful and fulfilling lives by opening their minds to opportunities and providing the tools to live with dignity.
Pamela Jones Mastrota, President & CEO
Barbara Travis, Vice President of Donor Development

6391 National MS Society: New York City Chapter
733 Third Avenue   212-463-7787
New York, NY 10017-2098   800-344-4867
                                         Fax: 212-989-4362
Committed to providing comprehensive support services to help people with MS and their families cope with the consequences of the disease. The goal is to empower people with MS and their loved ones so that they can better control their lives.
Ruth Brenner, Chapter President
Robin Einbinder, Executive Vice President Programs

6392 National MS Society: Northeastern New York Chapter
421 New Karner Road   585-271-0801
Albany, NY 12205-5156   800-344-4867
                                         Fax: 518-464-1232
                                         chapter@msupstateny.org
                                         www.nationalmssociety.org/chapters/NYR/i
Barbara R Milano, Chapter President
Elliey Kiale-Ingalsb, Chapter Chair

6393 National MS Society: Southern New York Chapter
2 Gannett Drive   914-694-1655
White Plains, NY 10604-2145   800-344-4867
                                             Fax: 914-345-3504
The mission of the National MS Society is to end the devastating
effects of multiple sclerosis. The Southern NY Chapter is commit-
ted to helping people with MS to live independently.
Andrea Maloney, Interim Chapter President
Christina Szeliga, Administrative Coordinator

6394 National MS Society: Upstate New York Chapter
457 State Street   585-271-0801
Binghamton, NY 13901-2341   800-344-4867
                                             Fax: 607-722-1485
                                     chapter@msupstateny.org
                          www.nationalmssociety.org/chapters/NYR/i
James Ahearn, Chapter President
Jonathan Smith, Program Coordinator

**6395 National MS Society: Western New York/ Northwestern
Pennsylvania Chapter**
4245 Union Road   585-271-0801
Buffalo, NY 14225-5040   800-344-4867
                                             Fax: 716-634-2979
                          www.nationalmssociety.org/chapters/NYR/i
Arthur V Cardella, Chapter President
Betsy Farkas, Director Chapter Programs

6396 National Multiple Sclerosis: Upstate New York Chapter
National Multiple Sclerosis Society
1650 S Avenue   716-271-0801
Rochester, NY 14620-3901   800-344-4867
                                             Fax: 716-442-2817
                                 CHAPTER@MSUPSTATENY.ORG
Randal A Simonetti, President & CEO
Stephanie Mincer, Senior Vice President of Programs

North Carolina

6397 National MS Society: Central North Carolina Chapter
2211 W Meadowview Road   336-299-4136
Greensboro, NC 27407-3400   800-344-4867
                                             Fax: 336-855-3039
                                           NCC@NMSS.ORG
Elizabeth Green, Chapter President
Davishia Baldwin, Volunteer Coordinator

6398 National MS Society: Eastern North Carolina Chapter
3101 Industrial Drive   919-834-0678
Raleigh, NC 27609-7577   800-344-4867
                                             Fax: 919-834-9822
                                           NCT@NMSS.ORG
Craig Robertson, Interim Chapter President
Debbie Hoffman, Vice President Operations

6399 National Multiple Sclerosis Society
9801-I Southern Pine Boulevard   704-525-2955
Charlotte, NC 28273-5561   800-344-4867
                                             Fax: 704-527-0406
                                           mac@nmss.org
                                     www.nationalmssociety.org/mac
The Mid-Atlantic chapter of the National MS Society serves
80,000 people with multiple sclerosis in South Carolina and western North Carolina. The Chapter is dedicated to helping people
with MS learn to manage and understand their disease and to
achieve maximum independence.
Allison Mertens, Chair Board of Trustees
Jennifer Lee, Chapter President

North Dakota

6400 National MS Society: Dakota Chapter
5990 14th Street S   701-235-2678
Fargo, ND 58104   800-344-4867
                                             Fax: 701-235-6358
Kelly Boeddeker, Senior Development Manager
Amanda Noce, Programs Manager

Ohio

6401 Columbus Center of the National Multiple Sclerosis Society
National Multiple Sclerosis Society
651 G Lakeview Plaza Boulevard   614-880-2290
Worthington, OH 43229-3626   800-344-4867
                                             Fax: 614-880-2296
                                     www.nationalmssociety.org
Stacey Wilko LSW, Program Coordinator
Tony Bernard LSW, Program Coordinator

**6402 National MS Soceity: Western Ohio Chapter The Woolpert
Building**
The Woolpert Building
409 E Monument Avenue   937-461-5232
Dayton, OH 45402-1261   800-344-4867
                                             Fax: 937-461-3500
                                     www.nationalmssociety.org
Providing accurate, up-to-date information to individuals with
MS, their families and healthcare providers is central to our
mission.
12 pages
Karen Joseph, Program Director
Judy LaMusga, Chapter Chair

6403 National MS Society: Southwestern Ohio/Northern Kentucky
4440 Lake Forest Drive   513-769-4400
Cincinnati, OH 45242-3755   800-344-4867
                                             Fax: 513-769-6019
                                           OHGinfo@nmss.org
                                     www.nationalmssociety.org
Tena Bunnell, Chapter President
Becky Wiehe, Service Director

6404 National MS Society: Northeast Ohio Chapter
The Hanna Building
6155 Rockside Road   216-696-8220
Independence, OH 44131-1901   800-344-4867
                                             Fax: 216-696-2817
                                     www.nationalmssociety.org
Janet Kramer, Chapter President
Greg Kovach, Director of Services

6405 National MS Society: Northwest Ohio Chapter
401 Tomahawk Drive   419-897-9533
Maumee, OH 43537-1633   800-344-4867
                                             Fax: 419-897-9733
                                   Maureen.Mohney@nmss.org
                          www.nationalmssociety.org/chapters/OHO/i
Jacque Pratt, Chapter Program Coordinator
Tonya Scherf, Program Director

Oklahoma

6406 National MS Society: Oklahoma Chapter
4604 E 67th Street   918-488-0882
Tulsa, OK 74136-4946   800-344-4867
                                             Fax: 918-488-0913
Paula Cortner, Chapter President
Denise Allen, Finance/HR Manager

Oregon

6407 National MS Society: Oregon Chapter
5331 SW Macadam Avenue   503-223-9511
Portland, OR 97239   800-344-4867
                                             Fax: 503-223-2912
The Pregon Chapter is aggressively pursuing the mission to end the
devastating effects of MS by providing programs designed to en-
hance the families throughout Oregon and Clark County,
Washington.
Wendy Allison, Office Coordinator
Sally Alworth, Director of Finance

Pennsylvania

6408   National MS Society: Central Pennsylvania Chapter
2040 Linglestown Road   717-652-2108
Harrisburg, PA 17110-1095   800-344-4867
                                                    Fax: 717-652-2590
                                                    PAC@NMSS.ORG
                                    www.nationalmssociety.org/chapters/PAC/i
Margie Adelmann, President
Debbie Rios, Executive Vice President

6409   National MS Society: Greater Delaware Valley Chapter
30 South 17th Street   215-271-1500
Philadelphia, PA 19103-5519   800-344-4867
                                                    Fax: 215-271-6122
                                                    PAE@NMSS.ORG
John H Scott, President
Randee Forstein, VP Programs & Community Outreach

Rhode Island

6410   National MS Society: Rhode Island Chapter
205 Hallene Road   401-738-8383
Warwick, RI 02886-2452   800-344-4867
                                                    Fax: 401-738-8469
                                                    christina.roche@nmss.org
                                    www.nationalmssociety.org/chapters/RIR/i
Provides local programs and services to people with MS and their
families. These services include information and referral, equipment loans, purchase assistance, programs for the newly diagnosed and education and support groups.
3M Members
Kathy Mechnig, Chapter President
Catie Dussault, Director of Special Events

South Carolina

6411   National MS Society: South Carolina Branch
2711 Middleburg Drive   803-799-7848
Columbia, SC 29204-2413   800-344-4867

Tennessee

6412   National MS Society: Southeast Tennessee/North Georgia Chapte
5720 Uptain Road   423-954-9700
Chattanooga, TN 37411-5642   800-344-4867
                                                    Fax: 423-855-9667
                                                    www.nationalmssociety.org
Jeanne Brice, Services Manager

6413   National MS Society: Mid-South Chapter
3100 Walnut Grove Road   901-755-4900
Memphis, TN 38111-3530   800-344-4867
                                                    Fax: 901-324-9668
                                                    www.nationalmssociety.org
The mission of the National Multiple Sclerosis Society is to end the
devastating effects of MS.
Dee Blake, Chapter President
Sherree Wilson, Services Director

6414   National MS Society: Mid-South Chapter, Nashville Office
4219 Hillsboro Road   615-269-9055
Nashville, TN 37215-3332   800-344-4867
                                                    Fax: 615-269-9470
                                                    TNS@NMSS.ORG
Jim Ward, Chapter President
Beth Smith, Vice President of Client Programs

Texas

6415   National MS Society: North Central Texas Chapter
4086 Sandshell Drive   817-306-7003
Fort Worth, TX 76137   800-344-4867
                                                    Fax: 817-877-1205
                                    www.nationalmssociety.org/chapters/TXH/i
Educational programs, self-help groups, and information and re-
ferral for persons and families diagnosed with multiple sclerosis.
12 pages Quarterly
Justin Martin, Coordinator Development
Lynette Jarvis-Barre, Senior Manager Programs & Services

6416   National MS Society: Panhandle Chapter
6222 Canyon Drive   806-468-8005
Amarillo, TX 79109-6730   800-344-4867
                                                    Fax: 806-468-8022
                                                    TXP@NMSS.ORG
Gail Lindsey, Programs and Services Coordinator
April Brownlee, Development Coordinator Special Events

6417   National MS Society: Southern Texas
8111 N Stadium Drive   713-526-8967
Houston, TX 77054   800-344-4867
                                                    Fax: 713-394-7422
                                                    TXH@NMSS.ORG
Mark Neagli, Chapter President
Deborah Pope, VP - Operations

6418   National MS Society: West Texas Division
1031 Andrews Highway   432-522-2143
Midland, TX 79701-4636   800-344-4867
                                                    Fax: 432-694-7970
                                                    TXQ@NMSS.ORG
Sharon Rader, Regional Development Manager
Rona Bowerman, Regional Programs and Services Manager

6419   National MS Socisty: Southeast Texas Chapter
8111 N Stadium Drive   713-526-8967
Houston, TX 77054-4051   800-344-4867
                                                    Fax: 713-394-7422
                                                    TXH@NMSS.ORG
                                                    www.nationalmssociety.org
Mark Neagli, Chapter President
Jim Tidwell, Chairman

Utah

6420   National MS Society: Utah State Chapter
1440 Foothill Drive   801-493-0113
Salt Lake City, UT 84108-3537   800-527-8116
                                                    Fax: 801-493-0122
                                                    utah.idaho@nmss.org
                                                    www.nationalmssociety.org
Our mission is to end the devastating effects of MS. Serving indi-
viduals with MS and their families through programs, research,
awareness and education.
Annette Royle, Chapter President
Dee Dee Fox, Director of Client Programs and Services

Vermont

6421   National MS Society: Vermont Division
75 Talcott Road   802-864-6356
Williston, VT 05495   800-344-4867
                                                    Fax: 802-864-6509
                                                    VTN@NMSS.ORG
Committed to ending the devastating effects of MS.
Christine Newberr, Programs and Services Coordinator
Lindsay Going, Development Coordinator Special Events

Virginia

6422   National MS Society: Blue Ridge Chapter
1020 Carrington Place   804-971-8010
Charlottesville, VA 22901   800-344-4867
                                                    Fax: 804-979-4475
                                                    VAB@NMSS.ORG
                                    www.nationalmssociety.org/chapters/VAB/i
Faith Painter, Chapter President
Delton Hanson, Operations Director

6423   National MS Society: Central Virginia Chapter
2112 W Laburnum Avenue   804-353-5008
Richmond, VA 23227   800-344-4867
                                                    Fax: 804-353-5595
Sherri Ellis, Chapter President
Andy Page, Director of Community Development

6424 National MS Society: Hampton Roads Chapter
760 Lynnhaven Parkway   757-490-9627
Virginia Beach, VA 23452-6311   800-344-4867
                                               Fax: 757-490-1617
www.nationalmssociety.org/chapters/VAX/i
Sharon Grossman, Chapter President
Michelle Derr, Vice President Finance/Administration

Washington

6425 National MS Society: Greater Washington Chapter
192 Nickerson Street   206-284-4254
Seattle, WA 98109   800-344-4867
                                               Fax: 206-284-4972
Patricia Shepherd-Ba, Chapter President
Erin Poznanski, Vice President Chapter Programs

6426 National MS Society: Inland Northwest Chapter
818 E Sharp Avenue   509-482-2022
Spokane, WA 99202-1935   800-344-4867
                                               Fax: 509-483-1077
                                               WAI@NMSS.ORG
Robert Hansen, Chapter President
Patty Mathias, Office Manager

Wisconsin

6427 National MS Society: Wisconsin Chapter
1120 James Drive   262-369-4400
Hartland, WI 53029   800-344-4867
                                               Fax: 262-369-4410
                                               info.wisms@nmss.org
Colleen Kalt, President & CEO
Melissa Palfery, Executive Assistant

Wyoming

6428 National MS Society: Wyoming Chapter
525 Randall Avenue   307-433-9590
Cheyenne, WY 82001-1627   800-344-4867
                                               Fax: 307-433-8657
                                               WYY@NMSS.ORG
Cheryl Seaberg, Programs and Services Coordinator
Stephanie Batson, Development Coordinator Special Events

Libraries & Resource Centers

6429 St. Agnes Hospital Medical: Health Science Library
305 North Street   914-681-4500
White Plains, NY 10605   Fax: 914-328-6408
Labe C Scheinberg MD, Director

Research Centers

6430 Brigham and Women's Hospital: Center for Neurologic Diseases
LMRC Building
75 Francis Street   617-732-5500
Boston, MA 02115   800-294-9999
                                               TTY: 617-732-6458
                                               www.brighamandwomens.org
Offers research relating to Multiple Sclerosis and other autoimmune diseases.
Dennis J. Selkoe, Co-Director
Howard L. Weiner, Co-Director

6431 Center for Neuroimmunology: University of Alabama at Birmingham
1720 7th Ave S   205-934-0683
Birmingham, AL 35294   Fax: 205-996-4039
                                               www.main.uab.edu/neurology
Evaluate and treat acute and chronic neurological and neuromuscular diseases which are caused by autoimmune mechanisms or linked to presumed abnormalities affecting the immune system.
Khurram Bashir, Director

6432 Jimmie Heuga Center
27 Main Street   970-926-1290
Edwards, CO 81632   800-367-3101
                                               Fax: 970-926-1295
                                               info@mscando.org
                                               www.mscando.org
Conducts research and studies on multiple sclerosis patients.
Kim Lennox Sharkey, Chief Executive Officer
Carrie Van Beek, Office Coordinator

6433 Neuromuscular Treatment Center: Univ. of Texas Southwestern Medical Center
Department of Neurology   214-648-3111
Dallas, TX 75390   www.utsouthwestern.edu
Basic and clinical studies of myasthenia gravis.
Daniel K Podolsky MD, President
Diane Jeffries, Director

6434 Rush University Multiple Sclerosis Center
1653 W. Congress Parkway   312-942-5000
Chicago, IL 60612   888-352-RUSH
                                               TTY: 312-942-2207
                                               complaint@jointcommission.org
                                               www.rush.edu
The Multiple Sclerosis Center combines comprehensive treatment with clinical and laboratory research to provide the highest quality patient care.
Floyd A Davis, Director

Support Groups & Hotlines

6435 MS Toll-Free Information Line
National Multiple Sclerosis Society
733 3rd Avenue   800-344-4867
New York, NY 10017-3288
Offers public and professional information, brochures and referrals to MS patients, their families and health care professionals.

6436 MSWorld
1943 Morrill Street   415-701-1117
Sarasota, FL 34236   877-710-0302
                                               msworld@msworld.org
                                               www.msworld.org/
MSWorld is for people with multiple sclerosis their families and friends, offer support via chat, e-mail, message boards, magazines.
Kathleen Wilson, Founder/President

6437 Multiple Sclerosis Action Group
National Multiple Sclerosis Society
733 3rd Avenue   409-883-2282
New York, NY 10017   800-344-4867
                                               www.nationalmssociety.org/index.aspx
Richard J Mengel, Treasurer
Fred J Lublin, Director

6438 National Health Information Center
Office of Disease Prevention & Health Promotion
1101 Wootton Pkwy   Fax: 240-453-8281
Rockville, MD 20852   odphpinfo@hhs.gov
                                               www.health.gov/nhic
Supports public health education by maintaining a calendar of National Health Observances; helps connect consumers and health professionals to organizations that can best answer questions and provide up-to-date contact information from reliable sources; updates on a yearly basis toll-free numbers for health information, Federal health clearinghouses and info centers.
Don Wright, MD, MPH, Director

6439 Traditional Tibetan Healing
13 Harrison Street   617-666-8635
Sommerville, MA 2143-6504   866-628-6504
                                               Kelob@gte.net
                                               www.tibetanherbalhealing.com/
To rid mankind from chronic illnesses using alternative methods.
Keyzon Bhutti, Chief Physician

Books

6440 300 Tips for Making Life with Multiple Sclerosis Easier
Demos Medical Publishing
11 West 42nd Street   212-683-0072
New York, NY 10036   Fax: 212-683-0118
                                   orderdept@demospub.com
                                   www.demosmedpub.com

Techniques for better living.
109 pages
ISBN: 1-888799-23-4
Shelley Peterman Schwarz, Author

6441 Alternative Medicine and Multiple Sclerosis
Demos Medical Publishing
11 West 42nd Street   212-683-0072
New York, NY 10036   Fax: 212-683-0118
                                   orderdept@demospub.com
                                   www.demosmedpub.com

These therapies are organized alphabetically so that readers can
readily pinpoint a specific treatment and learn about its origins,
merits, and possible uses in MS
272 pages
ISBN: 1-888799-52-8
Allen C. Bowling, Author

6442 Fall Down Seven Times Get Up Eight
Miramar Communications
PO Box 8987   800-543-4116
Malibu, CA 90265-8987
The second in Dr. Wolf's series on MS management: including
chapters on stress and fatigue, planning for serious disability and
lots more.
211 pages

6443 Living with Multiple Sclerosis
Demos Medical Publishing
11 West 42nd Street   212-683-0072
New York, NY 10036   Fax: 212-683-0118
                                   orderdept@demospub.com
                                   www.demosmedpub.com

ISBN: 1-888799-26-9
Dr. Diana M Schneider

6444 Living with Multiple Sclerosis: A Wellness Approach
Demos Vermande
11 West 42nd Street   212-683-0072
New York, NY 10036-8804   800-532-8663
The book incorporates recent developments in the management of
multiple sclerosis and includes strategies for patients who want to
optimize their health through exercise, stress management and
good nutrition.
112 pages
ISBN: 1-888799-00-5
George Kraft, Author
Marci Catanzaro,, Author

6445 Meeting the Challenge of Progressive Multiple Sclerosis
Demos Medical Publishing
11 West 42nd Street   212-683-0072
New York, NY 10036   Fax: 212-683-0118
                                   orderdept@demospub.com
                                   www.demosmedpub.com

This book is designed specifically for people who have been told
they have or are developing the progressive form of multiple sclerosis. It focuses on ways to not only manage the progressive disease and its symptoms but also to cope with the life changes that
may accompany it.
128 pages
ISBN: 1-888799-46-3
Patricia K. Coyle, Author
June Halper, Author

6446 Multiple Sclerosis
Demos Medical Publishing
11 West 42nd Street   212-683-0072
New York, NY 10036   800-532-8663
                                   Fax: 212-683-0118
                                   orderdept@demospub.com
                                   www.demosmedpub.com

This new comprehensive review of the many fields of basic and
clinical research that impact our understanding of multiple sclerosis has its basis in this premise
224 pages
ISBN: 1-888799-54-4
Robert Herndon, Author

6447 Multiple Sclerosis, The Questions you Have Answers You Need
Demos Medical Publishing
11 West 42nd Street   212-683-0072
New York, NY 10036   Fax: 212-683-0118
                                   orderdept@demospub.com
                                   www.demosmedpub.com

The Questions You Have, The Answers You Need continues to be
the definitive guide for everyone concerned with this disease those
who have MS, those who share their lives with someone who has it,
and all healthcare professionals involved with its management
592 pages
ISBN: 1-888799-43-9
Rosalind C. Kalb, Author

6448 Multiple Sclerosis: A Guide for Families
Demos Medical Publishing
11 West 42nd Street   212-683-0072
New York, NY 10036-8804   800-532-8663
                                   Fax: 212-683-0118
                                   orderdept@demospub.com
                                   www.demosmedpub.com

With its complex and unpredictable course, MS affects every area
of family life. This book covers a broad range of medical, psychological, social, vocational, economic and legal problems.
1997 207 pages Paperback
ISBN: 1-888799-14-5
Rosalind C. Kalb, Author

6449 Multiple Sclerosis: A Guide for Patients and Their Families
Raven Press
11 West 42nd Street   212-683-0072
New York, NY 10036-2601   800-777-2295
                                   orderdept@demospub.com
                                   www.demosmedpub.com

The Second Edition of this popular and highly acclaimed guide
features expanded coverage of the causes, epidemiology, and genetics of multiple sclerosis and contains many new illustrations
that make the rehabilitative techniques presented easier for the patient to understand and follow.
288 pages Paperback
ISBN: 0-881672-55-6
Labe C. Scheinberg, Author
Nancy J. Holland, Editor

6450 Multiple Sclerosis: A Personal Exploration
Demos Vermande
11 West 42nd Street   212-683-0072
New York, NY 10036-8804   800-532-8663
                                   Fax: 212-683-0118
                                   orderdept@demospub.com
                                   www.demosmedpub.com

As a doctor and psychiatrist who has MS, the author of this refresh-
ingly frank and practical book is able to draw on personal experience, as well as professional knowledge and insights.
1993 192 pages
ISBN: 0-285650-18-1
Alexander Burnfield, Author

6451 Multiple Sclerosis: Your Legal Rights
Demos Medical Publishing
11 West 42nd Street   212-683-0072
New York, NY 10036   Fax: 212-683-0118
                                   orderdept@demospub.com
                                   www.demosmedpub.com

This extensively revised third edition continues to provide reliable
basic information and possible solutions to the legal problems that
often affect people with multiple sclerosis (MS).
156 pages
ISBN: 1-888799-31-5
Lanny Perkins, Author
Sara Perkins, Author

6452 **The Comfort of Home Multiple Sclerosis Edition: A Guide for Caregivers**
Marie M. Meyer and Paula Derr, RN, author
CareTrust Publications
PO Box 10283   800-565-1533
Portland, OR 97296-0283   Fax: 415-673-2005
                                sales@comfortofhome.com
                                www.comfortofhome.com
Reviews caregiving options and discusses the financial and legal decisions you may encounterr. Readers will learn how to set up a safe and comfortable home for the person whose needs are changing and abilities declining. Comfort offers guidance through every caregiving stage and most decisions one will face in daily living, as well as in avoiding caregiver burnout. Valuable for the caregiver and the patient.
324 pages
ISBN: 0-966476-76-X
Paula Derr, Author
Maria M. Meyer, Author

6453 **Understanding Multiple Sclerosis**
Melissa Stauffer, author
University Press of Mississippi
3825 Ridgewood Road   601-432-6205
Jackson, MS 39211-6492   Fax: 601-432-6217
                                kburgess@ihl.state.ms.us
                                www.upress.state.ms.us
For patients and companions, an overview of all aspects of MS.
2006 144 pages Paperback
ISBN: 1-578068-03-7
Melissa Stauffer, Author

Magazines

6454 **Inside MS**
National Multiple Sclerosis Society
733 3rd Avenue   212-986-3240
New York, NY 10017-3288   800-344-4867
                                Fax: 212-986-7981
                                www.nationalmssociety.org
Full color quarterly magazine on living well with mutiple sclerosis. Articles by people with MS; daily living, achievments, news, treatments, research, advocacy, humor, travel, helpful resources, large type. The magazine is a benefit of membership.
64 pages 4x Year
Eli rubenstein, Chairman of the Board
Cynthia Zagieboylo, Chapter President

Newsletters

6455 **Inside MS Bulletin**
National Multiple Sclerosis Society
733 3rd Avenue   212-986-3240
New York, NY 10017-3288   800-344-4867
                                Fax: 212-986-7981
                                www.nationalmssociety.org
Newsletter offering information on the organization activities. Profiles of donors, and reports on MS research programs.
Eli Rubenstein, Chairman of the Board
Cynthia Zagieboylo, Chapter President

6456 **MS Connection**
National Multiple Sclerosis Society
3101 Industrial Drive   919-834-0678
Raleigh, NC 27609   Fax: 704-527-0406
                                mac@nmss.org
Provides education, support and information about Chapter activities for people living with multiple sclerosis in South Carolina and western North Carolina.
Quarterly
Eli Rubenstein, Chairman of the Board
Cynthia Zagieboylo, Chapter President

6457 **Motivator**
Multiple Sclerosis Foundation

6350 N Andrews Avenue   954-776-6805
Fort Lauderdale, FL 33309-2130   800-441-7055
                                www.msfacts.org
Reports on the latest advancements regarding medical treatments/therapies for MS, inspirational feature stories, coping skills, correspondence from readers, and ongoing MSAA programs, services, and activities.
BiMonthly

6458 **Multiple Sclerosis Quarterly Report**
Demos Vermande
11 West 42nd Street   212-683-0072
New York, NY 10036-8804   800-532-8663
                                Fax: 212-683-0118
                                orderdept@demospub.com
                                www.demosmedpub.com
This is the definitive newsletter for everyone who has MS, with feature articles, research updates, book reviews, and more. It is developed with the sponsorship of the Eastern Paralyzed Veterans of America and the National Multiple Sclerosis Society. The MSQR will keep you informed of new developments in the management of MS and strategies for living successfully with the disease.
1997 Quarterly

6459 **National Multiple Sclerosis Society: Allegheny District Chapter**
1501 Reedsdale Street   412-261-6347
Pittsburgh, PA 15233-6220   800-344-4867
                                Fax: 412-232-1461
                                www.nationalmssociety.org
12 pages 4 per year
Eli Rubenstein, Chairman of the Board
Cynthia Zagieboylo, President & CEO

Pamphlets

6460 **ADA and People with MS**
National Multiple Sclerosis Society
733 3rd Avenue   212-986-3240
New York, NY 10017-3288   800-344-4867
                                Fax: 212-986-7981
                                www.nationalmssociety.org
What the Americans with Disabilities Act means in employment, public accommodations, transportation, and telecommunications.
24 pages
Laura D. Cooper, Author
Mark Stolman, Volunteer

6461 **At Home with MS: Adapting Your Environment**
National Multiple Sclerosis Society
733 3rd Avenue   212-986-3240
New York, NY 10017-3288   800-344-4867
                                Fax: 212-986-7981
                                www.nationalmssociety.org
Modify a house or apartment to save energy, compensate for reduced vision or mobility, and live comfortably. Many do-it-yourself changes.
28 pages
Jane E. Harmon, Author
Donna M. Jensen, Assistant Writer

6462 **At Our House**
National Multiple Sclerosis Society
733 3rd Avenue   212-986-3240
New York, NY 10017-3288   800-344-4867
                                Fax: 212-986-7981
                                www.nationalmssociety.org
A coloring book for children, ages 5-8, about a Mama Bear with MS. contains some very basic facts with an afterword for parents on how to talk to young children about MS.
20 pages

6463 **Chapter Services at a Glance**
National Multiple Sclerosis Society
733 3rd Avenue   212-986-3240
New York, NY 10017-3288   800-344-4867
                                Fax: 212-986-7981
                                www.nationalmssociety.org
A summary of services offerred by local chapters. Contains membership form.

6464 Check Your Multiple Sclerosis Facts
National Multiple Sclerosis Society
733 3rd Avenue   212-986-3240
New York, NY 10017-3288   800-344-4867
                               Fax: 212-986-7981
                        www.nationalmssociety.org
A brief checklist of MS basics - definition, symptoms, and outlook.

6465 Choosing a Pharmacy Service
National Multiple Sclerosis Society
733 3rd Avenue   212-986-3240
New York, NY 10017-3288   800-344-4867
                               Fax: 212-986-7981
                        www.nationalmssociety.org
What to look for when choosing a prescription drug provider.
20 pages

6466 Clear Thinking About Alternative Therapies
National Multiple Sclerosis Society
733 3rd Avenue   212-986-3240
New York, NY 10017-3288   800-344-4867
                               Fax: 212-986-7981
                        www.nationalmssociety.org
Highlights facts and common misconceptions, compares alternative and conventional medicine, and suggests ways to evaluate benefits and risks.

6467 Controlling Spasticity
National Multiple Sclerosis Society
733 3rd Avenue   212-986-3240
New York, NY 10017-3288   800-344-4867
                               Fax: 212-986-7981
                        www.nationalmssociety.org
An overview of ways to control this common and sometimes disabling MS symtpom. Includes roles of self-help, medications, physical therapists, nurses, and physicians.

6468 Food for Thought: MS and Nutrition
National Multiple Sclerosis Society
733 3rd Avenue   212-986-3240
New York, NY 10017-3288   800-344-4867
                               Fax: 212-986-7981
                        www.nationalmssociety.org
A guide to healthy eating and coping with symptoms that may affect eating habits.
20 pages

6469 Getting a Grip on Gait
National Multiple Sclerosis Society
733 3rd Avenue   212-986-3240
New York, NY 10017-3288   800-344-4867
                               Fax: 212-986-7981
                               nat@nmss.org
                        www.nationalmssociety.org
Walking problems and how they can be addressed.

6470 Hiring Help at Home?
National Multiple Sclerosis Society
733 3rd Avenue   212-986-3240
New York, NY 10017-3288   800-344-4867
                               Fax: 212-986-7981
                               nat@nmss.org
                        www.nationalmssociety.org
Checklists and worksheets for people who need help at home. Forms for needs assessment, job description, and employment contract.

6471 Insight Into Eyesight
National Multiple Sclerosis Society
733 3rd Avenue   212-986-3240
New York, NY 10017-3288   800-344-4867
                               Fax: 212-986-7981
                               nat@nmss.org
                        www.nationalmssociety.org
Current therapy for MS-related eye disorders. Discusses low-vision aids.

6472 Living with MS
National Multiple Sclerosis Society

733 3rd Avenue   212-986-3240
New York, NY 10017-3288   800-344-4867
                               Fax: 212-986-7981
                               nat@nmss.org
                        www.nationalmssociety.org
Answers to 28 questions most often asked when the diagnosis is MS - from possible causes to advice on coping.
20 pages

6473 Moving with Multiple Sclerosis
National Multiple Sclerosis Society
733 3rd Avenue   212-986-3240
New York, NY 10017-3288   800-344-4867
                               Fax: 212-986-7981
                               nat@nmss.org
                        www.nationalmssociety.org
Step-by-step illustrations of passive and active stretching, balance, and conditioning exercises.
30 pages

6474 Multiple Sclerosis and Your Emotions
National Multiple Sclerosis Society
733 3rd Avenue   212-986-3240
New York, NY 10017-3288   800-344-4867
                               Fax: 212-986-7981
                               nat@nmss.org
                        www.nationalmssociety.org
How to manage some of the emotional challenges created by MS.
32 pages

6475 On the Question of Pregnancy
National Multiple Sclerosis Society
733 3rd Avenue   212-986-3240
New York, NY 10017-3288   800-344-4867
                               Fax: 212-986-7981
                               nat@nmss.org
                        www.nationalmssociety.org
Reassuring answers on pregnancy, delivery, and nursing.

6476 On: Alternative Therapies
National Multiple Sclerosis Society
733 3rd Avenue   212-986-3240
New York, NY 10017-3288   800-344-4867
                               Fax: 212-986-7981
                               nat@nmss.org
                        www.nationalmssociety.org
Checklist for people who are considering an alternative treatment.

6477 On: Diagnosis...Putting the Pieces Together
National Multiple Sclerosis Society
733 3rd Avenue   212-986-3240
New York, NY 10017-3288   800-344-4867
                               Fax: 212-986-7981
                               nat@nmss.org
                        www.nationalmssociety.org
Explains usual steps and tests. Includes how to prepare for an MRI.

6478 On: Energy Management
National Multiple Sclerosis Society
733 3rd Avenue   212-986-3240
New York, NY 10017-3288   800-344-4867
                               Fax: 212-986-7981
                               nat@nmss.org
                        www.nationalmssociety.org
Guidelines for budgeting your energy when it's limited by fatigue through prioritizing, delegating, and simplifying tasks.

6479 On: Fatigue
National Multiple Sclerosis Society
733 3rd Avenue   212-986-3240
New York, NY 10017-3288   800-344-4867
                               Fax: 212-986-7981
                               nat@nmss.org
                        www.nationalmssociety.org
The mystery of MS fatigue, practical tips for coping, and the medications sometimes prescribed.

6480 On: Genes
National Multiple Sclerosis Society

733 3rd Avenue   212-986-3240
New York, NY 10017-3288
    Fax: 212-986-7981
    nat@nmss.org
    www.nationalmssociety.org
Recent information on MS and heredity.

6481 On: Pain
National Multiple Sclerosis Society
733 3rd Avenue   212-986-3240
New York, NY 10017-3288   800-344-4867
    Fax: 212-986-7981
    nat@nmss.org
    www.nationalmssociety.org
Myths and facts about MS pain. Covers types of pain and possible treatment.

6482 Plaintalk: A Booklet About MS for Families
National Multiple Sclerosis Society
733 3rd Avenue   212-986-3240
New York, NY 10017-3288   800-344-4867
    Fax: 212-986-7981
    nat@nmss.org
    www.nationalmssociety.org
Discusses some of the more difficult physical and emotional problems families may face.
32 pages

6483 Rehab Outlook
National Multiple Sclerosis Society
733 3rd Avenue   212-986-3240
New York, NY 10017-3288   800-344-4867
    Fax: 212-986-7981
    nat@nmss.org
    www.nationalmssociety.org
What rehabilitation can do for mobility, fatigue, driving, speech, memory, bowel or bladder problems, sexuality, and more.
24 pages

6484 Research Directions in Multiple Sclerosis
National Multiple Sclerosis Society
733 3rd Avenue   212-986-3240
New York, NY 10017-3288   800-344-4867
    Fax: 212-986-7981
    nat@nmss.org
    www.nationalmssociety.org
An overview of current research on key areas of immunology, genetics, virology, and cell biology explained for nonscientists.
16 pages

6485 Sexual Problems Your Doctor Didn't Mention
National Multiple Sclerosis Society
733 3rd Avenue   212-986-3240
New York, NY 10017-3288   800-344-4867
    Fax: 212-986-7981
    nat@nmss.org
    www.nationalmssociety.org
How MS may affect sexuality and what can be done.

6486 Solving Cognitive Problems
National Multiple Sclerosis Society
733 3rd Avenue   212-986-3240
New York, NY 10017-3288   800-344-4867
    Fax: 212-986-7981
    nat@nmss.org
    www.nationalmssociety.org
Mental functions most likely to be affected by MS. Suggestions for self-help and information about cognitive rehabiitation.
20 pages

6487 Someone You Know Has MS: A Book for Families
National Multiple Sclerosis Society
733 3rd Avenue   212-986-3240
New York, NY 10017-3288   800-344-4867
    Fax: 212-986-7981
    nat@nmss.org
    www.nationalmssociety.org
For children ages 6-12 who have a parent with MS. Provides facts and explores children's fears and concerns.
32 pages

6488 Taking Care: A Guide for Well Partners
National Multiple Sclerosis Society
733 3rd Avenue   212-986-3240
New York, NY 10017-3288   800-344-4867
    Fax: 212-986-7981
    nat@nmss.org
    www.nationalmssociety.org
Introduces the concept of carepartnering to balance both partners' needs. Includes practical suggestions about getting and giving help.
16 pages

6489 Taming Stress in Multiple Sclerosis
National Multiple Sclerosis Society
733 3rd Avenue   212-986-3240
New York, NY 10017-3288   800-344-4867
    Fax: 212-986-7981
    nat@nmss.org
    www.nationalmssociety.org
Stress and depression, and how both relate to MS. Tips on simplifying daily life. Instructions on muscle relaxation, deep breathing, and visualization relaxation.
36 pages

6490 Things I Wish Someone Had Told Me
National Multiple Sclerosis Society
733 3rd Avenue   212-986-3240
New York, NY 10017-3288   800-344-4867
    Fax: 212-986-7981
    nat@nmss.org
    www.nationalmssociety.org
First-person story. A positive and practical approach to adjusting to life with MS.
20 pages

6491 Understanding Bladder Problems in Multiple Sclerosis
National Multiple Sclerosis Society
733 3rd Avenue   212-986-3240
New York, NY 10017-3288   800-344-4867
    Fax: 212-986-7981
    nat@nmss.org
    www.nationalmssociety.org
The three main types of bladder dysfunction explained. Guidelines for management.
12 pages

6492 Understanding Bowel Problems in MS
National Multiple Sclerosis Society
733 3rd Avenue   212-986-3240
New York, NY 10017-3288   800-344-4867
    Fax: 212-986-7981
    nat@nmss.org
    www.nationalmssociety.org
An exploration of ways to manage bowel problems in MS.
24 pages

6493 What Everyone Should Know About Multiple Sclerosis
National Multiple Sclerosis Society
733 3rd Avenue   212-986-3240
New York, NY 10017-3288   800-344-4867
    Fax: 212-986-7981
    nat@nmss.org
    www.nationalmssociety.org
Overview of MS, suitable for the whole family.
16 pages

6494 What Is Multiple Sclerosis?
National Multiple Sclerosis Society
733 3rd Avenue   212-986-3240
New York, NY 10017-3288   800-344-4867
    Fax: 212-986-7981
    nat@nmss.org
    www.nationalmssociety.org
For the newly diagnosed and others who need an overview of symptoms, disease patterns, diagnosis, prognosis, treatment, and research efforts.

6495 When a Parent Has MS: A Teenager's Guide
National Multiple Sclerosis Society

733 3rd Avenue
New York, NY 10017-3288

212-986-3240
800-344-4867
Fax: 212-986-7981
nat@nmss.org
www.nationalmssociety.org

For older children and teenagers who have a parent with MS. Discusses issues brought up by real kids.
24 pages

6496 **Win-Win Approach to Reasonable Accommodations**
National Multiple Sclerosis Society
733 3rd Avenue
New York, NY 10017-3288

212-986-3240
800-344-4867
Fax: 212-986-7981
nat@nmss.org
www.nationalmssociety.org

A practical guide to obtaining workplace accommodations.
20 pages

Audio & Video

6497 **Aqua Exercises for Multiple Sclerosis**
National Multiple Sclerosis Society
733 3rd Avenue
New York, NY 10017-3288

212-986-3240
800-344-4867
Fax: 212-986-7981
nat@nmss.org
www.nationalmssociety.org

A workout that cools and supports the body, with exercises to reduce spasticity, build muscles, and improve posture. With waterproof chart.
20 minutes

6498 **Clinical Trials in Multiple Sclerosis: Searching for New Therapies**
National Multiple Sclerosis Society
733 3rd Avenue
New York, NY 10017

212-986-3240
800-344-4867
Fax: 212-986-7981
nat@nmss.org
www.nationalmssociety.org

Describes studies to determine the safety and efficacy of new drugs to treat MS. Why studies are essential, how they are conducted, and the role of participants.
20 minutes

6499 **Now, More Than Ever: Progress in Multiple Sclerosis Research**
National Multiple Sclerosis Society
733 3rd Avenue
New York, NY 10017-3288

212-986-3240
800-344-4867
Fax: 212-986-7981
nat@nmss.org
www.nationalmssociety.org

Traces the National Multiple Sclerosis Society's historic role in propelling MS research and explains current approaches for nonscientists.
10 minutes

Web Sites

6500 **Healing Well**
www.healingwell.com
An online health resource guide to medical news, chat, information and articles, newsgroups and message boards, books, disease-related web sites, medical directories, and more for patients, friends, and family coping with disabling diseases, disorders, or chronic illnesses.

6501 **Health Finder**
www.healthfinder.gov
Searchable, carefully developed web site offering information on over 1000 topics. Developed by the US Department of Health and Human Services, the site can be used in both English and Spanish.

6502 **Healthlink USA**
www.healthlinkusa.com
Health information concerning treatment, cures, prevention, diagnosis, risk factors, research, support groups, email lists, personal stories and much more. Updated regularly.

6503 **MedicineNet**
www.medicinenet.com
An online resource for consumers providing easy-to-read, authoritative medical and health information.

6504 **Medscape**
www.medscape.com
Medscape offers specialists, primary care physicians, and other health professionals the Web's most robust and integrated medical information and educational tools.

6505 **Multiple Sclerosis Foundation**
www.msfocus.org
Dedicated to helping create a brighter tomorrow for those with MS, the foundation offers a wide array of free services including: national toll-free support, educational programs, homecare, support groups, assitive technology, publications, a comprehensive website and more to improve the quality of life for those affected by MS.

6506 **National Multiple Sclerosis Society**
www.nmss.org
The Society helps people affected by MS by funding cutting-edge research, driving change through advocacy, facilitating professional education, and providing programs and services that help people with MS and their families move their lives forward.

6507 **Neurology Channel**
www.healthcommunities.com
Find clearly explained, medically accurate information regarding conditions, including an overview, symptoms, causes, diagnostic procedures and treatment options. On this site it is possible to ask questions and get information from a neurologist and connect to people who have similar health interests.

6508 **WebMD**
www.webmd.com
Provides credible information, supportive communities, and in-depth reference material about health subjects. A source for original and timely health information as well as material from well known content providers.

Description

6509 Muscular Dystrophy

Muscular dystrophy is a group of genetic disorders marked by progressive weakness and degeneration of the skeletal, or voluntary, muscles that control movement. The muscles of the heart and other involuntary muscles may also be affected in some forms of muscular dystrophy, and a few forms of the disease involve other organs as well. Mutations in the DMD gene, which encodes the Dystrophin protein, are responsible for muscular dystrophy. Dystrophin helps anchor the contractile elements of the muscle to the cell membrane and to extracellular elements outside the muscle cells. Without functional Dystrophin, the muscle cells become damaged from normal use and degenerate.

Muscular dystrophy can affect people of all ages. The most common form, Duchenne, appears in childhood, but others may not appear until middle age or later.

Duchenne muscular dystrophy affects males almost exclusively. By age five, those with Duchenne experience progressive weakness and difficulty in climbing, jumping and hopping. By ages eight to ten, leg braces are often required, and eventually walking is impossible. Duchenne is also associated with heart problems, although without symptoms, and intellectual impairment that affects verbal ability more than performance. Death usually occurs in the third decade of life, often as a result of pneumonia. The less severe Becker muscular dystrophy is characterized by less severe muscular weakness that appears later (about age 12). Affected boys are typically able to walk until at least age 15 and can still walk into adulthood. Weakness eventually overtakes them, and they will become confined to a wheelchair. Most men with Becker muscular dystrophy survive into their fourth or fifth decade.

No specific treatment exists. Daily prednisone provides significant benefit but owing to the medication's numerous side effects, it should be reserved for patients with major functional decline. Other treatment includes physical therapy, which can help minimize the shortening of the muscles that occurs around joints; assistive devices; and avoidance of prolonged immobility. There are now techniques available to detect female carriers of the defective gene, enabling genetic counseling for families and couples considering conception.

Other forms of muscular dystrophy are myotonic, limb-girdle and facioscapulohumeral. Information about when and where muscle weakness first occurred, and its severity, is very helpful in classifying the type of muscular dystrophy. Studying a small piece of muscle tissue can indicate whether the disorder is muscular dystrophy and which form of the disease it is. Genetic tests are also available. Stem cell treatments in animals have shown some limited success, but this technology remains a future rather than present hope.

National Agencies & Associations

6510 Muscular Dystrophy Association
161 N Clark
Chicago, IL 60601
800-572-1717
resourcecenter@mdausa.org
www.mda.org
Supports scientific research on the causes and effective treatments for muscular dystrophy and related neuromuscular disorders.
Lynn O'Connor Vos, President & CEO
Adam Cotumaccio, MBA, Executive Vice President

6511 Muscular Dystrophy Canada
40 Eglinton Avenue E
Toronto, Ontario, M4P-3A2
800-567-2873
info@muscle.ca
www.muscle.ca
Dedicated to improving the quality of life of Canadians with neuromuscular disorders and funding leading research for the discovery of therapies and cures for neuromuscular disorders.

6512 Parent Project: Muscular Dystrophy
401 Hackensack Avenue
Hackensack, NJ 07601
201-250-8440
800-714-5437
Fax: 201-250-8435
info@parentprojectmd.org
www.parentprojectmd.org
Organization of families around the world who have children diagnosed with Duchenne, working together to raise funds for research and treatments.

Research Centers

6513 Baylor College of Medicine: Jerry Lewis Neuromuscular Disease Research
Methodist Neurological Institute
Department of Neurology
Houston, TX 77030
713-798-4333
Fax: 713-798-3854
neurochair@bcm.edu
www.bcm.edu/neurology
Offers research into biochemistry molecular genetics and neuromuscular disorders.
Eli M. Mizrahi, M.D., Chair, Department of Neurology
Travis G. Corwin, Department Administrator

6514 Columbia Presbyterian Medical Center Neurological Institute
Columbia University
710 W 168th Street
New York, NY 10032
212-305-2700
Fax: 212-058-98
www.cumc.columbia.edu
Neuromuscular clinical research center.
Hiroshi Mits MD, Division Head Neuromuscular Division

6515 Columbia University Clinical Research Center for Muscular Dystrophy
College of Physicians & Surgeons
116th and Broadway
New York, NY 10027
212-854-1754
Fax: 212-305-1343
www.columbia.edu

Salvatore DiMauro, Co Director

6516 Hospital of the University of Pennsylvania University of Pennsylvania
University of Pennsylvania

3400 Spruce Street
Philadelphia, PA 19104
215-662-4000
800-789-PENN
Fax: 215-903-09
pleasure@email.chop.edu
www.pennhealth.com

Research program centering its efforts on finding better ways to prevent and treat neuromuscular disorders.
David E Pleasure MD, Director

6517 Mayo Clinic and Foundation Mayo Foundation
Mayo Foundation
201 W Center Street
Rochester, MN 55905
507-284-2511
Fax: 507-284-0161
TTY: 507-284-9786
www.mayo.edu

Neuromuscular clinical research center with a primary research interest in neuropathies.
Peter J Dyck MD, Director Nerve Studies
Andrew G Engel MD, Director Muscle Studies

6518 Muscular Dystrophy Association
3300 E Sunrise Drive
Tucson, AZ 85718-3299
520-529-2000
800-572-1717
Fax: 520-529-5300
mda@mdausa.org
www.MDausa.org

Fights neuromuscular disease including all muscular dystrophies. Conducts extensive programs of research services and public education including 230 clinics.
Robert Ross, President/CEO

6519 University of Utah Utah Genome Depot University of Utah
University of Utah
20 S 2030 E
Salt Lake City, UT 84112
801-585-7606
Fax: 801-857-7177
bob.weiss@genetics.utah.edu
www.genome.utah.edu

Focuses research on human muscular dystrophies.
Robert Weiss, Principal Investigator
Jackie Tyce, Program Coordinator

Support Groups & Hotlines

6520 Facioscapulohumeral Muscular Dystrophy Society (FSH Society)
450 Bedford Street
Lexington, MA 02420
781-860-0501
Fax: 781-860-0599
solvefshd@fshsociety.org
www.fshsociety.org

The Facioscapulohumeral Muscular Dystrophy Society (FSH Society) serves as a resource for individuals and families with FSHD, representing them and advocating on their behalf. Purposes of the organization are to accumulate, disseminate and encourage the exchange of information about FSHD, including educating the general public, relevant governmental bodies, and the medical and scientific professions about the existence, diagnosis and treatment of FSHD.
Daniel Paul Perez, President/CEO
June Kinoshita, Executive Director

6521 National Health Information Center
Office of Disease Prevention & Health Promotion
1101 Wootton Pkwy
Rockville, MD 20852
Fax: 240-453-8281
odphpinfo@hhs.gov
www.health.gov/nhic

Supports public health education by maintaining a calendar of National Health Observances; helps connect consumers and health professionals to organizations that can best answer questions and provide up-to-date contact information from reliable sources; updates on a yearly basis toll-free numbers for health information, Federal health clearinghouses and info centers.
Don Wright, MD, MPH, Director

Books

6522 Clinical Evaluation and Diagnostic Tests for Neuromuscular Disorders
Butterworth-Heinemann Medical

3255 Bell Helicopter Blvd
Fort Worth, TX 76101
817-280-2011
Fax: 817-280-2321
custserv.bh@elsevier.com
www.bellhelicopter.com

Expert advice from leading authorities on how and when to use the numerous evaluation tests now available for diagnosis and management of neuromuscular disorders.
2002

6523 Everyday Life with ALS: A Practical Guide
Muscular Dystrophy Association
3300 E Sunrise Drive
Tucson, AZ 85718-3299
520-529-5317
800-572-1717
Fax: 520-529-5383
publications@mdausa.org
www.mda.org

Advice and information addressing degrees of affliction of those with ALS. Ways to conserve energy, to modifying your home space, to medical devices and equipment. Consider using the Guide with your care team.
2005
Christina Medvescek, Director of Editorial Services

6524 Journey of Love: Parent's Guide to Duchenne Muscular Dystrophy
Muscular Dystrophy Association
3300 E Sunrise Drive
Tucson, AZ 85718-3299
520-529-5317
800-572-1717
Fax: 520-529-5383
publications@mdausa.org
www.mda.org

Complete guide for parents with children diagnosed with DMD. Information includes explanation of the disease, treatments, research, services provided by MDA, guides to finding assistance and more.
170 pages Paperback
Bob Mackle, Director Public Information
Christina Medvescek, Director of Editorial Services

6525 MDA ALS Caregiver's Guide
Muscular Dystrophy Association
3300 E Sunrise Drive
Tucson, AZ 85718-3299
520-529-5317
800-572-1717
www.mda.org

A comprehensive guide to caring for a person with ALS at home. Covers everything from physical care to psychological and emotional concerns to getting financial assistance. Companion to Everyday Life with ALS: A Practical Guide.
2008 58 pages Paperback
Bob Mackle, Director Public Information
Christina Medvescek, Director of Editorial Services

6526 Moonrise: One Family, Genetic Identity, & Muscular Dystrophy
St. Martin's Press
175 5th Avenue
New York, NY 10010
212-674-5151
Fax: 212-677-7456
us.macmillan.com/smp

A mother writes about her teen-age son who has Duchenne muscular dystrophy, the life he leads, and the one he can look forward to.
2003

6527 Muscular Dystrophy & Other Neuromuscular Diseases: Psychological Issues
Leon Charash, Robert Lovelace, author
Haworth Press
10 Alice Street
Binghamton, NY 13904
607-722-5857
800-429-6784
Fax: 607-722-0012
www.haworthpress.com

Thoughtful book from professionals who assist people with neuromuscular disorders to help them adapt to lifestyle changes accompanying these disorders.
250 pages Hardcover
ISBN: 1-560240-77-0

6528 Muscular Dystrophy in Children: Guide for Families
Demos Medical Publishing

11 West 42nd Street
New York, NY 10036

212-683-0072
800-532-8663
Fax: 212-683-0118
support@demosmedical.com
www.demosmedical.com

Addresses emotional as well as physical challenges that families and caregivers will have to face and gives readers information on muscular dystrophy, how to adapt to a child's needs, and present research being conducted. In addition, it gives parents and caregivers sources for additional support and suggestions for further reading.
1999
Beth Kaufman Barry, Publisher
David D'Addona, Acquisitions Editor

6529 Neuromuscular Dis. of Infancy, Childhood & Adolescece: A Clinician's Approach
Butterworth-Heinemann Medical
3255 Bell Helicopter Blvd
Fort Worth, TX 76101

817-280-2011
Fax: 817-280-2321
custserv.bh@elsevier.com
www.bellhelicopter.com

Explains how childhood neuromuscular diseases differ from those in adult patients, and provides clinicians with all the knowledge they need to successfully diagnose and treat pediatric patients.
2003

6530 Noninvasive Mechanical Ventilation
John Bach, MD, author
Elsevier
Book Customer Service Dpt
St. Louis, MO 63146

800-545-2522
Fax: 800-535-9935
usbkinfo@elsevier.com
www.elsevier.com

Describes the use of inspiratory and expiratory muscle aids to prevent the pulmonary complications of lung disease and conditions with muscle weakness. It also describes treatment and rehabilitation interventions specific for patients with these conditions. This book is unique in presenting the use of entirely noninvasive management alternatives to eliminate respiratory morbidity and avoid the need to resort to tracheostomy for the majority of patients with lung or neuromuscular disease.
2002 348 pages Paperback
ISBN: 1-560535-49-0

6531 Physical Medicine & Rehabilitation
WB Saunders/Elsevier Science/Harcourt
200 Wheeler Road
Burlington, MA 01803

781-221-2212
Fax: 781-221-1615
custserv.bh@elsevier.com
www.us.elsevierhealth.com

Current aspects of physical medicine and rehabilitation in a single, readable volume. Completely updated and revised edition includes all the latest advances and techniques.
2001

Children's Books

6532 Abby & the South Seas Adventure Series
Tyndale House Publishers
PO Box 80
Wheaton, IL 60189

630-668-8300
Fax: 630-668-3245

Delightful new series, focusing on the travels of Abby Kendall, who has muscular dystrophy, is a sure-fire hit for 8 to 12 year old girls. Lots of surprises will keep them coming back for each new Abby title.
2000

6533 Heartsongs, Journey Through Heartsongs, Hope Through Heartsongs, Celebrate
Hyperion Books
1344 Crossman Avenue
Sunnyvale, CA 94089

408-744-9500
Fax: 408-744-0400
www.hyperion.com

By the 2002-2003 National Goodwill Ambassador for the Muscular Dystrophy Association. The first two books of inspiring poems were both on the New York Times bestseller list. Mattie's struggle with muscular dystrophy has never kept him from feeling deep love for his family, friends, country and faith — heartfelt emotions that are reflected throughout these pages by a precociously brilliant boy.
2001-2003
Carol Sowell, Director Publications

6534 Muscular Dystrophy
Enslow Publishers
40 Industrial Road
Berkeley Heights, NJ 07922-0398

800-398-2504
Fax: 908-771-0925
info@enslow.com
www.enslow.com

Written for children, this book follows two families with muscular dystrophy and describes various forms of the disease, who gets it, and how to learn to live with it.
2000

Magazines

6535 Quest Magazine
Muscular Dystrophy Association
3300 E Sunrise Drive
Tucson, AZ 85718-3299

520-529-5317
800-572-1717
Fax: 520-529-5300
publications@mdusa.org
www.mda.org

Quarterly magazine. Contains stories about vital concerns of people with meuromuscular diseases and their community. Find tips, hobbies, resources, treatments, findings, and products. Available online.
30 pages Paperback
Bob Mackle, Director Public Information
Christina Medvescek, Director of Editorial Services

Pamphlets

6536 Breathe Easy: Respiratory Care with Muscular Dystrophy
Muscular Dystrophy Association
3300 E Sunrise Drive
Tucson, AZ 85718-3299

520-529-5317
800-572-1717
Fax: 520-529-5383
publications@mdusa.org
www.mda.org

Members of a respiratory care team describe how muscular dystrophy can affect breathing, maintaining respiratory health and types of therapies. Also available in Spanish.
2006
Christina Medvescek, Director of Editorial Services

6537 Everybody's Different Nobody's Perfect
Muscular Dystrophy Association
3300 E Sunrise Drive
Tucson, AZ 85718-3299

520-529-5317
800-572-1717
Fax: 520-529-5300
publications@mdusa.org
www.mda.org

Children's Book. Explains how muscular dystrophy affects children and describes how people are different from each other in many ways. Emphasizing fun, friendship and caring, this booklet is ideal for heightening awareness and encouraging understanding of persons with disabilities. Also available in Spanish.
1999 11 pages Paperback
Bob Mackle, Director Public Information
Christina Medvescek, Director of Editorial Services

6538 Facts About Charcot-Marie-Tooth Disease
Muscular Dystrophy Association
3300 E Sunrise Drive
Tucson, AZ 85718-3299

520-529-5317
800-572-1717
Fax: 520-529-5383
publications@mdusa.org
www.mda.org

Covers the forms of the disease and outlines the characteristics and genetic patterns of the CMTs. Research efforts aimed at finding the

causes, treatments and cures are also described. Also available in Spanish.
15 pages
Christina Medvescek, Director of Editorial Services

6539   Facts About Duchenne & Becker Muscular Dystrophies
Muscular Dystrophy Association
3300 E Sunrise Drive   520-529-5317
Tucson, AZ 85718-3299   800-572-1717
                                         Fax: 520-529-5383
                                    publications@mdausa.org
                                             www.mda.org
Introductory booklet describes the two disorders, testing, inheritance and treatments. Also available in Spanish.
Christina Medvescek, Director of Editorial Services

6540   Facts About Facioscapulohumeral Muscular Dystrophy
Muscular Dystrophy Association
3300 E Sunrise Drive   520-529-5317
Tucson, AZ 85718-3299   800-572-1717
                                         Fax: 520-529-5383
                                    publications@mdausa.org
                                             www.mda.org
Introductory booklet describes FSHD in easy-to-understand terms and answers commonly asked questions about the disease. Also available in Spanish.
Christina Medvescek, Director of Editorial Services

6541   Facts About Friedreich's Ataxia
Muscular Dystrophy Association
3300 E Sunrise Drive   520-529-5317
Tucson, AZ 85718-3299   800-572-1717
                                         Fax: 520-529-5300
                                    publications@mdusa.org
                                             www.mda.org
Explains Friedreich's ataxia in layman's terms and answers commonly asked questions about the disease. Also available in Spanish.
15 pages Paperback
Bob Mackle, Director Public Information
Christina Medvescek, Director of Editorial Services

6542   Facts About Limb-Girdle Muscular Dystrophy
Muscular Dystrophy Association
3300 E Sunrise Drive   520-529-5317
Tucson, AZ 85718-3299   800-572-1717
                                         Fax: 520-529-5383
                                    publications@mdausa.org
                                             www.mda.org
Introductory booklet provides basic facts about LGMD and contains information regarding the many forms, diagnostic tests and current treatments. Also available in Spanish.
Christina Medvescek, Director of Editorial Services

6543   Facts About Metabolic Diseases of Muscle
Muscular Dystrophy Association
3300 E Sunrise Drive   520-529-5317
Tucson, AZ 85718-3299   800-572-1717
                                         Fax: 520-529-5300
                                    publications@mdusa.org
                                             www.mda.org
Provides an overview of the 11 inheritable metabolic diseases of muscle encompassed by MDA's program. Addresses commonly asked questions and highlights MDA's research efforts aimed at finding the causes of and effective treatments for these disorders. Also available in Spanish.
20 pages Paperback
Bob Mackle, Director Public Information
Christina Medvescek, Director of Editorial Services

6544   Facts About Mitochondrial Myopathies
Muscular Dystrophy Association
3300 E Sunrise Drive   520-529-5317
Tucson, AZ 85718-3299   800-572-1717
                                         Fax: 520-529-5300
                                    publications@mdusa.org
                                             www.mda.org

Explains mitochondrial myopathies in layman's terms and answers the most frequently asked questions about this disease. Also available in Spanish.
24 pages Paperback
Bob Mackle, Director Public Information
Christina Medvescek, Director of Editorial Services

6545   Facts About Myasthenia Gravis
Muscular Dystrophy Association
3300 E Sunrise Drive   520-529-5317
Tucson, AZ 85718-3299   800-572-1717
                                         Fax: 520-529-5300
                                    publications@mdusa.org
                                             www.mda.org
Explains myasthenia gravis and Lambert-Eaton syndrome in layman's terms and answers the most frequently asked questions about these diseases. Also available in Spanish.
19 pages Paperback
Bob Mackle, Director Public Information
Carol Sowall, Director Publications

6546   Facts About Myopathies
Muscular Dystrophy Association
3300 E Sunrise Drive   520-529-5317
Tucson, AZ 85718-3299   800-572-1717
                                         Fax: 520-529-5300
                                    publications@mdusa.org
                                             www.mda.org
Overview of the myopathies encompassed by MDA's program. Addresses commonly asked questions and highlights MDA's research efforts aimed at finding the causes of and effective treatments for these disorders. Also available in Spanish.
18 pages Paperback
Bob Mackle, Director Public Information
Christina Medvescek, Director of Editorial Services

6547   Facts About Myotonic Muscular Dystrophy
Muscular Dystrophy Association
3300 E Sunrise Drive   520-529-5317
Tucson, AZ 85718-3299   800-572-1717
                                         Fax: 520-529-5383
                                    publications@mdausa.org
                                             www.mda.org
Introductory booklet provides basic facts about the disorder and explains the causes and effects, as well as tests used to diagnose and MDA's search for treatments and cures. Also available in Spanish.
Christina Medvescek, Director of Editorial Services

6548   Facts About Plasmapheresis
Muscular Dystrophy Association
3300 E Sunrise Drive   520-529-5317
Tucson, AZ 85718-3299   800-572-1717
                                         Fax: 520-529-5300
                                    publications@mdusa.org
                                             www.mda.org
Describes plasmapheresis, a plasma exchange procedure often utilized as a treatment for autoimmune disease such as myasthenia gravis and Lambert-Eaton syndrome.
Paperback
Bob Mackle, Director Public Information
Christina Medvescek, Director of Editorial Services

6549   Facts About Polymyostis/Dermatomyositis
Muscular Dystrophy Association
3300 E Sunrise Drive   520-529-5317
Tucson, AZ 85718-3299   800-572-1717
                                         Fax: 520-529-5300
                                    publications@mdusa.org
                                             www.mda.org
Outlines these two front forms of inflammatory myopathy. Current approaches to treatment and MDA's efforts in continued research are described. Also available in Spanish.
13 pages Paperback
Bob Mackle, Director Public Information
Christina Medvescek, Director of Editorial Services

6550   Facts About Rare Muscular Dsytrophies
Muscular Dystrophy Association

3300 E Sunrise Drive
Tucson, AZ 85718-3299
520-529-5317
800-572-1717
Fax: 520-529-5300
publications@mdusa.org
www.mda.org

This brochure gives basic facts about four forms of muscular dystrophy (Congenital, Distal, Emery-Dreifuss and Oculopharyngeal) and addresses commonly asked questions. Also available in Spanish.
28 pages Paperback
Bob Mackle, Director Public Information
Christina Medvescek, Director of Editorial Services

6551 **Facts About Spinal Muscular Atrophy**
Muscular Dystrophy Association
3300 E Sunrise Drive
Tucson, AZ 85718-3299
520-529-5317
800-572-1717
Fax: 520-529-5300
publications@mdusa.org
www.mda.org

Covers the four forms of the disease and outlines the characteristics and genetic patterns of the SMAs. Research efforts aimed at finding the causes, treatments and cures are also described. Also available in Spanish.
15 pages Paperback
Bob Mackle, Director Public Information
Christina Medvescek, Director of Editorial Services

6552 **Genetics and Neuromuscular Diseases**
Muscular Dystrophy Association
3300 E Sunrise Drive
Tucson, AZ 85718-3299
520-529-5317
800-572-1717
Fax: 520-529-5383
publications@mdausa.org
www.mda.org

Booklet describes what a genetic disorder is and explains how genetic testing and counseling can help people understand how disorders that may affect them or their children are inherited. Also available in Spanish.
Christina Medvescek, Director of Editorial Services

6553 **Hey, I'm Here Too**
Muscular Dystrophy Association
3300 E Sunrise Drive
Tucson, AZ 85718-3299
520-529-5317
800-572-1717
Fax: 520-529-5383
publications@mdausa.org
www.mda.org

Help for siblings of boys with Duchenne muscular dystrophy. Explores how they feel about themselves, their brothers and their families. Also provides specific answers to some questions that siblings may wonder about. Also available in Spanish.
28 pages
Bob Mackle, Director Public Information
Christina Medvescek, Director of Editorial Services

6554 **Learning to Live with Neuromuscular Desease: A Message to Parents**
Muscular Dystrophy Association
3300 E Sunrise Drive
Tucson, AZ 85718-3299
520-529-5317
800-572-1717
Fax: 520-529-5383
publications@mdausa.org
www.mda.org

Helps parents and families cope with the fact that their child has a neuromuscular disease and with the impact the disease will have on everyday life. Also available in Spanish.
Christina Medvescek, Director of Editorial Services

6555 **MDA Camp: A Special Place**
Muscular Dystrophy Association
3300 E Sunrise Drive
Tucson, AZ 85718-3299
520-529-5317
800-572-1717
Fax: 520-529-5300

Highlights the activities of MDA dummer camps for youngsters diagnosed with one of the more than 40 diseases in MDA's program. Shares camper and volunteer reactions. Also available in Spanish.
Paperback
Bob Mackle, Director Public Information
Carol Sowall, Director Publications

6556 **MDA Fact Sheet**
Muscular Dystrophy Association
3300 E Sunrise Drive
Tucson, AZ 85718-3299
520-529-5317
800-572-1717
Fax: 520-529-5383
publications@mdausa.org
www.mda.org

Basic information on MDA's origins and purposes; the more than 40 neuromuscular diseases in MDA's program, and brief symptom descriptions by category. Also available in Spanish.
Christina Medvescek, Director of Editorial Services

6557 **MDA Services for the Individual, Family and Community**
Muscular Dystrophy Association
3300 E Sunrise Drive
Tucson, AZ 85718-3299
520-529-5317
800-572-1717
Fax: 520-529-5383
publications@mdausa.org
www.mda.org

Lists the diseases covered by MDA as well as eligibility criteria for MDA's services program, a list of MDA-sponsored clinics nationwide, and the services available through local MDA offices. Also available in Spanish.
Christina Medvescek, Director of Editorial Services

6558 **Teacher's Guide to Neuromuscular Disease**
Muscular Dystrophy Association
3300 E Sunrise Drive
Tucson, AZ 85718-3299
520-529-5317
Fax: 520-529-5383
publications@mdausa.org
www.mda.org

This publication provides a source of guidance and information to teachers, giving details about neuromuscular diseases, how they affect school participation, and ways that teachers can help meet the needs of students affected by these disorders.
2005
Christina Medvescek, Director of Editorial Services

6559 **Travis, I Got Lots of Neat Stuff Children Living with Muscular Dystrophy**
Muscular Dystrophy Association
3300 E Sunrise Drive
Tucson, AZ 85718-3299
520-529-5317
800-572-1717
Fax: 520-529-5383
publications@mdausa.org
www.mda.org

Booklet illustrates that a child with muscular dystrophy can do many things. Adapted for MDA's Hop-a-Thon program, the booklet heightens awareness and understanding of people with disabilities. It's suitable for youngsters in elementary school. Also available in Spanish.
24 pages
Christina Medvescek, Director of Editorial Services

Audio & Video

6560 **Muscular Dystrophy**
Films for the Humanities & Sciences
Box 2053
Princeton, NJ 08543-2053
609-419-8000
800-257-5126
Fax: 609-275-3767

Video deals with how Muscular Dystrophy sufferers deal with the disease that has no cure. Three life stories dealing with surgery, medicine, therapy and bracing as a means to survive. Dr. Betty Banke discusses the need to find a cure while Richard Nordgren from the Dartmouth-Hitchcock Medical Center discusses treatment.
20 Minutes

Web Sites

6561 **Healing Well**
www.healingwell.com
An online health resource guide to medical news, chat, information and articles, newsgroups and message boards, books, disease-related web sites, medical directories, and more for patients,

friends, and family coping with disabling diseases, disorders, or chronic illnesses.

6562   Health Finder

www.healthfinder.gov
Searchable, carefully developed web site offering information on over 1000 topics. Developed by the US Department of Health and Human Services, the site can be used in both English and Spanish.

6563   Healthlink USA

www.healthlinkusa.com
Health information concerning treatment, cures, prevention, diagnosis, risk factors, research, support groups, email lists, personal stories and much more. Updated regularly.

6564   MedicineNet

www.medicinenet.com
An online resource for consumers providing easy-to-read, authoritative medical and health information.

6565   Medscape

www.medscape.com
Medscape offers specialists, primary care physicians, and other health professionals the Web's most robust and integrated medical information and educational tools.

6566   Muscular Dystrophy Association

www.mdausa.org
Information on effective treatments for muscular dystrophy, related neuromuscular disorders and research programs. In addition, MDA offers a comprehensive program of patient and community services, with access to over 230 MDA-supported clinics nationwide.

6567   Parent Project: Muscular Dystrophy

www.parentprojectmd.org
Parent Project Muscular Dystrophy (PPMD) is the largest most comprehensive nonprofit organization in the United States focused on finding a cure for Duchenne muscular dystrophy. There mission is to end Duchenne. They invest deeply in treatments for this generation of young men affected by Duchenne and in research that will benefit future generations.

6568   WebMD

www.webmd.com
Provides credible information, supportive communities, and in-depth reference material about health subjects. A source for original and timely health information as well as material from well known content providers.

Description

6569 ## Myasthenia Gravis

Myasthenia gravis is an autoimmune disease that impairs proper communication between motor nerves and skeletal muscles, resulting in muscle weakness. The immune system attacks the acetylcholine receptors on the surfaces of muscle cells at the neuromuscular junction, which is the structure which receives the motor nerve chemical signal that tells the muscle to contract. Circulating antibodies attack this junction and destroy the acetylcholine receptor, leading to weakness of voluntary muscles and muscle fatigue after exercise. Any muscle may be involved, but muscles in the face and throat are especially susceptible. The disease therefore especially affects chewing, swallowing, coughing and facial expressions. Double vision (diplopia) and drooping of the eyelids (ptosis) are two of the most common manifestations of this disease. These manifestations fluctuate in intensity over hours to days. Myasthenia gravis usually develops in women between the ages of 20-40 and in older men, between the ages of 50-80. It may, however, affect men or women at any age, but it rarely begins during childhood.

Myasthenia gravis is diagnoses with an "ice pack test," blood tests to detect the anti-acetylcholine receptor-specific antibodies, and electromyography tests that measure muscle function. Because this disease is caused by an overactive immune system, most treatments target this system. These include corticosteroids, immunosuppressive drugs such as azathioprine, cyclosporine, plasmapheresis (filtration of the blood with retention of the cells and removal of the plasma), intravenous immunoglobulins and surgical removal of the thymus gland. In addition, anticholinesterase drugs like pyridostigmine or neostigmine increase the level of the neurotransmitter acetylcholine at the neuromuscular junction, thereby increasing muscle strength. These drugs relieve symptoms but do not alter the progression of the disease. Removal of the thymus gland (thymectomy) can cure the disease in some cases but should only be considered in elderly patients.

Because of the progressive weakness associated with this disease, physical therapy and assistive devices are generally required.

National Agencies & Associations

6570 **American Association for Pediatric Ophthalmology And Strabismus**
655 Beach Street   415-561-8505
San Francisco, CA 94109   Fax: 415-561-8531
aapos@aao.org
www.aapos.org
Promotes information about eye conditions for individuals worldwide and educational resources for ophthalmologists.

6571 **American Association of Neuromuscular & Electrodiagnostic Medicine**
2621 Superior Drive NW   507-288-0100
Rochester, MN 55901   Fax: 507-288-1225
aanem@aanem.org
www.aanem.org
The American Association of Neuromuscular & Electrodiagnostic Medicine (AANEM) is a nonprofit membership association dedicated to the advancement of neuromuscular, musculoskeletal, and electrodiagnostic medicine.
Shirlyn A. Adkins, JD, Executive Director
Millie Suk, JD, MPP, Health Policy Director

6572 **Myasthenia Gravis Foundation of America**
355 Lexington Avenue   800-541-5454
New York, NY 10017   Fax: 212-297-2159
mgfa@myasthenia.org
www.myasthenia.org
Funds research for better treatments and a cure for myasthenia gravis.
Linda L. Kusner, PhD, Board
Robert L. Ruff, MD, PhD, Board

State Agencies & Associations

Alaska

6573 **Pacific Northwest Chapter of the Myasthenia Gravis Foundation of America**
PO Box 58785   425-235-1435
Renton, WA 98058-6562   877-252-0677
Fax: 425-204-2070
washington@myasthenia.org
www.myasthenia.org

Arizona

6574 **Jim L Walker: Arizona Chapter of the Myasthenia Gravis Foundation of America**
PO Box 34173   480-451-3060
Phoenix, AZ 85067-4173   877-347-7905
Fax: 480-767-7029
arizona@myasthenia.org
www.azmgfa.org
Jim LoVecchio, Chairman
Stephane Borsk, Vice Chairman

Connecticut

6575 **Connecticut Chapter of the Myasthenia Gravis Foundation of America**
P.O. Box 2801   203-556-5012
Danbury, CT 06813-2801   866-329-8784
conn@myasthenia.org
www.myasthenia.org/connecticut_nutmeg
Irving Beck ED

Delaware

6576 **MD/DC/Delaware Chapter of Myasthenia Gravis Foundation of America**
PO Box 186   410-437-1157
Pasedena, MD 21123-0186   866-437-2881
maryland@myasthenia.org
www.myasthenia.org/LivingwithMG/MGFAChap

District of Columbia

6577 **MD/DC/Delaware Chapter of Myasthenia Gravis Foundation of America**
PO Box 186   410-437-1157
Pasedena, MD 21113-0186   866-437-2881
maryland@myasthenia.org

Florida

6578 Florida Chapter of the Myasthenia Gravis Foundation of America
14502 87 Avenue N
Seminole, FL 33776-0623
727-596-1491
877-596-1491
Fax: 727-596-1491
wcflorida@myasthenia.org
www.myasthenia.org

Georgia

6579 Georgia Chapter of the Myasthenia Gravis Foundation of America
P.O. Box 889085
Atlanta, GA 30356
770-427-3441
800-743-4339
Fax: 770-973-3269
georgia@myasthenia.org
www.mggeorgia.org

Hawaii

6580 Pacific Northwest Chapter of the Myasthenia Gravis Foundation of America
PO Box 58785
Renton, WA 98058-6562
425-235-1435
877-252-0677
Fax: 425-204-2070
washington@myasthenia.org
www.myasthenia.org

Idaho

6581 Pacific Northwest Chapter of the Myasthenia Gravis Foundation of America
PO Box 58785
Renton, WA 98058-6562
425-235-1435
877-252-0677
Fax: 425-204-2070
washington@myasthenia.org
www.myasthenia.org

Indiana

6582 Greater Indianapolis Chapter of the Myasthenia Gravis Foundation of America
8922 Haverstick Road
Indianapolis, IN 46240
317-846-1462
Spknke@aol.com
www.4-mga.org/?

Earl Zimmerman, Chair

Maine

6583 Connecticut Chapter of the Myasthenia Gravis Foundation of America
P.O. Box 2801
Danbury, CT 06813-2801
203-556-5012
866-329-8784
conn@myasthenia.org
www.myasthenia.org/connecticut_nutmeg

Irving Beck ED

Maryland

6584 MD/DC/Delaware Chapter of Myasthenia Gravis Foundation of America
PO Box 186
Pasadena, MD 21123-0186
410-437-1157
866-437-2881
maryland@myasthenia.org
www.myasthenia.org

Massachusetts

6585 Mass./New Hampshire Chapter of the Myasthenia Gravis Foundation of America
460 S. River St.
Marshfield, MA 02050
508-435-3808
www.ma-nhmgfa.org

Michigan

6586 Great Lakes Chapter of the Myasthenia Gravis Foundation of America
2660 Horizon Drive SE
Grand Rapids, MI 49546
616-956-0622
800-224-9180
Fax: 616-956-9234
myasthenia.info@gmail.com
www.myasthenia-mi.org
Autoimmune, neuromuscular disease manifest in weakness of voluntary muscles; arms, legs, eyes, facial expressions, severe cases of breathing.
Susan Richards, Executive Director
Paulus Heule, President

Minnesota

6587 Minnesota State Chapter of the Myasthenia Gravis Foundation of America
29234 Piney Way
Breezy Point, MN 56472-1715
218-562-4594
minnesota@myasthenia.org
www.myasthenia.org

Montana

6588 Pacific Northwest Chapter of the Myasthenia Gravis Foundation of America
PO Box 58785
Renton, WA 98058-6562
425-235-1435
877-252-0677
Fax: 425-204-2070
washington@myasthenia.org
www.myasthenia.org

New Hampshire

6589 Mass./New Hampshire Chapter of the Myasthenia Gravis Foundation of America
460 S River Street
Marshfield, MA 02050
508-435-3808
massachusetts@myasthenia.org
www.ma-nhmgfa.org

Marilyn Buckner, Chair
Virginia Pierce, RN, Treasurer

New Jersey

6590 Garden State Chapter of the Myasthenia Gravis Foundation of America
PO Box 4258
Wayne, NJ 07474-1362
973-835-4444
800-437-4949
Fax: 973-835-4452
www.mgnj.org

Robert Allen, Chairman
Kelley DeVincentis, Executive Director

New York

6591 Upstate NY Chapter of the Myasthenia Gravis Foundation of America
14 Summit Rd.
Delmar, NY 12054
518-439-5377
800-581-5377
Fax: 518-439-8783
upstatenewyork@myasthenia.org
www.myasthenia.org

Barry Levine, President/Chair

North Carolina

6592 Carolinas Chapter of the Myasthenia Gravis Foundation of America
506 E Forest Hills Boulevard
Durham, NC 27707-1801
919-966-4131
800-842-8711
Fax: 919-489-7564
tvassar56@aol.com

Oklahoma

6593 Oklahoma Chapter of the Myasthenia Gravis Foundation of America
4606 E 67th St S
Tulsa, OK 74136
918-494-4951
Fax: 918-494-4951
oklahoma@myasthenia.org
www.myasthenia.org
Peggy Foust, Executive Director
Margret Feller, Vice-President/Treasurer

Oregon

6594 Pacific Northwest Chapter of the Myasthenia Gravis Foundation of America
PO Box 58785
Renton, WA 98058-6562
425-235-1435
877-252-0677
Fax: 425-204-2070
washington@myasthenia.org
www.myasthenia.org

Rhode Island

6595 Connecticut Chapter of the Myasthenia Gravis Foundation of America
P.O. Box 2801
Danbury, CT 06813-2801
203-556-5012
866-329-8784
conn@myasthenia.org
www.myasthenia.org/connecticut_nutmeg
Irving Beck ED

South Carolina

6596 Carolinas Chapter of the Myasthenia Gravis Foundation of America
506 E Forest Hills Boulevard
Durham, NC 27707-1801
919-490-2937
800-842-8711
Fax: 919-489-7564
tvassar56@aol.com
www.myasthenia.org

Texas

6597 Northwest Texas Chapter of the Myasthenia Gravis Foundation of America
3406 Manioca Road
Lubbock, TX 79403
806-749-3126
Fax: 915-554-7044
nwtexas@myasthenia.org
www.nwtcmg.org
Lowell McBroom, Vice-Chairperson

Vermont

6598 Connecticut Chapter of the Myasthenia Gravis Foundation of America
P.O. Box 2801
Danbury, CT 06813-2801
203-556-5012
866-329-8784
conn@myasthenia.org
www.myasthenia.org/connecticut_nutmeg
Irving Beck ED

Washington

6599 Pacific Northwest Chapter of the Myasthenia Gravis Foundation of America
PO Box 58785
Renton, WA 98058-6562
425-235-1435
877-252-0677
Fax: 425-204-2070
washington@myasthenia.org
www.myasthenia.org

Wisconsin

6600 Wisconsin Chapter of the Myasthenia Gravis Foundation of America
2474 S 96 Street
W Allis, WI 53227
262-938-9800
800-541-5454
Fax: 262-789-3363
wisconsin@myasthenia.org
www.myasthenia.org
The Myasthenia Gravis Foundation of America is the only national volunteer health agency dedicated solely to fight against myasthenoia gravis.
Patricia Lamp, Chairperson
Ellie Burbach, Vice-Chairperson

Wyoming

6601 Pacific Northwest Chapter of the Myasthenia Gravis Foundation of America
PO Box 58785
Renton, WA 98058-6562
425-235-1435
877-252-0677
Fax: 425-204-2070
washington@myasthenia.org
www.myasthenia.org

Support Groups & Hotlines

6602 National Health Information Center
Office of Disease Prevention & Health Promotion
1101 Wootton Pkwy
Rockville, MD 20852
Fax: 240-453-8281
odphpinfo@hhs.gov
www.health.gov/nhic
Supports public health education by maintaining a calendar of National Health Observances; helps connect consumers and health professionals to organizations that can best answer questions and provide up-to-date contact information from reliable sources; updates on a yearly basis toll-free numbers for health information, Federal health clearinghouses and info centers.
Don Wright, MD, MPH, Director

Arizona

6603 Myasthenia Gravis Support Group of Arizona Jim L. Walker Chapter
Phoenix, AZ
520-889-6910
www.myasthenia.org
Serves patients and their families throughout the state. The goal is to help achieve the conquest of Myasthenia Gravis through research, education, public awareness, anf fundraising.

Connecticut

6604 Myasthenia Gravis Support Group of Connect icut (Nutmeg Group)
conn@myasthenia.org
www.myasthenia.org
Serves patients and their families throughout the state. The goal is to help achieve the conquest of Myasthenia Gravis through research, education, public awareness, anf fundraising.

Georgia

6605 Myasthenia Gravis Support Group of Atlanta
770-427-3441
mg.georgia@yahoo.com
www.myasthenia.org
Serves patients and their families throughout the state. The goal is to help achieve the conquest of Myasthenia Gravis through research, education, public awareness, anf fundraising.

Iowa

6606 Myasthenia Gravis Support Group of Ames
515-708-5386
amy.schindel@gmail.com
www.myasthenia.org

Serves patients and their families throughout the state. The goal is to help achieve the conquest of Myasthenia Gravis through research, education, public awareness, anf fundraising.

Kentucky

6607 Myasthenia Gravis Support Group of Louisvi lle
859-967-4117
jennifer-howard@hotmail.com
www.myasthenia.org
Serves patients and their families throughout the state. The goal is to help achieve the conquest of Myasthenia Gravis through research, education, public awareness, anf fundraising.

Louisiana

6608 Myasthenia Gravis Support Group of Louisia na
504-376-7474
tommy.santora@gmail.com
www.myasthenia.org
Serves patients and their families throughout the state. The goal is to help achieve the conquest of Myasthenia Gravis through research, education, public awareness, anf fundraising.

Massachusetts

6609 Myasthenia Gravis Support Group of Eastern Massachusetts and New Hampshire
508-435-3808
www.ma-nhmgfa.org
Serves patients and their families throughout the state. The goal is to help achieve the conquest of Myasthenia Gravis through research, education, public awareness, anf fundraising.

6610 Myasthenia Gravis Support Group of Western Massachusetts and New Hampshire
508-435-3808
www.ma-nhmgfa.org
Serves patients and their families throughout the state. The goal is to help achieve the conquest of Myasthenia Gravis through research, education, public awareness, anf fundraising.

Minnesota

6611 Myasthenia Gravis Support Group of Mid-Min n
218-563-4594
mgcorn@uslink.net
www.myasthenia.org
Serves patients and their families throughout the state. The goal is to help achieve the conquest of Myasthenia Gravis through research, education, public awareness, anf fundraising.

6612 Myasthenia Gravis Support Group of South East Minnesota
507-206-0625
mgwalleworld@gmail.com
www.myasthenia.org
Serves patients and their families throughout the state. The goal is to help achieve the conquest of Myasthenia Gravis through research, education, public awareness, anf fundraising.

6613 Myasthenia Gravis Support Group of the Twin Cities
651-633-5465
liannema@mac.com
www.myasthenia.org
Serves patients and their families throughout the state. The goal is to help achieve the conquest of Myasthenia Gravis through research, education, public awareness, anf fundraising.

New Hampshire

6614 Myasthenia Gravis Support Group of Eastern Massachusetts and New Hampshire
508-435-3808
www.ma-nhmgfa.org
Serves patients and their families throughout the state. The goal is to help achieve the conquest of Myasthenia Gravis through research, education, public awareness, anf fundraising.

6615 Myasthenia Gravis Support Group of Western Massachusetts and New Hampshire
508-435-3808
www.ma-nhmgfa.org
Serves patients and their families throughout the state. The goal is to help achieve the conquest of Myasthenia Gravis through research, education, public awareness, anf fundraising.

New Mexico

6616 Myasthenia Gravis Support Group of New Mex ico
505-934-2423
cormier87@q.com
www.myasthenia.org
Serves patients and their families throughout the state. The goal is to help achieve the conquest of Myasthenia Gravis through research, education, public awareness, anf fundraising.

New York

6617 Myasthenia Gravis Support Group of Manhatt an
namerican@myasthenia.org
www.myasthenia.org
Serves patients and their families throughout the state. The goal is to help achieve the conquest of Myasthenia Gravis through research, education, public awareness, anf fundraising.

6618 Myasthenia Gravis Support Group of Upstate New York
518-439-5377
www.myasthenia.org
Serves patients and their families throughout the state. The goal is to help achieve the conquest of Myasthenia Gravis through research, education, public awareness, anf fundraising.

North Carolina

6619 Myasthenia Gravis Support Group of Charlotte
704-536-9572
877-643-2221
www.cncmg.org
Serves patients and their families throughout the state. The goal is to help achieve the conquest of Myasthenia Gravis through research, education, public awareness, anf fundraising.

6620 Myasthenia Gravis Support Group of Central North Carolina
919-567-9313
Serves patients and their families throughout the state. The goal is to help achieve the conquest of Myasthenia Gravis through research, education, public awareness, anf fundraising.

6621 Myasthenia Gravis Support Group of Durham/ Chapel Hill
704-536-9572
877-643-2221
mmenold@gmail.com
www.myasthenia.org
Serves patients and their families throughout the state. The goal is to help achieve the conquest of Myasthenia Gravis through research, education, public awareness, anf fundraising.

6622 Myasthenia Gravis Support Group of Fayette ville
877-643-2221
www.myasthenia.org
Serves patients and their families throughout the state. The goal is to help achieve the conquest of Myasthenia Gravis through research, education, public awareness, anf fundraising.

Ohio

6623 Myasthenia Gravis Support Group of Columbu s
j.eickholt@aol.com
www.myasthenia.org
Serves patients and their families throughout the state. The goal is to help achieve the conquest of Myasthenia Gravis through research, education, public awareness, anf fundraising.

6624 Myasthenia Gravis Support Group of Summit- Stark
330-628-2148
ralberte@neo.rr.com
www.myasthenia.org

Serves patients and their families throughout the state. The goal is to help achieve the conquest of Myasthenia Gravis through research, education, public awareness, anf fundraising.

Oklahoma

6625 **Myasthenia Gravis Support Group of Tulsa and Oklahoma City**
918-494-4951
oklahoma@myasthenia.org
www.myasthenia.org
Serves patients and their families throughout the state. The goal is to help achieve the conquest of Myasthenia Gravis through research, education, public awareness, anf fundraising.

Pennsylvania

6626 **Myasthenia Gravis Support Group of Scranto n**
570-687-6009
vkrewsun@comcast.net
www.myasthenia.org
Serves patients and their families throughout the state. The goal is to help achieve the conquest of Myasthenia Gravis through research, education, public awareness, anf fundraising.

South Carolina

6627 **Myasthenia Gravis Support Group of Low Country**
843-388-1683
mgsupport11@comcast.net
www.myasthenia.org
Serves patients and their families throughout the state. The goal is to help achieve the conquest of Myasthenia Gravis through research, education, public awareness, anf fundraising.

6628 **Myasthenia Gravis Support Group of the Mountain and Up Country**
828-698-3928
wemtglen@bellsouth.net
www.myasthenia.org
Serves patients and their families throughout the state. The goal is to help achieve the conquest of Myasthenia Gravis through research, education, public awareness, anf fundraising.

Virginia

6629 **Myasthenia Gravis Support Group of Manassa s**
804-742-5149
agsteele@hughes.net
www.myasthenia.org
Serves patients and their families throughout the state. The goal is to help achieve the conquest of Myasthenia Gravis through research, education, public awareness, anf fundraising.

Washington

6630 **Myasthenia Gravis Support Group of Seattle , Olympia and Poulsbo**
425-271-5151
nwmg2012@gmail.com
www.myasthenia.org
Serves patients and their families throughout the state. The goal is to help achieve the conquest of Myasthenia Gravis through research, education, public awareness, anf fundraising.

6631 **Myasthenia Gravis Support Group of Spokane**
509-468-0507
www.myasthenia.org
Serves patients and their families throughout the state. The goal is to help achieve the conquest of Myasthenia Gravis through research, education, public awareness, anf fundraising.

Wisconsin

6632 **Myasthenia Gravis Support Group of Fox Valley**
262-938-9800
Fax: 262-789-3363
wisconsin@myasthenia.org
www.myasthenia.org

Serves patients and their families throughout the state of Wisconsin. The goal is to help achieve the conquest of Myasthenia Gravis through research, education, public awareness, anf fundraising.

6633 **Myasthenia Gravis Support Group of Milwaukee**
262-878-3866
Fax: 262-789-3363
mmcb1981@yahoo.com
www.myasthenia.org
Serves patients and their families throughout the state of Wisconsin. The goal is to help achieve the conquest of Myasthenia Gravis through research, education, public awareness, anf fundraising.

Newsletters

6634 **Alabama Chapter of the Myasthenia Gravis Foundation of America**
Alabama Chapter of the Myasthenia Gravis Found
300 Office Park Drive
Birmingham, AL 35223
205-868-1210
Fax: 205-868-1211
alchaptermgfa@aol.com
Three to four newsletters per year. Support Group Information, articles about MG and it's treatment, information about chapters operations.

6635 **Connecticut Nutmeg**
Myasthenia Gravis Foundation
113 Folly Brook Boulevard
Wethersfield, CT 06109
860-529-8784
Fax: 860-529-8784

6636 **Conquer**
Myasthenia Gravis Foundation of Illinois
2411 New Street
Blue Island, IL 60406-2328
708-385-3888
800-888-6208
Fax: 708-385-0447
myastheniaill@aol.com
myastheniagravis.org
A quarterly newsletter containing articles and stories relating to myasthenia gravis.
16 pages Quarterly
Gerald Tarka, Executive Director

6637 **East Central Florida Chapter of the Myasthenia Gravis Foundation of America**
PO Box 623
Ormond Beach, FL 32175-0623
904-672-2635
Published bi-monthly, and contains information about latest research. area meetings, and topics of concern for our readers.

6638 **Facts About Myasthenia Gravis for Patients and Families**
Myasthenia Gravis Foundation of America
5841 Cedar Lake Road
Minneapolis, MN 55416
952-545-9438
800-541-5454
Fax: 952-646-2028
myastheniagravis@msn.com
www.myasthenia.org
Offers information on the history, clinical symptoms and features, causes, diagnosis, treatment and prognosis of Myasthenia Gravis.
16 pages 4 per year
Debora K Boelz, CEO
Jennifer Heidelberger, Chapter Relations Manager

6639 **MG Communicator**
Great Lakes Chapter of the Myasthenia Gravis Found
2680 Horizon Drive SE
Grand Rapids, MI 49546
616-956-0622
800-224-9180
Fax: 616-956-9234
myasthenia.info@gmail.com
www.myasthenia-mi.org
3x/year
Susan Richards, Executive Director
Paulus Heule, President

6640 **Myasthenia Gravis Foundation: Geater South Texas**
10592 A Fuqua
Houston, TX 77089-1402
281-987-9393
Fax: 281-328-2430
Six issues per year. Support Group Information, articles about MG and it's treatment, information about Chapter operations.
Gary Owens, Chair

6641 Myasthenia Gravis Foundation: Northwest Texas Chapter
281 County Road 135   nwtxmg@hotmail.com
Ovalo, TX 79541
A quarterly newsletter containing articles and stories relating myasthenia gravis.
Jenne McVicker, Editor

6642 Puget Sound Chapter Newsletter
PO Box 587853   206-235-1435
Renton, WA 98058-1785   Fax: 206-204-2070
A quarterly newsletter containing the latest articles and stories relating to myasthenia gravis.

Web Sites

6643 Healing Well
www.healingwell.com
An online health resource guide to medical news, chat, information and articles, newsgroups and message boards, books, disease-related web sites, medical directories, and more for patients, friends, and family coping with disabling diseases, disorders, or chronic illnesses.

6644 Health Finder
www.healthfinder.gov
Searchable, carefully developed web site offering information on over 1000 topics. Developed by the US Department of Health and Human Services, the site can be used in both English and Spanish.

6645 Healthlink USA
www.healthlinkusa.com
Health information concerning treatment, cures, prevention, diagnosis, risk factors, research, support groups, email lists, personal stories and much more. Updated regularly.

6646 MedicineNet
www.medicinenet.com
An online resource for consumers providing easy-to-read, authoritative medical and health information.

6647 Medscape
www.medscape.com
Medscape offers specialists, primary care physicians, and other health professionals the Web's most robust and integrated medical information and educational tools.

6648 Myasthenia Gravis Foundation of America
www.myasthenia.org
The Myasthenia Gravis Foundation of America (MGFA) is a national volunteer health agency in the United States dedicated solely to the fight against myasthenia gravis. MGFA serves patients, their families and caregivers through a network of chapters, support groups and programs. Each chapter shares the vision of a world without MG.

6649 Neurology Channel
www.healthcommunities.com
Find clearly explained, medically accurate information regarding conditions, including an overview, symptoms, causes, diagnostic procedures and treatment options. On this site it is possible to ask questions and get information from a neurologist and connect to people who have similar health interests.

6650 WebMD
www.webmd.com
Provides credible information, supportive communities, and in-depth reference material about health subjects. A source for original and timely health information as well as material from well known content providers.

Description

6651 Neurofibromatosis

Neurofibromatosis, or von Recklinghausen disease, named after a German pathologist, is a cluster of related disorders with similar clinical manifestations and an inherited genetic basis. The more common form (type 1) occurs once in 2,500-3,000 births. Type 1 neurofibromatosis results from mutations in the NF1 gene, which encodes the Neurofibromin protein. Type 2 neurofibromatosis results from mutations in the NF2 gene, which encodes Merlin protein, and main causes acoustic neuromas. The third type of neurofibromatosis is called schwannomatosis and results from mutations in the SMARCB1 gene. Schwannomatosis is similar to type 2 neurofibromatosis, but it results from mutations in two distinct genes and the clinical profile of each disease is distinct. The skin and the nervous system are the primary target organs. Characteristic skin lesions are large, flat brown freckles, called cafe au lait spots, owing to their light coffee color. They are apparent at birth or in infancy in more than 90 percent of patients. Flesh-colored tumors appear in late childhood. Abnormal growths may be detectable in the brain, perhaps accounting for the seizures and learning difficulties commonly seen in this syndrome. Tumors may appear on the nerves from the eyes or the ears, sometimes causing hearing loss or visual disturbance. Skeletal deformities may also be present in type 1 neurofibromatosis, and children with type 1 neurofibromastosis may have juvenile myelomonocytic leukemia and muscle tumorscalled rhabdomysarcomas.

There is no specific therapy for this condition, but tumors that produce severe symptoms can be surgically removed or irradiated. Genetic counseling is important for the entire family.

National Agencies & Associations

6652 BC Centre for Ability
2805 Kingsway
Vancouver, BC, V5R-5H9
604-451-5511
778-328-1625
Fax: 604-451-5651
www.bc-cfa.org

Provides community-based services and resources to improve the lives of children, youth, and adults with disabilities and their families.
Joshua Myers, MSW, RSW, Executive Director
Paul McGuigan, President

6653 Children's Tumor Foundation
120 Wall Street
New York, NY 10005-3904
212-344-6633
800-323-7938
Fax: 212-747-0004
info@ctf.org
www.ctf.org

Dedicated to health and well being of individuals and families affected by the neurofibromatoses (NF).
Richard Horvitz, Chair
Annette Bakker, PhD, President

6654 Neurofibromatosis Network
213 S Wheaton Avenue
Wheaton, IL 60187
630-510-1115
800-942-6825
Fax: 630-510-8508
admin@nfnetwork.org
www.nfnetwork.org

A national non-profit organization providing support and services to NF families.
Ryan Geier, President
John Manth, Vice President

6655 Neurofibromatosis Society of Ontario
PO Box 91119 Bayview Village
Willowdale, Ontario, M2K-2Y6
866-843-6376
info@nfon.ca
www.nfon.ca

Supports individuals and families affected by NF, educates individuals, professionals, and the general public and supports NF research.
Lynne Leyland, Director
Gladys Hamilton, Director

State Agencies & Associations

Alabama

6656 NNFF Alabama Affiliate
1205 Branchwater Lane
Birmingham, AL 35216
205-529-8006
info@ctf.org
www.ctf.org

Jeff Albright, Chairperson

Arizona

6657 Neurofibromatosis Association of Arizona
Po Box 2718
Chandler, AZ 85244
480-945-9650
Fax: 480-945-9650
Nicole Hicks, Executive Director
Michael Sheedy, President

Arkansas

6658 NNFF Arkansas Affilaite
139 Rainbow Lne
Bigelow, AR 72016
501-759-2710
info@ctf.org
www.ctf.org

Lesley Oslica, Information and Support

Colorado

6659 NNFF Colorado Chapter
70 N Ranch Road
Littleton, CO 80127
303-734-9942
info@ctf.org
www.ctf.org

Mark Ebel, Chapter President

Connecticut

6660 NNFF Connecticut Chapter
8 S Barn Hill Road
Bloomfield, CT 06002-1622
860-286-2705
Fax: 860-286-2705
TTY: 860-286-2705
TDD: 860-286-2705
StevenSand@aol.com

Steve Sandler, Chapter President

Florida

6661 NNFF Florida Chapter
PO Box 410684
Melbourne, FL 32941
321-253-1622
800-540-5721
info@ctf.org
www.ctf.org

Suzanne Earle, Chapter President

Georgia

6662 NNFF Georgia Affiliate
5 Ardmore Circle
Cartersville, GA 30120

678-428-9711
info@ctf.org
www.ctf.org

Randy Watkins, Chairman

Idaho

6663 NNFF Idaho Chapter
4419 E Linden Street
Caldwell, ID 83605-8037

208-459-6022

Suzy Crici, Chapter President

Illinois

6664 Illinois Midwest Neurofibromatosis
Neurofibromatosis
473 Dunham Rd
St. Charles, IL 60174

630-945-3562
800-322-6363
Fax: 630-932-8119
info@nfmidwest.org
nfmidwest.org

Diana Haberkamp, Executive Director
Jenny Perkins, Development Director/ Great Steps

6665 NF Center: North Broward Medical Center Neurofibromatosis
Neurofibromatosis
213 S. Wheaton Ave.
Wheaton, IL 60187-3502

630-510-1115
800-942-6825
Fax: 630-510-8508
admin@nfnetwork.org
www.nfnetwork.org

6666 NNFF Illinois Chapter: Chicago Area
5604 W Henderson 3 W
Chicago, IL 60634

info@ctf.org
www.ctf.org

Debbi Callahan, Vice President

6667 NNFF Illinois Chapter: Silvis Area
513 16th Street
Silvis, IL 61282

309-792-4195

Sue Rockwell, Patient Information and Support

6668 NNFF Illinois Chapter: Springfield Area
5 Twilight Lane
Springfield, IL 62712

217-529-0834
info@ctf.org
www.ctf.org

Marcia Miller, Treasurer

6669 NNFF Illinois Chapter:Peoria Region
PO Box 213
Emden, IL 62635

217-732-8568
info@ctf.org
www.ctf.org

Paul Beach, President

Indiana

6670 NNFF Indiana Chapter
1173 Hague Court
Franklinolis, IN 46131

317-736-7577
info@ctf.org
www.ctf.org

Dottie Whitehurst, Chapter President

Iowa

6671 NNFF Iowa Chapter
321 Glenview Drive
De Moines, IA 50312

515-277-8494
info@ctf.org
www.ctf.org

Sheila Drevyanko, Chapter President

Kansas

6672 NNFF Kansas Affiliate
12606 E 49th Terrace
Independence, MO 64055

816-737-8378
info@ctf.org
www.ctf.org

Annette Novak, Chairperson

6673 Neurofibromatosis Kansas and Central Plains
Neurofibromatosis
9218 Metcalf
Overland Park, KS 66212-1792

620-669-8453
800-942-6825
nprieb@sbcglobal.net
www.nfnetwork.org

Louisiana

6674 NNFF Louisiana Chapter
PO Box 499
Baton Rouge, LA 70821

225-665-3547
info@ctf.org
www.ctf.org

Debbie Bouy, Chairperson

Maryland

6675 Neurofibromatosis: Mid-Atlantic
Neurofibromatosis
2 Village Square.
Baltimore, MD 21210-2924

443-423-0535
800-942-6825
Fax: 301-577-0016
www.nfmidatlantic.org

Mid-Atlantic Chapter serves the following states: Maryland Virginia District of Columbia Delaware New Jersey Pennsylvania West Virginia and North Carolina.
Barbra Levin, Executive Director
Beverly B Dobson, President

Massachusetts

6676 Neurofibromatosis: New England
Neurofibromatosis
9 Bedford Street
Burlington, MA 01803-3702

781-272-9936
Fax: 781-272-9937
info@nfincne.org
www.nfincne.org

Karen Peluso, Executive Director
Dr Paul Epstein, President

Minnesota

6677 Neurofibromatosis: Minnesota
Neurofibromatosis
PO Box 18246
Minneapolis, MN 55418

651-225-1720

John Everett, President
Steven Schutts, Vice-President

Nevada

6678 NNFF Nevada Affiliate: Reno Area
8065 White Falls Drive
Reno, NV 89506

775-972-1882
info@ctf.org
www.ctf.org

David Rice, Chairperson

Oregon

6679 NNFF Oregon Affiliate Kaiser Permanente Northwest
Kaiser Permanente Northwest
2806 SW Troy
Portland, OR 97227

503-331-6325
Fax: 503-331-6320
info@ctf.org
www.ctf.org

Katie Crow, Genetic Counselor

South Carolina

6680 NNFF South Carolina Chapter
111 Oakview Drive
Darlington, SC 29532

843-393-9672
info@ctf.org
www.ctf.org

Pat Chrisely, Chairperson

6681 NNFF Wisconsin Chapter
6562 W Glenbrook Road
Brown Deer, WI 53223
414-362-0211
info@ctf.org
www.ctf.org

Elaine Pankow, President

Support Groups & Hotlines

6682 Children's Tumor Foundation
95 Pine Street
New York, NY 10005
212-344-6633
800-323-7938
Fax: 212-747-0004
info@ctf.org
www.ctf.org

Sponsors critical research, public awareness and patient support services.
Allison Walsh, Communications Officer

6683 NF Support Group of West Michigan
Spectrum Health
PO Box 6026
Grand Rapids, MI 49516
616-451-3699
nfwestmich@aol.com
www.nfsupport.org

Rose Mary Anderson, Patient Advocate

6684 National Health Information Center
Office of Disease Prevention & Health Promotion
1101 Wootton Pkwy
Rockville, MD 20852
Fax: 240-453-8281
odphpinfo@hhs.gov
www.health.gov/nhic
Supports public health education by maintaining a calendar of National Health Observances; helps connect consumers and health professionals to organizations that can best answer questions and provide up-to-date contact information from reliable sources; updates on a yearly basis toll-free numbers for health information, Federal health clearinghouses and info centers.
Don Wright, MD, MPH, Director

6685 Neurofibromatosis
9320 Annapolis Road
Lanham, MD 20706-3123
301-918-4600
800-942-6825
Fax: 301-918-0009
www.nfnetwork.org
Dedicated to individuals and families affected by the neurofibromatosis through educational, support, clinical and research programs.
Miguell Lessing, President
Rosemary Anderson, Vice President

6686 Neurofibromatosis Foundation: Colorado
2505 18th Street, Denver
Denver, CO 80211
303-433-8383
800-323-7938
UsRKids@aol.com
www.unitedwaydenver.org
Offers a support group to persons affected by neurofibromatosis. Offers panel discussion, sharing, fundraising, and fun activities. Also provides new patient information.
Charles Taylor
Jane Cahn

6687 Neurofibromatosis Support Network
Parents Helping Parents
1400 Parkmoor Avenue
San Jose, CA 95126
408-727-5775
855-727-5775
Fax: 408-286-1116
www.php.com
Helping children with special needs receive the resources, love, hope, respect, health care, education and other services they need to achieve their full potential by providing them with strong families and dedicated professionals to serve them.
Sheri Sobrato, MA/MFC

6688 Neuroscience Institute at Mercy Hospital
4120N W Memorial Road
Oklahoma City, OK 73120
800-996-3729
Fax: 405-752-3977
Mike Patt, Chief Executive Officer

6689 Texas Neurofibromatosis Foundation
3030 Olive Street
Dallas, TX 75219
972-868-794
Fax: 972-868-7626
www.texasnf.org

Cindy Hahn, Executive Director
Emily Deutscher, Development Coordinator

Newsletters

6690 Neurofibromatosis
213 S. Wheaton Ave.
Wheaton, IL 60187-3123
630-510-1115
800-942-6825
Fax: 630-510-8508
admin@nfnetwork.org
www.nfnetwork.org

Provides a variety of resources for NF families, professionals and researchers.
SemiAnnual
Gwen Charest, Executive Director

Pamphlets

6691 Child with Neurofibromatosis 1
Children's Tumor Foundation
120 Wall Street
New York, NY 10005-1703
212-344-6633
800-323-7938
info@ctf.org
www.ctf.org
Offers information on the prognosis, management, complications, genetic implications, and sources of support for children with neurofibromatosis 1.
Allison Walsh, Communications Officer

6692 Guide for Teens
Children's Tumor Foundation
120 Wall Street
New York, NY 10005-1703
212-344-6633
800-323-7938
info@ctf.org
www.ctf.org
Offers information for teenagers on how to face neurofibromatosis on a daily basis.
Allison Walsh, Communications Officer

6693 How NF-1 Affects the Body
Neurofibromatosis
213 S. Wheaton Ave.
Wheaton, IL 60187-3123
630-510-1115
800-942-6825
Fax: 630-510-8508
admin@nfnetwork.org
www.nfnetwork.org
A graphic showing the parts of the body where symptoms of NF-1 can occur.
Gwen Charest, Executive Director

6694 How NF-2 Affects the Body
Neurofibromatosis
213 S. Wheaton Ave.
Wheaton, IL 60187-3123
630-510-1115
800-942-6825
Fax: 630-510-8508
admin@nfnetwork.org
www.nfnetwork.org
A graphic showing the parts of the body where symptoms of NF-2 can occur.
Gwen Charest, Executive Director

6695 National NF Medical Resource Listing
Neurofibromatosis
213 S. Wheaton Ave.
Wheaton, IL 60187-3123
630-510-1115
800-942-6825
Fax: 630-510-8508
admin@nfnetwork.org
www.nfnetwork.org
A listing of medical centers in the US where geneticists and NF experts are located.
Gwen Charest, Executive Director

6696 Neurofibromatosis
March of Dimes

1275 Mamaroneck Avenue
White Plains, NY 10605

914-997-4488
Fax: 212-254-3518
NY639@marchofdimes.com
www.marchofdimes.com

Located on the website.

6697 Neurofibromatosis Type 2: Information for Patients and Families
Children's Tumor Foundation
120 Wall Street
New York, NY 10005-1703

212-344-6633
800-323-7938
info@ctf.org
www.ctf.org

Offers extensive information on what NF2 is and answers the most asked about questions regarding the illness.
Allison Walsh, Communications Officer

6698 Understanding Neurofibromatosis
213 S. Wheaton Ave.
Wheaton, IL 60187-3123

630-510-1115
800-942-6825
Fax: 630-510-8508
admin@nfnetwork.org
www.nfnetwork.org

A handbook specifically designed for the newly diagnosed NF families.
Gwen Charest, Executive Director

Web Sites

6699 Healing Well

www.healingwell.com

An online health resource guide to medical news, chat, information and articles, newsgroups and message boards, books, disease-related web sites, medical directories, and more for patients, friends, and family coping with disabling diseases, disorders, or chronic illnesses.

6700 Health Finder

www.healthfinder.gov

Searchable, carefully developed web site offering information on over 1000 topics. Developed by the US Department of Health and Human Services, the site can be used in both English and Spanish.

6701 Healthlink USA

www.healthlinkusa.com

Health information concerning treatment, cures, prevention, diagnosis, risk factors, research, support groups, email lists, personal stories and much more. Updated regularly.

6702 MGH Neurology

www.mgh.harvard.edu

Provides both unmonderated message boards and chat rooms for specific neurological disorders including: amyloidosis, arachnoiditis, cerebellar ataxia, congenital fiber type disproportion, CFS leak, DeMorsiers syndrome, erythromealgia, Lewy body disease, meningitis, meralgia paresthetic, Norrie disease, periodic paralysis, phantom limb pain, Romberg disorder, Syndenhams chorea, tethered cord syndrome, and thoracic outlet syndrome.

6703 MedicineNet

www.medicinenet.com

An online resource for consumers providing easy-to-read, authoritative medical and health information.

6704 Medscape

www.medscape.com

Medscape offers specialists, primary care physicians, and other health professionals the Web's most robust and integrated medical information and educational tools.

6705 Neurology Channel

www.healthcommunities.com

Find clearly explained, medically accurate information regarding conditions, including an overview, symptoms, causes, diagnostic procedures and treatment options. On this site it is possible to ask questions and get information from a neurologist and connect to people who have similar health interests.

6706 WebMD

www.webmd.com

Provides credible information, supportive communities, and in-depth reference material about health subjects. A source for original and timely health information as well as material from well known content providers.

Description

6707 Obesity

Obesity refers to a condition in which there is an excessive accumulation of fat in subcutaneous and other tissues of the body. Being obese and being overweight are not necessarily synonymous, as people who are overweight may have increased body size as a result of increased muscle or skeletal tissue mass. Obesity may develop at any age, but peak development periods occur during the first 12 months of life, between the ages of five and six years, and during the adolescent years in children. In adults, obesity may develop at any time, but many people may find that weight gain progresses through the 3rd-6th decade. It is clear from numerous medial, public health and sociologic studies that obesity in the United States occurs in a staggering proportion of the population and many consider it to be an epidemic.

Obesity may result from an increase in the actual number of fat cells or from an increase in the size of the individual fat cells. Researchers believe that fat cells increase in number in proportion to caloric intake increase and that this increase is particularly evident in the first 12 months of life. As children grow, increases in fat cell populations continue at a slower rate. Because the number of fat cells cannot be decreased, except surgically, later weight loss must result from the reduction of fat in individual fat-storing cells (adipocytes).

Obesity usually results when caloric intake exceeds the energy demands of the body, thus increasing the storage of body fat. Fat accumulation is usually a progressive process, resulting from repeated episodes of food intake exceeding the body's demand for energy (calories). Many factors may influence appetite or obesity. Such factors may include environmental influences; psychosocial disturbances that may be induced by stress or emotional upset or trauma; brain lesions that may involve certain area of the brain such as the hypothalamus or the pituitary gland (both essential to hormone production); an overabundance of insulin in the body (hyperinsulinism); and genetic influences. In addition, in rare instances, obesity may be a feature of certain genetic disorders (see *Prader-Willi syndrome*). The most common cause in North America however, is the excessive intake of calories, particularly those from fats and sugars, and the concomitant lack of physical exercise and activity that uses calories.

Complications of obesity in the child and the adult may include respiratory difficulties such as shortness of breath and increased cardiovascular risk factors such as high blood pressure, elevated total cholesterol levels as well as increased bad or LDL cholesterol and decreased good or HDL cholesterol, and increased levels of fatty acid and glycerol compounds (triglycerides). These are risk factors for the development of coronary artery disease, one of the leading causes of morbidity and the mortality in North America. In addition, obesity may be associated with a resistance to the hormone insulin that aids in the metabolism of glucose, fats, carbohydrates, and proteins. This resistance may lead to excessive levels of circulating insulin in the body (hyperinsulinism); however, the body is not able to appropriately use insulin and high blood sugar (hyperglycemia) may occur. This condition is known as Type II diabetes mellitus and its incidence in the population is also increasing dramatically in both children and adults. The diagnosis of obesity in children, adolescents and adults is usually determined through the use of certain screening methods such as measurement of the body mass index (BMI) as well as the triceps skinfold thickness.

Patterns of behavior that may lead to obesity may be established as early as infancy. For example, if parents or caregivers persistently use a bottle to pacify a crying baby, the baby may learn that food is equivalent to relief of stress. Treatment for obesity should include the cooperation and support of the entire family and may be directed toward psychological considerations, as well as proper exercise and nutrition to psychological and emotional needs may include behavior modification, as well as individual and family counseling. Medications for weight loss can produce short-term weight loss and include orlistat, which inhibits fat digestion and absorption and appetite suppressants (phentermine/topiramate, loracaserin, bupropion/naltrexone, and liraglutide). Vagal blocking device, gastric aspiration device, and gastric balloons also produce short-term weight loss. Studies have shown that bariatric surgery is the most effective treatment for long-term weight loss and reduction of obesity-related comorbidities. See also *Eating Disorders*.

National Agencies & Associations

6708 Active Healthy Kids Canada

416-913-0238
888-446-7432
Fax: 416-913-1541
www.activehealthykids.ca

Advocates the importance of quality, accessible, and enjoyable physical activity participation exercises for children and youth.

6709 American Obesity Treatment Association

117 Anderson Court
Dothan, AL 36303

334-403-4057
info@americanobesity.org
americanobesity.org

Provides obesity awareness and prevention information.
Cesar Cuneo, President & Founder
Gonzalo Tovar, Vice President

6710 National Association to Advance Fat Acceptance (NAAFA)
PO Box 4662 916-558-6880
Foster City, CA 94404-0662 naafa@naafa.org
www.naafaonline.com/dev2/
Non-profit organization committed to improving the lives of fat individuals and reducing discrimination.
Darliene Howell, Board Chair & Secretary
Peggy Howell, Vice Chair & Public Relations Director

6711 Obesity Canada
2-126 Li Ka Shing Center for Health 780-492-8361
Edmonton, Alberta, T6G-2E1 info@obesitynetwork.ca
www.obesitycanada.ca
An organization of researchers, clinicians and other health professionals dedicated to reducing the mental, physical and economic burden of obesity in Canadians.
Kelly Isfan, President & CEO
Feria Bacchus, MHSc, Managing Director

6712 Overeaters Anonymous
6075 Zenith Court NE 505-891-2664
Rio Rancho, NM 87144-6424 Fax: 505-891-4320
www.oa.org
A fellowship of individuals who meet in order to help solve their eating behaviors.

6713 Research Chair in Obesity Universit, Laval
2725 Chemin Sainte-Foy 418-656-8711
Quebec, Canada, G1V-4G5 Fax: 418-656-4929
obesity.chair@crhl.ulaval.ca
www.obesity.ulaval.ca
Shares communication about nutrition, energy metabolism, obesity, lipid metabolism and cardiovascular research. Provides continuing education about obesity to health professionals, physicians and to the public regarding the causes, the complications and the treatment of obesity.
Denis Richard, PhD, Chair

6714 Weight-Control Information Network
National Institutes of Health
31 Center Drive 800-860-8747
Bethesda, MD 20892-2560 TTY: 866-569-1162
healthinfo@niddk.nih.gov
www.win.niddk.nih.gov
WIN provides the general public, health professionals, and the media with up-to-date, science-based information on obesity, weight control, physical activity, and related nutritional issues.

Libraries & Resource Centers

6715 Weight-Control Information Network
National Institutes of Health
31 Center Drive 800-860-8747
Bethesda, MD 20892-2560 TTY: 866-569-1162
healthinfo@niddk.nih.gov
www.win.niddk.nih.gov
WIN provides the general public, health professionals, and the media with up-to-date, science-based information on obesity, weight control, physical activity, and related nutritional issues. WIN provides tip sheets, fact sheets, and brochures for a range of audiences. Some of WIN's content is available in Spanish.

Research Centers

6716 Harvard Clinical Nutrition Research Center
Harvard Medical School 617-998-8803
Boston, MA 02215 Fax: 617-998-8804
allan_walker@hms.harvard.edu
nutrition.med.harvard.edu
Mission is to derive the benefit of continuity in assessing the effectiveness of the Center from year to year while still allowing flexibility for new insights as the Center's activities evolve.
W Allan Walker, Director
George Blackburn, Associate Director

6717 Minnesota Obesity Center
1334 Eckles Avenue 763-807-0559
St Paul, MN 55108 mnoc@tc.umn.edu

Mission is to find ways to prevent weight gain obesity and its complications. The Center incorporates 46 Participating Investigators who are studying the causes and treatments of obesity. Provides the general public with a source of information on the happenings of the Center and on the current developments in the field of obesity.
Catherine C Welch, Program Coordinator

6718 New York Obesity/Nutrition Research Center
31 Center Drive MSC 2560 301-496-3583
Bethesda, MD 20892-2560 www2.niddk.nih.gov
Griffin P Rodgers, Director

6719 Obesity Research Center St. Luke's-Roosevelt Hospital
St. Luke's-Roosevelt Hospital
1090 Amsterdam Avenue 212-523-4196
New York, NY 10025 Fax: 212-523-3416
dg108@columbia.edu
The mission of the New York Obesity Research Center is to help reduce the incidence of obesity and related diseases through leadership in basic research clinical research epidemiology and public health patient care and public education.
Dr Xavier Pi-Sunyer, Director
Janet Crane, Dietitians

Support Groups & Hotlines

6720 Greater New York Metro Intergroup of Overeaters Anonymous
Madison Square Station 212-946-4599
New York, NY 10159-1235 office@oanyc.org
www.oanyc.org

Tom M, Chairman
Raina M, Vice chairman

6721 National Health Information Center
Office of Disease Prevention & Health Promotion
1101 Wootton Pkwy Fax: 240-453-8281
Rockville, MD 20852 odphpinfo@hhs.gov
www.health.gov/nhic
Supports public health education by maintaining a calendar of National Health Observances; helps connect consumers and health professionals to organizations that can best answer questions and provide up-to-date contact information from reliable sources; updates on a yearly basis toll-free numbers for health information, Federal health clearinghouses and info centers.
Don Wright, MD, MPH, Director

6722 Office of Chronic Disease Prevention and Nutrition Services
Obesity Prevention Program
150 N. 18th Avenue 602-542-1025
Phoenix, AZ 85007 Fax: 602-542-0883
Mission is to improve the health and quality of life of Arizona residents by reducing the incidence and severity of chronic disease and obesity through physical activity and nutrition interventions.
Renae Cunnien, Program Manager

Books

6723 An Atlas of Obesity and Weight Control
George A. Bray, author

212-216-7800
Fax: 212-564-7854
odphpinfo@hhs.gov
www.health.gov/dietaryguidelines/
This informative guide is a clearly written, beautifully illustrated color atlas on obesity, including its etiology, development and treatment. Contains nearly 150 clinical pictures of obesity and its related conditions, as well as many pertinent clinical guidelines and up-to-the-minute data on assessment and treatment.
135 pages

6724 Dietary Guidelines for Americans 2005
U.S. Government Printing Office

200 Indep. Ave, S.W.
Washington, DC 20201

202-619-0257
877-696-6775
odphpinfo@hhs.gov
www.health.gov/dietaryguidelines/

80 pages
Tommy G. Thompson, HHS-Secretary
Ann M. Veneman, USDA-Secretary

6725 Encyclopedia of Obesity and Eating Disorders
Facts on File
11 Penn Plaza
New York, NY 10001

212-967-8800
800-322-8755
Fax: 800-678-3633

From abdominoplasty to Zung Rating Scale, this volume defines and explains these disorders, along with medical and other problems associated with them.
272 pages Hardcover

6726 Handbook of Obesity Treatment
Guilford Press
370 Seventh Avenue
New York, NY 10001

800-365-7006
Fax: 212-966-6708
info@guilford.com
www.guilford.com

This comprehensive handbook guides mental, medical, and allied health professionals through the process of planning and delivering individualized treatment services for those seeking help for Obesity.
2001 624 pages Hardcover
ISBN: 1-572307-22-6

6727 Obesity
National Academies Press
500 Fifth Street, NW
Washington, DC 20001

202-334-3313
888-624-8373
Fax: 202-334-2451
www.nap.edu

A ground breaking report on childhood obesity providing indepth background and instructive case studies that illustrate just how serious and widespread the problem is; gives honest, authorative, based advice that consitute our best weapons in this critical battle.
280 pages

6728 Overeaters Anonymous
World Service Office
6075 Zenith Court NE
Rio Rancho, NM 87144-6807

505-891-2664
Fax: 505-891-4320
www.oa.org

World Service Office offers literature, provides information or meetings world wide.
204 pages Hardcover

6729 Preventing Childhood Obesity: Health in the Balance
National Academies Press
500 Fifth Street NW
Washington, DC 20001

202-334-3313
888-624-8373
Fax: 202-334-2451
www.nap.edu

Provides a broad-based examination of the nature, extent, and consequences of obesity. Also explores the underlying causes of this serious health problem and the actions needed to initiate support, and sustain the societal and lifestyle changes that can reverse the trend among our children and youth.
436 pages
ISBN: 0-309091-96-9

6730 Shape Up America!
6707 Democracy Boulevard
Bethesda, MD 20817

www.shapeup.org

A high profile national initiative to promote healthy weight and increased physical activity in America. Involves a broad based coalition of industry, medical/health, nutrition, physical fitness, and related organizations and experts.
C. Everett Koop, Founder
Barbara J. Moore, President And CEO

6731 Understanding Childhood Obesity
J Clinton Smith, MD, author
University Press of Mississippi

3825 Ridgewood Road
Jackson, MS 39211-6492

601-432-6205
800-737-7788
Fax: 601-432-6217
press@ihl.state.ms.us
www.upress.state.ms.us

A clear explanation of causes, diagnosis, and treatment of childhood obesity.
1999 120 pages Paperback
ISBN: 1-578061-34-2
Kathy Burgess, Advertising/Marketing Services Manager

6732 Understanding Obesity: The Five Medical Causes
Lance Levy, author
Firefly Books Ltd
50 Staples Avenue
Richmond Hill, Ontario, L4B-1H1

416-499-8412
Fax: 416-499-1142
www.fireflybooks.com

An authoritative book that focuses on the causes of, and the treatment for, obesity. Obesity is usually related to other health problems and treatment for them is the first step.
200 pages

Children's Books

6733 I Was a Fifteen-Year-Old Blimp
Harper & Row
10 E 53rd Street
New York, NY 10022-5299

212-207-7000

This story focuses on Gabby, a teenage girl who overhears others discuss her weight and takes radical steps to become popular.
Grades 6-9

Magazines

6734 CheckUp
Medical University of South Carolina
67 President Street
Charleston, SC 29425

843-792-2273
800-424-6872
Fax: 843-792-5432
www.muschealth.com/weight

Provides health information about screenings, treatments, medical advances and services available through MUSC, as well as advice about nutrition and prevention.
Susan Kammeraad-Campbell, Managing Editor
Damon Simmons, Art Director

6735 Official Journal of NAASO
NAASO
8757 Georgia Avenue
Silver Spring, MD 20910

301-563-6526
Fax: 301-563-6595
www.obesity.org

Promotes research, education and advocacy to better understand, prevent and treat obesity and improve the lives of those affected.
Barbara E. Corkey, Editor-In-Chief
Deborah Moskowitz, Managing Editor

6736 Progress Notes
Medical University of South Carolina
67 President Street
Charleston, SC 29425

843-792-2273
800-922-5250
Fax: 843-792-5432
www.muschealth.com/weight

Designed to inform the medical community developments at the Medical University of South Carolina and as a continuing medical education resource for practicing physicians and faculty.
Susan Kammeraad-Campbell, Managing Editor
Lynne Barber Associate Editor, Alex Sargent, Associate Editor

Newsletters

6737 Trim & Fit
Obesity Foundation
5600 S Quebec Street
Englewood, CO 80111-2202

303-850-0328

Offers nutrition facts and articles, low-fat recipes, medical information on heart disease and cancer relating to nutrition and more.
James F Merker CAE, Editor

Pamphlets

6738 About Overeaters Anonymous
Metro Intergroup of Overeaters Anonymous
6075 Zenith Court NE   212-206-8621
Rio Rancho, NM 87144-6807   Fax: 505-891-4320
                                                          www.oa.org
World Service Office offers literature, provides information or meetings world wide.

6739 An Inside View
Metro Intergroup of Overeaters Anonymous
6075 Zenith Court NE   212-206-8621
Rio Rancho, NM 87144-6807   Fax: 505-891-4320
                                                          www.oa.org
World Service Office offers literature, provides information or meetings world wide.

6740 Anonymity
Metro Intergroup of Overeaters Anonymous
6075 Zenith Court NE   212-206-8621
Rio Rancho, NM 87144-6807   Fax: 505-891-4320
                                                          www.oa.org
World Service Office offers literature, provides information or meetings world wide.

6741 Before You Take That First...
Metro Intergroup of Overeaters Anonymous
6075 Zenith Court NE   212-206-8621
Rio Rancho, NM 87144-6807   Fax: 505-891-4320
                                                          www.oa.org
World Service Office offers literature, provides information or meetings world wide.

6742 Compulsive Overeaters in the Military
Metro Intergroup of Overeaters Anonymous
6075 Zenith Court NE   212-206-8621
Rio Rancho, NM 87144-6807   Fax: 505-891-4320
                                                          www.oa.org
World Service Office offers literature, provides information or meetings world wide.

6743 Compulsive Overeating & Overaters Anonymous
Metro Intergroup of Overeaters Anonymous
6075 Zenith Court NE   212-206-8621
Rio Rancho, NM 87144-6807   Fax: 505-891-4320
                                                          www.oa.org
World Service Office offers literature, provides information or meetings world wide.

6744 For the Obese Employee
Metro Intergroup of Overeaters Anonymous
6075 Zenith Court NE   212-206-8621
Rio Rancho, NM 87144-6807   Fax: 505-891-4320
                                                          www.oa.org
World Service Office offers literature, provides information or meetings world wide.

6745 Guide to the 12 Steps for You
Metro Intergroup of Overeaters Anonymous
6075 Zenith Court NE   212-206-8621
Rio Rancho, NM 87144-6807   Fax: 505-891-4320
                                                          www.oa.org
World Service Office offers literature, provides information or meetings world wide.

6746 Hazelden Step Pamphlets for Overeaters
Hazelden
15251 Pleasant Valley Rd   651-213-4200
Center City, MN 55012-9640   800-328-9000
                                                 Fax: 651-213-4793
               customersupport@hazelden.org; www.hazelden.org
A 12 pamphlet collection that offers one person's interpretation of the Twelve Steps for overeaters.

6747 If God Spoke to Overeaters Anonymous
Metro Intergroup of Overeaters Anonymous
6075 Zenith Court NE   212-206-8621
Rio Rancho, NM 87144-6807   Fax: 505-891-4320
                                                          www.oa.org
World Service Office offers literature, provides information or meetings world wide.

6748 Many Symptoms, One Disease
Metro Intergroup of Overeaters Anonymous
6075 Zenith Court NE   212-206-8621
Rio Rancho, NM 87144-6807   Fax: 505-891-4320; www.oa.org
World Service Office offers literature, provides information or meetings world wide.

6749 Members in Relapse
Metro Intergroup of Overeaters Anonymous
6075 Zenith Court NE   212-206-8621
Rio Rancho, NM 87144-6807   Fax: 505-891-4320; www.oa.org
World Service Office offers literature, provides information or meetings world wide.

6750 One Day at a Time
Metro Intergroup of Overeaters Anonymous
6075 Zenith Court NE   212-206-8621
Rio Rancho, NM 87144-6807   Fax: 505-891-4320
                                                          www.oa.org
World Service Office offers literature, provides information or meetings world wide.

6751 Overeaters Anonymous Cares
Metro Intergroup of Overeaters Anonymous
6075 Zenith Court NE   212-206-8621
Rio Rancho, NM 87144-6807   Fax: 505-891-4320
                                                          www.oa.org
World Service Office offers literature, provides information or meetings world wide.

6752 Overeaters Anonymous is Not a Diet Club
Metro Intergroup of Overeaters Anonymous
6075 Zenith Court NE   212-206-8621
Rio Rancho, NM 87144-6807   Fax: 505-891-4320
                                                          www.oa.org
World Service Office offers literature, provides information or meetings world wide.

6753 Person to Person
Metro Intergroup of Overeaters Anonymous
6075 Zenith Court NE   212-206-8621
Rio Rancho, NM 87144-6807   Fax: 505-891-4320
                                                          www.oa.org
World Service Office offers literature, provides information or meetings world wide.

6754 Program of Recovery
Metro Intergroup of Overeaters Anonymous
6075 Zenith Court NE   212-206-8621
Rio Rancho, NM 87144-6807   Fax: 505-891-4320
                                                          www.oa.org
World Service Office offers literature, provides information or meetings world wide.

6755 Questions and Answers
Metro Intergroup of Overeaters Anonymous
6075 Zenith Court NE   212-206-8621
Rio Rancho, NM 87144-6807   Fax: 505-891-4320
                                                          www.oa.org
World Service Office offers literature, provides information or meetings world wide.

6756 So You've Reached Goal Weight
Metro Intergroup of Overeaters Anonymous
6075 Zenith Court NE   212-206-8621
Rio Rancho, NM 87144-6807   Fax: 505-891-4320
                                                          www.oa.org
World Service Office offers literature, provides information or meetings world wide.

6757 Think First...
Metro Intergroup of Overeaters Anonymous

6075 Zenith Court NE
Rio Rancho, NM 87144-6807

212-206-8621
Fax: 505-891-4320
www.oa.org

World Service Office offers literature, provides information or meetings world wide.

6758 To the Family
Metro Intergroup of Overeaters Anonymous
6075 Zenith Court NE
Rio Rancho, NM 87144-6807

212-206-8621
Fax: 505-891-4320
www.oa.org

World Service Office offers literature, provides information or meetings world wide.

6759 To the Man
Metro Intergroup of Overeaters Anonymous
6075 Zenith Court NE
Rio Rancho, NM 87144-6807

212-206-8621
Fax: 505-891-4320
www.oa.org

World Service Office offers literature, provides information or meetings world wide.

6760 To the Newcomer
Metro Intergroup of Overeaters Anonymous
6075 Zenith Court NE
Rio Rancho, NM 87144-6807

212-206-8621
Fax: 505-891-4320
www.oa.org

World Service Office offers literature, provides information or meetings world wide.

6761 To the Teen
Metro Intergroup of Overeaters Anonymous
6075 Zenith Court NE
Rio Rancho, NM 87144-6807

212-206-8621
Fax: 505-891-4320
www.oa.org

World Service Office offers literature, provides information or meetings world wide.

6762 Tools of Recovery
Metro Intergroup of Overeaters Anonymous
6075 Zenith Court NE
Rio Rancho, NM 87144-6807

212-206-8621
Fax: 505-891-4320
www.oa.org

World Service Office offers literature, provides information or meetings world wide.

6763 Twelve Traditions of Overeaters Anonymous
Metro Intergroup of Overeaters Anonymous
6075 Zenith Court NE
Rio Rancho, NM 87144-6807

212-206-8621
Fax: 505-891-4320
www.oa.org

World Service Office offers literature, provides information or meetings world wide.

6764 Welcome Back
Metro Intergroup of Overeaters Anonymous
6075 Zenith Court NE
Rio Rancho, NM 87144-6807

212-206-8621
Fax: 505-891-4320
www.oa.org

World Service Office offers literature, provides information or meetings world wide.

Audio & Video

6765 Obesity Online
NAASO

301-563-6526
www.obesity-online.com

Educational resource for clinicians, researchers and educators with an interest in obesity and its related disorders.
Samuel Klein, Editor
Christie M. Ballantyne, Editor

Web Sites

6766 Boston Obesity Nutrition Research Center (BONRC)
www.bmc.org

Provides resources and support for studies in the area of obesity and nutrition. Comprised of four research cores located within the Boston area. In the areas of adipocytes, epidemiology and statistics, body composition, energy expenditure and genetic analyses, and transgenic animal models.

6767 Center for Human Nutrition
A interdisciplinary team encompassing basic and clinical research, post-graduate training and career development of nutrition professionals, and commuity outreach. The research conducted at the CHN focuses on obesity prevention and treatment, nutrient metabolism, and micronutrient status in children. Activities conducted aim to improve the quallity of life by promoting physical activity and nutritional awareness.

6768 Clinical Nutrition Research Unit (CNRU)
Promotes and enhances the interdisciplinary nutrition research and education at the Univeristy of Washington. By providing a number of Core Facilities, the CNRU attempts to integrate and coordinate the abundant ongoing activities with the goals of fostering new interdiscilinary research collaborations, stimulating new research activities, improving nutrition education at multiple levels, and facilitating the nutritional management of patients.

6769 MedicineNet
www.medicinenet.com

An online resource for consumers providing easy-to-read, authoritative medical and health information.

6770 New York Obesity/Nutrition Research Center (ONRC)
www.niddk.nih.gov

Funded by the National Institute of Diabetes and Digestive and Kidney Diseases (NIDDK). A combined effort of Columbia ane Cornell Universities. Provides participating investigators of funded projects relevant to obesity research with valuable laboratory, technical, and educational services that otherwise would not be available to them, thereby improving the productivity an efficiency of their operations.

6771 North American Association for the Study of Obesity
www.obesity.org

The leading scientific society dedicated to the study of obesity. Committed to encouraging research on the causes and treatment of obesity, and to keeping the medical community and public informed of new advances.

6772 Research Chair on Obesity
obesity.chair.ulaval.ca

Ever since 1997, the Research Chair in Obesity is dedicated to support and launch initiatives leading to a better understanding of obesity through research on the mechanisms of body weight regulation, to facilitate communication between researchers, to promote the training of highly qualified personnel, to contribute to continuing education for health professionals, and to inform the public on the causes, consequences, treatments, and prevention of obesity.

6773 University of Pittsburgh Obesity/Nutrition Research Center
Goal is to develop more effective interventions for the prevention and treatment of obesity. Exists to support research functions for investigators studying the broad areas of obesity and nutrition. Focuses on behavioral aspects of obesity and behavioral treatment of this disease.

6774 Vanderbilt Clinical Nutrition Research Unit (CNRU)
A core center grant funded by the National Institute of Diabetes and Digestive and Kidney Diseases (NIDDK). Nutrition research is carried out by faculty members i most academic departments and extends from basic laboratory research to clinical and applied research. Maintains service facilities to support both basic and clinical research. Supports research cores that bring nutrition investigators together to discuss their work.

6775 Weight-Control Information Network
www.win.niddk.nih.gov

The Weight-control Information Network (WIN) provides the general public, health professionals, and the media with up-to-date, science-based information on obesity, weight control, physical activity, and related nutritional issues. WIN provides tip sheets, fact sheets, and brochures for a range of audiences. Some of WIN's content is available in Spanish.

Description

6776 Osteogenesis Imperfecta

Osteogenesis imperfecta, OI, often called "brittle bone" disease, is a group of serious genetic disorders that are characterized by abnormally fragile bones that break or fracture easily. There are at least eight distinct forms of the disorder, with neonatal (congenital) being the most severe. A person with OI has either less collagen, the major protein of the connective tissue, including bone, or a poorer quality collagen. Infants born with OI may have multiple bone fractures and hearing loss, and routine vaginal delivery may lead to significant bone fractures, hemorrhage into the brain and other major problems. Survivors develop shortened extremities and other bony abnormalities. If no injury to the brain occurs then mental and intellectual function should be unaffected. Hearing loss may occur.

At present, there is no effective treatment for this disorder. Careful handling of these infants is essential. Gentle exercise and physical therapy are directed at preventing fractures and increasing function. Surgical implants can provide stability to the skeletal structure. Genetic counseling is also important. Stem cell transplantations in laboratory animals have improved bone density and architecture, but this approach remains experimental presently.

National Agencies & Associations

6777 NIH Osteoporosis and Related Bone Diseases National Resource Center
Bethesda, MD 20892   202-223-0344
800-624-2663
Fax: 202-293-2356
TTY: 202-466-4315
nihboneinfo@mail.nih.gov
www.bones.nih.gov
Provides patients, health professionals and the public with resources and information on osteoporosis, Paget's disease of bone, osteogenesis imperfecta, and other metabolic bone diseases.

6778 National Institute of Child Health and Human Development
PO Box 3006   800-370-2943
Rockville, MD 20847   Fax: 866-760-5947
TTY: 888-320-6942
www.nichd.nih.gov
NICHD seeks to better understand disabilities and important events that occur during pregnancy.
Diana W. Bianchi, MD, Director
Constantine Stratakis, Scientific Director

6779 Osteogenesis Imperfecta Foundation
804 W Diamond Avenue   301-947-0083
Gaithersburg, MD 20878   844-889-7579
Fax: 301-947-0456
BoneLink@oif.org
www.oif.org
Support and resources for families and medical professionals dealing with osteogenesis imperfecta.
Kenneth W. Gudek, Sr., President
Tracy Smith Hart, CEO

Libraries & Resource Centers

6780 NIH Osteoporosis and Related Bone Diseases - National Resource Center
2 AMS Circle   202-223-0344
Bethesda, MD 20892-3676   800-624-2663
Fax: 202-293-2356
TTY: 202-466-4315
niamsboneinfo@mail.nih.gov
www.osteo.org
Provides patients, health professionals and the public with an important link to resources and information on osteoporosis, Paget's disease of bone, osteogenesis imperfecta, and other metabolic bone diseases. The National Resource Center's mission is to expand awareness and enhance knowledge and understanding of the prevention, early detection, and treatment of these diseases.

Research Centers

6781 American Society for Bone and Mineral Research
2025 M Street NW   202-367-1161
Washington, DC 20036-3309   Fax: 202-672-2161
asbmr@asbmr.org
www.asbmr.org
The mission of the ASBMR is to be the premier society in the field of bone and mineral metabolism through promoting excellence in bone and mineral research fostering integration of clinical and basic science and facilitating the translation of that science to health care and clinical practice.
Ann Elderkin, Executive Director
Douglas Fesler, Associate Executive Director

6782 Children's Brittle Bone Foundation
7701 95th Street   773-236-2223
Pleasant Pride, WI 53158   866-694-2223
Fax: 262-947-0724
info@cbbf.org
www.cbbf.org
The mission of the Children's Brittle Bone Foundation is to provide for research into the causes diagnosis treatment prevention a eventual cure for Osteogenesis Imperfecta (OI) while supporting programs which improve the quality of life for people afflicted.

Support Groups & Hotlines

6783 National Health Information Center
Office of Disease Prevention & Health Promotion
1101 Wootton Pkwy   Fax: 240-453-8281
Rockville, MD 20852   odphpinfo@hhs.gov
www.health.gov/nhic
Supports public health education by maintaining a calendar of National Health Observances; helps connect consumers and health professionals to organizations that can best answer questions and provide up-to-date contact information from reliable sources; updates on a yearly basis toll-free numbers for health information, Federal health clearinghouses and info centers.
Don Wright, MD, MPH, Director

6784 Osteogenesis Imperfecta Foundation
804 W Diamond Avenue   301-947-0083
Gaithersburg, MD 20878   800-981-2663
Fax: 301-947-0456
TDD: 202-466-4315
BoneLink@oif.org
www.oif.org
Support and resources for families and medical professional dealing with osteogeneis imperfecta.
Marybeth Huber, Information Resource Director
Bill Bradner, Director Communication/Events

Books

6785 Children with Ostegogenesis Imperfecta: St raties to Enhance Performance
Holly Lea Cintas, Lynn Gerber, author
Osteogenesis Imperfecta Foundation
804 W Diamond Avenue
Gaithersburg, MD 20878
301-947-0083
800-981-2663
Fax: 301-947-0456
BoneLink@oif.org
www.oif.org
This guide covers the same issues, but has been written especially for elementary school readers.
252 pages Paperback
ISBN: 0-964218-95-X
Mary Beth Huber, Information/Resource Director

6786 Growing Up with OI: A Guide for Children
Ellen Painter Dollar, author
Osteogenesis Imperfecta Foundation
804 W Diamond Avenue
Gaithersburg, MD 20878
301-947-0083
800-981-2663
Fax: 301-947-0456
bonelink@oif.org
www.oif.org
This guide covers the same issues as the adult book, Growing Up with OI: A Guide for Families and Caregivers, but has been written especially for elementary school readers.
122 pages Paperback
ISBN: 0-964218-92-5
Mary Beth Huber, Information/Resource Director

6787 Growing Up with OI: A Guide for Families a nd Caregivers
Ellen Painter Dollar, author
Osteogenesis Imperfecta Foundation
804 W Diamond Avenue
Gaithersburg, MD 20878-1414
301-947-0083
800-981-2663
Fax: 301-947-0456
BoneLink@oif.org
www.oif.org
This guide covers common questions parents, family members and caregivers have about raising a child with OI. The focus is onmaximizing abilities and proactive problem solving. Chapters cover medical, financial, emotional and school related issues.
295 pages Paperback
ISBN: 0-964218-91-7
Mary Beth Huber, Information/Resource Director

6788 Managing Osteogenesis Imperfecta: A Medical Manual
Priscilla Wacaster, MD, author
Osteogenesis Imperfecta Foundation
804 W Diamond Avenue
Gaithersburg, MD 20878-1414
301-947-0083
800-981-2663
Fax: 301-947-0456
BoneLink@oif.org
www.oif.org
The manual is designed for physicians, physical and occupational therapists, orthopedic technologists, early intervention providers and others who come in contact with persons with OI. It covers a broad range of topics including genetics, diagnosis, pregnancy, arthritis, osteoperosis and rodding.
Mary Beth Huber, Information/Resource Director

6789 Therapeutic Strategies: A Guide for Occupational & Physical Therapists
Ellen Painter Dollar, author
Osteogenesis Imperfecta Foundation
804 W Diamond Avenue
Gaithersburg, MD 20878-1414
301-947-0083
800-981-2663
Fax: 301-947-0456
BoneLink@oif.org
www.oif.org
This booklet is intended for medical professionals, or for families to use as a resource while working with a medical professional.
14 pages
Mary Beth Huber, Information/Resource Director

Newsletters

6790 Breakthrough
Osteogenesis Imperfecta Foundation
804 W Diamond Avenue
Gaithersburg, MD 20878-1414
301-947-0083
800-981-2663
Fax: 301-947-0456
BoneLink@oif.org
www.oif.org
Newsletter of the Osteogenesis Imperfecta Foundation that provides information on current research and OIF fundraising activities as well as support features.
15 pages Quarterly
Mary Beth Huber, Information/Resource Director

Pamphlets

6791 Caring for Infants and Children with Osteogenesis Imperfecta
Osteogenesis Imperfecta Foundation
804 W Diamond Avenue
Gaithersburg, MD 20878-1414
301-947-0083
800-981-2663
Fax: 301-947-0456
BoneLink@oif.org
www.oif.org
A companion to the videotape You Are Not Alone. Presents some basic information and unique tips on caring for a baby with OI. Available in Spanish.
24 pages
Mary Beth Huber, Information/Resource Director

6792 Osteogenesis Imperfecta: A Guide for Medic al Professionals, Individuals & Families
Osteogenesis Imperfecta Foundation
804 W Diamond Avenue
Gaithersburg, MD 20878-1414
301-947-0083
800-981-2663
Fax: 301-947-0456
BoneLink@oif.org
www.oif.org
This pamphlet contains basic information about the types of OI, inheritance factors, diagnosis and treatment.
10 pages Paperback
Mary Beth Huber, Information/Resource Director

Audio & Video

6793 Going Places and Plan for Success: An Educ ator's Guide to Students with OI
Osteogenesis Imperfecta Foundation
804 W Diamond Avenue
Gaithersburg, MD 20878-1414
301-947-0083
800-981-2663
Fax: 301-947-0456
BoneLink@oif.org
www.oif.org
A 15-minute video with booklet that guides educators and parents through planning steps that will help children with OI fully participate in school activities.
Mary Beth Huber, Information/Resource Director

6794 Within Reach
Osteogenesis Imperfecta Foundation
804 W Diamond Avenue
Gaithersburg, MD 20878-1414
301-947-0083
800-981-2663
Fax: 301-947-0456
TDD: 202-466-4315
BoneLink@oif.org
www.oif.org
This 50-minute video features in-depth interviews with adults living with OI. They talk candidly about how they have achieved independent and satisfying lives, addressing such issues as travel, career, marriage and family.
VHS/DVD
Mary Beth Huber, Information/Resource Director

6795 You Are Not Alone
Osteogenesis Imperfecta Foundation

804 W Diamond Avenue
Gaithersburg, MD 20878-1414
301-947-0083
800-981-2663
Fax: 301-947-0456
TDD: 202-466-4315
BoneLink@oif.org
www.oif.org

Explores the emotional turmoil of dealing with the diagnosis of OI and offers practical and uplifting solutions for caring for infants with Type II to severe Type III OI. Also valuable for new families with the more mild forms of OI. Available open captioned or with Spanish subtitles (specify if needed). Add $5.00 per video for Canadian orders and $11.00 per video for overseas orders.
Mary Beth Huber, Information/Resource Director

Web Sites

6796 Healing Well

www.healingwell.com

An online health resource guide to medical news, chat, information and articles, newsgroups and message boards, books, disease-related web sites, medical directories, and more for patients, friends, and family coping with disabling diseases, disorders, or chronic illnesses.

6797 Health Finder

www.healthfinder.gov

Searchable, carefully developed web site offering information on over 1000 topics. Developed by the US Department of Health and Human Services, the site can be used in both English and Spanish.

6798 Healthlink USA

www.healthlinkusa.com

Health information concerning treatment, cures, prevention, diagnosis, risk factors, research, support groups, email lists, personal stories and much more. Updated regularly.

6799 MedicineNet

www.medicinenet.com

An online resource for consumers providing easy-to-read, authoritative medical and health information.

6800 Medscape

www.medscape.com

Medscape offers specialists, primary care physicians, and other health professionals the Web's most robust and integrated medical information and educational tools.

6801 Osteogenesis Imperfecta Foundation

www.oif.org

A website for those who want to learn more about Osteogenesis Imperfecta, the OI Foundation, and what they do.

6802 Osteoporosis and Related Bone Diseases: National Resource Center (NIGH)

www.niams.nih.gov/Health_Info/Bone

Provides patients, health professionals and the public with an important link to resources and information on osteoporosis and other metabolic bone diseases.

6803 WebMD

www.webmd.com

Provides credible information, supportive communities, and in-depth reference material about health subjects. A source for original and timely health information as well as material from well known content providers.

Description

6804 Osteoporosis

Osteoporosis is a general term for many conditions which result in a reduction in bone mass. Most cases occur in post-menopausal women because estrogen loss is associated with decreased bone mass. These women are at risk for fractures of the wrist, spine and hip. Post-menopausal osteoporosis may also cause marked reduction in a woman's height, as multiple vertebral bodies in the spine compress downwards over the years. Risk factors for osteoporosis include white race, cigarette smoking, thin body build and early menopause. Men can develop a similar condition, but it is generally much less severe. Excessive activity of the adrenal glands (Cushing's syndrome), the thyroid gland (thyrotoxicosis), the parathyroid glands (hyperparathyroidism), and the pituitary gland (hyperprolactinemia) cause bones to thin, as does underactivity of the testes or ovaries. Anorexia nervosa and prolonged administration of cortisone or heparin will also thin the bones.

Treatment is in part nonspecific and can include surgery or other immobilization to treat fractures of the hip or wrist, control of pain with medications and physical therapy to encourage return to pre-fracture function. Specific therapy includes calcium and Vitamin D supplementation and weight-bearing exercises. Bisphosphonates, such as alendronate, risendronate, ibandronate, and zoledronic acid inhibit osteoclasts, the cells that resorb bone, and are first-line treatment for osteoporosis. Other newer therapies have been developed, such as denosumab, which also decreases bone resorption, and parathyroid hormone mimics, such as teriparatide and abaloparatide, which increase bone deposition.

National Agencies & Associations

6805 American Association of Clinical Endocrinologists

904-353-7878
Fax: 240-547-0026
www.aace.com

A professional community of physicians specializing in endocrinology, diabetes, and metabolism. Referrals and patient information available.
Sandra L. Weber, MD, President
Felice A. Caldarella, MD, Vice President

6806 American Chronic Pain Association

PO Box 850
Rocklin, CA 95677

800-533-3231
ACPA@theacpa.org
www.theacpa.org

The ACPA facilitates peer support and education for individuals with chronic pain in its many forms, in order to increase quality of life. Also raises awareness among the healthcare community, and with policy makers.
Penney Cowan, Founder & CEO
Daniel Galia, Director, Global Support

6807 American Physical Therapy Association

1111 North Fairfax Street
Alexandria, VA 22314-1488

703-684-2782
800-999-2782
Fax: 703-684-7343
memberservices@apta.org
www.apta.org

The American Physical Therapy Association (APTA) is an individual membership professional organization representing more than 100,000 member physical therapists (PTs), physical therapist assistants (PTAs), and students of physical therapy.
Justin Moore, Chief Executive Officer
Mandy Frohlich, COO & EVP, Strategic Affairs

6808 National Association of Chronic Disease Directors

325 Swanton Way
Decatur, GA 30030

info@chronicdisease.org
www.chronicdisease.org

Non-profit public health organization committed to serving the chronic disease program directors of each state and jurisdiction in the United States.
Gabriel Kaplan, President
John W. Robitscher, MPH, CEO

6809 National Osteoporosis Foundation

251 18th Street S
Arlington, VA 22202

800-231-4222
info@nof.org
www.nof.org

The nation's leading resource for people seeking current and accurate medical information on the causes, prevention, detection and treatment of osteoporosis.
Elizabeth Thompson, CEO
Susan Greenspan, MD, President

6810 Osteoporosis Canada

1200 Eglinton Avenue E
Toronto, Ontario, M3C-1H9

416-696-2663
800-463-6842
Fax: 416-696-2673
www.osteoporosis.ca

National organization serving people who have, or are at risk for osteoporosis.
Cheryl Baldwin, Chair
Emily Bartens, Vice Chair

6811 Society For Post-Acute and Long-Term Care Medicine

10500 Little Patuxent Parkway
Columbia, MD 21044

410-740-9743
800-876-2632
Fax: 410-740-4572
info@paltc.org
www.paltc.org

Provides education, advocacy, information and professional development to promote the delivery of standardized post-acute and long-term care medicine.
Arif Nazir, MD, FACP, CMD, President
Karl Steinberg, MD, HMCD, CMD, Vice President

District of Columbia

6812 Nurse Practitioners in Women's Health

505 C Street NE
Washington, DC 20002

202-543-9693
info@npwh.org
www.npwh.org

Ensures the delivery and accessibility of primary and specialty healthcare to women of all ages by women's health and women's health focused nurse practitioners.
Gay Johnson, CEO
Aimee Chism Holland, DNP, Chair

Libraries & Resource Centers

6813 NIH Osteoporosis and Related Bone Diseases - National Resource Center

2 AMS Circle
Bethesda, MD 20892-3676

202-223-0344
800-624-2663
Fax: 202-293-2356
TTY: 202-466-4315

Provides patients, health professionals and the public with an important link to resources and information on osteoporosis, Paget's disease of bone, osteogenesis imperfecta, and other metabolic bone diseases. The National Resource Center's mission is to expand awareness and enhance knowledge and understanding of the prevention, early detection, and treatment of these diseases.

Research Centers

6814 Medical College of Pennsylvania Center for the Mature Woman
3300 Henry Avenue   215-842-6000
Philadelphia, PA 19129
our purpose is to provide consumers information to help them get high quality services and products at the best possible prices.
Jon Schneider,MD, Director

6815 Osteoporosis Center Memorial Hospital/Advanced Medical Diagn
Memorial Hospital/Advanced Medical Diagnostic
1700 Coffee Road   209-526-4500
Modesto, CA 95355   www.memorialmedicalcenter.org
Memorial Medical Center is part of Memorial Hospitals Association a not-for-profit organization that exists to maintain and improve the health status of citizens in the greater Stanislaus County.
David Benn, Director
Bev Finley, Director

6816 Regional Bone Center Helen Hayes Hospital
Helen Hayes Hospital
51-55 Route 9W   845-786-4000
W Haverstraw, NY 10993   1 8-8 7- 734
                                      Fax: 845-947-3097
                                      TTY: 845-947-3187
                                      info@helenhayeshospital.org
                                      www.helenhayeshospital.org
The mission of the Regional Bone conduct a broad-based research program focused on the elucidation of cellular mechanisms underlying metabolic bone disease and the development of new treatments for bone disease.
David W Dempster PhD, Director
Adrienne Tewksbury, Grants Administrator

6817 University of Connecticut Osteoporosis Center
263 Farmington Avenue   860-679-2000
Farmington, CT 06030   800-535-6232
                                      Fax: 860-679-1258
                                      www.uchc.edu

Jay R Lieberman, Director

Support Groups & Hotlines

6818 National Health Information Center
Office of Disease Prevention & Health Promotion
1101 Wootton Pkwy   Fax: 240-453-8281
Rockville, MD 20852   odphpinfo@hhs.gov
                                www.health.gov/nhic
Supports public health education by maintaining a calendar of National Health Observances; helps connect consumers and health professionals to organizations that can best answer questions and provide up-to-date contact information from reliable sources; updates on a yearly basis toll-free numbers for health information, Federal health clearinghouses and info centers.
Don Wright, MD, MPH, Director

6819 National Osteoporosis Foundation (NOF)
1232 22nd Street NW   202-223-2226
Washington, DC 20037-1292   Fax: 202-223-2237
                                webmaster@nof.org
                                www.nof.org
Dedicated to reducing the widespread prevalence of osteoporosis through programs of research, education and advocacy. Provides referrals to existing support groups, as well as free resources, training and materials to assist people to start groups.
Amy Porter, Executive Director & CEO
Robert R Recker, Chairman of the Board

Books

6820 One-Hundred-Fifty Most Asked Questions About Osteoporosis
Hearst Books
1350 Ave of the Americas   212-261-6500
New York, NY 10016   Fax: 212-261-6595
1993
ISBN: 0-688123-34-1

6821 Preventing & Reversing Osteoporosis: Every Woman's Guide
Prima Publishing
PO Box 1260   916-624-5718
Rocklin, CA 95677-1260
1993 275 pages
ISBN: 1-559582-98-7

6822 Preventing and Managing Osteoporosis
Springer Publishing Company
11 West 42nd Street   212-431-4370
New York, NY 10036-3955   877-687-7476
                                      Fax: 212-941-7842
                                      cs@springerpub.com
                                      www.springerpub.com
This book will raise awareness and inform health professionals about this often preventable and treatable disease. Written by a team of authors from medicine, nursing, nutrition, exercise physiology, and physical therapy, the book provides an overview of the disease process.
216 pages Hardcover
ISBN: 0-826113-18-4
M Susan Burke MD, Editor
Helen Wright PhD, Editor

Newsletters

6823 Osteoporosis Report
National Osteoporosis Foundation
1150 17th Street, NW   202-223-2226
Washington, DC 20036-1292   800-221-4222
                                      Fax: 202-223-2237
                                      communications@nof.org
                                      www.nof.org
A benefit to members of the National Osteoporosis Foundation (NOF), the Osteoporosis Report includes updates on recent research, strategies for bone health and other information. NOF is the only nonprofit, voluntary health organization dedicated to reducing the widespread prevalence of osteoporosis through programs of research, education and advocacy. Contact the foundation for membership information.
Quarterly

Pamphlets

6824 Boning Up on Osteoporosis
National Osteoporosis Foundation
1150 17th Street, NW   202-223-2226
Washington, DC 20036-1292   800-221-4222
                                      Fax: 202-223-2237
                                      info@nof.org
                                      www.nof.org
Risk factor card.

6825 How Strong Are Your Bones?
1150 17th Street, NW   202-223-2226
Washington, DC 20036-1292   800-221-4222
                                      Fax: 202-223-2237
                                      info@nof.org
                                      www.nof.org
Describes the various methods for determining bone mass, including types of equipment and how bone density testing is used in the diagnosis and treatment of osteoporosis.
12 pages

6826 Living with Osteoporosis
1150 17th Street, NW   202-223-2226
Washington, DC 20036-1292   800-221-4222
                                      Fax: 202-223-2237
                                      info@nof.org
                                      www.nof.org
A guide to preventing falls in the home and to protecting yourself from injury during your daily routine.

6827 Medications and Bone Loss
1150 17th Street, NW
Washington, DC 20036-1292
202-223-2226
800-221-4222
Fax: 202-223-2237
info@nof.org
www.nof.org

Designed for women dealing with menopause, this brochure provides information of estrogen replacement therapy and its relationship to bone health and osteoporosis prevention and treatment.

6828 Men with Osteoporosis: In Their Own Words
1150 17th Street, NW
Washington, DC 20036-1292
202-223-2226
800-221-4222
Fax: 202-223-2237
info@nof.org
www.nof.org

6829 Official Prevention Month Poster
1150 17th Street, NW
Washington, DC 20036-1292
202-223-2226
800-221-4222
Fax: 202-223-2237
info@nof.org
www.nof.org

Poster promotes public awareness about osteoporosis. It can be used as a compliment to the education kit, or by itself for exhibits, health fairs or community programs.

6830 Official Prevention Week Poster
1150 17th Street, NW
Washington, DC 20036-1292
202-223-2226
800-221-4222
Fax: 202-223-2237
info@nof.org
www.nof.org

Poster promotes public awareness about osteoporosis. It can be used as a compliment to the education kit, or by itself for exhibits, health fairs or community programs.

6831 Osteoporosis Education Kit
1150 17th Street, NW
Washington, DC 20036-1292
202-223-2226
800-221-4222
Fax: 202-223-2237
info@nof.org
www.nof.org

This kit is designed for preparing public and patient education programs. Updated annually and includes age-targeted materials, nutrition information and osteoporosis fact sheets that are easily duplicated.

6832 Osteoporosis Education Poster
1150 17th Street, NW
Washington, DC 20036-1292
202-223-2226
800-221-4222
Fax: 202-223-2237
info@nof.org
www.nof.org

Ideal for health care settings, the poster clearly illustrates the effect of osteoporosis on bone tissue and common fracture sites.

6833 Osteoporosis Information Package
NAMSIC/National Institutes of Health
1 AMS Circle
Bethesda, MD 20892-0001
301-495-4484
877-226-4267
Fax: 301-718-6366
TTY: 301-565-2966
niamsinfo@mail.nih.gov
www.nih.gov/niams

The National Institute of Arthritis and Musculoskeletal and Skin Diseases Information Clearinghouse serves the public, patients, and health professionals
19 pages

6834 Osteoporosis International
1150 17th Street, NW
Washington, DC 20036-1292
202-223-2226
800-221-4222
Fax: 202-223-2237
info@nof.org
www.nof.org

An international multidisciplinary, clinically oriented journal for the exchange of ideas concerning osteoporosis.

6835 Osteoporosis in Men Information Package
NAMSIC/National Institutes of Health
1 AMS Circle
Bethesda, MD 20892-0001
301-495-4484
877-226-4267
Fax: 301-715-6366
TTY: 301-565-2966
niamsinfo@mail.nih.gov
www.nih.gov/niams

The National Institute of Arthritis and Musculoskeletal and Skin Diseases Information Clearinghouse serves the public, patients, and health professionals
19 pages

6836 Osteoporosis: Clinical Updates
1150 17th Street, NW
Washington, DC 20036-1292
202-223-2226
800-221-4222
Fax: 202-223-2237
info@nof.org
www.nof.org

NOF's health profession newsletter provides an in depth focus on varying clinical topics.

6837 Osteoporosis: The Silent Disease-Slide Lecture Presentation
1150 17th Street, NW
Washington, DC 20036-1292
202-223-2226
800-221-4222
Fax: 202-223-2237
info@nof.org
www.nof.org

This 42-slide presentation is ideal for community, patient and worksite education progams. It covers basic bone biology, osteoporosis risk factors, diagnosis, prevention and treatment and concludes with a patient case history. A question and answer document is also provided to assist the presenter with audience questions.
Slide set

6838 Patient Education Sample Pack
1150 17th Street, NW
Washington, DC 20036-1292
202-223-2226
800-221-4222
Fax: 202-223-2237
info@nof.org
www.nof.org

This pack contains one of each of NOF's patient education brochures and a catalog; health professionals can select the brochures appropriate for their audience.
Ten brochures

6839 Risk Factor Card: Can It Happen to You?
National Osteoporosis Foundation
1150 17th Street, NW
Washington, DC 20036-1292
202-223-2226
800-221-4222
Fax: 202-223-2237
info@nof.org
www.nof.org

Explains osteoporosis, the causes, symptoms and preventions and high risk persons.

6840 Stand Up to Osteoporosis
National Osteoporosis Foundation
1150 17th Street, NW
Washington, DC 20036-1292
202-223-2226
800-221-4222
Fax: 202-223-2237
info@nof.org
www.nof.org

One of 25 educational brochures on all aspects of this chronic and debilitating disease. The National Osteoporosis Foundation (NOF) is the nation's only private, nonprofit organization dedicated to education, advocacy and public services. Memberships are available to health professionals and public. Quarterly newsletter and physician's guide.

6841 Strategies for People with Osteoporosis
1150 17th Street, NW
Washington, DC 20036-1292
202-223-2226
800-221-4222
Fax: 202-223-2237
info@nof.org
www.nof.org

This series of articles from NOF's newsletter helps patients learn how to cope with osteoporosis. Articles cover hip, vertebrae and wrist fracture recovery, fall-proofing your home, finding the right doctor, what to do after you've been diagnosed and more.

Audio & Video

6842 Be BoneWise: Exercise
National Osteoperosis Foundation
1150 17th Street, NW
Washington, DC 20036-1292

202-223-2226
800-221-4222
Fax: 202-223-2237
info@nof.org
www.nof.org

Take steps toward better bones, health, flexibility and balance with the offical weight bearing and strength training exercise video.

6843 Osteoperosis: The Silent Disease
National Osteoperosis Foundation
1150 17th Street, NW
Washington, DC 20036-1292

202-223-2226
800-221-4222
Fax: 202-223-2237
info@nof.org
www.nof.org

A scripted, visual presentation covers basic bone biology, osteoperosis risk factors, diagnosis, prevention and treatment. Available as a slide presentation or power point CD Rom.

6844 Patient Education Video
National Osteoperosis Foundation
1150 17th Street, NW
Washington, DC 20036-1292

202-223-2226
800-221-4222
Fax: 202-223-2237
info@nof.org
www.nof.org

Discusses treatment, exercise, nutrition and coping strategies for those already diagnoses with osteoporosis.
15 minutes

Web Sites

6845 Healing Well

www.healingwell.com
An online health resource guide to medical news, chat, information and articles, newsgroups and message boards, books, disease-related web sites, medical directories, and more for patients, friends, and family coping with disabling diseases, disorders, or chronic illnesses.

6846 Health Finder

www.healthfinder.gov
Searchable, carefully developed web site offering information on over 1000 topics. Developed by the US Department of Health and Human Services, the site can be used in both English and Spanish.

6847 Healthlink USA

www.healthlinkusa.com
Health information concerning treatment, cures, prevention, diagnosis, risk factors, research, support groups, email lists, personal stories and much more. Updated regularly.

6848 MedicineNet

www.medicinenet.com
An online resource for consumers providing easy-to-read, authoritative medical and health information.

6849 Medscape

www.medscape.com
Medscape offers specialists, primary care physicians, and other health professionals the Web's most robust and integrated medical information and educational tools.

6850 NIH Osteoporosis and Related Bone Disease

www.niams.nih.gov/Health_Info/Bone
Provides patients, health professionals, and the public with an important link to resources and information on metabolic bone diseases. The center is dedicated to increasing the awareness, knowledge, and understanding of physicians, health professionals, patients, underserved and at-risk populations, and the general public about the prevention, early detection, and treatment of osteoporosis and related bone diseases.

6851 National Osteoporosis Foundation

www.nof.org
The National Osteoporosis Foundation is dedicated to preventing osteoporosis, promoting strong bones, and reducing human suffering through education, advocacy and research.

6852 WebMD

www.webmd.com
Provides credible information, supportive communities, and in-depth reference material about health subjects. A source for original and timely health information as well as material from well known content providers.

Description

6853 Paget Disease

Paget disease is a disorder of the bone, which typically results in enlarged and deformed bones in one or more regions of the skeleton. Excessive bone breakdown and formation cause new bone to be dense but fragile. Paget disease occurs most frequently in the spine, skull, pelvis, and legs.

Early symptoms of Paget disease include bone and joint pain and fatigability, as well as headaches and hearing loss, when the skull is affected. Deformities of bone such as enlargement of the forehead, bowing of a limb, and curvature of the spine may occur as the disease progresses.

The cause of Paget disease is unknown. It is sometimes familial, but a specific genetic pattern is unclear. The risk for Paget disease increases with age.

The course of the disease varies greatly and may range from complete stability to rapid progression. Generally, symptoms progress slowly in affected bones with usually no spread to normal ones.

Although there is no cure for Paget disease at the present, treatments include drugs (bisphosphonates) that suppress disease activity. Orthopedic surgery for joint replacement or stabilization may also be beneficial.

National Agencies & Associations

6854 American Chronic Pain Association
PO Box 850
Rocklin, CA 95677

800-533-3231
ACPA@theacpa.org
www.theacpa.org

The ACPA facilitates peer support and education for individuals with chronic pain in its many forms, in order to increase quality of life. Also raises awareness among the healthcare community, and with policy makers.
Penney Cowan, Founder & CEO
Daniel Galia, Director, Global Support

Foundations

6855 Arthritis Foundation
1355 Peachtree Street NE
Atlanta, GA 30309

404-872-7100
800-283-7800
Fax: 404-872-0457
help@arthritis.org
www.arthritis.org

A nonprofit organization that depends on volunteers to provide services to help people with arthritis. Supports research to find ways to cure and prevent arthritis and provides services to improve the quality of life for those affected by arthritis. Provides help through information, referrals, speakers bureaus, forums, self-help courses, and various support groups and programs nationwide.
Ann M. Palmer, President & CEO
Guy S. Eakin, PhD, Sr Vice President, Scientific Strategy

Support Groups & Hotlines

6856 National Health Information Center
Office of Disease Prevention & Health Promotion

1101 Wootton Pkwy
Rockville, MD 20852

Fax: 240-453-8281
odphpinfo@hhs.gov
www.health.gov/nhic

Supports public health education by maintaining a calendar of National Health Observances; helps connect consumers and health professionals to organizations that can best answer questions and provide up-to-date contact information from reliable sources; updates on a yearly basis toll-free numbers for health information, Federal health clearinghouses and info centers.
Don Wright, MD, MPH, Director

Newsletters

6857 Update
Paget Foundation
120 Wall Street
New York, NY 10005-4001

212-509-5335
800-237-2438
Fax: 212-509-8492
PagetFdn@aol.com
www.paget.org

Provides information for consumers and health professionals on the following disorders: paget's disease of bone, primary hyperparathyroidism, fibrous dysplasia, osteopetrosis (not osteoporosis) and the complications of breast and prostate cancer metastic to the bone.
3 per year
Charlene Waldman, Executive Director

Pamphlets

6858 Questions & Answers About Paget's Disease of Bone
Paget Foundation
120 Wall Street
New York, NY 10005-4001

212-509-5335
800-237-2438
Fax: 212-509-8492
pagetfdn@aol.com
www.paget.org

The Paget Foundation provides this and other question and answer booklets and fact sheets on Paget's disease of bone, primary hyperparathyroidism,, fibrous dysplasia, osteopetrosis (not osteoporosis) and breast and prostate cancer metastic to bone. These publications are available on the foundation websit and in print.
Charlene Waldman, Executive Director

Web Sites

6859 Healing Well
www.healingwell.com

An online health resource guide to medical news, chat, information and articles, newsgroups and message boards, books, disease-related web sites, medical directories, and more for patients, friends, and family coping with disabling diseases, disorders, or chronic illnesses.

6860 Health Finder
www.healthfinder.gov

Searchable, carefully developed web site offering information on over 1000 topics. Developed by the US Department of Health and Human Services, the site can be used in both English and Spanish.

6861 Healthlink USA
www.healthlinkusa.com

Health information concerning treatment, cures, prevention, diagnosis, risk factors, research, support groups, email lists, personal stories and much more. Updated regularly.

6862 MedicineNet
www.medicinenet.com

An online resource for consumers providing easy-to-read, authoritative medical and health information.

6863 Medscape
www.medscape.com

Medscape offers specialists, primary care physicians, and other health professionals the Web's most robust and integrated medical information and educational tools.

6864   Paget Foundation for Paget's Disease of Bone & Related Disorders
Includes information for patients and health professionals on Paget's disease of bone, primary hyperparathyroidism, fibrous dysplasia, osteopetrosis (not osteoporosis) and the complications of certain cancers on the skeleton.

6865   WebMD

www.webmd.com
Provides credible information, supportive communities, and in-depth reference material about health subjects. A source for original and timely health information as well as material from well known content providers.

Description

6866 Parkinson Disease

Parkinson disease is a neurological condition characterized by slow and decreased movement. It affects about 1 percent of those over age 65. The cause of Parkinson disease is unknown, but both genetic and environmental factors may play a role. In a minority of cases, Parkinson disease develops after repeated head trauma, carbon monoxide poisoning, drug use, or viral infections that affect the brain.

In about 50 percent to 80 percent of patients, Parkinson disease begins with a slight tremor in the hands, resembling "pill-rolling" when at rest. With fatigue and stress, the tremor becomes more pronounced. As the disease progresses, voluntary movements, such as walking and eating, become more and more difficult. Rigidity and postural instability (difficulty standing up) develop. Dementia affects approximately one third of patients with advanced Parkinson disease.

Because Parkinson disease is characterized by reduced levels of neurotransmitter chemicals, notably dopamine, in certain parts of the brain, therapy has focused on restoring dopamine levels to normal. Monoamine oxidase type B inhibitors given early in the disease, may protect the cells that secrete these chemicals, and thus delay the need for other therapy. When it is necessary to directly manipulate the chemical levels because of progression of the disease, levodopa, related to dopamine, is the mainstay of treatment and is associated with improvement of all Parkinson symptoms. Levodopa is given with carbidopa, which inhibits the enzyme (peripheral decarboxylase) that degrades levodopa. This combination medication is marketed under the trade name Sinemet. This medication works well for the first 2-5 years, after which symptoms begin to return. The addition of further inhibitors of levodopa degradation (COMT inhibitors and MAO-B inhibitors) can augment the efficacy of levodopa for many more years. Anticholinergic medications are especially helpful in treating tremor and drooling. Dopamine agonists are often used as adjunct treatments with levodopa, particularly early in the course of the disease. These drugs decrease fluctuations in treatment efficacy.

Parkinson disease is the subject of intense research, and experimental surgical or drug treatments are frequently available to patients whose response to standard therapy has been unsatisfactory. General supportive care should not be neglected and includes physical therapy and an exercise program to help optimize mobility. Stem cells treatments have proven their efficacy in animal models and are human clinical trials are in process.

National Agencies & Associations

6867 American Parkinson Disease Association (APDA)

135 Parkinson Avenue — 800-223-2732
Staten Island, NY 10305 — Fax: 718-981-4399
apda@apdaparkinson.org
www.apdaparkinson.org

Funds research towards finding the cause and cure for Parkinson's Disease. Offers patient education, information, support groups nationwide.
Leslie A. Chambers, MSPH, President & CEO
Rebecca Gilbert, MD, PhD, Vice President

6868 International Parkinson and Movement Disorder Society

555 East Wells Street — 414-276-2145
Milwaukee, WI 53202-3823 — Fax: 414-276-3349
info@movementdisorders.org
www.movementdisorders.org

The MDS is comprised of clinicians, scientists, and other healthcare professionals interested in Parkinson's disease, as well as related neurodegenerative and neurodevelopmental disorders, hyperkinetic movement disorders, and abnormalities in muscle tone and motor control.
Jennie Socha, Executive Director
Erin Weileder, Director, Membership & Communications

6869 Michael J. Fox Foundation for Parkinson's Research

Grand Central Station — 800-708-7644
New York, NY 10163-4777 — www.michaeljfox.org

The Michael J. Fox Foundation is dedicated to ensuring the development of a cure for Parkinson's disease through funding for research.
Deborah W. Brooks, Co-Founder & Executive Vice Chairman
Todd Sherer, CEO

6870 National Institute of Neurological Disorders and Stroke

NIH Neurological Institute — 301-496-5751
Bethesda, MD 20824 — 800-352-9424
www.ninds.nih.gov

Seeks to reduce the burden of neurological disease affecting individuals from all walks of life.
Walter J. Koroshetz, MD, Director
Amy B. Adams, Director, Office of Scientific Liaison

6871 Parkinson Canada

4211 Yonge Street — 416-227-9700
Toronto, Ontario, M2P-2A9 — 800-565-3000
Fax: 844-440-8963
info@parkinson.ca
www.parkinson.ca

A non-profit, national charity raising money to find a cure for Parkinson's disease through corporate sponsorships, and public donations.
Judi Richardson, Chair
Lindsay Abbey, Director

6872 Parkinson's Foundation

200 SE 1st Street — 800-473-4636
Miami, FL 33131-1407 — contact@parkinson.org
www.parkinson.org

A non-profit organization dedicated to research, diagnosis, treatment and care for individuals suffering from Parkinson's and other related neurological diseases.
Howard D. Morgan, Chair
Andrew B. Albert, Vice Chair

6873 Parkinson's Institute and Clinical Center

2500 Hospital Drive — 408-734-2800
Mountain View, CA 94040 — 800-655-2273
Fax: 650-770-0204
www.thepi.org

Working for a cure for Parkinson's Disease and providing treatment to those afflicted with the disease.
Thomas D. Follett, BSE, MSE, MBA, Chair
Carrolee Barlow, MD, PhD, CEO

State Agencies & Associations

Arizona

6874 Arizona Chapter of the National Parkinson Foundation
20280 N 59th Avenue
Glendale, AZ 85308-6182
480-607-1960
866-637-8772
Fax: 480-607-1957
Affiliate chapter of The National Parkinson Foundation Inc.
Alan Marks, President
Kenneth Larkin, Vice President

California

6875 Los Angeles Alliance Against Parkinson's Disease
3251 Oakley Drive
Los Angeles, CA 90068-1315
323-851-3230
www.parkinson.org/chapters.htm#
Affiliate of the National Parkinson Foundation.

6876 National Parkinson Foundation: California Office
4929 Wilshire Boulevard
Los Angeles, CA 90010-3899
323-442-8434

6877 National Parkinson Foundation: Orange County Chapter
PO Box 2207
Newport Beach, CA 92659
949-945-6200
Fax: 949-548-4624
info@yahoo.com
www.npfocc.org
Affiliate of The National Parkinson Foundation.
George Strickland, President
Janet Buell, Vice president

6878 Northstate Parkinson's Chapter
1003 Yuba Street
Redding, CA 96001
530-229-0878
www.parkinson.org
Affiliate of The National Parkinson Foundation, Inc.
Craig Boyer

6879 Parkinson Association of the Sacramento Valley
900 Fulton Avenue
Sacramento, CA 96825-4502
916-534-7279
800-473-4636
Fax: 916-489-0241
parkanc@sbcglobal.net
www.parkinsonsacramento.org
Bernardine Ford, President
George Johnston, 2nd Vice President

6880 Parkinson Network of Mount Diablo
Po Box 3127
Walnut Creek, CA 94598-0127
925-284-2189
mmhansell@hotmail.com
www.parkinson.org
Affiliate of the National Parkinson Foundation.
Mary Hansell

Colorado

6881 Colorado Parkinson Foundation
1155 Kelly Johnson Boulevard
Colorado Springs, CO 90920-1494
719-884-0103
800-327-4545
Fax: 719-495-909
rpfarrer@msn.com
The mission of the National Parkinson Foundation if to find the cause of the cure for Parkinson disease through research. To improve the quality if life for persons with Parkinson and their caregivers. To also educate persons with Parkinson their carecar
Ric Pfarrer, Chairperson

Florida

6882 Alzheimer/Parkinson Association of Indian River County
2300 5th Avenue
Vero Beach, FL 32960
772-563-0505
alzsupport@fastmail.fm
www.parkinson.org
Toni Teresi, Chairperson

6883 Parkinson Association of Greater Daytona Beach
111 North Frederick Avenue
Daytona Beach, FL 32114
386-252-8959
goatie@cfl.rr.com
www.parkinson.org
Nancy Dawson, Chairperson

6884 Parkinson Association of Southwest Florida
1048 Goodlette-Frank Road
Naples, FL 34102
239-417-3465
Fax: 239-417-3469
pasfi@aol.com
www.pasfi.org
Affiliate of the National Parkinson Foundation.
Scott Leamon, Chair
Chris Spine, Executive Director

6885 South Palm Beach County Chapter of NFP
PO Box 880145
Boca Raton, FL 33433-0145
561-482-2867
www.parkinson.org
Irving Layton, Chairperson

6886 Southeast Parkinson Disease Association
6530 Metrowest Boulevard
Orlando, FL 32835-6520
407-489-4124
srh_pres@sepda.org
www.sepda.org
Steve Hochberger, Chairperson

Georgia

6887 Northwest Georgia Parkinson Disease Association
708 Glen Milner Boulevard
Rome, GA 30161
706-235-3164
webmaster@gaparkinsons.org
James Trussel, Chairperson

Hawaii

6888 Hawaii Parkinson Association Gwendolyn A Montibon President
Gwendolyn A Montibon, President
3375 Koapaka St.,
Honolulu, HI 96817
808-734-9398
Fax: 808-528-1897
kekim@hawaii.edu
www.parkinson.org
Affiliate of The National Parkinson Foundation.

Kansas

6889 Northeast Kansas Parkinson Association
PO Box 251
Topeka, KS 66601
785-228-1337
www.parkinson.org
Mary Hatke, Chairperson

6890 Parkinson Association of Greater Kansas City
8900 State Line Road
Leawood, KS 66206
913-341-8828
Fax: 913-341-8885
www.parkinsonheartland.org
Affiliate of The National Parkinson Foundation.
Kirk Gutekunst, President
Mary Lee Shucart, Secretary

Louisiana

6891 Eljay Foundation for Parkinson Syndrome Awareness
715 Ryan Street
Lake Charles, LA 70601
337-310-0083
info@eljayfd.org
www.eljayfd.org
Eligha Guillory, President
Anna C. Drake, Secretary

Massachusetts

6892 Cape Cod Chapter National Parkinson Foundation
33 Ships Way
Buzzards Bay, MA 02532-0584
508-385-2333
meacapecod@yahoo.com
www.parkinson.org
Affiliate of The National Parkinson Foundation.
Joseph Wimbrow, President

6893 National Parkinson Foundation:Cape Cod Chapter
33 Ships Way
Buzzards Bay, MA 02532-0584
508-385-2333
meacapecod@yahoo.com
www.parkinson.org
Garland Smith, Chairperson

6894 Northeast Parkinson's and Caregivers
27 Sutcliffe Road
Brimfield, MA 01010
508-756-7721
Richard Stake, Chairperson

Minnesota

6895 Parkinson Association of Minnesota
5905 Golden Valley Road,   763-545-1272
Golden Valley, MN 55422-4602   800-327-4545
                                             info@parkinsonmn.org
                                             www.parkinsonmn.org
Affiliate of The National Parkinson Foundation.
Paul Blom, President
Collen Crane, Therapy Representative

New Jersey

6896 Parkinson Alliance
PO Box 308   609-688-0870
Kingston, NJ 08528   800-579-8440
                                             Fax: 609-688-0875
                                             admin@parkinsonalliance.net
                                             www.parkinsonalliance.net
The Princeton-New Jersey based Parkinson Alliance is a National
nonprofit organization dedicated to raising funds to help finance
the most promising research to find the cause and curefor Parkin-
son's disease.
Martin Tuchman, Chairman
Margaret Tuchman, President

New York

6897 National Parkinson Foundation: New York Office
122 E 42nd Street   800-457-6676
New York, NY 10017-5622   www.parkinson.org/

6898 Parkinsons Wellness Group of Western New York
5140 Main Street   716-218-1027
Depew, NY 14221   coach71395@aol.com
                                             http://www.npfwny.org/
Site changed
Robert J Plunket, President
Gary Kurdziel, Vice President

Oklahoma

6899 Parkinson Foundation of the Heartland Oklahoma Branch
1000 W Wilshire   405-810-0695
Oklahoma City, OK 73116   www.parkinson.org
Satellite office of the Kansas Chapter
Jim Keating, Chairperson

Oregon

6900 Parkinsons Resources of Oregon
3975 Mercantile Drive   503-594-0901
Lake Oswego, OR 97035   800-426-6806
                                             Fax: 503-594-0547
                                             info@parkinsonsresources.org
                                             www.parkinsonsresources.org
Holly Chaimov, Executive Director

Pennsylvania

6901 Parkinson Chapter of Greater Pittsburgh
6507 Wilkins Avenue   412-365-2086
Pittsburgh, PA 15217
Doreen Grasso, Chairperson
Maggie Schmidt, Executive Director

6902 Parkinson Council
111 Presidential Boulevard   610-668-4292
Bala Cynwyd, PA 19004   Fax: 610-668-4275
                                             info@theparkinsoncouncil.org
                                             www.theparkinsoncouncil.org
The Parkinson Council is dedicated to promoting research initiat-
ing to find the causes and cure for Parkinson Disease educating patients their caregivers healthcare professionals and the general
public about Parkinson's and improving the quality of lif
Jeff Keefer, President
Jo Ann Zoll, Vice President

South Dakota

6903 Parkinson Association of South Dakota
PO Box 87952   605-328-4227
Sioux Falls, SD 57109-9938   Fax: 605-328-7150
Affiliate of The National Parkinson Foundation.
Elaine Spader, President
Lori Jones, Vice President

Virginia

6904 Parkinson Foundation of the National Capitol Area
7700 Leesburg Pike,   703-734-1017
Falls church, VA 22043-4201   Fax: 703-734-1241
                                             pfnca@parkinsonfoundation.org
                                             www.parkinsonfoundation.org
Daniel M Lewis, Chairperson
Donna Schena, Vice Chairman

Wisconsin

6905 Wisconsin Parkinson Association
945 N 12th Street   414-219-7061
Milwaukee, WI 53233   800-972-5455
                                             Fax: 414-219-6564
                                             www.wiparkinson.org
Chapter of The National Parkinson Foundation.
Keith Brewer, President

Foundations

6906 Parkinsons Disease Foundation
1359 Broadway   212-923-4700
New York, NY 10018   800-457-6676
                                             Fax: 212-923-4778
                                             info@pdf.org
                                             www.pdf.org
The foundation has been one of teh leaders in subsidizing research
into Parkinson's Disease. Offers many services including The
Summer Fellowship Program, The Postdoctoral Fellowship Program, support groups nationwide, grants for clinical and labora-
tory studies, public awareness and government promotion of the
disease.
Howard D. Morgan, chair/Co Preident
Constance Woodruff atwell, Vice Chair

Libraries & Resource Centers

6907 Parkinson's Resource Organization
74090 El Paseo   760-773-5628
Palm Desert, CA 92260-4135   877-775-4111
                                             Fax: 760-773-9803
                                             info@parkinsonsresource.org
                                             www.parkinsonsresource.org
Our mission is to help families affected by Parkinson's forge
through the journey of the disease's progression with as much
quality as life can provide. Working so no one is isolated because
of Parkinson's
Jo Rosen, Visionary, President, Founder
William R Remery, Treasurer

Research Centers

6908 California Institute for Medical Research
2260 Clove Drive   408-998-4554
San Jose, CA 95128   Fax: 408-998-2723
                                             www.cimr.org
Medical research including infectious diseases stroke and cancer
specializing in Parkinson's Disease related studies.
David A Stevens, President
John Hotson, Vice President

6909 Texas Tech University Tarbox Parkinson's Disease Institute
3601 4th Street   806-743-1000
Lubbock, TX 79430   www.ttuhsc.edu

The current objectives of the Tarbox Institute are to provide services for Parkinson's disease patients and their families in the underserved West Texas area; to maintain a Parkinson's Disease Information and Referral Center to enable both healthcare professionals and affected families to obtain the latest information on services available new developments in research support groups and educational literature.
Tedd L Mitchell, President
Pureza Martinez, Chief of Staff

6910 University of Alabama at Birmingham Parkinsons Disease Center
1720 7th Avenue S   205-934-4011
Birmingham, AL 35294   Fax: 205-346-78
          TDD: 205-934-4642
          apda@uab.edu
          www.uab.edu
Offers educational emotional and political support to Parkinson disease patients and their families.
Ray Watts, Interim CEO
David G Standaert, Director

6911 William T Gossett Parkinson's Disease Center
Henry Ford Hospital
Department of Neurology   313-972-1693
Detroit, MI 48202
Jay M Gorell MD, Director

Support Groups & Hotlines

California

6912 Parkinson's Disease Association of San Die go (PDASD)
8555 Areo Drive   858-273-6763
San Diego, CA 92123-1746   877-737-7576
          Fax: 858-273-6764
          info@pdasd.org
          www.pdasd.org
Information and referral research center for Parkinson's disease patients and their families.
Jerry Henberger, Executive Director
Rick Brydges, President

Florida

6913 Greater Daytona Area Parkinson Support Group
Bishop's Glen Retirement Center   904-322-4748
Daytona, FL   www.parkinson.org
Affiliate of the National Parkinson Foundation.

6914 National Parkinson Foundation Hotline
National Parkinson Foundation
1501 NW 9th Avenue Bob Hope Road   305-243-6666
Miami, FL 33136   800-327-4545
          Fax: 305-243-5595
          www.parkinson.org
Offers support and emergency information for persons with Parkinson's and their families.
Jose Garcia Pebrosa, Director

6915 Pembroke Pines Parkinson Support Group
Century Village, Club House   954-433-0947
Pembroke Pines, FL 33027   www.parkinson.org
Affiliate of the National Parkinson Foundation.

Hawaii

6916 Kuakini Parkinson Disease (PD) Information & Referral
Kuakini Medical Center
347 North Kuakini Street   808-536-2236
Honolulu, HI 96817   800-570-1101
          Fax: 808-528-1897
          pr@kuakini.org
The Kuakini Parkinson Disease (PD) Information & Referral Office provides referrals to neurologists and other special services for Parkinson disease patients; provides information about community services to assist PD patients and their caregivers in finding optimal care; distributes educational materials; conducts

educational conferences and other activities; and assists with support groups for PD patients and caregivers.
Gary K Kajiwara, President/Chief Executive Officer
Gregg Oishi, SVP/Chief Operating Officer

Illinois

6917 Rockford Parkinson's Support Group
5415 Watson Road   815-654-0614
Rockford, IL 61108   800-972-5455
Affiliate of The National Parkinson Foundation, Inc.

Maryland

6918 Parkinson Support Groups of America
11376 Cherry Hill Road   301-937-1545
Beltsville, MD 20705
Offers support networks and groups for persons with Parkinson's disease, families, friends and professionals.

Missouri

6919 APDA Center for Advanced Parkinson Disease Research
Washington University School of Medicine
660 South Euclid   314-362-6909
St Louis, MO 63110   Fax: 314-362-0168
          joel@npg.wustl.edu
          www.neuro.wustl.edu/parkinson/
Information and referral research center for Parkinson's disease patients and their families.
David m Holtzman, Chairman
Brad a Racette, Vice Chairman

6920 Ozarks Parkinson Support Group
Po Box 50595   417-885-9595
Springfield, MO 65805
Affiliate of the National Parkinson Foundation.
Monty Montgomery, Contact

New Jersey

6921 New Jersey Parkinson's Disease Information Center
Robert Wood Johnson University Hospital
One Robert Wood Johnson Place   732-828-3000
New Brunswick, NJ 08901   Fax: 732-745-3114
          elizabeth.schaaf@rwjuh.edu
          www.rwjuh.edu/medical_services/
The New Jersey Parkinson's Disease Information and Referral Center reaches out to persons affected by Parkinson's disease, including patients, families and healthcare professionals. This Information and Referral Center is committed to providing community education and information as well as support groups for caregivers and persons with Parkinson's disease.
Elizabeth Schaaf, Parkinson's Disease Center Coordinator

New York

6922 American Parkinson Disease Association Hotline
1250 Hylan Boulevard   800-908-2732
Staten Island, NY 10305   Fax: 718-981-4399
Offers information and physician referrals to patients and their families.
Joel Gerstel, Director

6923 New York College of Osteopathic Medicine
PO Box 8000   516-686-3747
Old Westbury, NY 11568-8000   800-345-6948
          Fax: 516-686-7613
          http://www.nyit.edu/medicine/
Information and referral research center for Parkinson's disease patients and their families.
Rosslee , Vice President

6924 Parkinson's Support Group of Upstate New York
PO Box 23204   716-377-6718
Rochester, NY 14692-3204
Affiliate of The National Parkinson Foundation, Inc.
David Look, President

6925 St. John's Episcopal Hospital
327 Beach 19th street
Smithtown, NY 11691   718-869-7000
                              www.ehs.org
Information and referral research center for Parkinson's disease patients and their families.
Nelson toebbe, Chief Executive Officer
Richard A Brown, Chief Operating Officer

6926 University of Rochester
500 Wilson Boulevard
Rochester, NY 14627   585-275-3221
                              888-822-2256
                              www.rochester.edu/
Information and referral research center for Parkinson's disease patients and their families.

Oregon

6927 Oregon Health Sciences University
3181 SW Sam Jackson Park Road   503-494-5285
Portland, OR 97239   888-222-6478
                                  www.ohsu.edu
Information and referral research center for Parkinson's disease patients and their families.

Pennsylvania

6928 University of Pittsburgh
4200 Fifth avenue   412-624-4141
Pittsburgh, PA 15260   Fax: 412-383-2264
                              webmaster@pitt.edu
                              www.pitt.edu
Information and referral research center for Parkinson's disease patients and their families.
Patricia E. Beeson, Vice Chancellor
John P Elliott, Director of Internal Affairs

Texas

6929 Presbyterian Hospital of Dallas
612 E. Lamar Boulevard   214-345-6789
Arlington, TX 76011   www.texashealth.org
Information and referral research center for Parkinson's disease patients and their families.
Phillip Moroneso, Chair
Brock Campton, Vice Chair

6930 University of Texas HSC at San Antonio
7703 Floyd Curl Drive   210-567-7000
San Antonio, TX 78229-3900   www.uthscsa.edu/
Information and referral research center for Parkinson's disease patients and their families.

Washington

6931 University of Washington
Box 355840   206-543-5369
Seattle, WA 98195-5840   uwvic@u.washington.edu
                              www.washington.edu/
Information and referral research center for Parkinson's disease patients and their families.

Books

6932 Coping with Parkinson's Disease
American Parkinson's Disease Association
135 Parkinson Avenue   718-981-8001
Staten Island, NY 10305-1944   800-223-2732
                            Fax: 718-981-4399
                              apda@apdaparkinson.org
                              www.apdaparkinson.org
Offers information on the illness, incidence, treatments, education and support for both patients and professionals.
88 pages

6933 Living with Parkinson's Disease
Demos Medical Publishing

386 Park Avenue S   212-683-0072
New York, NY 10016-8804   800-532-8663
                            Fax: 212-683-0118
Written specifically for anyone who has been diagnosed with Parkinson's disease, as well as family members and friends.
1996 150 pages
ISBN: 1-888799-10-2
Dr. Diana M Schneider, President

6934 Parkinson's - A Personal Story of Acceptance
Branden Publishing Company
17 Station Street Box 843   617-734-2045
Wellesley, MA 02482   Fax: 617-734-2046
                              www.brandenbooks.com

1993 162 pages Paperback
ISBN: 0-828319-49-9

6935 Parkinson's Disease & Movement Disorders
Williams & Wilkins
351 W Camden Street   301-528-4000
Baltimore, MD 21201-7912   800-638-0672
1993 640 pages
ISBN: 0-683043-80-3

6936 Parkinson's Disease Handbook
National Parkinson Foundation
200 SE 1st Street   305-547-6666
Miami, FL 33131-1407   800-473-4636
                            Fax: 305-537-9901
                              contact@parkinson.org
                              www.parkinson.org
A guide for patients and their families regarding the illness of Parkinson's.
Paperback

6937 Parkinson's Disease: A Guide for Patient and Family
Raven Press
1185 Ave of the Americas   212-930-9500
New York, NY 10036-2601   800-777-2295
Recommended by patients, the medical community and the leading medical journals, this guide offers information on the most recent medical advances in the field of Parkinson's disease and answers the patients most frequently asked questions about the illness.
224 pages Hardcover
ISBN: 0-781703-12-3

6938 Parkinsonian Syndromes
John H Dekker & Sons
2941 Clydon Avenue SW   616-538-5160
Grand Rapids, MI 49509-2403 Fax: 616-538-0720
1993 584 pages
ISBN: 0-824788-38-9

6939 The Comfort of Home for Parkinson Disease: A Guide for Caregivers
Marie Meyer & Paula Derr, RN with Susa Imke, RN/MS, author
CareTrust Publications
PO Box 10283   800-565-1533
Portland, OR 97296-0283   Fax: 415-673-2005
                              sales@comfortofhome.com
                              www.comfortofhome.com

Comfort will help caregivers be equipped with information about everything from the importance of and noticing wearing off signs to making difficult decisions to travel, equipment options, therapies and dietary guidelines. It offers caregivers mental and emotional support in coping with their challenging role, as well.
2007 298 pages
ISBN: 0-966476-77-8

Children's Books

6940 Journey to Almost There
Clarion Books
215 Park Avenue S   212-420-5800
New York, NY 10003-1603
An interesting tale that surrounds the relationship of Alison and her Granfather O'Brien when Alison's mother feels that he should enter an elderly home.
Grades 6-9

Newsletters

6941 APDA Newsletter
American Parkinson Disease Association
135 Parkinson Avenue
Staten Island, NY 10305-1943
718-981-8001
800-223-2732
Fax: 718-981-4399
apda@apdaparkinson.org
www.apdaparkinson.org
Current information on matters of interest for PD patients and families.
Joel A Miele, President
Joel Gerste, Executive Director

6942 American Parkinson Disease Association Newsletter
60 Bay Street
Staten Island, NY 10301-2514
718-981-8001
800-223-2732
Offers information on the association activities and events, convention and legislative information, medical updates and research reports for the Parkinson's patient and their families.
Quarterly

6943 News & Review
Parkinsons Disease Foundation
1359 Broadway
New York, NY 10018
212-923-4700
800-457-6676
Fax: 212-923-4778
info@pdf.org
www.pdf.org
In each issue we include reports on scientific research and discoveries, treatments and therapies, commentary from physicians and insight from Parkinson's specialists. We also provide practical suggestions, tips and articles from people who live with the disease and wish to share their experiences.
Quarterly
Lewis P Rowland, MD, President
Robin A Elliott, Executive Director

6944 Parkinson Report
National Parkinson Foundation
200 SE 1st Street
Miami, FL 33131-1407
305-547-6666
800-473-4636
Fax: 305-537-9901
contact@parkinson.org
www.parkinson.org
Offers association news and events, conference and symposia news, legislative and medical updates, research reports and more for the Parkinson's patient, their families and the general public.
Quarterly

6945 Parkinson's Disease Foundation Newsletter
Parkinson's Disease Foundation
650 W 168th Street
New York, NY 10032-3702
212-923-4700
800-457-6676
Provides information on Parkinson's Disease Foundation events, news stories of research findings, and technical advances in the field of patient care.

Pamphlets

6946 A One-Stop Shop for Parkinson's Informatio n
Parkinsons Disease Foundation
1359 Broadway
New York, NY 10018
212-923-4700
800-457-6676
Fax: 212-923-4778
info@pdf.org
www.pdf.org
An explanation of PDF's services and resources that are available to answer your most important questions about Parkinson's disease. These services include a toll-free helpline, our Ask the Expert web service and print/video materials.
Lewis P Rowland, MD, President
Robin A Elliott, Executive Director

6947 Adjustment, Adaptation and Accomodation: Psychological Approaches
National Parkinson Foundation
200 SE 1st Street
Miami, FL 33131-1407
305-547-6666
800-473-4636
Fax: 305-537-9901
contact@parkinson.org
www.parkinson.org
Coping strategies for Parkinson's disease.

6948 Akathisia in Parkinson's Disease
Parkinson United Foundation
833 W Washington Blvd
Chicago, IL 60607
312-733-1893
1990

6949 Answering Your Questions About PROPATH
525 Middlefield Road
Menlo Park, CA 94025-3447
800-776-7284
This brochure explains and offers an introduction to PROPATH, a program for Parkinson's disease patients.

6950 Autonomic Failure and Parkinson's Disease
United Parkinson Foundation
833 W Washington Blvd
Chicago, IL 60607-2316
312-733-1893
1990

6951 Balance Disturbances and Parkinson's Disease
United Parkinson Foundation
833 W Washington Blvd
Chicago, IL 60607-2316
312-733-1893
1990

6952 Basic Information About Parkinson's Disease
American Parkinson's Disease Association
135 Parkinson Avenue
Staten Island, NY 10305-1944
718-981-8001
800-223-2732
Fax: 718-981-4399
apda@apdaparkinson.org
www.apdaparkinson.org
Offers information on the illness, incidence, treatments, education and support for both patients and professionals.

6953 Deep Brain Stimulation for Parkinson's Disease
Parkinsons Disease Foundation
1359 Broadway
New York, NY 10018
212-923-4700
800-457-6676
Fax: 212-923-4778
info@pdf.org
www.pdf.org
This booklet addresses the newest area of surgical options in the treatment of PD symptoms _ deep brain stimulation (or DBS) surgery _ while also describing older surgical approaches used to treat PD.
Lewis P Rowland, MD, President
Robin A Elliott, Executive Director

6954 Dental Care for the Patient with Parkinson's Disease
United Parkinson Foundation
833 W Washington Blvd
Chicago, IL 60607-2316
312-733-1893
1987

6955 Depression and Dementia in Parkinson's Disease
United Parkinson Foundation
833 W Washington Blvd
Chicago, IL 60607-2316
312-733-1893
1993

6956 Diagnosis Parkinson's Disease: You Are Not Alone
Parkinsons Disease Foundation
1359 Broadway
New York, NY 10018
212-923-4700
800-457-6676
Fax: 212-923-4778
info@pdf.org
www.pdf.org
Designed for the person newly diagnosed with Parkinson's, this informational booklet serves as a reference for the many questions that may arise. It shares resources, medical expert testimony and

the experiences of people who have dealt with the diagnosis of Parkinson's disease.
Booklet
Lewis P Rowland, MD, President
Robin A Elliott, Executive Director

6957   Dietary Considerations for Parkinson's Disease Patients
United Parkinson Foundation
833 W Washington Blvd   312-733-1893
Chicago, IL 60607-2316

6958   Differential Diagnosis of Parkinsonism
United Parkinson Foundation
833 W Washington Blvd   312-733-1893
Chicago, IL 60607-2316
1984

6959   Driving and the Parkinson's Disease Patient: Some Considerations
United Parkinson Foundation
833 W Washington Blvd   312-733-1893
Chicago, IL 60607-2316
1994

6960   Efficacy of Antiparkinson Medications
United Parkinson Foundation
833 W Washington Blvd   312-733-1893
Chicago, IL 60607-2316
1983

6961   Equipment and Suggestions for Persons with Parkinson's Disease
American Parkinson's Disease Association
135 Parkinson Avenue   718-981-8001
Staten Island, NY 10305-1944   800-223-2732
                                             Fax: 718-981-4399
                                      apda@apdaparkinson.org
                                         www.apdaparkinson.org
Offers information on the illness, incidence, treatments, education and support for both patients and professionals.
19 pages

6962   Eyes and Parkinson's Disease
United Parkinson Foundation
833 W Washington Blvd   312-733-1893
Chicago, IL 60607-2316
1986

6963   Fighting Back Against PD: One Women's Story
National Parkinson Foundation
200 SE 1st Street   305-547-6666
Miami, FL 33131-1407   800-473-4636
                                             Fax: 305-537-9901
                                        contact@parkinson.org
                                            www.parkinson.org
One woman's battle against Parkinson's disease.

6964   Fulfilling the Hope: Our Commitment to the Parkinson's Community
Parkinsons Disease Foundation
1359 Broadway   212-923-4700
New York, NY 10018   800-457-6676
                                             Fax: 212-923-4778
                                                   info@pdf.org
                                                    www.pdf.org
This brochure provides an overview of Parkinsons Disease Foundations services and programs.
Lewis P Rowland, MD, President
Robin A Elliott, Executive Director

6965   Good Nutrition in Parkinson's Disease
American Parkinson Disease Association
60 Bay Street   800-223-2732
Staten Island, NY 10301-2514
Offers information on diet, nutrients, proteins and recipes for people with Parkinson's disease.

6966   How to Start a Parkinson's Disease Support Group
American Parkinson's Disease Association

135 Parkinson Avenue   718-981-8001
Staten Island, NY 10305-1944   800-223-2732
                                             Fax: 718-981-4399
                                      apda@apdaparkinson.org
                                         www.apdaparkinson.org
Offers information on the illness, incidence, treatments, education and support for both patients and professionals.
42 pages

6967   MR Imaging in Parkinson's Disease
United Parkinson Foundation
833 W Washington Blvd   312-733-1893
Chicago, IL 60607-2316
1990

6968   Micrographia
United Parkinson Foundation
833 W Washington Blvd   312-733-1893
Chicago, IL 60607-2316
1991

6969   Neuropsychology and Parkinson's Disease
United Parkinson Foundation
833 W Washington Blvd   312-733-1893
Chicago, IL 60607-2316
1992

6970   Neurotrophic Factors in Parkinson's Disease
United Parkinson Foundation
833 W Washington Blvd   312-733-1893
Chicago, IL 60607-2316
1992

6971   One Step at a Time Brochure
United Parkinson Foundationon
833 W Washington Blvd   312-733-1893
Chicago, IL 60607-2316
An exercise manual for the Parkinsonian patient.
1985

6972   Pain Syndromes and Parkinson's Disease
United Parkinson Foundation
833 W Washington Blvd   312-733-1893
Chicago, IL 60607-2316
1990

6973   Parkinson Handbook: A Guide for Patients and Their Families
National Parkinson Foundation
200 SE 1st Street   305-547-6666
Miami, FL 33131-1407   800-473-4636
                                             Fax: 305-537-9901
                                        contact@parkinson.org
                                            www.parkinson.org
Offers informative, up-to-date information on exercises, hobbies, treatments, speech impairments and psychological aspects.

6974   Parkinson's Advocacy: The Keys to Empowerment
Parkinsons Disease Foundation
1359 Broadway   212-923-4700
New York, NY 10018   800-457-6676
                                             Fax: 212-923-4778
                                                   info@pdf.org
                                                    www.pdf.org
Use this informational brochure to learn how to harness your power as a person living with Parkinson's and join the fight for a cure.
Lewis P Rowland, MD, President
Robin A Elliott, Executive Director

6975   Parkinson's Disease Handbook
American Parkinson's Disease Association
135 Parkinson Avenue   718-981-8001
Staten Island, NY 10305-1944   800-223-2732
                                             Fax: 718-981-4399
                                      apda@apdaparkinson.org
                                         www.apdaparkinson.org
Offers information on the illness, incidence, treatments, education and support for both patients and professionals.
40 pages

6976   Parkinson's Disease Q&A: A Guide for Patients
Parkinsons Disease Foundation
1359 Broadway   212-923-4700
New York, NY 10018   800-457-6676
                                           Fax: 212-923-4778
                                                  info@pdf.org
                                                  www.pdf.org
This booklet answers the most frequently asked questions about
Parkinson's disease. Movement disorder specialists from the Co-
lumbia University Medical Center address topics ranging from
signs of Parkinson's to treatment options to daily living issues.
Booklet
Lewis P Rowland, MD, President
Robin A Elliott, Executive Director

6977   Parkinson's Disease and the Menstrual Cycle
United Parkinson Foundation
833 W Washington Blvd   312-733-1893
Chicago, IL 60607-2316
1990

6978   Parkinson's Disease: The Patient Experience
United Parkinson Foundation
833 W Washington Blvd   312-733-1893
Chicago, IL 60607-2316
Booklet designed for patients with Parkinson's disease and their
families to explain medical terminology and offer suggestions on
how to deal with the disease more easily.
1986

6979   Parkinson's Patient: What You and Your Family Should Know
National Parkinson Foundation
200 SE 1st Street   305-547-6666
Miami, FL 33131-1407   800-473-4636
                                           Fax: 305-537-9901
                                           contact@parkinson.org
                                                www.parkinson.org
Offers a brief overview of Parkinson's Disease causes, symptoms
and treatments as well as offering an insight into statistical information on the illness.

6980   Patient Perspectives on Parkinson's
National Parkinson Foundation
200 SE 1st Street   305-547-6666
Miami, FL 33131-1407   800-473-4636
                                           Fax: 305-537-9901
                                           contact@parkinson.org
                                                www.parkinson.org
Offers a brief overview of Parkinson's disease, the onset of the illness, depression, sexuality, exercise, sleep and nutrition information for daily living.
45 pages

6981   Perioperative Management of Parkinson's Disease
United Parkinson Foundation
833 W Washington Blvd   312-733-1893
Chicago, IL 60607-2316
1989

6982   Pet Scans: A New Look at Parkinson's Disease
United Parkinson Foundation
833 W Washington Blvd   312-733-1893
Chicago, IL 60607-2316
1989

6983   Podiatry and Parkinson's Disease
United Parkinson Foundation
833 W Washington Blvd   312-733-1893
Chicago, IL 60607-2316
1983

6984   Postural Hypotension
United Parkinson Foundation
833 W Washington Blvd   312-733-1893
Chicago, IL 60607-2316
1988

6985   Practical Pointers for Parkinson Patients
National Parkinson Foundation

200 SE 1st Street   305-547-6666
Miami, FL 33131-1407   800-473-4636
                                           Fax: 305-537-9901
                                           contact@parkinson.org
                                                www.parkinson.org
Offers a brief overview of Parkinson's disease, the onset of the illness, depression, sexuality, exercise, sleep and nutrition information for daily living.

6986   Role of Physical Therapy in Parkinson's Disease
United Parkinson Foundation
833 W Washington Blvd   312-733-1893
Chicago, IL 60607-2316
1985

6987   Sexual and Bladder Difficulties in Parkinson's Disease
United Parkinson Foundation
833 W Washington Blvd   312-733-1893
Chicago, IL 60607-2316
1988

6988   Sleep Problems with Parkinson's Disease
United Parkinson Foundation
833 W Washington Blvd   312-733-1893
Chicago, IL 60607-2316
1992

6989   Speech & Swallowing Problems for Parkinsonians
National Parkinson Foundation
200 SE 1st Street   305-547-6666
Miami, FL 33131-1407   800-473-4636
                                           Fax: 305-537-9901
                                           contact@parkinson.org
                                                www.parkinson.org
Offers a brief overview of Parkinson's disease, the onset of the illness, depression, sexuality, exercise, sleep and nutrition information for daily living.

6990   Speech Problems & Swallowing Problems in Parkinson's Disease
American Parkinson Disease Association
60 Bay Street   800-223-2732
Staten Island, NY 10301-2514
Offers information on speech problems, swallowing problems,
hearing impairments and facial mobility for the person with
Parkinson's.

6991   Speech and Voice Impairment
United Parkinson Foundation
833 W Washington Blvd   312-733-1893
Chicago, IL 60607-2316
1983

6992   Stages of Parkinson's Disease
United Parkinson Foundation
833 W Washington Blvd   312-733-1893
Chicago, IL 60607-2316
1983

6993   Suggested Exercise Program for People with Parkinson's Disease
American Parkinson Disease Association
60 Bay Street   800-223-2732
Staten Island, NY 10301-2514
Exercise program pamphlet with full illustrations explaining each
exercise.
23 pages

6994   Treatment of Parkinson's Disease with Carbidopa-Levodopa
National Parkinson Foundation
200 SE 1st Street   305-547-6666
Miami, FL 33131-1407   800-473-4636
                                           Fax: 305-537-9901
                                                www.parkinson.org
Offers information on treating Parkinson's Disease.

Audio & Video

6995   Diagnosis Parkinson's Disease: You Are Not Alone
Parkinsons Disease Foundation

1359 Broadway
New York, NY 10018

212-923-4700
800-457-6676
Fax: 212-923-4778
info@pdf.org
www.pdf.org

Designed for the person newly diagnosed with Parkinson's, this informational booklet and video serve as a reference for the many questions that may arise. It shares resources, medical expert testimony and the experiences of people who have dealt with the diagnosis of Parkinson's disease.
Video & Booklet
Lewis P Rowland, MD, President
Robin A Elliott, Executive Director

6996 Motivating Moves for People with Parkinson's
Parkinsons Disease Foundation
1359 Broadway
New York, NY 10018

212-923-4700
800-457-6676
Fax: 212-923-4778
info@pdf.org
www.pdf.org

Motivating Moves is a unique program of 24 seated exercises designed especially for people with Parkinson's. Exercises address typical Parkinson's symptoms such as stability, flexibility, posture, vocal range and facial expressivity. The video is divided into three sections, How to Do Motivating Moves (45 minutes), The Exercise Class (36 minutes) and Practical Tips for Daily Living (4 minutes).
Video
Lewis P Rowland, MD, President
Robin A Elliott, Executive Director

6997 PDF Exercise Program
Parkinsons Disease Foundation
1359 Broadway
New York, NY 10018

212-923-4700
800-457-6676
Fax: 212-923-4778
info@pdf.org
www.pdf.org

This program consists of three sets of exercises specifically designed for PD patients. Each exercise is clearly illustrated in a 3-ring binder with flip-chart pages and includes two cassette tapes, which provide verbal cues and music for timing.
Cassettes
Lewis P Rowland, MD, President
Robin A Elliott, Executive Director

6998 Parkingson's: Lynda's Story
David Tucker, author

Fanlight Productions
32 Court Street
Brooklyn, NY 11201

718-488-8900
800-876-1710
Fax: 718-488-8642
info@fanlight.com
www.fanlight.com

Parkingson's disease is robbing Lynda McKenzie of normal coordination and movement. She's prepared to participate in a clinical study of surgery to transplant fetal cells directly into her brain, but she will have to live for a year not knowing whether she has received the actual cells or a placebo.
1999 46 Minutes
ISBN: 1-572954-22-1
Nicole Johnson, Publicity Coordinator

Web Sites

6999 Healing Well
www.healingwell.com
An online health resource guide to medical news, chat, information and articles, newsgroups and message boards, books, disease-related web sites, medical directories, and more for patients, friends, and family coping with disabling diseases, disorders, or chronic illnesses.

7000 Health Finder
www.healthfinder.gov
Searchable, carefully developed web site offering information on over 1000 topics. Developed by the US Department of Health and Human Services, the site can be used in both English and Spanish.

7001 Healthlink USA
www.healthlinkusa.com
Health information concerning treatment, cures, prevention, diagnosis, risk factors, research, support groups, email lists, personal stories and much more. Updated regularly.

7002 MedicineNet
www.medicinenet.com
An online resource for consumers providing easy-to-read, authoritative medical and health information.

7003 Medscape
www.medscape.com
Medscape offers specialists, primary care physicians, and other health professionals the Web's most robust and integrated medical information and educational tools.

7004 National Parkinson Foundation
www.parkinson.org
Information on research, diagnosis, treatment and care for men and women suffering from parkinson's and other related neurological diseases.

7005 Neurology Channel
www.healthcommunities.com
Find clearly explained, medically accurate information regarding conditions, including an overview, symptoms, causes, diagnostic procedures and treatment options. On this site it is possible to ask questions and get information from a neurologist and connect to people who have similar health interests.

7006 WebMD
www.webmd.com
Provides credible information, supportive communities, and in-depth reference material about health subjects. A source for original and timely health information as well as material from well known content providers.

Description

7007 Post-Polio Syndrome

Post-Polio syndrome (PPS), also known as the late effects of polio or post-polio sequelae, is characterized by new symptoms that occur in people with a history of polio after a long period of stability during which whatever strength they had recovered remained unchanged. PPS affects approximately 25-40 percent of polio survivors, 15 to 40 years after the initial episode. The hallmark of PPS is new weakness. Other symptoms include fatigue, pain, particularly in the joints, difficulty breathing and swallowing, intolerance to cold, and new muscle atrophy.

While the cause of PPS is not clearly understood, two theories exist. One suggests PPS is caused by the repeated overuse of muscle groups not previously known to have been affected by polio. This overuse weakens them, and it is this weakness that is the major indicator of PPS. A related, but distinct theory postulates that since polio virus attacks motor neurons in the spinal cord, nearby motor neuron axons sprout new nerve termini that innervate those muscle groups that are devoid of proper motor neuron innervation. This healing process restores neural control to the skeletal muscles, but these doubly loaded motor neurons, as a consequence of their heavier workload, simply begin to degenerate faster than their singly-load counterparts. A polio survivor with an affected leg may find that his or her arms become newly affected. Whether the arm problems are a result of undetected muscle damage that occurred at the time of the original polio or newer damage resulting from the overuse of the remaining good muscles, or a combination of the two, is not clearly understood.

PPS is frequently emotionally difficult for polio survivors. Many feel they have triumphed over their initial polio, or have come to terms with their resulting disabilities. To think that the polio is coming back is often terrifying. These emotional issues are frequently made more difficult by the fact that PPS is often mis-diagnosed as other conditions or normal aging. Also, patients are often given misinformation about PPS.

Post-polio syndrome, like most diseases classified as syndromes, does not have a specific diagnostic test, but a diagnosis of exclusion. This means that other medical conditions that may present with symptoms similar to those found in PPS should be considered and excluded, if possible. Once diagnosis of PPS is determined, treatment is individualized by primary symptoms and may include medications, supervised therapy, injections and, in some cases, surgery. Exercise programs have shown some benefit in many PPS patients.

National Agencies & Associations

7008 American Association of Neuromuscular & Electrodiagnostic Medicine
2621 Superior Drive NW
Rochester, MN 55901
507-288-0100
Fax: 507-288-1225
aanem@aanem.org
www.aanem.org

The American Association of Neuromuscular & Electrodiagnostic Medicine (AANEM) is a nonprofit membership association dedicated to the advancement of neuromuscular, musculoskeletal, and electrodiagnostic medicine.
Shirlyn A. Adkins, JD, Executive Director
Millie Suk, JD, MPP, Health Policy Director

7009 American Chronic Pain Association
PO Box 850
Rocklin, CA 95677
800-533-3231
ACPA@theacpa.org
www.theacpa.org

The ACPA facilitates peer support and education for individuals with chronic pain in its many forms, in order to increase quality of life. Also raises awareness among the healthcare community, and with policy makers.
Penney Cowan, Founder & CEO
Daniel Galia, Director, Global Support

7010 Chronic Syndrome Sufferers Association
1487 Redbud Drive
Huntington, NY 11743
www.cssa-inc.org

Educates the general population and health-care professionals on chronic immunological and neurological disorders.
Clair Flores, Head of Operations

7011 Orthopaedic Rehabilitation Association
3 Cooper Plaza
Camden, NJ 08103
856-968-7695
Fax: 856-968-8766
jaconetti-lauren@cooperhealth.edu
www.orthorehabassoc.org

Association whose membership consists of orthopaedic surgeons interested in the rehabilitation of patients with complex musculoskeletal problems.
David Fuller, MD, President
E. Byron Marsolais, MD, PhD, Secretary

7012 Polio Survivors Association
12720 La Reina Avenue
Downey, CA 90242
562-862-4508
Fax: 562-862-4508
info@polioassociation.org
www.polioassociation.org

Non-profit association to promote the well-being and improve the quality of life for polio survivors.
Richard Daggett, President

7013 Post-Polio Awareness & Support Society of British Columbia
2-2630 Ross Lane
Victoria, BC, V8T-5L5
250-477-8244
www.post-polio.org

A non-profit society that connects support groups.
Joan Toone, President

Support Groups & Hotlines

7014 National Health Information Center
Office of Disease Prevention & Health Promotion
1101 Wootton Pkwy
Rockville, MD 20852
Fax: 240-453-8281
odphpinfo@hhs.gov
www.health.gov/nhic

Supports public health education by maintaining a calendar of National Health Observances; helps connect consumers and health professionals to organizations that can best answer questions and provide up-to-date contact information from reliable sources; updates on a yearly basis toll-free numbers for health information, Federal health clearinghouses and info centers.
Don Wright, MD, MPH, Director

7015 PostPolio Health International
4207 Lindell Boulevard
Saint Louis, MO 63108-2915
314-534-0475
Fax: 314-534-5070
www.post-polio.org/

Post-Polio Health International's mission is to enhance the lives and independence of polio survivors and home ventilator users through education, advocacy, research and networking.
Willism G Stothers, President
Saul J Morse, Legal counsel

Books

7016 Managing Post-Polio: A Guide for Polio Survivors and Their Families
Yale University Press
4207 Lindell Boulevard
St. Louis, MO 63108-9040
314-534-0475
Fax: 314-534-5070
info@post-polio.org
www.post-polio.org
Diagnosis and management of polio-related health problems . Essential resources for polio survivors, their families and health care providers.

7017 Managing Post-Polio: A Guide to Living Well with Post-Polio Syndrome
ABI Professional Publications
PO Box 5243
Arlington, VA 22205
703-525-5488
Fax: 703-524-4105
Practical information resulting from a combination of professional knowledge and personal experience. A comprehensive array of topics are addressed: the diagnostic process, finding expert medical care, energy conservation, psychosocial aspects of disability, support groups, vocational strategies, managed care concerns, Social Security benefits, and internet resources.
256 pages

Newsletters

7018 Polio Network News
Post-Polio Health International
4207 Lindell Boulevard
St. Louis, MO 63108-2915
314-534-0475
Fax: 314-534-5070
info@ventusers.org
www.ventusers.org
The newsletter of the International Ventilator Users Network, an affiliate of Post-Polio Health International.
Joan Headley, Executive Director

7019 Post-Polio Health
Post-Polio Health International
4207 Lindell Boulevard
Saint Louis, MO 63108-2915
314-534-0475
Fax: 314-534-5070
info@ventusers.org
www.ventusers.org
The newsletter of the International Ventilator Users Network, an affiliate of Post-Polio Health International.
12 pages Quarterly
Joan Headley, Executive Director

7020 Post-Polio Health International
Joan L Headley, author
4207 Lindell Boulevard
St. Louis, MO 63108-2915
314-534-0475
Fax: 314-534-5070
info@post-polio.org
www.post-polio.org
Provides educational materials, advocacy, networking and support research to enhance the lives and independence of polio survivors and users of home mechanical ventilators. Minimum $25.00 with membership.
12 pages
Joan Headley, Executive Director

7021 Ventilator-Assisted Living
Joan L Headley, author
4207 Lindell Boulevard
St. Louis, MO 63108-2915
314-534-0475
Fax: 314-534-5070
info@post-polio.org
www.post-polio.org
Provides educational materials, advocacy, networking and support research to enhance the lives and independence of polio survivors

and users of home mechanical ventilators. Minimum $25.00 with membership.
12 pages
Joan Headley, Executive Director

7022 Ventilator: Assisted Living
Post-Polio Health International
4207 Lindell Boulevard
St. Louis, MO 63108-2915
314-534-0475
Fax: 314-534-5070
info@ventusers.org
www.ventusers.org
The newsletter of the International Ventilator Users Network, an affiliate of Post-Polio Health International.
12 pages Newsletter
Joan Headley, Executive Director

Pamphlets

7023 Guidelines for People Who Have Had Polio
March of Dimes
PO Box 1657
Wilkes-Barre, PA 18703
717-820-8104
800-367-6630
Fax: 570-825-1987
Located on website as a PDF file. Information based on March of Dimes International Conference on Post-Polio Syndrome.

7024 Post-Polio Syndrome: Identifying Best Practices in Diagnosis and Care
March of Dimes
1275 Mamaroneck Avenue
White Plains, NY 10605
914-997-4488
Fax: 212-254-3518
NY639@marchofdimes.com
www.marchofdimes.com
Located on website as PDF file.

Web Sites

7025 EMedicine
emedicine.medscape.com
EMedicine was launched in 1996 and is the largest and most current clinical knowledge base available to physicians and health professionals.

7026 International Rehabilitation Center for Polio
International Rehabilitation Center for Polio (IRCP) at Spaulding Rehabilitation HOspital website offers information about PPS and resources for polio survivors and others with an interest in post-polio syndrome.

7027 MedicineNet
www.medicinenet.com
An online resource for consumers providing easy-to-read, authoritative medical and health information.

7028 Polio Experience Network
www.polionet.org
The Polio Experience Network offers information, inspiration, ideas and resources for polio survivors and those seeking information on post-polio syndrome.

7029 Social Security Administration
www.ssa.gov/agency
Social Security delivers a broad range of services online at socialsecurity.gov and through a nationwide network of over 1,400 offices that include regional offices, field offices, card centers, teleservice centers, processing centers, hearing offices, the Appeals Council, and our State and territorial partners, the Disability Determination Services.

Description

7030 Post-Traumatic Stress Disorder

Post-Traumatic Stress Disorder, or PTSD, is one of the Anxiety Disorders receiving particular attention because it affects a significant number of individuals returning from war zones, as well as those affected by terrorism and natural disasters. PTSD has been recognized for at least a hundred years. During and after World War I, traumatized soldiers' symptoms of hypersensitivity, avoidance, and other characteristics of what we now call PTSD were called 'shell shock' in the past. PTSD continues to be identified with military service, but it is not limited to members of the military. It can affect adults and children exposed to terrifying and dangerous events in any circumstances: natural disasters, physical and/or sexual attacks, acts of terrorism and accidents, for example. By definition, the precipitating event must be outside the bounds of everyday human experience and the individual must feel helpless to protect him or herself from the event. Women appear to be somewhat more vulnerable to PTSD than men. PTSD has five main components that include experiencing the traumatic event, re-experiencing the event in the form of intrusive thoughts or memories, nightmares flashbacks, or waking dreams, engaging in avoidance of people, situations, or feelings associated with the event, suffering from these experiences, and having increased arousal or a feeling of always being on edge.

National Agencies & Associations

7031 Administration for Children and Families
330 C Street SW
Washington, DC 20201
202-205-8347
Fax: 202-205-9721
www.acf.hhs.gov
The Administration for Children & Families (ACF) is a division of the U.S. Department of Health & Human Services (HHS). ACF promotes the economic and social well-being of families, children, individuals and communities.
Lynn Johnson, Assistant Secretary
Jerry Milner, Acitng Commissioner, Children & Families

7032 African American Post Traumatic Stress Disorder Association
9129 Veterans Drive SW
Lakewood, WA 98498
253-589-0766
aaptsdassn.org
www.aaptsdassn.org
Non-profit organization supporting Post-Traumatic Stress Disorder (PTSD) research, and individuals with PTSD. Develops programs that encourage healthy living and provides assistance to individuals with PTSD.
Sidney A. Lee, President
Donald Curtis, Vice President

7033 Agency for Healthcare Research and Quality
5600 Fishers Lane
Rockville, MD 20857
301-427-1104
www.ahrq.gov
The Agency for Healthcare Research and Quality's (AHRQ) mission is to produce evidence to make health care safer, higher quality, more accessible, equitable, and affordable, and to work within the U.S. Department of Health and Human Services and with other partners to make sure that the evidence is understood and used.
Gopal Khanna, MBA, Director
Howard E. Holland, Director, Communications

7034 Agency for Toxic Substances and Disease Registry
4770 Buford Hwy NE
Atlanta, GA 30341-3717
770-488-0736
800-232-4636
Fax: 770-488-1547
TTY: 888-232-6348
jah8@cdc.gov
www.atsdr.cdc.gov
The Agency for Toxic Substances and Disease Registry (ATSDR), based in Atlanta, Georgia, is a federal public health agency of the U.S. Department of Health and Human Services. ATSDR serves the public by using the best science, taking responsive public health actions, and providing trusted health information to prevent harmful exposures and diseases related to toxic substances.
Patrick Breysse, PhD, CIH, Director
Jack Hanley, Acting Branch Chief, Central Branch

7035 American Academy of Child and Adolescent Psychiatry (AACAP)
3615 Wisconsin Avenue NW
Washington, DC 20016-3007
202-966-7300
Fax: 202-464-0131
clinical@aacap.org
Promotes the healthy development of children, adolescents, and families through advocacy, education, and research.
Karen Dineen Wagner, MD, PhD, President
Bennett L. Leventhal, MD, Treasurer

7036 American Chronic Pain Association
PO Box 850
Rocklin, CA 95677
800-533-3231
ACPA@theacpa.org
www.theacpa.org
The ACPA facilitates peer support and education for individuals with chronic pain in its many forms, in order to increase quality of life. Also raises awareness among the healthcare community, and with policy makers.
Penney Cowan, Founder & CEO
Daniel Galia, Director, Global Support

7037 American Medical Association (AMA)
330 N Wabash Ave.
Chicago, IL 60611-5885
312-464-4782
800-262-3211
www.ama-assn.org/ama
Committed to ensuring sustainable physician practices that result in better health outcomes for patients.
James L. Madara, MD, CEO & Executive Vice President
Howard C. Bauchner, MD, Senior Vice President & Editor-in-Chief

7038 American Psychiatric Association
800 Maine Avenue SW
Washington, DC 20024
202-559-3900
apa@psych.org
www.psychiatry.org
A medical specialty society representing a growing membership of psychiatrists. Offers information for psychiatrists, medical students, patients and families.

7039 American Psychological Association
750 First Street NE
Washington, DC 20002-4242
202-336-5500
800-374-2721
TTY: 202-336-6123
www.apa.org
Advancing the creation, communication and application of psychological knowledge to benefit society and improve people's lives.
Rosie Phillips Davis, PhD, President
Jean A. Carter, PhD, Treasurer

7040 American Public Health Association (APHA)
800 I Street NW
Washington, DC 20001
202-777-2742
Fax: 202-777-2534
TTY: 202-777-2500
www.apha.org
Aims to strengthen the public health profession and promote and advocate for public health issues and policies backed by science.
Pamela M. Aaltonen, PhD, President
Georges C. Benjamin, MD, Executive Director

7041 American Trauma Society (ATS)
201 Park Washington Court   703-538-3544
Falls Church, VA 22046   800-556-7890
                                         Fax: 703-241-5603
                                         info@amtrauma.org
                                         www.amtrauma.org
American Trauma Society (ATS) is committed to the elimination of
needless death and disability from injury. Advocates for trauma
prevention programs.
Christopher Michetti, MD, President
Suzanne M. Prentiss, Executive Director

7042 Anxiety Disorders Association of America
8701 Georgia Avenue   240-485-1001
Silver Spring, MD 20910   Fax: 240-485-1035
                                         information@adaa.org
                                         www.adaa.org
ADAA is a national non-profit organization dedicated to the prevention, treatment, and cure of anxiety, depression, OCD, PTSD,
and related disorders and to improving the lives of all people who
suffer from them through education, practice, and research.
Mary E. Beth Salcedo, MD, President
Luana Marques, PhD, President-Elect

7043 Association for Behavioral and Cognitive Therapies
305 7th Avenue   212-647-1890
New York, NY 10001   www.abct.org
Multidisciplinary organization committed to the advancement of
evidence-based approaches to treating and improving human
functioning.
Mary Jane Eimer, CAE, Executive Director
David Teisler, CAE, Director of Communications

7044 Association for Traumatic Stress Specialists
5000 Old Buncombe Road   864-294-4337
Greenville, SC 29617   admin@atss.info
                                         www.atss.info
Professional membership organization of individuals engaged in
and committed to excellence in trauma services, response, and
treatment.
Linda Hood, BA, CTSS, President
Brad Coulbeck, CTSS, Vice President

7045 Centers for Medicare & Medicaid Services
7500 Security Boulevard   410-786-3000
Baltimore, MD 21244   877-267-2323
                                         TTY: 866-226-1819
                                         www.cms.gov
U.S. federal agency which administers Medicare, Medicaid, and
the State Children's Health Insurance Program.
Seema Verma, Administrator
Tom Corry, Director

7046 Freedom From Fear
308 Seaview Avenue   718-351-1717
Staten Island, NY 10305   help@freedomfromfear.org
                                         www.freedomfromfear.org
Freedom From Fear is a national non-profit mental health advocacy organization providing community support and promoting research and education.
Mary Guardino, Founder & Executive Director

7047 Goodwill Industries International, Inc.
15810 Indianola Drive   800-466-3945
Rockville, MD 20855   contactus@goodwill.org
                                         www.goodwill.org
A nonprofit, community-based organization whose mission is to
help people achieve self-sufficiency through the dignity and
power of work, serving people who are disadvantaged, disabled or
elderly. The mission is accomplished through providing independent living skills, affordable housing, and training and placement in
community employment. The GoodWill Network includes 160 independent, local locations across the U.S. and Canada.
S. Dale Jenkins, Chair
Steven C. Preston, President & CEO

7048 International Society for Traumatic Stress Studies
1 Parkview Plaza   847-686-2234
Oakbrook Terrace, IL 60181   Fax: 847-686-2251
                                         info@istss.org
                                         www.istss.org
The International Society for Traumatic Stress Studies is dedicated
to sharing information about the effects of trauma and traumatic
stress.
Julian D. Ford, PhD, ABPP, President
Ananda Amsdatter, PhD, Vice President

7049 International Society for the Study of Trauma and Dissociation
1420 New York Avenue   202-803-6332
Washington, DC 20005   Fax: 202-747-2864
                                         info@isst-d.org
                                         www.isst-d.org
The International Society for the Study of Trauma and Dissociation is a non-profit, professional association organized to develop
clinically effective and empirically based resources and responses
to trauma and dissociation.
Christine Forner, BA, BSW, MSW, President
D. Michael Coy, MA, LICSW, Treasurer

7050 National Alliance on Mental Illness (NAMI)
3803 N Fairfax Drive   703-524-7600
Arlington, VA 22203   800-950-6264
                                         info@nami.org
                                         www.nami.org
Committed to building better lives for the millions of Americans
affected by mental illness by raising awareness and offering com-
munity support.
Adrienne Kennedy, MA, President
Lacey Berumen, PhD, LAC, MNM, First Vice President

7051 National Association of Social Workers (NASW)
750 First Street NE   202-408-8600
Washington, DC 20002   800-742-4089
                                         membership@socialworkers.org
                                         www.socialworkers.org
The National Association of Social Workers (NASW) is the largest
membership organization of professional social workers in the
world, working to enhance and maintain professional standards
and advance social policies.
Kathryn Conley Wehrmann, PhD, President
Angelo McClain, PhD, LICSW, CEO

7052 National Center for Complementary and Integrative Health
9000 Rockville Pike   888-644-6226
Bethesda, MD 20892   TTY: 866-464-3615
                                         info@nccih.nih.gov
                                         nccih.nih.gov
The National Center for Complementary and Integrative Health
(NCCIH) is the Federal Government's lead agency for scientific
research on the diverse medical and health care systems, practices,
and products that are not generally considered part of conventional
medicine.
Helene M. Langevin, MD, Director
David Shurtleff, Ph.D., Deputy Director

7053 National Human Genome Research Institute
Building 31, Room 4B09   301-402-0911
Bethesda, MD 20892-2152   Fax: 301-402-2218
                                         www.genome.gov
The National Human Genome Research Institute began as the Na-
tional Center for Human Genome Research (NCHGR), which was
established in 1989 to carry out the role of the National Institutes
of Health (NIH) in the International Human Genome Project
(HGP).
Eric D. Green, M.D., Ph.D., Director
Lawrence Brody, Ph.D., Director, Division of Genomics & Society

7054 National Institute of Environmental Health Sciences
105 T.W. Alexander Drive   919-541-3345
Research Triangle Park, NC 27709   webcenter@niehs.nih.gov
                                         www.niehs.nih.gov
The mission of the NIEHS is to discover how the environment af-
fects people in order to promote healthier lives.
Linda S. Birnbaum, PhD, Director
Richard Woychik, PhD, Deputy Director

7055 National Institute of General Medical Sciences
45 Center Drive MSC 6200
Bethesda, MD 20892-6200

301-496-7301
info@nigms.nih.gov
www.nigms.nih.gov

The National Institute of General Medical Sciences (NIGMS) supports basic research that increases understanding of biological processes and lays the foundation for advances in disease diagnosis, treatment and prevention.
Jon R. Lorsch, PhD, Director
Judith H. Greenberg, PhD, Deputy Director

7056 National Institute of Mental Health
6001 Executive Boulevard
Rockville, MD 20852

866-615-6464
Fax: 301-443-4279
TTY: 866-415-8051
nimhinfo@nih.gov
www.nimh.nih.gov

The National Institute of Mental Health works to transform the understanding and treatment of mental illnesses through basic and clinical research, paving the way for prevention, recovery, and cure.
Joshua A. Gordon, MD, PhD, Director

7057 Posttraumatic Stress Disorder (PTSD) Alliance

888-436-6306
www.ptsdalliance.org

Provides educational resources to individuals diagnosed with PTSD and their loved ones; those at risk for developing PTSD; and medical, healthcare and other frontline professionals.

7058 The Society of Federal Health Professionals (AMSUS)
12154 Darnestown Road
Gaithersburg, MD 20878-2206

301-897-8800
www.amsus.org

The Society of Federal Health Professionals (AMSUS) is a non-profit organization for federal and international health professionals committed to improving the health of all Americans.
John M. Cho, MD, Executive Director & CEO
Ken Canestrini, Deputy Executive Director & COO

State Agencies & Associations

District of Columbia

7059 Administration for Community Living
One Massachusetts Avenue
Washington, DC 20001

202-619-0724
800-677-1116
Fax: 202-357-3555
aclinfo@acl.hhs.gov
www.acl.gov

ACL brings together the efforts and achievements of the Administration on Aging, the Administration on Intellectual and Developmental Disabilities, and the HHS Office on Disability to serve as the Federal agency responsible for increasing access to community supports, while focusing attention and resources on the unique needs of older Americans and people with disabilities across the lifespan.
Kathy Greenlee, Administrator
Sharon Lewis, Principal Deputy Administrator

7060 Federal Emergency Management Agency
500 C Street S.W.
Washington, DC 20472

202-646-2500
800-621-3362
TTY: 800-427-5593
www.fema.gov

FEMA's mission is to support the citizens and first responders to ensure that as a nation we work together to build, sustain and improve our capability to prepare for, protect against, respond to, recover from and mitigate all hazards.
W. Craig Fugate, Administrator
Michael Coen, Jr., Chief of Staff

7061 U.S. Department of Health and Human Services
200 Independence Ave, SW
Washington, DC 20201

877-696-6775
www.hhs.gov

The U.S. Department of Health and Human Services (HHS) is the U.S. government's principal agency for protecting the health of all Americans and providing essential human services, especially for those who are least able to help themselves.
Sylvia M. Burwell, Secretary
Mary K. Wakefield, Acting Deputy Secretary

Florida

7062 Goodwill Industries-Suncoast
10596 Gandy Boulevard
St. Petersburg, FL 33702

727-523-1512
888-279-1988
TTY: 727-579-1068
www.goodwill-suncoast.org

A nonprofit, community-based organization whose mission is to help people achieve self-sufficiency through the dignity and power of work, serving people who are disadvantaged, disabled or elderly. The mission is accomplished through providing independent living skills, affordable housing, and training and placement in community employment.
Heather Ceresoli, CPA, Chair
Deborah A. Passerini, President & CEO

Maryland

7063 Center for Mental Health Services
Room 6-1057
Rockville, MD 20857

240-276-1310
www.samhsa.gov

The Center for Mental Health Services leads federal efforts to promote the prevention and treatment of mental disorders. Congress created CMHS to bring new hope to adults who have serious mental illness and children with emotional disorders.
Paolo del Vecchio, M.S.W., Director
Elizabeth Lopez, Ph.D., Deputy Director

Virginia

7064 National Science Foundation
4201 Wilson Blvd
Arlington, VA 22230

703-292-5111
TDD: 703-292-5090
info@nsf.gov
www.nsf.gov

NSF is the only federal agency whose mission includes support for all fields of fundamental science and engineering, except for medical sciences.
France A. Cordova, Director
Joan Ferrini-Mundy, Chief Operating Officer

Libraries & Resource Centers

7065 Anxiety Resource Center
312 Grandville Ave.
Grand Rapids, MI 49503

616-356-1614
director@anxietyresourcecenter.org
anxietyresourcecenter.org

The Anxiety Resource Center, Inc. of Grand Rapids, Michigan, was founded to educate the public and professional communities about anxiety disorders, including Obsessive-Compulsive Disorder and OCD Spectrum Disorders; to reduce the stigma associated with these illnesses; and to provide a place that offers support, hope and inspiration.

7066 Brain Injury Resource Center
P.O.BOX 84151
Seattle, WA 98124

206-621-8558
brain@headinjury.com
www.headinjury.com

Providing wealth of information, creative solutions and leadership on issues related to brain injury since 1985.

7067 BrainLine.org
2775 South Quincy Street
Arlington, VA 22206

703-998-2020
info@BrainLine.org

BrainLine is a national multimedia project offering information and resources about preventing, treating, and living with TBI.
Noel Gunther, Executive Director
Christian Lindstrom, Director, Learning Media

7068 Center for the Study of Traumatic Stress
4301 Jones Bridge Road
Bethesda, MD 20814

cstsinfo@usuhs.mil
www.cstsonline.org

There sustained mission is to advance scientific and academic knowledge, interventions, educational resources and outreach to mitigate the impact of trauma from exposure to war, disasters, terrorism, community violence and public health threats.
Robert J. Ursano, MD, Director

7069   Gift From Within
16 Cobb Hill Rd.
Camden, ME 4843
207-236-8858
Fax: 207-236-2818
JoyceB3955@aol.com
www.giftfromwithin.org
PTSD Resources for Survivors and Caregivers.

7070   Institute on Violence, Abuse and Trauma
10065 Old Grove Road
San Diego, CA 92131
858-527-1860
Fax: 858-527-1743
www.ivatcenters.org
The Institute on Violence, Abuse and Trauma (IVAT) is an international resource and training center at Alliant International University.
Robert Geffner, Ph.D., President
Sandi Capuano Morrison, M.A., Executive Director

7071   National Center for PTSD
802-296-6300
ncptsd@va.gov
www.ptsd.va.gov
The National Center for PTSD is dedicated to research and education on trauma and PTSD.

7072   National Center for Victims of Crime
2000 M Street NW
Washington, DC 20036
202-467-8700
Fax: 202-467-8701
webmaster@ncvc.org
www.victimsofcrime.org
The mission of the National Center for Victims of Crime is to forge a national commitment to help victims of crime rebuild their lives. They are dedicated to serving individuals, families, and communities harmed by crime.
Mai Fernandez, Executive Director
Jeffrey R. Dion, Deputy Executive Director

7073   National Headache Foundation
820 N. Orleans
Chicago, IL 60610
312-274-2650
info@headaches.org
www.headaches.org
The mission at the National Headache Foundation has been to further awareness of headache and migraine as legitimate neurobiological diseases.
Arthur H. Elkind, M.D., President
Vincent Martin, M.D., Vice President

7074   National Sexual Violence Resource Center
123 North Enola Drive
Enola, PA 17025
717-909-0710
877-739-3895
Fax: 717-909-0714
TTY: 717-909-0715
resources@nsvrc.org
www.nsvrc.org
The NSVRC's Mission is to provide leadership in preventing and responding to sexual violence through collaboration, sharing and creating resources, and promoting research.

7075   Posttraumatic Stress Disorder (PTSD) Alliance
www.ptsdalliance.org
The Posttraumatic Stress Disorder (PTSD) Alliance is a group of professional and advocacy organizations that have joined forces to provide educational resources to individuals diagnosed with PTSD and their loved ones; those at risk for developing PTSD; and medical, healthcare and other frontline professionals.

7076   RNtoBSN.org
1001 McKinney St.
Houston, TX 77002
505-221-6056
contact@rntobsn.org
www.rntobsn.org
RNtoBSN.org's mission is plain: Further the education of new and established nurses.
Caroline Porter Thomas, BSN, RN, Expert

7077   Sidran Institute
PO Box 436
Brooklandville, MD 21022
410-825-8888
Fax: 410-560-0134
help@sidran.org
www.sidran.org
Sidran (SID-run) began in 1986 out of a family tragedy when a beloved family member who had been abused in childhood was subsequently diagnosed with serious, debilitating psychiatric problems and a related life-threatening medical disorder.
Esther Giller, President/ Director
Tracy Howard, Book Sales/ Office Manager

7078   Suicide Prevention Resource Center
43 Foundry Avenue
Waltham, MA 2453
877-438-7772
Fax: 617-969-9186
TTY: 617-964-5448
info@sprc.org
www.sprc.org
SPRC is the nation's only federally supported resource center devoted to advancing the National Strategy for Suicide Prevention.
Jerry Reed, PhD, MSW, Director
Chris Miara, MS, Director of Operations & Resources

7079   Trauma Center
1269 Beacon Street
Brookline, MA 2446
617-232-1303
Fax: 617-232-1280
www.traumacenter.org
The Trauma Center is a program of Justice Resource Institute (JRI), a large nonprofit organization dedicated to social justice by offering hope and promise of fulfillment to children, adults, and families who are at risk of not receiving effective services essential to their safety, progress, and/or survival.
Dr. Bessel van der Kolk, Founder
Margaret Blaustein, Ph.D, Director of Training and Education

7080   Women's Resource Center
113 W. Wayne Avenue
Wayne, PA 19087
610-687-6391
Fax: 610-687-2967
info@womensrc.org
womensresourcecenter.net
Women's Resource Center (WRC) is a registered 501c3 nonprofit that supports women, strengthens families and builds communities through information, referral, counseling, legal, and educational services.
Shelley Potente, MA, President
Virginia Bowden, Vice President

Research Centers

7081   ChildTrauma Academy
866-943-9779
Fax: 713-513-5465
cta@childtrauma.org
childtrauma.org
CTA is a not-for-profit organization based in Houston, Texas working to improve the lives of high-risk children through direct service, research and education.
Bruce D. Perry, M.D., Ph.D., Founder/ Senior Fellow
Jana Rosenfelt, M.Ed., Executive Director

7082   National Center for PTSD
802-296-6300
ncptsd@va.gov
www.ptsd.va.gov
The National Center for PTSD is dedicated to research and education on trauma and PTSD.

Arizona

7083   Mayo Clinic
13400 E. Shea Blvd.
Scottsdale, AZ 85259
480-301-8000
800-446-2279
www.mayoclinic.org
Mayo Clinic is a not-for-profit organization and proceeds from Web advertising help support our mission. Mayo Clinic does not endorse any of the third party products and services advertised.
Sandhya Pruthi, M.D., Medical Director
Kenneth G. Berge, M.D., Senior Medical Editor

California

7084 Synergy Clinical Research Center
1908 Sweetwater Road   888-539-0282
National City, CA 91950   Fax: 619-327-0163
                        www.synergyresearchcenters.com
Synergy is dedicated to providing comprehensive and exemplary clinical research services to advance the science of medicine.
Dr. Bari , Medical Director, Principal Investigator
Dr. Ishaque , Medical Director, Principal Investigator

7085 The Center for Culture, Trauma and Mental Health Disparities
760 Westwood Plaza   310-794-9929
Los Angeles, CA 90024   www.semel.ucla.edu/cctmhd
The Center for Culture, Trauma, and Mental Health Disparities is a multi-ethnic and multi-disciplinary group promoting interdisciplinary research examining the prevalence and impact of traumatic experiences on PTSD, depression and concomitant cognitive/emotional, behavioral, psychological and biological processes in ethnic minority populations.
Gail Wyatt, Director

7086 UCLA Anxiety Disorders Research Center
Department of Psychology   310-825-9312
Los Angeles, CA 90094   rose@psych.ucla.edu
                               anxiety.psych.ucla.edu
The purpose of The ADRC is to further our understanding of the factors that place individuals at risk for developing phobias, anxiety disorders and related conditions, and to develop more effective treatments that have long lasting effects and are cost effective.
Michelle G. Craske, Ph.D., Director
Raphael Rose, Ph.D., Associate Director

Connecticut

7087 Yale Child Study Center
230 South Frontage Rd.   203-785-2540
New Haven, CT 6519   childstudycenter.yale.edu
At our core is the mission to improve the lives of children and families through research, service, and training.
Dr. Linda Mayes, Interim Director

District of Columbia

7088 Center for Mind-Body Medicine
5225 Connecticut Avenue   202-966-7338
Washington, DC 20015   cmbm.org
The Center for Mind-Body Medicine creates communities of hope and healing.
James S. Gordon, MD, President
James S. Gordon, MD, Founder/ Director

Florida

7089 Center for the Study of Emotion and Attention
University of Florida   Fax: 352-392-6047
Gainesville, FL 32611   csea.phhp.ufl.edu
The Center for the Study of Emotion & Attention is a facility for the scientific study of human emotion, highlighting emotion's foundation on survival circuits in the mammalian brain, and its motivational significance for attentional engagement and response mobilization.

Georgia

7090 Mood and Anxiety Disorders Program of Emory University
12 Executive Park Dr., NE   404-778-6663
Atlanta, GA 30329   studies@emoryclinicaltrials.com
                               www.psychiatry.emory.edu
The Mood and Anxiety Disorders Program of Emory Univeristy's School of Medicine is a dedicated research program within Emory's Department of Psychiatry and Behavioral Sciences.
Boadie Dunlop, M.D., Assistant Professor
Jeff Rakofsky, M.D., Associate Professor

Illinois

7091 International Society for Traumatic Stress Studies
111 Deer Lake Road   847-480-9028
Deerfield, IL 60015   Fax: 847-480-9282
                                        info@istss.org
                                        www.istss.org
The International Society for Traumatic Stress Studies is dedicated to sharing information about the effects of trauma and the discovery and dissemination of knowledge about policy, program and service initiatives that seek to reduce traumatic stressors and their immediate and long-term consequences.
Miranda Olff, PhD, President
Julian Ford, PhD, Vice President

Indiana

7092 GoldPoint Clinical Research
8902 North Meridian Strt.   317-229-6202
Indianapolis, IN 46260   Fax: 317-218-3347
GoldPoint Clinical Research of Indianapolis' team has 20 years of experience conducting more than 250 Phase II, III & IV neuroscience clinical trials. As one of the Midwest's leading research study centers, GoldPoint is led by medical director and board-certified addiction psychiatrist, Richard Saini, MD. - See more at: http://goldpointcr.com/about-us/leadership/#sthash.oaNpLa69.dpuf
Mary Newkerk, Director of Operations

Maryland

7093 Center for the Study of Traumatic Stress
Uniformed Services Uni.   cstsinfo@usuhs.mil
Bethesda, MD 20814   www.cstsonline.org
Robert J. Ursano, MD, Director

7094 National Institute of Mental Health
6001 Executive Boulevard   301-443-4536
Rockville, MD 20852   Fax: 301-443-4279
                                   NIMHinfo@mail.nih.gov
                                        www.nimh.nih.gov
The mission of NIMH is to transform the understanding and treatment of mental illnesses through basic and clinical research, paving the way for prevention, recovery, and cure.

Massachusetts

7095 Center for Anxiety and Related Disorders at Boston University
648 Beacon St.   617-353-9610
Boston, MA 2215   bonnieb@bu.edu
                                        www.bu.edu/card
The Center for Anxiety and Related Disorders (CARD) is an internationally known clinical and research center dedicated to advancing knowledge and providing care for anxiety, mood, eating, sleep, and related disorders.
David H. Barlow, Ph.D., Founder and Director Emeritus
Timothy A. Brown, Psy.D., Director of Research and Research Admin

7096 Trauma Center
1269 Beacon Street   617-232-1303
Brookline, MA 2446   Fax: 617-232-1280
                                     www.traumacenter.org
The Trauma Center is a program of Justice Resource Institute (JRI), a large nonprofit organization dedicated to social justice by offering hope and promise of fulfillment to children, adults, and families who are at risk of not receiving effective services essential to their safety, progress, and/or survival.
Dr. Bessel van der Kolk, Founder
Margaret Blaustein, Ph.D, Director of Training and Education

New York

7097 The Dana Foundation
505 Fifth Avenue   212-223-4040
New York, NY 10017   Fax: 212-317-8721
                                       danainfo@dana.org
                                        www.dana.org

The Dana Foundation is a private philanthropic organization that supports brain research through grants, publications, and educational programs.
Edward F. Rover, Chairman/ President
Burton M. Mirsky, EVP, Finance

Virginia

7098 Samueli Institute
1737 King Street   703-299-4800
Alexandria, VA 22314   Fax: 703-535-6752
www.samueliinstitute.org
Samueli Institute is advancing the science of healing worldwide by applying academic rigor to research on healing, well-being and resilience; translating evidence into action for the U.S. Military and large-scale health systems; and fostering wellness through self-care to create a flourishing society.
Susan Samueli, PhD, Co-Founder
Wayne B. Jonas, MD, President/ CEO

Washington

7099 Center for Anxiety and Traumatic Stress
Guthrie Annex 2   206-685-3617
Seattle, WA   faculty.washington.edu/zoellner/
Lori A. Zoellner, PhD, Director
Richard Ries, MD, Medical Director

Wisconsin

7100 Injury Research Center
8701 Watertown Plank Rd.   414-955-7670
Milwaukee, WI 53226   Fax: 414-955-6470
irc@mcw.edu
www.mcw.edu
The Injury Research Center (IRCInjury Research Center at the Medical College of Wisconsin) at the Medical College was established as a comprehensive federally funded injury control research center to address the burden of injury in the Great Lakes Region of the Midwest (WI, MN, IL, IN, MI and OH).
Stephen Hargarten, MD, MPH, Director
E. Brook Lerner, PhD, Deputy Director

Support Groups & Hotlines

7101 American Self-Help Group Clearinghouse
www.selfhelpgroups.org
American Self-Help Group Clearinghouse has a keyword-searchable database of over 1,100 national, international, model and online self-help support groups for addictions, bereavement, health, mental health, disabilities, abuse, parenting, caregiver concerns and many other stressful life situations.

7102 COPLINE
501 Iron Bridge Rd.   800-267-5463
Freehold, NJ 7728   Copline@optonline.net
www.copline.org
Copline is the first national law enforcement officers hotline in the country that is manned by retired law enforcement officers. Retired law enforcement officers are trained in active listening and bring the knowledge and understanding of the many psychosocial stre
Stephanie Samuels, M.A., MSW, LCSW, President/ Creator/ Founder
Dennis Cronin, Vice President

7103 Child Help
4350 E. Camelback Road   480-922-8212
Phoenix, AZ 85018   800-422-4453
www.childhelp.org
Michael Medoro, Child Development Officer
Jon Taylor, Chief Financial Officer

7104 Crime Survivors
PO Box 54552   949-872-7895
Irvine, CA 92619   844-853-4673
crimesurvivors@aol.com
www.crimesurvivors.org

Crime Survivors vision is for victims of crime to recover from their experience mentally, physically, emotionally, and financially, by receiving the respect, support, and protection from law enforcement, the judicial system, and the community.
Patricia Wenskunas, Founder / CEO
Janet Wilson Irving, Chairperson

7105 Heal My PTSD with Michele Rosenthal
healmyptsd.com
Offers information anyone would need to discover what there is to know about symptoms of PTSD, treatment options and the path to feeling better.
Michele Rosenthal, Founder

7106 MDJunction
800-273-8255
www.mdjunction.com
MDJunction is a meeting place for people who deal with health challenges, a comfort zone to help and get help by people who are in your spot.

7107 Mental Health America
2000 N. Beauregard Street   703-684-7722
Alexandria, VA 22311   800-969-6642
Fax: 703-684-5968
www.mentalhealthamerica.net
Mental Health America (MHA) - founded in 1909 - is the nation's leading community-based non-profit dedicated to helping all Americans achieve wellness by living mentally healthier lives.
Paul Gionfriddo, President/ CEO
Nathaniel Counts, Senior Policy Associate

7108 National Health Information Center
Office of Disease Prevention & Health Promotion
1101 Wootton Pkwy   Fax: 240-453-8281
Rockville, MD 20852   odphpinfo@hhs.gov
www.health.gov/nhic
Supports public health education by maintaining a calendar of National Health Observances; helps connect consumers and health professionals to organizations that can best answer questions and provide up-to-date contact information from reliable sources; updates on a yearly basis toll-free numbers for health information, Federal health clearinghouses and info centers.
Don Wright, MD, MPH, Director

7109 Out of the Storm
cptsd.org
Out of the Storm is a discussion group and resource site for those whose lives have been affected by Complex Post Traumatic Disorder (CPTSD).

7110 PTSD Family Support Group
2133 Upton Drive   757-222-2247
Virginia Beach, VA 23454
Love4Vets will ambitiously, humbly, and respectfully aim to become a proactive organization throughout the nation that military veterans will have as a first choice for empowerment and support.
April Krowel, Chairman
Ela Kelly, Founder/ CEO

7111 PTSD Hotline
800-273-8255
Info@PTSDHotline.Com
www.ptsdhotline.com/index.html
This Website deals primarily with PTSD as it relates to Veterans.

7112 PTSDanonymous.org
ptsda@comcast.net
www.ptsdanonymous.org
A nationwide network of community based, non-clinical, veteran lead support group meetings for those suffering from military trauma and seeking the fellowship of their peers.

7113 Pandora's Aquarium
www.pandys.org
A rape, sexual assault, and sexual abuse survivor message board and chat room.

7114 Panic Survivor
www.panicsurvivor.com
A community to sove anxiety disorder problem.

7115 Rape, Abuse & Incest National Network
1220 L Street, NW
Washington, DC 20005
202-544-3064
Fax: 202-544-3556
info@rainn.org
rainn.org
RAINN (Rape, Abuse & Incest National Network) is the nation's largest anti-sexual violence organization and was named one of America's 100 Best Charities by Worth magazine.
Scott Berkowitz, President/ Founder
Regan Burke, Chairperson

7116 Recovery International
105 W. Adams St.
Chicago, IL 60603
312-337-5661
866-221-0302
Fax: 312-726-4446
Christine@recoveryinternational.org
www.recoveryinternational.org
Recovery International offers meetings to men and women of all ages that ease the suffering from mental health issues by gaining skills to lead more peaceful and productive lives. In the last 76 years RI has equipped over 1 million people with tools to control behavior and change attitudes.
Christine Lewis, Executive Director
Caitlin Fahey, Project Coordinator

7117 Suicide.org
800-784-2433
Kevin@Suicide.org
www.suicide.org
If you are suicidal, have attempted suicide, or are a suicide survivor, you will find help, hope, comfort, understanding, support, love, and extensive resources here.
Kevin Caruso, Founder
Adam Sutherland, Vice President

7118 Support4Hope
PO Box 184
Deer Lodge, TN 37726
Admin@Support4hope.com
www.support4hope.com
Support4Hope is dedicated to support of various mental health issues such as Bipolar Disorder, Depression, Anxiety Disorders, Schizophrenia, Post Traumatic Stress Disorder (PTSD) and the problems that arise from them along with other problems such as Domestic Abuse.

7119 United States 211 Information and Referral Systems
www.211.org
Helps connect to a community resource specialist in an area to get in touch with local organizations that provide critical services.

7120 Veterans Crisis Line
800-273-8255
www.veteranscrisisline.net
The Veterans Crisis Line connects Veterans in crisis and their families and friends with qualified, caring Department of Veterans Affairs responders through a confidential toll-free hotline, online chat, or text.

7121 Vetwives Living With PTSD
livingwithptsd.yuku.com
Forum for people suffering with PTSD.

Books

**7122 A Practical Guide to PTSD Treatment:
Pharmacological&Psychotheraputic Aprch**
750 First St. NE
Washington, DC 20002
202-336-5500
800-374-2721
TTY: 202-336-6123
TDD: 202-336-6123
www.apa.org
The book is suitable for psychologists and social workers who may be unfamiliar with pharmacological approaches to PTSD, as well as psychiatrists and other medical personnel who may be less familiar with the best empirically-validated forms of psychotherapy.
Matthew J. Friedman, MD, PhD, Editor
Nancy C. Bernardy, PhD, Editor

7123 Caring for Veterans With Deployment-Related Stress Disorders
750 First St. NE
Washington, DC 20002
202-336-5500
800-374-2721
TTY: 202-336-6123
TDD: 202-336-6123
www.apa.org
Caring for Veterans With Deployment-Related Stress Disorders explores the myriad causes and consequences of these peculiar war-zone disorders, yet its emphasis is on prevention and treatment through better assessment, psychopharmacological and psychotherapeutic interventions (including couple/family therapy), and appropriate evidence-based treatments.
Matthew J. Friedman, MD, PhD, Editor
Jennifer J. Vasterling, PhD, Editor

7124 EMDR as an Integrative Psychotherapy Approach
750 First St. NE
Washington, DC 20002
202-336-5500
800-374-2721
TTY: 202-336-6123
TDD: 202-336-6123
www.apa.org
In EMDR as an Integrative Psychotherapy Approach, EMDR originator Francine Shapiro explores the latest developments and theoretical perspectives on, and clinical implications of, this complex psychotherapy approach originally developed to treat posttraumatic stress disorder.
Francine Shapiro, PhD, Editor

**7125 Ethnocultural Aspects of Posttraumatic Stress
Disorder:Issues,Rsrch, Clncl Appl**
750 First St. NE
Washington, DC 20002
202-336-5500
800-374-2721
TTY: 202-336-6123
TDD: 202-336-6123
www.apa.org
This richly documented, edited volume is the first systematic examination of ethnocultural aspects of PTSD. Leaders in the field of PTSD research and practice explore both universal and culture-specific reactions to trauma, and discusses implications for research, treatment, and prevention.
Raymond M. Scurfield, Editor
Ellen T. Gerrity, Editor

**7126 Hope for Recovery: Understanding Posttraumatic Stress
Disorder**
www.ptsdalliance.org
In clear and sympathetic language, Hope for Recovery seeks to dispel the myths about PTSD that keep many people from recognizing the problem and obtaining help.

7127 Personality-Guided Therapy for Posttraumatic Stress Disorder
750 First St. NE
Washington, DC 20002
202-336-5500
800-374-2721
TTY: 202-336-6123
TDD: 202-336-6123
www.apa.org
In Personality-Guided Therapy for Posttraumatic Stress Disorder, George S. Everly, Jr. and Jeffrey M. Lating shed light on the role personality factors play in the genesis and treatment of posttraumatic stress disorder (PTSD).
Jeffrey M. Lating, PhD, Editor
George S. Everly, Jr., PhD, Editor

**7128 Psychological Assessment Of Adult Post Traumatic
States:Phenomenolgy,Diag&Meas**
750 First St. NE
Washington, DC 20002
202-336-5500
800-374-2721
TTY: 202-336-6123
TDD: 202-336-6123
www.apa.org
This book is the second edition of the well-known Psychological Assessment of Adult Posttraumatic States, published in 1997. A major update from the first edition, it presents a detailed, yet practical summary of the major issues and instruments involved in the assessment of posttraumatic disturbance.
John Briere, PhD, Editor

7129 Psychology in the Service of National Security
750 First St. NE
Washington, DC 20002

202-336-5500
800-374-2721
TTY: 202-336-6123
TDD: 202-336-6123
www.apa.org

This volume highlights the diverse contributions of military psychologists toward U.S. security and toward the discipline of psychology itself.
A. David Mangelsdorff, PhD, Author

7130 Taking Control of Anxiety: Small Steps for Getting The Best Of Worry,Stress&Fear
750 First St. NE
Washington, DC 20002

202-336-5500
800-374-2721
TTY: 202-336-6123
TDD: 202-336-6123
www.apa.org

This straightforward guide, filled with compelling case examples and easy to use techniques, will teach you to identify, reduce, eliminate, and prevent the negative effects of anxiety.
Bret A. Moore, PsyD, Author

7131 Trauma Services for Women in Substance Abuse Treatment: An Integrated Approach
750 First St. NE
Washington, DC 20002

202-336-5500
800-374-2721
TTY: 202-336-6123
TDD: 202-336-6123
www.apa.org

This book is a hands-on guide for clinicians seeking to treat women who suffer from both a history of trauma and the effects of substance abuse.
Aimee Campbell, MSSW, Author
Gloria M. Miele, PhD, Author

7132 Trauma&Health:Physical Health Consequences Of Exposure To Extreme Stress
750 First St. NE
Washington, DC 20002

202-336-5500
800-374-2721
TTY: 202-336-6123
TDD: 202-336-6123
www.apa.org

This volume provides a comprehensive summary of existing literature and a refreshing look at current empirical work. It will stimulate research and support clinical practice by providing clinicians with solid information that can inform their work with patients. Trauma and Health clearly shows that poor physical health should be recognized, along with poor mental health as an outcome of traumatic exposure.
Bonnie L. Green, PhD, Editor
Paula P. Schnurr, PhD, Editor

7133 Trauma&Substance Abuse:Causes,Consequences and Treatment Of Comorbid Disorders
750 First St. NE
Washington, DC 20002

202-336-5500
800-374-2721
TTY: 202-336-6123
TDD: 202-336-6123
www.apa.org

Trauma and Substance Abuse: Causes, Consequences, and Treatment of Comorbid Disorders, Second Edition offers a broad overview of current trends in the field of co-occurring substance abuse and PTSD from both clinical and research perspectives.
Jennifer P. Read, PhD, Editor
Paige Ouimette, PhD, Editor

7134 Treating PTSD With Cognitive-Behavioral Therapies: Interventions That Work
750 First St. NE
Washington, DC 20002

202-336-5500
800-374-2721
TTY: 202-336-6123
TDD: 202-336-6123
www.apa.org

Explaining each approach's theoretical underpinnings as well as its step-by-step implementation, the authors cover both trauma-focused techniques such as prolonged exposure, cognitive processing therapy, and stress inoculation training, and non-trauma-focused or present-centered techniques such as breathing training, relaxation training, and positive self-talk. The

book also addresses depression and social isolation, symptoms that often accompany PTSD.
Philippe Shnaider, Author
Candice M. Monson, PhD, Author

7135 Wheels Down: Adjusting to Life After Deployment
750 First St. NE
Washington, DC 20002

202-336-5500
800-374-2721
TTY: 202-336-6123
TDD: 202-336-6123
www.apa.org

This book, written by military psychologists Moore and Kennedy, is a down-to-earth guide that's full of practical advice. The authors talk straight about both the joys and challenges of returning home, advising that one size does NOT fit all when it comes to making the transition. They share thoughtful, constructive tips for dealing with unwanted surprises like relationship break-ups, financial problems, and kids who are suddenly strangers.
Carrie H. Kennedy, PhD, ABPP, Author
Bret A. Moore, PsyD, ABPP, Author

7136 Why Are You So Scared? A Child's Book About Parents With PTSD
750 First St. NE
Washington, DC 20002

202-336-5500
800-374-2721
TTY: 202-336-6123
TDD: 202-336-6123
www.apa.org

When a parent has PTSD, children can often feel confused, scared, or helpless. Why Are You So Scared? explains PTSD and its symptoms in nonthreatening, kid-friendly language, and is full of questions and exercises that kids and parents can work through together.
Beth Andrews, LCSW, Author

7137 Your Life After Trauma
500 Fifth Avenue
New York, NY 10110

212-354-5500
Fax: 212-869-0856
books.wwnorton.com

In this book, the author applies her personal experience and professional wisdom to offer readers an invaluable roadmap to overcoming their own trauma, in particular the loss of sense of self that often accompanies it.
Michele Rosenthal, Author

Newsletters

7138 PTSD Research Quarterly

802-296-6300
ncptsd@va.gov
www.ptsd.va.gov

Each RQ contains a review article written by guest experts on a specific topic related to PTSD.

7139 The Post-Traumatic Gazette
P.O. Box 2757
High Springs, FL 32655

352-215-9251
www.patiencepress.com

Offers new perspectives, new ideas, new treatments, new resources and encourage people to find what works for people suffering with PTSD.

7140 The Post-Traumatic Stress Disorder Relationship

800-289-0963

Pamphlets

7141 PTSD: A Guide for the Frontline

www.ptsdalliance.org

This free, 20-page booklet is designed as a primer for "frontline" professionals who interact with trauma survivors and people suffering from Posttraumatic Stress Disorder.

Web Sites

7142 Aces Too High

acestoohigh.com

ACESTooHigh is a news site that reports on research about adverse childhood experiences, including developments in epidemiology, neurobiology, and the biomedical and epigenetic consequences of toxic stress.

7143 AdvocateWeb

www.advocateweb.org

AdvocateWeb is a nonprofit organization providing information and resources to promote awareness and understanding of the issues involved in the exploitation of persons by trusted helping professionals.

7144 AfterTheInjury.org

aftertheinjury@email.chop.edu
www.aftertheinjury.org

This website was developed by an interdisciplinary team of researchers and practitioners with expertise in pediatric injury, child health care, and traumatic stress.

7145 Athealth.com

athealth.com

Athealth.com was founded in 1997 by a psychiatrist to provide mental health information and services for mental health professionals and those they serve.

7146 Bright Side, The

The Bright Side was created as a means of support - whether you are dealing with depression, grief, suicide, mental illness, emotional crisis, or are just feeling overwhelmed with life, you are not alone!

7147 David Baldwin's Trauma Information Pages

www.trauma-pages.com

These Trauma Pages focus primarily on emotional trauma and traumatic stress, including PTSD (Post-traumatic Stress Disorder) and dissociation, whether following individual traumatic experience(s) or a large-scale disaster.

7148 Family Of a Vet

Info@FamilyofaVet.com
www.familyofavet.com

Family Of a Vet was started by the proud wife of an OIF Veteran who suffers from PTSD (Post Traumatic Stress Disorder) and TBI (Traumatic Brain Injury).

7149 Gift From Within

www.giftfromwithin.org

PTSD Resources for Survivors and Caregivers.

7150 Healing From Complex Trauma & PTSD/CPTSD

www.healingfromcomplextraumaandptsd.com

Assists people in their healing from complex trauma journey.
Lilly Hope Lucario, Survivor/Author/Writer/Blogger

7151 Hope for Healing.Org

865-471-8366
hopeforhealing.org

7152 Make the Connection

800-273-8255
maketheconnection.net

Make the Connection is a public awareness campaign by the U.S. Department of Veterans Affairs (VA) that provides personal testimonials and resources to help Veterans discover ways to improve their lives.

7153 Mental Health Matters

mental-health-matters.com

MHMatters was founded to supply information and resources to mental health consumers, professionals, students and supporters.

7154 Mental Health Today

mental-health-today.com

The purpose of Mental Health Today is to help stop the pain caused by mental health disorders.
Patty Fleener M.S.W., Owner/ Operator

7155 MentalHelp.net

800-273-TALK
www.mentalhelp.net

They provide online mental health and wellness education.

7156 MyPTSD

www.myptsd.com

PTSD Forum launched on the 06th Sep, 2005, with one simple aim, to provide quality PTSD information and support to all concerned.

7157 PTSD Support Services

888-335-8699

7158 PTSDinfo.org

www.ptsdinfo.org

7159 Psychguides.com

855-900-6733
www.psychguides.com

There goal is to shed light on psychological disorders, allowing you to recognize, understand and cope with these challenging diagnoses in yourself, friends and family members.

7160 VA Caregiver Support

www.caregiver.va.gov

Tips, tools, and other resources for caregivers of veterans.

Description

7161 Prader-Willi Syndrome

Prader-Willi syndrome, PWS, is a group of abnormalities first described by Drs. Prader, Labart, and Willi in 1956. This complex genetic, albeit uncommon condition occurs in about one in every 20,000 births. Normally, we inherit one copy of each chromosome from each parent; one from our mother (maternal copy), and one from our father (paternal copy). Some genes are active only on the paternal copy and other genes are only active on the maternal copy. This parent-specific gene activation is called genomic imprinting, and genomic imprinting plays a role in PWS. In about 70 percent of PWS patients, there is a missing piece (deletion) of part of the paternal copy of chromosome 15. In 25 percent of PWS cases, the patient has two copies of the maternal copy of chromosome 15 (i.e. both copies of chromosome 15 were inherited from the mother, a condition called uniparental disomy). In other cases, the paternal copy has had its genes inactivated by various mechanisms. A group of genes called the SNORD116 cluster seems to cause PES when it is inactivated on the paternal copy of chromosome 15.

PWS is characterized by obesity, short stature, small penis and testicles (hypogonadism), small hands and feet, mental disabilities and decreased muscle tone. During the toddler years, many patients begin to overeat. Some persons with PWS may show signs of obsessive-compulsive disorder, apart from their obsessions with food. In addition to insatiable hunger, other behavioral features include emotional highs and lows, poor motor skills and cognitive impairment. Sexual development is halted, and facial and skeletal abnormalities develop.

Therapies for PWS are aimed at symptoms with an emphasis on specialized diets and customized exercise programs and support.

National Agencies & Associations

7162 Foundation for Prader-Willi Research
340 S Lemon Avenue
Walnut, CA 91789

888-322-5487
Fax: 888-559-4105
info@fpwr.org
www.fpwr.org

Committed to finding treatments for Prader-Willi syndrome through the advancement of research.
Daniel Chorney, President
John Walter, CEO

7163 National Institute of Child Health and Human Development
PO Box 3006
Rockville, MD 20847

800-370-2943
Fax: 866-760-5947
TTY: 888-320-6942
www.nichd.nih.gov

NICHD seeks to better understand disabilities and important events that occur during pregnancy.
Diana W. Bianchi, MD, Director
Constantine Stratakis, Scientific Director

7164 Prader-Willi Syndrome Association
8588 Potter Park Drive
Sarasota, FL 34238

800-926-4797
www.pwsausa.org

Established in order to provide support and information about Prader-Willi syndrome for individuals, families, professionals, and other organizations.
James Kane, Chair
Tammie Penta, Vice Chair

State Agencies & Associations

Arizona

7165 Prader-Willi Syndrome Arizona Association: Phoenix Area
Prader-Willi Syndrome Association
3920 East Bronco Trail
Phoenix, AZ 85044

602-481-5314
www.pwsausa.org

Sheila McMahon, President

7166 Prader-Willi Syndrome Arizona Association
Prader-Willi Syndrome Association
13839 N Bentwater Drive
Tucson, AZ 85737

602-481-5314
www.pwsausa.org

Tammie Penta, President

Arkansas

7167 Prader-Willi Arkansas Association Prader-Willi Syndrome Association
Prader-Willi Syndrome Association
107 Jessica Drive
Sherwood, AR 72120-4245

501-920-6768
www.pwsausa.org

Jim Patton, President

California

7168 Prader-Willi California Foundation
514 N Prospect Avenue
Redondo Beach, CA 90277

310-372-5053
800-400-9994
Fax: 310-372-4329
PWCF1@aol.com
www.pwsausa.org

Lisa Graziano, Executive Director

Colorado

7169 Prader-Willi Colorado Association
Prader-Willi Syndrome Association
8290 S Yukon Way
Littleton, CO 80128

303-973-4780
hosler@dynamicsolutions.com
www.pwsausa.org

Lynette Hosler, President

Connecticut

7170 Prader-Willi Connecticut Association
Prader-Willi Syndrome Association
129 Way Road
Salem, CT 06420-3306

203-239-9902
pwsactchapter@yahoo.com
www.pwsausa.org

Vicki Knoph, President

Delaware

7171 Prader-Willi Delaware Association
Prader-Willi Syndrome Association
300 Bethel Circle Millwood
Middletown, DE 19709

302-378-7385
swede455@aol.com
www.pwsausa.org

Karen Swanson, President

Florida

7172 Prader-Willi Florida Association
Prader-Willi Syndrome Association
17777 S W 285 Street
Homestead, FL 33030

305-245-6484
pwfa2000@aol.com
www.pwsausa.org

Debbie Stallings, Co-President
John Stallings, Co-President

Georgia

7173 Prader-Willi Georgia Association
Prader-Willi Syndrome Association
562 Lakeland Plaza
Cumming, GA 30040
770-886-2334
877-866-2334
Fax: 770-886-2335
pwsaga@earthlink.net
www.pwsausa.org

Debbie Lang, Executive Director
Greg Talley, President

Hawaii

7174 Prader-Willi Hawaii Association
Prader-Willi Syndrome Association
269 Kaha Street
Hailua, HI 96734
808-263-8177
susanlundh@yahoo.com
www.pwsausa.org

Susan Lundh, President

Idaho

7175 Prader-Willi Idaho Association
Prader-Willi Syndrome Association
550 Lodgepole Road
Athol, ID 83801
208-683-2993
idaho4ts@aol.com
www.pwsausa.org

Susan Lundh, President
Gene Todhunter, Local Contact

Illinois

7176 Prader-Willi Illinois Association
Prader-Willi Syndrome Association
2128 N Sedgwick Street
Chicago, IL 60614
773-281-9170
www.pwsausa.org
Jeffrey Fender, President

Indiana

7177 Prader-Willi Indiana Association
Prader-Willi Syndrome Association
7536 Moonbeam Drive
Indianapolis, IN 46259
317-527-9173
pwsain@yahoo.com
www.pwsausa.org

Jacque McGuire, President

Iowa

7178 Prader-Willi Iowa Association
Prader-Willi Syndrome Association
15130 Holcomb Avenue
Clive, IA 50325-9695
515-987-0288
ktcaedav@netins.net
www.pwsausa.org

Tammi Davis, President
Edie Bogaczyk, President

Kentucky

7179 Prader-Willi Kentucky Association
Prader-Willi Syndrome Association
9213 Reigate Court
Louisville, KY 40222
502-339-7872
national@pwsausa.org
www.pwsausa.org

Frank Beckles, President
Rick Settles

Massachusetts

7180 Prader-Willi New England Association
Prader-Willi Syndrome Association
Andover, MA 01757
978-475-5570
pwsane@aol.com
www.pwsausa.org

Eileen Rullo, President

Michigan

7181 Prader-Willi Michigan Association
2155 Ascot Rd
Ann Arbor, MI 48103
734-998-3507
chrishendrick@cablespeed.com
www.pwsausa.org

Jon Hendrick, Co-Chairperson
Chris Hendrick, Co-Chairperson

Minnesota

7182 Prader-Willi Minnesota Association
Prader-Willi Syndrome Association
7209 Oaklawn Avenue
Woodbury, MN 55105
952-893-9318
national@pwsausa.org
www.pwsausa.org

Jey Behnken, President

Missouri

7183 Prader-Willi Missouri Association
Prader-Willi Syndrome Association
1465 S Grand Boulevard Missouri Str
Louis, MO 63104
314-268-4027
Fax: 314-935-7461
national@pwsausa.org
www.pwsausa.org

Barbara Whitman, President

Nebraska

7184 Prader-Willi Nebraska Association
Prader-Willi Syndrome Association
302 S 49th Avenue
Omaha, NE 68132
402-551-9168
national@pwsausa.org
www.pwsausa.org

Jennifer Varner, Local Contact

New Jersey

7185 Prader-Willi New Jersey Association
Prader-Willi Syndrome Association
514 Gatewod Road
Cherry Hill, NJ 08003
856-795-4229
national@pwsausa.org
www.pwsausa.org

Sybil Cohen, President
Judy Livny, Vice-President

New York

7186 Prader-Willi New York Association
Prader-Willi Syndrome Association
PO Box 1114
Niagara Falls, NY 14304
716-276-2211
800-442-1655
alliance@prader-willi.org
www.prader-willi.org

Nina Roberto, Executive Director
Amy McDougall, President

North Carolina

7187 Prader-Willi North Carolina Association
Prader-Willi Syndrome Association
1404 Sutton Drive
Kinston, NC 28501
252-527-1813
national@pwsausa.org
www.pwsausa.org

Becky Smith, President

North Dakota

7188 Prader-Willi North Dakota Association
Prader-Willi Syndrome Association
2902 S University Drive
Fargo, ND 58103-6032
701-232-3301
Fax: 701-237-5775
fraser@fraserltd.org
www.fraserltd.org

Sandra leyland, Executive Director
Michael Kirk, Vice President

Ohio

7189 Prader-Willi Ohio Association
Prader-Willi Syndrome Association
4075 W 226 Street
Fairview Park, OH 44126

440-716-0552
pwsaohio@aol.com
www.pwsausa.org

Jennifer Bolander, President

Oklahoma

7190 Prader-Willi Oklahoma Association
Prader-Willi Syndrome Association
3816 SE 89th Street
Oklahoma City, OK 74135-6222

405-677-8089
national@pwsausa.org
www.pwsausa.org

Daphne Mosley, President

Oregon

7191 Prader-Willi Oregon Association
Prader-Willi Syndrome Association
303 E Historic Columbia
Troutdale, OR 97060

503-669-7191
national@pwsausa.org
www.pwsausa.org

Lennae Elkington, President

Pennsylvania

7192 Prader-Willi Pennsylvania Association
Prader-Willi Syndrome Association
104 Persimmon Place
Cranberry Township, PA 16066

724-779-4415
national@pwsausa.org
www.pwsausa.org

Debbie Fabio, President

South Carolina

7193 Prader-Willi South Carolina Association
Prader-Willi Syndrome Association
912 Lake Spur Lane
Chapin, SC 29036

803-345-1379
national@pwsausa.org
www.pwsausa.org

Rhett Eleazer, Local Contact

Tennessee

7194 Prader-Willi Tennessee Association
Prader-Willi Syndrome Association
1200 Villa Place
Nashville, TN 37212

615-790-6659
national@pwsausa.org
www.pwsausa.org

Misti Love, President

Texas

7195 Prader-Willi Texas Association
Prader-Willi Syndrome Association
14427 Perchin Drive
San Antonio, TX 78247

210-946-6789
national@pwsausa.org
www.pwsausa.org

Amber Robenson, President

Utah

7196 Prader-Willi Utah Association
Prader-Willi Syndrome Association
2652 Nottingham Way
Salt Lake City, UT 84108

801-582-0998
Fax: 801-768-3924
national@pwsausa.org
www.pwsausa.org

Lisa Thornton, President

Washington

7197 Prader-Willi Washington Association
Prader-Willi Syndrome Association

16208 SE 46th Place
Bellevue, WA 98006

206-285-7679
www.pwsausa.org

Joanne Underwood, Co-President
Susan Lundh, Co-President

Wisconsin

7198 Prader-Willi Wisconsin Association
Prader-Willi Syndrome Association
2701 N Alexander Street
Appleton, WI 54911-2512

920-882-6371
866-797-2947
www.pwsausa.org

Mary Lynn Larson, Program Director
Mike Larson, President

Support Groups & Hotlines

7199 National Health Information Center
Office of Disease Prevention & Health Promotion
1101 Wootton Pkwy
Rockville, MD 20852

Fax: 240-453-8281
odphpinfo@hhs.gov
www.health.gov/nhic

Supports public health education by maintaining a calendar of National Health Observances; helps connect consumers and health professionals to organizations that can best answer questions and provide up-to-date contact information from reliable sources; updates on a yearly basis toll-free numbers for health information, Federal health clearinghouses and info centers.
Don Wright, MD, MPH, Director

7200 PraderWilli Syndrome Association
PraderWilli Syndrome Association
5700 Midnight Pass Road
Sarasota, FL 34242

941-312-0400
800-926-4797
Fax: 941-312-0142
pwsuasa@aol.com
www.pwsausa.org

John Heybatch, Co-Chair
Julie Doherty, Secretary

Books

7201 Child with Prader-Willi Syndrome: Birth to Three
Prader-Willi Syndrome Association (USA)
8588 Potter Park Drive
Sarasota, FL 34238

941-312-0400
800-926-4797
Fax: 941-312-0142
info@pwsausa.com
www.pwsausa.org

Discusses the common concerns of the first three years and offers specific recommendations for early intervention strategies. A helpful and positive resource for families, physicians, early intervention workers and other care providers. Booklet
2004 34 pages
Craig Pulhemus, Executive Director

7202 Early Years
Prader-Willi Syndrome Association (USA)
8588 Potter Park Drive
Sarasota, FL 34238

941-312-0400
800-926-4797
Fax: 941-312-0142
info@pwsausa.com
www.pwsausa.org

Collection of articles regarding young children with PWS — many from a parent's perspective.
1998 37 pages
Craig Polhemus, Executive Director

7203 Growing Up with Prader-Willi Syndrome: Personal Reflections of a Mother
Prader-Willi Syndrome Association (USA)
8588 Potter Park Drive
Sarasota, FL 34238

941-312-0400
800-926-4797
Fax: 941-312-0142
info@pwsausa.com
www.pwsausa.org

Collection of 15 articles. Tips for managing family life on a practical level. Booklet
2003 37 pages
Craig Polhemus, Executive Director

7204 Growth Hormone & Prader-Willi Syndrome: A Reference for Familes & Care Providers
Linda S. Keder, author
Prader-Willi Syndrome Association (USA)
8588 Potter Park Drive   941-312-0400
Sarasota, FL 34238   800-926-4797
                        Fax: 941-312-0142
                        info@pwsausa.com
                        www.pwsausa.org
Reference for families and care providers.
2001 52 pages
Craig Polhemus, Executive Director

7205 Handbook for Parents
Shirley Neason, author
Prader-Willi Syndrome Association (USA)
8588 Potter Park Drive   941-312-0400
Sarasota, FL 34238   800-926-4797
                        Fax: 941-312-0142
                        info@pwsausa.com
                        www.pwsausa.org
Parent-to-Parent handbook for understanding and managing issues related to PWS, from birth to adulthood.
1999 75 pages
Craig Polhemus, Executive Director

7206 Nutrition Care for Children with PWS: Infants and Toddlers
J. Hovasi & D. Doorlag, with J. Loker & C. Loker, author
Prader-Willi Syndrome Association (USA)
8588 Potter Park Drive   941-312-0400
Sarasota, FL 34238   800-926-4797
                        Fax: 941-312-0142
                        info@pwsausa.com
                        www.pwsausa.org
Provides answers to frequently asked questions about nutrition and feeding infants and toddlers with PWS.
2004 62 pages
Craig Polhemus, Executive Director

7207 Sometimes I'm Mad, Sometimes I'm Glad - A Sibling Booklet
Sarah Heinemann, author
Prader-Willi Syndrome Association (USA)
8588 Potter Park Drive   941-312-0400
Sarasota, FL 34238   800-926-4797
                        Fax: 941-312-0142
                        info@pwsausa.com
                        www.pwsausa.org
Explains sibling relationships and how they are affected by Prader-Willi syndrome. Written in the voice of a sibling of someone with PWS. Ages 5-13
32 pages
Craig Polhemus, Executive Director

7208 Supporting Adults with Prader-Willi Syndro me in a Residential Setting
B.J. Goff, Ed.D, author
Prader-Willi Syndrome Association (USA)
8588 Potter Pass Drive   941-312-0400
Sarasota, FL 34238   800-926-4797
                        Fax: 941-312-0142
                        info@pwsausa.com
                        www.pwsausa.org
Filling a large gap for care givers of those with Prader-Willi Sydrome, this is an extensive manual covering residential care issues; including management strategies, specifics for phase of life, and a number of additional ideas.
2002 121 pages
Craig Polhemus, Executive Director

Newsletters

7209 Gathered View
Prader-Willi Syndrome Association (USA)
8588 Potter Park Drive   941-312-0400
Sarasota, FL 34238   800-926-4797
                        Fax: 941-312-0142
                        info@pwsausa.com
                        www.pwsausa.org
The official newsletter of PWSA, mailed 6 time/year to members. Offers current research findings, behavior and weight management techniques, educational news, articles and more.
BiMonthly
Craig Polhemus, Executive Director

Pamphlets

7210 An Early Prader-Willi Syndrome Diagnosis & How to Make it Easier on Parents
Prader-Willi Foundation
40 Holly Lane   516-944-8136
Roslyn Hts, NY 11577-1533   800-253-7993
                        Fax: 516-944-3173
                        foundation@prader-willi.inter.net
                        www.prader-willi.org
A parent of a child with PWS and an advocate for others with the afflication speaks.
Rachel Johnson, President and Author

7211 Behavior Management: Collection of Articless
Prader-Willi Syndrome Association (USA)
8588 Potter Park Drive   941-312-0400
Sarasota, FL 34238   800-926-4797
                        Fax: 941-312-0142
                        info@pwsausa.com
                        www.pwsausa.org
Includes general articles of behavior concerns, use of psychotropic medications, skin picking and teaching social skills.
2003 49 pages
Craig Polhemus, Executive Director

7212 Educational Choices for Children with PWS
Prader-Willi Foundation
40 Holly Lane   516-944-8136
Roslyn Hts, NY 11577-1533   800-253-7993
                        Fax: 516-944-3173
                        www.prader-willi.org
Parents of young children with Prader-Willi syndrome discuss their individual philosophies of educational choice - inclusion vs. specialized setting.
Rachel Johnson, President and Author

7213 Nutrition Care for Adolescents and Adults with PWS
Karenn H. Borgie, MA, RD, author
Prader-Willi Syndrome Association (USA)
8588 Potter Park Drive   941-312-0400
Sarasota, FL 34238   800-926-4797
                        Fax: 941-312-0142
                        info@pwsausa.com
                        www.pwsausa.org
covers essential diet information for families, caregivers, and residential service providers.
Craig Polhemus, Executive Director

7214 Nutrition Care for Children with PWS, Ages 3-9
Karen H. Borgie, MA, RD, author
Prader-Willi Syndrome Association (USA)
8588 Potter Park Drive   941-312-0400
Sarasota, FL 34238   800-926-4797
                        Fax: 941-312-0142
                        info@pwsausa.com
                        www.pwsausa.org
Discusses calorie needs, supplements, diet planning, food management, and exchange lists. Softvcover.
Craig Polhemus, Executive Director

7215 What Educators Should Know About Prader-Willi Syndrome
Prader-Willi Syndrome Association (USA)

8588 Potter Park Drive
Sarasota, FL 34238

941-312-0400
800-926-4797
Fax: 941-312-0142
info@pwsausa.com
www.pwsausa.org

Offers guidelines and strategies for helping the student with PWS stay focused, develop skills and knowledge, and minimize problems associated with the syndrome in the school setting.
Craig Polhemus, Executive Director

Audio & Video

7216 Prader-Willi Syndrome: An Overview for Health Professionals
Prader-Willi Syndrome Association
5700 Midnight Pass Road
Sarasota, FL 34242-3000

941-312-0400
800-926-4797
Fax: 941-312-0142
info@pwsausa.com
www.pwsausa.org

Essential viewing for all health care professionals who are not experts on prader-willi syndrome. It deals with all major genetics and health care issues of the child with PWS.
2002

7217 Prader-Willi Syndrome: the Early Years
Prader-Willi Syndrome Association
5700 Midnight Pass Road
Sarasota, FL 34242-3000

941-312-0400
800-926-4797
Fax: 941-312-0142
www.pwsausa.org

Offers help and practical suggestions for those families with a young child newly diagnosed with PWS. Genetics, medical, early intervention and family issues are presented, personalized with family interviews. Although focusing on young children, this video is a wonderful resource for schools and families with children of all ages.
2002

Web Sites

7218 Healthlink USA

www.healthlinkusa.com

Health information concerning treatment, cures, prevention, diagnosis, risk factors, research, support groups, email lists, personal stories and much more. Updated regularly.

7219 MedicineNet

www.medicinenet.com

An online resource for consumers providing easy-to-read, authoritative medical and health information.

7220 Medscape

www.medscape.com

Medscape offers specialists, primary care physicians, and other health professionals the Web's most robust and integrated medical information and educational tools.

Description

7221 Raynaud's Disease

Raynaud's disease is the spasm of blood vessels to fingers and toes, resulting in restricted blood supply in response to cold or emotional upset. Symptoms include tingling and numbness. During an episode, which can last from minutes to hours, the arteries contract briefly and the skin, deprived of oxygen, turns pale and then blue. As arteries relax and blood begins to flow, reddening, tingling, or swelling may occur. While hands and feet are most commonly affected, the nose and ears can also be subject to Raynaud's.

Raynaud's most commonly affects women under 40, accounting for perhaps 90 percent of all cases. When the classic symptoms are present, without other complaints, the condition is referred to as Raynaud's disease (primary Raynaud's), and generally results in no serious consequences. The second form, Raynaud's phenomenon (secondary Raynaud's), is the result of other underlying medical conditions, including scleroderma, vascular disease, rheumatoid arthritis and lupus.

Certain drugs can also trigger Raynaud's, including ergotamine, birth control pills, over-the-counter cold medicines, and several different beta-blockers, which are drugs used in the treatment of heart disease. About 10 percent of Raynaud's cases are related to specific repetitive stress activities such as the operation of pneumatic drills and other hand-held vibrating machinery. In most Raynaud's cases, symptoms are discomforting but not serious. In extreme cases, Raynaud's can result in tissue atrophy and gangrene. Preventative measures include protection from cold, even when taking food out of the refrigerator or freezer and avoiding behavior that disrupts blood flow, for instance, smoking cigarettes.

Medical treatment of Raynaud's is directed toward improving blood flow to the extremities. In many cases, simple exercises are prescribed, and relaxation techniques, such as biofeedback, teach the body to ignore trivial or transient signals of cold. In other cases, vasodilator drugs (calcium channel blockers and alpha-adrenergic antagonists) which are designed to relax and open blood vessels to improve blood flow are prescribed. In the most extreme cases, surgery may be performed to cut nerves that may be inappropriately triggering the contraction of arteries, although relief may last only 1 to 2 years. Herbal remedies have been used in the treatment of Raynaud's and other circulatory conditions, especially the Chinese herb Dong quai, but there are no rigorous studies to confirm its efficacy. There is also evidence that foods rich in vitamin E, and fish oils, may help to reduce or moderate the vascular spasms that produce Raynaud's symptoms.

National Agencies & Associations

7222 American Chronic Pain Association
PO Box 850
Rocklin, CA 95677
800-533-3231
ACPA@theacpa.org
www.theacpa.org
The ACPA facilitates peer support and education for individuals with chronic pain in its many forms, in order to increase quality of life. Also raises awareness among the healthcare community, and with policy makers.
Penney Cowan, Founder & CEO
Daniel Galia, Director, Global Support

7223 Raynaud's Association
11 Topstone Road
Redding, CT 06896
800-280-8055
info@raynauds.org
www.raynauds.org
A non-profit organization providing support and education to individuals with Raynaud's Phenomenon.

Foundations

7224 Arthritis Foundation
1355 Peachtree Street NE
Atlanta, GA 30309
404-872-7100
800-283-7800
Fax: 404-872-0457
help@arthritis.org
www.arthritis.org
A nonprofit organization that depends on volunteers to provide services to help people with arthritis. Supports research to find ways to cure and prevent arthritis and provides services to improve the quality of life for those affected by arthritis. Provides help through information, referrals, speakers bureaus, forums, self-help courses, and various support groups and programs nationwide.
Ann M. Palmer, President & CEO
Guy S. Eakin, PhD, Sr Vice President, Scientific Strategy

Libraries & Resource Centers

7225 Arizona Telemedicine Program
University of Arizona, Health Science Center
PO Box 245105
Tucson, AZ 85724-5105
520-626-2493
Fax: 520-626-4774
kerps@email.arizona.edu
www.telemedicine.arizona.edu/index.html
The Arizona Telemedicine Program is a large, multidisciplinary, university-based program that provides telemedicine services, distance learning, informatics training, and telemedicine technology assessment capabilities to communities throughout Arizona, the sixth largest state in the United States, in square miles.
Ronald S Weinstein, MD, Director
Ana Maria Lopez, Medical Director

Support Groups & Hotlines

7226 National Health Information Center
Office of Disease Prevention & Health Promotion
1101 Wootton Pkwy
Rockville, MD 20852
Fax: 240-453-8281
odphpinfo@hhs.gov
www.health.gov/nhic
Supports public health education by maintaining a calendar of National Health Observances; helps connect consumers and health professionals to organizations that can best answer questions and provide up-to-date contact information from reliable sources; updates on a yearly basis toll-free numbers for health information, Federal health clearinghouses and info centers.
Don Wright, MD, MPH, Director

Books

7227 Raynaud's Phenomenon
Oxford University Press

PO Box 7669
Atlanta, GA 30357

404-872-7100
800-283-7800
Fax: 404-872-0457

This is a detailed and technical work on the physiology finger circulation, and on diagnosis and treatment of Raynaud's Phenomenon and Raynaud's Disease. Includes a chapter on Acrocyanosis and Livedo reticularis.

186 pages
ISBN: 0-195057-56-2

Pamphlets

7228 Raynaud's Phenomenon
Arthritis Foundation
PO Box 7669
Atlanta, GA 30357-0669

404-872-7100
800-283-7800
Fax: 404-872-0457

Web Sites

7229 Health Finder

www.healthfinder.gov

Searchable, carefully developed web site offering information on over 1000 topics. Developed by the US Department of Health and Human Services, the site can be used in both English and Spanish.

7230 MedicineNet

www.medicinenet.com

An online resource for consumers providing easy-to-read, authoritative medical and health information.

7231 Scleroderma Foundation

www.scleroderma.org

Offers materials and referrals, conducts workshops and support groups for those with Raynaud's and their families.

Description

7232 Sarcoidosis

Sarcoidosis is a chronic disease that can affect almost any part of the body. It is characterized by the deposition of small clumps of inflammatory cells (granulomas) in multiple organs. The cause is unknown, but there is a strong genetic contribution to the disease, and it is thought to be related to an immunologic defect or infection. Incidence varies widely between countries. In the United States, sarcoidosis is 10- to 18-fold higher in African-Americans than in whites. Most cases start between the ages of 30 and 50 years.

Clinical features vary considerably, depending on the site and extent of involvement. Systemic symptoms may include fatigue, weight loss, loss of appetite and fever. Local symptoms may involve any organ, but the most commonly affected are the lungs, skin, eyes and lymph nodes. If the disease becomes severe and life-threatening, it is usually because of lung involvement. Patients develop cough, wheeze, chest pain and difficulty breathing.

Both the severity and the long-term outlook are extremely variable. In most patients, the disease regresses within 2 years and does not recur. In approximately 25 percent of patients, the disease progresses and causes serious disability. If progressive symptoms require treatment, corticosteroids are usually given. If these are not effective or tolerated, immunosuppressive drugs may be used. Methotrexate in combination with corticosteroids is the first-line treatment for neurological sarcoidosis, but methotrexate must be given with folic acid to reduce its toxicity and can be toxic to the lungs if used long-long-term. Azathioprine is an appropriate alternative but is toxic to the liver. Biological agents like adalimumab are effective and well tolerated treatments, but they are more expensive. Approximately 5 percent of patients die of respiratory failure.

National Agencies & Associations

7233 American Chronic Pain Association
PO Box 850
Rocklin, CA 95677
800-533-3231
ACPA@theacpa.org
www.theacpa.org
The ACPA facilitates peer support and education for individuals with chronic pain in its many forms, in order to increase quality of life. Also raises awareness among the healthcare community, and with policy makers.
Penney Cowan, Founder & CEO
Daniel Galia, Director, Global Support

7234 Autoimmune Advocacy Alliance
509-630-5344
info@a3autoimmunity.org
www.a3autoimmunity.org
Organization working to achieve understanding and support for the needs of those living with autoimmune diseases.
Annie Holt, Co-Founder
Jennifer Berg, ND, Director

7235 National Sarcoidosis Resource Center
PO Box 1593
Piscataway, NJ 08855-1593
732-463-0497
Fax: 732-463-0467
www.nsrc-global.net
Provides resources, information, and referrals to individuals with sarcoidosis, and raises public awareness about the disease.
Sandra Conroy, President

7236 Sarcoidosis Networking Association
1820 W Webster Avenue
Chicago, IL 60614
312-341-0500
253-988-1528
lynn@sarcoidosisnetwork.org
Educates individuals, provides physician information and heightens public awareness about Sarcoidosis.
Reading Wilson, Co-Founder & President
Leslie Serchuck, MD, Vice President

Research Centers

7237 Sarcoidosis Center
6005 Park Avenue
Memphis, TN 38119
901-761-5877
866-727-2643
Fax: 901-761-2280
sarcoid@sarcoidcenter.com
www.sarcoidcenter.com
A nonprofit tax exempt organization dedicated to increasing knowledge of the disease sarcoidosis. This broad goal encompasses three main areas: Disseminating information to professionals who assist with treatment of the disease obtaining and dispersing funds to assist with investigation into the cause and treatment of the disease and providing support for individuals afflicted with the disease.

7238 Sarcoidosis Treatment and Research Center Thomas Jefferson University Hospital
Thomas Jefferson University Hospital
111 S 11th Street
Philadelphia, PA 19107-5092
215-955-6840
Fax: 215-923-5828
www.jeffersonhospital.org
Stephen K klasko, President/CEO
Sergio Jimen MD, Professor

Support Groups & Hotlines

7239 Better Breather's Clubs
American Lung Association of Virginia
1301 Pennsylvania Ave.
Richmond, DC 20004
202-785-3355
Fax: 202-452-1805
www.lungusa.org
Support Groups for those suffering from chronic obstructive pulmonary disease (COPD) such as emphysema, chronic bronchitis and asthma. In these meetings members give and receive support, and learn more about chronic lung disease from health care professionals who share trends in therapy, medication and other topics, or simply answer members' questions.
Catherine G Hamm, President/Chief Excutive Officer
Michelle LaRose, Development Director

7240 Let's Breathe Sarcoidosis Support Group
2225 Foster Street
Evanston, IL 60201-3353
708-328-9410
bharris354@aol.com
Brenda Harris, Facilitator

7241 Middle Tennessee Sarcoidosis Support Group
PO Box 1342
Cookesville, TN 38503   www.tennesseesarcoidosisawareness.org
931-528-7826
Becky Robertson, Group Leader

7242 Mount Sinai Sarcoidosis Support Group
One Gustave L. Levy Place
New York, NY 10029
212-241-6500
86- 67- 372
www.mountsinai.org

7243 National Health Information Center
Office of Disease Prevention & Health Promotion
1101 Wootton Pkwy
Rockville, MD 20852
Fax: 240-453-8281
odphpinfo@hhs.gov
www.health.gov/nhic

539

Supports public health education by maintaining a calendar of National Health Observances; helps connect consumers and health professionals to organizations that can best answer questions and provide up-to-date contact information from reliable sources; updates on a yearly basis toll-free numbers for health information, Federal health clearinghouses and info centers.
Don Wright, MD, MPH, Director

7244 Pacific NW Support Group
Providence Hospital
PO Box 58785   42- 2-5 14
Renton, WA 98058   877- 25- 067
                                                      Fax: 42- 2-4 20
                                         washington@myasthenia.org
                                                  www.myasthenia.org

Ed Girvan, Facilitator

7245 Sarcoidosis HelpNet
PO Box 022642   732-463-0497
Brooklyn, NY 11202   Fax: 732-463-0467
Soneni B Smith, Contact

7246 Sarcoidosis Research Institute (SRI)
3475 Central Avenue   901-766-6951
Memphis, TN 38111   Fax: 901-774-7294
                             www.sarcoidcenter.com/saradd.htm
The Sarcoidosis Research Institute is a non-profit, tax-exempt organization dedicated to increasing knowledge of the disease sarcoidosis. This broad goal encompasses three main areas: Disseminating information to professionals who assist with treatment of the disease; Obtaining and dispersing funds to assist with investigation into the cause and treatment of the disease; and, providing support for individuals afflicted with the disease.
Paula Yette Polite, Board of Directors President
Wayne Crook, Vice President Board of Directors

7247 Sarcoidosis Self-Help Group: New York
Nassau County Medical Center
2201 Hempstead Turnpike   516-483-2666
East Meadow, NY 11554
Robert Schoenfeld, Facilitator

7248 Sarcoidosis Self-Help Group: Virginia
American Lung Association of Northern Virginia
9735 Main Street   703-591-4131
Fairfax, VA 22031
Carolyn Thomas, Facilitator

7249 Sarcoidosis Support Group Delaware
American Lung Association of Delaware
1021 Gilpin Avenue   302-655-7258
Wilmington, DE 19806   800-548-8252
                                             Fax: 302-655-8546
                                              dbrown@alade.org
                                                  www.alade.org

Peter Shanley, Chairman
Harold P. Wimmer, President/CEO

7250 Sarcoidosis Support Group: New Jersey
268 Dr. ML King Boulevard   201-374-7570
Newark, NJ 07106
Jean Curlin-Miller, Facilitator

7251 Sarcoidosis Support Group: Washington DC
110 Irving Street   202-877-6286
Washington, DC 20010   Fax: 202-877-5779

7252 Triangle Area Sarcoidosis Support Group
Soapstone UM Church
12837 Norwood Road   919-676-6498
Raleigh, NC 27613
Priscilla Fairley, Facilitator

7253 Understanding Sarcoidosis Self-Help Group
2112 Highland Avenue   412-652-6089
New Castle, PA 16105

7254 University of North Carolina Sarcoidosis Support Group
UNC Chapel Hill Healthcare

130 Mason Farm Road   919-966-2531
Chapel Hill, NC 27599   sharikia_burt@med.unc.edu
Sharikia Burt, Clinical Coordinator

7255 West Tennessee Sarcoidosis Support Group
1670 McLemoresville Road   731-986-9832
Huntington, TN 38344
Patricia Coleman, Group Leader

Books

7256 Sarcoidosis Resource Guide and Directory
PC Publications
PO Box 1593   732-699-0733
Piscataway, NJ 08855-1593   800-223-6429
                                             Fax: 732-699-0882
                                                www.nsrc-global.net

1993 304 pages Paperback
ISBN: 0-963122-25-8

Newsletters

7257 Online Sarcoidosis Newsletter
National Sarcoidosis Resource Center
PO Box 1593   732-699-0733
Piscataway, NJ 08855-1593   800-223-6429
                                             Fax: 732-699-0882
                                                www.nsrc-global.net

Offers information on the center's activities and events, medical and legislative updates for the patients and their families.
Quarterly

Pamphlets

7258 Anemia of Sarcoidosis
PC Publications
PO Box 1593   732-699-0733
Piscataway, NJ 08855-1593   800-223-6429
                                             Fax: 732-699-0882
                                                www.nsrc-global.net

7259 Bronchoalveolar Lymphocytes in Sarcoidosis
PC Publications
PO Box 1593   732-699-0733
Piscataway, NJ 08855-1593   800-223-6429
                                             Fax: 732-699-0882
                                                www.nsrc-global.net

7260 Case Report: MR Imaging of Myocardial Sarcoidosis
PC Publications
PO Box 1593   732-699-0733
Piscataway, NJ 08855-1593   800-223-6429
                                             Fax: 732-699-0882
                                                www.nsrc-global.net

7261 Case Report: Osseous Sarcoidosis and Chronic Polyarthritis
PC Publications
PO Box 1593   732-699-0733
Piscataway, NJ 08855-1593   800-223-6429
                                             Fax: 732-699-0882
                                                www.nsrc-global.net

7262 Case Report: Overlap of Granulomatous Vasculitis and Sarcoidosis
PC Publications
PO Box 1593   732-699-0733
Piscataway, NJ 08855-1593   800-223-6429
                                             Fax: 732-699-0882
                                                www.nsrc-global.net

7263 Case Report: Rapidly Dev. Confusion, Impaired Memory and Unsteady Gait
PC Publications
PO Box 1593   732-699-0733
Piscataway, NJ 08855-1593   800-223-6429
                                             Fax: 732-699-0882
                                                www.nsrc-global.net

7264 Coping with Sarcoidosis
National Sarcoidosis Resource Center
PO Box 1593
Piscataway, NJ 08855-1593
732-699-0733
800-223-6429
Fax: 732-699-0882
www.nsrc-global.net

A pamphlet offering information on how to manage and live with sarcoidosis.

7265 Disability Law: A Legal Primer
PC Publications
PO Box 1593
Piscataway, NJ 08855-1593
732-699-0733
800-223-6429
Fax: 732-699-0882
www.nsrc-global.net

7266 Drugs That Have Been Used for the Treatment of Sarcoidosis
PC Publications
PO Box 1593
Piscataway, NJ 08855-1593
732-699-0733
800-223-6429
Fax: 732-699-0882
www.nsrc-global.net

7267 Effect of Corticosteroid or Methotrexate Therapy on Lung Lymphocytes
PC Publications
PO Box 1593
Piscataway, NJ 08855-1593
732-699-0733
800-223-6429
Fax: 732-699-0882
www.nsrc-global.net

7268 Effects of Sarcoid and Steroids on Angiotensin-Converting Enzyme
PC Publications
PO Box 1593
Piscataway, NJ 08855-1593
732-699-0733
800-223-6429
Fax: 732-699-0882
www.nsrc-global.net

7269 Evaluation of the Efficacy and Toxicity of the Cyclosporine
PC Publications
PO Box 1593
Piscataway, NJ 08855-1593
732-699-0733
800-223-6429
Fax: 732-699-0882
www.nsrc-global.net

7270 Gastrointestinal Presentation of Churg Strauss Syndrome
PC Publications
PO Box 1593
Piscataway, NJ 08855-1593
732-699-0733
800-223-6429
Fax: 732-699-0882
www.nsrc-global.net

7271 Governor New Jersey Proclamation: Sarcoidosis Awareness Day
PC Publications
PO Box 1593
Piscataway, NJ 08855-1593
732-699-0733
800-223-6429
Fax: 732-699-0882
www.nsrc-global.net

7272 How to Get the Most Out of Your Doctor: A Neurologist's Perspective
PC Publications
PO Box 1593
Piscataway, NJ 08855-1593
732-699-0733
800-223-6429
Fax: 732-699-0882
www.nsrc-global.net

7273 Ideas and Considerations for Starting a Self-Help Mutual Aid Group
PC Publications
PO Box 1593
Piscataway, NJ 08855-1593
732-699-0733
800-223-6429
Fax: 732-699-0882
www.nsrc-global.net

7274 Masqueraders of Sarcoidosis
PC Publications
PO Box 1593
Piscataway, NJ 08855-1593
732-699-0733
800-223-6429
Fax: 732-699-0882
www.nsrc-global.net

7275 Mayor Piscataway, NJ Proclamation: Sarcoidosis Awareness Day
PC Publications
PO Box 1593
Piscataway, NJ 08855-1593
732-699-0733
800-223-6429
Fax: 732-699-0882
www.nsrc-global.net

7276 Multidisciplinary Clinico-Pathologic Conference
PC Publications
PO Box 1593
Piscataway, NJ 08855-1593
732-699-0733
800-223-6429
Fax: 732-699-0882
www.nsrc-global.net

7277 National Sarcoidosis Resource Center
PC Publications
PO Box 1593
Piscataway, NJ 08855-1593
732-699-0733
800-223-6429
Fax: 732-699-0882
www.nsrc-global.net

A booklet offering a brief introduction to the illness and offers information on the role of the Center in finding a cure and educating the public on Sarcoidosis.

7278 Neurosarcoidosis
PC Publications
PO Box 1593
Piscataway, NJ 08855-1593
732-699-0733
800-223-6429
Fax: 732-699-0882
www.nsrc-global.net

7279 Neurosarcoidosis or Multiple Sclerosis?
National Sarcoidosis Resource Center
PO Box 1593
Piscataway, NJ 08855-1593
732-699-0733
800-223-6429
Fax: 732-699-0882
www.nsrc-global.net

7280 Paranoid Psychosis Due to Neurosarcoidosis
PC Publications
PO Box 1593
Piscataway, NJ 08855-1593
732-699-0733
800-223-6429
Fax: 732-699-0882
www.nsrc-global.net

7281 Patient Information Package
National Sarcoidosis Resource Center
PO Box 1593
Piscataway, NJ 08855-1593
732-699-0733
800-223-6429
Fax: 732-699-0882
www.nsrc-global.net

Contains various brochures and pamphlets offering information about Sarcoidosis.

7282 Physician Listings
PC Publications
PO Box 1593
Piscataway, NJ 08855-1593
732-699-0733
800-223-6429
Fax: 732-699-0882
www.nsrc-global.net

7283 Possible Association of Rheumatoid Arthritis & Sarcoidosis
PC Publications
PO Box 1593
Piscataway, NJ 08855-1593
732-699-0733
800-223-6429
Fax: 732-699-0882
www.nsrc-global.net

7284 Presidential Proclamation - National Sarcoidosis Awareness Day
PC Publications
PO Box 1593
Piscataway, NJ 08855-1593
732-699-0733
800-223-6429
Fax: 732-699-0882
www.nsrc-global.net

7285 Psychological Factors in Sarcoidosis
PC Publications
PO Box 1593
Piscataway, NJ 08855-1593
732-699-0733
800-223-6429
Fax: 732-699-0882
www.nsrc-global.net

Sarcoidosis / Pamphlets

7286 Public Law 102-94
PC Publications
PO Box 1593
Piscataway, NJ 08855-1593
732-699-0733
800-223-6429
Fax: 732-699-0882
www.nsrc-global.net

7287 Pulmonary Sarcoidosis: Evaluation with High Resolution
PC Publications
PO Box 1593
Piscataway, NJ 08855-1593
732-699-0733
800-223-6429
Fax: 732-699-0882
www.nsrc-global.net

7288 Pulmonary Sarcoidosis: What We Are Learning
PC Publications
PO Box 1593
Piscataway, NJ 08855-1593
732-699-0733
800-223-6429
Fax: 732-699-0882
www.nsrc-global.net

7289 Questionnaire Responses for Demographics and Symptoms from 1000 Patients
PC Publications
PO Box 1593
Piscataway, NJ 08855-1593
732-699-0733
800-223-6429
Fax: 732-699-0882
www.nsrc-global.net

7290 Right & Left Ventricular Function at Rest in Patients with Sarcoidosis
PC Publications
PO Box 1593
Piscataway, NJ 08855-1593
732-699-0733
800-223-6429
Fax: 732-699-0882
www.nsrc-global.net

7291 Role of Magnetic Resonance Imaging in Neurosarcoidosis
PC Publications
PO Box 1593
Piscataway, NJ 08855-1593
732-699-0733
800-223-6429
Fax: 732-699-0882
www.nsrc-global.net

7292 Sarcoidosis
PC Publications
PO Box 1593
Piscataway, NJ 08855-1593
732-699-0733
800-223-6429
Fax: 732-699-0882
www.nsrc-global.net
Offers information on the illness, causes, symptoms and treatments.

7293 Sarcoidosis Diagnosed in a Patient with Known HIV Infection
PC Publications
PO Box 1593
Piscataway, NJ 08855-1593
732-699-0733
800-223-6429
Fax: 732-699-0882
www.nsrc-global.net

7294 Sarcoidosis Patient Questionnaire
PC Publications
PO Box 1593
Piscataway, NJ 08855-1593
732-699-0733
800-223-6429
Fax: 732-699-0882
www.nsrc-global.net

7295 Sarcoidosis Questionnaire: Demographics and Symptomatology-The Patients Respond
PC Publications
PO Box 1593
Piscataway, NJ 08855-1593
732-699-0733
800-223-6429
Fax: 732-699-0882
www.nsrc-global.net

7296 Sarcoidosis and Pregnancy: Clinical Observation
PC Publications
PO Box 1593
Piscataway, NJ 08855-1593
732-699-0733
800-223-6429
Fax: 732-699-0882
www.nsrc-global.net

7297 Sarcoidosis and You: A Listing of Possible Symptoms
PC Publications
PO Box 1593
Piscataway, NJ 08855-1593
732-699-0733
800-223-6429
Fax: 732-699-0882
www.nsrc-global.net

7298 Sarcoidosis in India: A Review of 125 Biopsy-Proven Cases from India
PC Publications
PO Box 1593
Piscataway, NJ 08855-1593
732-699-0733
800-223-6429
Fax: 732-699-0882
www.nsrc-global.net

7299 Sarcoidosis of the Liver
PC Publications
PO Box 1593
Piscataway, NJ 08855-1593
732-699-0733
800-223-6429
Fax: 732-699-0882
www.nsrc-global.net

7300 Sarcoidosis: A Multisystem Disease
PC Publications
PO Box 1593
Piscataway, NJ 08855-1593
732-699-0733
800-223-6429
Fax: 732-699-0882
www.nsrc-global.net
Explains the effects of the illness on the lungs and joints.

7301 Sarcoidosis: International Review
PC Publications
PO Box 1593
Piscataway, NJ 08855-1593
732-699-0733
800-223-6429
Fax: 732-699-0882
www.nsrc-global.net

7302 Sarcoidosis: Pleural Involvement Mimicking a Coin Lesson
PC Publications
PO Box 1593
Piscataway, NJ 08855-1593
732-699-0733
800-223-6429
Fax: 732-699-0882
www.nsrc-global.net

7303 Sarcoidosis: Usual and Unusual Manifestations
PC Publications
PO Box 1593
Piscataway, NJ 08855-1593
732-699-0733
800-223-6429
Fax: 732-699-0882
www.nsrc-global.net

7304 Seasonal Clustering of Sarcoidosis
National Sarcoidosis Resource Center
PO Box 1593
Piscataway, NJ 08855-1593
732-699-0733
800-223-6429
Fax: 732-699-0882
www.nsrc-global.net

7305 Successful Treatment of Myocardial Sarcoidosis with Steriods
PC Publications
PO Box 1593
Piscataway, NJ 08855-1593
732-699-0733
800-223-6429
Fax: 732-699-0882
www.nsrc-global.net

7306 Support Group Listing
PC Publications
PO Box 1593
Piscataway, NJ 08855-1593
732-699-0733
800-223-6429
Fax: 732-699-0882
www.nsrc-global.net

7307 Use of Low Dose Methotrexate in Refractory Sarcoidosis
PC Publications
PO Box 1593
Piscataway, NJ 08855-1593
732-699-0733
800-223-6429
Fax: 732-699-0882
www.nsrc-global.net

7308 World Association Sarcoidosi Other Granulatomous
PC Publications

542

PO Box 1593
Piscataway, NJ 08855-1593

732-699-0733
800-223-6429
Fax: 732-699-0882
www.nsrc-global.net

Audio & Video

7309 Dialogue with Doris
PC Publications
PO Box 1593
Piscataway, NJ 08855-1593

732-699-0733
800-223-6429
Fax: 732-699-0882
www.nsrc-global.net

7310 Help with a Hidden Disease Update
PC Publications
PO Box 1593
Piscataway, NJ 08855-1593

732-699-0733
800-223-6429
Fax: 732-699-0882
www.nsrc-global.net

7311 Of Their Own: Person to Person Show
PC Publications
PO Box 1593
Piscataway, NJ 08855-1593

732-699-0733
800-223-6429
Fax: 732-699-0882
www.nsrc-global.net

7312 Sarcoidosis Conference 2
PC Publications
PO Box 1593
Piscataway, NJ 08855-1593

732-699-0733
800-223-6429
Fax: 732-699-0882
www.nsrc-global.net

7313 Sarcoidosis Conference 3
PC Publications
PO Box 1593
Piscataway, NJ 08855-1593

732-699-0733
800-223-6429
Fax: 732-699-0882
www.nsrc-global.net

7314 Sarcoidosis and Lyme Disease
PC Publications
PO Box 1593
Piscataway, NJ 08855-1593

732-699-0733
800-223-6429
Fax: 732-699-0882
www.nsrc-global.net

7315 Sarcoidosis: What's That?
PC Publications
PO Box 1593
Piscataway, NJ 08855-1593

732-699-0733
800-223-6429
Fax: 732-699-0882
www.nsrc-global.net

7316 XIV International World Conference on Sarcoidosis: Patient Symposium
PC Publications
PO Box 1593
Piscataway, NJ 08855-1593

732-699-0733
800-223-6429
Fax: 732-699-0882
www.nsrc-global.net

Cassette.

Web Sites

7317 Healing Well
www.healingwell.com
An online health resource guide to medical news, chat, information and articles, newsgroups and message boards, books, disease-related web sites, medical directories, and more for patients, friends, and family coping with disabling diseases, disorders, or chronic illnesses.

7318 Health Finder
www.healthfinder.gov
Searchable, carefully developed web site offering information on over 1000 topics. Developed by the US Department of Health and Human Services, the site can be used in both English and Spanish.

7319 Healthlink USA
www.healthlinkusa.com
Health information concerning treatment, cures, prevention, diagnosis, risk factors, research, support groups, email lists, personal stories and much more. Updated regularly.

7320 MedicineNet
www.medicinenet.com
An online resource for consumers providing easy-to-read, authoritative medical and health information.

7321 Medscape
www.medscape.com
Medscape offers specialists, primary care physicians, and other health professionals the Web's most robust and integrated medical information and educational tools.

7322 National Sarcoidosis Resource Center
www.nsrc-global.net
Provides the general public with sarcoidosis information, for patients to obtain medical and emotional help and to provide government officials with the information they need.

7323 WebMD
www.webmd.com
Provides credible information, supportive communities, and in-depth reference material about health subjects. A source for original and timely health information as well as material from well known content providers.

Description

7324 Scleroderma

Scleroderma, literally 'hard skin,' is a form of systemic sclerosis, a generalized disturbance of connective and vascular tissue which leads to scarring (sclerosis). Scleroderma is a rare disease, with about 20,000 new cases in the United States each year. Women are 4 times as likely as men to get the disease, which typically begins between the ages of 30 and 50 years. It is comparatively rare in children. While the precise cause of the disease is unknown, genetic factors play an important role. Variations in two genes in particular, IRF5 and STAT4, which encode proteins that regulate the immune response, increase the risk of scleroderma.

Since almost any organ may be involved, the list of possible symptoms is extensive. Important ones include weakness, fatigue, stiffness, weight loss, shortness of breath, abdominal bloating and pain, diarrhea and irritation of the eyes. Kidney involvement usually causes abrupt acceleration of high blood pressure. A very characteristic symptom, although not unique to this disease, is Raynaud's phenomenon. On exposure to cold, the arteries of the patient's hands and feet contract, causing the skin color to change from red, to white (blanch), to blue (cyanosis), accompanied by pain and numbness.

If the disease is limited to the skin the prognosis is good, but involvement of lung and kidney in the systemic form may be fatal. Use of the ACE inhibitor class of anti-hypertensive drugs helps preserve kidney function. Many immunosuppressive drugs have been tried without clear success. Clinical trials of new agents are often available to patients. Stem cell transplants have shown remarkable success in small clinical trials, but much more work remains before these treatments are feasible. When end-stage kidney disease cannot be prevented, dialysis and transplant can be used, although the death rate remains high.

National Agencies & Associations

7325 Canadian Dermatology Association
1385 Bank Street   613-738-1748
Ottawa, Ontario, K1H-8N4   800-267-3376
Fax: 866-267-2178
www.dermatology.ca
Ensures the Canadian public has access to timely dermatologic care and represents certified dermatologists.
Neil Shear, MD, President
Jason Rivers, Vice President

7326 Raynaud's Association
11 Topstone Road   800-280-8055
Redding, CT 06896   info@raynauds.org
www.raynauds.org
A non-profit organization providing support and education to individuals with Raynaud's Phenomenon.

7327 Scleroderma Foundation
300 Rosewood Drive   978-463-5843
Danvers, MA 01923   800-722-4673
Fax: 978-777-1313
sfinfo@scleroderma.org
www.scleroderma.org
A national non-profit organization serving individuals with Scleroderma. Support groups are available nationwide.
Cos M. Mallozzi, Chair
Carol Feghali-Bostwick, PhD, Vice Chair

7328 Scleroderma Society of Ontario
41 King William Street   888-776-7776
Hamilton, Ontario, L8R-1A2   info@sclerodermaontario.ca
www.sclerodermaontario.ca
Committed to increasing public awareness, advancing patient wellness and supporting research in scleroderma.
Karen Nielsen, President
David Sauv,, Vice President

State Agencies & Associations

Arizona

7329 Scleroderma Foundation: Arizona Chapter
18402 N 19th Avenue   623-847-3757
Phoenix, AZ 85023   carolnader@cox.net
www.scleroderma.org
Local chapter of the national Scleroderma Foundation in Byfield, Massachusetts. Please contact this group for information on area support groups.
Carol Nader, President

California

7330 Scleroderma Foundation: Greater San Diego Chapter
PO Box 502948   619-655-4342
San Diego, CA 92150   kellyd.sclerosd@gmail.com
www.scleroderma.org
Local chapter of the national Scleroderma Foundation in Byfield, Massachusetts. Please contact this group for information on area support groups.
Fletcher Diehl, President
Carol Ireland, Vice President

7331 Scleroderma Foundation: Northern California Chapter
PO Box 601313   916-832-1102
Sacramento, CA 95860   NoCAchapter@scleroderma.org
www.scleroderma.org
Local chapter of the national Scleroderma Foundation in Byfield, Massachusetts. Please contact this group for information on area support groups.
Cathy Eddy, President
Cheryl George, Vice President

7332 Scleroderma Foundation: Southern California Chapter
10319 Jefferson Blvd.   310-287-0793
Culver City, CA 90232   877-443-5755
Fax: 310-477-8774
SoCAchapter@scleroderma.org
www.scleroderma.org
Local chapter of the national Scleroderma Foundation in Byfield, Massachusetts. Please contact this group for information on area support groups.
Brian Ross Adams, Executive Director
Dan Furst, President

Colorado

7333 Scleroderma Foundation: Colorado Chapter
2280 S Albion Street   303-806-6686
Denver, CO 80222-0940   COchapter@scleroderma.org
www.scleroderma.org
Local chapter of the national Scleroderma Foundation in Danvers, Massachusetts. Please contact this group for information on area support groups.
Rita Miller, President
Fran Penk, Vice President

District of Columbia

7334 Scleroderma Foundation: Greater Washington DC Chapter
2010 Corporate Ridge   202-999-4562
McLean, VA 22102   888-233-4779
                    GWDCchapter@scleroderma.org
                              www.scleroderma.org
Local chapter of the national Scleroderma Foundation in Byfield,
Massachusetts. Please contact this group for information on area
support groups.
Carol Sodetz, President

Florida

7335 Scleroderma Foundation: Southeast Florida Chapter
3930 Oaks Clubhouse Drive   954-798-1854
Pompano Beach, FL 33069-3913   Fax: 954-255-8081
                    sclerodermasefl@gmail.com
                              www.scleroderma.org
Local chapter of the national Scleroderma Foundation in Byfield,
Massachusetts. Please contact this group for information on area
support groups.
Berna Falkoff, President
Ruth Greenspan, Vice - Chair

Georgia

**7336 Scleroderma Foundation: Georgia Chapter Scleroderma
Foundation**
Scleroderma Foundation
PO Box 522   770-925-7037
Liburn, GA 30048   800-722-4673
                    GAchapter@scleroderma.org
                              www.scleroderma.org
Local chapter of the national Scleroderma Foundation in Byfield,
Massachusetts. Call the national office for contact information on
the Georgia Chapter. Please contact this group for information on
area support groups.
Stacy Wright, Contact
Mary Haulk, Contact

Illinois

7337 Scleroderma Foundation: Greater Chicago Chapter
134 N. LaSalle St.   312-660-1131
Chicago, IL 60602   Fax: 312-660-1133
                    GCchapter@scleroderma.org
                              www.scleroderma.org
Local chapter of the national Scleroderma Foundation. Please con-
tact group for information on area support groups.
Mike Robbins, President

Maine

7338 Scleroderma Foundation: New England Chapter
462 Boston Street   978-887-0658
Topsfield, MA 01983   888-525-0658
                              Fax: 978-887-0659
                    newengland@scleroderma.com
                              www.scleroderma.org
Local chapter of the national Scleroderma Foundation in Byfield,
Massachusetts. Please contact this group for information on area
support groups. Includes MA, ME, NH, VT, & RI.
Marie Coyle, President
Peter L. Hart, Treasurer

Massachusetts

7339 Scleroderma Foundation: New England Chapter
462 Boston Street   978-887-0658
Topsfield, MA 01983   888-525-0658
                              Fax: 978-887-0659
                    newengland@scleroderma.com
                              www.scleroderma.org
Local chapter of the national Scleroderma Foundation in Byfield,
Massachusetts. Please contact this group for information on area
support groups.
Marie Coyle, President
Peter L. Hart, Treasurer

Michigan

7340 Scleroderma Foundation: Michigan Chapter
23999 Telegraph   248-595-8526
Southfield, MI 48033   800-716-6554
                              Fax: 248-595-8586
                    MIchapter@scleroderma.org
                              www.scleroderma.org
Local chapter of the national Scleroderma Foundation in Danvers,
Massachusetts. Please contact this group for information on area
support groups, medical referrals, confrence dates and fund rais-
ing activities.
Duane Maladecki, President
Paul Rybicki, Vice President

Minnesota

7341 Scleroderma Foundation: Minnesota Chapter
PO Box 385246   877-794-0347
Bloomington, MN 55438   877-794-0347
                    MNChapter@scleroderma.org
                              www.scleroderma.org
Local chapter of the national Scleroderma Foundation in Byfield,
Massachusetts. Please contact this group for information on area
support groups.
Bonnie Handmacher, President
Jordana Schmidt, Vice President

Missouri

7342 Scleroderma Foundation: Missouri Chapter
PO Box 4123   417-887-3269
Springfield, MO 65808   MOchapter@scleroderma.org
                              www.scleroderma.org
Local chapter of the national Scleroderma Foundation in Byfield,
Massachusetts. Please contact this group for information on area
support groups.
Mary Blades, President
Rhonda Costa, Vice President

Nevada

7343 Scleroderma Foundation: Nevada Chapter
6760 Surrey Street   702-368-1572
Las Vegas, NV 89119   NVchapter@scleroderma.org
                              www.scleroderma.org
Local chapter of the national Scleroderma Foundation in Byfield,
Massachusetts. Please contact this group for information on area
support groups.
Barbara Dempsey, President
Sheila Gray, VP Support Group

New Hampshire

7344 Scleroderma Foundation: New England Chapter
462 Boston Street   978-887-0658
Topsfield, MA 01983   888-525-0658
                              Fax: 978-887-0659
                    newengland@scleroderma.com
                              www.scleroderma.org
Local chapter of the national Scleroderma Foundation in Byfield,
Massachusetts. Please contact this group for information on area
support groups.
Marie Coyle, President
Peter L. Hart, Treasurer

New York

7345 Scleroderma Foundation: Tri-State Chapter
59 Front Street   800-867-0885
Binghamton, NY 13905   800-867-0885
                              Fax: 607-723-2039
                    chribar@scleroderma.org
                              www.scleroderma.org
Local chapter of the national Scleroderma Foundation in Byfield,
Massachusetts. Please contact this group for information on area
support groups.
Jeff Mace, President
Bruce Cowen, Vice President

7346 Scleroderma Foundation: Western New York Chapter
PO Box 708
Hamburg, NY 14075
716-627-2283
877-969-2478
wnychpt@aol.com
www.scleroderma.org
Local chapter of the national Scleroderma Foundation in Byfield, Massachusetts. Please contact this group for information on area support groups.
Laura Henry, Co-President

Ohio

7347 Scleroderma Foundation: Ohio Chapter
PO Box 105
Worthington, OH 43085-0846
614-334-0846
866-849-9030
OHchapter@scleroderma.org
www.scleroderma.org
Local chapter of the national Scleroderma Foundation in Byfield, Massachusetts. Please contact this group for information on area support groups.
Debbie Metz, President
Garry Lazenby, Vice President

Oregon

7348 Scleroderma Foundation: Oregon Chapter
PO Box 19296
Portland, OR 97280-0296
503-245-4588
ORchapter@scleroderma.org
www.scleroderma.org
Local chapter of the national Scleroderma Foundation in Byfield, Massachusetts. Please contact this group for information on area support groups.
Liz Orem-Bedel, President
Richard Bates, Vice President

Pennsylvania

7349 Scleroderma Foundation: Western Pennsylvania Chapter
3500 Terrace Street
Pittsburgh, PA 15261
800-603-8960
800-722-4673
WPAchapter@scleroderma.org
www.scleroderma.org
Local chapter of the national Scleroderma Foundation in Byfield, Massachusetts. Please contact this group for information on area support groups.
Betty Aquino, President
Thomas A Medsger Jr, Treasurer

Rhode Island

7350 Scleroderma Foundation: New England Chapter
462 Boston Street
Topsfield, MA 01983
978-887-0658
888-525-0658
Fax: 978-887-0659
newengland@scleroderma.com
www.scleroderma.org
Local chapter of the national Scleroderma Foundation in Byfield, Massachusetts. Please contact this group for information on area support groups.
Marie Coyle, President
Peter L. Hart, Treasurer

South Carolina

7351 Scleroderma Foundation: South Carolina Chapter
713-D east Greenvile Street
Anderson, SC 29621
864-617-0237
866-557-3729
SCchapter@scleroderma.org
www.scleroderma.org
Local chapter of the national Scleroderma Foundation in Byfield. Massachusetts. Please contact this group for information on area support groups.
Susan Melvin, President
Karen Kemper, Vice President

Tennessee

7352 Scleroderma Foundation: Tennessee Chapter
PO Box 281977
Nashville, TN 37228
615-792-4610
800-497-5193
Fax: 615-792-4610
TNchapter@scleroderma.org
www.scleroderma.org
Local chapter of the national Scleroderma Foundation in Byfield, Massachusetts. Please contact this group for information on area support groups.
April Simpkins, President
Charles Cowell, Vice President

Texas

7353 Scleroderma Foundation: Bluebonnet Chapter
PO Box 1836
Allen, TX 75013-1894
972-396-9400
866-532-7673
Fax: 972-649-7910
TXchapter@scleroderma.org
www.scleroderma.org
Local chapter of the national Scleroderma Foundation in Byfield, Massachusetts. Please contact this group for information on area support groups.
Cindi Brannum, President
Peggy Brown, Vice President

Vermont

7354 Scleroderma Foundation: New England Chapter
462 Boston Street
Topsfield, MA 01983
978-887-0658
888-525-0658
Fax: 978-887-0659
newengland@scleroderma.com
www.scleroderma.org
Local chapter of the national Scleroderma Foundation in Byfield, Massachusetts. Please contact this group for information on area support groups.
Marie Coyle, President
Peter L. Hart, Treasurer

Virginia

7355 Scleroderma Foundation: Greater Washington DC Chapter
2010 Corporate Ridge
McLean, VA 22102
202-999-4562
888-233-4779
GWDCchapter@scleroderma.org
www.scleroderma.org
Local chapter of the national Scleroderma Foundation in Byfield, Massachusetts. Please contact this group for information on area support groups.
Carol Sodetz, President
Solomon reed, Treasurer

Washington

7356 Scleroderma Foundation: Evergreen Chapter
PO Box 84506
Seattle, WA 98124-5806
206-285-9822
WAchapter@scleroderma.org
www.scleroderma.org
Local chapter of the national Scleroderma Foundation in Byfield, Massachusetts. Please contact this group for information on area support groups.
Bunny Garthe, President
Nic Evans, Vice President

Foundations

7357 Juvenile Scleroderma Network
1204 W 13th Street
San Pedro, CA 90731
310-519-9511
866-338-5892
www.jsdn.org
Organization that is working to provide educational programs about JSD, and to help children and their families to gain a better understanding.
Jerry Gaither, Chairman
Kathy Gaither, President

Research Centers

7358 Boston University University Medical Center
University Medical Center
One Boston Medical Center Place   617-638-8000
Boston, MA 02118   www.bmc.org
Ongoing clinical trials and studies in scleroderma. Office hours by appointment.
Kate Walsh, President/CEO
Melynn Nuite RN, Clinical Trails Contact

7359 Center for Rheumatology
1367 Washington Avenue   518-489-4471
Albany, NY 12206   cbarr@joint-docs.com
                                 www.joint-docs.com
This is a committed research facility as well as a medical practice. Our research practice is made up of seven physicians a certified physician's assistant and four research coordinators. We may have as many as 20 ongoing trails at a time in various indications within the study of rheumatology. Investigational treatment of interstitial lung disease associated with systemic sclerosis.
Norman R Romanoff, Practitioner
Joel M Kremer, Practitioner

7360 Georgetown University Hospital: Department of Rheumatology
3800 Reservoir Road NW   202-444-8233
Washington, DC 20007   Fax: 202-444-7584
Research is based on clinical trials and special interest in scleroderma and kidney pulmonary hypertension pregnancy epidemiology and natural history of scleroderma subsets.
Sherry Magrudar, Executive Assistant
Ann Nichols, Senior Adminstrator

7361 Johns Hopkins University: Scleroderma Center
Johns Hopkins Bayview Medical Center
5501 Hopkins Bayview Circle   410-550-7715
Baltimore, MD 21224   Fax: 410-550-1363
                                 www.scleroderma.jhmi.edu
Specializes in the management of systemic sclerosis (scleroderma) Raynaud's phenomenon and related disorders. In addition to patient care the center is involved in both basic and clinical research projects.
Frederick M Wigley MD, Director
Sheila Friend, medical office coordinator

7362 Mayo Clinic Scottsdale Center for Scleroderma Care & Research
Mayo Clinic
13400 E Shea Boulevard   480-301-8000
Scottsdale, AZ 85259   800-446-2279
                                Fax: 480-301-7006
                                newsbureau@mayo.edu
                                www.mayoclinic.org/rheumatology
Integrates multiple medical as well as surgical specialties under the direction of the Division of Rheumatology to provide coordinated and comprehensive evaluations and treatment. New clinical trails are in development.
John H. Noseworthy MD, President/CEO
April Chang-Miller, Assistant Professor of Medicine

7363 Medical University of South Carolina Medical University of South Carolina
Medical University of South Carolina
171 Ashley Avenue   843-792-1414
Charleston, SC 29425   800-424-6872
                                Fax: 843-792-2601
                                wickman@musc.edu
                                www.musc.edu
Actively engaged in basic and clinical research of scleroderma.
Raymond S Greenburg, President
Dr. Mark Sothman, Vice President

7364 Scleroderma Clinical & Research Center State University of New York at Stonybro
State University of New York at Stonybrook
26 Research Way   631-444-0580
E Setauket, NY 01173-9260   Fax: 631-444-0562
                                www.scleroderma.org
Ongoing research of scleroderma.
Joseph Camerino, chair
Carol Feghali-Bostwick, Vce Chair

7365 Scleroderma Research Foundation
220 Montgomery Street   415-834-9444
San Francisco, CA 94104   800-637-4005
                                Fax: 415-834-9177
                                info@sclerodermaresearch.org
                                www.srfcure.org
Mission is to find a cure for scleroderma a life threatening and degenerative illness by funding and facilitating the most promising highest quality research and placing the disease and its need for a cure in the public eye.
Alex Gonzalez, Director of Development
Amy Hewitt, Executive Director

7366 Thomas Jefferson University Hospital
111 S 11th Street   215-955-6840
Philadelphia, PA 19107   Fax: 215-923-5828
                                www.jeffersonhospital.org
Provides diagnostic evaluations treatment and access to the latest research studies for more than one thousand patients with scleroderma and related diseases.
Stephen K klasko, President/CEO
Sergio Jimen MD, Professor

7367 University of Alabama Birmingham
1720 second Av Soyth   205-934-4011
Birmingham, AL 35294   www.uab.edu
Located in the Clinical Immunology and Rheumatology department Oral Type 1 Collagen in Scleroderma is studied.
Carol Garrison, President
William Ferniany, CEO

7368 University of Chicago Center for Advanced Medicine Duchossis Center
University of Chicago hospital
5841 S Maryland Avenue   773-702-1000
Chicago, IL 60637   888-824-0200
                                Fax: 773-028-02
                                orogers@medicine.bsd.uchicago.edu
                                www.uchospitals.com
Scleroderma clinic.
Michael Ellm MD, Clinic Contact
Ornery Rogers, Clinic Contact

7369 University of Illinois at Chicago Medical Center Outpatient Clinical Center
University of Illinois
600 S Hoyne Avenue   312-996-7000
Chicago, IL 60612   800-842-1002
                                Fax: 312-633-3434
                                TTY: 312-413-0123
                                info@iMDc.org
                                www.uic.edu
Scleroderma clinic held on the first and third Thursdays of every month.
Paula Allen Meares, Chancellor
Lon S. Kauffman, Vice Chancellor

7370 University of Pittsburgh
4200 Fifth avenue   412-624-4141
Pittsburgh, PA 15260   Fax: 412-383-2264
                                webmaster@pitt.edu
                                www.pitt.edu
Clinic and research of scleroderma.
Patricia E. Beeson, Vice Chancellor
John P Elliott, Director of Internal Affairs

7371 University of Tennessee Medical Group
956 Court Avenue   901-866-8383
Memphis, TN 38103   Fax: 901-866-8380
Ongoing research protocols.
Charles E. Woeppel MD, CEO

7372 University of Texas Health Science Center
7000 Fannin   713-500-4472
Houston, TX 77030   Fax: 713-500-3026
                                sclerodermaregister@uth.tmc.edu
                                www.uthouston.edu
Clinic research and clinical trials concerning scleroderma.
Giuseppe N. Colasurdo, President

Support Groups & Hotlines

7373 National Health Information Center
Office of Disease Prevention & Health Promotion
1101 Wootton Pkwy
Rockville, MD 20852   Fax: 240-453-8281
                                       odphpinfo@hhs.gov
                                       www.health.gov/nhic

Supports public health education by maintaining a calendar of National Health Observances; helps connect consumers and health professionals to organizations that can best answer questions and provide up-to-date contact information from reliable sources; updates on a yearly basis toll-free numbers for health information, Federal health clearinghouses and info centers.
Don Wright, MD, MPH, Director

7374 Rhode Island Scleroderma Support Group
18 Talbot Manor   401-781-5013
Cranston, RI 02905   scleroderma@hotmail.com
                               www.angelfire.com/ri/scleroderma
Meets on the fourth Wednsday of every month at Roger Williams Hospital.
Carole Cowell, President

7375 Scleroderma Support Groups
Scleroderma Foundation
12 Kent Way   978-463-5843
Byfield, MA 01922   800-722-4633
                                       Fax: 978-463-5809
                                       sfinfo@scleroderma.org
                                       www.scleroderma.org
Please contact the Scleroderma Foundation or visit our web site for a listing of support groups in your area.

Books

7376 Best of the Beacon
Scleroderma Foundation
12 Kent Way   978-463-5843
Byfield, MA 01922   800-722-4673
                                       Fax: 978-463-5809
                                       sfinfo@scleroderma.org
                                       www.scleroderma.org
Interesting, readable and highly practical collection of articles of particular interest to those living with scleroderma. This mini encyclopedia includes 11 medical articles, 358 most frequently asked questions, 34 sharing stories, 62 articles of special interest on a variety of useful topics and a glossary that defines 240 words you may encounter when reading about scleroderma.
Marie Coyle, Editor
Bianca Podesta, Author

7377 Handout on Health: Scleroderma
NAMSIC/National Institutes of Health
9000 Rockville Pike   301-495-4484
Bethesda, MD 20892-0001   877-226-4267
                                       Fax: 301-718-6366
                                       TTY: 301-565-2966
                                       niamsinfo@mail.nih.gov
                                       www.nih.gov

143 pages

7378 Helpful Hints for Living with Scleroderma
Scleroderma Foundation
12 Kent Way   978-463-5843
Byfield, MA 01922   800-722-4673
                                       Fax: 978-463-5809
                                       sfinfo@scleroderma.org
                                       www.scleroderma.org
Booklet of helpful suggestions from our chapters and members, for the comfort and convienience of others who share the same challenges.
57 pages
Marie Coyle, Editor

7379 Perspectives on Living with Scleroderma
Scleroderma Foundation

12 Kent Way   978-463-5843
Byfield, MA 01922   800-722-4673
                                       Fax: 978-463-5809
                                       sfinfo@scleroderma.org
                                       www.scleroderma.org
Insightful articles on coping with scleroderma come from not only from Dr. Flapan's counseling and volunteer work, but also from his personal experience as a scleroderma patient.
233 pages

7380 Scleroderma Book
Scleroderma Foundation
12 Kent Way   978-463-5843
Byfield, MA 01922   800-722-4673
                                       Fax: 978-463-5809
                                       sfinfo@scleroderma.org
                                       www.scleroderma.org
Definitive guide to scleroderma for patients and their families, with easy to understand explanations.
182 pages
Maureen D. Mayes, Author

7381 Scleroderma: Surviving a Seventeen-Year Itch
Scleroderma Foundation
                                       978-463-5809
                                       800-722-4673
                                       Fax: 978-463-5809
                                       sfinfo@scleroderma.org
                                       www.scleroderma.org
Self-help manual including history, diagnosis, daily routines and exercise programs for persons with scleroderma.

7382 Scleroderma: a New Role for Patients and Families
Scleroderma Foundation
12 Kent Way   978-463-5843
Byfield, MA 01922   800-722-4673
                                       Fax: 978-463-5809
                                       sfinfo@scleroderma.org
                                       www.scleroderma.org
Provides an overview of key issues and offers resources that enable patients and their families to find more resources on thier own.
168 pages
Michael Brown, Author

7383 Understanding & Managing Scleroderma
Scleroderma Foundation
12 Kent Way   978-463-5843
Byfield, MA 01923   800-722-4633
                                       Fax: 978-463-5809
                                       sfinfo@scleroderma.org
                                       www.scleroderma.org
Booklet intended to help persons with scleroderma, their families and others interested in scleroderma to better understand what scleroderma is, what effects it may have, and what those with scleroderma can do to help themselves and their physicians manage the disease. It answers some of the most frequently asked questions about scleroderma.

Magazines

7384 Scleroderma Voice
Scleroderma Foundation
12 Kent Way   978-463-5843
Byfield, MA 01922   800-722-4673
                                       Fax: 978-463-5809
                                       sfinfo@scleroderma.org
                                       www.scleroderma.org
Feautures the latest information available on scleroderma treatments and research. Subscription to the Voice includes a one-year membership in the Scleroderma Foundation.
Quarterly

Pamphlets

7385 If You Have Scleroderma You Need Not Feel Alone
Scleroderma Foundation

12 Kent Way
Byfield, MA 01922

978-463-5843
800-722-4673
Fax: 978-463-5809
sfinfo@scleroderma.org
www.scleroderma.org

Scleroderma Foundation's membership brochure. Free of charge, also available in Spanish.

7386 Scleroderma: an Overview
Scleroderma Foundation
12 Kent Way
Byfield, MA 01922

978-463-5843
Fax: 978-463-5809
sfinfo@scleroderma.org
www.scleroderma.org

Concise genral overview of sytemic scleroderma. Also available in Spanish, and downloadable in Portugese.

7387 What Causes Scleroderma?
Scleroderma Foundation
12 Kent Way
Byfield, MA 01922

978-463-5843
800-722-4673
Fax: 978-463-5809
sfinfo@scleroderma.org
www.scleroderma.org

Discusses the puzzling nature of scleroderma. Also available in Spanish, and downloadable in Portugese.

Web Sites

7388 Healing Well

www.healingwell.com

An online health resource guide to medical news, chat, information and articles, newsgroups and message boards, books, disease-related web sites, medical directories, and more for patients, friends, and family coping with disabling diseases, disorders, or chronic illnesses.

7389 Health Finder

www.healthfinder.gov

Searchable, carefully developed web site offering information on over 1000 topics. Developed by the US Department of Health and Human Services, the site can be used in both English and Spanish.

7390 Healthlink USA

www.healthlinkusa.com

Health information concerning treatment, cures, prevention, diagnosis, risk factors, research, support groups, email lists, personal stories and much more. Updated regularly.

7391 MedicineNet

www.medicinenet.com

An online resource for consumers providing easy-to-read, authoritative medical and health information.

7392 Medscape

www.medscape.com

Medscape offers specialists, primary care physicians, and other health professionals the Web's most robust and integrated medical information and educational tools.

7393 Scleroderma Foundation

www.scleroderma.org

501 (c)3 national nonprofit organization serving the interests of persons with scleroderma. The Foundation's 26 chapters and 135 support groups nationwide help to carry out its three-fold mission of support, education and research. The Scleroderma Foundation is a leading nonprofit supporter of scleroderma research — funding over $1 million of new grants each year to find the cause and cure of scleroderma.

7394 WebMD

www.webmd.com

Provides credible information, supportive communities, and in-depth reference material about health subjects. A source for original and timely health information as well as material from well known content providers.

Description

7395 **Scoliosis**

Scoliosis is a lateral curvature of the spine, with 60 to 80 percent of the cases occurring in girls. It may first be suspected when one of the teenager's shoulders appears higher than the other or clothes don't hang straight. The spinal curve is more pronounced when the adolescent bends forward. More than 80 percent of scoliosis is idiopathic, that is, there is no known cause. There are 3 million cases of scoliosis per year in the U.S.

Symptoms include prominent shoulder blades, uneven hip levels, and fatigue in the lower back after sitting or standing for prolonged periods of time. In many cases there are no symptoms unless the scoliosis is severe.

The prognosis depends on the site and severity of the curve, and the age of onset of symptoms. Early detection through school screening provides more treatment options, and prompt referral to an orthopedist is indicated. The majority of cases require only observation for progression. Approximately 20 percent of those with scoliosis will require an orthopedic brace or spinal fusion surgery.

National Agencies & Associations

7396 **American Academy of Orthopaedic Surgeons**
9400 West Higgins Road
Rosemont, IL 60018-4262
847-823-7186
800-626-6726
Fax: 847-823-8125
customerservice@aaos.org
www.aaos.org
Provides education and practice management services for orthopaedic surgeons and allied health professionals. Also serves as an advocate for improved patient care, and to inform the public.
Thomas E. Arend, Jr., Chief Executive Officer
Will Shaffer, MD, Medical Director

7397 **American Chronic Pain Association**
PO Box 850
Rocklin, CA 95677
800-533-3231
ACPA@theacpa.org
www.theacpa.org
The ACPA facilitates peer support and education for individuals with chronic pain in its many forms, in order to increase quality of life. Also raises awareness among the healthcare community, and with policy makers.
Penney Cowan, Founder & CEO
Daniel Galia, Director, Global Support

7398 **Federation of Spine Associations**
9400 W Higgins Road
Rosemont, IL 60018-1628
414-918-9834
847-698-1628
Fax: 698-268-9540
info@csrs.org
www.csrs.org
Provides a forum for spine societies to produce scientific research. Comprised of members of 4 organizations: the American Spinal Injury Association, the Cervical Spine Research Society, the North American Spine Society, and the Scoliosis Research Society.
Kerri L. Mink, Executive Director

7399 **National Scoliosis Foundation**
5 Cabot Place
Stoughton, MA 02072
800-673-6922
Fax: 781-341-8333
NSF@scoliosis.org
www.scoliosis.org
Promotes school screening, raises public awareness, fosters public education, and maintains a resource center for professional information and scoliosis conferences. Offers support groups for people affected by the disease.
Joseph P. O'Brien, MBA, President & CEO
Robert M. Vincent, MBA, Treasurer

Research Centers

7400 **Scoliosis Research Society**
555 E Wells Street
Milwaukee, WI 53202
414-289-9107
Fax: 414-276-3349
info@srs.org
www.srs.org
This society provides an international forum for those interested in the management of spinal deformities. It holds a yearly meeting at which health professionals meet to share observations and results and to explore new avenues of research.
Kamal N. Ibrahim, President
Hubert Labelle, Treasurer

7401 **Shriners Hospital for Crippled Children Chicago Unit**
Chicago Unit
2211 N Oak Park Avenue
Chicago, IL 60707
813-281-0300
Fax: 773-855-88
www.shrinershospitalsforchildren.org
A 60-bed orthopedic hospital providing comprehensive spinal cord injury care to children. Provides care for spinal deformities Cerebral Palsy Osteoeneisis Imperfecta and Scoliosis as well as others.
John A. Cinotto, Chairman
Diether Sturm, Chief of Staff

Support Groups & Hotlines

7402 **National Health Information Center**
Office of Disease Prevention & Health Promotion
1101 Wootton Pkwy
Rockville, MD 20852
Fax: 240-453-8281
odphpinfo@hhs.gov
www.health.gov/nhic
Supports public health education by maintaining a calendar of National Health Observances; helps connect consumers and health professionals to organizations that can best answer questions and provide up-to-date contact information from reliable sources; updates on a yearly basis toll-free numbers for health information, Federal health clearinghouses and info centers.
Don Wright, MD, MPH, Director

Books

7403 **Adult Scoliosis Surgery...It Can Be Done**
St. Luke's Spine Center
555 East Wells Street
Milwaukee, WI 53202-3805
414-289-9107
Fax: 414-276-3349
info@srs.org
www.srs.org

21 pages
Ashtin Neuschaefer, Administrative Manager
Lily Atonio, Education and Program Manager

7404 **Coalition Index**
American School Health Association
7918 Jones Branch Drive
McLean, VA 22102
703-506-7675
800-445-2742
Fax: 703-506-3266
info@ashaweb.org
www.ashaweb.org

Linda Morse, President
Ty Oehrtman, Vice President

7405 **Getting Ready, Getting Well**
National Scoliosis Foundation

5 Cabot Place
Stoughton, MA 02072

781-341-6333
800-673-6922
Fax: 781-341-8333
NSF@scoliosis.org
www.scoliosis.org

73 pages
Joseph P O'Brien, President/CEO

7406 Handbook of Scoliosis
Scoliosis Research Society
555 East Wells Street
Milwaukee, WI 53202

414-289-9107
Fax: 414-276-3349
info@srs.org
www.srs.org

Ashtin Neuschaefer, Administrative Manager
Lily Atonio, Education and Program Manager

7407 Stopping Scoliosis
National Scoliosis Foundation
5 Cabot Place
Stoughton, MA 02072

781-341-6333
800-673-6922
Fax: 781-341-8333
NSF@scoliosis.org
www.scoliosis.org

Joseph P O'Brien, President/CEO

7408 Twenty Years at Hull House
New American Library
375 Hudson Street
New York, NY 10014

212-366-2000

Grades 7-12

Children's Books

7409 Deenie
Bradbury Press
866 3rd Avenue
New York, NY 10022-6221

212-702-2000
800-257-5755

Deenie, a beautiful thirteen-year-old girl, had a mother who was pushing her to become a model. The agency representatives told Deenie she had the looks but walked differently. Deenie's main wish was to become a cheerleader. Her close friend, Janet, made the cheerleading squad but Deenie didn't make the finalist list. After this her gym teacher noticed her posture and called her family. After seeing therapists, the diagnosis of adolescent idiopathic scoliosis was made.
159 pages Hardcover
ISBN: 0-027110-20-6

7410 Tina's Story...Scoliosis and Me
Alfred I DuPont Institute
555 East Wells Street
Milwaukee, WI 53202

414-289-9107
Fax: 414-276-3349
info@srs.org
www.srs.org

Ashtin Neuschaefer, Administrative Manager
Lily Atonio, Education and Program Manager

7411 What Young People and Parents Need to Know about Scoliosis
American Physical Therapy Association
5 Cabot Place
Stoughton, MA 02072

781-341-6333
800-673-6922
Fax: 781-341-8333
NSF@scoliosis.org
www.scoliosis.org

A physical therapist's perspective.

Newsletters

7412 Backtalk
Scoliosis Association
5 Cabot Place
Stoughton, MA 02072-1705

781-341-6333
800-673-6922
Fax: 781-341-8333
NSF@scoliosis.org
www.scoliosis.org

Information for families, patients and health care professionals.

Pamphlets

7413 1 in Every 10 Persons Has Scoliosis
National Scoliosis Foundation
5 Cabot Place
Stoughton, MA 02072

781-341-6333
800-673-6922
Fax: 781-341-8333
NSF@scoliosis.org
www.scoliosis.org

Explains what scoliosis is and illustrates how to screen for it. It also contains facts about the Foundation.
Joseph P O'Brien, President/CEO

7414 Adolescent Idiopathic Scoliosis: Prevelance, Natural History, Treatments
National Scoliosis Foundation
5 Cabot Place
Stoughton, MA 02072

781-341-6333
800-673-6922
Fax: 781-341-8333
NSF@scoliosis.org
www.scoliosis.org

Expert overview of a condition that affects many young people.
Joseph P O'Brien, President/CEO

7415 Boston Bracing System for Idiopathic Scoliosis
National Scoliosis Foundation
5 Cabot Place
Stoughton, MA 02072

781-341-6333
800-673-6922
Fax: 781-341-8333
NSF@scoliosis.org
www.scoliosis.org

Explaination of an available option.
Joseph P O'Brien, President/CEO

7416 Brace & Her Brace is No Handicap
National Scoliosis Foundation
5 Cabot Place
Stoughton, MA 02072

781-341-6333
800-673-6922
Fax: 781-341-8333
NSF@scoliosis.org
www.scoliosis.org

Contains two illustrated short stories, each about a teenage girl coping successfully with scoliosis.
Joseph P O'Brien, President/CEO

7417 Getting a Second Opinion
National Scoliosis Foundation
5 Cabot Place
Stoughton, MA 02072

781-341-6333
800-673-6922
Fax: 781-341-8333
NSF@scoliosis.org
www.scoliosis.org

Reprinted from Health Tips.
Joseph P O'Brien, President/CEO

7418 Going Home
University Hospital Spine Center
2074 Abington Road
Cleveland, OH 44106

216-844-1616

Instructions for pediatric and adult patients who have had a spinal fusion.

7419 Medical Update Column
National Scoliosis Foundation
5 Cabot Place
Stoughton, MA 02072

781-341-6333
800-673-6922
Fax: 781-341-8333
NSF@scoliosis.org
www.scoliosis.org

Reprints from past issues of the Spinal Connections Medical Update Column available on various topics.
Joseph P O'Brien, President/CEO

7420 NSF Packets
National Scoliosis Foundation
5 Cabot Place
Stoughton, MA 02072

781-341-6333
800-673-6922
Fax: 781-341-8333
NSF@scoliosis.org
www.scoliosis.org

Packet contains information for parents and young people, adults, and healthcare professionals.
Joseph P O'Brien, President/CEO

7421 Patient with Scoliosis
Educational Services, Division of AJV Company
555 East Wells Street
Milwaukee, WI 53202-2925

414-289-9107
Fax: 414-276-3349
info@srs.org
www.srs.org

A reprint from the American Journal of nursin.
Ashtin Neuschaefer, Administrative Manager
Lily Atonio, Education and Program Manager

7422 Postural Screening Program
National Scoliosis Foundation
5 Cabot Place
Stoughton, MA 02072

781-341-6333
800-673-6922
Fax: 781-341-8333
NSF@scoliosis.org
www.scoliosis.org

Guidelines for physicians and school nurses.
Joseph P O'Brien, President/CEO

7423 Questions Most Often Asked the NSF
National Scoliosis Foundation
5 Cabot Place
Stoughton, MA 02072

781-341-6333
800-673-6922
Fax: 781-341-8333
NSF@scoliosis.org
www.scoliosis.org

Answers the most frequently asked questions about scoliosis and the foundation in general.
Joseph P O'Brien, President/CEO

7424 Scoliosis
Scoliosis Research Society
555 East Wells Street
Milwaukee, WI 53202

414-289-9107
Fax: 414-276-3349
info@srs.org
www.srs.org

Brochure describing scoliosis, kyphosis, lordosis; causes, prevention, treatment and adult scoliosis.
Ashtin Neuschaefer, Administrative Manager
Lily Atonio, Education and Program Manager

7425 Scoliosis Patient Becomes a Model
National Scoliosis Foundation
5 Cabot Place
Stoughton, MA 02072

781-341-6333
800-673-6922
Fax: 781-341-8333
NSF@scoliosis.org
www.scoliosis.org

Reprinted from Children's Today.
Joesph P O'Brien, President/CEO

7426 Scoliosis Road Map
University Hospital Spine Center
555 East Wells Street
Milwaukee, WI 53202

414-289-9107
Fax: 414-276-3349
info@srs.org
www.srs.org

Written for teenagers affected by this illness.
Ashtin Neuschaefer, Administrative Manager
Lily Atonio, Education and Program Manager

7427 Scoliosis Screening: The Carlsbad Program
National Scoliosis Foundation
5 Cabot Place
Stoughton, MA 02072

781-341-6333
800-673-6922
Fax: 781-341-8333
NSF@scoliosis.org
www.scoliosis.org

Exceptional scoliosis screening program.
Joseph P O'Brien, President/CEO

7428 Scoliosis Surgery, What's It All About?
University Hospital Spine Center

555 East Wells Street
Milwaukee, WI 53202

414-289-9107
Fax: 414-276-3349
info@srs.org
www.srs.org

This pamphlet answers many of the questions patients ask before having surgery.
Ashtin Neuschaefer, Administrative Manager
Lily Atonio, Education and Program Manager

7429 Scoliosis and Kyphosis
Scoliosis Research Society
555 East Wells Street
Milwaukee, WI 53202

414-289-9107
Fax: 414-276-3349
info@srs.org
www.srs.org

Information and advice from parents.
Ashtin Neuschaefer, Administrative Manager
Lily Atonio, Education and Program Manager

7430 Scoliosis, Me?
North Dallas Scoliosis Center
555 East Wells Street
Milwaukee, WI 53202-3525

414-289-9107
Fax: 414-276-3349
info@srs.org
www.srs.org

Detailed answers to questions most asked by parents and teens.
Ashtin Neuschaefer, Administrative Manager
Lily Atonio, Education and Program Manager

7431 Scoliosis... Now it Can Be Treated in Adults as Well as Children
National Scoliosis Foundation
5 Cabot Place
Stoughton, MA 02072

781-341-6333
800-673-6922
Fax: 781-341-8333
NSF@scoliosis.org
www.scoliosis.org

Reprinted from Cleveland Magazine.
Joseph P O'Brien, President/CEO

7432 Scoliosis: Handbook for Patients
National Scoliosis Foundation
5 Cabot Place
Stoughton, MA 02072

781-341-6333
800-673-6922
Fax: 781-341-8333
NSF@scoliosis.org
www.scoliosis.org

Information on detection and treatment of adolescent scoliosis, kyphosis and lordosis and adult scoliosis.
Joseph P O'Brien, President/CEO

7433 Screening Procedure Guidelines for Spinal Deformity
Scoliosis Research Society
555 East Wells Street
Milwaukee, WI 53202

414-289-9107
Fax: 414-276-3349
info@srs.org
www.srs.org

Seven page brochure covers reasons, organizations and procedures for spinal screening. Signs of spinal deformity, as seen in both standing and forward bending positions are illustrated and discussed. Includes sample screening form.
7 pages
Ashtin Neuschaefer, Administrative Manager
Lily Atonio, Education and Program Manager

7434 Spinal Deformity: Congenital Scoliosis and Kyphosis
Scoliosis Research Society
555 East Wells Street
Milwaukee, WI 53202

414-289-9107
Fax: 414-276-3349
info@srs.org
www.srs.org

Discusses signs and causes of congenital spinal deformities, associated conditions, treatment options and a glossary of terms.
12 pages
Ashtin Neuschaefer, Administrative Manager
Lily Atonio, Education and Program Manager

7435 Spinal Deformity: Scoliosis and Kyphosis
Scoliosis Research Society

555 East Wells Street
Milwaukee, WI 53202

414-289-9107
Fax: 414-276-3349
info@srs.org
www.srs.org

Twelve page brochure discusses signs and causes of scoliosis and kyphosis, indications for treatment, treatment options, commonly asked questions and a glossary of terms.
12 pages
Ashtin Neuschaefer, Administrative Manager
Lily Atonio, Education and Program Manager

7436 What Young People & Their Parents Need to Know About Scoliosis
American Physical Therapy Association
555 East Wells Street
Milwaukee, WI 53202-1488

414-289-9107
Fax: 414-276-3349
info@srs.org
www.srs.org

A physical therapists' perspective.
Ashtin Neuschaefer, Administrative Manager
Lily Atonio, Education and Program Manager

7437 What if You Need an Operation for Scoliosis?
St. Luke's Spine Center
555 East Wells Street
Milwaukee, WI 53202-3805

414-289-9107
Fax: 414-276-3349
info@srs.org
www.srs.org

Ashtin Neuschaefer, Administrative Manager
Lily Atonio, Education and Program Manager

7438 When the Spine Curves
National Scoliosis Foundation
5 Cabot Place
Stoughton, MA 02072

781-341-6333
800-673-6922
Fax: 781-341-8333
NSF@scoliosis.org
www.scoliosis.org

Joseph P O'Brien, President/CEO

7439 You and Your Brace
University Hospital Spine Center
152 South Street
Bridgewater, MA 02324

508-279-3101
smilemaker@archorthodontics.com
www.archorthodontics.com

Audio & Video

7440 Cutting Edge Medical Report
National Scoliosis Foundation
5 Cabot Place
Stoughton, MA 02072

781-341-6333
800-673-6922
Fax: 781-341-8333
NSF@scoliosis.org
www.scoliosis.org

As seen on the Discovery Channel, this video is an indepth examination of the latest developments in the diagnosis and treatment of scoliosis.
Joseph P O'Brien, President/CEO

7441 Growing Straighter and Stronger
National Scoliosis Foundation
5 Cabot Place
Stoughton, MA 02072

781-341-6333
800-673-6922
Fax: 781-341-8333
NSF@scoliosis.org
www.scoliosis.org

Fifteen-minute presentation available in VHS video format, for the pre-screening education of students in grades 5 through 7.
Videotape
Joseph P O'Brien, President/CEO

7442 Preparing Yourself for Spinal Surgery for Teenagers with Severe Scoliosis
National Scoliosis Foundation

5 Cabot Place
Stoughton, MA 02072

781-341-6333
800-673-6922
Fax: 781-341-8333
NSF@scoliosis.org
www.scoliosis.org

Patient education video helping to reduce anxiety for teenagers facing surgery by giving a sense of what to expect before, during, and after surgery.
Joseph P O'Brien, President/CEO

7443 School Screening with Dr. Robert Keller
National Scoliosis Foundation
5 Cabot Place
Stoughton, MA 02072

781-341-6333
800-673-6922
Fax: 781-341-8333
NSF@scoliosis.org
www.scoliosis.org

Training video that teaches the proper technique for doing spinal screening. Defines scoliosis and kyphosis. Four teenagers, three with curves and one without, are examined and the findings explained.
Videotape
Joseph P O'Brien, President/CEO

7444 Scoliosis: An Adult Perspective
National Scoliosis Foundation
5 Cabot Place
Stoughton, MA 02072

781-341-6333
800-673-6922
Fax: 781-341-8333
NSF@scoliosis.org
www.scoliosis.org

Dr. Blackman and five women patients provide an overall perspective of what scoliosis is, who gets it, the types of devices, myths about the disorder, and options for treatment.
Joseph P O'Brien, President/CEO

7445 Sharing Scoliosis: You're Not Alone
National Scoliosis Foundation
5 Cabot Place
Stoughton, MA 02072

781-341-6333
800-673-6922
Fax: 781-341-8333
NSF@scoliosis.org
www.scoliosis.org

The Missouri chapter of the NSF, shares their experience with scoliosis including diagnosis, wearing a brace, surgery, and recovery. It is a good source of support for patients of all ages and their families.
Joseph P O'Brien, President/CEO

7446 Spinal Screening Program
Scoliosis Research Society
555 East Wells Street
Milwaukee, WI 53202

414-289-9107
Fax: 414-276-3349
info@srs.org

Twenty minute videotape designed to instruct screeners in the spinal screening program. It demonstrates methods of screening, showing adolescents with normal and abnormal spines. Includes sample screening form.
VHS Video Tape
Ashtin Neuschaefer, Administrative Manager
Lily Atonio, Education and Program Manager

7447 Taking the Mystery Out of Spinal Deformities
Children's Hospital of LA, Div. of Orthopaedics
1300 N. Vermont
Los Angeles, CA 90027

213-660-2450
800-841-7439
RWETZEL@chla.usc.edu
www.answers4families.org

Answers questions most often asked by screeners, patients and parents.
Videotape

7448 Understanding Scoliosis
National Scoliosis Foundation
5 Cabot Place
Stoughton, MA 02072

781-341-6333
800-673-6922
Fax: 781-341-8333
NSF@scoliosis.org
www.scoliosis.org

Kaiser Permanente's educational video clearly and positively addresses the patient community. In this video four teenagers at various stages of treatment talk about their life with scoliosis.
Joseph P O'Brien, President/CEO

7449 What's This Thing Called Scoliosis
National Scoliosis Foundation
5 Cabot Place
Stoughton, MA 02072

781-341-6333
800-673-6922
Fax: 781-341-8333
NSF@scoliosis.org
www.scoliosis.org

Comprehensive overview of scoliosis using the latest computer technology. The anatomical spine and animated model work together to truly show the 3D aspects of scoliosis and the corresponding impact on the patient.
Joseph P O'Brien, President/CEO

7450 You Are Not Alone
Minnesota Spine Center
606 24th Avenue S
Minneapolis, MN 55454-1438

612-332-3843

A video presenting two women's experiences with surgery. Personal life, concerns, hospital experience, recovery and improved lifestyle are openly discussed.
Videotape

Web Sites

7451 American Association of Neurological Surgeons
www.neurosurgery.org/
Official web site of the American Association of Neurological Surgeons and Congress of Neurological Surgeons. Whether you are a patient, physician, health care professional, or member of the media, this site is your online resource for neurosurgical information.

7452 British Scoliosis Research Society
This site contains: background to the meeting, Scoliosis Research Society review papers on the aetiology of idiopathic scoliosis, a list of participants, abstracts classified by discussion group and the chairman's conclusions for each group.

7453 Healing Well
www.healingwell.com
An online health resource guide to medical news, chat, information and articles, newsgroups and message boards, books, disease-related web sites, medical directories, and more for patients, friends, and family coping with disabling diseases, disorders, or chronic illnesses.

7454 Health Finder
www.healthfinder.gov
Searchable, carefully developed web site offering information on over 1000 topics. Developed by the US Department of Health and Human Services, the site can be used in both English and Spanish.

7455 Healthlink USA
www.healthlinkusa.com
Health information concerning treatment, cures, prevention, diagnosis, risk factors, research, support groups, email lists, personal stories and much more. Updated regularly.

7456 MedicineNet
www.medicinenet.com
An online resource for consumers providing easy-to-read, authoritative medical and health information.

7457 Medscape
www.medscape.com
Medscape offers specialists, primary care physicians, and other health professionals the Web's most robust and integrated medical information and educational tools.

7458 Patients Rate Their Scoliosis Doctors
This web site is a free internet service for communicating subjective impressions of medical doctor (MD) reputations among scoliosis patients. Please use this system to learn some of the subjective impressions of the treatment other patients have received from their doctors.

7459 Scoliosis Association
www.sauk.org.uk/
The Scoliosis Association (UK) was founded in 1981. It is the only independent support group for scoliosis in the UK. SAUK aims to provide information about scoliosis, eliminate fear and stigma, and offer contacts for shared experiences.

7460 WebMD
www.webmd.com
Provides credible information, supportive communities, and in-depth reference material about health subjects. A source for original and timely health information as well as material from well known content providers.

Description

7461 Seizure Disorders

There are two types of seizure disorders: an isolated, nonrecurring attack, such as may occur with high fevers in children, head trauma, or from other diseases (metabolic abnormalities or brain tumor) and epilepsy, which is characterized by recurrent, sudden, rapid changes in brain function caused by abnormalities in the electrical activity of the brain. Roughly 3.4 million Americans suffer from epilepsy (3 million adults and 470,000 children).

Seizures can be classified as generalized, affecting the whole brain at once, or focal (partial), affecting a part of the brain. Absence (petit mal) attacks are generalized seizures in which there is only a brief (10-30 second) loss of consciousness, with eye and muscle fluttering but no loss of muscle tone. Atonic seizure, also known as "drop attacks," all the patient's muscles go limp and he or she drops to the ground. These are almost always very brief (one-two seconds), but injuries may result from falls. Myoclonic seizures, or myoclonic jerks, are very short-lasting muscle jerks that may involve few or many muscles of the body. There is no loss of consciousness during myoclonic seizures. A generalized tonic-clonic seizure (grand mal) usually lasts 1-2 minutes, and includes loss of consciousness, falling, and involuntary contractions of the arms and legs. Some patients report that they see flashing lights and experience a heightened sense of taste and smell (known as an aura) that indicates they are about to have a seizure.

In many cases there is no apparent cause of the disorder, and it is therefore called idiopathic epilepsy.

Treatment aims primarily to control seizures. Causative or precipitating factors should be eliminated. Drug treatment is the mainstay of therapy for most types of seizures. In order to limit toxic effects, an attempt is made to use only a single drug. Some patients may need to take more than one drug. In most cases, acceptable control can be achieved with medications alone. Rarely, seizures will not respond to drugs, and surgery on the brain will be recommended. In this procedure, the surgeon tries to identify and destroy the part of the brain triggering the seizures.

National Agencies & Associations

7462 Administration for Children and Families
330 C Street SW 202-205-8347
Washington, DC 20201 Fax: 202-205-9721
www.acf.hhs.gov
The Administration for Children & Families (ACF) is a division of the U.S. Department of Health & Human Services (HHS). ACF promotes the economic and social well-being of families, children, individuals and communities.
Lynn Johnson, Assistant Secretary
Jerry Milner, Acitng Commissioner, Children & Families

7463 Agency for Healthcare Research and Quality
5600 Fishers Lane 301-427-1104
Rockville, MD 20857 www.ahrq.gov

The Agency for Healthcare Research and Quality's (AHRQ) mission is to produce evidence to make health care safer, higher quality, more accessible, equitable, and affordable, and to work within the U.S. Department of Health and Human Services and with other partners to make sure that the evidence is understood and used.
Gopal Khanna, MBA, Director
Howard E. Holland, Director, Communications

7464 Agency for Toxic Substances and Disease Registry
4770 Buford Hwy NE 770-488-0736
Atlanta, GA 30341-3717 800-232-4636
Fax: 770-488-1547
TTY: 888-232-6348
jah8@cdc.gov
www.atsdr.cdc.gov
The Agency for Toxic Substances and Disease Registry (ATSDR), based in Atlanta, Georgia, is a federal public health agency of the U.S. Department of Health and Human Services. ATSDR serves the public by using the best science, taking responsive public health actions, and providing trusted health information to prevent harmful exposures and diseases related to toxic substances.
Patrick Breysse, PhD, CIH, Director
Jack Hanley, Acting Branch Chief, Central Branch

7465 American Epilepsy Society
135 S LaSalle Street 312-883-3800
Chicago, IL 60603 Fax: 312-896-5784
info@aesnet.org
www.aesnet.org
Fosters treatment of epilepsy in its biological, clinical and social phases.
Paige B. Pennell, MD, President
William D. Gaillard, MD, First Vice President

7466 Centers for Medicare & Medicaid Services
7500 Security Boulevard 410-786-3000
Baltimore, MD 21244 877-267-2323
TTY: 866-226-1819
www.cms.gov
U.S. federal agency which administers Medicare, Medicaid, and the State Children's Health Insurance Program.
Seema Verma, Administrator
Tom Corry, Director

7467 Epilepsy Foundation
8301 Professional Place W 301-459-3700
Landover, MD 20785 800-332-1000
Fax: 301-557-2684
contactus@efa.org
www.epilepsyfoundation.org
A national, charitable, non-profit volunteer agency dedicated to the welfare of people with epilepsy. Goals include the prevention and cure of seizure disorders, the alleviation of their effects and the promotion of independence.
Phil Gattone, President & CEO
Lee Gaston, CFO

7468 National Association of Epilepsy Centers
600 Maryland Avenue SW 202-524-6767
Washington, DC 20024 Fax: 202-484-1244
info@naec-epilepsy.org
www.naec-epilepsy.org
A non-profit organization supporting professional education in the treatment of epilepsy. Referrals are made to over 50 centers nationwide.
Nathan B. Fountain, MD, President
Susan T. Herman, MD, Vice President

7469 National Center for Complementary and Integrative Health
9000 Rockville Pike 888-644-6226
Bethesda, MD 20892 TTY: 866-464-3615
info@nccih.nih.gov
nccih.nih.gov
The National Center for Complementary and Integrative Health (NCCIH) is the Federal Government's lead agency for scientific research on the diverse medical and health care systems, practices, and products that are not generally considered part of conventional medicine.
Helene M. Langevin, MD, Director
David Shurtleff, Ph.D., Deputy Director

7470 National Human Genome Research Institute
Building 31, Room 4B09   301-402-0911
Bethesda, MD 20892-2152   Fax: 301-402-2218
                                                www.genome.gov
The National Human Genome Research Institute began as the National Center for Human Genome Research (NCHGR), which was established in 1989 to carry out the role of the National Institutes of Health (NIH) in the International Human Genome Project (HGP).
Eric D. Green, M.D., Ph.D., Director
Lawrence Brody, Ph.D., Director, Division of Genomics & Society

7471 National Institute for Occupational Safety and Health
Patriots Plaza 1
395 E Street SW   202-245-0625
Washington, DC 20201   800-232-4636
                                                Fax: 513-533-8347
                                                TTY: 888-232-6348
                                                www.cdc.gov/niosh
The National Institute for Occupational Safety and Health (NIOSH) is the U.S. federal agency that conducts research and makes recommendations to prevent worker injury and illness.
John Howard, MD, Director
Frank Hearl, PE, Chief of Staff

7472 National Institute of Biomedical Imaging and Bioengineering
9000 Rockville Pike   301-496-8859
Bethesda, MD 20892   info@nibib.nih.gov
                                                www.nibib.nih.gov
The mission of the National Institute of Biomedical Imaging and Bioengineering (NIBIB) is to improve health by leading the development and accelerating the application of biomedical technologies.
Bruce J. Tromberg, PhD, Director
Jill Heemskerk, PhD, Deputy Director

7473 National Institute of Environmental Health Sciences
105 T.W. Alexander Drive   919-541-3345
Research Triangle Park, NC 27709   webcenter@niehs.nih.gov
                                                www.niehs.nih.gov
The mission of the NIEHS is to discover how the environment affects people in order to promote healthier lives.
Linda S. Birnbaum, PhD, Director
Richard Woychik, PhD, Deputy Director

7474 National Institute of General Medical Sciences
45 Center Drive MSC 6200   301-496-7301
Bethesda, MD 20892-6200   info@nigms.nih.gov
                                                www.nigms.nih.gov
The National Institute of General Medical Sciences (NIGMS) supports basic research that increases understanding of biological processes and lays the foundation for advances in disease diagnosis, treatment and prevention.
Jon R. Lorsch, PhD, Director
Judith H. Greenberg, PhD, Deputy Director

7475 National Institute of Neurological Disorders and Stroke
NIH Neurological Institute   301-496-5751
Bethesda, MD 20824   800-352-9424
                                                www.ninds.nih.gov
Seeks to reduce the burden of neurological disease affecting individuals from all walks of life.
Walter J. Koroshetz, MD, Director
Amy B. Adams, Director, Office of Scientific Liaison

7476 U.S. Food and Drug Administration
10903 New Hampshire Avenue   301-796-8240
Silver Spring, MD 20993-0002   888-463-6332
                                                www.fda.gov
FDA is responsible for protecting the public health by assuring the safety, efficacy and security of human and veterinary drugs, biological products, medical devices, the nation's food supply, cosmetics, and products that emit radiation.
Norman E. Sharpless, MD, Commissioner
Denise Hinton, Chief Scientist

State Agencies & Associations

California

7477 Epilepsy Foundation of Northern California
5700 Stoneridge Mall Road   415-677-4011
Pleasanton, CA 94588-2824   800-632-3532
                                                Fax: 415-677-4190
                                                efnca@epilepsynorcal.org
                                                www.epilepsynorcal.org
Nonprofit organization serving families affected by epilepsy.
Katherine Keene, President & CEO
Mary Lee Cascino, Programme Manager

Florida

7478 Epilepsy Association of Big Bend
1215 Lee Avenue   850-222-1777
Tallahassee, FL 32303-2651   Fax: 850-222-7440
                                                epilepsyassoc@embarqmail.com
                                                www.epilepsyassoc.org
Services include: Case management, prevention education, counseling and advocacy, information and referral.

7479 Epilepsy Foundation of South Florida
7300 N Kendall Drive   305-670-4949
Miami, FL 33156-7840   Fax: 305-670-0904
A twenty five year old nonprofit community based organization dedicated to enhancing the personal and social adjustments of individuals with seizure disorders and their families.
Karen Basha Egozi, Executive Director
Ana Alfonso, Executive Administrator

7480 Epilepsy Services Foundation
4618 N Armenia Avenue   813-374-8907
Tampa, FL 33603-2706   Fax: 813-443-5546
                                                info@epilepsysf.org
                                                www.epilepsysf.org
Information on medical and supportive services for persons affected by epilepsy living in West Central Florida. Raise funds to provide medical and supportive services and to build an endowment to make a difference in the lives of generations to come.
Thomas Orth, Executive Director

7481 Epilepsy Services of North Central Florida
11200 NW 8th Avenue   352-392-6449
Gainesville, FL 32601-4946   800-330-9746
                                                Fax: 352-392-5792
                                                jlyons@college.med.ufl.edu
                                                www.floridaepilepsy.org/northcentral.htm
Jim Lyons, Program Director
Mike Dorsey, PE Coordinator

7482 Epilepsy Services of Northeast Florida
5209 San Jose Boulevard   904-731-3751
Jacksonville, FL 32207-2267
Services include: Program case management, program prevention and education, employment services, children's summer camp, counseling and advocacy, and information and referrals.

7483 Epilepsy Services of Southwest Florida
1900 Main Street   941-953-5988
Sarasota, FL 34236   Fax: 941-366-5890
Dedicated to providing case management and medical services for individuals with seizure disorders who meet eligibility criteria. Provides employment education for individuals and families affected by seizure disorders and prevention education to the com
Thomas Garrity, Executive Director

7484 Manattee County Office Epilepsy Services of Southwest Florida
1701 14th Street W   941-746-6488
Bradenton, FL 34205-7132   Fax: 941-746-8382
                                                bardentonep@aol.com
Brian Larocque, Social Worker

New Jersey

7485 Epilepsy Foundation of New Jersey
429 River View Plaza
Trenton, NJ 08611-3420
800-336-5843
800-336-5843
Fax: 609-392-5621
TTY: 800-852-7899
TDD: 800-852-7899
efnj@efnj.com
www.efnj.com

Robert L. D'Avanzo, President
Michael P. Rinaldo, Chairman of the Board

New York

7486 Epilepsy Foundation of Long Island
506 Stewart Avenue
Garden City, NY 11530-4700
516-739-7733
888-672-7154
Fax: 516-794-2180
info@epil.org
www.efli.org

Jeffrey L. Nagel, President
Henry Klosowski, Vice President

Pennsylvania

7487 Epilepsy Foundation of Western Pennsylvania
1323 Forbes Avenue
Pittsburgh, PA 15219-4725
412-261-5880
Fax: 412-261-5361
staff@efwp.org
www.efwp.org

Judith K. Painter, Executive Director
Peggy Beem, Associate Director

Virginia

7488 National Science Foundation
4201 Wilson Blvd
Arlington, VA 22230
703-292-5111
TDD: 703-292-5090
info@nsf.gov
www.nsf.gov

NSF is the only federal agency whose mission includes support for all fields of fundamental science and engineering, except for medical sciences.
France A. Cordova, Director
Joan Ferrini-Mundy, Chief Operating Officer

Washington

7489 Epilepsy Foundation of North West Washington
2311 N 45th Street
Seattle, WA 98103
206-547-4551
800-752-3509
Fax: 206-547-4557
www.epilepsyfoundation.org

Brent Herrmann, President/CEO
Alta C Hancock, Associate Director

Research Centers

7490 Baylor College of Medicine: Epilepsy Research Center
Texas Medical Center
6550 Fannin
Houston, TX 77030
713-798-4333
Fax: 713-798-7533
neurochair@bcm.edu
www.bcm.edu/neurology

The clinical program at Baylor College of Medicine for the comprehensive evaluation of those with epilepsy or those suspected of having seizures or epilepsy.
Eli Mizrahi MD, Director

7491 Duke University Center for the Advanced Study of Epilepsy
Duke Neuroscience Clinic
200 Trent Drive
Durham, NC 27710
919-668-7600
888-ASK-DUKE
www.dukehealth.org

Clinical and research unit that experiments in limbic epilepsy.
James McNama MD, Director
William B Gallentine

7492 Neurology Research Center Helen Hayes Hospital
Helen Hayes Hospital
53-55 Route 9W
W Haverstraw, NY 10993
845-786-4535
888-70R-EHAB
Fax: 845-947-3097
info@helenhayeshospital.org
www.helenhayeshospital.org

Robert Linds MD, Chief Internal medicine
Jason P Greenberg, Assistant Clinical Professor of Neurolog

7493 University of Illinois at Chicago Consultation Clinic for Epilepsy
912 S Wood Street
Chicago, IL 60612-7330
312-996-7000
800-842-1002
Fax: 312-633-3434
TTY: 312-413-0123
www.uic.edu

Paula Allen Meares, Chancellor
Lon S. Kauffman, Vice Chancellor

7494 University of Tennessee: Center for Neuroscience
875 Monroe Avenue
Memphis, TN 38163-0001
901-448-5960
Fax: 901-448-4685
www.uthsc.edu/neuroscience/

Epilepsy research and studies.
William E Armstrong, Director
Anton J Reiner, Co-Director

7495 University of Wisconsin Madison Neurophysiology Laboratory
UW Hospital and Clinics
600 Highland Avenue
Madison, WI 53792
608-263-6400
800-323-8942
Fax: 608-265-5512
www.uwhealth.org

Epilepsy research.
Thomas P Sutula, Chairman of Neurology
Paul A Rutecki, Vice Chairman of Neurology

Support Groups & Hotlines

7496 Epilepsy Foundation of America Helpline
Epilepsy Foundation of America
4351 Garden City Drive
Landover, MD 20785-7223
866-330-1000
800-332-1000
Fax: 301-459-1569
postmaster@esa.org
www.epilepsyfoundation.org

A toll free information and referral service staffed by specially trained people who will answer questions and discuss concerns about seizure disorders and their treatment. Staff will direct callers to local affiliates of the EFA and tell about a broad range of medical services that respond to the needs of people with seizure disorders.
Phil Gattone, Chief Executive Officer

7497 National Health Information Center
Office of Disease Prevention & Health Promotion
1101 Wootton Pkwy
Rockville, MD 20852
Fax: 240-453-8281
odphpinfo@hhs.gov
www.health.gov/nhic

Supports public health education by maintaining a calendar of National Health Observances; helps connect consumers and health professionals to organizations that can best answer questions and provide up-to-date contact information from reliable sources; updates on a yearly basis toll-free numbers for health information, Federal health clearinghouses and info centers.
Don Wright, MD, MPH, Director

Books

7498 Americans with Disabilities Act
Epilepsy Foundation of America
200 Constitution Ave., NW
Washington, DC 20210-2267
301-459-3700
866-487-2365
Fax: 301-577-9056
www.dol.gov

Learn how the Americans With Disabilities Act of 1990 can benifit you. Excellent comprehensive resource for individuals with seizure disorders.
46 pages Softcover
ISBN: 0-802774-65-2

7499 Bomb in the Brain: A Heroic Tale of Science, Surgery and Survival
MacMillan Publishing Company
3651 Peachtree Parkway   678-802-1922
Suwanee, GA 30024   Fax: 678-802-1922
www.paperbackswap.com
The autobiographical account of this author's struggle with epilepsy and the debilitating effects it has on health, emotions, and mental stability.
Grades 10-12
Richard Pickering, Founder & President

7500 Brainstorms: Epilepsy in Our Words
8301 Prof PlaceE   301-459-3700
Landover, MD 20785-2267   800-332-1000
                                     Fax: 301-459-1569
                                     ContactUs@efa.org
                                     www.epilepsy.com
Patients describe their experiences with seizures. Sixty-eight in-depth personal accounts of actual seizures are followed by a short section on how epilepsy affects the lives of the patients.
197 pages Paperback
ISBN: 0-802774-65-2

7501 Children with Epilepsy
Epilepsy Foundation of America
8301 Prof PlaceE   301-459-3700
Landover, MD 20785-2267   800-332-1000
                                     Fax: 301-459-1569
                                     ContactUs@efa.org
                                     www.epilepsy.com
Offers direction and support to parents of a child with epilepsy, by first educating them about epilepsy and then helping them cope with the effects this disorder will have on their child and family.
314 pages Paperback
ISBN: 0-933149-19-0

7502 Does Your Child Have Epilepsy?
8301 Prof PlaceE   301-459-3700
Landover, MD 20785-2267   800-332-1000
                                     Fax: 301-459-1569
                                     ContactUs@efa.org
                                     www.epilepsy.com
This book establishes Ten Basic Rules for parents of children with epilepsy.
201 pages Softcover

7503 Embrace the Dawn
Epilepsy Foundation of America
8301 Prof PlaceE   301-459-3700
Landover, MD 20785-2267   800-332-1000
                                     Fax: 301-459-1569
                                     ContactUs@efa.org
                                     www.epilepsy.com
A moving biographical account of one person's lifelong experience with epilepsy.
127 pages Softcover

7504 Epilepsy A to Z
8301 Prof PlaceE   301-459-3700
Landover, MD 20785-2267   800-332-1000
                                     Fax: 301-459-1569
                                     ContactUs@efa.org
                                     www.epilepsy.com
This book is designed to give health-care personnel a convenient way to find brief answers to questions about epilepsy. It includes definitions of terms, ranging all the way from abdominal epilepsy to Zonisimide.
322 pages Softcover

7505 Epilepsy Diet Treatment: An Introduction to the Ketogenic Diet
Epilepsy Foundation of America

8301 Prof PlaceE   301-459-3700
Landover, MD 20785-2267   800-332-1000
                                     Fax: 301-459-1569
                                     ContactUs@efa.org
                                     www.epilepsy.com
The only book devoted exclusively to the ketogenic diet - a rigid, mathematically calculated, doctor-supervised diet that is high in fat and low in carbohydrate and protein with strictly limited calories and liquid intake. Gives all the facts about the diet, plus quotes from parents showing what the experience is really like and 30 sample recipes.
1996 200 pages
ISBN: 0-939957-86-8

7506 Epilepsy Surgery
Raven Press
Landover, MD 20785-2601   301-459-3700
                                          800-332-1000
                                     Fax: 301-459-1569
                                     ContactUs@efa.org
                                     www.epilepsy.com
The most complete and current references on surgical treatments of the epilepsies.
880 pages
ISBN: 0-881678-21-0

7507 Epilepsy and the Family: A New Guide
Harvard University Press
79 Garden Street   800-448-2242
Cambridge, MA 02138 www.hup.harvard.edu/catalog/LECEPF.html
ISBN: 0-674258-97-5

7508 Epilepsy: 199 Answers
Demos Medical Publishing
11 West 42nd Street   212-683-0072
New York, NY 10016-8804   800-532-8663
                                     Fax: 212-683-0118
                                     support@demosmedical.com
                                     www.demosmedpub.com
Addresses the needs of everyone with epilepsy. A helpful guide to the most common questions asked by people with epilepsy and will help the reader to work with his physician and take charge of the epilepsy.
1996 152 pages
ISBN: 1-888799-09-9
Dr. Diana M Schneider, President

7509 Epilepsy: A Behavior Medicine Approach to Assessment & Treatment in Children
Hogrefe & Huber Publications
PO Box 51   716-282-1610
Lewiston, NY 14092-0051   Fax: 716-484-4200
1993 200 pages
ISBN: 0-889371-06-7

7510 Epilepsy: Current Approaches to Diagnosis and Treatment
Raven Press
919 South Univ Ave   212-930-9500
Ann Arbor, MI 48109-2601   catalog.hathitrust.org
288 pages
ISBN: 0-881676-15-2

7511 Epilepsy: I Can Live with That
Landover, MD 20785-2267   301-459-3700
                                          800-332-1000
                                     Fax: 301-577-9056
                                     ContactUs@efa.org
                                     www.epilepsy.com
The experience of epilepsy as recorded by a group of ordinary men and women living in Australia. Each story focuses on personal growth, triumph over disability and emphasizes individual courage and hope.
Softcover
ISBN: 0-802774-65-2

7512 Epilepsy: Models, Mechanisms & Concepts
Cambridge University Press

40 W 20th Street
New York, NY 10011-4211

212-924-3900
800-221-4512
Fax: 212-691-3239
customerservice@cup.org

1993 400 pages
ISBN: 0-521392-98-5
Alice Ra, Assistant Marketing Manager

7513   Epilepsy: Patient and Family Guide
O Devinsky, MD, author

FA Davis Company
1915 Arch Street
Philadelphia, PA 19103

215-568-2172
800-523-4049
Fax: 215-568-5065
info@fadavis.com
www.fadavis.com

Epilepsy expert Dr. Orrin Devinsky provides an easy-to-read guide to understanding the disease so that patients can achieve — and maintain — a higher quality of life. This book will educate recently-diagnosed patients, as well as those who have been living with epilepsy for years.
434 pages Paperback
ISBN: 0-803604-98-X
Michael Torso, Marketing Manager

7514   Equal Partners

Epilepsy Foundation of America
7, Market Street
Floriana, MT 1083-2267

356-212-0400
800-332-1000
Fax: 356-212-0397
info@equalpartners.org.mt
www.equalpartners.org.mt

This book tells the story of a young Harvard-trained doctor whose experiences with seizures, brain surgery and subsequent epilepsy turns her from physician to patient.
257 pages Hardcover
ISBN: 0-802774-65-2
Louise Pisani, President
Elena Tanti Burlo, VP

7515   Guide to Understanding and Living with Epilepsy

8301 Prof PlaceE
Landover, MD 20785-2267

301-459-3700
800-332-1000
Fax: 301-577-9056
ContactUs@efa.org
www.epilepsy.com

Easy-to-understand resource for people with epilepsy and their families. Covers a wide range of medical, social and legal issues. Topics include expanation of seizures and epilepsy; information about medication, side effects and risks; and getting the best medical care.

7516   Ketogenic Diet: A Treatment for Epilepsy

Demos Medical Publishing
11 West 42nd Street
New York, NY 10036

212-683-0072
Fax: 212-683-0118
support@demosmedical.com
www.demosmedpub.com

256 pages
ISBN: 1-888799-39-0
Dr. Diana M Schneider

7517   Living Well with Epilepsy

Epilepsy Foundation of America
8301 Prof PlaceE
Landover, MD 20785-2267

301-459-3700
800-332-1000
Fax: 301-459-1569
ContactUs@efa.org
www.epilepsy.com

Designed to help both health-care professionals and patients to understand all aspects of diagnosis and of pharmacologic and surgical management; to enable patients to participate more knowledgeably in interactions with their health care team and to help steer them toward a more normal, fulfilling life.
166 pages Softcover
ISBN: 1-888799-11-0

7518   Managing Seizure Disorder

Epilepsy Foundation of America

8301 Prof PlaceE
Landover, MD 20785-2267

301-459-3700
800-332-1000
Fax: 301-459-1569
ContactUs@efa.org
www.epilepsy.com

Provides health professionals with detailed information, on a variety of subjects, designed to help them help people with epilepsy live the kind of life they desire.
276 pages Softcover
ISBN: 0-802774-65-2

7519   Miles to Go Before I Sleep

Epilepsy Foundation of America
8301 Prof PlaceE
Landover, MD 20785-2267

301-459-3700
800-332-1000
Fax: 301-459-1569
ContactUs@efa.org
www.epilepsy.com

This book tells the story of a hijacking in which the author sustained a severe brain injury that, among other things, affected her vision, her memory, and left her with epilepsy.
230 pages Hardcover
ISBN: 0-802774-65-2

7520   Students with Seizures: A Manual for School Nurses

Epilepsy Foundation of America
8301 Prof PlaceE
Landover, MD 20785-2267

301-459-3700
800-332-1000
Fax: 301-459-1569
ContactUs@efa.org
www.epilepsy.com

A professional text with the sole purpose of creating a more accepting and understanding school environment for children with seizure disorders.
131 pages Paperback

Children's Books

7521   Dotty the Dalmatian has Epilepsy

Epilepsy Foundation of America
8301 Prof PlaceE
Landover, MD 20785-2267

301-459-3700
800-332-1000
Fax: 301-459-1569
ContactUs@efa.org
www.epilepsy.com

This is the story of Dotty the Dalmatian who discovers she has epilepsy.
16 pages Softcover
ISBN: 0-802774-65-2

7522   Epilepsy

Franklin Watts Grolier
8301 Prof PlaceE
Landover, MD 20785-0001

301-459-3700
800-332-1000
Fax: 301-459-1569
ContactUs@efa.org
www.epilepsy.com

This book explains what epilepsy is, causes of epileptic seizures, diagnosis and treatments.
96 pages Grades 7-12
ISBN: 0-531108-07-4

7523   Lee the Rabbit with Epilepsy

8301 Prof PlaceE
Landover, MD 20785-2267

301-459-3700
800-332-1000
Fax: 301-459-1569
ContactUs@efa.org
www.epilepsy.com

Written for children ages 3-6, this illustrated picture book follows the adventures of a small rabbit who has seizures during a fishing trip with her Grandpa.
23 pages Hardcover

7524   Season of Secrets

Little, Brown & Company
3 Center Plz
Boston, MA 02108

617-227-0730
800-759-0190
Fax: 800-286-9471

Grades 4-6

Newsletters

7525 Epilepsia: Journal of the International League Against Epilepsy
Blackwell Publishing, Inc.
Commerce Place   201-748-6000
Hoboken, NJ 07030   800-862-6657
                                               Fax: 201-748-6088
                                                 info@wiley.com
                                        www.blackwellpublishing.com
The leading international journal on the epilepsies for more than
30 years, Epilepsia provides comprehensive coverage of current
clinical and research results.

7526 Epilepsy Services Foundation Newsletter
4618 N Armenia Avenue   813-870-3414
Tampa, FL 33603-2706   Fax: 813-870-1321
                                        eswcf@epilepsyservices.com
                                         www.epilepsyservices.com
Information on medical and supportive services for persons affected by epilepsy living in West Central Florida. Raise funds to
provide medical and supportive services to build and endowment
to make a difference in the lives of generations to come.
2 pages 2-3 x/year
Thomas Orth, Executive Director

Pamphlets

7527 Child with Epilepsy at Camp
Epilepsy Foundation of America
8301 Prof PlaceE   301-459-3700
Landover, MD 20785-2267   800-332-1000
                                               Fax: 301-459-1569
                                                ContactUs@efa.org
                                                 www.epilepsy.com
Helps to explain why the child with epilepsy should be included in
the camping experience.
14 pages Pamphlet

7528 Children and Seizures: Information for Babysitters
Epilepsy Foundation of America
8301 Prof PlaceE   301-459-3700
Landover, MD 20785-2267   800-332-1000
                                               Fax: 301-459-1569
                                                ContactUs@efa.org
                                                 www.epilepsy.com
Explains seizures, routine and special care, emergency aid and
first aid to babysitters. Also offers a graph to write down important
information about the child with seizure disorders for a quick
reference.

7529 Epilepsy Medicines and Dental Care
Epilepsy Foundation of America
8301 Prof PlaceE   301-459-3700
Landover, MD 20785-2267   800-332-1000
                                               Fax: 301-459-1569
                                                ContactUs@efa.org
                                                 www.epilepsy.com
Explains dental care and includes instructions for brushing and
flossing.

7530 Epilepsy: Legal Rights, Legal Issues
Epilepsy Foundation of America
8301 Prof PlaceE   301-459-3700
Landover, MD 20785-2267   800-332-1000
                                               Fax: 301-459-1569
                                                ContactUs@efa.org
                                                 www.epilepsy.com
Offers persons diagnosed with epilepsy information on their legal
rights in employment, education, insurance and general disability
benefits.
9 pages

7531 Epilepsy: Part of Your Life Series
Epilepsy Foundation of America
8301 Prof PlaceE   301-459-3700
Landover, MD 20785-2267   800-332-1000
                                               Fax: 301-459-1569
                                                ContactUs@efa.org
                                                 www.epilepsy.com

Provides information for staying healthy, describes various tests
and diagnostic procedures, includes information for parents of
children with epilepsy and provides general answers to questions
about epilepsy.
Series of 4

7532 Epilepsy: You and Your Child, a Guide for Parents
Epilepsy Foundation of America
8301 Prof PlaceE   301-459-3700
Landover, MD 20785-2267   800-332-1000
                                               Fax: 301-459-1569
                                                ContactUs@efa.org
                                                 www.epilepsy.com
This instructional booklet offers information on emotional aspects
of epilepsy, how to handle seizures, medication, diet and nutrition,
and offers referral organizations for parents.

7533 Epilepsy: You and Your Treatment
Epilepsy Foundation of America
8301 Prof PlaceE   301-459-3700
Landover, MD 20785-2267   800-332-1000
                                               Fax: 301-459-1569
                                                ContactUs@efa.org
                                                 www.epilepsy.com
Reviews medical tests and diagnostic procedures used by physi-
cians in diagnosing epilepsy.

7534 Facts About Epilepsy
Epilepsy Foundation of America
8301 Prof PlaceE   301-459-3700
Landover, MD 20785-2267   800-332-1000
                                               Fax: 301-459-1569
                                                ContactUs@efa.org
                                                 www.epilepsy.com
Designed for use by physicians and other health professionals with
an interest in or who deal with the problems of people with epilepsy.
16 pages Softcover

7535 Finding Out About Seizures: A Guide to Medical Tests
Epilepsy Foundation of America
8301 Prof PlaceE   301-459-3700
Landover, MD 20785-2267   800-332-1000
                                               Fax: 301-459-1569
                                                ContactUs@efa.org
                                                 www.epilepsy.com
Introduces adults and children with epilepsy to the types of tests
they may have to undergo.

7536 Kits for Adults with Epilepsy
Epilepsy Foundation of America
8301 Prof PlaceE   301-459-3700
Landover, MD 20785-2267   800-332-1000
                                               Fax: 301-459-1569
                                                ContactUs@efa.org
                                                 www.epilepsy.com
A variety of informative pamphlets for persons with epilepsy or
seizure disorders.

7537 Management by Common Sense
Epilepsy Foundation of America
8301 Prof PlaceE   301-459-3700
Landover, MD 20785-2267   800-332-1000
                                               Fax: 301-459-1569
                                                ContactUs@efa.org
                                                 www.epilepsy.com
Promotes the employability of people with seizure disorders. Provides employers with information about epilepsy, customer/client
reactions, workers' compensation issues, side effects of medication and other information relevant to employing a person with
epilepsy.
46 pages Paperback
ISBN: 0-802774-65-2

7538 Me and My World Packet for Children
Epilepsy Foundation of America
8301 Prof PlaceE   301-459-3700
Landover, MD 20785-2267   800-332-1000
                                               Fax: 301-459-1569
                                                ContactUs@efa.org
                                                 www.epilepsy.com

Collection of pamphlets designed for children with epilepsy.

7539 Medicines for Epilepsy
Epilepsy Foundation of America
8301 Prof PlaceE   301-459-3700
Landover, MD 20785-2267   800-332-1000
                                    Fax: 301-459-1569
                                    ContactUs@efa.org
                                    www.epilepsy.com
Offers information on medication and treatments, generic drugs, side effects, drug abuse and more. Contains a color chart with picyures of the most common medications for epilepsy.

7540 Mom I Have a Staring Problem
Epilepsy Foundation of America
8301 Prof PlaceE   301-459-3700
Landover, MD 20785-2267   800-332-1000
                                    Fax: 301-459-1569
                                    ContactUs@efa.org
                                    www.epilepsy.com
Tiffany, a seven-year-old, describes her experience with petit mal seizures; her feelings, wishes and fears. Written to help adults recognize a hidden problem that could be occuring with a child who has learning problems.
24 pages Softcover
ISBN: 0-802774-65-2

7541 My Brother Matthew
Woodbine House
8301 Prof PlaceE   301-459-3700
Landover, MD 20785-2267   800-332-1000
                                    Fax: 301-459-1569
                                    ContactUs@efa.org
                                    www.epilepsy.com
A picture and text book for children who have a brother or sister with developmental delay.
25 pages Harcoverr
ISBN: 0-802774-65-2

7542 My Friend Emily
Epilepsy Foundation of America
8301 Prof PlaceE   301-459-3700
Landover, MD 20785-2267   800-332-1000
                                    Fax: 301-459-1569
                                    ContactUs@efa.org
                                    www.epilepsy.com
A story about Emily and her best friend Katy. Emily, a self confident child who enjoys life, shows that kids with epilepsy are just like other kids.
35 pages Softcover
ISBN: 0-802774-65-2

7543 Patient's Guide to Everyday Life
Epilepsy Foundation of America
8301 Prof PlaceE   301-459-3700
Landover, MD 20785-2267   800-332-1000
                                    Fax: 301-459-1569
                                    ContactUs@efa.org
                                    www.epilepsy.com
Provides information for the newly diagnosed individual with epilepsy.

7544 Preventing Epilepsy
Epilepsy Foundation of America
8301 Prof PlaceE   301-459-3700
Landover, MD 20785-2267   800-332-1000
                                    Fax: 301-459-1569
                                    ContactUs@efa.org
                                    www.epilepsy.com
Examines some known causes of seizures and suggests precautionary measures which may prevent the occurrence of epilepsy.
16 pages

7545 Recognizing the Signs of Childhood Seizures
Epilepsy Foundation of America
8301 Prof PlaceE   301-459-3700
Landover, MD 20785-2267   800-332-1000
                                    Fax: 301-459-1569
                                    ContactUs@efa.org
                                    www.epilepsy.com
Explains what seizures are and what to look for in your child.

7546 Seizure Recognition and First Aid
Epilepsy Foundation of America
8301 Prof PlaceE   301-459-3700
Landover, MD 20785-2267   800-332-1000
                                    Fax: 301-459-1569
                                    ContactUs@efa.org
                                    www.epilepsy.com
Helps you recognize a seizure when it happens and give basic first aid.

7547 Surgery for Epilepsy
Epilepsy Foundation of America
8301 Prof PlaceE   301-459-3700
Landover, MD 20785-2267   800-332-1000
                                    Fax: 301-459-1569
                                    ContactUs@efa.org
                                    www.epilepsy.com
Describes current surgical treatment and the testing that precedes it.
12 pages

7548 Talking to Your Doctor About Seizure Disorders
Epilepsy Foundation of America
8301 Prof PlaceE   301-459-3700
Landover, MD 20785-2267   800-332-1000
                                    Fax: 301-459-1569
                                    ContactUs@efa.org
                                    www.epilepsy.com
Designed to help the patient talk with medical personnel about treatment of epilepsy.
Pamphlet

7549 Teacher's Role, A Guide for School Personnel
Epilepsy Foundation of America
8301 Prof PlaceE   301-459-3700
Landover, MD 20785-2267   800-332-1000
                                    Fax: 301-459-1569
                                    ContactUs@efa.org
                                    www.epilepsy.com
Provides tips on recognizing seizures and handling a seizure in the classroom.
14 pages

Audio & Video

7550 Comprehensive Clinical Management of the Epilepsies
Epilepsy Foundation of America
8301 Prof PlaceE   301-459-3700
Landover, MD 20785-2267   800-332-1000
                                    Fax: 301-459-1569
                                    ContactUs@efa.org
                                    www.epilepsy.com
Excellent reference on the treatment of epilepsy.
17 minutes

7551 How to Recognize and Classify Seizures
Epilepsy Foundation of America
8301 Prof PlaceE   301-459-3700
Landover, MD 20785-2267   800-332-1000
                                    Fax: 301-459-1569
                                    ContactUs@efa.org
                                    www.epilepsy.com
Discusses the classification of seizures and epileptic syndromes.
25 minutes

7552 Just Like You and Me
TASH
2013 H Street NW   202-540-9020
Washington, DC 20006   Fax: 202-637-0138
A video/print package on successful living with epilepsy.
Ralph Edwards, President
Jean Trainor, Vice President

7553 Meeting the Challenge: Employment Issues and Epilepsy
Epilepsy Foundation of America

8301 Prof PlaceE   301-459-3700
Landover, MD 20785-2267   800-332-1000
Fax: 301-459-1569
ContactUs@efa.org
www.epilepsy.com

This video answers the fquestions most often asked by emloyers. It covers issues such as driving, absenteeism, productivity, accidents and first aid, and emphasized that most people with epilepsy can be gainfully employed.
9 minutes

7554 Rest of the Family
Epilepsy Foundation of America
8301 Prof PlaceE   301-459-3700
Landover, MD 20785-2267   800-332-1000
Fax: 301-459-1569
ContactUs@efa.org
www.epilepsy.com

Presents the feelings and concerns of other family members including siblings, of children with epilepsy.
Video cassette

7555 Seizure First Aid
Epilepsy Foundation of America
8301 Prof PlaceE   301-459-3700
Landover, MD 20785-2267   800-332-1000
Fax: 301-459-1569
ContactUs@efa.org
www.epilepsy.com

This video combines footage of real seizures with reenactments to demonstrate proper first aid procedures. In addition, people with epilepsy talk about how they feel when they have a seizure, discuss how they would like friends, family and the general public to react when a seizure occurs.
10 minutes

7556 Understanding Seizure Disorders
Epilepsy Foundation of America
8301 Prof PlaceE   301-459-3700
Landover, MD 20785-2267   800-332-1000
Fax: 301-459-1569
ContactUs@efa.org
www.epilepsy.com

Provides an explanation of seizure disorders in everyday language and dispels many misconceptions about epilepsy with medically accurate information.
Video cassette

7557 Voices from the Workplace
Epilepsy Foundation of America
8301 Prof PlaceE   301-459-3700
Landover, MD 20785   800-332-1000
Fax: 301-459-1569
ContactUs@efa.org
www.epilepsy.com

Inspirational tape to help people with epilepsy cope with employment challenges. Individuals with epilepsy describe personal and social challenges in the workplace. They explain how they cope with their seizures and the reactions of co-workers and the public.

Web Sites

7558 American Epilepsy Society
www.aesnet.org
The Society seeks to promote interdisciplinary communications, scientific investigation and exchange of clinical information about epilepsy.

7559 Epilepsy Foundation of America
www.efa.org
Information on the prevention and cure of seizure disorders, the alleviation of their effects, and the promotion of independence and optimal quality of life for people who have these disorders.

7560 Healing Well
www.healingwell.com
An online health resource guide to medical news, chat, information and articles, newsgroups and message boards, books, disease-related web sites, medical directories, and more for patients, friends, and family coping with disabling diseases, disorders, or chronic illnesses.

7561 Health Finder
www.healthfinder.gov
Searchable, carefully developed web site offering information on over 1000 topics. Developed by the US Department of Health and Human Services, the site can be used in both English and Spanish.

7562 Healthlink USA
www.healthlinkusa.com
Health information concerning treatment, cures, prevention, diagnosis, risk factors, research, support groups, email lists, personal stories and much more. Updated regularly.

7563 MedicineNet
www.medicinenet.com
An online resource for consumers providing easy-to-read, authoritative medical and health information.

7564 Medscape
www.medscape.com
Medscape offers specialists, primary care physicians, and other health professionals the Web's most robust and integrated medical information and educational tools.

7565 Neurology Channel
www.healthcommunities.com
Find clearly explained, medically accurate information regarding conditions, including an overview, symptoms, causes, diagnostic procedures and treatment options. On this site it is possible to ask questions and get information from a neurologist and connect to people who have similar health interests.

7566 WebMD
www.webmd.com
Provides credible information, supportive communities, and in-depth reference material about health subjects. A source for original and timely health information as well as material from well known content providers.

Description

7567 **Sexually Transmitted Diseases**

Sexually transmitted diseases, STDs, are among the most common infectious diseases in the U.S. More than 30 different STDs have been identified, and roughly 13 million persons are affected. Fortunately, most STDs are curable with prompt treatment, and do not become chronic. These include bacterial vaginosis, gonorrhea, syphilis, trichomoniasis and chlamydia. People who suffer from these diseases over long periods almost always do so because of re-infection rather than treatment failure. HIV and hepatitis B are commonly transmitted through sexual intercourse; see also *AIDS* and *Hepatitis*.

Fortunately, behavioral changes in sexual practices can drastically reduce the risk of STDs. Abstinence from intercourse or having a long-term mutually faithful monogamous relationship with an uninfected partner give essentially complete protection. Risk rises with multiple partners, unprotected intercourse between males, anonymous sex and contact with high-risk individuals, such as prostitutes. Barrier methods, notably condoms, give significant but not complete protection.

Until recently, no vaccines were available for any common STD except hepatitis B. However, researchers developed a vaccine for human papilloma virus (HPV) that is, amazingly, 100 percent effective. The vaccine is such a critical discovery because one specific type of HPV causes cervical cancer. Common STDs which may become chronic despite treatment are described below.

Genital herpes is a virus of the herpes family characterized by blisters (vesicles) in the genital area. The appearance of the blisters is often preceded by low-grade fever and by burning pain in the affected area. The first episode is often the most painful. Specific anti-viral therapies (valacyclovir, acyclovir, and famciclovir) will shorten the duration and intensity of an attack. Herpes infections are self-limited but recurrent because the virus chronically infects nerves that radiate from the spinal column. Under certain conditions, such as febrile illness and physical or emotional stress, the virus reactivates and causes another outbreak. People with frequent recurrences can lower the risk of repeat attacks by taking a low dose of the anti-viral medication every day.

Genital warts are caused by the human papilloma virus (HPV.) There are roughly 750,000 new cases each year in the United States. The warts may appear anywhere in the genital and rectal area, making transmission difficult to prevent with a condom. Genital warts in the male, unless quite large, are often just a cosmetic nuisance, although a wart inside the urinary passage may cause discomfort. Women with genital warts not only need to have the warts removed, but to be observed for pre-cancerous changes in the cervix. Warts are generally destroyed by application of chemicals, but doctors have also used laser beams, freezing and electrical currents to destroy them. Recurrence after treatment is common, even in the absence of re-infection.

Pelvic inflammatory disease (PID) is not always sexually transmitted, but it is included here because chlamydia and gonorrhea, which are sexually transmitted, are commonly the cause of PID. In this condition, the sensitive pelvic reproductive organs are attacked, leading to fever and lower abdominal pain and occasionally collection of pus in a pelvic abscess. Even after the attack is treated with high doses of antibiotics, residual scarring may lead to chronic pelvic pain, pain with intercourse, infertility and ectopic pregnancy, in which the fertilized egg implants in other pelvic structures outside the uterus. Prompt recognition and vigorous treatment of the acute attack of PID are important.

National Agencies & Associations

7568 **American Sexual Health Association (ASHA)**
PO Box 13827   919-361-8400
Research Triangle Park, NC 27709   info@ashasexualhealth.org
                                                       www.ashasexualhealth.org
Provides resources to local communities to improve STD control programs through citizen action.
Lynn Barclay, President & CEO
Deborah Arrindell, Vice President

7569 **Centers for Disease Control & Prevention: Division of Adolescent & School Health**
1600 Clifton Road   800-232-4636
Atlanta, GA 30329-4027   TTY: 888-232-6348
                                          www.cdc.gov/HealthyYouth
CDC promotes the health and well-being of children and adolescents to enable them to become healthy and productive adults.

7570 **National Institute of Allergy and Infectious Diseases**
NIAID Office of Communications & Govt Relations
5601 Fishers Lane   301-496-5717
Bethesda, MD 20892-9806   866-284-4107
                                          Fax: 301-402-3573
                                          TDD: 800-877-8339
                                          ocpostoffice@niaid.nih.gov
                                          www.niaid.nih.gov
Conducts and supports research on allergies; focused on understanding what happens to the body during the allergic process. Educates patients and health care workers in controlling allergic disease; offers various research centers that conduct and evaluate educational programs focused on methods to control allergic diseases.
Anthony S. Fauci, MD, Director

Research Centers

7571 Herpes Resource Center
PO Box 13827
Research Triangle Park, NC 27709
919-361-8400
800-227-8922
Fax: 919-361-8425
www.ashastd.org
Offers information and referrals for persons affected by herpes and other sexually transmitted disease prevention.
Lynn Barclay, President and Chief Executive Officer
Deborah Arrindell, Vice President Health Policy

7572 International Union Against Venereal Diseases
New York Hospital - Cornell Medical Center
1153 York Avenue
New York, NY 10021
212-746-1200
Fax: 212-746-1202
Encourages campaigns medical and social against venereal disease.
Lewis Drusin MD, Director

7573 University of Chicago Committee on Virology
Marjorie B Kovler Viral Oncology Laboratories
910 E 58th Street
Chicago, IL 60637
773-702-1620
Fax: 773-702-1631
mgcb.bsd.uchicago.edu
Focuses research into the area of sexually transmitted disease.
Bernard Roizman, Chairman
Olaf Schneewind, Professor and Chairman

Support Groups & Hotlines

7574 National Health Information Center
Office of Disease Prevention & Health Promotion
1101 Wootton Pkwy
Rockville, MD 20852
Fax: 240-453-8281
odphpinfo@hhs.gov
www.health.gov/nhic
Supports public health education by maintaining a calendar of National Health Observances; helps connect consumers and health professionals to organizations that can best answer questions and provide up-to-date contact information from reliable sources; updates on a yearly basis toll-free numbers for health information, Federal health clearinghouses and info centers.
Don Wright, MD, MPH, Director

Books

7575 Herpes and Papilloma Viruses Volume I & II
Raven Press
1600 Clifton Road
Atlanta, GA 30329-2601
212-930-9500
800-232-4636
www.cdc.gov
382 pages
ISBN: 0-881671-95-9

7576 Sexually Transmitted Diseases
Raven Press
1600 Clifton Road
Atlanta, GA 30329-2601
212-930-9500
800-232-4636
www.cdc.gov
Focuses on the clinically important subject of the immune response to sexually transmitted diseases.
350 pages
ISBN: 0-881678-82-1

7577 Understanding Helps
University Press of Mississippi
3825 Ridgewood Road
Jackson, MS 39211-6492
601-432-6205
800-737-7788
Fax: 601-432-6217
press@ihl.state.ms.us
www.upress.state.ms.us
This book is for people who wish to learn about herpes simplex viruses, two remarkably complex microbes capable of causing a wide variety of infections. These include genital herpes, a very common chronic sexually transmitted disease.
120 pages Hardcover
ISBN: 1-578060-40-0
Kathy Burgess, Advertising Manager/Marketing Assistant

7578 Understanding Herpes: Revised Second Edition
Lawrence R Stanberry, MD; PhD, author
University Press of Mississippi
3825 Ridgewood Road
Jackson, MS 39211-6492
601-432-6205
Fax: 601-432-6217
kburgess@ihl.state.ms.us
www.upress.state.ms.us
A concise overview of advances and resources.
2006 144 pages Paperback
ISBN: 1-578068-68-1
Kathy Burgess, Advertising/Marketing Services Manager

7579 Women at Risk
Bristol Publishing
2790 44th St. SW
Wyoming, MI 49519-0811
415-895-4461
Fax: 415-895-4459
https://warinternational.org
1993 159 pages
ISBN: 0-917851-62-5

Children's Books

7580 Teen Guide to Safe Sex
Franklin Watts Grolier
90 Old Sherman Tpke
Danbury, CT 06816-0001
203-797-3500
800-621-1115
Fax: 203-797-3197
www.grolier.com
A basic book about sexually transmitted diseases. Describes what they are, what causes them, how to recognize them and how teenagers can protect against them.
64 pages Grades 9-12
ISBN: 0-531105-92-0

Newsletters

7581 Sexually Transmitted Diseases: Journal
Julius Scachter, PhD, author
Lippincott Wiliiams & Wilkins
2700 Lake CookRoad
Riverwoods, IL 60015-1600
847-580-5000
800-638-3030
Fax: 301-223-2400
orders@lww.com
www.lww.com
This timely, scholarly journal publishes original, peer-reviewed articles on clinical, laboratory, immunologic, epidemiologic, sociologic, and historical topics pertaining to sexually transmitted diseases and related fields.
Monthly

7582 Step Perspective
Seattle Treatment Education Project
127 Broadway E
Seattle, WA 98102-5711
206-329-4857
800-869-7837
www.quick-step.in
A publication of the Seattle Treatment Education Project. Published three times a year.
Michael Auch, Executive Director

Pamphlets

7583 AIDS...What We Need To Know Pamphlet
March of Dimes
1275 Mamaroneck Avenue
White Plains, NY 10605
914-997-4488
Fax: 212-254-3518
NY639@marchofdimes.com
www.marchofdimes.com

Discusses the facts about HIV Æinfection and AIDS and how you can reduce your risk.
Pkg of 50
ISBN: 0-923500- -

7584 Chlamydial Infection
National Institute of Allergy/Infectious Diseases
Nat Institutes of Health   301-496-5717
Bethesda, MD 20892-0001   www.nih.gov
Offers information on diagnosis, treatment, effects, prevention and research.

7585 Genital Herpes
National Institute of Allergy/Infectious Diseases
Nat Institutes of Health   301-496-5717
Bethesda, MD 20892-0001   www.nih.gov
Offers information on symptoms, causes, diagnosis and reccurences.

7586 Genital Herpes Fact Sheet
March of Dimes
1275 Mamaroneck Avenue   914-997-4488
White Plains, NY 10605   Fax: 212-254-3518
NY639@marchofdimes.com
www.marchofdimes.com
Fact Sheets: one to two page review written for the general public.

7587 Gonorrhea
National Institute of Allergy/Infectious Diseases
Nat Institutes of Health   301-496-5717
Bethesda, MD 20892-0001   www.nih.gov
Offers information on the symptoms, diagnosis, treatment, complications, prevention and research.

7588 Human Papillomavirus and Genital Warts
National Institute of Allergy/Infectious Diseases
Nat Institutes of Health   301-496-5717
Bethesda, MD 20892-0001   www.nih.gov
Offers information on diagnosis, treatment, complications and prevention of the diseases.

7589 Introduction to Sexually Transmitted Diseases
National Institute of Allergy/Infectious Diseases
Nat Institutes of Health   301-496-5717
Bethesda, MD 20892-0001   www.nih.gov
Offers information on STDs, various types and symptoms, research, and referral services.

7590 Other Important STD's
National Institute of Allergy/Infectious Diseases
Nat Institutes of Health   301-496-5717
Bethesda, MD 20892-0001   www.nih.gov
Lists over ten of the most common sexually transmitted diseases. Offers information on what they are, the causes and treatments, research being done in these areas and referral numbers of where to call for more information on the diseases.

7591 Pelvic Inflammatory Disease
National Institute of Allergy/Infectious Diseases
Nat Institutes of Health   301-496-5717
Bethesda, MD 20892-0001   www.nih.gov
Offers information on the causes, symptoms, risk factors, diagnosis, treatment, and prevention.

7592 Syphilis
National Institute of Allergy/Infectious Diseases

Nat Institutes of Health   301-496-5717
Bethesda, MD 20892-0001   www.nih.gov
Offers information on what syphilis is, the symptoms, complications, diagnosis, prevention and treatment methods available.

7593 Vaginal Infections
National Institute of Allergy/Infectious Diseases
Nat Institutes of Health   301-496-5717
Bethesda, MD 20892-0001   www.nih.gov
Lists three specific types of vaginitis, with information on their symptoms, prevention, complications and treatments.

Web Sites

7594 American Social Health Association
www.ashasexualhealth.org
The American Sexual Health Association promotes the sexual health of individuals, families and communities by advocating sound policies and practices and educating the public, professionals and policy makers, in order to foster healthy sexual behaviors and relationships and prevent adverse health outcomes.

7595 Centers for Disease Control
www.cdc.gov
Offers reprints, reports, public awareness and educational materials and research on sexually transmitted diseases.

7596 Healing Well
www.healingwell.com
An online health resource guide to medical news, chat, information and articles, newsgroups and message boards, books, disease-related web sites, medical directories, and more for patients, friends, and family coping with disabling diseases, disorders, or chronic illnesses.

7597 Health Finder
www.healthfinder.gov
Searchable, carefully developed web site offering information on over 1000 topics. Developed by the US Department of Health and Human Services, the site can be used in both English and Spanish.

7598 Healthlink USA
www.healthlinkusa.com
Health information concerning treatment, cures, prevention, diagnosis, risk factors, research, support groups, email lists, personal stories and much more. Updated regularly.

7599 MedicineNet
www.medicinenet.com
An online resource for consumers providing easy-to-read, authoritative medical and health information.

7600 Medscape
www.medscape.com
Medscape offers specialists, primary care physicians, and other health professionals the Web's most robust and integrated medical information and educational tools.

7601 WebMD
www.webmd.com
Provides credible information, supportive communities, and in-depth reference material about health subjects. A source for original and timely health information as well as material from well known content providers.

Description

7602 **Sickle Cell Disease**

Sickle cell disease (also called sickle cell anemia) is an inherited defect of hemoglobin, the oxygen-carrying element in the blood. Under some circumstances, the normally disc-shaped red blood cell takes on a crescent or sickle shape. It then becomes lodged in small capillaries and prevents normal oxygen flow to the tissues. This oxygen deprivation can cause sickle cell crises, with symptoms of severe pain in the back, joints, hands, and feet, and may even include neurologic changes. Severe abdominal pain and vomiting may also occur.

Sickle cell anemia occurs almost exclusively in African Americans. There are approximately 55,000 people in the United States with this condition. These children have sickle cell trait, occurring when one receives a copy of the sickle cell gene from only one parent. Only if a child receives a copy of the defective gene from both parents will the full-blown disease develop.

Therapy for sickle cell disease is aimed at preventing and treating infections, maintaining an adequate diet and fluid intake, and managing acute attacks with painkillers, oxygen, antibiotics and blood transfusion. Hydroxyurea has been shown to reduce the number of attacks by 50 percent as well as the need for transfusion. In the past, death typically occurred because of overwhelming infection or from organ destruction brought about by multiple sickling crises. Modern therapy has improved life expectancy dramatically, but some level of disability is common. Genetic counseling is important for the patient and all family members. Bone marrow transplants can cure sickle cell disease and gene therapy trials are presently in progress.

National Agencies & Associations

7603 **American Chronic Pain Association**
PO Box 850   800-533-3231
Rocklin, CA 95677   ACPA@theacpa.org
                                                                    www.theacpa.org
The ACPA facilitates peer support and education for individuals with chronic pain in its many forms, in order to increase quality of life. Also raises awareness among the healthcare community, and with policy makers.
Penney Cowan, Founder & CEO
Daniel Galia, Director, Global Support

7604 **American Sickle Cell Anemia Association**
10900 Carnegie Avenue   216-229-8600
Cleveland, OH 44106   Fax: 216-229-4500
                                                            irabragg@ascaa.org
                                                                  www.ascaa.org
Provides education, testing, counseling and supportive services forindividuals with sickle cell anemia and its hemoglobinopathy variants.
Ira Bragg-Grant, Executive Director
Gilberto Peña, Coordinator

7605 **Sickle Cell Association of Ontario**
1171 McCowan Road   416-789-2855
Toronto, Ontario, M1S-5G8   info@sicklecellontario.ca
                                                          www.sicklecellontario.ca

A voluntary, non-profit, charitable organization providing support and resources for individuals and families affected by Sickle Cell Disease.
Lillie Johnson, Founder
Ulysse Guerrier, Chair

7606 **Sickle Cell Disease Association of America**
3700 Koppers Street   410-528-1555
Baltimore, MD 21227   800-421-8453
                                                            Fax: 410-528-1495
                                                 admin@sicklecelldisease.org
                                                     www.sicklecelldisease.org
Advocates for individuals with sickle cell conditions and promotes public awareness while searching for a cure.
David N. Braxton, PhD, Chairman
Beverley Francis-Gibson, MA, President & CEO

7607 **Sickle Cell Information Center**
201 Dowman Drive   404-727-7857
Atlanta, GA 30322   Fax: 404-727-7880
                                                            aplatt@emory.edu
                                                                 www.scinfo.org
Provides sickle cell patients and their families with information, news, research updates and world wide sickle cell resources. Supports research for a cure.
Melissa Creary, PhD, MPH, Advisory Board Member
James R. Eckman, MD, Advisory Board Member

Foundations

7608 **James R Clark Memorial Sickle Cell Foundation**
1420 Gregg Street   803-765-9916
Columbia, SC 29201   800-506-1273
                                                            Fax: 803-799-6471
                                                            sicklecell@sc.rr.com
Genetic Blood Disorder Disease.
Melodie A Hunnicutt, Executive Director
Saundra Kidwell, Director Finance

7609 **Northeast Louisiana Sickle Cell Anemia Foundation**
1604 Winnsboro Road   318-322-0896
Monroe, LA 71202   Fax: 318-387-4740
                                                              sickle@bayou.com
The Foundation is a community-based non-profit, tax-exempt organization whose purpose is to provide services to sickle cell patients and their families, as well as be a resource in the communities we serve (12 northeast parishes) We provide education, trait counseling, patient assistance and social services. Our services are free.
Lasandre R Starks, Executive Director
Cheryl Minor, Registered Social Worker

7610 **Sickle Cell Foundation of Georgia**
2391 Benjamin E Mays Drive   404-755-1641
Atlanta, GA 30311   800-326-5287
                                                            Fax: 404-755-7955
                                              n_nichols@sicklecellatlaga.org
                                                      www.sicklecellatlaga.org
Our mission is dedicated to providing education, screening and counseling programs for Sickle Cell and other abnormal hemoglobin.
D Jean Brannan, President
Nesby Gibson, Project Director

7611 **Sickle Cell Foundation of Greater Montgomery**
3180 US Highway 8 West   334-286-9122
Montgomery, AL 36108   800-742-5534
                                                            sicklec2@aol.com
The main objectives of the Foundation are to give accurate information about sickle cell disease and related hemoglobinopathies, to provide testing and diagnostic services to interested persons, to counsel individuals with positive test results so they can make informed decisions about their lives and to provide supportive services for clients and their family members.
Willie Owens, Executive Director

Research Centers

7612 Boston Sickle Cell Center Boston Medical Center
Boston Medical Center
88 E Newton Street 617-414-1020
Boston, MA 02118-2999 Fax: 617-414-1021
mhsteinb@bu.edu
The treatment facility of choice for Boston-area patients with sickle cell disease. The Center also promotes interactive basic and clinical research and patient and professional educational activities.
Martin Steinberg, Director
Shawn H Eung, Program Manager

7613 Columbia University: Comprehensive Sickle Cell Center
Harlem Hospital
506 Lenox Avenue 212-939-1426
New York, NY 10037-1000
Research into sickle cell disease.
Dr Jeanne Smith, Director

7614 Comprehensive Sickle Cell Center Children's Hospital Research Foundation
Children's Hospital Research Foundation
3333 Burnet Avenue 513-636-4541
Cincinnati, OH 45229 800-344-2462
Fax: 513-636-5562
blood@cchmc.org
www.cincinnatichildrens.org
Offers research and statistical information in the area of sickle cell disease.
Clinton Joiner, Director
Karen Kalinyak, Clinical Director

7615 Howard University Center for Sickle Cell Disease
1840 7th Street NW 202-865-8284
Washington, DC 20001 Fax: 202-232-6719
sicklecell@howard.edu
www.sicklecell.howard.edu
Victor R Gordeuk, Director
Catherine Nwokolo, Clinical Staff Member

7616 Medical College of Georgia: Sickle Cell Center
1521 Pope Avenue 706-721-2171
Augusta, GA 30912-0002 Fax: 706-721-4575
Offers research into sickle cell disease.
Abdullah Kutlar, Director
Kavita Natarajan

7617 Philadelphia Biomedical Research Institute
100 Ross and Royal Road 610-962-0615
King of Prussia, PA 19406 Fax: 610-254-9332
stohmishi@aol.com
members.aol.com/stohinishi/phila_biomed
Study on the management of sickle cell anemia through nutrition.
S Tsuyoshi Ohinishi PhD, Director

7618 SUNY Health Science Center at Brooklyn Sickle Cell Center
450 Clarkson Avenue 718-270-1000
Brooklyn, NY 11203 Fax: 718-270-7592
John C LaRosa, President
Paul J Davis, Interim Chief Financial Officer

7619 Sickle Cell Anemia Research Foundation
2625 3rd Street 913-588-5000
Alexandria, VA 71309 877-722-7370
Fax: 318-487-9990
scarf@sicklecelldisease.org
www.kumc.edu
The Sickle Cell Anemia Research Foundation provides a comprehensive program on Sickle Cell Disease. We offer education training counseling and help with prescriptions.

7620 Sickle Cell Association of the Texas Gulf Coast
2626 S Loop W 713-666-0300
Houston, TX 77054-2649 Fax: 713-660-17
Rebecca Jasso, Executive Director

7621 University of California Northern Comprehensive Sickle Cell Center
Childrens Hospital Research Center
747 50 2nd Street 510-428-3651
Oakland, OK 94609-3594
Sickle cell disease research.
Elliot Vichinsky, Director

7622 University of Southern California: Comprehensive Sickle Cell Center
2025 Zonal Avenue 213-342-1259
Los Angeles, CA 90033-1034
Dr Cage S Johnson, Director

7623 University of Texas Southwestern Medical Center/Sickle Cell Management
Southwestern Medical Center
1935 Medical District Drive 214-456-7000
Dallas, TX 75235-7701 Fax: 214-648-3122
www.childrens.com
Focuses on the prevention of disease complications and management using the newest treatment strategies including hydroxyurea chronic transfusions stem cell (bone marrow) transplantation and state-of-the-art approaches to infection prevention pain management and treatment of specific organ-related complications (chest syndrome priapism avascular necrosis of the femoral head etc.).
George Bucha MD, Director
James F Amatruda

7624 Wayne State University: Comprehensive Sickle Cell Center
Curricular Affairs Office
Scott Hall 313-577-2424
Detroit, MI 48201 Fax: 313-577-8777
wayne.edu
Charles F Whitten MD, President

Support Groups & Hotlines

7625 Keon Paschal Perry Sickle Cell Anemia Disease Awareness
7510 Granby Street, Perry Building 888-406-5111
Norfolk, VA 23505 keon4u@aol.com
International Sickle Cell Anemia Disease Awareness Campaign.
Roy L Perry-Bey, CEO/Executive Director

7626 Lehigh Valley Sickle Cell Support Group
PO Box 1711 610-706-0636
Allentown, PA 18105-1711 SororW@aol.com
www.members.aol.com/SororW/index.html
Anyone affected/effected by Sickle Cell and all interested persons. Our mission is to educate the local community about Sickle Cell.

7627 National Health Information Center
Office of Disease Prevention & Health Promotion
1101 Wootton Pkwy Fax: 240-453-8281
Rockville, MD 20852 odphpinfo@hhs.gov
www.health.gov/nhic
Supports public health education by maintaining a calendar of National Health Observances; helps connect consumers and health professionals to organizations that can best answer questions and provide up-to-date contact information from reliable sources; updates on a yearly basis toll-free numbers for health information, Federal health clearinghouses and info centers.
Don Wright, MD, MPH, Director

7628 Sickle Cell Anemia Association of Austin: Marc Thomas Chapter
PO Box 201092 512-335-2306
Austin, TX 78720-1092
To raise awareness, resources and support for clients with sickle cell disease.
Linda L Thomas

7629 Sickle Cell Disease Association of America Philadelphia/Delaware Valley Chapter
4601 Market Street 215-471-8686
Philadelphia, PA 19139 Fax: 215-471-7441
scdaa.pdvc@verizon.net
www.sicklecelldisorder.com
The Philadelphia/Delaware Valley Chapter of the Sickle Cell Disease Association of America (SCDAA/PDVC) assists the sickle

cell community by serving as a vehicle and resource center for the psycho-social and social service needs of those individuals affected by the disease through the following services: case management; counseling; hospital/clinic visits; advocacy; career/vocational assistance; newborn screening follow-up; transportation; and outreach/community education.

Stanley A Simpkins, Executive Director
Karin Darius, Program Director

Pamphlets

7630 Sickle Cell Disease
March of Dimes
1275 Mamaroneck Avenue   914-997-4488
White Plains, NY 10605   Fax: 212-254-3518
                                          NY639@marchofdimes.com
                                          www.marchofdimes.com
Fact Sheets: one to two page review written for the general public.

Web Sites

7631 American Sickle Cell Anemia
                                          www.ascaa.org
Comprehensive services through diagnostic testing, evaluation, counseling and supportive services to individuals and families at risk for Sickle Cell Disease.

7632 Healing Well
                                          www.healingwell.com
An online health resource guide to medical news, chat, information and articles, newsgroups and message boards, books, disease-related web sites, medical directories, and more for patients, friends, and family coping with disabling diseases, disorders, or chronic illnesses.

7633 Health Finder
                                          www.healthfinder.gov
Searchable, carefully developed web site offering information on over 1000 topics. Developed by the US Department of Health and Human Services, the site can be used in both English and Spanish.

7634 Healthlink USA
                                          www.healthlinkusa.com
Health information concerning treatment, cures, prevention, diagnosis, risk factors, research, support groups, email lists, personal stories and much more. Updated regularly.

7635 MedicineNet
                                          www.medicinenet.com
An online resource for consumers providing easy-to-read, authoritative medical and health information.

7636 Medscape
                                          www.medscape.com
Medscape offers specialists, primary care physicians, and other health professionals the Web's most robust and integrated medical information and educational tools.

7637 Sickle Cell Disease Association of America
                                          sicklecelldisease.org
Purpose is to promote leadership on a national level in order to create awareness in all circles of the impact of sickle cell disease on emotional and economic well-being of families and the individual.

7638 WebMD
                                          www.webmd.com
Provides credible information, supportive communities, and in-depth reference material about health subjects. A source for original and timely health information as well as material from well known content providers.

Description

7639 **Sjogren's Syndrome**

Sjogren's syndrome (also called sicca syndrome) is a relatively common autoimmune disorder (0.1-4 percent or population) characterized by dryness of the mouth, eyes and mucous membranes. Variable enlargement of the lacrimal (tear) or salivary gland can occur. The disorder has no known cause, but genome-wide association studies have established that this disease has some genetic basis. Sjogren's syndrome is divided into primary (affecting only the eyes and mouth) and secondary (generalized) forms which may be associated with connective tissue diseases such as rheumatoid arthritis, systemic lupus erythematosus, polymyositis or scleroderma.

Patients who suffer from Sjogren's syndrome often complain initially of a gritty sensation in the eyes or severe dryness of the mouth. Patients may develop kidney, skin, neurologic, pulmonary or joint problems.

Treatment for Sjogren's is mainly symptomatic in the form of artificial tears, sipping fluids throughout the day, chewing gum and using special mouthwash. Pilocarpine or cevimeline may be used to stimulate saliva production. Severe cases, especially if they affect parts of the body outside of the glands, may require corticosteroid therapy, such as methylprednisolone or loteprednol, or immunosuppressive drugs like rituximab or hydroxychloroquine. Dental caries (cavities) are a complication of dry mouth, so close dental follow-up is important.

National Agencies & Associations

7640 **American Chronic Pain Association**
PO Box 850   800-533-3231
Rocklin, CA 95677   ACPA@theacpa.org
    www.theacpa.org
The ACPA facilitates peer support and education for individuals with chronic pain in its many forms, in order to increase quality of life. Also raises awareness among the healthcare community, and with policy makers.
Penney Cowan, Founder & CEO
Daniel Galia, Director, Global Support

7641 **Sj"gren's Syndrome Foundation**
10701 Parkridge Boulevard   301-530-4420
Reston, VA 20191   800-475-6473
    Fax: 301-530-4415
    info@sjogrens.org
    www.sjogrens.org
Provides patients with applicable medical information and coping strategies that minimize the effects of Sj"gren's syndrome.
Janet E. Church, Chairman
Steven Taylor, CEO

Support Groups & Hotlines

7642 **National Health Information Center**
Office of Disease Prevention & Health Promotion
1101 Wootton Pkwy   Fax: 240-453-8281
Rockville, MD 20852   odphpinfo@hhs.gov
    www.health.gov/nhic
Supports public health education by maintaining a calendar of National Health Observances; helps connect consumers and health professionals to organizations that can best answer questions and provide up-to-date contact information from reliable sources; updates on a yearly basis toll-free numbers for health information, Federal health clearinghouses and info centers.
Don Wright, MD, MPH, Director

Books

7643 **New Sjogren's Syndrome Handbook**
Sjogren's Syndrome Foundation
6707 Democracy Boulevard   301-530-4420
Bethesda, MD 20817-2025   800-475-6473
    Fax: 301-530-4415
    www.sjogrens.org
An authoritative guide for patients and health care providers on the many aspects of Sjogren's syndrome written by renowned experts, plus practical suggestions for living more comfortably with this chronic illness.
Hardcover
ISBN: 0-195117-24-7
Kenneth Economou, Chairman
Stephen Cohen, Chairman-Elect

Newsletters

7644 **Moisture Seekers Newsletter**
Sjogren's Syndrome Foundation
6707 Democracy Boulevard   301-530-4420
Bethesda, MD 20817-2025   800-475-6473
    Fax: 301-530-4415
    www.sjogrens.org
Contains up-to-date information on Sjogren's syndrome including new treatments, new products, and clinical trails; also features articles on the ways members cope with this chronic disease.
9x Year
Kenneth Economou, Chairman
Stephen Cohen, Chairman-Elect

Pamphlets

7645 **Dry Eyes? Dry Mouth? Dry Nose? Arthritis? If Two or More: Sjogren's Syndrome**
Sjogren's Syndrome Foundation
1 AMS Circle   301-495-4484
Bethesda, MD 20892-3136   877-226-4267
    Fax: 301-718-6366
    TTY: 301-565-2966
    NIAMSinfo@mail.nih.gov
    www.niams.nih.gov
Offers a brief overview of what the illness is, a history, statistical information, causes, symptoms and treatments.

7646 **Sjogren's Syndrome**
NAMSIC/National Institutes of Health
1 AMS Circle   301-495-4484
Bethesda, MD 20892-0001   877-226-4267
    Fax: 301-718-6366
    TTY: 301-565-2966
    NIAMSinfo@mail.nih.gov
    www.nih.gov/niams/
14 pages

Audio & Video

7647 **SjoGren's Syndrome Survival Guide**
6707 Democracy Boulevard   301-530-4420
Bethesda, MD 20817   800-475-6473
    Fax: 301-530-4415
    staylor@sjogrens.org
    www.sjogrens.org
A complete resource for Sjogren's sufferers providing the newest medical information, research results, and treatment methods available, as well as the most effective and practical self-help strategies. Sjogren's syndrome is an autoimmune disease in which the

body's immune system mistakenly attacks its own moisture producing glands.

Kenneth Economou, Chairman
Stephen Cohen, Chairman-Elect

Web Sites

7648   Healing Well

www.healingwell.com

An online health resource guide to medical news, chat, information and articles, newsgroups and message boards, books, disease-related web sites, medical directories, and more for patients, friends, and family coping with disabling diseases, disorders, or chronic illnesses.

Peter Waite, Founder & CEO

7649   Health Finder

www.healthfinder.gov

Searchable, carefully developed web site offering information on over 1000 topics. Developed by the US Department of Health and Human Services, the site can be used in both English and Spanish.

7650   Healthlink USA

www.healthlinkusa.com

Health information concerning treatment, cures, prevention, diagnosis, risk factors, research, support groups, email lists, personal stories and much more. Updated regularly.

7651   MedicineNet

www.medicinenet.com

An online resource for consumers providing easy-to-read, authoritative medical and health information.

7652   Medscape

www.medscape.com

Medscape offers specialists, primary care physicians, and other health professionals the Web's most robust and integrated medical information and educational tools.

7653   National Sjogren's Syndrome Association

www.sjogrens.org

Provides educational materials to members about medical developments and research concerning SS nationally and internationally. Membership also includes assorted discounts on additional materials and events.

7654   Sjogren's Syndrome Foundation

www.sjogrens.org

Information on Sjogren's Syndrome, the SS Foundation, and links to other related sites.

7655   WebMD

www.webmd.com

Provides credible information, supportive communities, and in-depth reference material about health subjects. A source for original and timely health information as well as material from well known content providers.

Description

7656 Skin Disorders

The three most common chronic skin disorders are acne, psoriasis and eczema. Although these conditions do not shorten one's life, or cause significant disability, they can have a profound effect on one's quality of life and self-esteem.

Acne is probably the most common skin disorder and can affect all age groups. It typically occurs in adolescents and young adults. Acne involves the sebaceous glands - glands that produce sebum, a substance that preserves the skin's natural oiliness. In acne, the glands' pores become plugged, trapping the sebum and bacteria. Inflammation follows, resulting in small red tender bumps with a corresponding blackhead or whitehead. These lesions can become pus-filled or even cystic ranging from 1 mm to 5 mm. Acne is seen most commonly on the face, neck, back and shoulders. Treatment starts with keeping affected areas clean. Locally-applied creams include retinoic acid, benzoyl peroxide and various antibiotics. Oral antibiotics (tetracycline) are especially effective for large, deep pimples. Oral tretinoin (Accutane) is very affective, but causes birth defects and other side effects and should be used only as a last resort and in consultation with a dermatologist. Oral contraceptives are often helpful in young women.

Psoriasis usually begins in early adult life and affects 2-4 percent of the white population. A family history is common. The disease is characterized by scaly patches, some as small rain drops, others a few inches in diameter. Typical locations are the scalp, knees and elbows, but any part of the body may be affected. The patches are extremely itchy, and compulsive scratching may further damage the skin. In roughly 10 percent there is an associated arthritis. Milder cases are treated with steroid creams applied to skin and tar preparations or oral psoralen drugs, is effective in more severe cases. The most severe cases may require immunomodulating drugs like methotrexate or cyclosporine.

Eczema is a catchall term for many diseases which involve skin inflammation in response to some irritant. The irritant may be a direct one, such as contact dermatitis from the metal in a belt buckle, or an indirect one, as in atopic dermatitis triggered by various environmental agents (inhalants) and factors (certain foods). Atopic dermatitis is frequently associated with a personal or family history of allergic disorders (hay fever, asthma). For either situation, treatment consists of identifying and eliminating the offending agent(if possible) and local application of corticosteroid creams or nonspecific soothing and hydrating substances. Topical tacrolimus, approved by the FDA in 2000, is an immunosuppressive ointment effective for severe eczema without damaging the skin in the way that long-term topical steroids sometimes do.

National Agencies & Associations

7657 American Academy of Dermatology
PO Box 1968
847-240-1280
Des Plaines, IL 60017
888-462-3376
Fax: 847-240-1859
www.aad.org
Largest dermatologic association in the world and represents all practicing dermatologists in the United States.
George J. Hruza, MD, MBA, FAAD, President
Jane M. Grant-Kels, MD, FAAD, Vice President

7658 American Skin Association
335 Madison Avenue
212-889-4858
New York, NY 10017
info@americanskin.org
www.americanskin.org
Organization whose membership includes patients, families, advocates, physicians and scientists working together to cure melanoma, skin cancer and disease.
David A. Norris, MD, President
Howard P. Milstein, Chairman

7659 American Society for Dermatologic Surgery
5550 Meadowbrook Drive
847-956-0900
Rolling Meadows, IL 60008
Fax: 847-956-0999
www.asds.net
Exclusively represents dermatologic surgeons to treat the health of skin.
Murad Alam, MD, MBA, President
Mathew Avram, MD, Vice President

7660 American Society of Plastic Surgeons
444 E Algonquin Road
847-228-9900
Arlington Heights, IL 60005
800-514-5058
memserv@plasticsurgery.org
www.plasticsurgery.org
Provides patients with free information about various surgical procedures and also provides the names of board certified plastic surgeons in the patient's area.
Alan Matarasso, MD, FACS, President
Michael D. Costelloe, Executive Vice President

7661 Dermatology Foundation
1560 Sherman Avenue
847-328-2256
Evanston, IL 60201-4808
Fax: 847-328-0509
dfgen@dermatologyfoundation.org
www.dermatologyfoundation.org
Raises funds for the control of skin diseases through research, improved education and better patient care. Supports basic clinical investigations.
Janet A. Fairley, MD, President
Bruce U. Wintroub, MD, Chairman

7662 International Society of Dermatology
85 High Street
386-437-4405
Waldorf, MD 20602
Fax: 386-437-4427
info@intsocderm.org
www.intsocderm.org
Promotes interest, education and research in dermatology.
George T. Reizner, MD, President
Marcia Ramos-e-Silva, Executive Vice President

7663 National Eczema Association
505 San Marin Drive
415-499-3474
Novato, CA 94945
info@nationaleczema.org
www.nationaleczema.org
Offers research and information to persons with eczema and other skin disorders.
Lisa Choy, Chair
Christina Crowley, Secretary

7664 National Institute of Arthritis & Musculoskeletal & Skin Diseases
National Institutes of Health
Bethesda, MD 20892-3675
301-495-4484
877-226-4267
Fax: 301-718-6366
TTY: 301-565-2966
NIAMSinfo@mail.nih.gov
www.niams.nih.gov

Supports research into the causes, treatment, and prevention of arthritis and musculoskeletal and skin diseases, the training of basic and clinical scientists to carry out this research, and the dissemination of information on research programs.
Robert H. Carter, MD, Director
Gahan Breithaupt, Assoc. Director, Management & Operations

Foundations

7665 National Psoriasis Foundation
6600 SW 92nd Avenue   503-244-7404
Portland, OR 97223-7195   800-723-9166
Fax: 503-245-0626
getinfo@psoriasis.org
www.psoriasis.org
Misson: To find a cure for psoriasis arthritis and to eliminate their devastating effects through research, advocacy, and education. Provides: patient services; public and professional education; community services; government affairs; research.
Randy Beranek, President/CEO
Bill Cardmon, Chief Field Operations

Research Centers

7666 Agromedicine Program Medical University of South Carolina
Medical University of South Carolina
171 Ashley Av.   843-792-1414
Charleston, SC 29425-0100   Fax: 843-792-1798
www.musc.edu
Does research into the effects of pesticides on humans including epidemiology and skin diseases.
Dr Stanley Schuman, Director
W Stuart Smith, Vice President for Clinical Operations a

7667 Duke University Plastic Surgery Research Laboratories
Medical Center
Box 3974   919-681-8555
Durham, NC 27710-1   elizabeth.yundt@duke.edu
plastic.surgery.duke.edu
Conducts studies on skin cancer and aging skin.
Gregory Georgiade, Chief Division of Plastic and Reconstru
Detlev Erdmann, Associate Professor of Surgery

7668 Laboratory of Dermatology Research Memorial Sloane-Kettering Cancer Center
Memorial Sloane-Kettering Cancer Center
1275 York Avenue   212-639-2000
New York, NY 10065-6007   Fax: 212-717-3363
www.mskcc.org/mskcc
Specific studies on the identification of skin disorders and dermatology.
Allan C Halpern, Chief Dermatology Service

7669 Massachusetts General Hospital: Harvard Cutaneous Biology Research Center
Massachusetts General Hospital
55 Fruit Street   617-726-5254
Boston, MA 02114   Fax: 617-726-1875
TTY: 617-724-8800
www.massgeneral.org
Dermatology research.
Peter L Flavin, President
John R Hinghman, Secretary

7670 National Institute of Arthritis & Musculoskeletal & Skin Diseases
National Institutes of Health
Bethesda, MD 20892-3675   301-495-4484
877-226-4267
Fax: 301-718-6366
TTY: 301-565-2966
NIAMSinfo@mail.nih.gov
www.niams.nih.gov
Supports research into the causes, treatment, and prevention of arthritis and musculoskeletal and skin diseases, the training of basic

and clinical scientists to carry out this research, and the dissemination of information on research programs.
Robert H. Carter, MD, Director
Gahan Breithaupt, Assoc. Director, Management & Operations

7671 Orentreich Foundation for the Advancement of Science
855 Route 301   212-606-0836
Cold Spring, NY 10516-4155   Fax: 845-265-4210
ofas@orentreich.org
http://www.orentreich.org/team
Conducts biomedical research on dermatology.
Norman Orentreich, Founder and Co-Director
David S Orentreich, Co-Director

7672 Psoriasis Research Institute
6600 SW 92nd Avenue   503-244-7404
Portland, OR 97223   800-723-9166
Fax: 503-245-0626
getinfo@psoriasis.org
www.psoriasis.org
Studies the causes symptoms and treatments of psoriasis.
Randy Beranek, President/CEO
Bill Cardmon, Chief Field Operations

7673 Rockefeller University Laboratory for Investigative Dermatology
Rockefeller University
1230 York Avenue   212-327-7458
New York, NY 10021-6399   Fax: 212-570-8232
www.rockefeller.edu
Research into skin disorders and the whole specialty of dermatology in general.
D Martin Carter MD, PhD, Head

7674 Rockefeller University, Laboratory for Investigative Dermatology
1230 York Avenue   212-327-7458
New York, NY 10021-6399   Fax: 212-570-8232
www.rockefeller.edu

D Martin Carter MD, PhD, Head

7675 Scripps Clinic and Research Foundation: Autoimmune Disease Center
10550 N Torrey Pines Road   858-784-1000
La Jolla, CA 92037-1092   Fax: 619-554-6805
www.scripps.edu
Research into dermatomyositis and polymyositis.
Eng Tan, Professor Emeritus

7676 Sulzberger Institute for Dermatologic Education
PO Box 94020   847-330-0230
Palatine, IL 60094-4020   Fax: 847-330-0050
http://www.aad.org/
A nonprofit research center whose sole goal is to enhance patient care through the development and promotion of quality educational programs on the care and disorders of the skin, hair, nails and mucous membranes.
Dirk M. Elston, President
Lisa A. Garner, Vice president

7677 Sulzberger Institute for Dermatologic Educ
PO Box 94020   847-330-0230
Palatine, IL 60094   Fax: 847-330-0050
http://www.aad.org/
A nonprofit research center whose sole goal is to enhance patient care through the development and promotion of quality educational programs on the care and disorders of the skin hair nails and mucous membranes.
Dirk M. Elston, President
Lisa A. Garner, Vice president

7678 University of California: San Francisco Dermatology Drug Research
515 Spruce   415-476-2001
San Francisco, CA 94143-0001   Fax: 415-221-4751
www.ucsf.edu
Conducts clinical testing of new or existing pharmalogic agents used in the treatment of skin disorders.
John Koo MD, Director
Susan Desmond, Chancellor

7679 University of Texas: Southwestern Medical Center at Dallas, Immunodermatology
5323 Harry Hines Boulevard
Dallas, TX 75390-7208
214-648-3111
Fax: 214-688-8275
www.utsouthwestern.edu
Provides a focus for research into the causes prevention and management of diseases such as immune deficiencies and infections. Studies are aimed at increasing basic-level understanding of immunologic skin diseases.
Daniel K Podolsky MD, President
Diane Jeffries, Director

Support Groups & Hotlines

7680 National Health Information Center
Office of Disease Prevention & Health Promotion
1101 Wootton Pkwy
Rockville, MD 20852
Fax: 240-453-8281
odphpinfo@hhs.gov
www.health.gov/nhic
Supports public health education by maintaining a calendar of National Health Observances; helps connect consumers and health professionals to organizations that can best answer questions and provide up-to-date contact information from reliable sources; updates on a yearly basis toll-free numbers for health information, Federal health clearinghouses and info centers.
Don Wright, MD, MPH, Director

Books

7681 Managing Your Psoriasis
MasterMedia
P.O. Box 4014
Schaumburg, IL 60168
847-240-1280
866-503-7546
Fax: 847-240-1859
www.aad.org
1993 Paperback
ISBN: 0-942361-83-0

7682 Psoriasis and Psoriatic Arthritis Pocket Guide
National Psoriasis Foundation
6600 SW 92nd Avenue
Portland, OR 97223-7195
503-244-7404
800-723-9166
Fax: 503-245-0626
getinfo@psoriasis.org
www.psoriasis.org
The Pocket Guide includes algorithms for therapy_including combination and biologic treatments_based on patient types. This second edition was revised to provide guidance for managing patients with severe psoriasis and to put the roll of new biologics into perspective.
2005 79 pages
Krista Kellogg, Chair
Pete Redding, Vice-Chair

7683 Q&A's About Psoriasis
NAMSIC/National Institutes of Health
1 AMS Circle
Bethesda, MD 20892-0001
301-495-4484
877-226-4267
Fax: 301-718-6366
TTY: 301-565-2966
niamsinfo@mail.nih.gov
Offers various information for the psoriasis patient and their family regarding treatments, risks, nutrition and more.
24 pages

7684 Therapy of Moderate-to-Severe Psoriasis
National Psoriasis Foundation
6600 SW 92nd Avenue
Portland, OR 97223-7195
503-244-7404
800-723-9166
Fax: 503-245-0626
getinfo@psoriasis.org
www.psoriasis.org

Edited by Gerald D. Weinstein, MD, and Alice Gottlieb, MD, PhD, this book includes information on state-of-the-art clinical management through contributions from national experts on psoriasis.
2002
Krista Kellogg, Chair
Pete Redding, Vice-Chair

7685 Treatment Guide for the Health Insurance Industry
National Psoriasis Foundation
6600 SW 92nd Avenue
Portland, OR 97223-7195
503-244-7404
800-723-9166
Fax: 503-245-0626
getinfo@psoriasis.org
www.psoriasis.org
This easy-to-read general overview is a valuable tool for the insurer or any health professional interested in detailed information about psoriasis and psoriatic arthritis, patient quality of life issues, and many available treatments.
Krista Kellogg, Chair
Pete Redding, Vice-Chair

Magazines

7686 International Journal of Dermatology
International Society of Dermatology
200 1st Street SW
Rochester, MN 55905-0001
507-284-3736
onlinelibrary.wiley.com
Focuses on information for dermatologists and the whole specialty of dermatology research and education.
10x Year

7687 Journal of Dermatologic Surgery and Oncology
International Society for Dermatologic Surgery
930 N Meachan Road
Schaumburg, IL 60173
847-240-1005
Fax: 847-240-0101
www.aad.org
Focuses on medical updates and information on dermatology.
Monthly
Terrie Duhadway, Executive Publisher

7688 Journal of the Academy of Dermatology
American Academy of Dermatology
930 E. Woodfield Road
Schaumburg, IL 60173-4020
847-240-1005
Fax: 847-240-0101
www.aad.org
A scientific publication serving the clinical needs of the specialty and provides a wide selection of articles on various topics important to continuing medical education of Academy members and the international dermatologic community.
Monthly
Terrie Duhadway, Executive Publisher

7689 Psoriasis Advance
National Psoriasis Foundation
6600 SW 92nd Avenue
Portland, OR 97223-7195
503-244-7404
800-723-9166
Fax: 503-245-0626
getinfo@npfusa.org
www.psoriasis.org
Written especially for the psoriatis community four times a year. Provides current articles to keep you up to date with treatmetnt and research information, pave the way to empowerment, and connect you with others.
40 pages BiMonthly
Krista Kellogg, Chair
Pete Redding, Vice-Chair

7690 Psoriasis Forum
National Psoriasis Foundation
6600 SW 92nd Avenue
Portland, OR 97223-7195
503-244-7404
800-723-9166
Fax: 503-245-0626
getinfo@psoriasis.org
www.psoriasis.org

Dedicated to providing up-to-date and practical information to health care providers on the frontline of psoriasis treatment. Professional Members only.
Quarterly
Krista Kellogg, Chair
Pete Redding, Vice-Chair

Newsletters

7691 Dermatology Focus
Dermatology Foundation
1560 Sherman Avenue   847-328-2256
Evanston, IL 60201-4808   Fax: 847-328-0509
                          dfgen@dermatologyfoundation.org
                                            www.dermfnd.org
Designed to communicate to practitioners the latest advances in medical and surgical dermatology. The publication also serves as the Foundation's newsletter, recognizing the accomplishments and activities of the many dermatologists who give not only their monetary support, but countless hours to develop the research and teaching careers of future leaders throughout the specialty.
Quarterly
Michael D. Tharp, President
Bruce U. Wintroub, Chairman

7692 Dermatology Focus
Dermatology Foundation
1560 Sherman Avenue   847-328-2256
Evanston, IL 60201-4808   Fax: 847-328-0509
                          dfgen@dermatologyfoundation.org
                                            www.dermfnd.org
Designed to communicate to practitioners the latest advances in medical and surgical dermatology. The publication also serves as the Foundation's newsletter recognizing the accomplishments and activities of the many dermatologists who give not only their monetary support, but countless hours to develop the research and teaching careers of future leaders throughout the specialty.
Quarterly
Michael D. Tharp, President
Bruce U. Wintroub, Chairman

7693 Dermatology World
American Academy of Dermatology
P.O. Box 4014   847-240-1280
Schaumburg, IL 60168-4020   866-503-7546
                                        Fax: 847-240-1859
                                              www.aad.org
Offers Academy members information outside the clinical realm. It carries news of government actions, reports of socioeconomic issues, societal trends and other events which impinge on the practice of dermatology.
Monthly

7694 Progress in Dermatology
Dermatology Foundation
1560 Sherman Avenue   847-328-2256
Evanston, IL 60201-4808   Fax: 847-328-0509
                          dfgen@dermatologyfoundation.org
                                            www.dermfnd.org
The journal provides in-depth coverage of clinically relevant topics as well as basic scientific advances affecting all of dermatology. Distributed exclusively to members of the Foundation.
Quarterly
Michael D. Tharp, President
Bruce U. Wintroub, Chairman

7695 Psoriasis Newsletter
Psoriasis Research Institute
6600 SW 92nd Avenue   503-244-7404
Portland, OR 97223   800-723-9166
                                        Fax: 503-245-0626
                                        getinfo@psoriasis.org
                                            www.psoriasis.org
Offers information and medical updates on the disease of psoriasis, events, fundraising and more.
4 pages Quarterly
Krista Kellogg, Chair
Pete Redding, Vice-Chair

Pamphlets

7696 Acne
American Academy of Dermatology
PO Box 4014   847-240-1280
Schaumburg, IL 60168-4014   866-503-7546
                                        Fax: 847-240-1859
                                              www.aad.org
Explains the causes of acne. Treatments are explored, including diet, medications, antibiotics, and sun exposure. Available in Spanish.
1996

7697 Allergic Contact Rashes
American Academy of Dermatology
PO Box 4014   847-240-1280
Schaumburg, IL 60168-4014   866-503-7546
                                        Fax: 847-240-1859
                                              www.aad.org
Lists the common causes of skin rashes, including jewelry and hidden ingredients in fabrics and household products.
1997

7698 Athlete's Foot
American Academy of Dermatology
PO Box 4014   847-240-1280
Schaumburg, IL 60168-4014   866-503-7546
                                        Fax: 847-240-1859
                                              www.aad.org
This common fungal infection is not only a problem for athletics. Discusses what causes it and how to treat it.
1994

7699 Black Skin
American Academy of Dermatology
PO Box 4014   847-240-1280
Schaumburg, IL 60168-4014   866-503-7546
                                        Fax: 847-240-1859
                                              www.aad.org
Explains the skin diseases common with black skin and how they are diagnosed and treated.
1996

7700 Conception, Pregnancy & Psoriasis
National Psoriasis Foundation
6600 SW 92nd Avenue   503-244-7404
Portland, OR 97223-7195   800-723-9166
                                        Fax: 503-245-0626
                                              www.aad.org
Explains pregnancy factors for persons with psoriasis.

7701 Cosmetics & Skin Care
American Academy of Dermatology
PO Box 4014   847-240-1280
Schaumburg, IL 60168-4014   866-503-7546
                                        Fax: 847-240-1859
                                              www.aad.org
Discusses skin reactions to fragrances, makeup, and bath and body care products.
1994

7702 Darker Side of Tanning
American Academy of Dermatology
PO Box 4014   847-240-1280
Schaumburg, IL 60168-4014   866-503-7546
                                        Fax: 847-240-1859
                                              www.aad.org
Discusses the dangers of ultraviolet radiation from the sun, tanning beds, and sun lamps. Includes descriptions of the different skin types and tips to help minimize the sun's damage to the skin and eyes.
1996

7703 Eczema/Atopic Dermatitis
American Academy of Dermatology
PO Box 4014   847-240-1280
Schaumburg, IL 60168-4014   866-503-7546
                                        Fax: 847-240-1859
                                              www.aad.org

Explains how to recognize and treat dermatitis.
1995

7704 For Parents
National Psoriasis Foundation
6600 SW 92nd Avenue
Portland, OR 97223-7195
503-244-7404
800-723-9166
Fax: 503-245-0626
getinfo@npfusa.org
www.psoriasis.org

Offers advice and resources on how to educate yourself about psoriasis and your child, as well as treatment information and summer camps.

7705 Genital Psoriasis
National Psoriasis Foundation
6600 SW 92nd Avenue
Portland, OR 97223-7195
503-244-7404
800-723-9166
Fax: 503-245-0626
getinfo@npfusa.org
www.psoriasis.org

Introduces the reader to the basics of genital psoriasis, and treatment options.

7706 Hand Eczema
American Academy of Dermatology
PO Box 4014
Schaumburg, IL 60168-4014
847-240-1280
866-503-7546
Fax: 847-240-1859
www.aad.org

Shows examples of hand rashes, explains causes, lists protective measures and treatments.
1993

7707 Hives
American Academy of Allergy, Asthma and Immunology
555 East Wells Street
Milwaukee, WI 53202-3889
414-272-6071
800-822-2762
Fax: 414-272-6070
www.aaaai.org

This brochure offers information on what causes hives, what is Angioedema, and how hives can be treated.

7708 Home Phototherapy
National Psoriasis Foundation
6600 SW 92nd Avenue
Portland, OR 97223-7195
503-244-7404
800-723-9166
Fax: 503-245-0626
getinfo@npfusa.org
www.psoriasis.org

Talks about the use of a home UVB unit to treat psoriasis.

7709 Methotrexate (MTX)
National Psoriasis Foundation
6600 SW 92nd Avenue
Portland, OR 97223-7195
503-244-7404
800-723-9166
Fax: 503-245-0626
getinfo@npfusa.org
www.psoriasis.org

An introductions to MTX treatment.

7710 Oral Retinoid Therapy (Soriatane)
National Psoriasis Foundation
6600 SW 92nd Avenue
Portland, OR 97223-7195
503-244-7404
800-723-9166
Fax: 503-245-0626
getinfo@npfusa.org
www.psoriasis.org

Explains Soriatane treatment options.

7711 PUVA (Psoralen Plus Ultraviolet Light A)
National Psoriasis Foundation
6600 SW 92nd Avenue
Portland, OR 97223-7195
503-244-7404
800-723-9166
Fax: 503-245-0626
getinfo@npfusa.org
www.psoriasis.org

Explains PUVA treatment options, pros, cons, and potential side-effects.

7712 Pityriasis Rosea
American Academy of Dermatology
PO Box 4014
Schaumburg, IL 60168-4014
847-240-1280
866-503-7546
Fax: 847-240-1859
www.aad.org

Discusses the appearance, symptoms, and causes of this common rash. Diagnosis and treatment are also explained.
1996

7713 Psoriasis on Specific Skin Sites
National Psoriasis Foundation
6600 SW 92nd Avenue
Portland, OR 97223-7195
503-244-7404
800-723-9166
Fax: 503-245-0626
getinfo@npfusa.org
www.psoriasis.org

Including nails, ears, eyelids, face, mouth and lips, hands and feet.

7714 Psoriasis: How It Makes You Feel
National Psoriasis Foundation
6600 SW 92nd Avenue
Portland, OR 97223-7195
503-244-7404
800-723-9166
Fax: 503-245-0626
getinfo@npfusa.org
www.psoriasis.org

7715 Psoriatic Arthritis
National Psoriasis Foundation
6600 SW 92nd Avenue
Portland, OR 97223-7195
503-244-7404
800-723-9166
Fax: 503-245-0626
getinfo@npfusa.org
www.psoriasis.org

7716 Rosacea
American Academy of Dermatology
PO Box 4014
Schaumburg, IL 60168-4014
847-240-1280
866-503-7546
Fax: 847-240-1859
www.aad.org

The condition, do's and don'ts for rosacea patients, and treatment are explained.
1995

7717 Scabies
American Academy of Dermatology
PO Box 4014
Schaumburg, IL 60168-4014
847-240-1280
866-503-7546
Fax: 847-240-1859
www.aad.org

Explains the nature of the scabies parasite, symptoms, at-risk groups, individual and large group treatments. Available in Spanish.
1997

7718 Scalp Psoriasis
National Psoriasis Foundation
6600 SW 92nd Avenue
Portland, OR 97223-7195
503-244-7404
800-723-9166
Fax: 503-245-0626
getinfo@npfusa.org
www.psoriasis.org

7719 Seborrheic Dermatitis
American Academy of Dermatology
PO Box 4014
Schaumburg, IL 60168-4014
847-240-1280
866-503-7546
Fax: 847-240-1859
www.aad.org

Answers the most frequently asked questions about this common, easily treatable skin condition.
1995

7720 Seborrheic Keratoses
American Academy of Dermatology
PO Box 4014
Schaumburg, IL 60168-4014
847-240-1280
866-503-7546
Fax: 847-240-1859
www.aad.org

Describes seborrheic keratosis growths, causes, and treatments.
1997

7721 Skin Cancer
American Academy of Dermatology
PO Box 4014   847-240-1280
Schaumburg, IL 60168-4014   866-503-7546
                                      Fax: 847-240-1859
                                           www.aad.org
Warning signs and how to perform self-examinations are discussed.
1994

7722 Skin Conditions Related to AIDS
American Academy of Dermatology
PO Box 4014   847-240-1280
Schaumburg, IL 60168-4014   866-503-7546
                                      Fax: 847-240-1859
                                           www.aad.org
What AIDS is, who's at risk, and other important information about this major health problem are discussed.
1997

7723 Specific Forms of Psoriasis
National Psoriasis Foundation
6600 SW 92nd Avenue   503-244-7404
Portland, OR 97223-7195   800-723-9166
                                      Fax: 503-245-0626
                                      getinfo@npfusa.org
                                        www.psoriasis.org
Pustular, Guttate, Inverse, and Erythrodermic.

7724 Spider Veins, Varicose Vein Therapy
American Academy of Dermatology
PO Box 4014   847-240-1280
Schaumburg, IL 60168-4014   866-503-7546
                                      Fax: 847-240-1859
                                           www.aad.org
Discusses the latest methods for removing unsightly and unwanted blood vessels that appear mostly on the legs.
1995

7725 Sun & Water Therapy
National Psoriasis Foundation
6600 SW 92nd Avenue   503-244-7404
Portland, OR 97223-7195   800-723-9166
                                      Fax: 503-245-0626
                                      getinfo@npfusa.org
                                        www.psoriasis.org

7726 Sun Protection for Children
American Academy of Dermatology
PO Box 4014   847-240-1280
Schaumburg, IL 60168-4014   866-503-7546
                                      Fax: 847-240-1859
                                           www.aad.org
Teaches parents how to protect their children from the sun's harmful rays.
1996

7727 Sun and Your Skin
American Academy of Dermatology
PO Box 4014   847-240-1280
Schaumburg, IL 60168-4014   866-503-7546
                                      Fax: 847-240-1859
                                           www.aad.org
Information on acute sunburn, premature aging of the skin, allergies, and skin cancer. Tips on how to be sun smart.
1994

7728 Sunlight, Ultraviolet Radiation and the Skin
National Cancer Institute
149 Madison Avenue   212-725-5176
New York, NY 10016-0001   800-422-6237
                                        www.skincancer.org

7729 Tinea Versicolor
American Academy of Dermatology

PO Box 4014   847-240-1280
Schaumburg, IL 60168-4014   866-503-7546
                                      Fax: 847-240-1859
                                           www.aad.org
Discusses the symptoms, diagnosis, and treatment of this often misunderstood fungal infection.
1995

7730 Treatment Overview
National Psoriasis Foundation
6600 SW 92nd Avenue   503-244-7404
Portland, OR 97223-7195   800-723-9166
                                      Fax: 503-245-0626
                                      getinfo@npfusa.org
                                        www.psoriasis.org
Discusses a number of available psoriasis treatments, what is considered by the doctor when developing a treatment plan, and treatment resources.

7731 Vascular Birthmarks
American Academy of Dermatology
PO Box 4014   847-240-1280
Schaumburg, IL 60168-4014   866-503-7546
                                      Fax: 847-240-1859
                                           www.aad.org
Includes descriptions and treatments for most common types of vascular birthmarks - macular stains, hemangiomas, and port-wine stains.
1997

7732 Vitiligo
American Academy of Dermatology
PO Box 4014   847-240-1280
Schaumburg, IL 60168-4014   866-503-7546
                                      Fax: 847-240-1859
                                           www.aad.org
Discusses lost skin pigmentation and what can be done about it, including repigmentation therapy.
1994

7733 Young People and Psoriasis
National Psoriasis Foundation
6600 SW 92nd Avenue   503-244-7404
Portland, OR 97223-7195   800-723-9166
                                      Fax: 503-245-0626
                                      getinfo@npfusa.org
                                        www.psoriasis.org
Infancy through adolescence.

7734 Your Diet & Psoriasis
National Psoriasis Foundation
6600 SW 92nd Avenue   503-244-7404
Portland, OR 97223-7195   800-723-9166
                                      Fax: 503-245-0626
                                        www.psoriasis.org
A discussion of particular diets, foods and supplements and the effect they have on psoriasis.

7735 Your Skin and Your Dermatologist
American Academy of Dermatology
PO Box 4014   847-240-1280
Schaumburg, IL 60168-4014   866-503-7546
                                      Fax: 847-240-1859
                                           www.aad.org
Explains why a dermatologist is the appropriate specialist for the care of diseases of the skin, hair, nails, and mucous membranes.
1997

Audio & Video

7736 Allergic Skin Reactions
American Academy of Allergy, Asthma and Immunology
555 East Wells Street   414-272-6071
Milwaukee, WI 53202-3889   800-822-2762
                                      Fax: 414-272-6070
                                           www.aaaai.org
In some people, allergy symptoms include itching redness, rashes, or hives. This video describes the symptoms, triggers, and treat-

ment for common skin reactions such as dermatitis, hives and angioedema.
10-13 minutes

7737 Basic Science Series
American Academy of Dermatology
PO Box 4014
Schaumburg, IL 60168-4014
847-240-1280
866-503-7546
Fax: 847-240-1859
www.aad.org

Combines high-quality 35mm slides and accompanying narration on audiocassette and features topics that underline and support clinical dermatology. The series is useful for residents in training as well as practicing dermatologists.
Slides

7738 CME Video Library
American Academy of Dermatology
PO Box 4014
Schaumburg, IL 60168-4014
847-240-1280
866-503-7546
Fax: 847-240-1859
www.aad.org

A series of video programs developed by AAD experts recognized for their continued efforts in dermatologic advancement.
Videotapes

7739 Facts About Acne
American Academy of Dermatology
PO Box 4014
Schaumburg, IL 60168-4014
847-240-1280
866-503-7546
Fax: 847-240-1859
www.aad.org

The etiology of acne and treatment choices are explained by consultants, with patient encounters.
13 minutes

7740 Mystery of Contact Dermatitis
American Academy of Dermatology
PO Box 4014
Schaumburg, IL 60168-4014
847-240-1280
866-503-7546
Fax: 847-240-1859
www.aad.org

The causes and treatment of some common forms of contact dermatitis are shown with consultation and commentary.
10 minutes

7741 National Library of Dermatologic Teaching Slides
American Academy Of Dermatology
PO Box 94020
Palatine, IL 60094-4020
847-240-1280
866-503-7546
Fax: 847-240-1859
www.aad.org

A collection of dermatologic teaching slides offering the most comprehensive series ever assembled. Each set offers a realistic presentation of classic clinical skin conditions encountered by the dermatologist.

7742 Skin Cancer: The Undeclared Epidemic
American Academy of Dermatology
PO Box 4014
Schaumburg, IL 60168-4014
847-240-1280
866-503-7546
Fax: 847-240-1859
www.aad.org

Examples of skin cancer lesions, interviews with patients at screenings, and comments from Academy members.
9 minutes

7743 Skin Care Under the Sun
American Academy of Dermatology
PO Box 4014
Schaumburg, IL 60168-4014
847-240-1280
866-503-7546
Fax: 847-240-1859
www.aad.org

Dramatization of the dangers of overexposure to the sun, providing explanations of the effects of ultraviolet radiation on the skin.
7 minutes

Web Sites

7744 American Academy of Dermatology
www.aad.org
Promotes and advances the science and art of medicine and surgery related to the skin, promotes the highest possible standards in clinical practice, education and research.

7745 American Society of Plastic and Reconstructive Surgeons
www.plasticsurgery.org
The mission of ASPS is to advance quality care to plastic surgery patients by encouraging high standards of training, ethics, physician practice and research in plastic surgery. The Society is a strong advocate for patient safety and requires its members to operate in accredited surgical facilities that have passed rigorous external review of equipment and staffing.

7746 Derma Doctor
www.dermadoctor.com
The most informative skin care site on the Web. An extensive library of newsletters to help answer your questions.

7747 Dermatology Foundation
Raises funds for the control of skin diseases through research, improved education and better patient care. Supports basic clinical investigations.

7748 Healing Well
www.healingwell.com
An online health resource guide to medical news, chat, information and articles, newsgroups and message boards, books, disease-related web sites, medical directories, and more for patients, friends, and family coping with disabling diseases, disorders, or chronic illnesses.

7749 Health Finder
www.healthfinder.gov
Searchable, carefully developed web site offering information on over 1000 topics. Developed by the US Department of Health and Human Services, the site can be used in both English and Spanish.

7750 Healthlink USA
www.healthlinkusa.com
Health information concerning treatment, cures, prevention, diagnosis, risk factors, research, support groups, email lists, personal stories and much more. Updated regularly.

7751 MedicineNet
www.medicinenet.com
An online resource for consumers providing easy-to-read, authoritative medical and health information.

7752 Medscape
www.medscape.com
Medscape offers specialists, primary care physicians, and other health professionals the Web's most robust and integrated medical information and educational tools.

7753 National Psoriasis Foundation
www.psoriasis.org
The National Psoriasis Foundation (NPF) is a non-profit, voluntary health agency dedicated to curing psoriatic disease and improving the lives of those affected.

7754 Skin Store
www.skinstore.com
Carries over 500 of the finest skincare products, available at the lowest prices, delivered immediately to your home.

7755 WebMD
www.webmd.com
Provides credible information, supportive communities, and in-depth reference material about health subjects. A source for original and timely health information as well as material from well known content providers.

Description

7756 Sleep Disorders

Sleep disorders are defined as disturbances that affect the ability to fall or stay asleep, that involve sleeping too much, or that result in abnormal sleep-related behavior. They can be categorized into primary sleep disorders; sleep disorders related to another mental disorder or a general medical condition; and substance induced sleep disorder. The two conditions discussed here, narcolepsy and obstructive sleep apnea, are both primary sleep disorders.

Narcolepsy is a rare disorder of abnormal and irresistible daytime drowsiness. Excessive daytime sleepiness with involuntary daytime sleep episodes, disturbed nighttime sleep, and cataplexy (sudden weakness or loss of muscle tone, often triggered by emotion), are the most common symptoms of narcolepsy. Generally, symptoms appear between the onset of puberty and age 25, and worsen as the patient ages. There are 100,000 people in the US with this condition.

Although the exact cause of narcolepsy is unknown, there appears to be a genetic link, since up to 10 percent of individuals diagnosed with narcolepsy with cataplexy have a close relative with similar symptoms. Almost everyone with narcolepsy who have cataplexy have extremely low levels of a brain chemical hypocretin, which promotes wakefulness and regulates REM sleep.

The initial line of treatment is central nervous system stimulants such as modafinil or methylphenidate. Alternative treatments include particular antidepressants or the sedative sodium oxybate (also known as gamma hydroxybutyrate). All drug treatments must be accompanied by lifestyle changes such as taking short naps, maintaining a regular sleep schedule, avoiding smoking throughout the day and caffeine or alcohol or large meals before bed, and daily exercise.

Obstructive sleep apnea is a serious and common sleep disorder that features heavy snoring and breathing irregularities. It is chronic and relapsing, and varies in severity from mild to lethal. Almost 90 percent of the estimated 12 million sleep apnea sufferers are male. Obstructive sleep apnea is biomechanical and usually occurs when tissues in the back of the throat collapse and close the breathing passage. Sufferers experience heavy snoring, periods during sleep when breathing halts for 10 seconds or more, and many short awakenings which they do not remember. In the worst cases, sufferers may cease breathing for more than half of total sleeping time, which can result in daytime fatigue, oxygen deprivation and hypertension.

Signs of sleep apnea or a related sleeping disorder include loud, habitual snoring, fatigue on waking, daytime sleepiness, and choking, gasping or holding one's breath while asleep. Overweight persons and smokers are more prone to develop this disorder. Heavy eating, late-night snacking, sedative use, and alcohol consumption are often contributing factors.

The diagnosis of sleep apnea often requires a polysomnography, or sleep study, which monitors brain waves, muscle tension, eye movement, respiration and blood-oxygen levels. Obviously, a partner can easily help to confirm these symptoms; single people can arrange for sleep observation in a hospital or clinic setting. Behavior modification is frequently sufficient to reduce or eliminate many snoring problems, as is sleeping on one's side and/or without a pillow. In addition to behavioral changes, mild cases are often responsive to oral devices that help to keep airways open by bringing the jaw forward, elevating the soft palate, or repositioning the tongue. More severe cases can be treated with a C-PAP (continuous positive airway pressure) machine, or a Bi-Level (Bi-PAP) machine, both of which blow air into the patient's airways in a regulated manner. Surgery is sometimes indicated, when facial or oral irregularities, such as jaw irregularities, small throat openings, enlarged tonsils, a large tongue or other tissue in front of the airway, or a deviated septum, impede proper airflow.

National Agencies & Associations

7757 American Chronic Pain Association
PO Box 850
Rocklin, CA 95677

800-533-3231
ACPA@theacpa.org
www.theacpa.org

The ACPA facilitates peer support and education for individuals with chronic pain in its many forms, in order to increase quality of life. Also raises awareness among the healthcare community, and with policy makers.
Penney Cowan, Founder & CEO
Daniel Galia, Director, Global Support

7758 American Sleep Apnea Association
641 S Street NW
Washington, DC 20001-5196

888-293-3650
Fax: 888-293-3650
asaa@sleepapnea.org
www.sleepapnea.org

Offers help and information to persons with sleep apnea and their families.
Adam Amdur, Chief Patient Officer
Andres Mendoza, Treasurer

7759 Narcolepsy Network
PO Box 2178
Lynnwood, WA 98036

401-667-2523
888-292-6522
NarNet@narcolepsynetwork.org
narcolepsynetwork.org

Offers help and information to persons with narcolepsy and their families.
Keith Harper, President
Sharon O'Shaughnessy, MA, SLP, Vice President

7760 National Institute of Neurological Disorders and Stroke
NIH Neurological Institute
Bethesda, MD 20824

301-496-5751
800-352-9424
www.ninds.nih.gov

Seeks to reduce the burden of neurological disease affecting individuals from all walks of life.
Walter J. Koroshetz, MD, Director
Amy B. Adams, Director, Office of Scientific Liaison

7761 National Sleep Foundation
Washington, DC   www.sleepfoundation.org
Non-profit organization dedicated to improving public health and understanding of sleep disorders by supporting education and sleep-related research.

7762 Sleep Research Society American Academy of Sleep Medicine
2510 N Frontage Road   630-737-9702
Darien, IL 60561   Fax: 630-737-9790
                    coordinator@srsnet.org
                    www.sleepresearchsociety.org
Facilitates communication among research workers in the field of sleep medicine.
Andrew D. Krystal, MD, President
Sara J. Aton, PhD, Secretary & Treasurer

Research Centers

7763 Baylor College of Medicine: Sleep Disorder and Research Center
6620 Main St   713-798-1000
Houston, TX 77030-3498   800-229-5671
                    Fax: 713-796-9718
                    baylorclinicweb@bcm.edu
                    www.baylorclinic.com
Internal unit of the College that focuses on research into sleep and sexual dysfunction in males.
Shyam Subramanian, Medical Director
Charlie Lan, Assistant Professor of Medicine

7764 Capital Regional Sleep-Wake Disorders Center
St. Peter's Hospital and Albany Medical Center
25 Hackett Boulevard   518-436-9253
Albany, NY 12208-3420
Cheryl Carlu MD

7765 Center for Narcolepsy Research at the University of Illinois at Chicago
University of Illinois
845 S Damen Avenue   312-996-5176
Chicago, IL 60612-7350   Fax: 312-996-7008
                    CNSHR@listserv.uic.edu
Provides information to health professionals and people with sleep disorders regarding diagnosis and treatment. Maintain national network with sleep professionals throughout the US.
6-8 pages 2 per year
David W Carley, Director
Julie Law, Center Administrator

7766 Center for Research in Sleep Disorders Affiliated with Mercy Hospital
Mercy Hospital of Hamilton/Fairfield
1275 E Kemper Road   513-671-3101
Cincinnati, OH 45246
Martin Schar PhD

7767 Center for Sleep & Wake Disorders: Miami Valley Hospital
One Wyoming Street   937-208-8000
Dayton, OH 45409-2722   www.miamivalleyhospital.org
Offering the largest variety of sleep disorder testing available in the area it also offers comprehensive sleep care and care of related issues with a sleep lab clinical treatment pulmonary treatment and behavioral treatment in the same facility.
Kevin Huban, Director
Amy Cline, Administrative Director

7768 Center for Sleep Medicine of the Mount Sinai Medical Center
One Gustave L.Levy Place   212-241-6500
New York, NY 10029-6500   Fax: 212-875-84
                    www.mountsinai.org
The Center for Sleep Medicine at The Mount Sinai Medical Center is a comprehensive program dedicated to the diagnosis and treatment of all aspects of sleep pathology including breathing related sleep disorders periodic limb movements in sleep insomnia and narcolepsy. Mechanical (CPAP BiPAP ventilator) surgical dental and pharmacologic therapies are available.
E Neil Schachter, Professor
Gwen S Skloot, Associates Professor

7769 Geisinger Wyoming Valley Medical Center: Sleep Disorders Center
1000 E Mountain Drive   570-819-5770
Wilkes-Barre, PA 18711   www.geisinger.org
Our dedicated sleep team operates service sleep centers and laboratories to diagnose and treat a broad range of sleep disorders.˜ Geisinger sleep centers are conveniently located in Danville Bloomsburg Shamokin Wilkes-Barre and Mt. Pocono.
Andrew Paul Matragrano, Director
Stephanie Schaefer, Nurse Practitioner

7770 Johns Hopkins University: Sleep Disorders Francis Scott Key Medical Center
Francis Scott Key Medical Center
601 N Caroline Street   410-550-0545
Baltimore, MD 21287   www.hopkinshospital.org
The Johns Hopkins University Sleep Disorders Center is a tertiary care center for patients with sleep/wake disorders and medical disorders associated with sleep.
Phillip L Smith, Director

7771 Knollwoodpark Hospital Sleep Disorders Center
5600 Girby Road   251-660-5120
Mobile, AL 36693-3398   Fax: 251-660-5245
                    71054.2530@compuserve.com
                    www.southalabama.edu/usakph

7772 Knollwoodpark Hospital Sleep Disorders Cen
5600 Girby Road   251-660-5120
Mobile, AL 36693   Fax: 251-660-5245
                    71054.2530@compuserve.com

7773 Loma Linda University Sleep Disorders Clinic
VA Hospital Medical Services Center
11201 Benton Street   909-825-7084
Loma Linda, CA 92357-1   800-741-8387
                    Fax: 909-963-64
Ralph Downey III MD, Director

7774 Methodist Hospital Sleep Center Winona Memorial Hospital
Rehab Centers
6565 Fannin Street   713-441-7854
Houston, TX 77030-8126   Fax: 713-790-2612
                    www.methodisthealth.com
Marc L Boom, President & CEO
David M Underwood, Vice Chairman

7775 MidWest Medical Center: Sleep Disorders Center
Winona Memorial Hospital
Indianapolis, IN 46208-4688   317-927-2100
                    Fax: 317-927-2914

7776 Northwest Ohio Sleep Disorders Center Toledo Hospital
Toledo Hospital
2142 N Cove Boulevard   419-471-5629
Toledo, OH 43606-3896
Frank O Horton III MD, Director

7777 Ohio Sleep Medicine Institute
4975 Bradenton Avenue   614-766-0773
Dublin, OH 43017-3521   Fax: 614-766-2599
                    info@sleepmedicine.com
                    www.sleepmedicine.com
A comprehensive accredited sleep disorders center that is dedicated to excellence in sleep medicine care. Offer evaluation, diagnosis and treatment for adults and children with sleep apnea, insomnia, restless legs syndrome, narcolepsy, parasomnias, circadian rhythms disorders, shift work, fatigue and other sleep problems.
Betty Palmer, Director

7778 Penn Center for Sleep Disorders: Hospital of the University of Pennsylvania
3400 Spruce Street   215-662-7772
Philadelphia, PA 19104-4204   Fax: 215-349-8038
Joanne Getsy MD, Director

7779 **Presbyterian-University Hospital: Pulmonary Sleep Evaluation Center**
DeSoto At O'Hara Street   412-647-3475
Pittsburgh, PA 15213
Mark Sanders MD, Director

7780 **Scripps Clinic Sleep Disorders Center Scripps Clinic**
Scripps Clinic
10666 N Torrey Pines Road   858-455-9100
La Jolla, CA 92037-1027   Fax: 858-828-64
                    malcoRN@scrippsclinic.com
                              www.scripps.org
The Scripps Clinic Sleep Center provides evaluation diagnosis and treatment of a full range of sleep disorders such as Circadian rhythm disorders Insomnia Narcolepsy Night terror Nightmares Restless legs syndrome Sleep apnea Sleepwalking and Snoring.
Dan Dworsky MD, Medical Director
Merrill M Mitler MD, Scientific Director

7781 **Sleep Alertness Center: Lafayette Home Hospital**
2400 S Street   765-447-6811
Lafayette, IN 47904-3027   glenda.eberhard@glhsi.org
Frederick Ro MD

7782 **Sleep Center: Community General Hospital**
750 East Adams Street   315-464-5540
Syracuse, NY 13210-5100   www.cgh.org
The Sleep Center at Community General Hospital is a specialized facility providing accurate diagnosis and recommending treatment of sleep-related problems.
Robert Westl MD, Medical Director
Antonio Cule MD, Neurology Consultant

7783 **Sleep Disorders Center Bethesda Oak Hospital**
619 Oak Street   513-569-5400
Cincinnati, OH 45206-1613   www.trihealth.com
Milton Krame MD

7784 **Sleep Disorders Center Columbia Presbyterian Medical Center**
The University Hospital of Columbia & Cornell
161 Fort Washington Avenue   212-305-1860
New York, NY 10032   Fax: 212-305-5496
                                   www.sleepnyp.com
A Highly specialized outpatient facility for the evaluation and treatment of patients with problems related to sleep and wakefulness.
Neil B Kavey, Medical Director
Andrew Tucker, Director

7785 **Sleep Disorders Center Dartmouth Hitchcock Medical Center**
Darthmouth Hitchcock medical Center
One Rope Ferry Road   603-650-1200
Hanover, NH 03755-1   877-367-1797
                                   Fax: 603-650-1202
                  Joanne.MacQuarrie@dartmouth.edu
                              dms.dartmouth.edu
Provides consultation and testing for all varieties of sleep-related disturbances including snoring sleep apnea narcolepsy restless legs syndrome periodic limb movement disorder insomnia parasomnias and circadian rhythm disorders.
Glen Greenough, Fellowship Director
Michael Sate MD, Director

7786 **Sleep Disorders Center Lankenau Hospital**
100 E Lancaster Avenue   610-645-3400
Wynnewood, PA 19096-3498   Fax: 610-645-2291

7787 **Sleep Disorders Center Ohio State University Medical Center**
410 W.10th Ave   614-257-2500
Columbus, OH 43210-1228   800-293-5123
                                   Fax: 614-257-2551
                         webmaster@osumc.edu
                              medicalcenter.osu.edu
Ulysses J Magalang MD, Medical Director

7788 **Sleep Disorders Center at California: Pacific Medical Center**
2340 Clay Street   415-923-3336
San Francisco, CA 94115-1932   Fax: 415-923-3584
                    76307.2221@compuserve.com

7789 **Sleep Disorders Center at California: Paci**
2340 Clay Street   415-923-3336
San Francisco, CA 94115   Fax: 415-923-3584
                    76307.2221@compuserve.com

7790 **Sleep Disorders Center of Metropolitan Toronto**
500 Alden Road   905-475-5155
Markham Ontario, CA M6B-4H6   888-401-5155
                                   Fax: 647-436-7607
                         sleep@compuserve.com
                              www.sdc.ca
Jeffrey Lips MD, Director

7791 **Sleep Disorders Center of Rochester: St. Mary's Hospital**
2110 Clinton Avenue S   716-442-4141
Rochester, NY 14618-2616
Donald Green MD

7792 **Sleep Disorders Center of Western New York Millard Fillmore Hospital**
726 Exchange Street   716-859-5600
Buffalo, NY 14210-1120   Fax: 716-887-5332
                         gates.kaleidahealth.org
Daniel Rifkin, Director

7793 **Sleep Disorders Center: Cleveland Clinic Foundation**
9500 Euclid Avenue   216-636-5860
Cleveland, OH 44195-0001   800-223-2273
                                   Fax: 216-445-1022
                                   TTY: 216-444-0261
                              my.clevelandclinic.org
Accredited by the American Academy of Sleep Medicine the Cleveland Clinic Sleep Disorders Center is staffed by physicians specializing in sleep disorders from a variety of disciplines including adult and child neurology pulmonary and critical care medicine psychology psychiatry otolaryngology and dentistry.
Nancy Foldva Schaefer DO, Director
Petra Podmor RPSGT, Laboratory Manager

7794 **Sleep Disorders Center: Community Medical Center**
1822 Mulberry Street   717-969-8931
Scranton, PA 18510-2375
John Goodnow, Director

7795 **Sleep Disorders Center: Crozer-Chester Medical Center**
Sleep Disorders Center
175 E Chester Pike   610-447-2689
Ridley Park, PA 19078-3975   www.crozer.org
A multidisciplinary facility for the investigation and treatment of sleep problems
Calvin Staff MD, Medical Director

7796 **Sleep Disorders Center: Good Samaritan Medical Center**
1020 Franklin Street   814-533-1661
Johnstown, PA 15905-4109
Richard Parc DO, Director

7797 **Sleep Disorders Center: Kettering Medical Center**
3935 Southern Boulevard   937-395-8805
Kettering, OH 45439-1295   Fax: 937-395-8821
                              www.kmcnetwork.org
Donna Arand PhD, Clinical Director
George G Burton MD, Medical Director

7798 **Sleep Disorders Center: Medical College of Pennsylvania**
3200 Henry Avenue   215-842-4250
Philadelphia, PA 19129-1137
June M Fry MD PhD, Director

7799 **Sleep Disorders Center: Newark Beth Israel Medical Center**
201 Lyons Avenue at Osborne Terrace   973-926-2973
Newark, NJ 07112-2027   www.sbhcs.com
Evaluates a wide range of disorders including sleep apnea snoring insomnia narcolepsy sleep-wake schedule disorders and male impotency. The center also provides board-certified consultants in sleep medicine neurology urology endocrinology psychiatry cardiology and ear nose and throat surgery in addition to certified sleep technologists.
Monroe S Karetzky MD

7800 **Sleep Disorders Center: Rhode Island Hospital**
70 Catamore Boulevard 401-431-5420
E Providence, RI 02914 Fax: 401-431-5429
www.lifespan.org
Richard Mill MD, Director

7801 **Sleep Disorders Center: St. Vincent Medical Center**
2213 Cherry Street 419-321-4980
Toledo, OH 43608-2691
Joseph Schaf PhD, Director

7802 **Sleep Disorders Center: University Hospital, SUNY at Stony Brook**
240 Middle Country Road 631-444-2500
Smithtown, NY 11787-0001 Fax: 631-444-2580
Wallace Mend MD

7803 **Sleep Disorders Center: Winthrop, University Hospital**
259 First Street 516-663-0333
Mineola, NY 11501-3808 www.winthrop.org
Steven H Feinsilver MD

7804 **Sleep Disorders Unit Beth Israel Deaconess Medical Center**
330 Brookline Avenue 617-667-3237
Boston, MA 02215-5400 www.bidmc.org
Jean K Matheson MD

7805 **Sleep Laboratory St Joseph's Hospital**
St Joseph's Hospital
301 Prospect Ave 315-703-2138
Syracuse, NY 13203 888-785-6371
Fax: 315-755-77
www.sjhsyr.org
The Sleep Lab focuses on diagnosing and treating Obstructive Sleep Apnea and sleep-related breathing disorders and has the largest number of sleep-credentialed physicians and registered sleep technologists of any sleep lab in the area.
Edward T Downing, Director

7806 **Sleep Laboratory, Maine Medical Center**
22 Bramhall Street 207-871-2279
Portland, ME 04102-3134

7807 **Sleep Medicine Associates of Texas**
5477 Glen Lakes Drive 214-750-7776
Dallas, TX 13210-4353 Fax: 214-750-4621
www.sleepmed.com
First largest and longest standing accredited sleep center in North Texas.
Philipp Becker, President and Founding Partner
Andrew O Jamieson MD, Chairman of the Board and Founding Partn

7808 **Sleep Research Foundation**
170 Morton Street 617-522-9270
Boston, MA 02130-3735
Ernest Hartm MD, Director

7809 **Sleep Wake Disorders Center Montefiore Sleep Disorders Center**
111 E 210th Street 718-920-4321
Bronx, NY 10467-2401 Fax: 718-798-4352
www.montefiore.org
Provide outstanding clinical care for patients with disorders that affect the sleep-wake cycle and are committed to performing high quality research and to making outstanding contributions to the areas of clinical research that includes the entire spectrum of sleep medicine.
Michael J Thorpy MD, Director
Karen Ballab MD, Associate Director

7810 **Sleep and Chronobiology Center: Western Psychiatric Institute and Clinic**
3811 Ohara Street 412-624-2246
Pittsburgh, PA 15213-2593
Charles F Reynolds III MD, Director

7811 **Sleep-Wake Disorders Center: New York Hospital-Cornell Medical Center**
520 E 70th Street 212-746-2623
New York, NY 10021-1504 Fax: 212-746-5509
www.weillcornell.org
Charles Poll MD, Director

7812 **Sleep/Wake Disorders Center: Community Hospitals of Indianapolis**
1500 N Ritter Avenue 317-355-4275
Indianapolis, IN 46219-3027 Fax: 317-351-2785
Marvin E Vollmer MD

7813 **Sleep/Wake Disorders Center: Hampstead Hospital**
E Road 603-329-5311
Hampstead, NH 03841
Deborah Sewi PhD

7814 **Stanford University Center for Narcolepsy Dept of Psychiatry & Behavioral Sciences**
450 Broadway Street 650-725-6517
Redwood City, CA 94063-5102 Fax: 650-498-7761
med.stanford.edu
Dr Emanuel Mignot, Director
Marlene Iry, Admin Associate

7815 **Thomas Jefferson University: Sleep Disorders Center**
Jefferson Medical College
1020 Walnut Street 215-955-6000
Philadelphia, PA 19107-5083 800-JEF-FNOW
Fax: 215-955-9783
www.jefferson.edu
A comprehensive clinical research and educational program in sleep and sleep disorders medicine.
Karl Doghram MD, Medical Director

7816 **University of Texas Sleep/Wake Disorders Center**
Southwestern Medical Center
5323 Harry Hines Boulevard 214-648-7350
Dallas, TX 75390-9070 Fax: 214-487-59
Studies sleep/wake disorders including insomnia apnea and narcolepsy.
Howard Roffw MD, Director

Support Groups & Hotlines

7817 **Narcolepsy Institute/Montefiore Medical Center**
111 E 210th Street 718-920-6799
Bronx, NY 10467-2490 Fax: 718-654-9580
MGoswami@aol.com
www.narcolepsyinstitute.org
The Narcolepsy Institute provides psychosocial support services for narcolepsy.
Dr. Meeta Goswami, Director

7818 **Narcolepsy Network**
129 Waterwheel Lane 401-667-2523
North Kingstown, RI 02852 888-292-6522
Fax: 401-633-6567
narnet@narcolepsynetwork.org
www.narcolepsynetwork.org
Provides advocacy and education, supports research. Newsletter, conferences, phone support and group development guidelines.
Patricia Higgins, President
Eveline V. Honig, Md, MPh, Executive Director

7819 **National Health Information Center**
Office of Disease Prevention & Health Promotion
1101 Wootton Pkwy Fax: 240-453-8281
Rockville, MD 20852 odphpinfo@hhs.gov
www.health.gov/nhic
Supports public health education by maintaining a calendar of National Health Observances; helps connect consumers and health professionals to organizations that can best answer questions and provide up-to-date contact information from reliable sources; updates on a yearly basis toll-free numbers for health information, Federal health clearinghouses and info centers.
Don Wright, MD, MPH, Director

Books

7820 ABC of ZZZs
National Sleep Foundation
1010 N. Glebe Road   703-243-1697
Arlington, VA 22201-1235   Fax: 202-347-3472
nsf@sleepfoundation.org
www.sleepfoundation.org
A primer on sleep basics, including getting enough sleep, why
sleep is important, and ' sleep stealers.'
Charles A. Czeisler, Chairman
Max Hirshkowitz, Vice Chairman

7821 Doctor, I Can't Sleep: Insomnia Training Manual
Narcolepsy Network
1010 N. Glebe Road   703-243-1697
Arlington, VA 22201-0460   Fax: 513-891-9936
nsf@sleepfoundation.org
www.sleepfoundation.org
Comprehensive course manual for primary care physicians and the
public. Outlines basic facts about epidemiology, sleep hygiene, relaxation techniques, diagnosis, and treatment.
100+ pages
Charles A. Czeisler, Chairman
Max Hirshkowitz, Vice Chairman

7822 International Classification of Sleep Disorders
American Academy of Sleep Medicine
2510 North Frontage Road   630-737-9700
Darien, IL 60561   Fax: 630-737-9790
www.aasmnet.org
A comprehensive manual for physicians and other healthcare professionals containing information on 84 sleep disorders. The extensive text describes the diagnostic features of each disorder and
includes specific diagnostic and severity criteria for each disorder.
396 pages Paperback
Timothy I. Morgenthaler, President
Nathaniel F. Watson, President-Elect

7823 Living with Narcolepsy
National Sleep Foundation
1010 N. Glebe Road   703-243-1697
Arlington, VA 22201-1235   Fax: 513-891-9936
nsf@sleepfoundation.org
www.sleepfoundation.org
Defines and describes narcolepsy and what can be expected after
diagnosis, including effects on education, career, social and family
life.
Charles A. Czeisler, Chairman
Max Hirshkowitz, Vice Chairman

7824 Melatonin: The Basic Facts
National Sleep Foundation
1010 N. Glebe Road   703-243-1697
Arlington, VA 22201-1235   Fax: 513-891-9936
nsf@sleepfoundation.org
www.sleepfoundation.org
If you're curious about melatonin, it's not suprising. There has
been a lot of attention paid to the hormone in popular magazines
and books, scholarly journals, and advertisements. You may habe
heard claims that malatonin cures everything from jet lag to insomnia to aging.
Charles A. Czeisler, Chairman
Max Hirshkowitz, Vice Chairman

7825 Narcolepsy Primer
Meeta Goswami, Michael Thorpy, author
Narcolepsy Institute/Montefiore Medical Center
111 E 210th Street   718-920-6799
Bronx, NY 10467-2401   Fax: 718-654-9580
MGsowami@aol.com
narcolepsyinstitute.org
A guide for physicians, patients and their families on the affects,
causes and prevention of narcolepsy.
Dr. Meeta Goswami, Director

7826 Narcolepsy Primer Package
Meeta Goswami, Michael Thorpy, author
Narcolepsy Institute/Montefiore Medical Center

111 E 210th Street   718-920-6799
Bronx, NY 10467-2401   Fax: 718-654-9580
MGsowami@aol.com
narcolepsyinstitute.org
The package includes: Narcolepsy Primer; Manuel on Narcolepsy
and A Counseling Service for Narcolepsy: A Sociomedical Model.
Dr. Meeta Goswami, Director

7827 Pain and Sleep
National Sleep Foundation
1010 N. Glebe Road   703-243-1697
Arlington, VA 22201-1235   Fax: 513-891-9936
nsf@sleepfoundation.org
www.sleepfoundation.org
Whether pain results from headache, backache, arthritis, or other
conditions, it frequently occurs with sleep difficulty. This overview of the pain and sleep connection describes behavioral and
pharmacological approaches to pain management.
Charles A. Czeisler, Chairman
Max Hirshkowitz, Vice Chairman

**7828 Sleep Aids: Everything You Wanted To Know But Were Too
Tired To Ask**
National Sleep Foundation
1010 N. Glebe Road   703-243-1697
Arlington, VA 22201-1235   Fax: 513-891-9936
nsf@sleepfoundation.org
www.sleepfoundation.org
If you have trouble falling or staying asleep, or you wake up feeling unrefreshed, you may be suffering from insomnia. Insomnia is
a symptom. It may be caused by stress, anxiety, depression, disease, pain, medications, sleep disorders or poor sleep habits.
Charles A. Czeisler, Chairman
Max Hirshkowitz, Vice Chairman

7829 Sleep Apnea
National Sleep Foundation
1010 N. Glebe Road   703-243-1697
Arlington, VA 22201-1235   Fax: 513-891-9936
nsf@sleepfoundation.org
www.sleepfoundation.org
A brochure about sleep apnea, a breathing disorder characterized
by brief interruptions of breathing during sleep. Brochure explains
what it is, who gets it, and how it is diagnosed and treated.
Charles A. Czeisler, Chairman
Max Hirshkowitz, Vice Chairman

7830 Snoring and Sleep Apnea
Demos Medical Publishing
11 West 42nd Street   212-683-0072
New York, NY 10036   Fax: 212-683-0118
A straightforward, jargon-free approach to dealing with snoring
and sleep problems.
222 pages
ISBN: 1-888799-29-3
Dr. Diana M Schneider, President

**7831 You Don't LOOK Sick!: Living Well with Invisible Chronic
Illness**
Joy Selak, Steven Overman, author
Haworth Press
10 Alice Street   607-722-5857
Binghamton, NY 13904-1580   800-429-6784
Fax: 607-722-0012
www.haworthpress.com
Chronicles a patient's true-life stories and her physician's compas-
sionate commentary as they take a journey through the three stages
of chronic illness - Getting Sick, Being Sick, and Living Well.
Hardcover $29.95 (ISBN): 978-0-7890-2488-0, Paperback $14.95
(ISBN): 978-0-7890-2499-7.
145 pages Hrdcover/Ppbck

Magazines

7832 SleepMatters
National Sleep Foundation

1010 N. Glebe Road
Arlington, VA 22201-1235

703-243-1697
Fax: 513-891-9936
nsf@sleepfoundation.org
www.sleepfoundation.org

Covering hot sleep news, profiles, advice from experts and much more!
Quarterly
Charles A. Czeisler, Chairman
Max Hirshkowitz, Vice Chairman

Newsletters

7833 Eye Opener
American Narcolepsy Association
425 Cal Strt, Suite 201
San Francisco, CA 94126-6230

415-788-4793

Offers information on sleep disorders including a question and answer column for persons suffering from disorders.

7834 Narcolepsy Institute/Montefiore Medical Center
Meeta Goswami, author
Narcolepsy Institute
111 E 210th Street
Bronx, NY 10467-2490

718-920-6799
Fax: 718-654-9580
MGsowami@aol.com
narcolepsyinstitute.org

The Narcolepsy Institute provides psychosocial support services for narcolepsy and has a newsletter, a video, and a primer on narcolepsy.
8 pages Bi-Annual
Dr. Meeta Goswami, Director

7835 Sleep Medicine Alert
Nationa Sleep Foundation
1010 N. Glebe Road
Arlington, VA 22201-1235

703-243-1697
Fax: 513-891-9936
nsf@sleepfoundation.org
www.sleepfoundation.org

This quearterly newsletter is for healthcare professionals. It offers updates on sleep research and its clinical implications, information on diagnosing and treating a variety of sleep disorders.
Charles A. Czeisler, Chairman
Max Hirshkowitz, Vice Chairman

7836 Wake-Up Call
American Sleep Apnea Association
1717 Penn Ave, NW
Washington, DC 20006

202-293-3650
888-293-3650
Fax: 202-293-3656
asaa@sleepapnea.org
www.sleepapnea.org

Contains information of interest to APNEA patients and their families.
Quarterly
Michael P Coppola MD, President and Chief Medical Officer
Nancy Rothstein, Secretary

Pamphlets

7837 Get the Facts About Sleep Apnea
American Sleep Apnea Association
1717 Penn Ave, NW
Washington, DC 20006

202-293-3650
888-293-3650
Fax: 202-293-3656
asaa@sleepapnea.org
www.sleepapnea.org

7838 Helping Yourself to a Good Night's Sleep
Nantional Sleep Foundation
1010 N. Glebe Road
Arlington, VA 22201-1253

703-243-1697
Fax: 513-891-9936
nsf@sleepfoundation.org
www.sleepfoundation.org

About half of Americans report sleep difficulty at least occasionally, according to National Sleep Foundation surveys. These woes-

called insomnia by doctors-have far reaching effects. This brochure details the many things you can do to improve your sleep.
Charles A. Czeisler, Chairman
Max Hirshkowitz, Vice Chairman

7839 Narcolepsy
American Academy of Sleep Medicine
2510 North Frontage Road
Darien, IL 60561

630-737-9700
Fax: 630-737-9790
www.aasmnet.org

Describes the causes, symptoms and treatments of a disorder characterized by excessive sleepiness.
Lot of 50
Timothy I. Morgenthaler, President
Nathaniel F. Watson, President-Elect

7840 Sleep Diary
National Sleep Foundation
1010 N. Glebe Road
Arlington, VA 22201-1235

703-243-1697
Fax: 513-891-9936
nsf@sleepfoundation.org
www.sleepfoundation.org

It includes sections on sleep schedules, quality and quantity of sleep, sleep disturbances, sleep hygiene and daytime sleepiness. It enables people to identify their sleep and health habits and note any sleep problems they may have.
Charles A. Czeisler, Chairman
Max Hirshkowitz, Vice Chairman

7841 Sleep Strategies for Shift Workers
National Sleep Foundation
1010 N. Glebe Road
Arlington, VA 22201-1235

703-243-1697
Fax: 513-891-9936
nsf@sleepfoundation.org
www.sleepfoundation.org

This brochure outlines the common effects of shift work on health, workplace alertness and productivity and offers tips about diet, sleep environment, medications, light therapy and sleep hygiene.
Charles A. Czeisler, Chairman
Max Hirshkowitz, Vice Chairman

7842 Wake Up! Brochure
National Sleep Foundation
1010 N. Glebe Road
Arlington, VA 22201-1235

703-243-1697
Fax: 513-891-9936
nsf@sleepfoundation.org
www.sleepfoundation.org

A blooklet dedicated to the drowsy driving problem, including the risks, the myths, the danger signals and recommendations.
Charles A. Czeisler, Chairman
Max Hirshkowitz, Vice Chairman

7843 When You Can't Sleep
Narcolepsy Network
1010 N. Glebe Road
Arlington, VA 22201-0460

703-243-1697
888-292-6522
Fax: 513-891-9936
nsf@sleepfoundation.org
www.sleepfoundation.org

A primer on sleep basics, including getting enough sleep, why sleep is important, and sleep stealers. Plus a sleep quotient quiz.
Charles A. Czeisler, Chairman
Max Hirshkowitz, Vice Chairman

7844 Women and Sleep
National Sleep Foundation
1010 N. Glebe Road
Arlington, VA 22201-1235

703-243-1697
Fax: 513-891-9936
nsf@sleepfoundation.org
www.sleepfoundation.org

A brochure dealing with the effects of sleep on women which explores reasons for tiredness, increased accidents, problems concentrating, and poor performance on the job and in school, and possible increased sickness.
Charles A. Czeisler, Chairman
Max Hirshkowitz, Vice Chairman

Audio & Video

7845 Narcolepsy
American Academy of Sleep Medicine
2510 North Frontage Road
Darien, IL 60561
630-737-9700
Fax: 630-737-9790
www.aasmnet.org
Addresses the etiology, pathophysiology, diagnosis and management of narcolepsy.
58 slides
Timothy I. Morgenthaler, President
Nathaniel F. Watson, President-Elect

7846 Narcolepsy: Fanlight Productions
Jason Margolis, author
Fanlight Productions
4196 Washington Street
Boston, MA 02131-1731
617-469-4999
800-937-4113
Fax: 617-469-3379
fanlight@fanlight.com
www.fanlight.com
This remarkable film presents the experiences of three individuals whose lives and relationships have been disrupted by narcolepsy.
2000 25 Minutes
ISBN: 1-572953-23-2

7847 Video on Narcolepsy
Narcolepsy Institute/Montefiore Medical Center
111 E 210th Street
Bronx, NY 10467
718-920-6799
Fax: 718-654-9580
MGsowami@aol.com
Clinical symptoms, genetics, diagnosis, effects of Narcolepsy, support groups.
Dr. Meeta Goswami, Director

Web Sites

7848 American Sleep Apnea Association
The American Sleep Apnea Association, founded in 1990, is a 501(c)(3) nonprofit organization that promotes awareness of sleep apnea, works for continuing improvements in treatments for this serious disorder, and advocates for the interests of sleep apnea patients.

7849 American Sleep Disorders Association
Provides full diagnostic and treatment services to improve the quality of care for patients with all types of sleep disorders.

7850 Healing Well
www.healingwell.com
An online health resource guide to medical news, chat, information and articles, newsgroups and message boards, books, disease-related web sites, medical directories, and more for patients, friends, and family coping with disabling diseases, disorders, or chronic illnesses.

7851 Health Finder
www.healthfinder.gov
Searchable, carefully developed web site offering information on over 1000 topics. Developed by the US Department of Health and Human Services, the site can be used in both English and Spanish.

7852 Healthlink USA
www.healthlinkusa.com
Health information concerning treatment, cures, prevention, diagnosis, risk factors, research, support groups, email lists, personal stories and much more. Updated regularly.

7853 MGH Neurology WebForums
Online. Provides both unmoderated message boards and chat rooms for specific neurological disorders.

7854 MedicineNet
www.medicinenet.com
An online resource for consumers providing easy-to-read, authoritative medical and health information.

7855 Medscape
www.medscape.com
Medscape offers specialists, primary care physicians, and other health professionals the Web's most robust and integrated medical information and educational tools.

7856 National Sleep Foundation
www.sleepfoundation.org
Information for millions of Americans who suffer from sleep disorders, and to prevent the catastrophic accidents that are related to poor or disordered sleep through research, education and the dissemination of information.

7857 Neurology Channel
www.healthcommunities.com
Find clearly explained, medically accurate information regarding conditions, including an overview, symptoms, causes, diagnostic procedures and treatment options. On this site it is possible to ask questions and get information from a neurologist and connect to people who have similar health interests.

7858 Sleep Research Society
www.sleepresearchsociety.org
Facilitates communication among research workers in this field, but does not sponsor research investigations on its own.

7859 WebMD
www.webmd.com
Provides credible information, supportive communities, and in-depth reference material about health subjects. A source for original and timely health information as well as material from well known content providers.

Description

7860 Spina Bifida

Spina bifida refers to conditions which result in an incomplete closure of the spinal column during the first few weeks of embryonic development. It is the most serious of a group of disorders called neural tube defects and occurs in one of every 2,00 live births. Most cases are sporadic, but a small percentage of cases run in families. The severity of spina bifida ranges from mild to severe.

Spina bifida is a complex condition that results from a complex interplay between multiple genetic and environmental factors. Mutations in the MTHFR (methylene tetrahydrofolate reductase) gene increase the risk of spina bifida. Maternal risk factors include diabetes mellitus, obesity, exposure to high temperatures during the early stages of pregnancy, and the use of antiseizure medications, such as valproic acid and carbamazepine.

Spina bifida occulta is an opening in one or more vertebrae without damage to the spinal cord. Meningocele is when the protective covering around the spinal cord (meninges) has protruded into the vertebrae, with little, if any, damage. Myelomeningocele, the most severe form of spina bifida, is when part of the actual spinal cord pushes through the back and exposes nerves and tissues.

The effects of spina bifida, in its most extreme state, are serious. They can include paralysis, loss of bowel and bladder control and hydrocephalus. Other inherited abnormalities may be present. Open spina bifida can be diagnosed in utero by finding elevations of a specific protein in maternal amniotic fluid. Prevention involves supplementation with folic acid. Treatments for spina bifida require a united effort by a team of specialists, and depend on the severity of the defects. With proper care, many children with spina bifida live fairly normal lives. See also *Birth Defects*.

National Agencies & Associations

7861 Canadian & American Spinal Research Organizations
90 Eglinton Avenue E
Toronto, Ontario, M4P-2Y3
905-508-4000
info@csro.com
www.csro.com
Dedicated to improving quality of life for individuals with spinal cord injuries and those with related neurological deficits, through research.
Barry Munro, Chair
Dave Lostchuk, Treasurer

7862 Easterseals
141 W Jackson Blvd
Chicago, IL 60604
312-726-6200
800-221-6827
Fax: 312-726-1494
info@easterseals.com
www.easterseals.com
Provides services to children and adults with disabilities as well as support to their families.
Angela F. Williams, President & CEO
Sharon Watson, Vice President, Communications/Marketing

7863 Spina Bifida Association of America
1600 Wilson Boulevard
Arlington, VA 22209
202-944-3285
800-621-3141
sbaa@sbaa.org
www.spinabifidaassociation.org
Advocates for research for the benefit of individuals living with Spina Bifida, and educates the community.
Nicole Gower, Chair
Maria Bournias, Secretary & Treasurer

7864 Spina Bifida and Hydrocephalus Association of Canada
472-167 Lombard Avenue
Winnipeg, Manitoba, R3B-0T6
204-925-3650
800-565-9488
Fax: 204-925-3654
info@sbhac.ca
www.sbhac.ca
Conducts research, promotes awareness, and educates in order to reduce the rate of neural tube defects. Provides support to families affected by spina bifida.
Susana Scott, President
Lorelai Fletcher, Vice President

State Agencies & Associations

Alabama

7865 Spina Bifida Association of Alabama
PO Box 13254
Birmingham, AL 35202-0538
256-617-1414
info@sbaofal.org
www.sbaofal.org
Betsy Hopson, President
Steven Horne, Vice President

Arizona

7866 Spina Bifida Association of Arizona
1001 E Fairmount Avenue
Phoenix, AZ 85014-4806
602-274-3323
Fax: 602-274-7632
www.sbaaz.org
Benjaman D Scanlan, President
Ron Whiteside, Treasurer

California

7867 Spina Bifida Association of Greater San Diego
PO Box 232272
San Diego, CA 92193-2272
619-491-9018
Fax: 619-275-3361
sbaofgsd@hotmail.com
www.spinabifidasandiego.com
Erika Jorquera, President

Colorado

7868 Spina Bifida Association of Colorado
PO Box 22994
Denver, CO 80222-0994
303-797-7870
Fax: 303-730-8032
sbacolorado@gmail.com
www.coloradospinabifida.org
Chris Mestas, Chairman
Lavon Birney, Executive Director

Connecticut

7869 Spina Bifida Association of Connecticut
370 Osgood Avenue
New Britain, CT 06053-2545
860-839-0115
800-574-6274
Fax: 860-832-6260
www.sbac.org
Mary Attardo, President
Kiley J Carlson, Executive Director

Spina Bifida / State Agencies & Associations

Delaware

7870 Spina Bifida Association of Delaware
PO Box 807
Wilmington, DE 19899-0807
302-478-4805
kbasar@aol.com
www.angelfire.com/de/sbaofde/

Blake Heath, Vice President
Andy Anderso Jr, Treasurer

Florida

7871 Spina Bifida Association of Florida Space Coast
100 W Lucerne Circle
Orlando, FL 32801-2549
407-248-9210
Fax: 321-454-9737
www.sbacentralflorida.org

Rob Roy, Chairman
Melisa Portnoy, Secretary

7872 Spina Bifida Association of Jacksonville
807 Childrens Way
Jacksonville, FL 32207-8426
904-697-3686
800-722-6355
Fax: 904-390-3466
www.sbaj.org

Michael Erhard, Chairperson

7873 Spina Bifida Association of Tampa
100 W Lucerne Circle
Orlando, FL 32801-1038
407-248-9210
Fax: 813-872-9845
sbatampabay@aol.com

Dianne Gore, President

Georgia

7874 Spina Bifida Association of Georgia
1448 Mclendon Drive
Decatur, GA 30033
770-939-1044
Fax: 770-939-1049
info@spinabifidaga.org
www.spinabifidaofgeorgia.org

Provides referrals, evaluation, treatment and therapeutic activities for children and teens afflicted with spina bifida. The goal of this center is to help children or teenagers prepare for life.

William Turnispeed, President
Judy Thibadeau, Vice President

Illinois

7875 Illinois Spina Bifida Association
8765 W Higgins Road
Chicago, IL 60631-1693
773-444-0305
800-969-4722
Fax: 630-637-1066
info@i-sba.org
www.sbail.org

Dedicated to improving the quality of life of people with spina bifida through direct services, information and referral and public awareness. Direct services include a residential summer camp for children with spina bifida over the age of seven.

Scott J Munkvold, President
Amy Maggio, CEO

Indiana

7876 Spina Bifida Association of Central Indiana
PO Box 19814
Indianapolis, IN 46279-0814
317-592-1630
Fax: 317-351-2010
pres@sbaci.org
www.sbaci.org

James Zetzl, President

Iowa

7877 Spina Bifida Association of Iowa
8525 Douglas Avenue
Urbandale, IA 50322-1456
515-278-7013
contact@sbaia.org
www.spinabifidaia.com

Rod Tressel, President

Kentucky

7878 Spina Bifida Association of Kentucky
Kosair Charities Center

982 Eastern Parkway
Louisville, KY 40217-1568
502-637-7363
866-340-7225
Fax: 502-637-1010
sbak@sbak.org
www.sbak.org

Angela Cosby, President
Patty Dissell, Executive Director

Louisiana

7879 Spina Bifida Association of Greater New Orleans
PO Box 1346
Kenner, LA 70063-1346
504-737-5181
Fax: 504-538-9046
sbagno@sbagno.com
www.sbagno.org

Al Hitt, President
Judy Otto, Vice-President

Maryland

7880 Spina Bifida Association of Maryland
2416 Lampost Lane
Baltimore, MD 21234-1460
410-665-1543
Fax: 410-833-1700
sbamaryland@comcast.net

7881 Spina Bifida Association of the Eastern Shore
316 Prospect Avenue
Easton, MD 21601-4046
410-822-8609
Fax: 410-822-5455
www.spinabifidaassociation.org

Massachusetts

7882 Spina Bifida Association of Massachusetts
321 Fortune Boulevard
Milford, MA 01757-2741
617-742-2574
888-479-1900
Fax: 978-649-8725

Brendan Sullivan, President
Cara Packard, Vice President

Michigan

7883 Spina Bifida Association of Grand Rapids
235 Wealthy Street SE
Grand Rapids, MI 49503-5299
616-240-9672
Fax: 616-222-1541
WMiSBA@hotmail.com
www.spinabifida.org

Carol Carpenter, President

7884 Spina Bifida Association of Upper Peninsula Michigan
1220 N 3rd Street
Ishpeming, MI 44849-1108
906-485-5127
Fax: 906-225-7230
cbengson@nmu.edu

Lois Bengson, President

7885 Spina Bifida and Hydrocephalus Association of Southwestern Michigan
PO Box 212
Mattawan, MI 49071-0212
269-385-3959
Fax: 269-392-9765
marenhorkness@yahoo.com

Richard Benthnin, President

Minnesota

7886 Spina Bifida Association of Minnesota
PO Box 29323
Minneapolis, MN 55429-0212
651-222-6395
Fax: 952-591-0246
sbamn@hotmail.com

Wendy Swanson, President
Jim Thayer, Executive Director

Missouri

7887 Spina Bifida Association of Greater St. Louis
8050 Watson Road
Saint Louis, MO 63119-2000
314-843-2244
800-784-0983
Fax: 314-353-1446
www.sbstl.com

Mark Abbott, President

Cara Packard, Vice President

Nebraska

7888 Spina Bifida Association of Nebraska
7612 Maple Street
Omaha, NE 68134-2153
LeAnn Karman, President
402-932-5826
Fax: 402-572-3002

New Jersey

7889 Spina Bifida Association of the Tri-State Region
84 Park Avenue
Flemington, NJ 08822-1174
908-782-7475
877-722-8774
Fax: 908-782-6102
info@thesbrn.org
Serves New Jersey, New York Metro Area and Southern Connecticut.
Jane Horowitz, Executive Director and President
K David Holmes, Chairman of the Board

New Mexico

7890 Spina Bifida Association of New Mexico
1127 University Boulevard NE
Albuquerque, NM 87102-1740
505-242-1184
Rey Garduno, Executive Director
Ann Beddingfield, Interim Treasurer

New York

7891 Spina Bifida Association of Albany/Capital District
100 Spring
Scotia, NY 12302-3312
518-399-9151
sbaalbany102@aol.com
Kevin Chamberlain, Co-President
Vanessa Chamberlain, Co-President

7892 Spina Bifida Association of Greater Rochester
PO Box 3
Fairport, NY 14450-0003
585-381-5471
Fax: 585-264-9547
jarmst4459@aol.com
JoAnn Armstrong, President

7893 Spina Bifida Association of Nassau County
12 Hampton Road
Sound Beach, NY 11789
631-821-9028
kid3418@optonline.net
www.spinabifidaassociation.org
Leslieann Sussman, President

North Carolina

7894 Spina Bifida Association of North Carolina
3915 Grace Court
Indian Trail, NC 28079
704-882-0988
800-847-2262
Fax: 704-882-0988
sbanc@mindspring.com
www.spinabifidaassociation.org
Julie Yindra, President
Kin Gates, Executive Director

Ohio

7895 Spina Bifida Association of Canton
S Cherokee Trail
Malvern, OH 44644
330-863-2531
Fax: 330-863-1172
www.spinabifidasupport.com
Connie Griffin, President

7896 Spina Bifida Association of Central Ohio
7239 Upper Cambridge Way
Westerville, OH 43082
614-818-3840
Laurie Schulze, Treasurer
Chrissy Zepfel, President

7897 Spina Bifida Association of Cincinnati
644 Linn Street
Cincinnati, OH 45203-0152
513-923-1378
www.sbacincy.org
Brady Sellet, President
Diane Burns, Executive Director

7898 Spina Bifida Association of Greater Dayton
4801 Springfield Street
Dayton, OH 45431
937-236-1122
Fax: 937-434-4899
mvspinabifida@yahoo.com
David Skinner, President
Lisa Maas, Vice President

7899 Spina Bifida Association of Northwest Ohio
302 Conant St
Maumee, OH 43537
419-794-0561
Fax: 419-533-3952
Ginnette Clark, President
Julie Harley, Vice President

Pennsylvania

7900 Spina Bifida Association of Central Pennsylvania
209 E State Street
Quarryville, PA 17566-1242
717-786-9280
888-770-SBPA
Fax: 717-786-8821
SBAofPA@aol.com
Patricia Fulvio, President
Amy Graver, Chairman

7901 Spina Bifida Association of Delaware Valley
Havertown, PA 19083-0289
610-584-5530
800-223-0222
Fax: 215-412-9396
info@sbadv.org
www.sbadv.org
Spina Bifida is the most common permanently disabling birth defect in the United States. An average of 8 babies every day are born with Spina Bifida or a similar birth defect of the brain and spine. There are over 60 million women in the U.S. who could become pregnant and each one is at risk of having a baby born with Spina Bifida. The mission of the Spina Bifida Association of Delaware Valley is to promote the prevention of Spina Bifida and to enhance the lives of all affected.
Marilyn Lieb, President
Keri Mascaro, Executive Director

7902 Spina Bifida Association of Greater Pennsylvania
209 E State Street
Quarryville, PA 17566-9614
717-786-9280
Fax: 717-786-8821
sbaofpa@aol.com
www.spinabifidaresource.weebly.com
The Spina Bifida Resource was started in the 1970's, when a group of Moms met while their children had therapy. As the needs and issues were discussed, the group decided to band together for support. Thus the Spina Bifida Association of Lancaster County was born. Our first public meeting had 45 parents and concerned professionals in attendance. After about 20 years, the Board felt the need to change our name to reflect all those we served in and around Pennsylvania. Thus we became the Spina
Amy Graver, President
Patricia Fulvio, Executive Director

Rhode Island

7903 Spina Bifida Association of Rhode Island
Warwick, RI 02887-6948
401-732-7862
Fax: 401-732-7862
www.spinabifidaassociation.org

Tennessee

7904 Spina Bifida Association of Tennessee
Nashville, TN 37202-5529
615-791-8117
Fax: 615-791-1518
lynnhess56@comcast.net
www.spinabifidasupport.com
Lynn Cook, President

Texas

7905 Spina Bifida Association of Austin
9301 Bradner Drive
Austin, TX 78748
512-292-6317
Fax: 512-479-3845
austinspinabifida@yahoo.com
www.spinabifidasupport.com
Kelley Hively, President

7906   Spina Bifida Association of Dallas
705 W Avenue B   972-238-8755
Garland, TX 75040   Fax: 972-414-3772
                                          sbdal@aol.com
                                          www.sbdallas.org

Robin Lee, President*
Ryan McCoy, Vice President

7907   Spina Bifida Association of Texas, Gulf Coast
440 Benmar   281-447-2707
Houston, TX 77060-2460   Fax: 281-997-2278
                                fandfsports@sbcglobal.net
                                          www.sbahgc.org

The mission of Spina Bifida Houston Gulf Coast is to promote public awareness and enrich the lives of individuals and families living with spina bifida.
Jennifer Franklin, Vice President
Joan Peck, Treasurer

Washington

7908   Spina Bifida Association of Washington State
611 2nd Street   253-589-3700
Snohomish, WA 98290   888-289-3702
                                     Fax: 775-766-1654
                                         sbaws@yahoo.com
                                          www.sbaws.org

The Spina Bifida Association of Washington State is an affiliated chapter of the national Spina Bifida Association.
Jason Lane, Chair
Ryan Callaway, Director

Wisconsin

7909   Spina Bifida Association of Northern Wisconsin
Schofield, WI 54476-0421   715-798-3944
David Blanchard, President

7910   Spina Bifida Association of Southeastern Wisconsin
830 N 109th Street   414-607-9061
Wauwatosa, WI 53226   Fax: 414-607-9602
                                          www.sbawi.org

Spina Bifida occurs when the spine of the baby fails to close. This creates an opening, or lesion, on the spinal column. Because of the opening on the spinal column, the nerves in the spinal column may be damaged and not work properly. This results in some degree of paralysis. The higher the lesion is on the spinal column, the greater the likelihood of increased paralysis. Surgery to close the spine is generally done within hours after birth. The surgery helps reduce the risk of infection and pr
Karen Drzewiecki, President
David G. Tucker, MSW, Executive Director

7911   Spina Bifida Association of the Greater Fox Valley
325 N John Street   920-687-0801
Kimberly, WI 54136   fus1234@athenet.net
                                www.spinabifidasupport.com

Kelly Richard, President

Foundations

7912   March of Dimes Foundation
1550 Crystal Drive   888-663-4637
Arlington, VA 22202   www.marchofdimes.org
Seeks to improve the health of babies by preventing birth defects, premature birth, and infant mortality through programs of research, community services, education, and advocacy.
Stacey D. Stewart, President

Support Groups & Hotlines

7913   National Health Information Center
Office of Disease Prevention & Health Promotion
1101 Wootton Pkwy   Fax: 240-453-8281
Rockville, MD 20852   odphpinfo@hhs.gov
                                          www.health.gov/nhic

Supports public health education by maintaining a calendar of National Health Observances; helps connect consumers and health professionals to organizations that can best answer questions and provide up-to-date contact information from reliable sources; updates on a yearly basis toll-free numbers for health information, Federal health clearinghouses and info centers.
Don Wright, MD, MPH, Director

Books

7914   Answering Your Questions About Spina Bifida
Spina Bifida Association of America
1600 Wilson Blvd.   202-944-3285
Arlington, VA 22209-4226   800-621-3141
                                     Fax: 202-944-3295
                                          sbaa@sbaa.org
                                          www.sbaa.org

Provides information to help people understand the basic medical, educational and social issues which commonly affect people with Spina Bifida.
Megan Sorensen, Chair
Wilson Neyland, Chair-Elect

7915   Bowel Continence and Spina Bifida
Spina Bifida Association of America
1600 Wilson Blvd.   202-944-3285
Arlington, VA 22209-4226   800-621-3141
                                     Fax: 202-944-3295
                                          sbaa@sbaa.org
                                          www.sbaa.org

An excellent book aimed at anyone (infant or adult) trying to attain bowel continence. Focuses on continence programs, bowel management development and techniques.
Megan Sorensen, Chair
Wilson Neyland, Chair-Elect

7916   Clinic Directory
Spina Bifida Association of America
1600 Wilson Blvd.   202-944-3285
Arlington, VA 22209-4226   800-621-3141
                                     Fax: 202-944-3295
                                          sbaa@sbaa.org
                                          www.sbaa.org

A directory of health care clinics throughout the United States for children and adults with spina bifida.
200 pages 3-Ring Binder
Megan Sorensen, Chair
Wilson Neyland, Chair-Elect

7917   Complete IEP Guide: How to Advocate for Your Special Ed Child
Spina Bifida Association
1600 Wilson Blvd.   202-944-3285
Arlington, VA 22209-4226   800-621-3141
                                          sbaa@sbaa.org
                                          www.sbaa.org

This all-in-one guide will help you understand special education law, identify your child's needs, prepare for meetings, develop the IEP and resolve disputes.
Megan Sorensen, Chair
Wilson Neyland, Chair-Elect

7918   Confronting the Challenges of Spina Bifida
Spina Bifida Association of America
1600 Wilson Blvd.   202-944-3285
Arlington, VA 22209-4226   800-621-3141
                                     Fax: 202-944-3295
                                          sbaa@sbaa.org
                                          www.sbaa.org

A group curriculum addressing self-care, self-esteem, and social skills in 8 to 13 year olds.
Megan Sorensen, Chair
Wilson Neyland, Chair-Elect

7919   Healthcare Guidelines
Spina Bifida Association of America

1600 Wilson Blvd.
Arlington, VA 22209-4226

202-944-3285
800-621-3141
Fax: 202-944-3295
sbaa@sbaa.org
www.sbaa.org

Megan Sorensen, Chair
Wilson Neyland, Chair-Elect

7920 Learning Disabilities and the Person with Spina Bifida
Spina Bifida Association of America
1600 Wilson Blvd.
Arlington, VA 22209-4226

202-944-3285
800-621-3141
Fax: 202-944-3295
sbaa@sbaa.org
www.sbaa.org

Megan Sorensen, Chair
Wilson Neyland, Chair-Elect

7921 Negotiating the Special Education Maze: A Guide for Parents and Teachers
Spina Bifida Association
1600 Wilson Blvd.
Arlington, VA 22209-4226

202-944-3285
800-621-3141
sbaa@sbaa.org
www.sbaa.org

An excellent aid for the development of an effective special education program.
Megan Sorensen, Chair
Wilson Neyland, Chair-Elect

7922 New Language of Toys: Teaching Communication Skills to Children...
Spina Bifida Association
1600 Wilson Blvd.
Arlington, VA 22209-4226

202-944-3285
800-621-3141
sbaa@sbaa.org
www.sbaa.org

A guide for parents and teachers, this reader-friendly resource guide provides a wealth of information on how play activities affect a child's language development (with a focus on special needs) and where to get the toys and materials to use in these activities.
Megan Sorensen, Chair
Wilson Neyland, Chair-Elect

7923 Nick Joins In
Spina Bifida Association
1600 Wilson Blvd.
Arlington, VA 22209-4226

202-944-3285
800-621-3141
sbaa@sbaa.org
www.sbaa.org

When Nick, who is in a wheelchair, enters a regular classroom, for the first time he realizes that he has much to contribute.
Megan Sorensen, Chair
Wilson Neyland, Chair-Elect

7924 Princess Pooh
Spina Bifida Association
1600 Wilson Blvd.
Arlington, VA 22209-4226

202-944-3285
800-621-3141
sbaa@sbaa.org
www.sbaa.org

Jealous of her disabled sister's royal treatment as she sits on her throne with wheels, Patty Jean borrows it and discovers that life in a wheelchair isn't so easy.
Megan Sorensen, Chair
Wilson Neyland, Chair-Elect

7925 SBAA General Information Packet
Spina Bifida Association of America
1600 Wilson Blvd.
Arlington, VA 22209-4226

202-944-3285
800-621-3141
Fax: 202-944-3295
sbaa@sbaa.org
www.sbaa.org

Megan Sorensen, Chair
Wilson Neyland, Chair-Elect

7926 Sexuality and the Person with Spina Bifida
Spina Bifida Association of America

1600 Wilson Blvd.
Arlington, VA 22209-4226

202-944-3285
800-621-3141
Fax: 202-944-3295
sbaa@sbaa.org
www.sbaa.org

Focuses on sexuality, sexual development, sexual activity, and other important issues.
Megan Sorensen, Chair
Wilson Neyland, Chair-Elect

7927 Social Development and the Person with Spina Bifida
Spina Bifida Association of America
1600 Wilson Blvd.
Arlington, VA 22209-4226

202-944-3285
800-621-3141
Fax: 202-944-3295
sbaa@sbaa.org
www.sbaa.org

Megan Sorensen, Chair
Wilson Neyland, Chair-Elect

7928 Steps to Independence: Teaching Everyday Skills to Children with Special Needs
Spina Bifida Association
1600 Wilson Blvd.
Arlington, VA 22209-4226

202-944-3285
800-621-3141
sbaa@sbaa.org
www.sbaa.org

A guide to help parents teach life skills to their disabled child.
Megan Sorensen, Chair
Wilson Neyland, Chair-Elect

7929 Taking Charge
Spina Bifida Association of America
1600 Wilson Blvd.
Arlington, VA 22209-4226

202-944-3285
800-621-3141
Fax: 202-944-3295
sbaa@sbaa.org
www.sbaa.org

Teenagers talk about life and physical disabilities.
Megan Sorensen, Chair
Wilson Neyland, Chair-Elect

7930 Unlocking Potential: College and Other Choices for People with LD and AD/HD
Spina Bifida Association
1600 Wilson Blvd.
Arlington, VA 22209-4226

202-944-3285
800-621-3141
sbaa@sbaa.org
www.sbaa.org

An indispensible tool for high school students with learning disabilities and AD/HD. Includes a comprehensive listing of resources.
Megan Sorensen, Chair
Wilson Neyland, Chair-Elect

Children's Books

7931 Margaret's Moves
Dutton Children's Books
2620 S. 7th St
Louisville, KY 40216-3658

502-584-5234
Fax: 502-371-0615
info@margaretsmoving.com
margaretsmoving.com

This story deals with all the nuances and impairments that children afflicted with spina bifida must encounter and succeed in overcoming.
Grades 4-6

7932 Rolling Along with Goldilocks and the Three Bears
Spina Bifida Association
1600 Wilson Blvd.
Arlington, VA 22209-4226

202-944-3285
800-621-3141
sbaa@sbaa.org
www.sbaa.org

The familiar folktale with a special-needs twist.
Megan Sorensen, Chair
Wilson Neyland, Chair-Elect

7933 Views from Our Shoes: Growing Up with a Brother or Sister with Special Needs
Spina Bifida Association
1600 Wilson Blvd.   202-944-3285
Arlington, VA 22209-4226   800-621-3141
                                           sbaa@sbaa.org
                                           www.sbaa.org
A balanced view of the positives and negatives of living with a disabled sibling. Written for siblings ages nine and up.
Megan Sorensen, Chair
Wilson Neyland, Chair-Elect

Newsletters

7934 Insights Into Spina Bifida
Spina Bifida Association of America
1600 Wilson Blvd.   202-944-3285
Arlington, VA 22209-4226   800-621-3141
                                           Fax: 202-944-3295
                                           sbaa@sbaa.org
                                           www.sbaa.org
Includes articles on the latest research, the latest up-dates on legislation, features and emotional aspects specific to Spina Bifida, educational information and information on the Association's national conference.
BiMonthly
Megan Sorensen, Chair
Wilson Neyland, Chair-Elect

7935 NASS News
1400 Indpndc Ave., SW   847-698-1628
Washington, DC 20250-4037   800-727-9540
                                           nass@nass.usda.gov
                                           www.nass.usda.gov
Association activities newsletter.
Sue King, Public Affairs Office Director
Kissy Young, Senior Public Affairs Specialist

Pamphlets

7936 Educational Issues Among Children with Spina Bifida
Spina Bifida Association of America
1600 Wilson Blvd.   202-944-3285
Arlington, VA 22209-4226   800-621-3141
                                           Fax: 202-944-3295
                                           sbaa@sbaa.org
                                           www.sbaa.org
1995
Megan Sorensen, Chair
Wilson Neyland, Chair-Elect

7937 Learning Among Children with Spina Bifida
Spina Bifida Association of America
1600 Wilson Blvd.   202-944-3285
Arlington, VA 22209-4226   800-621-3141
                                           Fax: 202-944-3295
                                           sbaa@sbaa.org
                                           www.sbaa.org
1995
Megan Sorensen, Chair
Wilson Neyland, Chair-Elect

7938 Monetary Allowance, Health Care and Vocational Training
National Veterans Services Fund
PO Box 2465   203-656-0003
Darien, CT 06820-0465   Fax: 203-656-1957
                                           NatVetSvc@aol.com
Monetary allowance, health care and vocational training and rehabilitation for Vietnam Veterans' children with spine bifida.
Pamphlet

7939 Sexual Issues in Spina Bifida
Spina Bifida Association of America

1600 Wilson Blvd.   202-944-3285
Arlington, VA 22209-4226   800-621-3141
                                           Fax: 202-944-3295
                                           sbaa@sbaa.org
                                           www.sbaa.org
1993
Megan Sorensen, Chair
Wilson Neyland, Chair-Elect

7940 Urologic Care of the Child with Spina Bifida
Spina Bifida Association of America
1600 Wilson Blvd.   202-944-3285
Arlington, VA 22209-4226   800-621-3141
                                           Fax: 202-944-3295
                                           sbaa@sbaa.org
                                           www.sbaa.org
1994
Megan Sorensen, Chair
Wilson Neyland, Chair-Elect

Audio & Video

7941 Protecting Against Latex Allergy
Spina Bifida Association of America
1600 Wilson Blvd.   202-944-3285
Arlington, VA 22209-4226   800-621-3141
                                           Fax: 202-944-3295
                                           sbaa@sbaa.org
                                           www.sbaa.org
Audio-visual resource focusing on the awareness of latex allergies.
Audio-Visual
Megan Sorensen, Chair
Wilson Neyland, Chair-Elect

7942 Raising a Child with Spina Bifida: An Introduction
Ajn Company
New York, NY 10019   212-582-8820
                                           800-226-6256
                                           Fax: 212-586-5462
Offers information parents need when their child is born with spina bifida. Uses clear explanations to define spina bifida and discuss its implications for the child. Covers procedures the child may face, such as a ventricular shunt. Emphasizes the importance of early intervention and contains footage of happy and healthy children and interviews with parents.
29 minutes

7943 The Challenge
Spina Bifida Association of America
1600 Wilson Blvd.   202-944-3285
Arlington, VA 22209-4226   800-621-3141
                                           Fax: 202-944-3295
                                           sbaa@sbaa.org
                                           www.sbaa.org
A human look of how people come to grips with and overcome the challenges related to living with Spina Bifida.
14 minutes
Megan Sorensen, Chair
Wilson Neyland, Chair-Elect

Web Sites

7944 Healing Well
                                           www.healingwell.com
An online health resource guide to medical news, chat, information and articles, newsgroups and message boards, books, disease-related web sites, medical directories, and more for patients, friends, and family coping with disabling diseases, disorders, or chronic illnesses.

7945 Health Finder
                                           www.healthfinder.gov
Searchable, carefully developed web site offering information on over 1000 topics. Developed by the US Department of Health and Human Services, the site can be used in both English and Spanish.

7946   Healthlink USA

www.healthlinkusa.com

Health information concerning treatment, cures, prevention, diagnosis, risk factors, research, support groups, email lists, personal stories and much more. Updated regularly.

7947   March of Dimes Foundation

www.marchofdimes.org

Online resources on birth defects.

7948   MedicineNet

www.medicinenet.com

An online resource for consumers providing easy-to-read, authoritative medical and health information.

7949   Medscape

www.medscape.com

Medscape offers specialists, primary care physicians, and other health professionals the Web's most robust and integrated medical information and educational tools.

7950   Spina Bifida Association of America

The Spina Bifida Association (SBA) serves adults and children who live with the challenges of Spina Bifida. Since 1973, SBA has been a national voluntary health agency solely dedicated to enhancing the lives of those with Spina Bifida and those whose lives are touched by this challenging birth defect. Its tools are education, advocacy, research, and service.

7951   WebMD

www.webmd.com

Provides credible information, supportive communities, and in-depth reference material about health subjects. A source for original and timely health information as well as material from well known content providers.

Description

7952 Spinal Cord Injuries

Spinal cord injury results from trauma to or disease of the spinal cord. Depending on where the spinal cord was injured, paraplegia (paralysis affecting the legs and lower part of the body) or quadriplegia (paralysis affecting all muscles below the neck and therefore all four limbs), may occur. Bladder and/or sexual function may be damaged. Each year, 17,000 people, mostly teenage males, sustain a spinal cord injury as a result of motor vehicle or sports-related accidents, or violent crimes.

Modern medical and surgical care has dramatically increased both long-term survival and quality of life in victims of spinal cord injury. This improvement reflects intensive medical care and appropriate surgical stabilization at the time of the injury, and in later years, attention to preventing the complications, such as skin breakdown, bladder infection and lung dysfunction. One of the greatest challenges is helping persons with spinal cord injuries to live as productive and independent a life as possible. Rehabilitation should begin as soon as possible after the injury. It usually starts with several weeks at a specialized inpatient facility, then transitions to family-assisted or independent living, depending on the extent of the disability. The multidisciplinary team provides education, emotional support, physical and occupational therapy, assistive devices, braces, and beds, and helps arrange special vans or modifications to the patient's home. Many voluntary societies and government agencies can help with the transition to life in the community. Stem cell treatments have produced very modest improvements in test subjects and much work remains to be done before such treatment can be brought to human patients.

National Agencies & Associations

7953 American Association of Spinal Cord Injury Nurses (AASCIN)
75-20 Astoria Boulevard   718-803-3782
Jackson Heights, NY 11370   Fax: 718-803-0414
aascin@unitedspinal.org
www.aascin.org
Comprised of nurses who specialize in spinal cord research, nursing and education.

7954 American Chronic Pain Association
PO Box 850   800-533-3231
Rocklin, CA 95677   ACPA@theacpa.org
www.theacpa.org
The ACPA facilitates peer support and education for individuals with chronic pain in its many forms, in order to increase quality of life. Also raises awareness among the healthcare community, and with policy makers.
Penney Cowan, Founder & CEO
Daniel Galia, Director, Global Support

7955 American Spinal Injury Association (ASIA)
2209 Dickens Road   804-565-6396
Richmond, VA 23230   Fax: 804-282-0090
asia@societyhq.com
www.asia-spinalinjury.org

Promotes and establishes standards for all aspects of health care of individuals with spinal cord injury from onset throughout life, and conducts research.
Andrei Krassioukov, MD, PhD, President
Suzanne Groah, MD, MSPH, President-Elect

7956 Association of Spinal Cord Injury Professionals, Inc.
6 Lawrence Square   217-321-2488
Springfield, IL 62704   Fax: 217-525-1271
Provides education and training opportunities for psychologists, social workers and counselors in order to meet the health care needs of individuals affected by spinal cord injury and dysfunction.
Jeff Johns, MD, President
Matt Davis, Chair

7957 National Spinal Cord Injury Statistical Center
University of Alabama, Dept. of Physical Medicine
1717 6th Avenue S   205-934-3342
Birmingham, AL 35233   Fax: 205-975-4691
TTY: 205-934-4642
nscisc@uab.edu

Directs analysis and management of the world's largest spinal cord injury research database.
Yuying Chen, MD, PhD, Director

7958 Paralyzed Veterans of America
801 Eighteenth Street NW   800-424-8200
Washington, DC 20006-3517   info@pva.org
www.pva.org

Dedicated to serving veterans with a spinal cord injury or disease by providing health care services, and funding research and education on spinal cord injury and dysfunction.
David Zurfluh, President
Carl Blake, Executive Director

7959 Rick Hansen Foundation
300-3820 Cessna Drive   800-213-2131
Richmond, B.C., V7B-0A2   info@rickhansen.com
www.rickhansen.com
Funds spinal cord injury research and care, and works to create a world accessible to all who have spinal cord injuries.
Rick Hansen, Founder
Doramy Ehling, CEO

7960 Spinal Cord Injury Network International
3911 Princeton Drive   800-548-2673
Santa Rosa, CA 95405-7013   Fax: 707-577-0605
contact@spinalcordinjury.org
www.spinalcordinjury.org
Provides information and referral services for individuals and their families experiencing spinal cord injury.

7961 Spinal Cord Society
19051 County Highway 1   218-739-5252
Fergus Falls, MN 56537-7609   Fax: 218-739-5262
www.scsus.org
Funds research for spinal cord injuries and provides physician referrals.

7962 The Reeve Foundation
636 Morris Turnpike   800-225-0292
Short Hills, NJ 07078   information@christopherreeve.org
www.christopherreeve.org
Funds research on spinal cord injuries and improves the quality of life for people living with paralysis through grants and advocacy.
Peter Wilderotter, President & CEO
Maggie Goldberg, COO

7963 United Spinal Association
120-34 Queens Boulevard   718-803-3782
Kew Gardens, NY 11415   Fax: 718-803-0414
www.unitedspinal.org
Created by paralyzed WWII veterans, the United Spinal Association continues to provide support for individuals living with spinal cord injuries. Rehabilitation, community, and informational resources are available.

State Agencies & Associations

Arizona

7964 Arizona Spinal Cord Injury Association
Samaritan Rehab Institute R-2
5025 E Washington St
Phoenix, AZ 85034

602-507-4209
888-889-2185
Fax: 602-507-4214
info@azspinal.org
www.azspinal.org

The Arizona Spinal Cord Injury Association is a nonprofit organization dedicated to enhancing the lives of individuals with spinal cord injuries. We also offer support and education to family members, professionals, and community members.
Don Price, President
Donna Powers, Vice President

California

7965 National Spinal Cord Injury Association: San Diego County Chapter
6645 Alvarado Road
San Diego, CA 92120

619-229-7001
rehabdsg@gte.net
www.users.erols.com

Organization dedicated to improving the quality of life for persons with spinal cord injury and related disorders and their families. Seeks to fufill this mission by raising awareness about spinal cord injury through education, injury prevention, improvement of medical, rehabilitative and supportive services, research and public policy formulation.
Royce Hamrick

7966 National Spinal Cord Injury Association: Los Angeles Chapter
311 Robertson Boulevard
Beverly Hills, CA 90211

310-553-4833
Fax: 310-659-5040
www.users.erols.com

Organization dedicated to improving the quality of life for persons with spinal cord injury and related disorders and their families. Seeks to fufill this mission by raising awareness about spinal cord injury through education, injury prevention, improvement of medical, rehabilitative and supportive services, research and public policy formulation.
Paul Berns MD, President

Connecticut

7967 National Spinal Cord Injury Association: Connecticut Chapter
Wallingford, CT 06492

203-284-1045

Organization dedicated to improving the quality of life for persons with spinal cord injury and related disorders and their families. Seeks to fufill this mission by raising awareness about spinal cord injury through education, injury prevention, improvement of medical, rehabilitative and supportive services, research and public policy formulation.
Bill Mancini, President
Liza Ethier, Contact

Georgia

7968 Shepherd Center
2020 Peachtree Road NW
Atlanta, GA 30309

404-352-2020
admissions@shepherd.org
www.shepherd.org

Shepherd Center is a 152-bed facility. Last year Shepherd had 965 admissions to its inpatient programs and 571 to its day patient programs. In addition, Shepherd sees more than 6,600 people annually on an outpatient basis.
Gary R. Ulicny, Ph.D, President/CEO
Brock K Bowman, Assistant Medical Director

Illinois

7969 Spinal Cord Injury Association of Illinois
1032 S LaGrange Road
LaGrange, IL 60525

708-352-6223
877-373-0301
Fax: 708-352-9065
sciinjury@aol.com
www.sci-illinois.org

Spinal Cord Injury Association of Illinois (formerly NSCIA, Illinois Chapter) is a 501(c)3 non-profit organization providing information and support resources for people paralyzed by trauma and medical conditions, family members, and health care and related professionals that serve the SCI community. Our office is located in LaGrange, IL, a suburb of Chicago, but we serve the entire state.
Kim Eberhardt Muir, MS, OTR, President
Vic Myers, Vice President

Indiana

7970 National Spinal Cord Injury Association: Central Indiana Chapter
2109 Cleveland Street
Garyanapolis, IN 46404

219-944-8037
Fax: 317-329-2530
rjackson@ci.gary.in.us

Organization dedicated to improving the quality of life for persons with spinal cord injury and related disorders and their families. Seeks to fufill this mission by raising awareness about spinal cord injury through education, injury prevention, improvement of medical, rehabilitative and supportive services, research and public policy formulation.
Lucille Hightower

Kentucky

7971 National Spinal Cord Injury Association: Derby City Area Chapter
Center for Accessible Living
305 W. Broadway
Louisville, KY 40202

502-588-8574
dallgood@calky.org

Derby City Area Spinal Cord Injury Association, the Louisville Kentucky Chapter of the (N.S.C.I.A.) National Spinal Cord Injury Association. Derby City Area Spinal Cord Injury Association is a organization for individuals with spinal cord injuries, their families, and health professionals across Kentucky. Founded in 1984 as a Charter Member of the N.S.C.I.A., it was incorporated under IRS Section 501 (c) 3 as a not for profit organization.
David Allgood, President
Adam Ford, Vice President

Louisiana

7972 National Spinal Cord Injury Association: Louisiana Chapter
3650 18th Street
Metairie, LA 70002

504-455-1178
Fax: 504-455-7315

Organization dedicated to improving the quality of life for persons with spinal cord injury and related disorders and their families. Seeks to fufill this mission by raising awareness about spinal cord injury through education, injury prevention, improvement of medical, rehabilitative and supportive services, research and public policy formulation.
Yadi Mark

Massachusetts

7973 National Spinal Cord Injury Association
545 Concord Avenue
Cambridge, MA 02138-1173

301-588-6959
800-962-9629
Fax: 301-588-9414
nscia2@aol.com
www.spinalcord.org

Organization dedicated to improving the quality of life for persons with spinal cord injury and related disorders and their families. Seeks to fufill this mission by raising awareness about spinal cord injury through education, injury prevention, improvement of medical, rehabilitative and supportive services, research and public policy formulation.

7974 National Spinal Cord Injury Association: Greater Boston Chapter
New England Rehabilitation Hospital
Two Rehabilitation Way
Woburn, MA 01801

781-933-8666
Fax: 781-933-0043
sciboston@aol.com
www.sciboston.com

Organization dedicated to improving the quality of life for persons with spinal cord injury and related disorders and their families.

Seeks to fulfill this mission by raising awareness about spinal cord injury through education and injury prevention.

Dave Estrada, Director
Kevin Gibson, Coordinator

New Hampshire

7975 **New Hampshire Chapter NSCIA**
Northeast Rehabilitation Hospital
21 Chenell Drive
Concord, NH 03301-3974

603-479-0560
800-826-3700
Fax: 928-438-9607
debbie@gsil.org
www.spinalcord.org

Lisa Thompson, President

New York

7976 **Greater Rochester Area Chapter NSCIA**
Rochester, NY 14602-0076

585-234-3269
rochesternscia@yahoo.com
www.spinalcord.org

Karen Genet, Contact
Cathy Flanagan, Contact

7977 **National Spinal Cord Injury Association**
75-20 Astoria Blvd
Jackson Heights, NY 11370

718-803-3782
800-962-9629
Fax: 301-990-0445
nscia2@aol.com
www.spinalcord.org

National Spinal Cord Injury Association, the membership division of United Spinal, was founded in 1948 to improve the lives of all paralyzed Americans. Our mission is to improve the quality of life of all people living with a spinal cord injury or disease. We provide active-lifestyle information, peer support and advocacy that empower individuals to achieve their highest potential in all facets of life

Steven A Towle, Contact

Pennsylvania

7978 **Shriners Hospital for Children**
3551 N Broad Street
Philadelphia, PA 19140

215-430-4000
800-281-4050
Fax: 215-430-4079
tdiamond@shrinenet.org
www.shrinershospitalsforchildren.org

Studies and research done on children with spinal cord injuries.

Scott . Kozin, M.D, Chief of Staff
Terry Diamond, Development Officer

7979 **Spinal Cord Injury Program at Harmarville Rehabilitation Center**
Pittsburgh, PA 15238

412-828-1300
800-624-4673

Most comprehensive center for the treatment of spinal cord injury and disease.

Texas

7980 **Rio Grande Chapter: NSCIA Rio Vista Rehabilitation Hospital**
Rio Vista Rehabilitation Hospital
1395 George Dieter
El Paso, TX 79936-2901

915-298-7241
riograndenscia@aol.com
www.spinalcord.org

Sukie Armendariz, Contact
Ron Prieto, Contact

Virginia

7981 **Old Dominion Area Chapter: NSCIA**
5206 Markel Road
Richmond, VA 23226

804-726-4990
Fax: 888-752-7857

Our mission is to enable people with spinal cord injuries and disease to achieve their highest level of health, independence and quality of life. We educate public officials, community leaders, and citizens to the needs of persons with spinal cord injury and disease, and the importance of creating an environment of greater in-

dependence for all. We offer a variety of services and a wealth of knowledge towards unlocking the door for active living with SCI.

Steve Fetrow, President
Craig Fabian, Vice President

Wisconsin

7982 **Southeastern Wisconsin Chapter of the Nati onal Spinal Cord Injury Association**
Sacred Heart Rehabilitation Hospital
540 South 1st Street
Milwaukee, WI 53204-1993

414-384-4022
Fax: 414-384-7820
office@spinalcordwi.org
www.spinalcord.org

The mission of the NSCIA-SWC is to assist people who have some degree of paralysis through injury or disease with a goal of returning them to a life of dignity, self-confidence and independence in a community that is all inclusive.

John Dzicwa, President

Research Centers

7983 **Miami Project to Cure Paralysis**
1095 NW 14th Terrace
Miami, FL 33101

305-243-6001
800-STA-NDUP
Fax: 205-243-6017
miamiproject@med.miami.edu
www.miamiproject.miami.edu

In 1985, Barth A. Green, M.D. and NFL Hall of Fame linebacker Nick Buoniconti helped found TheMiami Projectto Cure Paralysis after Nick's son, Marc, sustained a spinal cord injury during a college football game. Today, The Miami Project is the world's most comprehensive spinal cord injury research center, and is a designated Center of Excellence at the University of Miami Miller School of Medicine. The Miami Project's international team is housed in the Lois Pope LIFE Center and includes more t

Barth A. Green, M.D., Co-Founder and Chairman
Marc A Buoniconti, President

7984 **Pushin On: RRTC on Secondary Conditions of Spinal**
UAB Office of Research Services
1717 6th Avenue South
Birmingham, AL 35249-7330

205-934-3283
Fax: 205-975-4691
TDD: 205-934-4642
sciweb@uab.edu
www.spinalcord.uab.edu

Pushin' On is an enewsletter published to provide persons with SCI and their families with information of interest. The newsletter is offered 2 times per year and sent electronically to subscribers to the UAB-SCIMS Email List, and it is posted online for our follows on facebook and twitter.

8 pages 2 per year
Amie B McLain, MD., Program Director
Phil Klebine, Editor

7985 **RRTC on Aging with a Disability Los Amigos Research and Education Instit**
Los Amigos Research and Education Institute
7601 E Imperial Highway
Downey, CA 90242-3456

562-401-7402
Fax: 562-401-7011
www.agingwithdisability.org

A federally funded rehabilitation research and training center.

Bryan Kemp PhD, Director
Leanne Carro Pt PhD, Training Director

Support Groups & Hotlines

7986 **Georgia National Spinal Cord Injury Association Support Group Network**
Columbus, GA 31920

800-422-3352

Support group dedicated to improving the quality of life for persons with spinal cord injury and related disorders and their families. Seeks to fufill this mission by raising awareness about spinal cord injury through rehabilitative and supportive services, research and public policy formulation.

Andy Harp

7987 HEALTHSOUTH Rehabilitation Hospital of Tal lahassee
1675 Riggins Road 850-656-4800
Tallahassee, FL 32308 Fax: 850-656-4809
www.healthsouthtallahassee.com
Our hospital provides a wide range of physical rehabilitation services, a vast network of highly-skilled, independent private practice physicians and HealthSouth therapists and nurses, and the most innovative equipment and rehabilitation technology, ensuring that all patients have access to the highest quality care. Designed with our patient's care in mind, HealthSouth Rehabilitation Hospital of Tallahassee offers semi-private rooms, which promote social interaction and support throughout the re
Dale Neely, Chief Executive Officer
Robert Rowland, M.D., Medical Director

7988 Maryland National Spinal Cord Injury Association Support Group Network
Kerman Hospital
2200 Kerman Drive 410-448-6307
Baltimore, MD 21207 800-962-9629
mhenley@kernan.umm.edu
www.spinalcord.org
Open group for all caregivers and does not focus on a specific disability, disease or condition.

7989 National Health Information Center
Office of Disease Prevention & Health Promotion
1101 Wootton Pkwy Fax: 240-453-8281
Rockville, MD 20852 odphpinfo@hhs.gov
www.health.gov/nhic
Supports public health education by maintaining a calendar of National Health Observances; helps connect consumers and health professionals to organizations that can best answer questions and provide up-to-date contact information from reliable sources; updates on a yearly basis toll-free numbers for health information, Federal health clearinghouses and info centers.
Don Wright, MD, MPH, Director

7990 National Spinal Cord Injury Support Goups
Florida Rehabilitation and Sports Medicine
5165 Adanson Street 407-895-7991
Orlando, FL 32804
Support group dedicated to improving the quality of life for persons with spinal cord injury and related disorders and their families. Seeks to fufill this mission by raising awareness about spinal cord injury through rehabilitative and supportive services, research and public policy formulation.

7991 VIVA!
Health Enhancement Learning Programs
Dallas, TX 75354-3065 972-986-2977
800-334-4403
A computer-based patient education system on spinal cord injury.

7992 National Spinal Cord Injury Support Groups
Healthsouth Central Georgia Rehab Hospital
777 Hemlock Street 478-633-1000
Macon, GA 31201 800-491-3550
Fax: 478-633-5134
www.centralgarehab.com/
Support group dedicated to improving the quality of life for persons with spinal cord injury and related disorders and their families. Seeks to fufill this mission by raising awareness about spinal cord injury through rehabilitative and supportive services, research and public policy formulation.
Connie Cater, President
Starr H. Purdue, Chairman

7993 National Spinal Cord Injury Support Groups
HEALTHSOUTH, Sea Pines Rehabilitation Hospital
101 E Florida Avenue 407-984-4600
Melbourne, FL 32901 laura.leitz@healthsouth.com
www.spinalcord.org
In a support group, members provide each other with various types of help for shared purposes. The help can take the form of providing and evaluating relevant information, relating personal experiences, listening to and accepting others' experiences, educating and guiding, or for providing sympathetic understanding and establishing social networks. Support Groups may each have their

own way of accomplishing their mission but all of them share the same goal of improving the lives of participants.

7994 National Spinal Cord Injury Support Groups
115 Alpine Street 334-456-1768
Chickasaw, AL 36611
Support group dedicated to improving the quality of life for persons with spinal cord injury and related disorders and their families. Seeks to fufill this mission by raising awareness about spinal cord injury through rehabilitative and supportive services, research and public policy formulation.

Books

7995 Body Silent: An Anthropologist Embarks into the World of the Disabled
WW Norton Publishing
500 Fifth Avenue 212-354-5500
New York, NY 10110 Fax: 212-869-0856
www.wwnorton.com
Diagnosed at midlife in the early 1980s with an inoperable (and, at the time, untreatable) ependymona of the spine, an anthropologist frankly discusses his progressive disability.
ISBN: 0-393307-02-6

7996 Climbing Back
Miramar Communications
PO Box 8987 800-543-4116
Malibu, CA 90265-8987
The author broke his back after a climbing fall. With his sights at the top of the mountain he climbs back in this inspiring story.
256 pages Hardcover

7997 Occupational Therapy Practice Guidelines for Adults with Spinal Cord Injury
American Occupational Therapy Association
4720 Montgomery Lane 301-652-6611
Bethesda, MD 20814-1220 Fax: 240-762-5150
TDD: 800-377-8555
www.aota.org
31 pages
ISBN: 1-569001-54-5

7998 Options: Spinal Cord Injury and the Future
National Spinal Cord Injury Association
120-34 Queens Blvd. 718-803-3782
Kew Gardens, NY 11415-3243 800-404-2898
Fax: 718-803-0414
info@unitedspinal.org
www.spinalcord.org
A collection of conversations with people who have had spinal cord injuries who share some of their experiences and emotions.
150 pages
David C. Cooper, Chairman
Joseph Gaskins, President & CEO

7999 Spinal Cord Injury Home Care Manual
Santa Clara Valley Medical Center
751 S Bascom Avenue 408-885-5000
San Jose, CA 95128-2699 www.scvmed.org
Provides people with spinal cord injury, their families and professionals with information about physical care, independent living, psychosocial issues, attendant care and supplies.
Paul E. Lorenz, Chief Executive Officer
Benita McLarin, Chief Operating Officer

8000 Spinal Network
Miramar Communications
120-34 Queens Blvd. 718-803-3782
Kew Gardens, NY 11415 800-404-2898
Fax: 718-803-0414
info@unitedspinal.org
www.spinalcord.org

Total wheelchair resource book.
David C. Cooper, Chairman
Joseph Gaskins, President & CEO

Children's Books

8001 Follow Your Dreams
National Spinal Cord Injury Association
120-34 Queens Blvd.
Kew Gardens, NY 11415-3243
718-803-3782
800-404-2898
Fax: 718-803-0414
info@unitedspinal.org
www.spinalcord.org
JT, born with spina bifida, goes on an adventure. Written for and by children with SCI, for children ages 9-12.
30 pages
David C. Cooper, Chairman
Joseph Gaskins, President & CEO

8002 Tell it Like it is
National Spinal Cord Injury Association
120-34 Queens Blvd.
Kew Gardens, NY 11415-3243
718-803-3782
800-404-2898
Fax: 718-803-0414
info@unitedspinal.org
www.spinalcord.org
Written by teenagers with SCI for teenagers with SCI.
David C. Cooper, Chairman
Joseph Gaskins, President & CEO

Magazines

8003 SCI Life
National Spinal Cord Injury Association
120-34 Queens Blvd.
Kew Gardens, NY 11415-3243
718-803-3782
800-404-2898
Fax: 718-803-0414
info@unitedspinal.org
www.spinalcord.org
Official magazine of NSCIA. Updates on topics such as research, medical issues, prevention, new products, books, and Association activities.
Quarterly
David C. Cooper, Chairman
Joseph Gaskins, President & CEO

8004 Spinal Column
Shepherd Spinal Center
7075 Veterans Blvd.
Burr Ridge, IL 60527-1465
630-230-3600
www.spine.org
This quarterly magazine from the spinal center offers information on the newest treatments, therapies, referral centers, assistive devices and much more for persons living with spina bifida, multiple sclerosis and other chronic physical ailments.
Quarterly
Heidi Prather, President
Christopher Bono, First Vice President

Newsletters

8005 Progress in Research
American Paralysis Association
4400 Fifth Avenue
Pittsburgh, PA 15213-1020
412-268-1062
800-225-0292
Fax: 973-912-9433
http://www.chem.cmu.edu
Offers information on the association, news, reviews, books, and information on the latest medical and technological advances in spinal cord injury research.
Quarterly
Susan P Howley, Research Director
Mitchell R Stoller, President/CEO

8006 Pushing on: University of Alabama
Christopher Reeve Association
4400 Fifth Avenue
Pittsburgh, PA 15213
412-268-1062
800-225-0292
Fax: 973-912-9433
http://www.chem.cmu.edu

A research newsletter regarding spinal cord injuries.
Quarterly
Mitchell R Stoller, President/CEO

8007 Spinal Cord Society Newsletter
Spinal Cord Society
19051 County Highway 1
Fergus Falls, MN 56537
218-739-5252
Fax: 218-739-5262
www.members.aol.com/scsweb
Offers medical reports, articles, convention news, chapter news and more for persons with spinal cord injury.
Monthly

8008 Walking Tomorrow: University of Alabama
Christopher Reeve Association
4400 Fifth Avenue
Pittsburgh, PA 15213-1020
412-268-1062
800-225-0292
Fax: 973-912-9433
http://www.chem.cmu.edu
A research newsletter regarding spinal cord injuries.
Quarterly
Mitchell R Stoller, President/CEO

Pamphlets

8009 Autonomic Dysreflexia
National Spinal Cord Injury Association
120-34 Queens Blvd.
Kew Gardens, NY 11415-3243
718-803-3782
800-404-2898
Fax: 718-803-0414
info@unitedspinal.org
www.spinalcord.org
David C. Cooper, Chairman
Joseph Gaskins, President & CEO

8010 Choosing A Spinal Cord Injury Rehabilitation Program
National Spinal Cord Injury Association
120-34 Queens Blvd.
Kew Gardens, NY 11415-3243
718-803-3782
800-404-2898
Fax: 718-803-0414
info@unitedspinal.org
www.spinalcord.org
Includes a listing of programs accredited by CARF & Model Centers designated by NIDRR.
David C. Cooper, Chairman
Joseph Gaskins, President & CEO

8011 Fun and Games
National Spinal Cord Injury Association
120-34 Queens Blvd.
Kew Gardens, NY 11415-3243
718-803-3782
800-404-2898
Fax: 718-803-0414
info@unitedspinal.org
www.spinalcord.org
David C. Cooper, Chairman
Joseph Gaskins, President & CEO

8012 Functional Electrical Stimulation: Clinical Applications
National Spinal Cord Injury Association
120-34 Queens Blvd.
Kew Gardens, NY 11415-3243
718-803-3782
800-404-2898
Fax: 718-803-0414
info@unitedspinal.org
www.spinalcord.org
David C. Cooper, Chairman
Joseph Gaskins, President & CEO

8013 Importance of Basic Science in Research
National Spinal Cord Injury Association
120-34 Queens Blvd.
Kew Gardens, NY 11415-3243
718-803-3782
800-404-2898
Fax: 718-803-0414
info@unitedspinal.org
www.spinalcord.org
David C. Cooper, Chairman
Joseph Gaskins, President & CEO

8014 Male Reproductive Function After Spinal Cord Injury
National Spinal Cord Injury Association

120-34 Queens Blvd.　718-803-3782
Kew Gardens, NY 11415-3243　800-404-2898
Fax: 718-803-0414
info@unitedspinal.org
www.spinalcord.org

David C. Cooper, Chairman
Joseph Gaskins, President & CEO

8015　Medical Facilities and Resources for Ventilator Users
National Spinal Cord Injury Association
120-34 Queens Blvd.　718-803-3782
Kew Gardens, NY 11415-3243　800-404-2898
Fax: 718-803-0414
info@unitedspinal.org
www.spinalcord.org

David C. Cooper, Chairman
Joseph Gaskins, President & CEO

8016　Reading Resources on Spinal Cord Injury
National Spinal Cord Injury Association
120-34 Queens Blvd.　718-803-3782
Kew Gardens, NY 11415-3243　800-404-2898
Fax: 718-803-0414
info@unitedspinal.org
www.spinalcord.org

David C. Cooper, Chairman
Joseph Gaskins, President & CEO

8017　Sexuality After Spinal Cord Injury
National Spinal Cord Injury Association
120-34 Queens Blvd.　718-803-3782
Kew Gardens, NY 11415-3243　800-404-2898
Fax: 718-803-0414
info@unitedspinal.org
www.spinalcord.org

David C. Cooper, Chairman
Joseph Gaskins, President & CEO

8018　Spinal Cord Injury Awareness
National Spinal Cord Injury Association
120-34 Queens Blvd.　718-803-3782
Kew Gardens, NY 11415-3243　800-404-2898
Fax: 718-803-0414
info@unitedspinal.org
www.spinalcord.org

Understanding the importance of language and images.
David C. Cooper, Chairman
Joseph Gaskins, President & CEO

8019　Spinal Cord Injury: Statistical Information
National Spinal Cord Injury Association
120-34 Queens Blvd.　718-803-3782
Kew Gardens, NY 11415-3243　800-404-2898
Fax: 718-803-0414
info@unitedspinal.org
www.spinalcord.org

David C. Cooper, Chairman
Joseph Gaskins, President & CEO

8020　Starting a Support Group
National Spinal Cord Injury Association
120-34 Queens Blvd.　718-803-3782
Kew Gardens, NY 11415-3243　800-404-2898
Fax: 718-803-0414
info@unitedspinal.org
www.spinalcord.org

David C. Cooper, Chairman
Joseph Gaskins, President & CEO

8021　Tendon Transfer Surgery
National Spinal Cord Injury Association
120-34 Queens Blvd.　718-803-3782
Kew Gardens, NY 11415-3243　800-404-2898
Fax: 718-803-0414
info@unitedspinal.org
www.spinalcord.org

David C. Cooper, Chairman
Joseph Gaskins, President & CEO

8022　Travel After Spinal Cord Injury
National Spinal Cord Injury Association

120-34 Queens Blvd.　718-803-3782
Kew Gardens, NY 11415-3243　800-404-2898
Fax: 718-803-0414
info@unitedspinal.org
www.spinalcord.org

David C. Cooper, Chairman
Joseph Gaskins, President & CEO

8023　Understanding Spinal Muscular Atrophy
Families of Spinal Muscular Atrophy
PO Box 196　847-367-7620
Libertyville, IL 60048-0196　800-886-1762
Fax: 847-367-7623
info@fsma.org
www.curesma.com
Offers a brief overview of Spinal Muscular Atrophy, causes, treatments, symptoms and unknowns.
Kenneth Hobby, President
Richard Rubenstein, Chair

8024　What is Spinal Cord Injury?
National Spinal Cord Injury Association
120-34 Queens Blvd.　718-803-3782
Kew Gardens, NY 11415-3243　800-404-2898
Fax: 718-803-0414
info@unitedspinal.org
www.spinalcord.org

David C. Cooper, Chairman
Joseph Gaskins, President & CEO

8025　What is a Physiatrist?
National Spinal Cord Injury Association
120-34 Queens Blvd.　718-803-3782
Kew Gardens, NY 11415-3243　800-404-2898
Fax: 718-803-0414
info@unitedspinal.org
www.spinalcord.org

David C. Cooper, Chairman
Joseph Gaskins, President & CEO

8026　What's New in Spinal Cord Injury Research?
National Spinal Cord Injury Association
120-34 Queens Blvd.　718-803-3782
Kew Gardens, NY 11415-3243　800-404-2898
Fax: 718-803-0414
info@unitedspinal.org
www.spinalcord.org

David C. Cooper, Chairman
Joseph Gaskins, President & CEO

Audio & Video

8027　Living with Spinal Cord Injury
Barry Corbet, author

Fanlight Productions
4196 Washington Street　617-469-4999
Boston, MA 02131-1731　800-937-4113
Fax: 617-469-3379
fanlight@fanlight.com
www.fanlight.com
A series of three videos produced by an individual who has experienced spinal cord injury himself. Changes is about coming to terms with spinal cord injury and beginning rehabilitation. Outside looks at the life-long process by which some injured people have created active and rewarding lives. Survivors explores the problems of growing old with a disability.
1973 84 Minutes

8028　SCI and Lower Extremity Orthoses
Health Enhancement Learning Programs
292 Washington Ave, Ext　518-452-6898
Albany, NY 12203-3065　800-334-4403
lermagazine.com
A video presenting an overview of indications and use of HKAFO, KAFO and AFO. Perfect resource for medical presentations and professional workshops.
Richard Dubin, Founder and Publisher
Jordana Bieze Foster, Editor

8029   Spinal Cord Injury Video Access
Spinal Cord Injury Access International
292 Washington Ave, Ext   518-452-6898
Albany, NY 12203   800-548-2673
                                             lermagazine.com
Offers informational videotapes on spinal cord injury.
Richard Dubin, Founder and Publisher
Jordana Bieze Foster, Editor

8030   Spinal Injury Slide Series
Health Enhancement Learning Programs
292 Washington Ave, Ext   518-452-6898
Albany, NY 12203-3065   800-334-4403
                                             lermagazine.com
A slide series based on the VIVA program, a patient education system on spinal cord injury.
Richard Dubin, Founder and Publisher
Jordana Bieze Foster, Editor

Web Sites

8031   American Association of Spinal Cord Injury Nurses
www.aascin.org
Comprised of nurses who specialize in spinal cord research, nursing and education.

8032   American Paraplegic Society
www.apssci.org
A professional membership organization for physicians, scientists and allied health care professionals.

8033   Christopher Reeve Paralysis Foundation
www.christopherreeve.org
The Reeve Foundation is dedicated to curing spinal cord injury by funding innovative research, and improving the quality of life for people living with paralysis through grants, information and advocacy.

8034   Healing Well
www.healingwell.com
An online health resource guide to medical news, chat, information and articles, newsgroups and message boards, books, disease-related web sites, medical directories, and more for patients, friends, and family coping with disabling diseases, disorders, or chronic illnesses.

8035   Health Finder
www.healthfinder.gov
Searchable, carefully developed web site offering information on over 1000 topics. Developed by the US Department of Health and Human Services, the site can be used in both English and Spanish.

8036   Healthlink USA
www.healthlinkusa.com
Health information concerning treatment, cures, prevention, diagnosis, risk factors, research, support groups, email lists, personal stories and much more. Updated regularly.

8037   MedicineNet
www.medicinenet.com
An online resource for consumers providing easy-to-read, authoritative medical and health information.

8038   Medscape
www.medscape.com
Medscape offers specialists, primary care physicians, and other health professionals the Web's most robust and integrated medical information and educational tools.

8039   Miami Project to Cure Paralysis
www.miamiproject.miami.edu
Science and clinical research to restore function after spinal cord injury. The primary emphasis is on basic science research, under the direction of Dr. Richard Bunge, an eminent researcher.

8040   Sexual Health Network
Informative site dealing with disability, sexuality and fertility.

8041   Spinal Cord Injury Information Network Center
www.spinalcord.uab.edu
The University of Alabama at Birmingham Spinal Cord Injury Model System (UAB-SCIMS) maintains this Information Network as a resource to promote knowledge in the areas of research, health and quality of life for people with spinal cord injuries, their families, and SCI-related professionals. Here, you will find our educational materials and information on research activities of the UAB-SCIMS along with links to outside (Internet) information.

8042   Spinal Cord Injury Network International
www.sonic.net/~spinal
A non-profit organization that provides information and referral services and lends videos.

8043   University of Alabama, (UAB)
www.spinalcord.uab.edu
The University of Alabama at Birmingham Spinal Cord Injury Model System (UAB-SCIMS) maintains this Information Network as a resource to promote knowledge in the areas of research, health and quality of life for people with spinal cord injuries, their families, and SCI-related professionals. Here, you will find our educational materials and information on research activities of the UAB-SCIMS along with links to outside (Internet) information.

8044   WebMD
www.webmd.com
Provides credible information, supportive communities, and in-depth reference material about health subjects. A source for original and timely health information as well as material from well known content providers.

Description

8045 **Stroke**

Strokes are caused by an interruption of blood flow in the brain, and usually — 80 percent of cases — are the result of a blocked blood vessel. The incidence increases with age, is higher in men than in women, and is higher in blacks than in whites. Depending on the severity and location of the damage, symptoms of stroke may include sudden weakness or paralysis (especially on one side of the body), blurred vision, difficulty speaking, slurred speech, dizziness and falling, extreme headache, stiff neck, altered level of alertness, and loss of bladder control. High blood pressure, atherosclerosis (fatty deposits), heart disease, diabetes, cigarette smoking, and heavy alcohol use are the major risk factors predisposing someone to stroke.

Preventive therapy is aimed at treatment of high blood pressure, heart disease, and diabetes. If someone has had a stroke they may be treated with blood thinning agents and/or other medication to prevent brain swelling. Research has shown that patients who are given one of these agents within three hours of stroke symptoms may have some or total restoration of neurologic function. To that end, the Golden Hour program was developed in which emergency medical personnel can initiate therapy in certain patients on the way to the hospital. Rehabilitation after the stroke involves physical and occupational therapy. Many stroke survivors experience depression and difficulty regaining independence, so it is important to provide emotional support for both survivors and their families.

National Agencies & Associations

8046 **American Heart Association**
7272 Greenville Avenue
Dallas, TX 75231
888-478-7653
800-242-8721
www.heart.org
The American Heart Association is the nation's oldest, largest voluntary organization devoted to fighting cardiovascular diseases and stroke. Funds research and raises public awareness of heart diseases.
Nancy Brown, CEO
Ivor J. Benjamin, MD, FAHA, President

8047 **American Stroke Association**
7272 Greenville Avenue
Dallas, TX 75231
800-242-9872
888-478-7653
www.heart.org
Dedicated to the prevention, diagnosis, and treatment of stroke. Funds research on stroke and advises the public on how to detect and avoid stroke.
Nancy Brown, CEO
Ivor J. Benjamin, MD, FAHA, President

8048 **Heart and Stroke Foundation of Canada**
110-1525 Carling Avenue
Ottawa, Ontario, K1Z-8R9
888-473-4636
Fax: 613-727-1895
www.heartandstroke.ca
Leading authority on cardiovascular disease, providing resources for individuals and funding scientific research on heart disease and stroke.
Yves Savoie, CEO
Anne Simard, Chief Mission & Research Officer

8049 **March of Dimes Canada**
10 Overlea Boulevard
Toronto, Ontario, M4H-1A4
416-425-3463
800-263-3463
Fax: 416-425-1920
www.marchofdimes.ca
A national service offering support, education and community programs for stroke survivors, their caregivers and families.
Leonard Baker, President & CEO
Jerry Lucas, Vice President & COO

8050 **National Heart, Lung & Blood Institute**
31 Center Drive
Bethesda, MD 20892
nhlbiinfo@nhlbi.nih.gov
www.nhlbi.nih.gov
Trains, conducts research, and educates in order to promote the prevention and treatment of heart, lung, and blood disorders.
Gary H. Gibbons, MD, Director
Nakela Cook, MD, MPH, FACC, Chief of Staff

8051 **National Institute of Neurological Disorders and Stroke**
NIH Neurological Institute
Bethesda, MD 20824
301-496-5751
800-352-9424
www.ninds.nih.gov
Seeks to reduce the burden of neurological disease affecting individuals from all walks of life.
Walter J. Koroshetz, MD, Director
Amy B. Adams, Director, Office of Scientific Liaison

Foundations

8052 **American Stroke Foundation**
5916 Dearborn
Mission, KS 66202
913-649-1776
866-549-1776
Fax: 913-649-6661
www.americanstroke.org
The vision of the American Stroke Foundation is to reach out to stroke survivors and their families across America and empower them to reclaim hope for life after stroke
Joan McDowd, Executive Director
Jen Creed, Director of Programs and Outreach

Research Centers

8053 **Bowman Gray School of Medicine**
Medical Center Boulevard
Winston Salem, NC 27157-0001
919-716-7461
Fax: 919-716-5639
James Toole MD, Professor

8054 **Cerebral Blood Flow Laboratories Veterans Administration Medical Center**
Veterans Administration Medical Center
2002 Holcombe Boulevard
Houston, TX 77030-4211
713-795-5807
Fax: 713-957-01
Offers research in cerebrovascular disorders and risk factors for stroke.
John S Meyer MD, Director

8055 **Comprehensive Stroke Center of Oregon University of Oregon Health Sciences Cen**
University of Oregon Health Sciences Center
3181 SW Sam Jackson Park Road
Portland, OR 97239-3098
503-494-7225
www.ohsu.edu
The Oregon Stroke Center (OSC) was established over 20 years ago to provide comprehensive treatment and prevention services to stroke patients throughout the Northwest. Recognized as a national leader in acute stroke treatment, the OSC mobile stroke team provides novel stroke treatments to multiple Portland hospitals. In addition to clinical care, the OSC is actively involved in clinical and basic research and provides extensive stroke related education to the public and providers. Quick action
Wayne Clark, M.D., Professor
Helmi Lutsep, M.D., Professor

8056 **Departments of Neurology & Neurosurgery: University of California, San Francisco**
UCSF Medical Center

505 Parnassus Avenue
San Francisco, CA 94143
415-476-1537
Fax: 415-476-0616
bill.dillon@radiology.ucsf.edu
www.radiology.ucsf.edu

The Department of Radiology & Biomedical Imaging at the University of California, San Francisco combines clinical excellence, trailblazing research, and outstanding education in a leading academic health sciences institution. Our faculty includes some of the foremost names in diagnostic and interventional radiology today.
Dr. Ronald Arenson, Chairman
Catherine Garzio, Director of Administration

8057 Hospital of the University of Pennsylvania
3400 Spruce Street
Philadelphia, PA 19104
215-662-4000
800-789-PENN
Fax: 215-903-09
www.pennmedicine.org

The Hospital of the University of Pennsylvania (HUP) is world-renowned for its clinical and research excellence, forging the way for newer and better ways to diagnose and treat illnesses and disorders. The world-class faculty and staff of the Hospital of the University of Pennsylvania are dedicated to superior patient care, education and research for a better, healthier future. Their significant and groundbreaking contributions to medicine are recognized both nationally and internationally. The
David E Pleasure MD, Director

8058 Massachusetts General Departments of Neurology and Neurosurgery
Massachusetts General Hospital
55 Fruit Street
Boston, MA 02114
617-726-2000
www.massgeneral.org

Guided by the needs of our patients, our mission is to be the preeminent academic neurology department in the US by: providing outstanding clinical care while rapidly discovering new treatments to reduce and eliminate the devastating impact of neurological disorders; training the very best neurologists and scientists of the future, and improving the health and well-being of the diverse communities we serve.
Peter Slavin, Director
Robert Ackerman, Doctor

8059 Stroke Research and Treatment Center UAB Medical Center
Medical Center
1530 3rd Ave S
Birmingham, AL 35294-7
205-934-9999
800-822-6478
Fax: 205-996-4039

The nationally-ranked UAB Department of Neurology is home to eight comprehensive divisions and seven centers offering an array of clinical activities. Over 26,000 patients are cared for annually through state-of-the-art subspecialty care and innovative treatments. Our residents have the opportunity to work in various neurology fields with 50 clinical and research faculty members.
Andrei V Alexandrov MD, Director and Professor
Andrei V. Alexandrov, M.D., Director, Comprehensive Stroke Research

8060 University of Iowa College of Medicine
451 Newton Road
Iowa City, IA 52242
319-335-6707
www.medicine.uiowa.edu

The Roy J. and Lucille A. Carver College of Medicine is a highly ranked medical school where students learn to become accomplished clinicians and top-flight researchers and educators. Students come to Iowa to study medicine in a program that uses case-based learning as the basis of their education. With its emphasis on problem-solving skills, early exposure to patients, and enhanced community-based experiences, UI medical students typically earn impressive scores on Step 1 of the U.S. Medical Li
Debra A. Schwinn, MD, Dean
Donna L. Hammond, PhD, Executive Associate Dean

8061 University of Maryland Center for Studies of Cerebrovascular Disease & Stroke
16 S Utah Street
Baltimore, MD 21201
410-328-4323
Fax: 410-328-1149
Thomas R Price MD, Principal Investor

8062 University of Miami School of Medicine Department of Neurology
1120 NW 14th Street
Miami, FL 33136
305-243-6732
877-243-4340
Fax: 305-243-1632
RSacco@med.miami.edu
www.med.miami.edu
Ralph L Sacco MD, Chairman-Department of Neurology
Myron D Ginsberg MD, Professor

8063 Wake Forest University: Cerebrovascular Research Center
Department of Neurology
300 S Hawthorne Road
Winston-Salem, NC 27103-2732
336-748-2338
Fax: 336-748-5477
Cerebrovascular research.
Dr James Toole, Director

8064 Washington University School of Medicine
660 S Euclid Avenue
Saint Louis, MO 63110-1016
314-362-5000
www.medicine.wustl.edu

Washington University School of Medicine is a leader in improving human health throughout the world. As noted leaders in patient care, research and education, our outstanding faculty members have contributed many discoveries and innovations to the field of science since the founding of the School of Medicine in 1891. The School of Medicine is one of seven schools of Washington University in St. Louis.
Larry J. Shapiro, M.D, Executive Vice Chancellor for Medical Af

Support Groups & Hotlines

8065 National Health Information Center
Office of Disease Prevention & Health Promotion
1101 Wootton Pkwy
Rockville, MD 20852
Fax: 240-453-8281
odphpinfo@hhs.gov
www.health.gov/nhic

Supports public health education by maintaining a calendar of National Health Observances; helps connect consumers and health professionals to organizations that can best answer questions and provide up-to-date contact information from reliable sources; updates on a yearly basis toll-free numbers for health information, Federal health clearinghouses and info centers.
Don Wright, MD, MPH, Director

8066 Stroke Clubs International
805 12th Street
Galveston, TX 77550
409-762-1022
strokeclubs@earthlink.net
www.ninds.nih.gov

Organization of persons who have experienced strokes, their families and friends for the purpose of mutual support, education, social and recreational activities. Provides information and assistance to Stroke Clubs (which are usually sponsored by local organizations).
Ellis Williamson

Books

8067 Alzheimer's, Stroke and 29 Other Neurological Disorders Sourcebook
Omnigraphics
155 West Congress
Detroit, MI 48226-3993
313-961-1340
800-234-1340
Fax: 800-875-1340
contact@omnigraphics.com
omnigraphics.com

Provides vital information for the nontechnical reader focusing on Alzheimer's disease, stroke and various neurological disorders. Answers thousands of questions related to afflications of the central nervous system with each chapter reviwing a particular disorder and offers in-depth discussions.

8068 Courage: Poems & Positive Thoughts for Stroke Survivors
National Stroke Association
9707 E Easter Lane
Centennial, CO 80112-3747
303-649-9299
800-787-6537
Fax: 303-649-1328
info@stroke.org
www.stroke.org

Words of inspiration from survivors and caregivers.
83 pages
Matt Lopez, Chief Executive Officer
Sharon Januchowski, Executive Vice President

8069 Discovery Circles
National Stroke Association
9707 E Easter Lane
Centennial, CO 80112-3747
303-649-9299
800-787-6537
Fax: 303-649-1328
info@stroke.org
www.stroke.org
NSA's guide to organizing and facilitating stroke support groups. This detailed manual describes the support group structure and the facilitator's role.
213 pages
Matt Lopez, Chief Executive Officer
Sharon Januchowski, Executive Vice President

8070 Magic of Humor in Caregiving
National Stroke Association
9707 E Easter Lane
Centennial, CO 80112-3747
303-649-9299
800-787-6537
Fax: 303-649-1328
info@stroke.org
www.stroke.org
A dynamic researching tool focusing on the necessity of humor in daily caregiving interaction.
Matt Lopez, Chief Executive Officer
Sharon Januchowski, Executive Vice President

8071 November Days
National Stroke Association
9707 E Easter Lane
Centennial, CO 80112-3747
303-649-9299
800-787-6537
Fax: 303-649-1328
info@stroke.org
www.stroke.org
A caregiver's story of her struggle with a loved one's stroke.
225 pages
Matt Lopez, Chief Executive Officer
Sharon Januchowski, Executive Vice President

8072 Occupational Therapy Practice Guidelines for Adults with Stroke
American Occupational Therapy Association
4720 Montgomery Lane
Bethesda, MD 20814-1220
301-652-6611
Fax: 240-762-5150
TDD: 800-377-8555
www.aota.org

15 pages
ISBN: 1-569001-55-3

8073 Stroke Book
William Morrow & Company
P.O. Box 1181
Bloomington, IN 47402-4702
212-261-6500
mystrokeofinsight.com
1993
ISBN: 0-688090-55-9

8074 Stroke: A Clinical Approach
Butterworth-Heinemann
P.O. Box 1181
Bloomington, IN 47402-2079
617-928-2500
800-366-2665
mystrokeofinsight.com

1993 584 pages
ISBN: 0-750691-81-6

8075 Stroke: A Guide for Patient and Family
Raven Press
5323 Harry Hines Blvd
Dallas, TX 75390-2601
214-648-3111
info@strokecenter.org
www.strokecenter.org

224 pages
ISBN: 0-881672-79-3

8076 Stroke: Your Complete Exercise Guide
Human Kinetics Publishers

9707 E Easter Lane
Centennial, CO 80112-5076
217-351-1549
800-747-4457
Fax: 217-351-5076
info@stroke.org
www.stroke.org
Part of the Cooper Clinic and Research Institute Fitness Series providing exercise rehabilitation for persons suffering from strokes.
126 pages Paperback
ISBN: 0-873224-28-0
Matt Lopez, Chief Executive Officer
Sharon Januchowski, Executive Vice President

8077 Ted's Stroke: The Caregiver's Story
National Stroke Association
9707 E Easter Lane
Centennial, CO 80112-3747
303-649-9299
800-787-6537
Fax: 303-649-1328
info@stroke.org
www.stroke.org
Personal experiences, guidance and tips for caregivers.
175 pages
ISBN: 0-962487-61-9
Matt Lopez, Chief Executive Officer
Sharon Januchowski, Executive Vice President

8078 The Comfort of Home for Stroke: A Guide fo r Caregivers
Marie Meyer & Paula Derr, RN with Jon Caswell, author
CareTrust Publications
PO Box 10283
Portland, OR 97296-0283
800-565-1533
Fax: 415-673-2205
sales@comfortofhome.com
www.comfortofhome.com
Comfort guides readers through every caregiving stage, from understanding personality changes, preparing the home, equipment, the healthcare team, and the activities of daily living. It helps take the fear out of home care and assists caregivers in maintaining peace of mind.
2007 344 pages
ISBN: 0-966476-78-6

8079 Women in Your Life: Protect Yourself, Protect Your Family
National Stroke Association
9707 E Easter Lane
Centennial, CO 80112-3747
303-649-9299
800-787-6537
Fax: 303-649-1328
info@stroke.org
www.stroke.org
Valuable information about the unique toll stroke takes on women.
Matt Lopez, Chief Executive Officer
Sharon Januchowski, Executive Vice President

Magazines

8080 Stroke Connection
American Stroke Foundation
5916 Dearborn St
Mission, KS 66202
913-649-1776
Fax: 913-649-6661
www.americanstroke.org
Official magazine of the American Stroke Foundation. Supports stroke survivors, their families, caregivers and friends by providing resources, services, education and information that improves the quality of life.
Richard March, Chair
David Marshall, Vice Chairman

Pamphlets

8081 African-Americans and Stroke
National Stroke Association
9707 E Easter Lane
Centennial, CO 80112-3747
303-649-9299
800-787-6537
Fax: 303-649-1328
info@stroke.org
www.stroke.org

Matt Lopez, Chief Executive Officer
Sharon Januchowski, Executive Vice President

8082 **Aneurysm Answers**
National Stroke Association
9707 E Easter Lane
Centennial, CO 80112-3747

303-649-9299
800-787-6537
Fax: 303-649-1328
info@stroke.org
www.stroke.org

Matt Lopez, Chief Executive Officer
Sharon Januchowski, Executive Vice President

8083 **Check Your Pulse, America: Atrial Fibrillation**
National Stroke Association
9707 E Easter Lane
Centennial, CO 80112-3747

303-649-9299
800-787-6537
Fax: 303-649-1328
info@stroke.org
www.stroke.org

Matt Lopez, Chief Executive Officer
Sharon Januchowski, Executive Vice President

8084 **Cholesterol and Stroke**
National Stroke Association
9707 E Easter Lane
Centennial, CO 80112-3747

303-649-9299
800-787-6537
Fax: 303-649-1328
info@stroke.org
www.stroke.org

Matt Lopez, Chief Executive Officer
Sharon Januchowski, Executive Vice President

8085 **Facts on Heart Disease, Heart Attack, Stroke and Risk Factors**
American Heart Association
1600 Clifton Road
Atlanta, GA 30329-5129

214-373-6300
800-232-4636
Fax: 214-706-1341
www.cdc.gov

Offers information on how to recognize a heart attack or stroke, recovery and rehabilitation techniques and risk factors.

8086 **High Blood Pressure and Stroke**
National Stroke Association
9707 E Easter Lane
Centennial, CO 80112-3747

303-649-9299
800-787-6537
Fax: 303-649-1328
info@stroke.org
www.stroke.org

Matt Lopez, Chief Executive Officer
Sharon Januchowski, Executive Vice President

8087 **Mobility: Issues Facing Stroke Survivors and Their Families**
National Stroke Association
9707 E Easter Lane
Centennial, CO 80112-3747

303-649-9299
800-787-6537
Fax: 303-649-1328
info@stroke.org
www.stroke.org

Matt Lopez, Chief Executive Officer
Sharon Januchowski, Executive Vice President

8088 **Recurrent Stroke**
National Stroke Association
9707 E Easter Lane
Centennial, CO 80112-3747

303-649-9299
800-787-6537
Fax: 303-649-1328
info@stroke.org
www.stroke.org

Matt Lopez, Chief Executive Officer
Sharon Januchowski, Executive Vice President

8089 **Smoking Cessation: Be Smoke Free in 3 Minutes**
National Stroke Association
9707 E Easter Lane
Centennial, CO 80112-3747

303-649-9299
800-787-6537
Fax: 303-649-1328
info@stroke.org
www.stroke.org

Matt Lopez, Chief Executive Officer
Sharon Januchowski, Executive Vice President

8090 **Stroke: Hope Through Research**
Office of Scientific & Health Reports

P.O. Box 5801
Bethesda, MD 20824-0001

301-496-5751
800-352-9424
www.ninds.nih.gov

Offers information on stroke, research and advances in treatments and rehabilitation programs to help patients.

8091 **Transient Ischemic Attack**
National Stroke Association
9707 E Easter Lane
Centennial, CO 80112-3747

303-649-9299
800-787-6537
Fax: 303-649-1328
info@stroke.org
www.stroke.org

Matt Lopez, Chief Executive Officer
Sharon Januchowski, Executive Vice President

Audio & Video

8092 **Secret Life of the Brain**
PBS Home Video
PO Box 751089
Charlotte, NC 28275

877-727-7467
Fax: 703-739-8131
www.pbs.org/wnet/brain/about.html

Reveals the facinating processes involved in brain development across a lifetime. The five-part series informs viewers of exciting new information in the brain sciences, introduces the foremost researchers in the field, and utilizes dynamic visual imagry and compelling human stories to help a general audience understand otherwise difficult scientific concepts.
5 Tapes
Paula Kerger, President/CEO
Wayne Godwin, Chief Operating Officer

8093 **Stroke: Touching the Soul of Your Family**
National Stroke Association
9707 E Easter Lane
Centennial, CO 80112-3747

303-649-9299
800-787-6537
Fax: 303-649-1328
info@stroke.org
www.stroke.org

Fifteen minute video chronicling three stroke survivors and their courageous struggle to overcome daily challenges and educate others about stroke.
Matt Lopez, Chief Executive Officer
Sharon Januchowski, Executive Vice President

Web Sites

8094 **American Heart Association**
www.heart.org/HEARTORG

A national organization whose primary concern is the reduction of death and disability due to cardiovascular diseases and stroke.

8095 **Healing Well**
www.healingwell.com

An online health resource guide to medical news, chat, information and articles, newsgroups and message boards, books, disease-related web sites, medical directories, and more for patients, friends, and family coping with disabling diseases, disorders, or chronic illnesses.

8096 **Health Finder**
www.healthfinder.gov

Searchable, carefully developed web site offering information on over 1000 topics. Developed by the US Department of Health and Human Services, the site can be used in both English and Spanish.

8097 **Healthlink USA**
www.healthlinkusa.com

Health information concerning treatment, cures, prevention, diagnosis, risk factors, research, support groups, email lists, personal stories and much more. Updated regularly.

8098 **MedicineNet**
www.medicinenet.com

An online resource for consumers providing easy-to-read, authoritative medical and health information.

8099   Medscape

www.medscape.com

Medscape offers specialists, primary care physicians, and other health professionals the Web's most robust and integrated medical information and educational tools.

8100   National Heart, Lung & Blood Institute

www.nhlbi.nih.gov

Primary responsibility of this organization is the scientific investigation of heart, blood vessel, lung and blood disorders. Oversee research, demonstration, prevention, education and training activities in these fields and emphasizes the control of stroke.

8101   National Stroke Association

www.stroke.org

A national organization whose sole purpose is to reduce the incidence and impact of stroke through prevention, treatment, rehabilitation and research, and support for stroke survivors and their families. Educational resources on all aspects of stroke available on website.

8102   Neurology Channel

www.healthcommunities.com

Find clearly explained, medically accurate information regarding conditions, including an overview, symptoms, causes, diagnostic procedures and treatment options. On this site it is possible to ask questions and get information from a neurologist and connect to people who have similar health interests.

8103   WebMD

www.webmd.com

Provides credible information, supportive communities, and in-depth reference material about health subjects. A source for original and timely health information as well as material from well known content providers.

Description

8104 Substance Abuse Disorder

Substance abuse is a broad term that refers to any illegal, dangerous or destructive use of some substance. This use may be legal (binge drinking by an adult) or illegal (smoking crystal methamphetamine). Abused substances include alcohol, nicotine, marijuana, heroin, prescription painkillers and tranquilizers, stimulants such as amphetamines and cocaine, and hallucinogens such as LSD. The abuse may be a danger to the user, family members, business associates, close friends or even total strangers. Substance dependence refers to a state of strong compulsion to use the substance, in many cases accompanied by physical withdrawal symptoms if the substance is not regularly available.

The cause of substance abuse is very complex, and involves an interplay between the individual's behavioral choices, their genetic background and past and present social environment. Some substance abusers also have a definable psychiatric disorder such as depression or schizophrenia; treatment of these dual-disorder patients is especially challenging.

The consequences of substance abuse are well-known, and include job loss, arrest, family breakup, automobile and other accidents, birth defects (fetal alcohol syndrome), direct toxic effects (cirrhosis of the liver from alcohol or lung cancer from smoking), and infections (HIV or hepatitis B from sharing needles). Substance abuse, unless it occurs in extremely isolated persons, greatly affects family members and loved ones. Family members often deny the reality of the abuse, and may help, or enable, the abuser to cover up the problem and avoid its consequences.

There is no quick and universally effective treatment for substance abuse. Options range from inexpensive peer-based organizations such as Alcoholics Anonymous to very expensive long-term inpatient programs. Some peer-based programs appeal to a niche defined by sex, race, age or religious affiliation. Treatment is much more likely to succeed if it is freely chosen by the individual rather than mandated by a court. Dropout during treatment and relapse after initial success are common, but many people do achieve life-long cures with abstinence from further substance abuse. Family members should look for education and support through groups like Al-Anon, which bring them together with people facing similar situations.

National Agencies & Associations

8105 AAA Foundation for Traffic Safety
607 14th Street NW
Washington, DC 20005
202-638-5944
Fax: 202-638-5943
info@aaafoundation.org
www.aaafoundation.org

A non-profit foundation conducting research with the goal of preventing traffic deaths. Raises awareness on road safety measures and driver education.
C. Y. David Yang, Executive Director
Tara Kelley-Baker, Group Leader

8106 African American Family Services
310 Groveland Avenue S
Minneapolis, MN 55403
612-813-5034
Fax: 651-925-0044
www.aafs.net

African American Family Services works with individuals, families and communities affected by addiction and mental illness. Provides culturally-specific mental health services.
Freddie Davis-English, Chairman of the Board
Thomas Adams, PhD (ABD), MSW, Chief Executive Officer

8107 Al-Anon Family Group Headquarters
1600 Corporate Landing Parkway
Virginia Beach, VA 23454-5617
757-563-1600
888-425-2666
Fax: 757-563-1656
wso@al-anon.org
www.al-anon.org

At Al-Anon Family Group meetings, family members and friends of problem drinkers share their experiences and learn how to apply the principles of the Al-Anon program to their individual situations.
Robert Schneider, Director

8108 Alcoholics Anonymous
475 Riverside Drive at W 120th St
New York, NY 10115
212-870-3400
Fax: 212-870-3003
international@aa.org
www.aa.org

Alcoholics Anonymous is an international alliance of supportive individuals who have had a drinking problem. Membership is available to anyone wanting to improve their situation.

8109 American Chronic Pain Association
PO Box 850
Rocklin, CA 95677
800-533-3231
ACPA@theacpa.org
www.theacpa.org

The ACPA facilitates peer support and education for individuals with chronic pain in its many forms, in order to increase quality of life. Also raises awareness among the healthcare community, and with policy makers.
Penney Cowan, Founder & CEO
Daniel Galia, Director, Global Support

8110 American Council on Addiction & Alcohol Problems
2376 Lakeside Drive
Birmingham, AL 35244
205-989-8177
ccorley@alcap.com
sapacap.com

The American Council on Addiction and Alcohol Problems is a non-profit organization whereby state organizations, national religious bodies, and other concerned groups unite to solve the issues caused by addiction.
Rob Chambers, President
Joe Godfrey, President-Elect

8111 American Dental Association
211 E Chicago Avenue
Chicago, IL 60611-2678
312-440-2500
Fax: 312-440-2822
affiliates@ada.org
www.ada.org

The nation's largest dental association, representing dentists. A leading source of oral health related information for dentists and their patients.

8112 Association of Halfway House Alcoholism Programs of North America (AHHAP)
2360 Corporate Circle
Henderson, NV 89074
650-618-9889
888-843-8169
TTY: 650-618-1414
contact.omics@omicsonline.org
www.omicsonline.org

Open-access publisher running over 700 scientific journals in the medical, clinical, pharmaceutical, and engineering technology fields. Current literature and research on addictions can be ac-

cessed, as well as connections to halfway houses across North America.
Olivia Howard, President
David Logan, Vice President

8113 Center for Substance Abuse Prevention Substance Abuse & Mental Health Services
5600 Fishers Lane   877-726-4727
Rockville, MD 20857   www.samhsa.gov
Connects people and resources with strategies and programs designed to encourage efforts aimed at reducing and eliminating alcohol, tobacco and other drug problems in society. Works with federal, state, public and private organizations to develop prevention programs.

8114 Cocaine Anonymous World Services
21720 S Wilmington Avenue   310-559-5833
Long Beach, CA 90810-1641   Fax: 310-559-2554
                                    cawso@ca.org
                                    www.ca.org
Members are recovering from addiction, and offer support and maintain their sobriety by working together.

8115 Drug Abuse Resistance Education of America
PO Box 512090   310-215-0575
Los Angeles, CA 90051-0090   800-223-3273
                                    Fax: 310-215-0180
                                    www.dare.com
Provides information, resources, tips, warning signs and other information for parents and kids to help keep children off drugs.
Michele M. Leonhart, Chair
Robert J. Strang, Vice Chair

8116 Facing Addiction with NCADD
217 Broadway   212-269-7797
New York, NY 10007   800-622-2255
                                    Fax: 212-269-7510
                                    national@ncadd.org
                                    www.ncadd.org
Facing Addiction with the National Council on Alcoholism and Drug Dependence (NCADD) have merged to form into a national leading organization dedicated to fighting the addiction epidemic, providing awareness, support, and resources.
James L. Abernathy, Chairman & CEO
Michael Ballue, CADC II, BSBA, Director

8117 Families Anonymous, Inc. Recovery Fellowship
701 Lee Street   800-736-9805
Des Plaines, IL 60016   847-294-5877
                                    Fax: 847-294-5837
                                    info@familiesanonymous.org
                                    www.familiesanonymous.org
Addresses the needs of families who are concerned about a relative with a drug problem and with related behavioral problems. Offers informational packets, meetings and support networks for these families.

8118 Hazelden Betty Ford Foundation
PO Box 11   844-598-4521
Center City, MN 55012-0011   800-257-7810
                                    info@hazeldenbettyford.org
                                    www.hazelden.org
Helps individuals, families, and communities struggling with alcohol abuse, substance abuse, and drug addiction by offering prevention and recovery solutions nationwide.
James A. Blaha, Vice President, CFO & CAO
Debra Bauman, Vice President & CIO

8119 Indian Health Service Federal Health Program
5600 Fishers Lane   605-226-7456
Rockville, MD 20857   800-225-0241
                                    www.ihs.gov
Provides a comprehensive program of alcoholism and substance abuse prevention and treatment for Native Americans and Alaskan natives.

8120 Lawyers Concerned for Lawyers
2550 University Avenue W   651-646-5590
Saint Paul, MN 55114   866-525-6466
                                    help@mnlcl.org
                                    www.mnlcl.org

A non-profit organization of recovering lawyers, judges, law students, and concerned others. Educates and arranges interventions and offers lawyer-only AA meetings.
Howard Bolter, Chair
Warren Maas, Treasurer

8121 Marijuana Anonymous World Services
340 S Lemon Avenue   800-766-6779
Walnut, CA 91789-2706   office@marijuana-anonymous.org
                                    www.marijuana-anonymous.org
Non-profit fellowship of individuals with marijuana addiction, seeking sobriety and support.

8122 MindWise Innovations
270 Bridge Street   781-239-0071
Dedham, MA 02026   Fax: 781-320-9136
                                    info@mindwise.org
                                    www.mindwise.org
Formerly known as Screening For Mental Health, MindWise Innovations provides resources to schools, workplaces, and communities to address mental health issues, substance abuse, and suicide.
Bryan Kohl, Senior Vice President
Marjie McDaniel, Vice President

8123 Mothers Against Drunk Driving (MADD)
511 E John Carpenter Freeway   877-275-6233
Irving, TX 75062   www.madd.org
Founded by a small group of mothers and currently one of the largest crime victims organizations in the world. Resources available online.
Helen Witty, President
Adam Vanek, CEO

8124 Narcotics Anonymous World Services
PO Box 9999   818-773-9999
Van Nuys, CA 91409   Fax: 818-700-0700
                                    fsmail@na.org
                                    www.na.org
A fellowship of men and women who meet to help one another with their drug dependency. Support and resources are available.

8125 National Association for Children of Alcoholics (NACOA)
10920 Connecticut Avenue   301-468-0985
Kensington, MD 20895   888-554-2627
                                    nacoa@nacoa.org
                                    www.nacoa.org
Advocates for all children and families affected by alcohol and other drug dependencies. Programs, training, and other resources are available.
Peter Palanca, MD, Vice Chairman
Robert W. Denniston, Vice Chairman

8126 National Association of Alcoholism and Drug Abuse Counselors (NAADAC)
44 Canal Center Plaza   703-741-7686
Alexandria, VA 22314   Fax: 703-741-7698
                                    naadac@naadac.org
                                    www.naadac.org
Largest membership organization serving addiction counselors, educators and other addiction-focused health care professionals who specialize in addiction prevention, treatment and education.
Cynthia Moreno Tuohy, BSW, SAP, Executive Director
Jessica Gleason, JD, Deputy Director

8127 National Association on Drug Abuse Problems
355 Lexington Avenue   212-986-1170
New York, NY 10017   info@nadap.org
                                    www.nadap.org
Private non-profit corporation providing skills, evaluation, job training and job placement to recovering drug addicts in the metropolitan New York area.
John A. Darin, President & CEO
Tyler H. Beebe, Treasurer

8128 National Crime Prevention Council
2614 Chapel Lake Drive   443-292-4565
Gambrills, MD 21054   www.ncpc.org

Organization working to prevent crime and drug use by developing materials for parents and children, teaching strategies to communities, and raising awareness by coodinating with local agencies.

Ann M. Harkins, Esq., President & CEO
Brian Monks, Vice President & CSO

8129 National Families in Action (NFIA)
PO Box 133136   404-248-9676
Atlanta, GA 30333-3136   nfia@nationalfamilies.org
www.nationalfamilies.org
Non-profit organization that obtained the nation's first state laws banning the sale of drug paraphernalia. Leads a national effort to help parents replicate Georgia's laws in other states to prevent the marketing of drugs and drug use to children.

Sue Rusche, President
Carol S. Reeder, Treasurer

8130 National Organization on Fetal Alcohol Syndrome
1200 Eton Court NW   202-785-4585
Washington, DC 20007   information@nofas.org
www.nofas.org
Dedicated to eliminating birth defects caused by alcohol consumption during pregnancy by raising awareness of safe pregnancy measures, and the consequences of drinking during pregnancy.

Tom Donaldson, President
Kathleen Tavenner Mitchell, MHS, Vice President

8131 Office of Women's Services Substance Abuse & Mental Health Services
5600 Fishers Lane   877-726-4727
Rockville, MD 20857-0001   www.samhsa.gov
Provides leadership and guidance in creating and maintaining an agency-wide focus for addressing the substance abuse and mental health needs of women.

8132 Office on Smoking and Health: Centers for Disease Control & Prevention
1600 Clifton Road   800-232-4636
Atlanta, GA 30329-4027   TTY: 888-232-6348
tobaccoinfo@cdc.gov
www.cdc.gov/tobacco
Offers reference services to researchers through the Technical Information Center. Publishes and distributes a number of titles in the field of smoking and health.

8133 Partnership for Drug-Free Kids
633 Third Avenue   212-922-1560
New York, NY 10011-6706   855-378-4373
www.drugfree.org
Partnered with Center on Addiction, and dedicated to transforming how addiction is addressed by the nation, from prevention to recovery.

Creighton Drury, CEO
James G. Niven, Chair

8134 Remove Intoxicated Drivers (RID-USA)
PO Box 520   877-823-9235
Schenectady, NY 12301   888-283-5144
ridusa@verizon.net
rid-usa.org
Volunteers working to deter impaired driving, to help its victims obtain justice, restitution and peace of mind while navigating the criminal justice systems, and to curb the alcohol abuse which leads to drunk driving.

Doris Aiken, Founder & President
Bill Aiken, Vice President & Manager

8135 Students Against Destructive Decisions
1440 G Street NW   508-481-3568
Washington, DC 20005   info@sadd.org
www.sadd.org
Provides students with prevention tools to deal with the issues of underage drinking, drug use, risky and impaired driving, and other destructive decisions.

Rick Birt, President & CEO
Elizabeth Vermette, Managing Director

8136 Substance Abuse and Mental Health Services Administration (SAMHSA)
5600 Fishers Lane   877-726-4727
Rockville, MD 20857   Fax: 240-221-4292
TTY: 800-487-4889
findtreatment.samhsa.gov
www.samhsa.gov
Part of the U.S. Department of Health and Human Services, SAMHSA promotes, monitors, evaluates and coordinates programs for the prevention and treatment of alcoholism and alcohol abuse.

Thomas Clarke, PhD, Director
Elinore F. McCance-Katz, MD, PhD, Assistant Secretary

State Agencies & Associations

Alabama

8137 Division of Mental Illness and Substance Abuse Community Programs
Department of Mental Health
Montgomery, AL 36130-1410   334-242-3454
800-367-0955
Fax: 334-242-0725
Alabama.DMH@mh.alabama.gov
www.mh.alabama.gov

Kent Hunt, Associate Commissioner Substance Abuse
Susan P Chambers, Associate Commissioner Mental Illness

Alaska

8138 Office of Alcohol and Substance Abuse Department of Health and Social Services
Department of Health and Social Services
350 Main Street   907-465-3030
Juneau, AK 99811   800-465-4828
Fax: 907-465-3068
Stacy.Toner@Alaska.gov
dhss.alaska.gov/Pages/default.aspx

William J. Streuss, Commissioner
Tara Horton, Special Assistant

Arizona

8139 Alcoholism and Drug Abuse: Office of Community Behavioral Health
Department of Health Services
150 N 18th Avenue   602-364-4558
Phoenix, AZ 85007-3228   Fax: 602-364-4570
cancerlr@azdhs.gov
www.azdhs.gov
The Arizona Department of Health Services promotes and protects the health of Arizona's children and adults. Its mission is to set the standard for personal and community health through direct care, science, public policy, and leadership.

January Contreras, Acting Director

Arkansas

8140 Office of Alcohol and Drug Abuse Prevention
305 South Palm Street   501-686-9866
Little Rock, AR 72205   877-726-4727
Fax: 501-686-9035
SAMHSA's mission is to reduce the impact of substance abuse and mental illness on America's communities.

California

8141 California Women's Commission on Alcohol and Drug Dependencies
14622 Victory Boulevard   818-376-0470
Van Nuys, CA 91411
Dedicated to improving the quality and increasing the quantity of services to women with alcohol-related problems.

8142   Department of Alcohol and Drug Programs
1700 K Street
Sacramento, CA 95811-4037
916-445-0834
800-879-2772
Fax: 916-323-1270
www.colorado.gov/CDHS

Kathryn P Jett, Director

Colorado

8143   Alcohol and Drug Abuse Division Department of Human Services
Department of Human Services
4055 S Lowell Boulevard
Denver, CO 80236-3120
303-866-7480
Fax: 303-866-7481
jaqueline.enriques@state.co.us

Janet Wood, Director
Mary McCann, Acting Manager

Connecticut

8144   Connecticut Alcohol and Drug Abuse Commission
410 Capitol Avenue
Hartford, CT 06134
860-418-7000
800-446-7348
Fax: 860-418-6780
TTY: 860-418-6707
The mission of the Department of Mental Health and Addiction Services is to improve the quality of life of the people of Connecticut by providing an integrated network of comprehensive, effective and efficient mental health and addiction services that foster self-sufficiency, dignity and respect.
Patricia Rehmer, Commissioner

Delaware

8145   Delaware Division of Alcoholism, Drug Abuse and Mental Health
Alcohol And Drug Services
1901 North DuPont Highway
New Castle, DE 19720
302-255-9399
Fax: 302-255-4427
DHSSInfor@state.de.us
Our mission is to promote health and recovery by ensuring that Delawareans have access to quality prevention and treatment for mental health, substance use, and gambling conditions.
Renata J. Henry, Director

District of Columbia

8146   Health Planning and Development
825 N Capitol Street NE
Washington, DC 20002
202-727-8473
Fax: 202-727-8411
doh@dc.gov
doh.dc.gov/service/doh-substance-abuse

Florida

8147   Alcohol and Drug Abuse Program Department Of Children And Families
Department Of Children And Families
1317 Winewood Boulevard
Tallahassee, FL 32399-6570
850-487-2920
Fax: 850-414-7474
www.dcf.state.fl.us/mentalhealth/sa
The Substance Abuse and Mental Health (SAMH) Program, within the Florida Department of Children and Families, is the single state authority on substance abuse and mental health as designated by the federal Substance Abuse and Mental Health Services Administration (SAMHSA). The Department's SAMH Program oversees a statewide system of care for the prevention, treatment, and recovery of children and adults with serious mental illnesses and/or substance abuse disorders.
Cynthea Panzarino, Director

Georgia

8148   Alcohol and Drug Services Addictive Diseases Program
Addictive Diseases Program
Two Peachtree Street NW
Atlanta, GA 30303-3171
404-657-2331
Fax: 404-657-2160
www.mhddad.dhr.georgia.gov

DBHDD contracts with providers in all 6 regions to provide outpatient and residential substance abuse treatment to men and women who are struggling with the disease of addiction
Frank Berry, Commissioner

Hawaii

8149   Alcohol and Drug Abuse Division Department of Health
Department of Health
601 Kamokila Boulevard
Kapoleiu, HI 96707
808-692-7506
Fax: 808-692-7521
ATRINFO@doh.hawaii.gov
www.hawaii.gov/health
The mission of the Department of Health is to protect and improve the health and environment for all people in Hawai'i .
Loretta J. Fuddy, Director
Keith Yamamoto, Asst. Director

Idaho

8150   Department of Health and Welfare Department Of Health And Welfare
Department Of Health And Welfare
1720 Westgate Drive
Boise, ID 83704-0036
208-334-6747
800-926-2588
Fax: 208-334-6738
rossil@dhw.idaho.gov
www.healthandwelfare.idaho.gov

Landis Rossi, Regional Director
Richard Armstrong, Director

Illinois

8151   Department of Alcoholism and Substance Abuse
Department Of Human Services
100 W Randolph Street
Chicago, IL 60601
312-814-3840
800-843-6154
Fax: 312-814-2419
TTY: 800-447-6404
www.dhs.state.il.us

Theodora Binion-Tayl, Director

8152   Illinois Church Action on Alcohol Problems
1132 W Jefferson Street
Springfields, IL 62702
217-546-6871
Fax: 217-546-2814
www.ilcaaap.org
An interdenominational Christian agency representing church groups in Illinois. Works to prevent alcohol and other drug-related problems through education legislative action and public awareness.

8153   Parkside Medical Services Corporation
205 W Touhy Avenue
Park Ridge, IL 60068-4256
847-698-9866
800-727-5723
This establishment offers treatment and hope for the alcoholic/substance abuser. A resource center that provides information books and resources pertaining to substance abuse and offers treatment facilities in various states across the country.

Indiana

8154   Division of Addiction Services Department of Mental Health
Department of Mental Health
402 W Washington Street
Indianapolis, IN 46204-3614
317-232-7800
800-662-4357
Fax: 317-233-3472
www.in.gov/fssa

Gina Eckart, Director
Alma Burrus, Operations Manager

Iowa

8155   Department of Public Health: Division of Substance Abuse and Health
Lucas State Office Building
321 E 12th Street
Des Moines, IA 50319-0075
515-281-7689
866-227-9878
Fax: 515-281-4535
www.idph.state.ia.us

The Iowa Department of Public Health (IDPH) partners with local public health, policymakers, health care providers, business and many others to fulfill our mission of promoting and protecting the health of Iowans.
Kathy Stone, Director

Kansas

8156 Alcohol and Drug Abuse Services
915 Harrison Street
Topeka, KS 66612

785-296-3959
800-586-3690
Fax: 785-296-7275
TTY: 785-296-1491
dxmd@srskansas.org
www.srskansas.org

Don Jordan, Secretary
Laura Howard, Deputy Secretary/CFO

Kentucky

8157 Division of Substance Abuse: Department of Mental Health
Department For MH/MR Services
100 Fair Oaks Lane
Frankfort, KY 40621

502-564-2880
Fax: 502-564-7152
TTY: 502-564-5777

Louisiana

8158 Office of Human Services: Division of Alcohol and Drug Abuse
628 N 4th Street
Baton Rouge, LA 70802-2790

225-342-9500
855-229-6848
Fax: 225-342-3875
TTY: 225-342-5568
dhhwebinfo@la.gov
www.dhh.louisiana.gov

Maine

8159 Office of Alcohol and Drug Abuse Prevention
Ofice Of Substance Abuse
AMHI Complex, Marquardt Building
Augusta, ME 04333-0159

207-289-2595
Fax: 207-287-4334
www.maine.gov/dhhs/samhs/osa/

Kimberly A. Johnson, Director

Maryland

8160 Maryland State Alcohol and Drug Abuse Administration
55 Wade Avenue
Catonsville, MD 21228

410-402-8600
Fax: 410-402-8601
adaainfo@dhmh.state.md.us
www.maryland-adaa.org
The Alcohol and Drug Abuse Administration is committed to providing access to a quality and effective substance abuse prevention, intervention and treatment service system for the citizens of Maryland.
Kathleen Rebbert-Fra, Acting Director
Steve Bocian, Acting Deputy Director

Massachusetts

8161 Division of Substance Abuse
250 Washington Street
Boston, MA 02108-4619

617-624-5111
800-327-5050
Fax: 617-624-5185
TTY: 888-448-8321
bsas.questions@state.ma.us
www.mass.gov/eohhs/gov/departments/dph/p
Michael Botticelli, Director

Michigan

8162 Office of Substance Abuse Services Department of Public Health
Department of Public Health

320 S Walnut Street
Lansing, MI 48913

517-373-4700
888-736-0253
Fax: 517-335-2121
TTY: 517-373-3573
www.michigan.gov/mdch

Yvonne Blackmond, Director

Minnesota

8163 Chemical Dependency Program Division Department of Human Services
Department of Human Services
Saint Paul, MN 55164-3899

651-431-2460
800-627-3529
Fax: 651-582-1865
dhs.info@state.mn.us
mn.gov/dhs/about-dhs/
The Minnesota Department of Human Services, working with many others, helps people meet their basic needs so they can live in dignity and achieve their highest potential.

8164 Dentists Concerned for Dentists
450 N Syndicate   651-641-0730
Saint Paul, MN 55104   www.medhelp.org/amshc/amshc53.htm
A nonprofit organization for chemically dependent Minnesota dentists and concerned others.

Mississippi

8165 Division of Alcohol & Drug Abuse: Mississippi
Department of Mental Health
1101 Robert E Lee Building
Jackson, MS 39201

601-359-1288
877-210-8513
Fax: 601-359-6295
TTY: 601-359-6230
www.dmh.state.ms.us
Supporting a better tomorrow by making a difference in the lives of Mississippians with mental illness, substance abuse problems and intellectual/developmental disabilities one person at a time.
Rose Roberts, Chair
Jim Herzog, Vice Chair

8166 Division of Alcohol & Drug Abuse: South Department of Mental Health
1101 Robert E Lee Building
Jackson, MS 39201

601-359-1288
877-210-8513
Fax: 601-359-6295
TTY: 601-359-6230
www.dmh.state.ms.us
Supporting a better tomorrow by making a difference in the lives of Mississippians with mental illness, substance abuse problems and intellectual/developmental disabilities one person at a time.
Rose Roberts, Chair
Jim Herzog, Vice Chair

Missouri

8167 Missouri Division of Alcohol and Drug Abuse
Department of Mental Health
1706 E Elm Street
Jefferson City, MO 65102

573-751-4942
800-575-7480
Fax: 573-751-8224
TTY: 573-526-1201
dmhmail@dmh.mo.gov
dmh.mo.gov/ada/

Keith Schafer, Director
Heidi DiBiaso, Administrative Assistant

Montana

8168 Department of Institutions, Alcohol and Drug Abuse Division
Helena, MT 59620-2905   406-444-3964
Fax: 406-444-9389

Nebraska

8169 Department of Public Instruction: Division of Alcoholism and Drug Abuse
Division Of Behavioral Health

Lincoln, NE 68509-8925 402-471-7818
800-648-4444
Fax: 402-479-5162
www.hhs.state.ne.us

Scot Adams, Director
GibsonBlaine Shaffer, CEO

Nevada

8170 Alcohol and Drug Abuse Bureau: Department of Human Resources
4126 Technology Way 775-684-5943
Carson City, NV 89706 Fax: 775-684-5964
MHDS@MHDS.NV.GOV

Maria Canfield, Chief

New Hampshire

8171 Office of Alcohol and Drug Abuse Prevention
State Office Park South
129 Pleasant Street 800-804-0909
Concord, NH 03301-3852 Fax: 603-271-6105
www.dhhs.state.nh.us

New Jersey

8172 Department of Health
120 S Stockton Street 609-292-7837
Trenton, NJ 08625-0362 800-367-6543
Fax: 609-292-3816
georgene.rhodunda@dhs.state.nj.us
www.state.nj.us

Heather Howard, Commissioner
Mary E O'Dowd, Chief of Staff

8173 Division of Narcotic and Drug Abuse Control
120 S Stockton Street 609-292-5760
Trenton, NJ 08625-0362 800-238-2333
Fax: 609-292-3816
www.state.nj.us/humanservices

Jeffers, Director

New Mexico

8174 Substance Abuse Bureau
1190 Saint Francis Drive 505-827-2601
Santa Fe, NM 87502 800-362-2013
Fax: 505-827-0097

New York

8175 Division of Substance Abuse Services
Substance Abuse Services
1450 Western Avenue 518-473-3460
Albany, NY 12203-3526 877-846-7369
Fax: 518-457-5474
communications@oasas.ny.gov
www.oasas.ny.gov

Karen M Carpenter-Palumbo, Commissioner
Kathleen Caggiano-Si, Executive Deputy Commissioner

North Carolina

8176 Alcohol and Drug Abuse Section
Division of Mental Health & Mental Retardation
2001 Mail Service Center 919-733-7011
Raleigh, NC 27699-3007 800-662-7030
Fax: 919-508-0951
www.dhhs.state.nc.us

Leza Wainwright, Director
Michael S Lancaster, Director

North Dakota

8177 Division of Alcoholism & Drug Abuse: Department of Human Services
Department Of Human Services

1237 W Divide Avenue 701-328-8920
Bismarck, ND 58501 800-755-2719
Fax: 701-328-8969
www.nd.gov/dhs/services/mentalhealth/
The Mental Health and Substance Abuse Services Division provides leadership for the planning, development, and oversight of a system of care for children, adults, and families with severe emotional disorders, mental illness, and/or substance abuse issues.

Ohio

8178 Bureau on Alcohol Abuse and Recovery Ohio Department of Health
Ohio Department of Health
30 East Broad Street 614-466-3445
Columbus, OH 43215-2550 Fax: 614-752-8645
info@ada.ohio.gov
www.odadas.state.oh.us
The mission of the Ohio Department of Mental Health and Addiction Services (OhioMHAS) is to provide statewide leadership of a high-quality mental health and addiction prevention, treatment and recovery system that is effective and valued by all Ohioans.
Tracy J. Plouck, Director
Orman Hall, Director of the Governor's Cabinet Opiat

8179 Bureau on Drug Abuse: Ohio Department of Health
Ohio Department of Health
30 East Broad Street 614-466-3445
Columbus, OH 43215 Fax: 614-752-8645
info@ada.ohio.gov
The mission of the Ohio Department of Mental Health and Addiction Services (OhioMHAS) is to provide statewide leadership of a high-quality mental health and addiction prevention, treatment and recovery system that is effective and valued by all Ohioans.
Tracy J. Plouck, Director
Orman Hall, Director of the Governor's Cabinet Opiat

Oklahoma

8180 Oklahoma Department of Mental Health and Substance Abuse Services
Substance Abuse Program
1200 NE 13th Street 405-522-3908
Oklahoma City, OK 73117-3277 800-522-9054
Fax: 405-522-3650
TTY: 405-522-3851
jglover@odmhsas.org
www.odmhsas.org

J. Andy Sullivan, Chairperson
Larry McCauley, Vice Chair

Oregon

8181 Office of Alcohol and Drug Abuse Programs
500 Summer Street NE 503-945-5763
Salem, OR 97301-1118 Fax: 503-378-8467
TTY: 800-375-2863

Pennsylvania

8182 Drug and Alcohol Programs Department Of Health
Department Of Health
02 Kline Plaza 717-783-8200
Harrisburg, PA 17104-0090 877-724-3258
Fax: 717-787-6285
rkauffman@state.pa.us
www.ddap.pa.gov

Gary Tennis, Secretary
Kim Bowman, Deputy Secretary

Rhode Island

8183 Division of Substance Abuse: Department of Mental Health and Hospitals
Department Of Mental Health And Retardation
14 Harrington Road 401-462-2339
Cranston, RI 02920-0944 800-622-7422
Fax: 401-462-3204

Committed to assuring access to quality services and supports for Rhode Islanders with developmental disabilities, mental health and substance abuse issues, and chronic long term medical and psychiatric conditions. Our mission includes addressing the stigma attached to these disabilities as well as planning for the development of new services and prevention activities.
Craig S Stenning, Executive Director

South Carolina

8184 South Carolina Commission on Alcohol and Drug Abuse
Department Of Alcohol And Drug Abuse Services
2414 Bull Street
Columbia, SC 29201-9498
803-896-5555
Fax: 803-896-5557
The department's mission is to ensure the provision of quality services to prevent or reduce the negative consequences of substance use and addictions.
Bob Toomey, Director
Kaitlin Blanco-Silva, Project Manager

South Dakota

8185 Division of Alcohol & Drug Abuse: South Dakota
Department Of Human Services
3800 E Highway 34
Pierre, SD 57501-5070
605-773-5990
800-265-9684
Fax: 605-773-5483
TTY: 605-773-6412
infodhs@state.sd.us
www.dhs.sd.gov
Gilbert Sudbeck, Director

Tennessee

8186 Department of Mental Health and Mental Retardation, Alcohol & Drug Service
Bureau Of Alcohol And Drug Abuse Services
601 Mainstream Drive
Nashville, TN 37243-4401
615-532-6500
800-560-5767
Fax: 615-532-2419
www.state.tn.us
Michael A. Rabin, Director and Meida Contact
Lorene Lambert, Publications & Web Management

Texas

8187 Texas Commission on Alcohol and Drug Abuse Department Of State Health
Department Of State Health
Austin, TX 78714
512-206-5000
866-378-8440
Fax: 512-458-7477
TTY: 800-735-2989
TDD: 800-735-2989
web.master@dshs.state.tx.us
www.dshs.state.tx.us/mhsa/
Mission is to improve health and well-being in Texas.
David L. Lakey, Commissioner

Utah

8188 Department of Social Services: Division of Substance Abuse
Department Of Human Services
195 North 1950 West
Salt Lake City, UT 84116
801-538-3939
Fax: 801-538-9892
jemarrott@utah.gov
The Utah Division of Substance Abuse and Mental Health is the State agency responsible for ensuring that prevention and treatment services for substance abuse and mental health are available statewide. If you, a friend, or family member is struggling with a mental health problem or a problem with alcohol, tobacco, or other drugs there is help available. Hope and recovery are possible.
Paula Bell, Chairperson
Darryl Wagner, Vice Chairman

Vermont

8189 Alcohol and Drug Abuse Programs of Vermont Department Of Health
Department Of Health
108 Cherry Street
Burlington, VT 05402-1531
802-651-1550
Fax: 802-651-1573
www.healthvermont.gov

Virginia

8190 Substance Abuse Services Office of Virginia
Department of Mental Health & Mental Retardation
1220 Bank Street
Richmond, VA 23218-1797
804-786-3921
800-451-5544
Fax: 804-371-6638
TTY: 804-371-8977
Available to citizens statewide, Virginia's public mental health, intellectual disability and substance abuse services system is comprised of 16 state-operated facilities and 40 locally-run community services boards (CSBs) The CSBs and facilities serve children and adults who have-or who are at risk of-mental illness, serious emotional disturbance, intellectual disabilities, or substance abuse disorders.
Jim Stewart, Commissioner
Olivia Garland, Deputy Commissioner

Washington

8191 Washington Department of Social and Health Services, Alcohol and Drug Prog.
Department Of Social And Health Services
Olympia, WA 98504-5330
877-301-4557
800-737-0617
Fax: 360-438-8078
TTY: 877-301-4557
starkkd@dshs.wa.gov
www1.dshs.wa.gov

West Virginia

8192 West Virginia Division of Alcohol & Drug Abuse
Department Of Health And Human Resources
350 Capitol Street
Charleston, WV 25304-3702
304-356-4811
Fax: 304-558-1008
www.dhhr.wv.gov
The Division on Alcoholism and Drug Abuse, an operating division of the Bureau for Behavioral Health and Health Facilities (BBHHF) within the West Virginia Division of Health and Human Services is charged in code with being the Single State Authority (SSA) primarily responsible for prevention, control, treatment, rehabilitation, educational research and planning for substance abuse related services
Craig A. Richards, Deputy Commissioner

Wisconsin

8193 Office of Alcohol and Other Drug Abuse
1 W Wilson Street
Madison, WI 53703-7851
608-266-1865
Fax: 608-266-1533
TTY: 608-267-7371
dhswebmaster@wisconsin.gov
John Easterday, Administrator
Susan Gadacz, Contact

Wyoming

8194 Alcohol & Drug Abuse Programs of Wyoming Department Of Health
Department Of Health
401 Hathaway Building
Cheyenne, WY 82002-0480
307-777-7656
866-571-0944
Fax: 307-777-7439
Thomas O. Forslund, Director
Lee Clabots, Deputy Director

Libraries & Resource Centers

8195 National Clearinghouse for Alcohol and Drug Information
Rockville, MD 20847-2345
240-221-4019
800-729-6686
Fax: 240-221-4292
TDD: 800-487-4889
A resource for alcohol and other drug information. It carries a wide variety of publications dealing with alcohol and other drug abuse.
John Noble, Director

8196 Parents Resource Institute for Drug Education
160 Vanderbilt Court
Bowling Green, KY 42103
800-279-6361
Fax: 270-746-9598
info@pridesurveys.com
www.pridesurveys.com
Offers national information and educational materials pertaining to alcohol and drug dependency.
Thomas J Gleaton, EdD, President
Janie Pitcock, President

Research Centers

8197 Alcohol Disease Foundation
33 Eglantine Avenue
Pennington, NJ 08534-2308
609-737-0088
Founded in 1988 to promote research on testing systems that could diagnose the metabolic aspects of alcoholism. Seeks to educate the public on the validity of the disease concept of alcoholism.

8198 Alcohol Research Group Public Health Institute
Public Health Institute
6475 Christie Avenue
Emeryville, CA 94608-1324
510-597-3440
Fax: 510-985-6459
info@arg.org
www.arg.org
The Alcohol Research Group (ARG) of the Public Health Institute was established in 1959 to conduct and disseminate high-quality research in epidemiology of alcohol consumption and problems including alcohol use disorders, alcohol-related health services research, and analyses of alcohol policy and its impacts.
Dominique La MPH, Executive Director
Thomas K. Greenfield, Scientific Director

8199 Boston University Laboratory of Neuropsychology
Dept of Behavioral Neuroscience
80 E Concord Street M9
Boston, MA 02118
617-638-4803
Fax: 617-638-4806
www.bu.edu
Offers research and studies into the effects of Alcoholism pertaining to aphasia apraxia dementia memory disorders and various other neurological malfunctions.
Marlene Osca Berman PhD, Director

8200 Center for Alcohol & Addiction Studies Brown University
Brown University
121 South Main Street
Providence, RI 02903-0001
401-863-6600
Fax: 401-863-6697
caas@brown.edu
www.caas.brown.edu
The Center for Alcohol and Addiction Studies through its affiliation with the Brown Medical School occupies a unique position within the University. The Center brings together more that 90 faculty and professional staff members from 11 University departments and eight affiliated hospitals to promote the identification prevention and effective treatment of alcohol and other substance abuse.
Peter M Monti PhD, Center Director
Suzanne Colby Ph. D, Associate Director

8201 Cornerstone Medical Arts Center Hospital
Medical Arts Center Hospital
159-05 Union Turnpike
Fresh Meadows, NY 11366-2802
718-906-6700
800-233-9999
Fax: 718-906-6840
admin@cornerstoneny.com
www.cornerstoneny.com
Offers a complete integrated program for alcohol assessment alcohol and drug rehabilitation continuing care community education and comprehensive family recovery.
Norine Hurtado, Senior Vice President of Human Resources

8202 Do it Now Foundation
PO Box 27658
Tempe, AZ 85285-7658
480-736-0599
Fax: 480-736-0599
An information clearinghouse for service providers that publishes well-written pamphlets booklets and materials on chemical dependency and recovery.

8203 Dorothea Dix Hospital Clinical Research Unit
809 Ruggles Drive
Raleigh, NC 27603
919-733-5227
866-349-5627
Fax: 919-733-5351
www.med.unc.edu
Researches the biological risk factors of alcoholism using young adults without the disease but with history of familial alcoholism.
Terry Spell, Director
William L Roper, CEO

8204 Ernest Gallo Clinic and Research Center
5858 Horton Street
Emeryville, CA 94608
510-985-3100
Fax: 510-985-3101
ngreen@gallo.ucsf.edu
Alcoholism studies with a special emphasis on genetics.
John A. De Luca PHD, Chairman of the Board/President
Joseph E Gallo, President/Chief Executive Officer

8205 Families in Action National Drug Abuse Center
National Drug Abuse Center
PO Box 3553
Wilson, NC 27895
252-237-1242
Fax: 252-237-6544
phil@familiesinaction.org
www.familiesinaction.org
Publish prevention materials and serves as an information clearinghouse for families with a member suffering from a drug or alcohol addiction.
Phillip A Mooring, Executive Director
Anna Godwin, Coordinator

8206 Friends Medical Science Research Center
1229 West Mount Royal Avenue
Baltimore, MD 21217
410-752-4218
Fax: 310-477-9601
www.wellness.com
Studies narcotic addictions.
John Valenty, President
Rob Greenstein, President

8207 Hahnemann University Laboratory of Human Pharmacology
Department of Pharmacology
Broad and Vine
Philadelphia, PA 19102
215-762-7000
Fax: 215-762-8109
www.hahnemannhospital.com
Hahnemann University hospital is committed to providing quality patient care in an academic setting.
Benjamin Cal MD, Director

8208 Harvard Cocaine Recovery Project
1493 Cambridge Street
Cambridge, MA 02139-1099
617-498-1000
Fax: 617-642-58
Six-year study of relapse and recovery in cocaine addicts.
William McAu MD, Principal Investigator

8209 Interdisciplinary Program in Cell and Molecular Pharmacology
Medical University of South Carolina
173 Ashley Avenue BSB 358
Charleston, SC 29425
843-792-8975
Fax: 843-792-0481
Research into pharmacology and toxicology.
Kenneth D Tew, Ph.D., D.Sc., Professor and Chairman
Michelle Shorter, Administrative Coordinator

8210 Johns Hopkins University: Behavioral Pharmacology Research Unit
John Hopkins Bay View Campus
5510 Nathan Shock Drive
Baltimore, MD 21224-2735
410-955-5000
Fax: 410-550-0030
bigelow@jhmi.edu
www.hopkinsmedicine.org

An internationally recognized center of excellence in research on psychoactive drugs. As the name implies BPRU's orientation is behavioral and pharmacological emphasizing a behavioral analysis of drug action.
George E Bigelow PhD, Scientific Director
Eric C Strain MD, Medical Director

8211 Kettering-Scott Magnetic Resonance Laboratory
Wright State University, School of Medicine
PO Box 927   937-775-2934
Dayton, OH 45435-0927   www.med.wright.edu
No information found on the website.
Marjorie Bowman, MD and Dean
Betty Kangas, Assistant to the dean

8212 Marin Institute
24 Belvedere Street   415-456-5692
San Rafael, CA 94901-4817   Fax: 415-456-0491
                                               www.marinInstitute.org
The mission of this Institute is to reduce the toll of alcohol and other drug problems on Marin County and society in general. The Institute fulfills this mission by developing implementing evaluating and disseminating innovative approaches to prevention locally nationally and internationally.
Bruce Lee Livingston MPP, Executive Director
Michele Simo JD MPH, Research & Policy Director

8213 Narcotic and Drug Research
11 Beach Street   212-966-8700
New York, NY 10013-2429   Fax: 212-334-8058
Nonprofit organization that is devoted to drug abuse education treatment and prevention.
Douglas S Lipton PhD, Director

8214 National Center on Addiction and Substance Abuse
Columbia University
633 3rd Avenue   212-841-5200
New York, NY 10017-6706   800-622-4357
                                                Fax: 212-956-8020
                                               www.casacolumbia.org
The only nation-wide organization that brings together under one roof all the professional disciplines needed to study and combat abuse of all substances - alcohol nicotine as well as illegal prescription and performance enhancing drugs - in all sectors of society.
Lee C. Bollinger, President
Ursula M. Burns, Chairman and CEO

8215 National Prevention Resource Center CSAP Division of Communications Programs
CSAP Division of Communications Programs
5600 Fishers Lane   301-443-9936
Rockville, MD 20857-0001
Supports an array of prevention program evaluation approaches including individual grantee evaluations program evaluations and a National Evaluation Project. Also offers a National Data Base to provide information on programs for prevention of substance abuse.

8216 National Treatment Consortium for Alcohol and Other Drugs
PO Box 1294   202-434-4780
Washington, DC 20013   www.ntc-usa.org

8217 National Volunteer Training Center for Substance Abuse Prevention
CSAP Division of Communications Programs
5600 Fishers Lane   301-443-9936
Rockville, MD 20857
Volunteers are always on hand to provide answers, information, referrals and resources pertaining to alcohol, drugs and substance abuse.

8218 National Volunteer Training Center for Sub CSAP Division of Communications Programs
5600 Fishers Lane   301-443-9936
Rockville, MD 20857
Volunteers are always on hand to provide answers information referrals and resources pertaining to alcohol drugs and substance abuse.

8219 Ohio State University Clinical Pharmacology Division
College of Medicine
370 Western 9th Avenue   614-292-2220
Columbus, OH 43210-1239   800-252-3636
                                                Fax: 614-292-4293
Substance abuse and alcohol related research.
Robert Bornstein PHD, Vice dean for academic affairs
Glen Apsloss, Director

8220 RADAR Network National Clearinghouse for Alcohol & Dru
National Clearinghouse for Alcohol & Drug Info
PO Box 2345   301-468-2600
Rockville, MD 20847-2345   800-729-6686
                                                Fax: 240-221-4292
                                               TTY: 800-487-4889
                                               TDD: 800-487-4889
Consists of state clearinghouses specialized information centers of national organizations and the Department of Education Regional Training Centers. Each RADAR member can offer the public a variety of information services.
John Noble, Director

8221 Research Institute on Alcoholism State University of New York at Buffalo
State University of New York at Buffalo
1021 Main Street   716-887-2566
Buffalo, NY 14203   Fax: 716-872-52
                                              connors@ria.buffalo.edu
Integral part of the New York State Division of Alcoholism and Alcohol Abuse.
Kenneth E Leonard, PhD, Director
Kimberly S Walitzer, PhD, Deputy Director

8222 Rockefeller University Laboratory of Biology
1230 York Avenue   212-327-8000
New York, NY 10065   Fax: 212-327-7974
                                               www.rockefeller.edu
Marc Tessier Lavigne, President

8223 Rutgers University Center of Alcohol Studies
Busch Campus
607 Allison Road   732-445-2190
Piscataway, NJ 08854   Fax: 732-445-3500
                                              alclib@rci.rutgers.edu
                                             alcoholstudies.rutgers.edu
Causes and treatment of alcoholism.
Robert Pandi PhD, Director

8224 Rutgers University: Controlled Drug- Delivery Research Center
College of Pharmacy
PO Box 789   732-932-3834
Piscataway, NJ 08855-0789   Fax: 732-932-5767
Yie W Chien, Director

8225 Ruth E Golding Clinical Pharmacokinetics Laboratory
College of Pharmacy
1703 E Mabel   520-626-1938
Tucson, AZ 85721-1427   www.pharmacy.arizona.edu
Conducts studies of drugs in humans and animals.
Michael Maye MD, Head

8226 Southern California Research Institute
7065 Hayvenhurst Avenue   310-390-8481
Van Nuys, CA 90066   Fax: 310-390-8482
Effects of alcohol and drugs on behavior studies.
Dary Fiorent PhD, Executive Director
Bergetta Die BA, Research Associate

8227 Stanford Center for Research in Disease Prevention
Stanford University School of Medicine
1070 Arastradero Road   650-723-6254
Palo Alto, CA 94304   Fax: 650-723-6254
                                              prevention.stanford.edu
Prevention and control of alcohol and drug abuse related disorders.
John P.A Loannidis, MD, DSc, Director

8228 State University of New York at Buffalo Toxicology Research Center
3435 Main Street   716-831-2125
Buffalo, NY 14214   Fax: 716-829-2806
www.smbs.buffalo.edu
Toxicology-related research and services including the development of tests to evaluate toxins chemicals and drugs.
Michale E. Cain, Director
Dr James R Olson, Assistant Director

8229 University of California: Los Angeles Alcohol Research Center
405 Hilgard Ave   310-825-4321
Los Angeles, CA 90095-8353   Fax: 310-206-7309
www.ucla.edu
Causes of alcoholism including genetics.
Dr Ernest Noble, Director

8230 University of Michigan: Alcohol Research Center
400 E Eisenhower Parkway   734-764-1817
Ann Arbor, MI 48108-3318   Fax: 734-998-7994
www.umich.edu
Alcohol abuse studies among the elderly including the relationship between alcohol and aged disorders.
Robert A Zucker PhD, Contact

8231 University of Michigan: Psychiatric Center
4250 Plymouth road   734-936-5900
Ann Arbor, MI 48109-0001   Fax: 734-936-9761
www.umich.edu
Psychiatric disease research pertaining to the effects of alcoholism and drug abuse.
Gregory W Dalack, MD

8232 University of Minnesota: Program on Alcohol/Drug Control
Stadium Gate 27   612-624-6861
Minneapolis, MN 55455
Alcohol tobacco and drug research.
Dr James Schaefer, Director

8233 University of Missouri: Kansas City Drug Information Service
2464 Charlotte   816-235-5490
Kansas City, MO 64108-2640   Fax: 816-235-5491
umkcdruginformation@umkc.edu
Literature research and evaluation of clinical drug problems and questions.
Pat Bryant PhD, Director
Heather A Pace PhD, Assistant Director

8234 University of Tennessee Drug Information Center
875 Monroe Avenue   901-528-5555
Memphis, TN 38163-1   Fax: 901-448-5419
Katie Suda, Director
Camille Thornton, Assistant Professor

8235 University of Texas Health Science Center Neurophysiology Research Center
Speech & Hearing Institute
7000 Fannin   713-500-4472
Houston, TX 77030-3405   Fax: 713-792-4513
Conducts clinical and animal studies aimed at combating alcohol drug and tobacco dependence.
Giuseppe N Colasurdo, Director

8236 University of Texas at Austin: Drug Synamics Institute
1 University Station   512-475-9746
Austin, TX 78712   Fax: 512-471-2746
www.utexas.edu
Pharmaceutical and drug research.
Janet C Walkow PhD, Director
Carla Van Den Berg PhD, Associate Professor

8237 University of Utah: Center for Human Toxicology
30 South 2000 East   801-581-6731
Salt Lake City, UT 84112-1210   Fax: 801-581-3716
dwilkins@alanine.pharm.utah.edu
www.pharmacy.utah.edu
Clinical forensic and toxicology research.
Chris M . Ireland PHd, Dean
Dennis Crouch, Director

8238 University of Wisconsin Milwaukee Medicinal Chemistry Group
University of Wisconsin
PO Box 413   414-229-1122
Milwaukee, WI 53201-413   www4.uwm.edu
Research on drugs including studies of valium receptors.
Michael R. Lovell, Chancellor

Support Groups & Hotlines

8239 Al-Anon Alateen Family Group Hotline
1600 Corporate Landing Parkway   757-563-1600
Virginia Beach, VA 23454-970   888-425-2666
Fax: 757-563-1655
wso@alanon.org
www.al-anon.alateen.org
A mutual peer-to-peer support program with groups meeting worldwide to provide hope and help to the families of alcoholics. Although a seperate entity from Alcoholics Anonymous, our program is based upon the Twelve Steps.
Ric Buchanan, Executive Director

8240 Alcohol Drug Treatment Referral
1316 South Coast Highway   800-454-8966
Laguna Beach, CA 92651-3118   Fax: 949-281-1933
National Help and Referral Network, a nonprofit organization available 24 hours a day to assist people troubled by drug or alcohol abuse. Here to provide information on addiction treatment and support services and to help save lives and mend broken dreams.
Mike Cohan, Director

8241 Alcoholics Anonymous World Services
PO Box 459   212-870-3400
New York, NY 10163-4059   Fax: 212-870-3003
www.aa.org
Alcoholics Anonymous is a fellowship of men and women who share their experience, strength and hope with each other that they may solve their common problem and help others to recover from alcoholism. The only requirement for membership is a desire to stop drinking. There are no dues or fees for AA membership; they are self-supporting through their own contributions.
Greg M, General Manager

8242 Drug Free Workplace Hotline
Division of Workplace Programs
Samhsa Diagonal CSAP 1 Choke Cherry   240-276-2612
Rockville, MD 20857   877-726-4727
Fax: 240-276-1210
TDD: 800-457-4889
webmaster@samhsa.hhs.gov
A hotline for businesses to obtain information on a wide range of drug abuse related problems, issues and services.
Robert Stephenson II, Director

8243 Friday Night Live
California Dept of Drug & Alcohol Programs
1700 K Street   916-445-7456
Sacramento, CA 95814   Fax: 916-230-59
www.communitycounseling.org/fnl
These groups, located in California, are all run by students with a faculty adviser. They arrange local alcohol and drug free events, from dances and movies to visiting hospitalized children. Students not only have fun but they learn to have fun sober.
Jim Kooler, Administrator
Laura Purcellabuzo, Project Coordinator

8244 Images Within: A Child's View of Parental Alcoholism
Children of Alcoholics Foundation
PO Box 4185   212-595-5810
New York, NY 10163-4185   800-359-2623
www.coaf.org
An innovative program designed to teach all children about family alcoholism. Middle-school-aged children learn how to get help for themselves or give help to their friends.

8245 International Lawyers in Alcoholics Anonymous
39 Smith Neck Road   860-529-7474
Old Lyme, CT 6371   www.ilaa.org
Provides 40 independent local groups.
Scoot Huyghebaert, Chairman

8246 National Health Information Center
Office of Disease Prevention & Health Promotion
1101 Wootton Pkwy
Rockville, MD 20852
Fax: 240-453-8281
odphpinfo@hhs.gov
www.health.gov/nhic

Supports public health education by maintaining a calendar of National Health Observances; helps connect consumers and health professionals to organizations that can best answer questions and provide up-to-date contact information from reliable sources; updates on a yearly basis toll-free numbers for health information, Federal health clearinghouses and info centers.
Don Wright, MD, MPH, Director

8247 ToughLove International
PO Box 1069
Doylestown, PA 18901-0019
215-348-7090
800-333-1069

This national self-help group for parents, children and communities emphasizes cooperation, personal initiative and action. Publishes books, brochures and promotional information and holds workshops and seminars across the country.

8248 WFS' New Life Program
Women for Sobriety
PO Box 618
Quakertown, PA 18951-0618
215-536-8026
Fax: 215-538-9026
newlife@nni.com
www.womenforsobriety.org

A self-help program for women that can be used independent from AA or with AA. Groups are in many states in the United States. Donations suggested.
Rebecca M Fenner, Director

Books

8249 AA Comes of Age
Alcoholics Anonymous
PO Box 459
New York, NY 10163-0459
212-870-3400
Fax: 212-870-3137
www.aa.org

Tells how AA was started, how the Steps and Traditions evolved and how the AA Fellowship grew and spread overseas.

8250 AA in Prison: Inmate to Inmate
Alcoholics Anonymous
PO Box 459
New York, NY 10163-0459
212-870-3400
Fax: 212-870-3137
www.aa.org

Thirty-two stories that share the experience of men and women who found AA while in prison.
128 pages

8251 Accepting Ourselves & Others
Hazelden
15251 Pleasant Valley Rd
Center City, MN 55012-9640
651-213-4200
800-257-7810
Fax: 651-213-4426
www.hazelden.org

Fully revised and expanded second edition. Examines recovery as it affects the gay, lesbian, and bisexual community, as well as their friends, family, and therapists. Addresses the relationship between substance abuse and being a sexual minority, and discusses the impact of other issues such as anxiety, depression, sexual abuse, and learning disabilities.
379 pages Paperback
ISBN: 1-568381-20-4
Sharon Birnbaum, Corporate Director of Human Resources
Jim Blaha, VP CFO and CAO

8252 Addiction and Responsibility
The Crossroad Publishing Company
1001 N. Fairfax St.
Alexandria, VA 22314-6503
703-741-7686
800-548-0497
Fax: 703-741-7698
naadac@naadac.org
www.naadac.org

Anyone who has wrestled with such basic questions about addiction such as: Is drug addiction a behavior disorder or a character flaw? Is it genetic or learned? What is it like to be addicted? will find welcome answers in this groundbreaking philosophical inquiry into the addictive mind. The author helps readers understand addiction.
192 pages
ISBN: 0-824513-65-7
Kirk Bowden, President
Gerry Schmidt, President-Elect

8253 Addictions Counseling
The Crossroad Publishing Company
1001 N. Fairfax St.
Alexandria, VA 22314-6503
703-741-7686
800-548-0497
Fax: 703-741-7698
naadac@naadac.org
www.naadac.org

A practical guide to counseling people with chemical and other addictions.
144 pages Paperback
ISBN: 0-824513-86-0
Kirk Bowden, President
Gerry Schmidt, President-Elect

8254 Addictive Personality
Hazelden
15251 Pleasant Valley Rd
Center City, MN 55012-9640
651-213-4200
800-257-7810
Fax: 651-213-4426
www.hazelden.org

Understanding how an individual becomes an addict through examination of addiction's causes, stages of development, and consequences. Second edition further refines these ideas and includes the most recent information on the addictive process, cultural influences on addictive behaviors, recovery, genetic factors in addiction, mental health issues, and new research findings.
130 pages Paperback
ISBN: 1-568381-29-8
Sharon Birnbaum, Corporate Director of Human Resources
Jim Blaha, VP CFO and CAO

8255 Addictive Thinking Understanding Self-Deception
Hazelden
15251 Pleasant Valley Rd
Center City, MN 55012-9640
651-213-4200
800-257-7810
Fax: 651-213-4426
www.hazelden.org

Illustrates the irrational perspective and complicated, contradictory thinking patterns of addictive thinking, and demonstrates how they lead to low self-esteen, addiction, and relapse. Revised edition includes expanded information on depression and affective disorders, the relationship between addictive thinking and relapse, and the new research related to the origins of addictive thinking.
140 pages Paperback
ISBN: 1-568381-38-7
Sharon Birnbaum, Corporate Director of Human Resources
Jim Blaha, VP CFO and CAO

8256 Adult Children of Alcoholics
Hazelden
15251 Pleasant Valley Rd
Center City, MN 55012-9640
651-213-4200
800-257-7810
Fax: 651-213-4426
www.hazelden.org

Written to and for adult children of dysfunctional families.
138 pages Paperback
Sharon Birnbaum, Corporate Director of Human Resources
Jim Blaha, VP CFO and CAO

8257 Al-Anon Family Groups
Al-Anon Family Group Headquarters
1600 Corp Landing Pkwy
Virginia Beach, VA 23454-5617
757-563-1600
800-425-2666
Fax: 757-563-1655
wso@al-anon.org
www.al-anon.alateen.org

Basic book that explains the purpose of fellowship, how it works and how it is held in unity. Includes real life stories by husbands, wives, parents and children of those who suffer from alcoholism.
177 pages
ISBN: 0-910034-54-0
Caryn Johnson, Director Communications

8258 Al-Anon's Twelve Steps and Twelve Traditions
Al-Anon Family Group Headquarters
1600 Corp Landing Pkwy   757-563-1600
Virginia Beach, VA 23454-5617   800-425-2666
                                     Fax: 757-563-1655
                                          wso@al-anon.org
                                          www.al-anon.alateen.org
Written for people whose lives have been affected by alcoholism.
142 pages Hardcover
ISBN: 0-910034-24-9
Caryn Johnson, Director Communications

8259 Alateen: A Day at a Time
Al-Anon Family Group Headquarters
1600 Corp Landing Pkwy   757-563-1600
Virginia Beach, VA 23454-5617   800-425-2666
                                     Fax: 757-563-1655
                                          wso@al-anon.org
                                          www.al-anon.alateen.org
A collection of positive, daily sharings written by teenagers
around the world.
384 pages
ISBN: 0-910034-53-2
Caryn Johnson, Director Communications

8260 Alateen: Hope for Children of Alcoholics
Al-Anon Family Group Headquarters
1600 Corp Landing Pkwy   757-563-1600
Virginia Beach, VA 23454-5617   800-425-2666
                                     Fax: 757-563-1655
                                          wso@al-anon.org
                                          www.al-anon.alateen.org
A gold mine of information written by Alateens themselves. It cov-
ers the history of Alateen, understanding alcoholism and personal
stories.
115 pages
ISBN: 0-910034-20-6
Caryn Johnson, Director Communications

**8261 Alcohol and Other Drug Services: Dir. of California's
Community Services**
Department of Alcohol and Drug Programs
1501 Capitol Avenue   916-332-7012
Sacramento, CA 95899-4022   www.dhcs.ca.gov
A directory listing agencies, alcohol and drug providers, county
504 coordinators and county program administrators for the state
of California.
136 pages

**8262 Alcohol, Drug and Other Addictions: A Directory of Treatment
Centers**
Oryx Press
3100 East Commercial Blvd   602-265-2651
Fort Lauderdale, FL 33308-3397   800-279-4663
                                          www.recovery.org
Lists 18,000 federal, state and local addiction treatment regimens
that include public and private centers.

8263 Alcohol, Tobacco and Other Drugs May Harm the Unborn
National Clearinghouse for Alcohol and Drug Info.
PO Box 2345   800-729-6686
Rockville, MD 20847-2345
Presents the most recent findings of basic research and clinical
studies conducted on the effects of alcohol, drugs and tobacco on
the unborn.

8264 Alcoholics Anonymous
Alcoholics Anonymous
PO Box 459   212-870-3400
New York, NY 10163-0459   Fax: 212-870-3137
                                          www.aa.org
Third edition of the Big Book, basic text of AA. Chapters describe
the AA recovery program and personal histories have been added.

8265 Alcoholics Anonymous: The Big Book
Hazelden
15251 Pleasant Valley Rd   651-213-4200
Center City, MN 55012-9640   800-257-7810
                                     Fax: 651-213-4426
                                          www.hazelden.org

Classic text that guides Alcoholics Anonymous programs and describes how millions of men and women have recovered from alcoholism.
575 pages Paperback
Sharon Birnbaum, Corporate Director of Human Resources
Jim Blaha, VP CFO and CAO

**8266 American Academy of Psychiatrists in Alcoholism and Addiction
Directory**
400 Massasoit Avenue   401-524-3076
East Providence, RI 02914   Fax: 401-272-0922
                                          www.aaap.org
Lists 900 member professionals who are concerned with drug and
alcohol abuse.
Laurence M. Westreich, President
John A. Renner, Jr., President-Elect

**8267 An Annotated Bibliography of Recent Empirical Research In
Methadone**
National Clearinghouse for Alcohol and Drug Info.
PO Box 2345   800-729-6686
Rockville, MD 20847-2345
Provides guidelines and suggestions to investigators engaged in
the demanding and essential task of followup research on intrave-
nous drug users who have contracted AIDS.
97 pages

8268 As Bill Sees It
Alcoholics Anonymous
PO Box 459   212-870-3400
New York, NY 10163-0459   Fax: 212-870-3137
                                          www.aa.org
This collection of Bill W's writings offers a daily source of com-
fort and inspiration.

8269 As We Understood...
Al-Anon Family Group Headquarters
1600 Corp Landing Pkwy   757-563-1600
Virginia Beach, VA 23454-5617   800-425-2666
                                     Fax: 757-563-1655
                                          wso@al-anon.org
                                          www.al-anon.alateen.org
Al-Anon members share their understanding of a higher power,
fellowship, spiritual awakening, prayer, meditation and letting go.
269 pages
ISBN: 0-910034-56-7
Caryn Johnson, Director Communications

8270 Black, Beautiful and Recovering
African American Family Services
2616 Nicollet Avenue S   612-871-7878
Minneapolis, MN 55408
A helpful guide for Black people who are in the process of recovering from alcohol or other substance abuse problems.
10 pages

8271 Body, Mind, and Spirit
Hazelden
15251 Pleasant Valley Rd   651-213-4200
Center City, MN 55012-9640   800-257-7810
                                     Fax: 651-213-4426
                                          www.hazelden.org
Addressing such issues as self-esteem, fear, anger, and spirituality,
these 366 daily meditations and affirmations integrate the physi-
cal, mental, and spiritual aspects of healing from addiction.
410 pages Paperback
ISBN: 1-568380-77-1
Sharon Birnbaum, Corporate Director of Human Resources
Jim Blaha, VP CFO and CAO

8272 Came to Believe
Alcoholics Anonymous
PO Box 459   212-870-3400
New York, NY 10163-0459   Fax: 212-870-3137
                                          www.aa.org
A collection of stories by AA members who write about what the
phrase spiritual awakening means to them.
120 pages

8273 Chemically Dependent Older Adults
Hazelden
15251 Pleasant Valley Rd
Center City, MN 55012-9640
651-213-4200
800-257-7810
Fax: 651-213-4426
www.hazelden.org
Reviews the importance of considering the older adult's health, living conditions and social and economic resources when developing treatment and aftercare plans.
136 pages Paperback
Sharon Birnbaum, Corporate Director of Human Resources
Jim Blaha, VP CFO and CAO

8274 Childhood and Adolescent Drug Abuse: A Physician's Guide
American Council on Drug Education
6001 Executive Boulevard
Bethesda, MD 20892-4425
301-443-1124
800-488-3784
www.drugabuse.gov
A scientific monograph which educates and sensitizes doctors to the dimensions of drug problems.
68 pages

8275 Circle of Hope
Hazelden
15251 Pleasant Valley Rd
Center City, MN 55012-9640
651-213-4200
800-257-7810
Fax: 651-213-4426
www.hazelden.org
Spirituality, acceptance, and living one day at a time are show through personal stories of individuals living with HIV and AIDS and dealing with adiction and recovery.
364 pages Paperback
ISBN: 0-894866-10-9
Sharon Birnbaum, Corporate Director of Human Resources
Jim Blaha, VP CFO and CAO

8276 Citizen's Alcohol and Other Drug Prevention Directory
National Clearinghouse for Alcohol and Drug Info.
PO Box 2345
Rockville, MD 20847-2345
800-729-6686
National directory of over 3,000 state, local and government agencies dealing with alcohol and other drug-related topics.
276 pages

8277 Cocaine Today
American Council on Drug Education
6001 Executive Boulevard
Bethesda, MD 20892-4425
301-443-1124
800-488-3784
www.drugabuse.gov
A recent revision of this popular book. Cocaine Today takes a new look at cocaine and its derivative, crack.

8278 Codependent No More
Hazelden
15251 Pleasant Valley Rd
Center City, MN 55012-9640
651-213-4200
800-257-7810
Fax: 651-213-4793
info@hazelden.org
www.hazelden.org
Explains codependent behaviors in clear, simple terms.
208 pages Paperback
Mark Mishek, President and Chief Executive Officer
Joe Jaksha, Publisher

8279 Color of Light
Hazelden
15251 Pleasant Valley Rd
Center City, MN 55012-9640
651-213-4200
800-257-7810
Fax: 651-213-4793
info@hazelden.org
www.hazelden.org
These 366 meditations speak to both the practical and spiritual journey of living with HIV/AIDS, and demonstrate how to integrate personal values with those offered in chemical dependency recovery and the Twelve Steps.
400 pages Paperback
ISBN: 0-894865-11-0
Mark Mishek, President and Chief Executive Officer
Joe Jaksha, Publisher

8280 Confusion is a State of Grace
Hazelden
15251 Pleasant Valley Rd
Center City, MN 55012
651-213-4200
800-257-7810
Fax: 651-213-4793
info@hazelden.org
www.hazelden.org
Compilation of quotes that captures the wisdom, humor, and healing found in Al-Anon and other Twelve Step groups.
153 pages Paperback
ISBN: 1-568380-89-5
Mark Mishek, President and Chief Executive Officer
Joe Jaksha, Publisher

8281 Courage to Be Me: Living with Alcoholism
Al-Anon Family Group Headquarters
1600 Corp Landing Pkwy
Virginia Beach, VA 23454-5617
757-563-1600
800-425-2666
Fax: 757-563-1655
wso@al-anon.org
www.al-anon.alateen.org
Written for and by Alateens of all ages who will treasure the honesty and strength of recovery shown.
326 pages
ISBN: 0-910034-30-3
Caryn Johnson, Director Communications

8282 Daily Reflections: A Book of Reflections by AA Members for AA Members
Alcoholics Anonymous
PO Box 459
New York, NY 10163-0459
212-870-3400
Fax: 212-870-3137
www.aa.org
AAs reflect on favorite quotations from A.A. literature. A reading for each day of the year.

8283 Day at a Time: Daily Reflections for Recovering People
Hazelden
15251 Pleasant Valley Rd
Center City, MN 55012-9640
651-213-4200
800-257-7810
Fax: 651-213-4793
info@hazelden.org
www.hazelden.org
Offers inspiration and hope for people recovering from chemical dependency or other addictions. Each daily passage reinforces the message of Twelve Step recovery.
384 pages Paperback
ISBN: 1-568380-36-4
Mark Mishek, President and Chief Executive Officer
Joe Jaksha, Publisher

8284 Day by Day
Hazelden
15251 Pleasant Valley Rd
Center City, MN 55012
651-213-4200
800-257-7810
Fax: 651-213-4793
info@hazelden.org
www.hazelden.org
A book of daily meditations for recovering addicts that reinforce Narcotics Anonymous principles and objectives.
400 pages Paperback
Mark Mishek, President and Chief Executive Officer
Joe Jaksha, Publisher

8285 Days of Healing, Days of Joy
Hazelden
15251 Pleasant Valley Rd
Center City, MN 55012-9640
651-213-4200
800-257-7810
Fax: 651-213-4793
info@hazelden.org
www.hazelden.org
Three hundred and sixty-six daily quotes, meditations and affirmations to help adult children in their search for serenity.
400 pages Paperback
Mark Mishek, President and Chief Executive Officer
Joe Jaksha, Publisher

8286 Developing Chemical Dependency Services for Black People
African American Family Services

2616 Nicollet Avenue S
Minneapolis, MN 55408 612-871-7878
This manual has been developed to address many of the questions asked by new or expanding programs as they establish new culturally specific initiatives for African-American clients.
78 pages

8287 Dilemma of the Alcoholic Marriage
Al-Anon Family Group Headquarters
1600 Corp Landing Pkwy 757-563-1600
Virginia Beach, VA 23454-5617 800-425-2666
Fax: 757-563-1655
wso@al-anon.org
www.al-anon.alateen.org
This book explores the problem of alcoholism in marriage and includes questions for applying the twelve steps to relationships.
100 pages
ISBN: 0-910034-18-4
Caryn Johnson, Director Communications

8288 Dr. Bob and the Good Oldtimers
Alcoholics Anonymous
PO Box 459 212-870-3400
New York, NY 10163-0459 Fax: 212-870-3137
www.aa.org
The life story of the fellowship's co-founder, interwoven wth recollections of early AA in the Midwest.

8289 Drug Abuse and Addiction Information/Treatment Programs
American Business Directories
5711 S 86th Circle 402-593-4600
Omaha, NE 68127-4146 Fax: 402-331-1505
Number of entries is 9,425.

8290 Drug Use Among American High School Seniors, College Students & Youth
National Clearinghouse for Alcohol and Drug Info.
PO Box 2345 800-729-6686
Rockville, MD 20847-2345
Comprehensive reports presenting the results of the 16th national survey of the drug use and related attitudes of American high school seniors.
199 pages Volumes I & II

8291 Drugs and Pregnancy: It's Not Worth the Risk
American Council on Drug Education
204 Monroe Street 800-488-3784
Rockville, MD 20850
A scientific monograph for health care providers which teaches them to identify alcohol and drug problems in their patients.
48 pages

8292 Dual Diagnosis
Hazelden
15251 Pleasant Valley Rd 651-213-4200
Center City, MN 55012-9640 800-257-7810
Fax: 651-213-4793
info@hazelden.org
www.hazelden.org
Focuses on the issues surrounding the treatment of clients with co-existing chemical dependency and psychiatric conditions.
191 pages Paperback
Mark Mishek, President and Chief Executive Officer
Joe Jaksha, Publisher

8293 Dual Disorders
Hazelden
15251 Pleasant Valley Rd 651-213-4200
Center City, MN 55012-9640 800-257-7810
Fax: 651-213-4793
info@hazelden.org
www.hazelden.org
Presents case histories and analyses of psychiatric disorders.
140 pages Paperback
Mark Mishek, President and Chief Executive Officer
Joe Jaksha, Publisher

8294 Dual Disorders Recovery Book
Hazelden

15251 Pleasant Valley Rd 651-213-4200
Center City, MN 55012-9640 800-257-7810
Fax: 651-213-4793
info@hazelden.org
www.hazelden.org
Helps individuals with dual disorders develop a plan for daily living through a specially-designed Twelve-Step program.
242 pages Paperback
ISBN: 1-568380-34-8
Mark Mishek, President and Chief Executive Officer
Joe Jaksha, Publisher

8295 Each Day a New Beginning
Hazelden
15251 Pleasant Valley Rd 651-213-4200
Center City, MN 55012-9640 800-257-7810
Fax: 651-213-4793
info@hazelden.org
www.hazelden.org
Promotes the development of a significant spiritual core for recovery that can be enhanced throughout the rest of life.
400 pages Paperback
Mark Mishek, President and Chief Executive Officer
Joe Jaksha, Publisher

8296 Elephant in the Living Room: A Leader's Guide
Hazelden
15251 Pleasant Valley Rd 651-213-4200
Center City, MN 55012-9640 800-257-7810
Fax: 651-213-4793
info@hazelden.org
www.hazelden.org
The adult companion to the classic children's book. Caretakers learn how to explain addiction and its effect on the family to small children who's parents or siblings are chemically dependent.
129 pages Paperback
ISBN: 1-568380-34-8
Mark Mishek, President and Chief Executive Officer
Joe Jaksha, Publisher

8297 Encyclopedia of Drug Abuse
Facts on File
11 Penn Plaza 212-967-8800
New York, NY 10001 800-322-8755
Fax: 800-678-3633
www.ncjrs.gov
More that 500 entries explore: specific drugs, countries, organizations, treatment programs, laws, medical terms, and psychosocial concepts.
496 pages Hardcover

8298 Ethics for Addiction Professionals
Hazelden
15251 Pleasant Valley Rd 651-213-4200
Center City, MN 55012-9640 800-257-7810
Fax: 651-213-4793
info@hazelden.org
www.hazelden.org
Probes crucial, complex ethical issues including counselor relapse, paid referrals and discrimination.
60 pages
Mark Mishek, President and Chief Executive Officer
Joe Jaksha, Publisher

8299 Extent and Adequacy of Insurance Coverage for Substance Abuse I & II
National Clearinghouse for Alcohol and Drug Info.
PO Box 2345 800-729-6686
Rockville, MD 20847-2345
These volumes examine the extent to which the cost of alcohol and other drug treatments is covered by private insurance, public financing and other sources.

8300 Eye Opener
Hazelden
15251 Pleasant Valley Rd 651-213-4200
Center City, MN 55012-9640 800-257-7810
Fax: 651-213-4793
info@hazelden.org
www.hazelden.org

Daily meditations about understanding the Alcoholics Anonymous program, writen by a favorite early AA member and author.
380 pages Cloth
ISBN: 0-894860-23-2
Mark Mishek, President and Chief Executive Officer
Joe Jaksha, Publisher

8301 Fact Is...Hispanic Parents Can Help Their Children Avoid Alcohol/Drugs
National Clearinghouse for Alcohol and Drug Info.
PO Box 2345   800-729-6686
Rockville, MD 20852-2345

8302 Feeding the Hungry Heart, the Experience of Compulsive Eating
Gurze Books
PO Box 2238   888-346-8205
Carlsbad, CA 92018-2238   Fax: 760-434-5476
                                        gzcatl@aol.com
                                        www.bulimia.com
This is a widely respected, extremely readable book from Ms. Roth and the many participants of early breaking free workshops. It is an intimate, vulnerable sharing of experiences which continues to touch and change lives.
212 pages Paperback

8303 Food for Thought: Daily Meditations for Overeaters
Hazelden
15251 Pleasant Valley Rd   651-213-4200
Center City, MN 55012-9640   800-257-7810
                                        Fax: 651-213-4793
                                        info@hazelden.org
                                        www.hazelden.org
Offers guidance in the early days of living a Twelve Step program.
400 pages Paperback
ISBN: 0-894860-90-9
Mark Mishek, President and Chief Executive Officer
Joe Jaksha, Publisher

8304 Forum Favorites: Volumes 1, 2, 3 & 4
Al-Anon Family Group Headquarters
1600 Corp Landing Pkwy   757-563-1600
Virginia Beach, VA 23454-5617   800-425-2666
                                        Fax: 757-563-1655
                                        wso@al-anon.org
                                        www.al-anon.alateen.org
Personal sharings show how the fundamentals of the Al-Anon programs are applied to everyday situations.
428 pages Set of 4
ISBN: 0-910034-51-6
Caryn Johnson, Director Communications

8305 Freedom from Smoking at Work Program
American Lung Association
55 W. Wacker Drive   312-801-7630
Chicago, IL 60601   800-548-8252
                                        Fax: 202-452-1805
                                        www.lungusa.org
ALA program for organizations interested in creating a healthier workplace environment through a comprehensive, multicomponent smoking education, cessation and policy development program designed for the workplace.
Kathryn A. Forbes, Chairman
Harold Wimmer, President and CEO

8306 Future by Design/A Community Framework
National Clearinghouse for Alcohol and Drug Info.
PO Box 2345   800-729-6686
Rockville, MD 20847-2345
Provides communities with a manageable framework for getting involved in alcohol and other drug prevention.
234 pages

8307 Gentle Path Through the Twelve Steps
Hazelden
15251 Pleasant Valley Rd   651-213-4200
Center City, MN 55012-9640   800-257-7810
                                        Fax: 651-213-4793
                                        info@hazelden.org
                                        www.hazelden.org

This workbook provides a unique set of structured forms and exercises to help recoving people integrate the Twelve Steps in all aspects of their lives.
224 pages Paperback
ISBN: 1-568380-58-5
Mark Mishek, President and Chief Executive Officer
Joe Jaksha, Publisher

8308 Getting Started in AA
Hazelden
15251 Pleasant Valley Rd   651-213-4200
Center City, MN 55012-9640   800-257-7810
                                        Fax: 651-213-4793
                                        info@hazelden.org
                                        www.hazelden.org
Practical suggestions for staying sober, summaries of AA principles, concepts, and slogans, and a historical overview to help the reader understand the spirit of the program.
211 pages Paperback
ISBN: 1-568380-91-7
Mark Mishek, President and Chief Executive Officer
Joe Jaksha, Publisher

8309 Getting Tough on Gateway Drugs: A Guide for the Family
American Council On Drug Education
204 Monroe Street   301-294-0603
Rockville, MD 20850-4425   800-488-3784
Gateway drugs including marijuana, alcohol and tobacco are those which open doors into all drug abuse. This family survival guide helps parents understand the consequences of drug dependence and suggests actions the family can take to prevent and solve drug problems.
332 pages
William F Current, Executive Director

8310 Getting it Together: Promoting Drug Free Communities
National Clearinghouse for Alcohol and Drug Info.
PO Box 2345   800-729-6686
Rockville, MD 20847
Provides resources and step-by-step information on how local communities and organizations can work effectively with young people who are committed to preventing alcohol and other drug abuse.
71 pages

8311 God Grant Me the Laughter: A Treasury of Twelve Step Humor
Hazelden
15251 Pleasant Valley Rd   651-213-4200
Center City, MN 55012-9640   800-257-7810
                                        Fax: 651-213-4793
                                        info@hazelden.org
                                        www.hazelden.org
Hearty cartoons and humorous anecdotes clearly demonstrate how readers' lives today contrast with their drinking and drug using in the past.
200 pages Paperback
ISBN: 1-568380-38-0
Mark Mishek, President and Chief Executive Officer
Joe Jaksha, Publisher

8312 Good First Step
Hazelden
15251 Pleasant Valley Rd   651-213-4200
Center City, MN 55012-9640   800-257-7810
                                        Fax: 651-213-4793
                                        info@hazelden.org
                                        www.hazelden.org
Features a structured format and emphasis on the meaning of the First Step to help build a solid foundation for recovery.
60 pages Paperback
ISBN: 1-568381-13-1
Mark Mishek, President and Chief Executive Officer
Joe Jaksha, Publisher

8313 Goodbye Hangovers, Hello Life
Women for Sobriety
PO Box 618   215-536-8026
Quakertown, PA 18951-0618   Fax: 215-536-9026
                                        newlife@nni.com
                                        www.womenforsobriety.org

A book about recovery - how it happens, what problems arise and how to overcome these problems.
250 pages Paperback

8314 Grateful to Have Been There
Hazelden
15251 Pleasant Valley Rd
Center City, MN 55012

651-213-4200
800-257-7810
Fax: 651-213-4793
info@hazelden.org
www.hazelden.org

Aide and executive secretary to AA's co-founder Bill W. for 20 years, Wing shares her memories and impressions of 42 years of involvement with the Fellowship.
150 pages Paperback
ISBN: 0-942421-44-2
Mark Mishek, President and Chief Executive Officer
Joe Jaksha, Publisher

8315 Growing Up Drug Free: A Parent's Guide to Prevention
National Clearinghouse for Alcohol and Drug Info.
400 Maryland Ave, SW
Washington, DC 20202

202-260-3954
800-729-6686
www.jtnn.org

Offers information on what parents can do to prevent their child from becoming a substance abuser/alcoholic. Focuses on counseling, peer pressure issues, education, school-parent cooperation and offers an introduction to each drug, symptoms and how to spot the warning signs of drug addiction.
47 pages

8316 Handle with Care
Hazelden
15251 Pleasant Valley Rd
Center City, MN 55012-9640

651-213-4200
800-257-7810
Fax: 651-213-4793
info@hazelden.org
www.hazelden.org

A comprehensive look at how parents, teachers and other care givers of children ages 10 and younger can identify and meet their special needs.
Mark Mishek, President and Chief Executive Officer
Joe Jaksha, Publisher

8317 Help for Helpers: Daily Meditations for Counselors
Hazelden
15251 Pleasant Valley Rd
Center City, MN 55012-9640

651-213-4200
800-257-7810
Fax: 651-213-4793
info@hazelden.org
www.hazelden.org

Written by addiction treatment center staff members from across the country, these daily meditations encourage, comfort, and challenge helpers to understand others and themselves.
400 pages Paperback
ISBN: 1-568380-61-5
Mark Mishek, President and Chief Executive Officer
Joe Jaksha, Publisher

8318 Helping Homeless People with Alcohol and Other Drug Problems
National Clearinghouse for Alcohol and Drug Info.
PO Box 2345
Rockville, MD 20847

800-729-6686

Developed by professionals who work directly with homeless people, this manual provides basic information about homeless people with AOD problems.
50 pages

8319 Helping Your Students Say No Teacher's Guide
National Clearinghouse for Alcohol and Drug Info.
PO Box 2345
Rockville, MD 20847-2345

800-729-6686
TDD: 800-487-4489

Explains the effects of alcohol on the body, why children start to drink, how teachers can help their students refuse alcohol and deal with the first signs of drinking.
13 pages
Lynn Hallard, Author

8320 How to Manage Your Drug-Free Workplace Programs
American Council on Drug Education

204 Monroe Street
Rockville, MD 20850-4425

800-488-3784
www.ascicorp.com

Step-by-step process for introducing and managing a drug awareness program that includes a variety of additional tips to complement messages in the drug awareness pamphlet series.
48 pages

8321 I'm Black and I'm Sober
Hazelden
15251 Pleasant Valley Rd
Center City, MN 55012-9640

651-213-4200
800-257-7810
Fax: 651-213-4793
info@hazelden.org
www.hazelden.org

An autobiography written by a recovering African American woman who discusses the impact of discrimination and the obstacles faced through the journey back to sobriety.
279 pages Paperback
ISBN: 1-568380-71-2
Mark Mishek, President and Chief Executive Officer
Joe Jaksha, Publisher

8322 If Only I Could Quit
Hazelden
15251 Pleasant Valley Rd
Center City, MN 55012-9640

651-213-4200
800-257-7810
Fax: 651-213-4793
info@hazelden.org
www.hazelden.org

Promotes the Twelve Step process for recovery from nicotine addiction.
320 pages Paperback
Mark Mishek, President and Chief Executive Officer
Joe Jaksha, Publisher

8323 In God's Care
Hazelden
15251 Pleasant Valley Rd
Center City, MN 55012-9640

651-213-4200
800-257-7810
Fax: 651-213-4793
info@hazelden.org
www.hazelden.org

Excellent relaxation and education tool for clients working on their Second and Third Steps.
400 pages Paperback
Mark Mishek, President and Chief Executive Officer
Joe Jaksha, Publisher

8324 Keep Quit
Hazelden
15251 Pleasant Valley Rd
Center City, MN 55012-9640

651-213-4200
800-257-7810
Fax: 651-213-4793
info@hazelden.org
www.hazelden.org

Daily motivational guide to help the new nonsmoker understand the craving for nicotine and learn how to break the rituals and patterns associated with relapse.
300 pages Paperback
ISBN: 1-568381-04-2
Mark Mishek, President and Chief Executive Officer
Joe Jaksha, Publisher

8325 Keep it Simple
Hazelden
15251 Pleasant Valley Rd
Center City, MN 55012-9640

651-213-4200
800-257-7810
Fax: 651-213-4793
info@hazelden.org
www.hazelden.org

Daily prayers that help clients learn to ask for help and to turn their self-will over to a Higher Power.
400 pages Paperback
Mark Mishek, President and Chief Executive Officer
Joe Jaksha, Publisher

8326 Learning to Live Drug Free: A Curriculum Model for Prevention
National Clearinghouse for Alcohol and Drug Info.
PO Box 2345
Rockville, MD 20847-2345

800-729-6686

Provides a flexible framework for classroom-based prevention efforts for kindergarten through grade 12.
52 pages

8327 Let's Talk About Alcohol Abuse
Rosen Publishing Group's PowerKids Press
29 East 21st Street   212-777-3017
New York, NY 10010   800-237-9932
Fax: 888-436-4643
customerservice@rosenpub.com
www.rosenpublishing.com
In gentle and sensitive terms this book talks about when a parent drinks and what alcohol can do to the body. Kids are told about the illegality of drinking as minors. Recommended for grade K-4.
ISBN: 0-823923-03-7
Marianne Johnston, Author

8328 Life of My Own: Daily Meditations on Hope and Acceptance
Hazelden
15251 Pleasant Valley Rd   651-213-4200
Center City, MN 55012-9640   800-257-7810
Fax: 651-213-4793
info@hazelden.org
www.hazelden.org
Offers daily access to strength, serenity, and insight in our relationships with chemically dependent people.
400 pages Paperback
ISBN: 0-894868-63-2
Mark Mishek, President and Chief Executive Officer
Joe Jaksha, Publisher

8329 Little Red Book
Hazelden
15251 Pleasant Valley Rd   651-213-4200
Center City, MN 55012-9640   800-257-7810
Fax: 651-213-4793
info@hazelden.org
www.hazelden.org
A primer for members of Alcoholics Anonymous. Each page acts as a study guide to the Big Book and its teachings.
164 pages Paperback
ISBN: 0-894869-85-X
Mark Mishek, President and Chief Executive Officer
Joe Jaksha, Publisher

8330 Living Sober
Hazelden
15251 Pleasant Valley Rd   651-213-4200
Center City, MN 55012-9640   800-257-7810
Fax: 651-213-4793
info@hazelden.org
www.hazelden.org
Offers clients sound advice about how to stay sober.
88 pages Paperback
Mark Mishek, President and Chief Executive Officer
Joe Jaksha, Publisher

8331 Lois Remembers
Al-Anon Family Group Headquarters
1600 Corp Landing Pkwy   757-563-1600
Virginia Beach, VA 23454-5617 800-425-2666
Fax: 757-563-1655
wso@al-anon.org
www.al-anon.alateen.org
The memoirs of a co-founder of Al-Anon. Lois tells her personal story and recalls the eventful years before and after the founding of AA and Al-Anon.
204 pages
ISBN: 0-910034-23-0
Caryn Johnson, Director Communications

8332 Marijuana
Branden Publishing Company
PO Box 812094   617-734-2045
Wellesley, MA 02482   Fax: 617-734-2046
www.branden.com

Paperback
ISBN: 0-828319-49-9

8333 Marijuana Smoking Prevention Program for Schools
American Lung Association
1740 Broadway   212-315-8700
New York, NY 10017   education.drugfreeworld.org
Cast of the TV show FAME enlivens highly motivational program to inform parents about the dangers of pot and discourages 9-11 year olds from using it.

8334 Marijuana Today
American Council on Drug Education
204 Monroe Street   301-762-0505
Rockville, MD 20850-4425 800-488-3784
Fax: 301-762-0080
info@armstrongcheris.com
www.armstrongcheris.com
A revision of the long time bestseller, this book examines the history of marijuana, its use, the risks associated with use and the short and long-term effects of use.

8335 Marijuana and Reproduction
American Council on Drug Education
204 Monroe Street   301-762-0505
Rockville, MD 20850-4425 800-488-3784
Fax: 301-762-0080
info@armstrongcheris.com
A scientific monograph for physicians which describes marijuana, profiles the users and discusses the effects on the reproductive system.
30 pages

8336 Marketing Booze to Blacks
African American Family Services
2616 Nicollet Avenue S   612-871-7878
Minneapolis, MN 55408
This controversial book details how liquor industries target the black population with its advertising.
55 pages

8337 Mistaken Beliefs About Relapse
Hazelden
15251 Pleasant Valley Rd   651-213-4200
Center City, MN 55012-9640   800-257-7810
Fax: 651-213-4793
info@hazelden.org
www.hazelden.org
Examines mistaken beliefs people have about relapse.
30 pages Paperback
Mark Mishek, President and Chief Executive Officer
Joe Jaksha, Publisher

8338 My Mind is Out to Get Me: Humor and Wisdom in Recovery
Hazelden
15251 Pleasant Valley Rd   651-213-4200
Center City, MN 55012   800-257-7810
Fax: 651-213-4793
info@hazelden.org
www.hazelden.org
Five hundred inspirational sayings and slogans that reflect both the lighter side of living a sober life and the profound wisdom offered in recovery. Each quote has been drawn from the wisdom of Alcoholics Anonymous.
180 pages Paperback
ISBN: 1-568380-10-0
Mark Mishek, President and Chief Executive Officer
Joe Jaksha, Publisher

8339 Narcotics Anonymous
Hazelden
15251 Pleasant Valley Rd   651-213-4200
Center City, MN 55012-9640   800-257-7810
Fax: 651-213-4793
info@hazelden.org
www.hazelden.org
Men and women describe the N.A. program and how it works.
289 pages Paperback
Mark Mishek, President and Chief Executive Officer
Joe Jaksha, Publisher

8340 National Conference on Drug Abuse Researcg & Practice
National Clearinghouse for Alcohol and Drug Info.

PO Box 2345
Rockville, MD 20847   800-729-6686

Offers summaries of workshops, forums, dinner speeches and sessions presented at the National Conference on Drug Abuse Research and Practice.
275 pages
Alan I Leshner, Director
Donna E Shalala, secretary

8341   National Directory of Drug Abuse and Alcoholism Treatment and Programs
US National Institute On Drug Abuse
6001 Executive Boulevard   301-443-1124
Bethesda, ML 20892   NIDANEWS@list.nih.gov
                                                    www.nida.nih.gov

Eleven thousand listings of agencies that administer treatment and services on the federal, state and local levels.
Nora D. Volkow, Director

8342   Night Light: A Book of Nighttime Meditations
Hazelden
15251 Pleasant Valley Rd   651-213-4200
Center City, MN 55012-9640   800-257-7810
                                                    Fax: 651-213-4793
                                                    info@hazelden.org
                                                    www.hazelden.org

Three hundred and sixty-six meditations designed to help relax and encourage prayer. Reminds readers to look to their Higher Power for strength, reassurance, comfort, and guidance.
400 pages Paperback
ISBN: 0-894863-81-9
Mark Mishek, President and Chief Executive Officer
Joe Jaksha, Publisher

8343   Not God: A History of Alcoholics Anonymous
Hazelden
15251 Pleasant Valley Rd   651-213-4200
Center City, MN 55012-9640   800-257-7810
                                                    Fax: 651-213-4793
                                                    info@hazelden.org
                                                    www.hazelden.org

Documenting AA's philosophical and social development within the larger context of American culture, this book follows the remarkable story of the evolution of a small group of Depression-era alcoholics into a worldwide movement.
436 pages Paperback
ISBN: 0-894860-65-8
Mark Mishek, President and Chief Executive Officer
Joe Jaksha, Publisher

8344   Occupational Therapy Practice Guidelines for Adults with Substance Use Disorders
American Occupational Therapy Association
4720 Montgomery Lane   301-652-6611
Bethesda, MD 20814-1220   800-729-2682
                                                    Fax: 240-762-5150
                                                    TDD: 800-377-8555
                                                    praota@aota.org.
                                                    www.aota.org

22 pages
ISBN: 1-569001-60-X

8345   Of Course You're Angry
Hazelden
15251 Pleasant Valley Rd   651-213-4200
Center City, MN 55012-9640   800-257-7810
                                                    Fax: 651-213-4793
                                                    info@hazelden.org
                                                    www.hazelden.org

Revised edition dealing with the nature and resolution of anger. Demonstrates how to make anger work in a positive and effective way that can ease, rather than exacerbate, the challenges of early recovery.
120 pages Paperback
ISBN: 1-568381-41-7
Mark Mishek, President and Chief Executive Officer
Joe Jaksha, Publisher

8346   One Day at a Time in Al-Anon
Al-Anon Family Group Headquarters

1600 Corp Landing Pkwy   757-563-1600
Virginia Beach, VA 23454-5617   800-425-2666
                                                    Fax: 757-563-1655
                                                    wso@al-anon.org
                                                    www.al-anon.alateen.org

Inspirational daily readings cover various aspects of the Al-Anon philosopha and relate it to everyday situations.
376 pages
ISBN: 0-910034-21-4
Caryn Johnson, Director Communications

8347   Operation PAR
National Clearinghouse for Alcohol and Drug Info.
PO Box 2345   800-729-6686
Rockville, MD 20847-2345

Describes successful community alcohol and other drug abuse prevention and treatment programs.
40 pages

8348   Parent Training is Prevention
National Clearinghouse for Alcohol and Drug Info.
PO Box 2345   800-729-6686
Rockville, MD 20847-2345   www.sdsalarms.com

Contains information to help communities identify and carry out programs on parenting.
184 pages

8349   Pass it On
Alcoholics Anonymous
Grand Central Station   212-870-3400
New York, NY 10163   Fax: 212-870-3137
                                                    www.aa.org

The story of Bill Wilson, the co-founder of AA and the development of the Fellowship.

8350   Passages Through Recovery
Hazelden
15251 Pleasant Valley Rd   651-213-4200
Center City, MN 55012-9640   800-257-7810
                                                    Fax: 651-213-4793
                                                    info@hazelden.org
                                                    www.hazelden.org

Guides clients through the six stages of recovery.
130 pages Paperback
Mark Mishek, President and Chief Executive Officer
Joe Jaksha, Publisher

8351   Peer Pressure Reversal
Human Resource Development Press
22 Amherst Road   413-253-3488
Amherst, MA 01002-9730

8352   Pregnancy and Exposure to Alcohol and Other Drug Use
National Clearinghouse for Alcohol and Drug Info.
PO Box 2345   800-729-6686
Rockville, MD 20847-2345   www.health.org

This report is for health care professionals presenting the state-of-the-art information about preventing ATOD use among women of childbearing age.

8353   Preparing for the Drug-Free Years: A Family Activity Book
Developmental Research and Programs
130 Nickerson Street   206-286-1805
Seattle, WA 98145-1746   800-736-2630
                                                    Fax: 206-286-1462

8354   Presence at the Center
Hazelden
15251 Pleasant Valley Rd   651-213-4200
Center City, MN 55012-9640   800-257-7810
                                                    Fax: 651-213-4793
                                                    info@hazelden.org
                                                    www.hazelden.org

About a new way of life that addresses transformation, change, the presence of a Higher Power, letting go of reluctance and fear, and the freedom commitment can bring.
76 pages Paperback
ISBN: 1-568380-01-1
Mark Mishek, President and Chief Executive Officer
Joe Jaksha, Publisher

8355 Prevention Plus II: Tools for Creating & Sustaining a Drug-Free Community
National Clearinghouse for Alcohol and Drug Info.
PO Box 2345   800-729-6686
Rockville, MD 20847-2345   www.health.org
Provides a framework for organizing or expanding community alcohol and other drug problem prevention activities for youth into a coordinated, complimentary system.
541 pages

8356 Prevention Plus III: Assessing Alcohol & Other Prevention Programs
National Clearinghouse for Alcohol and Drug Info.
PO Box 2345   800-729-6686
Rockville, MD 20847-2345   www.health.org
Provides tools and techniques for alcohol and other drug prevention, planning and implementation.
470 pages

8357 Prevention Resource Guide: Alcohol and Other Drug Related Periodicals
National Clearinghouse for Alcohol and Drug Info.
PO Box 2345   800-729-6686
Rockville, MD 20847-2345   www.health.org
Provides a concise annotated bibliography of journals, newsletters and other publications related to the AOD prevention field.
12 pages

8358 Prevention Resource Guide: American Indian/Native Alaskans
National Clearinghouse for Alcohol and Drug Info.
PO Box 2345   800-729-6686
Rockville, MD 20847-2345   www.health.org
This resource guide is a survey of current data on alcohol abuse among American Indians and Native Alaskans.
24 pages

8359 Prevention Resource Guide: Asian and Pacific Islander Americans
National Clearinghouse for Alcohol and Drug Info.
PO Box 2345   800-729-6686
Rockville, MD 20847-2345   www.health.org
Contains facts and figures about Asian and Pacific Islander Americans and alcohol and other drug prevention.
13 pages

8360 Prevention Resource Guide: Elementary Youth
National Clearinghouse for Alcohol and Drug Info.
PO Box 2345   800-729-6686
Rockville, MD 20847-2345   www.health.org
This resource guide includes materials specifically developed for youth that may be used in an elementary school setting.
23 pages

8361 Prevention Resource Guide: Pregnant Postpartum Women and Their Infants
National Clearinghouse for Alcohol and Drug Info.
PO Box 2345   800-729-6686
Rockville, MD 20847-2345   www.health.org
This resource guide targets health care providers, prevention program planners and counselors of pregnant and postpartum women between the ages of 15 and 44.
30 pages

8362 Prevention Resource Guide: Secondary School Students
National Clearinghouse for Alcohol and Drug Info.
PO Box 2345   800-729-6686
Rockville, MD 20847-2345   www.health.org
This resource guide targets teachers, administrators and program leaders who come in contact with secondary school youth.
27 pages

8363 Prevention Resource Guide: Women
National Clearinghouse for Alcohol and Drug Info.
PO Box 2345   800-729-6686
Rockville, MD 20847-2345   www.health.org
This resource guide provides the latest information about the effects of drugs and alcohol on women.
32 pages

8364 Prevention in Action
National Clearinghouse for Alcohol and Drug Info.

PO Box 2345   800-729-6686
Rockville, MD 20847-2345
Provides descriptions selected by representatives of national organizations and State alcohol and drug agency representatives.
20 pages

8365 Program for You
Hazelden
15251 Pleasant Valley Rd   651-213-4200
Center City, MN 55012-9640   800-257-7810
                                                       Fax: 651-213-4793
                                                       info@hazelden.org
                                                       www.hazelden.org
Study guide interpreting the original AA program as described in Alcoholics Anonymous and helps apply the wisdom to everyday life.
183 pages Paperback
ISBN: 0-894867-41-5
Mark Mishek, President and Chief Executive Officer
Joe Jaksha, Publisher

8366 Promise of a New Day: A Book of Daily Meditations
Hazelden
15251 Pleasant Valley Rd   651-213-4200
Center City, MN 55012-9640   800-257-7810
                                                       Fax: 651-213-4793
                                                       info@hazelden.org
                                                       www.hazelden.org
Simple, inspiring wisdom about creating and maintaining inner peace. Each of the 366 daily meditations expresses the essence of Twelve Step spirituality without the program jargon.
400 pages Paperback
ISBN: 0-894862-03-0
Mark Mishek, President and Chief Executive Officer
Joe Jaksha, Publisher

8367 Quit & Stay Quit: A Personal Program to Stop Smoking
Hazelden
15251 Pleasant Valley Rd   651-213-4200
Center City, MN 55012-9640   800-257-7810
                                                       Fax: 651-213-4793
                                                       info@hazelden.org
                                                       www.hazelden.org
Guide to nicotine recovery offering an effective long-term program to quit by showing readers how smoking has subtly shaped their values, attitudes, and lives.
196 pages Paperback
ISBN: 1-568381-09-3
Mark Mishek, President and Chief Executive Officer
Joe Jaksha, Publisher

8368 Quit Smoking Manual
American Lung Association
1740 Broadway   212-315-8700
Silver Spring, MD 20907-4315   800-358-9295
                                                       www.tobaccoprogram.org
Original self-help smoking cessation manual showing the public how to quit smoking in 20 days.
64 pages

8369 Recovery Journal for Exploring Who I Am
Hazelden
15251 Pleasant Valley Rd   651-213-4200
Center City, MN 55012-9640   800-257-7810
                                                       Fax: 651-213-4793
                                                       info@hazelden.org
                                                       www.hazelden.org
Introduces clients to journal writing as an effective therapeutic adjunct for addiction recovery.
48 pages
Mark Mishek, President and Chief Executive Officer
Joe Jaksha, Publisher

8370 School Answers Back: Responding to Student Drug Use
American Council on Drug Education
204 Monroe Street   800-488-3784
Rockville, MD 20850
Provides teachers, counselors, administrators and parents with a model for schools to use in confronting drug and alcohol abuse.
145 pages

8371 Search for Serenity
Hazelden
15251 Pleasant Valley Rd
Center City, MN 55012-9640

651-213-4200
800-257-7810
Fax: 651-213-4793
info@hazelden.org
www.hazelden.org

Provides clients with practical inspiration to change their feelings toward people and situations.
152 pages Paperback
Mark Mishek, President and Chief Executive Officer
Joe Jaksha, Publisher

8372 Shame Faced
Hazelden
15251 Pleasant Valley Rd
Center City, MN 55012-9640

651-213-4200
800-257-7810
Fax: 651-213-4793
info@hazelden.org
www.hazelden.org

Discusses the relationship between shame and chemical dependency.
28 pages
Mark Mishek, President and Chief Executive Officer
Joe Jaksha, Publisher

8373 Skeptic's Guide to the 12 Steps
Hazelden
15251 Pleasant Valley Rd
Center City, MN 55012-9640

651-213-4200
800-257-7810
Fax: 651-213-4793
info@hazelden.org
www.hazelden.org

Investigates each of the 12 steps to gain a deeper understanding of a Higher Power.
241 pages Paperback
Mark Mishek, President and Chief Executive Officer
Joe Jaksha, Publisher

8374 Smoking and Pregnancy Kit for Health Care Providers
American Lung Association
1740 Broadway
New York, NY 10019-4315

212-315-8700

A program kit for health care providers designed to educate pregnant women not to smoke and to help them kick the habit.

8375 Smoking, Drinking & Illicit Drug Use
National Clearinghouse for Alcohol and Drug Info.
PO Box 2345
Rockville, MD 20847-2345

800-729-6686
www.healthieryou.com

Comprehensive reports representing the results of the 12th national survey on drug use and analyzing data collected from young Americans from 1975-1991.

8376 Sober But Stuck
Hazelden
15251 Pleasant Valley Rd
Center City, MN 55012-9640

651-213-4200
800-257-7810
Fax: 651-213-4793
info@hazelden.org
www.hazelden.org

Collection of personal stories by men and women who are long-time members of Alcoholics Anonymous. Each story shares the anecdotes and resources which helped members break through the barriers that limited their enjoyment of a sober life.
215 pages Paperback
ISBN: 1-568380-78-X
Mark Mishek, President and Chief Executive Officer
Joe Jaksha, Publisher

8377 Social Policy Prevention Handbook
African American Family Services
2616 Nicollet Avenue S
Minneapolis, MN 55408

612-871-7878

A manual that details IBCA's community based approach to the development of alcohol and drug abuse prevention strategies.
24 pages

8378 Staying Clean
Hazelden

15251 Pleasant Valley Rd
Center City, MN 55012-9640

651-213-4200
800-257-7810
Fax: 651-213-4793
info@hazelden.org
www.hazelden.org

Each section focuses on one of 33 proven ideas for staying drug-free, such as professional help, prayer, support groups and meditation.
76 pages Paperback
Mark Mishek, President and Chief Executive Officer
Joe Jaksha, Publisher

8379 Staying Sober
Hazelden
15251 Pleasant Valley Rd
Center City, MN 55012-9640

651-213-4200
800-257-7810
Fax: 651-213-4793
info@hazelden.org
www.hazelden.org

Discusses addictive diseases and its physical, psychological and social effects.
228 pages Paperback
Mark Mishek, President and Chief Executive Officer
Joe Jaksha, Publisher

8380 Step Zero: Getting to Recovery
Hazelden
15251 Pleasant Valley Rd
Center City, MN 55012-9640

651-213-4200
800-257-7810
Fax: 651-213-4793
info@hazelden.org
www.hazelden.org

Explains the concepts of Step Zero, when clients drop their defenses, begin to face themselves and start to assess their behavior and the reasons for it.
170 pages Paperback
Mark Mishek, President and Chief Executive Officer
Joe Jaksha, Publisher

8381 Stools and Bottles
Hazelden
15251 Pleasant Valley Rd
Center City, MN 55012-9640

651-213-4200
800-257-7810
Fax: 651-213-4793
info@hazelden.org
www.hazelden.org

Depicts the first Three steps using a three-legged stool and eight whiskey bottles representing character defects revealed when working Step Four.
160 pages Hardcover
Mark Mishek, President and Chief Executive Officer
Joe Jaksha, Publisher

8382 Substance Abuse and Physical Disability
Allen Heinemann, PhD, author
Haworth Press
9400 Universal Boulevard
Orlando, FL 32819-1580

607-722-5857
866-860-1971
Fax: 607-722-0012
www.haworthpress.com

This book offers information on alcohol and drug abuse being a contributing factor in traumatic and disabling injuries.
1993 289 pages Hardcover
ISBN: 1-560242-89-3
Amie Gilmore, Show Director
Kerry Cree, Sales Manager

8383 Success Stories from Drug-Free Schools
National Clearinghouse for Alcohol and Drug Info.
PO Box 2345
Rockville, MD 20847-2345

800-729-6686
www.health.org

Salutes the 107 schools honored by the US Department of Education's Drug-Free Recognition Program.
59 pages

8384 Tackling Alcohol Problems on Campus: Tools for Media Advocacy
National Clearinghouse for Alcohol and Drug Info.
PO Box 2345
Rockville, MD 20857-2345

800-729-6686
www.nacoa.org

Substance Abuse Disorder / Books

Reviews the role of alcohol on campus and shows how to use the media to get attention and support.
38 pages
Stephanie Loebs, Chairman
Peter Palanca, Vice Chairman

8385 Team Up for Drug Prevention with America's Young Athletes
Drug Enforcement Administration, Demand Reduction
1405 I Street NW   202-307-5550
Washington, DC 20537-0001   www.dea.gov
Michele M. Leonhart, DEA Administrator

8386 Ten Steps to Help Your Child Say No: A Parent's Guide
National Clearinghouse for Alcohol and Drug Info.
PO Box 2345   800-729-6686
Rockville, MD 20847-2345

8387 Things My Sponsors Taught Me
Hazelden
15251 Pleasant Valley Rd   651-213-4200
Center City, MN 55012-9640   800-257-7810
                                      Fax: 651-213-4793
                                      info@hazelden.org
                                      www.hazelden.org
Features AA philosophy, quotes, slogans and refreshing reminders.
76 pages Paperback
Mark Mishek, President and Chief Executive Officer
Joe Jaksha, Publisher

8388 Today I Will Do One Thing: Daily Readings for Awareness & Hope
Hazelden
15251 Pleasant Valley Rd   651-213-4200
Center City, MN 55012-9640   800-257-7810
                                      Fax: 651-213-4793
                                      info@hazelden.org
                                      www.hazelden.org
Specially designed to integrate recovery from addiction with the treatment of emotional or psychiatric illness. Each meditation focuses on a task or goal to be completed each day.
400 pages Paperback
ISBN: 1-568380-83-6
Mark Mishek, President and Chief Executive Officer
Joe Jaksha, Publisher

8389 Today's Gift
Hazelden
15251 Pleasant Valley Rd   651-213-4200
Center City, MN 55012-9640   800-257-7810
                                      Fax: 651-213-4793
                                      info@hazelden.org
                                      www.hazelden.org
Inspiring meditations bringing families together and strengthening family bonds.
400 pages Paperback
Mark Mishek, President and Chief Executive Officer
Joe Jaksha, Publisher

8390 Touchstones
Hazelden
15251 Pleasant Valley Rd   651-213-4200
Center City, MN 55012-9640   800-257-7810
                                      Fax: 651-213-4793
                                      info@hazelden.org
                                      www.hazelden.org
A book of daily meditations for men in the Twelve-Step program.
400 pages Paperback
Mark Mishek, President and Chief Executive Officer
Joe Jaksha, Publisher

8391 Turnabout
Women for Sobriety
14488 Old Stage Road   215-536-8026
Lenoir City, TN 37772-0618   Fax: 215-536-8026
                                      WFSobriey@aol.com
                                      www.mediapulse.com
This is the story of the founder of Women for Sobriety and her struggle to quit drinking.
183 pages

8392 Turning Awareness Into Action: What Your Community Can Do About Drug Use
National Clearinghouse for Alcohol and Drug Info.
PO Box 2345   800-729-6686
Rockville, MD 20847-2345   www.health.org
This bilingual booklet is designed to show leaders at the grassroots level how to make the most of their talents and their community's resources.
73 pages

8393 Twelve Step Sponsorship: How it Works
Hazelden
15251 Pleasant Valley Rd   651-213-4200
Center City, MN 55012-9640   800-257-7810
                                      Fax: 651-213-4793
                                      info@hazelden.org
                                      www.hazelden.org
Complete handbook for working with a newcomer. Based on Twelve Step traditions and knowledge passed orally through the generations, this working manual defines the sponsorship role and guides sponsors through the rewards and pitfalls of reaching out to help new program members.
260 pages Paperback
ISBN: 1-568381-22-0
Mark Mishek, President and Chief Executive Officer
Joe Jaksha, Publisher

8394 Twelve Steps and Traditions
Hazelden
15251 Pleasant Valley Rd   651-213-4200
Center City, MN 55012-9640   800-257-7810
                                      Fax: 651-213-4793
                                      info@hazelden.org
                                      www.hazelden.org
Outlines the core principles by which AA members recover and by which the fellowship functions.
192 pages Paperback
Mark Mishek, President and Chief Executive Officer
Joe Jaksha, Publisher

8395 Twelve Steps and Twelve Traditions
Alcoholics Anonymous
PO Box 459   212-870-3400
New York, NY 10163-0459   800-328-9000
                                      Fax: 212-870-3137
                                      info@hazelden.org
                                      www.hazelden.org
Twenty-four essays on the Steps and Traditions that discuss the principles of individual recovery and group unity.

8396 Twelve Steps and Twelve Traditions for Alateen
Al-Anon Family Group Headquarters
1600 Corp Landing Pkwy   757-563-1600
Virginia Beach, VA 23454-5617   800-425-2666
                                      Fax: 757-563-1655
                                      wso@al-anon.org
                                      www.al-anon.alateen.org
Questions, discussions and personal reflections of Alateen members.
60 pages
Caryn Johnson, Director Communications

8397 Twelve Steps for Everyone...Who Really Wants Them
Hazelden
15251 Pleasant Valley Rd   651-213-4200
Center City, MN 55012-9640   800-257-7810
                                      Fax: 651-213-4793
                                      info@hazelden.org
                                      www.hazelden.org
A basic primer outlining how spiritual and emotional health can be found by working and living the Twelve Steps. Emphasizes that the Twelve Steps are for anyone who wants to change.
208 pages Paperback
ISBN: 1-568380-47-X
Mark Mishek, President and Chief Executive Officer
Joe Jaksha, Publisher

8398 Twelve Steps of Alcoholics Anonymous
Hazelden

624

15251 Pleasant Valley Rd
Center City, MN 55012-9640
651-213-4200
800-257-7810
Fax: 651-213-4793
info@hazelden.org
www.hazelden.org

A series of short discussions that interpret each of the Twelve Steps, from admission of individual powerlessness outlined in Step One to the moral inventory of Step Four and the spiritual awakening of Step Twelve.
130 pages Paperback
ISBN: 0-894869-04-3
Mark Mishek, President and Chief Executive Officer
Joe Jaksha, Publisher

8399   Twenty Four Hours a Day
Hazelden
15251 Pleasant Valley Rd
Center City, MN 55012-9640
651-213-4200
800-257-7810
Fax: 651-213-4793
info@hazelden.org
www.hazelden.org

Offers a resource that serves as a solid foundation in a spiritual program. Simple, yet effective resource that helps clients relate to the Twelve-Step program.
400 pages Paperback
Mark Mishek, President and Chief Executive Officer
Joe Jaksha, Publisher

8400   Walk in Dry Places
Hazelden
15251 Pleasant Valley Rd
Center City, MN 55012-9640
651-213-4200
800-257-7810
Fax: 651-213-4793
info@hazelden.org
www.hazelden.org

Core-recovery book filled with practical spiritual advice and time-honored Twelve Step philosophy. Insightful explorations of the deeper issues of living in recovery address the daily concerns of those new to life without alcoholism, as well as those with long-term sobriety.
400 pages Paperback
ISBN: 1-568381-27-1
Mark Mishek, President and Chief Executive Officer
Joe Jaksha, Publisher

8401   Wasted Tales of a Gen X Drunk
Hazelden
15251 Pleasant Valley Rd
Center City, MN 55012-9640
651-213-4200
800-257-7810
Fax: 651-213-4793
info@hazelden.org
www.hazelden.org

Cynicism and black humor underscore this hard-edged memoir of a young journalist's alcoholism and subsequent recovery. Captures the ethos of a generation often suspicious and alienated by the Twelve-Step approach.
250 pages Cloth
ISBN: 1-568381-42-5
Mark Mishek, President and Chief Executive Officer
Joe Jaksha, Publisher

8402   What Works: Schools Without Drugs
National Clearinghouse for Alcohol and Drug Info.
PO Box 2345
Rockville, MD 20847-2345
800-729-6686

8403   What You Can Do About Drug Use in America
National Clearinghouse for Alcohol and Drug Info.
PO Box 2345
Rockville, MD 20847-2345
301-468-2600
800-729-6686
www.health.org

Offers information on what parents and professionals can do to prevent drug use in America.

8404   Why Am I Afraid to Tell You Who I Am?
Hazelden

15251 Pleasant Valley Rd
Center City, MN 55012-9640
651-213-4200
800-257-7810
Fax: 651-213-4793
info@hazelden.org
www.hazelden.org

Outlines types of interpersonal relationships.
Mark Mishek, President and Chief Executive Officer
Joe Jaksha, Publisher

8405   Woman's Way Through the Twelve Steps
Hazelden
15251 Pleasant Valley Rd
Center City, MN 55012-9640
651-213-4200
800-257-7810
Fax: 651-213-4793
info@hazelden.org
www.hazelden.org

How women understnad and work the Twelve Steps of AA, including reflections of spirituality, powerlessness, and the emergence of a sense of the feminine soul.
228 pages Paperback
ISBN: 0-894869-93-0
Mark Mishek, President and Chief Executive Officer
Joe Jaksha, Publisher

8406   Young Teens: Who They Are and How to Talk to Them About Alcohol & Drugs
National Clearinghouse for Alcohol and Drug Info.
PO Box 2345
Rockville, MD 20847-2345
800-729-6686

Offers information on how parents, educators and concerned citizens can work together to help youngsters avoid alcohol and other drugs by understanding the risks and dangers.
57 pages

Children's Books

8407   Alcoholism
Franklin Watts Grolier
90 Old Sherman Turnpike
Danbury, CT 06816-0001
203-797-3500
800-621-1115
Fax: 203-797-3197
www.grolier.com

This comprehensive overview describes the different types of alcoholism, the addictive personality and the warning signs.
112 pages Grades 7-12
ISBN: 0-531108-79-1

8408   Alcoholism and the Family
Franklin Watts Grolier
90 Old Sherman Turnpike
Danbury, CT 06816-0001
203-797-3500
800-621-1115
Fax: 203-797-3197
www.grolier.com

This book, after discussing what alcoholism is, its effects on health and behavior modifications through alcohol, starts addressing one of the most important aspects of alcoholism, the effects on the family.
32 pages Grades 3-5
ISBN: 0-531125-48-3

8409   America's War on Drugs
Franklin Watts Grolier
90 Old Sherman Turnpike
Danbury, CT 06816
203-797-3500
800-621-1115
Fax: 203-797-3197
www.grolier.com

An overview of the United States' attempts to combat illegal drugs on the supply side, from stopping the supply of drugs into the country.
160 pages Grades 7-12
ISBN: 0-531109-54-2

8410   Buzzy's Rebound
National Clearinghouse for Alcohol and Drug Info.
PO Box 2345
Rockville, MD 20847-2345
800-729-6686
www.sdsalarms.com

A Fat Albert comic book that describes the pressure on a new kid in town to drink.
18 pages

8411 Caffeine and Nicotine
Hazelden
15251 Pleasant Valley Rd   651-213-4200
Center City, MN 55012-9640   800-257-7810
                                    Fax: 651-213-4793
                                    info@hazelden.org
                                    www.hazelden.org
Simple, clear, and accurate presentation of nicotine and caffeine dependency. How to avoid these addictions, and why teens ought to do so.
64 pages Paperback
ISBN: 1-568381-68-9
Mark Mishek, President and Chief Executive Officer
Joe Jaksha, Publisher

8412 Christy's Chance
Crestridge Corporate Center
10155 York Road   410-628-0390
Hunt Valley, MD 21030   Fax: 410-628-0398
                                    www.networkpub.com
A story geared to younger teens that allows the reader to make a nonuse decision about marijuana.

8413 Cocaine
Hazelden
15251 Pleasant Valley Rd   651-213-4200
Center City, MN 55012-9640   800-257-7810
                                    Fax: 651-213-4793
                                    info@hazelden.org
                                    www.hazelden.org
The information that teens need to stay drug-free, promoting understanding of the ramifications, both social and personal.
64 pages Paperback
ISBN: 1-568381-64-6
Mark Mishek, President and Chief Executive Officer
Joe Jaksha, Publisher

8414 Coping with Codependency
Hazelden
15251 Pleasant Valley Rd   651-213-4200
Center City, MN 55012-9640   800-257-7810
                                    Fax: 651-213-4793
                                    info@hazelden.org
                                    www.hazelden.org
Explains the cycle of codependency, describes its destructive effects on all involved, and suggests ways to break free and live in more healthy relationships.
64 pages Paperback
ISBN: 1-568381-85-9
Mark Mishek, President and Chief Executive Officer
Joe Jaksha, Publisher

8415 Coping with Depression
Hazelden
15251 Pleasant Valley Rd   651-213-4200
Center City, MN 55012-9640   800-257-7810
                                    Fax: 651-213-4793
                                    info@hazelden.org
                                    www.hazelden.org
Practical ways to cope with depression. Provides clear suggestions for handling life's downers, and encourages readers to seek professional help when they feel they can't deal with problems themselves.
64 pages Paperback
ISBN: 1-568381-79-4
Mark Mishek, President and Chief Executive Officer
Joe Jaksha, Publisher

8416 Coping with Drinking and Driving
Hazelden
15251 Pleasant Valley Rd   651-213-4200
Center City, MN 55012-9640   800-257-7810
                                    Fax: 651-213-4793
                                    info@hazelden.org
                                    www.hazelden.org

Addressing teens' illusion of invulnerability, the author describes exactly how alcohol affects the body and one's driving skills, emphasizing that teens are not immune to alcohol's effects.
64 pages Paperback
ISBN: 1-568381-80-8
Mark Mishek, President and Chief Executive Officer
Joe Jaksha, Publisher

8417 Coping with Peer Pressure
Hazelden
15251 Pleasant Valley Rd   651-213-4200
Center City, MN 55012-9640   800-257-7810
                                    Fax: 651-213-4793
                                    info@hazelden.org
                                    www.hazelden.org
Discussion of the positive and negative effects that members of a peer group can have on each other and explores ways teens can handle the pressure they face.
64 pages Paperback
ISBN: 1-568381-83-2
Mark Mishek, President and Chief Executive Officer
Joe Jaksha, Publisher

8418 Coping with Stress
Hazelden
15251 Pleasant Valley Rd   651-213-4200
Center City, MN 55012-9640   800-257-7810
                                    Fax: 651-213-4793
                                    info@hazelden.org
                                    www.hazelden.org
Outlines positive strategies to help teens learn to cope more effectively with stress, rather than turning to destructive outlets such as drugs and even suicide.
64 pages Paperback
ISBN: 1-568381-76-X
Mark Mishek, President and Chief Executive Officer
Joe Jaksha, Publisher

8419 Coping with a Drug-Abusing Parent
Hazelden
15251 Pleasant Valley Rd   651-213-4200
Center City, MN 55012-9640   800-257-7810
                                    Fax: 651-213-4793
                                    info@hazelden.org
                                    www.hazelden.org
Describes steps that teens, powerless to stop a drug-abusing parent from continuing on that destructive path, can take to to learn to take better care of themselves. Includes coping strategies and who to call for help.
64 pages Paperback
ISBN: 1-568381-78-6
Mark Mishek, President and Chief Executive Officer
Joe Jaksha, Publisher

8420 Crack Down on Drugs
National Clearinghouse for Alcohol and Drug Info.
PO Box 2345   800-729-6686
Rockville, MD 20847   www.healthieryou.com
Coloring book for children featuring McGruff, the crime dog, that teaches young children the importance of refusing alcohol and drug abuse.
Ages 5-8

8421 Different Like Me: A Book for Teens Who Worry About Their Parents' Using
Johnson Institute
Ohms Lane   612-831-1630
Edina, MN   www.kineticvideo.com
Provides support and information for teens who are concerned, confused, scared and angry because their parents abuse alcohol and other drugs.
110 pages

8422 Drug Abuse: The Impact on Society
Franklin Watts Grolier
90 Old Sherman Turnpike   203-797-3500
Danbury, CT 06816   800-621-1115
                                    Fax: 203-797-3197
                                    www.grolier.com

Discusses all major aspects of illegal drug usage and the health and personality effects they cause.
144 pages Grades 7-12
ISBN: 0-531105-79-2

8423   Drugs and AIDS
Hazelden
15251 Pleasant Valley Rd   651-213-4200
Center City, MN 55012-9640   800-257-7810
                                 Fax: 651-213-4793
                                 info@hazelden.org
                                 www.hazelden.org
Covers many topics through case studies, including the effects of the disease on the body, transmission, homosexuality, condom use, drug treatment, and peer pressure.
64 pages Paperback
ISBN: 1-568381-72-7
Mark Mishek, President and Chief Executive Officer
Joe Jaksha, Publisher

8424   Drugs and Anger
Hazelden
15251 Pleasant Valley Rd   651-213-4200
Center City, MN 55012-9640   800-257-7810
                                 Fax: 651-213-4793
                                 info@hazelden.org
                                 www.hazelden.org
True-to-life scenarios and practical techniques found here can help teens cope constructively with their anger.
64 pages Paperback
ISBN: 1-568381-73-5
Mark Mishek, President and Chief Executive Officer
Joe Jaksha, Publisher

8425   Drugs and Depression
Hazelden
15251 Pleasant Valley Rd   651-213-4200
Center City, MN 55012-9640   800-257-7810
                                 Fax: 651-213-4793
                                 info@hazelden.org
                                 www.hazelden.org
Describes positive ways of handling depression, as well as suggesting resources for receiving assistance.
64 pages Paperback
ISBN: 1-568381-74-3
Mark Mishek, President and Chief Executive Officer
Joe Jaksha, Publisher

8426   Drugs and Domestic Violence
Hazelden
15251 Pleasant Valley Rd   651-213-4200
Center City, MN 55012-9640   800-257-7810
                                 Fax: 651-213-4793
                                 info@hazelden.org
                                 www.hazelden.org
Describes valuable coping tactics that can help teens stay safe in situations involving domestic violence and drug use.
64 pages Paperback
ISBN: 1-568381-75-1
Mark Mishek, President and Chief Executive Officer
Joe Jaksha, Publisher

8427   Drugs and Your Friends
Hazelden
15251 Pleasant Valley Rd   651-213-4200
Center City, MN 55012-9640   800-257-7810
                                 Fax: 651-213-4793
                                 info@hazelden.org
                                 www.hazelden.org
Helps teens make sound decisions on vital choices and provides many suggestions for resisting peer pressure.
64 pages Paperback
ISBN: 1-568381-70-0
Mark Mishek, President and Chief Executive Officer
Joe Jaksha, Publisher

8428   Drugs and Your Parents
Hazelden

15251 Pleasant Valley Rd   651-213-4200
Center City, MN 55012-9640   800-257-7810
                                 Fax: 651-213-4793
                                 info@hazelden.org
                                 www.hazelden.org
Practical advice for teenage children of parents addicted to alcohol or other drugs. How to cope initially with the situation as well as long-term survival strategies.
64 pages Paperback
ISBN: 1-568381-71-9
Mark Mishek, President and Chief Executive Officer
Joe Jaksha, Publisher

8429   Drugs in the Body: Effects of Abuse
Franklin Watts Grolier
90 Old Sherman Turnpike   203-797-3500
Danbury, CT 06816   800-621-1115
                                 Fax: 203-797-3197
                                 www.grolier.com
Traces the effects of cocaine and crack, opium, morphine, heroine, marijuana and hashish, LSD and PCP in a person's system. Special emphasis is placed on long-term adverse effects in the body.
144 pages Grades 7-12
ISBN: 0-531125-07-6

8430   Elephant in the Living Room: The Children's Book
Hazelden
15251 Pleasant Valley Rd   651-213-4200
Center City, MN 55012-9640   800-257-7810
                                 Fax: 651-213-4793
                                 info@hazelden.org
                                 www.hazelden.org
An activity book to help children understand and cope with the problem of chemical dependency in the family.
88 pages Paperback
ISBN: 1-568380-35-6
Mark Mishek, President and Chief Executive Officer
Joe Jaksha, Publisher

8431   Facts on Alcohol
Franklin Watts Grolier
90 Old Sherman Turnpike   203-797-3500
Danbury, CT 06816   800-621-1115
                                 Fax: 203-797-3197
                                 www.grolier.com
Offers various information on alcohol so young children can have an opportunity to form their own opinions and the ability to make their own decisions when it comes to alcoholism.
32 pages Grades 5-7
ISBN: 0-531108-21-0

8432   Facts on the Crack and Cocaine Epidemic
Franklin Watts Grolier
90 Old Sherman Turnpike   203-797-3500
Danbury, CT 06816   800-621-1115
                                 Fax: 203-797-3197
                                 www.grolier.com
Offers young children information on these deadly drugs to help them become informed.
32 pages Grades 5-7
ISBN: 0-531108-22-8

8433   Feed Your Head
Hazelden
15251 Pleasant Valley Rd   651-213-4200
Center City, MN 55012-9640   800-257-7810
                                 Fax: 651-213-4793
                                 info@hazelden.org
                                 www.hazelden.org
Offers practical guidance for young people.
137 pages Paperback
Mark Mishek, President and Chief Executive Officer
Joe Jaksha, Publisher

8434   Gangs and Drugs
Hazelden

15251 Pleasant Valley Rd
Center City, MN 55012-9640
651-213-4200
800-257-7810
Fax: 651-213-4793
info@hazelden.org
www.hazelden.org

Encouraging and helpful message that goes beyond Just say no.
240 pages Paperback
ISBN: 1-568381-35-2
Mark Mishek, President and Chief Executive Officer
Joe Jaksha, Publisher

8435 How to Say No and Keep Your Friends
Hazelden
15251 Pleasant Valley Rd
Center City, MN 55012-9640
651-213-4200
800-257-7810
Fax: 651-213-4793
info@hazelden.org
www.hazelden.org

Ideas to help teens deal with negative peer pressure.
112 pages
Mark Mishek, President and Chief Executive Officer
Joe Jaksha, Publisher

8436 I Can Talk About What Hurts
Hazelden
15251 Pleasant Valley Rd
Center City, MN 55012-9640
651-213-4200
800-257-7810
Fax: 651-213-4793
info@hazelden.org
www.hazelden.org

Written and illustrated for children whose lives have been affected by someone else's chemical dependency.
56 pages Paperback
Mark Mishek, President and Chief Executive Officer
Joe Jaksha, Publisher

8437 I Wish Daddy Didn't Drink So Much
Judith Vigna, author
Albert Whitman & Company
250 South NW Highway
Park Ridge, IL 60068-2723
847-232-2800
800-255-7675
Fax: 847-581-0039
mail@awhitmanco.com
www.albertwhitman.com

A young girl shres her feelings and frustrations about her alcoholic father's behavior.
1993 32 pages Grades P-3
ISBN: 0-807535-23-0
Pat McPartland, Sales
Joe Campbell, Customer Service

8438 If Drugs Are So Bad, Why Do So Many People Use Them?
Hazelden
15251 Pleasant Valley Rd
Center City, MN 55012-9640
651-213-4200
800-257-7810
Fax: 651-213-4793
info@hazelden.org
www.hazelden.org

Uses direct language to explain drugs and their effects.
29 pages Grades 5-9
Mark Mishek, President and Chief Executive Officer
Joe Jaksha, Publisher

8439 In a Perfect World
Hazelden
15251 Pleasant Valley Rd
Center City, MN 55012-9640
651-213-4200
800-257-7810
Fax: 651-213-4793
info@hazelden.org
www.hazelden.org

Kevin thinks his world will be perfect when his father stops drinking, but Kevin is in for a few surprises.
160 pages Softcover
Mark Mishek, President and Chief Executive Officer
Joe Jaksha, Publisher

8440 Inhalants
Hazelden
15251 Pleasant Valley Rd
Center City, MN 55012-9640
651-213-4200
800-257-7810
Fax: 651-213-4793
info@hazelden.org
www.hazelden.org

Clear, straightforward explanation of the dangers and consequences of using seemingly harmless chemicals, such as model airplane glue, hair spray, whipping cream, and cleaning and lighter fluids, as well as sources of help for those who need it.
64 pages Paperback
ISBN: 1-568381-69-7
Mark Mishek, President and Chief Executive Officer
Joe Jaksha, Publisher

8441 Inside Out
Hazelden
15251 Pleasant Valley Rd
Center City, MN 55012-9640
651-213-4200
800-257-7810
Fax: 651-213-4793
info@hazelden.org
www.hazelden.org

Offers open-ended sentences for readers to fill in their responses.
97 pages Paperback
Mark Mishek, President and Chief Executive Officer
Joe Jaksha, Publisher

8442 Kids and Alcohol: Get High on Life
Health Communications
1721 Blount Road
Pompano Beach, FL 33069
954-360-0909
www.hoffmanestates.com
A workbook designed to help children make important decisions in their lives and feel good about themselves.
Ages 11-14
Jamie Rattray, Author

8443 Let's Talk About Drug Abuse
Rosen Publishing Group's PowerKids Press
29 East 21st Street
New York, NY 10010
212-777-3017
800-237-9932
Fax: 888-436-4643
customerservice@rosenpub.com
www.rosenpublishing.com

A first step in a child's education about the dangers of drugs. Recommended for grade K-4.
ISBN: 0-823923-02-9
Anna Kreiner, Author

8444 McGruff's Surprise Party
National Clearinghouse for Alcohol and Drug Info.
PO Box 2345
Rockville, MD 20847-2345
800-729-6686
files.eric.ed.gov
A comic book that helps children understand the importance of refusing alcohol and other drugs.
14 pages Ages 8-10
Paula Stauffer, Author

8445 My Body is My House
Hazelden
15251 Pleasant Valley Rd
Center City, MN 55012
651-213-4200
800-257-7810
Fax: 651-213-4793
info@hazelden.org
www.hazelden.org

A coloring book about alcohol, drugs and health.
16 pages
Mark Mishek, President and Chief Executive Officer
Joe Jaksha, Publisher

8446 Sad Story of Mary Wanna or How Marijuana Harms You
Woodmere Press
PO Box 20
New York, NY 10025
A coloring book for children that contains pictures of the damage that marijuana does to the body.
40 pages Grades 1-4

8447 Should Drugs Be Legalized?
Franklin Watts Grolier
90 Old Sherman Turnpike
Danbury, CT 06816-0001
203-797-3500
800-621-1115
Fax: 203-797-3197
www.grolier.com

Presents a discussion of this controversial subject.
160 pages Grades 7-12

8448 **Smoking-At Issues Series**
Greenhaven Press
10650 Toebben Drive   800-354-9706
Independence, KY 41051-9187   Fax: 800-487-8488
                                       order.samples@cengage.com
                                       solutions.cengage.com/greenhaven
Written in a straightforward manner, this book answers questions
most young adults are asking regarding smoking and health.
ISBN: 0-737701-57-9

8449 **Stand Strong**
African American Family Services
2616 Nicollet Avenue S   612-871-7878
Minneapolis, MN 55408   888-786-6798
                                       www.rehabs.com
Comic book prevention for young adults. Profiles two African-American teens as they go through the hazards and risks of
drug use and sexual behavior.
16 pages

8450 **Summer of Sassy Jo**
Houghton Mifflin
Wayside Road   800-225-3362
Burlington, MA 01803
A story of a thirteen-year-old girl faced with reconciliation with
her recovered alcoholic mother after eight years of abandonment.
192 pages Grades 7+
ISBN: 0-395669-56-1

8451 **Teen Alcoholism-Teen Issues**
Lucent Books
Thomson Gale   800-877-4253
San Diego, CA 48333-9187   Fax: 800-414-5043
Offers readable interviews for reports and answers the most fre-
quently asked questions about alcohol.
ISBN: 1-590185-01-3

8452 **Teen Guide to Pregnancy, Drugs and Smoking**
Franklin Watts Grolier
90 Old Sherman Turnpike   203-797-3500
Danbury, CT 06816-0001   800-621-1115
                                       Fax: 203-797-3197
                                       www.grolier.com
Outlines the risks of smoking and drug taking while pregnant and
answers teenagers' questions about the use of legal, illegal and prescription drugs.
64 pages Grades 9-12
ISBN: 0-531108-35-0

8453 **Understanding Drugs**
Franklin Watts Grolier
90 Old Sherman Turnpike   203-797-3500
Danbury, CT 06816-0001   800-621-1115
                                       Fax: 203-797-3197
                                       www.grolier.com
This series of books explains the current drug phenomenon at a
high-interest, low-vocabulary level. Gives in-depth information
about all aspects of commonly abused substances, including their
negative mental, physical and social effects. Each book features
photographs, diagrams, a glossary, an index and list of addresses
for futher information and help. Set of seven volumes.
Grades 5-7

8454 **Violence and Drugs**
Franklin Watts Grolier
90 Old Sherman Turnpike   203-797-3500
Danbury, CT 06816-0001   800-621-1115
                                       Fax: 203-797-3197
                                       www.grolier.com
This informative book studies the fascinating link between drug
use and violent behavior.
112 pages Grades 9-12
ISBN: 0-531108-18-0

8455 **What's Drunk Mama?**
Al-Anon Family Group Headquarters

1600 Corp Landing Pkwy   757-563-1600
Virginia Beach, VA 23454-5617   800-425-2666
                                       Fax: 757-563-1655
                                       wso@al-anon.org
                                       www.al-anon.alateen.org
Large print illustrated booklet for use as a shared reading experi-
ence to help younger children understand alcoholism.
32 pages
Caryn Johnson, Director Communications

8456 **Whiskers Says No to Drugs**
Weekly Reader Skills Books
245 Long Hill Road   860-446-3355
Jefferson City, MO 65102-4063   Fax: 800-724-4911
                                       www.weeklyreader.com
This book contains stories and follow-up activities for students to
provide information and form attitudes before they face peer pres-
sure to experiment.
Grades 2-3

8457 **Why Do People Drink Alcohol?**
Franklin Watts Grolier
90 Old Sherman Turnpike   203-797-3500
Danbury, CT 06816-0001   800-621-1115
                                       Fax: 203-797-3197
                                       www.grolier.com
Answers young children's questions about alcoholism.
32 pages Grades 3-5
ISBN: 0-531171-34-5

8458 **Why Do People Smoke?**
Franklin Watts Grolier
90 Old Sherman Turnpike   203-797-3500
Danbury, CT 06816-0001   800-621-1115
                                       Fax: 203-797-3197
                                       www.grolier.com
Raises and answers questions of specific interest to seven-to-ten
year olds about smoking.
32 pages Grades 3-5
ISBN: 0-531171-92-2

8459 **Why Do People Take Drugs?**
Franklin Watts Grolier
90 Old Sherman Turnpike   203-797-3500
Danbury, CT 06816-0001   800-621-1115
                                       Fax: 203-797-3197
                                       www.grolier.com
Raises important questions and offers some answers for young
children on the aspects and everyday living with a drug addiction.
32 pages Grades 3-5
ISBN: 0-531171-13-2

8460 **Winning the Battle Against Drugs: Rehabilitation Programs**
Franklin Watts Grolier
90 Old Sherman Turnpike   203-797-3500
Danbury, CT 06816-0001   800-621-1115
                                       Fax: 203-797-3197
                                       www.grolier.com
Programs contained in this book will help adolescents see that drug
and alcohol addiction can be successfully treated.
160 pages Grades 7-12
ISBN: 0-531110-63-0

8461 **Young Person's Guide to the Twelve Steps**
Hazelden
15251 Pleasant Valley Rd   651-213-4200
Center City, MN 55012-9640   800-257-7810
                                       Fax: 651-213-4793
                                       info@hazelden.org
                                       www.hazelden.org
Explains the Twelve Steps in the best way young people can under-
stand: in their own language.
168 pages Paperback
Mark Mishek, President and Chief Executive Officer
Joe Jaksha, Publisher

8462 **Young, Sober & Free**
Hazelden

15251 Pleasant Valley Rd
Center City, MN 55012-9640

651-213-4200
800-257-7810
Fax: 651-213-4793
info@hazelden.org
www.hazelden.org

Features young peoples' personal experiences of living with addiction.
137 pages Paperback
Mark Mishek, President and Chief Executive Officer
Joe Jaksha, Publisher

Magazines

8463 ACAP Recap
American Council on Alcohol Problems
3426 Bridgeland Drive
Bridgeton, MO 63044-2603

314-739-5944
Fax: 314-739-0848
www.lifemanagement.com

Offers information on organization activities and events, updates on resources and publications and legislative information for affiliate executives.
Monthly
Dr. Curt Scarborough, Executive Director

8464 American Issue
American Council on Alcohol Problems
3426 Bridgeland Drive
Bridgeton, MO 63044-2603

314-739-5944
Fax: 314-739-0848

Offered to contributors of the organization.
Monthly
Dr. Curt Scarborough, Executive Director

8465 Drug Abuse Update
2296 Henderson Mill Road
Atlanta, GA 30345-2739

770-934-6364

A journal of news and information for persons interested in drug prevention.
Quarterly

8466 Forum Magazine
Al-Anon Alateen Family Group Headquarters
1600 Corp Landing Pkwy
Virginia Beach, VA 23454-970

757-563-1600
888-425-2666
Fax: 757-563-1655
www.al-anon.alateen.org

Contains many personal stories of inspiration, some of which are maade available each month on the Internet by authorization of Al-Anon Family Group Headquarters, Inc.
Ric Buchanan, Executive Director

8467 Lead Line
Grapevine
PO Box 1980
New York, NY 10163-1980

212-870-3400
Fax: 212-870-3301

AA members all over the world communicate with each other through the pages of this magazine. It contains: insight into how AAs stay sober; readers' views; old-timers corner, beginners meeting, youth enjoying sobriety, and spotlight on service.
Monthly

Newsletters

8468 ADPA Professional
Alcohol/Drug Problems Association of North America
307 N Main Street
St. Charles, MO 63301

314-589-6702
Fax: 314-940-2358

Offers information to members on events, conferences and activities, reviews the newest resources and technology pertaining to alcoholism and drug addiction.

8469 Drug-Free Workplace Educator
American Council on Drug Education
204 Monroe Street
Rockville, MD 20850-4425

301-294-0600
800-488-3784
www.ascicorp.com

Offers continuing education for employers and their supervisors responsible for substance abuse prevention. Practical articles feature information to help employers design, implement and maintain a drug-free workplace.
BiMonthly

8470 Just Say Notes
Just Say No International
2101 Webster Street
Oakland, CA 94612-3065

510-451-6666
800-258-2766

Offers information on the organizations, activities, programs, conferences and events.
BiMonthly

8471 RID-USA Newsletter
Remove Intoxicated Drivers (RID-USA)
PO Box 520
Schenectady, NY 12301-0520

518-393-4357
888-283-5144
Fax: 518-370-4917
www.rid-usa.org

Membership news.
3x Year
Doris Aiken, President & CEO

8472 Sobering Thoughts
Women for Sobriety
PO Box 618
Quakertown, PA 18951-0618

215-536-8026
800-333-1606
Fax: 215-536-9026
newlife@nni.com
www.womenforsobriety.org

A monthly membership newsletter for women with an addiction problem who wish for recovery and start a new life.
16 pages Monthly
Rebecca Fenner, Director

8473 Substance Abuse Funding News
CD Publications
2222 Sedwick Drive
Durham, NC 27713-4571

301-588-6380
855-237-1396
Fax: 800-508-2592

Detailed coverage of private and federal funding opportunities for alcohol, tobacco and drug abuse programs. Plus advice on successful grantseeking strategies and news affecting your programs.
18 pages BiWeekly
Mary Compton, Publisher
Amy Bernstein, Editor

Pamphlets

8474 AA Member: Medications and Other Drugs
Alcoholics Anonymous
PO Box 459
New York, NY 10163-0459

212-870-3400
Fax: 212-870-3137
www.aa.org

Report from a group of doctors in Alcoholics Anonymous.

8475 AA Service Manual: Twelve Concepts for World Service
Alcoholics Anonymous
PO Box 459
New York, NY 10163-0459

212-870-3400
Fax: 212-870-3137
www.aa.org

This manual opens with a history of AA services.

8476 AA and the Armed Services
Alcoholics Anonymous
PO Box 459
New York, NY 10163-0459

212-870-3400
Fax: 212-870-3137
www.aa.org

Personal stories tell how men and women in the military can beat a drinking problem.

8477 AA and the Gay/Lesbian Alcoholic
Alcoholics Anonymous
PO Box 459
New York, NY 10163-0459

212-870-3400
Fax: 212-870-3137
www.aa.org

Excerpts from experience, strength and hope of sober gay and lesbian alcoholics.

8478 AA as a Resource for Health Care Professionals
Alcoholics Anonymous
PO Box 459   212-870-3400
New York, NY 10163-0459   Fax: 212-870-3137
                                                        www.aa.org
Information about the Fellowship and describes some approaches
that health care professionals use in referring problem drinkers to
AA.

8479 AA for the Native North American
Alcoholics Anonymous
PO Box 459   212-870-3400
New York, NY 10163-0459   Fax: 212-870-3137
                                                        www.aa.org
Addressed to and contains stories by Native American AA mem-
bers.

8480 AA for the Woman
Alcoholics Anonymous
PO Box 459   212-870-3400
New York, NY 10163-0459   Fax: 212-870-3137
                                                        www.aa.org
Relates the experiences of alcoholic women, all ages and from all
walks of life.

8481 AA in Correctional Facilities
Alcoholics Anonymous
PO Box 459   212-870-3400
New York, NY 10163-0459   Fax: 212-870-3137
                                                        www.aa.org
Experience based on the functioning of AA groups in prisons, with
institutional opinions recommending AA as a helpful ally.

8482 AA in Treatment Facilities
Alcoholics Anonymous
PO Box 459   212-870-3400
New York, NY 10163-0459   Fax: 212-870-3137
                                                        www.aa.org
Shares experiences of treatment facility administrators and of
AA's who have carried the message into these facilities.

8483 Acceptance
Hazelden
15251 Pleasant Valley Rd   651-213-4200
Center City, MN 55012-9640   800-257-7810
                                                  Fax: 651-213-4793
                                                  info@hazelden.org
                                                  www.hazelden.org
Addresses issues such as facing life, the kindness of God, suffering
and contentment.
Mark Mishek, President and Chief Executive Officer
Joe Jaksha, Publisher

8484 Adult Children of Alcoholics Newcomer Packet
Al-Anon Family Group Headquarters
1600 Corp Landing Pkwy   757-563-1600
Virginia Beach, VA 23454-5617   800-425-2666
                                                  Fax: 757-563-1655
                                                  wso@al-anon.org
                                                  www.al-anon.alateen.org
For those who have grown up with parental alcoholism, this is a
loving introduction to Al-Anon and the twelve steps.
9 pieces
Caryn Johnson, Director Communications

8485 African Americans in Treatment
Hazelden
15251 Pleasant Valley Rd   651-213-4200
Center City, MN 55012   800-257-7810
                                                  Fax: 651-213-4793
                                                  info@hazelden.org
                                                  www.hazelden.org
Helps African American clients understand treatment from a cul-
tural standpoint.
23 pages
Mark Mishek, President and Chief Executive Officer
Joe Jaksha, Publisher

8486 Al-Anon Newcomers Packet
Al-Anon Family Group Headquarters

1600 Corp Landing Pkwy   757-563-1600
Virginia Beach, VA 23454-5617   800-425-2666
                                                  Fax: 757-563-1655
                                                  wso@al-anon.org
                                                  www.al-anon.alateen.org
Material specifically for the newcomer to Al-Anon packed in a
handsome sleeve.
8 pieces
Caryn Johnson, Director Communications

8487 Al-Anon Spoken Here
Al-Anon Family Group Headquarters
1600 Corp Landing Pkwy   757-563-1600
Virginia Beach, VA 23454-5617   800-425-2666
                                                  Fax: 757-563-1655
                                                  wso@al-anon.org
                                                  www.al-anon.alateen.org
Why are Al-Anon meetings the way they are? Questions and answers that lead to a better understanding of the importance of keeping Al-Anon principles.
8 pages
Caryn Johnson, Director Communications

8488 Al-Anon is for Men
Al-Anon Family Group Headquarters
1600 Corp Landing Pkwy   757-563-1600
Virginia Beach, VA 23454-5617   800-425-2666
                                                  Fax: 757-563-1655
                                                  wso@al-anon.org
                                                  www.al-anon.alateen.org
Straight forward questions to help men identify their reactions to
alcoholism in another person.
6 pages
Caryn Johnson, Director Communications

8489 Al-Anon, You and the Alcoholic
Al-Anon Family Group Headquarters
1600 Corp Landing Pkwy   757-563-1600
Virginia Beach, VA 23454-5617   800-425-2666
                                                  Fax: 757-563-1655
                                                  wso@al-anon.org
                                                  www.al-anon.alateen.org
Answers the most frequently asked questions about Al-Anon and
how it helps families deal with problems brought about by alcoholism.
12 pages
Caryn Johnson, Director Communications

8490 Alateen Newcomer Packet
Al-Anon Family Group Headquarters
1600 Corp Landing Pkwy   757-563-1600
Virginia Beach, VA 23454-5617   800-425-2666
                                                  Fax: 757-563-1655
                                                  wso@al-anon.org
                                                  www.al-anon.alateen.org
Helpful leaflets assembled in a sleeve ready to give to the new
young member.
13 pieces
Caryn Johnson, Director Communications

8491 Alateen Talk
Al-Anon Family Group Headquarters
1600 Corp Landing Pkwy   757-563-1600
Virginia Beach, VA 23454-5617   800-425-2666
                                                  Fax: 757-563-1655
                                                  wso@al-anon.org
                                                  www.al-anon.alateen.org
Al-Anon is a mutual support group of peers who share their experience in applying the Al-Anon principles to problems related to the
effects of a problem drinker in their lives. It is not group therapy
and is not led by a counselor or therapist
Robert Schneider, Director Communications

8492 Alcohol Alert #11: Estimating the Cost of Alcohol Abuse
National Clearinghouse for Alcohol and Drug Info.
1101 Wootton Parkway   800-729-6686
Rockville, MD 20852-2345   Fax: 240-453-8282
                                                  odphpinfo@hhs.gov
                                                  www.health.org

Discusses the various problems of estimating the cost of alcohol abuse.

8493   Alcohol Alert #15: Alcohol and AIDS
National Clearinghouse for Alcohol and Drug Info.
1101 Wootton Parkway   800-729-6686
Rockville, MD 20852-2345   Fax: 240-453-8282
                                   odphpinfo@hhs.gov
                                        www.health.org

Discusses the relationship between alcohol consumption and HIV infection and AIDS.

8494   Alcohol Alert #16: Moderate Drinking
National Clearinghouse for Alcohol and Drug Info.
1101 Wootton Parkway   800-729-6686
Rockville, MD 20852-2345   Fax: 240-453-8282
                                   odphpinfo@hhs.gov
                                        www.health.org

Defines moderate drinking and explores the benefits and risks associated with moderate drinking.

8495   Alcohol Alert #17: Treatment Outcome Research
National Clearinghouse for Alcohol and Drug Info.
1101 Wootton Parkway   800-729-6686
Rockville, MD 20852-2345   Fax: 240-453-8282
                                   odphpinfo@hhs.gov
                                        www.health.org

Discusses purpose, methodology, randomization, blinding, followup and what treatment outcome research reveals.

8496   Alcohol Alert #18: The Genetics of Alcoholism
National Clearinghouse for Alcohol and Drug Info.
1101 Wootton Parkway   800-729-6686
Rockville, MD 20852-2345   Fax: 240-453-8282
                                   odphpinfo@hhs.gov
                                        www.health.org

Presents the results of studies that investigate the role of genes and the environment in the development of alcoholism.

8497   Alcohol Alert #21: Alcohol and Cancer
National Clearinghouse for Alcohol and Drug Info.
1101 Wootton Parkway   800-729-6686
Rockville, MD 20852-2345   Fax: 240-453-8282
                                   odphpinfo@hhs.gov
                                        www.health.org

The Office of Disease Prevention and Health Promotion (ODPHP) plays a vital role in keeping the Nation healthy. Learn more about our work by exploring our national health initiatives

8498   Alcohol Alert #23: Alcohol and Minorities
National Clearinghouse for Alcohol and Drug Info.
1101 Wootton Parkway   800-729-6686
Rockville, MD 20852-2345   Fax: 240-453-8282
                                   odphpinfo@hhs.gov
                                        www.health.org

The Office of Disease Prevention and Health Promotion (ODPHP) plays a vital role in keeping the Nation healthy. Learn more about our work by exploring our national health initiatives

8499   Alcohol Alert #24: Animal Models in Alcohol Research
National Clearinghouse for Alcohol and Drug Info.
1101 Wootton Parkway   800-729-6686
Rockville, MD 20852-2345   Fax: 240-453-8282
                                   odphpinfo@hhs.gov
                                        www.health.org

The Office of Disease Prevention and Health Promotion (ODPHP) plays a vital role in keeping the Nation healthy. Learn more about our work by exploring our national health initiatives

8500   Alcohol Alert #25: Alcohol-Related Impairment
National Clearinghouse for Alcohol and Drug Info.
1101 Wootton Parkway   800-729-6686
Rockville, MD 20852-2345   Fax: 240-453-8282
                                   odphpinfo@hhs.gov
                                        www.health.org

The Office of Disease Prevention and Health Promotion (ODPHP) plays a vital role in keeping the Nation healthy. Learn more about our work by exploring our national health initiatives

8501   Alcohol Alert #26: Alcohol and Hormones
National Clearinghouse for Alcohol and Drug Info.

1101 Wootton Parkway   800-729-6686
Rockville, MD 20852-2345   Fax: 240-453-8282
                                   odphpinfo@hhs.gov
                                        www.health.org

The Office of Disease Prevention and Health Promotion (ODPHP) plays a vital role in keeping the Nation healthy. Learn more about our work by exploring our national health initiatives

8502   Alcohol Alert #27: Alcohol Medication Interactions
National Clearinghouse for Alcohol and Drug Info.
1101 Wootton Parkway   800-729-6686
Rockville, MD 20852-2345   Fax: 240-453-8282
                                   odphpinfo@hhs.gov
                                        www.health.org

The Office of Disease Prevention and Health Promotion (ODPHP) plays a vital role in keeping the Nation healthy. Learn more about our work by exploring our national health initiatives

8503   Alcohol and Drug Abuse in Black America: A Guide for Community Action
African American Family Services
2616 Nicollet Avenue S   612-871-7878
Minneapolis, MN 55408   855-522-3013
                                   findthebestrehab.org

A booklet giving a description of the history and the current manifestations of alcohol and drug problems in Black America with a discussion of strategies for fundamental change.
24 pages

8504   Alcohol and Pregnancy
March of Dimes
233 Park Avenue South   212-353-8353
New York, NY 10003   Fax: 212-254-3518
                              NY639@marchofdimes.com
                                   www.marchofdimes.com

8505   Alcoholics Anonymous and Employee Assistance Program
Alcoholics Anonymous
PO Box 459   212-870-3400
New York, NY 10163-0459   Fax: 212-870-3137
                                        www.aa.org

Of interest to management and union officials, this pamphlet gives concise descriptions of the help AA can offer to the alcoholic employee.

8506   Alcoholism Tends to Run in Families
National Clearinghouse for Alcohol and Drug Info.
1101 Wootton Parkway   800-729-6686
Rockville, MD 20852-2345   Fax: 240-453-8282
                                   odphpinfo@hhs.gov
                                        www.health.org

Provides answers and questions about how to help children of alcoholics and where to find resources for additional information.

8507   Alcoholism: A Merry-Go-Round Named Denial
Al-Anon Family Group Headquarters
1600 Corp Landing Pkwy   757-563-1600
Virginia Beach, VA 23454-5617   800-425-2666
                                   Fax: 757-563-1655
                                   wso@al-anon.org
                              www.al-anon.alateen.org

Dramatic explanations that help family members and friends see the roles they play in the problems of alcoholism.
18 pages
Caryn Johnson, Director Communications

8508   Alcoholism: The Family Disease
Al-Anon Family Group Headquarters
1600 Corp Landing Pkwy   757-563-1600
Virginia Beach, VA 23454-5617   800-425-2666
                                   Fax: 757-563-1655
                                   wso@al-anon.org
                              www.al-anon.alateen.org

A treasury of information and inspiration with the purpose of the Al-Anon program, actual stories of people who found serenity in Al-Anon, questions/answers, slogans, evaluations and thoughts to live by.
48 pages
Caryn Johnson, Director Communications

8509 Anabolic Steroids: A Threat to Body and Mind
National Clearinghouse for Alcohol and Drug Info.
PO Box 2345   800-729-6686
Rockville, MD 20847   files.eric.ed.gov
Summarizes the findings of recent studies on the use of anabolic
steroids in the United States.
11 pages

8510 Anonymity
Al-Anon Family Group Headquarters
1600 Corp Landing Pkwy   757-563-1600
Virginia Beach, VA 23454-5617   800-425-2666
                                                Fax: 757-563-1655
                                                wso@al-anon.org
                                                www.al-anon.alateen.org
Offers information on Al-Anon and Alateen traditions and what a
big factor anonymity plays for members.
6 pages
Caryn Johnson, Director Communications

8511 Are You Concerned About Someone's Drinking
Al-Anon Family Group Headquarters
1600 Corp Landing Pkwy   757-563-1600
Virginia Beach, VA 23454-5617   800-425-2666
                                                Fax: 757-563-1655
                                                wso@al-anon.org
                                                www.al-anon.alateen.org
Al-Anon is a mutual support group of peers who share their experience in applying the Al-Anon principles to problems related to the
effects of a problem drinker in their lives. It is not group therapy
and is not led by a counselor or therapist
12 pages
Caryn Johnson, Director Communications

8512 Be Kind to Nonsmokers
American Lung Association
1740 Broadway   212-315-8700
New York, NY 10019-4315
Explains why smoke hurts nonsmokers.

8513 Best of Public Outreach
Al-Anon Family Group Headquarters
1600 Corp Landing Pkwy   757-563-1600
Virginia Beach, VA 23454-5617   800-425-2666
                                                Fax: 757-563-1655
                                                wso@al-anon.org
                                                www.al-anon.alateen.org
Helps groups, committees and individuals carry out their PI institutions and CPC activities; includes suggested activities and open
letters to various professionals.
24 pages
Caryn Johnson, Director Communications

8514 Black, Beautiful and Recovering
Hazelden
15251 Pleasant Valley Rd   651-213-4200
Center City, MN 55012-9640   800-257-7810
                                                Fax: 651-213-4793
                                                info@hazelden.org
                                                www.hazelden.org
Hazelden, a part of the Hazelden Betty Ford Foundation, has been
saving lives and restoring families from substance abuse and ad-
diction for more than 60 years
20 pages
Mark Mishek, President and Chief Executive Officer
Joe Jaksha, Publisher

8515 Chemical Dependency and the African American
Hazelden
15251 Pleasant Valley Rd   651-213-4200
Center City, MN 55012-9640   800-257-7810
                                                Fax: 651-213-4793
                                                info@hazelden.org
                                                www.hazelden.org
Reviews the impact alcohol and other drug abuse has on African
American communities.
66 pages
Mark Mishek, President and Chief Executive Officer
Joe Jaksha, Publisher

8516 Chemical Dependency: An Acceptable Disease
Hazelden
15251 Pleasant Valley Rd   651-213-4200
Center City, MN 55012-9640   800-257-7810
                                                Fax: 651-213-4793
                                                info@hazelden.org
                                                www.hazelden.org
Help persons identify and acknowledge their chemical depend-
ency.
14 pages
Mark Mishek, President and Chief Executive Officer
Joe Jaksha, Publisher

8517 Chew or Snuff is Real Bad Stuff
National Cancer Institute
Building 31   301-496-4000
Bethesda, MD 20892   www.killthecan.org
A pamphlet describing the hazards of using smokeless tobacco.
8 pages

8518 Cigarette Smoking
American Lung Association
1740 Broadway   212-315-8700
New York, NY 10019-4315
Leaflet presenting the facts about how cigarette smoke is related to
lung disease.

8519 Communication Skills
Hazelden
15251 Pleasant Valley Rd   651-213-4200
Center City, MN 55012-9640   800-257-7810
                                                Fax: 651-213-4793
                                                info@hazelden.org
                                                www.hazelden.org
Helps clients discover how to become better listeners.
Mark Mishek, President and Chief Executive Officer
Joe Jaksha, Publisher

8520 Community Campaign Brochure
National Clearinghouse for Alcohol and Drug Info.
PO Box 2345   800-729-6686
Rockville, MD 20847-2345   files.eric.ed.gov
Information and promotional brochure discusses key prevention
concepts and messages and details how to plan campaign events.

8521 Crack
Hazelden
15251 Pleasant Valley Rd   651-213-4200
Center City, MN 55012-9640   800-257-7810
                                                Fax: 651-213-4793
                                                info@hazelden.org
                                                www.hazelden.org
Explains history, use and effects of crack cocaine.
Mark Mishek, President and Chief Executive Officer
Joe Jaksha, Publisher

8522 Crack Cocaine: The Big Lie
National Clearinghouse for Alcohol and Drug Info.
1101 Wootton Parkway   800-729-6686
Rockville, MD 20852-2345   Fax: 240-453-8282
                                                odphpinfo@hhs.gov
                                                www.health.org
Offers information on what crack and cocaine are, how strong the
addictions are from these drugs, how they affect the body and other
risks in taking cocaine and crack.

8523 Crossing the Line Between Social Drinking and Alcoholism
Hazelden
15251 Pleasant Valley Rd   651-213-4200
Center City, MN 55012-9640   800-257-7810
                                                Fax: 651-213-4793
                                                info@hazelden.org
                                                www.hazelden.org
Hazelden, a part of the Hazelden Betty Ford Foundation, has been
saving lives and restoring families from substance abuse and ad-
diction for more than 60 years
20 pages
Mark Mishek, President and Chief Executive Officer
Joe Jaksha, Publisher

8524 Denial
Hazelden
15251 Pleasant Valley Rd
Center City, MN 55012-9640
651-213-4200
800-257-7810
Fax: 651-213-4793
info@hazelden.org
www.hazelden.org
Describes denial and its role in the five-stage acceptance process.
Mark Mishek, President and Chief Executive Officer
Joe Jaksha, Publisher

8525 Depression and Recovery from Chemical Dependency
Hazelden
15251 Pleasant Valley Rd
Center City, MN 55012-9640
651-213-4200
800-257-7810
Fax: 651-213-4793
info@hazelden.org
www.hazelden.org
Outlines depression's warning signs.
Mark Mishek, President and Chief Executive Officer
Joe Jaksha, Publisher

8526 Detaching with Love
Hazelden
15251 Pleasant Valley Rd
Center City, MN 55012-9640
651-213-4200
800-257-7810
Fax: 651-213-4793
info@hazelden.org
www.hazelden.org
Addresses the essential recovery tools clients need to cope with addiction and detach from the problem.
Mark Mishek, President and Chief Executive Officer
Joe Jaksha, Publisher

8527 Detachment
Al-Anon Family Group Headquarters
1600 Corp Landing Pkwy
Virginia Beach, VA 23454-5617
757-563-1600
800-425-2666
Fax: 757-563-1655
wso@al-anon.org
www.al-anon.alateen.org
Everything you always wanted to know about detachment in an easy-to-use leaflet.
Caryn Johnson, Director Communications

8528 Did You Grow Up with a Problem Drinker?
Al-Anon Family Group Headquarters
1600 Corp Landing Pkwy
Virginia Beach, VA 23454-5617
757-563-1600
800-425-2666
Fax: 757-563-1655
wso@al-anon.org
www.al-anon.alateen.org
Twenty personal questions help individuals decide if they can benefit from Al-Anon.
Caryn Johnson, Director Communications

8529 Do You Think You're Different?
Alcoholics Anonymous
PO Box 459
New York, NY 10163-0459
212-870-3400
Fax: 212-870-3137
www.aa.org
Speaks to newcomers who may wonder how AA can work for someone different.

8530 Don't Let Your Dreams Go Up in Smoke
American Lung Association
1740 Broadway
New York, NY 10019-4315
212-315-8700
Photos, testimonials and clear language to deliver the message that everyone can and should stop smoking.

8531 Don't Lose a Friend to Drugs
National Crime Prevention Council
1201 Connecticut Ave NW
Washington, DC 20036-3802
202-466-6272
Fax: 202-296-1356
www.ncpc.org
Offers practical advice to teenagers on how to say no to drugs, how to help a friend who uses drugs and how to initiate community efforts to prevent drug use.
Ann M. Harkins, President and Chief Executive Officer

8532 Drinking Alcohol During Pregnancy
March of Dimes
1275 Mamaroneck Avenue
White Plains, NY 10605
212-353-8353
Fax: 212-254-3518
NY639@marchofdimes.com
www.marchofdimes.com
Fact Sheets: one to two page review written for the general public.

8533 Drug Free Zones: A Manual
African American Family Services
2616 Nicollet Avenue S
Minneapolis, MN 55408
612-871-7878
This booklet describes a variety of strategies concerned citizens are using to reclaim their neighborhoods from rampant drug abuse and dealing.
24 pages

8534 Drugs and Pregnancy
March of Dimes
1275 Mamaroneck Avenue
White Plains, NY 10605
212-353-8353
Fax: 212-254-3518
NY639@marchofdimes.com
www.marchofdimes.com
Brochures: 3 panel color brochures written for the general public.
pkg 50

8535 Employer's Guide to Dealing with Substance Abuse
National Clearinghouse for Alcohol and Drug Info.
1101 Wootton Parkway
Rockville, MD 20852-2345
800-729-6686
Fax: 240-453-8282
odphpinfo@hhs.gov
www.health.gov
Instructs employers in setting up comprehensive alcohol and other drug programs in the workplace.
18 pages

8536 Enabling
Hazelden
15251 Pleasant Valley Rd
Center City, MN 55012-9640
651-213-4200
800-257-7810
Fax: 651-213-4793
info@hazelden.org
www.hazelden.org
Describes problems families encounter when they focus their lives on their chemically dependent family member.
Mark Mishek, President and Chief Executive Officer
Joe Jaksha, Publisher

8537 Facts About Alateen
Al-Anon Family Group Headquarters
1600 Corp Landing Pkwy
Virginia Beach, VA 23454-5617
757-563-1600
800-425-2666
Fax: 757-563-1655
wso@al-anon.org
www.al-anon.alateen.org
Offers information on Alateen member services.
4 pages
Caryn Johnson, Director Communications

8538 Facts About Alcohol Abuse
Medical Arts Center Hospital
57 W 57th Street
New York, NY 10019-2802
212-838-2169
Fax: 212-755-0200
A question and answer pamphlet that offers information on alcohol abuse and the effects the abuse has on the family unit.

8539 Family Denial
Hazelden
15251 Pleasant Valley Rd
Center City, MN 55012-9640
651-213-4200
800-257-7810
Fax: 651-213-4793
info@hazelden.org
www.hazelden.org
Describes ways for families to recognize denial, examine common fears that cause denial and develop methods for overcoming it.
Mark Mishek, President and Chief Executive Officer
Joe Jaksha, Publisher

8540 Fetal Alcohol Syndrome
Hazelden

15251 Pleasant Valley Rd
Center City, MN 55012-9640

651-213-4200
800-257-7810
Fax: 651-213-4793
info@hazelden.org
www.hazelden.org

A source of information about the effects of drinking while pregnant.
Mark Mishek, President and Chief Executive Officer
Joe Jaksha, Publisher

8541 Fight Drug Abuse at Home, Work, School and in the Community
American Council for Drug Education
204 Monroe Street
Rockville, MD 20850-4425

800-488-3784
www.hoffmanestates.com

A catalog of print and video materials pertaining to substance abuse, alcoholism and drugs.

8542 For a Strong and Healthy Baby
National Clearinghouse for Alcohol and Drug Info.
1101 Wootton Parkway
Rockville, MD 20852-2345

800-729-6686
Fax: 240-453-8282
odphpinfo@hhs.gov
www.health.org

Recommends that women not drink or use other drugs if pregnant or planning to become pregnant.

8543 Free to Care
Hazelden
15251 Pleasant Valley Rd
Center City, MN 55012-9640

651-213-4200
800-257-7810
Fax: 651-213-4793
info@hazelden.org
www.hazelden.org

Explores today's definition of family and new attitudes about gender, technology, single-parents, relatives and friends.
Mark Mishek, President and Chief Executive Officer
Joe Jaksha, Publisher

8544 Freedom from Despair
Al-Anon Family Group Headquarters
1600 Corp Landing Pkwy
Virginia Beach, VA 23454-5617

757-563-1600
800-425-2666
Fax: 757-563-1655
wso@al-anon.org
www.al-anon.alateen.org

A message of hope for those faced with a problem they can't solve alone.
4 pages
Caryn Johnson, Director Communications

8545 Freedom from Smoking Flyer
American Lung Association
1740 Broadway
New York, NY 10019-4315

212-315-8700

4 color flyer describing all FFS programs.

8546 Getting in Touch with Al-Anon/Alateen
Al-Anon Family Group Headquarters
1600 Corp Landing Pkwy
Virginia Beach, VA 23454-5617

757-563-1600
800-425-2666
Fax: 757-563-1655
wso@al-anon.org
www.al-anon.alateen.org

A listing of Al-Anon information services throughout the world. Helps members, the public and professionals located nearby Al-Anon or Alateen groups.
Caryn Johnson, Director Communications

8547 Grieving
Hazelden
15251 Pleasant Valley Rd
Center City, MN 55012-9640

651-213-4200
800-257-7810
Fax: 651-213-4793
info@hazelden.org
www.hazelden.org

Outlines the five-phase grieving process for clients and the significance of each.
Mark Mishek, President and Chief Executive Officer
Joe Jaksha, Publisher

8548 Guidance on Our Journeys
Hazelden
15251 Pleasant Valley Rd
Center City, MN 55012-9640

651-213-4200
800-257-7810
Fax: 651-213-4793
info@hazelden.org
www.hazelden.org

Examines the relationship between the recovering person and his or her sponsor.
Mark Mishek, President and Chief Executive Officer
Joe Jaksha, Publisher

8549 Guide for the Family of the Alcoholic
Al-Anon Family Group Headquarters
1600 Corp Landing Pkwy
Virginia Beach, VA 23454-5617

757-563-1600
800-425-2666
Fax: 757-563-1655
wso@al-anon.org
www.al-anon.alateen.org

A clear and realistic look at alcoholism, problems encountered by those close to the alcoholic and choices available to the family.
16 pages
Caryn Johnson, Director Communications

8550 Have Fun! Figure Out the Smoking Puzzle
American Lung Association
1740 Broadway
New York, NY 10019-4315

212-315-8700

Crossword puzzles make stimulating points on the effects of smoking.

8551 Healthy Beginning, Promotional Flyers
American Lung Association
1740 Broadway
New York, NY 10019-4315

212-315-8700

Flyer offers tips to help protect newborn and young children from the harmful effects of passive smoking.

8552 Help a Friend to Stop Smoking
American Lung Association
1740 Broadway
New York, NY 10019-4315

212-315-8700

This original guide to helping family members and friends support a smoker who is trying to quit smoking.
12 pages

8553 Helping Smokers Get Ready to Quit
American Lung Association
1740 Broadway
New York, NY 10019-4315

212-315-8700

Offers suggestions on how to get smokers to think about quitting and how to open up a dialogue on the issue.

8554 Helping Your Child Say No: A Parent's Guide
National Clearinghouse for Alcohol and Drug Info.
PO Box 2345
Rockville, MD 20847-2345

800-729-6686
www.hoffmanestates.com

Explains to parents how alcohol affects the body, how to tell if your child has been drinking and why children start to drink.

8555 Homeward Bound
Al-Anon Family Group Headquarters
1600 Corp Landing Pkwy
Virginia Beach, VA 23454-5617

757-563-1600
800-425-2666
Fax: 757-563-1655
wso@al-anon.org
www.al-anon.alateen.org

A booklet designed to help beginners make the transition from the family treatment setting to Al-Anon. Contains forty members' personal sharings, a basic glossary of Al-Anon terms, brief explanations of Al-Anon slogans and helpful suggestions for newcomers.
48 pages
Caryn Johnson, Director Communications

8556 How Can I Help My Children?
Al-Anon Family Group Headquarters
1600 Corp Landing Pkwy
Virginia Beach, VA 23454-5617

757-563-1600
800-425-2666
Fax: 757-563-1655
wso@al-anon.org
www.al-anon.alateen.org

Parents can help their children achieve a healthier attitude. Improving our own attitudes and behavior will help the entire family.
20 pages
Caryn Johnson, Director Communications

8557 How Drug Abuse Takes Profit Out of Business
National Clearinghouse for Alcohol and Drug Info.
PO Box 2345   800-729-6686
Rockville, MD 20847-2345   www.hoffmanestates.com
Answers employers questions about substance abuse in the workplace.

8558 How to Get the Most Out of Group Therapy
Hazelden
15251 Pleasant Valley Rd   651-213-4200
Center City, MN 55012-9640   800-257-7810
                                                Fax: 651-213-4793
                                                info@hazelden.org
                                                www.hazelden.org
Answers clients' questions about going to and getting help from group therapy.
Mark Mishek, President and Chief Executive Officer
Joe Jaksha, Publisher

8559 How to Help a Friend Quit Smoking
American Lung Association
1740 Broadway   212-315-8700
New York, NY 10019-4315
Discusses how friends, family and co-workers can assist smokers with their concerns about quitting smoking.

8560 How to Take Care of Your Baby Before Birth
National Clearinghouse for Alcohol and Drug Info.
1101 Wootton Parkway   800-729-6686
Rockville, MD 20852-2345   Fax: 240-453-8282
                                                odphpinfo@hhs.gov
                                                www.health.org
A low-literacy brochure aimed at pregnant women that describes what they should and should not do during pregnancy.

8561 I Can't Be Addicted Because...
Hazelden
15251 Pleasant Valley Rd   651-213-4200
Center City, MN 55012-9640   800-257-7810
                                                Fax: 651-213-4793
                                                info@hazelden.org
                                                www.hazelden.org
Focuses on denial and elaborates on its most common forms.
Mark Mishek, President and Chief Executive Officer
Joe Jaksha, Publisher

8562 Ice Storm
Hazelden
15251 Pleasant Valley Rd   651-213-4200
Center City, MN 55012-9640   800-257-7810
                                                Fax: 651-213-4793
                                                info@hazelden.org
                                                www.hazelden.org
Prepares treatment professionals for the complications of one of the most recently synthesized drugs - ice.
Mark Mishek, President and Chief Executive Officer
Joe Jaksha, Publisher

8563 If Someone Close to You Has a Problem with Alcohol or Other Drugs
National Clearinghouse for Alcohol and Drug Info.
1101 Wootton Parkway   800-729-6686
Rockville, MD 20852-2345   Fax: 240-453-8282
                                                odphpinfo@hhs.gov
                                                www.health.org
This booklet is aimed at the general public and gives support and suggestions on coping with someone close who has an alcohol or drug problem.

8564 If You Are a Professional, AA Wants to Work with You
Alcoholics Anonymous
PO Box 459   212-870-3400
New York, NY 10163-0459   Fax: 212-870-3137
                                                www.aa.org
Directed at professionals of all types who deal with alcoholics.

8565 If Your Parents Drink Too Much
Al-Anon Family Group Headquarters
1600 Corp Landing Pkwy   757-563-1600
Virginia Beach, VA 23454-5617   800-425-2666
                                                Fax: 757-563-1655
                                                wso@al-anon.org
                                                www.al-anon.alateen.org
Alateen's cartoon booklet.
24 pages
Caryn Johnson, Director Communications

8566 Illicit Drug Use During Pregnancy
March of Dimes
1275 Mamaroneck Avenue   212-353-8353
White Plains, NY 10605   Fax: 212-254-3518
                                                NY639@marchofdimes.com
                                                www.marchofdimes.com
Fact Sheets: one to two page review for the general public. Also available electronically from the website www.marchofdimes.com

8567 Index to Alcoholics Anonymous
Hazelden
15251 Pleasant Valley Rd   651-213-4200
Center City, MN 55012-9640   800-257-7810
                                                Fax: 651-213-4793
                                                info@hazelden.org
                                                www.hazelden.org
Features page and line references to the topics discussed in Alcoholics Anonymous, the Big Book.
Mark Mishek, President and Chief Executive Officer
Joe Jaksha, Publisher

8568 Is AA for Me?
Alcoholics Anonymous
PO Box 459   212-870-3400
New York, NY 10163-0459   Fax: 212-870-3137
                                                www.aa.org
An illustrated easy to read version of the 12 questions in Is AA for You? pamphlet.
32 pages

8569 Is AA for You?
Alcoholics Anonymous
PO Box 459   212-870-3400
New York, NY 10163-0459   Fax: 212-870-3137
                                                www.aa.org
Symptoms of alcoholism are summed up in 12 questions most AA's had answered to identify themselves as alcoholics.

8570 Is There a Safe Tobacco?
American Lung Association
1740 Broadway   212-315-8700
New York, NY 10019-4315
Offers information on the health risks of cigarette smoking, pipes and cigars.

8571 Is There an Alcoholic in Your Life?
Alcoholics Anonymous
PO Box 459   212-870-3400
New York, NY 10163-0459   Fax: 212-870-3137
                                                www.aa.org
Explains the AA program as it affects anyone close to an alcoholic.

8572 It Happened to Alice
Alcoholics Anonymous
PO Box 459   212-870-3400
New York, NY 10163-0459   Fax: 212-870-3137
                                                www.aa.org
Easy to read comic-book style format for women alcoholics.

8573 It Sure Beats Sitting in a Cell
Alcoholics Anonymous
PO Box 459   212-870-3400
New York, NY 10163-0459   Fax: 212-870-3137
                                                www.aa.org
An illustrated pamphlet which presents the experience of seven inmates who found AA while in prison. It also offers suggested dos and don'ts for staying sober after release.

8574 Kids and Drugs: A Handbook for Parents & Professionals
PANDAA Press

4111 Watkins Trl
Annandale, VA 22003-2051
703-750-9285
www.sdsalarms.com

8575 Let's Solve the Smokeword Puzzle
American Lung Association
1740 Broadway
New York, NY 10019-4315
212-315-8700
Fifth graders will love getting an antismoking message through solving a crossword puzzle.

8576 Let's Talk
Hazelden
15251 Pleasant Valley Rd
Center City, MN 55012-9640
651-213-4200
800-257-7810
Fax: 651-213-4793
info@hazelden.org
www.hazelden.org
Offers 12 guidelines to promote effective communication between parent and child.
Mark Mishek, President and Chief Executive Officer
Joe Jaksha, Publisher

8577 Letter to a Woman Alcoholic
Alcoholics Anonymous
PO Box 459
New York, NY 10163-0459
212-870-3400
Fax: 212-870-3137
www.aa.org
Describes with sensitive understanding the problem of the alcoholic woman.

8578 Letting Go of the Need to Control
Hazelden
15251 Pleasant Valley Rd
Center City, MN 55012-9640
651-213-4200
800-257-7810
Fax: 651-213-4793
info@hazelden.org
www.hazelden.org
Discusses how control issues are common among chemically dependent people.
Mark Mishek, President and Chief Executive Officer
Joe Jaksha, Publisher

8579 Lifetime of Freedom from Smoking: Maintenance Manual
American Lung Association
1740 Broadway
New York, NY 10019-4315
212-315-8700
Companion manual helps persons stay quit once they have stopped smoking.
28 pages

8580 Little More About Alcohol
Alcohol Research Information Service
1120 E Oakland Avenue
Lansing, MI 48906-5513
517-485-9900
Fax: 517-485-1928
www.hoffmanestates.com
A cartoon character explains the facts about alcohol and its effects on the body.

8581 Living Sober
Alcoholics Anonymous
PO Box 459
New York, NY 10163-0459
212-870-3400
Fax: 212-870-3137
www.aa.org
Practical book demonstrating through simple examples, how AA members throughout the world live and stay sober one day at a time.
88 pages

8582 Living in a Shelter?
Al-Anon Family Group Headquarters
1600 Corp Landing Pkwy
Virginia Beach, VA 23454-5617
757-563-1600
800-425-2666
Fax: 757-563-1655
wso@al-anon.org
www.al-anon.alateen.org
Al-Anon is a mutual support group of peers who share their experience in applying the Al-Anon principles to problems related to the effects of a problem drinker in their lives. It is not group therapy and is not led by a counselor or therapist
100 pieces
Caryn Johnson, Director Communications

8583 Look at Cross-Addiction
Hazelden
15251 Pleasant Valley Rd
Center City, MN 55012-9640
651-213-4200
800-257-7810
Fax: 651-213-4793
info@hazelden.org
www.hazelden.org
Discusses cross-addiction, denial, coping skills and avoidance.
Mark Mishek, President and Chief Executive Officer
Joe Jaksha, Publisher

8584 Look at Relapse
Hazelden
15251 Pleasant Valley Rd
Center City, MN 55012-9640
651-213-4200
800-257-7810
Fax: 651-213-4793
info@hazelden.org
www.hazelden.org
Addresses emotional consequences of relapse, such as decreased feelings of self-esteem and self-confidence.
Mark Mishek, President and Chief Executive Officer
Joe Jaksha, Publisher

8585 Managing Cocaine Cravings
Hazelden
15251 Pleasant Valley Rd
Center City, MN 55012-9640
651-213-4200
800-257-7810
Fax: 651-213-4793
info@hazelden.org
www.hazelden.org
Offers clients hands-on plan to help them stay away from cocaine.
Mark Mishek, President and Chief Executive Officer
Joe Jaksha, Publisher

8586 Marijuana
Hazelden
15251 Pleasant Valley Rd
Center City, MN 55012-9640
651-213-4200
800-257-7810
Fax: 651-213-4793
info@hazelden.org
www.hazelden.org
Outlines the physical and psychological effects of marijuana unique to episodic and chronic use.
65 pages
Mark Mishek, President and Chief Executive Officer
Joe Jaksha, Publisher

8587 Media Kit
Al-Anon Family Group Headquarters
1600 Corp Landing Pkwy
Virginia Beach, VA 23454-5617
757-563-1600
800-425-2666
Fax: 757-563-1655
wso@al-anon.org
www.al-anon.alateen.org
An attractive silver folder containing information necessary to work with radio and TV stations.
Caryn Johnson, Director Communications

8588 Member's Eye View of Alcoholics Anonymous
Alcoholics Anonymous
PO Box 459
New York, NY 10163-0459
212-870-3400
Fax: 212-870-3137
www.aa.org
Designed to explain to people in the helping professionals how AA works.
30 pages

8589 Members of the Clergy Ask About Alcoholics Anonymous
Alcoholics Anonymous
PO Box 459
New York, NY 10163-0459
212-870-3400
Fax: 212-870-3137
www.aa.org
Introduction to AA for members of the clergy unfamiliar with the Fellowship.

8590 Memo to an Inmate Who May Be an Alcoholic
Alcoholics Anonymous
PO Box 459
New York, NY 10163-0459
212-870-3400
Fax: 212-870-3137
www.aa.org

A message from AA's who have themselves been inmates. Their personal stories offer a new outlook to inmate alcholics who want to know who AA can help.

8591 Men Newcomer Packet
Al-Anon Family Group Headquarters
1600 Corp Landing Pkwy
Virginia Beach, VA 23454-5617
757-563-1600
800-425-2666
Fax: 757-563-1655
wso@al-anon.org
www.al-anon.alateen.org
For men who are not sure Al-Anon is for them, this collection offers a realistic look at alcoholism and straight forward answers to frequently asked questions.
8 pieces
Caryn Johnson, Director Communications

8592 Message to Correctional Facilities Administrators
Alcoholics Anonymous
PO Box 459
New York, NY 10163-0459
212-870-3400
Fax: 212-870-3137
www.aa.org
Information about what AA is and can do, and how groups function in correctional facilities.

8593 Message to Teenagers
Alcoholics Anonymous
PO Box 459
New York, NY 10163-0459
212-870-3400
Fax: 212-870-3137
www.aa.org
This brochure offers a simple, 12-question quiz designed to help teenagers decide when drinking is becoming a problem in their lives.

8594 Military Packet
Al-Anon Family Group Headquarters
1600 Corp Landing Pkwy
Virginia Beach, VA 23454-5617
757-563-1600
800-425-2666
Fax: 757-563-1655
wso@al-anon.org
www.al-anon.alateen.org
For those in the armed services with loved ones or colleagues who are alcoholic, here's a collection that says, Al-Anon can help.
7 pieces
Caryn Johnson, Director Communications

8595 Moment to Reflect on Codependency
Hazelden
15251 Pleasant Valley Rd
Center City, MN 55012-9640
651-213-4200
800-257-7810
Fax: 651-213-4793
info@hazelden.org
www.hazelden.org
A collection of four booklets offering meditations that emphasize and reinforce self-esteem for young people recovering from addiction.
Mark Mishek, President and Chief Executive Officer
Joe Jaksha, Publisher

8596 Moment to Reflect on Self-Esteem
Hazelden
15251 Pleasant Valley Rd
Center City, MN 55012-9640
651-213-4200
800-257-7810
Fax: 651-213-4793
info@hazelden.org
www.hazelden.org
Focuses on the fundamental recovery issue of self-esteem.
4 Booklets
Mark Mishek, President and Chief Executive Officer
Joe Jaksha, Publisher

8597 Moving On! From Alateen to Al-Anon
Al-Anon Family Group Headquarters
1600 Corp Landing Pkwy
Virginia Beach, VA 23454-5617
757-563-1600
800-425-2666
Fax: 757-563-1655
wso@al-anon.org
www.al-anon.alateen.org

Former Alateen members experience the joy of continued recovery in Al-Anon.
12 pages
Caryn Johnson, Director Communications

8598 NIDA Capsules
National Clearinghouse for Alcohol and Drug Info.
1101 Wootton Parkway
Rockville, MD 20852-2345
800-729-6686
Fax: 240-453-8282
odphpinfo@hhs.gov
www.health.gov
The Office of Disease Prevention and Health Promotion (ODPHP) plays a vital role in keeping the Nation healthy. Learn more about our work by exploring our national health initiatives

8599 Newcomer Asks
Alcoholics Anonymous
PO Box 459
New York, NY 10163-0459
212-870-3400
Fax: 212-870-3137
www.aa.org
Gives straightforward answers on 15 points that once puzzled many of us.

8600 Nicotine Addiction and Cigarettes
American Lung Association
1740 Broadway
New York, NY 10019-4315
212-315-8700
Offers information on nicotine and cigarette smoking.

8601 No Smoking Coloring Book
American Lung Association
1740 Broadway
New York, NY 10019-4315
212-315-8700
Preschool and primary grade children will enjoy drawing and coloring while getting an antismoking message.

8602 No Smoking: Lungs At Work
American Lung Association
1740 Broadway
New York, NY 10019-4315
212-315-8700
Describes how lungs work and how they are affected by smoking.

8603 Now What Do I Do for Fun?
Hazelden
15251 Pleasant Valley Rd
Center City, MN 55012-9640
651-213-4200
800-257-7810
Fax: 651-213-4793
info@hazelden.org
www.hazelden.org
Explores the dilemma of finding new interests in recovery after completing treatment.
Mark Mishek, President and Chief Executive Officer
Joe Jaksha, Publisher

8604 Older Adults After Treatment
Hazelden
15251 Pleasant Valley Rd
Center City, MN 55012-9640
651-213-4200
800-257-7810
Fax: 651-213-4793
info@hazelden.org
www.hazelden.org
Discusses aftercare issues, such as family relations, health, medication and relapse.
Mark Mishek, President and Chief Executive Officer
Joe Jaksha, Publisher

8605 Older Adults in Treatment
Hazelden
15251 Pleasant Valley Rd
Center City, MN 55012-9640
651-213-4200
800-257-7810
Fax: 651-213-4793
info@hazelden.org
www.hazelden.org
Examines past beliefs about addiction and defines chemical dependency as a disease.
Mark Mishek, President and Chief Executive Officer
Joe Jaksha, Publisher

8606 On the Air: A Guide to Creating A Smoke-Free Workplace
American Lung Association

1740 Broadway
New York, NY 10019-4315 212-315-8700

A step-by-step guide for organizations interested in developing and implementing a successful workplace smoking control policy.
24 pages

8607 Parents Newcomer Packet
Al-Anon Family Group Headquarters
1600 Corp Landing Pkwy 757-563-1600
Virginia Beach, VA 23454-5617 800-425-2666
Fax: 757-563-1655
wso@al-anon.org
www.al-anon.alateen.org

For parents who realize their child is an alcoholic, this is a compassionate and reassuring welcome to Al-Anon.
9 pieces
Caryn Johnson, Director Communications

8608 Points for Parents Perplexed About Drugs
Hazelden
15251 Pleasant Valley Rd 651-213-4200
Center City, MN 55012-9640 800-257-7810
Fax: 651-213-4793
info@hazelden.org
www.hazelden.org

Clear guidelines to help adults recognize, evaluate and deal with adolescent drug abuse.
16 pages
Mark Mishek, President and Chief Executive Officer
Joe Jaksha, Publisher

8609 Preventing Relapse
Hazelden
15251 Pleasant Valley Rd 651-213-4200
Center City, MN 55012-9640 800-257-7810
Fax: 651-213-4793
info@hazelden.org
www.hazelden.org

Offers practical information and personal stories to help clients better understand the relapse process.
28 pages
Mark Mishek, President and Chief Executive Officer
Joe Jaksha, Publisher

8610 Program Booklet
Women for Sobriety
PO Box 618 215-536-8026
Quakertown, PA 18951-0618 Fax: 215-536-8026
www.womenforsobriety.org

Purse size booklet that explains the Thirteen Statements of Dr. Kirkpatrick's New Life program, statement by statement.

8611 Put on the Brakes Bulletin: Take a Look at College Drinking
National Clearinghouse for Alcohol and Drug Info.
1101 Wootton Parkway 800-729-6686
Rockville, MD 20852-2345 Fax: 240-453-8282
odphpinfo@hhs.gov
www.health.org

This second edition continues CSAP's campaign to raise awareness about the problems of college drinking.

8612 Q&A About Smoking and Health
American Lung Association
1740 Broadway 212-315-8700
New York, NY 10019-4315

Gives fact-crammed answers to questions on smoking and health.

8613 Quick List to Build Pride in Your Communities
National Clearinghouse for Alcohol and Drug Info.
PO Box 2345 800-729-6686
Rockville, MD 20847-2345 www.hoffmanestates.com

This parent guide is an adaptation of CSAP's Be Smart! Quick List: 10 Steps to Help Your Child Say No.

8614 Reducing the Health Risks of Secondhand Smoke
American Lung Association
1740 Broadway 212-315-8700
New York, NY 10019-4315

What a person can do at home, work and in public places to reduce the health risks of secondhand smoke.

8615 Relapse and the Addict
Hazelden
15251 Pleasant Valley Rd 651-213-4200
Center City, MN 55012-9640 800-257-7810
Fax: 651-213-4793
info@hazelden.org
www.hazelden.org

Identifies specific stages and triggers of relapse.
Mark Mishek, President and Chief Executive Officer
Joe Jaksha, Publisher

8616 Releasing Anger
Hazelden
15251 Pleasant Valley Rd 651-213-4200
Center City, MN 55012-9640 800-257-7810
Fax: 651-213-4793
info@hazelden.org
www.hazelden.org

Discusses anger as a normal feeling and how anger can endanger recovery.
Mark Mishek, President and Chief Executive Officer
Joe Jaksha, Publisher

8617 Research on Drugs and the Workplace
National Clearinghouse for Alcohol and Drug Info.
PO Box 2345 800-729-6686
Rockville, MD 20847-2345 www.hoffmanestates.com

Discusses prevalence and costs to society of drug use in the workplace, along with information on employee assistance programs, drug testing, grants and additional resources.

8618 Secondhand Smoke
American Lung Association
1740 Broadway 212-315-8700
New York, NY 10019-4315

Documents the effects of tobacco smoke on nonsmokers.

8619 Seven Reasons Not to Use Drugs and Alcohol
American Council On Drug Education
204 Monroe Street 800-488-3784
Rockville, MD 20850-4425 www.hoffmanestates.com

A series of five pamphlets offering information on the hazards of alcohol, crack, cocaine, steroids and tobacco products.
Grades 4-6

8620 Sexual Intimacy and the Alcoholic Relationship
Al-Anon Family Group Headquarters
1600 Corp Landing Pkwy 757-563-1600
Virginia Beach, VA 23454-5617 800-425-2666
Fax: 757-563-1655
wso@al-anon.org
www.al-anon.alateen.org

Sex and alcohol? Al-Anon members face this personal problem when they apply to the Al-Anon program indexed.
48 pages
Caryn Johnson, Director Communications

8621 Should Tobacco Advertising and Promotion Be Banned?
American Lung Association
1740 Broadway 212-315-8700
New York, NY 10019-4315

Answers many questions about tobacco advertising and promotion, and explains how ads are targeted to vulnerable populations.

8622 Smoke Free Family Promotional Leaflet
American Lung Association
1740 Broadway 212-315-8700
New York, NY 10019-4315

Leaflet and order form describe an entire range of ALA's smoking-related materials.

8623 Smokeless Tobacco: No Way
American Lung Association
1740 Broadway 212-315-8700
New York, NY 10019-4315

Written for junior and senior high school students, this booklet presents the facts about health risks of smokeless tobacco use.

8624 Smoking and Pregnancy
American Lung Association

1740 Broadway
New York, NY 10019-4315   212-315-8700

Written in a question/answer format, this pamphlet discusses many issues relating to smoking and pregnancy.

8625   Stop Smoking, Stay Trim
American Lung Association
1740 Broadway   212-315-8700
New York, NY 10019-4315

Outlines how to avoid gaining weight while quitting smoking.

8626   Stop Smoking: A Guide to Your Options
American Lung Association
1740 Broadway   212-315-8700
New York, NY 10019-4315

Describes a variety of approaches to smoking cessation. Offers guidance on how to choose a program.

8627   Straight Back Home
Hazelden
15251 Pleasant Valley Rd   651-213-4200
Center City, MN 55012-9640   800-257-7810
    Fax: 651-213-4793
    info@hazelden.org
    www.hazelden.org

Written for adolescents completing inpatient treatment and returning home.
Mark Mishek, President and Chief Executive Officer
Joe Jaksha, Publisher

8628   Stress in Recovery
Hazelden
15251 Pleasant Valley Rd   651-213-4200
Center City, MN 55012-9640   800-257-7810
    Fax: 651-213-4793
    info@hazelden.org
    www.hazelden.org

Outlines methods for clients to overcome stress in their daily lives.
Mark Mishek, President and Chief Executive Officer
Joe Jaksha, Publisher

8629   This Is AA
Alcoholics Anonymous
PO Box 459   212-870-3400
New York, NY 10163-0459   Fax: 212-870-3137
    www.aa.org

A pamphlet offering an introduction to the AA recovery program.

8630   Three Talks to Medical Societies
Alcoholics Anonymous
PO Box 459   212-870-3400
New York, NY 10163-0459   Fax: 212-870-3137
    www.aa.org

Contains Bill Wilson's, the co-founder of AA, principles borrowed from medicine and religion and a summary of AA's first 23 years.

8631   Time to Start Living
Alcoholics Anonymous
PO Box 459   212-870-3400
New York, NY 10163-0459   Fax: 212-870-3137
    www.aa.org

Addresses the older alcoholic, with nine stories of men and women who came to AA after the age of 60 (large print edition is also available).

8632   Too Many Young People Drink and Know Too Little About the Consequences
National Clearinghouse for Alcohol and Drug Info.
PO Box 2345   800-729-6686
Rockville, MD 20847-2345   www.hoffmanestates.com

Provides up-to-date resources and statistics on the widespread use of alcohol by youth under 21 years of age.

8633   Too Young?
Alcoholics Anonymous
PO Box 459   212-870-3400
New York, NY 10163-0459   Fax: 212-870-3137
    www.aa.org

This cartoon pamphlet speaks to teenagers in their own language, telling the varied drinking stories of six youn people (13 to 18).

8634   Treating Nicotine Addiction
Hazelden
15251 Pleasant Valley Rd   651-213-4200
Center City, MN 55012-9640   800-257-7810
    Fax: 651-213-4793
    info@hazelden.org
    www.hazelden.org

Describes the success of one chemical dependency treatment center that began treating nicotine as an addiction.
Mark Mishek, President and Chief Executive Officer
Joe Jaksha, Publisher

8635   Twelve Steps Illustrated
Alcoholics Anonymous
PO Box 459   212-870-3400
New York, NY 10163-0459   Fax: 212-870-3137
    www.aa.org

An easy-to-read version of AA's twelve steps.

8636   Twelve Steps for Tobacco Users
Hazelden
15251 Pleasant Valley Rd   651-213-4200
Center City, MN 55012-9640   800-257-7810
    Fax: 651-213-4793
    info@hazelden.org
    www.hazelden.org

Presents the Surgeon General's findings that classify nicotine as an addictive substance.
25 pages
Mark Mishek, President and Chief Executive Officer
Joe Jaksha, Publisher

8637   Understanding Depression and Addiction
Hazelden
15251 Pleasant Valley Rd   651-213-4200
Center City, MN 55012-9640   800-257-7810
    Fax: 651-213-4793
    info@hazelden.org
    www.hazelden.org

Hazelden, a part of the Hazelden Betty Ford Foundation, has been saving lives and restoring families from substance abuse and addiction for more than 60 years
29 pages
Mark Mishek, President and Chief Executive Officer
Joe Jaksha, Publisher

8638   Understanding Major Anxiety Disorders and Addiction
Hazelden
15251 Pleasant Valley Rd   651-213-4200
Center City, MN 55012-9640   800-257-7810
    Fax: 651-213-4793
    info@hazelden.org
    www.hazelden.org

Hazelden, a part of the Hazelden Betty Ford Foundation, has been saving lives and restoring families from substance abuse and addiction for more than 60 years
36 pages
Mark Mishek, President and Chief Executive Officer
Joe Jaksha, Publisher

8639   Understanding Ourselves and Alcoholism
Al-Anon Family Group Headquarters
1600 Corp Landing Pkwy   757-563-1600
Virginia Beach, VA 23454-5617   800-425-2666
    Fax: 757-563-1655
    wso@al-anon.org
    www.al-anon.alateen.org

Explains how compulsion, obsession and denial affect those close to an alcoholic as well as the alcoholic.
6 pages
Caryn Johnson, Director Communications

8640   Understanding Personality Problems and Addiction
Hazelden
15251 Pleasant Valley Rd   651-213-4200
Center City, MN 55012-9640   800-257-7810
    Fax: 651-213-4793
    info@hazelden.org
    www.hazelden.org

Describes common features of personality problems, such as self-centeredness and setting boundaries.
28 pages
Mark Mishek, President and Chief Executive Officer
Joe Jaksha, Publisher

8641 Understanding Post-Traumatic Stress Disorder and Addiction
Hazelden
15251 Pleasant Valley Rd   651-213-4200
Center City, MN 55012-9640   800-257-7810
                                         Fax: 651-213-4793
                                         info@hazelden.org
                                         www.hazelden.org
Hazelden, a part of the Hazelden Betty Ford Foundation, has been saving lives and restoring families from substance abuse and addiction for more than 60 years
17 pages
Mark Mishek, President and Chief Executive Officer
Joe Jaksha, Publisher

8642 Unpuffables Promotional Brochure
American Lung Association
1740 Broadway   212-315-8700
New York, NY 10019-4315
Describes the ALA Unpuffables program.

8643 What Are the Signs of Alcoholism?
Hazelden
15251 Pleasant Valley Rd   651-213-4200
Center City, MN 55012-9640   800-257-7810
                                         Fax: 651-213-4793
                                         info@hazelden.org
                                         www.hazelden.org
Self-test for clients to review the role of alcohol in their lives.
Mark Mishek, President and Chief Executive Officer
Joe Jaksha, Publisher

8644 What Happened to Joe?
Alcoholics Anonymous
PO Box 459   212-870-3400
New York, NY 10163-0459   Fax: 212-870-3137
                                         www.aa.org
Dramatic story of a young construction worker and his drinking problem, told in brightly colored comic book style.

8645 What Happens After Treatment?
Al-Anon Family Group Headquarters
1600 Corp Landing Pkwy   757-563-1600
Virginia Beach, VA 23454-5617   800-425-2666
                                         Fax: 757-563-1655
                                         wso@al-anon.org
                                         www.al-anon.alateen.org
Al-Anon is a mutual support group of peers who share their experience in applying the Al-Anon principles to problems related to the effects of a problem drinker in their lives. It is not group therapy and is not led by a counselor or therapist
100 pieces
Caryn Johnson, Director Communications

8646 What is AA?
Hazelden
15251 Pleasant Valley Rd   651-213-4200
Center City, MN 55012-9640   800-257-7810
                                         Fax: 651-213-4793
                                         info@hazelden.org
                                         www.hazelden.org
Answers the basic questions about Alcoholics Anonymous.
Mark Mishek, President and Chief Executive Officer
Joe Jaksha, Publisher

8647 What is NA?
Hazelden
15251 Pleasant Valley Rd   651-213-4200
Center City, MN 55012-9640   800-257-7810
                                         Fax: 651-213-4793
                                         info@hazelden.org
                                         www.hazelden.org

Helps clients evaluate their addiction to narcotics and answers their questions about N.A.
Mark Mishek, President and Chief Executive Officer
Joe Jaksha, Publisher

8648 What's Your Cigarette Smoking IQ?
American Lung Association
1740 Broadway   212-315-8700
New York, NY 10019-4315
Brief true-or-false quiz that tests a person's knowledge of the effects of smoking.

8649 When You Go Back to Work
Hazelden
15251 Pleasant Valley Rd   651-213-4200
Center City, MN 55012-9640   800-257-7810
                                         Fax: 651-213-4793
                                         info@hazelden.org
                                         www.hazelden.org
Stories demonstrating co-workers' attitudes clients may face upon their return to work.
Mark Mishek, President and Chief Executive Officer
Joe Jaksha, Publisher

8650 When Your Teen is in Treatment
Hazelden
15251 Pleasant Valley Rd   651-213-4200
Center City, MN 55012-9640   800-257-7810
                                         Fax: 651-213-4793
                                         info@hazelden.org
                                         www.hazelden.org
A guide for parents.
Mark Mishek, President and Chief Executive Officer
Joe Jaksha, Publisher

8651 Where Do I Go from Here?
Alcoholics Anonymous
PO Box 459   212-870-3400
New York, NY 10163-0459   Fax: 212-870-3137
                                         www.aa.org
For people leaving treatment facilities, single-sheet flyer tells of continuing help offered by outside AAs.

8652 Why Anonymity in Al-Anon?
Al-Anon Family Group Headquarters
1600 Corp Landing Pkwy   757-563-1600
Virginia Beach, VA 23454-5617   800-425-2666
                                         Fax: 757-563-1655
                                         wso@al-anon.org
                                         www.al-anon.alateen.org
Al-Anon is a mutual support group of peers who share their experience in applying the Al-Anon principles to problems related to the effects of a problem drinker in their lives. It is not group therapy and is not led by a counselor or therapist
12 pages
Caryn Johnson, Director Communications

8653 Workers at Risk: Drugs and Alcohol on the Job
National Clearinghouse for Alcohol and Drug Info.
PO Box 2345   800-729-6686
Rockville, MD 20847-2345   www.hoffmanestates.com
Gives facts about drugs in the workplace and suggests appropriate behavior for employees who are confronted with a coworker's use of alcohol or other drugs.

8654 You Can Help Your Community Get Rid of Drugs
National Clearinghouse for Alcohol and Drug Info.
PO Box 2345   800-729-6686
Rockville, MD 20847-2345   www.hoffmanestates.com
Supports drug abuse treatment and explains how drug use can create problems for your community.

8655 Young Children and Drugs: What Parents Can Do
Wisconsin Clearinghouse
1954 E Washington Avenue   www.hoffmanestates.com
Madison, WI 53704-5275
100 Brochures

8656 Youth and the Alcoholic Parent
Al-Anon Family Group Headquarters

1600 Corp Landing Pkwy
Virginia Beach, VA 23454-5617
757-563-1600
800-425-2666
Fax: 757-563-1655
wso@al-anon.org
www.al-anon.alateen.org

Questions and suggestions to help young people improve their own lives.
12 pages
Caryn Johnson, Director Communications

Audio & Video

8657 AA: Rap with Us
Alcoholics Anonymous
PO Box 459
New York, NY 10163-0459
212-870-3400
Fax: 212-870-3137
www.aa.org

Features four anonymous young AA members. Rap music and lyrics bridge these four young people's stories of alcoholic despair and A.A. recovery.
16 minutes

8658 Al-Anon Video
Al-Anon Family Group Headquarters
1600 Corp Landing Pkwy
Virginia Beach, VA 23454-5617
757-563-1600
800-425-2666
Fax: 757-563-1655
wso@al-anon.org
www.al-anon.org

Al-Anon is a mutual support group of peers who share their experience in applying the Al-Anon principles to problems related to the effects of a problem drinker in their lives. It is not group therapy and is not led by a counselor or therapist
12 pages
Caryn Johnson, Director Communications

8659 Al-Anon is for African Americans...and All People of Color
Al-Anon Family Group Headquarters
1600 Corp Landing Pkwy
Virginia Beach, VA 23454-5617
757-563-1600
800-425-2666
Fax: 757-563-1655
wso@al-anon.org
www.al-anon.alateen.org

Al-Anon is a mutual support group of peers who share their experience in applying the Al-Anon principles to problems related to the effects of a problem drinker in their lives. It is not group therapy and is not led by a counselor or therapist
12 pages
Caryn Johnson, Director Communications

8660 Al-Anon's Path to Recovery: Al-Anon is for Americans/Aboriginals
Al-Anon Family Group Headquarters
1600 Corp Landing Pkwy
Virginia Beach, VA 23454-5617
757-563-1600
800-425-2666
Fax: 757-563-1655
wso@al-anon.org
www.al-anon.alateen.org

Al-Anon is a mutual support group of peers who share their experience in applying the Al-Anon principles to problems related to the effects of a problem drinker in their lives. It is not group therapy and is not led by a counselor or therapist
12 pages
Caryn Johnson, Director Communications

8661 Alcoholics Anonymous: An Inside View
Alcoholics Anonymous
PO Box 459
New York, NY 10163-0459
212-870-3400
Fax: 212-870-3137
www.aa.org

Depicts alcoholics, recovering in A.A., going about their daily lives, attending A.A. meetings, and other gatherings.
28 minutes

8662 Art of Living with Change: Turning Your Good Intentions Into Progress...
Hazelden

15251 Pleasant Valley Rd
Center City, MN 55012-9640
651-213-4200
800-257-7810
Fax: 651-213-4793
info@hazelden.org
www.hazelden.org

Hazelden, a part of the Hazelden Betty Ford Foundation, has been saving lives and restoring families from substance abuse and addiction for more than 60 years
45 minutes
ISBN: 0-894868-40-3
Mark Mishek, President and Chief Executive Officer
Joe Jaksha, Publisher

8663 Bill Discusses the Twelve Traditions
Alcoholics Anonymous
PO Box 459
New York, NY 10163-0459
212-870-3400
Fax: 212-870-3137
www.aa.org

Bill W. tells how the principles safe-guarding A.A. unity developed.
60 minutes

8664 Bill's Own Story
Alcoholics Anonymous
PO Box 459
New York, NY 10163-0459
212-870-3400
Fax: 212-870-3137
www.aa.org

Co-founder Bill W. tells of his drinking and recovery.
60 minutes

8665 Caring for Ourselves: Hope for Healthy Relationships
Hazelden
15251 Pleasant Valley Rd
Center City, MN 55012-9640
651-213-4200
800-257-7810
Fax: 651-213-4793
info@hazelden.org
www.hazelden.org

Hazelden, a part of the Hazelden Betty Ford Foundation, has been saving lives and restoring families from substance abuse and addiction for more than 60 years
50 minutes
ISBN: 0-894866-38-9
Mark Mishek, President and Chief Executive Officer
Joe Jaksha, Publisher

8666 Hope: Alcoholics Anonymous
Alcoholics Anonymous
PO Box 459
New York, NY 10163-0459
212-870-3400
Fax: 212-870-3137
www.aa.org

Explains the principles of AA: what it is, steps, traditions, sponsorship, and basic recovery tools.
15 minutes

8667 It Sure Beats Sitting in a Cell
Alcoholics Anonymous
PO Box 459
New York, NY 10163-0459
212-870-3400
Fax: 212-870-3137
www.aa.org

Filmed inside correctional facilities in the United States and Canada, this film tells the story of four young AA's who were in prison as a result of drinking, yet today are sober.
17 minutes

8668 Markings on the Journey
Alcoholics Anonymous
PO Box 459
New York, NY 10163-0459
212-870-3400
Fax: 212-870-3137
www.aa.org

Videocassette depicts 45 years of AA history, using rare materials from our archives.
35 minutes

8669 Men's Work: How to Stop the Violence that Tears Our Lives Apart
Hazelden

15251 Pleasant Valley Rd
Center City, MN 55012-9640

651-213-4200
800-257-7810
Fax: 651-213-4793
info@hazelden.org
www.hazelden.org

Hazelden, a part of the Hazelden Betty Ford Foundation, has been saving lives and restoring families from substance abuse and addiction for more than 60 years
50 minutes
ISBN: 0-894868-28-4
Mark Mishek, President and Chief Executive Officer
Joe Jaksha, Publisher

8670 Secret to a Satisfied Life: The Way You Encounter Life Can Bring Happiness...
Hazelden
15251 Pleasant Valley Rd
Center City, MN 55012-9640

651-213-4200
800-257-7810
Fax: 651-213-4793
info@hazelden.org
www.hazelden.org

Hazelden, a part of the Hazelden Betty Ford Foundation, has been saving lives and restoring families from substance abuse and addiction for more than 60 years
45 minutes
ISBN: 0-894868-17-9
Mark Mishek, President and Chief Executive Officer
Joe Jaksha, Publisher

8671 Women: Coming Out of the Shadows
Elyse A Williams, author
Fanlight Productions
32 Court Street
Brooklyn, NY 11201-1731

718-488-8900
718-488-8642
Fax: 718-488-8642
info@fanlight.com
www.fanlight.com

Fanlight Productions is a leading distributor of innovative film and video works on the social issues of our time
1991 27 Minutes
ISBN: 1-572950-84-6

8672 Young People and AA
Alcoholics Anonymous
PO Box 459
New York, NY 10163-0459

212-870-3400
Fax: 212-870-3137
www.aa.org

Four young AA members describe what it is like drinking, what happened to bring them to AA, and what their lives are like sober today.
28 minutes

Web Sites

8673 AAA Foundation for Traffic Safety
www.aaafoundation.org
The AAA Foundation for Traffic Safety was founded in 1947 by AAA to conduct research to address growing highway safety issues. The organization's mission is to identify traffic safety problems, foster research that seeks solutions and disseminate information and educational materials.

8674 Al-Anon
www.al-anon.alateen.org
The single purpose of this organization is to help families and friends of alcoholics, whether the alcoholic is still drinking or not.

8675 Alateen
www.al-anon.org/for-alateen
A part of the Al-Anon program, Alateen is for teenagers who have been affected by someone else's drinking, whether it be a family member or a friend.

8676 American Council for Drug Education
www.acde.org/
This organization provides information on drug use, publishes books and offers films and curriculum materials for prevention.

8677 CSAP State Liason Program
www.samhsa.gov
This program is designed to support alcohol and other drug abuse prevention efforts in the States.

8678 Center for Substance Abuse Prevention
www.samhsa.gov
The mission of the Center for Substance Abuse Prevention is to improve behavioral health through evidence-based prevention approaches.

8679 Cocaine Anonymous
www.ca.org
A support group based on the twelve steps of Alcoholics Anonymous that focuses specifically on problems of cocaine addiction.

8680 Dentists Concerned for Dentists
A nonprofit organization for chemically dependent Minnesota dentists and concerned others.

8681 Families Anonymous
www.familiesanonymous.org/
Addresses the needs of families who are concerned about a relative with a drug problem and with related behavioral problems.

8682 Hazelden
www.hazelden.com
Organization dedicated to providing quality rehabilitation, education and professional services for chemical dependency and related addictive behaviors.

8683 Healing Well
www.healingwell.com
An online health resource guide to medical news, chat, information and articles, newsgroups and message boards, books, disease-related web sites, medical directories, and more for patients, friends, and family coping with disabling diseases, disorders, or chronic illnesses.

8684 Health Finder
www.healthfinder.gov
Searchable, carefully developed web site offering information on over 1000 topics. Developed by the US Department of Health and Human Services, the site can be used in both English and Spanish.

8685 Healthlink USA
www.healthlinkusa.com
Health information concerning treatment, cures, prevention, diagnosis, risk factors, research, support groups, email lists, personal stories and much more. Updated regularly.

8686 Indian Health Service
www.ihs.gov
Charged with providing a comprehensive program of alcoholism and substance abuse prevention and treatment for Native Americans and Alaskan natives.

8687 Lawyers Concerned for Lawyers
www.mnlcl.org/
Lawyers Concerned for Lawyers provides free, confidential peer and professional assistance to Minnesota lawyers, judges, law students, and their immediate family members on any issue that causes stress or distress.

8688 MedicineNet
www.medicinenet.com
An online resource for consumers providing easy-to-read, authoritative medical and health information.

8689 Medscape
www.medscape.com
Medscape offers specialists, primary care physicians, and other health professionals the Web's most robust and integrated medical information and educational tools.

8690 National Clearinghouse for Alcohol and Drug Information

8691 National Council on Alcoholism and Drug Dependence
www.ncadd.org
Provides education, information, help and hope in the fight against addictions. Nationwide network of affiliates, advocates preven-

tion, intervention and treatment, and is committed to ridding the disease of its stigma and its sufferers of their denial and shame.

8692   National Crime Prevention Council

www.ncpc.org

This organization works to prevent crime and drug use in many ways, including developing materials for parents and children.

8693   Office on Smoking and Health

www.cdc.gov/tobacco/

Offers reference services to researchers through the Technical Information Center. Publishes and distributes a number of titles in the field of smoking and health.

8694   Safe Homes

This national organization encourages parents to sign a contract stipulating that when parties are held in one another's homes they will adhere to a strict no-alcohol/no-drug-use rule.

8695   Substance Abuse and Mental Health Services Administration

www.samhsa.gov

The goal of this organization is to reduce incidence and prevalence of mental disorders and substance abuse and improve treatment outcomes for persons suffering from addictive and mental health problems and disorders.

8696   WebMD

www.webmd.com

Provides credible information, supportive communities, and in-depth reference material about health subjects. A source for original and timely health information as well as material from well known content providers.

Description

8697 Sudden Infant Death Syndrome

Sudden Infant Death Syndrome, SIDS, is the sudden death of an infant or young child that is unexpected and for which there is no demonstrable cause. It is the most common cause of death in children between 1 and 12 months of age, with a peak incidence between the second and fourth month of life. Almost all SIDS deaths occur when the infant is thought to be sleeping.

Despite extensive research, no cause for SIDS has been found, although evidence suggests that it may be related to malfunction of the mechanisms that control the heart function and breathing process. The diagnosis cannot be made without an adequate investigation of the infant after its death. The incidence of SIDS is 1 in 2,000, and is greater in premature babies, babies born to mothers who are young, unwed, smoke, have had many births, did not complete high school, and have had poor prenatal care. Other possible factors include exposure to cigarette smoke, cold months, soft bedding (lamb's wool), waterbed mattresses, an overheated environment, upper respiratory infections, and being a sibling of a SIDS victim.

Recent studies have indicated that having babies sleep on their backs reduces the risks of SIDS. The American Academy of Pediatrics recommends that infants be placed on their back for sleep. It further advises to avoid overwrapping the infant, remove soft bedding, and avoid smoking during and after pregnancy. In 1994, the Back to Sleep Campaign was launched, a national campaign that encourages that infants be placed to sleep on their backs. Between 1992 and 1996, the rate of SIDS dropped 38 percent and has continued to decrease since then.

Parents who lose a child to SIDS are grief-stricken and, because no definitive cause can be found for their seemingly healthy baby's death, usually have excessive guilt feelings. Bereavement support is necessary not only during the days immediately following the infant's death, but also for at least several months.

National Agencies & Associations

8698 American SIDS Institute
528 Raven Way
Naples, FL 34110
239-431-5425
800-232-7437
Fax: 239-431-5536
prevent@sids.org
www.sids.org
Dedicated to the prevention of sudden infant death and promotes infant health through research, clinical services, education, and family support.
Carl E. Hunt, MD, Chairman
Betty McEntire, PhD, Executive Director & CEO

8699 Compassionate Friends
1000 Jorie Boulevard, Suite 140
Oak Brook, IL 60523
630-990-0010
877-969-0010
Fax: 630-990-0246
nationaloffice@compassionatefriends.org
www.compassionatefriends.org

A national organization that offers over 600 local chapters that give support to parents and siblings who have experienced the death of a child. Offers monthly support meetings to learn how to cope.
Allie Sims-Franklin, President
Debbie Dullabaun, Vice President

8700 First Candle
49 Locust Avenue
New Canaan, CT 06840
203-966-1300
800-221-7437
info@firstcandle.org
www.sidsalliance.org
Promotes preventive measures to reduce the occurrence of Sudden Infant Death Syndrome (SIDS), and offers support to families grieving from the loss of an infant.
David Cunningham, Chair
Kelly Neal Mariotti, Treasurer

8701 National Center for Education in Maternal and Child Health
Box 571272
Washington, DC 20057-1272
www.ncemch.org
Leads the maternal and child health community by applying research to education and developmental programs with the goal of improving the well-being of families.
Rochelle Mayer, Ed D, Executive Director
John Richards, MA, AITP, Director

8702 National Institute of Child Health and Human Development
PO Box 3006
Rockville, MD 20847
800-370-2943
Fax: 866-760-5947
TTY: 888-320-6942
www.nichd.nih.gov
NICHD seeks to better understand disabilities and important events that occur during pregnancy.
Diana W. Bianchi, MD, Director
Constantine Stratakis, Scientific Director

8703 National Organization for Rare Disorders
55 Kenosia Avenue
Danbury, CT 06810-1968
203-744-0100
800-999-6673
Fax: 203-263-9938
www.rarediseases.org
NORD is a federation of voluntary health organizations dedicated to helping people with rare orphan diseases and assisting the organizations that serve them. It is committed to the identification, treatment, and cure of rare disorders through programs of education, advocacy, research, and service.
Peter Saltonstall, President & CEO
Pamela Gavin, Chief Strategy Officer

8704 Share Pregnancy and Infant Loss Support, Inc.
402 Jackson Street
Saint Charles, MO 63301-3468
636-947-6164
800-821-6819
Fax: 636-947-7486
dcochran@nationalshare.org
www.nationalshare.org
Offers support, resources, and education on miscarriage, stillborn and newborn death.
Debra L. Cochran, Executive Director

8705 Sudden Infant Death Syndrome (SIDS) Network
PO Box 267
Ledyard, CT 06339
Fax: 860-887-7309
sidsnet1@sids-network.org
www.sids-network.org
Dedicated to eliminate Sudden Infant Death Syndrome (SIDS) through the support of research on SIDS. Provides support for those grieving and raises public awareness of SIDS.
Chuck Mihalko, Co-founder & President

State Agencies & Associations

Alabama

8706 Bureau of Family Health Services: Alabama Department of Public Health
19 South Jackson Street

201 Monroe Street
Montgomery, AL 36104
334-206-5300
800-252-1818
Fax: 334-269-5200
llee@aap.net
www.adph.org

Linda P Lee, Executive Director

Alaska

8707 SIDS Information and Counseling Program: Alaska Department of Health
350 Main Street, Room 404
Juneau, AK 99811-3553
907-465-3030
Fax: 907-465-3068
william.hogan@alaska.gov
www.dhss.alaska.gov

Alaska Pioneer Homes assist older Alaskans to have the highest quality of life by providing assisted living in a safe home setting which promotes positive relationships, meaningful activities, physical, emotional and spiritual growth.
William J Streur, Commissioner
Jay Butler, Chief Medical Officer

Arizona

8708 Arizona SIDS Founation
PO Box 1111
Phoenix, AZ 85001
520-297-6013
800-597-7437

Vanessa Seaney, President

8709 Office of Womens And Childrens Health: Alabama Department of Health
State Dapartment of Healths Services
150 N 18th Avenue
Phoenix, AZ 85007-2602
602-542-1025
Fax: 602-542-0883
newbers@azdhs.gov
www.azdhs.gov

The Arizona Department of Health Services promotes and protects the health of Arizona's children and adults. Its mission is to set the standard for personal and community health through direct care, science, public policy, and leadership.
Susan Newber RN, Manager

Arkansas

8710 Arkansas Department of Health: SIDS Information & Counseling Program
4815 W Markham Street
Little Rock, AR 72205-3866
501-661-2000
www.healthyarkansas.com

To protect and improve the health and well-being of all Arkansans
Nathaniel Smith, MD, MPH
Dawn Graziani

California

8711 California SIDS Program
11344 Coloma Road
Gold River, CA 95670-6052
916-851-7437
800-369-7437
Fax: 916-851-5937
www.californiasids.com

IT is designed to serve the many individuals affected by a SIDS death, and to educate the public about SIDS.
Gwen Edelstein RN,PNP,MPA, Program Director
Cheryl McBride, Program Manager

8712 SIDS Alliance Of Northern California
1547 Palos Verdes Mall
Walnut Creek, CA 94597
925-274-1109
877-938-7437

A non-profit, completely volunteer group of SIDS parents and professionals dedicated to family support and community education regarding SIDS.
Lorie Gehrke, President

8713 SIDS Foundation of Southern California
10811 Washington Boulevard
Culver City, CA 90232
310-558-4511
Fax: 310-558-7075
sidsfsc@aol.com
sidsfoundationofsoutherncalifornia.org

Margot Stern Bennett, Executive Director

Colorado

8714 Colorado SIDS Program
425 S Cherry Street
Denver, CO 80224
303-320-7771
888-285-7437
Fax: 303-320-7827

Tena Saltzman, Executive Director

8715 Colordao Department of Health and Environment
4300 Cherry Creek Drive S
Denver, CO 80246-1530
303-692-2000
800-886-7689
Fax: 303-782-5576
TTY: 303-691-7700
cdphe.information@state.co.us
www.cdphe.state.co.us

Martha Rudolph, Director
Karin McGowan, Interim Executive Director

Connecticut

8716 Connecticut SIDS Alliance
PO Box 486
Torrington, CT 06790
860-626-1542
866-574-7437
Fax: 860-496-9919
ctsids@aol.com

Shannon Strandberg, Secretary

8717 SIDS Program: Connecticut Department of Health
410 Capitol Avenue
Hartford, CT 06134
860-509-8074
Fax: 860-509-7720

Marilyn Binns, Program Coordinator

Delaware

8718 SIDS Information & Counseling: Division of Public Health
1901 N DuPont Highway
New Castle, DE 19720
302-255-9040
Fax: 302-255-4429
www.dhss.delaware.gov

To improve the quality of life for Delaware's citizens by promoting health and well-being, fostering self-sufficiency, and protecting vulnerable populations.
Elaine Marke LCSW BCD, Program Coordinator

District of Columbia

8719 DC Department of Health Maternal and Family Health Administration
Maternal And Family Health Administration
899 North Capitol Street NE
Washington, DC 20002
202-442-5955
Fax: 202-442-4795
TTY: 711
doh@dc.gov
www.dchealth.dc.gov

The Mission of the Department of Health is to promote and protect the health, safety and quality of life of residents, visitors and those doing business in the District of Columbia.
Saul M. Levin, M.D., M.P.A., Interim Director
Rosie McLaren, Program Manager

8720 Department of Health and Human Services
200 Independence Avenue SW
Washington, DC 20201
919-715-8430
877-696-6775
www.hhs.gov

The Department of Health and Human Services (HHS) is the United States government's principal agency for protecting the health of all Americans and providing essential human services, especially for those who are least able to help themselves.
April Ellis, SIDS Program Manager

8721 Region III Office Program: Consultants for Maternal and Child Health
Public Ledger Building
2115 Wisconsin Avenue NW
Washington, DC 20007-3309
202-784-9771
Fax: 202-784-9777
OHRCinfo@georgetown.edu
www.mchoralhealth.org

The purpose of the National Maternal and Child Oral Health Resource Center (OHRC) is to respond to the needs of states and communities in addressing current and emerging public oral health issues. OHRC supports health professionals, program administra-

tors, educators, policymakers, and others with the goal of improving oral health services for infants, children, adolescents, and their families.
Jolene Bertness, Health Education Specialist
Katrina Holt, Director

8722 Region IV Office Program Consultants for Maternal and Child Health
2115 Wisconsin Avenue
Washington, DC 20007-8909
202-784-9771
Fax: 202-784-9777
OHRCinfo@georgetown.edu
www.mchoralhealth.org
The purpose of the National Maternal and Child Oral Health Resource Center (OHRC) is to respond to the needs of states and communities in addressing current and emerging public oral health issues.
E Joseph Alderman DDS MPH, Oral Health Consultant

8723 Region IX Office Program Consultants for Maternal and Child Health
2115 Wisconsin
Washington, DC 94103
202-784-9771
Fax: 202-784-9777
OHRCinfo@georgetown.edu
www.mchoralhealth.org
Katrina Holt, Director

8724 Region VIII Office Program Consultants for Maternal and Child Health
2115 Wisconsin Avenue
Washington, DC 80294-1961
202-784-9771
Fax: 202-784-9777
OHRCinfo@georgetown.edu
www.mchoralhealth.org
The purpose of the National Maternal and Child Oral Health Resource Center (OHRC) is to respond to the needs of states and communities in addressing current and emerging public oral health issues
Valerie Orla RDH BS, Oral Health Consultant

Florida

8725 Children's Medical Services Program: Florida SIDS Program
4052 Bald Cypress Way
Tallahassee, FL 32399
850-245-4444
Fax: 904-488-2341
Health@doh.state.fl.us
www.doh.state.fl.us
To protect, promote & improve the health of all people in Florida through integrated state, county, & community efforts.
Susan Potts, Coordinator

8726 Florida Department of Health
4052 Bald Cypress Way
Tallahassee, FL 32399
850-245-4444
Fax: 850-245-4047
www.floridahealth.gov
To protect, promote & improve the health of all people in Florida through integrated state, county, & community efforts.
Michelle Tallent, Deputy Secretary, Operations

8727 Florida SIDS Alliance
4044 W Lake Mary Boulevard
Lake Mary, FL 32746
305-232-1640
800-SID-SFLA
Fax: 407-444-5208
sidsfla@yahoo.com
Steve Bonwit, Officer
Roy Bagley, President

Georgia

8728 Georgia Department of Public Health: Center for Family Resource Planning
2 Peachtree Street NW
Atlanta, GA 30303
404-657-3550
Fax: 404-463-6729
dph.georgia.gov
Provides grief support for parents.
Kathleen E. Toomey, MD, MPH, Commissioner

8729 Georgia Department of Public Health: Infant and Child Health
2 Peachtree Street NW
Atlanta, GA 30303
404-651-7371
Fax: 404-463-6729
Kathleen E. Toomey, MD, MPH, Commissioner

8730 Georgia SIDS Project
4112-2 E Ponce De Leon Avenue
Clarkston, GA 30021
678-342-3360
Fax: 404-296-7211
gasids@mindspring.com
Sudden Infant Death Syndrome is the sudden death of an infant under one year of age which remains unexplained after a thorough case investigation.
Diane Manheim, Director

Hawaii

8731 Hawaii Department of Health: Family Health Division
Child Wellness Program
1250 Punchbowl Street
Honolulu, HI 96813
808-586-4400
Fax: 808-733-9032
Gwen Palmer, Coordinator

Idaho

8732 Idaho Department of Health and Welfare
590 W Washington Street
Boise, ID 83720
208-334-4000
800-632-8000
Fax: 208-334-4015
www.healthandwelfare.idaho.gov
Offers programs that deal with complex social, economic and individual issues, often helping people in crisis situations. Programs are designed to strengthen families and promote self-reliance.

Illinois

8733 SIDS of Illinois
6010 Route 53
Lisle, IL 60532
630-541-3901
Fax: 630-541-8246
www.sidsillinois.org
Marsha Cooper, President
Anita L. Jordan Johnson, Vice President

8734 Statewide SIDS Program: Illinois Department of Public Health
500 E Monroe Street
Springfield, IL 62761
217-557-2931
Fax: 217-524-2831
Babara Breidenbaugh, Program Specialist

Indiana

8735 Indiana State Department of Health Maternal And Child Health Services
Maternal And Child Health Services
2 N Meridian Street
Indianapolis, IN 46204
317-233-1325
800-457-8283
Fax: 317-233-1300
www.in.gov/hpb
Beth Johnson, Nurse Consultant

8736 SIDS Center of Indiana
1810 Broad Ripple Avenue
Indianapolis, IN 46220
317-254-9255
Fax: 317-254-9266
Our mission is to be a resource center that supports parents, families and friends in communities across the state whose lives are touched by sudden, unexpected infant death.
John Schutt, Chairperson

Iowa

8737 Iowa SIDS Alliance
406 SW School Street
Ankeny, IA 50023
515-965-7655
866-480-4741
Fax: 515-964-7506
info@iowasids.org
www.iowasids.org
The Iowa Sudden Infant Death Syndrome Foundation is a statewide, non-profit, voluntary health organization dedicated to providing emotional support to SIDS and SUID families residing in Iowa, educating professionals and the general public about SIDS and risk reduction, and funding medical research into the causes of SIDS.
Patty Keeley, Executive Director
Jennifer Atzen, President

8738 Iowa SIDS Program Iowa Department of Public Health
Iowa Department of Public Health

321 E 12th Street
Des Moines, IA 50319-0075   515-281-7689
    866-227-9878
Promoting and protecting the health of Iowans
Jane Borst, Bureau Chief
Sally Clausen

Kansas

8739 Kansas Department of Health & Environment: Bureau of Family Health
Bureau Of Children, Youth And Families
1000 SW Jackson Street   786-296-1500
Topeka, KS 66612-1274   800-332-6262
    Fax: 785-296-6553
    kdhe.info@ks.gov
    www.kdheks.gov
To protect and improve the health and environment of all Kansans.
Laura Kelly, Governor
Lee A. Norman, MD, Secretary

8740 SIDS Network of Kansas
1148 S Hillside   316-682-1301
Wichita, KS 67211   866-399-7437
    Fax: 316-682-1274
    www.kidsks.org

Christy Schunn, LSCSW, Executive Director
Amanda Yoder, Communications Assistant

Kentucky

8741 Department of Public Health: Adult and Child Health Division
275 E Main Street   502-564-3236
Frankfort, KY 40621   800-372-2973
    Fax: 502-564-8389
    TTY: 800-627-4702

Marcia Burkow, SIDS Coordinator

8742 SIDS Network of Kentucky
PO Box 186   800-928-7437
Caneyville, KY 42721-3555   Fax: 859-245-0717
Supporting family members and others who have been touched by the tragedy of a sids or other infants death.
Adrienne Grizzell, Executive Director

Louisiana

8743 Office of Public Health
628 N 4th Street   225-342-9500
Baton Rouge, LA 70802   Fax: 225-342-5568
    hhwebadmin@la.gov
    www.dhh.louisiana.gov/offices/?ID=79
Tracy Hubbard, Coordinator

8744 Public Health Services of Louisiana
628 N 4th Street   225-342-9500
Baton Rouge, LA 70802-0629   Fax: 225-342-5568
    dhhwebadmin@la.gov
    www.dhh.state.la.us/
The mission of the Department of Health and Hospitals is to protect and promote health and to ensure access to medical, preventive and rehabilitative services for all citizens of the State of Louisiana.
Jamie Roques RNC, SIDS Coordinator
Courtney Phillips, Deputy Secretary

Maine

8745 Department of Human Services
221 State Street   207-287-3707
Augusta, ME 04333-0001   Fax: 207-287-3005
    TTY: 800-606-0215
    www.state.me.us/dhs/
Brenda Harvey, Commissioner

8746 Maine SIDS Foundation
14 Charlonate Drive   207-657-2220
Gray, ME 04039   Fax: 207-657-3737
    roybagley@aol.com
    www.sidsalliance.org
Roy Bagley, Chairperson

8747 Maine SIDS Program Department Of Human Services
Department Of Human Services
200 Main Street   207-795-4450
Lewiston, ME 04240   Fax: 207-795-4445
Luanne Crinion, Program Coordinator

Maryland

8748 First Candle
2105 Laurel Bush Road   Fax: 651-310-2106
Bel Air, MD 21015   TTY: 800-221-7437
    info@firstcandle.org
    www.sidsalliance.org
First Candle is a leading national nonprofit organization dedicated to safe pregnancies and the survival of babies through the first years of life. Current priorities are to eliminate Stillbirth, Sudden Infant Death Syndrome (SIDS) and other Sudden Unexpected Infant Deaths (SUID) with programs of research, education and advocacy
Michael J. Schaffer, President
Kelly Neal Mariotti, Chief Executive Officer

8749 Maryland SIDS Information & Counseling Program
22 S Green Street   410-328-8667
Baltimore, MD 21201   800-492-5538
    TTY: 410-328-9600
    TDD: 410-328-9600
    webmaster@umm.edu
UMMC exists to serve the state and region as a tertiary/quaternary care center, to serve the local community with a full range of care options, to educate and train the next generation of health care providers, and to be a site for world-class clinical research.
Jeffrey A Rivest, President and Chief Executive Officer
R Keith Allen, Senior Vice President

Massachusetts

8750 Region I Office Program: Consultants for Maternal and Child Health
John F Kennedy Building   617-899-1355
Boston, MA 02203   Fax: 202-833-8288
    Mary.Foley@mcphs.edu
    www.mchoralhealth.org
Mary Foley RDH MPH, Oral Health Consultant

Michigan

8751 Apnea Identification Program Children's Hospital of Michigan
Children's Hospital of Michigan
3901 Beaubien Street   313-745-5437
Detroit, MI 48201-2196   888-DMC-2500
    www.childrensdmc.org
To provide the highest quality of care for children, to inform that care through research innovations, and to ensure that children have access to the care they need.
Karen Branif RN MSW, Nurse Specialist

8752 Genesee County Health Department
630 S Saignaw Street   810-257-3612
Flint, MI 48502-3915   Fax: 810-257-3147
    gchd-info@gchd.us
    www.gchd.us

Kay Doerr, Chairperson
Brenda Clack, Vice-Chairperson

8753 Kent County Health Department
300 Monroe Avenue NE   616-632-7590
Grand Rapids, MI 49503-1996   www.accesskent.com
The mission of Kent County government is to be an effective and efficient steward in delivering quality services for our diverse community. Our priority is to provide mandated services, which may be enhanced and supplemented by additional services to improve the quality of life for all our citizens within the constraints of sound fiscal policy.
Colleen Jill RN, SIDs Coordinator
David Kraker

8754 Michigan Department of Health & Human Services
3423 MLK Boulevard
Lansing, MI 48909
517-373-1820
Fax: 517-373-2129
lauberc@michigan.gov
www.michigan.gov
Cheryl Lauber, Coordinator

8755 Oakland County Health Division: SIDS Project
1200 N Telegraph
Pontiac, MI 48341-0482
248-858-1280
800-774-4542
Fax: 248-858-0178
TTY: 248-452-2247
TDD: 248-452-2247
www.oakgov.com
David Conklin, Librarian
George J Miller Jr MA, Director

8756 SIDS LEAD: Children's Special Health Care Services
Michigan Department of Public Health
201 Townsend Street
Lansing, MI 48913-2934
517-373-3740
TTY: 517-373-3573
TDD: 517-373-3573
norris@michigan.gov
www.michigan.gov/mdch
Improving the experience of care, improving the health of populations, and reducing per capita costs of health care
Janet Olszewski, Director
Ed Dore, Chief Deputy Director

Minnesota

8757 Minnesota Sudden Infant Death Center Minneapolis Children's Medical Center
Minneapolis Children's Medical Center
2525 Chicago Avenue
Minneapolis, MN 55404-4518
612-813-6000
Fax: 612-813-7344
Sara Schumacher, Project Coordinator

Mississippi

8758 Mississippi SIDS Alliance
5454 I-55 North
Jackson, MS 39211-2170
877-471-7437
www.sidsalliance.org
Scott Parrish, President
Brian Roach, Vice President

8759 Mississippi State Department of Health and Child Health Services
570 E Woodrow Wilson
Jackson, MS 39216
601-576-7400
866-458-4948
Fax: 601-576-7498
Linda.Proctor@msdh.state.ms.us
www.msdh.state.ms.us
Linda Proctor, Coordinator

Missouri

8760 Region VII Office Program: Consultants for Maternal and Child Health
Federal Building
10031 Perry Drive
Overland Park, KS 66212-2826
913-888-1377
Fax: 816-426-3633
www.mchoralhealth.org
Lawrence Wal DDS MPH, Oral Health Consultant

8761 SIDS Resources
1120 S Sixth Street
Saint Louis, MO 63104
314-822-2323
800-421-3511
Fax: 314-588-0850
The mission of SIDS Resources, Inc. is to promote safe practices which reduce the risk of infant death and to provide bereavement support for families who have lost babies.
Lori Behrens, Executive Director
Ellen Reynolds, Program Coordinator

8762 Western Region SIDS Resources
4051 Broadway
Kansas City, MO 64111
816-569-6956
Fax: 816-753-6906
www.sidsalliance.org

Provides free supportive services and education to those affected by the sudden and unexpected death of an infant - birth through 12 months. Provides education and support to professionals and communities regarding healthy and safe infant care practices and safe sleep for infants
Shay Logan, Program Coordinator

Montana

8763 Department of Public Health and Human Services
1400 Broadway
Helena, MT 59620
406-444-3565
800-232-4636
Fax: 406-444-2606
www.dphhs.mt.gov
Richard H. Opper, Director
Peggy Baker, Administrative Aide

Nebraska

8764 Nebraska Department of Health Perinatal Child and Adolescent Health
301 Centennial Mall South
Lincoln, NE 68509
402-471-0165
Fax: 402-471-7049
Jan Heusinkvelt, RN, BSN, Community Health Nurse

8765 Nebraska SIDS Foundation University of Nebraska Medical Center
University of Nebraska Medical Center
PO Box 460905
Papillion, NE 68046
402-431-8076

Nevada

8766 Nevada State Health Division Bureau of Family Health Services
Bureau Of Family Health Services
3427 Goni Road
Carson City, NV 89706
775-684-4285
Fax: 775-684-4245
Cynthia Huthht, Health Program Specialist

New Hampshire

8767 New Hampshire SIDS Program
New Hampshire Division of Public Health Services
29 Hazen Drive
Concord, NH 03301
603-271-4536
Fax: 603-271-4519
sidsnet1@sids-network.org
www.sids-network.org
Audrey Knigh MSN CPNP, SIDS Coordinator

New Jersey

8768 New Jersey Department of Health: Child Health Program
PO Box 360
Trenton, NJ 08625
609-292-7837
800-367-6543
www.state.nj.us/health
The mission of the department of health is to improve health through leadership and innovation.
Linda Jones Hicks, Director
Shirley White-Walker, Chair

8769 New Jersey SIDS Alliance
15 Meadowbrook Road
Boonton Township, NJ 07005
973-299-6523
njsids@yahoo.com
www.sidsalliance.org
Genny Elias-Warren, Chairperson

8770 SIDS Center of New Jersey
1 Robert Wood Johnson Place
New Brunswick, NJ 08903-1766
732-249-2160
800-704-7437
Fax: 732-235-6609
Provide public health education to reduce the risk of sudden infant death
Thomas Hegyi MD, Co-Medical Director
Barbara Ostf PhD, Program Director

New Mexico

8771 New Mexico SIDS Information and Counseling Program
University of New Mexico School of Medicine

2500 Marble NE
Albuquerque, NM 87131

505-277-3053
Fax: 505-272-3601
sidsnet1@sids-network.org
www.sids-network.org

Beverly Whit RN MS, Director

New York

8772 NYS Center for Sudden Infant Death: Eastern Satellite Office
Albany Medical College
47 New Scotland Avenue
Albany, NY 12208

518-262-5918
Fax: 518-262-7237
whittrm@mail.amc.edu

Mary Whittredge, Regional Coordinator

8773 New York City Center for SIDS
New York City Satellite Office
520 1st Avenue
New York, NY 10016

212-686-8854
800-522-5006
Fax: 212-532-6564
evelyne.longchamp@sids1.ssw.sunysb.edu

Judith Gaine CSW PhD, SIDS Program Director

8774 New York State Center for SIDS: School of Social Welfare
Stony Brook University
101 Nicolls Road
Stony Brook, NY 11794-0001

631-444-4000
800-336-7437
Fax: 631-444-6475

Stony Brook Medicine expresses our shared mission of research, clinical care and education - a mission embraced by our faculty, staff, researchers, and students. It is the embodiment of everything we do on behalf of the health of patients - not only here in our community, but also in the region and worldwide.

Marie Chandi CSW, Associate Project Director

8775 Region II Office Program: Consultants for Maternal and Child Health
345 E 24th Street
New York, NY 10010-0004

212-998-9654
Fax: 212-995-4364
ngh1@nyu.edu
www.mchoralhealth.org

Neal Herman DDS, Oral Health Consultant

8776 WNYS Center for SIDS
3580 Harlem Road
Buffalo, NY 14215

716-837-5189
Fax: 716-836-1578
www.sidsalliance.org

Jan Walkden, Family Service Coordinator

North Carolina

8777 SIDS Alliance of the Carolinas
306 Lucas Park Drive
Greensboro, NC 27455

336-545-3348
sandylkennedy@hotmail.com
www.sidsalliance.org

Sandy Kennedy, Chairperson

North Dakota

8778 North Dakota SIDS Alliance
128 Apollo Avenue
Bismarck, ND 58503

701-530-2507
Fax: 701-223-0440
ndsids@btinet.net
www.sidsalliance.org

Barb Delvo, Chairperson

8779 North Dakota SIDS Management Program
Division of Maternal and Child Health
600 E Boulevard Avenue
Bismarck, ND 58505-0200

701-328-2372
800-472-2286
Fax: 701-328-4727
www.ndhealth.gov

Provides support education and follow-up to parents/caregivers family and childcare providers suffering a sudden infant death
Kjersti Hintz, Program Director
Terry Dwelle, MD

Ohio

8780 District Board of Health: Mahoning County
50 Westchester Drive
Youngstown, OH 44515

330-270-2855
800-873-MCHD
Fax: 330-270-2860
TTY: 800-750-0750
www.mahoning-health.org

The mission of the District Board of Health is to promote and protect the health of individuals and communities, to create a safer, healthier environment, and to improve quality of life
Lisa Weiss MD, Forum Health
Bev Fisher, Manager

8781 Ohio Department of Health
Child Fatality Review
246 N High Street
Columbus, OH 43215

614-466-3543
866-634-7654
Fax: 614-564-2433
SmkInfo@odh.ohio.gov~
www.odh.ohio.gov

Theodore E. Wymyslo, Director
Frances Veverka, RS MPH, Ohio Health Commissioners

8782 SIDS Network of Ohio
421 Graham Road
Cuyahoga Falls, OH 44221

800-477-7437
Fax: 330-929-0593
SIDNetwork@sidsohio.org
www.sidsohio.org

The SID Network of Ohio promotes infant safety in an effort to reduce the rate of SIDS and Sudden Unexpected Infant Death (SUID). We accomplish this through the promotion of infant health and wellness, community education and medical research. We also provide supportive services to those who have been affected by the sudden loss of a child age 2 and under.
Leslie Redd, Executive Director
Jennifer Connolly, Development Coordinator

Oklahoma

8783 Oklahoma State Department of Health: Maternal and Child Health Services
1000 NE 10th Street
Oklahoma City, OK 73117-1207

405-524-3468
800-955-3468
Fax: 405-271-9202
www.ok.gov

As the official Internet gateway of Oklahoma, we are committed to providing citizens and businesses with efficient online access to government.
Paula Wood, Executive Assistant
Suzanna Dooley

Oregon

8784 Oregon Health Authority
500 Summer Street NE
Salem, OR 97301

503-947-2340
800-375-2863
Fax: 503-947-5461
TTY: 503-945-6214
www.oregon.gov

Patrick Allen, Director
Collette Young, Administrator, Public Health Practice

Pennsylvania

8785 Pennsylvania Department of Health Bureau of Family Health
Bureau of Family Health
625 Forster Street
Harrisburg, PA 17120

717-772-2762
877-PAH-EALT
Fax: 717-772-0323
bcaboot@state.pa.us
www.dsf.health.state.pa.us

Robert Torres, Deputy Secretary for Administration
Michael Wolf, Secretary

8786   SIDS of Pennsylvania
810 River Avenue
Pittsburgh, PA 15212
412-322-5680
800-721-7437
Fax: 412-481-5968
sidspa@aol.com
www.cribsforkids.org

Cribs for Kidsr has been making an impact on the rates of babies dying of accidental death due to unsafe sleeping environmentsby educating parents on the importance of safe sleep practices and by providing Graco Pack 'n Play portable cribs to families who, otherwise, cannot otherwise afford a safe place for their babies to sleep.
Judith A Bannon, Executive Director
Joseph T Dominick, RN, Chairman

Rhode Island

8787   Rhode Island Department of Health
3 Capitol Hill
Providence, RI 02908
401-222-5960
800-942-7434
Fax: 401-222-6548
TTY: 711
www.health.state.ri.us

David R Gifford MD MPH, Director
Donald L Carcieri, Governor

South Carolina

8788   Division of Perinatal Systems Mills Jarret Complex
Mills Jarret Complex
Box 101106
Columbia, SC 29211
803-898-0734
Fax: 803-898-2065
swansokm@dhec.sc.gov

Kathy Swanson, State FIMR Director

South Dakota

8789   South Dakota Department of Health
Health Building
600 E Capitol Avenue
Pierre, SD 57501
605-773-3361
800-738-2301
Fax: 605-773-5509
DOH.info@state.sd.us
www.doh.sd.gov

Nancy Shoup, Program Coordinator

Tennessee

8790   Tenessee Department of Health
Division of Maternal & Child Health
425 5th Avenue N
Nashville, TN 37243-4701
615-741-3111
Fax: 615-741-1063
tn.health@tn.gov
health.state.tn.us

The Department of Health works to promote, protect and improve the health and well-being of Tennesseans
John J. Dreyzehner, MD, MPH, Commissioner

8791   Tennessee SIDS Alliance
373 Woodcrest Drive
Kingsport, TN 37663
423- 23- 821
lisasids@cs.com
The SID Alliance of TN's mission is as a volunteer. non-profit organization dedicated to the support and service of all Tennessee SIDS families and friends.
Lisa Hunt, Chairperson

Texas

8792   Department of State Health Offices
Title V And Health Resources
100 West 49th Street
Austin, TX 78756
512-776-7111
888-963-7111
Fax: 512-458-7650
www.dshs.state.tx.us

To improve health and well-being in Texas
David L. Lakey, MD

8793   Greater Houston Chapter SIDS Alliance
916 Satsuma Street
Pasadena, TX 77506
713-924-1419
Fax: 281-541-5340
anita.carmona@us.rhodia.com
www.sidsalliance.org
Anita Carmona, Chairperson

8794   Harris County Public Health and Environmental Services
2223 W Lop S
Houston, TX 77027
713-439-6000
www.hcphes.org
Promoting a Healthy and Safe Community.
Herminia Palacio, Executive Director

8795   Region VI Office Program Consultants for Maternal and Child Health
1301 Young Street
Dallas, TX 75202-4325
214-767-3003
Fax: 214-767-3038
geurink@zeecon.com
www.mchoralhealth.org
Kathy Geurin RDH BS MA, Oral Health Consultant

8796   Southwest SIDS Research Institute
Brazosport Memorial Hospital
230 Parking Way
Lake Jackson, TX 77566
979-297-2101
www.swsids.com
Our mission is to end unexpected infant mortality through education, support, medical servicesandresearch.
ISBN: 9-792992-81-4
Richard A. Hardoin, MD
Judith A. Henslee, LMSW, Executive Director

Utah

8797   Utah Department of Health
Child Adolescent & School Health Program
288 N 1460 W
Salt Lake City, UT 84116-3231
801-538-6003
Fax: 801-538-6200
www.health.utah.gov
The mission of the Utah Department of Health is to protect the public's health through preventing avoidable illness, injury, disability and premature death; assuring access to affordable, quality health care; and promoting healthy lifestyles.
David Sundwa MD, Executive Director
A Richard Melton, Deputy Director

8798   Utah SIDS Alliance
1760 American Park Circle
W Valley City, UT 84119
801-487-7800
Fax: 801-487-4477
lisa.hughes@fnwmail.com
www.sidsalliance.org
Lisa Hughes, President
Troy Hughes, Co-President

Vermont

8799   Vermont Department of Health: SIDS Information and Counseling Program
108 Cherry Street
Burlington, VT 05402
802-652-2000
Fax: 802-652-2005
TTY: 800-253-0191
healthvermont.gov
Kathy Keleher, Assistant Director Public Health

Virginia

8800   SIDS Mid-Atlantic
PO Box 799
Haymarket, VA 20168
703-955-6899
Fax: 703-933-9101
bconnal@aol.com
Betty Connal, Executive Director

8801   Virginia SIDS Alliance
PO Box 752
Mechanicsville, VA 23111
Fax: 757-548-7074
Terri Newman, President
Mark Ferraro, Vice President

8802   Virginia SIDS Program: Virginia Department of Health
Virginia Department of Health

109 Governor Street
Richmond, VA 23219

804-846-7772
Fax: 804-973-9498
www.vdh.virginia.gov

Virginia Health Information' is a resource for patients and consumers looking to learn about and compare options on everything from obstetrical services, to heart care, to pricing information on commonly performed medical procedures.
Robert Stroube, Commissioner
Rosanne Kolesar, Deputy Commissioner Public Health

Washington

8803 Region X Office Program Consultants for Maternal and Child Health
2201 Sixth Avenue
Seattle, WA 98121-1857

206-615-2518
Fax: 206-615-2500
www.mchoralhealth.org

Rebecca Slay DDS PhD, Oral Health Consultant

8804 SIDS Foundation of Washington
4649 Sunnyside Avenue N
Seattle, WA 98103

206-548-9290
800-533-0376
Fax: 206-548-9445
info@nwsids.org
www.nisa-sids.org

The Northwest Infant Survival & SIDS Alliance is dedicated to reducing the risk of sudden unexpected infant death through education and supporting research while providing bereavement services.
Krista Cossa Sandberg, Executive Director
Lindsey Hulet, Office Administrator

8805 SIDS Northwest Regional Center
Washington Department of Health
111 Israel Rd SE
Olympia, WA 98501-7880

360-236-3502
800-533-0376
Fax: 360-236-2323
mch.support@doh.wa.gov
www.doh.wa.gov

The Department of Health works to protect and improve the health of people in Washington State.
Lorrie Grevstad

West Virginia

8806 Office of Maternal, Child & Family Health
Bureau For Public Health
350 Capitol Street
Charelston, WV 25301

304-558-7997
Fax: 304-558-3510

Ann Munson, SIDS Coordinator

Wisconsin

8807 Infant Death Center of Wisconsin
Childrens Hospital Of Wisconsin
620 S. 76th St
Milwaukee, WI 53214

414-292-4000
Fax: 414-213-4952
www.idcw.org

Karen Ordinana, Executive Director
Matt Crespin, Associate Director

Wyoming

8808 Wyoming Department of Health
Community & Family Health Section
401 Hathaway Building
Cheyenne, WY 82002

307-777-7656
Fax: 307-777-7439

Our mission is to promote, protect, and enhance the health of all Wyoming citizens. The Wyoming Department of Health is the primary state agency for providing health and human services. We administer programs maintaining the health and safety of all citizens of Wyoming and our primary approach in solving health problems is prevention.
Thomas O. Forslund, Director
Heather Babbitt, Senior Administrator

Research Centers

8809 Massachusetts Sudden Infant Death Syndrome Boston City Hospital
Boston City Hospital
1 Boston Medical Center Place
Boston, MA 02118

617-638-8000
Fax: 617-534-5555
www.bmc.org

A joint program of Boston City Hospital and Children's Hospital. Services provided include around-the-clock availability for consultation to health professionals and families counseling of families parent group meetings and supportive home visits.

8810 Pediatric Pulmonary Unit Massachusetts General Hospital
Massachusetts General Hospital
55 Fruit Street
Boston, MA 02114

617-726-2000
Fax: 617-242-03
TTY: 617-724-8800
www.massgeneral.org

Sudden infant death syndrome and childhood disorders research.
Paul S Russell, MD

8811 Sudden Infant Death Syndrome Institute of the University of Maryland
22 S Green Street
Baltimore, MD 21201

410-538-3363
800-492-5538
www.umm.edu

Dr M John O'Brien MB, Director
Jeffrey A Rivest, FACHE, President and Chief Executive Officer

8812 USC: Neonatology Research Units
1240 Mission Road
Los Angeles, CA 90033

213-226-3408
Fax: 213-226-3440

Focuses on clinical problems of the newborn and premature infant.
Paul YK Wu MD, Director

Support Groups & Hotlines

8813 National Center for the Prevention of SIDS
1314 Bedford Avenue
Baltimore, MD 21208-6605

800-638-7437

Offers medical updates and information on prevention of SIDS and other disorders to parents and professionals.

8814 National Health Information Center
Office of Disease Prevention & Health Promotion
1101 Wootton Pkwy
Rockville, MD 20852

Fax: 240-453-8281
odphpinfo@hhs.gov
www.health.gov/nhic

Supports public health education by maintaining a calendar of National Health Observances; helps connect consumers and health professionals to organizations that can best answer questions and provide up-to-date contact information from reliable sources; updates on a yearly basis toll-free numbers for health information, Federal health clearinghouses and info centers.
Don Wright, MD, MPH, Director

8815 Parents Helping Parents A Family Resource Center
1400 Parkmoor Avenue
San Jose, CA 95126

408-727-5775
855-727-5775
Fax: 408-286-1116
www.php.com

A group of parents and professionals committed to alleviating some of the problems, hardships and concerns of families with children having special needs.
Mary Ellen Peterson, Director

8816 SIDS Information and Referral Hotline
SIDS Alliance
2105 Laurel Bush Road
Baltimore, MD 21015

443-640-1049
800-221-7437
Fax: 410-653-8709
www.firstcandle.org

Twenty-four hour information and referral line for parents who wish to discuss their concerns with a SIDS counselor, request additional information about SIDS and to receive referrals to the local SIDS affiliate in their area.
Deborah Boyd, Director

8817 SIDS Support Group
Massachusetts Center for SIDS
Boston Medical Center 617-638-8000
Boston, MA 02118 800-641-7437
www.bmc.org
Aids in the resolution of the early trauma of grief experienced by parents following the sudden unexpected death of their infant. The purposes are to provide a safe environemnt for parents to express their feelings, to provide contact with others who share their grief and are at various stages of resolution, to provide a reliable source of information about SIDS and to provide the opportunity to go on to help others.

Books

8818 Apparent Life-Threatening Event and Sudden Infant Death Syndrome
National Maternal and Child Health Clearinghouse
2070 Chain Bridge Road 703-442-9051
Vienna, VA 22182-2588 888-275-4772
Fax: 703-821-2098
ask@hrsa.gov
www.ask.hrsa.gov
Provides information about ALTE and its relationship to SIDS.

8819 Hospice Care for Children
Oxford University Press
2001 Evans Road 212-726-6000
Cary, NC 27513-2010 800-445-9714
Fax: 919-677-1303
custserv.us@oup.com
www.oup-usa.org
A comprehensive book offering the most inclusive and up-to-date information about caring for terminally ill children and their families.
304 pages
ISBN: 0-195073-12-6
Ann Armstrong-Dailey, Editor

8820 Professional's Role in Sudden Infant Death Syndrome
National Maternal and Child Health Clearinghouse
2070 Chain Bridge Road 703-442-9051
Vienna, VA 22182-2588 888-275-4772
Fax: 703-821-2098
ask@hrsa.gov
www.ask.hrsa.gov
Contains abstracts of articles on the role of professionals in SIDS.

8821 Smoking and Sudden Infant Death Syndrome
National Maternal and Child Health Clearinghouse
2070 Chain Bridge Road 703-442-9051
Vienna, VA 22182-2588 888-275-4772
Fax: 703-821-2098
ask@hrsa.gov
www.ask.hrsa.gov
Contains abstracts of materials about tobacco use, its relationship to SIDS and the dangers to the unborn and the newly born from passive and secondary smoking.

Newsletters

8822 Newsletter: SIDS
Massachusetts Center For SIDS
1 Boston Medical Ctr Plc 617-638-8000
Boston, MA 02118-2905 www.bmc.org
Boston Medical Center (BMC) is a 482-bed academic medical center located in Boston's historic South End
Monthly

8823 Parent Care News Brief
Parent Care
303 Watts Branch Parkway 301-294-9338
Rockville, MD 20850-1210 Fax: 301-294-8848
Features articles and medical updates pertaining to the care of the critically ill child.
Quarterly

Pamphlets

8824 Crib Death: The Sudden Infant Death Syndrome
US Department Of Health & Human Services
202 Indp Avenue SW 202-619-0257
Washington, DC 20201-0001 877-696-6775
Offers information on the most frequently asked questions pertaining to SIDS and crib death.
Kristen Brett
Kathy McKnight

8825 Developmental Delays and Developmental Disorders
National Maternal and Child Health Clearinghouse
2070 Chain Bridge Road 703-442-9051
Vienna, VA 22182-2588 888-275-4772
Fax: 703-821-2098
ask@hrsa.gov
www.ask.hrsa.gov
Contains abstracts of selected articles on developmental delays and developmental disorders and the relationship to SIDS.
1997

8826 Facts About SIDS
Sudden Infant Death Syndrome Alliance
1227 Malvern Road 410-653-8226
Malvern, 3144-6605 800-221-7437
Fax: 410-653-8709
yvonne@sidsandkids.org
www.sidsandkids.org
Offers information on basic facts, answers to the most frequently asked questions about SIDS and information on numbers to call and referral centers for more help.
Graham Henderson, Chairman
Mr Craig Heatley, Deputy Chairman

8827 Grief of Children After the Loss of a Sibling or Friend
National Maternal and Child Health Clearinghouse
2070 Chain Bridge Road 703-442-9051
Vienna, VA 22182-2588 888-275-4772
Fax: 703-821-2098
ask@hrsa.gov
www.ask.hrsa.gov
Discusses some of the common expressions of childrens grief and offers ways adults can help during the grieving process.
1995

8828 Infant Positioning and Sudden Infant Death Syndrome
National Maternal and Child Health Clearinghouse
2070 Chain Bridge Road 703-442-9051
Vienna, VA 22182-2588 888-275-4772
Fax: 703-821-2098
ask@hrsa.gov
www.ask.hrsa.gov
Contains abstracts of selected articles on the topic of sleep position and SIDS.
1994

8829 Nationwide Survey of Sudden Infant Death Syndrome (SIDS) Service
National Maternal and Child Health Clearinghouse
2070 Chain Bridge Road 703-442-9051
Vienna, VA 22182-2588 888-275-4772
Fax: 703-821-2098
ask@hrsa.gov
www.ask.hrsa.gov
Analysis of availability of SIDS services.
1994

8830 Parents and the Grieving Process
National Maternal and Child Health Clearinghouse
2070 Chain Bridge Road 703-442-9051
Vienna, VA 22182-2588 888-275-4772
Fax: 703-821-2098
ask@hrsa.gov
www.ask.hrsa.gov
Defines grief, presents common reactions and emotions expressed by the bereaved.
1992

8831   SIDS Information for the EMT
National Maternal and Child Health Clearinghouse
2070 Chain Bridge Road   703-442-9051
Vienna, VA 22182-2588   888-275-4772
                                     Fax: 703-821-2098
                                        ask@hrsa.gov
                                       www.ask.hrsa.gov
Provides suggestions for first response of emergency medical technicians and others at the time of sudden infant death.
1983

8832   SIDS Research: An Analysis in Three Parts
National Maternal and Child Health Clearinghouse
2070 Chain Bridge Road   703-442-9051
Vienna, VA 22182-2588   888-275-4772
                                     Fax: 703-821-2098
                                        ask@hrsa.gov
                                       www.ask.hrsa.gov
Contains articles from a three part series on SIDS research.
1993

8833   SIDS: Toward Prevention and Improved Infant Health
American SIDS Institute
528 Raven Way   239-431-5425
Naples, FL 34110-8657   800-232-7437
                                     Fax: 239-431-5536
                                       prevent@sids.org
                                         www.sids.org
the American SIDS Institute, a national nonprofit health care organization, is dedicated to the prevention of sudden infant death and the promotion of infant health
Marc Peterzell, Chairman

8834   Selected Book on Sudden Infant Death Syndrome
National Maternal and Child Health Clearinghouse
2070 Chain Bridge Road   703-442-9051
Vienna, VA 22182-2588   888-275-4772
                                     Fax: 703-821-2098
                                        ask@hrsa.gov
                                       www.ask.hrsa.gov
Provides a list of selected titles on SIDS covering topics such as research, support information and the professionals role.
1993

8835   Selected Resources for Children Grieving the Loss of Another Child
National Maternal and Child Health Clearinghouse
2070 Chain Bridge Road   703-442-9051
Vienna, VA 22182-2588   888-275-4772
                                     Fax: 703-821-2098
                                        ask@hrsa.gov
                                       www.ask.hrsa.gov
Provides a list of materials suitable for grieving children and teenagers.
1995

8836   Sudden Infant Death Syndrome and Risk Reduction
National Maternal and Child Health Clearinghouse
2070 Chain Bridge Road   703-442-9051
Vienna, VA 22182-2588   888-275-4772
                                     Fax: 703-821-2098
                                        ask@hrsa.gov
                                       www.ask.hrsa.gov
Contains abstracts of selected articles on risk reduction.
1997

8837   What Every Parent Should Know About SIDS
SIDS Alliance
1227 Malvern Road   410-653-8226
Malvern, 3144-6605   800-221-7437
                                     Fax: 410-653-8709
                                   yvonne@sidsandkids.org
                                    www.sidsandkids.org
Pamphlet offering information on what SIDS is, causes, prevention techniques and what parents can do.
Graham Henderson, Chairman
Mr Craig Heatley, Deputy Chairman

8838   What is SIDS?
National Maternal and Child Health Clearinghouse

2070 Chain Bridge Road   703-442-9051
Vienna, VA 22182-2588   888-275-4772
                                     Fax: 703-821-2098
                                        ask@hrsa.gov
                                       www.ask.hrsa.gov
Provides basic facts about SIDS and answers some of the most commonly asked questions.
1993

8839   When Sudden Infant Death Syndrome Occurs in Childcare Settings
National Maternal and Child Health Clearinghouse
2070 Chain Bridge Road   703-442-9051
Vienna, VA 22182-2588   888-275-4772
                                     Fax: 703-821-2098
Presents information about SIDS for child care providers.
1993

Web Sites

8840   American SIDS Institute
                                         sids.org/
Dedicated to the prevention of sudden infant death and the promotion of infant health through research, clinical services, education and family support.

8841   Center for Research for Mothers & Children
                                       cdrwww.who.ch/
Mission is to make sure everyone is born healthy and wanted, that women suffer no harmful effects from reproductive processes, and that all children have the chance to achieve their full potential for healthy and productive lives, free from disease or disability, and to ensure the health, productivity, independence, and well-being of all people through optimal rehabilitation.

8842   Compassionate Friends
                                 www.compassionatefriends.org
The Compassionate Friends provides highly personal comfort, hope, and support to every family experiencing the death of a son or a daughter, a brother or a sister, or a grandchild, and helps others better assist the grieving family.

8843   Healing Well
                                     www.healingwell.com
An online health resource guide to medical news, chat, information and articles, newsgroups and message boards, books, disease-related web sites, medical directories, and more for patients, friends, and family coping with disabling diseases, disorders, or chronic illnesses.

8844   Healthlink USA
                                     www.healthlinkusa.com
Health information concerning treatment, cures, prevention, diagnosis, risk factors, research, support groups, email lists, personal stories and much more. Updated regularly.

8845   MedicineNet
                                     www.medicinenet.com
An online resource for consumers providing easy-to-read, authoritative medical and health information.

8846   Medscape
                                     www.medscape.com
Medscape offers specialists, primary care physicians, and other health professionals the Web's most robust and integrated medical information and educational tools.

8847   National Center for Education in Maternal and Child Health
                                       www.ncemch.org
The National Center for Education in Maternal and Child Health provides national leadership to the maternal and child health community in three key areas - program development, policy analysis and education, and state-of-the-art knowledge to improve the health and well-being of the nation's children and families.

8848   National Organization for Rare Disorders
                                     www.rarediseases.org
NORD is a federation of voluntary health organizations dedicated to helping people with rare orphan diseases and assisting the organizations that serve them. It is committed to the identification,

treatment, and cure of rare disorders through programs of education, advocacy, research, and service. Website features resources for patients and families, patient organizations, and clinicians and researchers.

8849 WebMD

www.webmd.com

Provides credible information, supportive communities, and in-depth reference material about health subjects. A source for original and timely health information as well as material from well known content providers.

Description

8850 Systemic Lupus Erythematosus

Systemic lupus erythematosus (SLE) is a chronic autoimmune disease characterized by inflammation that affects multiple organ systems and occurs predominantly in young women. The inflammation characteristically occurs in connective tissues that may involve the brain, skin, kidneys, joints, bowel, and eyes. Of SLE cases, 90 percent are women, and the disease usually begins during the child-bearing years. Although the cause is unclear, there is a strong genetic component to SLE, since variations in 23 different genes are associated with an increased risk of SLE. SLE causes its damage through autoimmune mechanisms. The immune system attacks protein complexes normally found inside cells. For this reason, it seems that people with SLE have experiences episodes of severe cell destruction. These dead cells may release a host of macromolecular assemblages that activate the immune system to react against them, which results in the signs and symptoms of SLE. The manifestations of SLE vary extensively from one patient to another. Milder forms of SLE, cutaneous lupus erythematosus (CLE), only manifest symptoms in the skin. CLE comes in acute, subacute, and chronic subtypes and all of which show photosensitivity. One of the most common forms of chronic CLE is called discoid lupus erythematosus (DLE), in which patches of skin may turn red and develop white scales, followed by thinning and scarring. About 10 percent of patients with DLE will go on to develop SLE and roughly 25 percent of patients with SLE also have the manifestations of DLE. Almost any organ system can be affected, and symptoms may include fatigue, ulcers in the mouth and nose, respiratory problems (pleuritis, pulmonary hemorrhage, pneumonitis), fever, loss of appetite, heart disease (endocarditis, pericarditis), skin rashes, sensitivity to light (photophobia), joint pain (arthritis), high blood pressure, anemia, headaches, personality change, eye irritation, and inflammation of the kidney and hematuria.

SLE is diagnosed by a combination of symptoms and blood tests that detect specific antibodies against the patient's own tissues, which include anti-nuclear antibody (ANA), antibodies against double-stranded DNA (anti-dsDNA), anti-Sm nuclear antigen antibodies (anti-Sm), antiphospholipid antibody, and anti-beta2-glycoprotein I antibodies. Patients must show 4 of 17 diagnostic criteria that were proposed by the Systemic Lupus International Collaborating Clinics (SLICC), a consensus group of experts on SLE, including at least 1 of the 11 clinical criteria and 1 of the 6 immunologic criteria to confirm a diagnosis of SLE.

In general, the course of SLE is chronic and relapsing, often with long periods (years) of remission. It may only be mild or progress towards more serious illness and death from infection, kidney failure or neurologic damage. Survival has improved markedly in the past two decades because, for most patients with SLE the disease can be controlled with proper medications. All patients with SLE are treated with hydroxychloroquine. Those with moderate SLE patients are treated with NSAIDs and antimalarials, and for those with severe disease, patients are treated with large, prolonged doses of corticosteroids and immunosuppressants, such as cyclophosphamide (with mensa to prevent drug-associated cystitis) or mycophenolate mofetil. Some of these therapies may be associated with long-term complications.

National Agencies & Associations

8851 American Autoimmune Related Diseases Association
22100 Gratiot Avenue
Eastpointe, MI 48021
586-776-3900
800-598-4668
Fax: 586-776-3903
aarda@aarda.org
www.aarda.org

Provides mutual support and education for patients with any type of autoimmune disease. Support includes advocacy, referral to support groups, literature and conferences.
Virginia T. Ladd, President & Executive Director
Laura Simpson, Assistant Director

8852 American Juvenile Arthritis Organization
Arthritis Foundation
1330 West Peachtree Street
Atlanta, GA 30309
404-872-7100
800-283-7800
Fax: 440-872-9559
help@arthritis.org
www.arthritis.org

A council of the Arthritis Foundation devoted to serving the special needs of children, teens and young adults with childhood rheumatic diseases (including systemic lupus erythematosus) and their families. Provides support groups, information, advocacy, research updates, and conferences.
Ann M. Palmer, President & CEO
Guy S. Eakin, PhD, Sr Vice President, Scientific Strategy

8853 Lupus Foundation of America
2121 K Street NW
Washington, DC 20037
202-349-1155
Fax: 202-349-1156
info@lupus.org
www.lupus.org

The nation's leading non-profit voluntary health organization dedicated to finding the causes and cure for lupus.
Susan M. Manzi, MD, MPH, Chair & Director
Stevan W. Gibson, President & CEO

State Agencies & Associations

Alaska

8854 Lupus Foundation of America: Alaska Chapter
PO Box 240628
Anchorage, AK 99524
907-338-6332
800-307-5878
Fax: 907-345-0695
LFA_Alaska@hotmail.com
www.lupus.org/webmodules/webarticlesnet/

Judy Powell, Chair of the Board
Anna Tillman, Executive Director

Arizona

8855 Lupus Foundation of America: Greater Arizona Chapter
2001 West Camelback Road 480-201-5334
Phoenix, AZ 85015-4908 juliano@lupus.org
www.lupus.org/webmodules/webarticlesnet/
David Juliano, Outreach Development Manager

8856 Lupus Foundation of America: Southern Arizona Chapter
2583 North 1st Avenue 480-201-5334
Tucson, AZ 85719 www.lupus.org/webmodules/webarticlesnet/
David Juliano, Outreach Development Manager

Arkansas

8857 Lupus Foundation of America: Arkansas Chapter
220 Mockingbird 501-525-9380
Hot Springs, AR 71913 800-294-8878
Fax: 501-525-9380
lupusarkhs@direclynx.net
www.lupus-arkansas.com
Jamesetta Smith, President

California

8858 Bay Area LE Foundation
2635 N 1st Street 408-954-8600
San Jose, CA 95134 800-523-3363
Chapter of the Lupus Foundation of America.

8859 Lupus Foundation of America: California Chapter
18000 Studebaker Road 562-467-8994
Cerritos, CA 90703 800-558-0121
Fax: 916-973-8124
www.lupus.org/webmodules/webarticlesnet/
Laurie Gray, National Manager of Walk Development
Luz Maria Hernandez, Health Educator

Colorado

8860 Lupus Foundation of Colorado
1211 S Parker Road 303-597-4050
Denver, CO 80231 800-858-1292
Fax: 303-597-4054
info@lupuscolorado.org
www.lupuscolorado.org
Chapter of the Lupus Foundation of America.
Carol Wright, Chair
Debbie Lynch, Chief Executive Officer

Connecticut

8861 Lupus Foundation of America: Connecticut Chapter
270 Farmington Avenue 860-269-6240
Farmington, CT 06032-2402 800-699-6967
Fax: 860-269-6243
www.lupus.org/webmodules/webarticlesnet/
A non-profit organization and a National Health Agency established for the purpose of enlightening the public by focusing professional and public attention on Lupus Erythematosus promotes research by providing financial assistance and serves as the support bond for patients and their families.
Ron Marek, Chair
Michael Tommasi, President & CEO

Delaware

8862 Lupus Foundation of America: Delaware Chapter
100 West 10th Street 302-622-8700
Wilmington, DE 19801 800-880-8686
www.lupus.org/webmodules/webarticlesnet/
Debra L Riegel Jepson, Chair
James Stewart, Treasurer

Florida

8863 Lupus Foundation of America: Northeast Florida Chapter
PO Box 10486 904-645-8398
Jacksonville, FL 32247-0486 800-853-8398
Lee, President
Jon Kagan, Vice President

8864 Lupus Foundation of America: Northwest Florida Chapter
PO Box 17841 904-444-7070
Pensacola, FL 32522-7841 800-458-8211
Brenda Barto, Executive Director
Kathleen Laca, Director of Operations

8865 Lupus Foundation of America: Southeast Florida Chapter
2300 High Ridge Road 561-279-8606
Boynton Beach, FL 33426 855-905-8787
Fax: 561-935-1435
info@lupusfl.org
www.lupusfl.com
John Apgar, Chair
Amy Kelly-Yalden, President & CEO

8866 Lupus Foundation of America: Suncoast Chapter
3637 4th Street N 727-447-7075
St Petersburg, FL 33704-7485 800-684-9276
Fax: 727-447-8925
info@lupusflorida.org
www.lupusfl.com

8867 Lupus Foundation of America: Tampa Area Chapter
Dibbs Plaza
4119-20A Gunn Highway 813-960-3992
Tampa, FL 33624 800-330-3992
www.milupus.org/southeast.htm

8868 Lupus Foundation of Florida
535 Central Avenue 727-447-7075
St. Petersburg, FL 33701 800-684-9276
Fax: 727-447-7075
rmccolllum@lupusflorida.org
Chapter of the Lupus Foundation of America.
Maggi McQueen, Chairman
Rick McCollum, President & CEO

Georgia

8869 Lupus Foundation of America: Columbus Chapter
233 12th Street 706-571-8950
Columbus, GA 31901 www.milupus.org/southeast.htm

8870 Lupus Foundation of America: Greater Atlanta Chapter
1850 Lake Park Drive 770-333-5930
Smyrna, GA 30080-2203 800-800-4532
Fax: 770-333-5932
www.lupus.org/webmodules/webarticlesnet/
Maria Myler, President & CEO
Teri Emond, Program Director

Hawaii

8871 Hawaii Lupus Foundation
1200 College Walk 808-538-1522
Honolulu, HI 96817 800-201-1522
Chapter of the Lupus Foundation of America.

Illinois

8872 Lupus Foundation of America: Illinois Chapter
525 W. Monroe Street 312-542-0002
Chicago, IL 60661 800-258-7872
Fax: 312-255-8020
charles@lupusil.org
www.lupus.org/webmodules/webarticlesnet/
Offers support to individuals and families affected by Lupus, and looks to improve the diagnosis of and treatment of Lupus.
Charles Brummell, President & CEO
Mary Dollear, Vice-President

Indiana

8873 Lupus Foundation of America: Northeast Indiana Chapter
5401 Keystone Drive · 219-482-8205
Fort Wayne, IN 46825
Largent, Director

8874 Lupus Foundation of America: Northwest Indiana Lupus Chapter
PO Box 2763 · 219-762-6575
Portage, IN 46368 · 800-948-8806
lupusnwichapter@aol.com

Tammie

8875 Lupus Foundation of Indiana
9302 N. Meridian Street · 317-225-4400
Indianapolis, IN 46260 · 800-948-8806
info@lupusindiana.org
www.lupus.org/webmodules/webarticlesnet/
Chapter of the Lupus Foundation of America.
Matthew Johnson, Chair
Jan Ferris, Chief Executive Officer

Iowa

8876 Lupus Foundation of America: Iowa Chapter
3839 Merle Hay Road · 515-279-3048
Des Moines, IA 50310-1044 · 888-279-3048
info@lupusia.org
www.lupus.org/webmodules/webarticlesnet/

Barb Logue, President
Marilyn Rumsey, Treasurer

Kansas

8877 Lupus Foundation of America: Heartland Chapter
PO Box 12204 · 316-262-6180
Wichita, KS 67277 · www.lupus.org/webmodules/webarticlesnet/
Ruth Busch, Board Chair
Sandy Blaylock, Recording Secretary

Kentucky

8878 Lupus Foundation of Kentuckiana
4004 Hillsboro Pike · 615-298-2273
Nashville, TN 37215 · 877-865-8787
Fax: 615-292-0520
info@lupusmidsouth.org
www.lupus.org/webmodules/webarticlesnet/
Chapter of the Lupus Foundation of America.
Tanisha Hall, Chair
Mike Singer, President & CEO

Louisiana

8879 Louisiana Lupus Foundation
7732 Goodwood Boulevard · 225-927-8052
Baton Rouge, LA 70806 · 800-355-7473
www.louisianalupusfoundation.org/
Chapter of the Lupus Foundation of America.
Linda B Perkins, President
Carolyn M Bajoie, Board Member

Maine

8880 Lupus Group of Maine
PO Box 8168 · 207-878-8104
Portland, ME 04104 · www.milupus.org/northeast.htm
Chapter of the Lupus Foundation of America.
Watson, Executive Director
Jessica Gilbart, Health Education Coordinator

Maryland

8881 Lupus Foundation of America: DC, Maryland and Central & Northern Virginia
2000 L Street NW · 202-787-5380
Washington, DC 20036 · 888-787-5380
Fax: 202-787-5399
www.lupus.org/webmodules/webarticlesnet/
Chapter of the Lupus Foundation of America.
Marguerete A Luter, Chair
Jessica Gilbart, President & CEO

Massachusetts

8882 Lupus Foundation of America: Massachusetts Chapter
425 Watertown Street · 617-332-9014
Newton, MA 02158 · info@lupusne.org

Michigan

8883 Lupus Foundation of America: Michigan Lupus Foundation
26507 Harper Avenue · 586-775-8310
Saint Clair Shores, MI 48081 · 800-705-6677
Fax: 586-775-8494
www.milupus.org

Judith A Sova, President
Frank Mortl, III, Executive Director

Minnesota

8884 Lupus Foundation of America: Minnesota Chapter
2626 E 82nd Street · 952-746-5151
Bloomington, MN 55425 · 800-645-1131
Fax: 942-746-5155
info@lupusmn.org
www.lupusmn.org

Scott Brown, Chair
Jennifer Monroe, President

Mississippi

8885 Lupus Foundation of America: Mississippi Chapter
PO Box 24292 · 601-366-5655
Jackson, MS 39225-4292 · 800-866-9606
www.milupus.org/southeast.htm

Missouri

8886 Lupus Foundation of America: Kansas City
4640 Shenandoah Avenue · 800-958-7876
St Louis, MO 63110 · info@LFAheartland.org
www.lupus.org/webmodules/webarticlesnet/
Kevin Cheung, Chair of the Board
Amy Ondr, President & CEO

8887 Lupus Foundation of America: Ozarks Chapter
3150 W Marty Street · 417-887-1560
Springfield, MO 65807 · www.lupus.org

Montana

8888 Lupus Foundation of America: Montana Chapter
29 1/2 Alderson · 406-254-2082
Billings, MT 59102 · www.lupus.org

Nebraska

8889 Lupus Foundation of America: Omaha Chapter
Community Health Plaza
7101 Newport Avenue · 402-572-3150
Omaha, NE 68152 · www.milupus.org/midwest.htm

8890 Lupus Foundation of America: Western Nebraska Chapter
HCR 72 Box 58 · 308-764-2474
Sutherland, NE 69165

8891 New Hampshire Lupus Foundation
PO Box 444   603-424-0111
Nashua, NH 03061-0444   www.milupus.org
Chapter of the Lupus Foundation of America.
Beck-Clemens, Interim President and CEO
Adam Gold, Development Associate

8892 Lupus Foundation of America: New Jersey Chapter
150 Morris Avenue, Suite 102   973-379-3226
Springfield, NJ 07081   800-322-5816
                                                  Fax: 973-379-1053
                           info@lupusnj.org
             www.lupus.org/webmodules/webarticlesnet/
Ranit C Shriky, Chairman
Leonard J Andriuzzi, President & CEO

8893 Lupus Foundation of America: South Jersey Chapter
One Greentree Center   856-988-5444
Marlton, NJ 08053   Fax: 856-596-8359

8894 Lupus Foundation of America: New Mexico Chapter
PO Box 9125   505-999-1981
Albuquerque, NM 87119   800-843-9081
             www.lupus.org/webmodules/webarticlesnet/
Quinn, Executive Director
Nancy Beder, Director of Resources

8895 Lupus Alliance of America LIQ Affiliate
2255 Centre Avenue   516-783-3370
Bellmore, NY 11710   800-850-9000
                                                  Fax: 516-826-2058
                           info@lupusliqueens.org
                           www.lupusliqueens.org
Carol Goldklang, President
Kate Anastasia, Executive Director

8896 Lupus Alliance of Upstate New York
3871 Harlem Road   716-835-7161
Cheektowaga, NY 14215   800-300-4198
                                                  Fax: 716-835-7251
                           info@lupusupstateny.org
                           www.lupusupstateny.org
Lynn Szubinski, President
Honi Kurzeja, Executive Director

8897 Lupus Foundation of America: Bronx Chapter
PO Box 1117   718-822-6542
Bronx, NY 10462   www.milupus.org/northeast.htm

8898 Lupus Foundation of America: Central New York Chapter
Pickard Office Building
5858 E Molloy Road   315-454-9886
Syracuse, NY 13211   www.milupus.org/northeast.htm
Aman, President/CEO
Bob Stewart, Chairperson

8899 Lupus Foundation of America: Genessee Valley Chapter
500 Helendale Road   585-288-2910
Rochester, NY 14609   Fax: 585-288-1608
                           lupusgvc@frontiernet.net
Eileen M Arntsen, President/CEO
James E Mitchell Jr, Vice President

8900 Lupus Foundation of America: Westchester
100 S Bedford Road   914-948-1032
Mt Kisco, NY 10549   888-57L-UPUS

8901 Lupus Foundation of Mid and Northern New York
PO Box 139   315-829-4272
Utica, NY 13503-4303   866-258-7874
                                                  Fax: 315-829-4272
                           lupusmidny@aol.com
                           www.nolupus.org
David L Arntsen, Chairman
Kathleen A Arntsen, President/CEO

8902 SLE Foundation
330 Seventh Avenue   212-685-4118
New York, NY 10001   800-74L-UPUS
                                                  Fax: 212-545-1843
                           lupus@lupusny.org
                           www.lupusny.org
Chapter of the Lupus Foundation of America.
Bruce Cronstein, Chairman
Richard K DeScherer, President

**8903 Lupus Foundation of America: Winston-Triad Lupus Chapter
NCLF**
2841 Foxwood Lane   910-768-1493
Winston Salem, NC 27103
Ruth John, President/CEO
Ginger Dickerson, Chairman of the Board

8904 Lupus Foundation of America: North Carolin a Chapter
4530 Park Road   704-716-5640
Charlotte, NC 28209   877-849-8271
                                                  Fax: 704-716-5641
             www.lupus.org/webmodules/webarticlesnet/
Christine John-Fuller, President/CEO
Lorna Denton, Administrative Assistant

8905 Lupus Foundation of America: Greater Ohio Chapter
12930 Chippewa Road   440-717-0183
Brecksville, OH 44141   888-665-8787
                                                  Fax: 440-717-0186
                           suzanne@lupusgreaterohio.org
                           www.lupuscleveland.org
John Sheldon, Chairman
Suzanne Tierney, President & CEO

8906 Oklahoma Lupus Association
4100 N Lincoln Boulevard   405-427-8787
Oklahoma City, OK 73105   Fax: 405-427-8778
                           oklupus@flash.net
                           www.oklupus.com
Chapter of the Lupus Foundation of America.
Katherine

8907 Lupus Foundation of America: Central Pennsylvania Chapter
Old Liberty Square
4813 Jonestown Road   717-671-9515
Harrisburg, PA 17109   800-800-5776
                           www.lupuspa.org
Cheston M Berlin, Branch Council
Douglas C Berlin, Branch Council

8908 Lupus Foundation of America: Northeast Pennsylvania Chapter
615 Jefferson Avenue   570-558-2008
Scranton, PA 18510   800-800-5776
                                                  Fax: 570-558-2009
                           www.lupuspa.org
Marilyn Deutsch, PhD, Branch Council
Devon Fawcett, Branch Council

8909 **Lupus Foundation of America: Northwestern Pennsylvania Chapter**
PO Box 885 724-962-0368
Erie, PA 16512-0885 800-800-5776
Fax: 724-962-0368
www.lupuspa.org

Jane Lippinc Myarick, CEO

8910 **Lupus Foundation of America: Western Pennsylvania Chapter**
Landmarks Building
100 West Station Square Drive 412-261-5886
Pittsburgh, PA 15219 800-800-5776
Fax: 412-261-5365
info@lupuspa.org
www.lupuspa.org

Deborah Nigro, Executive Director
Shelly Tonti, Branch Director

8911 **Lupus Foundation of Philadelphia**
500 Old York Road 215-517-5070
Jenkintown, PA 19046 866-517-5070
Fax: 215-517-8483
info@lupustristate.org
www.lupus.org/webmodules/webarticlesnet/
Chapter of the Lupus Foundation of America.
Debra L Riegel Jepson, Chair
Annette Myarick, CEO

Rhode Island

8912 **Lupus Foundation of America: Rhode Island Chapter**
#8 Fallon Avenue 401-421-7227
Providence, RI 02908 www.milupus.org

South Carolina

8913 **Lupus Foundation of America: South Carolina Chapter**
L.E. Support Club
8039 Nova Court 843-764-1769
Charleston, SC 29420-8934
Nelson, Executive Director

Tennessee

8914 **Lupus Foundation of America Memphis Area Chapter**
3181 Poplar Avenue 901-458-5302
Memphis, TN 38111 888-915-8787
Fax: 901-217-3193
info@memphislupus.org
www.lupus.org/webmodules/webarticlesnet/
To educate and support those affected by lupus and to assist in finsing its cure. The goal is to unite and provide moral support and group strength for those individuals who are suspected of or diagnosed victims of Systemic Lupus Erythematosus and related disorders.
Yvonne D

8915 **Lupus Foundation of America: East Tennessee Chapter**
5612 Kingston Pike 615-584-5215
Knoxville, TN 37919 lupustn@aol.com
Hammond, Executive Director
Renee Levay Stewart, President

8916 **Lupus Foundation of America: Mid-South Area Chapter**
4004 Hillsboro Pike 615-298-2273
Nashville, TN 37215 877-865-8787
Fax: 615-292-0520
info@lupusmidsouth.org
www.lupus.org/webmodules/webarticlesnet/

Tanisha Hall, Chair
Mike Singer, President & CEO

Texas

8917 **Lupus Foundation of America: North Texas Chapter**
15660 North Dallas Parkway 469-374-0590
Dallas, TX 75248 866-205-2369
Fax: 469-374-0794
www.lupus.org/webmodules/webarticlesnet/
Saundra Finley, Chair
Tessie Holloway, President & CEO

8918 **Lupus Foundation of America: South Central Texas Chapter**
9330 Corporate Drive 210-651-9480
Selma, TX 78154 866-205-2369
www.lupus.org/webmodules/webarticlesnet/
Sylvia Arcos, Chair
Amy Humphrey, Treasurer

8919 **Lupus Foundation of America: Texas Gulf Coast Chapter**
3701 Kirby Drive 713-529-0126
Houston, TX 77098 800-458-7870
Fax: 713-529-0780
info@lupustexas.org
www.lupus.org/webmodules/webarticlesnet/
Tamara Atkins, Chair
Rebecca Kramer, President & CEO

8920 **Lupus Foundation of America: West Texas Chapter**
1717 Avenue K 806-744-6666
Lubbock, TX 79401 800-580-5878
www.milupus.org/southwest.htm
Reymond, Executive Director
Katie Fillnow, President

Utah

8921 **Lupus Foundation of America Utah Chapter**
352 S Denver Street 801-364-0366
Salt Lake City, UT 84111 800-657-6398
www.lupus.org/webmodules/webarticlesnet/
Noelle Reymond, President & CEO
Annette Lee, Development Director

Vermont

8922 **Lupus Foundation of America: Vermont Chapter**
57 S Main Street 802-244-5988
Waterbury, VT 05676 877-735-8787
www.lupus.org/webmodules/webarticlesnet/

Virginia

8923 **Lupus Foundation of America: Eastern Virginia Chapter**
Pembroke One
281 Independence Boulevard 757-490-2793
Virginia Beach, VA 23462 www.lupus.org/webmodules/webarticlesnet/
Fletcher, President
Sarah Guy, Executive Assistant

Washington

8924 **Lupus Foundation of America: Pacific Northwest Chapter**
800 5th Avenue 877-774-2992
Seattle, WA 98104 Fax: 206-546-8946
info@lupuspnw.org
www.lupus.org/webmodules/webarticlesnet/
Kristi Thomsen, President
Celia Y Weisman, CEO

Wisconsin

8925 **Lupus Foundation of America: Wisconsin Chapter**
1109 N Mayfair Road 414-443-6400
Milwaukee, WI 53226 866-LUP-USWI
Fax: 414-443-6400
lupuswi@lupuswi.org
www.lupus.org/webmodules/webarticlesnet/
Mary E Cronin, MD, Chairperson
Dawn T Thomas-Semanko, Executive Director

Foundations

8926 SLE Lupus Foundation
330 Seventh Avenue
New York, NY 10001

212-685-4118
800-74L-UPUS
Fax: 212-545-1843
lupus@lupusny.org
www.lupusny.org

The Foundation helps people with lupus, as well as their families and friends, cope with the anxieties and frustrations that often accompany daily living with a chronic illness. Sharing information and networking among patients and their families further helps dispel myths and provides daily support to those learning to live with lupus.
Bruce Cronstein, MD, Chairman
Richard K DeScherer, President

Research Centers

8927 Alliance for Lupus Research
28 W 44th Street
New York, NY 10036

212-218-2840
800-867-1743
info@lupusresearch.org
www.lupusresearch.org

Research foundation dedicated to providing information about lupus.
Robert Wood Johnson IV, Chairman
Ira Akselrad, Director

8928 Hahnemann University Lupus Study Center Hahnemann University Medical Center
Hahnemann University Medical Center
Broad and Vine Street
Philadelphia, PA 19102

215-762-7000
866-884-4HUH
Fax: 215-762-8109
www.hahnemannhospital.com

Raphael J Gotthelf, President

8929 Terri Gotthelf Lupus Research Institute
3 Duke Place
S Norwalk, CT 06854

800-828-87
Fax: 203-852-9720

Founded to help millions of lupus victims in the world and to encourage coordinate and direct future progress in the etiology diagnosis and treatment of this disease.
Theodore

Support Groups & Hotlines

8930 National Health Information Center
Office of Disease Prevention & Health Promotion
1101 Wootton Pkwy
Rockville, MD 20852

Fax: 240-453-8281
odphpinfo@hhs.gov
www.health.gov/nhic

Supports public health education by maintaining a calendar of National Health Observances; helps connect consumers and health professionals to organizations that can best answer questions and provide up-to-date contact information from reliable sources; updates on a yearly basis toll-free numbers for health information, Federal health clearinghouses and info centers.
Don Wright, MD, MPH, Director

Books

8931 Coping with Lupus
Lupus Foundation of America
1300 Piccard Drive
Rockville, MD 20850-4303

301-670-9292
800-558-0121
lupusinfo@aol.com
www.lupus.org

A practicing psychologist offers sound, meaningful and compassionate advice to individuals who must deal with lupus.
276 pages Paperback
ISBN: 0-895294-75-3

8932 Disability Workbook for Social Security Disability Applicants
Lupus Foundation of America
1300 Piccard Drive
Rockville, MD 20850-4303

301-670-9292
800-558-0121
lupusinfo@aol.com
www.lupus.org

Helps people get their disability benefits promptly, without unnecessary appeals. Tells what you have to prove and how to prove it.
137 pages
Douglas M. Smith, Author

8933 Get to Sleep! How to Sleep Well...Despite Lupus
Lupus Foundation of America
1300 Piccard Drive
Rockville, MD 20850-4303

301-670-9292
800-558-0121
lupusinfo@aol.com
www.lupus.org

Written in a simple, straightforward style, this easy-to-follow action guide teaches you the most effective strategies for enabling you to get the sleep you want and need!
17 pages

8934 Lupus Book
Lupus Foundation of America
1300 Piccard Drive
Rockville, MD 20850-4303

301-670-9292
800-558-0121
lupusinfo@aol.com
www.lupus.org

Packed with useful, easy-to-understand information and practical guidance for people with lupus, their family members, friends and physicians. This hardcover book explains virtually every aspect of the disease and will help people better manage their day-to-day fight with lupus.
ISBN: 0-195084-43-8
Iris Carden, Author

8935 Lupus Erythematosus: A Handbook for Physicians, Patients & Families
Lupus Foundation of America
1300 Piccard Drive
Rockville, MD 20850-4303

301-670-9292
800-558-0121
lupusinfo@aol.com
www.lupus.org

Written for physicians, people with lupus, their families and friends, this is LFA's most popular publication. The handbook provides a brief, but detailed, overview of the disease and guide for living well with lupus.
60 pages

8936 Lupus: Everything You Need to Know
Lupus Foundation of America
1300 Piccard Drive
Rockville, MD 20850-4303

301-670-9292
800-558-0121
lupusinfo@aol.com
www.lupus.org

Resource written for patients that want to learn more about lupus than what their doctors may or may not tell them.
236 pages
Jean Luc, Author

8937 Sick and Tired of Feeling Sick and Tired
Lupus Foundation of America
1300 Piccard Drive
Rockville, MD 20850-4303

301-670-9292
800-558-0121
lupusinfo@aol.com
www.lupus.org

Written in simple terms, the authors offer all readers- people with invisible chronic illness (ICI's), spouses, friends, family members, employers or health care providers, both understanding and practical guidance. This is a very useful resource for all those who live with ICI's and those who care for and about them.
288 pages
Mary E. E. Siegel, Author
Paul J. Donoghue, Author

8938 We Are Not Alone: Learning to Live with Chronic Illness
Lupus Foundation of America
1300 Piccard Drive
Rockville, MD 20850-4303

301-670-9292
800-558-0121
lupusinfo@aol.com
www.lupus.org

Complete and comprehensive, this book is about redesigning your life... about how to live better, not just differently.
335 pages
Sefra Kobrin Pritzele, Author

Children's Books

8939 Embracing the Wolf: A Lupus Victim and Her Family Learn to Live
Cherokee Publishing Company
PO Box 1730   770-438-7366
Marietta, GA 30061-1730   800-653-3952
This book gives a very detailed account of the effects of the disease that include emotions and moods for the victim and the way in which these attributes affect loved ones.
192 pages Hardcover
ISBN: 0-877971-66-8
Kenneth W Boyd, Publisher

8940 In Search of the Sun: A Woman's Courageous Victory Over Lupus
Scribner
866 3rd Avenue   212-702-2000
New York, NY 10022-6221   800-257-5755
This book is a revision of Henrietta Aladjem's book, The Sun Is My Enemy. In this book, with Peter Schur she discusses her fight with this deadly and widespread disease.
Grades 10-12

8941 When Mom Gets Sick
Lupus Foundation of America
1300 Piccard Drive   301-670-9292
Rockville, MD 20850-4303   800-558-0121
                                                 lupusinfo@aol.com
                                                 www.lupus.org
Written and illustrated by a 9-year-old, this is a compelling story based on the experiences of a sensitive and insightful young girl who makes the best from what could be a devastating situation.
27 pages

Newsletters

8942 Heliogram
Lupus Network
230 Ranch Drive   203-372-5795
Bridgeport, CT 06606-1747
Includes book reviews, medical abstracts and resource listings of physicians.
Quarterly
ISBN: 0-887168-0 -
Linda Rosinsky, Editor

8943 Informer
Simon Foundation
PO Box 815   847-864-3913
Wilmette, IL 60091-0815   Fax: 847-864-9758
Offers information and the latest updates concerning incontinence treatments, cures, medical aspects, resources and more.
Quarterly

8944 Lupus Foundation of America Memphis Area Chapter Newsletter
Lupus Foundation of America Memphis Area Chapter
3181 Poplar Avenue   901-458-5320
Memphis, TN 38111   888-915-8787
                                                 Fax: 901-217-3193

Monthly
Yvonne D Nelson, Executive Director

8945 Lupus Informer
Lupus Foundation of America: Arkansas Chapter
220 Mockingbird   501-525-9380
Hot Springs, AR 71913   800-294-8878
                                                 Fax: 501-525-9380
                                                 lupusarkhs@direclynx.net
                                                 www.lupus-arkansas.com

Lupus Chapter membership dues annually
Jamesetta Smith, President/CEO

8946 Lupus News
Lupus Foundation of America
1300 Piccard Drive   301-670-9292
Rockville, MD 20850-4303   800-558-0121
Provides detailed news for physicians, patients, their families and friends on lupus.
Quarterly

8947 Pennsylvania Lupus News
Lupus Foundation of Pennsylvania
Landmarks Building   412-261-5886
Pittsburgh, PA 15219   Fax: 412-261-5365
                                                 www.lupuspa.org

Deborah Nigro, Executive Director
Marian Belotti RN, Patient Services Director

8948 The Loop
SLE Lupus Foundation
330 Seventh Avenue   212-685-4118
New York, NY 10001   Fax: 212-545-1843
                                                 www.lupusny.org

Richard K DeScherer, President
Margaret G Dowd, Executive Director

Pamphlets

8949 Control Your Pain!
Lupus Foundation of America
1300 Piccard Drive   301-670-9292
Rockville, MD 20850-4303   800-558-0121
                                                 lupusinfo@aol.com
                                                 www.lupus.org
This easy to read booklet offers 144 concrete strategies for reducing and managing the pain of lupus.
48 pages

8950 Facts About Lupus
Lupus Foundation of America
1300 Piccard Drive   301-670-9292
Rockville, MD 20850-4303   800-558-0121
                                                 lupusinfo@aol.com
                                                 www.lupus.org
A series of brochures on a wide range of lupus-related topics including lab tests, medications, joint and muscle involvement, skin involvement, lupus and the kidneys, central nervous system involvement, lupus in men, pregnancy, well/coping, etc.
21 Brochures

8951 Handout on Health: Systemic Lupus Erythematosus
NAMSIC/National Institutes of Health
1 AMS Circle   301-495-4484
Bethesda, MD 20892-0001   877-226-4267
                                                 Fax: 301-718-6366
                                                 TTY: 301-565-2966
                                                 niamsinfo@mail.nih.gov
                                                 www.nih.gov/niams

8952 Living Well, Despite Lupus!
Lupus Foundation of America
1300 Piccard Drive   301-670-9292
Rockville, MD 20850   800-558-0121
                                                 lupusinfo@aol.com
                                                 www.lupus.org
This booklet offers 204 sure-fire strategies for taking charge of your life to enable you to live well.
1996 50 pages
ISBN: 0-895294-75-3

8953 Lupus Eritematoso (Spanish Booklet)
Lupus Foundation of America
1300 Piccard Drive   301-670-9292
Rockville, MD 20850-4303   800-558-0121
                                                 lupusinfo@aol.com
                                                 www.lupus.org
Written for physicians, people with lupus, their families and friends, this is LFA's most popular publication. The handbook pro-

vides a brief, but detailed, overview of the disease and guide for living well with lupus.

8954 Lupus Erythematosus
Lupus Foundation of America
1300 Piccard Drive
Rockville, MD 20850-4303

301-670-9292
800-558-0121
lupusinfo@aol.com
www.lupus.org

This booklet is intended to help patients understand what lupus is, how it may affect their lives and what they can do to help themselves and their physician in the management of the illness.
Edmund L. Dubois, Author
Daniel J. Wallace, Author

8955 Lupus Information Package
NAMSIC/National Institutes of Health
1 AMS Circle
Bethesda, MD 20892-0001

301-495-4484
877-226-4267
Fax: 301-718-6366
TTY: 301-565-2966
niamsinfo@mail.nih.gov
www.nih.gov/niams

8956 Many Shades of Lupus: Information for Multicultural Communities
NAMSIC/National Institutes of Health
1 AMS Circle
Bethesda, MD 20892-0001

301-495-4484
877-226-4267
Fax: 301-587-4352
TTY: 301-565-2966
niamsinfo@mail.nih.gov
www.nih.gov/niams

Audio & Video

8957 For Life: More Stories of Lupus
Marcia Urbin Raymond, author
Fanlight Productions
4196 Washington Street
Boston, MA 02131

617-469-4999
800-937-4113
Fax: 617-469-3349
fanlight@fanlight.com
www.fanlight.com

Three years after 'Stories of Lupus', the filmmaker revisits five people from the earlier film, to explore the day-to-day challenges and gifts that come to people living with a chronic illness as it evolves over time.
2002 53 Minutes
ISBN: 1-572954-17-5
Nicole Johnson, Publicity Coordinator

8958 Stories of Lupus
Fanlight Productions
4196 Washington Street
Boston, MA 02131

617-469-4999
800-937-4113
Fax: 617-469-3379
fanlight@fanlight.com
www.fanlight.com

Recently diagnosed with lupus, the filmmakers go on the road to interview others enduring the precarious roller coaster of symptoms, treatment, flare-ups and recoveries which characterize this complex, mysterious, and often life-threatening disease.
1999 27 Minutes
ISBN: 1-572954-16-7
Nicole Johnson, Publicity Coordinator

Web Sites

8959 Healing Well
www.healingwell.com
An online health resource guide to medical news, chat, information and articles, newsgroups and message boards, books, disease-related web sites, medical directories, and more for patients, friends, and family coping with disabling diseases, disorders, or chronic illnesses.

8960 Health Finder
www.healthfinder.gov
Searchable, carefully developed web site offering information on over 1000 topics. Developed by the US Department of Health and Human Services, the site can be used in both English and Spanish.

8961 Healthlink USA
www.healthlinkusa.com
Health information concerning treatment, cures, prevention, diagnosis, risk factors, research, support groups, email lists, personal stories and much more. Updated regularly.

8962 Lupus Foundation of America
www.lupus.org
The LFA mission is to assist local chapters in their efforts to provide supportive services to individuals living with lupus, educate the public about lupus, and supports research into the cause and cure of lupus.

8963 MedicineNet
www.medicinenet.com
An online resource for consumers providing easy-to-read, authoritative medical and health information.

8964 Medscape
www.medscape.com
Medscape offers specialists, primary care physicians, and other health professionals the Web's most robust and integrated medical information and educational tools.

8965 WebMD
www.webmd.com
Provides credible information, supportive communities, and in-depth reference material about health subjects. A source for original and timely health information as well as material from well known content providers.

Description

8966 Tay-Sachs Disease

Tay-Sachs disease is a lysosomal storage disease that results from mutations in the HEXA gene, which encodes the enzyme (hexosaminidase A). Insufficient hexosaminidase A activity leads to an accumulation of a lipid called a GM2 ganglioside in the brain (cerebral neurons), which causes the progressive death of nerve cells in the brain. The disease is genetic and is autosomal recessive; if two carriers have children, the disease would have a 1 in 4 chance of being passed on. The disease is most prevalent in those of Jewish families, particularly those of Eastern European (Ashkenazi) background. Other mutations in the HEXA gene cluster in French-Canadian and Cajun populations.

Symptoms usually present between 3-6 months of age. After 6 months, the child begins to miss developmental milestones. Early symptoms include mild muscle weakness, muscle spasms, and feeding difficulties. As the disease progresses, the patient may experience vision loss, seizures and eventually paralysis. Death usually occurs by the age of 4 years.

Treatment for Tay-Sachs disease is supportive and there is no cure. Genetic and premarital counseling is important to those at high risk.

National Agencies & Associations

8967 Jewish Genetics Disease Center
1425 Madison Avenue
New York, NY 10029

212-659-6700
Fax: 212-360-1809
www.icahn.mssm.edu

International resource for the study, diagnosis, and treatment of Jewish genetic diseases.
Robert J. Desnick, PhD, MD, Director

8968 National Institute of Child Health and Human Development
PO Box 3006
Rockville, MD 20847

800-370-2943
Fax: 866-760-5947
TTY: 888-320-6942
www.nichd.nih.gov

NICHD seeks to better understand disabilities and important events that occur during pregnancy.
Diana W. Bianchi, MD, Director
Constantine Stratakis, Scientific Director

8969 National Institute of Neurological Disorders and Stroke
NIH Neurological Institute
Bethesda, MD 20824

301-496-5751
800-352-9424
www.ninds.nih.gov

Seeks to reduce the burden of neurological disease affecting individuals from all walks of life.
Walter J. Koroshetz, MD, Director
Amy B. Adams, Director, Office of Scientific Liaison

8970 National Organization for Rare Disorders
55 Kenosia Avenue
Danbury, CT 06810-1968

203-744-0100
800-999-6673
Fax: 203-263-9938
www.rarediseases.org

NORD is a federation of voluntary health organizations dedicated to helping people with rare orphan diseases and assisting the organizations that serve them. It is committed to the identification, treatment, and cure of rare disorders through programs of education, advocacy, research, and service.
Peter Saltonstall, President & CEO
Pamela Gavin, Chief Strategy Officer

8971 National Tay-Sachs and Allied Diseases Association
2001 Beacon Street
Brighton, MA 02135

617-277-4463
info@ntsad.org
www.ntsad.org

Patient advocacy group funding research, raising awareness to prevent diseases, and supporting families and individuals around the world.
Sue Kahn, Executive Director
Diana Pangonis, Director, Family Svcs & Communications

Support Groups & Hotlines

8972 National Health Information Center
Office of Disease Prevention & Health Promotion
1101 Wootton Pkwy
Rockville, MD 20852

Fax: 240-453-8281
odphpinfo@hhs.gov
www.health.gov/nhic

Supports public health education by maintaining a calendar of National Health Observances; helps connect consumers and health professionals to organizations that can best answer questions and provide up-to-date contact information from reliable sources; updates on a yearly basis toll-free numbers for health information, Federal health clearinghouses and info centers.
Don Wright, MD, MPH, Director

8973 National Tay-Sachs & Allied Diseases Association of Delaware Valley
PO Box 441
Jenkintown, PA 19046

215-887-0877
Fax: 215-887-1931
info@tay-sachs.org
www.tay-sachs.org

Rebecca Tantala, Executive Director

8974 National TaySachs & Allied Diseases Association
2001 Beacon Street
Boston, MA 2135

617-277-4463
800-906-8723
Fax: 617-277-0134
info@ntsad.org
www.ntsad.org

A mutual support group coordinated by staff and volunteers who are parents of affected children or affected adults. One of several programs supported and sponsored by the association.
Sue Kahn, Executive Director
Diana Pangonis, Director, Family Svcs & Communications

Books

8975 Home Care Book
National Tay-Sachs and Allied Diseases Association
2001 Beacon Street
Brighton, MA 02135

617-277-4463
800-906-8723
Fax: 617-277-0134
info@ntsad.org
www.ntsad.org

Written by parents for parents and professionals, the Home Care Book is a guide to caring for children with progressive neurological disorders at home.
Shari Ungerleider, President
Merle Adelman, Vice President Development

8976 Home-Care Book
National Tay-Sachs and Allied Diseases Association
2001 Beacon Street
Brookline, MA 02146

617-277-4463
800-906-8723
Fax: 617-277-0134
info@ntsad.org
www.ntsad.org

National Tay-Sachs & Allied Diseases Association (NTSAD) is one of the oldest patient advocacy groups in the country. We focus on funding research, supporting over 500 families and individuals worldwide, and raising awareness to prevent disease
Shari Ungerleider, President
Merle Adelman, Vice President Development

8977 Late Onset Tay-Sachs Disease Medical Bibliography
National Tay-Sachs and Allied Diseases Association

2001 Beacon Street
Brookline, MA 02146

617-277-4463
800-906-8723
Fax: 617-277-0134
info@ntsad.org
www.ntsad.org

National Tay-Sachs & Allied Diseases Association (NTSAD) is one of the oldest patient advocacy groups in the country. We focus on funding research, supporting over 500 families and individuals worldwide, and raising awareness to prevent disease
Shari Ungerleider, President
Merle Adelman, Vice President Development

8978 Lifting of Canavan's Carrier Testing Facilities
National Tay-Sachs and Allied Diseases Association
2001 Beacon Street
Brookline, MA 02146

617-277-4463
800-906-8723
Fax: 617-277-0134
info@ntsad.org
www.ntsad.org

National Tay-Sachs & Allied Diseases Association (NTSAD) is one of the oldest patient advocacy groups in the country. We focus on funding research, supporting over 500 families and individuals worldwide, and raising awareness to prevent disease
Shari Ungerleider, President
Merle Adelman, Vice President Development

8979 Monograph on Canavan's Disease
National Tay-Sachs and Allied Diseases Association
2001 Beacon Street
Brookline, MA 02146

617-277-4463
800-906-8723
Fax: 617-277-0134
info@ntsad.org
www.ntsad.org

National Tay-Sachs & Allied Diseases Association (NTSAD) is one of the oldest patient advocacy groups in the country. We focus on funding research, supporting over 500 families and individuals worldwide, and raising awareness to prevent disease
Shari Ungerleider, President
Merle Adelman, Vice President Development

8980 Tay-Sachs Carrier Testing Directory
National Tay-Sachs and Allied Diseases Association
2001 Beacon Street
Brookline, MA 02146

617-277-4463
800-906-8723
Fax: 617-277-0134
info@ntsad.org
www.ntsad.org

National Tay-Sachs & Allied Diseases Association (NTSAD) is one of the oldest patient advocacy groups in the country. We focus on funding research, supporting over 500 families and individuals worldwide, and raising awareness to prevent disease
Shari Ungerleider, President
Merle Adelman, Vice President Development

8981 Tay-Sachs: The Dreaded Inheritance
National Tay-Sachs and Allied Diseases Assocation
2001 Beacon Street
Brighton, MA 02135

617-277-4463
800-906-8723
Fax: 617-277-0134
info@ntsad.org
www.ntsad.org

Descriptive narrative on caring for a child with Tay-Sachs Disease.
Shari Ungerleider, President
Merle Adelman, Vice President Development

8982 There is Only One Child
National Tay-Sachs and Allied Diseases Association
2001 Beacon Street
Brookline, MA 02146

617-277-4463
800-906-8723
Fax: 617-277-0134
info@ntsad.org
www.ntsad.org

National Tay-Sachs & Allied Diseases Association (NTSAD) is one of the oldest patient advocacy groups in the country. We focus on funding research, supporting over 500 families and individuals worldwide, and raising awareness to prevent disease
Shari Ungerleider, President
Merle Adelman, Vice President Development

8983 What Every Family Should Know Sixth Edition
National Tay-Sachs & Allied Diseases Association
2001 Beacon Street
Brighton, MA 02135

617-277-4463
800-906-8723
Fax: 617-277-0134
info@ntsad.org
www.ntsad.org

Detailing lysosomal storage and leukodystrophy disorders, with sections on Tay-Sachs, Sandhoff, Niemann-Pick, Gaucher, Canavan, Fabry, Pompe, therapeutic approaches and unique disease table.
50 pages
Shari Ungerleider, President
Merle Adelman, Vice President Development

Newsletters

8984 Breakthrough
National Tay-Sachs and Allied Diseases Association
2001 Beacon Street
Boston, MA 02135

617-277-4463
800-906-8723
Fax: 617-277-0134
info@ntsad.org
www.ntsad.org

Each year NTSAD publishes a newsletter for friends and supporters that focuses on the latest advances in research, profiles of families and individuals helped by NTSAD and disease profiles.
Annual
Shari Ungerleider, President
Merle Adelman, Vice President Development

8985 Late Onset Community Newsletter
National Tay-Sachs and Allied Diseases Association
2001 Beacon Street
Brighton, MA 02135

617-277-4463
800-906-8723
Fax: 617-277-0134
info@ntsad.org
www.ntsad.org

PSG members dealing with chronic forms of the allied diseases receive this newsletter focused specifically on the issues and perspectives unique to adults struggling with long-term disability issues. Public editions of the newsletter are also available.
Bi-Monthly
Shari Ungerleider, President
Merle Adelman, Vice President Development

8986 Lifeline
National Tay-Sachs and Allied Diseases Association
2001 Beacon Street
Brighton, MA 02135

617-277-4463
800-906-8723
Fax: 617-277-0134
info@ntsad.org
www.ntsad.org

The editorial content is wide ranging: symptom management and home health care; new product reviews; guidance in benefits and services advocacy for families and affected individuals of all ages; science and medical research updates; coverage of NTSAD events, fundraising, programs and administrative activities. Members only.
Quarterly
Shari Ungerleider, President
Merle Adelman, Vice President Development

Pamphlets

8987 Late Onset Tay-Sachs Fact Sheet
National Tay-Sachs and Allied Diseases Association
2001 Beacon Street
Brighton, MA 02135

617-277-4463
800-906-8723
Fax: 617-277-0134
info@ntsad.org
www.ntsad.org

This quick reference information sheet on the chronic or late onset form of Tay-Sachs is available for no charge.
Shari Ungerleider, President
Merle Adelman, Vice President Development

8988 Services to Families
National Tay-Sachs and Allied Diseases Association
2001 Beacon Street   617-277-4463
Brookline, MA 02146   800-906-8723
                                  Fax: 617-277-0134
                                  info@ntsad.org
                                  www.ntsad.org
National Tay-Sachs & Allied Diseases Association (NTSAD) is one of the oldest patient advocacy groups in the country. We focus on funding research, supporting over 500 families and individuals worldwide, and raising awareness to prevent disease
Shari Ungerleider, President
Merle Adelman, Vice President Development

8989 Tay-Sachs Information Sheet
March of Dimes
1275 Mamaroneck Avenue   212-353-8353
White Plains, NY 10605   Fax: 212-254-3518
                                  NY639@marchofdimes.com
                                  www.marchofdimes.com
Offers a brief overview of the illness, causes, symptoms and treatments are covered. Availabe electronically on the website: www.marchofdimes.com

8990 Tay-Sachs is
National Tay-Sachs and Allied Diseases Association
2001 Beacon Street   617-277-4463
Brookline, MA 02146   800-906-8723
                                  Fax: 617-277-0134
                                  info@ntsad.org
                                  www.ntsad.org
National Tay-Sachs & Allied Diseases Association (NTSAD) is one of the oldest patient advocacy groups in the country. We focus on funding research, supporting over 500 families and individuals worldwide, and raising awareness to prevent disease
Shari Ungerleider, President
Merle Adelman, Vice President Development

8991 Understanding Lysosomal Storage Diseases
National Tay-Sachs and Allied Diseases Association
2001 Beacon Street   617-277-4463
Brookline, MA 02146   800-906-8723
                                  Fax: 617-277-0134
                                  info@ntsad.org
                                  www.ntsad.org
National Tay-Sachs & Allied Diseases Association (NTSAD) is one of the oldest patient advocacy groups in the country. We focus on funding research, supporting over 500 families and individuals worldwide, and raising awareness to prevent disease
Shari Ungerleider, President
Merle Adelman, Vice President Development

8992 What is Canavan Disease?
National Tay-Sachs and Allied Diseases Association
2001 Beacon Street   617-277-4463
Brighton, MA 02135   800-906-8723
                                  Fax: 617-277-0134
                                  info@ntsad.org
                                  www.ntsad.org
The educational pamphlet describing Canavan Disease.
Shari Ungerleider, President
Merle Adelman, Vice President Development

8993 What is Tay-Sachs? Russian Translation
National Tay-Sachs and Allied Diseases Association
2001 Beacon Street   617-277-4463
Brighton, MA 02135   800-906-8723
                                  Fax: 617-277-0134
                                  info@ntsad.org
                                  www.ntsad.org
This informative educational pamphlet describing Infantile Tay-Sachs, its inheritance and prevention is available for no charge.
Shari Ungerleider, President
Merle Adelman, Vice President Development

Audio & Video

8994 For My Sister, Elyssa
National Tay-Sachs & Allied Diseases Assocation
2001 Beacon Street   617-277-4463
Brighton, MA 02135   800-906-8723
                                  Fax: 617-277-0134
                                  info@ntsad.org
                                  www.ntsad.org
Moving and informative 15 minute presentation told by a teenager who baby siter died from Tay-Sachs Disease. Contains information on Tay-Sachs Disease and simple steps each individual can take to prevent the tragedy of Tay-Sachs.
Shari Ungerleider, President
Merle Adelman, Vice President Development

Web Sites

8995 Healing Well
                                  www.healingwell.com
An online health resource guide to medical news, chat, information and articles, newsgroups and message boards, books, disease-related web sites, medical directories, and more for patients, friends, and family coping with disabling diseases, disorders, or chronic illnesses.

8996 Health Finder
                                  www.healthfinder.gov
Searchable, carefully developed web site offering information on over 1000 topics. Developed by the US Department of Health and Human Services, the site can be used in both English and Spanish.

8997 Healthlink USA
                                  www.healthlinkusa.com
Health information concerning treatment, cures, prevention, diagnosis, risk factors, research, support groups, email lists, personal stories and much more. Updated regularly.

8998 MedicineNet
                                  www.medicinenet.com
An online resource for consumers providing easy-to-read, authoritative medical and health information.

8999 Medscape
                                  www.medscape.com
Medscape offers specialists, primary care physicians, and other health professionals the Web's most robust and integrated medical information and educational tools.

9000 National Organization for Rare Disorders
                                  www.rarediseases.org
NORD is a federation of voluntary health organizations dedicated to helping people with rare orphan diseases and assisting the organizations that serve them. It is committed to the identification, treatment, and cure of rare disorders through programs of education, advocacy, research, and service. Website features resources for patients and families, patient organizations, and clinicians and researchers.

9001 WebMD
                                  www.webmd.com
Provides credible information, supportive communities, and in-depth reference material about health subjects. A source for original and timely health information as well as material from well known content providers.

Description

9002 Thyroid Disease

Thyroid Disease refers to a number of conditions that affect the thyroid, a small, butterfly-shaped gland located in the middle of the lower neck. Hormones T3 and T4, produced by the thyroid, deliver energy to cells of the body, thus controlling the body's metabolism. Conditions that result from an imbalance of these hormones are hypothyroidism — not enough thyroid hormones that results in the body using energy slower than it should, and hyperthyroidism — too much thyroid hormones that results in the body using energy faster than it should. These conditions can be caused by an inflammation of the thyroid gland, too much or too little iodine (used to produce thyroid hormones), or autoimmune disease, in which antibodies gradually either destroy the thyroid gland or speed up its function. Other thyroid conditions are Goiter — an enlarged thyroid; Thyroid Nodules — cysts, lumps, bumps and tumors that can be cancerous or benign; and Thyroiditis — inflammation of the thyroid gland. More than 20 million Americans have thyroid disease, and it affects many more women than men. Treatment includes synthetic hormone medication to replace missing hormones, radioactive iodine to deactivate the thyroid, and surgery for some goiters and cancerous nodules. Early diagnosis is often the key in prescribing treatment even before the onset of symptoms. Although thyroid disease is a chronic condition, careful disease management allows affected individuals to live healthy, normal lives.

National Agencies & Associations

9003 American Thyroid Association
6066 Leesburg Pike thyroid@thyroid.org
Falls Church, VA 22041 www.thyroid.org
Worldwide medical society and organization committed to the prevention, diagnosis, and treatment of thyroid disorders and thyroid cancer.
Elizabeth N. Pearce, MD, MSc, President
Victor J. Bernet, MD, Secretary & COO

9004 HealthyWomen
1 Harding Road 732-530-3425
Red Bank, NJ 07701 877-986-9472
info@healthywomen.org
www.healthywomen.org
Independent, non-profit organization seeking to educate women in all areas of health, to allow them to make informed choices. The HealthyWomen website features numerous tools and health calculators, plus other media.
Beth Battaglino, RN, Chief Executive Officer
Phyllis E. Greenberger, Sr. VP, Science & Health Policy

9005 Thyroid Federation International
PO Box 471 tfi@thyroid-fed.org
Bath, Ontario, K0H-1G0 www.thyroid-fed.org
A global network of organizations supporting individuals with thyroid disorders by providing resources and raising awareness.
Ashok Bhaseen, President
Peter Lakwijk, Treasurer

9006 Thyroid Foundation of Canada
PO Box 298 800-267-8822
Bath, Ontario, K0H-1G0 www.thyroid.ca

Established in 1980, the Thyroid Foundation of Canada was the first thyroid foundation in the world, and continues to provide resources and information for individuals affected by thyroid disease.
Laz Bouros, President
Kim McNally, Vice President

Support Groups & Hotlines

9007 National Health Information Center
Office of Disease Prevention & Health Promotion
1101 Wootton Pkwy Fax: 240-453-8281
Rockville, MD 20852 odphpinfo@hhs.gov
www.health.gov/nhic
Supports public health education by maintaining a calendar of National Health Observances; helps connect consumers and health professionals to organizations that can best answer questions and provide up-to-date contact information from reliable sources; updates on a yearly basis toll-free numbers for health information, Federal health clearinghouses and info centers.
Don Wright, MD, MPH, Director

Books

9008 The Thyroid Gland
Joel I Hamburger MD & Michael M Kaplan, author
Thyroid Foundation of Canada
P.O. Box 298 613-544-8364
Bath, -1G1 800-267-8822
Fax: 613-544-9731
www.thyroid.ca
The Thyroid Foundation of Canada is a non-profit registered volunteer organization whose mission is to support thyroid patients across Canada through awareness, education, and research
Donna Miniely, President
Rinda Hartner, Treasurer

9009 Thyroid Disease: The Facts
RIS Bayliss & WMG Tunbridge MD, author
Thyroid Foundation of Canada
P.O. Box 298 613-544-8364
Bath, -1G1 800-267-8822
Fax: 613-544-9731
www.thyroid.ca
The Thyroid Foundation of Canada is a non-profit registered volunteer organization whose mission is to support thyroid patients across Canada through awareness, education, and research
Donna Miniely, President
Rinda Hartner, Treasurer

9010 Thyroid Sourcebook
Thyroid Foundation of Canada
P.O. Box 298 613-544-8364
Bath, -1G1 800-267-8822
Fax: 613-544-9731
www.thyroid.ca
The Thyroid Foundation of Canada is a non-profit registered volunteer organization whose mission is to support thyroid patients across Canada through awareness, education, and research
Donna Miniely, President
Rinda Hartner, Treasurer

9011 Your Thyroid: A Home Reference
Lawrence Wood MD & David S Cooper MD, author
Thyroid Foundation of Canada
P.O. Box 298 613-544-8364
Bath, -1G1 800-267-8822
Fax: 613-544-9731
www.thyroid.ca
The Thyroid Foundation of Canada is a non-profit registered volunteer organization whose mission is to support thyroid patients across Canada through awareness, education, and research
Donna Miniely, President
Rinda Hartner, Treasurer

Magazines

9012 Clinical Thyroidology
American Thyroid Association
6066 Leesburg Pike
Falls Church, VA 22041

703-998-8890
800-849-7634
Fax: 703-998-8893
thyroid@thyroid.org
www.thyroid.org

An online publication, available monthly, this is a broad-ranging look at clinical and preclinical thyroid literature. The Editor searches the world literature for excellent thyroid studies and then summarizes them along side his expert commentary.
Robert C. Smallridge, President
John C. Morris, Secretary/Chief Operating Officer

9013 THYROID
American Thyroid Association
6066 Leesburg Pike
Falls Church, VA 22041

703-998-8890
800-849-7643
Fax: 703-998-8893
thyroid@thyroid.org
www.thyroid.org

The Associations monthly journal that touches on topics from the molecular biology of the thyroid gland to clinical management of thyroid disorders. All Association members receive a suvscription, and it is available to non-members.
Robert C. Smallridge, President
John C. Morris, Secretary/Chief Operating Officer

9014 Clinical Thyroidology for Patients
American Thyroid Association
6066 Leesburg Pike
Falls Church, VA 22041

703-998-8890
800-849-7634
Fax: 703-998-8893
thyroid@thyroid.org
www.thyroid.org

A collection of summaries of recently published articles fromt the medical literature that covers the broad spectrum of thryroid disorders. Notes descxribing published research studies were prepared by THYROID Editor, Ernest Mazzaferri, MD.
Robert C. Smallridge, President
John C. Morris, Secretary/Chief Operating Officer

Newsletters

9015 SIGNAL
American Thyroid Association
6066 Leesburg Pike
Falls Church, VA 22041

703-998-8890
800-849-7643
Fax: 703-998-8893
thyroid@thyroid.org
www.thyroid.org

Covers Association news, meetings, policies, leaders, and important thyroid-related issues.
Robert C. Smallridge, President
John C. Morris, Secretary/Chief Operating Officer

Pamphlets

9016 Hypothyroidism Web Booklet
American Thyroid Association
6066 Leesburg Pike
Falls Church, VA 22041

703-998-8890
800-489-7643
Fax: 703-998-8893
thyroid@thyroid.org
www.thyroid.org

This online booklet introduces the thryoid and hypothyroidism to the reader, explains symptoms, treatments, causes, who's at risk, and more.
2003 25 pages
Robert C. Smallridge, President
John C. Morris, Secretary/Chief Operating Officer

Web Sites

9017 American Thyroid Association

www.thyroid.org
Promotes excellence and innovation in clinical care, research, education, and public policy.
David S Cooper MD, President
Gregory A Brent MD, Secretary

9018 HealthyWomen

www.healthywomen.org
Independent, non-profit organization seeking to educate women in all areas of health, to allow them to make informed choices. The HealthyWomen website features numerous tools and health calculators, plus other media.

9019 MedicineNet

www.medicinenet.com
An online resource for consumers providing easy-to-read, authoritative medical and health information.

9020 Thyroid Federation International

www.thyroid-fed.org
Aims to work for the benefit of those affected by thyroid disorders throughout the world.

9021 Thyroid Foundation of Canada

www.thyroid.ca
The Thyroid Foundation of Canada is a non-profit registered volunteer organization whose mission is to support thyroid patients across Canada through awareness, education, and research.

Description

9022 Tick-Borne Disease

Ticks transmit disease to humans by being carriers for a variety of microorganisms. The most common tick-borne illness is Lyme disease, first recognized and so named in 1975 because of a cluster of cases found in Lyme, Connecticut. Lyme disease is a bacterial infection caused by Borrelia burgdorferi and is spread by the bite of an infected deer tick. The disease in its earliest stages causes an expanding bull-eye rash in at least 75 percent of patients. Flu-like symptoms — headaches, fever, fatigue — are common. The rash may be followed by progressive joint pain and swelling. Dysfunction of the heart (8 percent) and nervous system (15 percent) develop weeks to months later. Further progression causes arthritis and more serious neurologic problems.

Although only one third of patients remember a tick bite, greater than 60 percent do develop the tell-tale rash. Diagnosis requires a blood test to confirm the physical symptoms.

Oral antibiotics may be sufficient for the disease caught in the early stages. Long-standing, disseminated disease responds best to intravenous antibiotics.

Rocky Mountain spotted fever, also known as tick fever, is transmitted by a bite from either a dog tick or wood tick, depending on the part of the country. Like Lyme disease, it begins with flu-like symptoms — chills, fever and loss of appetite. A rash of small, reddish bumps, which gives the disease its name, begins on the wrist and ankle and spreads to the rest of the body. Aggressive antibiotic treatment should begin as early as possible. If left untreated, Rocky Mountain spotted fever has a mortality rate of 10-80 percent.

Prevention of tick-borne disease requires avoidance of tick bites, by using insect repellants and protective clothing, plus daily checks for ticks during periods of exposure. A vaccine may provide partial protection from Lyme disease for those regularly engaged in high-risk activities (i.e. property maintenance), although other conditions may complicate this treatment.

National Agencies & Associations

9023 American Lyme Disease Foundation
PO Box 466
Lyme, CT 06371
questions@aldf.com
www.aldf.com
The American Lyme Disease Foundation is devoted to the education, treatment, and prevention of Lyme disease, and provides the public with scientifically accurate information.
Phillip J. Baker, PhD, Executive Director
Maria Aguero-Rosenfeld, MD, Associate Director

9024 Global Lyme Alliance
1290 E Main Street
Stamford, CT 06902
202-969-1333
info@GLA.org
globallymealliance.org
Formerly known as the Tick-Borne Disease Alliance, Global Lyme Alliance is a leading organization committed to fighting Lyme dis-

ease and other tick-borne illnesses through conducting research and raising public awareness.
Scott Santarella, CEO
Timothy J. Sellati, PhD, Chief Scientific Officer

9025 Infectious Diseases Society of America
1300 Wilson Boulevard
Arlington, VA 22209
703-299-0200
Fax: 703-299-0204
www.idsociety.org
The Infectious Diseases Society of America (IDSA) represents physicians, scientists and other health care professionals who specialize in infectious diseases, and promotes research and shares knowledge in order to reduce the prevalence of infectious diseases.
Cynthia L. Sears, MD, FIDSA, President
Thomas File, Jr., MD, FIDSA, Chair

9026 Lyme Disease Association, Inc.
PO Box 1438
Jackson, NJ 08527
888-366-6611
Fax: 732-938-7215
LDA@LymeDiseaseAssociation.org
www.lymediseaseassociation.org
Association formed in order to fund research and educate the public about Lyme disease. Offers resources and information on Lyme disease.
Patricia V. Smith, BA, President
Pamela Lampe, Vice President & Treasurer

9027 National Capital Lyme Disease Association
PO Box 8211
McLean, VA 22106-8211
703-821-8833
natcaplyme@natcaplyme.org
www.natcaplyme.org
The National Capital Lyme Disease Association is a non-profit organization operated by volunteers dedicated to helping patients diagnosed with tick-borne illnesses. The association raises awareness to educate the public.
Monte Skall, Executive Director
Gregg Skall, Legal Counsel

Libraries & Resource Centers

9028 California Lyme Disease Association
PO Box 1352
Chico, CA 95927
info@lymedisease.org
www.lymedisease.org
The California Lyme Disease Association (CALDA) is an affiliate of the Lyme Disease Association, Inc. CALDA, a non-profit organization, was originally founded in 1990 as The Lyme Disease Resource Center (LDRC). We provide services for Lyme disease patients, their families and friends; provide a forum for physicians and health professionals for the exchange of ideas and information about symptoms, diagnosis, and treatment of Lyme disease.
Marilynn Barkley, Board of Directors
Barbara Barsoschinni, Board of Directors

Research Centers

9029 Ball State University Public Health Entomology Laboratory
2000 University Avenue
Muncie, IN 47306
765-289-1241
800-382-8540
TTY: 7
www.bsu.edu
Offers information on mosquitoes and mosquito-born diseases specializing in Lyme Disease.
Bob Pinger, Director
Jeffrey Clark, Department Chair and Professor

9030 Centers for Disease Control Division of Vector Borne Infectious Diseases
US Public Health Service
1600 Clifton Rd.
Atlanta, GA 30333
800-232-4636
Fax: 970-216-76
TDD: 888-232-6348
www.cdc.gov
Research done into lyme disease tularemia bubonic plague and all vector-borne infectious diseases — including west nile virus.
Dr. Tom Frieden, Director

Support Groups & Hotlines

9031 Advocates 4 Health: Tick-borne Disease Self-Help Group
PALS
PO Box 1271   805-544-0984
San Luis Obispo, CA 93406   advocates4heatlh@yahoo.com
Advocacy and support group increasing awareness, education and understanding of tick-borne disorders and other zoonotic diseases. This group fosters a supportive network between human/animal sufferers, caregivers, health care professionals and the general community.
Sheryl Glidden

9032 American Lyme Disease Foundation
2518 Ridge Court   785-248-3504
Lawrence, CT 66046   Inquire@aldf.com
                                                     www.aldf.com
Supports research and plays a key role in providing reliable and scientifically accurate information to the public and health care providers.
David L Weld, Executive Director
Jeffery Black, Partner

9033 Lyme Alliance
PO Box 454   517-563-3582
Concord, MI 49237   www.lymealliance.org
Lyme Alliance volunteers will address your questions concerning the newsletter, website, or questions about doctor referrals, medical treatment options, or information about Lyme disease.

9034 Lyme Disease Network
43 Winton Road   651-644-7239
East Brunswick, NJ 08816
Lynn M Olivier

9035 Lyme Disease Network Support Group of Alabama: Mobile Chapter
Mobile, AL 35758   256-772-6482
                                                 alabamalyme@usa.com
Support information, and referrals for victims of Lyme disease and their families.
Kara Tyson

9036 Lyme Disease Network of New Jersey
43 Winton Road   carol@lymenet.org
East Brunswick, NJ 08816   www.lymenet.org
Support information, and referrals for victims of Lyme disease and their families. Maintains comuter information system.
Bill Stolow, President

9037 Lyme Disease Network of South Carolina
Po Box 6634   803-798-5963
Columbia, SC 29260-6634
Sue Fox

9038 National Health Information Center
Office of Disease Prevention & Health Promotion
1101 Wootton Pkwy   Fax: 240-453-8281
Rockville, MD 20852   odphpinfo@hhs.gov
                                                    www.health.gov/nhic
Supports public health education by maintaining a calendar of National Health Observances; helps connect consumers and health professionals to organizations that can best answer questions and provide up-to-date contact information from reliable sources; updates on a yearly basis toll-free numbers for health information, Federal health clearinghouses and info centers.
Don Wright, MD, MPH, Director

Books

9039 Coping with Lyme Disease: A Practical Guide
Henry Holt & Company
115 W 18th Street   212-886-9200
New York, NY 10011-4113   Fax: 212-633-0748
1993 288 pages Paperback
ISBN: 0-805026-50-9

9040 Ecology & Environment Management of Lyme Disease
Rutgers University Press

109 Church Street   201-932-7762
New Brunswick, NJ 08901-1242
1993 224 pages
ISBN: 0-813519-28-4

9041 Everything You Need to Know About Lyme Disease
John Wiley & Sons Publishing
111 River Street   212-850-6000
Hoboken, NJ 07030-0012   800-225-5945
                                                    Fax: 201-748-6088
                                                    info@wiley.com
                                                    www.wiley.com
Wiley's Professional Development business creates products and services that help customers become more effective in the workplace and achieve career success
237 pages
ISBN: 0-471160-61-X
Stephen M. Smith, President and Chief Executive Officer
John Kritzmacher, Executive Vice President

9042 Let's Talk About Having Lyme Disease
Rosen Publishing Group's PowerKids Press
29 East 21st Street   212-777-3017
New York, NY 10010   800-237-9932
                                                   Fax: 888-436-4643
                                        customerservice@rosenpub.com
                                                www.rosenpublishing.com
Kids are taught to take precautions when walking in the woods and how to inspect themselves for ticks. The illness and recovery are also explained.
Grades K-4
ISBN: 0-823950-29-8
Elizabeth Weitzman, Author

Children's Books

9043 Lyme Disease
Franklin Watts Grolier
90 Old Sherman Turnpike   203-797-3500
Danbury, CT 06816-0001   800-621-1115
                                                   Fax: 203-797-3197
                                                   www.grolier.com
This book discusses the symptoms, prevention, treatments and the role of the tick. This source will not only help readers become aware of Lyme Disease, it will help them become informed.
64 pages Grades 5-7
ISBN: 0-531109-31-3

9044 Lyme Disease and Other Pest-Borne Illnesses
Franklin Watts Grolier
90 Old Sherman Turnpike   203-797-3500
Danbury, CT 06816-0001   800-621-1115
                                                   Fax: 203-797-3197
                                                   www.grolier.com
Scientific, without being technical, this book explains what Lyme Disease is, symptoms, causes and what a person can do if they contract it.
112 pages Grades 7-12
ISBN: 0-531125-23-8

Magazines

9045 Vector Borne & Zoonotic Diseases
Mary Ann Liebert
140 Huguenot Street   914-740-2100
New Rochelle, NY 10801-1961   800-654-3238
                                                   Fax: 914-740-2101
                                             www.liebertpub.com/vbz
Essential multidisiplinary journal dedicated to all aspects of human diseases that occur as zoonoses or are transmitted by invertibrate vectors.
Quarterly

Newsletters

9046 Lymelight Newsletter
Lyme Disease Foundation
1 Financial Plaza   860-525-2000
Hartford, CT 06103-2608   800-886-5963
                                          Fax: 860-525-8425
Newsletter offering up to date information on Lyme Disease and
related disorders, Foundation activities, conference and fund-raising information and resources.
4x Year

Pamphlets

9047 Frequently Asked Questions
Lyme Disease Foundation
1 Financial Plaza   860-525-2000
Hartford, CT 06103-2608   800-886-5963
                                          Fax: 860-525-8425
Overview of testing, treatment, transmission, and pregnancy.

9048 Guide to Lyme Disease
Lyme Disease Foundation
1 Financial Plaza   860-525-2000
Hartford, CT 06103-2608   800-886-5963
                                          Fax: 860-525-8425
Detailed information about Lyme disease and the LDF.

9049 Guide to Tick Spread Diseases
Lyme Disease Foundation
1 Financial Plaza   860-525-2000
Hartford, CT 06103-2608   800-886-5963
                                          Fax: 860-525-8425
                                               www.lyme.org
Symptoms, diagnosis and treatment for a variety of diseases.
16 pages

9050 Guide to Tick-Borne Disorders
Lyme Disease Foundation
1 Financial Plaza   860-525-2000
Hartford, CT 06103-2608   800-886-5963
                                          Fax: 860-525-8425
Symptoms, diagnosis, and treatment for a variety of diseases.

9051 LD Alert Card
Lyme Disease Foundation
1 Financial Plaza   860-525-2000
Hartford, CT 06103-2608   800-886-5963
                                          Fax: 860-525-8425
LD symptoms and prevention information.

9052 LD Awareness Packet
Lyme Disease Foundation
1 Financial Plaza   860-525-2000
Hartford, CT 06103-2608   800-886-5963
                                          Fax: 860-525-8425
Educational letter-size posters, brochures listed above, case
counts, Spanish information, insurance problem information,
General Diagnostic poster, & more.

9053 Lyme Disease & Pets
Lyme Disease Foundation
1 Financial Plaza   860-525-2000
Hartford, CT 06103-2608   800-886-5963
                                          Fax: 860-525-8425
                                          lymefna@aol.com
                                               www.lyme.org
Offers information on Lyme Disease and other tick-borne disor-
ders, through pets and animal transmission.
T Forchaser, Executive Director

9054 Quick Guide to Lyme Disease
American Lyme Disease Foundation
Post Office Box 466   914-277-6970
Lyme, CT 06371   Fax: 914-277-6974
                                          Executivedir@aldf.com
                                               www.aldf.com

Epidemiology, the cause of the disease, recognizing the symptoms,
what to do if you are bitten, treatment, vaccine and other tick-borne
diseases are all covered. One free copy, quantity prices vary.
Phillip J. Baker, Executive Director
Robert A. Proctor, Managing Director

9055 Self-Help (S-H) Program
Lyme Disease Foundation
1 Financial Plaza   860-525-2000
Hartford, CT 06103-2608   800-886-5963
                                          Fax: 860-525-8425
How to establish and conduct a S-H Group. Video, instruction
manual, brochure masters, posters, and more.
28 minutes

9056 Understanding Lyme Disease: Entendiendo Lyme Disease
American Lyme Disease Foundation
Post Office Box 466   914-277-6970
Lyme, CT 06371   Fax: 914-277-6974
                                          Executivedir@aldf.com
                                               www.aldf.com
Only available in Spanish, this brochure is for children ages 10-15
years old. Includes a basic desription of Lyme disease, symptoms,
diagnosis, prevention and proper tick removal. One free copy,
quantity prices vary.
Phillip J. Baker, Executive Director
Robert A. Proctor, Managing Director

9057 Understanding Ticks and Lyme Disease
American Lyme Disease Foundation
Post Office Box 466   914-277-6970
Lyme, CT 06371   Fax: 914-277-6974
                                          Executivedir@aldf.com
                                               www.aldf.com
For children 10-15 years old, basic description of Lyme disease,
symptoms, diagnosis, prevention and proper tick removal. One
free copy, quantity prices vary.
Phillip J. Baker, Executive Director
Robert A. Proctor, Managing Director

Audio & Video

9058 Case of the Great Imitator
American Lyme Disease Foundation
Post Office Box 466   914-277-6970
Lyme, CT 06371   Fax: 914-277-6974
                                          Executivedir@aldf.com
                                               www.aldf.com
For children ages 9-14 years old. Educational video made in coop-
eration with the Centers for Disease Control and Prevention.
Phillip J. Baker, Executive Director
Robert A. Proctor, Managing Director

9059 LD: Diagnosis & Treatment
Lyme Disease Foundation
1 Financial Plaza   860-525-2000
Hartford, CT 06103-2608   800-886-5963
                                          Fax: 860-525-8425
Physicians discuss the challenges of diagnosing and treating LD.
60 minutes

9060 LD: Facts for Kids
Lyme Disease Foundation
1 Financial Plaza   860-525-2000
Hartford, CT 06103-2608   800-886-5963
                                          Fax: 860-525-8425
Targeted toward kindergarten to fourth grade children, these vid-
eos educate youngsters about Lyme Disease and ticks.

9061 Lyme Disease: What You Should Know
Lyme Disease Foundation
1 Financial Plaza   860-525-2000
Hartford, CT 06103-2608   800-886-5963
                                          Fax: 860-525-8425
Diagnosis, treatment, transmission, prevention, and research. Interviews with patients, doctors, school officials, researchers, and
health department officials.
60 minutes

9062 Tick Talk
American Lyme Disease Foundation
Post Office Box 466
Lyme, CT 06371

914-277-6970
Fax: 914-277-6974
Executivedir@aldf.com
www.aldf.com

For children ages 5-8 years old. Educational video made in cooperation with the Centers for Disease Control and Prevention.

Phillip J. Baker, Executive Director
Robert A. Proctor, Managing Director

Web Sites

9063 America's Doctor Online Consulting
www.americasdoctor.com
Provides pharmaceutical and biotech companies and contract research organizations an exclusive source for conducting phase II-IV clinical research.

9064 American Lyme Disease Foundation
www.aldf.com
Provides a wide range of information, both in English and in Spanish, on the diagnosis, treatment, prevention and control of lyme disease and other tick-borne infections.

9065 CDC Intro to Lyme Disease
www.cdc.gov/ncidod/dvbid/lyme/incex.htm
Accurate, evidence based information on symptoms, diagnosis, treatment and prevention of Lyme disease and other tick-borne illnesses. Includes vaccine information, late-braking news, frequently asked questions and related links.

9066 Healing Well
www.healingwell.com
An online health resource guide to medical news, chat, information and articles, newsgroups and message boards, books, disease-related web sites, medical directories, and more for patients, friends, and family coping with disabling diseases, disorders, or chronic illnesses.

9067 Health Finder
www.healthfinder.gov
Searchable, carefully developed web site offering information on over 1000 topics. Developed by the US Department of Health and Human Services, the site can be used in both English and Spanish.

9068 Healthlink USA
www.healthlinkusa.com
Health information concerning treatment, cures, prevention, diagnosis, risk factors, research, support groups, email lists, personal stories and much more. Updated regularly.

9069 Lyme Disease Foundation
www.lyme.org
Provides a wide range of services including information and referral network on Lyme disease.

9070 MGH Neurology WebForums
Provides both unmoderated message board and chat rooms for specific neurological disorders including: amyloidosis, asachnoiditis, cerebellar ataxia, congenital fiber type disproportion, CFS leak, DeMorsiers syndrome, erythomelalgia, Lewy body disease, meningitis, meralgia paresthetic, Norrie disease, periodic paralysis, phantom limb pain, Romber disorder, Syndenhams chorea, tethered cord syndrome, and thoracic outlet syndrome.

9071 MedicineNet
www.medicinenet.com
An online resource for consumers providing easy-to-read, authoritative medical and health information.

9072 Medscape
www.medscape.com
Medscape offers specialists, primary care physicians, and other health professionals the Web's most robust and integrated medical information and educational tools.

9073 Neurology Channel
www.healthcommunities.com
Find clearly explained, medically accurate information regarding conditions, including an overview, symptoms, causes, diagnostic procedures and treatment options. On this site it is possible to ask questions and get information from a neurologist and connect to people who have similar health interests.

9074 Pubmed
www.ncbi.nlm.nih.gov/PubMed
National institutes of Health search engine for published medical and scientific research.

9075 University of Rhode Island Tick Research Laboratory
www.tickencounter.org
The TickEncounter Resource Center promotes tick-bite protection and tickborne disease prevention by engaging, educating, and empowering people to take action.

9076 WebMD
www.webmd.com
Provides credible information, supportive communities, and in-depth reference material about health subjects. A source for original and timely health information as well as material from well known content providers.

Description

9077 Tourette Syndrome

Tourette syndrome, TS, is a neurological disorder characterized by tics - involuntary, rapid, sudden movements or vocalizations that occur repeatedly in the same way. Onset of the disorder occurs before 18 years of age, and usually before the age of 12. Roughly 3-8 persons in 1000 will demonstrate this behavior at some time in his life. Boys are 3 or 4 times as likely as girls to develop TS.

Multiple motor and vocal tics can appear separately or simultaneously as part of the syndrome. Tics may occur many times daily, or intermittently, with periodic changes in their number, frequency, type and location. Sometimes they may disappear for weeks.

Over time, symptoms can range from hand jerking and throat clearing in the syndrome's early stages to jumping and vocalizing socially unacceptable phrases. Movements may also occur in combination with each other.

Although the cause of TS is unknown, researchers have identified factors which may be involved in producing the disease. Persons with TS may show subtle abnormalities in the structure of certain parts of the brain. The disease may reflect abnormal metabolism of a neurotransmitter (a chemical that brain cells use to signal one another) called dopamine; drugs affecting dopamine levels may reduce symptoms. Relatives of affected persons have an increased risk of disease, suggesting a genetic component. Finally, in some cases the brain's function may be affected by antibodies triggered by infection with a bacterium called Streptococcus pyogenes. Children who are not bothered by their tics should not be treated with drugs. Medications are reserved for those whose tics lead to symptoms which impair behavioral, physiologic or social function. Simple tics respond to benzodiazepines (tranquilizers). For more severe cases, antipsychotics such as haloperidol, or other antipsychotics, or clonidine, as blood pressure medication, may be used, but both drugs should be started slowly. Unfortunately, some antipsychotics may cause other movement disorders after prolonged use. Whether drug treatment is used or not, patients and their families may need counseling to deal with the disease's secondary effects, which may include bullying at school or conflict within the family. Fortunately, the condition often becomes much less severe, without any treatment, after 10 or 15 years.

National Agencies & Associations

9078 **American Academy of Neurology: Tourette Syndrome**
201 Chicago Avenue   612-928-6000
Minneapolis, MN 55415   800-879-1960
Fax: 612-454-2746
memberservices@aan.com
www.aan.com

A medical specialty society established to advance knowledge of neurology and promote the best possible care for patients with neurological disorders.
James C. Stevens, MD, FAAN, President
Ann H. Tilton, MD, FAAN, Vice President

9079 **Goodwill Industries International, Inc.**
15810 Indianola Drive   800-466-3945
Rockville, MD 20855   contactus@goodwill.org
www.goodwill.org
A nonprofit, community-based organization whose mission is to help people achieve self-sufficiency through the dignity and power of work, serving people who are disadvantaged, disabled or elderly. The mission is accomplished through providing independent living skills, affordable housing, and training and placement in community employment. The GoodWill Network includes 160 independent, local locations across the U.S. and Canada.
S. Dale Jenkins, Chair
Steven C. Preston, President & CEO

9080 **National Institute of Neurological Disorders and Stroke**
NIH Neurological Institute   301-496-5751
Bethesda, MD 20824   800-352-9424
www.ninds.nih.gov
Seeks to reduce the burden of neurological disease affecting individuals from all walks of life.
Walter J. Koroshetz, MD, Director
Amy B. Adams, Director, Office of Scientific Liaison

9081 **Tourette Association of America**
42-40 Bell Boulevard   888-486-8738
Bayside, NY 11361   support@tourette.org
www.tourette.org
National organization dedicated to the research, diagnosis, education and treatments for individuals with Tourette Syndrome. Raises awareness and acceptance of Tourette Syndrome.
Randi Zemsky, Board Chair
Stephen Barron, First Vice Chair

9082 **Tourette Syndrome Foundation of Canada**
5955 Airport Road   905-673-2255
Mississauga, Ontario, L4V-1R9   800-361-3120
Fax: 800-387-0120
admin@tourette.ca
www.tourette.ca
National voluntary organization dedicated to improving the quality of life for those with or affected by Tourette Syndrome through programs of education, advocacy, self-help and research.
Ramona Jennex, President

State Agencies & Associations

Florida

9083 **Goodwill Industries-Suncoast**
10596 Gandy Boulevard   727-523-1512
St. Petersburg, FL 33702   888-279-1988
TTY: 727-579-1068
www.goodwill-suncoast.org
A nonprofit, community-based organization whose mission is to help people achieve self-sufficiency through the dignity and power of work, serving people who are disadvantaged, disabled or elderly. The mission is accomplished through providing independent living skills, affordable housing, and training and placement in community employment.
Heather Ceresoli, CPA, Chair
Deborah A. Passerini, President & CEO

Research Centers

9084 **Tourette Syndrome Clinic Yale Child Study Center**
Yale Child Study Center
300 George St.   203-785-6396
New Haven, CT 06511   Fax: 203-785-6196
www.medicine.yale.edu

Clinical care center offering research solely into the causes symptoms and treatments for persons with Tourette Syndrome.
Diane B Findley, Associate Research Scientist and Clinic
Robert King, Medical Director

Support Groups & Hotlines

9085 National Health Information Center
Office of Disease Prevention & Health Promotion
1101 Wootton Pkwy   Fax: 240-453-8281
Rockville, MD 20852   odphpinfo@hhs.gov
                                      www.health.gov/nhic
Supports public health education by maintaining a calendar of National Health Observances; helps connect consumers and health professionals to organizations that can best answer questions and provide up-to-date contact information from reliable sources; updates on a yearly basis toll-free numbers for health information, Federal health clearinghouses and info centers.
Don Wright, MD, MPH, Director

Books

9086 Children with Tourette Syndrome
Woodbine House
6510 Bells Mill Road   800-843-7323
Bethesda, MD 20817-1636
This book offers parents information on Tourette Syndrome, causes, symptoms and medications, as well as the other disorders which are commonly linked with it. Other chapters include information on family life, education, advocacy and legal rights.
340 pages Paperback
ISBN: 0-933149-44-1

9087 Children with Tourette Syndrome: A Parent's Guide
Adam Ward Seligman, Echolalia Press
35158 Annapolis Road   707-886-1972
Annapolis, CA 95412-9713   888-766-4233
                                      Fax: 707-547-2199
                                      seligman@sonic.net
                                      www.sonic.net/echolaliapress/
It Publishes and Distributes Books, Music and TwoOn-Line Magazines for the Following Healing Communities
Adam Ward Seligman, Publisher and Co-editor
John S Hilkevich, Co-editor

9088 Living with Tourette Syndrome
Simon & Schuster
611 W Bay Street   800-999-5479
Tampa, FL 33606-2703
Provides valuable advice for children and adults with TS, their families, co-workers, teachers and friends. Describes the symptoms and related disorders, exposes many myths surrounding the disease, and advises adults on business and personal relationships.
256 pages
ISBN: 0-684811-60-0

9089 Ryan: A Mother's Story of her TS/ADHD Child
Adam Ward Seligman, Echolalia Press
35158 Annapolis Road   707-886-1972
Annapolis, CA 95412-9713   888-766-4233
                                      Fax: 707-547-2199
                                      seligman@sonic.net
                                      www.sonic.net
It Publishes and Distributes Books, Music and TwoOn-Line Magazines for the Following Healing Communities
Softcover
Adam Ward Seligman, Publisher and Co-editor
John S Hilkevich, Co-editor

9090 Teaching the Tiger: An Educator's Guide to TS/OCD/ADHD
Adam Ward Seligman, Echolalia Press
35158 Annapolis Road   707-886-1972
Annapolis, CA 95412-9713   888-766-4233
                                      Fax: 707-547-2199
                                      seligman@sonic.net
                                      www.sonic.net

It Publishes and Distributes Books, Music and TwoOn-Line Magazines for the Following Healing Communities
Workbook
Adam Ward Seligman, Publisher and Co-editor
John S Hilkevich, Co-editor

9091 Tourette Syndrome and Human Behavior
Adam Ward Seligman, Echolalia Press
35158 Annapolis Road   707-886-1972
Annapolis, CA 95412-9713   888-766-4233
                                      Fax: 707-547-2199
                                      seligman@sonic.net
                                      www.sonic.net
Publishes and distributes books, music and two online magazines.
Softcover
Adam Ward Seligman, Publisher and Co-editor
John S Hilkevich, Co-editor

9092 Tourette Syndrome: Advances in Neurology
Tourette Syndrome Association
42-40 Bell Boulevard   718-224-2999
Bayside, NY 11361-2861   888-480-8737
                                      Fax: 718-279-9596
                                      www.tsa-usa.org
In this single-volume reference, more than 90 of the foremost research and clinical leaders in the field review the current state of knowledge about this disorder.
400 pages
Thomas N Chase MD, Editor
Arnold J Friedhoff MD, Editor

9093 What Makes Ryan Tic?
Adam Ward Seligman, Echolalia Press
35158 Annapolis Road   707-886-1972
Annapolis, CA 95412-9713   888-766-4233
                                      Fax: 707-547-2199
                                      seligman@sonic.net
                                      www.sonic.net
It Publishes and Distributes Books, Music and TwoOn-Line Magazines for the Following Healing Communities
Softcover
Adam Ward Seligman, Publisher and Co-editor
John S Hilkevich, Co-editor

Children's Books

9094 Adam and the Magic Marble
Adam Ward Seligman, Echolalia Press
35158 Annapolis Road   707-886-1972
Annapolis, CA 95412-9713   888-766-4233
                                      Fax: 707-547-2199
                                      seligman@sonic.net
                                      www.sonic.net
It Publishes and Distributes Books, Music and TwoOn-Line Magazines for the Following Healing Communities
Adam Ward Seligman, Publisher and Co-editor
John S Hilkevich, Co-editor

9095 Hi! I'm Adam!
Adam Ward Seligman, Echolalia Press
35158 Annapolis Road   707-886-1972
Annapolis, CA 95412-9713   888-766-4233
                                      Fax: 707-547-2199
                                      www.sonic.net
It Publishes and Distributes Books, Music and TwoOn-Line Magazines for the Following Healing Communities
Adam Ward Seligman, Publisher and Co-editor
John S Hilkevich, Co-editor

9096 Matthew and the Tics
Tourette Syndrome Association
42-40 Bell Boulevard   718-224-2999
Bayside, NY 11361-2861   888-480-8738
                                      Fax: 718-279-9596
                                      www.tsa-usa.org
A story for young children with TS and their peers.
2 pages

Newsletters

9097 **Tourette Syndrome Association Newsletter**
42-40 Bell Boulevard   718-224-2999
Bayside, NY 11361   888-480-8738
Fax: 718-279-9596
ts@tsa-usa.org
www.tsa-usa.org
Offers information, articles and news on the latest technology and
advancements for persons with Tourette Syndrome.
Quarterly

Pamphlets

9098 **Commentary on Alternative Therapies for TS**
Tourette Syndrome Association
42-40 Bell Boulevard   718-224-2999
Bayside, NY 11361-2861   888-480-8738
Fax: 718-279-9596
www.tsa-usa.org
Summarizes physician/patient reports of symptom management
through non-pharmacological interventions.
2 pages

9099 **Consumer's Guide to TS Medications**
Tourette Syndrome Association
42-40 Bell Boulevard   718-224-2999
Bayside, NY 11361-2861   888-480-8738
Fax: 718-279-9596
www.tsa-usa.org
Covers common medications used for the control of TS motor and
vocal ties as well as those traditionally prescribed for associated
behaviors.
1992 12 pages

9100 **Coping with TS in the Classroom**
Tourette Syndrome Association
42-40 Bell Boulevard   718-224-2999
Bayside, NY 11361-2820   Fax: 718-279-9596
www.tsa-usa.org
Includes practical guidelines for education developed from a study
about cognitive effects on learning.
18 pages

9101 **Coping with TS, A Parent's Viewpoint**
Tourette Syndrome Association
42-40 Bell Boulevard   718-224-2999
Bayside, NY 11361-2861   888-480-8738
Fax: 718-279-9596
www.tsa-usa.org
An accalaimed medical writer and mother of three children with
TS, the author sensitively addresses common concerns and feel-
ings of parents.
1994 23 pages

9102 **Coping with Tourette Syndrome in Early Adulthood**
Tourette Syndrome Association
42-40 Bell Boulevard   718-224-2999
Bayside, NY 11361-2861   888-480-8738
Fax: 718-279-9596
www.tsa-usa.org
Focuses on two fundamental challenges facing adults with TS: employment and interpersonal relationships. Provides specific techniques for overcoming barriers.

9103 **Current Pharmacology of TS**
Tourette Syndrome Association
42-40 Bell Boulevard   718-224-2999
Bayside, NY 11361-2861   888-480-8738
Fax: 718-279-9596
www.tsa-usa.org
Covers all current medications used to treat TS with specific information about clinical evaluations and diagnosis.
12 pages

9104 **Dental Treatment of Patients with Gilles de la Tourette Syndrome**
Tourette Syndrome Association

42-40 Bell Boulevard   718-224-2999
Bayside, NY 11361-2861   888-480-8738
Fax: 718-279-9596
www.tsa-usa.org
Discusses TS movements and possible adverse interactions of dentistry and TS medications.
5 pages

9105 **Development of Behavioral and Emotional Problems in TS**
Tourette Syndrome Association
42-40 Bell Boulevard   718-224-2999
Bayside, NY 11361-2861   888-480-8738
Fax: 718-279-9596
www.tsa-usa.org
Using the Child Behavior Checklist, 78 male children were as-
sessed for a variety of behavioral problems. Relation to tic severity
covered.
1989 3 pages

9106 **Discipline and the Child with TS**
Tourette Syndrome Association
42-40 Bell Boulevard   718-224-2999
Bayside, NY 11361   888-480-8738
Fax: 718-279-9596
www.tsa-usa.org
Helps children redirect impulses and compulsions through teaching cause and effect relationships.
15 pages

9107 **Educator's Guide to Tourette Syndrome**
Tourette Syndrome Association
42-40 Bell Boulevard   718-224-2999
Bayside, NY 11361-2861   888-480-8738
Fax: 718-279-9596
www.tsa-usa.org
Covers symptoms, treatments and techniques for classroom management, attentional, writing and language problems.
16 pages

9108 **Genetics of Tourette's Syndrome: Who it Affects and How it
Occurs in Families**
Tourette Syndrome Association
42-40 Bell Boulevard   718-224-2999
Bayside, NY 11361-2861   888-480-8738
Fax: 718-279-9596
www.tsa-usa.org
TSA, founded in 1972, is dedicated to education, service, and research to identify the cause of, find the cure for, and control the effects of Tourette Syndrome
10 pages

9109 **Getting Into College: Strategies for the Student with TS**
Tourette Syndrome Association
42-40 Bell Boulevard   718-224-2999
Bayside, NY 11361   888-480-8738
Fax: 718-279-9596
www.tsa-usa.org
TSA, founded in 1972, is dedicated to education, service, and research to identify the cause of, find the cure for, and control the effects of Tourette Syndrome
10 pages

9110 **Gift of Hope**
Tourette Syndrome Association
42-40 Bell Boulevard   718-224-2999
Bayside, NY 11361-2861   888-480-8738
Fax: 718-279-9596
www.tsa-usa.org
TSA Brain Bank Program registration information. Includes donor
cards.

9111 **Grandparents Club**
Tourette Syndrome Association
42-40 Bell Boulevard   718-224-2999
Bayside, NY 11361-2861   888-480-8738
Fax: 718-279-9596
www.tsa-usa.org
A flyer describing how to join with other grandparents to support
TS research to benefit future generations.

9112 Guide to Diagnosis & Treatment
Tourette Syndrome Association
42-40 Bell Boulevard   718-224-2999
Bayside, NY 11361-2861   888-480-8738
                                         Fax: 718-279-9596
                                              www.tsa-usa.org
Covers symptoms, pharmacology and clinical assessments.
30 pages

9113 Guide to Housing for Adults with TS
Tourette Syndrome Association
42-40 Bell Boulevard   718-224-2999
Bayside, NY 11361-2861   888-480-8738
                                         Fax: 718-279-9596
                                              www.tsa-usa.org
A guide to finding housing, housing laws that help people with TS
and ways to maximize living environments.
1991 16 pages

9114 Health Insurance & Tourette Syndrome
Tourette Syndrome Association
42-40 Bell Boulevard   718-224-2999
Bayside, NY 11361-2861   888-480-8738
                                         Fax: 718-279-9596
                                              www.tsa-usa.org
Detailed, up-to-date packet of medical information for obtaining
health insurance as well as information for submission to insurance carriers.

9115 Helpful Techniques to Aid the Student with TS
Tourette Syndrome Association
42-40 Bell Boulevard   718-224-2999
Bayside, NY 11361-2861   888-480-8738
                                         Fax: 718-279-9596
                                              www.tsa-usa.org
Helpful hints for teacher with specific suggestions for test taking,
math computation, and note taking.
1 pages

9116 Learning Problems & the Child with TS
Tourette Syndrome Association
42-40 Bell Boulevard   718-224-2999
Bayside, NY 11361-2861   888-480-8738
                                         Fax: 718-279-9596
                                              www.tsa-usa.org
Report on learning problems identified through a study of 200 children with TS.
1 pages

9117 Need to Know
Tourette Syndrome Association
42-40 Bell Boulevard   718-224-2999
Bayside, NY 11361-2861   888-480-8738
                                         Fax: 718-279-9596
                                              www.tsa-usa.org
Recollections of a young woman who was diagnosed with TS in her
20s.
4 pages

9118 Neuropsychological Performance in Adults with TS
Tourette Syndrome Association
42-40 Bell Boulevard   718-224-2999
Bayside, NY 11361-2861   888-480-8738
                                         Fax: 718-279-9596
                                              www.tsa-usa.org
Describes clinical and neuropsychological testing on learning and
memory with TS adults.
7 pages

9119 Peer Problems in Tourette's Disorder
Tourette Syndrome Association
42-40 Bell Boulevard   718-224-2999
Bayside, NY 11361-2861   888-480-8738
                                         Fax: 718-279-9596
                                              www.tsa-usa.org
Detailed research findings of peer problems in children with TS.
Includes statistical results obtained from these studies.
1991 7 pages

9120 Pharmacotherapy of TS and Associated Disorders
Tourette Syndrome Association
42-40 Bell Boulevard   718-224-2999
Bayside, NY 11361-2861   888-480-8738
                                         Fax: 718-279-9596
                                              www.tsa-usa.org
Overview with emphasis on the complexities of prescribing TS
medications.
19 pages

9121 Problem Behaviors & TS
Tourette Syndrome Association
42-40 Bell Boulevard   718-224-2999
Bayside, NY 11361-2861   888-480-8738
                                         Fax: 718-279-9596
                                              www.tsa-usa.org
Describes recent research and what is now known about the relationship of a variety of behaviors and TS.
21 pages

9122 Recognizing TS in the Classroom
Tourette Syndrome Association
42-40 Bell Boulevard   718-224-2999
Bayside, NY 11361-2861   888-480-8738
                                         Fax: 718-279-9596
                                              www.tsa-usa.org
Provides an overview offering detailed symptoms checklist,
post-diagnosis advice and covers special education needs.
4 pages

9123 Risperidone as a Treatment for TS
Tourette Syndrome Association
42-40 Bell Boulevard   718-224-2999
Bayside, NY 11361-2861   888-480-8738
                                         Fax: 718-279-9596
                                              www.tsa-usa.org
TSA, founded in 1972, is dedicated to education, service, and research to identify the cause of, find the cure for, and control the effects of Tourette Syndrome
6 pages

9124 Specific Classroom Strategies and Techniques for Students with TS
Tourette Syndrome Association
42-40 Bell Boulevard   718-224-2999
Bayside, NY 11361-2861   888-480-8738
                                         Fax: 718-279-9596
                                              www.tsa-usa.org
An educator with TS spells out concrete methods for managing students with TS. She outlines many valuable classroom interventions to help youngsters deal with tic symptons, ADHD, visual
motor and fine motor integration, and behavioral difficulties.
1994 2 pages

9125 TS and Other Tic Disorders
Tourette Syndrome Association
42-40 Bell Boulevard   718-224-2999
Bayside, NY 11361-2861   888-480-8738
                                         Fax: 718-279-9596
                                              www.tsa-usa.org
Comprehensive overview of the complexities of TS. Includes tic
syndrome classifications, epidemiology, genetics, behavioral aspects, and summary.
17 pages

9126 TS and the School Nurse
Tourette Syndrome Association
42-40 Bell Boulevard   718-224-2999
Bayside, NY 11361-2861   888-480-8738
                                         Fax: 718-279-9596
                                              www.tsa-usa.org
Comprehensive professional guide to educational, social and medical implications.
19 pages

9127 TS and the School Psychologist
Tourette Syndrome Association

42-40 Bell Boulevard
Bayside, NY 11361-2861
718-224-2999
Fax: 718-279-9596
www.tsa-usa.org

The role of the school psychologist is covered including testing procedures, counseling strategies and social implications.
1993 (rev.) 14 pages

9128 TS: A Look at the Interface Between TS & the Law
Tourette Syndrome Association
42-40 Bell Boulevard
Bayside, NY 11361-2861
718-224-2999
888-480-8738
Fax: 718-279-9596
www.tsa-usa.org

Summarizes important legislation protecting the rights of students with TS. Also covers resources and hints about how to prepare for dealing successfully with educators and school systems.
1 pages

9129 TSA Medical Letters
Tourette Syndrome Association
42-40 Bell Boulevard
Bayside, NY 11361-2861
718-224-2999
888-480-8738
Fax: 718-279-9596
www.tsa-usa.org

Annual publication of TSA's Medical Committe covering recent, significant findings from scientific articles.
16 pages

9130 Teens and Tourette Syndrome
Tourette Syndrome Association
42-40 Bell Boulevard
Bayside, NY 11361-2820
718-224-2999
Fax: 718-279-9596
ts@tsa-usa.org
www.tsa-usa.org

Covers self esteem, friends, dating, drugs and alcohol, stress, depression, academic and vocational planning, sibling relationships and medication.
16 pages

9131 Tourette Syndrome and the School Nurse
Tourette Syndrome Association
42-40 Bell Boulevard
Bayside, NY 11361-2820
718-224-2999
Fax: 718-279-9596
ts@tsa-usa.org
www.tsa-usa.org

Includes symptoms, epidemiology, associated beviors, developmental consequences, causes, treatments, role of the school nurse and additional resources.
20 pages

9132 Tourette: The Man and His Times
Tourette Syndrome Association
42-40 Bell Boulevard
Bayside, NY 11361-2861
718-224-2999
888-480-8738
Fax: 718-279-9596
www.tsa-usa.org

Rare historical biography of the famous French neurologist G. Gilles De La Tourette.
9 pages

9133 What School Bus Drivers Need to Know About Students with Tourette Syndrome
Tourette Syndrome Association
42-40 Bell Boulevard
Bayside, NY 11361-2820
718-224-2999
Fax: 718-279-9596
ts@tsa-usa.org
www.tsa-usa.org

Includes a description of the disorder, as well as related disorders and suggestions as to what school bus drivers can do for students with TS.
1 pages

Audio & Video

9134 A Regular Kid That's Me: Inservice Film for Educators
Tourette Syndrome Association

42-40 Bell Boulevard
Bayside, NY 11361
718-224-2999
888-480-8738
Fax: 718-279-9596
ts@tsa-usa.org
www.tsa-usa.org

Nineteen students with TS (ages 7-17) along with several educators are seen interacting in classroom settings. Includes the basic criteria for diagnosis, discussions of common associated behaviors, e.g. ADD with or without hyperactivity, obsessive compulsive symptoms and specific learning disabilities. Professionals describe the impact of having TS on educational placement and specific classroom strategies are presented. 45 minutes. May be purchased as part of a curriculum or separately. #AV-2
VHS 1/2 inch

9135 After the Diagnosis...the Next Steps
42-40 Bell Boulevard
Bayside, NY 11361
718-224-2999
888-480-8738
Fax: 718-279-9596
ts@tsa-usa.org
www.tsa-usa.org

When the diagnosis is Tourette Syndrome, what do you do first? How do you sort out the complexities of the disorder? Whose advice do you follow? What steps do you take to lead a normal life? Six people with TS—as different as any six people can be—relate the sometimes difficult, but finally triumphant path each took to lead the rich, fulfilling life they now enjoy. Narrated by Academy Award-winning actor, Richard Dreyfuss, the stories are blends of poignancy, fact and inspiration.

9136 Clinical Counseling: Towards a Better Understanding of TS
Tourette Syndrome Association
42-40 Bell Boulevard
Bayside, NY 11361
718-224-2999
888-480-8738
Fax: 718-279-9596
ts@tsa-usa.org
www.tsa-usa.org

Targeted to counselors, social workers, educators, psychologists and families, this video features expert physicians, allied professionals and several families summarizing key issues that can arise when counseling families with TS. 15 minutes. #AV-10A

9137 Complexities of TS Treatment: A Physician's Round Table
Tourette Syndrome Association
42-40 Bell Boulevard
Bayside, NY 11361
718-224-2999
888-480-8738
Fax: 718-279-9596
ts@tsa-usa.org
www.tsa-usa.org

Three internationally recognized TS experts provide colleagues with valuable information about the complexities of treating and advising families with TS. Emphasis is on different clinical approaches to patients with a broad range of symptom severity. Co-morbid and associated conditions are covered. 15 minutes. #AV-10

9138 Educator's In-Service Program
Tourette Syndrome Association
42-40 Bell Boulevard
Bayside, NY 11361
718-224-2999
888-480-8738
Fax: 718-279-9596
www.tsa-usa.org

A curriculum designed to train educators to recognize and understand TS and guide students with TS and associated disorders in a classroom setting. Developed by the Tourette Syndrome Association for the training of all educational personnel. Includes 2 videos, a particpant's guide, a set of 20 transparencies, 2 scripted curriculum modules and a comprehensive teacher's guide. Discounted for members.

9139 Gift of Hope
Tourette Syndrome Association
42-40 Bell Boulevard
Bayside, NY 11361
718-224-2999
888-480-8738
Fax: 718-279-9596
ts@tsa-usa.org
www.tsa-usa.org

The cause of TS lies in the brain. Because their are no animal models to study this disorder, human brain tissue is of vital importance for progress in research. Increased brain bank registration is a prime objective of the TSA. VHS 1/2 inch. 14 minutes. Available for shipping cost only. #AV- 7

9140 Guide to Diagnosis
Tourette Syndrome Association
42-40 Bell Boulevard   718-224-2999
Bayside, NY 11361-2861   888-480-8738
                              Fax: 718-279-9596
                              www.tsa-usa.org
A video and companion guide for interested medical professionals who have not seen a substantial number of TS patients.
30 minutes

9141 I'm a Person Too
Tourette Syndrome Association
42-40 Bell Boulevard   718-224-2999
Bayside, NY 11361   888-480-8738
                              Fax: 718-279-9596
                              ts@tsa-usa.org
                              www.tsa-usa.org
Narrated by Cliff Robertson, this video features 5 people with TS; 2 elementary school students and 3 adults from diverse social backgrounds. They talk about a broad variety of symptoms and their personal experiences living with the disorder. VHS 1/2 inch. 22 minutes. #AV1

9142 Panel of Experts
Tourette Syndrome Association
42-40 Bell Boulevard   718-224-2999
Bayside, NY 11361-2861   888-480-8738
                              Fax: 718-279-9596
                              www.tsa-usa.org
Five leading authorities bring their in-depth knowledge and experience to bear in a wide-ranging discussion that covers current strategies in TS diagnosis, and medication.
30 minutes

9143 Parent's Perspective: Diplomacy in Action
Tourette Syndrome Association
42-40 Bell Boulevard   718-224-2999
Bayside, NY 11361-2861   888-480-8738
                              Fax: 718-279-9596
                              www.tsa-usa.org
The child with TS faces a set of special problems in school. The level of achievement reached in large measure is dependent on the attitude of teachers and administrators. Therefore, educating the educators becomes a high priority with the parent.
45 minutes

9144 Stop It!... I Can't!
Tourette Syndrome Association
42-40 Bell Boulevard   718-224-2999
Bayside, NY 11361   888-480-8738
                              Fax: 718-279-9596
                              ts@tsa-usa.org
                              www.tsa-usa.org
Narrated by William Shatner, this video promotes sensitivity, education, acceptance and confidence for children with TS. Produced in the 1970's, but provides a valuable and classic message. VHS 1/2 inch. 13 minutes.

9145 TS-The Parent's Perspective: Diplomacy in Action
Tourette Syndrome Association
42-40 Bell Boulevard   718-224-2999
Bayside, NY 11361   888-480-8738
                              Fax: 718-279-9596
                              ts@tsa-usa.org
                              www.tsa-usa.org
The child with TS faces a set of special problems in school. The level of achievement reached in large measure is dependent on the attitude of teachers and administrators. Therefore educating the educators becomes a high priority for the parent. Special education professionals provide firm guidance to famillies on school advocacy issues. Concrete suggestions are offered to smooth the road to success in school for the student with TS. VHS 1/2 inch. 45 minutes. #AV-6

9146 TS: A Panel of Experts
Tourette Syndrome Association

42-40 Bell Boulevard   718-224-2999
Bayside, NY 11361   888-480-8738
                              Fax: 718-279-9596
                              ts@tsa-usa.org
                              www.tsa-usa.org
Five leading authorities bring their in-depth knowledge and experience to bear in a wide-ranging discussion that covers current strategies in TS diagnosis and medication, behavioral problems, predicted course and other aspects of this disorder. VHS 1/2 inch. 30 minutes. # AV-5

9147 Talking About Tourette Syndrome
Tourette Syndrome Association
42-40 Bell Boulevard   718-224-2999
Bayside, NY 11361   888-480-8738
                              Fax: 718-279-9596
                              ts@tsa-usa.org
                              www.tsa-usa.org
When the professional is also the patient, a unique perspective emerges. A psychiatrist leads a candid probing discussion with a brother and sister- all have Tourette syndrome. This free-wheeling exchange brings to the viewer many instructive and often surprising observations about TS and obsessive compulsive symptoms. VHS 1/2 inch. 45 minutes. #AV-8

9148 Tourette Syndrome: Guide to Diagnosis
Tourette Syndrome Association
42-40 Bell Boulevard   718-224-2999
Bayside, NY 11361   888-480-8738
                              Fax: 718-279-9596
                              ts@tsa-usa.org
                              www.tsa-usa.org
Video for interested medical professionals who have not seen substantial numbers of TS patients. Presents 7 patients with TS who exhibit the full range of movements, vocalizations and behavioral patterns associated with the disorder. Descriptions and demonstrations of other movement disorders are also presented for the purpose of differential diagnosis. VHS 1/2 inch. 30 minutes. A 29 page companion piece by Drs. Ruth Brunn, Donald Cohen and James Leckman is available at $6.00/3.50 shipping.#AV4

9149 Family Life with Tourette Syndrome... Personal Stories: Professor Peter
Tourette Syndrome Association
42-40 Bell Boulevard   718-224-2999
Bayside, NY 11361   888-480-8738
                              Fax: 718-279-9596
                              ts@tsa-usa.org
                              tsa-usa.org
Now a world class scientific research expert and a professor of biology at Harvard and Purdue, Professor Hollenbeck talks about growing up positively with TS, never hesitating to have children, and offering good advice for newly diagnosed families. 7 minutes, 27 seconds. If purchased together, the six videos in this series are $50.00. #AV-11A

9150 Family Life with Tourette Syndrome... Personal Stories: Reverend Mike
Tourette Syndrome Association
42-40 Bell Boulevard   718-224-2999
Bayside, NY 11361   888-480-8738
                              Fax: 718-279-9596
                              ts@tsa-usa.org
                              tsa-usa.org
Mike Higgins did not receive a diagnosis of TS until he was in the army! Mike overcame significant symptoms and childhood teasing. Reverend Mike talks about the value of strong family life, faith, support groups and acceptance of the person, and not the disorder as a good way to live positively with TS. If purchased together, the six videos in this series are $50.00. #AV-11B

9151 Family Life with Tourette Syndrome... Personal Stories: Rachel
Tourette Syndrome Association
42-40 Bell Boulevard   718-224-2999
Bayside, NY 11361   888-480-8738
                              Fax: 718-279-9596
                              ts@tsa-usa.org
                              tsa-usa.org
Challenged by TS, ADHD and OCD Rachel and her family endured difficult reactions, behavioral episodes, and at times, a great loss

of hope. Now seventeen years old, Rachel and family overcame stresses and strains by sticking together through the highs and lows to find Rachel today a confident and happy teen. 10 minutes. If purchased together, the six videos in this series are $50.00. #AV-11C

9152 Family Life with Tourette Syndrome... Personal Stories: The Turners
Tourette Syndrome Association
42-40 Bell Boulevard
Bayside, NY 11361

718-224-2999
888-480-8738
Fax: 718-279-9596
ts@tsa-usa.org
www.tsa-usa.org

Three of the four Turner daughters have TS in varying degrees. The family wondered how their symptoms came to be, how to dispense attention fairly, what to say to teachers and friends. They learned how to deal with sibling issues and low self esteem among the sisters. This determined family never gave up! 12 minutes. If purchased together, the six videos in this series are $50.00. #AV-11D

9153 Family Life with Tourette Syndrome... Personal Stories: Ryan
Tourette Syndrome Association
42-40 Bell Boulevard
Bayside, NY 11361

718-224-2999
888-480-8738
Fax: 718-279-9596
ts@tsa-usa.org
www.tsa-usa.org

Ryan's family first thought his behavior was a deliberate way to get attention. A school principal was harshly critical. The family soon learned to educate themselves and others about Ryan's TS. Things turned around as a result. A good teacher took a great interest, friends began to seek him out and Ryan grew into a young man with a positive outlook. 11 minutes, 28 seconds. If purchased together, the six videos in this series are $50.00. #AV-11E

9154 Family Life with Tourette Syndrome... Personal Stories: Dakota
Tourette Syndrome Association
42-40 Bell Boulevard
Bayside, NY 11361

718-224-2999
888-480-8738
Fax: 718-279-9596
ts@tsa-usa.org
www.tsa-usa.org

A happy 11 year old baseball playing, video game whiz, Dakota was initially diagnosed as having a brain tumor! He was actually affected by TS and AHD. This is a story of a child who developed a strong confidence and a good attitude, learning to believe in himself. He says the love of his grandparents was a special help! 7 minutes, 12 seconds. If purchased together, the 6 videos in this series are $50.00. #AV-11F

Web Sites

9155 American Academy of Neurology: Tourette Syndrome
www.aan.com
The American Academy of Neurology (AAN) is a worldwide professional association of more than 17,000 neurologists and neuroscience professionals dedicating to providing the best possible care for patients with neurological disorders.

9156 Healing Well
www.healingwell.com
An online health resource guide to medical news, chat, information and articles, newsgroups and message boards, books, disease-related web sites, medical directories, and more for patients, friends, and family coping with disabling diseases, disorders, or chronic illnesses.

9157 Health Finder
www.healthfinder.gov
Searchable, carefully developed web site offering information on over 1000 topics. Developed by the US Department of Health and Human Services, the site can be used in both English and Spanish.

9158 Healthlink USA
www.healthlinkusa.com
Health information concerning treatment, cures, prevention, diagnosis, risk factors, research, support groups, email lists, personal stories and much more. Updated regularly.

9159 MedicineNet
www.medicinenet.com
An online resource for consumers providing easy-to-read, authoritative medical and health information.

9160 Medscape
www.medscape.com
Medscape offers specialists, primary care physicians, and other health professionals the Web's most robust and integrated medical information and educational tools.

9161 WebMD
www.webmd.com
Provides credible information, supportive communities, and in-depth reference material about health subjects. A source for original and timely health information as well as material from well known content providers.

Description

9162 **Transplant-Related Conditions**

In recent decades, transplantation of solid organs (heart, liver, lung, kidney), bone marrow and stem cells has become an established part of medical care for advanced diseases in many patients who otherwise face end-organ failure and poor prognosis. While on one hand, transplantation may serve to cure the underlying disease it nonetheless often entails chronic medical therapy that will likely include the use of immunosuppressants, complications from chronic medications, frequent and long-term medical follow-up and diagnostic testing which may be invasive.

A number of clinical management protocols are utilized in the care of post-transplantation patient, and these vary depending on the type of transplant undertaken, the extent of the tissue match between donor and recipient, and the experience of the given transplantation center. In general, however, most patients who receive a transplanted organ or cells will require some chronic therapy (short or long-term) with immunosuppressive medications that, when given long-term, increase the risk of infections and cancer. These can be several or many and are given in an effort to control the patient's own immunologic response to receiving an organ or cells from another person. The body's natural response after recognizing such an exposure is to "fight" these cells and tissues with its own defense cells, which are designed to attack and kill foreign material. The immunosuppressive medications help modulate this response so that that the transplanted organ is not damaged, injured or "rejected" by the recipient who needs the organ or cells to function in a healthier manner. Immunosuppressive therapy and protection of the transplanted organ must be balanced against the adverse creation of an immunocompromised state in the patient placing him at greater risk for contracting infections that can be serious and even life threatening. Given these circumstances, transplant patients require close working relationships with their medical team along with a true commitment to be compliant with these potentially difficult and complicated medical regimens.

In addition to the medical therapy for patients who have received transplants, one must also consider the significant psychological and social aspects of having undergone such procedures. Strong social support systems and close attention to a healthy emotional and psychological status are important for successful management of these patients. Many transplant centers have extensive support services available to patients from which they and their families can benefit.

National Agencies & Associations

9163 **American Society of Transplantation (AST)**
1120 Route 73 · 856-439-9986
Mount Laurel, NJ 08054 · Fax: 856-581-9604
www.myast.org

The American Society of Transplantation is an organization of transplant professionals dedicated to advancing the field of transplantation through promoting research and education of organ transplantation, and by advocating for organ donations in order to improve patient care.
Dianne B. McKay, MD, FAST, President
John S. Gill, MD, MS, FAST, Treasurer

9164 **Association of Organ Procurement Organizations (AOPO)**
8245 Boone Boulevard · 703-556-4242
Vienna, VA 22182 · Fax: 703-556-4852
aopo@aopo.org
www.aopo.org
Non-profit organization involved in helping people find and obtain the organs they need for transplantation. Oversees 58 federally-designated Organ Procurement Organizations serving over 300 million Americans.
Diane Brockmeier, President
Kirk Mizelle, Secretary-Treasurer

9165 **Children's Organ Transplant Association (COTA)**
2501 W COTA Drive · 800-366-2682
Bloomington, IN 47403 · Fax: 812-336-8885
cota@cota.org
www.cota.org
Non-profit national charity dedicated to helping families and communities raise the necessary funds for transplant expenses.
Rick Lofgren, President & CEO
Lisa Fulkerson, Vice President & CFO

9166 **Donate Life America**
701 E Byrd Street · 804-377-3580
Richmond, VA 23219 · coalition@donatelife.net
www.donatelife.net
A non-profit alliance of national organizations and local coalitions across the United States that have joined forces to educate the public about organ, eye and tissue donation, correcting misconceptions about donation, and creating a greater willingness to donate.
G. David Fleming, President & CEO
Frank Wilton, Chair

9167 **Health Resources and Services Administration (HRSA)**
5600 Fishers Lane · 877-464-4772
Rockville, MD 20857 · www.hrsa.gov
Federal agency working to improve the quality and accessibility of health care for those in need. HRSA oversees organ, bone marrow, and cord blood donation, and protects individuals against malpractice, fraud, and abuse.
George Sigounas, MS, PhD, Administrator
Brian LeClair, JD, MBA, Deputy Administrator

9168 **Jewish Hospital Transplant Center KentuckyOne Health**
200 Abraham Flexner Way · 502-587-4011
Louisville, KY 40202 · 859-313-1000
www.kentuckyonehealth.org
Dedicated to providing care, education, and producing research, Jewish Hospital is a tertiary referral hospital federally designated to perform the 5 major solid organ transplants: heart, lung, liver, kidney, and pancreas.
Jane J. Chiles, Board Chair
Martha Jones, Board Vice Chair

9169 **National Foundation for Transplants**
5350 Poplar Avenue · 901-684-1697
Memphis, TN 38119 · 800-489-3863
Fax: 901-684-1128
info@transplants.org
www.transplants.org
Connects individuals seeking an organ transplant with donors and medical professionals, and provides financial assistance to transplant patients and their families.
Gina Castellaw, Chairlady
Bill Catlette, Vice Chairman

9170 **National Institute of Allergy and Infectious Diseases**
NIAID Office of Communications & Govt Relations

5601 Fishers Lane
Bethesda, MD 20892-9806
301-496-5717
866-284-4107
Fax: 301-402-3573
TDD: 800-877-8339
ocpostoffice@niaid.nih.gov
www.niaid.nih.gov

Conducts and supports research on allergies; focused on understanding what happens to the body during the allergic process. Educates patients and health care workers in controlling allergic disease; offers various research centers that conduct and evaluate educational programs focused on methods to control allergic diseases.
Anthony S. Fauci, MD, Director

9171   National Transplant Assistance Fund (NTAF)
2 Radnor Corporate Center
Radnor, PA 19087
800-642-8399
800-642-8399
www.helphopelive.org

Previously known as the National Transplant Assistance Fund, Help Hope Live supports transplant patients by providing financial assistance through sponsoring transplant patients in the community. Help Hope Live also serves those with catastrophic injuries by providing financial assistance.
Kelly L. Green, Executive Director
Marie O'Rourke, Director of Finance

9172   Organ Procurement and Transplantation Network (OPTN)
PO Box 2484
Richmond, VA 23218
800-292-9537
800-978-4334
www.optn.transplant.hrsa.gov

Links all professionals involved in the organ donation and transplantation system in the United States, and works to increase access to organ transplants and donors.
Sue Dunn, BSN, MBA, President & CEO
Maryl Johnson, MD, Vice President

9173   United Network for Organ Sharing (UNOS)
700 N 4th Street
Richmond, VA 23219
804-782-4800
800-292-9548
patientservices@unos.org
www.unos.org

Non-profit national scientific and educational organization that administers the Organ Procurement and Transplantation Network (OPTN), connecting organ transplantation professionals and volunteers with the goal of advancing donors nationwide.
Brian Shepard, CEO
Mary Ellison, PhD, MSHA, Chief External Relations Officer

9174   United Organ Transplant Association (UOTA)
6870 Jones Avenue
Riverside, CA 92505
951-785-5804
dmorgan@uota.org
www.uota.org

Non-profit charitable organization dedicated to providing educational, emotional, and financial support to the organ transplant community.
Don Goss, Founder

State Agencies & Associations

Alabama

9175   Alabama Organ Center
500 S 22 Street S
Birmingham, AL 35233
205-731-9200
800-252-3677
Fax: 205-731-9250
Rebecca.davis@ccc.uab.edu
alabamaorgancenter.org

A non-profit, independent organ procurement organization (OPO) serving the population of the Southeastern United States.
Devin E Eckhoff, Director
R Alan Hicks MPH CPTC, Associate Director

Arizona

9176   Donor Network of Arizona
201 W Coolidge
Phoenix, AZ 85013
602-222-2200
800-94D-ONOR
Fax: 602-222-2202
Contact.Us@dnaz.org
www.dnaz.org

Participates in the equitable distribution of organs, tissues, and corneas for transplant. Also offers donor family support services, community and health care education, and presentations.
Sara Pace Jones, Public Education Contact
Tim Brown, Chief executive officer

Arkansas

9177   Arkansas Regional Organ Recovery Agency
1701 Aldersgate Road
Little Rock, AR 72205
501-907-9150
800-727-6726
Fax: 501-372-6279
info@arora.org
www.arora.org

Makes every effort to provide organs and tissues for life-saving and life-enhancing transplantation. Goal will be accomplished through continuous hospital involvement which includes hospital training community involvement andpublic education.
Audrey Brown, Director of Community Education
Boyd Ward, Executive Director

California

9178   California Transplant Donor Network
1000 Broadway
Oakland, CA 94607
888-570-9400
888-570-9400
Fax: 510-444-8501
info@ctdn.org
www.ctdn.org

Helps patients in Northern and Central California and Northern Nevada receive organ and tissue transplants. Recovers organs from donors and matches them with the more than 6 000 people who are currently waiting for transplants in this region.
Cynthia Siljestrom, Chief Executive Officer
Sonia Salloum, Community Outreach Coordinator

9179   Golden State Donor Services
1760 Creekside Oaks Drive
Sacramento, CA 95833
916-567-1600
877-401-2546
Fax: 916-567-8300
info@gsds.org

Support, enhance, and provide for the recovery and allocation of anatomical gifts. Also work to educate the public regarding the critical need for organ and tissue doors.
Katherine Doolittle, Senior Public Education Coordinator
Helen Nelson, Executive Director

9180   LifeSharing Community Organ & Tissue Donation
3465 Camino Del Rio S
San Diego, CA 92108
619-521-1983
Fax: 619-521-2833
info@lifesharing.org
www.lifesharing.org

Non-profit unique and creative organ procurement organization that has centers at the University of California at San Diego Medical Center, Green Hospital of Scripps Clinic, Sharp Hospital.
Sharie Shipley, Public Education Contact
Bill Dawson, Chairman of Volunteer Action Committee

9181   One Legacy Transplant Donor Network
221 S Figueroa Street
Los Angeles, CA 90012
213-229-5600
800-786-4077
Fax: 213-229-5601
tmone@onelegacy.org
www.onelegacy.org

One Legacy is dedicaated to achieving the donation of life saving and life enhancing organs and tissues for those in need of transplants and to providing a sense of purpose and comfort to those families we serve.
Sandra Walla Blaydow, Human Resources Manager
Thomas Mone, Chief Executive Officer/EVP

Colorado

9182 Donor Alliance
720 S Colorado Boulevard — 303-329-4747
Denver, CO 80246 — 888-868-4747
Fax: 303-321-0366
www.donoralliance.org
In cooperation with others Donor Alliance facilitates the donation and recovery of organs and tissues for people needing transplantation. Donor Alliance is one of 58 not-for-profit organ recovery organizations federally designated by the U.S..
Jennifer Moe, Director of Community Relations/PR
Nancy Williams, Chairman

Connecticut

9183 NorthEast Organ Procurement Organization
80 Seymour Street — 860-545-5000
Hartford, CT 06102-5037 — Fax: 860-545-5066
www.harthosp.org/NEOPO/index.html
Assures that comprehensive organ and tissue donation services are provided to the community in an efficient and professional manner.
Ginger Van Nostrand, Public Education Contact

Florida

9184 LifeLink of Florida
409 Bayshore Boulevard — 813-253-2640
Tampa, FL 33606 — 800-262-5775
Fax: 813-348-0634
info@lifelinkfound.org
www.lifelinkfound.org
Independent, nonprofit community service organization dedicated to the recovery and transplantation of organs and tissues. Operates under the authority of the Social Security Act, and in accordance with the National Organ Transplant Act passed by Congress.
Dennis F Heinrichs, President
Dana L Shires Jr, Chairman of the Board

9185 LifeLink of Southwest Florida
409 Bayshore Boulevard — 813-253-2640
Tampa, FL 33906 — 800-262-5775
Fax: 813-348-0634
info@lifelinkfound.org
www.lifelinkfound.org
LifeLink of Southwest Florida and Florida Gulf Coast University joined forces to develop a survey instrument to assss student attitudes and opinions about donation. Worked to conduct and evaluate the impact of the multifaceted education campaign.
Dennis F Heinrichs, President
Dana L Shires Jr, Chairman of the Board

9186 TransLife/Florida Hospital
1560 Orange Avenue — 407-644-3770
Winter Park, FL 32789 — 800-443-6667
Fax: 407-303-2473
www.translife.org
Works closely with hospitals and donor families to coordinate the gift of life in Central Florida. Also a critical link between donors and possible recipients.
Carol Rumsey, Public Education Contact

Georgia

9187 LifeLink of Georgia
2875 Northwoods Parkway — 770-225-5465
Norcross, GA 30071 — 800-544-6667
info@lifelinkfound.org
The Foundation atempts to work in a sensitive diligent and compassionate manner with donor families to facilitate the donation of desperately needed organs and tissues for waiting patients.
Dennis F Heinrichs, President
Dana L Shires, Chairman of the Board

Hawaii

9188 Organ Donor Center of Hawaii
1149 Bethel Street — 808-599-7630
Honolulu, HI 96813 — 877-855-0603
Fax: 808-599-7631
www.organdonorhawaii.com
Non-profit organ procurement organization.
Stephen A Kula, Executive Director
Christine L Bogee, Administrative Services Director

Illinois

9189 Regional Organ Bank of Illinois, Inc.
5 Spring Lake Drive — 312-431-3600
Chicago, IL 60607 — 888-307-3668
Fax: 312-803-7643
info@robi.org
www.robi.org
ROBI'S mission is to save and enhance the lives of as many people as possible through organ and tissue donation.
Kim McCullough, Public Education Contact

Indiana

9190 Indiana Organ Procurement Organization,
3760 Guion Road — 317-685-0389
Indianapolis, IN 46222-1816 — 888-275-4676
Fax: 317-685-1687
info@iopo.org
www.iopo.org
Non-profit organ procurement organization designed to recover and distribute organ and tissues for transplantation.
Sam Davis, Director of Professional Services
Lynn Driver, President and CEO

Iowa

9191 Iowa Donor Network
550 Madison Avenue — 319-665-3787
N Liberty, IA 52317 — 800-831-4131
Fax: 319-665-3788
www.iowadonornetwork.org
Iowa Donor Network is dedicated to serving donow families potentialdonors and candidates doe transplantation through identifying potential donorssupporting and respecting donation decisions and maximizing the recovery of transplantable organs and tissues.
John Watson, Chair
Sara Drobnich, Vice-Chair

Kansas

9192 Midwest Transplant Network & Organ Bank
1900 W 47th Place — 913-262-1668
Westwood, KS 66205 — Fax: 913-262-5130
info@mwob.org
www.mwtn.org
Provides quality transplantation related services that will maximize the availability of organs and tissues to the comunities we serve. Provides procurement services for organ and tissue and laboratory services for HLA.
A. Michael Borkon, MD
Gary Duncan, CEO

Kentucky

9193 Kentucky Organ Donor Affiliates
106 E Broadway — 502-581-9511
Louisville, KY 40202 — 800-525-3456
Fax: 502-589-5157
info@kyorgandonor.org
www.kyorgandonor.org
Non-profit organ donor center that retrieves and distributes organs to qualified recipients.

Louisiana

9194 Louisiana Organ Procurement Agency
3545 N. I-10 Service Rd
Metairie, LA 70002-3626

800-521-4483
800-521-GIVE
Fax: 504-837-3587
info@lopa.org
www.lopa.org

Non-profit organ procurement organization federally-designated to increase the number of transplantable organs by providing families an opportunity to donate organs and tissues to support these families regardless of their decision.
John Egan, Public Education Contact

Maryland

9195 Transplant Resource Center of Maryland
1730 Twin Springs Road
Baltimore, MD 21227

410-242-7000
800-641-HERO
Fax: 410-242-1871
communications@TheLLF.org

Provides organ and tissue donation and recovery services hospital donor program development and community education to 42 hospitals and the citizens living in Maryland.
Ann Bromery, Chief Financial Officer
Charles Alexander, President & Chief Executive Officer

Massachusetts

9196 New England Organ Bank Massachusetts
One Gateway Center
Newton, MA 02158

800-446-NEOB
Fax: 617-244-8755
www.neob.org

Independent, not-for-profit agency whose mission is to recover, preserve, and distribute human organs and tissues for transplantation. A federally-designated organ procurement organization for all or part of the six New England states, it serves 177 acute care hospitals and 14 transplant centers.
Sean Fitzpatrick, Public Education Contact

Michigan

9197 Transplantation Society of Michigan
3861 Research Park Drive
Ann Arbor, MI 48108

734-973-1577
800-482-4881
Fax: 734-973-3133
info@giftoflifemichigan.org
www.giftoflifemichigan.org

Nonprofit independent corporation certified by Medicare and designated by the Centers for Medicare and Medicaid Services as an organ recovery organization for Michigan.
Tammie Harvermahl, Public Education Contact

Minnesota

9198 LifeSource, Upper Midwest Organ Procurement Organization, Inc.
2550 University Avenue West
St. Paul, MN 55114-1904

651-603-7800
Fax: 651-603-7801
info@life-source.org
www.life-source.org

Nonprofit, federally-designated organ procurement organization for the Upper Midwest, managing all organ donation activities in Minnesota.
Jill Halimi, Donor Family Services

Mississippi

9199 Mississippi Organ Recovery
12 River Bend Place
Flowood, MS 39232

601-933-1000
800-690-8878
Fax: 601-933-1006
www.msora.org

Not-for-profit organization coordinates the recovery of human organs for transplantation by working with and providing education to medical professionals donor families and the people of Mississippi.
Kelly Nations, Community Education Coordinator
Kevin Stump, Chief Executive Officer

Missouri

9200 Mid-America Transplant Services
1110 Highlands Plaza Drive E
Saint Louis, MO 63110-3205

314-735-8200
Fax: 314-991-2805
info@mts-stl.org

Community based not-for-profit organ procurement organization dedicated to enhancing the quality of human life. Coordinates the procurement of vital organs tissues and eyes in hospitals throughout its service area.
Diane Brockmeier, COO
Dean F Kappel, President and CEO

Nebraska

9201 Nebraska Organ Retrieval System
8502 W Center Road
Omaha, NE 68124

402-733-1800
877-633-1800
Fax: 402-733-9142
www.NEdonation.org

Responsible for retrieving the proper organs and distrbuting them to the recipients.
Kyle Herber, Executive Director
John Stallabaum, Client Services Manager

Nevada

9202 Nevada Donor Network
2059 E Sahara Avenue
Las Vegas, NV 89104

702-384-7616
Fax: 702-796-4225
ksatcher@nvdonor.org
www.nvdonor.org

Improving the quality of human life through the recovery of all available organs and tissues for transplantation education and research while maintaining the dignity of the donors and their families.
Liliana Arredondo, Public Education Coordinator
Ken Richardson, Executive Director

New Jersey

9203 Sharing Network Organ Tissue Donation Services
691 Central Avenue
New Providence, NJ 07974

908-516-5400
800-742-7365
Fax: 908-516-5501
tsn@sharenj.org
www.sharenj.org

Federally certified state-approved organ procurement organization responsible for recovering organ and tissue for New Jersey residents currently awaiting transplants.
Vito Pulito, Chair
Bruce I. Goldstein, Vice Chair

New Mexico

9204 New Mexico Donor Services
1609 University Blvd NE
Albuquerque, NM 87102

505-843-7672
877-401-2511
Fax: 505-343-1828
info@donatelifenm.org
www.donatelifenm.org

Transplant centers in the service area are: University of New Mexico Hospitals Presbyterian Hospital.
Wayne Dunlap, Interim Executive Director
Maria Sanders, Community Relations

New York

9205 Center for Donation & Transplantation
218 Great Oaks Boulevard
Albany, NY 12203

518-262-5606
800-256-7811
Fax: 518-262-5427
dfloeser@cdtny.org
www.cdtny.org

Dedicated to increasing organ and tissue donation by following procurement and equitable distribution of medically suitable organs and tissue for transplantation.
Michael Thiabault, Executive Director
Martin benoit, Director

9206 Finger Lakes Donor Recovery Network
Corporate Woods of Brighton
Rochester, NY 14623
585-272-4930
Fax: 585-272-4956
info@donorrecovery.org
www.donorrecovery.org
Nonprofit organization that covers the Finger Lakes Region Central and Upstate New York for transplant centers.
Diane Ashley, Executive Director
Julius Gene Lattore, Vice Chair

9207 New York Organ Donor Network, Inc
132 West 31st Street
New York, NY 10001
646-291-4444
Fax: 646-291-4600
The New York Organ Donor Network is dedicated to the recovery of organs and tissues for people in need of life-saving and life-improvving transplants.
Elaine Berg, President/CEO

9208 Upstate New York Transplant Services, Inc.
110 Broadway
Buffalo, NY 14203
716-853-6667
800-227-4771
Fax: 716-853-6674
info@unyts.org
www.unyts.org
An independent nonprofit organization that encourages and coordinates the donation of human organs and tissue for transplantation.
Richard A Grimm, Chairman
Michael Beecher, Vice Chairman

North Carolina

9209 Life Share of the Carolinas
5000 D Airport Center Parkway
Charlotte, NC 28208
704-512-3303
800-932-4483
Fax: 704-512-3056
lifeshare@carolinas.org
www.lifesharecarolinas.org
Mission is to improve the quality of human life through the provision of organs and tissues for transplantation and to serve our hospitals and their respective communities by rpoviding educational support services which enhance the donation process.
Dan Hayes, Medical Director
David Ugland, Bank Medical Director

Ohio

9210 Life Connection of Ohio
3661 Briarfield Boulevard
Maumee, OH 43537
419-893-1618
800-262-5443
Fax: 419-893-1827
ksteele@lcotro.org
www.lifeconnectionofohio.org
Life Connection of Ohio is committed to serving humanity by ending the wait for organ and tissue transplants in a manner that is beneficial to patients, donor families, health care professionals and the public.
Kara Steele, Director of Community Relations (Toledo)
Cathi Arends, Director of Community Relations (Dayton)

9211 LifeBanc
4775 Richmond Road,
Cleveland, OH 44128-5343
216-752-5433
888-558-LIFE
Fax: 216-751-4204
info@lifebanc.org
www.lifebanc.org
Non-profit organization that covers all of Northeast Ohio.
Monica Morgan, Public Education Contact

9212 Lifeline of Ohio Organ Procurement Agency, Inc.
770 Kinnear Road
Columbus, OH 43212
614-291-5667
800-525-5667
Fax: 614-291-0660
www.lifelineofohio.org
Lifeline of Ohio (LOOP) is an independent non-profit organization whose purpose is to promote and coordinate the donation of human organs and tissue dor transplantation.
Roger L Walker, Chairperson
Mark E Brainbridge, Treasurer

9213 Ohio Valley LifeCenter
2925 Vernon Place
Cincinnati, OH 45219-2430
513-558-5555
800-981-5433
Fax: 513-558-5556
info@lifepassiton.org
www.lifecnt.org
Encourages amd coordinates the donation of human organs and tissues in the Greater Cincinnati area. Provides educational and motivational progams to healthcare professionals regarding their important role in the donation of organs and tissues for transplant.
Mark Sommerville, Public Education Contact
Michael Edwards, Chairman

Oklahoma

9214 Oklahoma Organ Sharing Network
5801 N Broadway
Oklahoma City, OK 73118
888-580-5680
Fax: 405-840-9748
philvs@oosn.org ˜
LifeShare Transplant Donor Services of Oklahoma is committed to providing a better quality of life for those people who require organ or tissue transplantation while respecting and honoring those families who share the gift of life.
Harlan Wright, President

Oregon

9215 Pacific NW Transplant Bank
2611 SW 3rd Avenue
Portland, OR 97201-4952
503-494-5560
800-344-8916
Fax: 503-494-4725
pntb@ohsu.edu
www.pntb.org
Federally designated nonprofit organ procurement organization serving Oregon southwest Washington and western Idaho.
Mike Seeley, Executive Director
Craig Van De Walker, Director Of Operation

Pennsylvania

9216 Center for Organ Recovery & Education
RIDC Park
Pittsburgh, PA 15238
800-366-6777
Fax: 412-963-3563
hbulvony@core.org
www.core.org
Continues its efforts to lead the procurement field by becoming a full-service OPO.
Susan A Stuart, President & CEO
Karen Zumba, Executive Adminstratve Director

9217 Gift of Life Donor Program Pennsylvania
401 North 3rd Street
Philadelphia, PA 19123-3813
215-557-8090
888-366-6771
Fax: 215-963-0587
info@donors1.org
www.donors1.org
Formerly (Delaware Valley Transplant Program) is the region's nonprofit organ and tissue donor program serving eastern half of Pennsylvania, southern New Jersey and the state of Delaware. Also, considered a model program in the United States.
Glen D Moffet, Chair
Gerad J. Fulda, Vice Chair

Tennessee

9218 Mid-South Transplant Foundation, Inc. Tennessee
8001 Centerview Parkway
Corodova, TN 38018
901-328-4438
877-228-LIFE
Fax: 901-448-8126
www.midsouthtransplant.org
Mission is to provide the option of donation to all families of potential organ donors and to protect their rights and interest throughout the donation process.
Louis G Britt, President
Kenneth D Sellers, Medical Director

9219 Tennessee Donor Services
1600 Hayes Street
Nashville, TN 37203   423-915-0808
888-562-3774
Fax: 901-448-8126
info@donatelifetn.org
donatelifetn.org
Mission is to represent the interests of the people of our service area in the formulation of policies procedures and regulations concerning organ donation and transplantation.
Lisa Peoples, Public Education Contact
Jennifer Jenks, Contact

Utah

9220 Intermountain Donor Services
230 S 500 E
Salt Lake City, UT 84102   801-521-1755
800-833-6667
Fax: 801-364-8815
www.idslife.org
Provides high quality organ and tissue procurement services to the medical and public communities. Educating medical professionals and the poublic sector on the benefits of organ and tissue donation.
Alex McDonald, Public Education Director
Tracy C Schmidt, Executive Director

Virginia

9221 LifeNet
1864 Concert Drive
Virginia Beach, VA 23453   75- 46- 476
800-847-7831
Fax: 757-301-6582
lifenet@trans.org
An organ procurement agency and the largest full-service tissue bank in the United States providing musculoskeletal and cardiovascular tissues for transplant on a national and international basis.
Becky Lawson, Public Education Contact

9222 Washington Regional Transplant Consortium
7619 Little River Turnpike
Annandale, VA 22003   703-641-0100
866-232-3666
Fax: 703-658-0711
contactwrtc@wrtc.org
www.wrtc.org
Recently partnered with fellow Mid-Atlantic Coalition on Donation members and a company called Sports America to sponsor the second annual DeMatha Invitational. WRTC is the official link between organ and tissue donors and the patients who are waiting for transplant.
Sara Idler, Public Education Contact

Washington

9223 LifeCenter Northwest
11245 SE 6th Street
Bellevue, WA 98004   425-201-6563
877-275-5269
Fax: 425-688-7641
info@lcnw.org
www.lcnw.org
LifeCenter Northwest Organ Donation Network is a nonprofit organization that facilitates organ donation for a population of over 7.5 million people throughout Washington Montana Alasks and Nothern Idaho. Our mission is to fund education and outreach programs.
Megan Erwin, Vice President Community Relations
Diana Clark, President & CEO

Wisconsin

9224 University of Wisconsin Organ Procurement Organization
University of Wisconsin Hospital and Clinics
600 Highland Ave.   608-265-0356
Madison, WI 53972-1735   Fax: 608-262-9099
uwhcopo@uwhealth.org
www.uwhcopo.org
Located within a major academic center and is recognized as one of the most successful organ procurement programs in the nation.
Jill Ellefson, Public Education Contact

9225 Wisonsin Donor Network
638 North 18th Street?   41- 9-7 61
Milwaukee, WI 53233   1 -77 -32 4
Fax: 414-259-8059
labinfo@bcw.edu
www.bcw.edu
Recovers organs for transplant as well as provides public and professional education about the tremendous need for organ and tissue donors.
Richard S. Gallaghar, Chairman
Peter D. Zegler, Vice Chair

Foundations

9226 Musculoskeletal Transplant Foundation
125 May Street
Edison, NJ 08837   732-661-0202
800-946-9008
Fax: 732-661-2298
information@mtf.org
www.mtf.org
Non-profit service organization dedicated to providing quality tissue through a commitment to excellence in education, research, recovery and care for recipients, donors, and their families.
Bruce W Stroever, President/CEO
Martha Anderson, Executive Vice President

Research Centers

9227 Georgetown University Hospital Transplant Institute
3800 Reservoir Road, NW   202-444-2000
Washington, DC 20007   www.georgetownuniversityhospital.org
Founded to promote health through education, research, and patient care.

Support Groups & Hotlines

9228 National Health Information Center
Office of Disease Prevention & Health Promotion
1101 Wootton Pkwy   Fax: 240-453-8281
Rockville, MD 20852   odphpinfo@hhs.gov
www.health.gov/nhic
Supports public health education by maintaining a calendar of National Health Observances; helps connect consumers and health professionals to organizations that can best answer questions and provide up-to-date contact information from reliable sources; updates on a yearly basis toll-free numbers for health information, Federal health clearinghouses and info centers.
Don Wright, MD, MPH, Director

Books

9229 History of Organ and Cell Transplantation
Imperial College Press
57 Shelton St.
Lomdon, UK   207-836- 888
Fax: 207-836- 020
sales@wspc.co.uk
www.icpress.co.uk
Our aim is to create the highest quality, knowledge-based products and to enable continuous learning for the global scientific and professional communities
464 pages Hardcover
ISBN: 1-860942-09-1

9230 Legal and Ethical Aspects of Organ Transplantation
David P T Price, author
Cambridge University Press
40 West 20th Street
New York, NY 10011-4221   212-924-3900
Fax: 212-691-3239
www.cambridge.org/us
A comprehensive analysis of existing laws and policies governing transplantation practices around the world. Examines the meaning of death, cadaver organ procurement policies, use of living donors,

trading in human organs, experimental transplant procedures and xenotransplantation.
507 pages Hardcover
ISBN: 0-521651-64-6

9231 Organ Procurement and Transplantation:
Intitute of Medicine, author
National Academies Press
500 Fifth Street NW
Washington, DC 20001

202-334-3313
800-624-6242
Fax: 202-334-2451
Customer_Service@nap.edu
www.nap.edu

This book assesses the potential impact of the Final Rule on organ transplantation. Prensents new, original data, and assesses medical practices, social and economic observations, and other information.
232 pages Hardcover

9232 Organ Transplants from Executed Prisoners:
Louis J Palmer, author
McFarland & Company
960 NC Hwy 88W
Jefferson, NC 28640

336-246-4460
800-253-2187
Fax: 336-246-5018
info@mcfarlandpub.com
www.mcfarlandpub.com

A study of the utilitarian creation of death sentence organ removal statutes that would make legal the harvesting of transplantable organs from the cadavers of executed capital murders.
156 pages
ISBN: 0-786406-73-9

9233 Transplantation Ethics
Robert M. Veatch, author
Georgetown University Press
3240 Prospect Street, NW
Washington, DC 20007

202-687-5889
Fax: 202-687-6340
gupress@georgetown.edu
www.press.georgetown.edu

The first complete and systematic account of the ethical and policy controversies surrounding organ transplants.
2000 448 pages Paperback
ISBN: 0-878408-12-2
Richard Brown, Director
Donald Jacobs, Senior Acquisitions Editor

9234 Twice Dead: Organ Transplants and the Reinvention of Death
Margaret Lock, author
University of California Press
1445 Lower Ferry Road
Ewing, NJ 08618

609-883-1759
800-777-4726
Fax: 800-999-1958

Raises critically important questions about life and death in the modern world.
429 pages Paperback
ISBN: 0-520228-14-6
Alison Mudditt, Director

9235 US Organ Procurement System: A Prescription for Reform
David L. Kaserman, A.H. Barnett, author
American Enterprise Institute
1150 Seventeenth St, NW
Washington, DC 20036

202-862-5800
Fax: 202-862-7177
custserv@nbnbooks.com
www.aei.org

Isolates the procurement issue from others to make a compelling and persuasive case for markets in cadaveric organs.
177 pages Paperback
ISBN: 0-844741-71-X
Tully M. Friedman, Chairman and CEO
Daniel A. D'Aniello, Vice Chairman

Magazines

9236 Encore: Another Chance for Life
Chronimed Pharmacy

Po Box 59032
Minneapolis, MN 55459-9686

800-888-5753
www.transplantawareness.org

Published exclusively for transplant patients, their families, and friends, this publication provides a broad look at many issues surrounding transplantation and encourages personal stories and feedback from readers.
Quarterly

9237 Renalife
The American Association of Kidney Patients
100 S. Ashley Drive
Tampa, FL 33260

800-749-2257
aakpaz@enet.net

Provides articles, news items, and information of interest to kindey patients and their families, individuals, and organizations in the renal health care field.
3 Year

9238 Stadtlanders LifeTIMES
Stadtlanders Pharmacy
600 Penn Center Boulevard
Pittsburgh, PA 15235-5810

800-238-7828

Designed to be an educational, informative and supportive, focusing on a variety of health-care issues of concern to patients (including transplant patients).

Newsletters

9239 Advocate
National Foundation for Transplants
5350 Poplar Ave
Memphis, TN 38119

901-684-1697
800-489-3863
Fax: 901-684-1128
info@transplants.org
www.transplants.org

Linda J. Evans, Chairman
Matthew Schneider, Vice-Chairman

9240 Children's Organ Transplant Association (COTA)
2501 COTA Drive
Bloomington, IN 47403

800-366-2682
Fax: 812-336-8885
cota@cota.org
www.cota.org

Provides fundraising assistance to children and young adults needing life-saving transplants and promotes organ, marrow and tissue donation.
Rick Lofgren, President/CEO
Lisa Fulkerson, VP/CFO

9241 New Start News
National Transplant Assistance Fund (NTAF)
3475 West Chester Pike
Newtown Square, PA 19073

610-353-9684
800-642-8399
Fax: 610-353-1616
ntaf@transplantfund.org
m.helphopelive.org

Sidney P. Constien, Editor
Judy Walker, Editor

Web Sites

9242 American Society of Transplantation (AST)
An organization of transplant professionals dedicated to research, education, advocacy and patient care in transplantation science and medicine.

9243 Association of Organ Procurement Organizations (AOPO)
www.aopo.org

Organization involved in helping people find and obtain the organs they may need for transplantation.

9244 Children's Organ Transplant Association (COTA)
www.cota.org

Not-for-profit national chairty dedicated to helping families and communities raise the necessary funds for transplant expenses.

9245 Donate Life America
www.donatelife.net

A not-for-profit alliance of national organizations and local coalitions across the United States that have joined forces to educate the public about organ, eye and tissue donation, correcting misconceptions about donation and creating a greater willingness to donate.

9246 Georgetown University Hospital Transplant Institute

www.georgetownuniversityhospital.org

Founded to promote health through education, research, and patient care.

9247 Health Resources and Services Administration (HRSA)

www.hrsa.gov

Envisions optimal health for all, supported by a health care system that assures access to comprehensive, culturally competant, quality care. Provides national leadership, program resources and services needed to improve access to culturally competant, quality health care.

9248 Jewish Hospital Transplant Center

An elite group approved to perform five solid organ transplants and has been named a Federally Designated Medicare Heart, Lung, Kidney, Liver and Pancreas Transplant Center.

9249 MedicineNet

www.medicinenet.com

An online resource for consumers providing easy-to-read, authoritative medical and health information.

9250 National Foundation for Transplants

www.transplants.org

Mission is to reach out to help those who seek a new life through transplantation, by providing healthcare and financial support services and patient advocacy for transplant candidates families nationwide.

9251 National Transplant Assistance Fund (NTAF)

www.transplantfund.org

Helps to raise funds for transplant and catastrophic injury patients by providing compassionate support, education and expertise to them, their families and communities.

9252 Organ Procurement and Transplantation Network (OPTN)

A unified transplant network established by the United States Congress under the National Organ Transplant Act (NOTA) of 1984. A unique public-prvate partnership that links all of the professionals nvolved in the donation and transplantation system.

9253 Transweb: All About Transplantation and Donation

www.transweb.org

Non-profit educational website serving the world transplant community. Features news and events, real peoples experinces, the top 10 myths about donation, a donation quiz, and a large collection of questions and answers, as well as a reference area with everything from articles to videos.

9254 United Network for Organ Sharing (UNOS)

www.unos.org

Non-profit, scientific and educational organization that administers the nation's only Organ Procurement and Transplantation Network(OPTN). Mission is to advance organ availability and transplantation by uniting and supporting our communities for the benefit of patients through education, technology and policy development.

9255 United Organ Transplant Association (UOTA)

www.uota.org

Non-profit charitable Corporation dedicated to providing educational, emotional and financial support to pre- and post- transplant patients.

Description

9256 Tuberculosis

Tuberculosis, TB, is an infectious disease caused by Mycobacterium tuberculosis. It is spread through the air and normally affects the lungs (pulmonary tuberculosis). Extremely common in the United States early in the twentieth century, tuberculosis declined dramatically after 1950. This trend reversed itself after about 1985, due to immigration, the HIV epidemic, and the development of drug resistance by the M. tuberculosis.

The usual symptoms of TB infection of the lungs include persistent cough, chest pain and coughing up blood. TB infection can cause weight loss, night sweats and fatigue. Left untreated, TB may spread to the spine, causing bone breakdown with deformity, to the lining of the brain, causing tuberculous meningitis, or, in fact, to any organ of the body (extrapulmonary TB).

People who are otherwise healthy, and who are infected with a strain of mycobacterium that is sensitive to standard drugs, can almost always be cured after 6-9 months of therapy. Persons infected with HIV, because of their lowered resistance to disease, have trouble clearing their TB infection, even if they use effective drugs faithfully. Therefore, they should be treated for one year. Regardless of length of treatment, during this time the germ may become resistant to the drug being used. Therefore, treatment includes at least 4 drugs, so that a bacterium that develops resistance to one drug will still be killed by another one. Incomplete or interrupted treatment often leads todrug resistance. Bacteria that are resistant to multiple drugs may be passed to others and are now a serious public health menace. Unfortunately, the HIV-infected patient is an ideal breeding ground for drug-resistant TB germs.

Persons with drug-sensitive TB who are otherwise healthy and will cooperate with treatment are generally treated by community physicians. Those with complicated medical status (HIV, drug-resistant organisms) or social difficulties (alcoholism, substance abuse, homelessness) generally require specialized public health clinics that can combine medical expertise with nursing and social outreach support.

Many persons who have been infected by TB keep it successfully contained by their own immune systems. There is some risk that the initial infection may, even years later, overcoming the body's resistance and cause active disease. The tuberculin skin test (PPD) is used to widely screen certain high-risk populations, particularly those who have been exposed to an infectious individual. Prior, adequately treated infection may be diagnosed by a positive PPD and is sometimes treated with antibiotics to reduce the risk of future disease. BCG (Bacillus Calmette-Gu,rin) is an attenuated strain of M. tuberculosis that has been successfully used as a vaccine against tuberculosis. Unfortunately, it is not completely effective, and compromises the epidemiological usefulness of the PPD skin test.

National Agencies & Associations

9257 American Lung Association
55 W. Wacker Drive
Chicago, IL 60601

800-586-4872
info@lung.org
www.lung.org

The mission of the American Lung Association is to prevent lung disease and promote lung health by fighting disease in all its forms, with special emphasis on asthma, tobacco control and environmental health.
Harold P. Wimmer, National President & CEO
Albert Rizzo, MD, FACP, Chief Medical Officer

9258 Centers for Disease Control and Prevention
1600 Clifton Road
Atlanta, GA 30333-4027

800-232-4636
TTY: 888-232-6348
cdcinfo@cdc.gov
www.cdc.gov

The Centers for Disease Control and Prevention is dedicated to protecting and promoting health through the prevention and control of disease, injury, and disability.
Robert R. Redfield, MD, Director
Anne Schuchat, MD, Principal Deputy Director

9259 National Institute of Allergy and Infectious Diseases
NIAID Office of Communications & Govt Relations
5601 Fishers Lane
Bethesda, MD 20892-9806

301-496-5717
866-284-4107
Fax: 301-402-3573
TDD: 800-877-8339
ocpostoffice@niaid.nih.gov
www.niaid.nih.gov

Conducts and supports research on allergies; focused on understanding what happens to the body during the allergic process. Educates patients and health care workers in controlling allergic disease; offers various research centers that conduct and evaluate educational programs focused on methods to control allergic diseases.
Anthony S. Fauci, MD, Director

9260 Occupational Safety & Health Administration (OSHA)
200 Constitution Avenue NW
Washington, DC 20210

800-321-6742
TTY: 877-889-5627
www.osha.gov

Ensures the health and safety of America's workers by setting and enforcing guidelines and standards, training, and education in workplace safety measures. OSHA is part of the United States Department of Labor.
Loren Sweattwski, Deputy Assistant Secretary
Krisann Pearce, Chief of Staff

9261 Rutgers Global Tuberculosis Institute New Jersey Medical School
225 Warren Street
Newark, NJ 07103

973-972-3270
800-482-3627
Fax: 973-972-3268
www.globaltb.njms.rutgers.edu

Provides expert medical consultation, and trains health care providers and other health related professionals on the treatment of tuberculosis in an effort to prevent and cure tuberculosis worldwide.
Alfred A. Lardizabal, MD, Executive Director
Rajita Bhavaraju, MPH, PhD, Deputy Director

State Agencies & Associations

Alabama

9262 American Lung Association of Alabama
PO Box 3188   205-933-8821
Bessemer, AL 35023   800-LUN-GUSA
                                     Fax: 205-930-1717
Kim Perry, Director of Development

Alaska

9263 American Lung Association of Alaska
500 W International Airport Road   907-276-5864
Anchorage, AK 99518   800-LUN-GUSA
                                      Fax: 907-565-5587
                                      mlarson@aklung.org
                                      www.aklung.org
Marge Larson, Director

Arizona

9264 Northern Arizona Branch:Phoenix Area
102 W McDowell Road   602-258-7505
Phoenix, AZ 85003-1299   800-LUN-GUSA
                                      Fax: 602-258-7507
                                      www.lungarizona.org
Nancy Cohrs, Executive Director
Evelyn Frear, Office Manager

9265 Southern Arizona Branch: Tucson Area
2819 E Broadway   520-323-1812
Tuscon, AZ 85716   800-LUN-GUSA
                                      Fax: 520-323-1816
                                      www.lungarizona.org
Keith Kaback, Chairman
Heidi Miller, Vice Chairman

Arkansas

9266 American Lung Association of Arkansas
217 W 2nd Street   501-957-0758
Little Rock, AR 72201-1539   Fax: 501-978-5138
                                      inquiries@breathehealthy.org
                                      www.lung.org

California

9267 American Lung Association of California
424 Pendleton Way   510-638-LUNG
Oakland, CA 94621-2189   800-LUN-GUSA
                                      Fax: 510-638-8984
                                      www.lung.org
Linda Hinojosa, Chairman
Laura Keegan Boudreau, Acting CEO

Colorado

9268 American Lung Association of Colorado
5600 Greenwood Plaza Boulevard   303-388-4327
Greenwood Village, CO 80111-2305   800-LUN-GUSA
                                      Fax: 303-377-1102
                                      www.lung.org
Curt Huber, Executive Director
Connor Michael, Communications Manager

Connecticut

9269 American Lung Association of Connecticut
45 Ash Street   860-289-5401
E Hartford, CT 06108-3272   800-992-2263
                                      Fax: 860-289-5405
                                      info@lungne.org
                                      www.lung.org
Margaret LaCroix, Vice President Communications

Delaware

9270 American Lung Association of Delaware
630 Churchmans Rd   302-737-6414
Newark, DE 19806-3280   Fax: 302-737-126
                                      llyons@lunginfo.org
                                      www.lung.org
Peter Shanley, Chairman

District of Columbia

9271 American Lung Association of Washington
1301 Pennsylvania Ave NW   202-785-3355
Washington, DC 20004   800-732-9339
                                      Fax: 206-441-3277
                                      www.lung.org
Vivian Echavarria, Chair
Rick Weems, Secretary

9272 American Lung Association of the District of Columbia
1301 Pennsylvania Ave NW   202-785-3355
Washington, DC 20004-2617   Fax: 202-682-5607
                                      www.lung.org
Jan Morgan, Special Events Director
Phoebe Robinson, Administrative Coordinator

Florida

9273 American Lung Association of Florida
6852 Belfort Oaks Place   904-743-2933
Jacksonville, FL 32216-5216   800-940-2933
                                      Fax: 904-743-2916
                                      alaf@lungfla.org
                                      www.lung.org
Michael Diamond, President
Marilin K Glassberg, President-Elect

Georgia

9274 American Lung Association of Georgia
2452 Spring Road   770-434-5864
Smyrna, GA 30080   800-586-4872
                                      Fax: 770-319-0349
                                      www.lung.org
Charles J White, Chief Executive Officer
June Deen, VP Public Affairs

Hawaii

9275 American Lung Association of Hawaii
650 Iwilei Road   808-537-5966
Honolulu, HI 96817   Fax: 808-537-5971
                                      lung@ala-hawaii.org
                                      www.lung.org
Karen J Lee, President, Executive Director

Illinois

9276 American Lung Association of Illinois-Iowa
55 W Upper Wacker Dr   312-781-1100
Chicago, IL 60601   800-586-4872
                                      Fax: 217-787-5916
                                      info@lungil.org
                                      www.lung.org
Harold Wimmer, CEO
Lori Younker, Manager

Indiana

9277 **American Lung Association of Indiana: State Office & Support Office**
9445 Delegates Row,
Indianapolis, IN 46240

317-573-3900
800-LUN-GUSA
Fax: 317-819-1187
info@lungin.org
www.lung.org

Dana Pitts, VP Communications/Marketing

Kansas

9278 **American Lung Association of Kansas**
6701 W 64th Street
Overland Park, KS 66202-2419

913-912-7190
Fax: 866-575-1761
www.lung.org

Judy Keller, Executive Director

Kentucky

9279 **American Lung Association of Kentucky**
4100 Churchman Avenue
Louisville, KY 40209-0067

502-363-2652
800-LUN-GUSA
Fax: 502-363-0222
www.lung.org

Todd Adams, Development Director
Laura Collins, Executive Assistant

Louisiana

9280 **American Lung Association of Louisiana**
2325 Severn Avenue
Metairie, LA 70001-6918

504-828-5864
800-LUN-GUSA
Fax: 504-828-5867
www.lung.org

Aline Palmisano-Vita, Deputy Executive Director
Thomas P Lotz, Chief Executive Officer

Maine

9281 **American Lung Association of Maine**
122 State Street
Augusta, ME 04330

207-622-6394
800-LUN-GUSA
Fax: 639-426-2919
info@lungme.org
www.lung.org

Lee Scott, President of Health Promotion
Edward Miller, Executive Director/SVP

Maryland

9282 **American Lung Association of Maryland**
211 East Lombard St
Baltimore, MD 21202

443-451-4950
Fax: 410-560-0829
www.lung.org

Melina Davis-Martin, President and CEO
Krista Jennings, Chief Operations Officer

Massachusetts

9283 **American Lung Association of Massachusetts**
460 Totten Pond Road
Waltham, MA 02451

781-890-4262
Fax: 781-890-4280
info@lungma.org
www.lung.org

Michigan

9284 **American Lung Association of Michigan**
1475 E 12 Mile Road
Madison Heights, MI 48071

248-784-2000
800-543-5864
Fax: 248-784-2008
alam@alam.org
www.lung.org

Colette Scholzen, President

Minnesota

9285 **American Lung Association of Minnesota**
490 Concordia Avenue
Saint Paul, MN 55103-2441

651-227-8014
800-LUN-GUSA
Fax: 651-227-5459
info@alamn.org
www.lung.org

Bill Westhoff, President

Mississippi

9286 **American Lung Association of Mississippi**
731 Pear Orchard Road
Ridgeland, MS 39158

601-206-5810
800-586-4872
Fax: 601-206-5813
www.lung.org

Greg Wynne, Chairman
Jennifer Cofer, Deputy Executive Director

Missouri

9287 **American Lung Association of Missouri**
1118 Hampton Avenue
Saint Louis, MO 63139

314-645-5505
Fax: 314-645-7128
inquiries@breathehealthy.org
www.lung.org

Lori Pickens, Chief Executive Officer
Barry Freedman, VP Community Initiatives

Montana

9288 **American Lung Association of the Northern Rockies: Montana and Wyoming**
825 Helena Avenue
Helene, MT 59601-3459

406-442-6556
Fax: 406-442-2346
www.lung.org

Nebraska

9289 **American Lung Association of Nebraska**
8990 W Dodge Rd
Omaha, NE 68114

402-502-4950
Fax: 402-502-3012
www.lung.org

Nevada

9290 **American Lung Association of Idaho/Nevada**
10615 Double R Boulevard
Reno, NV 89521-7056

775-829-LUNG
800-LUN-GUSA
Fax: 775-829-5850
www.lung.org

Louise Martin, Executive Director
Gwen Bourne, Development Manager - Events

New Hampshire

9291 **American Lung Association of New Hampshire**
1800 Elm St
Manchester, NH 03104

603-369-3977
Fax: 603-369-3978
www.lung.org

Jeff Seyler, President & CEO
David Ales, Senior Vice President

New Jersey

9292 **American Lung Association of New Jersey**
1031 Route 22 West
Bridgewater, NJ 08807-3407

908-685-8040
800-LUN-GUSA
Fax: 908-851-2625
jgrinwald@lunginfo.org
www.lung.org

John A Rutkowski, President

New Mexico

9293 New Mexico Branch
7001 Menaul Boulevard NE
Albuquerque, NM 87110

505-265-0732
800-LUN-GUSA
Fax: 505-260-1739
www.lungusa.org

New York

9294 American Lung Association of Mid New York
155 Washington Avenue
Albany, NY 12210

518-465-2013
Fax: 518-465-2926
info@alany.org
www.lung.org

The mission of the American Lung Association and the American Lung Association of New York State is to prevent lung disease and promote lung health. The American Lung Association is the oldest voluntary health organization in the United States.
Deborah Carioto, President
Michael Seilback, Vice President Public Policy

North Carolina

9295 American Lung Association of North Carolina
514 Daniels St.
Raleigh, NC 27605

919-424-6069
800-892-5650
Fax: 919-856-8530
lungnc@lungusa.org
www.lung.org

Deborah C. Bryan, President

North Dakota

9296 American Lung Association of North Dakota
212 N 2nd Street
Bismarck, ND 58502

701-223-5613
Fax: 919-856-8530
dbryan@lungnc.org
www.lung.org

Deborah C Bryan, VP Advocacy & Donor Value
Mendi Nieters, Regional VP Development

Ohio

9297 American Lung Association of Ohio
1950 Arlingate Lane
Columbus, OH 43228

614-279-1700
800-LUN-GUSA
Fax: 614-279-4940
alao@ohiolung.org
www.lung.org

Tracy Ross, President / CEO

Oklahoma

9298 American Lung Association of Oklahoma
1010 E 8th Street
Tulsa, OK 74120

918-747-3441
Fax: 918-747-4629
www.lung.org

Sara Dreiling, Chief Executive Officer
Edward C Rosentel, Chief Financial and Operating Officer

Oregon

9299 American Lung Association of Oregon
7420 SW Bridgeport Road
Tigard, OR 97224

503-924-4094
Fax: 503-924-4120
info@lungoregon.org
www.lung.org

Jan Jensen, President
Dana Kaye, Executive Director

Pennsylvania

9300 American Lung Association of Pennsylvania
3001 Old Gettysburg Road
Camp Hill, PA 17011

717-541-5864
800-LUN-GUSA
Fax: 888-415-5757
dbrown@lunginfo.org
www.lung.org

South Carolina

9301 American Lung Association of South Carolina
1817 Gadsen Street
Columbia, SC 29201-2392

803-779-5864
800-849-5864
Fax: 803-254-2711
alasc@lungsc.org
www.lung.org

South Dakota

9302 American Lung Association of South Dakota
108 E 38th Street
Sioux Falls, SD 57105

605-336-7222
Fax: 803-254-2711
www.lung.org

Amanda Strickland, Regional Manager Special Events
Sharon Helps, Regional Manager Programs

Tennessee

9303 American Lung Association of Tennesse
One Vantage Way
Nashville, TN 37228

615-329-1151
800-LUN-GUSA
Fax: 615-329-1723
www.lung.org

Texas

9304 American Lung Association of Texas
8150 Brookriver Drive
Dallas, TX 75247-0460

512-467-6753
800-252-5864
Fax: 512-467-7621
www.lung.org

Phillip J Hanson, Senior VP Resource Development
Margaret Crump, Senior VP Community Initiatives

Utah

9305 American Lung Association of Utah
1930 S 1100 E
Salt Lake City, UT 84106-2317

801-484-4456
Fax: 801-484-5461
www.lung.org

Vermont

9306 American Lung Association of Vermont
372 Hurricane Lane
Williston, VT 05495-6196

802-876-6500
Fax: 802-876-6505
www.lung.org

Erin Hickey, Senior Manager Development
Margaret LaCroix, VP Marketing\Communications

Virginia

9307 American Lung Association of Virginia
9702 Gayton Rd
Richmond, VA 23238

804-955-4910
Fax: 804-267-5634
lungva@lungusa.org
www.lung.org

Melina Davis-Martin, President and CEO
Krista Jennings, Chief Operating Officer

West Virginia

9308 American Lung Association of West Virginia
2102 Kanawha Blvd
East Charleston, WV 25311-3980

304-342-6600
Fax: 304-342-6096
cfields@lunginfo.org
www.lung.org

Sara Crickenberger, Executive Director

Wisconsin

9309 American Lung Association of Wisconsin
13100 W Lisbon Road   262-703-4200
Brookfield, WI 53005-2508   800-586-4872
                                           Fax: 262-781-5180
                                           info@lungwi.org
                                           www.lung.org

Susan Gloede Swan, Executive Director
Dona Wininsky, Director of Public Policy

Research Centers

9310 University of Illinois at Chicago Lions
2035 W Taylor St   312-355-1715
Chicago, IL 60612   Fax: 312-355-2693
                                           www.uic.edu/pharmacy/research/itr
The Institute for Tuberculosis Research is comprised of approximately 30 individuals: biologists chemists pharmacologists and support staff - all working towards a single goal - the discovery of new drugs for tuberculosis.
Scott Franzblau, Director
Lorna Haubrich, ITR General Information

9311 University of Illinois at Chicago: Institute for Tuberculosis Research
833 S. Wood Street   312-355-1715
Chicago, IL 60612-7631   Fax: 312-355-2693
                                           www.uic.edu/pharmacy/research/itr
Scott Franzblau, Director
Lorna Haubrich, ITR General Information

Support Groups & Hotlines

9312 National Health Information Center
Office of Disease Prevention & Health Promotion
1101 Wootton Pkwy   Fax: 240-453-8281
Rockville, MD 20852   odphpinfo@hhs.gov
                                           www.health.gov/nhic
Supports public health education by maintaining a calendar of National Health Observances; helps connect consumers and health professionals to organizations that can best answer questions and provide up-to-date contact information from reliable sources; updates on a yearly basis toll-free numbers for health information, Federal health clearinghouses and info centers.
Don Wright, MD, MPH, Director

Pamphlets

9313 Classification of Tuberculosis and Other Mycobacterial Diseases
American Lung Association
1740 Broadway   212-315-8700
New York, NY 10019-4315
Chart listing different classes of tuberculosis and other mycobacterial diseases.

9314 Facts About Tuberculosis
American Lung Association
1740 Broadway   212-315-8700
New York, NY 10019-4315
Primary public information leaflet on TB as well as on its impact and treatment.
8 pages

9315 TB Skin Test
American Lung Association

1740 Broadway   212-315-8700
New York, NY 10019-4315
Primary public information leaflet on the TB skin test.
8 pages

9316 TB: What You Should Know
American Lung Association of Connecticut
45 Ash Street   860-289-5401
East Hartford, CT 06108-3294   800-586-4872
                                           Fax: 860-289-5405
                                           www.alact.org

Offers a brief overview of tuberculosis, how transmission is possible, and TB skin testing.
John E Zinn, President/CEO

9317 This is Mr. TB Germ
American Lung Association
1740 Broadway   212-315-8700
New York, NY 10019-4315
Lively booklet of drawings and very brief text giving a basic description of TB and its treatments.
20 pages

Web Sites

9318 American Lung Association
                                           www.lung.org
Offers research, medical updates, fund-raising, educational materials and public awareness campaigns relating to lung disease causes.

9319 Healing Well
                                           www.healingwell.org
An online health resource guide to medical news, chat, information and articles, newsgroups and message boards, books, disease-related web sites, medical directories, and more for patients, friends, and family coping with disabling diseases, disorders, or chronic illnesses.

9320 Health Finder
                                           www.healthfinder.gov
Searchable, carefully developed web site offering information on over 1000 topics. Developed by the US Department of Health and Human Services, the site can be used in both English and Spanish.

9321 Healthlink USA
                                           www.healthlinkusa.com
Health information concerning treatment, cures, prevention, diagnosis, risk factors, research, support groups, email lists, personal stories and much more. Updated regularly.

9322 MedicineNet
                                           www.medicinenet.com
An online resource for consumers providing easy-to-read, authoritative medical and health information.

9323 Medscape
                                           www.medscape.com
Medscape offers specialists, primary care physicians, and other health professionals the Web's most robust and integrated medical information and educational tools.

9324 WebMD
                                           www.webmd.com
Provides credible information, supportive communities, and in-depth reference material about health subjects. A source for original and timely health information as well as material from well known content providers.

Description

9325 **Tuberous Sclerosis Complex**

Tuberous sclerosis is a genetic disorder that causes benign, (non-cancerous) tumors (usually hamartomas or benign tumors formed from a mixture of different cells) to form in different locations - primarily in the brain, skin, kidneys, heart, lungs and even eyes. It occurs in 1 in 6,000 children. The name is derived from tuber-like growths on the brain that become hard. It usually shows itself in infancy or early childhood, and may cause seizures and/or mental disability. It is inherited by means of mutations in the TSC1 gene, which is on chromosome 9 or in the TSC2 gene, which is on chromosome 16. TSC1 encodes the Hamartin protein, and the TSC2 gene encodes the Tuberin protein. Both of these proteins control cell growth, and dysfunctional Harmartin or Tuberin cause uncontrolled cell proliferation. Tuberous sclerosis is inherited as an autosomal dominant mutation, meaning that the patient only needs one copy of the mutation to show the signs and symptoms of this disease. The severity of tuberous sclerosis is highly variable, even within the same family. Those with tuberous sclerosis can have mental disability as well as seizures.

There are various skin abnormalities that may provide a clue to the diagnosis when an infant or young child exhibits seizures or delayed development. The first is an area of decreased skin pigmentation, called an ash-leaf spot because of its shape. Multiple ash-leaf spots may appear on the trunk and limbs during infancy. At age 3 or 4, tiny red bumps, adenoma sebaceum, resembling acne may appear on the nose and cheeks. Finally, a roughened spot with the consistency of orange peel, shagren patch, may appear over the lower spine.

There is no cure so treatment is based on symptoms and can include anti-epileptic drugs for seizures, removal of skin lesions, treatment of high blood pressure caused by kidney problems, special education and, in some instances, surgery to remove growing tumors.

National Agencies & Associations

9326 **National Tuberous Sclerosis Association**
801 Roeder Road
Sliver Spring, MD 20910-4487

301-562-9890
800-225-6872
Fax: 301-562-9870
info@tsalliance.org
www.tsalliance.org

A voluntary non-profit organization that is dedicated to fostering and supporting tuberous sclerosis research; to provide education of the public, and to provide support of individuals with tuberous sclerosis.
Beth Dean, Chair
Chris Russell, Vice Chair

9327 **Rare Cancer Alliance**
1649 N Pacana Way
Green Valley, AZ 85614

800-345-6324
www.rare-cancer.org

Provides support to all children and adults diagnosed with rare cancer. Raises awareness and funding for rare cancer research.
Sharon Lane, Founder
MD Anderson

9328 **Tuberous Sclerosis Complex International**
801 Roeder Road
Silver Spring, MD 20708

301-562-9890
ksmith@tsalliance.org
www.tscinternational.org

Tuberous Sclerosis Complex International is a worldwide consortium of existing tuberous sclerosis complex associations and organizations. Tuberous Sclerosis Complex International exists to educate the public on tuberous sclerosis complex and develop improved treatments.

Support Groups & Hotlines

9329 **National Health Information Center**
Office of Disease Prevention & Health Promotion
1101 Wootton Pkwy
Rockville, MD 20852

Fax: 240-453-8281
odphpinfo@hhs.gov
www.health.gov/nhic

Supports public health education by maintaining a calendar of National Health Observances; helps connect consumers and health professionals to organizations that can best answer questions and provide up-to-date contact information from reliable sources; updates on a yearly basis toll-free numbers for health information, Federal health clearinghouses and info centers.
Don Wright, MD, MPH, Director

Books

9330 **Tuberous Sclerosis**
Oxford University Press
2001 Evans Road
Cary, NC 27513

800-445-9714
Fax: 919-677-1303
custserv.us@oup.com
www.oup-usa.org

A revision offering up-to-date medical information to families, researchers, and professionals on TS.
ISBN: 0-195122-10-0

Newsletters

9331 **NTSA Perspective**
National Tuberous Sclerosis Association
801 Roeder Road
Silver Spring, ML 20910-2226

301-562-9890
800-225-6872
Fax: 301-562-9870
info@tsalliance.org
www.ntsa.org

Offers the latest research and medical information on tuberous sclerosis to physicians and health care professionals.
Quarterly
Laura Lubbers, Chair
David Fitzmaurice, Vice Chair

Web Sites

9332 **Healing Well**

www.healingwell.com

An online health resource guide to medical news, chat, information and articles, newsgroups and message boards, books, disease-related web sites, medical directories, and more for patients, friends, and family coping with disabling diseases, disorders, or chronic illnesses.

9333 **Health Finder**

www.healthfinder.gov

Searchable, carefully developed web site offering information on over 1000 topics. Developed by the US Department of Health and Human Services, the site can be used in both English and Spanish.

9334 **Healthlink USA**

www.healthlinkusa.com

Health information concerning treatment, cures, prevention, diagnosis, risk factors, research, support groups, email lists, personal stories and much more. Updated regularly.

9335   MedicineNet
www.medicinenet.com
An online resource for consumers providing easy-to-read, authoritative medical and health information.

9336   Medscape
www.medscape.com
Medscape offers specialists, primary care physicians, and other health professionals the Web's most robust and integrated medical information and educational tools.

9337   National Tuberous Sclerosis Association
The Tuberous Sclerosis Alliance is dedicated to finding a cure for tuberous sclerosis complex (TSC) while improving the lives of those affected.

9338   WebMD
www.webmd.com
Provides credible information, supportive communities, and in-depth reference material about health subjects. A source for original and timely health information as well as material from well known content providers.

Description

9339 Turner Syndrome

Turner syndrome is a genetic disorder that occurs in 1 in 2,500 to 10,000 live female births. It only affects females because, rather than having two female sex (X) chromosomes, Turner syndrome patients have only one. The disease usually hinders sexual development and produces small stature. The intellectual capabilities of Turner Syndrome women as well within normal levels. There may be associated anomalies such as webbed neck and defects of the heart or aorta, which may occur in up to 25 percent of individuals.

Turner syndrome cannot be cured, but hormonal treatment may give the patient a more normal life. Growth hormone injections can help the patient reach a taller adult height, and estrogen replacement can encourage breast development and other sex characteristics. A few patients will develop menstrual periods spontaneously, and a few have become pregnant; most, however, are infertile. Psychological support for the patient and her family is important.

National Agencies & Associations

9340 Human Growth Foundation
997 Glencove Avenue
Glenhead, NY 11545
800-451-6434
Fax: 516-671-4055
hgf1@hgfound.org
www.hgfound.org
A non-profit, national organization committed to expanding and accelerating research into growth and growth disorders, provides education and support to those affected by growth disorders and their families and fosters the exchange of information.
Pisit Duke Pituckcheewanont, MD, President
Emily L. Germain-Lee, MD, Vice President

9341 The Magic Foundation
4200 Cantera Drive
Warrenville, IL 60555
630-836-8200
800-362-4423
Fax: 630-836-8181
contactus@magicfoundation.org
www.magicfoundation.org
A national non-profit organization created to provide support services for the families of children afflicted with a wide variety of chronic and/or critical disorders that affect a child's growth.
Rich Buckley, Chairman
Ken Dickard, Vice Chairman

9342 Turner Syndrome Society of the United States
11250 W Road
Houston, TX 77065
800-365-9944
info@turnersyndrome.org
www.turnersyndrome.org
A national non-profit organization in which members have available a host of informational and support services, including consultation services, and a resource center offering access to the most recently published articles on Turner's Syndrome.
Cindy Scurlock, President & CEO
Becky Brown, National Director

International

9343 Turner Syndrome Society of Canada
2100 Thurston Drive
Ottawa, K1G-4K8
613-321-2267
800-465-6744
info@turnersyndrome.ca
www.turnersyndrome.ca
International society providing support services, educational information and activities to persons with Turner's Syndrome, their families and the professionals who work with them.

State Agencies & Associations

California

9344 Northern California Turner Syndrome Resource Group
Sacramento, CA
800-365-9944
deborah@turnersyndrome.org
www.turnersyndrome.org
A resource group affiliated with the Turner Syndrome Society of the United States, focused on providing social support to all of the girls, women, and families affected by Turner Syndrome.
Rosemary Morris, Group Leader

Colorado

9345 Turner Syndrome Colorado
11269 Lamar Street
Westminster, CO 80020
720-628-6907
turnersyndromeco@gmail.com
www.turner-syndrome.org
Connects individuals and families touched by Turner Syndrome in an effort to create community, social support, and share local resources.
Marybel Good, Founder & President
Erica Haag, Board Member

Florida

9346 Northwest Florida Panhandle Turner Syndrome Resource Group
800-365-9944
deborah@turnersyndrome.org
www.turnersyndrome.org
Offers social support and shares resources for those affected by Turner Syndrome.
Carrie Odom, Group Leader

Illinois

9347 Illinois Turner Syndrome Resource Group
800-365-9944
deborah@turnersyndrome.org
www.turnersyndrome.org
Creates awareness of Turner Syndrome and provides members with social support.
Reenna Kaushik, Group Leader

Iowa

9348 Iowa Turner Syndrome Resource Group
800-365-9944
deborah@turnersyndrome.org
www.turnersyndrome.org
Offers social support for those afflicted with Turner Syndrome, and raises public awareness of Turner Syndrome.
Donna Rice, Group Leader

Kansas

9349 The Turner Syndrome Society: Kansas City Chapter
PO Box 7572
Overland Park, KS 66207-9998
tsskcpres@yahoo.ca
www.tsskc.org
Provides social support to those affected by Turner Syndrome, and shares resources.

Massachusetts

9350 Massachusetts Turner Syndrome Resource Group
800-365-9944
deborah@turnersyndrome.org
www.turnersyndrome.org
Fosters social support and raises awareness of Turner Syndrome.
Patricia Collins, Group Leader

Michigan

9351 The Turner Syndrome Society: Michigan Chapter
800-365-9944
deborah@turnersyndrome.org
www.turnersyndrome.org

Provides social support and shares local resources for those affected by Turner Syndrome.
Katie Visner, Group Leader

Minnesota

9352 The Turner Syndrome Society: Minnesota Chapter
800-365-9944
deborah@turnersyndrome.org
www.turnersyndrome.org
Provides support for all girls, women and their families in Minnesota affected by Turner Syndrome.
Colleen Daman, Chapter President
BilliJo Sielaff, Treasurer

New Jersey

9353 New Jersey Turner Syndrome Resource Group
800-365-9944
deborah@turnersyndrome.org
www.turnersyndrome.org
Raises awareness of Turner Syndrome and shares local resources with members affected by Turner Syndrome.
Nicole Boris, Group Leader

Oklahoma

9354 Northeast Oklahoma Resource Group (Tulsa)
Tulsa, OK
800-365-9944
deborah@turnersyndrome.org
www.turnersyndrome.org
Provides support and education to individuals wanting to learn moreabout Turner Syndrome, and those who are directly affected by Turner Syndrome.
Jenifur Davidson, Group Leader

Pennsylvania

9355 Pennsylvania Turner Syndrome Resource Group
800-365-9944
deborah@turnersyndrome.org
www.turnersyndrome.org
Provides social support, education, and resources for those affected by Turner Syndrome.
Audrie Noll, Group Leader

Texas

9356 The Turner Syndrome Society: Central Texas, Dallas/Ft.Worth, Houston
800-365-9944
deborah@turnersyndrome.org
www.turnersyndrome.org
The Central Texas, Dallas/Ft.Worth, and Houston chapters of the Turner Syndrome Society share support and local resources with others affected by Turner Syndrome.

Washington

9357 Washington Turner Syndrome Resource Group
800-365-9944
deborah@turnersyndrome.org
www.turnersyndrome.org
Offers support and information for all those touched by Turner Syndrome.
Deanna Carey-Crumpton, Group Leader

Libraries & Resource Centers

9358 Turner Syndrome Society Resource Center
Turner Syndrome Society of the United States
11250 W Road
Houston, TX 77065
832-912-6006
800-365-9944
Fax: 832-912-6446
tssus@turnersyndrome.org
www.turnersyndrome.org

The Turner Syndrome Society of the US creates awareness, promotes research, and provides support for all persons touched by Turner Syndrome.
Cindy Scurlock, Executive Director
Deborah Rios, Member Services Director

Support Groups & Hotlines

9359 National Health Information Center
Office of Disease Prevention & Health Promotion
1101 Wootton Pkwy
Rockville, MD 20852
Fax: 240-453-8281
odphpinfo@hhs.gov
www.health.gov/nhic
Supports public health education by maintaining a calendar of National Health Observances; helps connect consumers and health professionals to organizations that can best answer questions and provide up-to-date contact information from reliable sources; updates on a yearly basis toll-free numbers for health information, Federal health clearinghouses and info centers.
Don Wright, MD, MPH, Director

Newsletters

9360 Turner's Syndrome News
Turner's Syndrome Society of the United States
11250 West Road
Houston, TX 77065-4509
832-912-6006
800-365-9944
Fax: 832-912-6446
www.turner-syndrome-us.org
Includes articles addressing current issues in Turner's Syndrome, updates on national and local activities and letters from girls and women with Turner's syndrome and their families.
Quarterly
Trudy McCarthy, President
Emily Havrilak, Secretary

Pamphlets

9361 Answers to Some Commonly Asked Questions
Turner's Syndrome Society of the United States
11250 West Road
Houston, TX 77065-4509
832-912-6006
800-365-9944
Fax: 832-912-6446
www.turner-syndrome-us.org
Offers information on the Society's activities and the role they play in supporting people with Turner's syndrome.
Trudy McCarthy, President
Emily Havrilak, Secretary

9362 Facing the Challenges of Turner's Syndrome Together
Turner's Syndrome Society of the United States
11250 West Road
Houston, TX 77065-4509
832-912-6006
800-365-9944
Fax: 832-912-6446
www.turner-syndrome-us.org
A brochure offering information on Turner's syndrome, statistics on how widespread the disease is and the Society's role in conquering this disease and supporting their members.
Trudy McCarthy, President
Emily Havrilak, Secretary

9363 Facts About Turner's Syndrome
Turner's Syndrome Society of the United States
11250 West Road
Houston, TX 77065-4509
832-912-6006
800-365-9944
Fax: 832-912-6446
www.turner-syndrome-us.org
Offers statistical and factual information on the disease of Turner's syndrome, causes, symptoms, prevention and treatment.
Trudy McCarthy, President
Emily Havrilak, Secretary

9364 How to Start a Turner's Syndrome Support Group
Turner's Syndrome Society of the United States

11250 West Road   832-912-6006
Houston, TX 77065-4509   800-365-9944
      Fax: 832-912-6446
      www.turner-syndrome-us.org
Offers information to the lay person on how to obtain material from medical professionals, publicity aspects and funding aspects in pertaining to starting a support group.
Trudy McCarthy, President
Emily Havrilak, Secretary

9365 Turner's Syndrome Society Resource Bibliographies
Turner's Syndrome Society of the United States
11250 West Road
Houston, TX 77065-4509   832-912-6006
      800-365-9944
      Fax: 832-912-6446
      www.turner-syndrome-us.org
These fact sheets offer information on books, videos and other resources available on Turner's syndrome.
Trudy McCarthy, President
Emily Havrilak, Secretary

9366 Turner's Syndrome: A Guide for Families
Turner's Syndrome Society of the United States
11250 West Road   832-912-6006
Houston, TX 77065-4509   800-365-9944
      Fax: 832-912-6446
      www.turner-syndrome-us.org
Offers information to parents on the causes, symptoms, diagnosis and prognosis of Turner' syndrome, includes resources of where to go for help and support.
Trudy McCarthy, President
Emily Havrilak, Secretary

9367 Turner's Syndrome: A Personal Perspective
Turner's Syndrome Society of the United States
11250 West Road   832-912-6006
Houston, TX 77065-4509   800-365-9944
      Fax: 832-912-6446
      www.turner-syndrome-us.org
A reprint from the Adolescent and Pediatric Gynecology Journal offering a personal account of a woman with Turner's syndrome and her experiences.
Trudy McCarthy, President
Emily Havrilak, Secretary

9368 Turner's Syndrome: Hows and Whys of the Missing X Chromosome
Human Growth Foundation
997 Glencove Ave
Glen Head, NY 11545-1554   516-671-4041
      800-451-6434
      Fax: 516-671-4055
      hgf1@hgfound.org
      www.hgfound.org
Provides a brief overview for parents about Turner's Syndrome.
Pisit Pitukcheewanont, President
Patricia D Costa, Executive Director

Web Sites

9369 Healing Well
      www.healingwell.com

An online health resource guide to medical news, chat, information and articles, newsgroups and message boards, books, disease-related web sites, medical directories, and more for patients, friends, and family coping with disabling diseases, disorders, or chronic illnesses.

9370 Health Finder
      www.healthfinder.gov
Searchable, carefully developed web site offering information on over 1000 topics. Developed by the US Department of Health and Human Services, the site can be used in both English and Spanish.

9371 Healthlink USA
      www.healthlinkusa.com
Health information concerning treatment, cures, prevention, diagnosis, risk factors, research, support groups, email lists, personal stories and much more. Updated regularly.

9372 Human Growth Foundation
      hgfound.org
The focus and emphasis of the Foundation objectives vary with the opportunities to provide support, services, and education to children with disorders of growth and adults with growth hormone deficiency, and to the medical profession; and, with the availability of funding and communications media to support the programs and activities, and general office operations necessary to provide them.

9373 MAGIC Foundation for Children's Growth: Turner's Syndrome Division
      www.magicfoundation.org
National organization created to provide support services for the families of children afflicted with a wide variety of chronic and/or critical disorders that affect a child's growth.

9374 MedicineNet
      www.medicinenet.com
An online resource for consumers providing easy-to-read, authoritative medical and health information.

9375 Medscape
      www.medscape.com
Medscape offers specialists, primary care physicians, and other health professionals the Web's most robust and integrated medical information and educational tools.

9376 Turner's Syndrome Society of the United States
      www.turner-syndrome-us.org
Through this society, members have available a host of informational and support services including consultation services, a resource center offering access to the most recently published articles on Turner's syndrome, conferences, advocacy, information and referral services and public relations activities.

9377 WebMD
      www.webmd.com
Provides credible information, supportive communities, and in-depth reference material about health subjects. A source for original and timely health information as well as material from well known content providers.

Description

9378 Ulcerative Colitis

Ulcerative colitis is an inflammatory condition of the large bowel, or colon. The cause is unknown, but there is a strong genetic association. First degree relatives have a 3-9 percent lifetime risk of the disease, and the illness is much more common in certain racial groups.

Inflammation of the wall of the bowel leads to ulcerations of its surface. Symptoms include weight loss, fatigue, abdominal pain, and diarrhea, which may be bloody. Ulcerative colitis in patients who have a specific variation of particular cell surface proteins in their system (HLA-B27) has a strong association with an arthritis called ankylosing spondylitis. Several kinds of liver and biliary tract disease, inflammation of the eye, and certain characteristic skin rashes may occur.

Treatment depends on the severity of symptoms. Mild cases may respond to simple anti-diarrheal medicines. More severe cases are treated with either rectal or oral forms of 5-aminosalicylate (5-ASA), marketed under several trade names. Rectal corticosteroids, either as rectal foams or enemas, are sometimes necessary, and disease confined to the rectum can generally be managed with steroid enemas. Extensive disease may require oral steroid medication (prednisone or budesonide). Immunosuppressive drugs like azathioprine and 6-mercaptopurine are sometimes given if the disease is resistant to steroids or if steroid side effects are unacceptable. Biologic therapies, such as tumor necrosis factor-a inhibitors, such as infliximab, adalimumab, or golimumab are all quite effective and can be combined with other medications to drive the disease into remission. A newer drug, vendolizumab, has proven to work when other biologic therapies did not. Another newer oral medication, the JAK kinase inhibitor tofacitinib has also shown efficacy when steroids failed to treat the disease, but this drug has severe side effects. Twenty percent of patients will eventually have their entire colon removed, which cures the disease.

After many years of active ulcerative colitis there is an increased risk of colon cancer. It is usually preceded by warning signs visible on colonoscopy, so physicians generally begin an aggressive surveillance program after 8 to 10 years of disease.

National Agencies & Associations

9379 American Chronic Pain Association
PO Box 850
Rocklin, CA 95677

800-533-3231
ACPA@theacpa.org
www.theacpa.org

The ACPA facilitates peer support and education for individuals with chronic pain in its many forms, in order to increase quality of life. Also raises awareness among the healthcare community, and with policy makers.
Penney Cowan, Founder & CEO
Daniel Galia, Director, Global Support

9380 American Gastroenterological Association
National Office

4930 Del Ray Avenue
Bethesda, MD 20814

301-654-2055
Fax: 301-654-5920
member@gastro.org
www.gastro.org

AGA fosters the development and application of the science of gastroenterology by providing leadership and aid including patient care, research, teaching, continuing education, scientific communication and matters of national health policy.
Tom Serena, Executive Vice President
Sarah Fitzpatrick, Executive Office Coordinator

9381 National Institute of Diabetes & Digestive & Kidney Diseases
Office Of Communications and Public Liaison, NIH
31 Center Drive
Bethesda, MD 20892-2560

800-860-8747
TTY: 866-569-1162
healthinfo@niddk.nih.gov
www.niddk.nih.gov

Research areas include diabetes, digestive diseases, endocrine and metabolic diseases, hematologic diseases, kidney disease, liver disease, urologic diseases, as well as matters relating to nutrition and obesity.
Griffin P. Rodgers, MD, MACP, Director
Gregory Germino, MD, Deputy Director

9382 Reach Out for Youth with Ileitis and Colitis, Inc.
1250 Union Turnpike
New Hyde Park, NY 11040

631-293-3102
info@reachoutforyouth.org

Provides educational seminars, and individual and group support to patients and their families. Fundraising efforts support the Center's programs, and clinical and laboratory research.

9383 United Ostomy Associations of America, Inc
PO Box 525
Kennebunk, ME 04043

800-826-0826
www.ostomy.org

A national network for bowel and urinary diversion support groups in the United States. Its goal is to provide a non-profit association that will serve to unify and strengthen its member support groups, which are organized for the benefit of people who have, or will have intestinal or urinary diversions and their caregivers.
Christine Ryan, Executive Director
Jeanine Gleba, Advocacy Manager

Foundations

9384 Crohn's & Colitis Foundation
733 Third Avenue
New York, NY 10017

800-932-2423
info@crohnscolitisfoundation.org
www.crohnscolitisfoundation.org

CCF's mission is to cure and prevent Crohn's disease and ulcerative colitis through research, and to improve the quality of life of children and adults affected by the disease through education and support. The foundation offers patient and professional support.
Michael Osso, President & CEO
Caren Heller, MD, MBA, Chief Scientific Officer

Support Groups & Hotlines

9385 National Health Information Center
Office of Disease Prevention & Health Promotion
1101 Wootton Pkwy
Rockville, MD 20852

Fax: 240-453-8281
odphpinfo@hhs.gov
www.health.gov/nhic

Supports public health education by maintaining a calendar of National Health Observances; helps connect consumers and health professionals to organizations that can best answer questions and provide up-to-date contact information from reliable sources; updates on a yearly basis toll-free numbers for health information, Federal health clearinghouses and info centers.
Don Wright, MD, MPH, Director

Books

9386 Alive and Kicking
Rolf Benirschke Enterprises
PO Box 9922
Rancho Santa Fe, CA 92067-4922

800-571-4770
www.obrien.ie

Football star writes of his struggle with ulcerative colitis.

9387 Ask Audrey
7466 Pebble Lane   248-626-6960
West Bloomfield, MI 48322-3521
A compilation of material and the personal story of a medical psychotherapist who has inflammatory bowel disease. Includes practical tips on issues such as handling diarrhea, sexuality, relationships, traveling, coping with hospital stays, ostomies, and TPN.

9388 IBD Nutrition Book
John Wiley & Sons
1 Wiley Drive   800-225-5945
Somerset, NJ 08873-1222
Clinical dietitian/nutritionist's overview of the role of diet in IBD, including recipes and meal plans.

9389 Inflammatory Bowel Disease
Williams & Wilkins
351 W Camden Street   410-528-4398
Baltimore, MD 21201-7912   800-638-0672
                                                         Fax: 215-701-2407
liana.watson@wolterskluwer.com
www.wkadcenter.com
Detailed information on every aspect of IBD. Topics include medical and surgical management, epidemiology, fertility and pregnancy, psychosocial factors, and diagnostic techniques. Written for medical professionals and laypersons who are comfortable with medical terminology.
Liana Watson, Production Associate

Children's Books

9390 You're Bigger Than it
Hotel Dieu Hospital   613-544-3310
Ontario, Canada,
This cartoon book offers a lively, brief introduction to the basics of living with IBD. Contact can be reached at extension 2400.

Magazines

9391 Phoenix Magazine
United Ostomy Association of America
PO Box 512   800-826-0826
Northfield, MN 55057   Fax: 507-645-5168
info@uoaa.org
www.uoa.org
America's leading ostomy patient magazine providing colostomy, ileostomy, urostomy and continent diversion information, management techniques, new products and much more.
Quarterly
Susan Burns, President

Newsletters

9392 Inner Circle
Reach Out for Youth with Ileitis and Colitis
540 E. Canfield   631-293-3102
Detroit, MI 48025   bmawsu@gmail.com
www.reachoutforyouth.org
Newsletter for youth with ileitis and colitis.
Irwin Maltz, President
Carolyn King, Co-Founder

Pamphlets

9393 Bleeding in the Digestive Tract
Nat'l Digestive Diseases Information Clearinghouse
9000 Rockville Pike   301-496-6344
Bethesda, MD 20892-0001   www.medhelp.org
Informational fact sheet.

9394 Inside Story
Reach Out for Youth with Ileitis and Colitis

540 E. Canfield   631-293-2102
Detroit, MI 48025   bmawsu@gmail.com
www.reachoutforyouth.org
Educational brochure for youth with illeitis and colitis.
Irwin Maltz, President
Carolyn King, Co-Founder

9395 Ulcerative Colitis
National Organization For Rare Disorders
55 Kenosia Avenue   203-744-0100
Danbury, CT 06810-8923   Fax: 203-798-2291
orphan@rarediseases.org
www.rarediseases.org
The National Organization for Rare Disorders (NORD), a 501(c)(3) organization, is the leading voice of the rare disease community
Peter L. Saltonstall, President & CEO
Pamela Gavin, Chief Operating Officer

Web Sites

9396 Crohn's & Colitis Foundation
www.crohnscolitisfoundation.org
CCF's mission is to cure and prevent Crohn's disease and ulcerative colitis through research, and to improve the quality of life of children and adults affected by the disease through education and support. The foundation offers patient and professional support.

9397 Healing Well
www.healingwell.com
An online health resource guide to medical news, chat, information and articles, newsgroups and message boards, books, disease-related web sites, medical directories, and more for patients, friends, and family coping with disabling diseases, disorders, or chronic illnesses.

9398 Health Finder
www.healthfinder.gov
Searchable, carefully developed web site offering information on over 1000 topics. Developed by the US Department of Health and Human Services, the site can be used in both English and Spanish.

9399 Healthlink USA
www.healthlinkusa.com
Health information concerning treatment, cures, prevention, diagnosis, risk factors, research, support groups, email lists, personal stories and much more. Updated regularly.

9400 MedicineNet
www.medicinenet.com
An online resource for consumers providing easy-to-read, authoritative medical and health information.

9401 Medscape
www.medscape.com
Medscape offers specialists, primary care physicians, and other health professionals the Web's most robust and integrated medical information and educational tools.

9402 United Ostomy Associations of America, Inc
www.ostomy.org
A national network for bowel and urinary diversion support groups in the United States. Its goal is to provide a non-profit association that will serve to unify and strengthen its member support groups, which are organized for the benefit of people who have, or will have intestinal or urinary diversions and their caregivers.

9403 WebMD
www.webmd.com
Provides credible information, supportive communities, and in-depth reference material about health subjects. A source for original and timely health information as well as material from well known content providers.

Description

9404 Visual Impairment

Visual impairment encompasses a wide variety of disorders of the eye. It includes damage to the cornea or retina (macular degeneration or secondary to diabetes), cataracts, glaucoma, muscular imbalance, infections, congenital disorders and those associated with premature birth. Occasionally visual impairment reflects a disease behind the eye, involving some part of the brain that receives and processes images from the eyes.

Visual impairment covers a continuum from decreased visual acuity correctible by refractive means (glasses and contact lenses) to legal blindness, indicating less than 20/200 vision in the better eye, or an extremely limited field of vision. Totally blind represents the complete loss of sight.

Many health problems and eye injuries lead to visual impairment. Half a million Americans are visually impaired, and an additional 50,000 lose their sight each year. Cataracts account for one third of all visual impairments and cause 16 persons to lose their sight every day (over 24 million cases in 2016). Glaucoma causes vision impairment in 2.7 million persons. One thousand eye injuries resulting in some level of vision impairment occur in the workplace or home each day. Diabetic retinopathy is one of the leading causes of the new cases of blindness (over 7.6 million cases). Retinitis pigmentosa, a degeneration of the light-sensing tissue at the back of the eye, also causes vision (especially night vision) deterioration.

Depending on the cause of vision loss, the condition may be fully or partially correctible through surgery or visual aids. Sometimes treatment will not reverse prior losses, but will slow the progression of vision loss. When the visual loss cannot be reversed, a variety of supportive devices and services, improved over the past twenty years, can greatly enhance the person's functional status and quality of life.

Technology has played an increasing role in helping the visually impaired function in their daily lives. Recently, doctors implanted the first artificial retina, and relatively new laser technology allows eye specialists to surgically treat extreme degrees of nearsightedness and astigmatism (blurred vision caused by uneven curvature of the eye).

National Agencies & Associations

9405 Alliance for Aging Research
1700 K Street NW
Washington, DC 20006   202-293-2856
                              info@agingresearch.org
                              www.agingresearch.org

A non-profit organization dedicated to promoting scientific research on human aging and health.
Sue Peschin, President & CEO
Yvette Brown, Vice President

9406 American Academy of Ophthalmology
655 Beach Street   415-561-8500
San Francisco, CA 94109-7424   Fax: 415-561-8533
                                www.aao.org

The world's largest association of eye physicians and surgeons, who work to advance eyecare, and promote standards for ophthalmic education. The American Academy of Ophthalmology advocates for patients and provides medically accurate information for the public.

9407 American Association of the Deaf-Blind
PO Box 8064   301-495-4403
Kensington, MD 20891-2831   Fax: 301-495-4404
                                TTY: 301-495-4402
                                aadb-info@aadb.org
                                www.aadb.org

A non-profit organization that promotes better opportunities and services for deaf-blind people. Provides information, referrals, resources, and technical assistance to ensure increased independence for all deaf-blind people.
35-50 pages 600 Members
Ren, Pellerin, President
Mindy Dill, Vice President

9408 American Council of the Blind
1703 N Beauregard Street   202-467-5081
Alexandria, VA 22311   800-424-8666
                                 Fax: 703-465-5085
                                 info@acb.org
                                 www.acb.org

The American Council of the Blind supports all people who are blind or visually impaired by providing resources to increase their independence, security, equality of opportunity, and quality of life. The American Council of the Blind advocates for the visually impaired, and operates ACB Radio, offering news, information, and music from blind broadcasters.
Eric Bridges, Executive Director
Sharon Lovering, Editor

9409 American Foundation for the Blind
1401 S Clark Street   212-502-7600
Arlington, VA 22202   800-232-5463
                                 Fax: 212-502-7777
                                 info@afb.net
                                 www.afb.org

American Foundation for the Blind is a non-profit organization dedicated to improving the lives of people with vision loss and their families. American Foundation for the Blind promotes research and evidence-based technologies.
Kirk Adams, President & CEO
Megan Aragon, Director

9410 American Macular Degeneration Foundation
PO Box 515   413-268-7660
Northampton, MA 01061-0515   888-622-8527
                                 www.macular.org

The American Macular Degeneration Foundation is committed to preventing and curing macular degeneration by supporting research initiatives. The American Macular Degeneration Foundation offers support for individuals living with macular degeneration, and raises public awareness of the disease.
Chip Goehring, President & Trustee

9411 American Optometric Association
243 N Lindbergh Boulevard   314-991-4100
St. Louis, MO 63141-7881   800-365-2219
                                 www.aoa.org

The American Optometric Association represents more than 44,000 doctors of optometry, optometric professionals, and optometry students, and promotes care and advancements for eye health.
Samuel D. Pierce, OD, President
William T. Reynolds, OD, Vice President

9412 American Printing House for the Blind
1839 Frankfort Avenue   800-223-1839
Louisville, KY 40206   info@aph.org
                                 www.aph.org

The American Printing House for the Blind is a non-profit organization that provides materials, products, and services to people

who are blind and visually impaired, in order to further enhance their independence and education.
Craig Meador, President
Dorinda Rife, Vice President

9413 Associated Services for the Blind & Visually Impaired
919 Walnut Street   215-627-0600
Philadelphia, PA 19107   Fax: 215-922-0692
                                                          asbinfo@asb.org
                                                             www.asb.org
A private, non-profit organization dedicated to promote independence in people who are blind or visually impaired by providing public education and resources for clients.
Karla S. McCaney, President & CEO
Beth Deering, Director

9414 Association for Education & Rehabilitation of the Blind & Visually Impaired
1703 N Beauregard Street   703-671-4500
Alexandria, VA 22311   877-492-2708
                                                       Fax: 703-671-6391
                                                          aer@aerbvi.org
                                                            www.aerbvi.org
The only non-profit professional membership organization dedicated to the advancement of education and rehabilitation of blind and visually impaired children and adults.
Lou Tutt, Executive Director
Ginger Croce, Deputy Executive Director & CMO

9415 Association for Macular Diseases
210 E 64th Street   212-605-3719
New York, NY 10065   Fax: 212-605-3795
                                        association@retinal-research.org
                                                            www.macula.org
A nonprofit corporation promoting education and research in macular degeneration diseases. Provides a nationwide support group for individuals and their families adjusting to the life changes brought about by macular disease.
Bernard Landou, President
Mary Fern Breheney, Vice President

9416 Blinded Veterans Association
125 N West Street   800-669-7079
Alexandria, VA 22314   Fax: 202-371-8258
                                                            bva@bva.org
                                                              www.bva.org
Blinded Veterans Association is a voice for blinded veterans, and connects legally blind veterans to services, benefits, appropriate training, and opportunities in both the public and the private sectors.
Paperback
Tom Zampieri, National President
Joe McNeil, National Secretary

9417 Braille Institute of America
741 N Vermont Avenue   323-663-1111
Los Angeles, CA 90029   800-272-4553
                                                       Fax: 323-663-0867
                                                    la@brailleinstitute.org
                                                        www.brailleinstitute.org
The Braille Institute of America is a non-profit organization that offers a wide variety of programs and resources, all free of charge for the blind and visually impaired. The Braille Institute frequently sponsors nationwide programs that encourage further education, and the Braille Institute Library offers more than 1.4 million books in audio format, braille, and large-print.
Peter A. Mindrich, President
Gloria Coulston, Vice President

9418 Canine Companions for Independence
2965 Dutton Ave   866-224-3647
Santa Rosa, CA 95407   800-572-2275
                                                            info@cci.org
                                                              www.cci.org
A non-profit organization that enhances the lives of people with disabilities by uniting them with trained assistance dogs free of charge. Canine Companions offers four types of assistance dogs to meet the needs of adults with disabilities.
Paige Mazzoni, CEO
Jack Peirce, CFO & Corporate Treasurer

9419 Canine Helpers for the Handicapped, Inc.
5699 Ridge Road   716-433-4035
Lockport, NY 14094   chhdogs@aol.com
                                                       www.caninehelpers.org
A non-profit organization committed to training assistance dogs for people with disabilities. Dogs are trained for specific disabilities: hearing, mobility, seizure, and therapy.
Nick Underwood

9420 Council for Exceptional Children
2900 Crystal Drive   888-232-7733
Arlington, VA 22202-3557   TTY: 866-915-5000
                                                    service@cec.sped.org
                                                        www.cec.sped.org
Advocates appropriate policies, standards and development for individuals with special needs. Provides professional development for special educators.
Alexander T. Graham, Executive Director
Craig Evans, Director, Operations

9421 Council of Citizens with Low Vision International
6010 Lilywood Lane   865-766-0477
Knoxville, TN 37921   844-460-0625
                                                 business.office@cclvi.org
                                                            www.cclvi.org
A membership organization promoting the education of the general public of the capabilities of low vision people. Outreach programs are run by the Council in order to promote research and education.
Sarah Conrad, President
Kathy Farina, Vice President

9422 Diabetics Action Network
1501 Langford Road   410-215-8587
Gwynn Oak, MD 21207   bernienfb75@gmail.com
                                                              www.nfb.org
A resource of information for blind diabetics and individuals losing vision due to diabetes about non-visual techniques of independently managing diabetes and monitoring glucose levels.
Melissa Riccobono, President
Fredric K. Schroeder, First Vice President

9423 Fidelco Guide Dog Foundation
103 Vision Way   860-243-5200
Bloomfield, CT 06002   Fax: 860-769-0567
                                                         info@fidelco.org
                                                            www.fidelco.org
Fidelco Guide Dog Foundation breeds, trains, and places German shepherd guide dogs with the visually impaired, free of charge. Fidelco offers lifetime support and service to their clients with annual follow-up visits.
Karen C. Tripp, Chairman
G. Kenneth Bernhard, Esq., Vice Chairman

9424 Fight for Sight
381 Park Avenue S   212-679-6060
New York, NY 10016   Arthur@fightforsight.org
                                                        www.fightforsight.org
Charity that supports scientific research into blindness by providing grants to scientists working in vision research.
Norman J. Kleiman, PhD, Board President
Gaby Kressly, Board Secretary & Treasurer

9425 Foundation Fighting Blindness
7168 Columbia Gateway Drive   410-423-0600
Columbia, MD 21046   800-683-5555
                                                       TTY: 800-683-5551
                                                info@FightBlindness.org
                                                         www.blindness.org
Foundation Fighting Blindness is a private funder of research that provides insight into retinal degenerative diseases, specifically macular degeneration. The foundation is dedicated to discovering preventions, treatments and vision restoration for individuals.
David Brint, Chairman, Co-Founder & Principal
Gordon Gund, Co-Founder, Director & CEO

9426 Glaucoma Research Foundation
251 Post Street 415-986-3162
San Francisco, CA 94108 800-826-6693
question@glaucoma.org
www.glaucoma.org
Founded in 1978, Glaucoma Research Foundation continues to search for a cure for glaucoma, and works to restore vision through conducting research. The Foundation conducts and supports research that contributes to improved patient care and a better understanding of the disease process.
Andrew Iwach, MD, Executive Director
Thomas M. Brunner, President & CEO

9427 Guide Dog Users, Inc.
3603 Morgan Way 866-799-8436
Imperial, MO 63052 www.guidedogusersinc.org
Guide Dog Users, Inc. works to protect civil rights and enhance the quality of life for working guide dog teams and users by providing peer support and accessible information.
Laurie Mehta, President
Mary Beth Randall, Vice President

9428 Guide Dogs for the Blind
PO Box 151200 800-295-4050
San Rafael, CA 94915-1200 information@guidedogs.com
www.guidedogs.com
Entirely operated by volunteers and donors, Guide Dogs for the Blind connects individuals who are blind or visually impaired with trained guide dogs across the United States and Canada. Services are provided at no cost to the clients.
Christine Benninger, CEO
Cathy Martin, Treasurer & CFO

9429 Helen Keller National Center for Deaf-Blind Youths and Adults
141 Middle Neck Road 516-944-8900
Sands Point, NY 11050 hkncinfo@hknc.org
www.hknc.org
Helen Keller National Center for Deaf-Blind Youths and Adults gives individuals who are blind, visually-impaired, or deaf-blind, the tools needed to thrive. Instructors with firsthand experience of living with vision or combined vision and hearing loss train and guide each student with hands-on learning using advanced technology.
Joseph F. Bruno, President & CEO
Marc Feldman, CPA, CFO

9430 Learning Ally
20 Roszel Road 866-221-4792
Princeton, NJ 08540 info@learningally.org
www.learningally.org
Originally known as Recording for the Blind and Dyslexic, Learning Ally is one of the largest not-for-profit providers of audio textbooks and materials for all people who cannot effectively read standard print.
Andrew Friedman, President & CEO
Cynthia Hamburger, COO & Chief Information Officer

9431 Lighthouse Guild GuildCare
250 W 64th Street 212-769-6200
New York, NY 10023 800-284-4422
www.lighthouse.org
A leading resource worldwide on vision impairment and vision rehabilitation, Lighthouse Guild aims to prevent vision loss through the promotion of well-coordinated vision and healthcare services.
Alan R. Morse, President & CEO
James M. Dubin, Chairman

9432 National Alliance of Blind Students American Council of the Blind
1703 N Beauregard Street 202-467-5081
Alexandria, VA 22311 800-424-8666
info@acb.org
www.acb.org
Works to facilitate progress toward full accessibility of college programs and facilities, provides opportunities for discussion of issues important to students and assists with National Student Seminars.
Sara Conrad, President
Kerri Regan, Chair

9433 National Association for Parents of Children with Visual Impairments
15 W 65th Street 800-562-6265
New York, NY 10023 napvi@lighthouseguild.org
www.nei.nih.gov
An organization that strives to serve families with children of all ages and ranges with visual loss by providing information, assistance, and resources. Refers parents to community groups and other national and international agencies.
Linda Gerra, Executive Director

9434 National Association of Blind Lawyers
1660 S Albion Street 303-504-5979
Denver, CO 80222-4046 Fax: 303-757-3640
blindlaw@nfbnet.org
www.nfb.org
Membership organization of blind attorneys, law students, judges, and others in the law field. Provides support, information, and mentorship to prospective blind law students.
Scott C. LaBarre, President

9435 National Association of Blind Office Professionals
7001 Hamilton Avenue 513-931-7070
Cincinnati, OH 45231 Lhall007@cinci.rr.com
www.nfb.org
Membership organization of blind secretaries and transcribers at all levels. Addresses issues such as technology, accommodation and caregivers.
Lisa Hall, President

9436 National Association of Blind Students
PO Box 29623 203-273-8463
Winston-Salem, NC 27109 nabs.president@gmail.com
www.nfb.org
Provides support, information, and encouragement to blind college and university students. Offers resources on issues such as national testing, and accessible textbooks.
Kathryn Webster, President

9437 National Association of Guide Dog Users
1003 Papaya Drive 813-626-2789
Tampa, FL 33619 800-624-3841
president@nagdu.org
www.nagdu.org
Provides information and support for guide dog users and works to secure high standards in guide dog training. Addresses issues of discrimination of guide dog users and offers public education about guide dog use.
Marion Gwizdala, President

9438 National Association to Promote the Use of Braille
5805 Kellogg Avenue 952-927-7694
Edena, MN 55424 www.visionaware.org
Dedicated to securing improved Braille instruction, increasing the number of Braille materials available to the blind and providing information about the importance of Braille in securing independence, education, and employment for the blind. Affiliated with the National Federation of the Blind.

9439 National Braille Association
95 Allens Creek Road 585-427-8260
Rochester, NY 14618 Fax: 585-427-0263
www.nationalbraille.org
Provides transcription service for the creation of braille materials and maintains a depository of braille books. Provides continuing education for those who create braille materials.
Heidi Lehmann, President
David Shaffer, Executive Director

9440 National Braille Press
88 Saint Stephen Street 617-266-6160
Boston, MA 02115-4312 888-965-8965
Fax: 617-437-0456
contact@nbp.org
www.nbp.org
The National Braille Press is a non-profit publisher, and promotes literacy by providing literature in braille for blind children, and by

providing access to original braille works written by and for blind individuals.
Julie Pierog, Chair
Shelly O'Neill, Vice-Chair

9441 National Eye Institute (NEI): National Institutes of Health (NIH)
31 Center Drive MSC 2510 301-496-5248
Bethesda, MD 20892-2510 2020@nei.nih.gov
www.nei.nih.gov
The National Eye Institute conducts and supports research, and the education of blindness, eye diseases, and visual disorders. NEI coordinates international research into the causes of impaired vision.
Paul A. Sieving, MD, PhD, Director

9442 National Federation of the Blind
200 E Wells Street 410-659-9314
Baltimore, MD 21230 Fax: 410-685-5653
nfb@nfb.org
www.nfb.org
The oldest and largest organization of blind Americans, providing public education about blindness, support services to the newly blinded, and scholarships, among other programs.
50M Members
Mark A. Riccobono, President
Pam Allen, First Vice President & Chair

9443 National Federation of the Blind in Computer Science
406 Palm Street 650-213-1311
Santa Cruz, CA 95060-4722 buhrow@nfbcal.org
www.nfb.org
National organization of blind individuals knowledgeable in the computer science and technology fields. Works to develop new technologies, to secure access to current technology, and to develop new ways of using current or new technologies by the blind.
Brian Buhrow, President

9444 National Federation of the Blind: Deaf-Blind Division
216 W McNeal Street 856-765-0601
Millville, NJ 08332 cheiro_alice@aol.com
www.nfb.org
Deaf-blind individuals working to improve services, training and independence for the deaf-blind. Offer personal contact with other deaf-blind individuals knowledgeable in advocacy, education, employment, technology, discrimination and other issues surrounding deaf-blindness.
Alice Eaddy, President

9445 National Federation of the Blind: Human Services Division
661 Permenter Road 601-201-1602
Carthage, MS 39051 chapman.candicel@gmail.com
www.nfb.org
An organization of blind individuals working in counseling, psychology, social work, psychiatry, rehabilitation, and other social sciences. Dedicated to improving employment opportunities and advancement for blind individuals, and mentorship for aspiring professionals.
Candice Chapman, President

9446 National Federation of the Blind: Public Employees Division
Ivan Weich
4301 Clogston Avenue NE 360-731-9782
Bremerton, WA 98310 ieweich@budworks.net
www.nfb.org
Organization of blind individuals holding local, state or federal jobs. Focuses on issues such as changes in governmental hiring and retention practices, new job skills needed for the future, new electronic means of finding employment and more.
Ivan Weich, President

9447 National Federation of the Blind: Science and Engineering Division
10955 Deering Street 858-527-1727
San Diego, CA 92126 johnmillerphd@hotmail.com
www.nfb.org
Blind individuals with expertise and experience in fields such as genetics, telecommunications, biology, chemistry, physics and nuclear physics or mechanical electronic and chemical engineering support other blind individuals in excelling in their respective fields.
John Miller, PhD, President

9448 National Federation of the Blind: Writers Division
208-339-2430
thirdeyeonlyinaz@gmail.com
www.writers.nfb.org
Blind writers of all genres offer encouragement and support to blind writers and authors.
Eve Sanchez, President

9449 National Industries for the Blind
3000 Potomac Avenue 703-310-0500
Alexandria, VA 22305 www.nib.org
The largest non-profit organization and employer of blind individuals in the United States. Maintains, creates, and sustains employment for blind individuals by providing career training and industry connections.
Kevin A. Lynch, President & CEO
Angela Hartley, Executive Vice President & CPO

9450 National Library Service for the Blind and Physically Handicapped
1291 Taylor Street NW 202-707-5100
Washington, DC 20542 800-424-8567
Fax: 202-707-0712
TTY: 888-657-7323
nls@loc.gov
www.loc.gov
A national library service providing braille and recorded books and magazines to anyone who cannot read standard print because of visual or physical disabilities in the United States.
12 pages Quarterly
Frank Kurt Cylke, Director
Michael M. Moodie, Research and Development Officer

9451 National Organization of Parents of Blind Children
1026 E 36th Street 717-658-9894
Baltimore, MD 21218 NOPBCpres@gmail.com
www.nopbc.org
Organization offering support, information, and advocacy for parents of blind or visually impaired children. Affiliated with the National Federation of the Blind.
Carlton Anne Cook Walker, President
Penny Duffy, First Vice President

9452 New Eyes for the Needy
549 Millburn Avenue 973-376-4903
Short Hills, NJ 07078 info@new-eyes.org
www.new-eyes.org
A non-profit organization that provides new and recycled glasses for those with low vision who may not be able to afford them.
Susan Dyckman, President
Marie Cavanaugh, Managing Director

9453 Prevent Blindness
225 W Wacker Drive 800-331-2020
Chicago, IL 60606 info@preventblindness.org
www.preventblindness.org
Information and referral services provided on specific eye disorders. Publishes literature and supports community screening and testing programs.
Torrey Van Antwerp DeKeyser, Chair & Executive Director
Charles Garcia, Treasurer

9454 Randolph-Sheppard Vendors of America
940 Parc Helene Drive 504-328-6373
Marrero, LA 70072-2421 800-467-5299
Fax: 504-328-6372
rsva@randolph-sheppard.org
www.randolph-sheppard.org
Seeks proper implementation of the Randolph-Sheppard Act that protects the interests of blind vendors, and encourages good business practices for blind businessmen and businesswoman by promoting the opening of locations in more visible and profitable areas.
Dan Sippl, President
Richard Bird, First Vice President

9455 Research to Prevent Blindness
360 Lexington Avenue   212-752-4333
New York, NY 10017-6528   800-621-0026
                                  inforequest@rpbusa.org
                                            www.rpbusa.org
National voluntary health foundation established to foster research into the causes, prevention, and treatment of blindness and other diseases of the eye.
Brian F. Hofland, PhD, President
Diana Friedman, Director

9456 Second Sense: Beyond Vision Loss
65 E Wacker Place   312-236-8569
Chicago, IL 60601   Fax: 312-236-8128
                                     info@second-sense.org
                                         www.second-sense.org
Second Sense delivers programs that instruct daily living skills, orientation and mobility training, communication skills, and more to adults with vision loss.
Brett Christenson, President
Michael P. Wagner, Treasurer

9457 Seeing Eye
PO Box 375   973-539-4425
Morristown, NJ 07963-0375   info@seeingeye.org
                                          www.seeingeye.org
A non-profit training school for seeing eye dogs to guide blind people. Dogs are bred and trained by qualified instructors.
James A. Kutsch, Jr., PhD, President & CEO
Peggy Gibbon, Director

9458 Smith-Kettlewell Eye Research Institute
2318 Fillmore Street   415-345-2000
San Francisco, CA 94115-1813   Fax: 415-345-8455
                                      TTY: 415-345-2290
                                               www.ski.org
Dedicated to research on human vision in order to facilitate diagnosis, understanding, and rehabilitation of eye disorders.
Art Jampolsky, MD, Founder
John Brabyn, PhD, Executive Director

9459 The Metropolitan Washington Ear, Inc.
12061 Tech Road   301-681-6636
Silver Spring, MD 20904   Fax: 301-625-1986
                                    information@washear.org
                                            www.washear.org
A non-profit organization offering reading and information services for the blind, visually impaired and physically disabled individuals who cannot effectively read print, see plays, watch television programs, or view museum exhibits, all at no cost.
Margaret Pfanstiehl, President
Neely Oplinger, Executive Director

9460 United States Association for Blind Athletes
1 Olympic Plaza   719-866-3224
Colorado Springs, CO 80909   Fax: 719-866-3400
                                               www.usaba.org
National governing body for blind athletes in the United States.
Michael Bina, PhD, President
Larry Dickerson, Vice President

9461 World Services for the Blind
2811 Fair Park Boulevard   501-664-7100
Little Rock, AR 72204   800-248-0734
                                      Fax: 501-664-2743
                                       training@wsblind.org
                                             www.wsblind.org
Rehabilitation center for individuals who are blind or visually impaired, offering a great variety of resources from teaching life skills to career training.
Sharon Giovinazzo, President & CEO
Duane Clausen, CFO

9462 National Association of Blind Merchants
7450 Chapman Highway   888-687-6226
Knoxville, TN 37920   www.blindmerchants.org
Membership organization of blind persons employed in either self-employment work or the Randolph-Sheppard vending program. Provides information on issues that directly affect blind

merchants and their businesses, from social security tax, to rehabilitation.
Nicholas P. Gacos, President

State Agencies & Associations

Alabama

9463 Alabama Council of the Blind
1018 E Street S   256-362-5649
Talladega, AL 35160
David Trott, President

9464 National Federation of the Blind: Alabama
4905 Brooke Court   251-344-7960
Mobile, AL 36618-2708   mwkoger21@bellsouth.net
Minnie K Walker, President

Alaska

9465 National Federation of the Blind: Alaska
1169 Hess Avenue   907-479-6118
Fairbanks, AK 99709   jnhburton@gci.net
                                                 www.nfb.org

Jim Burton, President

Arizona

9466 Arizona Center for the Blind and Visually Impaired
3100 E Roosevelt Street   602-273-7411
Phoenix, AZ 85008-5036   Fax: 602-273-7410
                                        jlamay@acbvi.org
                                              www.acbvi.org
Provides services for individuals to enhance the quality of life of people who are blind or otherwise visually impaired. Services are available to adults who are either legally blind or visually impaired as well as those who have a degenerative eye condition.
Steve Walker, Chair
Stanton Stipes, Vice Chair

9467 Arizona Industries for the Blind
515 N 51st Avenue   602-771-9100
Phoenix, AZ 85043   Fax: 602-353-5703
                                       LHudspeth@azdes.gov
                                          www.azdes.gov/aib
Arizona Industries for the Blind was established in 1952 to provide employment and training opportunities for Arizonans who are legally blind.
Lorraine Hudspeth, Controller
Letty Cerpa, Senior Accountant

9468 National Federation of the Blind: Arizona
9014 E Bellevue Street   520-733-5894
Tucson, AZ 85715-5652   krezguy@cox.net
Bob Kresmer, President
Vicki Hodges, 1st Vice President

9469 Region 6 of the National Association for Parents of the Visually Impaired
Walnut Creek, CA 85282-5724   602-730-8282
                                   mebphillips@comcast.net
                                       www.spedex.com/napvi

Susan LaVenture, Executive Director
Julie Urban, President

Arkansas

9470 Arkansas Lighthouse for the Blind
6818 Murray Street   510-562-2222
Little Rock, AR 72209-2666   Fax: 501-568-5275
                                   www.arkansaslighthouse.org

Pat Smith, President
Jim Shenep, Vice President

9471 National Federation of the Blind: Arkansas
2360 Wedington Drive   479-582-0091
Fayetteville, AR 72701-2304   tosheeler@cox.net
                                                 www.nfb.org

Terry Sheeler, President

California

9472 Lighthouse for the Blind and Visually Impaired
Lighthouse Industries
214 Van Ness Avenue   415-431-1481
San Francisco, CA 94102   Fax: 415-863-7568
TTY: 415-431-4572
info@lighthouse-sf.org
www.lighthouse-sf.org
The LightHouse promotes the independence, equality and self-reliance of people who are blind or visually impaired through rehabilitation training and relevant services, such as access to employment, education, government, information, recreation and transportation.
Chuck Godwin, Executive Support
Anthony Fletcher, Associate Executive Director and COO

9473 National Federation of the Blind: California
3934 Kern Court   818-342-6524
Pleasonton, CA 94588   877-558-6524
Fax: 818-344-7930
nfbcal@sbcglobal.net
http://www.nfbcal.org/
Mary Willows, President
Ever Lee Harriston, Vice President

9474 Northwest Regional Training Center: Canine Companions for Independence
2965 Dutton Avenue   707-577-1000
Santa Rosa, CA 95407-0446   800-572-2275
TTY: 707-577-1756
info@cci.org
www.cci.org
Canine Companions for Independence is a non-profit organization that enhances the lives of people with disabilities by providing highly trained assistance dogs and ongoing support to ensure quality partnerships.
Corey Hudson, CEO
Kathy Pierson, Northwest Regional Executive Director

9475 Southwest Regional Training Center: Canine Companions for Independence
124 Rancho del Oro Drive   760-901-4300
Oceanside, CA 92057   800-572-2275
Fax: 760-901-4350
TTY: 760-901-4326
TDD: 760-901-4350
www.cci.org
Canine Companions for Independence is a non-profit organization that enhances the lives of people with disabilities by providing highly trained assistance dogs and ongoing support to ensure quality partnerships.
Linda Valliant, Executive Director
Chuck Contreras, Director of Development

Colorado

9476 National Federation of the Blind: Colorado
2233 W Shepperd Avenue   303-778-1130
Littleton, CO 80120   800-401-4NFB
slabarre@labarrelaw.com
www.nfbco.org
Scott LaBarre, President
Kevan Worley, 1st Vice President

Connecticut

9477 National Federation of the Blind: Connecticut
477 Connecticut Boulevard,   860-289-1971
East Hartford, CT 06108-3579   http://www.nfbct.org/
Alfonse DeLucia, President

9478 Prevent Blindness Tri-State
101 Whitney Avenue   800-850-2020
New Haven, CT 06510   info@preventblindnesstristate.org
Kathryn Garre-Ayars, President & CEO
Maria Giarratana, Grants Manager

Delaware

9479 Delaware Assocation for the Blind Department of Health & Social Services
Department of Health & Social Services
2915 Newport Gap Pike   302-655-2111
Wilmington, DE 19801-1526   888-777-3925
Fax: 302-655-1442
contact@dabdel.org
www.dabdel.org

9480 National Federation of the Blind: Delaware
2215 Bradmoor Road   302-652-6761
Wilmington, DE 19803-2646   lynne.majewski@gmail.com
www.nfb.org
Lynne Majewski, President

District of Columbia

9481 Columbia Lighthouse for the Blind
1825 K Street NW   301-589-0894
Washington, DC 20006   877-324-5252
Fax: 877-595-9228
info@clb.org
www.clb.org
Columbia Lighthouse for the blind offers programs and services that enable individuals who are blind or visually impaired to obtain and maintain independence at home, school and in the community.
Anthony Cancelosi, President/CEO

9482 National Federation of the Blind: DC
2354 13th Place, N.E.   202-352-1511
Washington, DC 20018-1841   callaway.shawn@gmail.com
www.nfb.org
Shawn M. Callaway, President

Florida

9483 National Federation of the Blind: Florida
3708 West Bay to Bay Blvd   386-677-6886
Tampa, FL 33629-4266   888-282-5972
president@nfbflorida.org
www.nfbflorida.org
Dan Hicks, President
Gloria Mills Hicks, Treasurer

9484 Southeast Regional Center: Canine Companions for Independence
Anheuser-Busch/SeaWorld Campus
8150 Clarcona Ocoee Road   407-522-3300
Orlando, FL 32818-0388   Fax: 407-522-3347
mager@cci.org
www.cci.org
Canine Companions for Independence is a non-profit organization that enhances the lives of people with disabilities by providing highly trained assistance dogs and ongoing support to ensure quality partnerships.
Margaret S Ager, Executive Director
Nancy Baumann, President

9485 Tampa Lighthouse for the Blind
1106 W Platt Street   813-251-2407
Tampa, FL 33606-2142   866-251-2407
Fax: 813-254-4305
TLH@tampalighthouse.org
www.tampalighthouse.org
Tampa Lighthouse for the Blind provides comprehensive rehabilitation programs for persons who are blind or visually impaired.
Cliff Olstrom, Executive Director

Georgia

9486 Georgia Industries for the Blind
700 Faceville Highway   229-248-2666
Bainbridge, GA 39818-0218   www.vocrehabga.org
The primary mission of the Georgia Industries for the Blind (GIB) is to provide employment opportunities for people who are visually impaired or blind.

9487 National Federation of the Blind: Georgia
315 Ponce de Leon Avenue 404-371-1000
Decatur, GA 30030 Fax: 404-371-1002
gscott@nfbga.org
www.nfb.org

Garrick Scott, President

9488 Southeastern Region: Helen Keller National Center
1003 Virginia Avenue 404-766-9625
Atlanta, GA 30354-1365 Fax: 404-766-3447
TTY: 404-766-2820
bc4hknc@aol.com
www.hknc.org

Barbara Chandler, Regional Representative

Hawaii

9489 Division of Vocational Rehabilitation and Services for the Blind
Department of Human Services
601 Kamokila Boulevard 808-692-7715
Kapolei, HI 96707 Fax: 808-692-7727
TTY: 808-692-7715
www.hawaiivr.org
The American Macular Degeneration Foundation is committed to the prevention and cure of macular degeneration and offers hope and support to those afflicted and their families. The Foundation is a major voice in establishing national research.
Joe Cordova, Administrator

9490 Ho'opono Workshop for the Blind
1901 Bachelor Street 808-586-5286
Honolulu, HI 96817 Fax: 808-586-5288
TTY: 808-586-5269

Dave Eveland, Administrator

9491 National Federation of the Blind: Hawaii
PO Box 4482 808-391-1214
Honolulu, HI 96812 nanifife@aol.com
hawaii.nfb.org

Nani Fife, President
Charlene Ota, Vice-President

Idaho

9492 National Federation of the Blind: Idaho
300 Willard Avenue 208-377-9825
Pocatello, ID 83201 Fax: 208-232-5416
ElsieLamp@yahoo.com
www.nfbidaho.org

Elsie H Lamp, President

Illinois

9493 Aid to the Aged, Blind or Disabled
Department of Human Services
100 South Grand Avenue, East 800-252-8635
Springfield, IL 62762 TTY: 800-447-6404
www.macular.org/stagency/state_il.html
The American Macular Degeneration Foundation is committed to the prevention and cure of macular degeneration and offers hope and support to those afflicted and their families. The Foundation will be a major voice in establishing the national research agenda for macular degeneration through promoting an alliance among the scientific community, government, and victims of the disease and their families to ensure the prevention and cure of the disease.

9494 Chicago Lighthouse for People Who are Blind and Visually Impaired
1850 W Roosevelt Road 312-666-1331
Chicago, IL 60608-1298 Fax: 312-243-8539
TTY: 312-666-8874
TDD: 312-666-8874
helpdesk@chicagolighthouse.org
www.thechicagolighthouse.org
The Chicago Lighthouse is a comprehensive private rehabilitation and educational facility dedicated exclusively to assisting children youth and adults who are blind visually impaired or multi-disabled.
Janet P Szlyk, Executive Director
William L Conaghan, Chairman

9495 Helen Keller National Center Regional Representatives
485 Avenue of the Cities 309-755-0018
E Moline, IL 61244 Fax: 309-755-0025
TTY: 309-755-0018
TDD: 309-755-0021
HKNC5LJT@aol.com
www.hknc.org

Laura J Thomas, Regional Representative

9496 National Federation of the Blind: Illinois
6919 W Berwyn Avenue 773-307-6440
Chicago, IL 60656-2040 www.nfbofillinois.org
Patti Gregory-Chang, President
Deborah Kent Stein, First Vice-President

Indiana

9497 Bosma Industries for the Blind
8020 Zionsville Road 317-684-0600
Indianapolis, IN 46268-3876 800-362-5463
Fax: 317-684-1946
info@bosma.org
www.bosma.org
It is the mission of Bosma Industries for the Blind to enhance opportunities for individuals who are blind or visually impaired to achieve their potential in vocational, economic, social and personal independence.
Lou Moneymaker, CEO
Connie F Campbell, CFO/COO

9498 National Federation of the Blind: Indiana
6010 Winnpeny Lane 317-205-9226
Indianapolis, IN 46220-5253 rb15@iquest.net
www.nfb.org

Ron Brown, President

Iowa

9499 National Federation of the Blind: Iowa
2721 34th Street 515-771-8348
Des Moines, IA 50310 www.nfb.org
Michael D Barber, President
April Enderton, First Vice-President

Kansas

9500 Kansas Industries for the Blind
425 MacVicar Street 785-296-3211
Topeka, KS 66606 Fax: 785-296-0728

9501 National Federation of the Blind: Kansas
11405 W Grant 913-339-9341
Wichita, KS 67209-3621 donnajwood@cox.net
www.nfbks.org

Donna Wood, President
Susan L Stanzel, First Vice President

Kentucky

9502 Kentucky Industries for the Blind
1900 Brownsboro Road 502-893-0211
Louisville, KY 40206-2102 Fax: 502-893-3885

9503 National Federation of the Blind: Kentucky
210 Cambridge Drive 502-366-2317
Louisville, KY 40214-2809
Cathy Jackson, President
Pamela Roark-Glisson, Vice President

Louisiana

9504 Industries for the Blind and Visually Impaired of Louisiana
PO Box 366 318-878-8171
Delhi, LA 71232-0366

9505 Louisiana Association for the Blind
1750 Claiborne Avenue   318-635-6471
Shreveport, LA 71103   877-913-6471
Fax: 318-635-8902
labstore@lablind.com
www.lablind.com
LAB employs people who are blind in manufacturing administrative training and a variety of job positions that match an individual's goals and potential.
Shelly Taylor, President/CEO
Doug Young, Vice President Administration

9506 National Federation of the Blind: Louisana
605 University Boulevard   318-251-1511
Ruston, LA 71270-4862   800-234-4166
www.nfbla.org
Pam Allen, President

Maine

9507 Maine Center for the Blind and Visually Impaired
189 Park Avenue   207-774-6273
Portland, ME 04102-2909   Fax: 207-774-0679
info@theiris.org
www.theiris.org
Leonard Cole, Chairman
Katherine Ray, Vice Chair

9508 National Federation of the Blind: Maine
33 Morse Avenue   207-212-1455
Lewiston, ME 04240-9707   leonproctorjr@yahoo.com
www.nfb.org
Leon Proctor, Jr, President

Maryland

9509 Blind Industries and Services of Maryland
3345 Washington Boulevard   410-737-2600
Baltimore, MD 21227   888-322-4567
Fax: 410-737-2665
www.bism.org
Blind Industries and Services of Maryland provides innovative rehabilitation services training and stable employment opportunities to our state's citizens who are blind or visually impaired.
Don Morris, Chairperson
Walter Brown, Vice-Chairperson

9510 National Federation of the Blind: Maryland
1026 E 36th Street   41- 6-5 06
Baltimore, MD 21218   president@nfbmd.org
www.nfbmd.org/
Melissa Riccobono, President
Debbie Brown, First Vice President

Massachusetts

9511 Carroll Center for the Blind
770 Centre Street   617-969-6200
Newton, MA 02458-2597   800-852-3131
Fax: 617-969-6204
TTY: 617-969-6204
info@carroll.org
www.carroll.org
Assists blind and visually impaired adults and adolescents to adjust to loss of vision. The goal of this dynamic program is to encourage independence, restore self-confidence, prepare for employment and improve the quality of life.
Dina Rosenbaum, Marketing Director

9512 Massachusetts Commission for the Blind
600 Washington St.   617-748-2000
Boston, MA 02111-4718   www.state.ma.us/mcb
Provides services to blind citizens of Massachusetts, enabling them to lead more fulfilling and independent lives. Offers vocational rehabilitation, independent living, social services, home care and respite assistance, radio reading programs and print resources.
Cheryl Standley, Contact
Janet LaBreck, Commissioner

9513 National Federation of the Blind: Massachusetts
140 Wood Street   508-679-8543
Somerset, MA 02726-5225   nfbmass@earthlink.net
http://www.nfbmass.org/
Priscilla Ferris, President

9514 New England Region: Helen Keller National Center
152 Lincoln Road   781-259-7100
Lincoln, MA 01773   Fax: 781-259-4014
www.hknc.org
Mary Ellen Barbiasz, Regional Representative
Peg Ouellette, Administrative Assistant

9515 Region 1 of the National Association for Parents of the Visually Impaired
Hudson, MA 06016-9560   860-623-4129
sue.rawley@verizon.net

Michigan

9516 Association for the Blind & Visually Impaired
456 Cherry Southeast   616-458-1187
Grand Rapids, MI 49503   800-466-8084
Fax: 616-458-7113
abvi@abvimichigan.org
www.abvimichigan.org
To advance the independence of people who are visually impaired and to promote the prevention of blindness.
Richard A Stevens, Executive Director
George Kremer, Director of Rehabilitation Services

9517 Greater Detroit Agency for the Blind and Visually Impaired
16625 Grand River Avenue   313-272-3900
Detroit, MI 48227-1419   Fax: 313-272-6893
information@gdabvi.org
www.gdabvi.org
We are a non-profit organization dedicated to preventing blindness reducing the impact of blindness and advocating for those with severe vision loss.
Frederick J Simpson, Chairman
Charles L Cone, Vice Chair

9518 National Federation of the Blind: Michigan
1212 N Foster Avenue   517-482-1800
Lansing, MI 48912-3309   f.wurtzel@comcast.net
www.nfbmi.org
Fred Wurtzel, President
Mary Ann Rojek, State Braille Coin Project Coordinator

Minnesota

9519 Duluth Lighthouse for the Blind
4505 W Superior Street   218-624-4828
Duluth, MN 55807-2728   800-422-0833
Fax: 218-624-4479
info@lighthousefortheblind-duluth.org
www.lighthousefortheblind-duluth.org
The LightHouse for the blind is a teaching facility providing employment, training and rehab instruction for blind and visually-impaired individuals.
Mary Junnila, Executive Director
Debbie , Book keeper

9520 National Federation of the Blind: Minnesota
100 East 22nd street   612-872-9363
Minneapolis, MN 55404-2217   joyce.scanlan@earthlink.net
http://www.nfbmn.org/
Jennifer Dunmann, President

Mississippi

9521 Mississippi Industries for the Blind
2501 N W Street   601-984-3200
Jackson, MS 39216-4417   866-859-4461
Fax: 601-987-3892
bcoy@msblind.org
www.msblind.org

The Mississippi Industries for the Blind seeks to provide jobs for the blind and visually-impaired.
Michael Chew, Executive Director
Bob Coy, Sales Manager

9522 National Federation of the Blind: Mississippi
PO Box 1515   601-969-3352
Jackson, MS 39215-5431   samgleese@earthlink.net
                                                      www.nfbofmississippi.org
rev Sam Gleese, President
Barbara Hadnot, Vice President

Missouri

9523 Alphapointe Association for the Blind
7501 Prospect   816-421-5848
Kansas City, MO 64132   Fax: 816-237-2019
                                                      www.alphapointe.org
The Alphapointe Association for the Blind has a Braille library a Senior Adult Services Program and a dedication to finding employment for the blind and visually-impaired.
Paulette Markel, Chairman
Ken Roberson, Secretary

9524 Kansas City Association for the Blind
1844 Broadway Street   816-333-2173
Kansas City, MO 64108-2007

9525 National Federation of the Blind: Missouri
3910 Tropical Lane   573-874-1774
Columbia, MO 65202-6205   info@nfbmo.org
                                                      www.nfbmo.org
Gary Wunder, President
Shelia Wright, First Vice President

Montana

9526 National Federation of the Blind: Montana
408 W Sussex Avenue   406-546-8546
Missoula, MT 59801   burk.dall@gmail.com
                                                      www.mt-blind.org
Daniel Burke, President
Dick Howse, 1st Vice President

Nebraska

9527 National Federation of the Blind: Nebraska
1033 O Street   402-477-7711
Lincoln, NE 68508-2468   866-254-6347
Amy Buresh, President
Jeff Altman, First Vice President

Nevada

9528 National Federation of the Blind: Nevada
1344 N. Jones Boulevard   702-228-4217
Las Vegas, NV 89108   realhappygirl1@gmail.com
Terri Rupp, President

9529 Southern Nevada Sightless
1001 N Bruce Street   702-642-6000
Las Vegas, NV 89101-1247   Fax: 702-649-6739
                                                      info@blindcenter.org
                                                      www.blindcenter.org
Neal Marek, Chairman
Veronica Wilson, President/CEO

New Hampshire

9530 National Federation of the Blind: New Hampshire
12 Summer St.   603-357-4080
Keene, NH 03431   cemcnabb21@yahoo.com
                                                      www.nfbnh.org/
Marie Johnson, President

New Jersey

9531 Bestwork Industries for the Blind
801 E Clements Bridge Road   856-939-5220
Runnemede, NJ 08078   800-370-9560
                                                      Fax: 856-939-5022
                                                      www.bestworkindustries.org
Bestwork Industries for the Blind is dedicated to providing employment opportunities for those with visual impairments.
James Varsaci, Founder

9532 National Federation of the Blind: New Jersey
254 Spruce Street   973-743-0075
Bloomfield, NJ 07003   nfbnj@yahoo.com
                                                      http://www.nfbnj.org/
Joe Ruffalo, President

New Mexico

9533 National Federation of the Blind: New Mexico
10315 Props dr. NE   505-268-3895
Albuquerque, NM 87112   http://www.nfbnm.org/
Arthur Schreiber, President

9534 New Mexico Industries for the Blind
2200 Yale Boulevard SE   505-841-8844
Albuquerque, NM 87106-4212   888-513-7958
                                                      Fax: 505-841-8850
                                                      Greg.Trapp@state.nm.us
                                                      www.state.nm.us/cftb
Greg Trapp, Executive Director
Dallas Allen, Commissioner

9535 State of New Mexico Commission for the Blind
2905 Rodeo Park Drive E   505-476-4479
Santa Fe, NM 87505   888-513-7968
                                                      Greg.Trapp@state.nm.us
The mission of the New Mexico Commission for the Blind is to encourage and enable blind citizens to achieve vocational economic and social equality. It provides career preparation and training in the skills of blindness.
Greg Trapp, Executive Director
Arthur A Schreiber, Chairman

New York

9536 Association for the Blind & Visually Impaired of Greater Rochester
422 South Clinton Avenue   585-232-1111
Rochester, NY 14620-1198   www.raen.org
Our mission is to assist people who are blind or visually impaired to achieve their highest level of independence in all aspects of their lives.
A Gidget Hopf, EdD, President/CEO

9537 Blind Association of Western New York
1170 Main Street   716-882-1025
Buffalo, NY 14209-2331   www.olmstedcenter.org
Patricia Clabeaux, Chairwomen
Phil Catanese, Vice Chairman

9538 Blind Work Association
55 Washington Street   607-724-2428
Binghamton, NY 13901-3770   Fax: 607-771-8045
                                                      bobh@clarityconnect.com

9539 Central Association for the Blind and Visually Impaired
507 Kent Street   315-797-2233
Utica, NY 13501-2317   877-719-9996
                                                      Fax: 315-797-2244
                                                      www.cabvi.org
Edward P. Welsch, Chairman
James B. Turnbill IV, Vice Chairman

9540 National Federation of the Blind: New York
PO Box 205666   718-567-7821
Brooklyn, NY 11220-4617   Fax: 718-765-1843
                                                      office@nfbny.org
                                                      www.nfbny.org
Carl Jacobsen, President
Mindy Jacobson, Vice President

9541 Northeastern Association of the Blind of Albany
301 Washington Avenue 518-463-1211
Albany, NY 12206-3012 Fax: 51- 4-3 35
www.naba-vision.org
NABA offers a wide range of services to those with visual impairments from its free vision screening service for children to training and placing legally blind adults in professional employment. Also provides rehabilitation services to seniors with age-related conditions.
Mark J McKarthy, Chair
david P. Quinn, Vice Chairman

9542 Southern Tier Association for the Visually Impaired
719 Lake Street 607-734-1554
Elmira, NY 14901-2538 Fax: 607-734-9467
info@st-avi.org
www.st-avi.org

Brian Bleiler, President
John Luce, Vice President

North Carolina

9543 Lions Industries for the Blind
4126 Berkeley Avenue 252-523-1019
Kinston, NC 28504-8321 Fax: 252-523-7090
customerser@lionsindustries.org
www.lionsindustries.com
The Lions Industries for the Blind provides employment opportunities for the blind and visually-impaired.
ray Amette, Executive Director
Marc Camnitz, General Manager

9544 National Federation of the Blind: North Carolina
128 Summerlea Drive 704-491-1486
Charlotte, NC 28214-1324 Fax: 704-391-3204
http://www.nfbofnc.org/
Gary Ray, President

9545 Winston-Salem Industries for the Blind
7730 N Point Drive 336-759-0551
Winston-Salem, NC 27106-3310 800-242-7726
Fax: 336-759-0990
info@wsifb.com
www.wsifb.com
The Winston-Salem Industries for the Blind provides employment opportunities for the blind and visually-impaired.
david Byler, Chair
Mike Faircloth, Vice Chairman

North Dakota

9546 National Federation of the Blind: North Dakota
301 4th St. East 701-572-3477
Williston, ND 58101 www.nfb.org
Duane Iverson, President

Ohio

9547 Cincinnati Association for the Blind
2045 Gilbert Avenue 513-221-8558
Cincinnati, OH 45202-1490 888-687-3935
Fax: 513-221-2995
info@cincyblind.org
www.cincyblind.org
Persons who are blind visually impaired or print impaired may choose from a wide range of services to help them live more independently. Our services are provided by qualified certified instructors and staff with highly specialized skills.
John Mitchell, Executive Director
Ginny Backschreider, Director of Program services

9548 Cleveland Sight Center
1909 E 101st Street 216-791-8118
Cleveland, OH 44106-8696 Fax: 216-791-1101
sfriedman@clevelandsightcenter.org
www.clevelandsightcenter.org

Mission is to enable people with vision impairment to reach their full potential and assure that adequate services are available to make a normal life possible.
William L. Spring, Chair
Thomas P. Furnas, Vice Chairman

9549 Cleveland Skilled Industries
2239 E 55th Street 216-431-8085
Cleveland, OH 44103-4451 Fax: 216-431-5123

9550 National Federation of the Blind: Ohio
P.O. Box 82055, 440-775-2216
Columbus, OH 43202-1517 www.nfbohio.org
Duffy Eric, President
Payne Richard, Vice President

Oklahoma

9551 National Federation of the Blind: Oklahoma
457 N. Blackwelder Avenue 405-600-0695
Edmond, OK 73034 jmassay1@cox.net
www.nfb.org

Jeannie Massay, President

9552 Oklahoma League for the Blind
501 N Douglas Avenue 405-232-4644
Oklahoma City, OK 73106 Fax: 405-236-5438
swright@newviewoklahoma.org
www.newviewoklahoma.org
The mission of the Oklahoma League for the Blind is to facilitate independence and improve the quality of life for people who are blind or vision impaired by providing employment opportunities and services.
Thomas Larson, Director
Elijha Straw, Business Manager

Oregon

9553 Blind Enterprises of Oregon
6540 SE Foster Road 503-774-6387
Portland, OR 97206 Fax: 503-774-0585
blindent@aol.com
www.blindenterprises.com

Tami Foss, Executive Director
Bill Smith, Operator

9554 National Federation of the Blind: Oregon
5005 Main Street 541-726-6924
Springfield, OR 97478 800-422-7093
admin@mainstreetmontessori.org
www.nfb.org

Carla McQuillan, President

Pennsylvania

9555 Association for the Blind & Visually Impaired of Lehigh County
845 Wyoming Street 610-433-6018
Allentown, PA 18103-2199 Fax: 610-433-4856
info@abvi.org
www.abvi.org
The ABVI mission is to strive to be our community's foremost provider and coordinator of preventative, educational, social and rehabilitative programs concerning vision loss. Our goal is to assist each individual and his/her family to achieve their greatest potential.
Kathleen Meckes, Executive Director

9556 Beaver County Association for the Blind
616 Fourth Street 724-843-1111
Beaver Falls, PA 15010 Fax: 724-843-8886
bcab@forcomm.net
The Beaver County Association for the Blind conducts educational programs about blindness or vision problems by request and provides opportunities to learn experience share and celebrate in the lives of the blind and visually impaired in Beaver County.
Fay Lentz, Executive Director
Linda Borghi, Controller/Business Manager

9557 Cambria County Association for the Blind and Handicapped
211 Central Avenue   814-536-3531
Johnstown, PA 15902   Fax: 814-539-3270
                                                            ccabh@ccabh.com
                                                            www.ccabh.com

The mission of the Cambria County Association for the Blind and Handicapped is to develop and support an environment for persons with disabilities which promotes vocational and employment training, independence and community involvement through rehabilitative programs.
Richard C Bosserman, President

9558 Chester County Association for the Blind
71 S First Avenue   610-384-2767
Coatesville, PA 19320   Fax: 610-384-8005
                                                            info@chescoblind.org
                                                            www.chescoblind.org

Anita Cavuto, Executive Director
John W Esworthy, President

9559 Delaware County Branch of the Pennsylvania Association for the Blind
100-106 W 15th Street   610-874-1476
Chester, PA 19013   Fax: 610-874-6454
                                                            www.libertynet.org

9560 Greater Wilkes-Barre Association for the Blind
1825 Wyoming Avenue   570-693-3555
Exeter, PA 18643   877-693-3555
                                                            Fax: 570-823-4841
                                                            info@wilkesbarreblind.com
                                                            www.wilkesbarreblind.com

Our mission is to address the needs of those with limited vision and we also take an active role in the prevention of blindness.
Ronald V Petrilla, Executive Director
Denise Culver, Office Manager

9561 Indiana County Association for the Blind
31 S 10th Street   724-465-5549
Indiana, PA 15701-2649

9562 Keystone Blind Association
1230 Stambaugh Avenue   724-347-5501
Sharon, PA 16146   800-837-4122
                                                            Fax: 724-347-2204
                                                            kba@keystoneblind.org
                                                            www.keystoneblind.org

The Keystone Blind Association is dedicated to maintaining and improving the quality of life for blind and/or visually impaired persons preventing blindness and providing employment opportunities and advocacy for persons who are disabled.
Jonathan G Fister, President/CEO
Perry Templeton, Vice President of Operations

9563 Lancaster County Association for the Blind
244 N Queen Street   717-291-5951
Lancaster, PA 17603-3512
Dennis L Steiner, President/CEO
Kay L Macsi, VP Rehabilitation and Education

9564 Montgomery County Association for the Blind
212 N Main Street   215-661-9800
North Wales, PA 19454-3117   Fax: 215-661-9888
                                                            mcab@mcab.org
                                                            www.mcab.org

MCAB's mission is to enhance the quality of life and independence of people coping with blindness and vision impairment through rehabilitation education support and advocacy.
Douglas Yingling, Executive Director
Sharon Zislis, Director of Development

9565 National Federation of the Blind: Pennsylvania
42 South 15th Street   215-988-0888
Philadelphia, PA 19102-2206   Fax: 215-988-0879
                                                            http://www.nfbp.org/

James Antonacci, President

9566 North Central Sight Services
2121 Reach Road   570-323-9401
Williamsport, PA 17701-0292   866-320-2580
                                                            Fax: 570-323-8194
                                                            ncss@ncsight.org
                                                            www.ncsight.org

Our agency philosophy focuses on helping people help themselves and emphasizes the abilities and capabilities of the blind and visually impaired people we serve.
Robert B Garrett, President/CEO
Barbara Snauffer, Administrative Assistant

9567 Pittsburgh Vision Services
1800 W Street   412-368-4400
Homestead, PA 15120   800-706-5050
                                                            Fax: 412-368-4090
                                                            TTY: 412-368-4095
                                                            www.bvrspittsburgh.org/

Pittsburgh Vision Services is a private non-profit United Way agency whose mission is to reduce the limitations that may result from loss of vision.
Dennis J Farkos, Chairman
louis A Lobes, Vice Chairman

9568 Somerset County Blind Center
748 S Center Avenue   814-445-1310
Somerset, PA 15501   Fax: 814-445-3184

The Somerset Blind Center offers a number of services to those who are blind or visually impaired, including work opportunities, eyeglass prescription programs, free vision screenings, and training facilities.
Rob Stemple, Executive Director
Anna Hope, Finance Manager

9569 Tri-County Association for the Blind
1130 S 19th Street   717-238-2531
Harrisburg, PA 17104-2200   Fax: 717-238-0710
                                                            info@vrocp.org
                                                            www.vrocp.org/

The Tri-County Association for the Blind works to improve the quality of life for people who are visually-impaired in the Tri-County region, by helping each person achieve his or her full potential and maximum independence.
Danette Blank, Executive Director
Laurie Thompson, Public Relations/Development Director

9570 VIABL Services of Northampton County
845 West Wyoming Street   610-433-6018
Allentown, PA 18103   Fax: 610-866-8730
                                                            viabl@viablservices.org
                                                            www.viablservices.org

Our mission is to promote the social economic and physical self-sufficiency of blind deaf-blind and visually impaired individuals by providing them with the resources and skills needed to live rewarding productive and independent lives.
Jan Leon, Executive Director

9571 Washington-Greene County Branch for the Pennsylvania Association for Blind
555 Gettysburg Pike,   71- 7-6 20
Mechanicsberg, PA 17055-3720   Fax: 71- 7-6 20
                                                            neal.carrigan@pablind.org
                                                            www.pablind.org

Neal J Carrigan, President/CEO
Willard D Brown, Vice-President for Finance

9572 York Industries for the Blind: Division of York County Blind Center
A Division of York County Blind Center
1380 Spahn Avenue   717-848-1690
York, PA 17403-5711   Fax: 717-845-3889
                                                            www.forsight.org

William H Rhinesmith, President

Rhode Island

9573 IN-SIGHT
43 Jefferson Boulevard
Warwick, RI 02888
401-941-3322
Fax: 401-941-3356
insightri@gmail.com
www.in-sight.org
IN-SIGHT is a private non-profit agency which has been serving the blind and visually impaired since 1925.
Gerard Goulet, President
Eleanor Acton, Director of Communications

9574 National Federation of the Blind: Rhode Island
PO Box 14404
East Providence, RI 02914
401-433-2606
Fax: 877-383-3682
info@nfbri.org
www.nfbri.org
Richard Gaffney, President

South Carolina

9575 National Federation of the Blind: South Carolina
1293 Professional Drive
Myrtle Beach, SC 29577
803-254-3777
http://www.nfbsc.net/
Parnell Diggs, President

South Dakota

9576 National Federation of the Blind: South Dakota
903 Fulton Street
Rapid City, SD 57701
605-791-3939
Kenneth Rollman, President

Tennessee

9577 Ed Lindsey Industries of the Blind
4110 Charlotte Avenue
Nashville, TN 37209-3749
615-627-4012
Fax: 615-741-5024
www.elifortheblind.org/
Allen Broughton, Executive Vice President
Patrick Broughton, Administrative Assistant

9578 National Federation of the Blind: Tennessee
1226 Goodman Circle West
Memphis, TN 38111-6524
901-452-6596
http://www.nfb-tennessee.org/
Michael Seay, President

Texas

9579 American Foundation for the Blind
11030 Ables Lane
Dallas, TX 75229
214-352-7222
Fax: 646-478-9260
dallas@afb.net
www.afb.org
Leads initiatives in the areas of aging and education. Nationally offers consultation, technical assistance and support and undertakes local and national efforts such as training programs, public education and coalition building in the areas of aging and elder care.

9580 Dallas Lighthouse for the Blind
4306 Capitol Avenue
Dallas, TX 75204
214-821-2375
Fax: 214-824-4612
www.dallaslighthouse.org
The Dallas Lighthouse for the Blind provides work opportunities for the blind and visually impaired.
Nancy J Perkins, President/CEO
Gordon Spark, Executive Vice president

9581 East Texas Lighthouse for the Blind
500 N Bois D'Arc
Tyler, TX 75702
903-595-3444
888-595-3444
Fax: 903-595-3447
customerservice@horizonind.com
www.horizonind.com

9582 El Paso Lighthouse for the Blind
200 Washington Street
El Paso, TX 79905
915-532-4495
Fax: 915-532-6338
www.lighthouse-elpaso.com

Lighthouse is guided by the unwavering belief that its rehabilitative and employment services can help any person overcome his or her disability and enable them to reach their fullest potential for self-sufficiency and independence.
Harry Tyler, President/CEO
Rusty Hooten, CFO

9583 Lighthouse for the Blind of Houston
3602 W Dallas
Houston, TX 77019-0435
713-527-9561
Fax: 713-284-8451
Founded in 1839 the Lighthouse of Houston is a private nonprofit rehabilitation center dedicated to helping blind and visually impaired people live independently.
Gibson M DuTerroil, President

9584 Lighthouse of the Blind of Fort Worth
912 W Broadway Street
Fort Worth, TX 76104
817-332-3341
Fax: 817-332-3456
www.lighthousefw.org
The Lighthouse of the Blind of Fort Worth offers many services including skills assessment orientation and mobilty training assisted employment and senior services.
Dr. Shannon Ship, Chairman
W.B. Zim Zimmerman, Vice Chair

9585 National Federation of the Blind: Texas
314 E Highland Mall Boulevard
Austin, TX 78752-3123
512-323-5444
866-636-3289
Fax: 512-420-8160
president@nfbtx.org
www.nfb-texas.org
Tommy Craig, President

9586 South Texas Lighthouse for the Blind
PO Box 9697
Corpus Christi, TX 78469
361-883-6553
888-255-8011
Fax: 361-883-1041
Regisb@stlb.net
www.stlb.net
Regis Barber, President/CEO
Nicky Ooi, VP/COO

9587 Texas Association of Retinitis Pigmentosa
PO Box 8388
Corpus Christi, TX 78468-8388
361-852-8515
Fax: 361-852-8515
tarpmail@homebiz101.com
A nonprofit organization based in Texas serving as a national information-sharing center to provide human services to persons with progressive vision loss from retinitis pigmentosa and other retinal degenerative disorders.
Dorothy H Stiefel, Executive Director

9588 Travis Association for the Blind
2307 Business Center Drive
Austin, TX 78764-3297
512-442-2329
Fax: 512-442-5498
info@austinlighthouse.org
www.austinlighthouse.org
Travis Association for the Blind (aka Austin Lighthouse) is a service oriented non-profit organization with the mission to assist people who are blind or vision impaired to attain the skills they need to become gainfully employed in the community.
Jerry A Mayfield, Executive Director
Benny Galloway, Chief Financial Officer

9589 West Texas Lighthouse for the Blind
2001 Austin Street
San Angelo, TX 76903-8705
325-653-4231
Fax: 325-657-9367
www.lighthousefortheblind.org
The West Texas Lighthouse for the Blind is a sheltered facility providing employment for blind and visually impaired individuals.
Steve Cecil, Chairman
Barbara Rogers, Vice Chair

Utah

9590 National Federation of the Blind: Utah
1751 Park St
Salt Lake City, UT 84105-7634
801-631-8108
801-463-6632
Fax: 801-294-6000
Baconev@yahoo.com
www.nfbutah.org

Everrete Bacon, President
Cheralyn Bra Creer, First Vice President

9591 Utah Industries for the Blind
PO Box 258
Salt Lake Cty, UT 84110-1258
801-533-9689

Vermont

9592 National Federation of the Blind: Vermont
561 East Hill Rd.
Middlesex, VT 05602
802-272-0087
deannaljones@comcast.net
www.nfbvt.org

Franklin Shiner, President

Virginia

9593 National Federation of the Blind: Virginia
3230 Grove Avenue
Richmond, VA 23221
703-319-9226
fschroeder@sks.com
www.nfbv.org

Fredric K Schroeder, President
Seville Allen, First Vice President

9594 Virginia Industries for the Blind
1102 Monticello Road
Charlottesville, VA 22902
434-295-5168
Fax: 434-977-0122
Our mission is to be a self-sufficient and self-supporting industry enhance the quality of life for blind and visually impaired individuals through providing gainful employment; and provide opportunities in career development and employment related services.
Robert C Berrang, Deputy Commissioner
Richard C Bohrer, Plant Manager

Washington

9595 Lighthouse for the Blind of Washington
2501 South Plum Street
Seattle, WA 98114
206-322-4200
Fax: 206-329-3397
www.seattlelighthouse.org

Kirk Adams, President
Tami berk, Director

9596 Northwestern Region: Helen Keller National Center
1620 18th Avenue
Seattle, WA 98122-6501
206-324-9120
Fax: 206-324-9159
TTY: 206-324-1133
nwhknc@juno.com
www.hknc.org

Dorothy Walt, Regional Representative

9597 Washington State Department of Services for the Blind
402 Legion Way
Olympia, WA 98504-0933
360-725-3830
800-552-7103
Fax: 360-407-0679
information@dsb.wa.gov
www.dsb.wa.gov
The Washington State Department of Services for the Blind (DSB) is a state rehabilitation agency that offers assistance to persons who are blind or visually impaired. We also provide various services for employers interested in accomodating or hiring workers with visual impairments.
Bill Palmer, Director

West Virginia

9598 AFB Technology & Employment Center
1000 Fifth Avenue
Huntington, WV 25701
304-523-8651
800-824-2184
Fax: 646-478-9260
AFBTECH@afb.net
www.afb.org

AFB Technology runs AFB's CareerConnect and the AFB TECH Product Evaluation Laboratory. Nationally offers consultation, technical assistance and support and undertakes local and national efforts in employment and technology.
Brad Hodges, National Technology Associate

9599 National Federation of the Blind: West Virginia
401 East Olive Street,
Bridgeport, WV 26330
304-622-0626
cs.nfbwv@verizon.net
www.nfbwv.org

Charlene Smyth, President

Wisconsin

9600 National Federation of the Blind: Wisconsin
27824 Nuthatch Road
Kendall, WI 54638
608-758-4800
johnfritz@centurytel.net
www.nfbwis.org/

John Fritz, President

9601 National Federation of the Blind: Writers
27824 Nuthatch Road
Kendall, WI 54638
608-758-4800
johnfritz@centurytel.net
www.nfbwis.org

John Fritz, President

9602 Wiscraft: Wisconsin Enterprises for the Blind
5316 W State Street
Milwaukee, WI 53208-2686
414-778-5800
Fax: 414-778-5805
sales@wiscraft.com
www.wiscraft.com

Wiscraft provides long-term supportive employment for people who are blind. It is a manufacturing company that operates as a non-profit with the clear mission of employing people who are blind by sellng blind-made products and services.
Jim Kerlin, President
Ron Hutchinson, Chair

Wyoming

9603 National Federation of the Blind: Wyoming
4808 Ontario Ave.
Cheyenne, WY 82009-0347
307-421-8522
kthornbury@bresnan.net
www.nfb.org

Kelly Thornbury, President

Foundations

9604 Foundation Fighting Blindness
7168 Columbia Gateway Drive,
Columbia, MD 21046-2220
410-568-0150
800-683-5555
TDD: 800-683-5551
info@FightBlindness.org
www.fightblindness.org
For a $25.00 annual membership fee, FFB offers information and referral services for affected individuals and their families as well as for doctors and eye care professionals. The Foundation also provides comprehensive information kits on retinitis pigmentosa, macular degeneration, and usher syndrome. Their newsletter, InFocus, and their e-newsletter, InSight, present articles on coping research updates, and Foundation news. A national conference is usually held every other year.
Gordon Gund, Chairman
Edward H. Gollob, President

9605 Glaucoma Research Foundation
251 Post Street
San Francisco, CA 94108
415-986-3162
800-826-6693
Fax: 415-986-3763
question@glaucoma.org
www.glaucoma.org
The Glaucoma Research Foundation is a nationa nonprofit dedicated to curing glaucoma. We receive no government funding. Your contribution is tax-deductible as allowed by law.
Thomas M Brunner, President/CEO

Libraries & Resource Centers

9606 District of Columbia Public Library Librarian for the Deaf Community
901 G Street North West
Washington, DC 20001
202-727-1111
www.dclibrary.org
Offers reference services through TDD, portable TDD for public use at pay phone, signers for library programs, sign language classes, information about deafness, print and non-print materials for persons who are deaf.
John W Hill, Jr, President
James W Lewis, Vice President

Alabama

9607 Alabama Radio Reading Service Network
WBHM
650 11th Street South
Birmingham, AL 35233-4530
205-934-2606
800-444-9246
Fax: 205-934-5075
philip@wbhm.org
www.wbhm.org/ARRS
Services and readings are relayed over the radio to three-quarters of Alabama for the benefit of the visually impaired.
sarah Delia, producer
Will Dahlberg, Manager

9608 Alabama Regional Library for the Blind and Physically Handicapped
Alabama Public Library Service
6030 Monticello Drive
Montgomery, AL 36130-6000
334-213-3906
800-392-5671
Fax: 334-213-3993
fzaleski@apls.state.al.us
http://statelibrary.alabama.gov
To promote and support equitable access to library and information resources and services to enable all Alabamians to satisfy their educational, working, cultural, and leisure-time interests. These resources and services will be provided through APLS's statewide programs and through direct grants and assistance to libraries and library systems to meet user's needs.
Fara Zaleski, Regional Librarian
Rebecca Mitchell, Director (APLS)

9609 Houston Love Memorial Library
212 West Burdeshaw Street
Dothan, AL 36303
334-793-9767
bforbus@yahoo.com
www.houstonlovelibrary.org
Offers magnifiers, summer reading programs and more for the blind and physically handicapped. Scanner, software and jaws for windows.
Steve Roy, Chair
Cindy Aman, Board

9610 Huntsville Subregional Library for the Blind and Physically Handicapped
P.O. Box 443
Huntsville, AL 35804
256-532-5980
Fax: 256-532-5994
bphdept@hpl.lib.al.us
www.hpl.lib.al.us/departments/bph
The Subregional Library for the Blind and Physically Handicapped is located in the Main branch of the Huntsville-Madison County Public Library. It is also part of a Library of Congress administered nationwide network of libraries serving persons who cannot use conventional printed materials.
Joyce Welch, Librarian

9611 Library and Resource Center for the Blind and Physically Handicapped
Alabama Institute for Deaf and Blind
205 South Street
Talladega, AL 35160
256-761-3237
800-848-4722
Fax: 256-761-3561
lacy.teresa@aidb.state.al.us
http://www.aidb.org
Using federal and state funds, the Resource Center purchases or produces braille textbooks and other necessary materials for students. The Resource Center also loans equipment, like braillewriters, to help students learn alternative methods of communication.
Dr,John Macia, President
Dr. Freida Meichan, Vice President

9612 Tuscaloosa Subregional Library for the Blind & Physically Handicapped
1801 Jack Warner Parkway
Tuscaloosa, AL 35401
205-345-5820
Fax: 205-752-8300
bjordan@tuscaloosa-library.org
www.tuscaloosa-library.org
Provide talking books to patrons who are unable to use standard print because of a visual or physical limitation. Deliver playback equipment to qualified patrons. Provides reference and referral service to this special population also.
Dr. Horace Allen, Chairman
Dr. Marcia Burke, Vice Chair

Alaska

9613 Alaska State Library Talking Book Center
National Library Services
344 W 3rd Avenue
Anchorage, AK 99501-2337
907-269-6575
800-776-6566
Fax: 907-269-6580
TDD: 907-269-6575
www.library.state.ak.us
The Alaska State Library Talking Book Center is a cooperative effort between the National Library Service and the Alaska State Library to provide print handicapped Alaskans with talking book and Braille service.
Bev Griffin, Library Assistant II
Stephanie Schott, Administrative Clerk I

Arizona

9614 Arizona State Braille and Talking Book Library
1030 N 32nd Street
Phoenix, AZ 85008-5108
602-255-5578
800-255-5578
Fax: 602-255-4312
Closed-circuit TV, summer reading programs, volunteer-produced cassette books, braille writer, films, large-print photocopier and more.
Catherine May, Chair
Ruth Solomon, Vice Chair

9615 Flagstaff City Coconino County Public Library
300 W Aspen Avenue
Flagstaff, AZ 86001-5304
520-779-7670
www.flagstaffpubliclibrary.org
Reference materials on blindness and other handicaps, braille writer, magnifiers and large-print photocopier.

9616 Phoenix Public Library: Special Needs Section
Burton Barr Central Library
1221 North Central Avenue
Phoenix, AZ 85004
602-262-4636
TDD: 602-254-8205
specialneeds@phxlib.org
www.phoenixpubliclibrary.org
The Special Needs Center is designed to make the services and resources of the Phoenix Public Library accessible to people with disabilities.
Toni Garvey, City Librarian

Arkansas

9617 Arkansas Regional Library for the Blind and Physically Handicapped
900 W Capitol
Little Rock, AR 72201-1049
501-682-2053
866-660-0885
Fax: 501-682-1529
TDD: 501-682-1002
nlsbooks@asl.lib.ar.us
www.asl.lib.ar.us
Public library books in recorded or braille format. Popular fiction and nonfiction books for all ages, books and players are on free loan, sent to patrons by mail and may be returned postage free. Anyone who cannot see well enough to read regular print with glasses on or who has a disability that makes it difficult to hold a book or turn the pages is eligible.
John D Hall, Coordinator

9618   Library for the Blind and Handicapped, Southwest
Columbia County Library
2057 North Jackson St   870-234-0399
Magnolia, AR 71754   866-234-8273
                                          Fax: 870-234-5077
                                          lbph@hotmail.com
The mission of the Columbia County Library is to help the people
of our community in their pursuits of information and education ,
as well as vocational and recreational endeavors, by providing current materials, services, and programs. Our inviting public libraries are the cornerstone of our diverse communities where all
people, regardless of age, race, or socio-economic circumstances
can experience personal enrichment and literary growth.
Laura Cleaveland, Director
Dana Thornton, Assistant Director

California

9619   Blind Childrens Center
4120 Marathon Street   323-664-2153
Los Angeles, CA 90029-3584   Fax: 323-665-3828
                                          www.blindchildrenscenter.org
The Blind Childrens Center is a family-centered agency which
serves children with visual impairments from birth to school-age.
The center-based and home-based programs and services help the
children acquire skills and build their independence. The Center
utilizes its expertise and experience to serve families and professionals worldwide through support services, education, and
research.
Midge Horton, Executive Director
Muriel Scharf, Director Development

9620   Braille Institute Library Services
741 North Vermont Avenue   323-663-1111
Los Angeles, CA 90029-3594   800-808-2555
                                          Fax: 323-662-2440
                                          TDD: 323-660-3880
                                          dls@braillelibrary.org
                                          www.braillelibrary.org
The Braille Institute is a non-profit organization whose mission is
to eliminate barriers to a fulfilling life caused by blindness and severe sight loss. The Institute provides an environment of hope and
encouragement for people who are blind and visually impaired
through integrated educational, social and recreational services
and programs.
Henry C. Chang, Librarian

9621   California State Library Braille and Talking Book Library
National Library Service
PO Box 942837   916-654-0640
Sacramento, CA 94237-0001   800-952-5666
                                          Fax: 916-654-1119
                                          btbl@library.ca.gov
                                          www.library.ca.gov
Library services in braille and recorded formats. Free to residents
of Northern California who are unable to read ordinary print on
hold a printed book.
Michael Marlin, Manager
Mary Jane Kayes, Outreach Coordinator

9622   Fresno County Public Library: Talking Book Library for the Blind
2420 Mariposa Street   559-488-3217
Fresno, CA 93721-3640   800-742-1011
                                          Fax: 559-488-1971
                                          TDD: 559-488-1642
                                          wendy.eisenberg@fresnolibrary.org
                                          www.fresnolibrary.org/tblb
We provide books and magazines on cassette tape and in Braille to
people of all ages who are blind, visually impaired, or have physi-
cal disabilities preventing the reading of standard print.
Karen Bosch Cobb, County Librarian
Wendy Eisenberg, Librarian

9623   San Francisco Public Library for the Blind and Print Disabled
100 Larkin Street   415-557-4253
San Francisco, CA 94102-4733   TTY: 415-557-4433
                                          citylibrarian@sfpl.org

Foreign-language books on cassette, children's books on cassettes
and more.
Luis Herrera, City Librarian
Marcia Schneider, Chief, Communications/Adult Services

9624   San Jose State University Library
1 Washington Square   408-924-1000
San Jose, CA 95192-0001   www.library.sjsu.edu
Information on physical disabilities, accessibility and learning
disabilities.

Colorado

9625   Boulder Public Library
1001 Arapahoe Avenue   303-441-3100
Boulder, CO 80302-1326   Fax: 303-442-1808
                                          ask@boulder.lib.co.us
                                          www.boulder.lib.co.us
Offers braille books, cassettes, talking books, large print photo-
copier, large print books and more for the visually impaired.
Tony Tallent, Library & Arts Director

9626   Colorado Talking Book Library
201 East Colfax Ave.   303-727-9277
Denver, CO 80203-8101   800-685-2136
                                          Fax: 303-727-9281
                                          ctbl.info@cde.state.co.us
                                          www.cde.state.co.us
Take advantage of the services offered by the Colorado Talking
Book Library (CTBL). CTBL provides postage-free recorded,
braille, and large print library materials to eligible residents in
Colorado.
Debbi MacLeod, Director

Connecticut

9627   Connecticut State Library for the Blind and Physically Handicapped
198 W Street   860-721-2020
Rocky Hill, CT 06067-3554   800-842-4516
                                          Fax: 860-721-2056
                                          lbph@cslib.org
Free audio cassettes and braille books and magazines along with
reference materials on blindness and other handicaps. Necessary
playback equipment for eligible residents of Connecticut.
Carol Taylor, Director

Delaware

9628   Delaware Division of Libraries: Library for the Blind and Physically Handicapped
43 South DuPont Highway   302-739-4748
Dover, DE 19901   800-282-8676
                                          Fax: 302-739-6787
                                          TDD: 302-739-4847
                                          john.phillos@state.de.us
                                          www.state.lib.de.us
Since 1971, the Delaware Library for the Blind and Physically
Handicapped has provided books in Braille and audio books on re-
cord and cassette for the blind and physically handicapped resi-
dents of Delaware.
John Phillos, Librarian

District of Columbia

9629   Council of Families with Visual Impairment
American Council of the Blind
1155 15th Street NW   202-467-5081
Washington, DC 20005   800-424-8666
                                          Fax: 202-467-5085
                                          info@acb.org
                                          www.acb.org
Members are sighted parents of blind or visually impaired children. Offers a forum for support and outreach, sharing of experiences in parent-child relationships, and educational and cultural
information about child development. Monitors developments in
technical and legislative arenas.
Melanie Brunson, Executive Director

9630 DC Public Library Adaptive Services Division
901 G Street NW, Room 215
Washington, DC 20001
202-727-2142
Fax: 202-727-1129
TTY: 202-727-2255
TDD: 202-727-1129
lbph.dcpl@dc.gov
www.dclibrary.org
The DC Public Library has a special Adaptive Technology Program to help older adults, the deaf, and those with visual and physical disabilities use library materials and resources.
Venetia V. Demson, Librarian

9631 National Library Service for the Blind and Physically Handicapped
1291 Taylor Street,
Washington, DC 20011
202- 70- 510
Fax: 202-707-0712
TDD: 202-707-0744
raj@loc.gov
www.loc.gov/nls
The NLS, Library of Congress, administers the free programs that loans recorded and braille books and magazines, music scores in braille and large print, and specially designed playback equipment to residents of the United States who are unable to read or use standard print materials due to visual or physical impairment.
Yealuri Rathan Raj, Librarian

Florida

9632 Brevard County Libraries: Talking Books Library
2725 Judge Fran Jamieson Way
Viera, FL 32940-7781
32- 6-3 20
Fax: 32- 9-2 63
dmartin@brev.org
www.brev.org
The Talking Books/Homebound Services has many devices and special materials to assist blind, physically handicapped and/or homebound citizens to access library services.
Debra A. Martin, Librarian

9633 Broward County Talking Book Library
100 S Andrews Avenue
Fort Lauderdale, FL 33301-1830
954-357-7555
Fax: 954-577-20
talkingbooks@browardlibrary.org
Reference materials on blindness and other handicaps, closed-circuit TV, Talking Book cassettes, print/Braille and descriptive videos.
William Forbes, Librarian

9634 Florida Bureau of Braille and Talking Book Library Services
421 Platt Street
Daytona Beach, FL 32114-2803
386-239-6000
800-226-6075
Fax: 386-239-6069
mike.gunde@dbs.fldoe.org
The Florida Bureau of Braille and Talking Book Library Services provides information and reading materials needed by Florida residents who are unable to use standard print as the result of visual, physical, or reading disabilities.
Michael Gunde, Librarian

9635 Hillsborough County Talking Book Library
Jan Kaminis Platt Regional Library
900 N ashley drive
Tampa, FL 33602-1214
813-273-3652
www.hcplc.org
This free program provides recorded and braille books and magazines to people who are blind, visually impaired or physically handicapped.
Ann Palmer, Librarian
Ann Palmer, Librarian

9636 Jacksonville Public Library
303 North Laura Street
Jacksonville, FL 32202
904-630-2665
http//jpl.coj.net
Discs, cassettes, reference materials on blindness and other handicaps and children's books on cassettes.
Dr Brenda Simmons Hutchins, Chairperson
Erin Skinner, Vice Chair

9637 Lee County Talking Books Library
13240 North Cleveland Avenue, #5-6
North Ft. Myers, FL 33903-4855
239-995-2665
800-854-8195
Fax: 239-995-1681
TDD: 2399952665
talkingbooks@leegov.com
www.lee-county.com/library
Talking Books are books and magazines that are recorded for people who need to hear their reading. The books are played on special players provided free by the National Library Service for the Blind and Physically Handicapped.
Sheldon Kaye, Librarian

9638 Miami Dade Talking Book Library
Miami Dade Public Library System
101 W flagler street
Miami, FL 33130
305- 37- 266
800-451-9544
Fax: 305-757-8401
TDD: 305-474-7258
talkingbooks@mdpls.org
www.mdpls.org
The Talking Books Library loans books and magazines on cassette tapes or in Braille FREE by mail to persons who have difficulty seeing or using standard small print.
Raymond Santiago, Director
Barbara Moyer, Librarian

9639 Orange County Library System: Orlando Public Library
101 E Central Boulevard
Orlando, FL 32801-2462
407-835-7323
Fax: 407-425-6779
www.ocls.info
The library's collection consists of a wide variety of print materials, including fiction, nonfiction, world languages, genealogy, and special materials that comprise the Florida and Disney collections. The library also has audiovisual materials and electronic resources to meet customer needs.
Mary Anne Hodel, Library Director/CEO

9640 Palm Beach County Library Annex: Talking Books
Mil-Lake Plaza
3650 Summit Blvd.
West Palm Beach,, FL 33406
561-233-2600
888-780-5151
Fax: 561-233-2627
talkingbooks@pbclibrary.org
www.pbclibrary.org
The Talking Books Library is a special service of the Palm Beach County Library and a part of the Library of Congress National Library Service for the Blind and Physically Handicapped.
Pat Mistretta, Librarian

9641 Pinellas Talking Book Library for the Blind and Physically Handicapped
1330 Cleveland Street
Clearwater, FL 33755-5103
727-441-9958
86- 6-9 95
Fax: 727-441-9068
TDD: 727-441-3168
www.pplc.us/tbl/
The Pinellas Talking Book Library's mission is to encourage and support reading by providing free library services to Pinellas County residents for whom conventional print is a barrier. The Pinellas Talking Book Library is part of a nationwide network of cooperating libraries serving people who have difficulty using or reading regular print.
Marilyn Stevenson, Access Services Librarian

9642 Sub Regional Talking Book Library
1755 Edgewood Avenue West
Jacksonville, FL 32208-7206
904-765-5588
Fax: 904-768-7822
TDD: 904-768-7822
Susan V Arthur, Librarian
Laurie Baumgardner, Librarian

9643 West Florida Public Library: Talking Book Library
239 North Spring Street
Pensacola, FL 32502-4822
850-436-5060
Fax: 850-436-5039
talkingbooks@ci.pensacola.fl.us
As a subregional Talking Book Library, the Pensacola Public Library offers free service by mail to blind and physically handi-

capped adults and children who have difficulty reading ordinary print or holding or turning the pages of a book.
Rodney L Kendig, Chairman
Dr. Rebecca Temple, Vice Chairman

Georgia

9644 Albany Library for the Blind and Physically Handicapped
Dougherty County Public Library
1180 Washington Avenue 478-744-0840
Macon, GA 31201 800-805-7613
Fax: 478-744-0840
lbph@docolib.org
www.docolib.org/libblind.html
The Library for the Blind and Physically Handicapped provides resources to individuals who are blind, visually impaired, physically handicapped or learning disabled in a thirteen-county area.
Kathryn Sinquefield, Librarian

9645 Atlanta Metro Subregional Library
1800 Century Place 404-235-7200
Atlanta, GA 30345 800-248-6701
Fax: 404-756-4618
glass@georgialibraries.org
www.georgialibraries.org/public.glass
Through Georgia's Regional Library for the Blind and Physically Handicapped and cooperating local libraries, Georgians have access to a free national library program that offers books and magazines on cassette tape and in Braille.
Linda B Stetson, Director

9646 Augusta Regional Library Talking Book Center
425 James Brown Boulevard 706-821-2625
Augusta, GA 30901 Fax: 706-724-5403
talkbook@ecgrl.org
Through the Georgia Library for Accessible Services, Georgians have access to a free national library program that offers books and magazines on cassette tape and in Braille.
Gary Swint, Librarian

9647 Bainbridge Subregional Library for the Blind and Physically Handicapped
Southwest Georgia Regional Library
301 South Monroe Street 229-248-2680
Bainbridge, GA 39819-4029 800-795-2680
Fax: 229-248-2670
TDD: 229-248-2665
lbph@swgrl.org
www.swgrl.org
The library houses a large collection of recorded materials as well as reference materials.
Susan S. Whittle, Director

9648 Columbus Library for Accessible Services (CLASS)
The Columbus Public Library
3000 Macon Road 706-243-2686
Columbus, GA 31906-2201 800-652-0782
Fax: 706-243-2710
sbarnes@cvrls.net
www.thecolumbuslibrary.org
CLASS serves as one of the Georgia subregional distribution centers for books and magazines on audiocassettes published by the National Library Service for the Blind and Physically Handicapped.
Suzanne Barnes, Librarian

9649 Georgia Library for Accessible Services (GLASS)
1800 Century Place 404-235-7200
Atlanta, GA 30345-3803 800-248-6701
Fax: 404-756-4618
glass@georgialibraries.org
www.georgialibraries.org
Georgians have access to a free national library program that offers books and magazines on cassette tape and in Braille. These materials are provided by the Library of Congress, National Library Service for the Blind & Physically Handicapped (NLS),), to eligible persons with a visual or physical disability. All reading material and playback equipment is sent to borrowers and returned by postage-free mail.
Linda B Stetson, Director

9650 Hall County Library System: East Hall Branch and Special Needs Library
2434 Old Cornelia Highway 770-532-3311
Gainesville, GA 30507 Fax: 770-531-2502
TDD: 770-531-2530
kevans@hallcountylibrary.org
The East Hall Branch and Special Needs Library goal is to provide excellent service to those with disabilities including the blind, handicapped, mobility impaired and deaf.
Kathy Evans, Branch Manager

9651 Middle Georgia Subregional Library for the Blind and Physically Handicapped
Washington Memorial Library
1180 Washington Avenue 478-744-0877
Macon, GA 31201-1790 800-805-7613
Fax: 478-744-0840
www.co.bibb.ga.us/library/TBC.htm
Books, magazines, newspapers, radio programs and various publications are available. Assistive technology equipment is also available at the library.
Thomas Jones, Director
Karen Monroe, Finance Officer

9652 Oconee Regional Library for the Blind and Physically Handicapped
801 Bellevue Avenue 478-275-5382
Dublin, GA 31040 800-453-5541
Fax: 478-275-3821
Through the Georgia Library for Accessible Services and cooperating local libraries, Georgians have access to a free national library program which offers braille and recorded materials.
Wanda Daniel, Librarian

9653 Rome Subregional Library for People with Disabilities
205 Riverside Parkway NE 706-236-4618
Rome, GA 30161-2911 888-263-0769
Fax: 706-236-4631
TDD: 706-236-4618
Provides free library service to the disabled in eleven counties of Northwest Georgia.
Delana Hickman, Coordinator

9654 Special Needs Library of Northeast Georgia
Athens-Clarke County Regional Library
2025 Baxter Street 706-613-3655
Athens, GA 30606-6331 800-531-2063
Fax: 706-613-3660
TDD: 706-613-3655
The Special Needs Library of Northeast Georgia provides free library services for patrons with visual, physical, and reading disabilities.
Claudia L. Markov, Librarian

9655 Subregional Library for the Blind and Physically Handicapped
Live Oak Public Libraries, Thunderbolt Branch
2002 Bull Street 912-652-3600
Savannah, GA 31401 800-342-4455
Fax: 912-354-5534
www.liveoakpl.org
Library for the blind and physically handicapped.
LaTrelle Mobley, Manager

9656 Three Rivers Regional Library
Brunswick-Glynn County Regional Library
208 Gloucester Street 912-267-1212
Brunswick, GA 31520-5324 866-833-2878
Fax: 912-267-9597
www.threeriverslibraries.org
The Talking Book Center serves 12 counties with over 1200 patrons. The center provides talking books which are recorded at a slower speed which requires the use of a special player.
Betty D. Ransom, Librarian

9657 Valdosta Talking Book Library
South Georgia Regional Library
300 Woodrow Wilson Drive 229-333-0086
Valdosta, GA 31602-2592 800-246-6515
Fax: 229-333-7669
www.sgrl.org

The Talking Book Center is available to blind persons with visual difficulty or physical handicaps which prevent them from using printed material.
Diane Jernigan, Librarian

9658   Hawaii State Library for the Blind and Physically Handicapped
402 Kapahulu Avenue
Honolulu, HI 96815

808-733-8444
800-559-4096
Fax: 808-733-8449
TDD: 808-733-8444
olbcirc@librarieshawaii.org
www.librarieshawaii.org

The Library for the Blind and Physically Handicapped serves as the regional library and machine lending agency for the blind and physically disabled throughout the state and the outlying Pacific Islands in cooperation with the Library of Congress and the National Library Service for the Blind and Physically Handicapped.
Fusako Miyashiro, Librarian

9659   Idaho Commission for Libraries Talking Book Service
325 West State Street
Boise, ID 83702-6072

208-334-2150
800-458-3271
Fax: 208-334-4016
TDD: 800-377-1363
talkingbooks@libraries.idaho.gov
http://libraries.idaho.gov/tbs

The Idaho Talking Book Service provides books and magazines in cassette format for individuals who are unable to read standard print.
Sue Walker, Librarian

9660   Illinois State Library Talking Book and Braille Service
401 East Washington
Springfield, IL 62701-1207

217-782-9435
800-665-5576
Fax: 217-558-4723
TDD: 888-261-7863

The Illinois State Library Talking Book and Braille Service plays a supporting rols for the Illinois Network of Libraries Serving the Blind and Physically Handicapped.

9661   Mid-Illinois Talking Book Center
125 Tower Drive
Burr Ridge, IL 60527

217-224-6619
800-426-0709
Fax: 217-224-9818
info@illinoistalkingbooks.org
www.illinoistalkingbooks.org

We provide free library service for anyone unable to read regular print because of low vision, blindness, or a physical disability. We provide recorded and Braille books and popular magazines. There are over 60,000 titles available including popular fiction and non-fiction, bestsellers, classics, history, biographies, children's books and more.
Karen Bershe, Director
Valerie Brandon, PR/Outreach Coordinator

9662   Shawnee Library System: Southern Illinois Talking Book Center
607 South Greenbriar Road
Carterville, IL 62918

618-985-8375
800-445-2665
Fax: 618-985-4211
TDD: 618-985-8375
imsastaff@imsa.lib.il.us
www.imsa.lib.il.us/

The Talking Book Program is a free library service for anyone who has difficulty reading print or holding books and turning pages due to any visual or physical limitation or medically diagnosed reading disability. Participants are loaned cassette players along with unabridged books and magazines on tape and in Braille.
Diana Brawley Sussman, Director/Librarian

9663   Skokie Accessible Library Services
Skokie Public Library
5215 Oakton Street
Skokie, IL 60077-3634

847-673-7774
Fax: 847-673-7797
www.skokie.lib.il.us

Library services for people with disabilities, including electronic aids, materials in special formats, programs and special services, and access to the North Suburban Library System.
Carolyn A Anthony, Director

9664   Voices of Vision Talking Book Center
125 Tower Drive
Burr Ridge, IL 60527

630-208-0398
800-426-0709
Fax: 630-208-0399
info@illinoistalkingbooks.org
www.illinoistalkingbooks.org.

Voices of Vision is part of a statewide and national network of libraries which provide the talking book and braille service. We provide free library service to persons unable to read or use conventional print material due to a visual or physical disability. There is no cost to eligible readers.
Karen Odean, Director

9665   Bartholomew County Public Library
National Library Services
536 Fifth Street
Columbus, IN 47201

812-379-1255
800-685-0524
Fax: 812-791-75
talkingbooks@barth.lib.in.us
www.barth.lib.in.us

Talking Books for the Blind and Physically Handicapped is a free library service for visually or physically challenged persons of all ages. Anyone who is unable to use regular printed materials as the result of a temporary or permanent visual or physical limitation is eligible.
Sharon Thompson, Librarian

9666   Evansville-Vanderburgh County Public Library
200 SE Martin Luther King Jr Blvd
Evansville, IN 47713

812-428-8200
Fax: 812-428-8397
www.evpl.org

The Evansville-Vanderburgh County Public Library, an essential provider of shared information and a core community service, promotes reading, lifelong learning, and economic vitality through its resources, services and programs to the residents of Vanderburgh County.
Mike Russ, President
Brenda Schiedler, Vice President

9667   Indiana Talking Book & Braille Library
315 West Ohio Street
Indianapolis, IN 46202

317-232-3697
800-622-4970
lbph@statelib.lib.in.us
www.in.gov/library/tbbl.htm

The TBBL provides large print books, braille books, and books on tape to Indiana residents who are unable to read regular print.
Roberta L Brooker, Interim Director

9668   Lake County Public Library
1919 W 81st Street
Merrillville, IN 46410

219-769-3541
Fax: 219-769-0690
www.lcplin.org/

Talking books provides cassette books, descriptive videos, magazines and large print books to people who are blind and physically handicapped. Materials are sent through the mail and the service is free to those who qualify.
Renee Lewis, Director

9669   Iowa Department for the Blind
524 Fourth Street
Des Moines, IA 50309-2364

515-281-1333
800-362-2587
Fax: 515-281-1263
TTY: 515-281-1355
www.blind.state.ia.us/?

Our program offers the specialized, integrated services that blind and severely visually impaired Iowans need to live independently and work competitively.
Allen Harris, Director

Kansas

9670 CKLS Headquarters
1409 Williams Street
Great Bend, KS 67530-4090
620-792-4865
800-362-2642
Fax: 620-793-7270
www.ckls.org
Offers direct services to rural residents and those who need special services because of disability.
Chris Rippel, Department Head Continuing Education
Kathy Rippel, Department Head

9671 Manhattan Subregional Library of the Kansas Talking Books Service
629 Poyntz Avenue
Manhattan, KS 66502-6006
785-776-4741
800-432-2796
Fax: 785-776-1545
www.manhattan.lib.ks.us
Books and magazines in braille and recorded format and playback equipment are provided to any Kansas citizen residing in the twelve county area of the North Central Kansas Libraries System who is unable to use standard print as a result of temporary or permanent visual or physical impairments.
Ann Pearce, Department Manager
Wandean Rivers, Assistive Technology Center Instructor

9672 Northwest Kansas Library System
Northwest Kansas Library System
2 Washington Square
Norton, KS 67654
785-877-5148
800-432-2858
Fax: 785-877-5697
www.nwkls.mykansaslibrary.org/
The Kansas Library Network for the Blind and Physically Handicapped, in cooperation with the Library of Congress, National Library Service for the Blind and Physically Handicapped, provides library services and materials to Kansans unable to use conventional print.
Leslie Bell, Director
Clarice Howard, BPH Librarian

9673 South Central Kansas Library System
321A North Main Street
South Hutchinson, KS 67505
620-663-3211
800-234-0529
Fax: 313-663-9797
phawkins@sckls.info
www.sckls.info/
Summer reading programs, braille writer, magnifiers, closed-circuit TV, large-print photocopier, cassette books and magazines, children's books on cassette, home visits and other reference materials on blindness and other handicaps.
Paul Hawkins, Director
Tram Nguyen, Technology Services Coordinator

9674 Talking Books Service
Topeka and Shawnee County Public Library
1515 SW 10th Avenue
Topeka, KS 66604-1304
785-580-4530
800-432-2925
Fax: 785-580-4530
www.tscpl.org/services/talkingbooks
Summer reading programs, braille writer, magnifiers, closed-circuit TV, large-print photocopier, cassette books and magazines, children's books on cassette, home visits and other reference materials on blindness and other handicaps.
Suzanne Bundy, Librarian

9675 Wichita Public Library
223 S Main
Wichita, KS 67202
316-261-8500
Fax: 316-262-4540
TDD: 316-262-3972
admin@wichita.lib.ks.us
Talking books provides cassette books, descriptive videos, magazines adn large print books to people who are blind and physically handicapped. Materials are sent through the mail and the service is free to those who qualify.
Brad Reha, Talking Books Manager

Kentucky

9676 Kentucky Talking Book Library
PO Box 537
Frankfort, KY 40602-0537
502-564-8300
800-372-2968
Fax: 502-564-5773
www.kdla.ky.gov
Our mission is to provide library service to individuals who have a visual or physical disability that prevents them from using standard print materials. We send books on tape and Braille books through the mail at no cost to our patrons.
Katherine K. Adelberg, E-Rate Coordinator,Field Services
Jackie Arnold, Local Records Regional Administrator

9677 Louisville Talking Book Library for the Blind and Physically Handicapped
301 York Street
Louisville, KY 40203-2205
502-574-1611
www.lfpl.org/tbl
The Louisville Talking Book Library offers recorded books and other materials to eligible visually and physically handicapped Jefferson County, KY residents. All recorded books & equipment may be sent to borrowers and returned by postage-free mail.
Linda Atzinger, Supervisor Accessibility Services

9678 Northern Kentucky Talking Book Library
502 Scott Boulevard
Covington, KY 41011
859-962-4095
866-491-7610
Fax: 859-962-4096
Our library provides books and magazines on specially recorded cassettes for people who are visually impaired and/or physically handicapped and live in Boone, Campbell, Carroll, Gallatin, Grant, Kenton, Owen and Pendleton counties.
Dave Schroeder, Director

Louisiana

9679 State Library of Louisiana
701 N 4th Street
Baton Rouge, LA 70802
225-342-4913
Fax: 225-219-4804
admin@state.lib.la.us
www.state.lib.la.us
Talking books provides cassette books, descriptive videos, magazines and large print books to people who are blind and physically handicapped. Materials are sent through the mail and the service is free to those who qualify.

Maine

9680 Bangor Public Library
145 Harlow Street
Bangor, ME 04401-4900
207-947-8336
Fax: 207-945-6694
bplill@bpl.lib.me.us
www.bpl.lib.me.us
Summer reading programs, braille writer, magnifiers, closed-circuit TV, large-print photocopier, cassette books and magazines, children's books on cassette, home visits and other reference materials on blindness and other handicaps.
Barbara McDade, Director

9681 Cary Library
107 Main Street
Houlton, ME 04730-2196
207-532-1302
Fax: 207-532-4350
www.cary.lib.me.us
Summer reading programs, braille writer, magnifiers, closed-circuit TV, large-print photocopier, cassette books and magazines, children's books on cassette, home visits and other reference materials on blindness and other handicaps.
Linda Faucher, Librarian

9682 Lewiston Public Library
200 Lisbon Street
Lewiston, ME 04240-7203
207-513-3004
Fax: 207-784-3011
TTY: 207-784-3123
www.lplonline.org
Summer reading programs, braille writer, magnifiers, closed-circuit TV, large-print photocopier, cassette books and magazines, children's books on cassette, home visits and other reference materials on blindness and other handicaps.
Rick Speer, Director
Jake Paris, Adult Services Librarian

9683 Maine State Library
64 State House Station
Augusta, ME 04333-0064
207-287-5650
800-452-8793
Fax: 207-287-5624
www.state.me.us/msl
Large Print Books is a service through Outreach Services for residents of Maine who are certified as visually impaired and public libraries who serve the visually impaired.
Chris Boynton, Outreach/Special Services Coordinator
Alan Fecteau, Media Coordinator

9684 Portland Public Library
5 Monument Square
Portland, ME 04101-4072
207-871-1700
Fax: 207-871-1715
reference@portland.lib.me.us
www.portlandlibrary.com
Portland Public Library's Outreach Services brings library resources to those who are unable to visit the library in person. For people living in nursing homes or assisted living facilities, or for those confined to home due to illness or disability, the library will deliver print and audio books right to your doorstep.
Stephen J Podgajny, Director

9685 Waterville Public Library
73 Elm Street
Waterville, ME 04901-6027
207-872-5433
Fax: 207-873-4779
www.watervillelibrary.org
Summer reading programs, braille writer, magnifiers, closed-circuit TV, large-print photocopier, cassette books and magazines, children's books on cassette, home visits and other reference materials on blindness and other handicaps.
Sarah Sugden, Director

Maryland

9686 American Action Fund for Blind Children and Adults
1800 Johnson Street, Suite 100
Baltimore, MD 21230
410-659-9315
actionfund@actionfund.org
www.actionfund.org
Our mission is to assist blind persons in securing reading matter, to educate the public about blindness, to give aid to the deaf-blind, to provide specialized aids and appliances to the blind, to give consultation to governmental and private agencies serving the blind, to offer assistance to older blind persons, to offer services to blind children and their parents, and to do any other lawful thing which it can to improve the quality of life for blind persons.
Barbara Loos, President
Ramona Walhof, First Vice President

9687 Disability Resource Center of Montgomery County Public Libraries
Rockville Library
21 Maryland Avenue
Rockville, MD 20850
240-777-0311
TTY: 240-773-3556
county.council@montgomerycountymd.gov
www.montgomerycountymd.gov
The Disability Resource Center (DRC) is the focal point within the Montgomery County Public Libraries (MCPL) for library and literacy services to people with disabilities, their families, caretakers and professionals.
Kay Bowman, Agency Manager

9688 International Braille and Technology Center for the Blind
National Federation of the Blind
1026 East 36th Street
Baltimore, MD 21218-4998
410-645-0632
Fax: 410-685-5653
melissa@riccobono.us
www.nfb.org
A comprehensive and complete evaluation and demonstration center for assistive technology used by the blind worldwide. Includes all Braille, synthetic speech, print-to-speech scanning, internet and portable devices and programs. Available for tours by appointment to blind persons, employers, technology manufacturers, teachers, parents and those working in the assistive technology field.
Melissa Riccobono, President

9689 Maryland State Library for the Blind and Physically Handicapped
415 Park Avenue
Baltimore, MD 21201
410-230-2424
800-964-9209
Fax: 410-333-2095
TTY: 800-934-2541
The basic mission of the Maryland State Library for the Blind and Physically Handicapped is to provide comprehensive library services to the eligible blind and physically handicapped residents of the State of Maryland.
Jill Lewis, Director

9690 Prince George's County Memorial Library: Talking Book Center
6532 Adelphi Road
Hyattsville, MD 20782-2098
301-699-3500
TTY: 301-808-2061
kathleen.teaze@pgcmls.info
www.prge.lib.md.us
Talking books provides cassette books, descriptive videos, magazines and large print books to people who are blind and physically handicapped. Materials are sent through the mail and the services are free to those who qualify.
Kathleen Teaze, Director

Massachusetts

9691 Caption Center
125 Western Avenue
Allston, MA 02134-1008
617-492-9225
Fax: 617-562-0590
Provides closed captioning for videos, including training, safety, instructional and educational films. Maintains a consumer information service for overcoming communications barriers in the workplace.
Lori Kay, Co-Director
Tom Apone, Co-Director

9692 Laboure College Library
2120 Dorchester Avenue
Boston, MA 02124-5617
617-296-8300
library@laboure.edu
www.laboure.edu
Offers information on physical disabilities, independent living, peer counseling and advocacy.
Maryann O'Toole, Director

9693 Perkins Braille and Talking Book Library
175 N Beacon Street
Watertown, MA 02472-2751
617-924-3434
800-852-3133
Fax: 617-972-7315
TTY: 617-972-7690
Info@Perkins.org
www.perkins.org
The Perkins Braille & Talking Book Library, funded in part by the Massachusetts Board of Library Commissioners, provides free services to Massachusetts residents of any age who are unable to read traditional print materials due to a visual or physical disability.
Kim Charlson, Director

9694 Talking Book Library at Worcester Public Library
3 Salem Square
Worcester, MA 1608-2074
508-799-1655
800-762-0085
Fax: 508-799-1676
Adapted computers, braille embosser, magnifiers, closed circuit TV, large print books, cassette books and magazines, children's books on cassette, reference materials on blindness and other disabilities. Summer reading programs.
James L Izatt, Librarian

Michigan

9695 Detroit Subregional Library for the Blind and Physically Handicapped
Detroit Public Library
3666 Grand River Avenue
Detroit, MI 48208
313-833-5494
Fax: 313-325-97
TDD: 313-833-5492
dmiddle@detroitpubliclibrary.org
www.detroit.lib.mi.us
Talking books along with talking book machines are available to eligible residents who live in a 14 ZIP code area of Detroit and Highland Park. Loans of the books and machines are made to indi-

viduals and to institutions such as schools, nursing homes and senior residences. Over 45,000 books are available. Magazines available in recorded format include Ebony, Good Housekeeping, and Sports Illustrated.
Dori V. Middleton, LBPH Specialist

9696 Grand Traverse Area Library for the Blind and Physically Handicapped
322 6th Street   616-935-6520
Traverse City, MI 49684-2414   Fax: 616-922-0904
    TDD: 616-922-0901

Evelyn Welty

9697 Kent County Library for the Blind
775 Ball Avenue NE   616-336-3250
Grand Rapids, MI 49503-1397   Fax: 616-336-3256
Summer reading programs, braille writer, magnifiers, closed-circuit TV, large-print photocopier, cassette books and magazines, children's books on cassette, home visits and other reference materials on blindness and other handicaps.
Claudya Muller, Librarian

9698 Library of Michigan Service for the Blind
PO Box 30007   517-373-5614
Lansing, MI 48909-7507   Fax: 517-735-65
    sbph@michigan.gov
    www.michigan.gov/sbth
Braille writer, magnifiers, closed circuit TV, large print photocopier, cassette books and magazines, children's books on cassette, reference materials on blindness and other handicaps. Books on cassette and braille books and cassette players will be loaned and sent through the mail at no charge. For blind and those physically unable to read standard print or turn the pages.
Susan Thinault, Manager

9699 Macomb Library for the Blind and Physically Handicapped
35891 South Gratiot   586-226-5072
Clinton Township, MI 48035-1132   Fax: 810-286-0634
    TDD: 8102869940
    www.cmpl.org/MLBPH/?
Summer reading programs, braille writer, closed-circuit TV, cassette books and magazines, children's books on cassette, reference materials on blindness and other handicaps.
Beverlee Babcock, Librarian

9700 Midwestern Michigan Library Cooperative
G4195 West Pasadena Avenue   810-732-1120
Flint, MI 48504   Fax: 810-321-15
    www.mideasteRN.lib.mi.us

Roger Mendell, Director

9701 Muskegon County Library for the Blind
635 Ottawa Street   616-724-6248
Muskegon, MI 49442-1016   Fax: 616-724-6675
    TDD: 616-722-4103
Summer reading programs, braille typewriter, magnifiers, closed-circuit TV, large-print photocopier, cassette books and magazines, children's books on cassette, home visits and other reference materials on blindness and other handicaps, The Reading Edge, Perkins Brailler and large print books.
Linda Clapp, Librarian

9702 Northland Library Cooperative
220 W. Clinton St.   231-855-2206
Charlevoix, MI 49720-2892   Fax: 517-354-3939
    www.nlc.lib.mi.us/
Summer reading programs, braille writer, magnifiers, closed-circuit TV, large-print photocopier, cassette books and magazines, children's books on cassette, home visits and other reference materials on blindness and other handicaps.
Catherine Glomski, Librarian

9703 Oakland County Library for the Visually and Physically Impaired
1200 N Telegraph Road   248-858-5050
Pontiac, MI 48341-1032   800-774-4542
    Fax: 248-858-9313
    www.co.oakland.mi.us/lVPi

Free cassette book service to eligible visually or physically impaired Oakland County residents; demonstrations, CCTV and hand held magnifiers and a large print collection.
David Conklin, Head Librarian

9704 St. Clark County Library for the Blind and Physically Handicapped
210 McMorran Boulevard   810-982-3600
Port Huron, MI 48060-4014   800-272-8570
    Fax: 810-987-7327
    lbph@sccl.lib.mi.us
    www.sccl.lib.mi.us/LBPH.aspx
Offers library services to the blind and visually impaired.
Jackie Skinner, Librarian

9705 Upper Peninsula Library for the Blind and Physically Handicapped
1615 Presque Isle Avenue   906-228-7697
Marquette, MI 49855-2811   Fax: 906-285-27
Summer reading programs, braille writer, magnifiers, closed-circuit TV, large-print photocopier, cassette books and magazines, children's books on cassette, home visits and other reference materials on blindness and other handicaps.
Susan Thinault, Manager

9706 Washtenaw County Library for the Blind and Physically Disabled
PO Box 8645   734-971-6059
Ann Arbor, MI 48107-8645   Fax: 734-971-3892
    comnet.org/cgi-bin/helpnet/viewitem?290+
Book lovers club.adaptive technology,cassette equipment, cassette books and magazines, described videos, low vision aids reference and referral services.
Margaret Wolfe, Cordinator

9707 Wayne County Regional Library for the Blind and Physically Handicapped
41365 Vincenti Court   248-536-3100
Novi, MI 48375-5310   888-968-2737
    Fax: 248-536-3098
    TDD: 313-326-3008
    www.tln.lib.mi.us
Summer reading programs, braille writer, magnifiers, closed-circuit TV, large-print photocopier, cassette books and magazines, children's books on cassette, home visits and other reference materials on blindness and other handicaps.
Pat Klemans, Librarian

Minnesota

9708 Duluth Public Library
City of Duluth Department
520 W Superior Street   218-730-4200
Duluth, MN 55802-1578   Fax: 218-233-15
    webmail@duluthmn.gov
    www.duluth.lib.mn.us
Adapted access to Apple computer, adapted toys and adapted library equipment.
Randall Deth Kelly, Director

9709 Minnesota Library for the Blind
1500 Highway 36 West   507-333-4828
Roseville, MN 55113   800-722-0550
    Fax: 507-333-4832
    mn.lbph@state.mn.us
    www.education.state.mn.us
Summer reading programs, braille writer, magnifiers, closed-circuit TV, large-print photocopier, cassette books and magazines, children's books on cassette, home visits and other reference materials on blindness and other handicaps.
Catherine Durivage, Director

Mississippi

9710 Christian Resource for People Who Are Blind
Care Ministries Inc
PO Box 1830   662-323-4999
Starkville, MS 39760-1830   800-366-2232
    careministries@bellsouth.net
    www.careministries.org

Offers braille and large print books and cassettes for the visually impaired.
B J LeJeune, Director

9711 Mississippi Library Commission
3881 Eastwood Drive
Jackson, MS 39211-7328

601-432-4486
800-647-7542
Fax: 601-961-4113
TDD: 601-354-6411
www.mlc.lib.ms.us

Summer reading programs, braille writer, magnifiers, closed-circuit TV, large-print photocopier, cassette books and magazines, children's books on cassette, home visits and other reference materials on blindness and other handicaps.
Larry Mc Millan, Director

Missouri

9712 Adriene Resource Center for Blind Children
Assembly of God Center for Blind
1445 Boonville Avenue
Springfield, MO 65802

417-862-2781
Fax: 417-625-20
info@ag.org
www.blind.ag.org

Offers braille and cassette lending library, braille and cassette Sunday school materials for all ages, braille and cassette periodicals and resource assistance, and resources for blind children and children of blind parents.
Paul Weingariner, Director
Caryl Weingariner, Co-Director

9713 Assemblies of God National Center for the Blind
1445 Boonville Avenue
Springfield, MO 65802

417-831-1964
Fax: 417-627-66

Offers braille and cassette lending library, braille and cassette Sunday school materials for all ages, braille and cassette periodicals and resource assistance, and resources for blind children and children of blind parents.
Paul Weingariner, Director

9714 Church of the Nazarene
Nazarene Publishing House
PO Box 419527
Kansas City, MO 64141-6527

816-931-1900
800-877-0700
www.nph.com

Offers braille and large print books. Also offers a lending library and cassettes for the blind.

9715 Lutheran Library for the Blind
Lutheran Church - Missouri Synod
1333 S Kirkwood Road
Saint Louis, MO 63122-7295

314-965-9000
800-248-1930
Fax: 314-996-1016
www.lcms.org

Offers braille and large print books and cassettes for the blind and visually impaired.

9716 Whitney Library for the Blind: Assemblies of God
1445 N Boonville Avenue
Springfield, MO 65802-1894

417-862-2781
800-641-4310
Fax: 417-862-5881
www.gospelpublishing.com

Offers braille and cassette lending library, braille and cassette Sunday school materials for all ages, braille and cassette periodicals and resource assistance.
Paul Weingariner, Librarian

9717 Wolfner Memorial Library for the Blind
PO Box 387
Jefferson City, MO 65102-387

573-751-8720
800-392-2614
Fax: 573-526-2985
TDD: 800-347-1379
wolfner@sos.mo.gov
www.sos.mo.gov/wolfner

Summer reading programs, braille writer, closed circuit TV, large print photocopier, cassette books and magazines, children's books on cassette, home visits and other reference materials on blindness and other handicaps.
Richard J Smith, Director Wolfner Library
Debbie Musselman, Administrative Program Coordinator

Montana

9718 Montana State Library
1515 E 6th Avenue
Helena, MT 59620-1800

406-444-3009
Fax: 406-444-0266
home.montanastatelibrary.org/?

Summer reading programs, braille writer, magnifiers, closed-circuit TV, large-print photocopier, cassette books and magazines, children's books on cassette, home visits and other reference materials on blindness and other handicaps.
Darlene Staffeldt, Director

Nebraska

9719 Nebraska Library Commission Talking Book and Braille Services
1200 N Street, Suite 120
Lincoln, NE 68508-2023

402-471-4038
800-742-7691
nlc.talkingbook@nebraska.gov
www.nlc.nebraska.gov/tbbs

Free loan of books and magazines on flash cartridge, cassette, and in Braille, including children's materials, along with specially designed playback equipment. Summer reading program for children and young adults, Braille embossing, closed circuit TV, large-print copier. Reference materials on blindness and other disabilities.
David Oertli, Director
Kay Goehring, Reader Services Coordinator

9720 North Platte Public Library
120 W 4th Street
North Platte, NE 69101-3901

308-535-8036
Fax: 308-535-8296
www.ci.north-platte.ne.us/library

Summer reading programs, braille writer, magnifiers, closed-circuit TV, large-print photocopier, cassette books and magazines, children's books on cassette, home visits and other reference materials on blindness and other handicaps.
Cecelia Lawrence, Library Director

Nevada

9721 Las Vegas Clark County Library District
7060 W. Windmill Lane
Las Vegas, NV 89113-5256

702-734-7323
www.lvccld.org

Summer reading programs, braille writer, magnifiers, closed-circuit TV, large-print photocopier, cassette books and magazines, children's books on cassette, home visits and other reference materials on blindness and other handicaps.
Daniel Walters, Executive Directors

9722 Nevada State Library and Archives
100 North Stewart Street
Carson City, NV 89701-4285

775-684-3360
800-922-2880
Fax: 775-684-3330
TDD: 775-687-8338
nslref@clan.lib.nv.us

Summer reading programs, braille writer, magnifiers, closed-circuit TV, large-print photocopier, cassette books and magazines, children's books on cassette, home visits and other reference materials on blindness and other handicaps.
Kevin E Putnam, Librarian

New Hampshire

9723 New Hampshire State Library
117 Pleasant Street
Concord, NH 03301-3852

603-271-3429
Fax: 603-271-8370

Summer reading programs, braille writer, magnifiers, closed-circuit TV, large-print photocopier, cassette books and magazines, children's books on cassette, home visits and other reference materials on blindness and other handicaps.
Eileen Keim, Librarian

9724 Voices for the Blind
PO Box 781
Barrington, NH 3825

603-332-9355

Tape library and depository for people with visual and learning disabilities. Recording services available by request.
Connie Hindman, Director

New Jersey

9725 New Jersey Library for the Blind and Handicapped
2300 Stuyvesant Avenue   609-530-4000
Trenton, NJ 08618-3226   800-792-8322
                                       Fax: 609-530-6384
                                       TDD: 877-882-5593
Summer reading programs, large print, cassette, braille books and
magazines, children's books on cassette and brailles and other reference materials on blindness and other handicaps.
Deborah Toomey, Director

New Mexico

**9726 New Mexico State Library for the Blind and Physically
Handicapped**
National Library Services
1209 Camino Carlos Rey   505-476-9770
Santa Fe, NM 87507   800-456-5515
                                       Fax: 505-476-9776
                                       lbph@state.nm.us
                                       www.nmstatelibrary.org/lbph?
Summer reading programs, braille writer, magnifiers, closed-cir-
cuit TV, large-print photocopier, cassette books and magazines,
children's books on cassette, home visits and other reference materials on blindness and other handicaps.
John Mugford, Library Manager

New York

9727 Choice Magazine Listening
85 Channel Drive   516-883-8280
Port Washington, NY 11050-2216   888-724-6423
                                       Fax: 516-944-6849
                                       choicemag@aol.com
                                       www.choicemagazinelistening.org
A free recorded spoken word magazine anthology for anyone college level and older unable to read large print because of visual or
physical handicaps. Produced on special speed cassette format,
playable on free library of congress player.
Sondra Mochson, Editor

9728 JGB Cassette Library International
Jewish Guild for the Blind
15 W 65th Street   212-769-6331
New York, NY 10023-6601   Fax: 212-769-6266
                                       bemass@aol.com
Summer reading programs, braille writer, magnifiers, closed-circuit TV, large-print photocopier, cassette books and magazines,
children's books on cassette, home visits and other reference materials on blindness and other handicaps.
Bruce Massis

9729 Nassau Library System
900 Jerusalem Avenue   516-292-8920
Uniondale, NY 11553-3039   Fax: 516-481-4777
                                       www.nassaulibrary.org/?
Summer reading programs, braille writer, magnifiers, closed-circuit TV, large-print photocopier, cassette books and magazines,
children's books on cassette, home visits and other reference materials on blindness and other handicaps.
Dorothy Pruyear, Librarian

**9730 New York State Talking Book & Braille Library, New York State
Library, DOE**
Empire State Plaza, CEC   518-474-5935
Albany, NY 12230-0001   800-342-3688
                                       Fax: 518-486-2142
                                       tbbl@mail.nysed.gov
                                       www.nysl.nysed.gov/tbbl/
Books on audio cassette, cassette players, braille books, summer
reading programs, braille writer, magnifiers, closed-circuit TV,
large-print photocopier, cassette books and magazines, children's
books on cassette, reference materials on blindness and other disabilities. Library is part of the National Service Network serving
those with print disabilities. Available: audio and braille books
sent post-free by mail, euipment loans, services to schools and institutions. Serves 55 New York counties.
Sharon B. Phillips, Program Director

9731 Suffolk Cooperative Library System
627 N Sunrise Service Road   631-286-1600
Bellport, NY 11713-9000   Fax: 631-286-1647
                                       gateway.suffolklibrarysystem.org
Talking books services.
Julie Klauber, Adjunct Professor

9732 Xavier Society for the Blind
154 E 23rd Street   212-473-7800
New York, NY 10010-4501   800-637-9193
                                       Fax: 212-473-7801
                                       info@xaviersocietyfortheblind.org
                                       www.XavierSocietyfortheBlind.org
Provides spiritual and inspirational reading material to visually
impaired persons in suitable format: Braille, large print and cassette, throughout the USA and Canada. Services provided by way
of regular periodicals which are non-returnable, and through our
lending library where books are returned. All services are provided
free of charge, and interested persons can write or phone.
Fr. John R. Sheehan, SJ, Chairman
Margie Montenegro, Client Services Representative

North Carolina

9733 North Carolina Library for the Blind
1841 Capital Boulevard   919-733-4376
Raleigh, NC 27635   888-388-2460
                                       Fax: 919-733-6910
                                       TDD: 919-733-1462
                                       nclbph@ncdcr.gov
                                       statelibrary.ncdcr.gov/lbph
A general interest library offering books and magazines at no cost
in large print, in braille on audio cassette for anyone who cannot
use regular print in North Carolina due to physical or visual disability. Summer reading programs, braille writer, magnifiers,
closed circuit TV, large print photocopier, cassette books and magazines, children's books on cassette, digital, cartridges and large
print and other reference materials.
Carl Keehn, Director

North Dakota

9734 North Dakota State Library Services for the Disabled
North Dakota State Library
604 E Boulevard Avenue   701-328-4622
Bismarck, ND 58505-800   800-843-9948
                                       Fax: 701-328-2040
                                       TDD: 800-892-8622
                                       statelib@nd.gov
                                       www.library.nd.gov

Stella Cone, Regional Librarian

9735 Services for the Visually Impaired
8720 Georgia Avenue   301-589-0894
Silver, MD 20910   Fax: 301-589-7281
Eligible readers of North Dakota receive library service from the
regional library in Pierre, South Dakota.
Betty Bender

Ohio

9736 Case Western Reserve University
10900 Euclid Avenue   216-368-2000
Cleveland, OH 44117-2620   www.cwru.edu
Research in electrical stimulation and rehabilitation technology.
Barbara R. Snyder, President
W. A. Bud Baeslack III, Executive Vice President

9737 Ohio Regional Library for the Blind and Physically Handicapped
800 Vine Street   513-369-6999
Cincinnati, OH 45202   800-528-0335
                                       Fax: 513-369-3111
                                       TDD: 513-369-6072
Summer reading programs, braille writer, magnifiers, closed-circuit TV, large-print photocopier, cassette books and magazines,
children's books on cassette, home visits and other reference materials on blindness and other handicaps.
Donna Foust, Librarian

9738 **State Library of Ohio Talking Book Program**
274 E First Avenue 614-644-6895
Columbus, OH 43201-3673 800-686-1531
Fax: 614-995-2186
A machine-lending agency for the visually impaired.
Roger Verney, Head Supervisor

Oklahoma

9739 **Oklahoma Library for the Blind and Physically Handicapped**
300 NE 18th Street 405-521-3514
Oklahoma City, OK 73105-3212 Fax: 405-214-82
Summer reading programs, braille writer, magnifiers, closed-circuit TV, large-print photocopier, cassette books and magazines, children's books on cassette, home visits and other reference materials on blindness and other handicaps.
Geraldine Adams, Director

9740 **Tulsa City: County Library System**
400 Civic Center 918-596-7977
Tulsa, OK 74103-3830 Fax: 918-596-7990
www.tulsalibrary.org
Summer reading programs, braille writer, magnifiers, closed-circuit TV, large-print photocopier, cassette books and magazines, children's books on cassette, home visits and other reference materials on blindness and other handicaps.
Ellen Ontko, Librarian

Oregon

9741 **Oregon State Library**
250 Winter Street NE 503-378-4243
Salem, OR 97301-3950 800-452-0292
Fax: 503-588-7119
TDD: 503-378-4276
www.oregon.gov/osl
Summer reading programs, braille writer, magnifiers, closed-circuit TV, large-print photocopier, cassette books and magazines, children's books on cassette, home visits and other reference materials on blindness and other handicaps.
Jim Scheppke, Head Librarian

Pennsylvania

9742 **Carnegie Library of Pittsburgh**
4724 Baum Boulevard 412-687-2440
Pittsburgh, PA 15213-1321 800-242-0586
Fax: 412-687-2442
Provides on loan recorded books and magazines, large print books, and described videos to Western Pennsylvannia residents unable to use standard printed materials due to visual, physical, or physically-based reading disabilities. Also loans special cassette and disc machines; does not loan equipment to play described videos. Information about disabilities and related agencies is also available.
Sue Murdock, Director
Kathleen Kappel, Assistant Director

9743 **Free Library of Philadelphia**
919 Walnut Street 215-925-3213
Philadelphia, PA 19107-5237 Fax: 215-928-0856
Summer reading programs, braille writer, magnifiers, closed-circuit TV, large-print photocopier, cassette books and magazines, children's books on cassette, home visits and other reference materials on blindness and other handicaps.
Vickie Lange Collins, Librarian

Rhode Island

9744 **Rhode Island Department of State Library for the Blind and Physically Handicapped**
1 Capitol Hl 401-277-2726
Providence, RI 02908-5803 Fax: 401-277-4195
Offers information and services for the visually impaired including reference materials, braille printers, braille writers, large-print books and more.
Richard Ledue, Librarian

South Carolina

9745 **South Carolina State Library**
PO Box 11469 803-734-8666
Columbia, SC 29202-0821 Fax: 803-734-8676
TDD: 803-734-7298
Summer reading programs, braille writer, magnifiers, closed-circuit TV, large-print photocopier, cassette books and magazines, children's books on cassette, home visits and other reference materials on blindness and other handicaps.
Guynell Williams, Librarian

South Dakota

9746 **South Dakota State Library**
800 Governors Drive 605-773-3131
Pierre, SD 57501-2235 Fax: 605-734-50
TDD: 605-773-4950
www.sdstatelibrary.com
Summer reading programs, braille writer, magnifiers, closed-circuit TV, large-print photocopier, cassette books and magazines, children's books on cassette, home visits and other reference materials on blindness and other handicaps.
Daniel Boyd, Librarian

Tennessee

9747 **LRC for Students with Disabilities**
MSU Library Reference Department
Memphis State University 901-678-2208
Memphis, TN 38152-0001 800-669-2267
Fax: 901-678-3070
www.memphis.edu
Information on physical disabilities, blindness and visual impairments.
Ross Johnson, Reference Librarian

9748 **Tennessee Library for the Blind and Physically Handicapped**
National Library Services
403 7th Avenue N 615-741-3915
Nashville, TN 37243-1409 800-342-3308
Fax: 615-532-8856
Offers free public library services to those unable to hold, read, or turn the pages of books and magazines due to physical or visual impairment. Collections include books and magazines in large print, braille and audio format. Players loaned for the audio books and magazines. All items are delivered and returned via the US Postal Service free matter mailing.
Ruth Hemphill, Director
Janie Murphee, Assistant Director

Texas

9749 **Houston Public Library Access Center**
500 McKinney Street 832-393-1313
Houston, TX 77002-2534 Fax: 832-931-83
website@hpl.lib.tx.us
www.houstonlibrary.org
Offers Kurzweil Reading Machine 400, closed-circuit TV, braille writer, reference materials on visual impairments and other handicaps.
Heidi Miller, Supervisor

9750 **Texas State Library**
1201 Brazos Street 512-463-5460
Austin, TX 78711-2927 800-252-9605
Fax: 512-936-0685
TDD: 512-463-5449
www.tsl.state.tx.us
Summer reading programs, braille writer, magnifiers, closed-circuit TV, large-print photocopier, cassette books and magazines, children's books on cassette, home visits and other reference materials on blindness and other handicaps.
Dale Propp, Librarian

9751 Texas State Library: Talking Book Program
1201 Brazos Street   512-463-5460
Austin, TX 78711-2927   800-252-9605
                                       Fax: 512-936-0685
                               tbp.services@tsl.state.tx.us
                                          www.tsl.state.tx.us
Part of the free National Library Services. Provides equipment and
books in alternate formats to qualified individuals who cannot read
standard print. Certified applications required. Disabilities and information referral services available.
Ava Smith, Librarian
Dina Abramson, Disabilities/Information Referral

Utah

9752 Utah State Library Division
Program for the Blind and Disabled
250 North 1950 West, Suite A   801-715-6789
Salt Lake City, UT 84116-7901   800-662-5540
                                       Fax: 801-715-6767
                                       TDD: 801-715-6721
                                          blind@utah.gov
                                  http://blindlibrary.utah.gov
Library providing services to individuals with visual impairments
who cannot read standard print.
Bessie Y. Oakes, Director

Vermont

9753 Vermont Department of Libraries Special Services Unit
109 State Street   80- 8-8 32
montpelier, VT 05609   800-479-1711
                                       Fax: 802-828-2199
                                ssu@mail.dol.state.vt.us
                                          dol.state.vt.us
Summer reading programs, braille writer, magnifiers, closed-circuit TV, large-print photocopier, cassette books and magazines,
children's books on cassette, home visits and other reference materials on blindness and other handicaps.
Theresa Faust, Librarian

Virginia

9754 Arlington County Department of Libraries
1015 N Quincy Street   703-228-5959
Arlington, VA 22201-4603   Fax: 703-358-5962
                                       TDD: 703-358-6320
                                www.library.arlingtonva.us/
Summer reading programs, braille writer, magnifiers, closed-circuit TV, large-print photocopier, cassette books and magazines,
children's books on cassette, home visits and other reference materials on blindness and other handicaps.
Roxanne Barnes, Librarian

9755 Central Rappahannock Regional Library
1201 Caroline Street   540-372-1144
Fredericksburg, VA 22401-3701   Fax: 540-373-9411
                                       TDD: 540-371-9165
Offers reference materials on blindness and other disabilities.
Nancy Schiff, Librarian

9756 Division for the Visually Handicapped
2900 Crystal Drive   703-620-3660
Arlington, VA 22202   888-232-7733
                                       Fax: 703-264-9494
                                       TTY: 866-915-5000
                                     service@cec.sped.org
                                          www.cec.sped.org
Members are teachers, college faculty members, administrators,
supervisors and others concerned with the education and welfare
of visually handicapped and blind children and youth. This is a di-
vision of the Council For Exceptional Children.
Stephanie Ineh, Customer Service Manager
Anitra Davis, Senior Customer Services Representative

9757 Fairfax County Public Library
12000 Government Center Parkway   703-660-6943
Fairfax, VA 22035-0012   Fax: 703-765-5893
                                       TDD: 703-660-8524

Summer reading programs, braille writer, magnifiers, closed-circuit TV, large-print photocopier, cassette books and magazines,
children's books on cassette, home visits and other reference materials on blindness and other handicaps.
Jeanette Studley, Librarian

9758 Hampton Subregional Library for the Blind
4207 Victoria Blvd.   75- 7-7 11
Hampton, VA 23669-4243   Fax: 75- 7-7 11
                                  www.hamptonpubliclibrary.org
Summer reading programs, braille writer, magnifiers, closed-circuit TV, large-print photocopier, cassette books and magazines,
children's books on cassette, home visits and other reference materials on blindness and other handicaps.
Douglas Perry, Director

9759 Newport News Public Library System
110 Main Street   757-591-4858
Newport News, VA 23601-4105   Fax: 757-591-7425
Summer reading programs, braille writer, magnifiers, closed-circuit TV, large-print photocopier, cassette books and magazines,
children's books on cassette, home visits and other reference materials on blindness and other handicaps.
Sue Balswin, Librarian

9760 Roanoke City Public Library System
2607 Salem Tpke NW   540-853-2648
Roanoke, VA 24017-5333   Fax: 540-853-1030
Summer reading programs, braille writer, magnifiers, closed-circuit TV, large-print photocopier, cassette books and magazines,
children's books on cassette, home visits and other reference materials on blindness and other handicaps.
Rebecca Cooper, Librarian

9761 Staunton Public Library: Talking Book Center
1291 Taylor Street,   20- 7-7 51
Washington, DC 20011-3229   20- 7-7 07
                                       Fax: 540-332-3906
                                          www.loc.gov/nls
Sub-regional library for those who are unable to use standard print
materials due to visual, physical, or reading disability.
Oakley Pearson, Librarian

9762 University Library Services
Virginia Commonwealth University
901 Park Avenue   804-828-1105
Richmond, VA 23284-2033   Fax: 804-828-0150
Library services for the visually disabled.
Sally Jacobs, Reference Librarian

9763 Virginia Beach Public Library
936 Independence Boulevard   757-460-7518
Virginia Beach, VA 23455-6006   Fax: 757-460-6741
                                          vb311@vbgov.com
                                          vbgov.com/libraries
Summer reading programs, braille writer, magnifiers, closed-circuit TV, large-print photocopier, cassette books and magazines,
children's books on cassette, home visits and other reference materials on blindness and other handicaps.
Susan Head, Librarian

Washington

9764 Washington Talking Book & Braille Library
2021 9th Avenue   206-615-0400
Seattle, WA 98121   Fax: 206-615-0437
                                       TTY: 206-615-0418
                                     wtbbl@spl.lib.wa.us
                                          www.wtbbl.org
Summer reading programs, braille writer, magnifiers, closed-circuit TV, large-print photocopier, cassette books and magazines,
children's books on cassette, home visits and other reference materials on blindness and other handicaps.
Danielle Miller, Director

West Virginia

9765 Cabell County Public Library
455 9th Street
Huntington, WV 25701-1417
304-528-5700
Fax: 304-285-5701
www.cabell.lib.wv.us
Summer reading programs, braille writer, magnifiers, Arkenstone reader/scanner, cassette books and magazines, children's books on cassette, home visits and other reference materials on blindness and other handicaps.
Judy K Ruke, Director
Angela Strait, Assistant Director

9766 Kanawha County Public Library
1900 Kanawha Boulevard E
Charleston, WV 25305-2609
304-558-2041
800-642-9021
Fax: 304-558-2044
kanawha.lib.wv.us
Summer reading programs, braille writer, magnifiers, closed-circuit TV, large-print photocopier, cassette books and magazines, children's books on cassette, home visits and other reference materials on blindness and other handicaps.
Francis Fesenmainer, Librarian

9767 Ohio County Public Library Services for the Blind and Physically Handicapped
52 16th Street
Wheeling, WV 26003-3671
304-232-0244
Fax: 304-232-6848
llnicholson@hotmail.com
Lori Nicholson, Subregional Librarian BIPH

9768 Parkersburg and Wood County Public Library
3100 Emerson Avenue
Parkersburg, WV 26104-2414
304-420-4587
800-642-8674
Fax: 304-420-4589
parkersburg.lib.wv.us
Services for the bind and physically handicapped.
Michael Hickman

9769 West Virginia Library Commission
1900 Kanawha Boulevard E
Charleston, WV 25305-0009
304-558-2041
800-642-9021
Fax: 304-558-2044
librarycommission.lib.wv.us
Summer reading programs, braille writer, magnifiers, closed-circuit TV, large-print photocopier, cassette books and magazines, children's books on cassette, home visits and other reference materials on blindness and other handicaps.
Francis Fesenmainer, Librarian

9770 West Virginia School for the Blind
301 E Main Street
Romney, WV 26757-1828
304-822-4800
Fax: 304-822-3377
cjohn@access.mountain.net
Summer reading programs, braille writer, magnifiers, closed-circuit TV, large-print photocopier, cassette books and magazines, children's books on cassette, home visits and other reference materials on blindness and other handicaps.
Cynthia Johnson, Librarian

Wisconsin

9771 Brown County Library
P.O box 23600
Green Bay, WI 54305-5194
920-448-4035
Fax: 920-448-4036
www.co.brown.wi.us
Summer reading programs, braille writer, magnifiers, closed-circuit TV, large-print photocopier, cassette books and magazines, children's books on cassette, home visits and other reference materials on blindness and other handicaps.
Moyninhan Jr Patrick, Chair
Lund Thomas, Vice Chair

9772 Wisconsin Regional Library for the Blind Talking Book Program
813 W Wells Street
Milwaukee, WI 53233-1436
414-286-3045
800-242-8822
Fax: 414-286-3102
TDD: 414-286-3548
mvalne@mpl.org

Circulates recorded materials, playback equipment and braille materials to print-handicapped Wisconsin residents.
Marsha Valance, Regional Librarian

Wyoming

9773 Wyoming Services for the Visually Disabled
State Department of Education
2300 Capitol Avenue Hathaway Buildi
Cheyenne, WY 82002-50
307-777-7690
Fax: 307-776-34
Eligible readers of Wyoming receive library service from the regional library in Salt Lake City, Utah.
Duane Edmonds, Chairman
Ruby Calvert, Vice Chairman

Research Centers

9774 Baylor College of Medicine: Cullen Eye Institute
6565 Fannin
Houston, TX 77030-2703
713-798-6100
800-229-5676
Fax: 713-798-4231
ant@bcm.edu
www.bcm.edu/eye
Research activities focus on restoring vision and preventing blindness through a better understanding of the disease.
Dan B Jones, Professor and Chair
Milton Boniuk, Professor

9775 BermanGund Laboratory for the Study of Retinal Degenerations
Massachusetts Eye & Eye Infirmary
243 Charles Street
Boston, MA 02114-3002
617-573-3600
Fax: 617-733-44
directors@meei.harvard.edu
The Berman-Gund Laboratory for the Study of Retinal Degenerations of Harvard Medical School continues multidisciplined research on retinitis pigmentosa, Usher syndrome, macular degeneration, and other related degenerative diseases of the retina.
Eliot L. Berson, M.D.,, Director
Eric A. Pierce, M.D., Ph.D.,, Associate Director

9776 Braille Institute Desert Center
70-251 Ramon Rd
Rancho Mirage, CA 92270-5203
760-321-1111
800-212-4533
Fax: 760-321-9715
dc@brailleinstitute.org
www.brailleinstitute.org
Dedicated to providing blind and visually impaired men women and children with the training programs and services they need to enjoy productive lives. Services offered include child development youth programs library services and adult education.
Leslie E Stocker Jr, President
Sally H Jameson, VP of Programs and Services

9777 Braille Institute Orange County Center
527 N Dale Avenue
Anaheim, CA 92801-4899
714-821-5000
Fax: 714-527-7621
oc@brailleinstitute.org
www.brailleinstitute.org
Offers services publications information and programs to blind and visually impaired persons.
Sheila F Daily, Orange County Regional Director
Gene Mathiowetz, Assistant Regional Director

9778 Braille Institute Santa Barbara Center Braille Institute of Los Angeles
Braille Institute of Los Angeles
2031 De La Vina Street
Santa Barbara, CA 93105-3895
805-682-6222
800-272-4553
Fax: 805-687-6141
sb@brailleinstitute.org
www.brailleinstitute.org
Offers classes type library services and information for persons with visual impairments.
Angela Nowlin, Assistant Regional Director
Michael Lazarovits, Santa Barbara Regional Director

9779 Braille Institute Sight Center
741 N Vermont Avenue
Los Angeles, CA 90029
323-663-1112
800-272-4553
Fax: 323-663-0867
la@brailleinstitute.org
www.brailleinstitute.org/los_angeles
Offers help programs services and information to the blind and visually impaired children and adults.
Dr Henry C Chang, Director of Library Services
Anita Wright, Los Angeles Regional Program Director

9780 Braille Institute Youth Center
741 N Vermont Avenue
Los Angeles, CA 90029-1381
323-663-1112
800-272-4553
Fax: 323-663-0867
la@brailleinstitute.org
Offers various youth programs and services for the blind and visually impaired youngster.
Leslie E Stocker Jr, President
Sally H Jameson, Vice President of Programs and Services

9781 Braille Textbook Assignment Service National Braille Association
National Braille Association
95 Allens Creek Road
Rochester, NY 14618-2537
585-427-8260
Fax: 585-427-0263
nbaoffice@nationalbraille.org
www.nationalbraille.org
National Braille Association, founded in 1945, is a non-profit organization dedicated to providing continuing education to those who prepare braille, and to providing braille materials to persons who are visually impaired.
Jan Carroll, President
David W Shaffer, Executive Director

9782 Carroll Center for the Blind
770 Centre Street
Newton, MA 02458-2597
617-969-6200
800-852-3131
Fax: 617-969-6204
TTY: 617-969-6204
info@carroll.org
www.carroll.org
The Carroll Center serves the needs of blind and visually-impaired persons by providing rehabilitation, skills training, and educational opportunities to achieve independence, self-sufficiency, and self-fulfillment and by educating the public regarding the potential of persons who are blind and visually-impaired.
Joseph Abely, President
Brian Charlson, Director of Computer Training Services

9783 Clearinghouse for Specialized Media and Translation
California Department of Education/CSMT
1430 N Street
Sacramento, CA 95814
916-445-5103
Fax: 916-323-9732
csmt@cde.ca.gov
www.cde.ca.gov/re/pn/sm
Assists schools and students in the identification and acquisition of textbooks reference books and study materials in aural media, braille, large print, and electronic media access technology.
Tom Torlakson, State Superintendent of Public Instructi
Jonn Paris-Salb, Administrator

9784 Clovernook Center for the Blind and Visually Impaired
7000 Hamilton Avenue
Cincinnati, OH 45231-5240
513-522-3860
888-234-7156
Fax: 513-728-3946
www.clovernook.org
Innovative programs including community living support and a youth initiative with a focus on developing the skills people with visual impairments need to become independent in the community. An array of employment services help individuals maximize their earning potential and job satisfaction, both on site in our manufacturing center and in the local job market.
Robin L Usalis, President/CEO
Jacqueline L Conner, VP of Multi-State Center East

9785 Dean A McGee Eye Institute
608 Stanton L Young Boulevard
Oklahoma City, OK 73104-5065
405-271-6060
800-787-9012
Fax: 405-271-4442
www.dmei.org

The Dean McGee Eye Institute is the first center in Oklahoma to offer a new treatment for dry eyes that can last up to a year and frees patients from time-consuming warm compresses and lubricating eye drops. The LipiFlow Thermal Pulsation System combines precisely administered heat and pressure to open and clear clogged oil glands in the eyelids, allowing lubricating oils to flow naturally again.
Edward L. Gaylord, Professor and Chair
Gregory L. Skuta, MD, President

9786 Emory University: Laboratory for Ophthalmic Research
1365B Clifton Road, N.E.
Atlanta, GA 30322-1013
404-778-2020
www.eyecenter.emory.edu
Various studies into the aspects of blindness.
Timothy W. Olsen, MD, Chair/Director
Joy H. Bell, Director of Public Relations

9787 Florida Ophthalmic Institute
7106 NW 11th Pl
Gainesville, FL 32605-3157
352-331-2020
Fax: 352-331-2019
afn22025@gmail.com
www.sites.google.com/site/flophthalmicin
Nonprofit organization that understands and treats ocular diseases including glaucoma.
Norman S Levy MD, Director
Trudy K. Ramjattan, MD, Surgeon

9788 Glaucoma Laser Trabeculoplasty Study Sinai Hospital of Detroit
Sinai Hospital of Detroit
6767 W Outer Drive
Detroit, MI 48235-2899
313-966-3256
Fax: 313-966-4296
Examines the effectiveness and safety of the treatments of glaucoma.
Hugh Beckman, Chairman

9789 Glaucoma Research Foundation
251 Post Street
San Francisco, CA 94108
415-986-3162
800-826-6693
Fax: 415-986-3763
question@glaucoma.org
www.glaucoma.org
Our mission is to prevent vision loss from glaucoma by investing in innovative research, education, and support with the ultimate goal of finding a cure.
Thomas M Brunner, Chief Executive Officer/President
Nancy Graydon, Executive Director of Development

9790 Harvard University Howe Laboratory of Ophthalmology
Massachusetts Eye & Ear Infirmary
243 Charles Street
Boston, MA 02114-3002
617-523-7900
www.masseyeandear.org
Established in 1926, the Howe Laboratory is comprised of investigators working on both basic research, focused on retinal development, structure and function in various organisms, and translational research, focused on developing treatments for glaucoma and conditions affecting the cornea.
Dr. Mack Cheney, Director
Wendy Williams, Associate Director

9791 Helen Keller International
352 Park Avenue S
New York, NY 10010
212-532-0544
877-535-5374
Fax: 212-532-6014
info@hki.org
www.hki.org
Nonprofit organization for the blind.
Kathy Spahn, President/CEO
Shawn K Baker, VP/Regional Director-Africa

9792 Helen Keller National Center for Deaf/Blind Youths and Adults
141 Middle Neck Road
Sands Point, NY 11050-1299
516-944-8900
Fax: 516-944-7302
TTY: 516-944-8637
hkncinfo@hknc.org
www.hknc.org
We enable all those who are deaf-blind to live and work in the community of their choice. We provide comprehensive vocational rehabilitation training at our headquarters in NY and assistance with job and residential placements when training is completed.
Joseph McNulty, Executive Director

9793 Institute for Visual Sciences
1 E 71st Street   212-305-2919
New York, NY 10021-4102
Ophthalmology with emphasis on the development of care for the eye.
Melissa Mount, Executive Director

9794 Institute of Ophthalmology and Visual Scie nce New Jersey Medical School
New Jersey Medical School
PO Box 1709   973-972-2036
Newark, NJ 07101-2425   Fax: 973-723-94
www.njms.rutgers.edu
The Institute comprises ophthalmic surgeons, researchers, ophthalmic surgeons-in-training, administrators, and ancillary staff (such as ophthalmic technicians). We are dedicated to providing outstanding compassionate patient care, teaching current and future providers of eye care, and developing cures for blindness. This site provides comprehensive information on our faculty members, eye-care professionals, patient-care services, research, residency training programs, and continuing education cu
Marco A Zarbin, MD, PhD, FACS, Chair
Robert D. Fechtner, Professor

9795 Jerusalem Center for Multi-Handicapped Blind Children
350 7th Avenue   212-279-4070
New York, NY 10001-7903   Fax: 212-279-4043
info@keren-or.org
keren-or.org
Maintains the Keren-Or Center for the Multiply Handicapped Blind Child in Jerusalem for rehabilitation and training. Funds acquired through contributions bequests and legacies.
Madelyn Cohen, Executive Director
Tamara Silberberg, Director Keren-Or Center

9796 Johns Hopkins University: Dana Center for Preventive Ophthalmology
Wilmer Ophthalmology Institute
600 N Wolfe Street   410-955-2777
Baltimore, MD 21287-0001
Research at the Dana Center focuses on national and international public health prevention of blinding eye disease.
Harry A Quigley, Director

9797 New Beginnings: The Blind Children's Center
4120 Marathon Street   213-664-2153
Los Angeles, CA 90029-3505   800-222-3566
The purpose of the Center is to turn initial fears into hope. Helps children and their families become independent by creating a climate of safety and trust. Children learn to develop self confidence and to master a wide range of skills. Services include an infant stimulation program, educational preschool, interdisciplinary assessment services, family services, correspondence program, toll free national hotline and a publication and research service.

9798 New Beginnings: The Blind Children's Cente
4120 Marathon Street   323-664-2153
Los Angeles, CA 90029   800-222-3566
Fax: 323-665-3828
www.blindchildrenscenter.org
The purpose of the Center is to turn initial fears into hope. Helps children and their families become independent by creating a climate of safety and trust. Children learn to develop self confidence and to master a wide range of skills. Services include an infant stimulation program educational preschool interdisciplinary assessment services family services correspondence program toll free national hotline and a publication and research service.

9799 Oregon Health Sciences University: Elk's Children's Eye Clinic
Casey Eye Institute
3375 SW Terwilliger Boulevard   503-494-3000
Portland, OR 97239-4197   Fax: 503-494-5347
www.ohsucasey.com
Our mission at the Casey Eye Institute is to provide excellent eye care in a quality cost-effective environment that combines education research clinical leadership and service to the community.
Earl Palmer, Director

9800 Reader-Transcriber Registry National Braille Association
National Braille Association

3 Townline Circle   716-427-8260
Rochester, NY 14623-2537
Certified braillists fill requests for college textbooks and other technical works through this service of the National Braille Association.

9801 Smith-Kettlewell Eye Research Institute
2318 Fillmore Street   415-345-2000
San Francisco, CA 94115-1821   Fax: 415-345-8455
www.ski.org
Dedicated to research on human vision. The Institute was founded to encourage a productive collaboration between the medical clinic and scientific laboratory. Research is conducted with clinical studies which relate directly to the diagnosis and treatment of eye diseases the development of devices and vocational programs to aid the partially sighted and basic research to understand how the eye and brain work for both the clinical and rehabilitation programs.
Arthur Jampolsky, Executive Director
Ruth S Poole, COO

9802 University of Illinois Eye and Ear Infirma ry
1855 W Taylor Street   312-996-6591
Chicago, IL 60612-7242   Fax: 312-996-7770
eyeweb@uic.edu
www.uic.edu/com/eye
Offers help support information and research for persons with vision problems including Retinitis Pigmentosa.
Dr. Rohit Verma, Department Chair
Elmer Tu, Director of Cornea Service

9803 University of Illinois at Chicago Lions of Illinois Eye Research Institute
UIC Eye Center
1905 W Taylor Street   312-996-1466
Chicago, IL 60612-7245   Fax: 312-355-4248
www.uic.edu/com/eye/Lions
Visual impairments and blindness research including glaucoma studies.
Janet Szlyk, President~
Julie Daraska, Secretary

9804 University of Miami: Bascom Palmer Eye Institute
Department of Ophthalmalogy
900 NW 17th Street   305-326-6000
Miami, FL 33136-1015   800-329-7000
Fax: 305-326-6306
www.bpei.med.miami.edu/site/default.asp
Clinical and basic research into blindness and visual impairments.
John G Clarkson, Dean Emeritus

9805 Visually Impaired Center
1422 W Court Street   810-767-4014
Flint, MI 48503   Fax: 810-767-0020
info@vicflint.org
www.vicflint.org
A private non-profit agency which offers special programs and some very practical help to people who are blind or partially sighted. Offers rehabilitation low vision aids orientation and mobility vocational training reading and information recreation counseling services volunteer services and community awareness.
Fharon Reigle, Director

9806 Warren Grant Magnuson Clinical Center National Institute of Health
National Institute of Health
9000 Rockville Pike   301-496-4000
Bethesda, MD 20892   800-411-1222
Fax: 301-480-9793
TTY: 866-411-1010
prpl@mail.cc.nih.gov
www.cc.nih.gov
Established in 1953 as the research hospital of the National Institutes of Health. Designed so that patient care facilities are close to research laboratories so new findings of basic and clinical scientists can be quickly applied to the treatment of patients. Upon referral by physicians patients are admitted to NIH clinical studies.
John I Gallin, Director
David Henderson, Deputy Director for Clinical Care

9807 Yale University: Vision Research Center
330 Cedar Street
New Haven, CT 06510-3218

203-785-5687
800-395-7949
Fax: 203-785-7401
sarah.gelo@yale.edu

Vision including studies on growth and development.
Bruce Shields, Chair
Sarah Gelo, Administrator

Kansas

9808 Kansas Services for the Blind and Visually Impaired
Social Rehabilitation Services
915 SW Harrison
Topeka, KS 66612-2445

785-368-7471
800-547-5789
Fax: 785-368-7467
TTY: 785-368-7478
rehab@srs.ks.gov

Instructional employment oriented services for blind adults.
Laura Howard, Deputy Secretary and Chief Financial Off
Theresa Addington, Accounting and Administrative Operations

Support Groups & Hotlines

9809 1-800-BRAILLE
Braille Institute
741 N Vermont Avenue
Los Angeles, CA 90029-3594

323-663-1111
800-272-4553
Fax: 323-663-0867
la@brailleinstitute.org
www.brailleinstitute.org

A toll free information and referral service where callers can obtain information about community programs and referrals to organizations serving the blind in their local areas.
Lester M. Straussman, Director
James B. Boyle, Boardmember

9810 AFB Toll-Free Hotline
American Foundation for the Blind
2 Penn Plaza
New York, NY 10121-2018

212-502-7600
800-232-5463
Fax: 888-545-8331
afbinfo@afb.net
www.afb.org

Supplies information on visual impairment and blindness, answers queries regarding AFB services, products, publications, technology, the Careers and Technology Information Bank (a national data bank) and much more.
Carl R. Augusto, President & CEO
Rick Bozeman, CFO

9811 Aurora of Central New York
518 James Street
Syracuse, NY 13203

315-422-7263
Fax: 315-422-4792
TTY: 315-422-9746
TDD: 315-422-9746
auroracny@auroraofcny.org
www.auroraofcny.org/

Professional counseling services to assist individuals and their families deal with the trauma of hearing or vision loss.
Earleen Foulk, President Board of Directors
Debra Chaiken, Executive Director

9812 Carroll Center for the Blind
770 Centre Street
Newton, MA 2458-2597

617-969-6200
800-852-3131
Fax: 617-969-6204
www.carroll.org

We have developed many methods for people with low vision to learn the skills to be independent in their homes, in class settings, and in their work places. Our services for the blind include vision rehabilitation services, vocational and transition programs, assistive technology training, educational support and recreation opportunities for individuals who are visually impaired of all ages
Dina Rosenbaum, VP Marketing

9813 Department of Ophthalmology Information Line
Illinois Eye & Ear Infirmary

1855 W Taylor Street m/c 648
Chicago, IL 60612-7242

312-996-6500
Fax: 312-996-7770
eyeweb@uic.edu
www.uic.edu/com/eye/

Offers eye clinic and physician referrals to persons suffering from vision disorders as well as offers emergency information.
Dimitri Azar, Director

9814 Job Opportunities for the Blind
National Federation of the Blind
200 E Wells St
Baltimore, MD 21230-4998

410-659-9314
Fax: 410-685-5653
nfb@nfb.org
www.nfb.org

A specialized service that provides free support, resources and information to blind persons seeking employment and to employers interested in hiring the blind. A partnership program with the US Department of Labor, this is the most successful program of it's kind in helping blind persons find competitive work.
Anthony Cobb, Dircetor

9815 National Association for Parents of the Visually Impaired
Watertown, MA 2471

617-972-7441
800-562-6265
Fax: 617-972-7444
napvi@perkins.org
www.napvi.org

Susan Laventure, Executive Director

9816 National Center for Sight
National Society to Prevent Blindness
211 Wacker Drive
Chicago, IL 60606

312-363-6001
800-331-2020
Fax: 312-363-6052

A toll-free line offering information on a broad range of vision, eye health and safety topics including sports eye safety, lazy eye, diabetic retinopathy, glaucoma, cataracts, children's eye disorders, and more.

9817 National Eye Health Education Program
1855 W Taylor Street
Chicago, IL 60612-7242

312-996-6590
800-786-3937
Fax: 312-996-9967
www.uic.edu

Offers information and support for persons with vision disorders, including Retinitis Pigmentosa.
Mary Go, Supervisor

9818 National Health Information Center
Office of Disease Prevention & Health Promotion
1101 Wootton Pkwy
Rockville, MD 20852

Fax: 240-453-8281
odphpinfo@hhs.gov
www.health.gov/nhic

Supports public health education by maintaining a calendar of National Health Observances; helps connect consumers and health professionals to organizations that can best answer questions and provide up-to-date contact information from reliable sources; updates on a yearly basis toll-free numbers for health information, Federal health clearinghouses and info centers.
Don Wright, MD, MPH, Director

9819 National Service Dog Center
Delta society
875 124th Avenue, NE
Bellevue, WA 98005

425-679-550
Fax: 425-679-5539
info@petpartners.org
www.petpartners.org

Pet Partners is the leader in demonstrating and promoting positive human-animal interaction to improve the physical, emotional and psychological lives of those we serve.
Brenda Bax, Chair
Mary Craig, Vice Chair/Treasurer

9820 PXE International
4301 Connecticut Avenue NW
Washington, DC 20008-2369

202-362-9599
Fax: 202-966-8553
info@pxe.org
www.pxe.org

Initiates, funds and conducts research; provides support for individuals and families affected by pseudoxanthoma elasticum; and provides resrouces for healthcare professionals.
Sharon Terry, CEO
Terry Dermaid, Executive Director

9821 Recorded Periodicals
Associated Services for the Blind
919 Walnut Street 215-627-0600
Philadelphia, PA 19107-5237 Fax: 215-922-0692
asbinfo@asb.org
www.asb.org
A subscription service of Associated Services for the Blind, these periodicals provide 21 magazines through this subscription service. A magazine list can be sent, in both large print and on audio cassette.
Richard Forsythe, Director
David Goldfield, Computer Instructor

9822 Recording for the Blind Helpline
20 Roszel Road 609-750-1830
Princeton, NJ 08540-6294 800-221-4792
PrincetonStudio@LearningAlly.org
www.learningally.org
An organization dedicated to helping people with print disabilities.
Andrew Friedman, President & CEO
Jim Halliday, Executive VP

9823 Vision Use in Employment
Carroll Center for the Blind
770 Centre Street 617-969-6200
Newton, MA 02458-2597 800-852-3131
Fax: 617-969-6204
www.carroll.org
We have developed many methods for people with low vision to learn the skills to be independent in their homes, in class settings, and in their work places. Our services for the blind include vision rehabilitation services, vocational and transition programs, assistive technology training, educational support and recreation opportunities for individuals who are visually impaired of all ages
Joseph Abely, President
Diana Rosenbaum, Director of Marketing

9824 Washington Connection
American Council of the Blind
1155 15th Street NW 202-467-5081
Washington, DC 20005-2706 800-424-8666
Fax: 202-467-5085
info@acb.org
www.acb.org
Coverage of issues affecting blind people via legislative information, participates in law-making, legislative training seminars and networking of support resources across the US.
Melanie Brunson, Executive Director

Books

9825 AFB Directory of Services for Blind/Vis. Impaired Persons in the US & Canada
AFB Press: American Foundation for the Blind
2 Penn Plaza 212-502-7600
New York, NY 10121 800-232-3044
Fax: 888-545-8331
literacy@afb.net
www.afb.org/store
Provides the most comprehensive collection of information available on services for blind and visually impaired individuals. Over 800 pages of revised and updated information on more than 1,500 agencies and 45 new indexes. Includes complete descriptions of services offered by organizations and web sites and e-mail addresses. Available online on a subscription basis.
Carl R Augusto, President & CEO
Rick Bozeman, Chief Financial Officer

9826 APH Catalog of Accessible Books for People Who are Visually Impaired
American Printing House for the Blind

1839 Frankfort Avenue 502-895-2405
Louisville, KY 40206-3148 800-223-1839
Fax: 502-899-2284
info@aph.org
www.aph.org
Offers thousands of selections and publishers of large type and braille books for persons with visual impairments.

9827 Access to Mass Transit for Blind & Visually Impaired Travelers
AFB Press: American Foundation for the Blind
2 Penn Plaza 212-502-7600
New York, NY 10121 800-232-3044
Fax: 888-545-8331
literacy@afb.net
www.afb.org/store
Addresses several travel issues vital to the independence of blind and visually impaired persons from serveral perspectives — those of the blind and visually impaired persons who use mass transit, orientation and mobility instructors and transportation professionals. Focusing on national and international issues, this information filled manual covers approaches to making mass transit available in several cities in the US and Canada, the United Kingdom and Japan.
192 pages Paperback
ISBN: 0-891281-66-5
Carl R Augusto, President & CEO
Rick Bozeman, Chief Financial Officer

9828 An Orientation and Mobility Primer for Families and Young Children
American Foundation for the Blind
2 Penn Plaza 212-502-7600
New York, NY 10121-2018 800-232-3044
Fax: 888-545-8331
literacy@afb.net
www.afb.org
Practical information for helping a child learn about his or her environment right from the start. Covers sensory training, concept development and orientation skills.
48 pages Papberback
ISBN: 0-891281-57-6
Carl R Augusto, President & CEO
Rick Bozeman, Chief Financial Officer

9829 Art Beyond Sight: Resource Guide to Art, Creativity and Visual Impairment
AFB Press: American Foundation for the Blind
2 Penn Plaza 212-502-7600
New York, NY 10121 800-232-3044
Fax: 888-545-8331
literacy@afb.net
www.afb.org/store
AFB and Art Education for the Blind have joined together to co-publish this one-of-a-kind resource that provides vital information on all aspects of exploring art and creativity by people who are blind or visually impaired. Includes a section of reproducible pages for classroom or workshop activities.
504 pages Paperback
ISBN: 0-891288-50-3
Carl R Augusto, President & CEO
Rick Bozeman, Chief Financial Officer

9830 Art and Science of Teaching Orientation to the Visually Impaired
AFB Press: American Foundation for the Blind
2 Penn Plaza 212-502-7600
New York, NY 10121 800-232-3044
Fax: 888-545-8331
literacy@afb.net
www.afb.org/store
Updated and comprehensive description of the techniques of teaching orientation and mobility, presented along with strategies for sensitive and effective teaching. Such factors as individual needs, environmental features and ethical issues are discussed in this important text.
200 pages Paperback
ISBN: 0-891282-59-9
Carl R Augusto, President & CEO
Rick Bozeman, Chief Financial Officer

9831 Beginning with Braille: Balanced Approach to Literacy
AFB Press: American Foundation for the Blind
2 Penn Plaza   212-502-7600
New York, NY 10121   800-232-3044
                                           Fax: 888-545-8331
                                          literacy@afb.net
                                          www.afb.org/store

Exciting resource from a skilled practitioner, this book provides a wealth of effective activitoes for promoting literacy at the early stages of braille instruction. The text includes creative and practical strategies for designing and delivering quality braille instruction and offers teacher-friendly suggestions for many areas, such as reading aloud to young children, selecting and making early tactile books and teaching tactile and hand movement skills. Tips on lessons and worksheets.
ISBN: 0-891283-23-4
Carl R Augusto, President & CEO
Rick Bozeman, Chief Financial Officer

9832 Behavioral Vision Approaches for Persons with Physical Disabilities
William V. Padula, author
Optometric Extension Program Foundation
1921 E. Carnegie Ave.   949-250-8070
Santa Ana, CA 92705-5510   Fax: 949-250-8157
                                          Kelin.Kushin@oep.org
                                          www.oepf.org

A discussion of the behavioral vision/neuro-motor approach to providing directions for prescriptive and therapeutic services for the visually handicapped child or adult.
197 pages
ISBN: 0-943599-04-0
Paul A. Harris, President
Robin Lewis, Vice President

9833 Blindness and Early Childhood Development
AFB Press: American Foundation for the Blind
2 Penn Plaza   212-502-7600
New York, NY 10121   800-232-3044
                                           Fax: 888-545-8331
                                          literacy@afb.net
                                          www.afb.org/store

Reviews knowledge of motor and locomotor development, language and cognitive processes and social, emotional and personality development. It is a classic resource for teachers and those who work with children who are blind or visually impaired.
384 pages Paperback
ISBN: 0-891281-23-1
Carl R Augusto, President & CEO
Rick Bozeman, Chief Financial Officer

9834 Braille Book Bank: Music Catalog
National Braille Association
95 Allens Creek Road   585-427-8260
Rochester, NY 14618   Fax: 585-427-0263
                                          NBAOffice@nationalbraille.org
                                          www.nationalbraille.org
Offers hundreds of musical titles in print form, braille and on cassette.
62 pages
Whitney Williams, President
Jana Hertz, Vice President

9835 Building Blocks: Foundations for Learning for Young Blind & Vis. Impaired Children
AFB Press: American Foundation for the Blind
2 Penn Plaza   212-502-7600
New York, NY 10121   800-232-3044
                                           Fax: 888-545-8331
                                          literacy@afb.net
                                          www.afb.org/store

Available in English and Spanish, this work presents the essential components of a successful early intervention program, including collaboration with family members, positive relationships between parents and professionals, public education, and attention to important programming components such as space exploration, braille readiness, orientation and mobility, play, cooking and music. VHS video also available.
149 pages Paperback
ISBN: 0-891281-87-8
Carl R Augusto, President & CEO
Rick Bozeman, Chief Financial Officer

9836 Burns Braille Transcription Dictionary
AFB Press: American Foundation for the Blind
2 Penn Plaza   212-502-7600
New York, NY 10121   800-232-3044
                                           Fax: 888-545-8331
                                          literacy@afb.net
                                          www.afb.org/store

A handy, portable guide that is a quick reference for anyone who needs to check print-to-braille and braille-to-print meanings and symbols. This easy-to-use listing provides readers with the essential alphabet, contractions, punctuation and signs and symbols for braille, as well as brief descriptions of rules for thier use. Organized into four clear sections aimed at providing information at a glance, this valuable tool is an ideal reference for teachers, rehabilitation professionals and others.
96 pages Paperback
ISBN: 0-891292-32-7
Carl R Augusto, President & CEO
Rick Bozeman, Chief Financial Officer

9837 Business Owners Who Are Blind or Visually Impaired
AFB Press: American Foundation for the Blind
2 Penn Plaza   212-502-7600
New York, NY 10121   800-232-3044
                                           Fax: 888-545-8331
                                          literacy@afb.net
                                          www.afb.org/store

Demonstrates the wide range of careers and talents that can be pursued by persons with visual impairments. Each profile features a successful individual who has accomplised his or her dream of business ownership and who shares important insights. Available in paperback, audio cassette or ASCII disk.
148 pages
ISBN: 0-891283-24-2
Carl R Augusto, President & CEO
Rick Bozeman, Chief Financial Officer

9838 Career Perspectives: Interviews with Blind & Visually Impaired Professionals
AFB Press: American Foundation for the Blind
2 Penn Plaza   212-502-7600
New York, NY 10121   800-232-3044
                                           Fax: 888-545-8331
                                          literacy@afb.net
                                          www.afb.org/store

Profiles of 20 successful archivers who describe in their own words what it takes to pursue and attain professional success in a sighted world. From all around the country and representing a wide range of professions, including law, science, journalism, management and medicine, the blind and visually impaired individuals featured serve as role models for others who wnat to follow career paths.
96 pages Paperback
ISBN: 0-891281-70-3
Carl R Augusto, President & CEO
Rick Bozeman, Chief Financial Officer

9839 Childhood Glaucoma: A Reference Guide for Families
NAPVI
15 West 65th Street   212-769-7819
New York, NY 10023-0317   800-284-4422
                                           Fax: 617-972-7444
                                          napvi@lighthouseguild.org
                                          www.napvi.org
Lighthouse Guild is the leading not-for-profit vision + healthcare organization, with a long-standing heritage of addressing the needs of people who are blind or visually impaired as well as those with multiple disabilities or chronic medical conditions.
James A Dubin, Chairman
Susan LaVenture, Executive Director

9840 Communication Skills for Visually Impaired
Charles C Thomas Publisher

2600 S 1st Street
Springfield, IL 62704-4730

217-789-8980
Fax: 217-789-9130
books@ccthomas.com
www.ccthomas.com

322 pages
ISBN: 0-398066-92-2

9841   Concept Development for Visually Impaired Children: Resource Guide
AFB Press: American Foundation for the Blind
2 Penn Plaza
New York, NY 10121

212-502-7600
800-232-3044
Fax: 888-545-8331
literacy@afb.net
www.afb.org/store

Program for integrating such concepts as body imagery, gross motor movement, posture and tactile discrimination into the curriculum from kindergarten on.
80 pages Paperback
ISBN: 0-891280-18-9
Carl R Augusto, President & CEO
Rick Bozeman, Chief Financial Officer

9842   Coping with Vision Loss
Bill Chapman, EdD, author
Hunter House Publishing
PO Box 2914
Alameda, CA 94501

510-865-5282
800-266-5592
Fax: 510-865-4295
ordering@hunterhouse.com
www.hunterhouse.com

Maximizing what you can see and do. The Author explains the five leading causes of vision loss, and how to use new skills and vision aids.
2001 304 pages Paperback
Cristina Sverdrup, Customer Service Manager

9843   Development of Social Skills by Blind and Visually Impaired Students
AFB Press: American Foundation for the Blind
2 Penn Plaza
New York, NY 10121

212-502-7600
800-532-3044
Fax: 888-545-8331
literacy@afb.net
www.afb.org/store

Examination of the social interactions of children with visual impairments, theory and research are combined to explore how these children can be helped to succeed socially. Innovative practical strategies are provided for educators, researchers and families on how to assist children in the development of social skills. Qualitative ethnographic approaches demonstrate how classroom teachers can work effectively with individual children and present valuable insights about children's interactions.
232 pages Paperback
ISBN: 0-891282-17-3
Carl R Augusto, President & CEO
Rick Bozeman, Chief Financial Officer

9844   Early Focus: Working with Young Children Who Are Blind or Visually Impaired
AFB Press: American Foundation for the Blind
2 Penn Plaza
New York, NY 10121

212-502-7600
Fax: 888-545-8331
literacy@afb.net
www.afb.org/store

Early intervention has increasingly been recognized as critical in the development and growth of children with visual impairments and other disabilities. Federal regulations have mandated early indentifacation and assesment, underscoring its importance for children's well being. This revised and updated edition of Early Focus provides the important information you need to know including serving culturally diverse families with children who have multiple disabilities and practical tips.
376 pages Paperback
ISBN: 0-891282-15-7
Carl R Augusto, President & CEO
Rick Bozeman, Chief Financial Officer

9845   Encyclopedia of Blindness and Vision Impairment
Facts on File

2 Penn Plaza
New York, NY 10121

212-967-8800
800-322-8755
Fax: 888-545-8331
literacy@afb.net
www.afb.org

Designed to provide both laymen and professionals with concise, practical information on the second most common disability in the US.
340 pages Hardcover
Carl R Augusto, President & CEO
Rick Bozeman, Chief Financial Officer

9846   Equals in Partnership: Basic Rights for Families of Children with Blindness
NAPVI
15 West 65th Street
New York, NY 10023-0317

212-769-7819
800-284-4422
Fax: 617-972-7444
napvi@lighthouseguild.org
www.napvi.org

Lighthouse Guild is the leading not-for-profit vision + healthcare organization, with a long-standing heritage of addressing the needs of people who are blind or visually impaired as well as those with multiple disabilities or chronic medical conditions.
James A Dubin, Chairman
Susan LaVenture, Executive Director

9847   Essential Elements in Early Intervention: Visual Impairment & Multiple Disability
AFB Press: American Foundation for the Blind
2 Penn Plaza
New York, NY 10121

212-502-7600
800-232-3044
Fax: 888-545-8331
literacy@afb.net
www.afb.org/store

Latest comprehensive resource from an outstanding early childhood specialist, this guide provides a range of information on effective early intervention with young children who are visually impaired and have other disabilities.
503 pages Paperback
ISBN: 0-891283-05-6
Carl R Augusto, President & CEO
Rick Bozeman, Chief Financial Officer

9848   Eye and Your Vision
Dr Lorrain H Marchi, author
National Association for Visually Handicapped
111 E 59th St
New York, NY 10022-6904

212-821-9497
800-284-4422
Fax: 212-727-2931
kcampbell@lighthouse.org
lighthouse.org/navh

A large booklet offering information, with illustrations, on the eye. Includes information on protection of eyesight, how the eye works and vision disorders.
19 pages $5.00 n/members
Lorraine Marchi LHD, Founder/CEO
Cesar Gomez, Executive Director

9849   First Steps
Blind Children's Center
4120 Marathon Street
Los Angeles, CA 90029-3584

213-664-2153
Fax: 213-665-3828
info@blindcntr.org
www.blindcntr.org

A handbook for teaching young children who are visually impaired. Designed to assist students, professionals and parents working with children who are visually impaired.
203 pages

9850   Foundations of Education
AFB Press: American Foundation for the Blind
2 Penn Plaza
New York, NY 10121

212-502-7600
800-232-3044
Fax: 888-545-8331
literacy@afb.net
www.afb.org/store

Complete revision of landmark text. Comprehensive compilation of state-of-the-art information is the essential resource on educating visually impaired students, the essential theory forming the knowledge base, and methodology of teaching visually impaired students in all areas.

2000
ISBN: 0-891283-49-8
Carl R Augusto, President & CEO
Rick Bozeman, Chief Financial Officer

9851 Foundations of Orientation and Mobility
AFB Press: American Foundation for the Blind
2 Penn Plaza   212-502-7600
New York, NY 10121   800-232-3044
                              Fax: 888-545-8331
                              literacy@afb.net
                              www.afb.org

Updated and revised, this new edition of the field's founding classics includes current research fom a variety of disiplines, an international perspective, and expanded contents on low vision, aging, multiple disabilities, accessibility, program design and adaptive technology from more than 30 eminent subject experts. Divided into four main sections, the book explores every of Orientation and Mobility learning and instruction.

800 pages Hardcover
ISBN: 0-891289-46-1
Carl R Augusto, President & CEO
Rick Bozeman, Chief Financial Officer

9852 Foundations of Rehabilitation Counseling with Persons Who Are Blind/Visually Imp.
AFB Press: American Foundation for the Blind
2 Penn Plaza   212-502-7600
New York, NY 10121   800-232-3044
                              Fax: 888-545-8331
                              literacy@afb.net
                              www.afb.org/store

Rehabilitation professionals have long recognized that the needs of people who are blind or visually impaired are unique and require a special knowledge and expertise for the provision and coordination of effective rehabilitation services. Contributions to this text from more than 25 experts provide essential information on subjects as functional, medical, vocational and phychological assessments, demographic and cultural issues, pacement and employment issues, and the rehabilitation team.

464 pages Hardcover
ISBN: 0-891289-45-3
Carl R Augusto, President & CEO
Rick Bozeman, Chief Financial Officer

9853 Get a Wiggle On
American Alliance For Health, Phys. Ed. & Dance
1900 Association Drive   703-476-3400
Reston, VA 20191-1598   800-213-7193
                              Fax: 703-476-9527
                              www.aahperd.org/

Gives teachers and parents practical suggestions for helping blind and visually impaired infants grow and learn like other children.

80 pages
ISBN: 0-883140-77-2
Steve Jefferies, President
E. Paul Roetert, Chief Executive Officer

9854 Guide to Independence for the Visually Impaired and Their Families
Demos Medical Publishing
11 West 42nd Street   212-683-0072
New York, NY 10036-8804   800-532-8663
                              Fax: 212-683-0118
                              support@demosmedical.com
                              www.demosmedical.com

This first comprehensive, hands-on book for the newly visually impaired and their families presents detailed instructions to deal with emotional reactions and fioght depression; contact organizations and get information; obtain federal and other types of financial aid; use the other senses more effectively; adapt their homes and do household chores; handle paperwork and become socially active.

248 pages Paperback
ISBN: 0-939957-61-2
David D'Addona, Acquisitions Editor

9855 Guidelines and Games for Teaching Efficient Braille Reading
AFB Press: American Foundation for the Blind
2 Penn Plaza   212-502-7600
New York, NY 10121   800-232-3044
                              Fax: 888-545-8331
                              literacy@afb.net
                              www.afb.org/store

Based on research in the areas of rapid reading and precision teaching, these effective guidelines and games represent a unique adaptation of a general reading program to the needs of braille readers.

116 pages Paperback
ISBN: 0-891281-05-3
Carl R Augusto, President & CEO
Rick Bozeman, Chief Financial Officer

9856 Hammond Large Type World Atlas
American Map-Langensceidt Publishing Group
15 Tyger River Drive   864-486-0214
Duncan, SC 29334   800-432-6277
                              Fax: 888-773-7979
                              www.hammondmap.com

100 maps.
ISBN: 0-816159-11-4

9857 Handbook for Itinerant and Resource Teachers of Blind Students
National Federation of the Blind
200 East Wells Street   410-659-9314
Baltimore, MD 21230-4998   Fax: 410-685-5653
                              nfb@nfb.org
                              www.nfb.org

The Handbook provides help to teachers, school administrators or other school personnel that have experience with blind or visually impaired students. The Handbook devotes 45 pages to Braille and how to teach Braille for parents and teachers; other chapters iclude law, physical education, fitting in socially, testing and evaluation, home economics, daily living skills and more.

533 pages Softcover
Mark Riccobono, President
James Gashel, Secretary

9858 Health Care Professionals Who are Blind or Visually Impaired
AFB Press: American Foundation for the Blind
2 Penn Plaza   212-502-7600
New York, NY 10121   800-232-3044
                              Fax: 888-545-8331
                              literacy@afb.net
                              www.afb.org/store

Exciting career possibilities for people who are visually impaired as well as those who are sighted. Inspirational profiles of 15 sucessful role models. Written in an accesible, easy-to-read style, this book documents the stories and stategies of professionals ranging from a forensic psychiatrist to a radiology dark room technician. Information on technology and tactics that are used to perform demanding jobs are also included. Available in paperback, audio casette, or ASCII disk.

2001 166 pages
ISBN: 0-891283-88-9
Carl R Augusto, President & CEO
Rick Bozeman, Chief Financial Officer

9859 I Keep Five Pairs of Glasses in a Flower Pot
Henrietta Levner, author
National Association for Visually Handicapped
111 E 59th St   212-821-9497
New York, NY 10022-6904   800-284-4422
                              Fax: 212-727-2931
                              kcampbell@lighthouse.org
                              lighthouse.org/navh

A short story, printed in 18 point type, is the saga of one womans struggle with low vision.
Lorraine Marchi LHD, Founder/CEO
Cesar Gomez, Executive Director

9860 If Blindness Comes
National Federation of the Blind
200 East Wells Street   410-659-9314
Baltimore, MD 21230-4998   Fax: 410-685-5653
                              nfb@nfb.org
                              www.nfb.org

An introduction to issues relating to vision loss and provides a positive, supportive philosophy about blindness. It is a general information book which includes answers to many common questions about blindness, information about services and programs for the blind and resource listings.

Mark Riccobono, President
James Gashel, Secretary

9861 Independence Without Sight or Sound: Suggestions for Practitioners
AFB Press: American Foundation for the Blind
2 Penn Plaza · 212-502-7600
New York, NY 10121 · · · · · · · · · · · · · · 800-232-3044
· Fax: 888-545-8331
· literacy@afb.net
· www.afb.org/store

Written in a personal and informal style, this practical guidebook covers the essential aspects of communicating and working with deaf-blind persons. Full of valuable information on subjects such as how to talk with deaf-blind people, adapt orientation and mobility techniques for deaf-blind travelers, and interact with deaf-blind individuals socially, this useful manual also contains a substantial resource section detailing sources of information and adapted equipment. Also available in braille.

193 pages Paperback
ISBN: 0-891282-46-7

Carl R Augusto, President & CEO
Rick Bozeman, Chief Financial Officer

9862 Jewish Heritage for the Blind
1655 E 24th Street · · · · · · · · · · · · · · · 718-338-4999
Brooklyn, NY 11229-2401 · · · · · · · · · · 800-995-1888
· Fax: 718-338-0653
· services@jhbinternational.org
· www.jhbinternational.org

Offers large print traditional prayer books for the High Holy days, festivals, fast days and daily rituals for those finding it difficult or impossible to read small print.

9863 Kernel Book Series
National Federation of the Blind
200 East Wells Street · · · · · · · · · · · · · · 410-659-9314
Baltimore, MD 21230-4998 · · · · · · · · Fax: 410-685-5653
· nfb@nfb.org
· www.nfb.org

A series of books written by the blind themselves. Each book is a collection of articles and stories about the real life experiences of blind persons. These books help educate the blind and the sighted alike about a positive philosophy regarding blindness.

Mark Riccobono, President
James Gashel, Secretary

9864 King James Bible: Large Print
Science Products
PO Box 888 · · · · · · · · · · · · · · · · · · · 800-888-7400
Southeastern, PA 19399-0888

24 point type easily seen with 20/200 acuity. Makes bible reading for children easier too.

9865 Knotholes are for Seeing: Therapy Through Poetry, Prose & Other Writings
Business of Living Publications
PO Box 8388 · · · · · · · · · · · · · · · · · · 512-852-8515
Corpus Christi, TX 78468-8388
ISBN: 1-879518-08-2

9866 Large Print American Heritage Dictionary
Houghton Mifflin Harcourt
222 Berkeley Street · · · · · · · · · · · · · · · 617-351-5000
Boston, MA 02116 · · · · · · · · · · · · · · · 800-888-7400
· www.hmco.com

More than 35,000 easy to read entries for those who prefer large type.
ISBN: 0-395929-32-6

Lawrence K. Fish, Director and Chairman of the Board
Sheru Chowdhry, Director

9867 Legislative Handbook for Parents
NAPVI

PO Box 317 · · · · · · · · · · · · · · · · · · · 617-972-7441
Watertown, MA 02471-0317 · · · · · · · · · 800-562-6265
· Fax: 617-972-7444
· www.spedex.com

Written by parents for parents in dealing with legislative processes that ultimately affect their children's lives.
Susan LaVenture, Executive Director

9868 Library Resources for the Blind and Physically Handicapped
National Library Service for the Blind
1291 Taylor Street NW · · · · · · · · · · · · · 202-707-5100
Washington, DC 20542-0002 · · · · · · · · Fax: 202-707-0712
· TDD: 202-707-0744
· nls@loc.gov
· www.loc.gov/nls

The mission of this web site is to provide program users, librarians, and the public a wide range of access to NLS publications, program information, and bibliographic data

9869 Low Vision: Reflections of the Past, Issues for the Future
AFB Press: American Foundation for the Blind
2 Penn Plaza · · · · · · · · · · · · · · · · · · · 212-502-7600
New York, NY 10121 · · · · · · · · · · · · · · 800-232-3044
· Fax: 888-545-8331
· literacy@afb.net
· www.afb.org/store

Research report based on a multiphase survey of professionals. Identifies important trends that will shape the field of low vision services into the next century. Designed for administrators, policy planners and university instructors, as well as for direct service providers, Low Vision includes overview papers by six eminent leaders in the low vision field.

181 pages Paperback
ISBN: 0-891282-18-1

Carl R Augusto, President & CEO
Rick Bozeman, Chief Financial Officer

9870 Madness of Usher's: Coping with Vision & Hearing Loss
Richard A. Lewis, Dorothy H. Stiefel, author
Business of Living Publications
PO Box 8388 · · · · · · · · · · · · · · · · · · 512-852-8515
Corpus Christi, TX 78468-8388
Paperback
ISBN: 1-879518-06-6
Dorothy H Stiefel, Author

9871 Mainstreaming & the American Dream: Soc. Logical Perspectives on Parental Coping
AFB Press: American Foundation for the Blind
2 Penn Plaza · · · · · · · · · · · · · · · · · · · 212-502-7600
New York, NY 10121 · · · · · · · · · · · · · · 800-232-3044
· Fax: 888-545-8331
· literacy@afb.net
· www.afb.org/store

Based on in-depth interviews with parents and professionals, this research monograph presents a sociological framework for looking at the needs and aspirations of parents of blind and visually impaired children.

256 pages Paperback
ISBN: 0-891281-91-6

Carl R Augusto, President & CEO
Rick Bozeman, Chief Financial Officer

9872 Mainstreaming the Visually Impaired Child
NAPVI
15 West 65th Street · · · · · · · · · · · · · · · 212-769-7819
New York, NY 10023-0317 · · · · · · · · · · 800-284-4422
· Fax: 617-972-7444
· napvi@lighthouseguild.org
· www.napvi.org

Lighthouse Guild is the leading not-for-profit vision + healthcare organization, with a long-standing heritage of addressing the needs of people who are blind or visually impaired as well as those with multiple disabilities or chronic medical conditions.
James A Dubin, Chairman
Susan LaVenture, Executive Director

9873 Making Life More Livable: Adaptations for Living at Home After Vision Loss
AFB Press: American Foundation of the Blind

2 Penn Plaza
New York, NY 10121

212-502-7600
800-232-3044
Fax: 888-545-8331
literacy@afb.net
www.afb.org/store

Essential guide for adults experiencing vision loss and an invaluable resource for their family and friends. Full of practical tips and illustrated by numerous photographs, this easy-to-use resource shows how people who are visually impaired can continue living independent, productive lives at home on their own. Useful general guidelines and room-by-room specifics provide simple and effective solutions for making homes accessible and everyday activities doable for visually impaired individuals.

132 pages Cassette avail.
ISBN: 0-891281-15-0
Carl R Augusto, President & CEO
Rick Bozeman, Chief Financial Officer

9874 Occupational Therapy Practice Guidelines for Adults with Low Vision
American Occupational Therapy Association
4720 Montgomery Lane
Bethesda, MD 20814-1220

301-652-6611
800-729-2682
Fax: 240-762-5150
TDD: 800-377-8555
www.aota.org

25 pages
ISBN: 1-569001-50-2

9875 Perkins Activity and Resource Guide: A Handbook for Teachers
Perkins School for the Blind Publications
175 N Beacon Street
Watertown, MA 02472-2790

617-924-3434
877-473-7546
Fax: 617-972-7334
publications@perkins.org
www.perkins.org

This is a comprehensive, two volume guide with over 1,000 pages of activities, resources and instructional strategies for teachers and parents of students with visual and multiple disabilities.
Kathy Heydt, Author
Monica Allon, Author

9876 Preschool Learning Activities for the Visually Impaired Child
NAPVI
15 West 65th Street
New York, NY 10023-0317

212-769-7819
800-284-4422
Fax: 617-972-7444
napvi@lighthouseguild.org
www.napvi.org

Lighthouse Guild is the leading not-for-profit vision + healthcare organization, with a long-standing heritage of addressing the needs of people who are blind or visually impaired as well as those with multiple disabilities or chronic medical conditions.
James A Dubin, Chairman
Susan LaVenture, Executive Director

9877 Prescriptions for Independence: Working with Older People Who Are Visually Imp.
AFB Press: American Foundation for the Blind
2 Penn Plaza
New York, NY 10121

212-502-7600
800-232-3044
Fax: 888-545-8331
literacy@afb.net
www.afb.org/store

Easy-to-read manual on how older persons with visual impairments can pursue their interests and activities in community residences, senior centers, long-term care facilities and other community settings. Topics covered include signs of vision loss, recreation, personal care, orientation and mobility and modifications in the environment.
87 pages Paperback
ISBN: 0-891282-44-0
Carl R Augusto, President & CEO
Rick Bozeman, Chief Financial Officer

9878 Providing Services for People with Vision Loss: Multidisciplinary Perspective
Resources For Rehabilitation

22 Bonad Road
Winchester, MA 01890

781-368-9080
Fax: 781-368-9096
info@rfr.org
www.rfr.org

A collection of articles by ophthalmologists and rehabilitation professionals, including chapters on operating a low vision service, starting self-help programs, mental health services, aids and techniques that help people with vision loss.
136 pages
ISBN: 0-929718-02-X
Susan L. Greenblatt, Editor

9879 Psychoeducational Assessment of Visually Impaired Students
Pro-Ed, Inc.
8700 Shoal Creek Blvd
Austin, TX 78757-6897

512-451-3246
800-897-3202
Fax: 800-397-7633
info@proedinc.com
www.proedinc.com

Professional reference book that addresses the problems specific to assessment of visually impaired children. Of particular value to the practitioner are the extensive reviews of available tests, including ways to adapt those not designed for use with the visually handicapped.
140 pages Paperback
Lindy Jordaan, Marketing Coordinator

9880 Resources Family Centered Intervention for Infants, Toddlers & Preschoolers
Hope
1856 N 1200 E
North Logan, UT 84341

435-245-2888
Fax: 435-245-2888

Describes children with vision impairment in terms of characteristics, needs, and parent concerns.
Hardcover

9881 Show Me How: Manual for Parents Preschool Visually Impaired & Blind Children
AFB Press: American Foundation for the Blind
2 Penn Plaza
New York, NY 10121

212-502-7600
800-232-3044
Fax: 888-545-8331
literacy@afb.net
www.afb.org/store

Practical guide for parents, teachers and others who help preschool children attain age-related goals. Includes activities for growing and learning, building self-concept, moving around, playing, perfecting daily living skills and developing sensory awareness. It also covers such issues as observing safety precautions, choosing appropriate toys and facilitating relationships with playmates.
56 pages Paperback
ISBN: 0-891281-13-4
Carl R Augusto, President & CEO
Rick Bozeman, Chief Financial Officer

9882 Starting Points
Blind Children's Center
4120 Marathon Street
Los Angeles, CA 90029-3584

213-664-2153
Fax: 213-665-3828

Basic information for the clasroom teacher of 3 to 8 year olds whose multiple disabilities include visual impairment.
160 pages

9883 Tactile Graphics
AFB Press: American Foundation for the Blind
2 Penn Plaza
New York, NY 10121

212-502-7600
800-232-3044
Fax: 888-545-8331
literacy@afb.net
www.afb.org/store

Easy-to-read encyclopedia handbook on translating visual information into a three-dimensional form that the blind and visually impaired persons can understand. This heavily illustrated guide covers theory, techniques, materials and step-by-step instructions for educators, rehabilitators, graphic artists, museum and busines

personnel, employers and anyone involved in producing tactile material for visually impaired persons.
544 pages Paperback
ISBN: 0-891281-94-0
Carl R Augusto, President & CEO
Rick Bozeman, Chief Financial Officer

9884 Teachers Who Are Blind or Visually Impaired
AFB Press: American Foundation for the Blind
2 Penn Plaza   212-502-7600
New York, NY 10121   800-232-3044
                               Fax: 888-545-8331
                                 literacy@afb.net
                                www.afb.org/store

First volume in the Jobs That Matter series, this book profiles 18 visually impaired individuals who have successfully fulfilled their dreams of becoming teachers. These engaging individuals demonstrate how visually impaired teachers can be effective in their jobs and achieve classroom success and satisfaction. Available in paperback, audio cassette or braille.
1998 176 pages
ISBN: 0-891283-06-4
Carl R Augusto, President & CEO
Rick Bozeman, Chief Financial Officer

9885 Textbook Catalog
National Braille Association
95 Allens Creek Road   585-427-8260
Rochester, NY 14618   Fax: 585-427-0263
                              www.nationalbraille.org
Lists hundreds of scholarly, college and professional textbooks offered in large print, braille or on cassette for visually impaired readers.
80 pages
Whitney Williams, President
Jana Hertz, Vice President

9886 To Love This Life: Quotations by Helen Keller
AFB Press: American Foundation for the Blind
2 Penn Plaza   212-502-7600
New York, NY 10121   800-232-3044
                               Fax: 888-545-8331
                                 literacy@afb.net
                                www.afb.org/store

Beautiful and moving souvenir of one of the world's most admired women. This memorable collection of quotations from Helen Keller brings words of wisdom, courage and inspiration from a remarkable individual who above all wanted to make a difference in the lives of her fellow men and women. The thought captured here — many from unpublished letters and speeches — offer profound statements on the meaning of being human and on life in all its complexity. Available in hardcover and audio cassette.
2000 118 pages
ISBN: 0-891283-47-1
Carl R Augusto, President & CEO
Rick Bozeman, Chief Financial Officer

9887 Unseen Minority: Social History of Blindness in the US
Frances A. Koestler, author

David McKay Company/AFB Press, Distributor
2 Penn Plaza   412-741-1398
New York, NY 10121   800-232-3044
                               Fax: 888-545-8331
                                 literacy@afb.net
                                   www.afb.org
Lively narrative, peppered with anecdotes, recounts how the blind overcame discrimination to gain full participation in the social, educational, economic and legislative spheres. Here are the gripping stories: Why it took a century for braille to become a universal medium in English, how america's first school for the blind began with a chance encounter on a Boston street, and how the talking book came into existence.
573 pages Hardcover
ISBN: 0-679505-39-3
Carl R Augusto, President & CEO
Rick Bozeman, Chief Financial Officer

9888 Vision and Aging: Crossroads for Service Delivery
AFB Press: American Foundation for the Blind

2 Penn Plaza   212-502-7600
New York, NY 10121   800-232-3044
                               Fax: 888-545-8331
                                 literacy@afb.net
                                www.afb.org/store
This overview of the service delivery systems in the aging and blindness fields covers the essential issues concerning vision loss among older persons in this country, the growth of visual impairment among the increasing number of elderly people in the US, and the policy and service questions that will demand national attention throughout this and the coming decades.
392 pages Paperback
ISBN: 0-891282-16-5
Carl R Augusto, President & CEO
Rick Bozeman, Chief Financial Officer

9889 Visual Aids and Informational Material
National Association for Visually Handicapped
111 E 59th St   212-821-9497
New York, NY 10022-6904   800-284-4422
                               Fax: 212-727-2931
                            kcampbell@lighthouse.org
                              lighthouse.org/navh
A large reference guide offering a list of visual aids and resources for persons with visual impairments.
65 pages
Lorraine Marchi LHD, Founder/CEO
Cesar Gomez, Executive Director

9890 Visual Handicaps and Learning
Pro-Ed, Inc.
8700 Shoal Creek Blvd   512-451-3246
Austin, TX 78757-6897   800-897-3202
                               Fax: 800-397-7633
                              info@proedinc.com
                               www.proedinc.com
This text covers a range of topics associated with visual impairment, from past practices to up-to-date research, and from legal responsibilities to personal beliefs, without losing sight of the individual child.
180 pages
ISBN: 0-890795-15-0
Lindy Jordaan, Marketing Coordinator

9891 Visual Impairment: An Overview
AFB Press: American Foundation for the Blind
2 Penn Plaza   212-502-7600
New York, NY 10121   800-232-3044
                               Fax: 888-545-8331
                                 literacy@afb.net
                                www.afb.org/store
Down-to-earth look at the common forms of vision loss and their impact on the individual. Explains the different aspects of visual impairment, describes adaptive techniques and devices and provides information on available resources and services in a conscise and easy-to-understand manner for professionals and visually impaired people and their families.
56 pages Paperback
ISBN: 0-891281-74-6
Carl R Augusto, President & CEO
Rick Bozeman, Chief Financial Officer

9892 Walking Alone and Marching Together
Floyd Matson, author
National Federation of the Blind
200 East Wells Street   410-659-9314
Baltimore, MD 21230-4998   Fax: 410-685-5653
                                    nfb@nfb.org
                                   www.nfb.org
The history of the organized blind movement, this book spans more than 50 years of civil rights, social issues, attitudes and experiences of the blind. Published in 1990, it has been read by thousands of blind and sighted persons and is used in colleges, libraries and programs across the country as an important tool in understanding blindness and it's impact on both personal lives and the society at large.
1100 pages
Mark Riccobono, President
James Gashel, Secretary

9893 **Webster Large Print Dictionary**
Random House
1745 Broadway, 15-3
New York, NY 10019
212-782-9000
800-888-7400
www.penguinrandomhouse.com
They are committed to helping authors realize their very best work and to finding innovative new ways of bringing stories and ideas to audiences worldwide
880 pages
ISBN: 0-375722-32-7

9894 **What Museum Guides Need to Know: Access for Blind & Visually Impaired Visitors**
AFB Press: American Foundation for the Blind
2 Penn Plaza
New York, NY 10121
212-502-7600
800-232-3044
Fax: 888-545-8331
literacy@afb.net
www.afb.org/store
Provides practical, easy-to-use guidelines on how to greet and help blind and visually impaired museum goers. With numerous photographs taken at the High School Museum of Art and the Atlanta Historical Society, this handbook also covers aesthetics and visual impairment, legal requirements for accessibility, resources, a training outline for museum requirements for accessibility, a bibliography on art and museum access for blind and visually impaired persons, and guidelines for preparing media.
64 pages Paperback
ISBN: 0-891281-58-4
Carl R Augusto, President & CEO
Rick Bozeman, Chief Financial Officer

Children's Books

9895 **Belonging**
Dial Books
375 Hudson Street
New York, NY 10014-3658
212-366-2000
www.penguin.com
Meg attended special schools for the blind until she was ready for high school. She decided that she wanted to go to a regular high school. She and her mother practiced her walks to school and studied the layout of the building prior to school starting, but Meg was unprepared for the trip when there were 1,500 students. She adjusted quickly to the crowds and the pace of the new school.
200 pages Hardcover
ISBN: 0-803705-30-1

9896 **Beside Me**
Leader Dogs For The Blind
1039 S. Rochester Road
Rochester Hills, MI 48307
248-651-9011
888-777-5332
Fax: 248-651-5812
TTY: 248-651-3713
leaderdog@leaderdog.org
www.leaderdog.org
Marion became blind as an adult. She was totally dependent on her parents to move around and go places she wanted to be. Marion decided to go to the leader-dog program and learn to use a leader dog. Particularly she wanted the independence she would need to go to college. Marion enrolled at the Leader-Dog-For-The-Blind program in Rochester, Michigan. After weeks of training she was given a German Shepherd named Heidi. Marion and Heidi trained together until they were a team and ready.
Films
Susan Daniels, President & CEO
Lorene Suidan, Chief Financial Officer

9897 **Guide Dog Goes to School**
William Morrow and Company
105 Madison Avenue
New York, NY 10016-7418
212-889-3050
800-843-9389
Cinderena is a golden retriever. As a puppy Cindy is outgoing and not afraid of things in her environment. This disposition is ideal for a guide dog to the blind, and Cindy is selected to be in a program for guide dogs. Follow Cindy as we focus on the guide dog training.
51 pages Hardcover
ISBN: 0-688068-44-8

9898 **How Do You Kiss a Blind Girl?**
Charles C Thomas Publisher
2600 S First Street
Springfield, IL 62704-4730
217-789-8980
Fax: 217-789-9130
books@ccthomas.com
www.ccthomas.com
Focuses, in a humorous way, on the attitudes toward persons with visual impairments.
126 pages
ISBN: 0-398052-62-X

9899 **Living with Blindness**
Franklin Watts Grolier
90 Old Sherman Turnpike
Danbury, CT 06816-0001
203-797-3500
800-621-1115
Fax: 203-797-3197
www.grolier.com
Shows how persons with visual impairments and blindness can overcome their disability and lead productive lives.
32 pages Grades 5-7
ISBN: 0-531108-43-0

9900 **Man Who Sang in the Dark**
Eth Clifford, author
Houghton, Mifflin & Company
1 Beacon Street
Boston, MA 02108-3107
617-725-5000
The story of a girl and a man who is blind and how they both come to an understanding about certain prejudices.
Grades 3-5

9901 **Out of the Corner of My Eye**
American Foundation for the Blind
15 W 16th Street
New York, NY 10011-6301
212-502-7600
Fax: 212-502-7777
A personal account of students' vision loss and subsequent adjustment that is full of practical advice and cheerful encouragement, told by an 87 year old retired college teacher who has maintained her independence and zest for life.
ISBN: 0-891281-93-2

9902 **She'll Never Walk Alone**
Leader Dog For The Blind
1964 Park Street
Regina, SK, S4P 3G4,
306-565-8211
Leader dogs for the blind require many weeks of training before they are ready to work with the blind individual. Two courses, basic and advanced, are provided for each dog.
Films

Magazines

9903 **Access World: Technology and People with Visual Impairments**
AFB Press: American Foundation for the Blind
2 Penn Plaza
New York, NY 10121
212-502-7600
800-232-3044
Fax: 888-545-8331
literacy@afb.net
www.afb.org/store
Comprehensive and reader friendly online magazine covering every aspect of assistive technology and visual impairment.
Bimonthly
Carl R Augusto, President & CEO
Rick Bozeman, Chief Financial Officer

9904 **Blind Educator**
National Federation of the Blind
200 East Wells Street
Baltimore, MD 21230-4998
410-659-9314
Fax: 410-685-5653
nfb@nfb.org
www.nfb.org
The articles in this newsletter are written by people who are blind. Blind people can teach. In fact, this newsletter captures a glimpse of the range of subjects and grade levels in which blind people are engaged.
Mark Riccobono, President
James Gashel, Secretary

9905 Braille Forum
Penny Reeder, author
American Council of the Blind
2200 Wilson Boulevard   202-467-5081
Arlington, VA 22201-2706   800-424-8666
Fax: 703-465-5085
info@acb.org
www.acb.org
Offered in large print, braille, half speed cassette, via email and on the website.
32 pages 10x/year
Kim Charlson, President
Melanie Brunson, Executive Director

9906 Braille Monitor
National Federation of the Blind
200 East Wells Street   410-659-9314
Baltimore, MD 21230-4998   Fax: 410-685-5653
nfb@nfb.org
www.nfb.org
The leading publication in the blindness field, with a circulation of 30,000, this publication addresses issues of concern to the blind and the philosophy and activities of the National Federation of the Blind.
100 pages Monthly
Mark Riccobono, President
James Gashel, Secretary

9907 Dialogue Magazine
Blindskills
PO Box 5181   503-581-4224
Salem, OR 97304-0181   800-860-4224
Fax: 503-518-0178
blindsici@teleport.com
Publishes quarterly magazine in braille, large-type, cassette and disk of news items, fiction and articles of special interest.
Quarterly

9908 Future Reflections
Barbara Cheadler, author
National Federation of the Blind
200 East Wells Street   410-659-9314
Baltimore, MD 21230-4998   Fax: 410-685-5653
nfb@nfb.org
www.nfb.org
National magazine written specifically for parents and educators of blind children. Each issue addresses various topics important to blind children, their families and to school personnel.
Quarterly
Mark Riccobono, President
James Gashel, Secretary

9909 Illinois Braille Messenger
Illinois Council of the Blind
PO Box 1336   217-523-4967
Springfield, IL 62705-1336   888-698-1862
Fax: 217-523-4302
icb@fgi.net
Quarterly
Laura Booker, Editor

9910 Journal of Vision Rehabilitation
Media Productions & Marketing
2440 O Street   402-474-2676
Lincoln, NE 68510-1125
Multidisciplinary journal containing articles and papers dealing with low vision, its evaluation, instrumentation and rehabilitation.

9911 Journal of Visual Impairment & Blindness
AFB Press: American Foundation for the Blind
2 Penn Plaza   212-502-7600
New York, NY 10121   800-232-3044
Fax: 888-545-8331
literacy@afb.net
www.afb.org/store

Peer-reviewed journal reporting on the cutting-edge research, innovative practice and news on all aspects of visual impairment. Available online, on cassette and ASCII disk.
10 Issues
Carl R Augusto, President & CEO
Rick Bozeman, Chief Financial Officer

9912 Recorded Periodicals
Associated Services for the Blind
919 Walnut Street   215-627-0600
Philadelphia, PA 19107-5237   Fax: 215-922-0692
asbinfo@asb.org
www.asb.org
A subscription service of Associated Services for the Blind, this service provides 26 recorded magazines for blind and visually impaired individuals.
Audio Cassette
Patricia C Johnson, President/CEO
Brian Rusk, Public Relations Officer

9913 Review
AER
206 N Washington Street   703-823-9690
Alexandria, VA 22314-2528   Fax: 703-823-9695
The Association's practice-oriented journal.

9914 Tactic
Clovernook Ctr. for the Blind & Visually Impaired
7000 Hamilton Avenue   513-522-3860
Cincinnati, OH 45231-5240   888-224-7156
Fax: 513-728-3946
www.clovernook.org
Clovernook recognizes that each person who comes to us for services brings their own unique set of experiences and expectations. Consequently our services are never one size fits all, but individually designed to reflect your preferences and goals.
Quarterly
Jeffrey D Brasie, President

9915 Voice of the Diabetic
National Federation of the Blind
200 East Wells Street   410-659-9314
Baltimore, MD 21230-4998   Fax: 410-685-5653
nfb@nfb.org
www.nfb.org
The leading publication in the diabetes field. Each issue addresses the problems and concerns of diabetes, with a special emphasis for those who have lost vision due to diabetes. Available in print and on cassette.
30 pages Quarterly
Mark Riccobono, President
James Gashel, Secretary

Newsletters

9916 ACB Reports
American Council of the Blind
2200 Wilson Boulevard   202-467-5081
Arlington, VA 22201-2706   800-424-8666
Fax: 703-465-5085
info@acb.org
www.acb.org
Radio news feature program for radio information services.
Monthly
Kim Charlson, President
Melanie Brunson, Executive Director

9917 AER Report
AER
1703 N. Beauregard Street   703-671-4500
Alexandria, VA 22311   877-492-2708
Fax: 703-671-6391
lou@aerbvi.org
www.aerbvi.org
Contains organizational news, conference dates and information concerning services to visually impaired people.
28 pages BiMonthly
Jackie Fairbarns, Assistant Director
Lou Tutt, Executive Director

9918 AFB News
American Foundation for the Blind
2 Penn Plaza
New York, NY 10121-2018
212-502-7600
800-232-3044
Fax: 888-545-8331
literacy@afb.net
www.afb.org

National newsletter for general readership about blindness and visual impairments featuring people, programs, services and activities.
12 pages Quarterly
Carl R Augusto, President & CEO
Rick Bozeman, Chief Financial Officer

9919 Aging and Vision News
National Center for Vision and Aging
800 2nd Avenue
New York, NY 10017
212-808-0077
800-334-5497
3x Year

9920 Awareness
NAPVI
15 West 65th Street
New York, NY 10023-0317
212-769-7819
800-284-4422
Fax: 617-972-7444
napvi@lighthouseguild.org
www.napvi.org

Lighthouse Guild is the leading not-for-profit vision + healthcare organization, with a long-standing heritage of addressing the needs of people who are blind or visually impaired as well as those with multiple disabilities or chronic medical conditions.
Quarterly
James A Dubin, Chairman
Susan LaVenture, Executive Director

9921 Braille Book Review
National Library Service for the Blind
1291 Taylor Street NW
Washington, DC 20542-0002
202-707-5100
Fax: 202-707-0712
TDD: 202-707-0744
nls@loc.gov
www.loc.gov/nls

The mission of this web site is to provide program users, librarians, and the public a wide range of access to NLS publications, program information, and bibliographic data
BiMonthly

9922 Bulletin
National Association for Visually Handicapped
111 E 59th St
New York, NY 10022-6904
212-821-9497
800-284-4422
Fax: 212-727-2931
kcampbell@lighthouse.org
lighthouse.org/navh

Annual report offering information on association activities and events, conferences, vision aids and resources for the visually impaired.
Lorraine Marchi LHD, Founder/CEO
Cesar Gomez, Executive Director

9923 DVH Quarterly
University of Arkansas At Little Rock
2801 S University Avenue
Little Rock, AR 72204-1000
501-569-3000
Fax: 501-663-3536
ualr.edu/www

Offers information on upcoming events, conferences and workshops on and for visual disabilities. Book reviews, information on the newest resources and technology, educational programs, want ads and more.
Quarterly
Bob Brasher, Editor

9924 Eye Research News
645 Madison Avenue
New York, NY 10022-1010
212-752-4333
800-621-0026
Fax: 212-688-6231
www.rpbusa.org

Newsletter on the latest development in eye research
Annual
David Weeks, Chairman
Diane S Swift, President

9925 Focus
Visually Impaired Center
1422 West Court Street
Flint, MI 48503
810-767-4014
Fax: 810-767-0020
info@vicflint.org
www.vicflint.org

Newsletter offering information for the visually impaired person in the forms of legislative and law updates, ADA information, support groups, hotlines, and articles on the newest technology in the field.
Quarterly
Laurie MacArthur, Executive Director

9926 Gleams Newsletter
Glaucoma Research Foundation
251 Post Street
San Francisco, CA 94108
415-986-3162
800-826-6693
Fax: 415-986-3763
question@glaucoma.org
www.glaucoma.org

It includes information about glaucoma, new treatments, updates on research findings, and more.
3x/year
Thomas M Brunner, President/CEO
Andrew L Jackson, Director Communications

9927 Guide Dog Foundation for the Blind Newsletter
371 E Jericho Turnpike
Smithtown, NY 11787-2976
631-930-9000
800-548-4337
Fax: 631-930-9009
info@guidedog.org
www.guidedog.org

This organization relies on voluntary public contributions to provide persons with blindness the gift of second sight through the eyes of a guide dog. This nonprofit organization furnishes guide dogs, free of charge, to qualified people who seek independence, mobility and companionship.
James C. Bingham, Chair
Alphonce J. Brown, Vice Chair

9928 Guide Dog News
Guide Dogs for the Blind
PO Box 151200
San Rafael, CA 94915
415-499-4000
800-298-4050
Fax: 415-499-4035
information@guidedogs.com
www.guidedogs.com

About graduates, volunteers and donors of Guide Dogs for the Blind.
Quarterly
Bob Burke, Board Chair
Chris Benninger, President and CEO

9929 Guideway
Guide Dog Foundation for the Blind
371 E Jericho Turnpike
Smithtown, NY 11787-2976
631-930-9000
800-548-4337
Fax: 631-930-9009
info@guidedog.org
www.guidedog.org

Offers updates and information on the foundation's activities and guide dog programs. In print form but is also available on cassette.
6 pages Monthly
James C. Bingham, Chair
Alphonce J. Brown, Vice Chair

9930 Hearsay
Radio Information Service
600 Forbes Avenue
Pittsburgh, PA 15282
412-488-3944
Fax: 412-488-3953
info@readingservice.org
www.readingservice.org

Newsletter for persons interested in radio reading services.
Quarterly

9931 Hub
SPOKES Unlimited
1006 Main Street
Klamath Falls, OR 97601   541-883-7547
                                      Fax: 541-885-2469
                                   www.spokesunlimited.org
Newsletter on rehabilitation, peer counseling, blindness, visual
impairments, information and referral.
Meg Graf, Resource Librarian

9932 InSight
Foundation Fighting Blindness
7168 Columbia Gateway Dr   410-423-0600
Columbia, MD 21046-2220   800-683-5555
                                      Fax: 410-363-2393
                                      TDD: 800-683-5551
                                   info@fightblindness.org
                                      www.blindness.org
The Foundation Fighting Blindness newsletter, delivered to members monthly. The major emphasis is to report on research and science news, and FDA approved clinical trials around retinal
degenerative dieseases.
20 pages 3 per year
William T. Schmidt, CEO
Stephen M. Rose, Chief Research Officer

9933 Lion
Lions Clubs International
300 W 22nd Street   630-571-5466
Oak Brook, IL 60523-8815   www.lionsclubs.org
Publication for the blind.

9934 Listen Up
Recording for the Blind & Dyslexic (RFB&D)
20 Roszel Road   609-452-0606
Princeton, NJ 08540-6294   800-221-4792
                                      Fax: 609-987-8116
                                      custserv@rfbd.org
                                     www.learningally.org
RFB&D's bi-monthly newsletter for members.

Andrew Friedman, President & CEO
Jim Halliday, Executive Vice President

9935 Long Cane News
American Foundation for the Blind
15 West 16th Street   212-294-8301
New York, NY 10011-6301   800-232-5463
                                      Fax: 212-502-7777
                                          www.cjh.org

Semiannual
Amy Goldman Fowler, Chair
Kenneth J. Bialkin, Vice Chair

9936 Musical Mainstream
National Library Service for the Blind
1291 Taylor Street NW   202-707-5100
Washington, DC 20542-0002   Fax: 202-707-0712
                                      TDD: 202-707-0744
                                         nls@loc.gov
                                          www.loc.gov

Articles selected from print music magazines.
Quarterly

9937 NAVH UPDATE
National Association for Visually Handicapped
111 E 59th St   212-821-9497
New York, NY 10022-6904   800-284-4422
                                      Fax: 212-727-2931
                                   kcampbell@lighthouse.org
                                      lighthouse.org/navh
This newsletter offers vision news, medical updates, assistive de-
vice information, resources and more for the visually impaired.
4 pages Quarterly
Lorraine Marchi LHD, Founder/CEO
Cesar Gomez, Executive Director

9938 NLS News
National Library Service for the Blind

1291 Taylor Street NW   202-707-5100
Washington, DC 20542-0002   Fax: 202-707-0712
                                      TDD: 202-707-0744
                                         nls@loc.gov
                                          www.loc.gov
Newsletter on current program developments.
Quarterly

9939 NLS Update
National Library Service for the Blind
1291 Taylor Street NW   202-707-5100
Washington, DC 20542-0002   Fax: 202-707-0712
                                      TDD: 202-707-0744
                                         nls@loc.gov
                                          www.loc.gov
Newsletter on the services volunteer activities.
Quarterly

9940 NOAH News
National Organization for Albinism
PO Box 959   603-887-2310
E. Hampsted, NH 03826-0959   800-473-2310
                                      Fax: 800-648-2310
                                      info@albinism.org
                                       www.albinism.org
NOAH serves the albinism community by providing information
and support. NOAH is a not-for-profit corporation chartered in
Pennsylvania
BiAnnually

9941 Newsline for the Blind
National Federation of the Blind
200 East Wells Street   410-659-9314
Baltimore, MD 21230-4998   Fax: 410-685-5653
                                         nfb@nfb.org
                                          www.nfb.org

Nation's only digital talking newspaper service for the blind. Allows the blind to read the full text of leading national and local
newspapers by using a touch-tone telephone. Service is free of
charge and available 24 hours a day, 7 days per week.
Mark Riccobono, President
James Gashel, Secretary

9942 Open Windows
Sunday School Board of the Southern Baptists
127 9th Avenue N   800-458-2772
Nashville, TN 37234-0001
Guide for personal devotions on audio cassette tape, using Bible
references, devotional readings, and prayer calendar of popular
Open Windows devotional guide for visually handicapped adults.
Quarterly

9943 Personal Reader Update
Personal Reader Department
9 Centennial Drive   978-977-2000
Peabody, MA 01960-7906   800-343-0311
                                      Fax: 978-977-2437
Offers information on new services, assistive devices and technol-
ogy for the blind.

9944 Prevent Blindness America News
Prevent Blindness America
211 West Wacker Drive   847-843-2020
Chicago, IL 60606   800-331-2020
                                   www.preventblindness.org
Offers information and articles on eye safety, programs, and ser-
vices of the Society.
Quarterly
Parry Hugh, President & CEO
Bilazer Arzu, Creative Director

9945 RP Messenger
Texas Association of Retinitis Pigmentosa
PO Box 8388   361-852-8515
Corpus Christi, TX 78468-8388   Fax: 361-852-8515
A bi-annual newsletter offering information on Retinitis
Pigmentosa.
BiAnnual

9946 Raised Dot Computing Newsletter
Raised Dot Computing
211 S Paterson Street 608-257-9595
Madison, WI 53703-3789
Discusses braille computer techniques and devices for blind persons.

9947 SCENE
Braille Institute
741 N Vermont Avenue 213-663-1111
Los Angeles, CA 90029-3594 800-272-4553
Fax: 323-663-0867
la@brailleinstitute.org
www.brailleinstitute.org
Offers information on the organization, question and answer column, articles on the newest technology and more for visually impaired persons.
Peter A. Mindnich, President
Paul J Porelli, Managing Editor

9948 Smith-Kettlewell Technical File
Smith-Kettlewell Eye Research Foundation
2318 Fillmore Street 415-345-2125
San Francisco, CA 94115-1821 Fax: 415-561-1610
www-test.ski.org/Rehab/sktf/
The Rehabilitation Engineering Research Center published the Smith-Kettlewell Technical File, a quarterly newsletter, in braille, large print, and recorded form, to serve as a guide to the current technology as applied to the needs of blind and low vision people, both electronics professionals and hobbyists. A survey of readers showed that this narrowed the existing gaps and allowed technically-minded visually impaired people to pursue their interests.
Quarterly

9949 Student Advocate
National Alliance of Blind Students
1155 15th Street NW 202-467-5081
Washington, DC 20005 800-424-8666
president@acbstudents.org
A communication forum covering issues of concern to postsecondary students who are blind.

Cammie Vloedman, President
Olivia Norman, First Vice President

9950 Talking Book Topics
National Library Services For The Blind
1291 Taylor Street NW 202-707-5100
Washington, DC 20542-0002 Fax: 202-707-0712
TDD: 202-707-0744
nls@loc.gov
www.loc.gov
Offers hundreds of listings of books, fiction and nonfiction, for adults and children on cassette. Also offers listings on foreign language books on cassette, talking magazines and reviews.
Bimonthly

9951 Tarheel Talk
North Carolina Library for the Blind
1841 Capital Boulevard 919-733-4376
Raleigh, NC 27635 888-388-2460
Fax: 919-733-6910
TDD: 919-733-1462
nclbph@ncdcr.gov
statelibrary.ncdcr.gov/lbph
Quarterly
Carl Keehn, Director

9952 The Macula Foundation Manhattan Eye, Ear & Throat Hospital
American Macular Degeneration Foundation
P.O. Box 515 413-268-7660
Northampton, MA 01061-0515 888-622-8527
Fax: 212-605-3795
foundation@retinal-research.org
www.macular.org/spotlite.html
Newsletter of the American Macular Degeneration Foundation, a nationwide support group for individuals and their families to ad-

just to the restrictions and changes brought about by macular disease.
Quarterly
Nikolai Stevenson, President
Walter Ross, VP

9953 The Pioneer Projects and Programs Periodic al
TelecomPioneers
1801 California Street 303-571-1200
Denver, CO 80202 800-872-5995
Fax: 303-572-0520
info@pioneersvolunteer.org
We're a dedicated, diverse network of current and retired telecommunications employees across the US and Canada
Monthly
Gloria Pazel, Chairman
Charlene Hill, Executive Director

9954 Viva Vital News
5016 Silk Oak Drive 941-371-2153
Sarasota, FL 34232-5410
Membership service organization offering information for veterans and is an affiliate of the American Council of the Blind.

9955 Voice of Vision
GW Micro
725 Airport N Office Park 802-362-3612
Fort Wayne, IN 46825-4229 Fax: 260-489-2608
sales@aisquared.com
www.gwmicro.com
Offers product reviews, product announcements, tips for making systems or applications more accessible, or explanations of concepts of interest to any computer user or would-be computer user. This association newsletter is available in braille, in large print, on audio cassette and on 3.5 or 5.25 IBM format diskette.
Quarterly

9956 What's Line
Alabama Regional Library for the Blind
6030 Monticello Drive 334-213-3906
Montgomery, AL 36130-6000 800-392-5671
Fax: 334-213-3993
fzaleski@apls.state.al.us
http://statelibrary.alabama.gov
Informational 4 page newsletter in large print. Also available in braille and e-text formats.
4 pages Quarterly
Fara Zaleski, Division
Rebecca Mitchell, Director

Pamphlets

9957 About Children's Vision: Guide for Parents
National Association for Visually Handicapped
111 E 59th St 212-821-9497
New York, NY 10022-6904 800-284-4422
Fax: 212-727-2931
kcampbell@lighthouse.org
lighthouse.org/navh
Offers a better understanding of the normal and possible abnormal development of a childs eyesight.
Lorraine Marchi LHD, Founder/CEO
Cesar Gomez, Executive Director

9958 Age Related Macular Degeneration
National Association for Visually Handicapped
111 E 59th St 212-821-9497
New York, NY 10022-6904 800-284-4422
Fax: 212-727-2931
kcampbell@lighthouse.org
lighthouse.org/navh
Describes various conditions which affect the macular area and how to best maximize the use of residual peripheral vision.
Lorraine Marchi LHD, Founder/CEO
Cesar Gomez, Executive Director

9959 Are You Looking for a Few Good Workers?
AFB Press: American Foundation for the Blind

2 Penn Plaza
New York, NY 10121

212-502-7600
800-232-3044
Fax: 888-545-8331
literacy@afb.net
www.afb.org/store

Helpful pamphlet explores both the importance and the advantage of hiring workers who are blind or visually impaired. Designed for human resource and other professionals responsible for hiring, it answers critical questions about hiring blind or visually impaired applicants. This enlightening guide to employment practices relating to these individuals offers insights on interviewing, job performance, tax incentives for businesses, insurance issues and more.
7 pages Pack of 20
ISBN: 0-891283-60-9
Carl R Augusto, President & CEO
Rick Bozeman, Chief Financial Officer

9960 BVA Bulletin
Blinded Veterans Association
477 H Street NW
Washington, DC 20001-2694

202-371-8880
800-669-7079
Fax: 202-371-8258
bva@bva.org
www.bva.org

The Bulletin informs blinded veterans, their families, and those of the general public with an interest in BVA issues, about the organization. The publication includes current information relating to technology for the blind, legislation affecting blinded veterans, and news about the people who have overcome the challenges of blindness and are doing amazing work in their lives.
32 pages Quarterly
Thomas Miller, Executive Director
Stuart Nelson, Coordinator Public Relations

9961 Books are Fun for Everyone
National Library Service for the Blind
1291 Taylor Street NW
Washington, DC 20542

202-707-5100
Fax: 202-707-0712
TDD: 202-707-0744
nls@loc.gov
www.loc.gov

The mission of this web site is to provide program users, librarians, and the public a wide range of access to NLS publications, program information, and bibliographic data

9962 Braille Alphabet and Numbers
AFB Press: American Foundation for the Blind
2 Penn Plaza
New York, NY 10121

212-502-7600
800-232-3044
Fax: 888-545-8331
literacy@afb.net
www.afb.org/store

Embossed with the braille alphabet and numbers, this 9 x 4 inch display card includes an explanation of braille and a short history of its development.
Pack of 25
ISBN: 0-891281-98-3
Carl R Augusto, President & CEO
Rick Bozeman, Chief Financial Officer

9963 Braille Literacy: Blind Persons, Families, Prof. & Producers of Braille
AFB Press: American Foundation for the Blind
2 Penn Plaza
New York, NY 10121

212-502-7600
800-232-3044
Fax: 888-545-8331
literacy@afb.net
www.afb.org/store

Vigorous defece of the use of braille and an explanation of the importance of positive attitudes toward it that states: Braille is an assertion of equality between blind and sighted persons with respect to written communication. For everyone who uses or teaches braille and is interested in its future.
12 pages Pack of 25
ISBN: 0-891289-28-3
Carl R Augusto, President & CEO
Rick Bozeman, Chief Financial Officer

9964 Braille: An Extraordinary Volunteer Opportunity
National Library Service for the Blind

1291 Taylor Street NW
Washington, DC 20542-0002

202-707-5100
Fax: 202-707-0712
TDD: 202-707-0744
nls@loc.gov
www.loc.gov

The mission of this web site is to provide program users, librarians, and the public a wide range of access to NLS publications, program information, and bibliographic data

9965 Cataracts
National Eye Institute, Information Office
31 Center Drive MSC 2510
Bethesda, MD 20892-2510

301-496-5248
2020@nei.nih.gov
www.nei.nih.gov

As part of the federal government's National Institutes of Health (NIH), the National Eye Institute's mission is to "conduct and support research, training, health information dissemination, and other programs with respect to blinding eye diseases
Paul A. Sieving, Executive Director

9966 Classification of Impaired Vision
National Association for Visually Handicapped
111 E 59th St
New York, NY 10022-6904

212-821-9497
800-284-4422
Fax: 212-727-2931
kcampbell@lighthouse.org
lighthouse.org/navh

Describes various degrees of impaired vision.
Lorraine Marchi LHD, Founder/CEO
Cesar Gomez, Executive Director

9967 Communicating with People Who Have Trouble Hearing & Seeing: A Primer
National Association for Visually Handicapped
111 E 59th St
New York, NY 10022-6904

212-821-9497
800-284-4422
Fax: 212-727-2931
kcampbell@lighthouse.org
lighthouse.org/navh

Line drawings that depict problems for those with both deficiencies.
Lorraine Marchi LHD, Founder/CEO
Cesar Gomez, Executive Director

9968 Dancing Cheek to Cheek
Blind Children's Center
4120 Marathon Street
Los Angeles, CA 90029-3584

213-664-2153
Fax: 213-665-3828

Discusses beginning social, play and language interactions.
33 pages

9969 Diabetes, Vision Impairment and Blindness
AFB Press: American Foundation for the Blind
2 Penn Plaza
New York, NY 10121

212-502-7600
800-232-3044
Fax: 888-545-8331
literacy@afb.net
www.afb.org/store

Presentation of how chronic diabetes affects vision and how diabetes can be managed at home by blind and visually impaired individuals.
32 pages
ISBN: 0-891289-02-0
Carl R Augusto, President & CEO
Rick Bozeman, Chief Financial Officer

9970 Diabetic Retinopathy
National Association for Visually Handicapped
111 E 59th St
New York, NY 10022-6904

212-821-9497
800-284-4422
Fax: 212-727-2931
kcampbell@lighthouse.org
lighthouse.org/navh

Describes types of this disease and methods of treatment.
Lorraine Marchi LHD, Founder/CEO
Cesar Gomez, Executive Director

9971 Directory of Radio Reading Services
Radio Information Service

600 Forbes Avenue
Pittsburgh, PA 15282

412-488-3944
Fax: 412-488-3953
info@readingservice.org
www.readingservice.org

Annually

9972 Don't Lose Sight of Age-Related Macular Degeneration
National Eye Institute, Information Office
31 Center Drive MSC 2510
Bethesda, MD 20892-2510

301-496-5248
2020@nei.nih.gov
www.nei.nih.gov

As part of the federal government's National Institutes of Health (NIH), the National Eye Institute's mission is to conduct and support research, training, health information dissemination, and other programs with respect to blinding eye diseases
Paul A. Sieving, Executive Director

9973 Don't Lose Sight of Cataracts
National Eye Institute, Information Office
31 Center Drive MSC 2510
Bethesda, MD 20892-2510

301-496-5248
2020@nei.nih.gov
www.nei.nih.gov

As part of the federal government's National Institutes of Health (NIH), the National Eye Institute's mission is to conduct and support research, training, health information dissemination, and other programs with respect to blinding eye diseases
Paul A. Sieving, Executive Director

9974 Don't Lose Sight of Glaucoma
National Eye Institute, Information Office
31 Center Drive MSC 2510
Bethesda, MD 20892-2510

301-496-5248
2020@nei.nih.gov
www.nei.nih.gov

As part of the federal government's National Institutes of Health (NIH), the National Eye Institute's mission is to conduct and support research, training, health information dissemination, and other programs with respect to blinding eye diseases
Paul A. Sieving, Executive Director

9975 Eye-Q Test
National Association for Visually Handicapped
111 E 59th St
New York, NY 10022-6904

212-821-9497
800-284-4422
Fax: 212-727-2931
kcampbell@lighthouse.org
lighthouse.org/navh

Five questions and answers to assist in knowing more about vision.
Lorraine Marchi LHD, Founder/CEO
Cesar Gomez, Executive Director

9976 Facts: Books for Blind and Physically Handicapped Individuals
National Library Service for the Blind
101 Independence Ave, SE
Washington, DC 20540-0002

202-707-5000
Fax: 202-707-0712
www.loc.gov

The Library of Congress is the nation's oldest federal cultural institution and serves as the research arm of Congress. It is also the largest library in the world, with millions of books, recordings, photographs, maps and manuscripts in its collections.
Annual
James H. Billington, Librarian

9977 Facts: Music for Blind and Physically Handicapped Individuals
National Library Service for the Blind
101 Independence Ave, SE
Washington, DC 20540-0002

202-707-5000
Fax: 202-707-0712
www.loc.gov

The Library of Congress is the nation's oldest federal cultural institution and serves as the research arm of Congress. It is also the largest library in the world, with millions of books, recordings, photographs, maps and manuscripts in its collections.
Annual
James H. Billington, Librarian

9978 Facts: Playback Machines and Accessories Provided on Free Loan
National Library Service for the Blind
101 Independence Ave, SE
Washington, DC 20540-0002

202-707-5000
Fax: 202-707-0712
www.loc.gov

The Library of Congress is the nation's oldest federal cultural institution and serves as the research arm of Congress. It is also the largest library in the world, with millions of books, recordings, photographs, maps and manuscripts in its collections.
James H. Billington, Librarian

9979 Facts: Sources for Purchase of Cassette & Disc Players From NLS
National Library Service for the Blind
101 Independence Ave, SE
Washington, DC 20540-0002

202-707-5000
Fax: 202-707-0712
www.loc.gov

The Library of Congress is the nation's oldest federal cultural institution and serves as the research arm of Congress. It is also the largest library in the world, with millions of books, recordings, photographs, maps and manuscripts in its collections.
James H. Billington, Librarian

9980 Family Guide to Vision Care
American Optometric Association
243 N Lindbergh Boulevard
Saint Louis, MO 63141-7881

314-991-4100
Fax: 314-991-4101
www.aoanet.org

Offers information on the early developmental years of your vision, finding a family optometrist and how to take care of your eyesight through the learning years, the working years and the mature years.

9981 Family Guide: Growth & Development of the Partially Seeing Child
National Association for Visually Handicapped
111 E 59th St
New York, NY 10022-6904

212-821-9497
800-284-4422
Fax: 212-727-2931
kcampbell@lighthouse.org
lighthouse.org/navh

Offers information for parents and guidelines in raising a partially seeing child.
Lorraine Marchi LHD, Founder/CEO
Cesar Gomez, Executive Director

9982 General Facts and Figures on Blindness
National Society to Prevent Blindness
500 Remington Road
Schaumburg, IL 60173-5624

800-331-2020

9983 General Interest Catalog
National Braille Association
3 Townline Circle
Rochester, NY 14623-2537

716-427-8260

Lists hundreds of titles of fiction and non-fiction books offered in large print, braille or on cassette to visually impaired readers.
19 pages

9984 Glaucoma
Foundation For Glaucoma Research
490 Post Street
San Francisco, CA 94102-1409

415-986-3162

Offers information on what glaucoma is, the causes, treatments, types of glaucoma, eye exams and prevention.

9985 Glaucoma: Sneak Thief of Sight
National Association for Visually Handicapped
111 E 59th St
New York, NY 10022-6904

212-821-9497
800-284-4422
Fax: 212-727-2931
kcampbell@lighthouse.org
lighthouse.org/navh

A pamphlet describing the disease, treatment and medications.
Lorraine Marchi LHD, Founder/CEO
Cesar Gomez, Executive Director

9986 Guide Dog Foundation Flyer
Guide Dog Foundation for the Blind
371 E Jericho Turnpike
Smithtown, NY 11787-2976

631-930-9000
800-548-4337
Fax: 631-930-9009
info@guidedog.org
www.guidedog.org

Offers information on the programs and services provided by the foundation.
James C. Bingham, Chair
Alphonce J. Brown, Vice Chair

9987 Guidelines for Comprehensive Low Vision Care
National Association for Visually Handicapped
111 E 59th St
New York, NY 10022-6904
212-821-9497
800-284-4422
Fax: 212-727-2931
lighthouse.org/navh
A description of the proper method to conduct a low vision evaluation.
Lorraine Marchi LHD, Founder/CEO
Cesar Gomez, Executive Director

9988 Guidelines for Helping Deaf/Blind Persons
Helen Keller National Center for Deaf/Blind
141 Middle Neck Road
Sands Point, NY 11050-1299
516-944-8900
Fax: 516-944-7302
TTY: 516-944-8637
www.hknc.org
The mission of the Helen Keller National Center for Deaf-Blind Youths and Adults is to enable each person who is deaf-blind to live and work in his or her community of choice.
Joseph McNulty, Executive Director

9989 Heart to Heart
Blind Children's Center
4120 Marathon Street
Los Angeles, CA 90029-3584
213-664-2153
Fax: 213-665-3828
Parents of blind and partially sighted children talk about their feelings.
12 pages

9990 Heartbreak of Being a Little Bit Blind
National Association for Visually Handicapped
111 E 59th St
New York, NY 10022-6904
212-821-9497
Fax: 212-727-2931
nvah@navh.org
lighthouse.org/navh
Summary of what it means to have impaired vision with illustrations. Free for members.
Lorraine Marchi LHD, Founder/CEO
Cesar Gomez, Executive Director

9991 Helen Keller
AFB Press: American Foundation for the Blind
2 Penn Plaza
New York, NY 10121
212-502-7600
800-232-3044
Fax: 888-545-8331
www.afb.org/store
Brief biography that focuses on the major events of Helen Keller's life, from her birth in Tuscumbia, Alabama on June 27, 1880 to her death in Connecticut on June 1, 1968.
6 pages Pack of 25
ISBN: 0-891282-03-3

9992 How Does a Blind Person Get Around?
AFB Press: American Foundation for the Blind
2 Penn Plaza
New York, NY 10121
212-502-7600
800-232-3044
Fax: 888-545-8331
www.afb.org/store
Offers information on daily living as a blind person.

9993 How to Develop a Self-Help Group for Elders Losing Eyesight
National Association for Visually Handicapped
111 E 59th St
New York, NY 10022-6904
212-821-9497
Fax: 212-727-2931
navh@navh.org
lighthouse.org/navh
The pioneer for development of self-help groups, using the NAVH model, this publication is designed to help start and facilitate self-help groups.
Lorraine Marchi LHD, Founder/CEO
Cesar Gomez, Executive Director

9994 How to Use Your Low Vision Glasses
National Association for Visually Handicapped

111 E 59th St
New York, NY 10022-6904
212-821-9497
Fax: 212-727-2931
navh@navh.org
lighthouse.org/navh
A line drawing showing the correct way to benefit from low vision glasses.
Lorraine Marchi LHD, Founder/CEO
Cesar Gomez, Executive Director

9995 Information on Glaucoma
Foundation for Glaucoma Research
251 Post Street
San Francisco, CA 94108-1409
415-986-3162
800-826-6693
question@glaucoma.org
www.glaucoma.org

9996 Information on Macular Degeneration
American Council of the Blind
2200 Wilson Boulevard
Arlington, VA 22201-2706
202-467-5081
800-424-8666
Fax: 202-467-5085
info@acb.org
www.acb.org
Melanie Brunson, Executive Director

9997 It's All Right to Be Angry
National Association for Visually Handicapped
111 E 59th St
New York, NY 10022-6904
212-821-9497
Fax: 212-727-2931
navh@navh.org
lighthouse.org/navh
A helpful pamphlet describing reactions to learning to live with vision impairment.
Lorraine Marchi LHD, Founder/CEO
Cesar Gomez, Executive Director

9998 Large Print Loan Library Catalog
National Association for Visually Handicapped
111 E 59th St
New York, NY 10022-6904
212-821-9497
Fax: 212-727-2931
navh@navh.org
lighthouse.org/navh
Listing of over 9,000 commercially published and NAVH large print books available through NAVH on a loan basis. Includes a limited selection of titles available for purchase.
Lorraine Marchi LHD, Founder/CEO
Cesar Gomez, Executive Director

9999 Learning to Play
Blind Children's Center
4120 Marathon Street
Los Angeles, CA 90029-3584
213-664-2153
Fax: 323-665-3828
www.blindchildrenscenter.org/index.php
Discusses how to present play activities to the visually impaired preschool child.
12 pages
Susan L. Recchia, M.A., Author

10000 Let's Eat
Blind Children's Center
4120 Marathon Street
Los Angeles, CA 90029-3584
213-664-2153
Fax: 323-665-3828
www.blindchildrenscenter.org/index.php
Teaches competent feeding skills to children with visual impairments.
28 pages
Jill Brody, M.A., O.T.R., Co-Author
Lynne Webber, Co-Author

10001 Low Vision Questions and Answers
AFB Press: American Foundation for the Blind
2 Penn Plaza
New York, NY 10121
212-502-7600
800-232-3044
Fax: 888-545-8331
www.afb.org/store
What does low vision mean? What do low vision services cost? What diseases cause low vision? Answers to these and other questions are presented in a straightfoward yet comprehensive format.

Photographs show how objects appear to people with low vision, what low vision devices look like, and how they are used.
21 pages Pack of 25
ISBN: 0-891281-96-7

10002 Magnifier
Macular Degeneration Foundation
P.O. Box 531313   702-450-2908
Henderson, NV 89053-0752   888-633-3937
liz@eyesight.org
www.eyesight.org

Large-font publication.

10003 Magnifier Highlights
Independent Living Aids
137 Rano Rd   800-537-2118
Buffalo, NY 14207-2341   Fax: 516-937-3906
indlivaids@aol.com
www.independentliving.com
Full line of magnifiers, ranging from high-powered vision aids to instruments and accessories
Marvin Sandler, President

10004 Move with Me
Blind Children's Center
4120 Marathon Street   213-664-2153
Los Angeles, CA 90029-3584   Fax: 323-665-3828
www.blindchildrenscenter.org/index.php
A parent's guide to movement development for visually impaired babies.
12 pages
Doris Hug, M.S., R.P.T., Co-Author
Nancy Chernus-Mansfield, M.A., Co-Author

10005 Music Is for Everyone
National Library Service for the Blind
1291 Taylor Street NW   202-707-5100
Washington, DC 20542-0002   Fax: 202-707-0712
nls@loc.gov
www.loc.gov/nls

10006 Parenting Preschoolers: Raising Young Blind & Visually Impaired Child
AFB Press: American Foundation for the Blind
2 Penn Plaza   212-502-7600
New York, NY 10121   800-232-3044
Fax: 888-545-8331
www.afb.org/store
Why is my baby so quiet? Why does my child seem slower than other children? What will happen when my child goes to school? This primer provides practical answers to the questions most frequently asked by parents and gives advice on what to expect, how to adapt to the child's situation and needs, and what to look for in early education programs.
28 pages Pack of 25
ISBN: 0-891289-98-4

10007 Patient's Guide to Visual Aids and Illumination
National Association for Visually Handicapped
111 E 59th St   212-821-9497
New York, NY 10022-6904   Fax: 212-727-2931
navh@navh.org
lighthouse.org/navh
A reference booklet offering information on aids for the visually impaired.
Lorraine Marchi LHD, Founder/CEO
Cesar Gomez, Executive Director

10008 Puppy Walker Brochure
Guide Dog Foundation for the Blind
371 E Jericho Turnpike   631-930-9000
Smithtown, NY 11787-2976   800-548-4337
Fax: 631-930-9009
info@guidedog.org
www.guidedog.org
Offers information on being a volunteer puppy walker family.
Wells B Jones CAE CFRE, CEO
Alphonce J. Brown, Jr., ACFRE, Vice Chair - Development

10009 Reaching, Crawling, Walking-Let's Get Moving
Blind Children's Center

4120 Marathon Street   213-664-2153
Los Angeles, CA 90029-3584   Fax: 323-665-3828
www.blindchildrenscenter.org/index.php
Orientation and mobility for visually impaired preschool children.
24 pages
Susan S. Simmons, Ph.D., Co-Author
Sharon O'Mara Maida, M.Ed., Co-Author

10010 Reading is for Everyone
National Library Service for the Blind
1291 Taylor Street NW   202-707-5100
Washington, DC 20542-0002   Fax: 202-707-0712
nls@loc.gov
www.loc.gov/nls

10011 Reading with Low Vision
National Library Service for the Blind
1291 Taylor Street NW   202-707-5100
Washington, DC 20542-0002   Fax: 202-707-0712
nls@loc.gov
www.loc.gov/nls

10012 Reference and Information Services from NLS
National Library Service for the Blind
1291 Taylor Street NW   202-707-5100
Washington, DC 20542-0002   Fax: 202-707-0712
nls@loc.gov
www.loc.gov/nls

10013 Resource List for Persons with Low Vision
American Council of the Blind
2200 Wilson Boulevard   202-467-5081
Arlington, VA 22201-2706   800-424-8666
Fax: 202-467-5085
info@acb.org
www.acb.org

Melanie Brunson, Executive Director

10014 Seeing Eye to Eye: An Administrator's Guide
AFB Press: American Foundation for the Blind
2 Penn Plaza   212-502-7600
New York, NY 10121   800-232-3044
Fax: 888-545-8331
www.afb.org/store
Visual impairment often has a profound impact on a child's ability to learn language and basic communication concepts. This easy-to-read booklet explains the student's needs and the practical services essential for helping them become literate and successful. An ideal tool for administrators and educators, it includes clear explanations of common terminology, the impact of visual impairment on learning, specialized services for visually impaired students, and in-service training for teachers.
72 pages Pack of 10
ISBN: 0-891283-59-5

10015 Selecting a Program
Blind Children's Center
4120 Marathon Street   213-664-2153
Los Angeles, CA 90029-3584   Fax: 323-665-3828
www.blindchildrenscenter.org/index.php
A guide for parents of infants and preschoolers with visual impairments.
28 pages
Deborah Chen, Ph.D., Co-Author
Mary Ellen McCann, M.A., Co-Author

10016 Standing on My Own Two Feet
Blind Children's Center
4120 Marathon Street   213-664-2153
Los Angeles, CA 90029-3584   Fax: 323-665-3828
www.blindchildrenscenter.org/index.php
A step-by-step guide to designing and constructing simple, individually tailored adaptive mobility devices for preschool-age children who are visually impaired.
36 pages
Lorie Lynn LaPrelle, M.A., Author

10017 Talk to Me
Blind Children's Center

4120 Marathon Street 213-664-2153
Los Angeles, CA 90029-3584 Fax: 323-665-3828
www.blindchildrenscenter.org/index.php
A language guide for parents of deaf children.
11 pages
Nancy Chernus-Mansfield, M.A., Co-Author
Linda Kekelis, M.A., Co-Author

10018 Talk to Me II
Blind Children's Center
4120 Marathon Street 213-664-2153
Los Angeles, CA 90029-3584 Fax: 323-665-3828
www.blindchildrenscenter.org/index.php
A sequel to Talk To Me, available in English and Spanish.
15 pages
Nancy Chernus-Mansfield, M.A., Co-Author
Dori Hayashi, M.A., Co-Author

10019 Talking Books for Senior Adults
National Library Service for the Blind
1291 Taylor Street NW 202-707-5100
Washington, DC 20542-0002 Fax: 202-707-0712
nls@loc.gov
www.loc.gov/nls

10020 Touch the Baby: Blind & Visually Impaired Children as Patients
American Foundation for the Blind
2 Penn Plaza 212-502-7600
New York, NY 10121-2018 800-232-3044
Fax: 888-545-8331
www.afb.org/store
How-to manual for health care professionals working in hospitals, clinics and doctors' offices that teaches the special communication and touch-related techniques needed to prevent blind and visually impaired patients from withdrawing from healthcare staff and the outside world. includes how to talk to infants and how to signal to children that a procedure may cause discomfort.
13 pages Pack of 25
ISBN: 0-891281-97-5

10021 Volunteer at Your Braille and Talking Book Library
National Library Service for the Blind
1291 Taylor Street NW 202-707-5100
Washington, DC 20542-0002 Fax: 202-707-0712
nls@loc.gov
www.loc.gov/nls

Brochure

10022 What Do You Do When You See a Blind Person — and What Don't You Do?
AFB Press: American Foundation for the Blind
2 Penn Plaza 212-502-7600
New York, NY 10121 800-232-3044
Fax: 888-545-8331
www.afb.org/store
Examples of real-life situations that teach sighted persons how to interact effectively with blind persons. Topics covered include how to help someone across the street, how not to distract a guide dog and how to take leave of a blind person.
8 pages Pack of 25
ISBN: 0-891281-95-9

10023 Wings for the Future
American Printing House for the Blind
1839 Frankfort Avenue 502-895-2405
Louisville, KY 40206-3148 800-223-1839
Fax: 502-899-2284
info@ahp.org
www.aph.org
This booklet offers an introduction to the American Printing House For The Blind's programs, services, tools, aids and more.
13 pages

10024 Without Sight and Sound
Helen Keller National Center for Deaf/Blind
141 Middle Neck Road 516-944-8900
Sands Point, NY 11050-1299 Fax: 516-944-7302
TTY: 516-944-8637
hkncinfo@hknc.org
www.hknc.org

Pamphlet offering facts, causes, types and descriptions of deaf/blindness.
Joseph McNulty, Executive Director

10025 You Seem Like a Regular Kid to Me
AFB Press: American Foundation for the Blind
2 Penn Plaza 212-502-7600
New York, NY 10121 800-232-3044
Fax: 888-545-8331
www.afb.org/store
An interview with Jane, a blind child, allows other children to understand what it's like to be blind. Jane explains how she gets around, takes care of herself, does her school work, spends her leisure time and even pays for things when she can't see money. Photographs show Jane engaged in various activities.
16 pages Pack of 25
ISBN: 0-891289-21-6
Chrissy Cowan, M.Ed., Author

Audio & Video

10026 Adult Bible Study
Sunday School Board of the Southern Baptists
127 9th Avenue N 800-458-2772
Nashville, TN 37234-0001
Unabridged Sunday School lessons recorded on audio cassette as printed in Adult Bible Study.
Quarterly

10027 Aging and Vision: Declarations of Independence
AFB Press: American Foundation for the Blind
2 Penn Plaza 212-502-7600
New York, NY 10121 800-232-3044
Fax: 888-545-8331
www.afb.org/store
Very personal look at five older people who have successfully coped with visual impairment and continue to lead active, satisfying lives. Their stories are not only inspirational, they also provide paractical, down-to-earth suggestions for adapting to vision loss later in life.
18 Minutes VHS
ISBN: 0-891282-20-3

10028 Bible Alliance
PO Box 621 941-748-3031
Bradenton, FL 34206-0621 aurora@auroraministries.org
www.auroraministries.org
Offers the Christian bible on cassettes in over 52 languages for those finding it impossible to read small print.

10029 Blindness: A Family Matter
AFB Press: American Foundation for the Blind
2 Penn Plaza 212-502-7600
New York, NY 10121 800-232-3044
Fax: 888-545-8331
www.afb.org/store
Frank exploration of the effects of an individual's visual impairment on other members of the family and how family members can play a positive role in the rehablitation process. Features three families whose success stories provide advice and encouragement, as well as interviews with newly blinded adults currently involved in a rehabilitation program. Also available in PAL.
23 Minutes VHS
ISBN: 0-891282-22-X

10030 Braille Documents
Metrolina Sight Services
P. O. Box 1830 662-323-4999
Starkville, MS 39760-2128 800-336-2232
careministries@bellsouth.net
This production shop creates Braille and large-print documents.

10031 Brief Encounters of the Right Kind: How to Make Your Point in 10 Minutes or Less
AFB Press: American Foundation for the Blind
2 Penn Plaza 212-502-7600
New York, NY 10121 800-232-3044
Fax: 888-545-8331
www.afb.org/store

Humorous and instructional tour through the do's and don'ts of lobbying at the local, state and national levels. Three seasoned lobbyists discuss how professionals, families, consumers and volunteer advocates can use their expert knowledge to influence public policy. A Toolkit for Advocates, the accompanying manual, complements the video by providing a summary of the legislative process and key points on how to meet successfully with legislators.
VHS & PAL
ISBN: 0-891282-83-1

10032 Destination Unlimited
Leader Dog For The Blind
1964 Park Street   306-565-8211
Regina, SK, S4P 3G4,
This is a documentary about Leader-Dog-For-The-Blind Program. The needs of various people and how their dog fulfills their needs are shown. In addition, the overall leader-dog program is reviewed. This training program would be of interest to many teenagers.
Films

10033 Employed Ability: Blind Persons on the Job
AFB Press: American Foundation for the Blind
2 Penn Plaza   212-502-7600
New York, NY 10121   800-232-3044
      Fax: 888-545-8331
      www.afb.org/store
Blind and visually impaired people from a wide variety of occupations talk about career opportunities and their experiences in the workplace. Employers and coworkers are also interviewed and speak openly about supervising and working alongside visually impaired employees.
14 Minutes VHS
ISBN: 0-891282-24-6

10034 Focused On: Importance and Need for Skills
AFB Press: American Foundation for the Blind
2 Penn Plaza   212-502-7600
New York, NY 10121   800-232-3044
      Fax: 888-545-8331
      www.afb.org/store
Provides an overview of the importance of social competence and details the course of social skills development in children in general and in children who are blind or visually impaired in particular. This study guide examines both the development of social skills in general and how this process applies to children who are blind or who have visual impairments.
VHS & PAL
ISBN: 0-891283-25-0

10035 Hand in Hand: It Can Be Done
AFB Press: American Foundation for the Blind
2 Penn Plaza   212-502-7600
New York, NY 10121   800-232-3044
      Fax: 888-545-8331
      www.afb.org/store
One hour introduction to working effectively with individuals who are deaf-blind. Designed as both an overview and a reinforcer of the self-study text, this video can be used as a whole or in sections for parents and regular educators, as well as in the community. Includes a discussion guide. Available in audioscribed or open captioned VHS and PAL.
ISBN: 0-891283-25-0

10036 Heart to Heart
Blind Children's Center
4120 Marathon Street   213-664-2153
Los Angeles, CA 90029-3584   Fax: 323-665-3828
      www.blindchildrenscenter.org/index.php
Parents of blind and partially sighted children talk about their feelings.
Videotape
Nancy Chernus-Mansfield, M.A., Co-Author
Dori Hayashi, M.A., Co-Author

10037 Helen Keller in Her Story
AFB Press: American Foundation for the Blind

2 Penn Plaza   212-502-7600
New York, NY 10121   800-232-3044
      Fax: 888-545-8331
      www.afb.org/store
Patty Duke, who portrayed the young Helen Keller on stage and on screen in The Miracle Worker, introduces this Oscar-winning documentary about the extraordinary lives of Ms. Keller, her teacher Anne Sullivan Macy and her friend and companion Polly Thompson. Includes vintage still photographs as well as early movie footage and newsreel footage.
VHS & PAL
ISBN: 0-891282-25-4
Nancy Hamilton, Author

10038 Let's Eat
Blind Children's Center
4120 Marathon Street   213-664-2153
Los Angeles, CA 90029-3584   Fax: 323-665-3828
      www.blindchildrenscenter.org/index.php
Teaches competent feeding skills to children with visual impairments.
Videotape
Jill Brody, M.A., O.T.R., Co-Author
Lynne Webber, Co-Author

10039 Making the Most of Early Communication: Strategies for Supporting Communication
AFB Press: American Foundation for the Blind
2 Penn Plaza   212-502-7600
New York, NY 10121   800-232-3044
      Fax: 888-545-8331
      www.afb.org/store
Demonstrates selected interventions to assist infants and toddlers with multiple disabilities, including vision and hearing loss, in developing early communication and other skills. Emphasizing the critical importance of early intervention, this video is designed to help service providers and families create effective communication straegies that encourage cognitive development and funtional abilities in young children with multiple disabilities and those who are deaf-blind. 37 minutes.
VHS & PAL
ISBN: 0-891282-96-3
Deborah Chen, Ph.D., Co-Author
Pamela Haag Schachter, MS.Ed., Co-Author

10040 New What Do You Do When You See a Blind Person?
AFB Press: American Foundation for the Blind
2 Penn Plaza   212-502-7600
New York, NY 10121   800-232-3044
      Fax: 888-545-8331
      www.afb.org/store
Engaging remake of the 1971 classic brings a fresh perspective on how to interact comfortably with someone who is visually impaired. The entertaining experiences of Mark Johnson, a computer programmer who is blind, and Dave Simon, a computer salesman who is not, show the simple ways to provide assistance, if it is needed, to someone who is blind or visually impaired. 16 minutes.
VHS & PAL
ISBN: 0-891283-13-7

10041 Oh, I See
AFB Press: American Foundation for the Blind
2 Penn Plaza   212-502-7600
New York, NY 10121   800-232-3044
      Fax: 888-545-8331
      www.afb.org/store
Lively and entertaining video provides practical suggestions on helping students who are blind and visually impaired adapt to the mainstream classroom. The modifacations shown can easily be used by teachers, students, or anyone working with blind and visually impaired students. Seven minutes.
VHS & PAL
ISBN: 0-891282-52-1

10042 Out of Left Field
AFB Press: American Foundation for the Blind
2 Penn Plaza   212-502-7600
New York, NY 10121   800-232-3044
      Fax: 888-545-8331
      www.afb.org/store

Illustrates how youngsters who are blind or visually impaired are integrated with their sighted peers in a variety of recreational and athletic activites. 17 minutes.
VHS & PAL
ISBN: 0-891282-28-9

10043 Profiles in Aging and Vision
AFB Press: American Foundation for the Blind
2 Penn Plaza   212-502-7600
New York, NY 10121   800-232-3044
                                                      Fax: 888-545-8331
                                                      www.afb.org/store
Can be used on its own or in conjunction with the text, this is an informative overview of the common eye conditions that affect older people, with a detailed description of the vision-related services that help older people who are visually impaired continue to lead independent lives. Experienced professionals provide valuable information on crucial issues, and older visually impaired persons offering their own revealing perspectives. 33 minutes.
VHS
ISBN: 0-891289-48-8
Alberta L. Orr, MSW, Executive Producer

10044 Reaching Out: A Creative Access Guide for Designing Exhibits & Cultural Programs
AFB Press: American Foundation for the Blind
2 Penn Plaza   212-502-7600
New York, NY 10121   800-232-3044
                                                      Fax: 888-545-8331
                                                      www.afb.org/store
Video and accompanying manual are a creative package for making information on cultural programs and facilities accessable to people who are blind or visually impaired. Created especially for libraries, museums, historical societies, outdoor cultural facilities, corporations and everyone whose mission involves providing information to the community, this video offers practical design and program solutions. 22 minutes.
VHS & PAL
ISBN: 0-891289-49-6
Elga Joffee, Co-Author
May Ann Siller, Co-Author

10045 Seven Minute Lesson
AFB Press: American Foundation for the Blind
2 Penn Plaza   212-502-7600
New York, NY 10121   800-232-3044
                                                      Fax: 888-545-8331
                                                      www.afb.org/store
Introduction to the basic techniques used when acting as a sighted guide for a person who is blind or visually impaired.
VHS & PAL
ISBN: 0-891282-29-7

10046 Solutions for Everyday Living for Older People with Visual Impairments
AFB Press: American Foundation for the Blind
2 Penn Plaza   212-502-7600
New York, NY 10121   800-232-3044
                                                      Fax: 888-545-8331
                                                      www.afb.org/store
Presents a positive and helpful view of how older people who have lost some or all of their vision can continue to lead satisfying lives within supportive environments. This engaing video shows how staff members in continuing care communities and other living settings for older people can help residents function as independently as possible. Different types of vision loss are explained, and simple solutions are offered for carrying out everyday activities. 34 minutes.
VHS & PAL
ISBN: 0-891288-52-X
Priscilla Rogers, Author

10047 Strategies for Community Access: Braille & Raised Large Print Facility Signs
AFB Press: American Foundation for the Blind
2 Penn Plaza   212-502-7600
New York, NY 10121   800-232-3044
                                                      Fax: 888-545-8331
                                                      www.afb.org/store

Brief and effective advocacy tool that can be used to educate architects, planners, facility managers, sign makers and consumers about the value of accessible signs. Topics covered include ADA requirements for accessible signs, samples of signs designed to be compatible with an organization's interior design, demonstrations of how blind and print signs are a cost-effective way to provide access. Reproducible fact sheets on ADA signage guidelines are enclosed. Seven minutes.
VHS & PAL
ISBN: 0-891282-56-4

10048 Understanding Braille Literacy
AFB Press: American Foundation for the Blind
2 Penn Plaza   212-502-7600
New York, NY 10121   800-232-3044
                                                      Fax: 888-545-8331
                                                      www.afb.org/store
Motovational and intructional video covers all aspects of a successful braille education program. Teachers and students demonstate how braille is learned and used from preschool through high school and describes how braille skills contribute to literacy, independence, mastery of academic skills and successful education experiences in the regular classroom. Parents, classroom teachers and school administrators also speak out about the importance of braille. 25 minutes.
VHS & PAL
ISBN: 0-891282-61-0
Diane P. Wormsley, Ph.D., Author

10049 We Can Do it Together: Mobility for Students with Multiple Disabilities
AFB Press: American Foundation for the Blind
2 Penn Plaza   212-502-7600
New York, NY 10121   800-232-3044
                                                      Fax: 888-545-8331
                                                      www.afb.org/store
Illustrates a transdisiplinary team approach to teaching orientation and mobility to students with severe visual and multiple impairments, covering both adapted communication systems that are used to teach mobility skills and basic indoor mobility in the school. For mobility instructors, administrators, teachers of visually impaired and severely disabled students, occupational, physical and speech therapists and parents. Discussion guide included, 13 minutes.
VHS & PAL
ISBN: 0-891282-13-0

10050 What Can Baby See? Vision Tests & Intervention Strategies for Infants
AFB Press: American Foundation for the Blind
2 Penn Plaza   212-502-7600
New York, NY 10121   800-232-3044
                                                      Fax: 888-545-8331
                                                      www.afb.org/store
Presents common vision tests and methods of gathering information that can be used with infants and very young children to help indentify visual impairments that require early intervention services. Effective ways of working with families and early intervention strategies for encouraging infants with multiple disabilities to use their vision in functional ways are demonstrated to help families and service providers contribute to children's growth and development.
VHS & PAL
ISBN: 0-891282-99-8

Web Sites

10051 ACB Government Employees
                                                      www.acb.org
Concerns of the organization include recruitment, placement and advancement of blind and visually impaired employees.

10052 ACB Radio Amateurs
                                                      www.acb.org
A radio amateur network of blind, visually impaired and sighted members who gather and share common problems and solutions to help members improve radio amateurs in getting started, provides access to educational materials in special media and publishes a directory for the visually impaired.

10053 ACB Social Service Providers

www.acb.org

Information on blind and visually impaired social workers, social service professionals, students pursuing careers in social work, and other interested persons.

10054 American Blind Lawyers Association

www.acb.org

Information on law school admission tests and bar exams, private sector and government employment relations and specialized work techniques for the blind and visually impaired.

10055 American Council of Blind Lions

www.acb.org

Information concerning Club activities in the field of work for the blind and encourages blind people to join Lions Clubs and other civic activities.

10056 American Council of the Blind

www.acb.org

Information for the visually impaired and fully sighted individuals who are concerned about the dignity and well-being of blind people throughout America.

10057 American Foundation for the Blind

www.afb.org

Our web site unique in that it combines state-of-the-art features, an attractive visual environment and an accessible design for people with all types of disabilities. Features include a searchable database of vision services nationwide, community message boards and the largest collection of Helen Keller memorbilia on the web. It meets the stringent AAA guidelines of the Web Accessibility Initiative of the World Wide Web Consortium, established to help organizations build accessible websites.

10058 American Printing House for the Blind

www.aph.org

This organization promotes the independence of blind persons by providing special media, tools and materials needed for education and life.

10059 Blinded Veterans Association

www.bva.org

Offers two main service programs without cost to blinded veterans. Field service program provides counseling to veterans and families, and information on benefits and rehabilitation.

10060 Braille Revival League

www.acb.org

Information for people to read and write in braille, advocates for mandatory braille instruction in educational facilities for the blind, strives to make available a supply of braille materials from libraries and printing houses and more.

10061 Council of Families with Visual Impairment

www.acb.org

Offers support and outreach, shares experiences in parent/child relationships, exchanges educational, cultural and medical information about child development and more.

10062 Fidelco Guide Dog Foundation

www.fidelco.org

Fidelco breeds, raises, trains, and places German shepherd guide dogs with men and women who are visually impaired, primarily in the Northeast.

10063 Guide Dog Foundation for the Blind

www.guidedog.org

Furnishes guide dogs, free of charge, to qualified people who seek independence, mobility and companionship.

10064 Guide Dog Users

www.acb.org

Promotes the acceptance of blind people and their dogs, works for enforcement and expansion of laws admitting guide dogs into public places, advocates for quality training and follow-up services.

10065 Healing Well

www.healingwell.com

An online health resource guide to medical news, chat, information and articles, newsgroups and message boards, books, disease-related web sites, medical directories, and more for patients, friends, and family coping with disabling diseases, disorders, or chronic illnesses.

10066 Health Finder

www.healthfinder.gov

Searchable, carefully developed web site offering information on over 1000 topics. Developed by the US Department of Health and Human Services, the site can be used in both English and Spanish.

10067 Healthlink USA

www.healthlinkusa.com

Health information concerning treatment, cures, prevention, diagnosis, risk factors, research, support groups, email lists, personal stories and much more. Updated regularly.

10068 Independent Visually Impaired Enterprises

www.acb.org

Information on rehabilitation facilities for all types of business enterprises and publicizes the capabilities of blind and visually impaired business persons.

10069 Library Users of America

www.acb.org

Provides for chapters in states through the US to encourage the development, acquisition and use of technology which enables blind and visually impaired persons to use printed material independently in library settings and elsewhere.

10070 Lighthouse International

www.lighthouse.org

Offers information about vision impairment and vision rehabilitation, and provides referrals to services and support groups nationwide.

10071 MedicineNet

www.medicinenet.com

An online resource for consumers providing easy-to-read, authoritative medical and health information.

10072 Medscape

www.medscape.com

Medscape offers specialists, primary care physicians, and other health professionals the Web's most robust and integrated medical information and educational tools.

10073 National Alliance of Blind Students

www.acb.org

Works to facilitate progress toward full accessibility of college programs and facilities, provides opportunities for discussion of issues important to students and assists with National Student Seminars.

10074 National Association of Blind Educators

www.nfb.org

Provides support and information regarding professional responsibilities, classroom techniques, national testing methods and career obstacles. Publishes The Blind Educator, national magazine specifically for blind educators.

10075 National Association of Blind Lawyers

www.nfb.org

Provides support and information regarding employment, techniques used by the blind, advocacy, laws affecting the blind, current information about the American Bar Association and other issues for blind lawyers.

10076 National Association of Blind Secretaries and Transcribers

www.nfb.org

Addresses issues such as technology, accomodation, career planning and job training.

10077 National Association of Blind Students

nabslink.org

The mission of the National Association of Blind Students is to promote equal access to educational and life opportunities for the blind.

10078 National Association of Blind Teachers

www.acb.org

Works to advance the teaching profession for blind and visually impaired people, protects the interest of teachers, presents discussions and solutions for special problems encountered by blind teachers and publishes a directory of blind teachers in the US.

10079 National Association of Guide Dog Users

www.nagdu.org

Provides information and support for guide dog users and works to secure high standards in guide dog training. Addresses issues of discrimination of guide dog users and offers public education about guide dog use.

10080 National Association to Promote the Use of Braille

NAPUB exists to promote the use of braille.

10081 National Braille Association

www.nationalbraille.org/

National Braille Association, founded in 1945, is a non-profit organization dedicated to providing continuing education to those who prepare braille, and to providing braille materials to persons who are visually impaired.

10082 National Federation of the Blind: Blind/Deaf Division

www.nfb.org

Offers personal contact with other deaf-blind individuals knowledgeable in advocacy, education, employment, technology, discrimination and other issues surrounding deaf-blindness.

10083 National Federation of the Blind

www.nfb.org

Provides public education about blindness, support services to the newly blinded, scholarships, publications about blindness, adaptive equipment for the blind, advocacy services, Newsline for the Blind, assistive technology information and Job Opportunities for the Blind.

10084 National Federation of the Blind in Computer Science

www.nfb.org

New technologies, to secure access to current technology and to develop new ways of using current or new technologies by the blind.

10085 National Federation of the Blind: Blind Merchants Division

www.nfb.org

Provides information regarding rehabilitation, social security, tax and other issues which directly affect blind merchants. Serves as advocacy and support group.

10086 National Federation of the Blind: Human Services Division

www.nfb.org

Organization of blind persons working in counseling, personnel, psychology, social work, psychiatry, rehabilitation and other social science and human resource fields. Provides resources regarding blindness-related techniques and methods used in these fields.

10087 National Federation of the Blind: Music Division

www.nfb.org

Offers support and information regarding copyright, publishing, promotion and other career details.

10088 National Federation of the Blind: Public Employees Division

www.nfb.org

Focuses on issues such as changes in governmental hiring and retention practices, new job skills needed for the future, government employment downsizing, new electronic means of finding public sector jobs, self-advocacy and career planning strategies.

10089 National Federation of the Blind: Science and Engineering Division

www.nfb.org

This is a strong support group to encourage blind persons in pursuit of these careers, many of which have been considered not possible for the blind in the past.

10090 National Federation of the Blind: Writers Division

www.nfb.org

Covers various aspects of this business, including selling your work, publishing, technology, motivation and discovering writing and publishing resources.

10091 National Library Service for the Blind

www.loc.gov/nls

Administers a national library service that provides braille and recorded books and magazines on free loan to anyone who cannot read standard print because of visual or physical disabilities who are eligible residents of the United States or American citizens living abroad.

10092 National Organization of Parents of Blind Children

www.nfb.org

Addresses issues ranging from help to parents of a newborn blind infant, mobility and Braille instruction, education, social and community participation, development of self-confidence and other vital factors involved in the growth of a blind child.

10093 National Organization of the Senior Blind

www.nfb.org

Provides support and information to other blind seniors. Issues include concerns such as remaining active in community and social life, maintaining private homes or living in retirement communities or nursing homes, learning the techniques used by the blind, independently caring for oneself and maintaining a positive approach to vision loss.

10094 Randolph-Sheppard Vendors of America

www.acb.org

Protects the interests of blind vendors, seeks proper implementation of the Randolph-Sheppard Act and encourages facility locations in more visible and profitable areas.

10095 Visually Impaired Data Processors International

www.acb.org

Provides for the exchange of work technique ideas and works with agencies to increase the availability of braille and recorded materials.

10096 Visually Impaired Piano Tuners International

www.acb.org

Works to preserve, advance and enrich the skilled professional piano tuning for competent, well-trained blind and visually impaired persons.

10097 Visually Impaired Veterans of America

www.acb.org

Promotes the rights of visually impaired veterans to receive all benefits, encourages research and development of new products for blind people.

10098 WebMD

www.webmd.com

Provides credible information, supportive communities, and in-depth reference material about health subjects. A source for original and timely health information as well as material from well known content providers.

Description

10099 War Syndromes

War syndromes have plagued soldiers for centuries. Though symptoms may vary, soldiers may become affected by various postulated physiological diseases as well as psychological illnesses. Agent Orange and the Gulf War Syndrome are two of the conditions still prevalent today.

Agent Orange is the common name for a mix of chemicals developed by the military during the Vietnam War to destroy vegetation that concealed the enemy. During the war, some soldiers were exposed heavily to this chemical; years later, many of them contracted a variety of conditions. There has been an intense controversy about whether Agent Orange caused these conditions, with medical scientists, patients, politicians and advocacy groups all involved.

Among the conditions sometimes attributed to Agent Orange exposure are a variety of cancers, an acne-like skin condition called chloracne, neurological diseases, repeated infections, sterility, and birth defects in the children of exposed persons.

To further understand this condition, the Department of Veterans Affairs has been established a registry of Vietnam veterans concerned that they may have been exposed to Agent Orange. Veterans who suspect their symptoms are related to this exposure can contact the Department's Medical Administrative Services to request the Agent Orange Registry Examination, a complete health evaluation. The Department offers service-connected compensation for those veterans who develop a condition believed to be related to exposure to Agent Orange.

Gulf War Syndrome, GWS, or Persian Gulf War Syndrome is a constellation of illnesses experienced by 5,000 to 80,000 US veterans after returning from the Persian Gulf Wars in the 1990's and 2000's. Symptoms are predominately neurologic and consist of impaired cognition, with problems of attention, memory, reasoning, insomnia, depression and headaches. Complaints of muscle and joint pain, gastrointestinal difficulties, vertigo and weakness are also common. As veterans resumed family life, various birth defects were added to the list. The cause of GWS is unknown.

A 1997 study funded by the Centers for Disease Control shows that Gulf War personnel are more likely than others to report depression, symptoms similar to post-traumatic stress disorder, chronic fatigue, cognitive difficulties, bronchitis, asthma, fibromyalgia, alcohol abuse, anxiety and sexual dysfunction.

Many causes of GWS have been suggested, but none have been definitely identified or eliminated. These include: effects of chemical and/or biological weapons; exposure to pesticides; smoke from oil well fires; airborne contamination from munitions plants destroyed in Iraq, exposure to depleted uranium used as a material in some US munitions and exposure to volatile solvents used in the normal course of equipment maintenance. None of these exposures have been convincingly linked to a cause of the illness.

Given the range of reported GWS effects, treatment is highly individualized and symptomatic. A number of specialized support groups and websites have been established by members of the Persian Gulf War Community.

National Agencies & Associations

10100 Agent Orange Registry Department of Veterans Affairs

Department of Veterans Affairs Headquarters
810 Vermont Avenue NW   877-222-8387
Washington, DC 20420   800-827-1000
    TTY: 800-829-4833
    www.publichealth.va.gov

A resource for veterans who have been exposed to chemical herbicides which might be causing a variety of ill effects. Contains information on exposure locations, available benefits, research studies on Agent Orange, and more. Services available to any eligible veteran who had active military service.
Robert Wilkie, Acting Secretary
James Byrne, Acting Deputy Secretary

10101 Centers for Disease Control

1600 Clifton Road   800-232-4636
Atlanta, GA 30329-4027   TTY: 888-232-6348
    cdcinfo@cdc.gov
    www.cdc.gov

Offers reprints from the CDC Health Status of Vietnam veterans and the Journal of the American Medical Association. Also offers reports from the Centers for Disease Control Vietnam Experience Study, which was a multidimensional assessment of the health of Vietnam War veterans. Contains survey results of Gulf War veterans, and background information on the health concerns of veterans, symptoms, and related diagnoses, as well as documentation on hospitalizations.
Sherri A. Berger, MSPH, Chief Operating Officer
Robert R. Redfield, MD, Director

10102 Goodwill Industries International, Inc.

15810 Indianola Drive   800-466-3945
Rockville, MD 20855   contactus@goodwill.org
    www.goodwill.org

A nonprofit, community-based organization whose mission is to help people achieve self-sufficiency through the dignity and power of work, serving people who are disadvantaged, disabled or elderly. The mission is accomplished through providing independent living skills, affordable housing, and training and placement in community employment. The GoodWill Network includes 160 independent, local locations across the U.S. and Canada.
S. Dale Jenkins, Chair
Steven C. Preston, President & CEO

10103 HonorBound Foundation

PO Box 2465   800-521-0198
Darien, CT 06820   www.honorboundfoundation.org

Previously known as the National Veterans Services Fund, the HonorBound Foundation has expanded their support to all veterans in need. HonorBound provides support to those who were exposed to the defoliant Agent Orange while serving the US in the conflict in Vietnam by providing medical and financial assistance to veterans.Veterans are assisted by social workers, who ensure that veterans are better able to navigate the VA system.

Phil Kraft, Executive Director
Cathie Greene, Vice President & Secretary

10104 VA Austin Information Technology Center
1615 E Woodward Street
Austin, TX 78772-0001
512-389-5380
webmaster@va.gov
www.oit.va.gov

Helps veterans register after receiving the Agent Orange examination through the Veterans Affairs Department.

State Agencies & Associations

Alabama

10105 Gulf War Veterans of Alabama
2344 Glendale Avenue
Montgomery, AL 36107
205-265-7723
Don Reeves
Shannon Reeves

10106 Veterans Administration Medical Center: Alabama
3701 Loop Road E
Tuscaloosa, AL 35404
205-554-2000
888-651-2685
Fax: 205-554-2034
TTY: 711
www.tuscaloosa.va.gov

The Tuscaloosa VA Medical Center (TVAMC) is located in West Alabama. The medical center provides primary and long-term healthcare to eligible veterans in the VA Southeast Network. Mental health services are also provided.

John F. Merkle, FACHE, Director
Amir Farooqi, FACHE, Associate Director

10107 Veterans Association Medical Center
700 S 19th Street
Birmingham, AL 35233-1927
205-933-8101
866-487-4243
Fax: 205-933-4484
TTY: 711
www.birmingham.va.gov

The Birmingham VA Medical Center provides acute tertiary care for eligible veterans in the VA Southeast Network.The medical centre provides a wide range of medical care, and is also a referral center for veterans and their beneficiaries.

Stacy J. Vasquez, Director
Mary Mitchell, Associate Director

Alaska

10108 Alaska VA Healthcare System
1201 N Muldoon Road
Anchorage, AK 99504
907-257-4700
888-353-7574
Fax: 907-257-6774
www.alaska.va.gov

The Alaska VA Healthcare System provides primary healthcare services to veterans. The facility offers specialty care, as well as mental health outpatient care. The facility has a partnership with the United States Air Force at Elmendorf Base, and provides assistance to homeless veterans, and those undergoing therapy.

Timothy Ballard, MD, MS, Director
Thomas A. Steinbrunner, FACHE, Associate Director

Arizona

10109 Phoenix VA Health Care System
Phoenix VA Health Care System
650 E Indian School Road
Phoenix, AZ 85012-1892
602-277-5551
800-554-7174
TTY: 711
www.phoenix.va.gov

The Phoenix VA Health Care System serves veterans at its main medical center in central Arizona. In addition, the Phoenix VA Health Care System has nine outpatient clinics for veterans. The Phoenix VA Health Care System offers community-based, patient-focused care with their PACT system, Patient Aligned Care

Team; ensuring that communication between patient and health care providers is uncomplicated.

RimaAnn Nelson, Director
Shawn Bransky, Deputy Director

10110 Southern Arizona VA Health Care System
Southern Arizona VA Health Care System
3601 S 6th Avenue
Tucson, AZ 85723
520-792-1450
800-470-8262
Fax: 520-629-1820
www.tucson.va.gov

The Southern Arizona VA Health Care System located in Tucson, Arizona, serves eligible veterans across seven counties in Southern Arizona, and one county in New Mexico. The Southern Arizona VA Health Care System offers specialized treatment programs to serve veterans.

William J. Caron, FACHE, Director
Katie A. Landwehr,MBA, FACHE, Associate Director

Arkansas

10111 Eugene J. Towbin Healthcare Center Central Arkansas VA Healthcare System
Eugene J. Towbin Healthcare Center
2200 Fort Roots Drive
North Little Rock, AR 72114-1706
501-257-1000
800-224-8387
TTY: 711
www.littlerock.va.gov

The Eugene J. Towbin Healthcare Center operates within the Central Arkansas VA Healthcare System. Located in North Little Rock and Little Rock (John L. McClellan Memorial Veterans Hospital), the Healthcare Center is able to address a large variety of health concerns for eligible veterans, offering community-based care through eight outpatient clinics.

Margie A. Scott, MD, Director
Cyril O. Ekeh, MHA, VHA-CM, Associate Director

10112 Gulf War Veterans of Arkansas
11127 Eglia Valley Drive
Little Rock, AR 72212
501-225-9437
Lydia Pace

California

10113 California Association of Persian Gulf Veterans
PO Box 3661
Santa Cruz, CA 95063
408-476-6684
Fax: 415-227-0848
CAGulfVets@aol.com
Erika Lundholm

10114 Northern California Association of Persian Gulf Veterans
9141 E Stockton Boulevard
Elk Grove, CA 95624
916-684-1693
Fax: 916-684-1693
NCAPGV@aol.com
Debbie Judd

10115 Sacramento Veterans Center
1111 Howe Avenue
Sacramento, CA 95825
916-566-7430
877-927-8387
Fax: 916-566-7433
Sandra Moreno, Acting Director
Albert Revives, Outreach Specialist

10116 San Francisco VA Medical Center
4150 Clement Street
San Francisco, CA 94121
415-221-4810
877-487-2838
www.sanfrancisco.va.gov

The San Francisco VA Health Care System provides health care to veterans through the San Francisco VA Medical Center, as well as through six outpatient clinics based in the community. The San Francisco VA Health Care System conducts research, and develops treatment programs aimed at improving the health of eligible veterans.

Bonnie S. Graham, MBA, Director
Jia F. Li, MBA, Associate Director

10117 VA Central California Health Care System
2615 E Clinton Avenue
Fresno, CA 93703
559-225-6100
888-826-2838
www.fresno.va.gov

The VA Central California Health Care System provides general and acute care to its patients. The VA Central California Health Care System serves veterans located in six counties in the San Joaquin Valley, and currently operates three outpatient clinics.
Charles Benninger, Acting Director
Demitric Franklin, Associate Director

10118 VA Greater Los Angeles Healthcare System
11301 Wilshire Boulevard   310-478-3711
Los Angeles, CA 90073   877-252-4866
    TTY: 711
    www.losangeles.va.gov
The VA Greater Los Angeles Healthcare System is comprised of three main centers; the West Los Angeles Medical Center, the Sepulveda Ambulatory Care Center, and the Los Angeles Ambulatory Care Center. The VA Greater Los Angeles Healthcare System is responsible for providing care to veterans located in five counties: Los Angeles, Ventura, Kern, Santa Barbara, and San Luis Obispo.
Ann Brown, FACHE, Director
Robert W. McKenrick, Executive Director

10119 VA Loma Linda Healthcare System
11201 Benton Street   909-825-7084
Loma Linda, CA 92357   800-741-8387
    Fax: 909-422-3106
    TTY: 711
    www.lomalinda.va.gov
The VA Loma Linda Healthcare System serves veterans within the San Bernardino and Riverside 2-county area. The main medical center is located in Loma Linda, where veterans are cared for.
Karandeep Sraon, MBA, FACHE, Director
Shane M. Elliott, MBA, Associate Director

10120 VA Northern California Health Care System
10535 Hospital Way   916-843-7000
Mather, CA 95655   844-698-2311
    www.northerncalifornia.va.gov
The VA Northern California Health Care System offers health care services to veterans in the form of general medical care, surgery, rehabilitative care, and mental health care. The VA Northern California Health Care System achives these goals through one medical center in Sacramento, one outpatient clinic in Martinez, and seven other outpatient clinics.
David Stockwell, Director
Timothy Graham, Associate Director

10121 VA Palo Alto Health Care System
3801 Miranda Avenue   650-493-5000
Palo Alto, CA 94304   800-455-0057
    Fax: 925-449-6522
    TTY: 711
The VA Palo Alto Health Care System provides care to veterans through three inpatient centers located at Palo Alto, Menlo Park, and Livermore, with seven outpatient clinics in San Jose, Fremont, Capitola, Monterey, Stockton, Modesto, and Sonora. The VA Palo Alto Health Care System offers engaged and extensive health care to all eligible veterans.
Thomas J. Fitzgerald III, CHESP, Director
Daniel Kulenich, Deputy Director

Colorado

10122 VA Western Colorado Health Care System
2121 N Avenue   970-242-0731
Grand Junction, CO 81501   866-206-6415
    www.grandjunction.va.gov
The VA Western Colorado Health Care System provides veterans with primary and secondary care, acute care, surgery, and psychiatric care. The main medical center is located in Grand Junction, with one community-based outpatient clinic, and one telehealth outreach clinic.
Michael T. Kilmer, Director
Srinivas Ginjupalli, Chief of Staff

Delaware

10123 Wilmington VA Medical Center
1601 Kirkwood Highway   302-994-2511
Wilmington, DE 19805   800-461-8262
    www.wilmington.va.gov
The Wilmington VA Medical Center offers eligible veterans a wide range of health services, from preventative care to long-term care. The Wilmington VA Medical Center overlooks community-based outpatient clinics which operate in Delaware.
Vince Kane, Director
George Tzanis, Chief of Staff

District of Columbia

10124 Disabled American Veterans Organization
807 Maine Avenue SW   202-554-3501
Washington, DC 20024   www.dav.org
The Disabled American Veterans Organization (DAV) is a non-profit charity that guides veterans as they transition back to civilian life. The DAV helps veterans navigate the VA health care system, and assists veterans in accessing their benefits through legislative work. The DAV is an advocate for veterans, and expands their assistance to veterans through the establishment of voluntary community programs.
Dennis R. Nixon, National Commander
J. Marc Burgess, National Adjutant

10125 US Department Of Veterans Affairs
810 Vermont Avenue NW   202-273-5400
Washington, DC 20420   844-698-2311
    TTY: 711
    www.va.gov
Provides a wide range of services for those who have been in the military and their dependents as well as offering information on driver assessment and education programs. Health care and disability records can be created and accessed. The US Department of Veterans Affairs has a complete directory of VA locations listed for veterans.
Robert Wilkie, Secretary of Veterans Affairs
James Byrne, Deputy Secretary

10126 Washington DC VA Medical Center
50 Irving Street NW   202-745-8000
Washington, DC 20422   877-328-2621
    Fax: 202-754-8530
    www.washingtondc.va.gov
Veterans can acquire a great variety of health care services at the Washington DC VA Medical Center, which serves veterans of the national capital area. The Medical Center oversees a Community Resource and Referral Center for homeless and at-risk veterans, which operates 24 hours a day, 7 days a week.
Michael S. Heimall, Director
Christopher J. Irwin, Associate Director

Florida

10127 Bay Pines VA Healthcare System
10000 Bay Pines Boulevard   727-398-6661
Bay Pines, FL 33744   888-820-0230
    Fax: 727-398-9442
    www.baypines.va.gov
Provides health care services to eligible veterans within ten counties in central southwest Florida. Also offers a telehealth service, so that veterans can access health care at their convenience.
Paul M. Russo, FACHE, RD, Director & CEO
Kristine Brown, MPH, Associate Director

10128 Desert Storm Justice Foundation: Florida
10 Marlow Road   813-635-3261
Frostproof, FL 33843-9321   Fax: 813-635-3261
    BillCarpenter@cjewel.com

William Carpenter

10129 Desert Storm Veterans of Florida, Inc.
PO Box 6081   407-269-3453
Titusville, FL 32782   PersianVet@aol.com
Kevin Knight

10130 Goodwill Industries-Suncoast
10596 Gandy Boulevard 727-523-1512
St. Petersburg, FL 33702 888-279-1988
TTY: 727-579-1068
www.goodwill-suncoast.org
A nonprofit, community-based organization whose mission is to help people achieve self-sufficiency through the dignity and power of work, serving people who are disadvantaged, disabled or elderly. The mission is accomplished through providing independent living skills, affordable housing, and training and placement in community employment.
Heather Ceresoli, CPA, Chair
Deborah A. Passerini, President & CEO

10131 James A. Haley Veterans' Hospital
13000 Bruce B. Downs Boulevard 813-972-2000
Tampa, FL 33612 888-716-7787
www.tampa.va.gov
A tertiary care facility that offers veterans a wide variety of health care services, from primary care to long-term care. Dentistry and extended care is also made available to eligible veterans.
Joe D. Battle, Director
Melissa Sundin, Acting Deputy Director

10132 Lake City VA Medical Center North Florida/South Georgia
Lake City VA Medical Center
619 S Marion Avenue 386-755-3016
Lake City, FL 32025 800-308-8387
www.northflorida.va.gov
Operated by the North Florida/South Georgia Veterans Health System, the Lake City VA Medical Center serves eligible veterans within the area, providing them with multiple health services.
Thomas Wisnieski, MPA, FACHE, Director
Wende Dottor, Deputy Director

10133 Malcom Randall VA Medical Center North Florida/South Georgia
1601 SW Archer Road 352-376-1611
Gainesville, FL 32608 800-324-8387
TTY: 711
www.northflorida.va.gov
Operated by the North Florida/South Georgia Veterans Health System, the Malcom Randall VA Medical Center serves eligible veterans within the area, providing them with multiple health services.
Thomas Wisnieski, MPA, FACHE, Director
Wende Dottor, Deputy Director

10134 Miami VA Healthcare System
1201 NW 16th Street 305-575-7000
Miami, FL 33125 888-276-1785
Fax: 305-575-3232
www.miami.va.gov
Serves veterans located in three countries in South Florida: Miami-Dade, Broward, and Monroe. Miami VA Healthcare System provides veterans with general medical care, as well as specialty care, such as open-heart surgery, a specialization that they provide to other VA facilities.
David J. VanMeter, FACHE, Acting Director
Loyman R. Marin, Associate Director

10135 Vietnam and All Veterans of Brevard
1125 W King Street 321-690-0805
Cocoa, FL 32922-0929 Fax: 321-690-0106
www.vietnamandallveteransofbrevard.com
A not-for-profit organization based in Brevard county that assists homeless veterans with transitional housing. Veterans help fellow veterans, and raise awareness of homelessness within the community.
Richard Russo, President
Richard Hendrick, Vice President

10136 West Palm Beach VA Medical Center
7305 N Military Trail 561-422-8262
West Palm Beach, FL 33410 800-972-8262
www.westpalmbeach.va.gov
The West Palm Beach VA Medical Center consists of one major medical facility, and provides general medical care, in addition to psychiatric and surgical care. A Blind Rehabilitation Center is operated by the major medical facility, and serves as a referral center for blind and visually impaired veterans.
Donna Katen-Bahensky, MSPH, Director & CEO
Cynthia O'Connell, MHA, FACHE, Associate Director

Georgia

10137 Atlanta VA Medical Center Atlanta VA Health Care System
Atlanta VA Medical Center
1670 Clairmont Road 404-321-6111
Decatur, GA 30033 844-698-2311
www.atlanta.va.gov
Part of the VA Southeast Network (VISN 7), the Atlanta VA Medical Center fulfills the health care needs of eligible veterans within the area.
Ajay Dhawan, MD, Director
Stephanie Repasky, Deputy Director

10138 Carl Vinson VA Medical Center Dublin VA Medical Center
1826 Veterans Boulevard 912-272-1210
Dublin, GA 31021 800-595-5229
TTY: 711
www.dublin.va.gov
The Carl Vinson VA Medical Center provides health care to veterans within the Middle Georgia area. Additionally, six community-based outpatient clinics exist to better serve veterans.
David L. Whitmer, FACHE, Director
Connie Hampton, DNP, RN, Interim Director

10139 Charlie Norwood VA Medical Center
950 15th Street Downtown 706-733-0188
Augusta, GA 30904 800-836-5561
Fax: 706-823-3934
TTY: 711
www.augusta.va.gov
Charlie Norwood VA Medical Centre is separated into two divisions to better serve the uptown and the downtown core. The uptown division provides psychiatric care, and rehabilitation, whereas the downtown core provides general medicine and surgical care for veterans.
Robin E. Jackson, Director
Srinivas Ginjupalli, Chief of Staff

10140 VA Southeast Network
3700 Crestwood Parkway 678-924-5700
Duluth, GA 30096 844-698-2311
www.southeast.va.gov
The VA Southeast Network (VISN 7) is the largest integrated health care system in America, and focuses on meeting the health care needs of veterans within the 244-county area.
Leslie Wiggins, Director
Ajay K. Dhawan, MD, FACHE, Chief Medical Officer

Hawaii

10141 Spark M. Matsunaga VA Medical Center VA Pacific Islands Health Care System
VA Pacific Islands Health Care System
459 Patterson Road 808-433-0600
Honolulu, HI 96819-1522 800-214-1306
www.hawaii.va.gov
Existing within the VA Pacific Islands Health Care System, Spark M. Matsunaga VA Medical Center covers a wide range of health care needs for veterans across Hawaii and the Pacific Islands. In addition, the health care system oversees seven outpatient clinics: West Oahu, Hawaii, Maui, Kauai, American Samoa, and Guam.
Jennifer S. Gutowski, MHA, FACHE, Director
Chandra S. Lake, MPA, ACHE, HCLDP, Associate Director

Idaho

10142 Boise VA Medical Center
500 Fort Street 208-422-1000
Boise, ID 83702 866-437-5093
www.boise.va.gov
Boise VA Medical Center serves veterans in Boise, and also operates outpatient clinics in the surrounding areas.
David Wood, Director
Nate Stewart, Associate Director

10143 Idaho Persian Gulf Veterans
2055 S Colorado Street
Boise, ID 83706   208-344-3028
Vaughn Kidwell
Teresa Kidwell

Illinois

10144 Captain James A. Lovell Federal Health Care Center
3001 Green Bay Road   847-688-1900
North Chicago, IL 60064   800-393-0865
                                   www.lovell.fhcc.va.gov
The Captain James A. Lovell Federal Health Care Center (FHCC)
fulfills the health care needs of active and retired veterans, and
their families.
Robert Buckley, Director
CAPT Gregory T. Thier, Deputy Director & Commanding Officer

10145 Desert Storm Justice Foundation: Illinois
Rural Route 4   618-457-2621
Carbondale, IL 62901
Shan Now

10146 Edward Hines Jr. VA Hospital
5000 S 5th Avenue   708-202-8387
Hines, IL 60141   888-598-7793
                                   richard.fox@va.gov
                                   www.hines.va.gov
Edward Hines Jr. VA Hospital provides veterans with primary care
and specialty care. The hospital also operates as a tertiary care re-
ferral center for the VISN 12.
Steven E. Braverman, MD, Director
Elaine Adams, MD, Chief of Staff

10147 Jesse Brown VA Medical Center
820 S Damen Avenue   312-569-8387
Chicago, IL 60612   888-569-5282
                                   www.chicago.va.gov
The Jesse Brown VA Medical Center cares for veterans in the city
of Chicago, Cook County in Illinois, and four counties in northwestern Indiana. In addition to addressing the health care needs of
veterans, the medical center is engaged in an outreach program
with the goal of informing veterans of the health benefits they are
entitled to.
Marc A. Magill, MS, Director
James Brunner, Acting Chief of Staff

10148 Marion VA Medical Center
Marion VA Medical Center
2401 W Main Street   618-997-5311
Marion, IL 62959   www.marion.va.gov
Marion VA Medical Center provides general and surgical care to
eligible veterans within several counties in Illinois, southwestern
Indiana, and northwest Kentucky.
Jo-Ann M. Ginsberg, MSN, RN, Director
Seth W. Barlage, Associate Director

10149 VA Great Lakes Health Care System
Four Westbrook Corporate Tower   708-492-3900
Westchester, IL 60154   www.visn12.va.gov
The VA Great Lakes Health Care System consists of eight VA medi-
cal centers, all focused around the goal of fulfilling the health care
needs of veterans.
Renee Oshinski, Director
Lynette J. Taylor, Deputy Director

10150 VA Illiana Health Care System
1900 E Main Street   217-554-3000
Danville, IL 61832   800-320-8387
                                   www.danville.va.gov
VA Illiana Health Care System is focused on improving the health
of veterans throughout 34 counties in Illinois and Indiana.
Kelley A. Sermak, Acting Director
Diana Carranza, FACHE, Associate Director

Indiana

10151 Fort Wayne Campus VA Northern Indiana Health Care System
2121 Lake Avenue   260-426-5431
Fort Wayne, IN 46805   800-360-8387
                               VHANINPublicAffairs@va.gov
                               www.northernindiana.va.gov
The Fort Wayne Campus provides veterans with primary and
seconday cmedical services, as well as surgical care.
Michael E. Hershman, Director
Jay Miller, Associate Director of Operations

10152 Marion Campus VA Northern Indiana Health Care System
1700 E 38th Street   765-674-3321
Marion, IN 46953   800-360-8387
                               VHANINPublicAffairs@va.gov
                               www.northernindiana.va.gov
The Marion Campus focuses on improving the mental health of
veterans, and provides extended care. Marion Campus offers nurs-
ing home care as an alternative.
Michael E. Hershman, Director
Jay Miller, Associate Director of Operations

Iowa

10153 Iowa City VA Health Care System
601 Highway 6 W   319-338-0581
Iowa City, IA 52246   800-637-0128
                                   www.iowacity.va.gov
Iowa City VA Health Care System provides a wide range of health
care services to veterans within 50 counties in Eastern Iowa, West-
ern Illinois, and Northern Missouri.
Judith Johnson-Mekota, Director
Javed H. Tunio, Chief of Staff

10154 VA Central Iowa Health Care System
3600 30th Street   515-699-5999
Des Moines, IA 50310   800-294-8387
                                   www.centraliowa.va.gov
The VA Central Iowa Health Care System provides acute and specialized health care to veterans. The medical facility operates an
extensive range of mental health services, including specialized
treatments for substance abuse and post-traumatic stress.
Gail Graham, Director
Jerry Blow, MD, Chief of Staff

Kansas

10155 Colmery-O'Neil VA Medical Center VA Eastern Kansas Health Care System
2200 SW Gage Boulevard   785-350-3111
Topeka, KS 66622   800-574-8387
                                   www.leavenworth.va.gov
Part of the Heartland Network (VISN 15), the Colmery-O'Neil VA
Medical Center improves the health of veterans living in Topeka,
Kansas.
A. Rudy Klopfer, Director
Lisa Curnes, Associate Director

10156 Dwight D. Eisenhower VA Medical Center VA Eastern Kansas Health Care System
4101 4th Street Trafficway   913-682-2000
Leavenworth, KS 66048   800-952-8387
                                   www.leavenworth.va.gov
Located within the VA Heartland Network (VISN 15), the Dwight
D. Eisenhower VA Medical Center improves the health of veterans
in Leavenworth, Kansas.
A. Rudy Klopfer, Director
Lisa Curnes, Associate Director

10157 Robert J. Dole VA Medical Center
5500 E Kellogg Avenue   316-685-2221
Wichita, KS 67218   888-878-6881
                                   www.wichita.va.gov
Located in the largest city in Kansas, Robert J. Dole VA Medical
Center addresses the health of veterans by providing a large range
of primary health services. The medical center offers specialty care

in the form of rehabilitation programs, and houses a prosthetic laboratory.
Rick A. Ament, FACHE, Director
Dana Foley, PhD, Associate Director

Kentucky

10158 Lexington VA Health Care System
1101 Veterans Drive   859-233-4511
Lexington, KY 40502   www.lexington.va.gov
The Lexington VA Health Care System is comprised of two main campuses, the Troy Bowling Campus, and the Franklin R. Sousley Campus. The Lexington VA Health Care System offers inpatient care for veterans.
Emma Metcalf, MSN, RN, Director
Patricia Breeden, MD, Chief of Staff

10159 Robley Rex VA Medical Center Louisville VA Medical Center
800 Zorn Avenue   502-287-4000
Louisville, KY 40206   800-376-8387
                                             www.louisville.va.gov
Robley Rex offers health care services to veterans within the 35-county area of Kentuckiana.
Stephen D. Black, Director
Larry D. Roberts, Associate Director

Louisiana

10160 Alexandria VA Healthcare System
2495 Shreveport Highway   318-466-4000
Pineville, LA 71360   800-375-8387
                                             www.alexandria.va.gov
Alexandria VA Healthcare System provides health care services to veterans in need. Alexandria offers a number of specialized programs for eligible veterans, some of which include home-based primary care, an adult day care program, and a homeless program.
Peter C. Dancy, Jr., Director
Lisa M. Hamilton, Associate Director

10161 Overton Brooks VA Medical Center
510 E Stoner Avenue   318-221-8411
Shreveport, LA 71101   800-863-7441
                                             www.shreveport.va.gov
A medical facility serving veterans in the South Central VA Health Care Network (VISN 16). Overton Brooks VA Medical Center is a primary receiving center for military casualties, and accepts referrals from the southeast Lousiana Veterans Healthcare System and the Alexandria VA Health Science Center.
Richard L. Crockett, Director
Zachary Sage, Associate Director

10162 Southeast Louisiana Veterans Health Care System
2400 Canal Street   800-935-8387
New Orleans, LA 70119   www.neworleans.va.gov
Southeast Louisiana Veterans Health Care System (SLVHCS) improves the health of veterans. SLVHCS offers specialty care in the form of respite care and community adult day care programs. In addition, SLVHCS operates a telehealth system, ensuring any veteran can access health care services from the comfort of their home.
Fernando O. Rivera, Director
Ralph Schapira, MD, Chief of Staff

Maine

10163 Maine VA Medical Center VA Maine Healthcare System
1 VA Center   207-623-8411
Augusta, ME 04330   877-421-8263
                                             TTY: 711
                                             TDD: 800-829-4833
                                             www.maine.va.gov
A medical facility offerring general medical, surgical, and mental health services to veterans.
Tracey B. Davis, Director
Russell Armstead, CGFM, Acting Associate Director

Maryland

10164 Baltimore VA Medical Center VA Maryland Health Care System
10 N Greene Street   410-605-7000
Baltimore, MD 21201-1524   www.maryland.va.gov
The Baltimore VA Medical Center offers health care services to veterans, and is home to the world's first filmless radiology department, allowing medical professionals to view radiology imaging almost instantly.
Adam M. Robinson, Jr., MD, Director
Sandra Marshall, MD, Chief of Staff

10165 Loch Raven VA Community Living & Rehabilitation Center
3901 The Alameda   410-605-7000
Baltimore, MD 21218-2100   www.maryland.va.gov
The Loch Raven VA Community Living & Rehabilitation Center works to restore independence for Maryland's veterans by providing a wide variety of physical therapies and rehabilitation programs.
Adam M. Robinson, Jr., MD, Director
Sandra Marshall, MD, Chief of Staff

10166 Perry Point VA Medical Center VA Maryland Health Care System
515 Broad Street   410-642-2411
Perry Point, MD 21902-9998   www.maryland.va.gov
The largest medical facility in the VA Maryland Health Care System, Perry Point provides long-term care, nursing home care, and hospice care for veterans.
Adam M. Robinson, Director
Sandra Marshall, Chief of Staff

10167 VA Capitol Health Care Network
849 International Drive   410-691-1131
Linthicum, MD 21090   www.va.gov
The VA Capitol Health Care Network (VISN 5) serves veterans from within Maryland, the District of Columbia, select areas of Virginia, West Virginia, and Pennsylvania.
Robert Walton, Director
Raymond Chung, MD, Chief Medical Officer

Massachusetts

10168 Brockton Division VA Boston Healthcare System
940 Belmont Street   508-583-4500
Brockton, MA 02301   800-865-3384
                                             www.boston.va.gov
The Brockton Division of the VA Boston Healthcare System is dedicated to providing health care to veterans located in Boston.
Vincent Ng, Director
Michael E. Charness, MD, Chief of Staff

10169 Edith Nourse Rogers Memorial Veterans Hospital: Bedford VA
200 Springs Road   781-687-2000
Bedford, MA 01730   800-838-6331
                                             www.bedford.va.gov
Bedford VA is a long-term care facility specializing in psychiatric care. Bedford VA provides inpatient and outpatient care.
Joan Clifford, Director
Ed Koetting, Associate Director

10170 Jamaica Plain Division VA Boston Healthcare System
150 S Huntington Avenue   617-232-9500
Boston, MA 02130   800-865-3384
                                             www.boston.va.gov
The Jamaica Plain Division of the VA Boston Healthcare System is dedicated to providing health care to veterans located in Boston.
Vincent Ng, Director
Michael E. Charness, MD, Chief of Staff

10171 West Roxbury Division VA Boston Healthcare System
1400 VFW Parkway   617-323-7700
West Roxbury, MA 02132   800-865-3384
                                             www.boston.va.gov
The West Roxbury Division of the VA Boston Healthcare System is dedicated to providing health care to veterans located in Boston.
Vincent Ng, Director
Michael E. Charness, MD, Chief of Staff

Michigan

10172 Aleda E. Lutz VA Medical Center: Saginaw, Michigan
1500 Weiss Street   989-497-2500
Saginaw, MI 48602   800-406-5143
www.saginaw.va.gov
Aleda E. Lutz VA Medical Center provides services for veterans living in all 35 counties located in central and northern Michigan's Lower Peninsula.
Barbara Bates, MD, Director
Thomas Campana, Acting Chief of Staff

10173 Battle Creek VA Medical Center
5500 Armstrong Road   269-966-5600
Battle Creek, MI 49037   888-214-1247
www.battlecreek.va.gov
A medical facility offering both inpatient and outpatient care. Each veteran enrolling for care is assigned their own primary care provider and team, who manage their case and provide consistent and coordinated care.
James Doelling, Director
Edward Dornoff, MPH, FACHE, Associate Director

10174 John D. Dingell VA Medical Center
4646 John R. Street   313-576-1000
Detroit, MI 48201   800-511-8056
www.detroit.va.gov
Part of the VA Healthcare System serving Ohio, Indiana, and Michigan (VISN 10), John D. Dingell VA Medical Center provides health care services to all veterans located in the Wayne, Oakland, Macomb and St. Clair counties.
Pamela J. Reeves, MD, Director
Michelle S. Werner, Associate Director

10175 Oscar G. Johnson VA Medical Center
325 E H. Street   906-774-3300
Iron Mountain, MI 49801   800-215-8262
www.ironmountain.va.gov
A primary and secondary level care facility providing veterans with acute care and general medicine care. The facility offers rehabilitation, extended care, and emergency services.
James W. Rice, Director
Drew A. DeWitt, FACHE, Associate Director

10176 VA Ann Arbor Healthcare System
2215 Fuller Road   734-769-7100
Ann Arbor, MI 48105   800-361-8387
www.annarbor.va.gov
VA Ann Arbor is a medical facility that doubles as a referral center for specialty care for veterans located within the 15-county area of Michigan and northwest Ohio.
Ginny Creasman, Pharm D, FACHE, Director
Chris Cauley, FACHE, Associate Director

Minnesota

10177 Desert Storm Justice Foundation: Minnesota
PO Box 186   218-258-3685
Buhl, MN 55713
Jeff Zakula

10178 Minneapolis VA Health Care System
1 Veterans Drive   612-725-2000
Minneapolis, MN 55417   866-414-5058
www.minneapolis.va.gov
Minneapolis VA Health Care System is a teaching hospital serving veterans with a broad range of medical services.
Patrick J. Kelly, FACHE, Director
Kent Crossley, MD, MHA, Chief of Staff

10179 St. Paul Regional Office
1 Federal Drive   800-827-1000
St. Paul, MN 55111-4050   Fax: 612-970-5415
VBADirectorStPaulRO@va.gov
www.benefits.va.gov
St. Paul Regional Office serves veterans in accessing their benefits. St. Paul's assists veterans in acquiring loans, pensions, and offers counseling services to determine eligibility for additional benefits and services.
Kim Graves, Director
Kay Anderson, Assistant Director

Mississippi

10180 G.V. (Sonny) Montgomery VA Medical Center
1500 E Woodrow Wilson Avenue   601-362-4471
Jackson, MS 39216   800-949-1009
TTY: 711
www.jackson.va.gov
A medical center providing veterans with primary, secondary, and tertiary medical care. In addition, G.V. (Sonny) Montgomery offers inpatient mental health care, as well as comprehensive health care for female veterans.
David M. Walker, Director
Kai D. Mentzer, Associate Director

10181 Gulf Coast Veterans Health Care System
400 Veterans Avenue   228-523-5000
Biloxi, MS 39531   800-296-8872
www.biloxi.va.gov
Part of the South Central VA Health Care Network (VISN16), Gulf Coast serves veterans in the region by providing medical care, and readjustment counseling centers.
Bryan C. Matthews, MBA, Director
Adam G. Bearden, MBA, FACHE, Acting Associate Director

10182 Jackson Regional Office
1600 E Woodrow Wilson Avenue   800-827-1000
Jackson, MS 32916   www.benefits.va.gov
Jackson Regional Office aids veterans in accessing their benefits, and provides information about health care services available to them.
Darryl Brady, Director
Tammy Fowler, Assistant Director

10183 South Central VA Health Care Network
715 S Pear Orchard Road   601-206-6900
Ridgeland, MS 39157   800-639-5137
Fax: 601-206-7018
www.visn16.va.gov
The South Central VA Health Care Network is a Veterans Integrated Service Network (VISN) serving veterans in Arkansas, Louisiana, Mississippi, parts of Texas, Missouri, Alabama, Oklahoma, and Florida.
Skye McDougall, PhD, Director
Shannon C. Novotny, MPA, FACHE, Deputy Director

Missouri

10184 Harry S. Truman Memorial Veterans' Hospital
800 Hospital Drive   573-814-6000
Columbia, MO 65201   800-349-8262
www.columbiamo.va.gov
Part of the Heartland Network (VISN 15), Harry S. Truman Memorial Veterans' Hospital specializes in providing medical care to veterans in 43 counties in Missouri and Pike County, Illinois.
David Isaacks, FACHE, Director
Lana Zerrer, MD, Chief of Staff

10185 John J. Pershing VA Medical Center
1500 N Westwood Boulevard   573-686-4151
Poplar Bluff, MO 63901   888-557-8262
www.poplarbluff.va.gov
A medical center providing primary care to veterans across 29 counties of southeast Missouri and northeast Arkansas. Outpatient clinics provide mental health services.
Patricia L. Hall, RN, MSN, PhD, Director
Libby J. Johnson, Associate Director

10186 Kansas City VA Medical Center
4801 Linwood Boulevard   816-861-4700
Kansas City, MO 64128   800-525-1483
www.kansascity.va.gov
Part of the Heartland Network (VISN 15), Kansas City VA Medical Center provides veterans with health care services.
Kathleen Fogarty, Director
Paula Roychaudhuri, FACHE, Associate Director

10187 VA Heartland Network
1201 Walnut Street 816-701-3002
Kansas City, MO 64106 www.visn15.va.gov
The VA Heartland Network (VISN 15) provides health care services to veterans in Kansas and Missouri, as well as parts of Illinois, Indiana, Kentucky and Arkansas. The Heartland Network is comprised of 7 medical facilities.

10188 VA St. Louis Health Care System John Cochran & Jefferson Barracks
915 N Grand Boulevard 314-652-4100
St. Louis, MO 63106 800-228-5459
www.stlouis.va.gov
Part of the Heartland Network (VISN 15), the St. Louis Health Care System offers medical care to veterans in east central Missouri and southwestern Illinois. The John Cochran Division provides surgical care, ambulatory medicine, and houses intensive care units, while the Jefferson Barracks Division provides psychiatric treatment and a nursing home care unit.
Keith D. Repko, Director
Michael D. Crittenden, MD, Chief of Staff

Montana

10189 Medical Center & Ambulatory Care Clinic Montana VA Health Care System
3687 Veterans Drive 406-442-6410
Fort Harrison, MT 59636 877-468-8387
www.montana.va.gov
The medical center and ambulatory care clinic operated by the Montana VA Health Care System provides care to veterans through an acute medical center, and multiple community-based clinics.
Paul Gregory, Acting Director
Anthony Giljum, Associate Director

10190 Miles City VA Clinic & Community Living Center
210 S Winchester Avenue 406-874-5600
Miles City, MT 59301-4798 877-468-8387
Fax: 406-874-5696
www.montana.va.gov
Serving veterans in southeastern Montana in Miles City, the Miles City VA Clinic and Community Living Center also operates a community based outpatient clinic.

Nevada

10191 North Las Vegas VA Medical Center VA Southern Nevada Healthcare System
6900 North Pecos Road 702-791-9000
North Las Vegas, NV 89086 888-633-7554
www.lasvegas.va.gov
Medical facility serving veterans in Las Vegas, with community-based outpatient clinics located across Nevada.
Tracy L. Skala, Acting Director
John L. Stelsel, Assistant Director

10192 VA Sierra Nevada Health Care System
975 Kirman Avenue 775-786-7200
Reno, NV 89502 888-838-6256
www.reno.va.gov
The VA Sierra Nevada Health Care System provides primary and secondary care to veterans across 20 counties in northern Nevada and northeastern California.
Lisa Howard, Director
Jack R. Smith, Associate Director

New Hampshire

10193 Manchester VA Medical Center VAMC Manchester, New Hampshire
718 Smyth Road 603-624-4366
Manchester, NH 03104 800-892-8384
www.manchester.va.gov
Since 1950, Manchester VA Medical Center has been providing veterans with health care services across the VA New England Healthcare System Network (VISN 1).
Alfred A. Montoya, Jr., MHA, FACHE, Director
Paul Zimmerman, DDS, Chief of Staff

New Jersey

10194 East Orange Campus VA New Jersey Health Care System
385 Tremont Avenue 973-676-1000
East Orange, NJ 07018 www.newjersey.va.gov
Part of the VA New Jersey Health Care System, the East Orange Campus provides primary care to veterans, in addition to a great variety of specialized programs.
Vincent F. Immiti, MBA, FACHE, Director
Mara Davis, Associate Director

10195 Lyons Campus VA New Jersey Health Care System
151 Knollcroft Road 908-647-0180
Lyons, NJ 07939 www.newjersey.va.gov
Part of the VA New Jersey Health Care System, the Lyons Campus provides primary care to veterans, in addition to a great variety of specialized programs.
Vincent F. Immiti, MBA, FACHE, Director
Mara Davis, Associate Director

New Mexico

10196 Raymond G. Murphy VA Medical Center New Mexico VA Health Care System
1501 San Pedro Drive SE 505-265-1711
Albuquerque, NM 87108 800-465-8262
www.albuquerque.va.gov
Provides medical care to veterans, and specializes in delivering rural health care in New Mexico.
Andrew M. Welch, MHA, FACHE, Director
Sonja Brown, Associate Director

New York

10197 Albany Stratton VA Medical Center
113 Holland Avenue 518-626-5000
Albany, NY 12208 800-223-4810
www.albany.va.gov
Albany Stratton VA Medical Center in Albany, New York, serves veterans in 22 counties of upstate New York, western Massachusetts and Vermont.
Darlene DeLancey, Director
Mary Ann Witt, Associate Director

10198 Batavia VA Medical Center VA Western New York Healthcare System
222 Richmond Avenue 585-297-1000
Batavia, NY 14020 www.buffalo.va.gov
Batavia houses separate residential post-traumatic stress disorder units for men and women veterans, and is part of the VA Western New York Healthcare System.
Michael J. Swartz, Director
Grace L. Stringfellow, MD, Chief of Staff

10199 Bath VA Medical Center
76 Veterans Avenue 607-664-4000
Bath, NY 14810 877-845-3247
www.bath.va.gov
A medical center serving veterans with a comprehensive range of health care services, including mental health care provided by community-based outpatient clinics located in Coudersport, Elmira, Mansfield, and Wellsville.
Bruce Tucker, Director
Susan Herson, MD, Chief of Staff

10200 Brooklyn Campus VA NY Harbor Health Care System
800 Poly Place 718-836-6600
Brooklyn, NY 11209 www.nyharbor.va.gov
The NY Harbor Healthcare System delivers health care services to veterans living in the 5 boroughs of New York City at their Brooklyn and Manhattan Campuses, and at the St. Albans Community Living Center.
Martina A. Parauda, Director
Cynthia Caroselli, PhD, RN, Associate Director

10201 Buffalo VA Medical Center VA Western New York Healthcare System
3495 Bailey Avenue 716-834-9200
Buffalo, NY 14215 800-532-8387
www.buffalo.va.gov

The Buffalo VA Medical Center provides a broad range of inpatient and outpatient long term care services for veterans. In addition, it is the main referral center for cardiac surgery, cardiology and comprehensive cancer care in the VA Western New York Healthcare System.
Michael J. Swartz, Director
Grace L. Stringfellow, MD, Chief of Staff

10202 Canandaigua VA Medical Center VA Health Care Upstate New York
400 Fort Hill Avenue　　　　585-394-2000
Canandaigua, NY 14424　　　800-204-9917
　　　　　　　　　www.canandaigua.va.gov
The Canandaigua VA Medical Center, part of VA Health Care Upstate New York provides inpatient and outpatient care to veterans. Canadaigua VA Medical Center is known for its focus on mental health issues, and conducts research on mental health.
Bruce Tucker, Director
Kenneth Piazza, Associate Director

10203 Manhattan VA Medical Center VA NY Harbor Health Care System
423 E 23rd Street　　　　212-686-7500
New York, NY 10010-5011　www.nyharbor.va.gov
Medical facility serving veterans in the NY Harbor area. Provides a full range of medical services.
Martina A. Parauda, Director
Cynthia Caroselli, PhD, RN, Associate Director

10204 Montrose Campus: Franklin Delano Roosevelt VA Hudson Valley Health Care System
2094 Albany Post Road　　914-737-4400
Montrose, NY 10548-1454　www.hudsonvalley.va.gov
The Montrose Campus of the VA Hudson Valley Health Care System is a provider of urgent health care services to veterans.
Margaret B. O'Shea Caplan, Director
Dawn M. Schaal, Associate Director

10205 New York/New Jersey VA Health Care Network
130 W Kingsbridge Road　　718-741-4134
Bronx, NY 10468　　　　　718-741-4134
　　　　　　　　　www.visn2.va.gov
The New York/New Jersey VA Health Care Network, or VISN 2, consists of 10 medical centers, and 59 community-based outpatient clinics to better serve the veteran population in New York and New Jersey.
Joan E. McInerney, MD, MBA, MA, Director

10206 Northport VA Medical Center
79 Middleville Road　　　631-261-4400
Northport, NY 11768　　www.northport.va.gov
The Northport VA Medical Center specializes in providing health care services to veterans in need.
Cathy Cruise, MD, Acting Director
Colleen Luckner, MBA, Associate Director

10207 Syracuse VA Medical Center
800 Irving Avenue　　　315-425-4400
Syracuse, NY 13210　　800-792-4334
　　　　　　　　www.syracuse.va.gov
The Syracuse VA Medical Center provides a full range of patient care services, education and research to serve veterans.
Judy Hayman, PhD, Director
Richard W. Salgueiro, Associate Director

North Carolina

10208 Charles George VA Medical Center
1100 Tunnel Road　　　828-298-7911
Asheville, NC 28805　　800-932-6408
　　　　　　　　www.asheville.va.gov
Part of the VA Mid-Atlantic Healthcare Network (VISN 6), Charles George VA Medical Center has been serving veterans since 1922. Outpatient clinics are located in Franklin, Rutherford County, and Hickory.
Stephanie Young, Director
Robert Evans, Associate Director

10209 Durham VA Health Care System
508 Fulton Street　　　919-286-0411
Durham, NC 27705　　　888-878-6890
　　　　　　　　www.durham.va.gov
Durham Veterans Affairs Medical Center serves the health care needs of eligible veterans living within 27 counties of central and eastern North Carolina.
Paul S. Crews, MPH, CPHQ, FACHE, Director
Kenneth C. Goldberg, MD, Chief of Staff

10210 Fayetteville VA Medical Center
2300 Ramsey Street　　910-488-2120
Fayetteville, NC 28301　800-771-6106
　　　　　　　　　TTY: 711
　　　　　　　www.fayettevillenc.va.gov
The Fayetteville Veterans Affairs Medical Center provides general medicine, surgery, and mental health care to veterans across nineteen counties located in the Southeastern Northern Carolina area.
Webster C. Bazemore, Interim Director
Gregory A. Antoine, Chief of Staff

10211 W. G. (Bill) Hefner VA Medical Center
1601 Brenner Avenue　　704-638-9000
Salisbury, NC 28144　　800-469-8262
　　　　　　　　www.salisbury.va.gov
A medical center offering primary and secondary inpatient health care to veterans living in 21 counties of the Central Piedmont Region of North Carolina.
Joseph Vaughn, MBA, FACHE, Director
Subbarao Pemmaraju, MD, Chief of Staff

North Dakota

10212 Fargo VA Health Care System
2101 N Elm Street　　701-239-3700
Fargo, ND 58102　　　800-410-9723
　　　　　　　　www.fargo.va.gov
Fargo VA provides health care services to veterans, and operates 10 community-based outpatient clinics to better serve veterans in need.
Lavonne K. Liversage, FACHE, Director
Breton M. Weintraub, MD, FACP, Chief of Staff

Ohio

10213 Chalmers P. Wylie Ambulatory Care Center VA Central Ohio Healthcare System
420 N James Road　　614-257-5200
Columbus, OH 43219　888-615-9448
　　　　　　　　www.columbus.va.gov
Chalmers P. Wylie Ambulatory Care Center provides veterans with medical care, from surgery to rehabilitation. Four community-based clinics focused on outpatient care are located in Grove City, Marion, Newark, and Zanesville.
Vivian T. Hutson, Director
Jamie Kuhne, LISW-S, Associate Director

10214 Chillicothe VA Medical Center
17273 State Route 104　　740-773-1141
Chillicothe, OH 45601　　800-358-8262
　　　　　　　　www.chillicothe.va.gov
The Chillicothe VA Medical Center provides acute and chronic mental health services, primary and secondary medical care, among other services. Chillicothe houses a specialized women veterans health clinic and serves as a chronic mental health referral center for other VA Medical Centers in southern Ohio and parts of West Virginia and Kentucky.
Kathy W. Berger, MHA, DNP, Director
James V. Zeigler, MA, CCP-SLP, Acting Associate Director

10215 Cincinnati VA Medical Center
3200 Vine Street　　513-861-3100
Cincinnati, OH 45220　www.cincinnati.va.gov
Cincinnati VA Medical Center consists of 2 divisions located in Cincinnati, Ohio and Fort Thomas, Kentucky. Services are provided for 15 counties in Ohio, Kentucky, and Indiana. Cincinnati also acts as a referral center for neurosurgery.
Mark Murdock, MHA, FACHE, Director
Gregory Goins, Associate Director

10216 Cleveland VA Medical Center VA Northeast Ohio Healthcare System
10701 E Boulevard · 216-791-3800
Cleveland, OH 44106 · 877-838-8262
www.cleveland.va.gov
Cleveland VA Medical Center is part of VISN 10, and provides a full range of primary, secondary and tertiary care services offered to an eligible veteran population covering 24 counties in northeast Ohio.
Susan M. Fuehrer, Director
Brian Cmolik, MD, FACS, Chief of Staff

10217 Dayton VA Medical Center
4100 W 3rd Street · 937-268-6511
Dayton, OH 45428 · 800-368-8262
TTY: 800-829-4833
www.dayton.va.gov
A medical facility offering comprehensive health care to veterans in Dayton, Ohio. A variety of specialized programs from an Alzheimer's unit to sleep disorder programs exist to better serve veterans.
Jill Dietrich, JD, MBA, FACHE, Director
Mark E. Butler, RPh, Acting Associate Director

10218 VA Healthcare System of Ohio
11500 Northlake Drive · 513-247-4621
Cincinnati, OH 45249 · www.visn10.va.gov
The VA Healthcare System (VISN 10) serves Ohio, Indiana, and Michigan. VISN 10 consists of 10 medical centers and 63 community-based outpatient clinics to better serve veterans.
Shella D. Stovall, Acting Director
Ronald Stertzbach, Deputy Director

Oklahoma

10219 Jack C. Montgomery VA Medical Center Eastern Oklahoma VA Health Care System
1011 Honor Heights Drive · 918-577-3000
Muskogee, OK 74401 · 888-397-8387
www.muskogee.va.gov
Medical facility serving veterans in 25 counties in eastern Oklahoma. Comprehensive health care services are offered.
Mark Morgan, MHA, FACHE, Director
Jonathan M. Plasencia, MBA, FACHE, Associate Director

10220 Oklahoma City VA Health Care System
921 NE 13th Street · 405-456-1000
Oklahoma City, OK 73104 · 866-835-5273
www.oklahoma.va.gov
The Oklahoma City VA Medical Center is a tertiary care facility and a referral center. The medical center provides a full range of patient care services for veterans.
Kristopher Wade Vlosich, Director
Paul Gregory, Associate Director

Oregon

10221 National Association of State Directors of Veterans Affairs
700 Summer Street NW · www.nasdva.us
Salem, OR 97301
The National Association of State Directors of Veterans Affairs (NASDVA) is an organization operating in each state of the United States, with its headquarters in Oregon. The State Directors at NASDVA work to ensure that veterans receive their benefits and entitlements regardless of their age, gender, and era of service.
Alfie Alvarado-Ramos, President

10222 Portland VA Medical Center VA Portland Health Care System
3710 SW U.S. Veterans Hospital Road · 503-220-8262
Portland, OR 97239 · 800-949-1004
www.portland.va.gov
The Portland VA Medical Center serves veterans in Oregon and southwest Washington. In addition to comprehensive medical and mental health services, the medical center supports ongoing research and medical education.
Darwin G. Goodspeed, Director
Cheryl L. Thieschafer, Deputy Director

10223 Roseburg VA Health Care System
913 NW Garden Valley Boulevard · 541-440-1000
Roseburg, OR 97471 · 800-549-8387
www.roseburg.va.gov
The Roseburg VA Health Care System consists of one main facility located in Roseburg and four community-based outpatient clinics. Roseburg offers primary care and hospital services in medicine, surgery and mental health for veterans.
Keith M. Allen, Director
Ryan Baker, CDFM, MBA, Associate Director

10224 White City VA Rehabilitation Center VA Southern Oregon
8495 Crater Lake Highway · 541-826-2111
White City, OR 97503 · 800-809-8725
Fax: 541-830-3500
www.southernoregon.va.gov
White City VA Rehabilitation Center is the only freestanding residential rehabilitation center, and provides veterans with short-term rehabilitative and long-term health care. The center maintains a focus on patient-centered care.
Philip G. Dionne, Director
Sharee Taylor, Associate Director

Pennsylvania

10225 Coatesville VA Medical Center
1400 Blackhorse Hill Road · 610-384-7711
Coatesville, PA 19320 · 800-290-6172
Coatesville VA Medical Center provides primary, urgent, and specialty care to veterans in Spring City and Newtown Square, Pennsylvania. In addition, Coatesville offers mental health care and operates a pharmacy.
Carla Sivek, Director
Michael F. Gliatto, MD, Chief of Staff

10226 Corporal Michael J. Crescenz VA Medical Center
3900 Woodland Avenue · 215-823-5800
Philadelphia, PA 19104 · 800-949-1001
www.philadelphia.va.gov
Provides medical care for veterans in the city of Philadelphia including six surrounding counties in southeastern Pennsylvania and southern New Jersey.
Patricia O'Kane, MSS, Director
John J. Kelly, MD, Chief of Staff

10227 Erie VA Medical Center
135 E 38th Street Boulevard · 814-868-8661
Erie, PA 16504 · 800-274-8387
www.erie.va.gov
Medical center serving veterans across 9 counties within northwestern Pennsylvania, eastern Ohio, and southwestern New York.
John A. Gennaro, Director
David M. Lavin, Chief of Staff

10228 H.J. Heinz Campus VA Pittsburgh Healthcare System
1010 Delafield Road · 412-822-2222
Pittsburgh, PA 15215 · 866-482-7488
www.pittsburgh.va.gov
VA Pittsburgh Healthcare System is composed of two main campuses: University Drive and H.J. Heinz. The healthcare system serves veterans living in the tri-state area of Pennsylvania, Ohio, and West Virginia. H.J. Heinz campus is a community living center and an ambulatory care center providing outpatient services, including dental care.
Barbara Forsha, MSN, RN, ET, Director
Ali Sonel, MD, Chief of Staff

10229 Lebanon VA Medical Center
1700 S Lincoln Avenue · 717-272-6621
Lebanon, PA 17042 · 800-409-8771
www.lebanon.va.gov
Lebanon VA Medical Center is located at the heart of Pennsylvania Dutch country and provides a comprehensive range of medical care for eligible veterans within the area. Additionally, Lebanon VA offers telehealth services, making health care accessible to veterans from their homes.
Robert W. Callahan Jr., Director
Jeffrey A. Beiler, Associate Director

10230 University Drive Campus VA Pittsburgh Healthcare System
University Drive C · · · · · · · · · · · · · · · 412-822-2222
Pittsburgh, PA 15240-1003 · · · · · · · · 866-482-7488
www.pittsburgh.va.gov
VA Pittsburgh Healthcare System is composed of two main campuses: University Drive and H.J. Heinz. The healthcare system serves veterans living in the tri-state area of Pennsylvania, Ohio, and West Virginia. University Drive campus serves as an acute care facility.
Barbara Forsha, MSN, RN, ET, Director
Ali Sonel, MD, Chief of Staff

10231 Wilkes-Barre VA Medical Center
1111 E End Boulevard · · · · · · · · · · · · 570-824-3521
Wilkes-Barre, PA 18711 · · · · · · · · · · 877-928-2621
www.wilkes-barre.va.gov
Wilkes-Barre VA Medical Center offers comprehensive health care to veterans residing in 18 counties in Pennsylvania and one county in New York.
Russell E. Lloyd, Director
Mirza Z. Ali, MD, Chief of Staff

Rhode Island

10232 Providence VA Medical Center
830 Chalkstone Avenue · · · · · · · · · · · 401-273-7100
Providence, RI 02908 · · · · · · · · · · · · 866-363-4486
www.providence.va.gov
The Providence VA Medical Center provides comprehensive outpatient and inpatient health care to veterans in Rhode Island and southeastern Massachusetts. Personalized care is offered to every veteran.
Susan MacKenzie, PhD, Director
Erin Clare Sears, MBA, MSW, Associate Director

South Carolina

10233 Columbia VA Health Care System
6439 Garners Ferry Road · · · · · · · · · · 803-776-4000
Columbia, SC 29209 · · · · · · · · · · · · · 888-651-2683
www.columbiasc.va.gov
Columbia VA Health Care System serves veterans by providing a full range of patient care services, including primary, secondary, and tertiary care. 7 community-based outpatient clinics located throughout South Carolina serve veterans residing in 36 counties.
David L. Omura, Director & CEO
Jeffrey Soots, Associate Director

10234 Ralph H. Johnson VA Medical Center
109 Bee Street · · · · · · · · · · · · · · · · · 843-577-5011
Charleston, SC 29401 · · · · · · · · · · · · 888-878-6884
www.charleston.va.gov
The Ralph H. Johnson VA Medical Center serves veterans in 22 counties along the South Carolina and Georgia coastline. Six community-based outpatient clinics exist to better serve the veteran population.
Scott R. Isaacks, MBA, FACHE, Director & CEO
Sharon Castle, PharmD, BCPS, Acting Associate Director & COO

South Dakota

10235 Fort Meade Campus VA Black Hills Health Care System
113 Comanche Road · · · · · · · · · · · · · 605-347-2511
Fort Meade, SD 57741 · · · · · · · · · · · · 800-743-1070
www.blackhills.va.gov
VA Black Hills Health Care System is comprised of two campuses: Fort Meade and Hot Springs. Both facilities provide primary and secondary medical and surgical care, residential rehabilitation treatment programs, extended nursing home care and psychiatric inpatient services for veterans living in South Dakota, portions of Nebraska, North Dakota, Wyoming and Montana.
Sandra L. Horsman, MBM, Director
C.B. Alexander, FACHE, Associate Director

10236 Hot Springs Campus VA Black Hills Health Care System
500 N 5th Street · · · · · · · · · · · · · · · · 605-745-2000
Hot Springs, SD 57747 · · · · · · · · · · · 800-764-5370
www.blackhills.va.gov

VA Black Hills Health Care System is comprised of two campuses: Fort Meade and Hot Springs. Both facilities provide primary and secondary medical and surgical care, residential rehabilitation treatment programs, extended nursing home care and psychiatric inpatient services for veterans living in South Dakota, portions of Nebraska, North Dakota, Wyoming and Montana.
Sandra L. Horsman, MBM, Director
C.B. Alexander, FACHE, Associate Director

10237 Sioux Falls VA Health Care System
2501 W 22nd Street · · · · · · · · · · · · · 605-336-3230
Sioux Falls, SD 57105-5046 · · · · · · · · 800-316-8387
www.siouxfalls.va.gov
Sioux Falls VA Health Care System provides inpatient and outpatient care for veterans in eastern South Dakota, southwestern Minnesota, and northwestern Iowa. Services include primary and specialty medical care, mental health care, and rehabilitation.
Barbara Teal, Acting Director
Timothy L. Pendergrass, MD, Chief of Staff

Tennessee

10238 Alvin C. York VA Medical Center Tennessee Valley Healthcare System
3400 Lebanon Pike · · · · · · · · · · · · · · 615-867-6000
Murfreesboro, TN 37129-1237 · · · · · · 800-228-4973
www.tennesseevalley.va.gov
Alvin C. York VA Medical Center is part of the Tennessee Healthcare System. Tennessee Valley Healthcare System provides primary and secondary care, general medicine, surgery and specialized care to veterans. The Alvin C. York VA Medical Center is a referral center for mental health services, geriatrics, and extended care.
Jennifer Vedral-Baron, MN, FAANP, Director
Suzanne L. Jen,, MBA, VHA-CM, Deputy Director

10239 James H. Quillen VA Healthcare System Mountain Home VA Healthcare System
Corner Of Lamont & Veterans Way · · · 423-926-1171
Mountain Home, TN 37684 · · · · · · · · 877-573-3529
www.mountainhome.va.gov
As part of the VA Midsouth Healthcare Network (VISN 9), James H. Quillen VA Healthcare System provides services available to veterans residing in the 41-county area of Tennessee, Virginia, Kentucky, and North Carolina.
Dean B. Borsos, MHSA, Director
David S. Hecht, MD, MBA, Chief of Staff

10240 Memphis VA Medical Center
1030 Jefferson Avenue · · · · · · · · · · · 901-523-8990
Memphis, TN 38104 · · · · · · · · · · · · · 800-636-8262
www.memphis.va.gov
Memphis VA Medical Center improves the health of veterans residing in 53 counties in western Tennessee, northern Mississippi, and northwest Arkansas.
David K. Dunning, MPA, Director & CEO
Frank W. Kehus, Associate Director & COO

10241 Nashville VA Medical Center Tennessee Valley Healthcare System
1310 24th Avenue S · · · · · · · · · · · · · 615-327-4751
Nashville, TN 37212-2637 · · · · · · · · · 800-228-4973
www.tennesseevalley.va.gov
Nashville VA Medical Center is part of the Tennessee Healthcare System. Tennessee Valley Healthcare System provides primary and secondary care, general medicine, surgery and specialized care to veterans. The Nashville VA Medical Center is the only VA facility supporting solid organ transplant programs, including total in-house kidney and bone marrow transplants.
Jennifer Vedral-Baron, MN, FAANP, Director
Suzanne L. Jen,, MBA, VHA-CM, Deputy Director

10242 VA MidSouth Healthcare Network (VISN 9)
1801 W End Avenue · · · · · · · · · · · · · 615-695-2200
Nashville, TN 37203 · · · · · · · · · · · · · 877-291-5311
Fax: 615-321-2721
www.visn9.va.gov
VA MidSouth Healthcare Network (VISN 9) is an integrated healthcare delivery system consisting of 9 medical centers located in Lexington and Louisville in Kentucky; and Memphis, Mountain Home, Murfreesboro and Nashville in Tennessee. In total, VISN 9

provides medical care to veterans in 238 counties within the MidSouth.
Cynthia Breyfogle, FACHE, Director
Todd D. Burnett, PsyD, Deputy Director

Texas

10243 Audie L. Murphy Memorial VA Hospital South Texas Veterans Health Care System
7400 Merton Minter   210-617-5300
San Antonio, TX 78229   877-469-5300
                            www.southtexas.va.gov
Part of the VA Heart of Texas Veterans Integrated Service Network (VISN 17), the South Texas Veterans Health Care System is comprised of two inpatient campuses: the Audie L. Murphy Memorial VA Hospital in San Antonio and the Kerrville VA Hospital in Kerrville, Texas. Audie L. Murphy is a quaternary care facility.
Christopher R. Sandles, MBA, FACHE, Director
Julianne Flynn, MD, Chief of Staff

10244 Central Texas Veterans Health Care System
1901 Veterans Memorial Drive   254-778-4811
Temple, TX 76504   800-423-2111
                                deborah.meyer@va.gov
                                www.centraltexas.va.gov
The Central Texas Veterans Health Care System consists of two VA medical centers located in Temple and Waco, one outpatient clinic in Austin, four community-based outpatient clinics in Brownwood, Bryan/College Station, Cedar Park, and Palestine, with a rural outreach clinic in La Grange.
Andrew T. Garcia, MHA, Director
Olawale O. Fashina, MD, MHSA, CPE, Chief of Staff

10245 El Paso VA Health Care Center
5001 N Piedras   915-564-6100
El Paso, TX 79930   800-672-3782
                        Fax: 915-564-7920
                        www.elpaso.va.gov
The El Paso VA Health Care System serves Veterans in southwest Texas and Doña Ana County, New Mexico. The El Paso VA Health Care System provides primary and specialized ambulatory care services at its main campus, and operates two outpatient clinics.
Michael L. Amaral, Director
Jamie D. Park, Associate Director

10246 George H. O'Brien, Jr. VA Medical Center West Texas VA Health Care System
300 Veterans Boulevard   432-263-7361
Big Spring, TX 79720   800-472-1365
                            www.bigspring.va.gov
George H. O'Brien, Jr. VA Medical Center fulfills the health care needs of veterans residing in Big Spring, Texas. This medical center maintains a domiciliary program, and provides mental health and dental care.
Kalautie S. JangDhari, Director
Manuel M. Davila, Associate Director

10247 Kerrville VA Hospital South Texas Veterans Health Care System
3600 Memorial Boulevard   830-896-2020
Kerrville, TX 78028   866-487-7653
                            www.southtexas.va.gov
Part of the VA Heart of Texas Veterans Integrated Service Network (VISN 17), the South Texas Veterans Health Care System is comprised of two inpatient campuses:the Audie L. Murphy Memorial VA Hospital in San Antonio and the Kerrville VA Hospital in Kerrville, Texas. Kerrville provides primary care along with palliative care.
Christopher R. Sandles, MBA, FACHE, Director
Julianne Flynn, MD, Chief of Staff

10248 Michael E. DeBakey VA Medical Center
2002 Holcombe Boulevard   713-791-1414
Houston, TX 77030-4298   800-553-2278
                            www.houston.va.gov
Provides medical services for the veteran population of southeast Texas, and operates a post-traumatic stress disorder clinic.
Francisco Vasquez, MBA, Director
J. Kalavar, MD, Chief of Staff

10249 Thomas E. Creek VA Medical Center Amarillo VA Health Care System
6010 Amarillo Boulevard W   806-355-9703
Amarillo, TX 79106   800-687-8262
                            www.amarillo.va.gov
The Amarillo VA Health Care System, a division of the Southwest VA Health Care Network (VISN 18), provides primary, specialty, and extended care to veterans throughout the Texas and Oklahoma panhandles, eastern New Mexico, and southern Kansas.
Michael L. Kiefer, MHA, FACHE, Director
Elizabeth Lowery, Associate Director

10250 VA Austin Outpatient Clinic
7901 Metropolis Drive   512-823-4000
Austin, TX 78744   www.centraltexas.va.gov
VA Austin Outpatient Clinic is the largest clinic in the nation, offering numerous specialty services from chemotherapy to gastroenterology.
Andrew T. Garcia, MHA, Director
Olawale O. Fashina, MD, MHSA, CPE, Chief of Staff

10251 VA Heart of Texas Health Care Network Dallas VA Medical Center
4500 S Lancaster Road   214-742-8387
Dallas, TX 75216   800-849-3597
                            www.northtexas.va.gov
The VA Heart of Texas Health Care Network provides health care services to veterans in 38 counties in Texas, and 2 counties in southern Oklahoma.
Stephen R. Holt, Director
Kendrick Brown, Associate Director

Utah

10252 George E. Wahlen Medical Center VA Salt Lake City Health Care System
500 Foothill Drive   801-582-1565
Salt Lake City, UT 84148   800-613-4012
                            www.saltlakecity.va.gov
The George E. Wahlen Department of Veterans Affairs Medical Center is a tertiary care facility and provides a comprehensive range of patient care services, from general medicine to surgery.
Shella Stovall, MNA, RN, NE-BC, Director
Warren E. Hill, Associate Director

Vermont

10253 White River Junction VA Medical Center
215 N Main Street   802-295-9363
White River Junction, VT 05009 866-687-8387
                            www.whiteriver.va.gov
The White River Junction VA Medical Center provides health care services to eligible Veterans in Vermont and the 4 counties in New Hampshire. The medical center is affiliated with the Geisel School of Medicine, formerly known as Dartmouth Medical School.
Brett Rusch, MD, Executive Director
Becky Rhoads, Au.D, Associate Director

Virginia

10254 Hampton VA Medical Center
100 Emancipation Drive   757-722-9961
Hampton, VA 23667   866-544-9961
                            www.hampton.va.gov
Hampton VA Medical Center provides comprehensive primary and specialty care at its main facility for veterans in southeastern Virginia and northeastern North Carolina. Two community-based outpatient clinics are located in Elizabeth City, Chesapeake, and Virginia Beach.
Taquisa K. Simmons, PhD, Director
Priscilla Hankins, MD, Chief of Staff

10255 Hunter Holmes McGuire VA Medical Center
1201 Broad Rock Boulevard   804-675-5000
Richmond, VA 23249   800-784-8381
                            www.richmond.va.gov
With its main facility located in Richmond, Virginia, Hunter Holmes provides medical services available to eligible veterans

from 52 cities and counties in central and southern Virginia, and parts of North Carolina.
J. Ronald Johnson, FACHE, Director
James W. Dudley, Associate Director

10256 Roanoke Vet Center
350 Albemarle Avenue SW   540-342-9726
Roanoke, VA 24016   877-927-8387
                                 www.va.gov
A medical facility serving the health needs of veterans in Roanoke, Virginia.
Michael Jenkins, Director
John Whitlock, Counselor

10257 Salem VA Medical Center
1970 Roanoke Boulevard   540-982-2463
Salem, VA 24153   888-982-2463
                                 www.salem.va.gov
Medical facility located in Salem, Virginia, with services available to eligible veterans living in 26 counties in southwestern Virginia.
Rebecca J. Stackhouse, MA, CTRS, Director
Allen R. Moye, MS, Associate Director

Washington

10258 Jonathan M. Wainwright Memorial VA MC Walla Walla VA Medical Center
77 Wainwright Drive   509-525-5200
Walla Walla, WA 99362   888-687-8863
                                 www.wallawalla.va.gov
Jonathan M. Wainwright Memorial VA Medical Center in Walla Walla serves the health care needs of veterans living in eastern Washington, Oregon, and western Idaho.
Christopher R. Bjornberg, Director
Marvin R. Crawford, MBA, Associate Director

10259 Spokane VA Medical Center Mann-Grandstaff VA Medical Center
4815 N Assembly Street   509-434-7000
Spokane, WA 99205   800-325-7940
                                 www.spokane.va.gov
The Spokane VA Medical Center serves the health care needs of veterans in Spokane, Washington, providing primary and secondary care, with a focus on preventive health and chronic disease management.
Robert J. Fischer, MD, FACOG, CPE, Director
Richard Rick Richards, MS, MBA, FACHE, Associate Director

10260 Tacoma Vet Center
4916 Center Street   253-565-7038
Tacoma, WA 98409   Fax: 253-254-0079
                                 www.va.gov
Medical facility serving veterans, and part of the VISN 20 Northwest Network.
William Philadelphia, PhD, LPC, Director
Audrey Dangtwu, Counselor

10261 VA Puget Sound Health Care System
1660 S Columbian Way   206-762-1010
Seattle, WA 98108   800-329-8387
                                 www.pugetsound.va.gov
VA Puget Sound Health Care System provides medical services for veterans residing in 14 counties around the Puget Sound in the Pacific Northwest, in addition to operating two main divisions located at American Lake, and Seattle.
Michael Tadych, FACHE, Director
Kathryn Sherrill, MSW, LCSW, BSN, Deputy Director

West Virginia

10262 Beckley VA Medical Center
200 Veterans Avenue   304-255-2121
Beckley, WV 25801   877-902-5142
                                 www.beckley.va.gov
Beckley VA Medical Center is a rural access facility, offering nursing care, post-acute rehabilitation care, palliative care, and respite care for veterans. A home based primary care program is also available.
Stacy J. Vasquez, Director
John D. Stout, MBA, Associate Director

10263 Hershel Woody Williams VA Medical Center
1540 Spring Valley Drive   304-429-6741
Huntington, WV 25704   800-827-8244
                                 www.huntington.va.gov
Hershel Woody Williams VA Medical Center provides medical care to veterans in its main facility in Huntington. Two community-based outpatient clinics and two rural health outreach clinics exist to better serve veterans. Services are available to veterans living in southwestern West Virginia, southern Ohio, and eastern Kentucky.
J. Brian Nimmo, Director
Kenneth Mortimer, FACHE, Associate Director

10264 Louis A. Johnson VA Medical Center
1 Medical Center Drive   304-623-3461
Clarksburg, WV 26301   800-733-0512
                                 www.clarksburg.va.gov
A medical facility serving the health care needs of veterans in Clarksburg, West Virginia since 1950.
Glenn R. Snider, Jr., MD, FACP, Director
Terry Massey, Associate Director

10265 Martinsburg VA Medical Center
510 Butler Avenue   304-263-0811
Martinsburg, WV 25405   800-817-3807
                                 www.martinsburg.va.gov
The Martinsburg VA Medical Center offers medical services made available to veterans living in 22 counties in Western Maryland, West Virginia, South Central Pennsylvania, and Northwest Virginia.
Timothy J. Cooke, Director
Kenneth W. Allensworth, FACHE, Associate Director

Wisconsin

10266 Milwaukee VA Medical Center (Zablocki)
5000 W National Avenue   414-384-2000
Milwaukee, WI 53295-1000   888-598-7793
                                 www.milwaukee.va.gov
The medical center in Milwaukee delivers primary, secondary, and tertiary medical care to eligible veterans. In addition, the medical center operates a mobile clinic that serves veterans four days a week.
Daniel Zomchek, PhD, Director
Michael Erdmann, MD, Chief of Staff

10267 Tomah VA Medical Center
500 E Veterans Street   608-372-3971
Tomah, WI 54660   800-872-8662
                                 TTY: 888-598-7793
                                 www.tomah.va.gov
As part of the VA Great Lakes Health Care System (VISN 12), Tomah VA Medical Center provides medical care available to veterans living in Western and Central Wisconsin.
Victoria P. Brahm, Director
Staci Williams, Associate Director

10268 William S. Middleton Memorial Veterans Hospital
2500 Overlook Terrace   608-256-1901
Madison, WI 53705   888-478-8321
                                 TTY: 888-598-7793
                                 www.madison.va.gov
The William S. Middleton Memorial Veterans Hospital provides tertiary medical, surgical, neurological, and psychiatric care. Outpatient services are also available to eligible veterans within 15 counties in south-central Wisconsin and 5 counties in northwestern Illinois.
John J. Rohrer, Director
Christine M. Kleckner, Associate Director

Wyoming

10269 Cheyenne VA Medical Center
2360 E Pershing Boulevard   307-778-7550
Cheyenne, WY 82001   888-483-9127
                                 www.cheyenne.va.gov

The Cheyenne VA Medical Center provides health care services to veterans residing in the tri-state area of southeastern Wyoming, northeastern Colorado and southwestern Nebraska.
Paul L. Roberts, Director
Michael Chad Cartwright, Associate Director

10270 Sheridan VA Medical Center
1898 Fort Road   307-672-3473
Sheridan, WY 82801   866-822-6714
                                    www.sheridan.va.gov
The Sheridan VA Medical Center provides medical care to eligible veterans. Additionally, 8 community-based outpatient clinics exist to better serve veterans across Wyoming.
Pamela S. Crowell, MPA, Director
Donald T. McGraw, Associate Director

Libraries & Resource Centers

10271 American GI Forum NVOP
611 N. Flores   210-212-4088
San Antonio, TX 78205   Fax: 210-223-4970
                                    nvopweb@agif-nvop.org
                                    www.agif-nvop.org
Our Mission is to establish and maintain a comprehensive community service agency with a diversified funding source that will serve the needs of veterans, their families, and other needy individuals of the community.

10272 COPIN Foundation
2644 North Avenue   716-283-5622
Niagara Falls, NY 14305   Fax: 716-283-5721

10273 Kennedy-Krieger Institute
707 N Broadway   443-923-9200
Baltimore, MD 21205   800-873-3377
                                    Fax: 443-923-9405
                                    www.kennedykrieger.org
Kennedy Krieger Institute is an internationally recognized institution dedicated to improving the lives of individuals with disorders of the brain, spinal cord, and musculoskeletal system through Patient Care, Research and Professional Training, Special Education and Community. We at the Kennedy Krieger Institute dedicate ourselves to helping children and adolescents with disorders of the brain, spinal cord and musculoskeletal system achieve their potential and participate as fully as possible i
Jennifer Accardo, M.D., Neurologist
Adrianna Amari, Ph.D., Training and research coordinator

10274 Shriver Center University Affiliated Program
Eunice Kennedy Shriver Center
200 Trapelo Road   781-642-0001
Waltham, MA 02452-6319   shriver.center@umassmed.edu
The Eunice Kennedy Shriver Center has a four-decade history of pioneering research, education, and service for people with intellectual and developmental disabilities (IDD) and their families. Founded in 1970, the Center was one of twelve original Intellectual and Developmental Disabilities Research Centers (IDDRCs) established by US Congress at that time and also one of the earliest-established University Centers of Excellence in Developmental Disabilities (UCEDD). The Center was named after Mr
William McIlvane, Director
Charles Hamad, Associate Director

10275 Veterans Benefits Clearinghouse
38 Dudley Street   617-541-8846
Roxbury, MA 02119-1707

Support Groups & Hotlines

10276 National Health Information Center
Office of Disease Prevention & Health Promotion
1101 Wootton Pkwy   Fax: 240-453-8281
Rockville, MD 20852   odphpinfo@hhs.gov
                                    www.health.gov/nhic
Supports public health education by maintaining a calendar of National Health Observances; helps connect consumers and health professionals to organizations that can best answer questions and provide up-to-date contact information from reliable sources; up-

dates on a yearly basis toll-free numbers for health information, Federal health clearinghouses and info centers.
Don Wright, MD, MPH, Director

10277 National Veterans Services Fund
Darien, CT 06820-0465   203-656-0003
                                         800-521-0198
                                    Fax: 203-656-1957
                                    NatVetSvc@aol.com
                                    www.nvsf.org
NVSF, Inc. provides an integrated program of services managed by veterans that include the following: a national hotline for veterans and their families that responds to hundreds of inquiries each month from throughout the country; an extensive repository of free information on topics ranging from the history of the Agent Orange lawsuit to the most recent Gulf War legislation; a special fund that offers limited emergency economic assistance and relief for families in crisis; business partnership
Phil Kraft, President

Books

10278 An Assessment of Technical Issues Raised in RW Haley's Critique of Health Studies
Gus Haggstrom, author
Rand Corporation
1776 Main Street   310-393-0411
Santa Monica, CA 90407-2138   Fax: 310-393-4818
                                    www.rand.org
The monograph/report was a product of the RAND Corporation from 1993 to 2003. RAND monograph/reports presented major research findings that addressed the challenges facing the public and private sectors.
ISBN: 0-833027-52-2
Gus Haggstrom, Author

10279 Gulf War and Health
National Academy Press
500 5th Street NW   202-334-3313
Washington, DC 20001   800-624-6242
                                    Fax: 202-334-2793
                                    Customer_Service@nap.edu
                                    www.nap.edu

Lyla M Hernandez, Editor
Merwyn R Greenlick, Editor

10280 Natural Attenuation for Groundwater Remediation
National Academy Press
500 5th Street NW   202-334-3313
Washington, DC 20001   800-624-6242
                                    Fax: 202-334-2793
                                    Customer_Service@nap.edu
                                    www.nap.edu

10281 Yes, You Can
Demos Medical Publishing
11 West 42nd Street   212-683-0072
New York, NY 10036   Fax: 212-683-0118
                                    support@demosmedical.com
                                    www.demosmedical.com

112 pages
ISBN: 1-888799-48-x
Dr. Diana M Schneider

Newsletters

10282 Agent Orange Briefs
Department of Veterans Affairs
810 Vermont Avenue NW   202-233-4000
Washington, DC 20420-0002
Designed to answer questions regarding Agent Orange and related matters. This fact sheet series is prepared and updated annually.
Monthly

10283 Agent Orange Review
Department of Veterans Affairs
810 Vermont Avenue NW   202-233-4000
Washington, DC 20420-0002

Published periodically to provide information on Agent Orange to concerned veterans and their families. The most recent issues include updated information about Federal government studies and activities related to Agent Orange and the Vietnam experience.

Pamphlets

10284 Agent Orange Anxiety: The Human Response to Possable Oncogenicity and Mutagencity
National Veterans Services Fund
PO Box 2465   203-656-0003
Darien, CT 06820-0465   800-521-0198
                                    Fax: 203-656-1957
                                    support@NVSF.org
                                    www.nvsf.org

Erwin R. Parson, Ph.D., Author

10285 Agent Orange Fact Sheet: A Historical Perspective
Veterans Of The Vietnam War
805 South Township Blvd   570-603-9740
Pittston, PA 18640-3327   Fax: 570-603-9741
                                    www.vvnw.org

Fact sheet designed to bring an awareness of Agent Orange and related herbicides to the American public, includes a bibliography for the professional.
10 pages

10286 Agent Orange and Birth Defects
Veterans Health Adminstration
810 Vermont Avenue NW   202-273-8580
Washington, DC 20420-3517   Fax: 202-273-9080
                              www.tpromo2.com/usvi/index2.htm
Letters to the editor, New England Journal of Medicine articles.

10287 Agent Orange and Chloracme
National Veterans Services Fund
PO Box 2465   203-656-0003
Darien, CT 06820-0465   800-521-0198
                                    Fax: 203-656-1957
                                    support@NVSF.org
                                    www.nvsf.org

10288 Agent Orange and Hodgkin's Disease
Veterans Health Administration
810 Vermont Avenue NW   203-273-8580
Washington, DC 20420-3517   Fax: 203-273-9080
                              www.tpromo2.com/usvi/index2.htm

10289 Agent Orange and Mutiple Myeloma
National Veterans Services Fund
PO Box 2465   203-656-0003
Darien, CT 06820-0465   800-521-0198
                                    Fax: 203-656-1957
                                    support@NVSF.org
                                    www.nvsf.org

10290 Agent Orange and Non-Hodgkin's Lymphoma
Veterans Health Administration
810 Vermont Avenue   203-273-8580
Washington, DC 20420-3517   Fax: 203-273-9080
                              www.tpromo2.com/usvi/index2.htm

10291 Agent Orange and Peripheral Neuropathy
Veterans Health Administration
810 Vermont Avenue   203-273-8580
Washington, DC 20420-3517   Fax: 203-273-9080

10292 Agent Orange and Porphyria Cutanea Tarda
National Veterans Services Fund
PO Box 2465   203-656-0003
Darien, CT 06820-0465   800-521-0198
                                    Fax: 203-656-1957
                                    support@NVSF.org
                                    www.nvsf.org

10293 Agent Orange and Prostate Cancer
National Veterans Services Fund

PO Box 2465   203-656-0003
Darien, CT 06820-0465   800-521-0198
                                    Fax: 203-656-1957
                                    support@NVSF.org
                                    www.nvsf.org

10294 Agent Orange and Respiratory Cancers
National Veterans Services Fund
PO Box 2465   203-656-0003
Darien, CT 06820-0465   800-521-0198
                                    Fax: 203-656-1957
                                    support@NVSF.org
                                    www.nvsf.org

10295 Agent Orange and Soft Tissue Sarcomas
National Veterans Services Fund
PO Box 2465   203-656-0003
Darien, CT 06820-0465   800-521-0198
                                    Fax: 203-656-1957
                                    support@NVSF.org
                                    www.nvsf.org

10296 Agent Orange and Spina Bifida
National Veterans Services Fund
PO Box 2465   203-656-0003
Darien, CT 06820-0465   800-521-0198
                                    Fax: 203-656-1957
                                    support@NVSF.org
                                    www.nvsf.org

10297 Agent Orange: It is Part of Your Life
National Veterans Services Fund
PO Box 2465   203-656-0003
Darien, CT 06820-0465   800-521-0198
                                    Fax: 203-656-1957
                                    support@NVSF.org
                                    www.nvsf.org

Dr. Arthur Galston, Author

10298 Brief History of the Agent Orange Lawsuit
National Veterans Services Fund
PO Box 2465   203-656-0003
Darien, CT 06820-0465   800-521-0198
                                    Fax: 203-656-1957
                                    support@NVSF.org
                                    www.nvsf.org

10299 Case Control Study: Soft-Tissue Sarcomas and Exposure to Phenoxyacetic Acids
National Veterans Services Fund
PO Box 2465   203-656-0003
Darien, CT 06820-0465   800-521-0198
                                    Fax: 203-656-1957
                                    support@NVSF.org
                                    www.nvsf.org

Case control study: soft-tissue sarcoma and exposure to phenoxyacetic acids or chlorophenols.
L. Hardell, Co-Author
A. Sandstrom, Co-Author

10300 Children of Vietnam Veterans: Complex Concerns and Innovative Solutions
National Veterans Services Fund
PO Box 2465   203-656-0003
Darien, CT 06820-0465   800-521-0198
                                    Fax: 203-656-1957
                                    support@NVSF.org
                                    www.nvsf.org

7 pages
Phillip R. Kraft, Author

10301 Dioxin, A Case in Point
National Veterans Services Fund
PO Box 2465   203-656-0003
Darien, CT 06820-0465   800-521-0198
                                    Fax: 203-656-1957
                                    support@NVSF.org
                                    www.nvsf.org

Luke G. Tedeschi, M.D., Author

10302 Enviromental Chloracne
National Veterans Services Fund
PO Box 2465   203-656-0003
Darien, CT 06820-0465   800-521-0198
Fax: 203-656-1957
support@NVSF.org
www.nvsf.org

10303 History of the Agent Orange Litigation
National Veterans Services Fund
PO Box 2465   203-656-0003
Darien, CT 06820-0465   800-521-0198
Fax: 203-656-1957
support@NVSF.org
www.nvsf.org

10304 List of Agent Orange-Related Illnesses Recognized By the VA
National Veterans Services Fund
PO Box 2465   203-656-0003
Darien, CT 06820-0465   800-521-0198
Fax: 203-656-1957
support@NVSF.org
www.nvsf.org

10305 List of Diseases Accepted by the VA for Presumptive Service-Connection
National Veterans Services Fund
PO Box 2465   203-656-0003
Darien, CT 06820-0465   800-521-0198
Fax: 203-656-1957
support@NVSF.org
www.nvsf.org
List of diseases accepted by the VA for presumptive service-connection that are associated with exposure to certain herbicide agents including Agent Orange.

10306 Relation of Soft-Tissue Sarcome, Malignant Lymphoma & Colon Cancer
National Veterans Services Fund
PO Box 2465   203-656-0003
Darien, CT 06820-0465   800-521-0198
Fax: 203-656-1957
support@NVSF.org
www.nvsf.org
Relation to soft-tissue sarcomas, malignant lymphoma and colon cancer to phenoxy acids, chlorphenois and other agents.

10307 Spina Bifida Benefits Guide
National Veterans Services Fund
PO Box 2465   203-656-0003
Darien, CT 06820-0465   800-521-0198
Fax: 203-656-1957
support@NVSF.org
www.nvsf.org

4 pages

Audio & Video

10308 Agent Orange Videotapes
Regional Learning Resources Service
915 N. Grand Boulevard   314-652-4100
St. Louis, MO 63106
Produces several Agent Orange videotape programs that explain what Agent Orange is, where, when and how it was used, why persons are concerned about exposure to it and what VA and other departments and agencies are doing in response to these concerns. These videotapes are maintained at all VA medical centers across the country.

Web Sites

10309 Gulf War Syndrome Database
www.louisville.edu/library/ekstrom
This is a substantial database of relevant documents and studies kept by University of Louisville, Ekstrom Library.

10310 Gulf War Veteran Resource Pages
www.gulfweb.org

This page is administered by Gulf War veterans and provides a great range of information on a variety of Gulf War-related items, including GWS. The site includes many links to other groups interested in GWS and to GWS studies.

10311 Healing Well
www.healingwell.com
An online health resource guide to medical news, chat, information and articles, newsgroups and message boards, books, disease-related web sites, medical directories, and more for patients, friends, and family coping with disabling diseases, disorders, or chronic illnesses.

10312 Health Finder
www.healthfinder.gov
Searchable, carefully developed web site offering information on over 1000 topics. Developed by the US Department of Health and Human Services, the site can be used in both English and Spanish.

10313 Healthlink USA
www.healthlinkusa.com
Health information concerning treatment, cures, prevention, diagnosis, risk factors, research, support groups, email lists, personal stories and much more. Updated regularly.

10314 Heatlhcentral.com
www.healthcentral.com
The HealthCentral Network has a collection of owned and operated web sites and multimedia affiliate properties providing timely, in-depth, trusted medical information, personalized tools and resources for people seeking to manage and improve their health.

10315 InteliHealth
InteliHealth's mission is to empower people with trusted solutions for healthier lives. They accomplish this by providing credible information fromt he most trusted sources.
Brian Berkenstock, Writer/Editor

10316 MedicineNet
www.medicinenet.com
Medicine Net is an online healthcare media publishing company. It provides easy-to-read, in-depth, authoritative medical information for consumers via its robust, user-friendly, interactive web site.

10317 Medscape
www.medscape.com
Medscape offers specialists, primary care physicians, and other health professionals the Web's most robust and integrated medical information and educational tools.

10318 National Veterans Services Fund
www.nvsf.org
Supports and informs those who were exposed to the defoliant Agent Orange, or dioxin, while serving the US in the conflict in Vietnam.

10319 Office of the Special Assistant for Gulf War Illnesses
www.gulflink.osd.mil
This is a page sponsored by the Defense Department's Special Assistant for Gulf War Illnesses. It provides information on and linkes to Federal and State-funded studies of Gulf War Illnesses.

10320 VA Caregiver Support
www.caregiver.va.gov
Tips, tools, and other resources for caregivers of veterans.

10321 WebMD
www.webmd.com
Provides credible information, supportive communities, and in-depth reference material about health subjects. A source for original and timely health information as well as material from well known content providers.

Description

10322 Wilson Disease

Wilson disease is a rare genetic disorder that results from an inability to adequately excrete copper. In the United States, approximately one person in 40,000 has this condition. The resulting accumulation of copper in the body's tissues and organs leads to disease of the brain and liver, and to a lesser extent, the kidney and red blood cells. The disease is genetic; it is caused by mutations in the ATP7B gene and if two carriers have children, the disease has a 1 in 4 chance of being passed on.

Build-up of copper in the liver causes a hepatitis-like illness with loss of appetite, low grade fever, abdominal discomfort and jaundice. If not detected and treated, this process can lead to cirrhosis and fatal liver failure. In 40-50 percent of patients, the illness affects the brain and can include unsteadiness, tremors, slurred speech and intellectual deterioration. Copper rings may appear in the eye (Kayser-Fleischer rings) in up to 10 percent of patients. Although they do not cause any symptoms, their appearance may help establish the diagnosis.

In untreated Wilson, the disease is fatal, generally before the age of 30. Continual, lifelong treatment is mandatory for any patient with confirmed Wilson disease, whether symptomatic or not. The critical therapy is to administer a drug that helps the body release its copper stores. D-penicillamine is the most common copper-chelating drug, and trientine is an alternative drug. Once copper levels are normalized, zinc supplements can help copper levels remain normal. Some patients, however, have required liver transplantation.

National Agencies & Associations

10323 American Liver Foundation
39 Broadway   212-668-1000
New York, NY 10006   800-465-4837
Fax: 212-483-8179
info@liverfoundation.org
www.liverfoundation.org
ALF raises awareness of liver disease through education, advocacy, and research for the prevention, treatment, and cure of liver disease, and provides support services to those affected.
Tom Nealon, President & CEO
Lynn Gardiner Seim, Executive Vice President & COO

10324 Wilson's Disease Association
1732 First Avenue   414-961-0533
New York, NY 10128   866-961-0533
info@wilsonsdisease.org
www.wilsonsdisease.org
WDA serves as an international non-profit health organization that funds research, provides support, and promotes awareness and education of Wilson's disease through the development of more precise diagnostic methods, and the creation of a network connecting patients to their families and healthcare providers.
8 pages
Jean P. Perog, President
Mary L. Graper, Vice President of Scientific Affairs

Foundations

10325 Hepatitis B Foundation
3805 Old Easton Road   215-489-4900
Doylestown, PA 18902   Fax: 215-489-4920
info@hepb.org
www.hepb.org
The Hepatitis B Foundation is a national non-profit organization committed to finding a cure for hepatitis B. The Hepatitis B Foundation supports immunization, research, and education, and is a primary resource for those affected by hepatitis B, the medical community and the general public.

Joel Rosen, Chairman
Timothy M. Block, PhD, Co-Founder & President

Support Groups & Hotlines

10326 National Health Information Center
Office of Disease Prevention & Health Promotion
1101 Wootton Pkwy   Fax: 240-453-8281
Rockville, MD 20852   odphpinfo@hhs.gov
www.health.gov/nhic
Supports public health education by maintaining a calendar of National Health Observances; helps connect consumers and health professionals to organizations that can best answer questions and provide up-to-date contact information from reliable sources; updates on a yearly basis toll-free numbers for health information, Federal health clearinghouses and info centers.
Don Wright, MD, MPH, Director

Pamphlets

10327 Wilson's Disease
American Liver Foundation
39 Broadway   212-668-1000
New York, NY 10006   800-465-4837
info@liverfoundation.org
www.liverfoundation.org
A brochure offering information on the causes, symptoms and treatments of Wilson's Disease.
Tom Nealon, President & CEO
Lynn Gardiner Seim, MSN, RN, Executive Vice President & COO

Web Sites

10328 Healing Well
www.healingwell.com
An online health resource guide to medical news, chat, information and articles, newsgroups and message boards, books, disease-related web sites, medical directories, and more for patients, friends, and family coping with disabling diseases, disorders, or chronic illnesses.
Peter Waite, MS, MA, Founder & CEO

10329 Health Finder
www.healthfinder.gov
Searchable web site offering information on over 1000 topics. Developed by the US Department of Health and Human Services, the site can be used in both English and Spanish.

10330 Healthlink USA
www.healthlinkusa.com
Health information web site and online discussion forum. Covers topics concerning treatment, cures, prevention, diagnosis, risk factors, research, support groups, email lists, personal stories and much more. Updated regularly.

10331 MedicineNet
www.medicinenet.com
An online resource for consumers providing easy-to-read, authoritative medical and health information produced and written by medical professionals. Includes a symptom checker, and a dictionary that defines and explains medical terms. MedicineNet is part of the WebMD Network.

10332 Medscape

www.medscape.com

Medscape offers medical professionals with the latest medical news, including advancements in drug treatments, and new journal articles. Medscape is part of the WebMD Network.

10333 WebMD

www.webmd.com

Provides up-to-date medical news and information, supportive communities, and in-depth reference material on a wide variety of health and wellness topics.

Tony G. Holcombe, President
John Whyte, MD, MPH, Chief Medical Officer

National Agencies & Associations

10334 ACLU National Prison Project
125 Broad Street   212-549-2500
New York, NY 10004   media@aclu.org
                                                     www.aclu.org
National Prison Project seeks to create constitutional conditions of confinement and strengthen prisoners' rights through class action litigation and public education. Policy priorities include reducing prison overcrowding and improving prisoner medical care.
Susan Herman, President
Anthony Romero, Chief Executive Officer

10335 AbleData
103 W. Broad Street   800-227-0216
Falls Church, VA 22046   Fax: 703-356-8314
                                                 TTY: 703-992-8313
                                          abledata@neweditions.net
                                               abledata.acl.gov
An information and referral service that uses computer listings and a large file system to answer requests related to assistive devices. Houses a large file system library and contacts with other sources which enables them to answer just about any question.

10336 Access Unlimited
570 Hance Road   800-849-2143
Binghamton, NY 13903   Fax: 607-669-4595
                                          tom@accessunlimited.com
                                           www.accessunlimited.com
We celebrate the rich diversity of our customers' needs by creating products that allow easy access to any vehicle, from cars and vans to trucks and SUVs. We believe that adaptive equipment should be unobtrusive and should meet the needs of its user with a minimum of modification to vehicle or lifestyle. We believe every person should be able to choose the vehicle they like best, regardless of their disability. Access Unlimited products empower people with disabilities to regain control of thei
Tom Cole, Owner

10337 American Academy of Pediatrics
141 NW Point Boulevard   847-434-4000
Elk Grove Village, IL 60007-1098   800-433-9016
                                                 Fax: 847-434-8000
                                                     www.aap.org
To attain optimal physical, mental, and social health and well-being for all infants, children, adolescents, and young adults.
Thomas K. McInerny, President
Errol T Alden MD FAAP, Executive Director

10338 American Association for the Advancement of Science
1200 New York Avenue NW   202-326-6400
Washington, DC 20005   Fax: 202-371-9526
                                             webmaster@aaas.org
                                                    www.aaas.org
The non-profit AAAS is open to all and fulfills its mission to advance science and serve society through initiatives that include science policy, international programs, science education, and public understanding of science.
William Press, Chair
Phillip A. Sharp, President

10339 American Association of People with Disabilities
2013 H Street, NW   202-457-0046
Washington, DC 20006   800-840-8844
                                                 Fax: 866-536-4461
                                                 TTY: 202-457-0046
                                                    www.aapd.com
The American Association of People with Disabilities is the nation's largest disability rights organization. We promote equal opportunity, economic power, independent living, and political participation for people with disabilities. Our members, including people with disabilities and our family, friends, and supporters, represent a powerful force for change.
Mark Perriello, President/CEO
Henry Claypool, Executive VP

10340 American Autoimmune Related Diseases Association
22100 Gratiot Avenue   586-776-3900
Eastpointe, MI 48021   800-598-4668
                                              Fax: 586-776-3903
                                                  aarda@aarda.org
                                                    www.aarda.org
Awareness, education, referrals for patients with any type of autoimmune disease.
Virginia T. Ladd, President & Executive Director
Laura Simpson, Assistant Director

10341 American Bar Association Commission on Mental and Physical Disability Law
1050 Connecticut Ave. N.W.   202-662-1000
Washington, DC 20036   800-285-2221
                                              Fax: 202-442-3439
                                          campdl@americanbar.org
                                             www.americanbar.org
The Commission's mission is to promote the ABA's commitment to justice and the rule of law for persons with mental, physical, and sensory disabilities and to promote their full and equal participation in the legal profession.
John W Parry, Director
Laurel G. Bellows, President

10342 American Camp Association
5000 State Road 67 N   765-342-8456
Martinsville, IN 46151-7902   800-428-2267
                                              Fax: 765-342-2065
                                                 www.acacamps.org
Formerly the American Camping Association, a community of camp professionals who have joined together to share the knowledge and experience and to ensure the quality of camp programs.
Tisha Bolger, President
Melanie Lock Herman, Treasurer

10343 American Counseling Association
5999 Stevenson Avenue   800-347-6647
Alexandria, VA 22304   Fax: 703-823-0252
                                              ryep@counseling.org
                                                www.counseling.org
A not-for-profit, professional and educational organization that is dedicated to the growth and enhancement of the counseling profession. Represents professional counselors in various practice settings.
Marcheta Evans, President
Richard Yep, Executive Director

10344 American Foundation for The Blind
2 Penn Plaza   212-502-7600
New York, NY 10121   800-232-5463
                                              Fax: 888-545-8331
                                                 afbinfo@afb.net
                                                     www.afb.org
AFB's priorities include broadening access to technology; elevating the quality of information and tools for the professionals who serve people with vision loss by providing them and their families with relevant and timely resources.
Carl R Augusto, President/CEO
Rick Bozeman, Chief Financial Officer

10345 American Institute for Preventive Medicine
30445 NW Highway   248-539-1800
Farmington Hills, MI 48334   800-345-2476
                                              Fax: 248-539-1808
                                             aipm@healthylife.com
                                                www.healthylife.com
An award winning, internationally recognized authority on th development and implementation of health promotion, wellness, medical self-care, and disease management programs and publications.
Larry Chapman, President
Dee Edington, Director

10346 American Institute for Preventive Medicine
30445 NW Highway   248-539-1800
Farmington Hills, MI 48334   800-345-2476
                                              Fax: 248-539-1808
                                             aipm@healthylife.com
                                                www.healthylife.com

The institute provides health promotion programs disease management guides and self-care publications to hospitals HMOs corporations and government agencies. Programs are designed to lower health care costs, decrease absenteeism and improve productivity.
Larry Chapman, President
Dee Edington, Director

10347 American Organ Transplant Association
PO Box 418   713-344-2402
Stilwell, KS 66085   Fax: 281-617-4274
                          aotaonline@gmail.com
                          www.aota.online.org
Helps patients with free transportation to and from their transplant center, many times hundreds of miles away. Also provides transplant patients and their loved ones with resources regarding transplantation.
Pamela H Terry, Board President
Kenneth Klingensmith, Immediate Past Board President

10348 American Red Cross National Headquarters
2025 E Street NW   202-303-5000
Washington, DC 20006   800-733-2767
                          www.redcross.org
The nation's premier emergency response organization that aids victims of devastating natural disasters; community services that help the needy; support and comfort for military members and their families; the collection, processing and distribution of lifesaving blood and blood products; educational programs that promote health and safety; and international relief and development programs.
Gail J McGovern, President/CEO
Bonnie McElveen-Hunt, Chairman

10349 American Rehabilitation Counseling Association
5999 Stevenson Avenue   800-347-6647
Alexandria, VA 22304-3300   Fax: 800-473-2329
                            TTY: 703-823-6862
                            TDD: 7038236862
                          webmaster@counseling.org
                          www.counseling.org
Mission of ARCA is to enhance the development of persons with disabilities throughout their life span and to promote excellence in the rehabilitation counseling professional.
Colleen Logan, President
Richard Yep, Executive Office

10350 American Society of Dermatology
Port St Lucie, FL 34984   561-873-8335
                            Fax: 561-344-8388
                          www.asd.org
The mission of this organization is to facilitate optimal dermatologic care being available to all citizens of this country by preserving, promoting and enhancing the private practice of dermatology. It shall represent its members in those scientific, educational, socioeconomic and legislative areas that affect the practice of dermatology and shall endeavor to cooperate with other organizations of similar purpose.
W Gerald Klinger MD, President
Don Printz, MD, Secretary

10351 Americas Association for the Care of the Children
PO Box 2154   303-527-2742
Boulder, CO 80306   aaccchildren.org
Carries out a variety of programs to promote the health of children. Publishes educational materials on child health of interest to parents, educators and health professionals.
Deborah Young, Executive Director & Founder
Judi Jackson, President

10352 Asbestos Information Association/North America
1745 Jefferson Davis Highway   703-412-1150
Arlington, VA 22202   Fax: 703-412-1586
                          aiabjpigg@aol.com
Founded to represent the interests of the asbestos industry and to collect and disseminate information about asbestos and asbestos products with emphasis on safety health and environmental issues.

10353 Beach Center on Disability
University of Kansas

1200 Sunnyside Avenue   785-864-7600
Lawrence, KS 66045   Fax: 786-864-7605
                          beachcenter@ku.edu
                          www.beachcenter.org
The Beach Center on Disability is a multi-disciplinary research and training center committed to making a significant and sustainable positive difference in the quality of life of individuals and families affected by disability and the professionals who support them. Its staff of approximately 40 professors, researchers, educators, doctoral students, and support personnel carry out research, technical assistance, and undergraduate, masters, and doctoral training. Its staff focuses on families, f
Ann Turnbull, Co-Founder, Co-Director, Distinguished P
Rud Turnbull, Co-Founder, Co-Director, Distinguished P

10354 Breaking New Ground Resource Center
2255 S University Street   765-494-5088
W Lafayette, IN 47907   800-825-4264
                            Fax: 765-496-1356
Has become internationally recoginzed as the primary source for information and resources on rehabilitation technology for persons working in agriculture.
Prof William Field, Project Leader

10355 Center for Children with Chronic Illness and Disability
University of Minnesota School of Public Health
2525 Chicago Avenue   612-813-6000
Minneapolis, MN 55404   Get.Well@childrensmn.org
                          www.childrensmn.org
Serving as Minnesota's children's hospitalSM since 1924, we provide 347 staffed beds at our two hospital campuses in St. Paul and Minneapolis. An independent, not-for-profit health care system, Children's provides care through more than 12,000 inpatient visits and more than 200,000 emergency room and other outpatient visits each year.
Alan L. Goldbloom, MD, Chief Executive Officer
David A. Brumbaugh, SPHR, Vice President Human Resources

10356 Center for Chronic Disease Prevention and Centers for Disease Control
1600 Clifton Road   404-639-3311
Atlanta, GA 30333   800-232-4636
                            TTY: 888-232-6348
                          cdcinfo@cdc.gov
                          www.cdc.gov
Chronic diseases such as heart disease cancer and diabetes are the leading causes of death and disability in the United States. These diseases account for 7 of every 10 deaths and affect the quality of life of 90 million Americans.
Richard E Besser, Director

10357 Center for Developmental Disabilities University of South Carolina
8301 Farrow Road   803-935-5231
Columbia, SC 29208   Fax: 803-935-5059
                          steve.wilson@uscmed.sc.edu
                          www.uscm.med.sc.edu/cdrhome
The vision of The Center for Developmental Disabilities is to work as a team to create a quality environment in which the following values are embraced: Everyone is treated with dignity and respect. Individual strengths and abilities are recognized.

10358 Center for Disability Resources
University of South Carolina
8301 Farrow Road   803-935-5231
Columbia, SC 29208   Fax: 803-935-5059
                          steve.wilson@uscmed.sc.edu
To enhance the well-being and quality of life of persons with disabilities and their families. Collaborates with persons with disabilities and their families to develop new knowledge and best practices, train leaders, and effect systems change.

10359 Center for Disease Control and Prevention
1600 Clifton Rd   800-232-4636
Atlanta, GA 30333   TTY: 888-232-6348
                          cdcinfo@cdc.gov
                          www.cdc.gov
To collaborate to create the expertise, information, and tools that people and communities need to protect their health - through

769

health promotion, prevention of disease, injury and disability, and preparedness for new health threats.
Thomas R Frieden MD MPH, Director

10360 Center for Health Research
Kaiser Permanente Northwest
3800 N Interstate Avenue
Portland, OR 97227-1098

503-335-2400
information@kpchr.org
www.kpchr.org

Conducts professionally independent, public domain research and idsseminates its findings in the scholarly literature and scientific community.
Mary L Durham PhD, Director
Donald R Freel, Executive Director COO

10361 Center for Medical Consumers
239 Thompson Street
New York, NY 10012

212-674-7105
centerformedicalconsumers@gmail.com
www.medicalconsumers.org

A non-profit advocacy organization that was founded with the philosophy: Whenever long-term drug therapy, elective surgery, or any other major treatment is prescribed, the question of whether the treatment has been proven safe and effective should come up.
Arthur Aaron Levin MPH, Director
Maryann Napoli, Associate Director

10362 Center for Parent Information & Resources
SPAN
35 Halsey Street
Newark, NJ 07102

973-642-8100
www.parentcenterhub.org

Serves as a central hub of information and products for Parent Centers that serve children with disabilities. Coordinates training, provides an e-newsletter twice a month, and produces specially designed databases.
Debra A. Jennings, Director
Jessica Wilson, Communications Director

10363 Center for Universal Design North Carolina State University
North Carolina State University
Campus Box 7701
Raleigh, NC 27695-8613

919-515-8302
800-647-6777
Fax: 919-515-8951
nilda_cosco@ncsu.edu
www.design.ncsu.edu

National research information and technical assistance center that evaluates develops and promotes accessible and universal design in housing buildings outdoor and urban environments and related products.
Nilda Cosco PhD, Education Specialist
Leslie Young, Director of Design

10364 Child Center
3995 Marcola Road
Springfield, OR 97477

541-726-1465
Fax: 541-726-5085
www.thechildcenter.org

To provide individualized, diagnostic, therapeutic and educational services for the emotional and behavioral problems children exhibit in the home, school and community; provide integreated community based psychiatric and support services that are child centered, family driven and culturally competent
Jeffrey Miller, President
Chris Dunnington, Vice President

10365 Children's Hospice International
500 Montgomery Street
Alexandria, VA 22314

703-684-0330
800-242-4453
Fax: 703-684-0226
info@chionline.org
www.chionline.org

To ensure medical, psychological, social and spiritual support to all children with life-threatening conditions and their families by providing a network of resources and care.
Ann Armstrong-Dailey, Founding Director/CEO
Richard Larkin, Secretary/Treasurer

10366 Children's National Medical Center
111 Michigan Avenue NW
Washington, DC 20010

202-476-5000
888-884-2327
TTY: 800-855-1155
tbear@childrensnational.org
www.childrensnational.org

The only exclusive provider of pediatric care in the metropolitan Washington area and is the only freestanding children's hospital between Philadelphia, Pittsburgh, Norfolk, and Atlanta; the leader in the development and application of innovative new treatments for childhood illness and injury.
Kurt Newman MD, President/CEO
Roberta Alessi, Senior VP

10367 Christian Horizons
25 Sportsworld Crossing Road
Kitchener, N2P 0

519-650-0966
866-362-6810
Fax: 519-650-8984
info@christian-horizons.org
www.christian-horizons.org

Empowers individuals with exceptional needs, enabling them to embrace their God-given potential and enjoy hope and opportunity in everyday living.
Nigel Wilford, Chair
Greg Wilson, Secretary

10368 Clearinghouse on Disability Information Office of Special Education & Rehab Svcs
US Department of Education
550 12th Street SW
Washington, DC 20202-2550

202-245-7307
Fax: 202-245-7636
TTY: 202-205-5637
TDD: 2022055637
customerservice@inet.ed.gov
www.health.gov/nhic/NHICScripts/Entry.cf

Provides information to people with disabilities or anyone requesting information by doing research and providing documents in response to inquiries. Information provided includes areas of federal funding for disability-related programs.
Carolyn Corlett, Contact

10369 Council for Learning Disabilities (CLD)
11184 Antioch Road
Overland Park, KS 66210

913-491-1011
Fax: 913-491-1012
CLDInfo@cldinternational.org
www.cldinternational.org

The Council for Learning Disabilities (CLD) is an international organization that promotes evidence-based teaching, collaboration, research, leadership, and advocacy. CLD is comprised of professionals who represent diverse disciplines and are committed to enhancing the education and quality of life for individuals with learning disabilities and others who experience challenges in learning.
Slivana Watson, President
Steve Chamberlain, President Elect

10370 Disabled & Alone: Life Services for the Handicapped
1440 Broadway
New York, NY 10018

212-532-6740
800-995-0066
Fax: 212-532-3588
info@disabledandalone.org
www.disabledandalone.org

A non-profit organization established to help families provide a secure future for their loved ones with a disability. Also believes that no person should have to live his life in loneliness and isolation because of a disability.
Leslie D Park, Chairman
Lee Alan Ackerman, Executive Director

10371 Distance Education and Training Council
1601 18th Street NW
Washington, DC 20009

202-234-5100
Fax: 202-332-1386
brianna@detc.org
www.detc.org

A voluntary, non-governmental, educational organization that operates a nationally recognized accrediting association, the DETC Accrediting Commission.
Michael P Lambert, Executive Director
Patrice Wall, General Information

10372 Educational Equity Center at The Academy for Educational Development
71 Fifth Avenue 212-243-1110
New York, NY 10003 Fax: 212-627-0407
lcolon@aed.org
www.edequity.org
A national non-profit organization promoting educational excellence for children.
Merle Froschl, Co-Director
Barbara Sprung, Co-Director

10373 Equal Opportunity Employment Commission
131 M Street NE 202-663-4900
Washington, DC 20507 TTY: 202-663-4494
info@eeoc.gov
www.eeoc.org
The U.S. Equal Employment Opportunity Commission (EEOC) is responsible for enforcing federal laws that make it illegal to discriminate against a job applicant or an employee because of the person's race, color, religion, sex (including pregnancy), national origin, age (40 or older), disability or genetic information. It is also illegal to discriminate against a person because the person complained about discrimination, filed a charge of discrimination, or participated in an employment discrimina
Jacqueline A Berrien, Chair
Constance S. Barker, Commissioner

10374 Estate Planning for the Disabled
2232 W Avenue 133 510-352-4127
San Leandro, CA 94577-1050 Fax: 510-352-4127
EFM@EFMOODY.com
www.efmoody.com
Counsels and assists parents of children with special needs to develop viable estate plans, letters of intent, wills and special needs trusts. EPD will work with the appropriate professionals and agencies to help put together an effective comprehensive plan.

10375 Extensions for Independence
555 Saturn Boulevard 619-618-2154
San Diego, CA 92154 866-632-7149
Fax: 866-632-7149
info@mouthstick.net
Designer and manufacturer of home and office related equipment for the functional independence of the most physically challenged.
Arthur Heyer, President

10376 Favarh
225 Commerce Drive 860-693-6662
Canton, CT 06019-1099 Fax: 860-693-8662
www.favarh.org
Provides a variety of programs and services to adults with developmental, physical or mental disabilities and their families, throughout the Farmington Valley communities of Avon, Burlington and more.
Stephen Morr MPA, Executive Director

10377 Federation for Children with Special Needs
529 Main Street 617-236-7210
Boston, MA 02129 800-331-0688
Fax: 617-241-0330
fcsninfo@fcsn.org
www.fcsn.org
A center for parents and parent organizations to work together on behalf of children with special needs.
Pam Nourse, Executive Director
Marilyn Favreau, Director, Statewide Family Engagement

10378 Florida Disabled Outdoor Association
2475 Apalachee Parkway 850-201-2944
Tallahassee, FL 32301 Fax: 850-201-2945
www.fdoa.org
Enriches lives through accessible inclusive recreation and active leisure for all.
David Jones, Director
Laurie LoRe-Gussak, Execcutive Director

10379 Genetic Alliance
4301 Connecticut Avenue NW 202-966-5557
Washington, DC 20008-2369 Fax: 202-966-8553
info@geneticalliance.org
www.geneticalliance.org
Non-profit organization seeks to transform healthcare for the better for individuals, families, and communities.
Sharon Terry, MA, President & CEO
Natasha Bonhomme, Chief Strategy Officer

10380 Goodwill Industries International, Inc.
15810 Indianola Drive 800-466-3945
Rockville, MD 20855 contactus@goodwill.org
www.goodwill.org
A nonprofit, community-based organization whose mission is to help people achieve self-sufficiency through the dignity and power of work, serving people who are disadvantaged, disabled or elderly. The mission is accomplished through providing independent living skills, affordable housing, and training and placement in community employment. The GoodWill Network includes 160 independent, local locations across the U.S. and Canada.
S. Dale Jenkins, Chair
Steven C. Preston, President & CEO

10381 HEATH Resource Center
George Washington University
2134 G Street NW 202-939-9329
Washington, DC 20052-0001 800-544-3284
Fax: 202-994-3365
AskHEATH@gwu.edu
www.heath.gwu.edu
Serves as a national clearinghouse on postsecondary education for individuals with disabilities.
Dr Joan Kester, Principal Investigator
Christopher Nace, Research

10382 Health Care For All
30 Winter Street 617-350-7279
Boston, MA 02108 Fax: 617-451-5838
TTY: 617-350-0974
aslemmer@hcfama.org
www.hcfama.org
HCFA seeks to create a consumer-centered health care system that provides comprehensive, affordable, accessible, culturally competent, high quality care and consumer education for everyone, especially the most vulnerable.
Amy Whitcomb Slemmer, Executive Director

10383 HealthyWomen
1 Harding Road 732-530-3425
Red Bank, NJ 07701 877-986-9472
info@healthywomen.org
www.healthywomen.org
Independent, non-profit organization seeking to educate women in all areas of health, to allow them to make informed choices. The HealthyWomen website features numerous tools and health calculators, plus other media.
Beth Battaglino, RN, Chief Executive Officer
Phyllis E. Greenberger, Sr. VP, Science & Health Policy

10384 Heart Touch Project™
3400 Airport Avenue 310-391-2558
Santa Monica, CA 90405 Fax: 310-391-2168
www.hearttouch.org
Non-profit, educational and service organization devoted to the delivery of compassionate and healing touch to home or hospital-bound men, women, and children.
Shawnee Isaac Smith, Co-Founder
Rene Russo, Co-Founder

10385 International Association for the Study of Pain
1510 H Street NW 202-856-7400
Washington, DC 20005 Fax: 202-856-7401
iaspdesk@iasp-pain.org
www.iasp-pain.org
The International Association for the Study of Pain is the leading professional forum for science, practice, and education in the field of pain.
Matthew D'Uva, Executive Director
Colleen Eubanks, Chief Operating Officer

10386 International Council on Disability
1012 14th Street NW   202-347-0102
Washington, DC 20005   Fax: 202-347-0315
                                               info@usicd.org
                                               www.usicd.org
To promote the rights and full participation of persons with disabilities through global engagement and United States foreign affairs.
Marca Bristo, President
Barbara LeRoy, Secretary

10387 LAUNCH Department of Special Education
Department of Special Education
Commerce, TX 75428   903-886-5932
Provides resources for learning disabled individuals coordinates efforts of other local state and national LD organizations acts as a communication channel for people with learning disabilities through a monthly newsletter and provides programs.

10388 Learning Disabilities Association of America
PO Box 10369   412-341-1515
Pittsburgh, PA 15234-1349   Fax: 412-344-0224
                                               info@LDAAmerica.org
                                               www.ldaamerica.org
An information and referral center for parents and professionals dealing with learning disabilities.
Stephanie Fedro-Byrom, Operations Manager
Maureen Swanson, Director, Healthy Children Project

10389 Learning How
1583 Sulphur Spring Road   410-242-7100
Baltimore, MD 21227   Fax: 410-242-5246
                                               www.learninghow.com
To provide educational materials for parents, teachers, and daycare providers that will encourage the learning process and help children reach their fullest potential.

10390 Life Development Institute
18001 N 79th Avenue   623-773-2774
Glendale, AZ 85308   866-736-7811
                                          Fax: 623-773-2788
                          info@life-development-inst.org
                          www.lifedevelopmentinstitute.org
LDI's mission to inspire individuals to experience success while optimizing their potential for an enhanced quality of life in a challenging and supportive learning environment. LDI is a nonprofit private organization based in Glendale Arizona.
Rob Crawford, CEO
Veronica Crawford, Vice President

10391 Lions Quest
300 W 22nd Street   630-571-5466
Oak Brook, IL 60523-8842   Fax: 630-571-5735
                                               www.lions-quest.org
To empower and support adults throughout the world to nuture caring and responsibility in young people.
Matthew Kiefer, Manager
Michael Di Maria, Educational Program Specialist

10392 Lymphatic Research Foundation
40 Garvies Point Road   516-625-9675
Glen Cove, NY 11542   Fax: 516-625-9410
                                               www.lymphaticresearch.org
A not-for-profit organization whose mission is to advance research of the lymphatic system and to find the cause and cure for lymphatic diseases, lymphedema, and related disorders.
Roy E. Reichbach, Executive Director
Phillip Braginsky, Chair

10393 MedEscort International ABE International Airport
ABE International Airport
PO Box 8766   610-792-3111
Allentown, PA 18105-8766   800-255-7182
                                          Fax: 610-791-9189
                                          service@medescort.com
                                          www.medescort.com
Offers specially trained escorts for individuals who cannot travel alone due to age or disability.
David M Stein DO, Medical Director
Sherry L Sefcik RN/BSN, Senior Flight Nurse

10394 MedicAlert Foundation International
2323 Colorado Avenue   888-633-4298
Turlock, CA 95382-2018   Fax: 800-863-3429
                          customer_service@medicalert.org
                                               www.medicalert.org
We protect the health and well-being of more than 4 million members worldwide through our trusted emergency support network. We educate emergency responders and medical personnel - our partners in everyday emergency situations. And we communicate your health information, your wishes, and your directives to ensure you receive the best care possible
Andrew B Wigglesworth, President/CEO
Karen M. Lamoree, COO

10395 Mental Health Services Training Center
University of Maryland
3700 Koppers Street   410-646-7758
Baltimore, MD 21227   Fax: 410-646-7849
                                wbaysmor@psych.umaryland.edu
Formerly the Mental Health Services Training Collaborative, assists Mental Hygiene Administration in planning, organizing and implementing conference and training activities to support the continued growth and development of the public mental health system.
Eileen Hansen MSSW, Director
Wendy Baysmore MSHSA, Assistant Director

10396 National Association of Councils on Developmental Disabilities
1825 K Street NW   202-506-5813
Washington, DC 20006   Fax: 202-506-5846
                                               info@nacdd.org
                                               www.nacdd.org
Serves as the national voice of State and Territorial Councils on Dvelopment Disabilities. Supports Councils in implementing the Developmental Disabilities Assistance and Bill of Rights Act and promoting the interests and rights of people with developmental disabilities and their familes.
Claire Mantonya, President
Brett Cunnigham, VP

10397 National Center for Family-Centered Care
695 Park Avenue   212-772-4000
New York, NY 10021   Fax: 212-452-7475
                                          gmallon@hunter.cuny.edu
                          www.hunter.cuny.edu/socwork/nrcfcpp//tra
Goals are to promote implementation of a family-centered care approach for children with special health care needs.
Karen Lawrence

10398 National Chronic Pain Outreach Association
Millboro, VA 24460   540-862-9437
                                          Fax: 540-862-9485
                                               www.chronicpain.org
Purpose is to lessen the suffering of people with chronic pain by educating pain sufferers, health care professionals, and the public about chronic pain and its management.

10399 National Clearinghouse of Rehabilitation Training Materials
Utah State University
6524 Old Main Hill   866-821-5355
Logan, UT 84322-6524   Fax: 435-797-7537
                                               ncrtm@usu.edu
                                               www.ncrtm.org
Offers reference materials on rehabilitation for professionals and the disabled.
Jared Schultz, Principal Investigator
Joshua Southwick, Interim Director

10400 National Council on Disability
1331 F Street NW   202-272-2004
Washington, DC 20004   Fax: 202-272-2022
                                          TTY: 202-272-2074
                                               ncd@ncd.gov
                                               www.ncd.gov
The National Council on Disability is an independent federal agency that works with the President and Congress to increase the inclusion independence and empowerment of Americans with disabilities. They are involved in policy making issues.
Jonathan Young, Ph.D., Chairman
Aaron Bishop, Executive Director

10401 National Council on Independent Living
1710 Rhode Island Avenue NW 202-207-0334
Washington, DC 20036 877-525-3400
Fax: 202-207-0341
TTY: 202-207-0340
ncil@ncil.org
www.ncil.org
A membership organization that advanced independent living and the rights of people with disabilities through consumer-driven advocacy.
Kelly Buckland, Executive Director
Dan Kessler, President

10402 National Digestive Diseases Information Clearinghouse
2 Information Way 800-891-5389
Bethesda, MD 20892-3570 Fax: 703-738-4929
TTY: 866-569-1162
nddic@info.niddk.nih.gov
www.digestive.niddk.nih.gov
Established to increase knowledge and understanding about digestive diseases among people with these conditions and their families, health care professionals, and the general public. To carry out this mission, NDDIC works closely with a coordinating panel of representatives from Federal agencies, voluntary organizations on the national level, and professional groups to identify and respond to informational needs about digestive diseases.

10403 National Endowment for the Arts: Office for Accessability
1100 Pennsylvania Avenue NW 202-682-5400
Washington, DC 20506 TTY: 202-682-5496
Since 1957, the YAI Network has been providing hope and opportunity to people of all ages with developmental disabilities and their families. Our organization includes more than 450 programs and serves more than 20,000 people every day.
Stephen E. Freeman, CEO
Thomas A. Dern, COO

10404 National Institute for People with Disabilities
460 W 34th Street 212-273-6100
New York, NY 10001-2382 www.yai.org
To create hope and opportunity for people with developmental and learning disabilities and their families.
Philip H Levy PhD, President/CEO

10405 National Institute of Child Health and Human Development
PO Box 3006 800-370-2943
Rockville, MD 20847 Fax: 866-760-5947
TTY: 888-320-6942
www.nichd.nih.gov
NICHD seeks to better understand disabilities and important events that occur during pregnancy.
Diana W. Bianchi, MD, Director
Constantine Stratakis, Scientific Director

10406 National Institute of Disability and Rehabilitation Research
US Department of Education
400 Maryland Avenue SW 202-245-7640
Washington, DC 20202 Fax: 202-245-7323
TTY: 202-245-7316
provides leadership and support for a comprehensive program and research related to the rehabilitation of individuals with disabilities. All of the programmatic efforts are aimed at improving the lives of individuals with disabilities from birth through adulthood.

10407 National Job Accommodation Network
Morgantown, WV 26506-6080 304-293-7186
800-526-7234
Fax: 304-293-5407
TTY: 877-781-9403
jan@askjan.org
www.askjan.org
The JAN is an international information service for people with disabilities and their employers. They have information about implementation of workplace accommodations as well as resources to promote an awareness of functional limitations.
Anne Hirsh, Co-Director
Louis Orslene, Co-Director

10408 National Legal Center for the Medically Dependent & Disabled
50 S Meridian Street 317-632-6245
Indianapolis, IN 46204-3537
Committed to defending the rights of vulnerable persons threatened by infanticide, euthanasia, assisted suicide, non-voluntary withdrawal/withholding of essential medical treatment and care and discrimination in health care financing.
Marilyn Bove, President

10409 National Network of Learning Disabled Adults
808 N 82nd Street 602-941-5112
Scottsdale, AZ 85257
Provides information and referral for LD adults involved with or in search of support groups and networking opportunities.

10410 National Organization for Rare Disorders
55 Kenosia Avenue 203-744-0100
Danbury, CT 06810-1968 800-999-6673
Fax: 203-263-9938
www.rarediseases.org
NORD is a federation of voluntary health organizations dedicated to helping people with rare orphan diseases and assisting the organizations that serve them. It is committed to the identification, treatment, and cure of rare disorders through programs of education, advocacy, research, and service.
Peter Saltonstall, President & CEO
Pamela Gavin, Chief Strategy Officer

10411 National Organization on Disability
77 Water Street 646-505-1191
New York, NY 10005 Fax: 646-505-1184
info@nod.org
www.nod.org
The National Organization on Disability (NOD) is a private, non-profit organization that promotes the full participation of America's 56 million people with disabilities in all aspects of life.
Carol Glazer, President
Aleysha Anderson, Administrative Assistant

10412 National Parent Network on Disabilities
1130 17th Street NW 202-434-8686
Washington, DC 20036 Fax: 202-638-7299
www.npnd.org
To provide a presence and national voice for all families of children, youth and adults with disabilities.
Linda Shepard, Executive Director
Jill Foss, Office Manager

10413 National Rehabilitation Information Center
8400 Corporate Drive 800-346-2742
Landover, MD 20785 Fax: 301-459-4263
TTY: 301-459-5984
www.naric.com
One of the three components of the office of Special Education and Rehabilitative Services. Operates in concert with the Rehabilitation Services Administration and the Office of Special Education Programs.
Mark X. Odum, Project Director
Jessica H. Chaiken, Media and Information Services Manager

10414 North American Society for Pediatric Gastroenterology, Hepatology & Nutrition
714 N. Bethlehem Pike 215-641-9800
Ambler, PA 19002 Fax: 215-641-1995
naspghan@naspghan.org
www.naspghan.org
Promotes research and provides a forum for professionals in the areas of pediatric GI liver disease, gastroenterology, and nutrition. Associated with fellow organizations in Europe and Australia (ESPGAN, AUSPGAN).
Margaret K. Stallings, Executive Director
Kim Rose, Associate Director

10415 Office of Civil Rights
US Department of Education

S/OCR, Room 7428 202-647-9295
Washington, DC 20520-1100 800-421-3481
Fax: 202-647-4969
TTY: 877-521-2172
socr_direct@state.gov
www.state.gov/s/ocr/

To ensure equal access to education and to promote educational excellence throughout the nation through vigorous enforcement of civil rights.
Russlynn Ali, Assistant Secretary

10416 Office of Policy Planning and Legislation
200 Independence Avenue SW 202-619-0257
Washington, DC 20201-0004 877-696-6775
www.hhs.gov/about/referlst.html

Administers grants to the states for social services under Title XX of the Social Security Act to welfare recipients and others likely to become welfare recipients.
G Barry Nielsen, Director

10417 Office of Special Education Programs
Department of Education
400 Maryland Avenue SW 202-245-7459
Washington, DC 20202 www2.ed.gov/about/offices/list/osers

Dedicated to improving results for infants, toddlers, children and youth with disabilities ages birth through 21 by providing leadership and financial support to assist states and local districts.
Melody Musgrove, Director
Bill Wolf, Acting Deputy Director

10418 Office on Smoking and Health
Centers for Disease Control and Prevention
4770 Buford Highway 404-639-3311
Atlanta, GA 30341-3717 800-232-4636
TTY: 888-232-6348
tobaccoinfo@cdc.gov

The leading federal agency for comprehensive tobacco prevention and control, the Office develops, conducts, and supports strategic efforts to protect the public's health from the harmful effects of tobacco use.
Tim McAfee MD MPH, Director

10419 Option Institute
2080 South Undermountain Road 413-229-2100
Sheffield, MA 01257 800-714-2779
Fax: 413-229-8931
participantsupport@option.org
www.option.org

Self-defeating beliefs, along with attitudes and judgments, can lead to a host of physical and psychological challenges. The Option Institute offers programs designed to help people gain new perspectives on the attitudes and judgments that may be affecting their lives.
Barry Kaufman, Co-Founder
Samahria Lyte Kaufman, Co-Founder

10420 Pediatric Neurology Georgetown University Hospital
Georgetown University Hospital
3800 Reservoir Road NW 202-444-2000
Washington, DC 20007 www.georgetownuniversityhospital.org

provides a wide range of consultative services, neurodiagnostic studies and therapies for children with neurodevelopmental disorders.
Cesar Santos MD, Chief

10421 People-to-People Committee for the Handicapped
Washington, DC 20036-8131 301-774-7446

Individuals concerned about the circumstances of handicapped people throughout the world. Disseminates information acts as a consultant in promoting exchange activities coordinates special assistance projects in developing countries and more.
David Brigham, Chairman

10422 President's Committee on the Employment of People with Disabilities
200 Constitution Avenue NW 202-693-6000
Washington, DC 20210 866-633-7365
Fax: 202-693-7888
TTY: 877-889-5627
webmaster@dol.gov
www.dol.gov

Independent federal agency to facilitate the communication coordination and promotion of public and private efforts to empower Americans with disabilities through employment.
Seth D. Harris, Secretary of Labour
Ana M. Ma, Chief of Staff

10423 Rehabilitation International
25 E 21st Street 212-420-1500
New York, NY 10010 Fax: 212-505-0871
ri@riglobal.org
www.riglobal.org

RI and its members work to protect the rights of people with disabilities, including ensuring access to and the improvement of crucial services for persons with disabilities and their families
Jan A. Monsbakken, President
Megan Brinster, Development/Program Officer

10424 Rehabilitation Services Administration
US Department of Education
1125 15th Street, NW 202-730-1843
Washington, DC 20005-2800 Fax: 202-730-1843
TTY: 202-730-1516
dds@dc.gov
www.dc.gov/DC/DDS/Rehabilitation+Service

Oversees grant programs that help individuals with physical or mental disabilities to obtain employment and live more independently through the provision of such supports as counseling, medical and psychological services, job training and other individualized services.
Lynnae M Ruttledge, Commissioner

10425 Social Security Administration Office of Public Inquiries
Office of Public Inquiries
Windsor Park Building 800-772-1213
Baltimore, MD 21235 TTY: 800-325-0778
www.ssa.gov

Administers old age survivors and disability insurance programs under Title II of the Social Security Act. Also administers the federal income maintenance program under Title XVI of the Social Security Act. Maintains networks of local/regional offices.
Michael J Astrue, Commissioner
James A Winn, Chief of Staff

10426 US Department of Justice
950 Pennsylvania Avenue NW 202-514-2000
Washington, DC 20530-0001 askdoj@usdoj.gov
www.usdoj.gov

To enforce the law and defend the interests of the United States according to the law; to ensure public safety against threats foreign and domestic; to provide federal leadership in preventing and controlling crime; to seek just punishment for those guilty of unlawful behavior; and to ensure fair and impartial administration of justice for all Americans.
Eric Holder, Attorney General
James Cole, Deputy Attorney General

10427 US Department of Transportation
1200 New Jersey Avenue SE 202-366-4000
Washington, DC 20590 866-377-8642
TTY: 800-877-8339
dot.comments@dot.gov
www.dot.gov

Serves the United States by ensuring a fast, safe, efficient, accessible and convenient transportation system that meets the vital national interests and enhances the quality of life of the American people, today and into the future.
Anthony Foxx, Secretary of Transportation
John D. Porcari, Deputy Secretary of Transport

10428 US Office of Personnel Management
1900 E Street NW
Washington, DC 20415   202-606-1800
TTY: 202-606-2532
General@opm.gov
www.opm.gov
Recruiting, retaining and honoring a world-class workforce to serve the American people.
Elaine Kaplan, Acting Director

10429 World Institute on Disability
3075 Adeline Street   510-225-6400
Berkeley, CA 94703-1520   Fax: 510-225-0477
TTY: 510-225-0478
wid@wid.org
www.wid.org
WID's mission in communities and nations worldwide is to eliminate barriers to full social integration and increase employment, economic security, and health care for persons with disabilities
Anita Shafer Aaron, Executive Director
Rebecca Palmer, Executive Assistant

State Agencies & Associations

Alabama

10430 Division of Rehabilitation: Montgomery
Montgomery, AL 36111-0586   334-281-8780
Marilyn Bove, President

Alaska

10431 Client Assistance Program: Anchorage
3330 Arctic Boulevard   907-333-2211
Anchorage, AK 99503   800-478-1234
Fax: 907-565-1000
akpa@dlcak.org

James Shine, President
Julie Renwick, Vice President

Arizona

10432 HPV Support Groups: Arizona
7331 E Osborn Drive   602-994-8330
Scottsdale, AZ 85251-6422   800-223-2159
sthf@home.com

Arkansas

10433 Disability Rights Center of Arkansas
1100 N University   501-296-1775
Little Rock, AR 72207   800-482-1174
Fax: 501-296-1779
www.arkdisabilityrights.org
Protection and advocacy system for people with disabilities in Arkansas.
Traci Perrin, President

California

10434 Disability Rights California
1831 K Street   916-504-5800
Sacramento, CA 95811   800-776-5746
Fax: 916-504-5801
TTY: 800-719-5798
services@disabilityrightsca.org
www.disabilityrightsca.org
Mission is to advance the rights of Californians with disabilities.
Catherine Blakemore, Executive Director
Andrew Murdryk, Deputy Director

Colorado

10435 Disability Careers
5760 E Evans Avenue   303-757-3070
Denver, CO 80222-5305   Fax: 303-757-3392
This is a non profit corporation that provides employee and employer services. Founder and Executive Director Ted Pavakis is a former commercial real estate broker with multiple sclerosis.

10436 Legal Center for People with Disabilities and Older People
455 Sherman Street   303-722-0300
Denver, CO 80203   800-288-1376
Fax: 303-722-0720
TTY: 303-722-3619
www.thelegalcenter.org
An independent public interest non-profit specializing in civil rights and discrimination issues. We protect the human, civil and legal rights of people with mental and physical disabilities, people with HIV, and older people throughout Colorado.
Mary Anne Harvey, Executive Director
Peter Lindquist, President

Connecticut

10437 Office of Protection and Advocacy for Persons with Disabilities
60B Weston Street   860-297-4300
Hartford, CT 06120-1551   800-842-7303
TTY: 860-297-4380
www.ct.gov
To advance the cause of equal rights for persons with disabilities and their families by: increasing the ability of individuals, groups and systems to safeguard rights; exposing instances and patterns of discrimination and abuse; seeking individual and systemic remediation when rights are violated; increasing public awareness of unjust situations and of means to address them; and empowering people with disabilities and their families to advocate effectively.

Delaware

10438 Client Assistance Program: Delaware
13 SW Front Street   302-422-6744
Milford, DE 19963-1900
Marilyn Bove, President

District of Columbia

10439 Client Assistance Program: District of Columbia
Rehabilitation Services Administration
605 G Street NW   202-727-0977
Washington, DC 20001-3705
Jim Tolbert, Director

10440 Information Protection & Advocacy Center for Handicapped Individuals
Center for Handicapped Individuals
4455 Connecticut Avenue NW   202-966-8081
Washington, DC 20008-2328
Marilyn Bove, President

Florida

10441 Disability Rights: Florida
2728 Centerview Drive   850-488-9071
Tallahassee, FL 32301   800-342-0823
Fax: 850-488-8640
TDD: 800-346-4127
www.disabilityrightsflorida.org
To advance the quality of life, dignity, equality, self-determination, and freedom of choice of persons with disabilities through collaboration, education, advocacy, as well, as legal and legislative issues.
Catherine Piecora, Chair
Minerva Bailey, Vice-Chair

10442 Goodwill Industries-Suncoast
10596 Gandy Boulevard   727-523-1512
St. Petersburg, FL 33702   888-279-1988
TTY: 727-579-1068
www.goodwill-suncoast.org
A nonprofit, community-based organization whose mission is to help people achieve self-sufficiency through the dignity and power of work, serving people who are disadvantaged, disabled or elderly. The mission is accomplished through providing independent living skills, affordable housing, and training and placement in community employment.
Heather Ceresoli, CPA, Chair
Deborah A. Passerini, President & CEO

10443 North Florida: HPV Support Group
126 Salem Court
Tallahassee, FL 32301-2810   850-877-3183

Georgia

10444 Division of Rehabilitation Service
148 Andrew Young Int'l Blvd NE   404-232-3910
Atlanta, GA 30303-1751   TTY: 404-232-3911
rehab@dol.state.ga.us
Operates five integrated and interdependent programs that share a primary goal — to help people with disabilities to become fully productive members of society by achieving independence and meaningful employment.

Hawaii

10445 Protection & Advocacy Agency
1132 Bishop Street   808-949-2922
Honolulu, HI 96813-9607   800-882-1057
Fax: 808-949-2928
TTY: 808-949-2922
info@hawaiidisabilityrights.org
www.hawaiidisabilityrights.org
Hawaii Disability Rights Center is the State of Hawaii's designated client assistance program and designated protection and advocacy system for people with disabilities.
Gary L Smith, Executive Director

Idaho

10446 Co-Ad
4477 Emerald St   208-336-5353
Boise, ID 83706-2017   800-632-5125
Fax: 208-336-5396
TTY: 208-336-5353
Marilyn Bove, President

Illinois

10447 Illinois Client Assistance Program
Illinois Department of Human Services
100 N 1st Street   800-641-3929
Springfield, IL 62702   TTY: 800-447-6404
dhs.cap@illinois.gov
www.dhs.state.il.us
Helps people with disabilities receive quality services by advocating for their interests and helping them identify resources, understand procedures, resolve problems, and protect their rights in the rehabilitation process, employment and home services.

10448 Legal Council for Health Justice
17 N State Street   312-427-8990
Chicago, IL 60602   Fax: 312-427-8419
legalcouncil.org
Provides legal advice and services for persons who are HIV positive or have AIDS, as well as their families. Also serves individuals with disabilities and chronic illnesses, senior citizens, and the homeless.
Tom Yates, Executive Director
Ruth Edwards, Senior Director, Program Services

Indiana

10449 Indiana Protection and Advocacy Services
4701 N Keystone Avenue   800-622-4845
Indianapolis, IN 46205   TTY: 800-838-1131
kpedevilla@ipas.in.gov
www.in.gov/ipas
To protect and promote the rights of individuals with disabilities, through empowerment and advocacy.
Karen Pedevilla, Education/Training Director

Iowa

10450 Client Assistance Program: Iowa Division on Persons with Disabilities
Division on Persons with Disabilities

Lucas State Office Building   515-281-3656
Des Moines, IA 50310   800-652-4298
Fax: 515-242-6119
TTY: 800-652-4298
dhr.disabilities@iowa.gov
The Division of Persons with Disabilities exists to promote the employment of Iowans with disabilities and reduce barriers to employment by providing information, referral, assessment and guidance, training, and negotiation services to employers and citizens with disabilities.
Marilyn Bove, President

Kansas

10451 Disability Rights Center of Kansas
635 SW Harrison   785-273-9661
Topeka, KS 66603-3726   877-776-1541
Fax: 785-273-9414
TTY: 877-335-3725
rocky@drckansas.org
www.icdri.org
A public interest legal advocacy agency empowered by federal law to advocate for the civil and legal rights of Kansans with disabilities.
Rocky Nichols MPA, Executive Director
Debbie White, Deputy Director

Kentucky

10452 Client Assistance Program: Kentucky
275 E Main Street   502-564-4440
Frankfort, KY 40621   800-633-6283
www.ovr.ky.gov
David Beach, Executive Director
Jane Smith, Director of Program Services

Louisiana

10453 Advocacy Center
8325 Oak Street   504-522-2337
New Orleans, LA 70118   800-960-7705
Fax: 504-522-5507
TTY: 855-861-3577
advocacycenter@advocacyla.org
www.advocacyla.org
Serves people with disabilities and senior citizens.
Lois Simpson, Executive Director

Maine

10454 Disability Rights Center: Maine
24 Stone St   207-626-2774
Augusta, ME 04330-2007   800-452-1948
Fax: 207-621-1419
advocate@drcme.org
www.drcme.org
To enhance and promote the equality, self-determination, independence, productivity, integration, and inclusion of people with disabilities through education, strategic advocacy and legal intervention.
Kim Moody, Executive Director
Kristin Aiello, Managing Attourney

Maryland

10455 Client Assistance Program: Maryland
Maryland State Department of Education
2301 Argonne Drive   410-554-9442
Baltimore, MD 21218   888-554-0334
Fax: 410-554-9362
TTY: 410-554-9360
cap@dors.state.md.us
www.dors.state.md.us
Helps individuals who have concerns or difficulties when applying for or receiving rehabilitation services funded under the Rehabilitation Act.
Beth Lash, Director

Massachusetts

10456 Client Assistance Program: Massachusetts
250 Washington Street   617-727-7440
Boston, MA 02108-1518   800-322-2020
                                   james.aprea@state.ma.us
                                              www.mass.gov
If you have a disability and want to work but are having trouble getting vocational rehabilitation services, or want a lifestyle which is more self-reliant but are having trouble getting independent living services, contact the Client Assistance Program (CAP).
Barbara E Lybarger Esq, Director

10457 Merrimack Valley HPV Support Group Holy Family Hospital
Holy Family Hospital
70 E Street   978-687-0156
Methuen, MA 01844-4597

10458 Neurosurgical Service
Massachusetts General Hospital
55 Fruit Street   617-726-2937
Boston, MA 02114   Referral@Neurosurgery.MassGeneral.org
                                   neurosurgery.mgh.harvard.edu
Uses a multidisciplinary approach to provide a complete range of services for the diagnosis, treatment and rehabilitation of patients with neurological disorders.

Michigan

10459 Client Assistance Program: Michigan
Michigan Protection and Advocacy Service
4095 Legacy Parkway   517-487-1755
Lansing, MI 48911-7508   800-292-5896
                                          Fax: 517-487-0827
                                           molson@mpas.org
                                              www.mpas.org
Assists people who are seeking or receiving services from Michigan Rehabilitation Services, Consumer Choice Programs, Michigan Commission for the Blind, Centers for Independent Living, and Supported Employment and Transition Programs.
Mark R Lezotte, President

10460 Commission for the Blind
201 N Washington 2nd Floor   517-373-2062
Lansing, MI 48909   800-292-4200
                                          Fax: 517-335-5140
                                          TDD: 517-373-4025
                                      heibeckc@michigan.gov
                                       www.michigan.gov/mcb
To provide opportunity to individuals who are blind or visually impaired to achieve employability and/or function independently in society.
Patrick Cannon, Director

Minnesota

10461 Minnesota Disability Law Center
430 1st Avenue N   612-334-5970
Minneapolis, MN 55401-1780   Fax: 612-334-5755
                                          TTY: 612-332-4668
                                              www.mndlc.org
Addresses the unique legal needs of Minnesotans with disabilities. Provides free civil legal assistance to individuals with disabilities statewide on legal issues related to their disabilities.
Cathy Madouken, Executive Director
Lisa Cohen, Deputy Director of Operations

Mississippi

10462 Mississippi Client Assistance Program
Mississippi Society for Disabilities
Jackson, MS 39296   601-362-2585
                                               800-962-2400
                                          Fax: 601-982-1951
                                               www.icdri.org
A federal grant to the State of Mississippi to provide advocacy services for clients and client applicants of the Office of Vocational Rehabilitation, Vocational Rehabilitation for the Blind, and the Independent Living programs.
Johnny McGinn, Director

Missouri

10463 Missouri Protection and Advocacy Services
925 S Country Club Drive   573-893-3333
Jefferson City, MO 65109   866-777-7199
                                          Fax: 573-893-4231
                                          TDD: 800-735-2966
                                          www.moadvocacy.org
To protect the rights of individuals with disabilities by providing advocacy and legal services.
Joe Wrinkle, Chair
Lawrence O. Daniels, Vice-Chair

Montana

10464 Disability Rights Montana
1022 Chestnut Street   406-449-2344
Helena, MT 59601   800-245-4743
                                          Fax: 406-449-2418
                                          TDD: 406-449-2344
                                advocate@disabilityrightsmt.org
                                       www.disabilityrightsmt.org
Protects and advocates for the human, legal, and civil rights of Montanans with disabilities while advancing dignity, equality, and self-determination.
Bernadette Franks-Ongoy, Executive Director
Alexandra Volkerts, Staff Attourney

Nebraska

10465 Client Assistance Program: Nebraska Division of Rehabilitative Services
Division of Rehabilitative Services
301 Centennial Mall S   402-471-3656
Lincoln, NE 68509   800-742-7594
The Nebraska Client Assistance Program is a free service to help you find solutions if you are having problems with any of the following programs: Vocational Rehabilitation, Nebraska Commission for the Blind and Visually Impaired or Centers for Independent Living.

10466 Omaha HPV Support Group: PP of Omaha
Planned Parenhood
4610 Dodge Street   402-397-2739
Omaha, NE 68132-3234   www.aad.org

Nevada

10467 Client Assistance Program: Nevada
2800 E Saint Louis Avenue   775-684-3849
Las Vegas, NV 89104   800-633-9879
                                          Fax: 775-684-3850
                                          TTY: 800-326-6868
                                     InternetHelp@nvdetr.org
                                         www.detr.state.nv.us
Designed to assist individuals with disabilities resolve problems they may experience with any of Nevada's rehabilitation programs.
Maureen Cole, Rehabilitation Administrator

New Hampshire

10468 Client Assistance Program: New Hampshire
Governor's Commission for the Handicapped
57 Regional Drive   603-271-2773
Concord, NH 03301-8518   800-852-3405
                                          Fax: 603-271-2837
                                          disability@nh.gov
                                www.nh.gov/disability/about/cap.htm
CAP provides information about vocational rehabilitation services; advises you of your rights and responsibilities; investigate your complaint; helps resolve problems with your vocational plan; and represents you at administratove reviews and fair hearings.
John Richards, Executive Director

New Jersey

10469 Disability Rights New Jersey
210 S Broad Street
Trenton, NJ 08608
609-292-9742
800-922-7233
Fax: 609-777-0187
TTY: 609-633-7106
adocate@drnj.org
www.drnj.org
To protect, advocate for and advance the rights of persons with disabilities in pursuit of a society in hich persons with disabilities exercise self-determination and choice, and are treated with dignity.
Walter A. Woodberry, Chair
Kathleen F. Wood, Vice Chair

New Mexico

10470 Protection and Advocacy System of Alburque rque
1720 Louisiana Boulevard NE
Albuquerque, NM 87110-7070
505-256-3100
800-432-4682
Fax: 505-256-3184
info@drnm.org
www.drnm.org
Disability Rights New Mexico - DRNM - is a private, non-profit organization whose mission is to protect, promote and expand the rights of persons with disabilities.
Marilyn Bove, President

New York

10471 Client Assistance Program: NY State Commission of Quality of Care
Advocacy Bureau
One Commerce Plaza
Albany, NY 12234-2810
518-459-6422
800-222-5627
Fax: 518-473-6296
accesadm@mail.nysed.gov
The Client Assistance Program (CAP) is a statewide network of skilled advocates that assist New Yorkers with disabilities in getting the training, equipment and services needed for employment.
Marilyn Bove, President

North Carolina

10472 North Carolina Client Assistance Program
805 Ruggles Drive
Raleigh, NC 27603-2806
919-855-3600
800-215-7227
Fax: 919-715-2456
nccap@dhhs.nc.gov
Helping people understand and access rehabilitation services.
John Marens, Director
Sharon Wisner, Client Advocate

North Dakota

10473 Client Assistance Program: North Dakota
400 East Broadway
Bismarck, ND 58501-1208
701-328-2950
800-472-2670
Fax: 701-328-3934
TDD: 707-328-8968
panda@nd.gov
www.ndpanda.org/cap
Assists clients and client applicants of North Dakota Vocational Rehabilitation services, Tribal Vocational Rehabilitation, or Independent Living services.

Ohio

10474 Cincinnati HPV Support Group: PP of Cincin nati
Planned Parenthood
PO Box 12407
Cincinnati, OH 45212-0407
513-357-7300
www.dermconsultants.com

10475 Disability Rights Center at Ohio Legal Rights Service
50 W Broad Street
Columbus, OH 43215-5923
614-466-7264
800-282-9181
TTY: 614-728-2553
www.disabilityrightsohio.org

To protect and advocate, in partnership with people with disabilities, for their human, civil and legal rights.
Kalpana Yalamanchili, Chair

10476 Richland County HPV Support Group
Mansfield, OH 44907-3881
419-525-3075
www.skinpatient.com

10477 Technology Resource Center
2140 Arbor Boulevard
Dayton, OH 45439
937-294-8086

Oklahoma

10478 Client Assistance Program: Oklahoma Office of Handicapped Concerns
Oklahoma Ofice of Handicapped Concerns
2401 NW 23rd
Oklahoma City, OK 73107-5106
405-521-3756
Fax: 405-522-6695
Marilyn.Burr@ohc.state.ok.us
www.icdri.org
Marilyn Bove, President

10479 Oklahoma City HPV Support Group: PP of Cen tral Oklahoma
Planned Parenthood of Central Oklahoma
Oklahoma City, OK 73103-1415
405-528-0221
www.aad.org

Oregon

10480 Resources for Seniors and People with Disabilities
Department of Human Services
500 Summer Street NE
Salem, OR 97301-1097
503-947-5811
800-282-8096
Fax: 503-378-2897
TTY: 800-282-8096
spd.web@state.or.us
www.oregon.gov
To secure economic, social, legal and political justice for individuals with disabilities through systems change
Dr Bruce Goldberg, Director
Margaret Carter, Deputy Director Human Services Program

Pennsylvania

10481 Client Assistance Program: Philadelphia
1515 Market Street
Philadelphia, PA 19102
215-557-7112
888-745-2357
Fax: 215-557-7602
TDD: 215-557-7112
www.equalemployment.org
Ensuring that vocation rehabilitation is open and responsive to your needs. Provides information and advice about rehabilitation programs; to advise you of your legal rights and responsibilities; to help resolve probelms that may arise while you are seeking services from rehabilitation programs; to help you pursue administrative and legal remedies to protect your rights.
Stephen S Pennington, Executive Director
Jamie C Ray- Leonetti, Assistant Director

Rhode Island

10482 Rhode Island Disability Law Center
275 Westminster Street
Providence, RI 02903-3434
401-831-3150
800-733-5332
Fax: 401-274-5568
TTY: 401-831-5335
info@ridlc.org
www.ridlc.org
Provides free legal assistance to persons with disabilities. Services include individual representation to protect rights or to secure benefits and services; self-help information; educational programs; and administrative and legislative advocacy.

South Carolina

10483 South Carolina Protection & Advocacy System for the Handicapped
3710 Landmark Drive 803-782-0639
Columbia, SC 29204-4034 866-275-7273
TTY: 866-232-4525
info@pandasc.org
www.pandasc.org

Marilyn Bove, President

10484 Tri County HPV Support Group
Mt Pleasant, SC 29465-1997 843-884-7333
www.aad.org

South Dakota

10485 South Dakota Advocacy Services
221 S Central Avenue 605-224-8294
Pierre, SD 57501 800-658-4782
Fax: 605-224-5125
TTY: 800-658-4782
sdas@sdadvocacy.com
www.sdadvocacy.com
To protect and advocate the rights of South Dakotans with disabilities through legal, administrative, and other remedies.

Tennessee

10486 Disability Law & Advocacy Center of Tennessee
2416 21st Avenue S 615-298-1080
Nashville, TN 37212 800-342-1660
Fax: 615-298-2046
gethelp@dlactn.org
www.dlactn.org
Advocates for the rights of Tennesseans with disabilities to ensure they have an equal opportunity to be productive and respected members of the society.
Jerry Gonzalez, Chair
Shalani Rose, Vice Chair

Texas

10487 Dallas/Ft.Worth Metroplex HPV Support Group
8215 Westchester Drive 214-363-6733
Dallas, TX 75225-6116

10488 Disability Rights Texas
Advocacy Inc
2222 W Braker Lane 512-454-4816
Austin, TX 78758-1024 866-362-2851
Fax: 512-323-0902
Protecting and advocating the rights of Texans with disabilities - because all people have dignity and worth.
Mary Faithfull, Executive Director

Utah

10489 Legal Center for People with Disabilities
205 North 400 West 801-363-1347
Salt Lake City, UT 84103-3076 800-662-9080
Fax: 801-363-1437
www.disabilitylawcenter.org
We enforce and strengthen laws that protect the opportunities, choices and legal rights of people with disabilities in Utah.
Kevin Murphy, President
Barbara M. Campbell, Senior VP

Vermont

10490 Citizen Advocacy of Burlington
Chase Mill 1 Mill Street 802-655-0329
Burlington, VT 05401
Marilyn Bove, President

10491 Client Assistance Program: Vermont Ladd Hall
Ladd Hall

57 N Main Street 802-775-0021
Rutland, VT 05701-8409 800-769-7459
Fax: 802-775-0022
nbreiden@vtlegalaid.org
www.icdri.org

Marilyn Bove, President

Virginia

10492 Richmond HPV Support Group: Fan Free Clini c
Fan Free Clinic
PO Box 5669 804-358-6343
Richmond, VA 23220-0669

10493 Virginia Office for Protection and Advocacy
1910 Byrd Avenue 804-225-2042
Richmond, VA 23230 800-552-3962
Fax: 804-662-7057
general.vopa@vopa.virginia.gov
www.vopa.state.va.us
Helps with disability-related problems like abuse, neglect, and discrimination. Also help people with disabilities obtain services and treatment.
Coleen Miller, Executive Director
Eric Berthiaume, Administrator

Washington

10494 Seattle HPV Support Group
Seattle, WA 98103-1171 425-619-7190
www.aad.org

10495 Washington State Client Assistance Program
2531 Rainer Avenue S 206-721-5999
Seattle, WA 98144-9510 800-544-2121
Fax: 206-721-5980
TTY: 888-721-6072
www.washingtoncap.org

Jerry Johnson, Director
Bob Huven, Rehabilitation Coordinator

West Virginia

10496 Northcentral West Virginia HPV Support Group
Monongalia County Health Department
453 Van Voorhis Road 304-598-5100
Morgantown, WV 26505-3408

10497 West Virginia Advocates
1207 Quarrier Street 304-346-0847
Charleston, WV 25301 800-950-5250
Fax: 304-346-0867
contact@wvadvocates.org
www.wvadvocates.org
Protects and advocates for the human and legal rights of persons with disabilities.
Clarice Hausch, Executive Director
Barbara Criner, Administrative Director

Wisconsin

10498 Governor's Committee for People with Disabilities
Wisconsin Department of Health Services
1 W Wilson Street 608-261-7816
Madison, WI 53703 Fax: 608-266-3386
TTY: 888-701-1251
sarah.lincoln@wisconsin.gov
In 1948, a Governor's Committee was established with one goal: to improve employment opportunities for people with disabilities.
Sarah Lincoln, Director

Wyoming

10499 Wyoming Protection & Advocacy System
7344 Stockman Street 307-632-3496
Cheyenne, WY 82009 Fax: 307-638-0815
wypanda@wypanda.com
www.wypanda.com

To establish, expand, protect and enforce the human and civil rights of persons with disabilities through administrative, legal, and other appropriate remedies.
Mary Carson Barks, President
Jeanne A Thobro, CEO

Libraries & Resource Centers

Alabama

10500 Horizons Schools
2018 15th Avenue South   205-322-6606
Birmingham, AL 35205   800-822-6242
                                           Fax: 205-322-6605
                                           www.horizonsschool.org
The Horizons School offers a non-degree postsecondary program specifically designed to facilitate personal, social and career independence for students with mild learning disabilities and other mild handicapping conditions.
Don Lutomski, President
Bayard Tynes, Treasurer

Arizona

10501 Life Development Institute
18001 N 79th Avenue   623-773-2774
Glendale, AZ 85308   866-736-7811
                                           Fax: 623-773-2788
                                           info@life-development-inst.org
                                           www.lifedevelopmentinstitute.org
Make the special wishes of children with life-threatening or terminal illnesses come true.
Rob Crawford, CEO
Veronica Crawford, Vice President

California

10502 Center for Adaptive Learning
3227 Clayton Road   925-827-3863
Concord, CA 94519   Fax: 925-827-4080
Committed to creating and maintaining a living and working environment for neurologically impaired individuals, which will promote dignity and support a sense of community. The CAL program provides each participant with an individual program for growth. CAL is committed to maintaining the highest quality of living possible, which will allow each client to develop a sense of pride, to augment self-esteem and to foster a sense of self-worth.
Robert L. Edwards, President
Barry Chinn, VP

10503 Independence Center
3640 S Sepulveda Boulevard   310-202-7102
Los Angeles, CA 90034   Fax: 310-202-7180
                                           judym@independencecenter.com
                                           www.independencecenter.com
A mainstreamed transitional residential program for young adults (18-30) with learning disabilities. Program highlights include training in independent living, social and vocational skills, counseling and more.
Judith Maizlish, Executive Director
Gloria Ogletree, Administrative Director

Connecticut

10504 Chapel Haven
1040 Whalley Avenue   203-397-1714
New Haven, CT 06515   Fax: 203-937-2466
                                           admissions@chapelhaven.org
                                           www.chapelhaven.org
Providing an array of lifelong individualized support services for adults (18+) on the autism spectrum and those with developmental and social disabilities, enabling them to lead independent and productive lives.
Betsey Parlato, CEO/Executive Director

District of Columbia

10505 ERIC Clearinghouse on Disabilities and Gifted Education
ERIC Project
C/O Computer Sciences Corporation   800-538-3742
Washington, DC 20008   Fax: 703-620-4334
                                           TTY: 703-264-9449
                                           www.eric.ed.gov
The ERIC mission is to provide a comprehensive, easy-to-use, searchable, Internet-based bibliographic and full-text database of education research and information. The simple version of that is that it provides an enormous amount of print materials online, for easy access to important research and journal materials.
Cheryl Racey, Director

Georgia

10506 Creative Community Services (CCS)
4487 Park Drive   770-469-6226
Norcross, GA 30093   866-618-2823
                                           Fax: 770-469-6210
                                           info@ccsgeorgia.org
                                           www.ccsgeorgia.org
Provides therapeutic foster care services for children and home-based support for adults with developmental disabilities. CCS improves the quality of life for children, adults and families through its community-based support and services. CCS gives both kids and adults hope by encouraging independent living resulting in involved, engaged citizens and community members.
Nicolette Lee, President
Henri Munyengano, Secretary

Massachusetts

10507 Berkshire Center
18 Park Street   413-243-2576
Lee, MA 01238   Fax: 413-243-3351
The College Internship Program at the Berkshire Center provides individualized, post-secondary academic, internship and independent living experiences for young adults with Asperger's Syndrome and other Learning Differences.
Lucy Gosselin MSBM, Program Director

Minnesota

10508 National Resource Library on Youth with Disabilities
University of Minnesota
Minneapolis, MN 55455   612-626-3087
                                                800-276-8642
                                           Fax: 612-626-2134
                                           TTY: 612-624-3939
                                           kdwb-var@umn.edu
                                           www.peds.umn.edu
Offers comprehensive sources of information related to adolescents, disability and transition. The database contains bibliographic, programs, training/education and technical assistance files for the medical community, families, parents and children with chronic illnesses.
Peggy Mann Reinhart, Director
Elizabeth Latts, Resource Coordinator

New Hampshire

10509 Camp Allen
56 Camp Road   603-622-8471
Bedford, NH 03110-6606   Fax: 603-626-4295
                                           www.campallennh.org
Camp Allen welcomes about 600 campers each summer. They are persons of all ages with special needs and extraordinary challenges, including cerebral palsy, autism, muscular dystrophy, Down syndrome, and other developmental disabilities.
Sebastian Grasso, President & CEO
Thomas Aites, Treasurer

10510 Center for Medical Consumers
239 Thompson Street   212-674-7105
New York, NY 10012   Fax: 212-674-7100
                       centersformedicalconsumers@gmail.com
                                www.medicalconsumers.org
A non-profit advocacy organization that was founded with the philosophy of: Whenever long-term drug therapy, elective surgery, or
any other major treatment is prescribed, the question of whether
the treatment has been proven safe and effective should come up.
And the prescribing physician should be expected to cite the
relevant studies.
Arthur Aaron Levin MPH, Director
Maryann Napoli, Associate Director

Support Groups & Hotlines

10511 Behavioral Pediatrics Program
KDWP Variety Family Center
200 Oak Street SE   612-626-4260
Minneapolis, MN 55455-2002   800-276-8642
                                         Fax: 612-624-0997
                                         TTY: 612-624-3939
                                www.peds.umn.edu/pedsadol
Behavioral Pediatrics Staff help children, teen and their families
with a wide variety of behavioral concerns including adjustment to
coping with chronic illness. Treatments vary depending on the age,
developmental state and needs of each child and family. Often,
children are taught to self-regulate their behavior.
Daniel Kohen MD, Director

10512 Caregiver Action Network
1150 Connecticut Avenue NW   202-454-3970
Washington, DC 20036-3904   info@caregiveraction.org
                                          caregiveraction.org
Aims to improve quality of life for Americans who care for loved
ones facing chronic illnesses, disabilities, diseases, or old age.
John Schall, Chief Executive Officer
Chance Browning, Senior Director, Programs

10513 Fetal Alcohol Network
KDWP Variety Family Center
200 Oak Street SE   612-626-4260
Minneapolis, MN 55455-2002   800-276-8642
                                         Fax: 612-624-0997
                                         TTY: 612-624-3939
                                         kdwb-var@umn.edu
                                www.peds.umn.edu/peds-adol
Staff provide assessment, intervention and consultation regarding
the physical, developmental learning, behavioral and emotional
well-being of children and individuals affected by prenatal exposure to alcohol and drugs.
Daniel Kohen MD, Director

10514 Friends Health Connection
New Brunswick, NJ 08903   732-418-1811
                                              800-483-7436
                                         Fax: 732-249-9897
                           info@friendshealthconnection.org
                               www.friendshealthconnection.org
Enhances mind, body and soul through our personalized support
network and dynamic educational and motivational programs.
Works with hospitals and other nonprofit organizations to complement their program offerings and connect people with resources
and support that can enrich their lives.

10515 Hospice and Homecare
3801 Vanesta Drive   785-537-0688
Manhattan, KS 66503   Fax: 785-537-1309
                                            info@hcandh.org
                               www.homecareandhospice.org
Aims to be the premier non-profit Homecare & Hospice provider
of compassionate, affordable health, wellness and support services.

10516 KDWB Family Resource Center
200 Oak Street SE   612-626-3087
Minneapolis, MN 55455-2002   800-276-8642
                                         Fax: 612-624-0997
                                         TTY: 612-624-3939
                                         kdwb-var@umn.edu
                                www.peds.umn.edu/peds-adol
A place families can visit to learn about their child's chronic illness
or disability, identify psychological and developmental issues, and
link-up with program and community resources. Information will
be available by telephone and via the web site.
Elizabeth Latts, Resource Coordinator

10517 KDWB Variety Family Canter
200 Oak Street SE   612-626-3087
Minneapolis, MN 55455-2002   800-276-8642
                                         Fax: 612-624-0997
                                         TTY: 612-624-3939
                                         kdwbvar@umn.edu
                               www.peds.umn.edu/pedsadol/
University-Community pertnership that provides family-centered
services that promote physical, emotional, psychological and social health and well being for children and youth at risk, including
children and youth with disabilities. The Center is dedicated to
teaching, research, outreach, and community services.
Peggy Mann Reinhart, Director
Elizabeth Latts, Resource Coordinator

10518 National Alliance for Caregiving
4720 Montgomery Lane   301-718-8444
Bethesda, MD 20814   Fax: 301-951-9067
                                          info@caregiving.org
                                           www.caregiving.org
Advocates on behalf of caregivers, as well as conducting research
and offering support services.
C. Grace Whiting, JD, President & CEO
Michael Wittke, BSW, MPA, Senior Director, Public Policy

10519 National Association for Home Care
228 Seventh Street SE   202-547-7424
Washington, DC 20003   Fax: 202-547-3540
                                                www.nahc.org
Promotes the concepts of hospice, a philosophy of health care
which is expressed through the provision of a variety of medical
and nonmedical services to terminally ill patients and their
families.
Val J. Halamandaris, President
Andrea Devoti, Chair

10520 National Family Caregivers Association
10400 Connecticut Avenue   301-942-6430
Kensington, MD 20895-3944   800-896-3650
                                         Fax: 301-942-2302
                              info@thefamilycaregiver.org
                                www.thefamilycaregiver.org
Educates, supports, empowers and speaks up for the more than 65
million Americans who care for loved ones with a chronic illness
or disability or the frailties of old age. Reaches across the boundaries of diagnosis, relationships and life stages to help transform
family caregivers' lives by removing barriers to health and well
being
Suzanne Mintz, President/CEO

10521 National Health Information Center
Office of Disease Prevention & Health Promotion
1101 Wootton Pkwy   Fax: 240-453-8281
Rockville, MD 20852   odphpinfo@hhs.gov
                                           www.health.gov/nhic
Supports public health education by maintaining a calendar of National Health Observances; helps connect consumers and health
professionals to organizations that can best answer questions and
provide up-to-date contact information from reliable sources; updates on a yearly basis toll-free numbers for health information,
Federal health clearinghouses and info centers.
Don Wright, MD, MPH, Director

10522 National Parent to Parent Support and Information System
3805 Presidential Parkway 770-451-5484
Atlanta, GA 30340 Fax: 770-458-4091
info@p2pga.org
www.p2pusa.org
NPPSIS is a nonprofit organization established to support, strengthen, and empower families through one-on-one parent contacts. They link families nationally whose children have special health care needs and rare disorders. They provide parents with heath care information, resources and referrals to allow them to identify appropriate services.
Dana Yarbrough, President
Debra S. Tucker, Executive Director

10523 Okizu Foundation Camps
16 Digital Drive 415-382-9083
Novato, CA 94949-6115 Fax: 415-382-8384
info@okizu.org
www.okizu.org
This foundation runs family camp programs for children who have cancer and their families, and for children who have or had a parent with cancer.
Suzie Randall, Executive Director
Heather Ferrier, Asst. Executive Director

10524 Parent to Parent of New York State
500 Balltown Road 518-381-4350
Schenectady, NY 12304-2247 800-305-8817
Fax: 518-393-9607
staciap2p@verizon.net
www.parenttoparentnys.org
Parent to Parent programs provide informational and emotional support to parents who have a child, adolescent or adult family member with special needs. Offers an important connection for a parent who is seeking support for special disability issues, by matching him or her with a trained veteran parent who has already been there. Because the two parents share so many common concerns and interests, the support given and received is often uniquely meaningful. Also helps families locate information
Jenni Austen, Regional Coordinator
Holly Bartczak, Coordinator

10525 Pediatric Psychology
KDWP Variety Family Center
200 Oak Street SE 612-626-4260
Minneapolis, MN 55455-2002 800-276-8642
Fax: 612-624-0997
TTY: 612-624-3939
kdwbvar@umn.edu
www.peds.umn.edu/pedsadol
Staff provide assessment, intervention and consultation regarding the physical, developmental, learning, behavioral and emotional well-being of children and individuals affected by prenatal exposure to alcohol and drugs.
Daniel Kohen MD, Director

10526 STAR Center for Family Health
KDWB University Pediatrics Family Center
200 Oak St, SE, 612-626-4260
Minneapolis, MN 55455-2002 Fax: 612-624-0997
TTY: 6126243939
kdwb-var@umn.edu
www.peds.umn.edu/peds-adol/
Helps children, youth and families develop new and enhanced ways of coping with stress, learn strategies for adjusting to living with a chronic illness, and discover new ways of finding health, balance and well-being.
Lavon Anderson, M.A., Administrator
Linda Boche, Executive Secretary to Division Director

10527 U Special Kids
KDWB Variety Family Center
200 Oak Street SE 612-626-3081
Minneapolis, MN 55455-2002 800-276-8642
Fax: 612-624-0997
TTY: 6126243939
uspclkid@umn.edu
www.peds.umn.edu/peds-adol/

A program that provides care coordinators for children with complex medical conditions. A team of health care providers advocates for children and their families within the health care system.
Anne Kelly MD, Director

10528 Visiting Nurse Association of America
601 Thirteenth St NW 202-384-1420
Washington, DC 20005 888-866-8773
Fax: 202-384-1444
webadmin@vnaa.org
www.vnaa.org
The VNAA will support, promote and advance nonprofit providers of home and community-based healthcare, hospice and health promotion services to ensure quality care for their communities.
Mary B. DeVeau, Chair
Ellen Rothberg, Vice Chair

10529 Well Spouse Association
63 W Main Street 732-577-8899
Freehold, NJ 07728 www.wellspouse.org
This association is a nonprofit national self-help organization serving the well spouse of the chronically ill. Members help each other develop coping and survival skills through local support groups (including bereavement), letter and telephone networks, and personal outreach and a quarterly newsletter.
Marilyn Kamp, Executive Director

Books

10530 A History of Childhood and Disability
Philip Safford and Elizabeth Safford, author
Teachers College Press
1234 Amsterdam Avenue 212-678-3929
New York, NY 10027 Fax: 212-678-4149
tcpress@tc.columbia.edu
www.teacherscollegepress.com
This book presents an interdisciplinary perspective on children considered exceptional and how services have evolved in reponse to their diverse neeeds.
1996 352 pages
ISBN: 0-807734-85-3
Philip Safford, Co-Author
Elizabeth Safford, Co-Author

10531 Art of Getting Well
David Spero, RN, author
Hunter House Publishing
424 Church Street 615-255-2665
Nashville, TN 37219 800-266-5592
Fax: 615-255-5081
ordering@hunterhouse.com
www.turnerpublishing.com
A five step plan for maximazing health when you have a chronic illness.
224 pages Paperback
David Spero, Author

10532 Assisstive Technology for Young Children: A Guide to Family-Centered Services
Sharon Lesar Judge and Howard P Parette, author
Brookline Books
8 Trumbull Rd 413-584-0184
Northampton, MA 01060 800-666-2665
Fax: 413-584-6184
brbooks@yahoo.com
brooklinebks.com
Explores the wide range of considerations involved in evaluating children's needs, selecting and prescribing devices, and training children, families, and teachers to use the technology.
1998 Softcover
ISBN: 1-571290-51-6

10533 Awaking to Disability
Volcano Press

PO Box 270
Volcano, CA 95689-0270

209-296-7989
800-879-9636
Fax: 209-296-4995
sales@volcanopress.com
www.volcanopress.com

From the disability activist whose columns have been avidly followed by readers of the Albuquerque Journal and Miami Herald comes this revealing compedium of her thoughts. It offers a perspective for parents of children with disabilites, or for newly disabled people.
1997 288 pages
ISBN: 1-884244-14-9

10534 Blood Pressure Book: How to Get it Down & Keep it Down
Bull Publishing
PO Box 1377
Boulder, CO 80306

303-545-6350
800-676-2855
Fax: 303-545-6354
www.bullpub.com

Provides basic information on the causes and treatment of high blood pressure includes check up charts and illustrations that will help readers find out where they stand and lead them to practical advice tailored to their own needs.
1996
ISBN: 0-923521-97-6

10535 Building Partnerships in Hospital Care
Bull Publishing
PO Box 1377
Boulder, CO 80306

303-545-6350
800-676-2855
Fax: 303-545-6354
www.bullpub.com

Aims to desensetize patients and families to their fears of illness, hospital machinery and authority figures at the same time resensitize institution weary professionals to the feelings, instincts and emotions that brought them into the field in the first place.
304 pages
ISBN: 0-923521-07-0

10536 Child of Mine: Feeding with Love and Good Sense
Bull Publishing
PO Box 1377
Boulder, CO 80306

303-545-6350
800-676-2855
Fax: 303-545-6354
www.bullpub.com

Parents need to learn how to provide a nutritionally wholesome diet, but they also need to know how to feed in a way that nurtures a child's senses of autonomy and trust in themselves and their bodies.
470 pages
ISBN: 0-923521-51-8
Ellyn Satter, Author

10537 Childhood Emergencies: What to Do A Quick Refrence Guide
Bull Publishing
PO Box 1377
Boulder, CO 80306

303-545-6350
800-676-2855
Fax: 303-545-6354
www.bullpub.com

Handy book contains clear and quick referance for most common injuries including cuts and wounds, broken bones, abdominal pain, burns, toothaches, convulsion, eye and ear injuries, abrasions, bites insect and animal, bleeding, choking, seizures, freezing and frostbite, CPR, etc.
44 pages
ISBN: 0-923521-62-3

10538 Chiropractor's Self-Help Back and Body Book
Samuel Homola, DC, author
Hunter House Publishers
424 Church Street
Nashville, TN 37219

615-255-2665
800-266-5592
Fax: 615-255-5081
ordering@hunterhouse.com
www.turnerpublishing.com

How to relieve common aches and pains at home and on the job.
2002 320 pages Paperback
ISBN: 0-897933-76-6
Samuel Homola, Author

10539 Choose the Right Long Term Care
NOLO
950 Parker Street
Berkeley, CA 94710-2524

800-728-3555
Fax: 800-645-0895
cs@nolo.com
www.nolo.com

You can use this book to figure out how to choose a nursing home, or find a viable alternative. Covers how to get the most out of Medicare and other benefit programs.
336 pages
ISBN: 0-873375-15-7
Chris Braun, President
Janet Portman, Executive Editor

10540 Chronic Physical Illness
S. Newman, E. Steed, K. Mulligan, author
McGraw-Hill Companies
Returns Department
Dubuque, IA 52002

877-833-5524
Fax: 609-308-4484
pbg.ecommerce_custserv@mcgraw-hill.com
www.mcgraw-hill.com

Provides an overview of self-management in chronic physical illness, theoretical and conceptual background, and examines issues related to the delivery of self-management. Discussion of a range of chronic conditions including: asthma, coronary artery disease, heart failure, COPD, hypertension, diabetes and rheumatoid arthritis. Authored by a number of leading international experts in the diseases they discuss. Hardcover also available for $136.95.
2008 240 pages
ISBN: 0-335217-86-9

10541 Directory of Health Grants
Research Grant Guides
PO Box 1214
Loxahatchee, FL 33470-1214
1000 foundation profiles.
Second edition
ISBN: 0-945078-19-6

561-795-6129
Fax: 561-795-7794

10542 Directory of Social Service Grants
Research Grant Guides
PO Box 1214
Loxahatchee, FL 33470-1214
1100 foundation profiles.
Second edition
ISBN: 0-945078-18-8

561-795-6129
Fax: 561-795-7794

10543 Disabled Woman's Guide to Pregnancy and Birth
Judith Rogers OTR, author
Demos Medical Publishing
11 W 42nd Street
New York, NY 10036

212-683-0072
800-532-8663
Fax: 212-683-0118
support@demosmedical.com
www.demosmedical.com

Based on the experiences of ninety women with disabilities who chose to have children. Contains in-depth interviews with women with 22 different types of disabilities and with a total of 143 pregnancies.
528 pages
ISBN: 1-932603-08-8
Beth Kaufman Barry, Publisher
David D'Addona, Acquisitions Editor

10544 Family Interventions Throughout Chronic Illness and Disability
Springer Publishing Company
536 Broadway
New York, NY 10012-3955

212-431-4370
Fax: 212-941-7842
marketing@springerpub.com
www.springerpub.com

This book provides usable methods for professionals to help families deal with the reality of chronic illness of disability of a family member. Included at the end of each section are study questions and suggested activities for those working with the disabled, as well as for students.
336 pages Hardcover
ISBN: 0-826155-80-1
Annette Imperati, Marketing Director

10545 Get Fit While You Sit: Easy Workouts From Your Chair
Charlene Torkelson, author

Hunter House Publishing
424 Church Street   615-255-2665
Nashville, TN 37219   800-266-5592
                                          Fax: 615-255-5081
                               ordering@hunterhouse.com
                               www.turnerpublishing.com

A total body workout that can be done right from your chair, anywhere. Perfect for office workers, travelers, and those with age-related movement limitations or special conditions.
Paperback
ISBN: 0-897932-53-0
Charlene Torkelson, Author

10546 Good Bones: Complete Guide to Building and Maintaining the Healthiest Bones
Barbara Luke, author

Bull Publishing
PO Box 1377   303-545-6350
Boulder, CO 80306   800-676-2855
                                          Fax: 303-545-6354
                                            www.bullpub.com

Examines 17 major risks in bone health with women. Author offers nutrional advice and preventative nutritional advice and prevenative measures in this comprehensive and scientifically sound guide for woman of all ages.
192 pages
ISBN: 0-923521-44-5

10547 Grants for Organizations Serving People with Disabilities
Research Grant Guides
PO Box 1214   Fax: 561-795-7794
Loxahatchee, FL 33470-1214
800 foundation profiles, including funding for all types of nonprofits. Also two key articles on winning grant strategies.
Tenth edition
ISBN: 0-945078-17-X

10548 Habits Not Diets: Secret to Lifetime Weight Control
James M Ferguson MD, Cassandra Ferguson, author

Bull Publishing
PO Box 1377   303-545-6350
Boulder, CO 80306   800-676-2855
                                          Fax: 303-545-6354
                                            www.bullpub.com

This sensible approach puts the emphasis on how to eat rather than what. Uses the cognitive aspects of weight management including thinking skills, stress management and problem solving to help analyze individual eating habits , break undesirable patterns and establish new ones.
352 pages
ISBN: 0-923521-70-7

10549 Health
Sage Publications
2455 Teller Road   805-499-9774
Thousand Oaks, CA 91320   800-818-7243
                                          Fax: 805-499-0871
                                   journals@sagepub.com
                                 www.sagepublications.com

A interdisciplinary and international journal committed to the social and cultural study of health, illness and medicine with a particular focus on the changing place of health matters in modern society and in public onsciousness.
Quarterly

10550 I Can't Chew Cookbook
J Randy Wilson, author

Hunter House Publishing
424 Church Street   615-255-2665
Nashville, TN 37219   800-266-5592
                                          Fax: 615-255-5081
                               ordering@hunterhouse.com
                               www.turnerpublishing.com

Delicious soft-diet recipes for people with chewing, swallowing and dry-mouth disorders.
224 pages Paperback
ISBN: 0-897934-00-8
J. Randy Wilson, Author

10551 Informed Woman's Guide to Breast Health
Kerry McGinn RN, author

Bull Publishing
PO Box 1377   303-545-6350
Boulder, CO 80306   800-676-2855
                                          Fax: 303-545-6354
                                            www.bullpub.com

Covers all elements of self-examination, mammography, medical exams and tests; includes new information about the genes BRCA 1 and BRCA 2, possible early predictors of cancer
ISBN: 0-923521-61-5

10552 Insider's Guide to HMOs
Penguin Putnam
PO Box 999   800-526-0275
Bergenfield, NJ 07621-0903   Fax: 800-227-9604
ISBN: 0-452276-91-8

10553 Journel to Pain Relief
Phyllis Berger, author

Hunter House Publishing
424 Church Street   615-255-2665
Nashville, TN 37219   800-266-5592
                                          Fax: 615-255-5081
                               ordering@hunterhouse.com
                               www.turnerpublishing.com

Hands-on guide to breakthroughs in pain treatment.
2007 288 pages Paperback
Cristina Sverdrup, Customer Service Manager

10554 Joy of Laziness
Peter Axt, PhD, Michaela Axt-Gardermann, author

Hunter House Publishing
424 Church Street   615-255-2665
Nashville, TN 37219   800-266-5592
                                          Fax: 615-255-5081
                               ordering@hunterhouse.com
                               www.turnerpublishing.com

Explains that every human being has a limited amount of energy at his or her disposal.
160 pages Paperback
ISBN: 0-897934-01-5
Peter Axt, Author

10555 Just Like Everyone Else
World Institute on Disability
3075 Adeline Street   510-225-6400
Berkeley, CA 94703-1520   Fax: 510-225-0477
                                    TTY: 510-225-0478
                                              wid@wid.org
                                                  wid.org

Provides perspective, inspiration and information about the Independent Living Movement and the Americans with Disabilities Act.
16 pages
Anita Shafer Aaron, Executive Director

10556 Laurel's Kitchen Caring: Recipes for Everyday Home Caregiving
Ten Speed Press
1745 Broadway   212-782-9000
New York, NY 10019-0123   800-841-2665
                                          Fax: 510-524-4588
                       CrownOSM@penguinrandomhouse.com
                                       crownpublishing.com

A cookbook tailored to the nutritional needs of recovering patients as well as morale booster, caregiving primer, and resource book.
1997 158 pages
ISBN: 0-898159-51-2

10557 Living a Healthy Life with Chronic Conditions
Kate Lorig, Halsted Holman, David Sobel, author

Bull Publishing

PO Box 1377
Boulder, CO 80306 303-545-6350
800-676-2855
Fax: 303-545-6354
www.bullpub.com

Full of tips, suggestions, and strategies to deal with chronic illness and common symptoms, such as fatigue, pain, shortness of breath, disability, and depression. Encourages readers to develop individual approaches to setting goals, making decisions, and finding resources and support so they are able to do the things they want, and need, to accomplish.
292 pages
ISBN: 1-933503-01-1
Kate Lorig, DrPH, Co-Author
Halsted Holman, MD, Co-Author

10558 Maximize Your Body Potential
Joyce D Nash PhD, author
Bull Publishing
PO Box 1377
Boulder, CO 80306 303-545-6350
800-676-2855
Fax: 303-545-6354
www.bullpub.com

Using selftests, checklists, and fill-in forms, shows readers how to make a committment, how to set realistic goals, and how to design an individualized exercise and eating program.
640 pages
ISBN: 0-923521-71-4
Joyce D. Nash, Ph.D., Author

10559 Menopause Without Medicine
Linda Ojeda, author
Hunter House Publishing
424 Church Street
Nashville, TN 37219 615-255-2665
800-266-5592
Fax: 615-255-5081
ordering@hunterhouse.com
www.turnerpublishing.com

Provides complete information on the symptoms of menopause - hot flashes, sexual changes, deperssion and osteoporosis - and how to alleviate them.
400 pages Paperback
ISBN: 0-897934-05-3

10560 Nolo's Guide to Soc. Security Disability: Getting and Keeping Your Benefits
David Morton MD, author
NOLO
950 Parker Street
Berkeley, CA 94710-2524 800-728-3555
Fax: 800-645-0895
cs@nolo.com
www.nolo.com

The essential book for anyone dealing with a long-term or permanent disability. Written both for first-time applicants and existing recipients of Social Security disability, this guide demystifies the program and tells you everything you need to know about qualifying and applying for benefits, maintaining your benefits, and appealing the denial of a claim.
512 pages
ISBN: 1-413311-04-4
David Morton, M.D., Author

10561 Ostomy Book: Living Comfortably with Colostomies, Ileostomies and Urostomies
Barbara Dorr Mullen, Kerry Anne McGinn, author
Bull Publishing
PO Box 1377
Boulder, CO 80306 303-545-6350
800-676-2855
Fax: 303-545-6354
www.bullpub.com

For people who have a colostomy, ileostomy or urinary diversion (utostomy), either permanent or temporary, as well as for family, friends and health professionals.
ISBN: 0-933503-13-4

10562 Psychological Management of Chronic Pain: A Treatment Manual
Springer Publishing Company

11 West 42nd Street
New York, NY 10036-3955 212-431-4370
877-687-7476
Fax: 212-941-7842
cs@springerpub.com
www.springerpub.com

This volume provides the clinician with a practical guide to help clients manage and alleviate problems associated with chronic pain and places an emphasis on the cognitive components of treatment. The manual illustrates a time-limited, therapist-guide/self-management program.
1996 80 pages Softcover
ISBN: 0-826161-12-X

10563 Self Help: Your Strategy for Living with COPD
Bull Publishing
PO Box 1377
Boulder, CO 80306 303-545-6350
800-676-2855
Fax: 303-545-6354
www.bullpub.com

Contains vital information for patients suffering from asthma, emphysema, or chronic bronchitis. Colorful charts, graphs and illustrations highlight major concepts and help make the booklet user friendly.
1997 32 pages
ISBN: 0-923521-40-2

10564 ShapeWalking
Marilyn Bach, PhD, Lorie Schleck, author
Hunter House Publishing
424 Church Street
Nashville, TN 37219 615-255-2665
800-266-5592
Fax: 615-255-5081
ordering@hunterhouse.com
www.turnerpublishing.com

An easy low cost total fitness program that is suited for exercisers of all levels.
144 pages Paperback
ISBN: 0-897933-73-5
Marilyn L. Bach, Author

10565 Social Security, Medicare and Government Pensions
Dorothy Matthews Berman, author
NOLO
950 Parker Street
Berkeley, CA 94710-2524 800-728-3555
Fax: 800-645-0895
cs@nolo.com
www.nolo.com

Gets you the most out of your retirement benefits
496 pages
ISBN: 1-413310-97-9
Dorothy Matthews Berman, Co-Author
Joseph Matthews, Co-Author

10566 Strength Training for Seniors
Michael Fekete, CSCS; ACE, author
Hunter House Publishing
424 Church Street
Nashville, TN 37219 615-255-2665
800-266-5592
Fax: 615-255-5081
ordering@hunterhouse.com
www.turnerpublishing.com

How to rewind your biological clock. Reduce a person's biological age by 10-20 years.
2006 160 pages Paperback
Cristina Sverdrup, Customer Service Manager

10567 Succeeding Against the Odds: Strategies and Insights from the Learning Disabled
Jeremy P Tarcher
5858 Wilshire Boulevard
Los Angeles, CA 90036-4521 213-935-9980

Filled with information on adults with learning disabilities, including the hidden handicaps, the definition of learning disabilities, and characteristics of individuals with learning disabilities. The book also looks at the responsibility of preparing for adulthood, and includes information for parents and teachers.
Lex Frieden, Program Director

10568 Taking Care of Caregivers
D Jeanne Roberts MA, author
Bull Publishing
PO Box 1377
Boulder, CO 80306

303-545-6350
800-676-2855
Fax: 303-545-6354
www.bullpub.com

Covers the needs of caregivers; their feelings; stress management techniques; communication; grief; sharing and support
ISBN: 0-923521-09-7
D. Jeanne Roberts, M.A., Author

10569 Tax Options and Strategies for People with Disabilities
Demos Vermande
11 West 42nd Street
New York, NY 10036-8804

212-683-0072
800-532-8663
Fax: 212-683-0118
support@demosmedical.com
www.demosmedical.com

1996 288 pages
ISBN: 0-939957-85-

10570 Teens Face to Face with Chronic Illness
Asthma and Allergy Foundation of America
8201 Corporate Drive
Landover, MD 20785-2330

202-466-7643
800-727-8462
Fax: 202-466-8940
Info@aafa.org
www.aafa.org

Young people easily relate to this book, which uses anecdotes from teens dealing with chronic illness. Teens address issues such as peer pressure and feeling different.
129 pages Paperback

10571 The Personal Care Attendant Guide: The Art of Finding, Keeping, or Being One
Katie Rodriguez Banister, author
Program Development Associates
11 West 42nd Street
New York, NY 10036-9576

212-683-0072
800-543-2119
Fax: 315-452-0710
support@demosmedical.com
www.demosmedical.com

To live independently, many people with chronic illness and/or disabilitiy hire a personal attendant to assist with day-to-day tasks. Finding a qualified caregiver can be challenging, but not impossible. The Guide teaches readers how to find a competent caregiver, and gives prospective attendants vital information and real-life examples to help them succeed. Includes easy-to-use forms and worksheets to make the search easy and organized, anecdotes, and resources.
2007 160 pages

10572 Time for Healing: Relaxation for Mind and Body
Bull Publishing
PO Box 1377
Boulder, CO 80306

303-545-6350
800-676-2855
Fax: 303-545-6354
www.bullpub.com

Helps and guides listeners release tension and acheive deep muscular relaxation, heightened self-awareness and total relaxation.
Catherine Regan, Ph.D., Author

10573 Understanding Addiction
Elizabeth Connell Henderson MD, author
University Press of Mississippi
3825 Ridgewood Road
Jackson, MS 39211

601-432-6205
800-737-7788
Fax: 601-432-6217
www.upress.state.ms.us

A concise overview of this complex affliction for all those affected by addiction — addicts, family members, and even employers
224 pages Paperback
ISBN: 1-578062-40-9
Elizabeth Connell Henderson, M.D., Author

10574 Understanding Anemia
Ed Uthman, MD, author
University Press of Mississippi

3825 Ridgewood Road
Jackson, MS 39211

601-432-6205
800-737-7788
Fax: 601-432-6217
www.upress.state.ms.us

Gently builds upon elementary knowledge of biology to provide the general reader with a fairly sophisticated understanding of the various causes of anemia, of the methods used to make diagnoses, and of the principles of treatment.
160 pages Paperback
ISBN: 1-578060-39-9
Ed Uthman, M.D., Author

10575 Understanding Child Sexual Abuse
Edward L Rowan, MD, author
University Press of Mississippi
3825 Ridgewood Road
Jackson, MS 39211

601-432-6205
800-737-7788
Fax: 601-432-6217
www.upress.state.ms.us

For those looking to comrephend and to prevent child sexual abuse, a succinct guidebook of advice and resources.
96 pages Paperback
ISBN: 1-578068-07-X
Edward L. Rowan, M.D., Author

10576 Understanding Cosmetic Laser Surgery
Robert Langdon, MD, author
University Press of Mississippi
3825 Ridgewood Road
Jackson, MS 39211

601-432-6205
800-737-7788
Fax: 601-432-6217
www.upress.state.ms.us

A description of the processes and procedures available in cosmetic laser surgery.
112 pages
ISBN: 1-578065-87-9
Robert Langdon, M.D., Author

10577 Understanding Dental Health
Francis G Serio, DMD; MS, author
University Press of Mississippi
3825 Ridgewood Road
Jackson, MS 39211

601-432-6205
800-737-7788
Fax: 601-432-6217
www.upress.state.ms.us

A user-friendly manual on the basics of dental health.
128 pages Paperback
ISBN: 1-578060-10-9
Francis G. Serio, D.M.D., M.S., Author

10578 Understanding Dietary Supplements
Jenna Hollenstein, author
University Press of Mississippi
3825 Ridgewood Road
Jackson, MS 39211

601-432-6205
800-737-7788
Fax: 601-432-6217
www.upress.state.ms.us

A handy guide to the evaluation and use of vitamins, minerals, herbs, botanicals, and more.
96 pages Paperback
ISBN: 1-578069-81-5
Jenna Hollenstein, MS, RD, ELS, Author

10579 Understanding Stuttering
Nathan Lavid, MD, author
University Press of Mississippi
3825 Ridgewood Road
Jackson, MS 39211

601-432-6205
800-737-7788
Fax: 601-432-6217
www.upress.state.ms.us

Insight into an ailment that impairs more than sixty million in the world population.
112 pages Paperback
ISBN: 1-578065-73-9
Nathan Lavid, M.D., Author

10580 Understanding Your Learning Disability
Cheri Warner, author
Ohio State University at Newark
1179 University Drive 740-366-3321
Newark, OH 43055 800-963-9275
newark.osu.edu
Provides tips for students based on the author's experience as a Learning Disability Specialist. Offers definitions, characteristics, and suggestions related to reading, math, note taking, test taking, social interactions, and organizational strategies.

10581 Writing from Within
Bernard Selling, author
Hunter House Publishers
424 Church Street 615-255-2665
Nashville, TN 37219 800-266-5592
Fax: 615-255-5081
www.turnerpublishing.com
A guide to creativity and life story writing
320 pages Paperback
ISBN: 0-897932-17-2

10582 Yes, You Can!: Go Beyond Physical Adversity and Live Life to Its Fullest
Janis Dietz PhD, author
Demos Medical Publishing
11 W 42nd Street 212-683-0072
New York, NY 10036 800-532-8663
support@demosmedical.com
Based on the premise that life should be lived to the fullest extent possible, disability or no disability.
102 pages Paperback
ISBN: 1-888799-48-x

Children's Books

10583 Are You Tired Again?...I Understand: An Activities Workbook for Children
Marilyn W Deutsch PhD, author
Western Psychological Services
625 Alaska Avenue 424-201-8800
Torrance, CA 90503-1251 800-648-8857
Fax: 424-201-6950
customerservice@wpspublish.com
www.wpspublish.com
This reassuring activity and coloring book is for children with a chronically ill parent—children who often feel guilty, neglected, lonely, helpless, and afraid. It gives these youngsters the tools they need to work through their feelings, while gently explaining why Mom isn't getting better, why she's always tired, and how the family can still enjoy life and function as a family. It can be used with individuals or with support groups.

10584 In the Hospital
Peter Alsop, Bill Harley, author
Compassion Books
7036 State Highway 80 S 828-675-5909
Burnsville, NC 28714-7569 800-970-4220
Fax: 828-675-9687
orders@compassionbooks.com
www.compassionbooks.com
Wonderful songs and entertaining stories dealing with being sick, being different, being scared and finding strength and hope.
Audiotape/Book
Bruce Greene, Director

10585 Zink the Zebra
Gareth Stevens, Inc
330 West Olive Street 414-332-3520
Milwaukee, WI 53212-3952 800-542-2595
Fax: 877-542-2596
customerservice@gspub.com
www.garethstevens.com
Zink is a zebra with spots instead of stripes. Here is an inspiring and touching tale about being different in ways that don't matter and shouldn't get in the way when it comes to making friends and enjoying companionship and respect. Written by 11-year-old

Kelly Weil in the last year of a battle she bravely fought, but ultimately lost, against cancer.
1997
ISBN: 0-836816-26-9

Magazines

10586 Advance: for Directors in Rehabilitation
Merion Publications
2900 Horizon Drive 215-265-7812
King of Prussia, PA 19406-2651 800-355-5627
webmaster@advanceweb.com
www.advanceweb.com
An informational magazine designed to provide a balance of material concerning all aspects of a rehabilitation manager's job.
Scott Huelskamp, Editor
Johnathan Bassett, Senior Associate Editor

10587 Closing the Gap
526 Main Street 507-248-3294
Henderson, MN 56044 Fax: 507-248-3810
info@closingthegap.com
www.closingthegap.com
Strives to provide parents and educators alike, the information and training necessary to locate, compare, and implement assistive technology.
BiMonthly
Budd Hagen, Co-Founder
Connie Kneip, VP/General Manager

10588 Exceptional Parent Magazine
209 Harvard Street 617-730-5800
Brookline, MA 02446-5005 800-852-2884
Fax: 617-730-8742

Lex Frieden, Program Director

Newsletters

10589 Asbestos Watch
PO Box 1483 301-243-5864
Baltimore, MD 21203-1483 Fax: 301-243-5234
www.whitelung.org
A national nonprofit organization dedicated to the education of the public to the hazards of asbestos exposure. The association developed programs of public education and consults with victims of asbestos exposure, school boards, building owners, government agencies, and others interested in identifying asbestos hazards and developing control programs.
Annual

10590 Chronic Pain Letter
Dolak
Old Chelsea Station 718-797-0015
New York, NY 10011
Brings current information on the management of chronic pain to the sufferer and the health professional.

Dorothy Fabian, Circulation Manager

10591 Health Facts
Center for Medical Consumers
237 Thompson Street 917-836-7596
New York, NY 10012-1017 Fax: 212-674-7100
centerformedicalconsumers@gmail.com
www.medicalconsumers.org
Analyses of topics such as cancer, nutrition, depression, exercise, prescription drugs and nonmedical therapies.
6 pages Monthly

10592 In Confidence
American Health Information Management Association
233 N Michigan Avenue 312-233-1100
Chicago, IL 60601 800-335-5535
Fax: 312-233-1090
info@ahima.org
www.ahima.org

Provides medical, legal and other professionals with a forum to exchange ideas and share knowledge about the confidentiality of health information and people's rights to privacy.
12 pages BiMonthly
Linda Kloss, Chief Executive Officer
Becky Perry, Executive Vice President & CFO

10593 Johns Hopkins Health Insider
Intelihealth
960C Harvest Drive   800-988-1127
Blue Bell, PA 19422   Fax: 800-676-3299
                                   www.jhinsider.com
Expert advice and information from America's leading health institution. The most authoritative, cutting-edge health information available today, straight from the leading specialists and experts.
David B Hellmann MD, Associate Editor
Linda A Lewandowski PhD, RN, Associate Editor

10594 Learning Disability Quarterly
Council for Learning Disabilities
11184 Antioch Road   913-491-1011
Overland Park, KS 66210   Fax: 913-491-1011
                                   www.cldinternational.org
Steve Chamberlain, President
Diane Bryant, President Elect

10595 Lifelines
Disabled & Alone/Life Services for the Handicapped
1440 Broadway   212-532-6740
New York, NY 10018   800-995-0066
                                   Fax: 212-532-6740
                                   info@disabledandalone.org
                                   www.disabledandalone.org
8 pages Quarterly
Leslie D Park, Chairman
Lee Alan Ackerman BA, Executive Director

10596 Lymphatic Research Matters
Lymphatic Research Foundation
261 Madison Avenue   516-625-9675
New York, NY 10016   Fax: 516-625-9410
                                   info@lymphaticnetwork.org
Reporting information about LRF activities and current research. The newsletters are sent to registrants in our data base: patients, their families, the scientific community and health care providers.
Bi-Annual
Philip Braginsky, Esq., Chair
Kenneth R. Cerini, Treasurer

10597 Mainstay
Well Spouse Association
63 W Main Street   732-577-8899
Freehold, NJ 7728   800-838-0879
                                   Fax: 732-577-8644
                                   info@wellspouse.org
                                   www.wellspouse.org
The Well Spouse Association quarterly newsletter featuring articles written by WSA members.

10598 NHF Head Lines
National Headache Foundation
820 N Orleans   312-274-2650
Chicago, IL 60610   888-643-5552
                                   Fax: 312-640-9049
                                   info@headaches.org
                                   www.headaches.org
Up-to-date information on the latest developments in headache treatment; breaking news about newly-approved drugs; reviews of topical books; reader's mail feature, where the nation's leading medical experts answer questions about headaches; and a list of support group meetings where you can learn how to make a positive change in your life.
Bimonthly
Robert R Dalton, Executive Director

10599 National Networker
National Network of Learning Disabled Adults
808 N 82nd Street   602-941-5112
Scottsdale, AZ 85257-3850

For adults with learning disabilities.
Quarterly
Lex Frieden, Program Director

10600 Orphan Disease Update
National Organization for Rare Disorders
55 Kenosia Avenue   203-744-0100
Danbury, CT 06810-8923   800-999-6673
                                   Fax: 203-798-2291
                                   orphan@rarediseases.org
                                   www.rarediseases.org
Information about rare disorders for families with similar disorders.

10601 VSA Arts
JFK Center for the Performing Arts
1300 Connecticut Ave NW   202-628-2600
Washington, DC 20036-1715   800-933-8721
                                   Fax: 202-737-0725
                                   TDD: 202-737-0645
VSA arts is an international, nonprofit organization dedicated to promoting artistic excellence and providing educational opportunities through the arts for children and adults with disabilities. The Creative Spirit is a quarterly newsletter that features VSA arts special events throughout the world, interviews with artistd and articles relating to disability and the arts.
8 pages
D Dixon, CEO
S Datton-Kumins, Writer/Research Coordinator

10602 Wheel Life News
University of Virginia, Rehab Engineering Centers
3363 University Station   804-924-0311
Charlottesville, VA 22903
Features tie downs and other adaptive technology for persons with disabilities.

10603 Worklife: A Publication of Employment and People with Disabilities
Office of Disability Employment Policy
200 Constitution Ave NW   202-693-7880
Washington, DC 20210   Fax: 202-693-7888
                                   TDD: 202-376-6205
Quarterly

Pamphlets

10604 Campus Opportunities for Students with Learning Differences
Judith & Stephen Crooker, author
Octameron Associates
PO Box 2748   703-836-5480
Alexandria, VA 22301   Fax: 703-836-5650
                                   octameron@aol.com
Tells learning disabled students what questions to ask when selecting a school, how to prepare for the more rigorous academic schedule and when to get special assistance.
36 pages
ISBN: 1-575090-52-x
Judith Crooker, Co-Author
Stephen Crooker, Co-Author

10605 Issues in Independent Living
Independent Living Research Utilization
2323 S Shepherd Drive   713-520-0232
Houston, TX 77019-7024   Fax: 713-520-5785
This booklet is a report of the National Study Group on the Implications of Health Care Reform for Americans with Disabilities and Chronic Health Conditions.
30 pages
Lex Frieden, Program Director

10606 OSERS News in Print: Office of Special Education & Rehabilitative Services
US Department of Education
400 Maryland Avenue SW   202-205-8241
Washington, DC 20202-0001   800-872-5327
                                   www.ed.gov

Provides information, research, and resources in the area of special learning needs.
Quarterly
Lex Frieden, Program Director

Audio & Video

10607 Assisting Parents Through the Mourning Process
Hope
5632 Van Nuys Blvd.   818-989-7221
Van Nuys, CA 91401-4648   800-405-8942
                                                Fax: 818-989-7826
Describes the mourning process experienced by some parents of children with disabilities and ways in which the professional can help them through the process.
20 minutes

10608 No Fears, No Tears
Leora Kuttner, PhD, author

Fanlight Productions
32 Court Street   718-488-8900
Brooklyn, NY 11201-1731   800-876-1710
                                                Fax: 718-488-8642
                                                info@fanlight.com
                                                www.fanlight.com
Dr. Leora Kuttner explores the effects of childrens pain management.
1985 28 Minutes

10609 No Fears, No Tears: 13 Years Later
Leora Kuttner, PhD, author

Fanlight Productions
32 Court Street   718-488-8900
Brooklyn, NY 11201-1731   800-876-1710
                                                Fax: 718-488-8642
                                                info@fanlight.com
                                                www.fanlight.com
Dr. Leora Kutner explores the effects of childrens pain management therapies 13 years after their use.
1998 47 Minutes
ISBN: 1-572952-77-6

Web Sites

10610 AbleData
                                                abledata.acl.gov
An information and referral service that uses computer listings and a large file system to answer requests related to assistive devices. Houses a large file system library and contacts with other sources which enables them to answer just about any question.

10611 Access Unlimited
                                          www.accessunlimited.com
Assists educators, health care providers and parents in discovering how personal computers help children and adults with disabilities compensate for some of the barriers imposed by their conditions.

10612 American Academy of Pediatrics
                                                www.aap.org
Committed to the attainment of optimal physical, mental and social health and well-being for all infants, children, adolescents and yound adults.

10613 American Association for the Advancement of Science
                                                www.aaas.org
An international non-profit organization dedicated to advancing science around the world by serving as an educators, leader, spokesperson and professional association.

10614 American Bar Association Commission
                                                www.americanbar.org
The ABA's Commission on the Mentally Disabled was established in 1973 to respond to the advocacy needs of persons with mental disabilities.

10615 American Camp Association
                                                www.acacamps.org

The American Camp Association (formerly known as the American Camping Association) is a community of camp professionals who, for over 100 years, have joined together to share our knowledge and experience and to ensure the quality of camp programs.

10616 American Counseling Association
                                                www.counseling.org
Dedicated to the growth and development of the counseling profession and those who are served.

10617 American Institute for Preventive Medicine
                                                www.healthylife.com
An award winning, internationally recognized authority on the development and implementation of health promotion, wellness, medical self-care and disease management programs and publications.

10618 American Organ Transplant Association
                                                www.aotaonline.org
To help transplant patients lead happy, productinve lives by helping them obtain and sustain transplantation.

10619 American Red Cross
                                                www.redcross.org
In addition to domestic disaster relief, the American Red Cross offers compassionate services in five other areas: community services that help the needy; support and comfort for military members and their families; the collection, processing and distribution of lifesaving blood and blood products; educational programs that promote health and safety; and international relief and development programs.

10620 American Self-Help Group Clearinghouse
A keyword-searchable database of over 1,100 national, international, model and online self-help support groups for addictions, bereavement, health, mental health, disabilities, abuse, parenting, caregiver concerns and many other stressful life situations.

10621 American Society of Dermatology
                                                www.asd.org
A non-partisan professional association of dematologists across the country whose mission is to facilitate optimal dermatologic care being available to all citizens of this country by preserving, promoting and enhancing the private practice of dermatology.

10622 Beach Center on Families and Disability
                                                www.beachcenter.org
Makes a significant and sustainable difference in the quality of life of families and individuals affected by disability and of those who are closely involved with them.

10623 Caring.com
                                                www.caring.com
Online portal for family caregivers who are caring for aging loved ones.

10624 Center for Chronic Disease Prevention and Health Promotion
                                                www.cdc.gov/nccdphp
The forefront of the nation's efforts to prevent and control chronic diseases. Leads efforts that promote health and well-being through prevention and control of chronic diseases.

10625 Center for Developmental Disabilities
                                                www.centerfor.com
Committed to its mission of helping children and adults with differing abilities achieve their dreams by overcoming barriers to living, working, learning and enjoying recreational opportunities in the community of their choice.

10626 ChiroWeb.com
                                                www.chiroweb.com
Chiropractic news source for chiropractors, students, patients and health care professionals. Over 7,000 articles are available.

10627 Commission on Accreditation of Rehabilitation Facilities
                                                www.carf.org
CARF reviews and grants accreditation services nationally and internationally at the request of a facility or program. Standards are applied to service areas and business practices, and accreditation is ongoing in an effort to encourage service providers to continuously improve services. The CARF group also includes CARF Canada and CARF Europe.

10628 Disabled & Alone/Life Services for the Handicapped
www.disabledandalone.org
A non-profit organization established to help families provide a secure future for their loved ones with a disability. Believes that no person should have to live his life in loneliness and isolation because of a disability.

10629 Discovery Health
www.discoverylife.com
A large website covering various health topics; such as male and female health, senior health, children's health, mental health, alternative medicine, nutrition, fitness, and more.

10630 Educational Equity Center at AED
www.edequity.org
EEC at AED is an outgrowth of Educational Equity Concepts, a national not-for-profit organization with a 22-year history of promoting educational excellence for all children.

10631 Healing Well
www.healingwell.com
A social network and support community for patients, caregivers, and families coping with the daily struggles of diseases, disorders and chronic illness.

10632 Health Care For All
www.hcfama.org
HCFA seeks to create a consumer-centered health care system that provides comprehensive, affordable, accessible, culturally competent, high quality care and consumer education for everyone, especially the most vulnerable.

10633 Health Finder
www.healthfinder.gov
A government website that contains information and tools to help you and those you care about stay healthy.

10634 Health on the Net Foundation
www.hon.ch
Promotes and guides the deployment of useful and reliable online health information, and its appropriate and efficient use.

10635 Healthcentral.com
www.healthcentral.com
Empower millions of people to improve and take control of their health and well-being.

10636 Healthlink USA
www.healthlinkusa.com
Discussion forum for treatments, symptoms and causes of 700 health conditions, diseases and topics.

10637 HealthyWomen
www.healthywomen.org
Independent, non-profit organization seeking to educate women in all areas of health, to allow them to make informed choices. The HealthyWomen website features numerous tools and health calculators, plus other media.

10638 Life Development Institute
discoverldi.com
Serving men and women between the ages of 18-30 who have Asperger's Syndrome, ADHD, learning disabilities, anxiety, depression and other disorders

10639 Lotsa Helping Hands
lotsahelpinghands.com
Platform for creating communities that assist in caring for loved ones, intended for caregivers, friends and family, and volunteers.

10640 MedicineNet
www.medicinenet.com
An online resource for consumers providing easy-to-read, authoritative medical and health information.

10641 Medscape
www.medscape.com
Medscape offers specialists, primary care physicians, and other health professionals the Web's most robust and integrated medical information and educational tools.

10642 Medtronic
www.medtronic.com
Medtronic is changing the face of chronic disease. By working closely with physicians around the world, they create therapies to help patients do things they never thought were possible.

10643 National Clearinghouse of Rehabilitation Training Materials
The mission of the NCRTM is to advocate for the advancement of best practice in rehabilitation counseling through the development, collection, dissemination, and utilization of professional knowledge, information and skill.

10644 National Council on Disability
www.ncd.gov
The National Council on Disability is an independent federal agency that works with the President and Congress to increase the inclusion, independence and empowerment of Americans with disabilities.

10645 National Digestive Diseases Information Clearinghouse
www.digestive.niddk.nih.gov
Offers various educational information, resources and reprints focusing on Colitis, Ulcerative Colitis and Crohn's disease.

10646 National Organization for Rare Disorders
www.rarediseases.org
NORD is a federation of voluntary health organizations dedicated to helping people with rare orphan diseases and assisting the organizations that serve them. It is committed to the identification, treatment, and cure of rare disorders through programs of education, advocacy, research, and service. Website features resources for patients and families, patient organizations, and clinicians and researchers.

10647 Next Step in Care
www.nextstepincare.org
Online platform with videos and guides for family caregivers and healthcare providers, as well as other resources. A program of United Hospital Fund.

10648 North American Society for Pediatric Gastroenterology, Hepatology & Nutrition
714 N. Bethlehem Pike   215-641-9800
Ambler, PA 19002   Fax: 215-641-1995
naspghan@naspghan.org
www.naspghan.org
Promotes research and provides a forum for professionals in the areas of pediatric GI liver disease, gastroenterology, and nutrition. Associated with fellow organizations in Europe and Australia (ESPGAN, AUSPGAN).
Margaret K. Stallings, Executive Director
Kim Rose, Associate Director

10649 Office of Special Education and Rehabilitative Services
www2.ed.gov/osers
The Office of Special Education and Rehabilitative Services (OSERS) is committed to improving the results and outcomes for people with disabilities of all ages.

10650 VA Caregiver Support
www.caregiver.va.gov
Tips, tools, and other resources for caregivers of veterans.

10651 WebMD
www.webmd.com
Provides credible information, supportive communities, and in-depth reference material about health subjects. A source for original and timely health information as well as material from well known content providers.

10652 World Institute on Disability
www.wid.org
A public policy center that is run by persons with disabilities. Conducts research, public education, and advocacy campaigns.

National Agencies & Associations

10653 A Kid Again
777-G Dearborn Park Lane   614-797-9500
Columbus, OH 43085   800-543-9735
        Fax: 614-797-9600
        customerservice@akidagain.org
        www.akidagain.org
Enriches the lives of children with life threatening illnesses and their families by providing year round fun-filled group activities and destination events by fostering joy, laughter, normalcy and supportive networking opportunities. Includes regional chapters.
Jeffrey Damron, CFRE, CEO
Kathy Fredericka, COO

10654 A Wish with Wings, Inc.
3751 West Freeway   817-469-9474
Fort Worth, TX 76107   Fax: 817-275-6005
        wish@awishwithwings.org
        www.awishwithwings.org
Grants the wishes of Texas children with life-threatening diseases.
Clarissa Hernandez, Program Manager
Judy Youngs, Executive Director

10655 BASE Camp Children's Cancer Foundation
650 North Wymore Road   407-673-5060
Winter Park, FL 32789-3679   Fax: 407-673-5095
        info@basecamp.org
        www.basecamp.org
Supports children and their families who are facing the challenge of living with cancer or other life-threatening hematological illnesses. Offers year round programs, monthly overnight camps, support groups, and weekly events.
Terri Jones, President/Founder
Cindy Whitaker, Parent & Program Coordinator

10656 Believe In Tomorrow Children's Foundation
6601 Frederick Road   410-744-1984
Baltimore, MD 21228   800-933-5470
        Fax: 410-744-1984
        info@believeintomorrow.org
        www.believeintomorrow.org
Formerly Grant-A-Wish Foundation, this Foundation provides exceptional hospital and retreat housing services to critically ill children and their families. The Foundation also believes that keeping families together during a child's medical crisis, and that the gentle caring environment is crucial.
Brian R Morrison, Founder
Richard E McCready, Chairman

10657 Camp Good Days
1332 Pittsford-Mendon Road   585-624-5555
Mendon, NY 14506   800-785-2135
        Fax: 585-624-5799
        www.campgooddays.org
A non-profit organization that provides a camping experience and more for children and adults facing the toughest challenges of life. Accepts the wishes of terminal ill children through age eighteen.
Gary Mervis, Founder/Chairman
Wendy Bleier-Mervis, Executive Director

10658 Children's Wish Foundation International
8615 Roswell Road   770-393-9474
Atlanta, GA 30350-7526   800-323-9474
        Fax: 770-393-0683
        arthurs@childrenswish.org
        www.childrenswish.org
Committed to bringing joy and happiness to seriously ill children throughout the world and this dedication has created special experiences for children around the globe. Our commitment is also developing hospital enrichment programs.
Linda Dozoretz, Executive Director
Cassie Sheets, Wish Coordinator

10659 Cure Our Children Foundation
711 S Carson Street   310-355-6046
Carson City, NV 89701   Fax: 310-454-9592
        barry@cureourchildren.org
        www.cureourchildren.org
Support medical approaches to treatment of Ewings Sarcoma. Alternate and complimentary treatment information is provided only for use in conjunction with traditional approaches.
Barry Sugarman, President

10660 Dream Come True
PO Box 21167   610-865-3475
Lehigh Valley, PA 18002   Fax: 610-865-4710
        RVasko@aol.com
        www.dreamcometrue.org
Seeks to fulfill the dreams of children ages 4 - 17 who are seriously, chronically and terminally ill and whom live in the Lehigh Valley area. Includes regional offices.
Rayann Vasko, Executive Director
Scott Griesemer, President

10661 Dream Factory, Inc.
National Headquarters
410 W. Chestnut Street   502-561-3001
Louisville, KY 40202   800-456-7556
        Fax: 502-561-3004
        dfinfo@dreamfactoryinc.org
        www.dreamfactoryinc.org
Grants wishes to children and young adults ages 3 - 18 with a critical or chronic illness.
Daniel Forrest, President
Todd Fairbanks, National Director/CEO

10662 Dream Foundation
1528 Chapala Street   805-564-2131
Santa Barbara, CA 93101   888-437-3267
        Fax: 805-564-7002
        www.dreamfoundation.org
Enhances the quality of life for individuals and families battling terminal illnesses ages 18 and over.
Kisa Heyer, CEO
Birgit Gutscher, Chief of Staff

10663 Friends of Karen
118 Titicus Road   914-277-4547
North Salem, NY 10560   info@friendsofkaren.org
        www.friendsofkaren.org
Provides financial, emotional and advocacy support to children with life-threatening illnesses and their families.
Judith Factor, Executive Director
Nancy Mariano, Regional Director

10664 Give Kids the World Village
210 S Bass Road   407-396-1114
Kissimmee, FL 34746   800-995-KIDS
        Fax: 407-396-1207
        dream@gktw.org
        www.gktw.org
An 84-acre non-profit resort in Central Florida that creates magical memories for children with life-threatening illnesses and their families. GKTW provides accommodations at its whimsical resort, donated attractions, tickets, meals and more for a week-long stay.
Pamela Landwirth, President
Tabrei Scott, Chief People Officer

10665 High Hopes Foundation
Everett Executive Suites
12 Murphy Drive   603-966-3483
Nashua, NH 03062   800-639-6804
        Fax: 603-429-0037
        highhopesfoundation.org
Grants wishes for severely and chronically ill children and young adults ages 3-18 who live in New Hampshire.
Jay Welch, President
Cheryl Paquette, Administrative Coordinator

10666 Hopes & Dreams Foundation, Inc.
517 Cedarbrook Road   215-264-2859
Southampton, PA 18966 info@hopesanddreamsfoundation.org
        www.hopesanddreamsfoundation.org
For children and young adults with disabilities such as down syndrome and other specific challenges. Helps to promote education and community involvement through social activities.
Vick Franklin, President

10667 Hopes & Dreams for Children
One Woodland Avenue   201-265-5400
Paramus, NJ 07652   www.hopesanddreamsforchildren.org
Provides funds to support local programs and activities in NJ for
handicapped children and their families.

10668 Kidd's Kids
220 E Las Colinas Boulevard   972-432-8595
Irving, TX 75039   866-541-5437
                                                Fax: 214-853-5212
                                                 www.kiddskids.com
Founded by nationally syndicated morning show personality Kidd
Kraddick. Provides chronically ill and/or physically challenged
children between the ages of 5 to 12 with an unforgettable
adventure.
Caroline Kraddick, Chief Executive Officer
Lyndsay Davis, Director of Operations

10669 Kids Wish Network
4060 Louis Avenue   727-937-3600
Holiday, FL 34691   888-918-9004
                                                Fax: 727-937-3688
                                          info@kidswishnetwork.org
                                          www.kidswishnetwork.org
A nationally recognized charitable organization dedicated to in-
fusing hope creating happy memories and improving the quality of
life for children. The Network also fulfills the wishes of children
ages 3 to 18 with life threatening medical conditions.
David Clevenger, President
Andrew Gottlieb, Treasurer

10670 Magic Moments
2112 11th Ave S   205-638-9372
Birmingham, AL 35205   Fax: 205-939-6717
                                            info@magicmoments.org
                                            www.magicmoments.org
Grants wishes to children 4 to 18 living or being treated in Alabama
who have chronic life-threatening diseases or who have severe
trauma (burn, spinal cord or head trauma).
Sandy Naramore, Executive Director
Amy Cowling, Program Coordinator

10671 Make-A-Wish Foundation of America
4742 N. 24th Street   602-279-9474
Phoenix, AZ 85016-4862   800-722-9474
                                                Fax: 602-279-0855
                                                   mawfa@wish.org
                                                      www.wish.org
A national organization that grants wishes for children with terminally or life threatening diseases and who are 18 years of age or
younger. Includes regional chapters.
David Williams, President/CEO

10672 Marty Lyons Foundation, Inc.
354 Veterans Memorial Highway   631-543-9474
Commack, NY 11725   Fax: 631-543-9479
                                      mac@martylyonsfoundation.org
                                      www.martylyonsfoundation.org
A national organization that grants wishes of children between the
ages of three and seventeen who have life-threatening diseases or
terminal illnesses. Those interested can submit applications for
their wish fulfillment.
Sandra White, Executive Director
Krystal DeWitt Monroy, Program Coordinator

10673 New Hope for Kids Wish Program
544 Mayo Avenue   407-331-3059
Maitland, FL 32751   Fax: 407-331-3063
                                      information@newhopeforkids.org
                                            www.newhopeforkids.org
Grants wishes to children ages 3-18 who have been diagnosed with
a life-threatening illness.
Dave Joswick, Executive Director
Dana Duffie, Office Manager

10674 Rainbow Connection
621 W University   248-601-9474
Rochester, MI 48307   877-649-4743
                                                Fax: 248-601-0086
                                          info@rainbowconnection.org
                                          www.rainbowwishconnection.org
Make the special wishes of children with life-threatening or termi-
nal illnesses come true.
George Miller, Executive Director
Kristen McKelvey, Wish Coordinator & Events Specialist

10675 Special Wish Foundation
1250 Memory Lane   614-258-3186
Columbus, OH 43209   800-486-9474
                                                Fax: 614-258-3518
                                          www.aspecialwishfoundation.org
A Special Wish Foundation Inc. is a non-profit charitable organi-
zation dedicated to granting the wishes of children under the age of
21 who have been diagnosed with a life-threatening disorder.
Laura Marchetta, Contact/Chicago Chapter
Patti Piening, Contact/Cincinnati

10676 Starlight Children's Foundation
400 Corporate Pointe   310-479-1212
Culver City, CA 90230   800-274-7827
                                                  info@starlight.org
                                                    www.starlight.org
A non-profit organization dedicated to brightening the lives of se-
riously ill children and their families.
Chris Helfrich, CEO
Samantha Martinez, Director, Programs

10677 Sunshine Foundation National Headquarters
1041 Mill Creek Drive   215-396-4770
Feasterville, PA 19053   Fax: 215-396-4774
                                        philly@sunshinefoundation.org
                                          www.sunshinefoundation.org
Answers the dreams of seriously ill physically challenged and
abused children aged three to eighteen whose families cannot fulfill their requests due to financial strain that the child's illness may
cause.
Kate Sample, President
Nicci Yu, Director, Program Services

10678 Wish Upon A Star
Visalia, CA 93278   559-733-7753
                                                     800-821-6805
                                                Fax: 559-733-0962
                                            info@wishuponastar.org
                                              www.wishuponastar.org
A non-profit law enforcement effort designed to grant the wishes
of children afflicted with high-risk and life threatening illnesses.
Carmen Perez, Executive Director

10679 Wishing Star Foundation
139 S Sherman   509-744-3411
Spokane, WA 99202   Fax: 509-744-3414
                                                  www.wishingstar.org
Grants wishes to children with life threatening illnesses. Ages
3-21 in Eastern Washington and all of Idaho.
Dan Curley, Executive Director
Veronica Smet, Program Director/Development

10680 Wishing Well Foundation USA, Inc.
PO Box 1554   504-510-5379
Marrero, LA 70073   888-663-9474
                                          wellfoundation52@gmail.com
To bring joy to children with life threatening illnesses by providing
them with their fondest wish in life.
Elwin Lebeau, President

Foundations

10681 Angelwish, Inc.
Rutherford, NJ 07070   201-672-0722
                                                Fax: 201-672-0733
                                                  info@angelwish.org
                                                    www.angelwish.org

Provides the public with an easy way to grant wishes to the millions of children that are living with HIV/AIDS around the world. Infected or affected by the disease, their opportunities for a normal childhood are virtually impossible. By harnessing the power of the Internet, Angelwish helps donors add a ray of hope to their lives.
Shimmy Mehta, Founder/CEO
Tom Fuller, Director

10682 Chef David's Kids
1100 E Oakland Park Boulevard 954-594-1024
Fort Lauderdale, FL 33334 chefdavidmitchell@gmail.com
www.chefdavidskids.com
Helps children afflicted with any form of terminal illness such as cancer, leukemia, and pediatric HIV. Also helps neglected and abused children.
Chef David Mitchell, Founder/Director of Operations
Laurie Amber, National Hospital Events Director

10683 Children's Wish Foundation of Canada
1101 Kingston Rd 905-427-5353
Pickering, L1V 1-7J7 800-267-9474
Fax: 905-427-0536
on@childrenswish.ca
www.childrenswish.ca
Works with the community to provide children living with high risk life threatening illnesses the opportunity to realize their most heartfelt wish.
Chris Kotsopoulos, Director
Jeannette Wakelin, Chair

10684 Dreams Come True
6803 Southpoint Parkway 904-296-3030
Jacksonville, FL 32216 Fax: 904-296-4244
www.dreamscometrue.org
Grants the dreams of children with life-threatening illnesses.
Jeffrey Conn, President
Eddie Allen, Managing Director

10685 Dreams for Seniors Charity Inc
512 Court Street 309-353-7300
Pekin, IL 61554 Fax: 309-353-7311
info@dreamsforseniorscharity.org
www.dreamsforseniorscharity.org
Dreams for Seniors Charity (Dreams for Seniors) is a 501(c)(3) non-profit organization focused on celebrating seniors, granting their wishes and making dreams come true.
Debbie Davison, President/Founder

10686 Jason's Dreams for Kids Foundation, Inc.
20 Monmouth Street 732-758-0060
Red Bank, NJ 07701 Fax: 732-758-0070
jasonsdreams@comcast.net
www.jasonsdreamsforkids.com
Devoted to granting wishes to children diagnosed with life-threatening illnesses. Holds a variety of fundraising events to meet the cost of fulfilling these childrens' wishes.

10687 Little Star Foundation
256 Rancho Milagro Way 800-543-6565
Hesperus, CO 81326 info@littlestar.org
www.littlestar.org
Provides lifetime opportunities for children with cancer to enhance the quality of their lives.
Andrea Jaeger, Co-Founder & President

10688 Starlight Children's Foundation
400 Corporate Pointe 310-479-1212
Culver City, CA 90230 info@starlight.org
www.starlight.org
Helps seriously ill children and their families cope with their pain, fear and isolation through entertainment, education and family activities.
Chris Helfrich, CEO
Samantha Martinez, Director, Programs

10689 Sunshine Dreams for Kids
300 Wellington St 519-642-0990
London, Ontario, N6B 2-5A9 800-461-7935
Fax: 519-642-1201
info@sunshine.ca
www.sunshine.ca
Grants dreams to children who are between the ages of 3 and 19 who are challenged by severe physical disabilities or life threatening illnesses.
Patrick DeMeester, MBA, President
Adam Jean, Treasurer

10690 United Special Sportsman Alliance
7864 Shotwell Lane 715-884-2256
Pittsville, WI 54466 800-518-8019
Fax: 715-884-7388
www.childswish.com
A dream wish granting charity that specializes in sending critically ill and disabled youth on the outdoor adventure of their dreams.
Brigid O'Donoghue, CEO/Founder
Ron Johnson, President

National Agencies & Associations

10691 Children's Hospice International
500 Montgomery Street
703-684-0330
Alexandria, VA 22314
800-24C-HILD
info@chionline.org
www.chionline.org
This organization was founded to provide a network of support and care for children with life threatening conditions and their families. The hospice is a team effort which provides medical, psychological, social and spiritual expertise in the US and abroad.
Ann Armstrong-Dailey, Founding Director/CEO
Rebecca Brant, Director

10692 Compassionate Friends
1000 Jorie Blvd
630-990-0010
Oak Brook, IL 60523
877-969-0010
Fax: 630-990-0246
nationaloffice@compassionatefriends.org
www.compassionatefriends.org
A national organization that gives support to people who have experienced the death of a child. Offers monthly support meetings to get through the difficult times and learn how to cope.
Alan Pedersen, Executive Director
Terry Novy, Chapter Services Coordinator

10693 HOSPICELINK Hospice Education Institute
Hospice Education Institute
3 Unity Square
207-255-8800
Machiasport, ME 04655-0098
800-331-1620
Fax: 207-255-8008
info@hospiceworld.org
Provides educational and informational services to health professionals and the public on subjects such as hospice care, death and dying and bereavement counseling.

10694 Helping Other Parents in Normal Grief
Underwood Memorial Hospital
509 N Broad Street
856-845-0100
Woodbury, NJ 08096
www.umhospital.org
Offers support to newly bereaved parents through trained parents who have suffered a similar loss and resolved their grief.
Eileen K. Cardile, RN, MS, CNA, President/CEO
John Graham, FACHE, Executive Vice President/COO

10695 National Association for Home Care and Hospice
228 7th Street SE
202-547-7424
Washington, DC 20003-4306
Fax: 202-547-3540
hospice@nahc.org
www.nahc.org
Promotes the concepts of hospice, a philosophy of health care which is expressed through the provision of a variety of medical and nonmedical services to terminally ill patients and their families.
Val J. Halamandaris, President
Andrea Devoti, Chair

10696 National Hospice & Palliative Care Organization (NHPCO)
1731 King Street
703-837-1500
Alexandria, VA 22314
800-646-6460
Fax: 703-837-1233
www.nhpco.org
The organization seeks to improve end-of-life care, widen access to hospice care, and improve quality of life for the dying and their loved ones.
Edo Banach, JD, President & CEO
Hannah Yang Moore, MPH, Chief Advocacy Officer

10697 National Institute for Jewish Hospice
732 University Street
516-791-9888
North Woodmere, NY 11581
800-446-4448
Fax: 516-791-6999
www.nijh.org
Serves as a resource center that seeks to help terminal patients and their families deal with their grief by providing information on traditional Jewish views on death, dying and managing the loss of a loved one.
Shirley Lamm, Executive Director
Maurice Lamm, Founder/President

10698 Share Pregnancy and Infant Loss Support, Inc.
The National Share Office
402 Jackson Street
636-947-6164
St. Charles, MO 63301
800-821-6819
Fax: 636-947-7486
info@nationalshare.org
www.nationalshare.org
Serving those whose lives have been touched by the tragic death of a baby through pregnancy loss, stillbirth or the first few months of life.
Cathie Lammert, Executive Director
Rose Carlson, Program Director

Support Groups & Hotlines

10699 Bereavement Group for Children
Corstone Center
250 Camino Alto
415-338-6161
Mill Valley, CA 94941-2535
Fax: 415-338-6165
info@corstone.org
www.corstone.org
The CorStone Center for Personal Resilience (CPR) develops and implements resilience-based interventions and research initiatives to improve the health, education, and self-sufficiency of marginalized adults and youth around the world.
Steve Leventhal, Executive Director
Brenda Rivas-Camarena, Program Coordinator

10700 Grief & Loss Support Group
First Love Outreach Ministries
Milwaukee, WI 53206
414-263-1323
Fax: 414-263-1148
zelodius@aol.com

Pr Zelodius Morton, CEO

10701 National Hospice Helpline
1731 King Street
703-837-1500
Alexandria, VA 22314
800-646-6460
Fax: 703-837-1233
nhpco_info@nhpco.org
www.nhpco.org
Offers more information on hospice in general and offers referrals to a hospice program in your area.
J. Donald Schumacher, President & CEO
Galen Miller, Executive VP

10702 Rainbows for All God's Children
1360 Hamilton Parkway
847-952-1770
Itasca, IL 60143
800-266-3206
Fax: 847-952-1774
info@rainbows.org
www.rainbows.org
A support program for children who have suffered a significant loss in their lives due to death, divorce or any other painful transition.
Bob Thomas, Executive Director
Laurie Olbrisch, Executive VP

Books

10703 A Good Death: Conversations with East Londoners
Lesley Cullen and Michael Young, author
Routledge
8th Floor, 711 3rd Avenue
212-216-7800
New York, NY 10016
800-634-7064
Fax: 212-564-7854
orders@taylorandfrancis.com
www.routledge.com
Based on a survey in East London and provides a wide range of fascinating and helpful insights into all aspects of experiencing death and surviving grief. The voices in the book are those of people who have managed to cope despite being under the shadow of impending death. Their experience could be a comfort to anybody in a similar situation. A Good Death is intended for people who are dying, and for student doctors, nurses, and social workers.
272 pages
ISBN: 0-415137-97-3

10704 Anatomy of Bereavement
Beverly Raphael, author
Rowman & Littlefield Publishers, Inc.
15200 NBN Way   717-794-3800
Blue Ridge Summit, PA 17214   800-462-6420
                                       Fax: 717-794-3803
                                       orders@rowman.com
                                       customercare@rowman.com
In this comprehensive book, Dr. Raphael describes all the stages of mourning and healing.
454 pages Softcover
ISBN: 1-568212-70-4

10705 Bereaved Children: A Support Guide for for Parents And Professionals
Earl A. Grollman, author
Beacon Press
24 Farnsworth Street   617-742-2110
Boston, MA 02210-2824   Fax: 617-723-3097
                                       www.beacon.org
Comprehensive guide that helps children and teens cope with the loss of a loved one.
256 pages
ISBN: 0-807023-07-5

10706 Bereaved Parent
Harriet Sarnoff Schiff, author
Penguin USA
375 Hudson Street   212-366-2372
New York, NY 10014   800-847-5515
                                       Fax: 212-366-2933
                                       insidesales@us.penguingroup.com
                                       www.penguingroup.com
Supportive advice for bereaved parents and professionals who work with them.
146 pages
ISBN: 0-140050-43-4

10707 Concerning Death: A Practical Guide for the Living
Earl A. Grollman, author
Beacon Press
24 Farnsworth Street   617-742-2110
Boston, MA 02210-2824   Fax: 617-723-3097
                                       www.beacon.org
A guide for people to learn how to cope with death and dying, and the many decisions involved in the process.
265 pages
ISBN: 0-807027-65-0

10708 Conversations At Midnight
William Morrow & Company/Order Department
39 Plymouth Street   973-227-7200
Fairfield, NJ 07004-1633   800-821-1513
Herbert Kramer is dying of cancer. For him, as for everyone someday, death is now an unavoidable companion. This book tells how Herb learns to acknowledge this presence and come to terms with human mortality. This book is a powerful way to look at death and to deal with losing a loved one.
256 pages Hardcover
ISBN: 0-688120-84-9

10709 Death and the Quest for Meaning
Stephen Strack & Herman Feifel, author
Rowman & Littlefield Publishers, Inc.
4501 Forbes Blvd.   301-459-3366
Lanham, MD 20706   800-462-6420
                                       Fax: 301-429-5748
                                       rowman.com
This work covers all aspects of the study of death and dying and the care of the bereaved.
Hardcover
ISBN: 0-765700-14-x
Stephen Strack, Co-Editor
Herman Feifel, Co-Editor

10710 Death: The Final Stage of Growth
Elisabeth Kubler-Ross, author
Simon & Schuster

1230 Ave of the Americas   212-698-7000
New York, NY 10020   www.simonandschuster.com
This books shows readers how to come to terms with death as a part of human development, and how death can provide us with a key meaning of human existence.
208 pages

10711 Difference in the Family
Penguin Putnam
PO Box 999   201-387-0600
Bergenfield, NJ 07621-0903   800-526-0275
                                       Fax: 800-227-9604
A frank chronicle of the grief, rage and guilt everyone in a family suffers after a death, and the adjustments each make to cope.
Helen Featherstone, Editor

10712 Dying and Disabled Children
Haworth Press
10 Alice Street   607-722-5857
Binghamton, NY 13904-1580   800-429-6784
                                       Fax: 607-722-0012
                                       www.haworthpress.com
In this sensitive and compassionate look at terminally ill and disabled children, professionals from the medical community examine the stresses faced by their parents and siblings. They address crucial element of communication in dealing with a child's serious illness. Ethical decision making, learning to recognize the child's suffering, and talking to children about death are honestly and clearly discussed.
153 pages Hardcover
ISBN: 0-866567-59-0

10713 For Those Who Live: Helping Children Cope with Death of a Brother or Sister
Centering Corporation
7230 Maple Street   402-553-1200
Omaha, NE 68134   866-218-0101
                                       Fax: 402-553-0507
                                       danni@centeringcorp.com
                                       www.centering.org
Deals with the grieving family as a whole and offers references for further help.
122 pages
Kathy LaTour, Editor

10714 Grief, Dying and Death: Clinical Intervention for Caregivers
Research Press
2612 N Mattis Avenue   217-352-3273
Champaign, IL 61822-1053   800-519-2707
                                       Fax: 217-352-1221
                                       rp@researchpress.com
                                       www.researchpress.com
In this comprehensive manual, the author provides both the theoretical background and the practical treatment interventions necessary for working with those who are bereaved or dying. Important topics such as anticipatory grief, postdeath mourning and the stress of grief are described in detail. Grief reactions, both normal and abnormal, as well as their causes are analyzed. Special attention is given to grief caused by death of a child or spouse, death by suicide, and children's grief.
488 pages Softcover
ISBN: 0-878222-32-4
Therese A. Rando, Author

10715 Helper's Journey
Dr. Dale G. Larson, author
Research Press
2612 N Mattis Avenue   217-352-3273
Champaign, IL 61822   800-519-2707
                                       Fax: 217-352-1221
                                       orders@researchpress.com
                                       www.researchpress.com
This groundbreaking work, written for both professional and volunteer caregivers, provides exercises, activities and specific strategies for more successful caregiving, increased personal growth and effective stress management. In this thoughtfully written book, Dr. Larson explores the theory and practice of helping. He includes numerous case examples and verbatim disclosures of fel-

low caregivers that powerfully convey the joys and sorrows of the helpers journey.
292 pages Softcover
ISBN: 0-878223-44-4
Dale G. Larson, Author

10716 On Death & Dying
Dr. Elizabeth Kubler-Ross, author
MacMillan Publishing Company
175 Fifth Avenue   646-307-5151
New York, NY 10010   customerservice@mpsvirginia.com
                                          www.macmillan.com
Offers a new perspective on the terminally ill by refocusing on the patient as a human being and teacher, in hopes of learning from him or her about the final stages of life.
277 pages Paperback
Elisabeth Kubler-Ross, Author

10717 On Death and Dying
MacMillan Publishing Company
175 Fifth Avenue   646-307-5151
New York, NY 10010
A wonderful book offering information on how to deal and cope with death and dying.
Paperback

10718 Recovery from Bereavement
Rowman & Littlefield Publishers, Inc.
4501 Forbes Blvd.   301-459-3366
Lanham, MD 20706   800-462-6420
                                          Fax: 301-429-5748
                                          orders@rowman.com
                                          www.rowmanlittlefield.com
Outstanding authorities on loss and bereavement discuss the factors that play a role in successful recovery.
344 pages Softcover
ISBN: 1-568213-61-1

10719 Talking About Death - A Dialog Between Parent and Child
Earl A. Grollman, author
Beacon Press
24 Farnsworth Street   617-742-2110
Boston, MA 02210-2824   Fax: 617-723-3097
                              bp_information@beacon.org
                                          www.beacon.org
A compassionate guide for children and adults. Also includes listings of resources and organizations.
128 pages

10720 Treatment of Complicated Mourning
Dr. Therese A. Rando, author
Research Press
2612 N Mattis Avenue   217-352-3273
Champaign, IL 61822   800-519-2707
                                          Fax: 217-352-1221
                                          orders@researchpress.com
                                          www.researchpress.com
This is the first book to focus specifically on complicated mourning, often referred to as pathological, unresolved, or abnormal grief. It provides caregivers with practical therapeutic strategies with and specific interventions that are necessary when traditional grief counseling is insufficient. The author provides critically important information on the prediction, identification, assessment, classification and treatment of complicated mourning.
768 pages Hardcover
ISBN: 0-878223-29-0
Therese A. Rando, Author

10721 What Helped Me When My Loved One Died
Beacon Press
24 Farnsworth Street   617-742-2110
Boston, MA 02210-2824   Fax: 617-723-3097
                                          www.beacon.org

Children's Books

10722 Aarvy Aardvark Finds Hope
Donna O'Toole, author
Centering Corporation
7230 Maple Street   402-553-1200
Omaha, NE 68134   866-218-0101
                                          Fax: 402-553-0507
                                          www.centering.org
A best selling, illustrated, read-aloud story of the pain and sadness of loss and the hope of grief recovery.
80 pages Paperback
Donna O'Toole, Author

10723 Badger's Parting Gifts
Susan Varley, author
Compassion Books, Inc.
7036 State Highway 80 S   828-675-5909
Burnsville, NC 28714-7569   800-970-4220
                                          Fax: 828-675-9687
                              orders@compassionbooks.com
                                          www.compassionbooks.com
A story of the death of old Badger. As the animals talk about Badger they remember the gift of skills and kindnesses he taught them.
23 pages Paperback
Susan Varley, Author

10724 Compassion Books, Inc.
7036 State Highway 80 S   828-675-5909
Burnsville, NC 28714-7569   800-970-4220
                                          Fax: 828-675-9687
                              orders@compassionbooks.com
                                          www.compassionbooks.com
Hand picked resources to help people through loss, grief and changes of all kinds. Carry over 400 books and videos on death and dying, bereavement and change, comfort and healing, hope and much more.
Bruce Greene, VP

10725 Fire in My Heart: Ice in My Veins
Enid Samuel Traisman, author
Compassion Books, Inc.
7036 State Highway 80 S   828-675-5909
Burnsville, NC 28714-7569   800-970-4220
                                          Fax: 828-675-9687
                              orders@compassionbooks.com
                                          www.compassionbooks.com
A fill in scrapbook/journal to help teenagers experiencing a loss express feelings, sort out their thoughts and gather memories.
70 pages Paperback
Enid Samuel Traisman, Author

10726 Gentle Willow: A Story for Children About Dying
Joyce C. Mills, PhD, author
Magination Press (American Psychological Assoc.)
750 First Street NE   202-336-5500
Washington, DC 20002-4242   800-374-2721
                                          TTY: 202-336-6123
                                          TDD: 202-336-6123
                                          order@apa.org
                                          www.apa.org
This book is written for children who may not survive their own illness or for children who know them. This tender and touching tale helps address feelings of disbelief, anger, and sadness, along with love and compassion.
2003 32 pages Hardcover
ISBN: 1-591470-71-7
Joyce C. Mills, PhD, Author
Cary Pillo, Illustration

10727 Great Change
Compassion Books, Inc.
7036 State Highway 80 S   828-675-5909
Burnsville, NC 28714-7569   800-970-4220
                                          Fax: 828-675-9687
                              orders@compassionbooks.com
                                          www.compassionbooks.com

In this deeply moving Native American story, grandmother uses nature to explain death, the great change, to a grieving granddaughter.
32 pages Hardcover
Bruce Greene, Director

10728 Let's Talk About When A Parent Dies
Rosen Publishing Group's PowerKids Press
29 E 21st Street — 212-777-3017
New York, NY 10010 — 800-237-9932
Fax: 888-436-4643
customerservice@rosenpub.com
www.rosenpublishing.com
This book guides children through the grieving process in a language they can understand. Recommended for grades K-4.
ISBN: 0-823923-09-6
Elizabeth Weitzman, Author

10729 Nana Upstairs and Nana Downstairs
Compassion Books
7036 State Highway 80 S — 828-675-5909
Burnsville, NC 28714-7569 — 800-970-4220
Fax: 828-675-9687
orders@compassionbooks.com
www.compassionbooks.com
This charming picture book recognizes that even after a family member dies the love connections continue in heart and home.
32 pages Paperback
Bruce Greene, Director

Magazines

10730 Compassion Books Catalog
Compassion Books
7036 State Highway 80 S — 828-675-5909
Burnsville, NC 28714-7569 — 800-970-4220
Fax: 828-675-9687
orders@compassionbooks.com
www.compassionbooks.com
More than 400 books and videos to help with serious illness, death and dying, and losses of all kinds.
32 pages
Bruce Greene, VP

Pamphlets

10731 Approaching Grief
Richard Deitrick/Ann Armstrong Dailey, author
Children's Hospice International
500 Montgomery Street — 703-684-0330
Alexandria, VA 22314 — 800-242-4453
info@chionline.org
www.chionline.org
Delves into the different stages of grief, guilt, depression, fear and anger. Also tells how children approach grief and ways in which to help your children get past the sorrow.
Ann Armstrong-Dailey, Founding Director/CEO
Rebecca Brant, Director

10732 Pregnancy After a Loss
Abbott Northwestern Hospital Parent Education
800 E 28th Strt — 612-863-4000
Minneapolis, MN 55407
This booklet is written by a group of parents that have experienced a pregnancy after a loss, sensitively written with suggestions for coping with the fears and anxieties of the new pregnancy.

10733 Pregnancy Heartbreak: Unfulfilled Promises
Abbott Northwestern Hospital Parent Education
800 E 28th Strt — 612-863-4000
Minneapolis, MN 55407
This handbook is written for parents who had to face the reality of the diagnosis and birth of a baby with life-threatening conditions.

Audio & Video

10734 Encounters with Grief
Fanlight Productions
C/O Icarus Films — 718-488-8900
Brooklyn, NY 11201 — 800-876-1710
Fax: 718-488-8642
info@fanlight.com
www.fanlight.com
A mother who lost her teenage son, a woman widowed in her sixties and a man whose wife died at fifty-two discuss the emotional upheaval that followed and their moving perspectives on the process of recovery.
1992 13 Minutes
ISBN: 1-572950-91-9

10735 Grave Words: Tools for Discussing End of Life Choices
Maren Monson, MD, author
Fanlight Productions
C/O Icarus Films — 718-488-8900
Brooklyn, NY 11201 — 800-876-1710
Fax: 718-488-8642
info@fanlight.com
www.fanlight.com
Blends humor, music and insightful interviews to confront the issues that arise in discussions between physicians and healthcare providers and patients about end-of-life care decisions.
1996 25 Minutes
ISBN: 1-572952-24-5
Maren Monsen, MD, Author

10736 Pitch of Grief
Eric Strange, author
Fanlight Productions
C/O Icarus Films — 718-488-8900
Brooklyn, NY 11201 — 800-876-1710
Fax: 718-488-8642
info@fanlight.com
www.fanlight.com
Explores the process of grieving through interviews with four bereaved men and women, and is helpful to not only the grieving person, but for others within the family who have faced the loss of a loved one.
1985 28 Minutes
ISBN: 1-572950-18-8
Eric Stange, Author

10737 There Was a Child
Fred Simon, author
Fanlight Productions
C/O Icarus Film — 718-488-8900
Brooklyn, NY 11201 — 800-876-1710
Fax: 718-488-8642
info@fanlight.com
www.fanlight.com
Demonstrates the impact that losing a pregnancy, or the birth of a stillborn child, has had on three mothers and a father. Validates the emotions of parents who feel alone with their loss, while helping health care workers and families to give appropriate, meaningful support.
1991 32 Minutes
ISBN: 1-572950-48-X
Fred Simon, Author

10738 We Will Remember
Compassion Books, Inc.
7036 State Highway 80 S — 828-675-5909
Burnsville, NC 28714-7569 — 800-970-4220
Fax: 828-675-9687
orders@compassionbooks.com
www.compassionbooks.com
A video meditation that uses the beauty of natural photography, soothing music and gentle words to give permission and encouragement in using the memories of the past for healing in the present.
11 minutes
James Miller, Author

10739 When the Bough Breaks
Fanlight Productions
32 Court Street
Brooklyn, NY 11201-1731

718-488-8900
800-876-1710
Fax: 718-488-8642
info@fanlight.com
www.fanlight.com

Based on the real story of a patient who experienced a stillbirth, these ten vignettes dramatically recreate her interactions with health care providers during the final weeks of pregnancy. Study guide included.
1992 71 Minutes
ISBN: 1-572951-08-7

Web Sites

10740 Compassionate Friends

www.compassionatefriends.org

Gives support to people who have experienced the death of a child.

10741 Hospice Association of America

www.nahc.org

Promotes the concepts of hospice, a philosophy of health care which is expressed through the provision of a variety of medical and nonmedical services to terminally ill patients and their families.

10742 National Hospice & Palliative Care Organization (NHPCO)

www.nhpco.org

The organization seeks to improve end-of-life care, widen access to hospice care, and improve quality of life for the dying and their loved ones. NHPCO's website offers information on regulations, advocacy, quality and performance, education, and a variety of other resources.

10743 Share Pregnancy and Infant Loss Support, Inc.

www.nationalshare.org

Offers studies, information, statistics, help and support to parents who have suffered the loss of a child.

A

AA and the Armed Services, 8476
AA and the Gay/Lesbian Alcoholic, 8477
AA as a Resource for Health Care Professionals, 8478
AA Comes of Age, 8249
AA for the Native North American, 8479
AA for the Woman, 8480
AA in Correctional Facilities, 8481
AA in Prison: Inmate to Inmate, 8250
AA in Treatment Facilities, 8482
AA Member: Medications and Other Drugs, 8474
AA Service Manual: Twelve Concepts for World
  Service, 8475
AA: Rap with Us, 8657
AAA Foundation for Traffic Safety, 8105, 8673
AAAD Bulletin, 4724
AABA Newsletter, 3768
AABA Support Group, 3710
AAGL - Elevating Gynecologic Surgery, 3789
aakpRENALIFE, 5683
AAO-HNS Foundation, 4360
Aaron Diamond AIDS Research Center, 412
AARP Alabama, 43
AARP Alaska, 44
AARP Arizona, 45
AARP Arkansas, 46
AARP Bulletin, 193
AARP California: Pasadena, 47
AARP California: Sacramento, 48
AARP Colorado, 49
AARP Connecticut, 50
AARP Delaware, 51
AARP Florida: Doral, 53
AARP Florida: St. Petersburg, 54
AARP Florida: Tallahassee, 55
AARP Foundation, 108
AARP Georgia, 57
AARP Hawaii, 58
AARP Idaho, 59
AARP Illinois: Chicago, 60
AARP Illinois: Springfield, 61
AARP Indiana, 63
AARP Iowa, 64
AARP Kansas, 65
AARP Kentucky, 66
AARP Louisiana: Baton Rouge, 67
AARP Louisiana: New Orleans, 68
AARP Magazine, 188
AARP Maine, 69
AARP Maryland, 70
AARP Massachusetts, 71
AARP Michigan, 72
AARP Minnesota, 73
AARP Mississippi, 74
AARP Missouri, 75
AARP Montana, 76
AARP Nebraska: Lincoln, 77
AARP Nebraska: Omaha, 78
AARP Nevada, 79
AARP New Hampshire, 80
AARP New Jersey, 81
AARP New Mexico, 82
AARP New York: Albany, 83
AARP New York: New York City, 84
AARP New York: Rochester, 85
AARP North Carolina, 86
AARP North Dakota, 87
AARP Ohio, 88
AARP Oklahoma, 89
AARP Oregon, 90
AARP Pennsylvania: Harrisburg, 91
AARP Pennsylvania: Philadelphia, 92
AARP Rhode Island, 93
AARP South Carolina, 94
AARP South Dakota, 95
AARP Tennessee, 96
AARP Texas: Austin, 97
AARP Texas: Dallas, 98
AARP Texas: Houston, 99
AARP Texas: San Antonio, 100
AARP Utah, 101
AARP Vermont, 102
AARP Virginia, 103
AARP Washington, 104

AARP Washington DC, 52
AARP West Virginia, 105
AARP Wisconsin, 106
AARP Wyoming, 107
Aarvy Aardvark Finds Hope, 10722
ABA Commission on Law and Aging, 22
Abby & the South Seas Adventure Series, 6532
ABC of AIDS, 455
ABC of ZZZs, 7820
ABC's of Finger Spelling, 4641
ABC's of Pediatric Inflammatory Bowel Disease,
  3058
ABCD: After Breast Cancer Diagnosis, 2088
AbleData, 4285, 4830, 10335, 10610
Abnormal Uterine Bleeding, 5508
About Asthma, 1447
About Children's Vision: Guide for Parents, 9957
About Head Injuries, 4221
About Headaches, 6308
About High Blood Pressure, 4940
About Hydrocephalus: A Book for Families, 5219
About Kidney Stones, 5688
About Kids GI Disorders, 3711
About Normal Pressure Hydrocephalus: A Book for
  Adults & Their Families, 5220
About Overeaters Anonymous, 6738
Abramson Cancer Center of the University of
  Pennsylvania, 2363
Abstracts in Social Gerontology, 189
Academic Acceptance of ASL, 4423
Academy for Eating Disorders, 3667, 3706
Academy for Gerontology in Higher Education, 23,
  113
Academy of Doctors of Audiology, 4286
Academy of Nutrition & Dietetics, 625, 728, 2625,
  2652, 3668, 3774, 3915, 3990
Academy of Rehabilitative Audiology, 4287
ACAP Recap, 8463
ACB Government Employees, 10051
ACB Radio Amateurs, 10052
ACB Reports, 9916
ACB Social Service Providers, 10053
Acceptance, 8483
Accepting Ourselves & Others, 8251
Access for All: Integrating Deaf, Hard of Hearing and
  Hearing Preschoolers, 4424
Access to Mass Transit for Blind & Visually Impaired
  Travelers, 9827
Access Unlimited, 10336, 10611
Access World: Technology and People with Visual
  Impairments, 9903
ACDS Infant, Toddler & Pre-school Curriculum for
  Children, 3604
Aces Too High, 7142
ACG Institute for Clinical Research and Education,
  3939
Achondroplasia, 4058
Ackerman Institute for the Family, 2337
ACLU National Prison Project, 10334
ACMH Newsletter, 6155
Acne, 7696
ACPA Facilitator Guide & Materials, 2920
ACPA Family Manual, 2921
ACPA Family Services, 1850
ACPA Journal Reflections of You, 2922
ACPA Relaxation Tapes, 2932
ACPA Video: 10 Steps from Patient to Person, 2933
ACSM's Exercise Management for Persons with
  Chronic Disease & Disabilities, 2923
Act Against AIDS, 249
Action Autonomie, 5903
Active Healthy Kids Canada, 6708
Activities for Developing Pre-Skill Concepts In
  Children with Autism, 1731
Activities for the Disabled, Elderly and Adults, 154
Acute Intermittent Porphyria, 3976
ADA and People with MS, 6460
ADA Clinical Education Series on CD-Rom, 3515
Adam and the Magic Marble, 9094
Adaptation to the Initial Crisis, 3642
ADARA Updated, 4725
ADD Stepping Out of the Dark, 1645
Addiction and Responsibility, 8252
Addictions Counseling, 8253
Addictive Personality, 8254

Addictive Thinking Understanding Self-Deception,
  8255
Addison News, 11
ADHD, 1640
ADHD in Adults, 1646
ADHD in Schools: Assessment and Intervention
  Strategies, 1615
ADHD in the Classroom: Strategies for Teachers,
  1647
ADHD Parenting Handbook: Practical Advice for
  Parents from Parents, 1614
ADHD Report, 1636
ADHD: Handbook for Diagnosis & Treatment, 1616
ADHD: What Do We Know?, 1648
Adjustment, Adaptation and Accomodation:
  Psychological Approaches, 6947
Administration for Children and Families, 1370,
  3536, 3669, 4288, 5728, 7031, 7462
Administration for Community Living, 7059
Adolescent Idiopathic Scoliosis: Prevelance, Natural
  History, Treatments, 7414
Adolescents with Closed Head Injuries: A Report of
  Initial Cognitive Deficits, 4222
Adopt the Baby You Want, 5443
Adopt-A-Special-Kid America, 5558
Adopting After Infertility: The Decision, the
  Commitment, the Experience, 5444
Adoption, 5509
Adoption Directory, 5445
Adoption Fact Book, 5446
Adoption Resource Book, 5447
ADPA Professional, 8468
Adriene Resource Center for Blind Children, 9712
Adult Bible Lessons for the Deaf, 4727
Adult Bible Study, 10026
Adult Children and Aging Parents, 155
Adult Children of Alcoholics, 8256
Adult Children of Alcoholics Newcomer Packet, 8484
Adult Congenital Heart Association, 2946
Adult Down Syndrome Center of Lutheran General
  Hospital, 3575
Adult Research Opportunities, 367
Adult Scoliosis Surgery...It Can Be Done, 7403
Advance, 1441
Advance Directives: A Guide for Patients and Their
  Families, 5689
Advance: for Directors in Rehabilitation, 10586
Advanced Cancer: Living Each Day, 2498
Advances in Cardiac and Pulmonary Rehabilitation,
  4924
Advances: Progress in Alzheimer Research and Care,
  1033
Adventures of Maxx, 5079
Adverse Reactions to Foods, 696
Advice From Your Allergist, 693
Advice to Parents of Children with HBV, 5161
Advocacy Center, 10453
Advocate, 6156, 9239
Advocates 4 Health: Tick-borne Disease Self-Help
  Group, 9031
AdvocateWeb, 7143
AEGIS AIDS Education Global Information System,
  438
AER Report, 9917
AFB Directory of Services for Blind/Vis. Impaired
  Persons in the US & Canada, 9825
AFB News, 9918
AFB Technology & Employment Center, 9598
AFB Toll-Free Hotline, 9810
Affiliated Children's Arthritis Centers of New
  England, 1240
Affirmation Tape, 2934
Affording Your Infertility, 5510
African American Family Services, 8106
African American Post Traumatic Stress Disorder
  Association, 7032
African Americans in Treatment, 8485
African-Americans and Stroke, 5276, 8081
After Breast Cancer: A Guide to Followup Care, 2499
After School...Then What? The Transition to
  Adulthood, 1877
After the Diagnosis...the Next Steps, 9135
AfterTheInjury.org, 7144
Age and Fertility, 5511
Age Related Macular Degeneration, 9958

Agency for Healthcare Research and Quality, 626, 1371, 3537, 3670, 4289, 5729, 7033, 7463
Agency for Healthcare: Research Facility, 4269
Agency for Toxic Substances and Disease Registry, 627, 1372, 4290, 5730, 7034, 7464
Agent Orange and Birth Defects, 1878, 10286
Agent Orange and Chloracme, 10287
Agent Orange and Hodgkin's Disease, 10288
Agent Orange and Mutiple Myeloma, 10289
Agent Orange and Non-Hodgkin's Lymphoma, 10290
Agent Orange and Peripheral Neuropathy, 10291
Agent Orange and Porphyria Cutanea Tarda, 10292
Agent Orange and Prostate Cancer, 10293
Agent Orange and Respiratory Cancers, 10294
Agent Orange and Soft Tissue Sarcomas, 10295
Agent Orange and Spina Bifida, 10296
Agent Orange Anxiety: The Human Response to Possable Oncogenicity and Mutagencity, 10284
Agent Orange Briefs, 10282
Agent Orange Fact Sheet: A Historical Perspective, 10285
Agent Orange Registry Department of Veterans Affairs, 10100
Agent Orange Review, 10283
Agent Orange Videotapes, 10308
Agent Orange: It is Part of Your Life, 10297
Aging and Alzheimer's Disease Center Newsletter, 1034
Aging and Alzheimer's Disease Center Oregon Health Sciences University, 948
Aging and Family Therapy, 156
Aging and Hearing Loss: Some Commonly Asked Questions, 4750
Aging and Our Families, 157
Aging and Vision News, 9919
Aging and Vision: Declarations of Independence, 10027
Aging In America, 109
Agromedicine Program Medical University of South Carolina, 7666
AHEPAN Magazine, 2979
Aid to the Aged, Blind or Disabled, 9493
AIDS & HIV Related Diseases, 456
AIDS & Other Manifestations of HIV Infection, 457
AIDS Alabama, 439
AIDS Alert, 458, 511, 524
AIDS and Hemophilia: Protecting Yourself and Others, 572
AIDS and HIV Related Diseases, 459
AIDS and Persons with Developmental Disabilities, 460
AIDS Awareness Library, 496
AIDS Clinical Care, 512
AIDS Clinical Trials Unit CARES Clinic, 366
AIDS Coalition of Cape Breton, 239
AIDS Committee of Durham Region, 240
AIDS Committee of North Bay & Area, 241
AIDS Committee of Ottawa, 242
AIDS Committee of Toronto, 243
AIDS Committee of York Region, 244
AIDS Education and Training Center National Multicultural Center, 605
AIDS Healthcare Foundation, 350
AIDS Hotline of Central New York, 440
AIDS in the Twenty-First Century: Disease and Globalization, 461
AIDS Library of Philadelphia, 361
AIDS Link, 525
AIDS Medicines in Development, 571
AIDS New Brunswick, 245
AIDS News, 526
AIDS Outreach Center (AOC), 338
AIDS Overview Series, 495
AIDS Policy and Law, 527
AIDS Resource Center of Wisconsin, 347
AIDS School Health Education Database Centers for Disease Control, 390
AIDS Support Group of Cape Cod, 441
AIDS To the Point: Confronting Youth Issues, 497
AIDS Treatment Data Network, 528
AIDS Treatment News, 529
AIDS United, 246, 606
AIDS Update, 530
AIDS Weekly Plus, 531

AIDS Work: Six Healthcare Workers Face the AIDS Crisis, 600
AIDS, Revised Edition, 462
AIDS, the Law & You, 573
AIDS...What We Need To Know Pamphlet, 7583
AIDS.ORG, 607
AIDS/STD News Report, 532
AIDS: A Communication Perspective, 463
AIDS: A Year In Review, 513
AIDS: Distinguishing Between Fact and Opinion, 464
AIDS: How it Works in the Body, 465, 498
AIDS: International Monthly Journal, 514
AIDS: The Disease State Management Resource, 515
AIDS: Trading Fears for Facts a Guide for Teens, 499
AIDS: Trading Fears for Facts: A Guide for Young People, 466
AIDS: Trading Fears for Facts: A Guide for Young People, 500
AIDSinfo, 247, 442
AIDSVu, 608
AJAO Newsletter, 1283
AJMR, 6148
Akathisia in Parkinson's Disease, 6948
Al-Anon, 8674
Al-Anon Alateen Family Group Hotline, 8239
Al-Anon Family Group Headquarters, 8107
Al-Anon Family Groups, 8257
Al-Anon is for African Americans...and All People of Color, 8659
Al-Anon is for Men, 8488
Al-Anon Newcomers Packet, 8486
Al-Anon Spoken Here, 8487
Al-Anon Video, 8658
Al-Anon's Path to Recovery: Al-Anon is for Americans/Aboriginals, 8660
Al-Anon's Twelve Steps and Twelve Traditions, 8258
Al-Anon, You and the Alcoholic, 8489
Alabama Ambassador: National Ataxia Foundation, 1523
Alabama Chapter of the American Association of Kidney Patients, 5581
Alabama Chapter of the Arthritis Foundation, 1192
Alabama Chapter of the Myasthenia Gravis Foundation of America, 6634
Alabama Council of the Blind, 9463
Alabama Department of Public Health, 284
Alabama Education of Homeless Children and Youth Program, 6048
Alabama Head Injury Foundation, 4082
Alabama Head Injury Foundation Helpline, 4145
Alabama Institute for Deaf and Blind, 4337
Alabama Organ Center, 9175
Alabama Radio Reading Service Network, 9607
Alabama Regional Library for the Blind and Physically Handicapped, 9608
Alaska Department of Health and Social Services: HIV/STD Program, 285
Alaska State Library Talking Book Center, 9613
Alaska VA Healthcare System, 10108
Alaskan Statewide AIDS Helpline, 443
Alateen, 8675
Alateen Newcomer Packet, 8490
Alateen Talk, 8491
Alateen: A Day at a Time, 8259
Alateen: Hope for Children of Alcoholics, 8260
Albany Library for the Blind and Physically Handicapped, 9644
Albany Medical College Joint Center for Cancer and Blood Disorders, 2338
Albany Medical College Pediatric Pulmonary & Cystic Fibrosis Center, 3144
Albany Medican Center, 5013
Albany Stratton VA Medical Center, 10197
Albert Einstein Cancer Center Albert Einstein College of Medicine, 2339
Albert Einstein Medical Center Hemophilia Program, 5014
Alberta Reappraising AIDS Society, 250
Alcohol & Drug Abuse Programs of Wyoming Department Of Health, 8194
Alcohol Alert #11: Estimating the Cost of Alcohol Abuse, 8492
Alcohol Alert #15: Alcohol and AIDS, 8493
Alcohol Alert #16: Moderate Drinking, 8494

Alcohol Alert #17: Treatment Outcome Research, 8495
Alcohol Alert #18: The Genetics of Alcoholism, 8496
Alcohol Alert #21: Alcohol and Cancer, 8497
Alcohol Alert #23: Alcohol and Minorities, 8498
Alcohol Alert #24: Animal Models in Alcohol Research, 8499
Alcohol Alert #25: Alcohol-Related Impairment, 8500
Alcohol Alert #26: Alcohol and Hormones, 8501
Alcohol Alert #27: Alcohol Medication Interactions, 8502
Alcohol and Drug Abuse Bureau: Department of Human Resources, 8170
Alcohol and Drug Abuse Division Department of Health, 8149
Alcohol and Drug Abuse Division Department of Human Services, 8143
Alcohol and Drug Abuse in Black America: A Guide for Community Action, 8503
Alcohol and Drug Abuse Program Department Of Children And Families, 8147
Alcohol and Drug Abuse Programs of Vermont Department Of Health, 8189
Alcohol and Drug Abuse Section, 8176
Alcohol and Drug Abuse Services, 8156
Alcohol and Drug Services Addictive Diseases Program, 8148
Alcohol and Other Drug Services: Dir. of California's Community Services, 8261
Alcohol and Pregnancy, 8504
Alcohol and the Liver: Myth vs. Facts, 5784
Alcohol Disease Foundation, 8197
Alcohol Drug Treatment Referral, 8240
Alcohol Research Group Public Health Institute, 8198
Alcohol, Drug and Other Addictions: A Directory of Treatment Centers, 8262
Alcohol, Tobacco and Other Drugs May Harm the Unborn, 8263
Alcoholics Anonymous, 8108, 8264
Alcoholics Anonymous and Employee Assistance Program, 8505
Alcoholics Anonymous World Services, 8241
Alcoholics Anonymous: An Inside View, 8661
Alcoholics Anonymous: The Big Book, 8265
Alcoholism, 8407
Alcoholism and Drug Abuse: Office of Community Behavioral Health, 8139
Alcoholism and the Family, 8408
Alcoholism Tends to Run in Families, 8506
Alcoholism: A Merry-Go-Round Named Denial, 8507
Alcoholism: The Family Disease, 8508
ALDA News, 4726
Aleda E. Lutz VA Medical Center: Saginaw, Michigan, 10172
ALEH Israel Foundation, 3573, 3657
ALEH Rehabilitation of Canada, 3574
Alert, 1569
Alerting and Communication Devices for Deaf and Hard of Hearing People, 4751
Alex: The Life of a Child, 3196
Alexander Graham Bell Association, 4831
Alexander Graham Bell's Life, 4752
Alexander, the Elephant Who Couldn't Eat Peanuts, 719
Alexandria VA Healthcare System, 10160
Alive and Kicking, 9386
All About Allergies, 686
All About Asthma, 1424
All About Fibromyalgia, 3871
All About the New Generation of Hearing Aids, 4753
All Access Mental Health, 5985
All Ages Support Group, 1959
Allegheny Singer Research Institute West Penn Allegheny Health System, 2364
Allergic Contact Rashes, 7697
Allergic Diseases, 697
Allergic Rhinitis, 720
Allergic Rhinitis: Nothing to Sneeze At!, 721
Allergic Skin Reactions, 722, 7736
Allergies, 687
Allergies A to Z, 673
Allergies and You, 698, 1448
Allergies to Animals, 699
Allergy & Asthma, 1449

Allergy & Asthma ADVOCATE Newsletter, 1442
Allergy & Asthma Network, 628, 729, 1373, 1505
Allergy & Asthma Today, 689, 1438
Allergy Alerts from Living with Allergies, 674
Allergy Plants that Cause Sneezing and Wheezing, 675
Alliance Brochure, 1578
Alliance for Aging Research, 215, 9405
Alliance for Lupus Research, 8927
Alliance for the Mentally Ill in Delaware (AMID), 5940
Alliance of Genetic Support Groups, 3847, 4063, 5213
Allies with Families, 6080
Alphabet of Animal Signs, 4642
Alphapointe Association for the Blind, 9523
ALS Association Free Standing Support Groups, 1149
ALS Association National Office, 1088
ALS Association: Alabama Chapter, 1091
ALS Association: Arizona Chapter, 1092
ALS Association: Arkansas Chapter, 1093
ALS Association: Central & Southern Ohio Chapter, 1121
ALS Association: Connecticut Chapter, 1101
ALS Association: East Michigan Chapter, 1111
ALS Association: Evergreen Chapter, 1133
ALS Association: Florida Chapter, 1103
ALS Association: Georgia Chapter, 1104
ALS Association: Golden West Chapter, 1094
ALS Association: Golden West Chapter - Greater Los Angeles Office, 1095
ALS Association: Golden West-Greater Bay, 1096
ALS Association: Greater Houston Office, 1129
ALS Association: Greater New York Chapter, 1119
ALS Association: Greater Philadelphia Chapter, 1124
ALS Association: Greater Sacramento Chapte r, 1097
ALS Association: Greater San Diego Chapter, 1098
ALS Association: Indiana Chapter, 1106
ALS Association: Kentucky Chapter, 1109
ALS Association: Massachusetts Chapter, 1110
ALS Association: Mid America Chapter Centr al Kansas Office, 1108
ALS Association: Mid America Chapter Kansas City Metro Area, 1107
ALS Association: Mid America Chapter- Southern Missouri Office, 1114
ALS Association: MidAmerica Chapter - Nebr aska Office, 1116
ALS Association: Minnesota, South Dakota, North Dakota Chapter, 1113, 1127
ALS Association: National Capital Area Chapter, 1102
ALS Association: New Mexico Chapter, 1118
ALS Association: Northern New England Chapter, 1117
ALS Association: Northern Ohio Chapter, 1122
ALS Association: Orange County Chapter, 1099
ALS Association: Oregon & SW Washington Chapter, 1123, 1134
ALS Association: Rocky Mountain Chapter, 1100
ALS Association: South Carolina Chapter, 1126
ALS Association: South Texas Chapter, 1130
ALS Association: Southeast Wisconsin Chapter, 1135
ALS Association: St. Louis Regional Chapter, 1115
ALS Association: Tennessee Chapter, 1128
ALS Association: Texas Chapter - Austin, 1131
ALS Association: Texas Chapter- Dallas, 1132
ALS Association: Upstate New York Chapter, 1120
ALS Association: West Michigan Chapter, 1112
ALS Association: Western Pennsylvania Chapter, 1125
ALS Center at UCSF, 1136
ALS Clinic at Penn Neurological Institute ALS Association Greater Philadelphia Cha, 1137
ALS Clinical Department of Neurology, 1138
ALS News & Views, 1168
ALS Today, 1162
Alta Bates Summit Medical Center, 6026
Alternative Medicine and Multiple Sclerosis, 6441
Alternatives for Women with Endometriosis Guide by Women for Women, 3808
Alvin C. York VA Medical Center Tennessee Valley Healthcare System, 10238
Alzheimer Disease and Associated Disorders, 1035

Alzheimer Disease and Associated Disorders: An International Journal, 1030
Alzheimer Early Stages, 988
Alzheimer Research Forum, 1075
Alzheimer Society of Alberta and Northwest Territories, 743
Alzheimer Society of B.C., 744
Alzheimer Society of Canada, 745
Alzheimer Society of Manitoba, 746
Alzheimer Society of New Brunswick, 747
Alzheimer Society of Newfoundland & Labrador, 748
Alzheimer Society of Nova Scotia, 749
Alzheimer Society of Ontario, 750
Alzheimer Society of Prince Edward Island, 751
Alzheimer Society of Saskatchewan, 752
Alzheimer Support, 1076
Alzheimer's & Related Dementias Education & Referral Center, 753
Alzheimer's Alliance: Texarkana Area, 910
Alzheimer's Arkansas Programs and Services, 768
Alzheimer's Association, 754, 1077
Alzheimer's Association Autopsy Assistance Network, 984
Alzheimer's Association Caregiver Resources, 1068
Alzheimer's Association Dementia Care Conference, 1069
Alzheimer's Association of Vermont and New Hampshire, 861
Alzheimer's Association Safe Return Police Training Video, 1070
Alzheimer's Association San Diego/Imperial Chapter, 770
Alzheimer's Association: Atlanta Chapter, 802
Alzheimer's Association: Augusta Chapter, 803
Alzheimer's Association: Big Sioux Chapter, 822
Alzheimer's Association: Broward County Chapter, 789
Alzheimer's Association: California Central Chapter: Ventura County Office, 771
Alzheimer's Association: Canton Chapter, 879
Alzheimer's Association: Capital of Texas Chapter, 911
Alzheimer's Association: Cascade/Coast Chapter, 890
Alzheimer's Association: Central Georgia Chapter, 804
Alzheimer's Association: Central Illinois Chapter, 813
Alzheimer's Association: Central Indiana Chapter, 820
Alzheimer's Association: Central Maryland Chapter, 836
Alzheimer's Association: Central New York Chapter, 866
Alzheimer's Association: Central Ohio Chapter, 880
Alzheimer's Association: Central Virginia Chapter, 925
Alzheimer's Association: Clark/Champaign, Miami Valley Chapter, 881
Alzheimer's Association: Cleveland Area Chapter, 882
Alzheimer's Association: Columbia-Willamet Chapter, 889
Alzheimer's Association: Connecticut Chapter, 785
Alzheimer's Association: Delaware Chapter, 787
Alzheimer's Association: Delaware Valley Chapter, 893
Alzheimer's Association: Desert Southwest Chapter, 763
Alzheimer's Association: East Central Florida Chapter, 790
Alzheimer's Association: East Central Illinois Chapter, 814
Alzheimer's Association: East Central Iowa Chapter, 823
Alzheimer's Association: East Central Michigan Chapter, 841
Alzheimer's Association: Eastern North Carolina Chapter, 876
Alzheimer's Association: Eastern Shore Chapter, 837
Alzheimer's Association: Eastern Tennessee Chapter, 904
Alzheimer's Association: El Paso Chapter, 912
Alzheimer's Association: Fargo/Moorhead Regional Center, 878

Alzheimer's Association: Florida Gulf Coast Chapter, 791
Alzheimer's Association: Four Rivers Chapter, 815
Alzheimer's Association: Great Plains Chap ter, 856
Alzheimer's Association: Greater Beaumont Area Chapter, 913
Alzheimer's Association: Greater Billings Area Chapter, 855
Alzheimer's Association: Greater Cincinnati Chapter, 883
Alzheimer's Association: Greater Columbus Chapter, 805
Alzheimer's Association: Greater Dallas Chapter, 914
Alzheimer's Association: Greater East Ohio Chapter: Greater Youngstown Office, 884
Alzheimer's Association: Greater East Texas Chapter, 915
Alzheimer's Association: Greater Georgia Chapter, 806
Alzheimer's Association: Greater Grand Junction Area Chapter, 782
Alzheimer's Association: Greater Idaho Chapter, 811
Alzheimer's Association: Greater Illinois Chapter, 816
Alzheimer's Association: Greater Illinois Chapter: Carbondale Office, 817
Alzheimer's Association: Greater Iowa Chapter, 824
Alzheimer's Association: Greater Miami Chapter, 792
Alzheimer's Association: Greater Michigan Chapter, 842
Alzheimer's Association: Greater Michigan Chapter: Upper Peninsula Region, 843
Alzheimer's Association: Greater Mid-Ohio, 895
Alzheimer's Association: Greater Mid-Ohio Valley Chapter, 934
Alzheimer's Association: Greater New Jersey Chapter, 862
Alzheimer's Association: Greater New Orleans Chapter, 832
Alzheimer's Association: Greater North Valley Chapter, 773
Alzheimer's Association: Greater Orlando Area Chapter, 793
Alzheimer's Association: Greater Palm Beach Area Chapter, 794
Alzheimer's Association: Greater Pennsylvania Chapter: SW Regional Office, 894
Alzheimer's Association: Greater Richmond Chapter, 926
Alzheimer's Association: Greater Sacramento, 772
Alzheimer's Association: Greater Washington DC Chapter, 788
Alzheimer's Association: Greater Wichita Falls Chapter, 916
Alzheimer's Association: Greater Wisconsin Chapter, 937
Alzheimer's Association: Heart of America Chapter, 827
Alzheimer's Association: Heart of Iowa Chapter, 825
Alzheimer's Association: Highland Rim Chapter, 905
Alzheimer's Association: Honolulu Chapter, 809
Alzheimer's Association: Houston and Southeast Texas Chapter, 917
Alzheimer's Association: Hudson Valley/ Rockland/Westchester NY Chapter, 867
Alzheimer's Association: Indianhead Chapter, 938
Alzheimer's Association: Inland Northwest Chapter, 932
Alzheimer's Association: Lake Superior Chapter, 939
Alzheimer's Association: Land of Lincoln Chapter, 818
Alzheimer's Association: Laurel Mountains Chapter, 896
Alzheimer's Association: Lexington/ Bluegrass Chapter, 829
Alzheimer's Association: Lincoln/Greater Nebraska Chapter, 857
Alzheimer's Association: Long Island Chapter, 868
Alzheimer's Association: Los Angeles Chapter, 774
Alzheimer's Association: Louisville Chapter, 830
Alzheimer's Association: Low Country Chapter, 901
Alzheimer's Association: Maine Chapter, 834
Alzheimer's Association: Mary's Peak Chapter, 891
Alzheimer's Association: Massachusetts Chapter, 839
Alzheimer's Association: Memphis Area Office, 906

Alzheimer's Association: Miami Valley Chapter, 885
Alzheimer's Association: Michigan Great Lakes Chapter: West Shore Region, 844
Alzheimer's Association: Mid-Michigan Chapter, 845
Alzheimer's Association: Mid-Missouri Chapter, 851
Alzheimer's Association: Mid-State South Carolina Chapter, 902
Alzheimer's Association: Mid-Willamette Chapter, 892
Alzheimer's Association: Middle Tennessee Chapter, 907
Alzheimer's Association: Midstate Wisconsin Chapter, 940
Alzheimer's Association: Minnesota/Dakotas, 848
Alzheimer's Association: Mississippi Chapter, 849
Alzheimer's Association: Monterey County Chapter, 775
Alzheimer's Association: N Central West Virginia Chapter, 935
Alzheimer's Association: National Capital Area Chapter, 927
Alzheimer's Association: New Mexico Chapter, 864
Alzheimer's Association: New York City Chapter, 869
Alzheimer's Association: North Alabama Chapter, 759
Alzheimer's Association: North Bay Chapter, 776
Alzheimer's Association: North Central Wisconsin Chapter, 941
Alzheimer's Association: Northeast Florida, 795
Alzheimer's Association: Northeast Michigan Chapter, 846
Alzheimer's Association: Northeast Pennsylvania Chapter, 897
Alzheimer's Association: Northeast Tennessee Chapter, 908
Alzheimer's Association: Northeast Texas Chapter, 918
Alzheimer's Association: Northeast Wisconsin Chapter, 942
Alzheimer's Association: Northeast/Central Louisiana Chapter, 831
Alzheimer's Association: Northeastern New York Chapter, 870
Alzheimer's Association: Northern Arizona, 764
Alzheimer's Association: Northern Central Florida Chapter, 796
Alzheimer's Association: Northern Idaho Chapter, 812
Alzheimer's Association: Northern Indiana Chapter, 821
Alzheimer's Association: Northern Nevada, 765
Alzheimer's Association: Northern Nevada Chapter, 859
Alzheimer's Association: Northwest Florida Chapter, 797
Alzheimer's Association: Northwest Michigan Chapter, 847
Alzheimer's Association: Northwest Missouri-Chapter, 852
Alzheimer's Association: Northwest Ohio Chapter, 886
Alzheimer's Association: Northwest Pennsylvania Chapter, 898
Alzheimer's Association: Oklahoma Chapter, 888
Alzheimer's Association: Omaha/Eastern Nebraska Chapter, 858
Alzheimer's Association: Orange County Chapter, 777
Alzheimer's Association: Piedmont-Valley Area Chapter, 928
Alzheimer's Association: Putnam County Chapter, 871
Alzheimer's Association: Rhode Island Chapter, 900
Alzheimer's Association: Rio Grande Valley Region, 919
Alzheimer's Association: Riverside/San Bernardino Counties Chapter, 778
Alzheimer's Association: Roanoke Salem Chapter, 929
Alzheimer's Association: Rochester Chapter, 872
Alzheimer's Association: Rocky Mountain Chapter, 783
Alzheimer's Association: San Francisco Bay Area Chapter, 779

Alzheimer's Association: Santa Barbara Central Coast Chapter, 780
Alzheimer's Association: Santa Cruz County Chapter, 781
Alzheimer's Association: South Central Connecticut Chapter, 786
Alzheimer's Association: South Central Pennsylvania Chapter, 899
Alzheimer's Association: South Central Texas, 921
Alzheimer's Association: South Central Wisconsin Chapter, 943
Alzheimer's Association: South Jersey Chapter, 863
Alzheimer's Association: South West Virginia Chapter, 936
Alzheimer's Association: Southeast Alabama Chapter, 760
Alzheimer's Association: Southeast Georgia Chapter, 807
Alzheimer's Association: Southeast Tennessee Chapter, 909
Alzheimer's Association: Southeast Wisconsin Chapter, 944
Alzheimer's Association: Southeastern Virginia Chapter, 930
Alzheimer's Association: Southern Arizona, 766
Alzheimer's Association: Southern Arizona Region, 767
Alzheimer's Association: Southern Nevada Chapter, 860
Alzheimer's Association: Southern Tier Chapter, 873
Alzheimer's Association: Southside Virginia Chapter, 931
Alzheimer's Association: Southwest Alabama Chapter, 761
Alzheimer's Association: Southwest Florida Chapter, 798
Alzheimer's Association: Southwest Georgia Chapter, 808
Alzheimer's Association: Southwest Missouri Chapter, 853
Alzheimer's Association: St. Louis Chapter, 854
Alzheimer's Association: STAR Chapter, Midland Region, 920
Alzheimer's Association: Sullivan/Delaware Chapter, 865
Alzheimer's Association: Sunflower Chapter, 828
Alzheimer's Association: Tampa Bay Chapter, 799
Alzheimer's Association: Tarrant County Chapter, 922, 1036
Alzheimer's Association: Upstate South Carolina Chapter, 903
Alzheimer's Association: Utah Chapter, 923
Alzheimer's Association: Vermont Chapter, 924
Alzheimer's Association: Volusia/Flagler Branch, 800
Alzheimer's Association: Waves of Stone Video and Documentary, 1071
Alzheimer's Association: West Central Florida Chapter, 801
Alzheimer's Association: West Central Ohio Chapter, 887
Alzheimer's Association: West Hawaii Chapter, 810
Alzheimer's Association: Western & Central Washington Chapter, 933
Alzheimer's Association: Western Arkansas Chapter, 769
Alzheimer's Association: Western Maryland Chapter, 838
Alzheimer's Association: Western New York Chapter, 874
Alzheimer's Association: Western North Car olina Chapter, 877
Alzheimer's Association: Western Regional Office: Massachusetts Chapter, 840
Alzheimer's Disease, 989, 1039
Alzheimer's Disease and Down Syndrome, 3634
Alzheimer's Disease Center Emory University/VA Medical Center, 949
Alzheimer's Disease Center Kentucky University, 950
Alzheimer's Disease Center Mayo Clinic Mayo Medical School, 951
Alzheimer's Disease Center Pennsylvania University School of Medicine, 952
Alzheimer's Disease Center: Boston University, 953
Alzheimer's Disease Center: Johns Hopkins University School of Medicine, 954

Alzheimer's Disease Center: University of Alabama at Birmingham, 956
Alzheimer's Disease Center: University of California, Davis, 955
Alzheimer's Disease Center: Washington University, 957
Alzheimer's Disease International, 1078
Alzheimer's Disease Orientation Kit, 990
Alzheimer's Disease Research Center Duke University, 959
Alzheimer's Disease Research Center Washington University School of Medicine, 958
Alzheimer's Disease Resource Agency of Alaska, 762
Alzheimer's Disease: A Guide to Federal Programs, 991
Alzheimer's Disease: Activity-Focused Care, 992
Alzheimer's Disease: Advances in Neurology, 993
Alzheimer's Disease: Questions and Answers, 994
Alzheimer's Disease: The Basics, 1040
Alzheimer's Disease: Thesaurus, 995
Alzheimer's Disease: Treatment and Family Stress: Directions for Research, 996
Alzheimer's Foundation of Staten Island, 875
Alzheimer's Foundation of the South: Mississippi Division, 850
Alzheimer's Services of the Capital Area, 833
Alzheimer's Support Group, 985
Alzheimer's Wyoming, 945
Alzheimer's, Stroke and 29 Other Neurological Disorders Sourcebook, 997, 8067
Alzheimer/Parkinson Association of Indian River County, 6882
AMC Cancer Research Center, 2287
America's Doctor Online Consulting, 9063
America's War on Drugs, 8409
American Academy for Cerebral Palsy and Developmental Medicine, 2665, 2811
American Academy of Allergy, Asthma & Immunology, 629, 653, 730, 1374, 1396, 1506
American Academy of Audiology, 4291, 4832
American Academy of Audiology Foundation, 4361
American Academy of Child and Adolescent Psychiatry (AACAP), 5904, 7035
American Academy of Dermatology, 2586, 7657, 7744
American Academy of Environmental Medicine, 630
American Academy of Neurology, 6286, 6325
American Academy of Neurology: Tourette Syndrome, 9078, 9155
American Academy of Ophthalmology, 9406
American Academy of Orthopaedic Surgeons, 2604, 7396
American Academy of Otolaryngology - Head and Neck Surgery, 4292, 4833
American Academy of Pediatrics, 10337, 10612
American Academy of Psychiatrists in Alcoholism and Addiction Directory, 8266
American Academy of Sleep Medicine, 2822
American Action Fund for Blind Children and Adults, 9686
American Annals of the Deaf, 4701
American Anorexia Bulimia Association of Philadelphia, 3699
American Anorexia Bulimia Association: New Jersey Chapter, 3695
American Association for Chronic Fatigue Syndrome, 2895
American Association for Pediatric Ophthalmology And Strabismus, 6570
American Association for Respiratory Care, 5810
American Association for the Advancement of Science, 10338, 10613
American Association for the Study of Liver Diseases, 5731, 5778, 5800
American Association of Caregiving Youth, 146
American Association of Clinical Endocrinologists, 6805
American Association of Diabetes Educators, 3208, 3524
American Association of Endocrine Surgeons, 2
American Association of Kidney Patients, 5577, 5597, 5718
American Association of Kidney Patients: Piney Woods Chapter, 5650

American Association of Kidney Patients: Tulsa Chapter, 5638

American Association of Neurological Surgeons, 7451

American Association of Neuromuscular & Electrodiagnostic Medicine, 1089, 6571, 7008

American Association of People with Disabilities, 10339

American Association of Retired Persons, 24, 216

American Association of Spinal Cord Injury Nurses, 7953, 8031

American Association of the Deaf-Blind, 4293, 9407

American Association on Intellectual and Developmental Disabilities, 5905

American Auditory Society, 4294

American Autoimmune Related Diseases Association, 251, 4859, 8851, 10340

American Bar Association Commission, 10614

American Bar Association Commission on Mental and Physical Disability Law, 10341

American Blind Lawyers Association, 10054

American Brain Tumor Association, 1901, 1963, 2078, 4075, 4155, 4270

American Camp Association, 10342, 10615

American Cancer Society, 2089, 2587

American Cancer Society Cancer Book, 2419

American Cancer Society Santa Clara County / Silicon Valley / Central Coast Region, 2122

American Cancer Society's Guide to Complementary/Alternative Cancer Methods, 2420

American Cancer Society's Guide to Pain Control, 2421

American Cancer Society's Healthy Eating Cookbook: A Celebration of Food..., 2422

American Cancer Society: Alabama, 2114

American Cancer Society: Alaska, 2116

American Cancer Society: Arizona, 2117

American Cancer Society: Arkansas, 2120

American Cancer Society: Boston, 2180

American Cancer Society: Central Los Angeles, 2123

American Cancer Society: Central New England Region-Weston MA, 2181

American Cancer Society: Central New York Region/East Syracuse, 2203

American Cancer Society: Colorado, 2145

American Cancer Society: Connecticut, 2146

American Cancer Society: Delaware, 2149

American Cancer Society: District of Columbia, 2151

American Cancer Society: Duluth, 2183

American Cancer Society: East Bay/Metro Region, 2124

American Cancer Society: Florida, 2154

American Cancer Society: Fresno/Madera Counties, 2125

American Cancer Society: Georgia, 2160

American Cancer Society: Harrisburg Capital Area Unit, 2228

American Cancer Society: Hawaii, 2163

American Cancer Society: Idaho, 2164

American Cancer Society: Illinois, 2165

American Cancer Society: Indiana, 2167

American Cancer Society: Inland Empire, 2126

American Cancer Society: Iowa, 2169

American Cancer Society: Jackson, 2188

American Cancer Society: Kansas City, 2171

American Cancer Society: Kentucky, 2174

American Cancer Society: Long Island, 2204

American Cancer Society: Louisiana, 2176

American Cancer Society: Maine, 2177

American Cancer Society: Maryland, 2178

American Cancer Society: Mendota Heights Mendota Heights, 2184

American Cancer Society: Montana, 2191

American Cancer Society: Nebraska, 2192

American Cancer Society: Nevada, 2194

American Cancer Society: New Hampshire Gail Singer Memorial Building, 2195

American Cancer Society: New Jersey, 2197

American Cancer Society: New Mexico, 2201

American Cancer Society: New York City, 2205

American Cancer Society: North Carolina, 2216

American Cancer Society: North Dakota, 2219

American Cancer Society: Ohio, 2220

American Cancer Society: Oklahoma, 2224

American Cancer Society: Orange County, 2127

American Cancer Society: Oregon, 2226

American Cancer Society: Philadelphia, 2229

American Cancer Society: Pittsburgh, 2230

American Cancer Society: Queens Region / Rego Park, 2206

American Cancer Society: Rhode Island, 2234

American Cancer Society: Rochester, 2185

American Cancer Society: Sacramento County, 2128

American Cancer Society: Saint Cloud, 2186

American Cancer Society: Saint Louis, 2190

American Cancer Society: San Diego County, 2129

American Cancer Society: San Francisco County, 2130

American Cancer Society: San Jose Prostate Cancer Support Group, 2388

American Cancer Society: Santa Maria Valley, 2131

American Cancer Society: Sonoma County, 2132

American Cancer Society: South Carolina, 2236

American Cancer Society: South Dakota, 2239

American Cancer Society: Tennessee, 2240

American Cancer Society: Texas, 2242

American Cancer Society: Utah, 2246

American Cancer Society: Vermont, 2247

American Cancer Society: Virginia, 2248

American Cancer Society: Washington, 2251

American Cancer Society: West Virginia, 2253

American Cancer Society: Westchester Region/White Plains, 2207

American Cancer Society: Wisconsin, 2254

American Cancer Society: Wyoming, 2256

American Celiac Society, 2626, 2653

American Childhood Cancer Organization, 2090

American Chronic Pain Association, 252, 1186, 1518, 2091, 2605, 2666, 2823, 2908, 2993, 3790, 3859, 4076, 6191, 6287, 6806, 6854, 7009, 7036, 7222, 7233

American Civil Liberties Union LGBT & AIDS Project, 253

American Cleft Palate - Craniofacial Association, 1824

American College of Allergy, Asthma & Immunology, 631, 654, 731, 1375, 1397, 1507

American College of Gastroenterology, 3916, 3991

American Council for Drug Education, 8676

American Council for Headache Education (ACHE), 6326

American Council of Blind Lions, 10055

American Council of the Blind, 9408, 10056

American Council on Addiction & Alcohol Problems, 8110

American Counseling Association, 6192, 10343, 10616

American Deaf Culture, 4425

American Deaf Culture: An Anthology, 4426

American Deafness and Rehabilitation Association, 4295

American Dental Association, 8111

American Diabetes Association, 3209, 3407, 3525

American Diabetes Association: Alabama, 3213

American Diabetes Association: Alaska, 3215

American Diabetes Association: Arizona, 3216

American Diabetes Association: Arizona, Border Area, 3217

American Diabetes Association: Arkansas, 3221

American Diabetes Association: Atlanta Met, 3218

American Diabetes Association: Atlanta Met ro, 3251

American Diabetes Association: Boston, 3277

American Diabetes Association: California, 3223

American Diabetes Association: Cedar Rapid s District, 3263

American Diabetes Association: Connecticut, 3234

American Diabetes Association: Delaware, 3238

American Diabetes Association: Denver, 3231

American Diabetes Association: District of Columbia, 3240

American Diabetes Association: Greater Ill inois, 3256

American Diabetes Association: Hawaii, 3254

American Diabetes Association: Kansas, 3266

American Diabetes Association: Kentucky, 3267

American Diabetes Association: Louisana, 3269

American Diabetes Association: Maine, 3273

American Diabetes Association: Maryland, 3275

American Diabetes Association: Michigan, 3279

American Diabetes Association: Minnesota, 3282

American Diabetes Association: Mississippi, 3284

American Diabetes Association: Missouri, 3285

American Diabetes Association: Montana, 3287

American Diabetes Association: Nashville, 3316, 3341

American Diabetes Association: Nebraska, 3288

American Diabetes Association: Nevada, 3291

American Diabetes Association: New Hampshire, 3294

American Diabetes Association: New Jersey, 3296

American Diabetes Association: New Mexico, 3301

American Diabetes Association: New York, 3303

American Diabetes Association: North Carolina, 3312

American Diabetes Association: North Dakota, 3317

American Diabetes Association: Northeast F lorida/Southeast Georgia, 3242

American Diabetes Association: Northern Arizona, 3219

American Diabetes Association: Northern Il linois, 3257

American Diabetes Association: Northern In diana/Northern Ohio, 3259

American Diabetes Association: Ohio, 3318

American Diabetes Association: Oklahoma, 3324

American Diabetes Association: Oregon, 3327

American Diabetes Association: Pennsylvania, 3329

American Diabetes Association: Rhode Island, 3336

American Diabetes Association: Richmond, 3353

American Diabetes Association: Savannah, 3252

American Diabetes Association: Seattle, 3243, 3356

American Diabetes Association: South Carolina, 3337

American Diabetes Association: South Coast Regional/Central Florida, 3244

American Diabetes Association: Tennessee, 3342

American Diabetes Association: Texas, 3345

American Diabetes Association: Utah, 3351

American Diabetes Association: Vermont, 3352

American Diabetes Association: Virginia, 3354

American Diabetes Association: Washington, 3357

American Diabetes Association: West Virginia, 3361

American Diabetes Association: Western Pennsylvania, 3330

American Diabetes Association: Wisconsin, 3363

American Epilepsy Society, 7465, 7558

American Federation for Aging Research, 110

American Fibromyalgia Research Association, 3902

American Fibromyalgia Syndrome Association, 2824, 3860

American Foundation for AIDS Research, 351

American Foundation for Children with AIDS, 352

American Foundation for Surgery of the Hand, 2609

American Foundation for The Blind, 10344

American Foundation for the Blind, 9409, 9579, 10057

American Foundation for Urologic Disease, 5320, 5365

American Foundation for Urologic Disease: Us Too Line, 2389

American Gastroenterological Association, 3992, 9380

American Gastroenterological Association National Office, 3917

American GI Forum NVOP, 10271

American Head and Neck Society, 4077

American Headache Society, 6288, 6327

American Hearing Research Foundation, 4362

American Heart Association, 4860, 4950, 8046, 8094

American Heart Association Diet, 4941

American Heart Association News, 4936

American Hellenic Educational Progressive Association, 2956

American Hemochromatosis Society, 3918, 3993

American Homes for the Aging: Midwest Regional Office, 819

American Homes for the Aging: Western, 784

American Institute for Cancer Research, 2152, 2390

American Institute for Preventive Medicine, 10346, 10617

American Institute for Preventive Medicine, 10345

American Institutes for Research Center on Aging, 114

American Issue, 8464

American Journal of Audiology, 4702

American Journal of Clinical Oncology: Cancer Clinical Trials, 2478

American Journal of Gastroenterology, 3950
American Journal of Gastrointestinal Surgery, 3951
American Journal of Hypertension, 5271
American Journal of Psychiatry, 6149
American Journal of Speech-Language Pathology, 4703
American Juvenile Arthritis Organization, 1187, 1360, 8852
American Kidney Fund, 5578, 5719
American Kidney Fund Helps When Nobody Else Will, 5690
American Liver Foundation, 5732, 10323
American Liver Foundation Arizona Chapter, 5744
American Liver Foundation Delaware Valley Chapter, 5760
American Liver Foundation Greater Kansas City Chapter, 5757
American Liver Foundation Greater Los Angeles Chapter, 5745
American Liver Foundation Greater New York Chapter, 5758
American Liver Foundation Gulf Coast Chapter, 5750
American Liver Foundation Illinois Chapter, 5751
American Liver Foundation Indiana Chapter, 5752
American Liver Foundation Michigan Chapter, 5755
American Liver Foundation Midsouth Chapter, 5762
American Liver Foundation Minnesota Chapte r, 5756
American Liver Foundation Northern CA Chapter, 5746
American Liver Foundation Pacific Northwest Chapter, 5764
American Liver Foundation Rocky Mountain Division, 5748
American Liver Foundation San Diego Chapte r, 5747
American Liver Foundation Western New York Chapter, 5759
American Liver Foundation Western Pennsylv ania, 5761
American Liver Foundation Wisconsin Chapter, 5765
American Liver Foundation: Connecticut Chapter, 5749
American Liver Foundation: Progress Newsletter, 5154
American Lung Association, 1376, 1508, 5811, 5892, 9257, 9318
American Lung Association Family Guide to Asthma and Allergies, 5876
American Lung Association HelpLine, 5873
American Lung Association of Alabama, 5817, 9262
American Lung Association of Alaska, 5818, 9263
American Lung Association of Arizona, 5819
American Lung Association of Arkansas, 5820, 9266
American Lung Association of California, 5821, 9267
American Lung Association of Colorado, 5822, 9268
American Lung Association of Connecticut, 5823, 9269
American Lung Association of Delaware, 5824, 9270
American Lung Association of Eastern Missouri, 5843
American Lung Association of Florida, 5826, 9273
American Lung Association of Georgia, 5827, 9274
American Lung Association of Hawaii, 5828, 9275
American Lung Association of Idaho, 5829
American Lung Association of Idaho/Nevada, 9290
American Lung Association of Illinois, 5830
American Lung Association of Illinois-Iowa, 9276
American Lung Association of Indiana, 5831
American Lung Association of Indiana: State Office & Support Office, 9277
American Lung Association of Iowa, 5832
American Lung Association of Kansas, 5833, 9278
American Lung Association of Kentucky, 5834, 9279
American Lung Association of Louisiana, 5835, 9280
American Lung Association of Maine, 5836, 9281
American Lung Association of Maryland, 5837, 9282
American Lung Association of Massachusetts, 5838, 9283
American Lung Association of Michigan, 5839, 9284
American Lung Association of Mid New York, 9294
American Lung Association of Minnesota, 5840, 9285
American Lung Association of Mississippi, 5841, 9286
American Lung Association of Missouri, 5842, 9287
American Lung Association of Nebraska, 5846, 9289

American Lung Association of Nevada, 5847
American Lung Association of New Hampshire, 9291
American Lung Association of New Hampshire, 5848
American Lung Association of New Jersey, 5849, 9292
American Lung Association of New Mexico, 5850
American Lung Association of New York State, 5851
American Lung Association of North Carolina, 5852, 9295
American Lung Association of North Dakota, 5853, 9296
American Lung Association of Northern Rockies, 5845
American Lung Association of Ohio, 5854, 9297
American Lung Association of Oklahoma, 5855, 9298
American Lung Association of Oregon, 5856, 9299
American Lung Association of Pennsylvania, 9300
American Lung Association of Rhode Island, 5859
American Lung Association of South Carolina, 5860, 9301
American Lung Association of South Dakota, 5861, 9302
American Lung Association of Tennesse, 9303
American Lung Association of Tennessee, 5862
American Lung Association of Texas, 5863, 9304
American Lung Association of the District of Columbia, 5825, 9272
American Lung Association of the Northern Rockies: Montana and Wyoming, 9288
American Lung Association of Utah, 5864, 9305
American Lung Association of Vermont, 9306
American Lung Association of Virginia, 5865, 9307
American Lung Association of Washington, 5866, 9271
American Lung Association of West Virginia, 5867, 9308
American Lung Association of Wisconsin, 5868, 9309
American Lung Association: Kansas City Office, 5844
American Lyme Disease Foundation, 9023, 9032, 9064
American Macular Degeneration Foundation, 9410
American Medical Association, 6328
American Medical Association (AMA), 7037
American Migraine Foundation, 6289
American Motility Society, 3919
American Myalgic Encephalomyelitis and Chronic Fatigue Syndrome Society, 2825
American Obesity Treatment Association, 6709
American Optometric Association, 9411
American Organ Transplant Association, 10347, 10618
American Osteopathic Association, 2909
American Pain Society, 2910, 2936
American Pancreatic Association, 3920
American Paraplegic Society, 8032
American Parkinson Disease Association (APDA), 6867
American Parkinson Disease Association Hotline, 6922
American Parkinson Disease Association Newsletter, 6942
American Perceptions of Aging in the 21st Century, 208
American Physical Therapy Association, 2911, 6807
American Porphyria Foundation, 3932, 3994
American Pregnancy Association, 5375
American Printing House for the Blind, 9412, 10058
American Pseudo-Obstruction and Hirschsprung's Disease Society, 3995
American Psychiatric Association, 5906, 6193, 7038
American Psychological Association, 5907, 6175, 7039
American Psychologist, 6150
American Public Health Association (APHA), 7040
American Red Cross, 10619
American Red Cross Blood Services, 4959, 5130
American Red Cross Hemophilia Center, 5015
American Red Cross National Headquarters, 10348
American Rehabilitation Counseling Association, 10349
American Respiratory Alliance of Western Pennsylvania, 5857

American Self-Help Group Clearinghouse, 7101, 10620
American Sexual Health Association (ASHA), 7568
American Sickle Cell Anemia, 7631
American Sickle Cell Anemia Association, 7604
American SIDS Institute, 8698, 8840
American Sign Language: A Beginning Course, 4427
American Skin Association, 7658
American Sleep Apnea Association, 7758, 7848
American Sleep Disorders Association, 7849
American Social Health Association, 7594
American Society for Bone and Mineral Research, 6781
American Society for Deaf Children, 4296, 4834
American Society for Dermatologic Surgery, 7659
American Society for Gastrointestinal Endoscopy, 3921, 3996
American Society for Parenteral and Enteral Nutrition (ASPEN), 3922
American Society for Reproductive Medicine, 3791, 3819, 5376, 5559
American Society for Reproductive Medicine: Clinic Specific Annual Report, 5500
American Society for Surgery of the Hand, 2606
American Society of Abdominal Surgeons, 3997
American Society of Colon and Rectal Surgeons, 2092, 2588
American Society of Dermatology, 10350, 10621
American Society of Hematology, 2957
American Society of Human Genetics, 1150
American Society of Hypertension, 5286
American Society of Plastic and Reconstructive Surgeons, 7745
American Society of Plastic Surgeons, 7660
American Society of Transplantation (AST), 9163, 9242
American Society on Aging, 217
American Speech-Language-Hearing Association, 4297
American Spinal Injury Association (ASIA), 7955
American Stroke Association, 8047
American Stroke Foundation, 8052
American Thyroid Association, 9003, 9017
American Tinnitus Association, 4298, 4835
American Trauma Society (ATS), 7041
Americans with Disabilities Act, 7498
Americans with Disabilities Act Resource Manual, 1299
Americans with Disabilities Act: CFS and Employment, 2865
Americans with Disabilities Act: What it Means for People with AIDS, 574
Americas Association for the Care of the Children, 2093, 10351
Amfar AIDS Handbook: The Complete Guide to Understanding HIV and AIDS, 467
Amyotrophic Lateral Sclerosis Toll Free Hotline, 1151
Amyotrophic Lateral Sclerosis: Guide for Patients and Families, 1154
An Annotated Bibliography of Recent Empirical Research In Methadone, 8267
An Assessment of Technical Issues Raised in RW Haley's Critique of Health Studies, 10278
An Atlas of Obesity and Weight Control, 6723
An Early Prader-Willi Syndrome Diagnosis & How to Make it Easier on Parents, 7210
An Educational Challenge: Meeting the Needs of Students with Brain Injury, 4191
An Inside View, 6739
An Introduction to Your Child Who Has Cerebral Palsy, 2797
An Invisible Condition: The Human Side of Hearing Loss, 4428
An Orientation and Mobility Primer for Families and Young Children, 9828
An Overview of Allergy, 723
Anabolic Steroids: A Threat to Body and Mind, 8509
Analgesic Rebound Headaches: Fact Sheet, 6309
Anaphylaxis, 700
Anatomy of a Psychiatric Illness, 6088
Anatomy of Bereavement, 10704
And After Tomorrow, 6173
And the Beat Goes On, 4937
Anemia of Sarcoidosis, 7258

Aneurysm Answers, 5277, 8082
Angels and Outcasts: An Anthology of Deaf Characters in Literature, 4429
Angels in the Sun Brain Tumor Support Group, 1951
Angelwish, Inc., 10681
Animal Signs: A First Book of Sign Language, 4643
ANKORS: Kootenay & Boundary HIV/AIDS and Hepatitis C Support Services, 248
Ankylosing Spondylitis, 1300
Ann Whitehill Down Syndrome Program, 3576
Anonymity, 6740, 8510
Anorexia Nervosa & Recovery: A Hunger for Meaning, 3723
Anorexia Nervosa & Related Eating Disorders, 3775
Another Handful of Stories, 4644
Another Home for Mom, 1072
Answering Your Questions About PROPATH, 6949
Answering Your Questions About Spina Bifida, 7914
Answers to Some Commonly Asked Questions, 9361
Answers to the Most Asked Questions About Impotence, 5312
Anxiety Disorders Association of America, 6194, 7042
Anxiety Disorders Center University of Wisconsin, 6030
Anxiety Resource Center, 7065
Anyone Can Have a Bleeding Problem, 5100
APDA Center for Advanced Parkinson Disease Research, 6919
APDA Newsletter, 6941
APF Newsletter, 3964
APH Catalog of Accessible Books for People Who are Visually Impaired, 9826
Aphasia: Struggling for Understanding, 214
APICHA News, 533
APLA Update, 534
Apnea Identification Program Children's Ho spital of Michigan, 8751
Apparent Life-Threatening Event and Sudden Infant Death Syndrome, 8818
Applying New Attitudes & Directions, 3772
Approaching Equality, 4430
Approaching Grief, 10731
Aqua Exercises for Multiple Sclerosis, 6497
Archstone Foundation, 111
Are You Concerned About Someone's Drinking, 8511
Are You Looking for a Few Good Workers?, 9959
Are You Tired Again?...I Understand: An Activities Workbook for Children, 10583
Arizona Association of the Deaf, 4338
Arizona Brain Tumor Support Group, 1916
Arizona Center for the Blind and Visually Impaired, 9466
Arizona Chapter of the National Parkinson Foundation, 6874
Arizona Department of Health Services: HIV Prevention Program, 286
Arizona Heart Institute, 4865
Arizona Industries for the Blind, 9467
Arizona Kidney Foundation, 5582
Arizona SIDS Founation, 8708
Arizona Spinal Cord Injury Association, 7964
Arizona State Braille and Talking Book Library, 9614
Arizona Telemedicine Program, 7225
Arkansas Association of the Deaf, 4339
Arkansas Cystic Fibrosis Center Arkansas Children's Hospital, 3089
Arkansas Department of Health: HIV Prevention Program, 289
Arkansas Department of Health: SIDS Information & Counseling Program, 8710
Arkansas FFCMH Jane Burgan, 5930
Arkansas Lighthouse for the Blind, 9470
Arkansas Regional Library for the Blind and Physically Handicapped, 9617
Arkansas Regional Organ Recovery Agency, 9177
Arlin J Brown Information Center, 2249
Arlington County Department of Libraries, 9754
Armond V Mascia Cystic Fibrosis Center NY Medical College, 3145
Around the Clock, 1649
Around the Clock with COPD, 5880
Art and Science of Teaching Orientation to the Visually Impaired, 9830

Art Beyond Sight: Resource Guide to Art, Creativity and Visual Impairment, 9829
Art of Getting Well, 10531
Art of Living with Change: Turning Your Good Intentions Into Progress..., 8662
ART-Assisted Reproductive Technologies, 5507
Artery, 5087
Arthritis, 1278
Arthritis & Autoimmunity Research Centre, 1188
Arthritis 101: Questions You Have, Answers You Need, 1261
Arthritis Accent, 1284
Arthritis and Diet Information Package, 1304
Arthritis and Employment: You Can Get the Job You Want, 1305
Arthritis and Inflammatory Bowel Disease, 1306
Arthritis and Musculoskeletal Center: UAB Shelby Interdisciplinary Biomedical Rese, 1241
Arthritis and Pregnancy, 1307
Arthritis and Vocational Rehabilitation, 1308
Arthritis Answers: Basic Information About Arthritis, 1301
Arthritis Foundation, 1238, 1361, 6855, 7224
Arthritis Foundation Information Helpline, 1257
Arthritis Foundation: Arkansas Chapter, 1194
Arthritis Foundation: Carolinas Chapter, 1222
Arthritis Foundation: Central Arizona Chapter, 1193
Arthritis Foundation: Central New York Chapter, 1218
Arthritis Foundation: Central Ohio Chapter, 1223
Arthritis Foundation: Central Pennsylvania Chapter, 1229
Arthritis Foundation: Eastern Missouri Chapter, 1214
Arthritis Foundation: Florida Chapter, Gulf Coast Branch, 1201
Arthritis Foundation: Georgia Chapter, 1202
Arthritis Foundation: Greater Chicago Chapter, 1203
Arthritis Foundation: Greater Illinois Chapter, 1204
Arthritis Foundation: Indiana Chapter, 1205
Arthritis Foundation: Iowa Chapter, 1206
Arthritis Foundation: Kansas Chapter, 1207
Arthritis Foundation: Kentucky Chapter, 1208
Arthritis Foundation: Long Island Chapter, 1219
Arthritis Foundation: Maryland Chapter, 1209
Arthritis Foundation: Massachusetts Chapter, 1210
Arthritis Foundation: Metropolitan Washington Chapter, 1200
Arthritis Foundation: Michigan Chapter Chapter and Metro Detroit, 1211
Arthritis Foundation: Mississippi Chapter, 1213
Arthritis Foundation: Nebraska Chapter, 1216
Arthritis Foundation: New Jersey Chapter, 1217
Arthritis Foundation: New York Chapter, 1220
Arthritis Foundation: Newsletter of Nebraska Chapter, 1285
Arthritis Foundation: North Central Chapter, 1212
Arthritis Foundation: North Texas Chapter, 1232
Arthritis Foundation: Northeastern Ohio Chapter, 1224
Arthritis Foundation: Northern California Chapter, 1195
Arthritis Foundation: Northern New England Chapter, 1234
Arthritis Foundation: Northwestern Ohio Chapter, 1225
Arthritis Foundation: Ohio River Valley Chapter, 1226
Arthritis Foundation: Oklahoma Chapter, 1228
Arthritis Foundation: Rockland/Orange Unit, 1221
Arthritis Foundation: Rocky Mountain Chapter, 1198
Arthritis Foundation: San Diego Area Chapter, 1196
Arthritis Foundation: Southeast Region, 1231
Arthritis Foundation: Southern Arizona Chapter, 1286
Arthritis Foundation: Southern California Chapter, 1197
Arthritis Foundation: Southern New England Chapter, 1199
Arthritis Foundation: Southern New England Chapter, 1230
Arthritis Foundation: Utah/Idaho Chapter, 1233
Arthritis Foundation: Virginia Chapter, 1235
Arthritis Foundation: Washington/Alaska Chapter, 1236
Arthritis Foundation: Western Missouri, Greater Kansas City, 1215

Arthritis Foundation: Wisconsin Chapter Foundation, 1237
Arthritis Foundation; Great Lakes Region, Northeastern Ohio, 1227
Arthritis Helpbook: A Tested Self-Management Program for Coping, 1262
Arthritis in Children and La Artritis Infantojuvenil, 1310
Arthritis in Children Information Package, 1309
Arthritis Information: Advocacy and Government Affairs, 1302
Arthritis Information: Children, 1303
Arthritis News, 1287
Arthritis Observer, 1288
Arthritis on the Job: You Can Work With It, 1311
Arthritis Reporter, 1289
Arthritis Self-Help Products, 1263
Arthritis Self-Management, 1264
Arthritis Society, 1189
Arthritis Today, 1282
Arthritis Trust of America, 2607
Arthritis Update of Rhode Island, 1290
Arthritis Volunteer, 1291
Arthritis: Do You Know?, 1312
Arthritis: What Exercises Work, 1265
Arthritis: Your Complete Exercise Guide, 1266
Article Reprint Exchange, 5101
As Bill Sees It, 8268
As We Understood..., 8269
ASAP Capsule, 3965
ASAP Digest, 3966
ASAP Forum, 3949
Asbestos in Your Home, 5881
Asbestos Information Association/North America, 10352
Asbestos Watch, 10589
Ask Audrey, 9387
ASL in Schools: Policies and Curriculum, 4422
ASL PAH! Deaf Students' Essays About their Language, 4421
ASL Poetry: Selected Works of Clayton Valli, 4786
Asperger Syndrome or High-Functioning Autism?, 1732
Asperger's Syndrome: A Guide for Parents and Professionals, 1733
Aspirin and Other Nonsteroidal Anti-Inflamatory Drugs, 1313
Assemblies of God National Center for the Blind, 9713
Assessing Psychopathology and Behavior Problems: Mentally Ill Persons, 6089
Assessment & Management of Mainstreamed Hearing-Impaired Children, 4431
Assessment of Hearing Impaired People, 4432
Assisstive Technology for Young Children: A Guide to Family-Centered Services, 10532
Assisting Parents Through the Mourning Process, 10607
Assistive Devices Demonstration Centers, 4754
Associated Services for the Blind & Visually Impaired, 9413
Association for Behavioral and Cognitive Therapies, 7043
Association for Children with Down Syndrome, 3566
Association for Children's Mental Health, 5969
Association for Education & Rehabilitation of the Blind & Visually Impaired, 9414
Association for Glycogen Storage Disease, 5733
Association for Macular Diseases, 9415
Association for Neuro-Metabolic Disorders, 3833
Association for Research of Childhood Cancer, 2340
Association for the Blind & Visually Impaired, 9516
Association for the Blind & Visually Impaired of Lehigh County, 9536, 9555
Association for the Cure of Cancer of the Prostate, 2589
Association for Traumatic Stress Specialists, 7044
Association of Children's Residential Centers, 5908
Association of Gastrointestinal Motility D isorders, 3712
Association of Halfway House Alcoholism Programs of North America (AHHAP), 8112
Association of Late-Deafened Adults, 4299
Association of Organ Procurement Organizations (AOPO), 9164, 9243

Association of Spinal Cord Injury Professionals, Inc., 7956
Asthma, 1425
Asthma Alert, 1450
Asthma and Allergies in Seniors, 1453
Asthma and Allergy Foundation of America, 655, 732, 1398, 1509
Asthma and Allergy Foundation of America: Alaska Chapter, 649, 1390
Asthma and Allergy Foundation of America: Michigan Chapter, 651, 1393
Asthma and Allergy Foundation of America: New England Chapter, 650, 1392
Asthma and Allergy Foundation of America: St. Louis Chapter, 652, 1394
Asthma and Pregnancy, 1454
Asthma and the Athlete, 1495
Asthma and the School Child, 1455
Asthma Canada, 632, 1377
Asthma Care Training for Kids, 1411
Asthma Challenge, 1426
Asthma Handbook, 1451
Asthma Handbook Slides, 1493
ASTHMA Hotline, 671
Asthma in the School: Improving Control with Peak Flow Monitoring, 1415
Asthma in the Workplace, 1416
Asthma Lifelines, 1452
Asthma Management, 1494
Asthma Organizer, 1412
Asthma Resources Directory, 1413
Asthma Self-Help Book, 1414
Asthma: The Complete Guide, 1417
At Grandma's House, 4645
At Home Among Strangers, 4433
At Home with AAKP, 5691
At Home with MS: Adapting Your Environment, 6461
At Our House, 6462
Ataxia Canada - Claude St-Jean Foundation, 1520
Ataxia Fact Sheet, 1579
Athealth.com, 7145
Athlete's Foot, 7698
Atlanta Georgia Chapter of the American Association of Kidney Patients, 5602
Atlanta Metro Subregional Library, 9645
Atlanta VA Medical Center Atlanta VA Health Care System, 10137
Atomz, 4064
Atopic Dermatitis, 1456
Attention, 1635
Attention Deficit Disorder, 1650
Attention Deficit Disorder Association, 1600
Attention Deficit Disorder: A Different Perception, 1617
Attention Deficit Disorder: Learning Disabilities, 1618
Attention Deficit Disorders and Hyperactivity, 1641
Attention Deficit Hyperactivity Disorder: What Every Parent Wants to Know, 1619
Attention Deficit Information Network, 1611
Attention Deficit/Hyperactivity Disorder, 1632
Audie L. Murphy Memorial VA Hospital South Texas Veterans Health Care System, 10243
Audio Cassette Program on Fibromyalgia, 3897
Audiology Express, 4728
Audiology Today, 4704
Augusta Regional Library Talking Book Center, 9646
Auricle, 4705
Aurora of Central New York, 4409, 9811
Autism and Asperger Syndrome Preparing for Adulthood, 1737
Autism Chapter of Bluegrass Chapter, 1684
Autism in Adolescents and Adults, 1738
Autism Research Institute, 1661, 1809
Autism Research Review International, 1784
Autism Resources, 1810
Autism Services Center, 1662
Autism Society of Alabama, 1670
Autism Society of Albany, 1698
Autism Society of America, 1663, 1725, 1811
Autism Society of Baltimore-Chesapeake, 1688
Autism Society of Black Hills, 1708
Autism Society of California, 1672
Autism Society of Central Oklahoma, 1703

Autism Society of Colorado, 1673
Autism Society of Dallas, 1710
Autism Society of District Columbia, 1674
Autism Society of East Tennessee, 1709
Autism Society of Florida, 1675
Autism Society of Gateway Chapter, 1692
Autism Society of Greater Cincinnati, 1701
Autism Society of Greater Georgia, 1677
Autism Society of Greater Harrisburg, 1705
Autism Society of Hawaii, 1678
Autism Society of Illinois, 1680
Autism Society of Indiana, 1681
Autism Society of Iowa, 1682
Autism Society of Kansas Autism Society of America, 1683
Autism Society of Louisiana, 1686
Autism Society of Maine, 1687
Autism Society of Massachusetts, 1689
Autism Society of Michigan, 1690
Autism Society of Minnesota, 1691
Autism Society of Nebraska, 1693
Autism Society of New Hampshire, 1695
Autism Society of New Mexico, 1697
Autism Society of North Carolina, 1699
Autism Society of North Carolina Bookstore, 1734
Autism Society of North Dakota, 1700
Autism Society of Northern Nevada, 1694
Autism Society of Northern Virginia, 1712
Autism Society of Ohio Tri-County Chapter, 1702
Autism Society of Oregon, 1704
Autism Society of Rhode Island, 1706
Autism Society of South Carolina, 1707
Autism Society of Southern Arizona, 1671
Autism Society of Southwest New Jersey, 1696
Autism Society of Treasure Valley, 1679
Autism Society of Vermont Autism Society of America, 1711
Autism Society of Washington, 1713
Autism Society of Western Kentucky, 1685
Autism Society of Wisconsin, 1715
Autism Socity of West Virginia, 1714
Autism Spectrum Disorders: The Complete Guide, 1780
Autism Through the Lifespan: The Eden Model, 1735
Autism Treatment Center of America, 1664, 1812
Autism Treatment Guide, 1736
Autism...Nature, Diagnosis and Treatment, 1739
Autism: A Strange, Silent World, 1795
Autism: A World Apart, 1796
Autism: Explaining the Enigma, 1740
Autism: Identification, Education and Treatment, 1741
Autism: The Facts, 1742
Autistic Adults at Bittersweet Farms, 1743
Autoimmune Advocacy Alliance, 7234
Autonomic Dysreflexia, 8009
Autonomic Failure and Parkinson's Disease, 6950
Avoiding Carpal Tunnel Syndrome, 2616
Avoiding Indecision and Hesitation with Hemophilia-Related Emergencies, 5074
Avoiding Unfortunate Situations, 1785
Awaking to Disability, 10533
Awareness, 9920

B

B Connected, 5155
B-Informed Newsletter, 5156
BABES Network-YWCA, 444
Babies with Down Syndrome, 3605
Baby of Your Own: New Ways to Overcome Infertility, 5448
Back Pain, 1314
Background on Functional Gastrointestinal Disorders, 3998
Backtalk, 7412
Badger's Parting Gifts, 10723
Bainbridge Subregional Library for the Blind and Physically Handicapped, 9647
Balance Disturbances and Parkinson's Disease, 6951
Balance Your Act: A Book for Adults with Diabetes, 3411
Ball State University Public Health Entomology Laboratory, 9029

Baltimore Headache Institute, 6293
Baltimore VA Medical Center VA Maryland Health Care System, 10164
Bangor Public Library, 9680
Barbara Davis Center for Childhood Diabetes, 3377
Bartholomew County Public Library, 9665
BASE Camp Children's Cancer Foundation, 10655
BASH Magazine, 3765
Basic Course in American Sign Language Vid eotape Package, 4787
Basic Course in Manual Communication, 4434
Basic Family Library, 2500
Basic Home Care for ALS Patients, 1169
Basic Information About Parkinson's Disease, 6952
Basic Questions About Head Injury & Disability, 4223
Basic Science Series, 7737
Basic Sign Communication: Student Materials, 4435
Basic Sign Communication: Vocabulary, 4436
Basic Vocabulary and Language Thesaurus for Hearing Impaired Children, 4437
Basic Vocabulary: American Sign Language for Parents and Children, 4438
Basics of HIV Disease: Questions and Answers, 575, 5102
Bassett Research Institute, 2341
Batavia VA Medical Center VA Western New York Healthcare System, 10198
Bath VA Medical Center, 10199
Baton Rouge Regional Tumor Registry Mary Bird Perkins Cancer Center, 2315
Battle Creek VA Medical Center, 10173
Baxter Hyland Division, 4960
Bay Area LE Foundation, 8858
Bay Pines VA Healthcare System, 10127
Baylor College of Medicine: Children's General Clinical Research Center, 3378
Baylor College of Medicine: Cullen Eye Institute, 9774
Baylor College of Medicine: Debakey Heart Center, 4866
Baylor College of Medicine: Epilepsy Research Center, 7490
Baylor College of Medicine: General Clinical Research Center for Adults, 3940
Baylor College of Medicine: Jerry Lewis Neuromuscular Disease Research, 6513
Baylor College of Medicine: Sleep Disorder and Research Center, 7763
Baylor University Bone Marrow Transplantation Research Center, 2374
Bayou Area Chapter of the American Association of Kidney Patients, 5613
Baystate Medical Center Wesson Memorial Unit, 3125
BC Centre for Ability, 6652
Be BoneWise: Exercise, 6842
Be Happy, Not Sad, 4646
Be Kind to Nonsmokers, 8512
Be Smart About HIV, 576
Beach Center on Disability, 10353
Beach Center on Families and Disability, 10622
Bearly Any Fat Cookbook, 3724
Beaver County Association for the Blind, 9556
Beckley VA Medical Center, 10262
Bees-Stealy Research Foundation, 4867
Before You Take That First..., 6741
Beginning Reading and Sign Language Video, 4788
Beginning with Braille: Balanced Approach to Literacy, 9831
Beginnings for Parents of Children Who are Deaf or Hard of Hearing, 4410
Behavior Management: Collection of Articless, 7211
Behavioral and Circadian Sleep Problems of Infancy and Childhood, 2885
Behavioral and Psychosocial Sequelae of Pediatric Head Injury, 4224
Behavioral Pediatrics Program, 10511
Behavioral Vision Approaches for Persons with Physical Disabilities, 9832
Behaviors, 1041
Behcet's Disease, 1315
Being Alive, 536
Being Alive Newsletter, 537
Being Close, 1457

Being in Touch, 4439
Believe In Tomorrow Children's Foundation, 10656
Belonging, 4647, 9895
Benaroya Research Institute Virginia Mason Medical Center, 3379
Bendectin Report, 1868
Bereaved Children: A Support Guide for for Parents And Professionals, 10705
Bereaved Parent, 10706
Bereavement Group for Children, 1918, 10699
Berkshire Center, 10507
BermanGund Laboratory for the Study of Retinal Degenerations, 9775
Bernardsville Beginnings, 3643
Beside Me, 9896
Best of Public Outreach, 8513
Best of Superstuff Activity Booklet, 1427
Best of the Beacon, 7376
Best Practices, 194
Best Practices in Educational Interpreting, 4440
Bestwork Industries for the Blind, 9531
BETA, 535
Bethy and the Mouse: God's Gifts in Special Packages, 3606
Better Breather's Clubs, 7239
Better Breathing Bulletin, 3188
Better Hearing News, 4729
Between Friends, 4441
Beyond Gentle Teaching, 1744
Beyond the Loss of the Breast, 2582
BIAW News, 4215
Bible Alliance, 10028
Bibliography, 5512
Big Red Factor, 5088
Biliary Atresia, 5785
Bill Discusses the Twelve Traditions, 8663
Bill's Own Story, 8664
Billy's Story, 3763
Biology of Reproduction, 5501
Biology of the Autistic Syndromes, 1745
Bipolar Disorder, 6160
Birmingham Support Group: National Ataxia Foundation, 1524
Birmingham VA Medical Center: Research and Development, 2268
Birth Defect News, 1874
Birth Defect Research for Children, Inc., 633, 733, 1378, 1825, 1892
Birth Defects & Genetics: The Genetics Revolution, 1879
Birth Defects of the Female Reproductive System, 5513
Bittersweet Waltz, 3644
Black and Deaf in America, 4442
Black Coalition for AIDS Prevention, 254
Black Death: AIDS in Africa, 468
Black Experience, 3516
Black Lung, 5882
Black Skin, 7699
Black, Beautiful and Recovering, 8270, 8514
Bladder Control for Women, 5353
Blank Childrens Hospital Pediatric Pulmonology Clinic, 3113
Bleeding Disorder Foundation of Washington, 5009
Bleeding in the Digestive Tract, 9393
Blick Clinic for Developmental Disabilities, 3577
Blind Association of Western New York, 9537
Blind Childrens Center, 9619
Blind Educator, 9904
Blind Enterprises of Oregon, 9553
Blind Industries and Services of Maryland, 9509
Blind Work Association, 9538
Blinded Veterans Association, 9416, 10059
Blindness and Early Childhood Development, 9833
Blindness: A Family Matter, 10029
Blood Pressure Book: How to Get it Down & Keep it Down, 10534
Bloodlines, 5089
Blueprint for Conversational Competence, 4443
Bockus Research Institute Graduate Hospital, 4868
Body Betrayed, 3725
Body Silent: An Anthropologist Embarks into the World of the Disabled, 7995
Body, Mind, and Spirit, 8271
Boise VA Medical Center, 10142

Bomb in the Brain: A Heroic Tale of Science, Surgery and Survival, 7499
Bone Marrow & Cancer Foundation, 2257, 2590
Bone Up on Arthritis, 1267
Boning Up on Osteoporosis, 6824
Book of Name Signs, 4444
Books are Fun for Everyone, 9961
Books for Parents of Deaf and Hard of Hearing Children, 4755
Bosma Industries for the Blind, 9497
Boston Bracing System for Idiopathic Scoliosis, 7415
Boston Hemophilia Center Fegan 5 Children's Hospital, 5016
Boston Obesity Nutrition Research Center (BONRC), 6766
Boston Sickle Cell Center Boston Medical Center, 7612
Boston University Arthritis Center, 1242
Boston University Cancer Research Center, 2321
Boston University Center for Human Genetics, 1836
Boston University Laboratory of Neuropsychology, 8199
Boston University Medical Campus General Clinical Research Center, 1243
Boston University University Medical Center, 7358
Boston University, Whitaker Cardiovascular Institute, 4869
Boulder Public Library, 9625
Bowel Cancer, 2423
Bowel Continence and Spina Bifida, 7915
Bowman Gray School of Medicine, 8053
Bowman Grey School of Medicine: Hemophilia Diagnostic Center, 5017
Boys Town National Research Hospital, 4369
Brace & Her Brace is No Handicap, 7416
Brachytherapy and IMRT, 2501
Brady Institute Jamaica Hospital Medical Center, 4129
Braille Alphabet and Numbers, 9962
Braille Book Bank: Music Catalog, 9834
Braille Book Review, 9921
Braille Documents, 10030
Braille Forum, 9905
Braille Institute Desert Center, 9776
Braille Institute Library Services, 9620
Braille Institute of America, 9417
Braille Institute Orange County Center, 9777
Braille Institute Santa Barbara Center Braille Institute of Los Angeles, 9778
Braille Institute Sight Center, 9779
Braille Institute Youth Center, 9780
Braille Literacy: Blind Persons, Families, Prof. & Producers of Braille, 9963
Braille Monitor, 9906
Braille Revival League, 10060
Braille Textbook Assignment Service National Braille Association, 9781
Braille: An Extraordinary Volunteer Opportunity, 9964
Brain & Behavior Research Foundation, 6195, 6255
Brain Cancer Support Group, 1991
Brain Cancer Support Group: Port Orchard, 2034
Brain Cancer Support Group: Seattle, 2035
Brain Damage is a Family Affair, 4225
Brain Injuries: A Guide for Families & Caretakers, 4226
Brain Injury Alliance of Iowa Helpline, 4158
Brain Injury Alliance of Kentucky, 4160
Brain Injury Alliance of Minnesota, 4166
Brain Injury Alliance of Montana, 4169
Brain Injury Alliance of New Jersey, 4171
Brain Injury Alliance of New Mexico, 4172
Brain Injury Alliance of Oregon, 4180
Brain Injury Alliance of Utah, 4183
Brain Injury Alliance of Wisconsin, 4189
Brain Injury Alliance of Wyoming, 4190
Brain Injury Association of America, 4078, 4271
Brain Injury Association of America's National Family Helpline, 4122
Brain Injury Association of Arizona, 4083, 4146
Brain Injury Association of Arkansas, 4084
Brain Injury Association of Arkansas Helpl ine, 4147
Brain Injury Association of California Hel pline, 4148
Brain Injury Association of Colorado, 4085

Brain Injury Association of Colorado Helpline, 4150
Brain Injury Association of Connecticut, 4086
Brain Injury Association of Connecticut Helpline, 4151
Brain Injury Association of Delaware, 4087
Brain Injury Association of Delaware Helpl ine, 4152
Brain Injury Association of Florida, 4088, 4153
Brain Injury Association of Hawaii, 4091, 4154
Brain Injury Association of Idaho, 4092
Brain Injury Association of Illinois, 4093
Brain Injury Association of Illinois Helpline, 4156
Brain Injury Association of Indiana, 4094
Brain Injury Association of Indiana Helpli ne, 4157
Brain Injury Association of Iowa, 4095
Brain Injury Association of Kansas and Greater Kansas City Helpline, 4096, 4159
Brain Injury Association of Kentucky, 4097
Brain Injury Association of Louisiana Help line, 4161
Brain Injury Association of Maine, 4098
Brain Injury Association of Maryland, 4099
Brain Injury Association of Maryland Helpl ine, 4162
Brain Injury Association of Massachusetts, 4100
Brain Injury Association of Massachusetts Helpline, 4163
Brain Injury Association of Michigan, 4101
Brain Injury Association of Michigan Helpline, 4165
Brain Injury Association of Minnesota, 4102
Brain Injury Association of Mississippi, 4103
Brain Injury Association of Mississippi Helpline, 4167
Brain Injury Association of Missouri, 4104
Brain Injury Association of Missouri Helpline, 4168
Brain Injury Association of Montana, 4105
Brain Injury Association of New Hampshire, 4106, 4170
Brain Injury Association of New Jersey, 4107
Brain Injury Association of New Mexico, 4108
Brain Injury Association of New York State, 4109
Brain Injury Association of New York State Helpline, 4173
Brain Injury Association of North Carolina, 4111
Brain Injury Association of North Carolina Helpline, 4176
Brain Injury Association of North Dakota, 4177
Brain Injury Association of Ohio, 4112, 4178
Brain Injury Association of Oklahoma, 4113
Brain Injury Association of Oklahoma Helpl ine, 4179
Brain Injury Association of Oregon, 4114
Brain Injury Association of Pennsylvania, 4115
Brain Injury Association of Rhode Island, 4116
Brain Injury Association of Rhode Island H elpline, 4181
Brain Injury Association of South Carolina, 4117
Brain Injury Association of Tennessee, 4118
Brain Injury Association of Tennessee Help line, 4182
Brain Injury Association of Texas, 4119
Brain Injury Association of Utah, 4120
Brain Injury Association of Vermont, 4121
Brain Injury Association of Vermont Helpli ne, 4184
Brain Injury Association of Virginia, 4123
Brain Injury Association of Virginia Helpline, 4185
Brain Injury Association of Washington, 4124
Brain Injury Association of Washington Hel pline, 4186
Brain Injury Association of West Virginia, 4125
Brain Injury Association of West Virginia Helpline, 4188
Brain Injury Association of Wisconsin, 4126
Brain Injury Association of Wyoming, 4127
Brain Injury Glossary, 4192
Brain Injury Resource Center, 4187, 7066
Brain Injury Source, 4216
Brain Injury/Brain Tumor Support Group, 1995
Brain Injury: A Home Based Cognitive Rehabilitation Program, 4227
Brain Research Center Children s Hospital National Medical Cen, 1909
Brain Research Foundation, 1910
Brain Research Institute: Medicine School University of California, Los Angeles, 4272
Brain Tissue Resource Center McLean Hospital, 1911
Brain Trauma Foundation, 4128
Brain Tumor Community Group, 2013
Brain Tumor Education & Support Group, 2011

Brain Tumor Foundation of Canada, 1904
Brain Tumor Networking Club, 1987
Brain Tumor Networking Group, 1977
Brain Tumor Patient and Caregiver Support Group, 1982
Brain Tumor Resource and Vital Encouragement, 1946
Brain Tumor Resource Directory, 2041
Brain Tumor Society, 1919, 2079
Brain Tumor Support and Networking Group, 1993
Brain Tumor Support Group, 1952, 1964, 1966, 1975
Brain Tumor Support Group for Patients and Families, 2000
Brain Tumor Support Group for Patients & Families, 1988
Brain Tumor Support Group of Maine, 1976
Brain Tumor Support Group: Ann Arbor, 1989
Brain Tumor Support Group: Charleston, 2021
Brain Tumor Support Group: Cincinnati, 2008
Brain Tumor Support Group: Duarte, 1920
Brain Tumor Support Group: El Paso, 2027
Brain Tumor Support Group: Florence, 2022
Brain Tumor Support Group: Fresno, 1921
Brain Tumor Support Group: Fullerton, 1922
Brain Tumor Support Group: John Sierzant Lutheran Hospital, Gunderson Clinic, 2039
Brain Tumor Support Group: Johnstown, 2014
Brain Tumor Support Group: Kansas City, 1992
Brain Tumor Support Group: Lahey, 1983
Brain Tumor Support Group: Long Island, 2001
Brain Tumor Support Group: Maryland, 1978
Brain Tumor Support Group: New Jersey, 1996
Brain Tumor Support Group: Newport Beach, 1923
Brain Tumor Support Group: Orange, 1924
Brain Tumor Support Group: Philadelphia, 2015
Brain Tumor Support Group: Pittsburgh, 2016
Brain Tumor Support Group: Providence, 2019
Brain Tumor Support Group: Raleigh Area, 2005
Brain Tumor Support Group: Redding, 1925
Brain Tumor Support Group: Richmond, 2032
Brain Tumor Support Group: Sacramento, 1926
Brain Tumor Support Group: San Diego, 1927
Brain Tumor Support Group: San Francisco, 1928
Brain Tumor Support Group: Santa Barbara, 1929
Brain Tumor Support Group: Southern West Virginia, 2038
Brain Tumor Support Group: Stanford, 1930
Brain Tumor Support Group: Toms River, 1997
Brain Tumor Support Group: West Bloomfield, 1990
Brain Tumor Support Group: Westlake Village, 1931
Brain Tumor Support Group: Worcester, 1984
Brain Tumor/Pituitary Patient Support Group, 1932
Brain Waves, 4217
Brainiacs, 1979
Brainlash, 4193
BrainLine.org, 7067
Brainstorm, 4218
Brainstorms: Epilepsy in Our Words, 7500
Brave Kids, 4027
Breaking New Ground Resource Center, 10354
Breakthrough, 6790, 8984
Breast Biopsy: What You Should Know, 2502
Breast Cancer, 2424
Breast Cancer Action, 2094
A Breast Cancer Journey: Your Personal Guidebook, 2418
Breast Cancer Resource Foundation of Alabama, 2269
Breast Cancer Society of Canada, 2095
Breast Cancer: Understanding Treatment Options, 2503
Breast Exams: What You Should Know, 2504
Breast Feeding the Baby with Down Syndrome, 3607
BReATHE, 1443
Breathe Easy: Respiratory Care with Muscular Dystrophy, 6536
Breathe Pennsylvania, 5858
Breathing Disorders: Your Complete Exercise Guide, 1418
Brevard County Libraries: Talking Books Library, 9632
Brief Encounters of the Right Kind: How to Make Your Point in 10 Minutes or Less, 10031
Brief History of the Agent Orange Lawsuit, 10298

Brigham and Women's Hospital: Center for Neurologic Diseases, 6430
Brigham and Women's Hospital: Rheumatology Immunology, and Allergy Division, 1399
Brigham and Women's Orthopedica and Arthritis Center, 1244
Brigham Young University Cancer Research Center, 2380
Bright Side, The, 7146
British Scoliosis Research Society, 7452
Brockton Division VA Boston Healthcare System, 10168
Broken Ears: Wounded Hearts, 4445
Bronchial Asthma: Principles of Diagnosis and Treatment, 1419
Bronchoalveolar Lymphocytes in Sarcoidosis, 7259
Bronkie the Bronchiasaurus, 1428
Brooklyn Campus VA NY Harbor Health Care System, 10200
Broward County Talking Book Library, 9633
Brown County Library, 9771
Brown University Division of Biology and Medicine, 2369
Buffalo VA Medical Center VA Western New York Healthcare System, 10201
Building Blocks: Foundations for Learning for Young Blind & Vis. Impaired Children, 9835
Building Partnerships in Hospital Care, 10535
Bulimia Anorexia Nervosa Association, 3671
Bulimia: A Guide to Recovery, 3726, 3773
Bulletin, 195, 9922
Bureau of Family Health Services: Alabama Department of Public Health, 8706
Bureau on Alcohol Abuse and Recovery Ohio Department of Health, 8178
Bureau on Drug Abuse: Ohio Department of Health, 8179
Burnham Institute Cancer Center The Burnham Institute for Medical Resear, 2273
Burns Braille Transcription Dictionary, 9836
Bursitis, Tendionitis and Other Soft Tissue Rheumatic Syndromes, 1316
Business Owners Who Are Blind or Visually Impaired, 9837
Butterfly Bulletin, 2049
Buyer's Guide, 3412
Buzzy's Rebound, 8410
BVA Bulletin, 9960

C

Cabell County Public Library, 9765
Cafe Plus, 4174
Caffeine and Nicotine, 8411
California Ambassador: National Ataxia Foundation, 1527
California Association of Persian Gulf Veterans, 10113
California Center for Population Research, 5433
California Collaborative Treatment Group, 290
California Department of Public Health: Office of AIDS, 291
California Institute for Medical Research, 6908
California Lyme Disease Association, 9028
California SIDS Program, 8711
California State Library Braille and Talking Book Library, 9621
California Teratogen Information Service UC San Diego School of Medicine Dept of, 1837
California Transplant Donor Network, 9178
California Women's Commission on Alcohol and Drug Dependencies, 8141
Cambria County Association for the Blind and Handicapped, 9557
Came to Believe, 8272
Camp Allen, 10509
Camp Good Days, 10657
Camps for Children with Cancer and their Siblings, 2505
Campus Opportunities for Students with Learning Differences, 10604
Can't You Be Still?, 2802
Can't Your Child Hear?, 4447

Canadian & American Spinal Research Organizations, 7861
Canadian Addison Society, 3
Canadian ADHD Resource Alliance, 1601
Canadian Adult Congenital Heart Network, 4861
Canadian Breast Cancer Network (CBCN), 2096
Canadian Cancer Society, 2097
Canadian Celiac Association, 2627
Canadian Cerebral Palsy Sports Association, 2667
Canadian Dermatology Association, 7325
Canadian Down Syndrome Society, 3538
Canadian Fabry Association, 3834
Canadian Federation of Mental Health Nurses, 5909
Canadian Foundation for AIDS Research, 353
Canadian Hard of Hearing Association, 4300
Canadian Hemophilia Society, 4961
Canadian Mental Health Association (CMHA), 5910
Canadian National Seniors Council, 25, 218
Canadian Pain Society, 2912
Canadian Society of Allergy and Clinical Immunology, 634, 1379
Canandaigua VA Medical Center VA Health Care Upstate New York, 10202
Cancer, 2460
Cancer and Leukemia Group B, 2300
Cancer Caring Center, 2098
Cancer Center of Wake Forest University at Bowman Gray School of Medicine, 2351
Cancer Control Society and Cancer Book House, 2133
Cancer Detection and Prevention Journal, 2479
Cancer Dictionary, 2425
Cancer Facts and Figures, 2426
Cancer Federation, 2264
Cancer in the Family: Helping Children Cope with a Parent's Illness, 2430
Cancer Information Service, 2265, 2391
Cancer Institute of Brooklyn, 2342
Cancer Nursing: An International Journal for Cancer Care, 2480
Cancer of the Bladder: Research Report, 2507
Cancer of the Colon and Rectum: Research Report, 2508
Cancer of the Ovary: Research Report, 2509
Cancer of the Pancreas: Research Report, 2510
Cancer of the Uterus: Endometrial Cancer, 2511
Cancer of the Uterus: Research Report, 2512
Cancer Patient/Caregiver Support Group, 1994
Cancer Prevention Institute of California, 2274
Cancer Rates and Risks, 2427
Cancer Research Center, 2331
Cancer Research Foundation of America, 2383
Cancer Research Institute: New York, 2343
Cancer Sourcebook, 2428
Cancer Support Community, 2392
Cancer Support Group, 2023
Cancer Support Group: Knoxville, 2024
Cancer Support Group: Nashville, 2025
Cancer Tests You Should Know About: A Guide for People 65 and Over, 2506
Cancer Therapy and Research Center, 2375
Cancer Therapy: Ind. Consumer's Guide to Non-Toxic Treatment & Prevention, 2429
Cancer Wellness House, 2031
Cancer: Overview Series, 2461
CancerCare, 2099
Cancervive, 2393
Candid Talk About Loss in Adoption, 5552
Candlelighters Guide to Bone Marrow Transplants in Children, 2513
Candlelighters' Quarterly, 2486
Candlelighters' Youth Newsletter, 2487
CANDU Parent Group, 6056
CanHelp, 2198
Canine Companions for Independence, 9418
Canine Helpers for the Handicapped, Inc., 9419
Canine Listener, 4730
Cape Cod Chapter National Parkinson Foundation, 6892
Capital Advantage, 197
Capital Regional Sleep-Wake Disorders Center, 7764
CAPSule, 196
Captain James A. Lovell Federal Health Care Center, 10144
Caption Center, 9691

Caption Center News, 4731
Captioned Films/Videos, 4363
Captioned Media Program, 4364
Cara: Growing with a Retarded Child, 3608
Cardiovascular Research and Training Center University of Alabama, 4870
Care of Alzheimer's Patients: A Manual for Nursing Home Staff, 999
Care of the Ears and Hearing for Health, 4756
Care of the Elderly in America, 209
Care That Works: A Relationship Approach to Persons with Dementia, 998
Career Perspectives: Interviews with Blind & Visually Impaired Professionals, 9838
Caregiver Action Network, 147, 10512
Caregiver Helpbook, 1000
Caregiver Stress, 1042
Caregiver Support Services, 148
Caregivers' Roller Coaster, 158
Caregiving: A Step-By-Step Resource for Caring for the Person w/Cancer at Home, 2431
Caring for Alzheimer's Patients, 1043
Caring for Alzheimer's Patients: A Guide for Family & Healthcare Providers, 1001
Caring for Infants and Children with Osteogenesis Imperfecta, 6791
Caring for Ourselves: Hope for Healthy Relationships, 8665
Caring for People with Severe Mental Disorders: A National Plan, 6090
Caring for the Diabetic Soul, 3413
Caring for Those You Love: A Guide to Compassionate Care for the Aged, 159
Caring for Veterans With Deployment-Related Stress Disorders, 7123
Caring for Your Liver, 5162
Caring Hand, 2050
Caring...Sharing: The Alzheimer's Caregiver, 1073
Caring.com, 219, 10623
Carl Vinson VA Medical Center Dublin VA Medical Center, 10138
Carnegie Library of Pittsburgh, 9742
Carolinas Chapter of the Myasthenia Gravis Foundation of America, 6592, 6596
Carolinas Support Group: National Ataxia National Ataxia Foundation, 1558
Carpal Tunnel Syndrome, 2615
Carpal Tunnel Syndrome Home Page, 2618
Carroll Center for the Blind, 9511, 9782, 9812
Cary Library, 9681
Cascade AIDS Project Hotline, 446
Case Control Study: Soft-Tissue Sarcomas and Exposure to Phenoxyacetic Acids, 10299
Case of the Great Imitator, 9058
Case Report: MR Imaging of Myocardial Sarcoidosis, 7260
Case Report: Osseous Sarcoidosis and Chronic Polyarthritis, 7261
Case Report: Overlap of Granulomatous Vasculitis and Sarcoidosis, 7262
Case Report: Rapidly Dev. Confusion, Impaired Memory and Unsteady Gait, 7263
Case Western Reserve University, 9736
Case Western Reserve University: Bolton Brush Growth Study Center, 4051
Case Western Reserve University: Center on Aging and Health, 115
Case Western Reserve University: Cystic Fibrosis Center, 3154
Case Western Reserve University: Ireland Cancer Center, 2354
Cataracts, 9965
Catastrophic Injury Cases: The Relationship of Traumatic Brain Injury, 4228
Caution! Treating Children with Acetaminophen, 5163
CCFA Alabama Chapter, 3001
CCFA California: Greater Los Angeles Chapter, 3003
CCFA Carolinas Chapter, 3025
CCFA Central Connecticut Chapter, 3005
CCFA Central Ohio Chapter, 3027
CCFA Florida Chapter, 3007
CCFA Georgia Chapter, 3008
CCFA Greater New York Chapter: National Headquarters, 3020

CCFA Greater Washington DC/Virginia Chapter, 3036
CCFA Houston Gulf Coast/South Texas Chapter, 3034
CCFA Illinois: Carol Fisher Chapter, 3009
CCFA Indiana Chapter, 3010
CCFA Iowa Chapter, 3011
CCFA Long Island Chapter, 3021
CCFA Louisiana Chapter, 3013
CCFA Maryland Chapter, 3014
CCFA Michigan Chapter: Farmington Hills, 3016
CCFA Mid-America Chapter: Kansas, 3012
CCFA Mid-America Chapter: Missouri, 3018
CCFA Minnesota Chapter, 3017
CCFA New England Chapter: Massachusetts, 3015
CCFA New Jersey Chapter, 3019
CCFA North Texas Chapter, 3035
CCFA Northeast Ohio Chapter, 3028
CCFA Northern Connecticut Affiliate Chapter, 3006
CCFA Oklahoma Chapter, 3030
CCFA Philadelphia/Delaware Valley Chapter, 3031
CCFA Rochester/Southern Tier Chapter, 3022
CCFA Rocky Mountain Chapter, 3004
CCFA South Carolina Chapter, 3026
CCFA Southwest Chapter: Arizona, 3002
CCFA Southwest Ohio Chapter, 3029
CCFA Tennessee Chapter, 3033
CCFA Upstate/Northeastern New York Chapter, 3023
CCFA Washington State Chapter, 3037
CCFA Western New York Chapter, 3024
CCFA Western Pennsylvania/West Virginia Chapter, 3032
CCFA Wisconsin Chapter, 3038
CCFA: A Case for Support, 3059
CD-A NIH Consensus Conference, 2651
CDC Intro to Lyme Disease, 9065
CDC National Prevention Information Network, 255, 391
Celebrate! Healthy Entertaining for Any Occasion, 2432
Celiac Disease, 2644
Celiac Disease & Gluten-Free Diet Online Resource Center, 2654
Celiac Disease Foundation, 2632, 2633, 2655
Celiac Disease: A Hidden Epidemic, 2645
Celiac Society, 2628
Center for Adaptive Learning, 10502
Center for Aging Research and Education at the UW-Madison School of Nursing, 116
Center for AIDS Prevention Studies, 540
Center for AIDS Prevention Studies AIDS Research Institute University of C, 368
Center for AIDS Research: Emory University Rollins School of Public Health, 392
Center for AIDS Research: Harvard Medical School, Division of AIDS, 404
Center for AIDS Research: Johns Hopkins University School of Medicine, 399
Center for Alcohol & Addiction Studies Brown University, 8200
Center for ALS and Related Diorders The Cleveland Clinic DepartmentOf Neurol, 1139
Center for Anxiety and Related Disorders at Boston University, 7095
Center for Anxiety and Traumatic Stress, 7099
Center for Blood Research Harvard Medical School/CBR, 405
Center for Cancer Survival, 2394
Center for Children with Chronic Illness and Disability, 10355
Center for Chronic Disease Prevention and Centers for Disease Control, 10356
Center for Chronic Disease Prevention and Health Promotion, 10624
Center for Developmental Disabilities, 10625
Center for Developmental Disabilities University of South Carolina, 10357
Center for Disabilities and Development, 3578
Center for Disability Resources, 10358
Center for Disease Control, 5560
Center for Disease Control and Prevention, 10359
Center for Donation & Transplantation, 9205
Center for Health Research, 10360
Center for Hearing and Communication, 4349

Center for Hearing Loss in Children Boystown National Research Hospital, 4370
Center for Human Nutrition, 6767
Center for Interdisciplinary Research in Immunology and Diseases at UCLA, 369
Center for Medical Consumers, 10361, 10510
Center for Mental Health Services, 7063
Center for Mind-Body Medicine, 7088
Center for Narcolepsy Research at the University of Illinois at Chicago, 7765
Center for Neurodevelopmental Studies, 1718
Center for Neuroimmunology: University of Alabama at Birmingham, 6431
Center for Organ Recovery & Education, 9216
Center for Parent Information & Resources, 1602, 3539, 4301, 10362
Center for Reconstructive Urology, 5299
Center for Research for Mothers & Children, 8841
Center for Research in Sleep Disorders Affiliated with Mercy Hospital, 7766
Center for Rheumatology, 7359
Center for Science in the Public Interest, 2153
Center for Sleep & Wake Disorders: Miami Valley Hospital, 7767
Center for Sleep Medicine of the Mount Sinai Medical Center, 7768
Center for Substance Abuse Prevention, 8678
Center for Substance Abuse Prevention Substance Abuse & Mental Health Services, 8113
Center for the Disabled, 2749
Center for the Study of Aging Newsletter, 198
Center for the Study of Anorexia and Bulimia, 3707
Center for the Study of Emotion and Attention, 7089
Center for the Study of Traumatic Stress, 7068, 7093
Center for Universal Design North Carolina State University, 10363
Center on Employment: Rochester Institute of Technology, 4302
Centers for AIDS Research: Albert Einstein College of Medicine, 413
Centers for AIDS Research: Baylor College of Medicine, 433
Centers for AIDS Research: Brown University, 429
Centers for AIDS Research: Case Western University, 424
Centers for AIDS Research: Columbia University College of Physicians, 414
Centers for AIDS Research: North-Central California, 370
Centers for AIDS Research: NYU School of Medicine, 415
Centers for AIDS Research: Univeristy of North Carolina at Chapel Hill, 423
Centers for AIDS Research: University of Alabama at Birmingham, 363
Centers for AIDS Research: University of California, Los Angeles, 372
Centers for AIDS Research: University of Colorado Health Sciences Center, 383
Centers for AIDS Research: University of Massachusetts Medical School, 406
Centers for AIDS Research: University of Pennsylvania, 425
Centers for AIDS Research: University of Washington, Harborview Medical Center, 436
Centers for AIDS Research: USCD Center for AIDS Research, 371
Centers for AIDS Research: Vanderbilt University Medical Center, 431
Centers for Disease Control, 7595, 10101
Centers for Disease Control & Prevention Hepatitis Branch, 5139
Centers for Disease Control & Prevention: Division of Adolescent & School Health, 635, 1380, 3540, 3672, 7569
Centers for Disease Control and Prevention, 2832, 9258
Centers for Disease Control and Prevention, 2897
Centers for Disease Control Division of Vector Borne Infectious Diseases, 9030
Centers for Medicare & Medicaid Services, 636, 1381, 3541, 3673, 4303, 5734, 7045, 7466
Central Arizona Chapter of the American Association of Kidney Patients, 5583

Central Association for the Blind and Visually Impaired, 9539
Central Brain Tumor Registry of the US, 1912
Central California Chapter National Multiple Sclerosis Society, 6350
Central California Chapter of the National Hemophilia Foundation, 4968
Central Florida Chapter, 6361
Central Institute for the Deaf, 4371
Central Louisiana State Hospital Medical and Professional Library, 6027
Central Maine Cystic Fibrosis Center, 3120
Central Missouri Regional Arthritis Center Stephen's College Campus, 1245
Central New Jersey Brain Tumor Support Group, 1998
Central New York Male Sexual Dysfunction Center, 5302
Central NY Area Support Group: National Ataxia Foundation, 1550
Central Ohio Chapter of the National Hemophilia Foundation, 4993
Central Ohio Support Group: National Ataxia Foundation, 1553
Central Oregon Brain Tumor Support Group, 2012
Central Rappahannock Regional Library, 9755
Central Texas Brain Tumor Support Group, 2028
Central Texas FFCMH, 6009
Central Texas Veterans Health Care System, 10244
Cerebral Blood Flow Laboratories Veterans Administration Medical Center, 8054
Cerebral Palsy, 2803
Cerebral Palsy Associations of New York State, 2750
Cerebral Palsy of Virginia, 2788
Cerebral Palsy: Facts & Figures, 2809
CF & Pediatric Pulmonary Care Center, 3146
CFIDS Association of America, 2896
CFIDS Chronicle, 2856
CFIDS in Children, 2867
CFIDS in Children Packet, 2835
CFIDS Membership Packet, 2866
CFS and Self-Esteem, 2886
CFS Cookbook, 2836
CFS in the Workplace, 2868
CFS: Addressing the Realities of a Chronic Illness, 2887
CFS: Unraveling the Mystery, 2888
Chadder, 1637
Challenge, 1638
Chalmers P. Wylie Ambulatory Care Center VA Central Ohio Healthcare System, 10213
Chapel Haven, 10504
Chapter Services at a Glance, 6463
Charles George VA Medical Center, 10208
Charlie Norwood VA Medical Center, 10139
Check Your Multiple Sclerosis Facts, 6464
Check Your Pulse, America: Atrial Fibrillation, 5278, 8083
CheckUp, 6734
Chef David's Kids, 10682
Chelsea: The Story of a Signal Dog, 4448
Chemical Dependency and the African American, 8515
Chemical Dependency Program Division Department of Human Services, 8163
Chemical Dependency: An Acceptable Disease, 8516
Chemically Dependent Older Adults, 8273
Chemotherapy and You: A Guide to Self-Help During Treatment, 2514
Chemotherapy Foundation, 2258
Chesapeake Area Support Group: National Ataxia Foundation, 1542
Chester County Association for the Blind, 9558
Chew or Snuff is Real Bad Stuff, 2515, 8517
Cheyenne VA Medical Center, 10269
Chicago Area Support Group: National Ataxia Foundation, 1537
Chicago Department of Public Health, 305
Chicago Lighthouse for People Who are Blind and Visually Impaired, 9494
Chicago Metro Support Group: National Ataxia Foundation, 1538
Chicagoland Chapter of the American Association of Kidney Patients, 5607
Child & Adolescent Behavioral Health, 6074

Child Center, 10364
Child Help, 7103
Child of Mine: Feeding with Love and Good Sense, 10536
Child with Epilepsy at Camp, 7527
A Child with Hearing Loss in Your Classroom? Don't Panic!, 4418
Child with Neurofibromatosis 1, 6691
Child with Prader-Willi Syndrome: Birth to Three, 7201
Childhood and Adolescent Drug Abuse: A Physician's Guide, 8274
Childhood Asthma, 1458
Childhood Asthma: A Guide for Parents, 1459
Childhood Asthma: A Matter of Control, 1460
Childhood Asthma: Learning to Manage, 1429
Childhood Brain Tumor Foundation Newsletter, 2051
Childhood Cancer Canada, 2100
Childhood Emergencies: What to Do A Quick Refrence Guide, 10537
Childhood Glaucoma: A Reference Guide for Families, 9839
Childhood Illnesses in Pregnancy: Chicken Pox & Fifth Disease, 1880
Childhood Liver Disease Research Network, 3083
Children & Adults with Attention Deficit /Hyperactivity Disorder, 1603
Children Affected by AIDS Foundation, 609
Children and Kidney Disease, 5692
Children and Seizures: Information for Babysitters, 7528
Children and the AIDS Virus: A Book for Children, Parents, and Teachers, 469
Children Living with Illness, 1933
Children of Aging Parents, 149
Children of Deaf Adults, 4411
Children of Vietnam Veterans: Complex Concerns and Innovative Solutions, 10300
Children with AIDS: Guidelines for Parents and Caregivers, 577
Children with Asthma: A Manual for Parents, 1420
Children with Autism, 1746
Children with Cerebral Palsy, 2798
Children with Disabilities: Understanding Sibling Issues, 4229
Children with Epilepsy, 7501
Children with Ostegogenesis Imperfecta: St raties to Enhance Performance, 6785
Children with Tourette Syndrome, 9086
Children with Tourette Syndrome: A Parent's Guide, 9087
Children's AIDS Fund International, 256
Children's Brain Tumor Foundation, 1905
Children's Brittle Bone Foundation, 6782
Children's Center for Cancer and Blood Disorders, 2371
Children's Gaucher Research Fund, 4024
Children's Heart Institute of Texas, 4871
Children's Heart Society, 4862
Children's Hemophilia Book, 5080
Children's Hospice International, 10365, 10691
Children's Hospital Hemophilia Treatment Center, 5018
Children's Hospital of Los Angeles, 3090
Children's Hospital of Orange County, 3087
Children's Hospital of Philadelphia, 3579
Children's Hospital Research Foundation, 2355
Children's Hydrocephalus Support Group, 5207
Children's Liver Alliance, 5801
Children's Liver Association for Support S ervices Newsletter, 5772, 5780
Children's Liver Association For Support Services (CLASS), 5735
Children's Lung Specialists, 3139
Children's Medical Services Program: Florida SIDS Program, 8725
Children's Mental Health Coalition of WNY, Inc., 5991
Children's Mercy Hospital Children's Mercy Hospitals & Clinics, 3135
Children's Motility Disorder Foundation, 3999
Children's National Medical Center, 10366
Children's Neurodevelopment Center, 3580
Children's Organ Transplant Association (COTA), 9165, 9240, 9244

Children's Rights Program, 4412
Children's Tumor Foundation, 6653, 6682
Children's Wish Foundation International, 10658
Children's Wish Foundation of Canada, 10683
Childrens Hospital at Oakland, 3091
Childrens Hospital Immunology Division Children's Hospital, 1400
Childrens Hospital Medical Center Cystic Fibrosis Center, 3126
Childrens Hospital of Philadelphia Hemophilia Program, 5019
Childrens Lung and Cystic Fibrosis Center, 3147
ChildTrauma Academy, 7081
Chillicothe VA Medical Center, 10214
Chiropractor's Self-Help Back and Body Book, 10538
ChiroWeb.com, 10626
Chlamydial Infection, 7584
Choice Magazine Listening, 9727
Choices for Work Program Goodwill Industries-Suncoast, 4089
Choices in Deafness, 4449
Choices: Realistic Alternatives in Cancer Treatment, 2433
Cholesterol and Stroke, 5279, 8084
Cholesterol and Your Heart, 4942
Choose the Right Long Term Care, 10539
Choosing a Pharmacy Service, 6465
Choosing A Spinal Cord Injury Rehabilitation Program, 8010
Choosing a Treatment for Kidney Failure, 5693
Chris Gets Ear Tubes, 4648
Christ Hospital Hepatitis C Support Group, 5147
Christian Horizons, 10367
Christian Resource for People Who Are Blind, 9710
Christopher Reeve Paralysis Foundation, 8033
Christus Santa Rosa Health System, 5020
Christy's Chance, 8412
Chronic Fatigue Syndrome & Fibromyalgia Support, 2833
Chronic Fatigue Syndrome & School Success, 2869
Chronic Fatigue Syndrome and the Yeast Connection, 2838
Chronic Fatigue Syndrome Cookbook: Delicious & Wellness-Enhancing Recipes, 2837
Chronic Fatigue Syndrome in Children, 2870
Chronic Fatigue Syndrome in Men, 2871
Chronic Fatigue Syndrome: A Pamphlet for Physicians, 2872
Chronic Fatigue Syndrome: For Those Who Care, 2889
Chronic Fatigue Syndrome: Information for Physicians, 2839
Chronic Fatigue Syndrome: Information, Relaxation/Healing Exercise, 2890
Chronic Fatigue Syndrome: The Limbic Hypothesis, 2840
Chronic Fatigue Syndrome: The Thief of Vitality, 2873
Chronic Fatigue: Your Complete Exercise Guide, 2841
Chronic Pain Association of Canada, 2913
Chronic Pain Letter, 10590
Chronic Physical Illness, 10540
Chronic Syndrome Sufferers Association, 7010
Chronic Viral Hepatitis Backgrounder, 5164
Chuck Baird, 4450
Church of the Nazarene, 9714
Cigarette Smoking, 8518
Cincinnati Association for the Blind, 9547
Cincinnati HPV Support Group: PP of Cincin nati, 10474
Cincinnati VA Medical Center, 10215
Circle of Hope, 8275
Cirrhosis: Many Causes, 5165
Citizen Advocacy of Burlington, 10490
Citizen's Alcohol and Other Drug Prevention Directory, 8276
City of Hope Comprehensive Cancer Research Center, 2275
City of Hope National Medical Center Beckman Research Institute, 2134
City of Hope National Medical Center Drug Discover/AIDS Group, 373

City University of New York Center for Research in Speech and Hearing, 4372
Civitan International Research Center, 4373
CKLS Headquarters, 9670
Classification of Impaired Vision, 9966
Classification of Tuberculosis and Other Mycobacterial Diseases, 9313
Classroom Notetaker, 4451
Clear Thinking About Alternative Therapies, 6466
Clearing the Air: A Guide to Quitting Smoking, 2516
Clearinghouse for Specialized Media and Translation, 9783
Clearinghouse on Disability Information Office of Special Education & Rehab Svcs, 10368
Cleft Lip & Palate, 1881
Clerc: The Story of His Early Years, 4649
Cleveland Clinic Lerner Research Institute, 4872
Cleveland Clinic Teaching Conference, 3986
Cleveland Hearing and Speech Center, 4374
Cleveland Sight Center, 9548
Cleveland Skilled Industries, 9549
Cleveland VA Medical Center VA Northeast Ohio Healthcare System, 10216
Client Assistance Program: Anchorage, 10431
Client Assistance Program: Delaware, 10438
Client Assistance Program: District of Columbia, 10439
Client Assistance Program: Iowa Division o n Persons with Disabilities, 10450
Client Assistance Program: Kentucky, 10452
Client Assistance Program: Maryland, 10455
Client Assistance Program: Massachusetts, 10456
Client Assistance Program: Michigan, 10459
Client Assistance Program: Nebraska Division of Rehabilitative Services, 10465
Client Assistance Program: Nevada, 10467
Client Assistance Program: New Hampshire, 10468
Client Assistance Program: North Dakota, 10473
Client Assistance Program: NY State Commission of Quality of Care, 10471
Client Assistance Program: Oklahoma Office of Handicapped Concerns, 10478
Client Assistance Program: Philadelphia, 10481
Client Assistance Program: Vermont Ladd Hall, 10491
Climbing Back, 7996
Clinic Directory, 7916
Clinical Care in the Rheumatic Disease, 1268
Clinical Counseling: Towards a Better Understanding of TS, 9136
Clinical Diabetes, 3494
Clinical Evaluation and Diagnostic Tests for Neuromuscular Disorders, 6522
Clinical Focus, 578
Clinical Focus on Primary Immune Deficiency Diseases, 354, 541, 579
Clinical Immunology, Allergy, and Rheumatology, 1401
Clinical Nutrition Research Unit (CNRU), 6768
Clinical Perspectives in Gastroenterology, 3952
Clinical Practice Recommendations, 3414
Clinical Presentation of the Primary Immunodeficiency Diseases, 580
Clinical Research Center Northwestern Center for Clinical Researc, 396
Clinical Research Center: Pediatrics Children's Hospital Research Foundation, 5767
Clinical Thyroidology, 9012
Clinical Thyroidology for Patients, 9014
Clinical Trial Fact Sheet, 2056
Clinical Trials in Multiple Sclerosis: Searching for New Therapies, 6498
Clinical Trials: Talking it Over, 581
Clinical Updates, 3967
Closer Look: The English Program at the Model Secondary School for the Deaf, 4452
Closing the Gap, 10587
Clotting Agents Are Lifesavers, 5103
Clovernook Center for the Blind and Visually Impaired, 9784
Club Foot and Other Foot Deformities, 1882
Clubhouse Kids Learn About Asthma, 1430
Cluster Headache: Fact Sheet, 6310
Cluster Headaches, 6329
CME Video Library, 7738

Co-Ad, 10446
Coalition for Advanced Cancer Treatment and Prevention, 2101
Coalition Index, 7404
Coalition of Voluntary Mental Health Agencies, 6176
Coatesville VA Medical Center, 10225
Cocaine, 8413
Cocaine Anonymous, 8679
Cocaine Anonymous World Services, 8114
Cocaine Today, 8277
Cochlear Implant Auditory Training Guidebook, 4453
Cochlear Implantation for Infants and Children, 4454
Coconut Creek Eating Disorders Support Group, 3713
Code V, 3968
Codependent No More, 8278
Cognition, Education and Deafness, 4455
Cognitive Neurology and Alzheimer's Disease Center, 960
COGREHAB, 1642
Colin and Ricky, 3645
Collaborative Medicine Center, 2395
Colmery-O'Neil VA Medical Center VA Eastern Kansas Health Care System, 10155
Colon and Rectal Surgery, 3049
Color of Light, 8279
Colorado Brain Tumor Support Group, 1947
Colorado Cancer Research Program, 2288
Colorado Chapter National Hemophilia Foun dation, 4972
Colorado Chapter of the American Association of Kidney Patients, 5591
Colorado FFCMH, 5934
Colorado Parkinson Foundation, 6881
Colorado SIDS Program, 8714
Colorado Talking Book Library, 9626
Colordao Department of Health and Environment, 8715
Colorectal Cancer Canada, 2102
Colorectal Cancer: A Compassionate Resource for Patients and Their Families, 2434
Coloring Book on Thalassemia, 2978
Columbia Lighthouse for the Blind, 9481
Columbia Presbyterian Medical Center Neurological Institute, 6514
Columbia University Clinical Research Center for Muscular Dystrophy, 6515
Columbia University Complete Home Guide to Mental Health, 6208
Columbia University Comprehensive Cancer Center, 2344
Columbia University Irving Center for Clinical Research Adult Unit, 4873
Columbia University Robert N. Butler Aging Center, 117
Columbia University: Comprehensive Sickle Cell Center, 7613
Columbia VA Health Care System, 10233
Columbus Center of the National Multiple Sclerosis Society, 6401
Columbus Children's Hospital: Cystic Fibrosis Center, 3155
Columbus Children's Research Institute, 658
Columbus Library for Accessible Services (CLASS), 9648
Come Sign With Us, 4789
Come Sign with Us: Sign Language Activities for Children, 4650
Comer Children's Hospital at the Universit, 3107
Comer Children's Hospital at the University of Chicago, 3106
Coming Home: A Discharge Manual for Families of Persons with a Brain Injury, 4194
Commentary on Alternative Therapies for TS, 9098
Commission for the Blind, 10460
Commission on Accreditation of Rehabilitation Facilities, 26, 10627
Commitment, 3189
Committee of Ten Thousand, 257, 610
Common Questions About Porphyria, 3977
Common Voice for Pierce County Parents, 6084
Commonwealth Cancer Help Program, 2396
Communicate with Me: Conversation Skills for Deaf Students, 4456

Communicating with People Who Have Trouble Hearing & Seeing: A Primer, 9967
Communication Access for Persons with Hearing Loss, 4457
Communication and Adult Hearing Loss, 4461
Communication Disorders Following Traumatic Brain Injury, 4195
Communication Issues Among Deaf People, 4458
Communication Issues Among Deaf People: Eyes, Hands and Voices, 4459
Communication Rules for Hard of Hearing People, 4460
Communication Skills, 8519
Communication Skills for Visually Impaired, 9840
Communication Skills in Children with Down Syndrome, 3609
Communication Unbound: How Facilitated Communication Is Challenging Views, 1747
Community Access, 6177
Community Access, Inc., 5911
Community Campaign Brochure, 8520
Community Health Funding Report, 542
Community Mental Health Foundation, 5986
Community Service Delivery for Children with HIV Infection and Families, 470
Community Services for Autistic Adults & Children, 1665, 1813
COMPASS Program, 445
Compassion Books Catalog, 10730
Compassion Books, Inc., 6147, 6230, 10724
Compassionate Friends, 8699, 8842, 10692, 10740
Complete Bedside Companion: No-Nonsense Advice to Caring for the Seriously Ill, 1155
Complete Book of Children's Allergies, 676
Complete Guide to Alzheimer's Proofing Your Home, 1002
Complete IEP Guide: How to Advocate for Your Special Ed Child, 7917
Complete Mental Health Directory, 6091
Complete Weight Loss Workbook, 3415
Complexities of TS Treatment: A Physician's Round Table, 9137
Comprehensive Care, 5104
Comprehensive Clinical Management of the Epilepsies, 7550
Comprehensive Gaucher Treatment Center at Tower Hematology Oncology, 4025
Comprehensive Hemophilia Diagnostic and Treatment Center, 5021
Comprehensive Pediatric Hemophilia Center University of South Florida, 5022
Comprehensive Services for Persons with Hemophilia, 5105
Comprehensive Sickle Cell Center Children's Hospital Research Foundation, 7614
Comprehensive Signed English Dictionary, 4462
Comprehensive Stroke Center of Oregon University of Oregon Health Sciences Cen, 8055
Compulsive Overeaters in the Military, 6742
Compulsive Overeating & Overaters Anonymous, 6743
Computer Planned Menus for Health Professionals, 3416
Computer-Related Repetitive Strain Injury, 2619
Concentrate, 5090
Concept Development for Visually Impaired Children: Resource Guide, 9841
Conception, Pregnancy & Psoriasis, 7700
Concerned Parent Coalition, 6086
Concerning Death: A Practical Guide for the Living, 10707
Condoms and Sexually Transmitted Diseases, Especially AIDS, 582
Conference Audiotapes, 2076
Confronting Alzheimer's Disease, 1003
Confronting the Challenges of Spina Bifida, 7918
Confusion is a State of Grace, 8280
Congenital Heart Defects, 4943
Congenital Heart Disease, 4925
Congenital Heart Disease Anomalies Support, Education & Resources CHASER, 4874
Congratulations: An Introduction to Down Syndrome for Parents/Family/Friends, 3646
Connecticut Alcohol and Drug Abuse Commission, 8144

Connecticut Brain Tumor Support Group, 1948
Connecticut Chapter of the Myasthenia Gravis Foundation of America, 6575, 6583, 6595, 6598
Connecticut Department of Health Services AIDS Programs, 297
Connecticut Down Syndrome Congress, 3557
Connecticut Nutmeg, 6635
Connecticut Pregnancy Exposure Information Service, 1852
Connecticut SIDS Alliance, 8716
Connecticut State Library for the Blind and Physically Handicapped, 9627
Conquer, 6636
Conquering Asthma, 1421
Conquering Headache, 6296
Conquering Infertility: A Guide for Couples, 5449
Consumer Bill of Rights and Responsibilities for Healthcare Service, 5106
Consumer Fact Sheet, 3190
Consumer Guide to Health Care Plans, 1461
Consumer Handbook on Dizziness and Vertigo, 4463
Consumer's Guide to Cancer Drugs, 2435
Consumer's Guide to Hearing Aids, 4757
Consumer's Guide to Insurance, 5450
Consumer's Guide to TS Medications, 9099
Consumer's Legal Guide to Today's Health Care, 5451
Continuing Care Retirement Community Directory, 160
Control Diabetes the Easy Way, 3417
Control Your Pain!, 8949
Controlling Asthma, 1439
Controlling Spasticity, 6467
Convenience Food Facts, 3418
Convention of American Instructors of the Deaf, 4304
Conversational Sign Language II: An Intermdiate Advanced Manual, 4464
Conversations At Midnight, 10708
Conversations with Anorexics, 3727
Cook Children's Medical Center: Cystic Fibrosis Clinic, 3169
Cooking a la Heart, 3419
Cooking for the Allergic Child, 677
Cooley's Anemia Foundation, 2972
Cooley's Anemia Foundation (CAF): Buffalo, 2965
Cooley's Anemia Foundation (CAF): California, 2959
Cooley's Anemia Foundation (CAF): Capital Area, 2961
Cooley's Anemia Foundation (CAF): Illinois Oakbrook Towers, 2960
Cooley's Anemia Foundation (CAF): Long Island, 2966
Cooley's Anemia Foundation (CAF): Massachusetts Chapter, 2962
Cooley's Anemia Foundation (CAF): New Jersey Chapter, 2963
Cooley's Anemia Foundation (CAF): Queens, 2967
Cooley's Anemia Foundation (CAF): Rochester, 2964
Cooley's Anemia Foundation (CAF): Staten Island, 2968
Cooley's Anemia Foundation (CAF): Suffolk Chapter Office, 2969
Cooley's Anemia Foundation (CAF): Texas, 2971
Cooley's Anemia Foundation (CAF): Westches ter/Rockland Chapter, 2970
Cooperative Gluten-Free Commercial Products Listing, 2636
COPIN Foundation, 10272
Coping Skills, 2874
Coping When You or a Friend is HIV-Positive, 471
Coping with a Drug-Abusing Parent, 8419
Coping with ADD/ADHD, 1620
Coping with Asthma, 1422
Coping With CFS, 2842
Coping with Codependency, 8414
Coping with Crohn's and Colitis is Tough, 3060
Coping with Depression, 8415
Coping with Depression and Mood Disorders, 6209
Coping with Drinking and Driving, 8416
Coping with Eating Disorders, 3728
Coping with Endometriosis, 3809
Coping with Infertility, 5553
Coping with Lupus, 8931
Coping with Lyme Disease: A Practical Guide, 9039
Coping with Mental Illness in the Family, 6161

Coping with Parkinson's Disease, 6932
Coping with Peer Pressure, 8417
Coping with Sarcoidosis, 7264
Coping with Stress, 8418
Coping with the Holidays, 5514
Coping with Tourette Syndrome in Early Adulthood, 9102
Coping with TS in the Classroom, 9100
Coping with TS, A Parent's Viewpoint, 9101
Coping with Vision Loss, 9842
Coping with Your Loved One's Brain Tumor, 2057
Coping: A Young Woman's Guide to Breast Cancer Prevention, 2436
COPLINE, 7102
Cornelia de Lange Syndrome Foundation, Inc, 1834
Cornell University: Winifred Masterson Burke Medical Research-Dementia, 961
Cornerstone Medical Arts Center Hospital, 8201
Corporal Michael J. Crescenz VA Medical Center, 10226
Corporate Angel Network, 2397
CORPUS, 538
Corticosteriod Medications, 1318
Cosmetics & Skin Care, 7701
COTT News, 539
Cott Washington Update, 543
Council for Exceptional Children, 1604, 1666, 1826, 3542, 9420
Council for Learning Disabilities (CLD), 10369
Council of Citizens with Low Vision International, 9421
Council of Families with Visual Impairment, 9629, 10061
Counseling Head Injured Patients: Guidelines for Community Health Workers, 4230
Countdown, 3487
Countdown to a Cure, 5107
County of Los Angeles Public Health: Division of HIV And STD Programs, 292
Courage to Be Me: Living with Alcoholism, 8281
Courage: Poems & Positive Thoughts for Stroke Survivors, 5264, 8068
Court-Related Needs of the Elderly and Persons with Disabilities, 161, 1004
CPPD Crystal Deposition Disease, 1317
Crack, 8521
Crack Cocaine: The Big Lie, 8522
Crack Down on Drugs, 8420
Creating a Circle of Learning: The Church and the Mentally Ill, 6093
Creating New Options, 6092
Creative Community Services (CCS), 10506
Creative Movements for Older Adults, 162
Creighton University Allergic Disease Center, 659
Creighton University Cardiac Center, 4875
Creighton University Midwest Hypertension Research Center, 5253
Crib Death: The Sudden Infant Death Syndrome, 8824
Crime Survivors, 7104
Critical Path AIDS Project, 516
Crohn's & Colitis Foundation, 3039, 3072, 9384, 9396
Crohn's Disease, 3061
Crohn's Disease and Ulcerative Colitis Fact Book, 3043
Crohn's Disease, Ulcerative Colitis and Your Child, 3071
Crohn's Disease, Ulcerative Colitis, and School, 3053
Crossing the Line Between Social Drinking and Alcoholism, 8523
CSA/USA Cookbook Series, 2635
CSAP State Liason Program, 8677
CTD Resource Network, 2617
CUED Speech Resource Book for Parents of Deaf Children, 4446
Cult of Thinness, 3729
Culture and the Restructuring of Community Mental Health, 6094
CUNY: Teratogen Information Service, 1851
Cure Our Children Foundation, 10659
Current Approaches to Down's Syndrome, 3610
Current Pharmacology of TS, 9103
Cutaneous Melanoma of the Head and Neck, 2517
Cutting Edge Medical Report, 7440

Cyclic Vomiting Syndrome Association, 3923, 4000
Cystic Fibrosis Canada, 3084
Cystic Fibrosis Care and Teaching Center Children's Medical Center, 3170
Cystic Fibrosis Center St. Vincent's Hospital & Medical Center, 3148
Cystic Fibrosis Center: All Children's Hospital, 3101
Cystic Fibrosis Center: Cedars-Sinai Medical Center, 3092
Cystic Fibrosis Center: Childrens Memorial Hospital, 3108
Cystic Fibrosis Center: National Institute of Health NIDDK, 3123
Cystic Fibrosis Center: Park Ridge Lutheran General Children's Hospital, 3109
Cystic Fibrosis Center: Phoenix Childrens Hospital, 3088
Cystic Fibrosis Center: Polyclinic Medical Center, 3161
Cystic Fibrosis Center: University of California at San Francisco, 3093
Cystic Fibrosis Foundation, 3086, 3124
Cystic Fibrosis Research, 3094
Cystic Fibrosis Worldwide, 3085
Cystic Fibrosis-Lung Disease Center: Santa Rosa Children's Hospital, 3171
Cystic Fibrosis: A Guide for Parents, 3191
Cystic Fibrosis: A Guide for Patient and Family, 3183
Cystic Firbrosis Center: Tufts New England Medical Center, 3127

D

Daddy's Girl, 3647
Daily Reflections: A Book of Reflections by AA Members for AA Members, 8282
Dallas Lighthouse for the Blind, 9580
Dallas/Ft.Worth Metroplex HPV Support Group, 10487
Dana Alliance for Brain Initiatives, 4130
Dana Farber Cancer Institute National Drug Discovery Group for AIDS Treatment, 407
Dana-Farber Institute: Department of Biostatistics and Computational Biology, 2322
Dancing Against the Darkness: A Journey Through America in the Age of AIDS, 472, 501
Dancing Cheek to Cheek, 9968
Dancing Without Music, 4465
Dano Cerebral: Guia Para Familias y Cuidadores, 4196
Darker Side of Tanning, 7702
Dartmouth Medical School: Microbiology Department, 3800
Dartmouth-Hitchcock Medical Center - Genetics and Development, 3581
David Baldwin's Trauma Information Pages, 7147
David H. Koch Institute for Integrative Ca ncer Research, 2323
David T Siegel Institute for Communicative Disorders, 4375
A Day At A Time, 2810
Day at a Time: Daily Reflections for Recovering People, 8283
Day by Day, 8284
A Day in the Life of a Child, 3985
Day We Met Cindy, 4651
Days of Healing, Days of Joy, 8285
Dayton VA Medical Center, 10217
DC Department of Health Maternal and Family Health Administration, 8719
DC Public Library Adaptive Services Division, 9630
DC Threshold Alliance for the Mentally Ill, 5943
de Tornyay Center For Healthy Aging at University of Washington, 145
Deadly Diet: Recovering from Anorexia & Bulimia, 3730
Deaf and Hard of Hearing Individuals, 4478
Deaf Artists of America, 4732
Deaf Association of Wyoming, 4359
Deaf Children in Public Schools Placement, Context, and Consequences, 4466
Deaf Children Signers, 4790
Deaf Culture Autobiographies, 4791
Deaf Culture Series, 4792

Deaf Culture Videotapes, 4758
Deaf Culture, Our Way, 4467
Deaf Culture: Suggested Readings, 4759
Deaf Empowerment, Emergence, Struggle and
	Rhetoric, 4468
Deaf Episcopalian, 4733
Deaf Heritage: A Narrative History of Deaf America,
	4469
Deaf Heritage: Student Text and Workbook, 4470
Deaf History Unveiled: Interpretations from the New
	Scholarship, 4471
Deaf in America: Voices from a Culture, 4479
Deaf Life, 4706
Deaf Like Me, 4472
Deaf Mosaic Series, 4793
Deaf President Now! The 1988 Revolution at
	Gallaudet University, 4473
Deaf Sport: The Impact of Sports Within the Deaf
	Community, 4474
Deaf Sports Review, 4707
Deaf Students and the School-to-Work Transition,
	4475
Deaf Studies Curriculum Guide, 4476
Deaf USA, 4708
Deaf Women: A Parade Through the Decades, 4477
Deaf Work, 4734
Deaf-Blind American, 4709
DeafEd.net, 4836
Deafness and Child Development, 4480
Deafness: 1993-2013, 4481
Deafness: A Fact Sheet, 4760
Deafness: A Personal Account, 4482
Deafness: An Autobiography, 4483
Deafness: Historical Perspectives, 4484
Deafness: Life and Culture II, 4485
Deafpride Advocate, 4735
Dealing with Mental Incapacity, 6095
Dean A McGee Eye Institute, 9785
Death and the Quest for Meaning, 10709
Death Be Not Proud: A Memoir, 2042
Death: The Final Stage of Growth, 10710
Deenie, 7409
Deep Brain Stimulation for Parkinson's Disease, 6953
Delaware Assocation for the Blind Department of
	Health & Social Services, 9479
Delaware County Branch of the Pennsylvania
	Association for the Blind, 9559
Delaware Department of Health and Social: Services
	HIV Prevention Program, 298
Delaware Division of Alcoholism, Drug Abuse and
	Mental Health, 8145
Delaware Division of Libraries: Library for the Blind
	and Physically Handicapped, 9628
Delaware FFMCH, 5941
Delaware Valley Chapter of the National Hemophilia
	Foundation, 4999
Delicate Balance: Living Successfully with Chronic
	Illness, 3872
Delware Valley Brain Tumor Support Group at
	Jefferson, 2017
Dementia Care Practice Recommendations Phases 1
	and 2, 1044
Denial, 8524
Dental Care for the Patient with Parkinson's Disease,
	6954
Dental Tips for Diabetics, 3499
Dental Treatment of Patients with Gilles de la
	Tourette Syndrome, 9104
Dentists Concerned for Dentists, 8164, 8680
Denver Childrens Hospital, 3097
Denver Support Group: National Ataxia Foundation,
	1532
Department of Alcohol and Drug Programs, 8142
Department of Alcoholism and Substance Abuse,
	8151
Department of Epidemiology and Health Policy
	Research: University of Florida, 387
Department of Health, 8172
Department of Health and Human Services, 8720
Department of Health and Welfare Department Of
	Health And Welfare, 8150
Department of Human Services, 8745
Department of Institutions, Alcohol and Drug Abuse
	Division, 8168

Department of Mental Health and Mental Retardation,
	Alcohol & Drug Service, 8186
Department of Ophthalmology Information Line,
	9813
Department of Pediatrics Medical College of Georgia,
	3104
Department of Pediatrics, Division of Rheumatology,
	1246
Department of Public Health and Human Services,
	8763
Department of Public Health: Adult and Child Health
	Division, 8741
Department of Public Health: Division of Substance
	Abuse and Health, 8155
Department of Public Instruction: Division of
	Alcoholism and Drug Abuse, 8169
Department of Reproductive Genetics: Magee
	Women's Hospital, 1838
Department of Social Services: Division of Substance
	Abuse, 8188
Department of State Health Offices, 8792
Departments of Neurology & Neurosurgery:
	University of California, San Francisco, 8056
Depression and Bipolar Support Alliance, 6206
Depression and Dementia in Parkinson's Disease,
	6955
Depression and its Treatment, 6211
Depression and Recovery from Chemical
	Dependency, 8525
Depression is a Treatable Illness: A Patients Guide,
	6232
Depression Sourcebook, 6210
Depressive Illnesses: Treatments Bring New Hope,
	6212
Derma Doctor, 7746
Dermatitis Herpetiformis, 2646
Dermatology Focus, 7692
Dermatology Foundation, 2259, 7661, 7747
Dermatology World, 7693
Desert Storm Justice Foundation: Florida, 10128
Desert Storm Justice Foundation: Illinois, 10145
Desert Storm Justice Foundation: Minnesota, 10177
Desert Storm Veterans of Florida, Inc., 10129
Desferal Q&A, 2981
Design of Rehabilitation Services in Psychiatric
	Hospital Settings, 6096
Designs on Life, 5452
Destination Unlimited, 10032
Detaching with Love, 8526
Detachment, 8527
Detroit Subregional Library for the Blind and
	Physically Handicapped, 9695
Detroit Support Group: National Ataxia Foundation,
	1544
Developing a Functional and Longitudinal Individual
	Plan, 1786
Developing Chemical Dependency Services for Black
	People, 8286
Developing Cognition in Young Children Who are
	Deaf, 4761
Developing IEPs Under the New Idea Regulations,
	1797
Developing Support Groups for Individuals with
	Early-Stage Alzheimer's Disease, 1005
Development of Behavioral and Emotional Problems
	in TS, 9105
Development of Social Skills by Blind and Visually
	Impaired Students, 9843
Developmental Delays and Developmental Disorders,
	8825
Developmental Evaluation Clinic, 3582
Developmental Medicine Center (DMC), 3583
Developmental Medicine Center Children's Hospital
	Boston, 408
Diabetes, 3478, 3488
Diabetes & Exercise Video, 3517
Diabetes & Pregnancy: What to Expect, 3420
Diabetes A to Z, 3421
Diabetes Action Network for the Blind, 3210
Diabetes Advisor, 3495
Diabetes and Brief Illness, 3501
Diabetes and Exercise, 3502
Diabetes and Kidney Disease, 5694
Diabetes Care, 3489
Diabetes Care Made Easy, 3422

Diabetes Control Program, 3369
Diabetes Dateline, 3496, 3500
Diabetes Dictionary, 3526
Diabetes Education and Research Center The Franklin
	House, 3380
Diabetes Education Goals, 3423
Diabetes Educator, 3497
Diabetes Exercise, 3527
Diabetes Forecast, 3490
Diabetes in Pregnancy, 3503
Diabetes Low-Fat & No-Fat Meals in Minutes, 3424
Diabetes Medical Nutrition Therapy, 3425
Diabetes Mellitus: A Practical Handbook, 3426
Diabetes Research and Training Center: University of
	Alabama at Birmingham, 3381
Diabetes Self-Management, 3427
Diabetes Society, 3408
Diabetes Society of Santa Clara Valley, 3224
Diabetes Sourcebook, 3428
Diabetes Spectrum: From Research to Practice, 3491
Diabetes Teaching Guide for People Who Use Insulin,
	3429
Diabetes Youth Curriculum: A Toolbox for Educators,
	3430
Diabetes Youth Foundation of Indiana, 3260
Diabetes, Vision Impairment and Blindness, 9969
Diabetes: A Guide to Living Well, 3431
Diabetes: Your Complete Exercise Guide, 3432
Diabetes: Your Questions Answered, 3433
Diabetic Foot Care, 3504
Diabetic Gourmet, 3434
Diabetic Retinopathy, 9970
Diabetic's Guide to Health and Fitness, 3435
Diabetics Action Network, 9422
Diagnosis and Treatment, 5166
Diagnosis and Treatment of Old Age, 163
Diagnosis and Treatment of Unilateral Hearing Loss,
	4794
Diagnosis Autism: Now What? 10 Steps to Improve
	Treatment Outcomes, 1748
Diagnosis Parkinson's Disease: You Are Not Alone,
	6956, 6995
Dial-a-Hearing Screening Test, 4413
Dialogue Magazine, 9907
Dialogue with Doris, 7309
Dialysis Patient: An Informative Guide for the
	Dentist, 5695
Dictionary for Brain Tumor Patients, 2058
Did You Grow Up with a Problem Drinker?, 8528
Diet and Arthritis, 1319
Diet and Headache: Fact Sheet, 6311
Diet and Nutrition in Porphyria, 3978
Diet and Your Liver, 5786
Diet Guide for the CAPD Patient, 5696
Diet Guide for the Hemodialysis Patient, 5697
Diet, Nutrition and Cancer Prevention: A Guide to
	Food Choices, 2519
Diet, Nutrition and Cancer Prevention: The Good
	News, 2518
Dietary Considerations for Parkinson's Disease
	Patients, 6957
Dietary Guidelines for Americans 2005, 6724
Diets to Help Gluten and Wheat Allergy, 678, 2637
Difference in the Family, 10711
Differences in Common: Straight Talk on Mental
	Retardation/Down Syndrome, 3611
Different Like Me: A Book for Teens Who Worry
	About Their Parents' Using, 8421
Differential Diagnosis of Parkinsonism, 6958
Digestive Disease National Coalition, 3924
Digestive Disorders Associates Ridgely Oaks
	Professional Center, 3941
Digestive Health Matters, 3050, 3953, 5346
Dilemma of the Alcoholic Marriage, 8287
Dilemmas of Providing Help in a Crisis: The Role of
	Friends & Parents, 2520
Dimensions of State Mental Health Policy, 6097
Dinosaur Tamer, 3479
Dioxin, A Case in Point, 10301
Direct and Indirect Costs of Diabetes in the US, 3436
Directory of Alzheimer's Disease Treatment Facilities
	& Home Health Care, 1006
Directory of Auditory-Oral Programs, 4486
Directory of Health Grants, 10541

Directory of National Genetic Voluntary Organizations, 1565
Directory of Neurosurgeons Who Treat Adults, 5221
Directory of Pediatric Neurosurgeons, 5222
Directory of Radio Reading Services, 9971
Directory of Social Service Grants, 10542
Disability and Chronic Fatigue Syndrome, 2843
Disability Careers, 10435
Disability Law & Advocacy Center of Tennessee, 10486
Disability Law: A Legal Primer, 7265
Disability Packet, 2875
Disability Resource Center of Montgomery County Public Libraries, 9687
Disability Rights California, 10434
Disability Rights Center at Ohio Legal Rights Service, 10475
Disability Rights Center of Arkansas, 10433
Disability Rights Center of Kansas, 10451
Disability Rights Center: Maine, 10454
Disability Rights Montana, 10464
Disability Rights New Jersey, 10469
Disability Rights Texas, 10488
Disability Rights: Florida, 10441
Disability Workbook for Social Security Disability Applicants, 8932
Disabled & Alone/Life Services for the Handicapped, 10628
Disabled & Alone: Life Services for the Handicapped, 10370
Disabled American Veterans Organization, 10124
Disabled Woman's Guide to Pregnancy and Birth, 10543
Discipline and the Child with TS, 9106
Discipline Under the New Idea: Practical Methods and Procedures, 1798
Discoveries, 5347
Discovering Sign Language, 4487
Discovery Book, 2799
Discovery Circles, 5265, 8069
Discovery Health, 2937, 10629
Diseases of the Colon and Rectum, 2481
Dissociation, 6272
Distance Education and Training Council, 10371
District Board of Health: Mahoning County, 8780
District of Columbia Public Library Librarian for the Deaf Community, 9606
Division for the Visually Handicapped, 9756
Division of Addiction Services Department of Mental Health, 8154
Division of Alcohol & Drug Abuse: Mississippi, 8165
Division of Alcohol & Drug Abuse: South Dakota, 8185
Division of Alcohol & Drug Abuse: South Department of Mental Health, 8166
Division of Alcoholism & Drug Abuse: Department of Human Services, 8177
Division Of Developmental and Behavioral Pediatrics, 1839
Division of Diabetes Translation, 3370
Division of Digestive & Liver Diseases of Cloumbia University, 3708
Division of Mental Illness and Substance Abuse Community Programs, 8137
Division of Narcotic and Drug Abuse Control, 8173
Division of Perinatal Systems Mills Jarret Complex, 8788
Division of Rehabilitation Service, 10444
Division of Rehabilitation: Montgomery, 10430
Division of Substance Abuse, 8161
Division of Substance Abuse Services, 8175
Division of Substance Abuse: Department of Mental Health and Hospitals, 8157, 8183
Division of Vocational Rehabilitation and Services for the Blind, 9489
Division on Endocrinology Northwestern University Feinberg School, 3382
Division TEACCH University of North Carolina at Chapel H, 1719
Do it Now Foundation, 8202
Do the Right Thing: Get a Mammogram, 2521
Do You Hear That?, 4795
Do You Think You're Different?, 8529
Doctor's Guide to Chronic Fatigue Syndrome, 2844

Doctor, I Can't Sleep: Insomnia Training Manual, 7821
Does Anyone Die of AIDS Anymore?, 601
Does Your Child Have Epilepsy?, 7502
Dogs for Better Lives, 1667, 4305
Don't Feel Sorry for Paul, 1872
Don't Let Your Dreams Go Up in Smoke, 8530
Don't Lose a Friend to Drugs, 8531
Don't Lose Sight of Age-Related Macular Degeneration, 9972
Don't Lose Sight of Cataracts, 9973
Don't Lose Sight of Glaucoma, 9974
Donate Life America, 9166, 9245
Donor Alliance, 9182
Donor Insemination, 5515
Donor Network of Arizona, 9176
Dorothea Dix Hospital Clinical Research Unit, 8203
Dotty the Dalmatian has Epilepsy, 7521
Douglas Tilden, the Man and His Legacy, 4488
Down Syndrome, 3635, 3658
Down Syndrome Association of Atlanta, 3560
Down Syndrome Association of Greater Cinci nnati, 3567, 3599
Down Syndrome Association of Hampton Roads, 3571
Down Syndrome Association of Los Angeles, 3555
Down Syndrome Association of Middle Tennessee, 3568
Down Syndrome Association of Minnesota, 3565
Down Syndrome Association of Wisconsin, 3572
Down Syndrome Center of Western Pennsylvania, 3584
Down Syndrome Clinic of Houston, 3585
Down Syndrome Guild of Dallas, 3569
Down Syndrome News, 3630
Down Syndrome Today, 3631
Down Syndrome, Papers and Abstracts for Professionals, 3628
Down Syndrome: A Review of Current Knowledge, 3612
Down Syndrome: An Update and Review for Primary Care Physicians, 3613
Down Syndrome: See the Potential, 3648
Down Syndrome: The Facts, 3614
Dr. Bernstein's Diabetes Solution, 3437
Dr. Bob and the Good Oldtimers, 8288
Dr. Dean Ornish's Program for Reversing Heart Disease, 4926
Dr. Gertrude A Barber National Institute, 3586
Dream Come True, 10660
Dream Factory, Inc., 10661
Dream Foundation, 10662
Dreams Come True, 10684
Dreams for Seniors Charity Inc, 10685
Drinking Alcohol During Pregnancy, 8532
Driving and the Parkinson's Disease Patient: Some Considerations, 6959
Driving Force: A Story of Life, 1171
Drug Abuse and Addiction Information/Treatment Programs, 8289
Drug Abuse Resistance Education of America, 8115
Drug Abuse Update, 8465
Drug Abuse: The Impact on Society, 8422
Drug and Alcohol Programs Department Of Health, 8182
Drug Free Workplace Hotline, 8242
Drug Free Zones: A Manual, 8533
Drug Use Among American High School Seniors, College Students & Youth, 8290
Drug-Free Workplace Educator, 8469
Drugs and AIDS, 8423
Drugs and Anger, 8424
Drugs and Depression, 8425
Drugs and Domestic Violence, 8426
Drugs and Porphyria, 3979
Drugs and Pregnancy, 8534
Drugs and Pregnancy: It's Not Worth the Risk, 8291
Drugs and Your Friends, 8427
Drugs and Your Parents, 8428
Drugs in the Body: Effects of Abuse, 8429
Drugs That Have Been Used for the Treatment of Sarcoidosis, 7266
Dry Eyes? Dry Mouth? Dry Nose? Arthritis? If Two or More: Sjogren's Syndrome, 7645
Dual Diagnosis, 8292

Dual Diagnosis of Major Mental Illness and Substance Disorder, 6098
Dual Diagnosis: Substance Abuse and Mental Illness, 6162
Dual Disorders, 8293
Dual Disorders Recovery Book, 8294
Duke Asthma, Allergy and Airway Center, 1402
Duke Comprehensive Cancer Center, 2352
Duke Pediatric Brain Tumor Family Support Program, 2006
Duke University Center for the Advanced Study of Epilepsy, 7491
Duke University Center for the Study of Aging and Human Development, 118, 962
Duke University Clinical Research Institute, 963
Duke University Pediatric Cardiac Catheterization Laboratory, 4876
Duke University Plastic Surgery Research Laboratories, 7667
Duluth Lighthouse for the Blind, 9519
Duluth Public Library, 9708
Dunshee House, 447
Durham VA Health Care System, 10209
Dursban Report, 1869
DVH Quarterly, 9923
Dwarf Athletic Association of America, 4042
Dwight D. Eisenhower VA Medical Center VA Eastern Kansas Health Care System, 10156
Dying and Disabled Children, 10712

E

E is for Exercise, 4944
Each Day a New Beginning, 8295
Ear and Hearing, 4762
Ear Book, 4489
EAR Foundation, 4306, 4837
Ear Gear: A Student Workbook on Hearing and Hearing Aids, 4490
Early Childhood Technical Assistance Center, 1827, 3543
Early Focus: Working with Young Children Who Are Blind or Visually Impaired, 9844
Early Menopause (Premature Ovarian Failure), 5516
Early Years, 7202
Early-Onset Alzheimer's: I'M Too Young to Have Alzheimer's Disease, 1045
Early-Stage Alzheimer's: If You Have Alzheimer's Disease What You Should Know, 1046
East Central Florida Chapter of the Myasthenia Gravis Foundation of America, 6637
East Lansing Cystic Fibrosis Center Michigan State University, 3130
East Orange Campus VA New Jersey Health Care System, 10194
East Texas Lighthouse for the Blind, 9581
Eastern Cooperative Oncology Group, 2365
Eastern Michigan Hemophilia Center St. Joseph Hospital, 5023
Eastern Virginia Medical School Children's Hospital of The King's Daught, 3176
Easterseals, 1828, 2668, 7862
Easterseals UCP North Carolina & Virginia, 2763
Easy & Elegant Entrees, 3438
Easy Food Tips for Heart Healthy Eating, 4945
Easy-to-Swallow, Easy-to-Chew Cookbook, 1156
Eat Well, But Wisely, 4946
Eating Defensively: Food Safety Advice for Persons with AIDS, 583
Eating Diorders Resource Catalogue, 3731
Eating Disorder Resource Center, 3714
Eating Disorder Sourcebook, 3732
Eating Disorders Anonymous, 3674
Eating Disorders Association of New Jersey, 3715
Eating Disorders Coalition for Research, Policy and Action, 3675
Eating Disorders Resource Catalogue, 3733
Eating Disorders Review, 3769
Eating Disorders-Overview Series, 3734
Eating Disorders: When Food Turns Against You, 3735
Eating Hints: Recipes and Tips for Better Nutrition During Cancer Treatment, 2522
Eating Without Packet, 701

Eaton-Peabody Laboratory of Auditory Physiology, 4376
Eau Claire Hemophilia Center, 5024
Ecology & Environment Management of Lyme Disease, 9040
Ectopic Pregnancy, 5517
Eczema/Atopic Dermatitis, 7703
Ed Lindsey Industries of the Blind, 9577
Edith Nourse Rogers Memorial Veterans Hospital: Bedford VA, 10169
Educating Deaf Children Bilingually, 4491
Educating Deaf Children: An Introduction, 4763
Educating Inattentive Children, 1651
Educating Patients and Families About Mental Illness: A Practical Guide, 6099
Educating the Deaf: Psychology, Principles and Practices, 4492
Education and Deafness, 4493
Education Concerns for the Traumatically Head Injured Student, 4231
Educational and Development Aspects of Deafness, 4494
Educational Choices for Children with PWS, 7212
Educational Equity Center at AED, 10630
Educational Equity Center at The Academy for Educational Development, 10372
Educational Issues Among Children with Spina Bifida, 7936
Educational Materials Database Centers for Disease Control, 393
Educational Rights for Children with Arthritis: A Parents Manual, 1269
Educator's Guide to Tourette Syndrome, 9107
Educator's In-Service Program, 9138
Edward Hines Jr. VA Hospital, 10146
Effect of Corticosteroid or Methotrexate Therapy on Lung Lymphocytes, 7267
Effective Teaching Methods for Autistic Children, 1749
Effects of Sarcoid and Steroids on Angiotensin-Converting Enzyme, 7268
Efficacy of Antiparkinson Medications, 6960
Efficacy of Asthma Education, Selected Abstracts, 1462
Ehlers-Danlos Syndrome, 1320
El Paso Lighthouse for the Blind, 9582
El Paso VA Health Care Center, 10245
Elder Care, 164
Eldercare Locator, 220
Elderly Health Services Letter, 199
Elderly in Modern Society, 165
Elderly with Chronic Mental Illness, 6100
Elders Assert Their Rights, 6101
Elephant in the Living Room: A Leader's Guide, 8296
Elephant in the Living Room: The Children's Book, 8430
Elevate NWO, 258
Elizabeth Glaser Pediatric AIDS Foundation, 355
Eljay Foundation for Parkinson Syndrome Awareness, 6891
Embers of the Fire, 3197
Embrace the Dawn, 7503
Embracing Play: Teaching Your Child with Autism, 1799
Embracing the Wolf: A Lupus Victim and Her Family Learn to Live, 8939
EMDR as an Integrative Psychotherapy Approach, 7124
EMedicine, 7025
Emory Autism Resource Center, 1716
Emory Brain Tumor Support Group, 1960
Emory University: Cystic Fibrosis Center, 3105
Emory University: Georgia Center for Cancer Statistics, 2296
Emory University: Laboratory for Ophthalmic Research, 9786
Emory University: National Cooperative Drug Discovery for AIDS Treatment, 394
Emory University: Winship Cancer Institute, 2297
Emotional Aspects of Infertility, 5518
Emotional Eating: A Practical Guide to Taking Control, 3736
Emotional Health Anonymous, 6062
Emphysema, 5883

Employed Ability: Blind Persons on the Job, 10033
Employer's Guide to Dealing with Substance Abuse, 8535
Empowerment and Black Deaf Persons, 4495
Enabling, 8536
Enabling Communication in Children with Autism, 1787
Encore: Another Chance for Life, 9236
Encounters with Autistic States, 1750
Encounters with Grief, 10734
Encyclopedia of Blindness and Vision Impairment, 9845
Encyclopedia of Deafness and Hearing Disorders, 4496
Encyclopedia of Depression, 6213
Encyclopedia of Drug Abuse, 8297
Encyclopedia of Mental Health, 6102
Encyclopedia of Obesity and Eating Disorders, 3737, 6725
Encyclopedia of Phobias, Fears, and Anxieties, 6103
Encyclopedia of Schizophrenia and the Psychotic Disorders, 6265
Endeavor, 4736
Ending Infertility Treatment, 5519
Endocrine News, 10
Endocrine Society, 4
Endocrinology Research Laboratory Cabrini Medical Center, 3383
Endometriosis, 5520
Endometriosis and Infertility and Traditional Chinese Medicine, 3811
Endometriosis Association, 3820
Endometriosis Association International, 3792, 3805
Endometriosis Association Newsletter, 3816
Endometriosis Association Research Program : Vanderbuilt University, 3801
Endometriosis Reseach Center and Women's Hospital, 3802
Endometriosis Research Center, 3793, 3803, 3821
Endometriosis Sourcebook, 3810
Endometriosis Support Group, 3822
Endometriosis: A Key to Healing through Nutrition, 3812
Endometriosis: A Natural Approach, 3813
Endometriosis: Advanced Management and Surgical Techniques, 3814
Endometriosis: Complete Reference for Taking Charge of Your Health, 3815
Endorphins: Eating Disorders & Other Addictive Behavior, 3738
Endoscopic Third Ventriculotomy, 5223
Enviromental Chloracne, 10302
Environmental Birth Defect Digest, 1870
Environmental Control Measures, 1496
Environmental Toxins and Fertility, 5521
Enzymology Research Laboratory Dept. of Veterans Affairs Medical Center, 5869
Ependymoma, 2059
Epilepsia: Journal of the International League Against Epilepsy, 7525
Epilepsy, 7522
Epilepsy A to Z, 7504
Epilepsy and the Family: A New Guide, 7507
Epilepsy Association of Big Bend, 7478
Epilepsy Diet Treatment: An Introduction to the Ketogenic Diet, 7505
Epilepsy Foundation, 7467
Epilepsy Foundation of America, 7559
Epilepsy Foundation of America Helpline, 7496
Epilepsy Foundation of Long Island, 7486
Epilepsy Foundation of New Jersey, 7485
Epilepsy Foundation of North West Washington, 7489
Epilepsy Foundation of Northern California, 7477
Epilepsy Foundation of South Florida, 7479
Epilepsy Foundation of Western Pennsylvania, 7487
Epilepsy Medicines and Dental Care, 7529
Epilepsy Services Foundation, 7480
Epilepsy Services Foundation Newsletter, 7526
Epilepsy Services of North Central Florida, 7481
Epilepsy Services of Northeast Florida, 7482
Epilepsy Services of Southwest Florida, 7483
Epilepsy Surgery, 7506
Epilepsy: 199 Answers, 7508
Epilepsy: A Behavior Medicine Approach to Assessment & Treatment in Children, 7509

Epilepsy: Current Approaches to Diagnosis and Treatment, 7510
Epilepsy: I Can Live with That, 7511
Epilepsy: Legal Rights, Legal Issues, 7530
Epilepsy: Models, Mechanisms & Concepts, 7512
Epilepsy: Part of Your Life Series, 7531
Epilepsy: Patient and Family Guide, 7513
Epilepsy: You and Your Child, a Guide for Parents, 7532
Epilepsy: You and Your Treatment, 7533
Equal Opportunity Employment Commission, 10373
Equal Partners, 7514
Equals in Partnership: Basic Rights for Families of Children with Blindness, 9846
Equipment and Suggestions for Persons with Parkinson's Disease, 6961
ERIC Clearinghouse on Disabilities and Gifted Education, 10505
Erie VA Medical Center, 10227
Ernest Gallo Clinic and Research Center, 8204
Ernest N Morial Asthma, Allergy & Respiratory Disease Center, 3119
Erythropoietic Protoporphyria, 3980
Essential Elements in Early Intervention: Visual Impairment & Multiple Disability, 9847
Essential Guide to Chronic Illness: The Active Patient's Handbook, 2924
Essential Guide to Psychiatric Drugs, 6214
Estate Planning for the Disabled, 10374
Ethics for Addiction Professionals, 8298
Ethnicity & Disease, 5272
Ethnicity Disease, 5273
Ethnocultural Aspects of Posttraumatic Stress Disorder:Issues,Rsrch, Clncl Appl, 7125
Etiology and Treatment of Bulimia Nervosa, 3739
Eugene J. Towbin Healthcare Center Central Arkansas VA Healthcare System, 10111
Evaluation and Management of Eating Disorders, 3740
Evaluation and Treatment of the Psychogeriatric Patient, 6104
Evaluation of the Efficacy and Toxicity of the Cyclosporine, 7269
Evansville-Vanderburgh County Public Library, 9666
Even Little Kids Get Diabetes, 3480
Everybody's Different Nobody's Perfect, 6537
Everyday Life with ALS: A Practical Guide, 6523
Everyone Likes to Eat, 3481
Everyone's Guide to Cancer Therapy, 2437
Everything You Need to Know About AIDS, 473
Everything You Need to Know About Being HIV Positive, 474
Everything You Need to Know About Depression, 6215
Everything You Need to Know About Lyme Disease, 9041
Everything You Need to Know When a Parent Has AIDS, 502
Everything You Need to Know When a Parent has AIDS, 475
Exceptional Cancer Patients/ECaP, 2398
Exceptional Cancer Patients/ECaP Newsletter, 2488
Exceptional Parent Magazine, 3629, 10588
Exchanges for All Occasions, 3439
Exercise and Your Arthritis, 1321
Exercise and Your Heart, 4947
Exercise Beats Arthritis, 1270
Exercise Guidelines for the Person with Lung Disease, 5884
Exercise-Induced Asthma & Bronchospasm, 1463
Exercising Your Pelvic Muscles, 5354
Expanding the Horizon of Hope: 50 Years of Progress, 3198
Experiences of Schizophrenia, 6266
Expert Guide to Beating Heart Disease: What You Absolutely Must Know, 4927
Exploring Care Options for a Relative with Alzheimer's Disease, 210
Extensions for Independence, 10375
Extent and Adequacy of Insurance Coverage for Substance Abuse I & II, 8299
Eye and Your Vision, 9848
Eye Opener, 7833, 8300
Eye Problems Associated with Hydrocephalus in Children, 5224

Eye Research News, 9924
Eye-Centered: A Study of Spirituality of Deaf People, 4497
Eye-Q Test, 9975
Eyes and Parkinson's Disease, 6962

F

FAAN Flashbacks, 702
Fabry Support & Information Group, 3844, 3848
Faces of Cystic Fibrosis, 3199
Facing Addiction with NCADD, 8116
Facing Forward: A Guide for Cancer Survivors, 2523
Facing the Challenges of Turner's Syndrome Together, 9362
Facioscapulohumeral Muscular Dystrophy Soc iety (FSH Society), 6520
Fact Is...Hispanic Parents Can Help Their Children Avoid Alcohol/Drugs, 8301
Fact Sheet: Attention Deficit Hyperactivity Disorder, 1643
Fact Sheet: Hydrocephalus, 5225
Factor Fax, 1292
Factor Nine News, 5091
Facts About AAT Deficiency-Related Emphysema, 5885
Facts About Acne, 7739
Facts About Alateen, 8537
Facts About Alcohol Abuse, 8538
Facts About Asbestos, 5886
Facts About Asthma, 1464, 5887
Facts About Charcot-Marie-Tooth Disease, 6538
Facts About Chronic Fatigue Syndrome, 2876
Facts About Duchenne & Becker Muscular Dystrophies, 6539
Facts About Epilepsy, 7534
Facts About Facioscapulohumeral Muscular Dystrophy, 6540
Facts About Friedreich's Ataxia, 6541
Facts About Hearing Aids, 4764
Facts About Kidney Diseases and Their Treatment, 5698
Facts About Kidney Stones, 5699
Facts About Limb-Girdle Muscular Dystrophy, 6542
Facts About Lung Cancer, 2524
Facts About Lupus, 8950
Facts About Metabolic Diseases of Muscle, 6543
Facts About Mitochondrial Myopathies, 6544
Facts About Myasthenia Gravis, 6545
Facts About Myasthenia Gravis for Patients and Families, 6638
Facts About Myopathies, 6546
Facts About Myotonic Muscular Dystrophy, 6547
Facts About Peak Flow Meters, 1465
Facts About Plasmapheresis, 6548
Facts About Polymyositis/Dermatomyositis, 6549
Facts About Radon, 2525
Facts About Rare Muscular Dsytrophies, 6550
Facts About SIDS, 8826
Facts About Spinal Muscular Atrophy, 6551
Facts About Tuberculosis, 9314
Facts About Turner's Syndrome, 9363
Facts and Fancies About Hearing Aids, 4765
Facts on Alcohol, 8431
Facts on Heart Disease, Heart Attack, Stroke and Risk Factors, 8085
Facts on Liver Transplantation, 5787
Facts on the Crack and Cocaine Epidemic, 8432
Facts: Books for Blind and Physically Handicapped Individuals, 9976
Facts: Music for Blind and Physically Handicapped Individuals, 9977
Facts: Playback Machines and Accessories Provided on Free Loan, 9978
Facts: Sources for Purchase of Cassette & Disc Players From NLS, 9979
Fairfax County Public Library, 9757
Fairview-University Hemophilia & Thrombosis Center, 5025
Fall Down Seven Times Get Up Eight, 6442
Falling in Old Age, 166
Familial Spastic Paraplegia, 1580
Families Anonymous, 8681

Families Anonymous, Inc. Recovery Fellowship, 8117
Families in Action National Drug Abuse Center, 8205
Families Together in New York State, 5992
Families United For CMH, Inc., 5938
Family, 1322
Family Action Network, 5955
Family Advocacy and Support Association, 5944
Family and ADPKD: A Guide for Children and Parents, 5673
Family Bonds: Adoption and the Politics of Parenting, 5453
Family Building Magazine, 5502
Family Carebook, 167
Family Caregiver Alliance/National Center on Caregiving, 27, 4079
Family Caregiving in Mental Illness, 6105
Family Cookbook: Volumes I-IV, 3440
Family Denial, 8539
Family Focus, 5684
Family Guide to Vision Care, 9980
Family Guide: Growth & Development of the Partially Seeing Child, 9981
Family Interventions Throughout Chronic Illness and Disability, 10544
Family Life with Tourette Syndrome... Personal Stories: Dakota, 9149, 9150, 9151, 9152, 9153, 9154
Family Meds, 5321
Family Of a Vet, 7148
Family Service Foundation, Inc., 6025
Family Support Bulletin, 2808
Family Support Network, 2795, 5979
Family Teaching Conference, 3987
Family: Making the Difference, 1323
Fanconi Anemia Research Fund, 2973
Fantastic Series, 4796
Fargo VA Health Care System, 10212
A Fate Better than Death, 4264
Fatty Liver, 5788
Favarh, 10376
Fayetteville VA Medical Center, 10210
Fear of Being Fat, 3741
Federal Emergency Management Agency, 7060
Federal Law of the Mentally Handicapped, 6106
Federal Medicaid Drug Program, 5075
Federation for Children with Special Needs, 1829, 10377
Federation of Families for Children's Mental Health, 6178
Federation of Families of South Carolina, 6077
Federation of Quebec Alzheimer Societies, 755
Federation of Spine Associations, 7398
Feed Your Head, 8433
Feeding the Hungry Heart, the Experience of Compulsive Eating, 8302
Feel Good Catalog, 2857
Feingold Association of the US, 1605
Fertilethoughts.com, 5561
Fertility After Cancer Treatment, 5522
Fertility and Pregnancy Guide for DES Daughters and Sons, 5454
Fertility and Women's Health Care Center, 5435
Fertility Clinic at the Shepherd Spinal Center, 5434
Fertility Research Foundation, 3798, 5431
Fetal Alcohol Network, 10513
Fetal Alcohol Syndrome, 8540
FFCMH: Denver/Aurora Chapter, 5935
FFCMH: Idaho Chapter, 5950
FFCMH: Indiana Chapter, 5954
FFCMH: Iowa Chapter, 5957
Fibromyalgia, 2877, 2891, 3873
Fibromyalgia & Other Central Pain Syndromes, 3874
Fibromyalgia and Chronic Myofascial Pain Syndrome: a Survivor Manual, 3880
Fibromyalgia AWARE, 3888
Fibromyalgia Clinic Kentfield Rehabilitation Newsletter, 3891
Fibromyalgia Frontiers, 3889
Fibromyalgia Guidelines: The Concensus Diagnosis & Treatment Protocols, 3875
Fibromyalgia Interval Training, 3898
Fibromyalgia Network, 3868
Fibromyalgia Relief Book: 213 Ideas for Improving Your Quality of Life, 3876

Fibromyalgia Resources Group, 3867
Fibromyalgia Stretch Video & Strength and Toning Video, 3899
Fibromyalgia Supporter, 3877
Fibromyalgia Survivor, 3878
Fibromyalgia Syndrome and Chronic Fatigue Syndrome in Young People, 3879
Fibromyalgia, Managing the Pain, 3881
Fibromyalgia: Face to Face, 3900
Fidelco Guide Dog Foundation, 9423, 10062
Fifty Things You Should Know About the Chronic Fatigue Syndrome Epidemic, 2845
Fight Drug Abuse at Home, Work, School and in the Community, 8541
Fight for Sight, 9424
Fight Hemophilia with Facts Not Fiction, 5108
Fighting Back Against PD: One Women's Story, 6963
Finding Out About Seizures: A Guide to Medical Tests, 7535
Finger Alphabet, 4652
Finger Lakes Donor Recovery Network, 9206
Fingers that Tickle and Delight, 4797
Fingerspelling and Numbers Software, 4798
Fire in My Heart: Ice in My Veins, 10725
First Candle, 8700, 8748
First Ohio Chapter: FFCMH, 6075
First Presbyterian Church in the City of New York Support Groups, 3716
First Steps, 9849
FIT Video, 1354
Fitness Book: For People with Diabetes, 3441
52 Proven Stress Reducers, 6307
Flagstaff City Coconino County Public Library, 9615
Florida Alliance for the Mentally Ill, 5945
Florida Ambassador: National Ataxia Foundation, 1533
Florida Association of the Deaf, 4341
Florida Brain Tumor Association, 1953
Florida Brain Tumor Support Group, 1954
Florida Brain Tumor Support Group: Deerfield Beach, 1955
Florida Bureau of Braille and Talking Book Library Services, 9634
Florida Chapter of the Myasthenia Gravis Foundation of America, 6578
Florida Department of Health, 8726
Florida Department of Health: HIV/AIDS Section, 300
Florida Disabled Outdoor Association, 10378
Florida FFCMH: Tampa Chapter, 5946
Florida Fibromyalgia News, 3892
Florida Gulf Coast Chapter National Multiple Sclerosis Society, 6362
Florida Heart Research Institute, 4877
Florida Hemophilia Association, 4973
Florida Institute for Family Involvement (FIFI), 6052
Florida Ophthalmic Institute, 9787
Florida SIDS Alliance, 8727
Flying Fingers Club, 4653
FM Auditory Trainers: A Winning Choice for Students, Teachers and Parents, 4498
FM Monograph, 3887
Focal Group Psychotherapy for Mental Health Professionals, 6107
FOCUS, 544
Focus, 1293, 9925
Focused On: Importance and Need for Skills, 10034
Follow Your Dreams, 8001
Fondation quebecoise du sida, 356
Food & Nutrition, 690, 2639, 3766, 3954
Food Allergy and Atopic Dermatitis, 703
Food Allergy News, 694
Food Allergy Research & Education, 637, 734
Food Allergy: A Primer for People, 679
Food for Thought: Daily Meditations for Overeaters, 8303
Food for Thought: MS and Nutrition, 6468
Food Safety and Inspection Service, 638
For a Strong and Healthy Baby, 8542
For Adults with Cystic Fibrosis: Facts on Reproduction, 3192
For Life: More Stories of Lupus, 8957
For My Sister, Elyssa, 8994
For Parents, 7704
For Teachers of the Hearing Impaired, 4499

For the Obese Employee, 6744
For Those Who Live: Helping Children Cope with Death of a Brother or Sister, 10713
For Those Who Take Care: An Alzheimer's Disease Training Program for Nurses, 1074
For Want of a Child: A Psychologist and His Wife Explore Infertility, 5455
Fort Meade Campus VA Black Hills Health Care System, 10235
Fort Wayne Campus VA Northern Indiana Health Care System, 10151
Forum Favorites: Volumes 1, 2, 3 & 4, 8304
Forum Magazine, 8466
Foundation Facts, 3193
Foundation Fighting Blindness, 9425, 9604
Foundation Focus, 3051
Foundation for Advancement in Cancer Therapy, 2208
Foundation for Prader-Willi Research, 7162
Foundations of Education, 9850
Foundations of Orientation and Mobility, 9851
Foundations of Rehabilitation Counseling with Persons Who Are Blind/Visually Imp., 9852
Foundations of Spoken Language for Hearing Impaired Children, 4500
Four Lives: A Portrait of Manic Depression, 6243
Fox Chase Cancer Center, 2366
Framingham Heart Study, 4878
Frat, 4737
Fred Hutchinson Cancer Research Center, 2385
Frederick Cancer Research Center, 2317
Free Hand: Education of the Deaf, 4501
Free Library of Philadelphia, 9743
Free to Care, 8543
Freedom from Despair, 8544
Freedom From Fear, 7046
Freedom from Headaches, 6297
Freedom from Smoking at Work Program, 8305
Freedom from Smoking Flyer, 8545
Frenkel's Exercises, 1581
Frequently Asked Questions, 9047
FreshAAIR, 1444
Fresno County Public Library: Talking Book Library for the Blind, 9622
Friday Night Live, 8243
Friedrich's Ataxia, 1582
Friends Health Connection, 10514
Friends Medical Science Research Center, 8206
Friends of Karen, 10663
Friends of Libraries for Deaf Action USA, 4365
From 16 Months to 17 Years...A Look at Down Syndrome, 3615
From One Family Member to Another, 4232
From Patient to Person: First Steps, 2925
From the Ashes, 4197
From Theory to Therapy: The Development of Drugs for Alzheimer's Disease, 168
Fulfilling the Hope: Our Commitment to the Parkinson's Community, 6964
Fun and Games, 8011
Functional Behavioral Assessments: How to Do Them Right!, 1800
Functional Electrical Stimulation: Clinical Applications, 8012
Funding Database Centers for Disease Control, 395
Future by Design/A Community Framework, 8306
Future Reflections, 9908

G

G.V. (Sonny) Montgomery VA Medical Center, 10180
GA and SK Etiquette, 4502
GA-SK Newsletter, 4738
Gallaudet Encyclopedia of Deaf People and Deafness, 4503
Gallaudet Today, 4739
Gallaudet University: Center for Auditory and Speech Sciences, 4377
Gallstones, 5789
Gangs and Drugs, 8434
Garden State Chapter of the Myasthenia Gravis Foundation of America, 6590
Garrett Mountain Chapter of the American Association of Kidney Patients, 5625

Gastro-Intestinal Research Foundation, 3933, 3942
Gastroenterology, 3955
Gastroenterology Nursing, 3956
Gastroenterology Therapy Online, 3777
Gastrointestinal Endoscopy, 3957
Gastrointestinal Presentation of Churg Strauss Syndrome, 7270
Gastrointestinal Research Foundation, 4001
Gateway Hemophilia Association, 4986
Gathered Fragments, 7209
Gaucher Disease Fact Sheet, 4030
Gaucher Disease Homepage, 4033
Gaucher Disease Newsletter, 4029
Gay Men's Health Crisis, 545
Gazoontite, 1510
Geisinger Wyoming Valley Medical Center: Sleep Disorders Center, 7769
Gene Clinics, 3849
Gene Testing for Ataxia, 1583
General Clinical Research Center at Beth Israel Hospital, 4879
General Clinical Research Center Mount Sinai School of Medicine, 416
General Clinical Research Center: UAB, 364
General Clinical Research Center: University of California at LA, 4880
General Facts and Figures on Blindness, 9982
General Interest Catalog, 9983
Generations, 1571
GENES Information Services, 1570
Genes, Blood & Courage, 2975
Genesee County Health Department, 8752
Genetic Alliance, 1726, 4043, 10379
Genetic and Rare Diseases Information Center, 3835
Genetic Counseling, 1883
Genetics and Deafness, 4766
Genetics and Inherited Traits, 1890
Genetics and Neuromuscular Diseases, 6552
Genetics of Tourette's Syndrome: Who it Affects and How it Occurs in Families, 9108
Genexus, 1572
Genital Herpes, 7585
Genital Herpes Fact Sheet, 7586
Genital Psoriasis, 7705
Gentle Path Through the Twelve Steps, 8307
Gentle Willow: A Story for Children About Dying, 10726
George E. Wahlen Medical Center VA Salt Lake City Health Care System, 10252
George H. O'Brien, Jr. VA Medical Center West Texas VA Health Care System, 10246
George Washington National Cooperative: Drug Discovery/AIDS Treatment, 385
George Washington University Center for Aging, Health and Humanities, 119
Georgetown University Center for Hypertension and Renal Disease Research, 5595
Georgetown University Child Development Center, 1840
Georgetown University Hospital Transplant Institute, 9227, 9246
Georgetown University Hospital: Department of Rheumatology, 7360
Georgetown University: Vincent T Lombardi Cancer Research Center, 2291
Georgia Alliance for the Mentally Ill, 5948
Georgia Association of the Deaf, 4342
Georgia Chapter of the Myasthenia Gravis Foundation of America, 6579
Georgia Department of Public Health: Center for Family Resource Planning, 8728
Georgia Department of Public Health: Infan t and Child Health, 8729
Georgia Department of Public Health: Office Of HIV/AIDS, 302
Georgia Industries for the Blind, 9486
Georgia Library for Accessible Services (GLASS), 9649
Georgia National Spinal Cord Injury Association Support Group Network, 7986
Georgia Parent Support Network (GPSN), 6054
Georgia SIDS Project, 8730
Georgia Support Group: National Ataxia Foundation, 1536

Geraldine Brush Cancer Research Institute California Pacific Medical Center, 2276
GERD Information Resource Center, 3776
Geriatric Care News, 200
Geriatric Rehabilitation Preview, 169
Geriatrics, 201
Gerontological Society of America, 28, 221
Gerontology News, 202
Gershenson Radiation Oncology Center Barbara Ann Karmanos Cancer Institute, 2324
Gestational Diabetes: What To Expect, 3505
Get a Wiggle On, 9853
Get Fit While You Sit: Easy Workouts From Your Chair, 10545
Get Real and Be Safe!, 5109
Get the Facts About Sleep Apnea, 7837
Get to Sleep! How to Sleep Well...Despite Lupus, 8933
Getting a Grip on Gait, 6469
Getting a Second Opinion, 7417
Getting Better Bit(e) by Bit(e), 3742
Getting Help to Hepatitis, 5790
Getting in Touch, 4799
Getting in Touch with Al-Anon/Alateen, 8546
Getting Into College: Strategies for the Student with TS, 9109
Getting it Together: Promoting Drug Free Communities, 8310
Getting Pregnant When You Thought You Couldn't, 5456
Getting Ready, Getting Well, 7405
Getting Started in AA, 8308
Getting Started with Facilitated Communication, 1801
Getting Started: How Do I Know If I'm Infertile?, 5523
Getting Tough on Gateway Drugs: A Guide for the Family, 8309
Gift From Within, 7069, 7149
Gift of Hope, 9110, 9191
Gift of Life Donor Program Pennsylvania, 9217
Gift of the Girl Who Couldn't Hear, 4654
Gifts of Love, 3649
GIG Quarterly Magazine, 2641
Gilda's Club: Grand Rapids, 2399
Gilda's Club: New York City, 2400
Gilda's Club: Quad Cities, 2401
Gilda's Club: South Florida, 2402
Ginny: A Love Remembered, 1007
Give Kids the World Village, 10664
Give Me One Wish, 3185
Glaucoma, 9984
Glaucoma Laser Trabeculoplasty Study Sinai Hospital of Detroit, 9788
Glaucoma Research Foundation, 9426, 9605, 9789
Glaucoma: Sneak Thief of Sight, 9985
Gleams Newsletter, 9926
Glendale Adventist Medical Center Brain Tumor Support Group, 1934
Glioblastoma Multiforme and Anaplastic Astrocytoma, 2060
Global AIDS: Myths and Facts, Tools for Fighting the AIDS Pandemic, 476
Global Lyme Alliance, 9024
Glomerulonephritis, 5700
Gluten Intolerance Group, 2629, 2656
God Grant Me the Laughter: A Treasury of Twelve Step Humor, 8311
God, the Universe and Hot Fudge Sundaes, 1873
Going Backwards, 3743
Going Home, 7418
Going Places and Plan for Success: An Educator's Guide to Students with OI, 6793
Going to School with Facilitated Communication, 1802
Gold Coast Down Syndrome Organization, 3558
Gold Treatment, 1324
Golden Cage: The Enigma of Anorexia Nervosa, 3744
Golden State Donor Services, 9179
Goldilocks and the Three Bears, 4655
GoldPoint Clinical Research, 7092
Gonorrhea, 7587
Good Bones: Complete Guide to Building and Maintaining the Healthiest Bones, 10546

A Good Death: Conversations with East Londoners, 10703
Good First Step, 8312
Good Nutrition in Parkinson's Disease, 6965
Goodbye Hangovers, Hello Life, 8313
Goodwill Industries International, Inc., 29, 1606, 1668, 1830, 3544, 4044, 5912, 7047, 9079, 10102, 10380
Goodwill Industries-Suncoast, 56, 1609, 1676, 1833, 3559, 4047, 5947, 7062, 9083, 10130, 10442
Gospel of Luke, 4800
Gout, 1325
Governor New Jersey Proclamation: Sarcoidosis Awareness Day, 7271
Governor's Committee for People with Disabilities, 10498
Grains and Flours, 2647
Grand Traverse Area Library for the Blind and Physically Handicapped, 9696
Grandfather Moose, 4656
Grandpa Doesn't Know It's Me, 1023
Grandpa's Music: A Story About Alzheimer's, 1024
Grandparents Club, 9111
Granite State FFCMH, 5983
Granny Good's Sign of Christmas, 4801
Grants for Organizations Serving People with Disabilities, 10547
Grateful to Have Been There, 8314
Grave Words: Tools for Discussing End of Life Choices, 10735
Gray Matters Support: Kansas City, 1971
Great Change, 10727
Great Lakes Chapter of the Myasthenia Gravis Foundation of America, 6586
Great Lakes Genetic News, 1573
Great Lakes Hemophilia Foundation, 5011
Great Plains Regional Hemophilia Center University of Iowa Hospitals, 5026
Great Starts & Fine Finishes, 3442
Greater Daytona Area Parkinson Support Group, 6913
Greater Detroit Agency for the Blind and Visually Impaired, 9517
Greater Grand Rapids Pediatric Hemophilia Program, 5027
Greater Houston Chapter SIDS Alliance, 8793
Greater Indianapolis Chapter of the Myasthenia Gravis Foundation of America, 6582
Greater Iowa Chapter Alzheimer's Association Quadcity Office, 826
Greater New York Metro Intergroup of Overeaters Anonymous, 6720
Greater New York Pull-Thru Network, 5338
Greater Rochester Area Chapter NSCIA, 7976
Greater Wilkes-Barre Association for the Blind, 9560
Green-Field Library-Alzheimer's Association, 947
Grief & Loss Support Group, 10700
Grief of Children After the Loss of a Sibling or Friend, 8827
Grief, Dying and Death: Clinical Intervention for Caregivers, 10714
Grieving, 8547
Grilled Cheese, 3482
Group Psychotherapy for Eating Disorders, 3745
Growing Children: A Parent's Guide, 4056
Growing Straighter and Stronger, 7441
Growing Together: Information for Parents of Deaf & Hard of Hearing Children, 4504
Growing Up Drug Free: A Parent's Guide to Prevention, 8315
Growing Up with OI: A Guide for Children, 6786
Growing Up with OI: A Guide for Families a nd Caregivers, 6787
Growing Up with Prader-Willi Syndrome: Personal Reflections of a Mother, 7203
Growth Hormone & Prader-Willi Syndrome: A Reference for Familes & Care Providers, 7204
Growth Hormone Testing, 4059
Guidance on Our Journeys, 8548
Guide Dog Foundation Flyer, 9986
Guide Dog Foundation for the Blind, 10063
Guide Dog Foundation for the Blind Newsletter, 9927
Guide Dog Goes to School, 9897
Guide Dog News, 9928
Guide Dog Users, 10064

Guide Dog Users, Inc., 9427
Guide Dogs for the Blind, 9428
Guide for Children and Teenagers to Crohn's Disease/Ulcerative Colitis, 3062
Guide for Teens, 6692
Guide for the Childless Couple, 5457
Guide for the Family of the Alcoholic, 8549
Guide to Diagnosis, 9140
Guide to Diagnosis & Treatment, 9112
Guide to Effective Volunteer Lobbying, 1326
Guide to Gluten-Free Diets, 704, 2648
Guide to Housing for Adults with TS, 9113
Guide to In Vitro Fertilization & Other Assisted Reproduction Methods, 5458
Guide to Independence for the Visually Impaired and Their Families, 9854
Guide to Insurance Coverage for People with Hemophilia, 5076
Guide to Living With HIV Infection, 477
Guide to Lyme Disease, 9048
Guide to Selecting and Monitoring Head Injury Rehabilitation Services, 4233
Guide to the 12 Steps for You, 6745
Guide to Tick Spread Diseases, 9049
Guide to Tick-Borne Disorders, 9050
Guide to Understanding and Living with Epilepsy, 7515
Guidelines and Games for Teaching Efficient Braille Reading, 9855
Guidelines for Comprehensive Low Vision Care, 9987
Guidelines for Finding Childcare, 5110
Guidelines for Helping Deaf/Blind Persons, 9988
Guidelines for People Who Have Had Polio, 7023
Guideway, 9929
Gulf Coast Veterans Health Care System, 10181
Gulf States Hemophilia Diagnostic and Treatment Center, 5028
Gulf War and Birth Defects, 1884
Gulf War and Health, 10279
Gulf War Syndrome Database, 10309
Gulf War Veteran Resource Pages, 10310
Gulf War Veterans of Alabama, 10105
Gulf War Veterans of Arkansas, 10112
Gundersen Clinic Comprehensive Hemophilia Treatment Center, 5029

H

H.J. Heinz Campus VA Pittsburgh Healthcare System, 10228
Habits Not Diets: Secret to Lifetime Weight Control, 10548
Hahnemann University Hospital, Orthopedic Wellness Center, 1247
Hahnemann University Laboratory of Human Pharmacology, 8207
Hahnemann University Likoff Cardiovascular Institute, 4881
Hahnemann University Lupus Study Center Hahnemann University Medical Center, 8928
Hahnemann University, Krancer Center for Inflammatory Bowel Disease Research, 3041
Hahnemann University: Division of Surgical Research, 5254
Hall County Library System: East Hall Branch and Special Needs Library, 9650
Hammond Large Type World Atlas, 9856
Hampton Subregional Library for the Blind, 9758
Hampton VA Medical Center, 10254
Hand Eczema, 7706
Hand in Hand: It Can Be Done, 10035
Handbook for Itinerant and Resource Teachers of Blind Students, 9857
Handbook for Parents, 7205
Handbook of Autism and Pervasive Developmental Disorders, 1751
Handbook of Head Truma: Acute Care to Recovery, 4198
Handbook of Headache Disorders, 6298
Handbook of Headache Management: A Practic al Guide to Diagnosis & Treatment, 6299
Handbook of Mental Health and Mental Disor der Among Black Americans, 6108

Handbook of Obesity Treatment, 6726
Handbook of Scoliosis, 7406
Handful of Stories, 4657
Handle with Care, 8316
Handmade Alphabet, 4658
Handout on Health: Scleroderma, 7377
Handout on Health: Systemic Lupus Erythematosus, 8951
Hands & Voices, 4307
Hands Organization: Advocacy Network for the Deaf and Hearing Impaired, 4308
Handtalk Zoo, 4505
Harbor-South Bay Orange County Chapter of the American Assoc. of Kidney Patients, 5585
Harold Talks About How He Inherited Hemophilia, 5081
Harold's Secret: A Boy with Hemophilia, 5082
Harris Center for Education and Advocacy in Eating Disorders, 3709
Harris County FFCMH, 6079
Harris County Public Health and Environmental Services, 8794
Harry S. Truman Memorial Veterans' Hospital, 10184
Harvard Clinical Nutrition Research Center, 6716
Harvard Cocaine Recovery Project, 8208
Harvard Throndike Laboratory Harvard Medical Center, 4882
Harvard University Howe Laboratory of Ophthalmology, 9790
Harvey A Friedman Center for Aging Washington University, 120
Hasta Luego, San Diego, 4659
Have Fun! Figure Out the Smoking Puzzle, 8550
Having Your Baby By Donor Insemination, 5459
Hawaii Department of Health: Family Health Division, 8731
Hawaii Department of Health: Harm Reduction Services Branch, 303
Hawaii Down Syndrome Congress, 3561
Hawaii Families As Allies (HFAA), 6055
Hawaii Lupus Foundation, 8871
Hawaii Parkinson Association Gwendolyn A Montibon President, 6888
Hawaii State Library for the Blind and Physically Handicapped, 9658
Hazelden, 8682
Hazelden Betty Ford Foundation, 8118
Hazelden Step Pamphlets for Overeaters, 6746
Head Injury and the Family: A Life and Living Perspective, 4199
Head Injury Survivor on Campus: Issues & Resources, 4234
Head Injury: A Booklet for Families, 4235
Head Injury: A Guide for Families, 4236
Headache, 6305
Headache Facts: What Everyone Should Know, 6312
Headache Handbook, 6313
Headache in Children: Fact Sheet, 6314
Headaches and Hydrocephalus, 5226
Headinjury.Com, 4273
Heads Up!, 1935
Headstrong Brain Tumor Support Group, 1972
HEAL, 448
Heal My PTSD with Michele Rosenthal, 7105
Healing From Complex Trauma & PTSD/CPTSD, 7150
Healing the Infertile Family, 5460
Healing Well, 13, 222, 612, 735, 1079, 1177, 1362, 1592, 1654, 1814, 1893, 2080, 2591, 2657, 2812, 2898, 2938, 2986, 3073, 3201, 3528
Healingwell, 1511
Health, 10549
Health After 50: Johns Hopkins Medical Letter, 203
Health Care For All, 10382, 10632
Health Care of the Aged, 170
Health Care Professionals Who are Blind or Visually Impaired, 9858
Health Central, 5894
Health Consequences of Smoking: Cancer & Chronic Lung Disease in the Workplace, 2438, 5877
Health Facts, 10591
Health Finder, 14, 223, 613, 736, 1080, 1178, 1363, 1512, 1593, 1655, 1815, 1894, 2081, 2592, 2620, 2658, 2813, 2899, 2939, 2987, 3074
Health Information Network, 260

Health Insurance, 1584, 5167
Health Insurance & Tourette Syndrome, 9114
Health Link USA, 15
Health on the Net Foundation, 10634
Health Planning and Development, 8146
Health Points, 1294, 2860, 2931, 3893
Health Resource, 2121
Health Resources and Services Administration (HRSA), 9167, 9247
Health Science Library, 3371
Health, Life and Disability Insurance for People with Arthritis, 1327
Healthcare Guidelines, 7919
Healthcentral.com, 10635
Healthlink USA, 224, 614, 737, 1081, 1179, 1364, 1513, 1594, 1656, 1816, 1895, 2082, 2593, 2659, 2814, 2900, 2940, 2988, 3075, 3203, 3530
HEALTHSOUTH Rehabilitation Hospital of Tallahassee, 7987
Healthwatch, 3894
Healthy Aging: Good Investment & Together We Care: Helping Caregivers Find Supp., 171
Healthy and Hearty Diabetic Cooking, 2439
Healthy Beginning, Promotional Flyers, 8551
Healthy Breathing, 1466
Healthy Eater's Guide to Family & Chain Restaurants, 3443
Healthy Eating, 3506
Healthy Food Choices, 3507
Healthy Homestyle Cookbook, 3444
Healthy Lives, 5190
Healthy Weight Network, 3676
HealthyWomen, 3794, 3826, 5377, 5565, 9004, 9018, 10383, 10637
Hear, 4740
Hear Center, 4378
Hear Now, 4841
Hear Now: Starkey Hearin Foundation, 4309
Hearing Aid Handbook, 4506
Hearing Education and Awareness for Rocker, 4842
Hearing Education and Awareness for Rocker s, 4310
Hearing Health, 4710
Hearing Health Foundation, 4311, 4843
Hearing Impaired Children and Youth and Developmental Disabilities, 4507
Hearing Industries Association, 4312, 4844
Hearing Loss, 4660
Hearing Loss and Hearing Aids: A Bridge to Healing, 4509
Hearing Loss and Rehabilitation, 4802
Hearing Loss Association of America, 4313
Hearing Loss Following Head Injury, 4237
Hearing Loss Help, 4508
Hearing Loss: Information for Professionals in the Aging Network, 4767
Hearsay, 9930
Heart and Down Syndrome, 3636
Heart and Stroke Foundation of Canada, 8048
Heart Defects, 4948
Heart Disease, 4928
Heart Disease Research Foundation, 4883
Heart of a Child: What Families Need to Know About Heart Disorders, 4929
Heart of America News, 2861
Heart Research Foundation of Sacramento, 4884
Heart to Heart, 9989, 10036
Heart Touch Project™, 30, 261, 10384
Heartbreak of Being a Little Bit Blind, 9990
Heartpoint, 2951
Hearts and Minds, 1961
Heartsongs, Journey Through Heartsongs, Hope Through Heartsongs, Celebrate, 6533
Heartstyle, 4938
HEATH Resource Center, 1610, 10381
Heatlhcentral.com, 10314
Helen Keller, 9991
Helen Keller in Her Story, 10037
Helen Keller International, 9791
Helen Keller National Center for Deaf-Blind Youths and Adults, 9429
Helen Keller National Center for Deaf/Blind Youths and Adults, 4314, 9792
Helen Keller National Center Regional Representatives, 9495
Heliogram, 8942

Help a Friend to Stop Smoking, 8552
Help for Headaches, 6290
Help for Helpers: Daily Meditations for Counselors, 8317
Help with a Hidden Disease Update, 7310
Help Yourself Cookbook, 1271
Help Yourself: Tips for Teenagers with Cancer, 2462
Help, Hope, Believe, 2526
Helper's Journey, 10715
Helpful Hints for Living with Scleroderma, 7378
Helpful Hints for the Allergic Patient, 705
Helpful Techniques to Aid the Student with TS, 9115
Helpful Tips for Carriers of HBV, 5168
Helping Adolescents with ADHD and Learning Disabilities, 1644
Helping Athletes with Eating Disorders, 3746
Helping Children Cope While a Sibling Undergoes Bone Marrow Transplant, 2527
Helping Children with Autism Learn: Treatment Approaches for Parents, 1752
Helping Families Understand PTSD, 6163
Helping Hand, 2052
Helping Homeless People with Alcohol and Other Drug Problems, 8318
Helping Other Parents in Normal Grief, 10694
Helping Others Breathe Easier, 1467
Helping Smokers Get Ready to Quit, 8553
Helping Your ADD Child With or Without Hyperactivity, 1621
Helping Your Child Say No: A Parent's Guide, 8554
Helping Your Students Say No Teacher's Guide, 8319
Helping Yourself to a Good Night's Sleep, 7838
HEMALOG, 5084
Hematin, 3981
Hematology Treatment Center of the Great Lakes Hemophilia Foundation, 5030
HemAware, 5085
Hemochromatosis, 5791
Hemochromatosis Awareness, 3969
Hemochromatosis Foundation, 4005
Hemodialysis, 5701
Hemophilia and Bleeding Disorders of Alaba ma, Inc., 4966
Hemophilia Association of San Diego County, 4969
Hemophilia Association of South Carolina, 5002
Hemophilia Association of the Capital Area, 5007
Hemophilia Association of the Huntington Area, 5031
Hemophilia Camp Directory, 5077
Hemophilia Center of Central Pennsylvania Penn State Milton S Hershey Medical Cent, 5032
Hemophilia Center of Rhode Island Rhode Island Hospital, 5033
Hemophilia Center of the Huntington Hospital, 5036
Hemophilia Center of West Virginia University Health Sciences Center, 5034
Hemophilia Center of Western New York, 4990
Hemophilia Center of Western New York Erie County Medical Center, 5035
Hemophilia Clinic: Childrens' Rehabilitation Service, 5037
Hemophilia Foundation of Arkansas, 4967
Hemophilia Foundation of Georgia, 4974
Hemophilia Foundation of Hawaii Kapiolani Medical Center, 4975
Hemophilia Foundation of Idaho, 4976
Hemophilia Foundation of Illinois, 4977
Hemophilia Foundation of Indiana, 4978
Hemophilia Foundation of Maryland, 4981
Hemophilia Foundation of Michigan, 4983
Hemophilia Foundation of Minnesota and the Dakotas, 4984
Hemophilia Foundation of Nevada, 4988
Hemophilia Foundation of New Mexico, 4989
Hemophilia Foundation of North Carolina, 4992
Hemophilia Foundation of Northern California, 4970
Hemophilia Foundation of Oregon, 4998
Hemophilia Foundation of Southern California, 4971
Hemophilia Health Services, 4962
Hemophilia NewsBriefs, 5092
Hemophilia Treatment Center at Children's National Medical Center, 5038
Hemophilia: Current Medical Management, 5113
Henry Ford Hospital: Hypertension and Vascular Research Division, 5255

Henry Vogt Cancer Research Institute James Graham Brown Cancer Center, 2311
Hepatitis, 5169
Hepatitis A and B Vaccination, 5170
Hepatitis A, B & C, 5171, 5792
Hepatitis A, B & C: Liver Disease You Should Know About, 5172
Hepatitis Alert, 5157
Hepatitis B Coalition, 5191
Hepatitis B Coalition News, 5158
Hepatitis B Foundation, 5145, 10325
Hepatitis B Prevention, 5173
Hepatitis B Prevention: A Resource Guide, 5150
Hepatitis B Video, 5184
Hepatitis B: Your Child at Risk, 5793
Hepatitis C: A Viral Mystery, 5185
Hepatitis Education Project, 5146, 5148
Hepatitis Fact Sheet, 5174
Hepatitis Foundation International, 5141
Hepatitis Information Network, 5192
Hepatitis Magazine, 5153
Hepatology, 5779
Here's Everything You'll Need to Save Money with the CFF Health Services, 3194
Here's What I Mean To Say, 2804
Hereditary Ataxia: Brochure, 1585
Hereditary Ataxia: Fact Sheets, 1586
Hereditary Ataxia: Guidebook for Managing Speech & Swallowing, 1566
Herpes and Papilloma Viruses Volume I & II, 7575
Herpes Resource Center, 7571
Hers Newsletter, 5505
Hershel Woody Williams VA Medical Center, 10263
Hey, I'm Here Too, 6553
HHS Satelite Video on Chronic Fatigue Syndrome and Fibromyalgia Association, 2892
Hi! I'm Adam!, 9095
Hidden Child: The Linwood Method for Reaching the Autistic Child, 1753
High Blood Pressure and its Effects on the Kidneys, 5703
High Blood Pressure and Stroke, 5280, 8086
High Blood Pressure and Your Kidneys, 5702
High Hopes Foundation, 10665
Hillsborough County Talking Book Library, 9635
Hiring Help at Home?, 6470
Hiring Persons with a Brain Injury: What to Expect, 4238
Hirsutism and Polycystic Ovarian Syndrome, 5524
Hispanic Deaf, 4510
A History of Childhood and Disability, 10530
History of Organ and Cell Transplantation, 9229
History of Special Education: From Isolation to Integration, 4511
History of the Agent Orange Litigation, 10303
HIV and AIDS During Pregnancy, 585
HIV Center for Clinical and Behavioral Studies, 417
HIV Counselor PERSPECTIVES, 546
HIV Disease in People with Hemophilia: Your Questions Answered, 5111
HIV Frontline, 547
HIV Infection and AIDS, 584
HIV Infection and Hemophilia, 5112
HIV Prevention Trials Unit University of Washington/Seattle HPTU Si, 437
HIV West Yellowhead Services, 259
Hiv.gov, 615
HIV/AIDS in the Workplace, 586
HIV/AIDS Prevention Program, 449
HIV/Hepatitis C in Prison (HIP) Committee, 611, 5140, 5186
Hives, 7707
Ho'opono Workshop for the Blind, 9490
Holliswood Hospital Psychiatric Care, Serv ices and Self-Help/Support Groups, 3717
Hollywood Area Brain Tumor Support Group, 1956
Hollywood Speaks, 4512
Home Care Book, 8975
Home Care Guide for Cancer, 2440
Home Control of Allergies and Asthma, 1468
Home Instead Center for Successful Aging University of Nebraska Medical Center, 121
Home Line, 3195
Home Phototherapy, 7708

Home Safety for People with Alzheimer's Disease, 1047
Home-Care Book, 8976
Hometown Heroes: Successful Deaf Youth in America, 4513
Homeward Bound, 8555
HonorBound Foundation, 10103
Hope and Help for Chronic Fatigue Syndrome, 2846
Hope and Recovery: A Mother-Daughter Story About Anorexia Nervosa & Bulimia, 3747
Hope for Children with AIDS, 587
Hope for Healing.Org, 7151
Hope for Recovery: Understanding Posttraumatic Stress Disorder, 7126
Hope Heart Institute, 4885
Hope: Alcoholics Anonymous, 8666
Hopes & Dreams for Children, 10667
Hopes & Dreams Foundation, Inc., 10666
Horizons Schools, 10500
Hormone Foundation, 16
Hormones, 5461
Hormones and Migraines: Fact Sheet, 6315
Hospice Alternative, 1008
Hospice and Homecare, 150, 10515
Hospice Association of America, 10741
Hospice Care for Children, 8819
Hospice Care for Patients with Advanced Progressive Dementia, 1009
HOSPICELINK Hospice Education Institute, 10693
Hospital Days: Treatment Ways, 2463
Hospital of the University of Pennsylvania, 8057
Hospital of the University of Pennsylvania University of Pennsylvania, 6516
Hospitalization Tips, 5227
Hot Springs Campus VA Black Hills Health Care System, 10236
House Ear Institute, 4315, 4845
Housing Works, 262
Houston Area Brain Tumor Network, 2029
Houston Ear Research Foundation, 4379
Houston Health Department: HIV-STD Viral Hepatitis Prevention, 339
Houston Love Memorial Library, 9609
Houston Public Library Access Center, 9749
Houston Support Group: National Ataxia Foundation, 1559
How Can I Help My Children?, 8556
How Can I Help?: A Handbook for Practical Suggestions for Infertility, 5462
How Can You Love Me, 5794
How Do You Kiss a Blind Girl?, 9898
How Does a Blind Person Get Around?, 9992
How Does Your Child Hear and Talk?, 4768
How Drug Abuse Takes Profit Out of Business, 8557
How Hearing Impacts Relationships, 4514
How Many Times a Day Do You Risk Being Infected with Hepatitis B?, 5175
How NF-1 Affects the Body, 6693
How NF-2 Affects the Body, 6694
How Strong Are Your Bones?, 6825
How the Student with Hearing Loss Can Succeed in College, 4515
How to Be a Successful Fertility Patient, 5463
How to Be an Assertive Parent on the Treatment Team, 5228
How to Control Bleeds: Inspired by Vince, an 8-year-old Boy with Hemophilia, 5114
How to Cook for People with Diabetes, 3445
How to Develop a Self-Help Group for Elders Losing Eyesight, 9993
How to Find More About Your Child's Birth Defect or Disability, 1885
How to Get the Most Out of Group Therapy, 8558
How to Get the Most Out of Your Doctor: A Neurologist's Perspective, 7272
How to Have Your Cake and Eat It Too, 4949
How to Help a Friend Quit Smoking, 8559
How to Keep an Infusion Log, 588
How to Live with a Mentally Ill Person: A Handbook of Day-to-Day Strategies, 6109
How to Manage Your Drug-Free Workplace Programs, 8320
How to Recognize and Classify Seizures, 7551
How to Say No and Keep Your Friends, 8435

How to Start a Parkinson's Disease Support Group, 6966
How to Start a Turner's Syndrome Support Group, 9364
How to Survive a Hearing Loss, 4516
How to Take Care of Your Baby Before Birth, 8560
How to Talk to Your Doctor About Headaches, 6316
How to Use Your Low Vision Glasses, 9994
Howard University Cancer Center, 2292
Howard University Center for Sickle Cell Disease, 7615
HPV Support Groups: Arizona, 10432
Hub, 9931
Hug Just Isn't Enough, 4517
Human Exposure Assessment for Airborne Pollutants: Advances & Opportunity, 680
Human Factor, 5086
Human Growth Foundation, 4048, 4068, 9340, 9372
Human Papillomavirus and Genital Warts, 7588
Hungry Self: Women, Eating and Identity, 3748
Hunter Holmes McGuire VA Medical Center, 10255
Huntsman Cancer Institute University of Utah School of Medicine, 2381
Huntsville Subregional Library for the Blind and Physically Handicapped, 9610
Husband Insemination, 5525
Huxley Insititute-American Schizophrenic Association, 6258
Hy Feinstein Clubhouse, 4175
Hydrocephalus Association, 5197, 5202, 5243
Hydrocephalus Association Newsletter, 5214
Hydrocephalus Association of North Texas, 5206
Hydrocephalus Association of Philadelphia, 5204
Hydrocephalus Association of Rhode Island, 5205
Hydrocephalus Center, 5244
Hydrocephalus Parents Support Group, 5208
Hydrocephalus Parents Support Group Newsletter, 5215
Hydrocephalus Support Group Newsletter, 5216
Hydrocephalus Support Group of Michigan Children's Hospital of Michigan, 5203
Hydrocephalus: A Guide for Patients, Families, and Friends, 5210
Hydrocephalus: A Neglected Disease, 5239
Hydroxychloroquine, 1328
Hyperactive Children Grown Up, 1622
Hypertension: Journal of the American Heart Association, 5290
Hypoglycemia The Other Sugar Disease, 3508
HypoPARAthyroidism Association, 5
Hypothyroidism Web Booklet, 9016
Hysterectomy Educational Resources & Services (HERS) Foundation, 3799, 5432

I

I Can Cope, 2403
I Can Hear!, 4803
I Can Hear!: II, 4804
I Can Talk About What Hurts, 8436
I Can't Be Addicted Because..., 8561
I Can't Chew Cookbook, 10550
I Choose to Fight: Tom Harper's Courageous Victory Over Cancer, 2441
I Didn't Hear the Dragon Roar, 4518
I Have a Sister, My Sister is Deaf, 4661
I Keep Five Pairs of Glasses in a Flower Pot, 9859
I See What You Say: Self Help Lip Reading Program, 4805
I Want My Little Boy Back, 1803
I Was a Fifteen-Year-Old Blimp, 3764, 6733
I Was So Mad!, 4662
I Wish Daddy Didn't Drink So Much, 8437
I'm a Meter Reader, 1431, 1497
I'm a Person Too, 9141
I'm Black and I'm Sober, 8321
I'm Just Not Myself Anymore: A Family Guide to Alzheimer's Disease, 1010
I'm Not Autistic on the Typewriter, 1754, 1804
IBD File, 3054
IBD Nutrition Book, 9388
Ice Storm, 8562
ID Card for Third Ventriculostomy Patients, 5229
Ida and Joseph Friend Cancer Resource Center, 2277

Idaho Alliance for the Mentally Ill, 5951
Idaho Commission for Libraries Talking Book Service, 9659
Idaho Department of Health and Welfare, 8732
Idaho Department of Health and Welfare: The STD/AIDS Program, 304
Idaho Persian Gulf Veterans, 10143
IDEA Advocacy for Children Who are Deaf or Hard of Hearing, 4519
Ideas and Considerations for Starting a Self-Help Mutual Aid Group, 7273
IDF Advocate, 548
IDF Guide for Nurses on Immune Globulin Therapy for Primary Immunodeficiency, 589
IDF Patient and Family Handbook, 590
If Blindness Comes, 9860
If Drugs Are So Bad, Why Do So Many People Use Them?, 8438
If God Spoke to Overeaters Anonymous, 6747
If Only I Could Quit, 8322
If Someone Close to You Has a Problem with Alcohol or Other Drugs, 8563
If You Are a Professional, AA Wants to Work with You, 8564
If You are Having Trouble Conceiving, 5527
If You Have Alzheimer's Disease: What You Should Know, What You Should Do, 1048
If You Have Scleroderma You Need Not Feel Alone, 7385
If You're Over 65 and Feeling Depressed..., 6233
If You've Thought About Breast Cancer, 2528
If Your Child Has Diabetes: An Answer Book for Parents, 3446
If Your Parents Drink Too Much, 8565
Ileostomy Guide, 3063
Illicit Drug Use During Pregnancy, 8566
Illinois Alliance for the Mentally Ill, 5952
Illinois Association of the Deaf, 4343
Illinois Braille Messenger, 9909
Illinois Church Action on Alcohol Problems, 8152
Illinois Client Assistance Program, 10447
Illinois Department of Public Health: Division of Infectious Diseases, 306
Illinois Federation of Families, 5953
Illinois Midwest Neurofibromatosis, 6664
Illinois Spina Bifida Association, 7875
Illinois State Library Talking Book and Braille Service, 9660
Illinois Teratogen Information Service (IT IS), 1853
Illinois Turner Syndrome Resource Group, 9347
Images Within: A Child's View of Parental Alcoholism, 8244
Immune Deficiency Foundation, 357, 591, 616, 656, 738
Immune Deficiency Foundation Newsletter, 549
Immune System: How it Works, 2529
Immunitherapy, 706
Immunization Action Coalition, 5142
Immunization Division Centers for Disease Control, 450
Immunotherapy, 724
Impact of AIDS, 503
Impact of Migraine: A Disabling and Costly Condition, 6317
Implications and Complications for Deaf Students of Full Inclusion Movement, 4520
Importance of Basic Science in Research, 8013
Impotence Causes and Treatments, 5313
Impotence Information Center, 5305
Impotence Resource Center of the Geddings Osbon Sr Foundation, 5325
Impotence Specialists.com, 5326
Impotence Treatment Options, 5316
Impotence World Association, 5327
Impotence Worldwide, 5310
Impotence: How to Overcome It, 5308
Impotents Anonymous, 5306
Improving Muscle Tone and Strength, 3901
In a Perfect World, 8439
In Confidence, 10592
In Control, 1355
In Focus, 550
In God's Care, 8323
In Our House, 4663
In Pursuit of Fertility, 5464

In Search of the Sun: A Woman's Courageous Victory Over Lupus, 8940
In Silence: Growing Up Hearing in a Deaf World, 4521
In the Hospital, 10584
In This Sign, 4522
In Vitro Fertilization, 5465
IN-SIGHT, 9573
Inclusion?, 4523
Incorporating Consumers into Regional Genetics Networks, 1587
Independence Center, 10503
Independence Without Sight or Sound: Suggestions for Practitioners, 9861
Independent Living Research Utilization Project, 2669
Independent Visually Impaired Enterprises, 10068
Index to Alcoholics Anonymous, 8567
Indian Health Service, 8686
Indian Health Service Federal Health Program, 8119
Indiana County Association for the Blind, 9561
Indiana Down Syndrome Foundation, 3562
Indiana Organ Procurement Organization,, 9190
Indiana Protection and Advocacy Services, 10449
Indiana Resource Center for Autism (IRCA), 1717
Indiana State Department of Health Maternal And Child Health Services, 8735
Indiana Talking Book & Braille Library, 9667
Indiana Teratogen Information Service, 1854
Indiana University Center for Aging Research, 964
Indiana University School of Medicine Center for Aging Research, 122
Indiana University: Area Health Education Center, 3384
Indiana University: Center for Diabetes Research, 3385
Indiana University: Human Genetics Center of Medical & Molecular Genetics, 965
Indiana University: Hypertension Research Center, 5256
Indiana University: Pharmacology Research Laboratory, 3386
Individual Psychotherapy with the Brain Injured Adult, 4239
Individuals with Arthritis, 1329
Individuals with Cerebral Palsy, 2800
Indoor Allergens: Assessing & Controlling Adverse Health Effects, 681
Industries for the Blind and Visually Impaired of Louisiana, 9504
Infant Death Center of Wisconsin, 8807
Infant Formulas for Allergic Infants and Dietetic Concerns for Toddlers, 682
Infant Motor Development: A Look at the Phases, 3650
Infant Positioning and Sudden Infant Death Syndrome, 8828
Infections Linked to AIDS, 592
Infectious Diseases Society of America, 9025
Infertility and Adoption, 5503
Infertility Book: A Comprehensive Medical & Emotional Guide, 5466
Infertility Books, 5566
Infertility Insurance, 5528
Infertility: A Comprehensive Text, 5467
Infertility: An Overview, 5529
Infertility: Causes and Treatment, 3817, 5530
Infertility: Coping and Decision Making, 5531
Infertility: Exploring the Male Factor, 5554
Infertility: The Emotional Roller Coaster, 5532
Inflammatory Bowel Disease, 3055, 9389
Inflammatory Bowel Disease Program, 2994
Information About the Sweat Test, 3200
Information General Sobre: Lesion Cerebral, 4240
Information on Glaucoma, 9995
Information on Macular Degeneration, 9996
Information Protection & Advocacy Center for Handicapped Individuals, 10440
Informed Consent: Does the Current Process Reflect Current Treatments, 2530
Informed Consent: Participation In Genetic Research Studies, 1588
Informed Decisions: The Complete Book of Cancer Diagnosis, Treatment and Recovery, 2442
Informed Woman's Guide to Breast Health, 10551

Informer, 5348, 8943
Infusion, 5093, 5099
Inhalants, 8440
Inhaled Medications for Asthma, 1469
Initiatives, 5094
Injury Research Center, 7100
Inland Empire Bleeding Disorders, 5010
Inner Circle, 3056, 9392
Innovations, 190
Inside Fibromyalgia, 3882
Inside Manic Depression, 6216
Inside MS, 6454
Inside MS Bulletin, 6455
Inside Out, 8441
Inside Story, 3057, 9394
Insider's Guide to HMOs, 10552
InSight, 9932
Insight Into Eyesight, 6471
Insights in the Dynamic Psychotherapy of Anorexia and Bulimia, 3749
Insights Into Infertility, 5533
Insights Into Spina Bifida, 7934
Institute for Basic Research in Developmental Disabilities, 966, 1720, 3597
Institute for Clinical Research Weill Cornell Medical College, 418
Institute for Life Course and Aging, 31
Institute for Rehabilitation and Research, 660, 4131
Institute for Visual Sciences, 9793
Institute of Ophthalmology and Visual Scie nce New Jersey Medical School, 9794
Institute of Psychiatry and Human Behavior: University of Maryland, 6031
Institute on Communication and Inclusion at Syracuse University, 1721
Institute on Health Care for the Poor and Underserved at Meharry Medical College, 517
Institute on Violence, Abuse and Trauma, 7070
Insulin-Dependent Diabetes, 3509
Insurance Articles, 2531
Integrating Community Resources, 4200
InteliHealth, 10315
Intensified Insulin Management for You, 3447
Intensive Diabetes Management, 3448
Inter-American Society of Hypertension, 5291
Inter-Provincial Roof Consultants, Ltd., 5143
Interdisciplinary Program in Cell and Molecular Pharmacology, 8209
Intermountain Donor Services, 9220
International Association for Chronic Fati gue Syndrome/Myalgic Encephalomyelitis, 2826
International Association for the Study of Pain, 2914, 10385
International Association of Cancer Victors and Friends, 2404
International Association of Eating Disorders Professionals Foundation, 2594, 3703
International Association of Laryngectomees, 2103
International Braille and Technology Center for the Blind, 9688
International Brain Injury Association, 4080
International Center for Fabry Disease, 3836, 3841
International Classification of Sleep Disorders, 2847, 7822
International Council of AIDS Service Organization, 263
International Council on Disability, 10386
International Council on Infertility Information Dissemination, 5378, 5567
International Diabetes Center at Nicollet, 3387
International Directory of Periodicals Related to Deafness, 4524
International Federation on Ageing, 32
International Foundation for Functional Gastrointestinal Disorders (IFFGD), 3040, 3934, 4006, 5337
International Foundation for Research and Education for Depression (iFred), 6196
International Health Guide for Senior Citizen Travelers, 172
International Hearing Dog, 4316
International Hearing Society, 4317, 4414
International Holistic Center, 2118
International Journal of Dermatology, 7686
International Journal of Technology and Aging, 191

International Lawyers in Alcoholics Anonymous, 8245
International Myopain Society, 3861
International Parkinson and Movement Disorder Society, 1519, 6868
International Pelvic Pain Society, 2915, 2941, 3795, 3827
International Rehabilitation Center for Polio, 7026
International Skeletal Dysplasia Registry Medical Genetics Institute, 4052
International Society for Adult Congenital Heart Disease (ISACHD), 2947
International Society for the Study of Dissociation, 6279
International Society for the Study of Trauma and Dissociation, 6256, 7049
International Society for Traumatic Stress Studies, 7048, 7091
International Society of Dermatology, 7662
International Storage Disease Collaborative, 3850
International Telephone Directory for TDD Users, 4525
International Union Against Venereal Diseases, 7572
Internet Health Resources, 5568
Internet Mental Health, 6182
Interpreters in Public Schools Kit, 4806
Interpreting Your PSA and Related Prostate Cancer Blood Tests, 2532
Interventions for Alzheimer's Disease: A Caregiver's Complete Reference, 1011
Interview with Kirsten Gonzales, 4807
Intestinal Fortitude, 5349
Intrauterine Growth Retardation, 4060
Introduction to Communication, 4526
Introduction to Infertility: The First Steps, 5534
Introduction to Sexually Transmitted Diseases, 7589
Introductory Information for Families, 4241
Invisible Condition: The Human Side of Hearing Loss, 4527
Invisible Inc #4, 4664
Invisible People: How the U.S. Has Slept Through the Global AIDS Pandemic, 478
Invisible Wall: Autism, 1805
Iowa Brain Tumor Support Group, 1968
Iowa Chapter of the Association of Kidney Patients, 5610
Iowa City VA Health Care System, 10153
Iowa Department for the Blind, 9669
Iowa Donor Network, 9191
Iowa Federaion of Families for Children's Mental Health (FFCMH), 6060
Iowa Oncology Research Association, 2308
Iowa SIDS Alliance, 8737
Iowa SIDS Program Iowa Department of Public Health, 8738
Iowa Turner Syndrome Resource Group, 9348
Iron Overload Alert, 3982
Ironic Blood, 3970
Is AA for Me?, 8568
Is AA for You?, 8569
Is There a Safe Tobacco?, 8570
Is There an Alcoholic in Your Life?, 8571
Is Your Liver Giving You the Silent Treatment?, 5176
ISSD News, 6274
Issues in Independent Living, 10605
Issues in Reproductive Management, 5468
Issues in Women's Gastrointestinal Health, 3983
It Happened to Alice, 8572
It Sure Beats Sitting in a Cell, 8573, 8667
It's All Right to Be Angry, 9997
It's Just Attention Disorder, 1652
It's Just Part of My Life, 5716
It's Not All in Your Head, 5309
It's Not Just Hearing AIDS: Deaf People and the Epidemic, 4808
It's Not Your Fault, 3750
Its Your Turn Now: Using Dialogue Journals with Deaf Students, 4528
IVF & GIFT: A Guide to Assisted Reproductive Technologies, 5526
Ivf.com, 5569

J

Jack C. Montgomery VA Medical Center Eastern Oklahoma VA Health Care System, 10219
Jackson Regional Office, 10182
Jacksonville Public Library, 9636
Jamaica Plain Division VA Boston Healthcare System, 10170
James A. Haley Veterans' Hospital, 10131
James H. Quillen VA Healthcare System Mountain Home VA Healthcare System, 10239
James R Clark Memorial Sickle Cell Foundation, 7608
JamesCare For Life Support Groups & Services, 2405
Jane & Terry Semel Institute for Neuroscie nce & Human Behavior, 6032
Jane and Richard Thomas Center for Down Syndrome, 3587
Jason's Dreams for Kids Foundation, Inc., 10686
Jean Mayer USDA Human Nutrition Research Center on Aging at Tufts University, 123
Jerusalem Center for Multi-Handicapped Blind Children, 9795
Jesse Brown VA Medical Center, 10147
Jessie's Legacy, 3677
Jewish Genetics Disaese Center, 4020
Jewish Genetics Disease Center, 8967
Jewish Heritage for the Blind, 9862
Jewish Hospital Transplant Center, 9248
Jewish Hospital Transplant Center KentuckyOne Health, 9168
JGB Cassette Library International, 9728
Jim L Walker: Arizona Chapter of the Myasthenia Gravis Foundation of America, 6574
JIMHO Affiliated Centers (Justice in Mental Health Organization), 5970
Jimmie Heuga Center, 6432
Job Opportunities for the Blind, 9814
Job Seeker Involvment in Securing Employment, 1788
Jodi House, 4149
Joey and Sam, 1781
John A. Hartford Foundation, 112
John D. Dingell VA Medical Center, 10174
John Douglas French Alzheimer's Foundation, 756
John J. Pershing VA Medical Center, 10185
John L McClellan Memorial Veterans' Hospital Research Office, 4886
John Tracy Clinic, 4318, 4846
John Tracy Clinic on Deafness, 4415
Johns Hopkins Brain Tumor Education Group, 1980
Johns Hopkins Center on Aging and Health, 124
Johns Hopkins Health Insider, 10593
Johns Hopkins University: Asthma and Allergy Center, 1403
Johns Hopkins University: Behavioral Pharmacology Research Unit, 8210
Johns Hopkins University: Center for Communication Programs, 400
Johns Hopkins University: Dana Center for Preventive Ophthalmology, 9796
Johns Hopkins University: Scleroderma Center, 7361
Johns Hopkins University: Sleep Disorders Francis Scott Key Medical Center, 7770
Johns Hopkins University: Sydney Kimmel Comprehensive Cancer Center, 2318
Jonathan M. Wainwright Memorial VA MC Walla Walla VA Medical Center, 10258
Jonsson Comprehensive Cancer Center University of California At Los Angeles, 2278
Joslin Center at University of Maryland Medicine, 3372
Joslin Diabetes Center, 3388
Joslin Magazine, 3492
Journal of AAA, 4711
Journal of Acquired Immune Deficiency Syndrome, 518
Journal of Chronic Fatigue Syndrome, 2901
Journal of Clinical Psychology, 6151
Journal of Dermatologic Surgery and Oncology, 7687
Journal of Head Trauma Rehabilitation, 4213
Journal of Musculoskeletal Medicine, 3895
Journal of Musculoskeletal Pain, 3890
Journal of Occupational & Environmental Medicine, 5504

Journal of Parenteral and Enteral Nutrition, 3958
Journal of Pediatric Gastroenterology and Nutrition, 3959
Journal of Speech-Language-Hearing Research, 4712
Journal of the Academy of Dermatology, 7688
Journal of the Academy of Nutrition and Dietetics, 691, 2640, 3767, 3960
Journal of the Chronic Fatigue Syndrome, 2859
Journal of the Medical Library Association, 519
Journal of Vision Rehabilitation, 9910
Journal of Visual Impairment & Blindness, 9911
Journal SLEEP, 2858
Journel to Pain Relief, 10553
Journey Into the Deaf World, 4529
Journey of Love: Parent's Guide to Duchenne Muscular Dystrophy, 6524
Journey Out of Silence, 4530
Journey to Almost There, 6940
Journeys with ALS, 1157
Joy of Laziness, 10554
Joy of Signing, 4531, 4809
JRA and Me, 1279
Just for Children: Helping You Understand Alzheimer's Disease, 1025
Just for Teens: Helping You Understand Alzheimer's Disease, 1049
Just Kids, 551
Just Like Everyone Else, 10555
Just Like You and Me, 7552
Just One Little Bite Can Hurt! Important Facts About Anaphylaxis, 707
Just Say Notes, 8470
Juvenile Dermatomyositis, 1330
Juvenile Diabetes Research Foundation, 3304
Juvenile Diabetes Research Foundation Cana da, 3368
Juvenile Diabetes Research Foundation International, 3367
Juvenile Diabetes Research Foundation/JDRF, 3319
Juvenile Diabetes Research Foundation: Akr on/Canton Chapter, 3321
Juvenile Diabetes Research Foundation: Albuquerque, 3302
Juvenile Diabetes Research Foundation: Bakersfield Chapter, 3225
Juvenile Diabetes Research Foundation: Bat on Rouge Chapter, 3270
Juvenile Diabetes Research Foundation: Ber ks County Chapter, 3332
Juvenile Diabetes Research Foundation: Birmingham, 3214
Juvenile Diabetes Research Foundation: Buf falo/Western New York Chapter, 3306
Juvenile Diabetes Research Foundation: Cap itol Chapter, 3241
Juvenile Diabetes Research Foundation: Cen tral Florida Chapter, 3245
Juvenile Diabetes Research Foundation: Cen tral Jersey Chapter, 3298
Juvenile Diabetes Research Foundation: Cen tral Oklahoma Chapter, 3325
Juvenile Diabetes Research Foundation: Central Pennsylvania Chapter, 3331
Juvenile Diabetes Research Foundation: Cha rlotte Chapter, 3314
Juvenile Diabetes Research Foundation: Colorado Springs Chapter, 3232
Juvenile Diabetes Research Foundation: Dal las Chapter, 3347
Juvenile Diabetes Research Foundation: Del aware, 3239
Juvenile Diabetes Research Foundation: Eas tern Iowa Chapter, 3264
Juvenile Diabetes Research Foundation: East Tennessee Chapter, 3343
Juvenile Diabetes Research Foundation: Fai rfield County Chapter, 3236
Juvenile Diabetes Research Foundation: Flo rida Sun Coast Chapter, 3246
Juvenile Diabetes Research Foundation: Geo rgia Chapter, 3253
Juvenile Diabetes Research Foundation: Gre ater Blue Ridge Chapter, 3355
Juvenile Diabetes Research Foundation: Gre ater Cincinnati Chapter, 3258, 3322

Juvenile Diabetes Research Foundation: Gre ater Fort Worth/ Arlington Chapter, 3348
Juvenile Diabetes Research Foundation: Gre ater Iowa Chapter, 3265
Juvenile Diabetes Research Foundation: Gre ater Madison Chapter, 3365
Juvenile Diabetes Research Foundation: Gre ater Palm Beach County Chapter, 3247
Juvenile Diabetes Research Foundation: Greater New Haven Chapter, 3235
Juvenile Diabetes Research Foundation: Haw aii Chapter, 3255
Juvenile Diabetes Research Foundation: Hou ston/Gulf Coast Chapter, 3349
Juvenile Diabetes Research Foundation: Hud son Valley Chapter, 3307
Juvenile Diabetes Research Foundation: Hun tington Chapter, 3362
Juvenile Diabetes Research Foundation: Ind iana State Chapter, 3261
Juvenile Diabetes Research Foundation: Inl and Empire Chapter, 3226
Juvenile Diabetes Research Foundation: Kentuckiana Chapter, 3268
Juvenile Diabetes Research Foundation: Lin coln Chapter, 3289
Juvenile Diabetes Research Foundation: Long Island/South Shore Chapter, 3305
Juvenile Diabetes Research Foundation: Los Angeles Chapter, 3227
Juvenile Diabetes Research Foundation: Lou isiana Chapter, 3271
Juvenile Diabetes Research Foundation: Low Country Chapter, 3339
Juvenile Diabetes Research Foundation: Mar yland Chapter, 3276
Juvenile Diabetes Research Foundation: Metropolitan Detroit/SE Michigan, 3280
Juvenile Diabetes Research Foundation: Mid -Jersey Chapter, 3299
Juvenile Diabetes Research Foundation: Mid dle Tennessee Chapter, 3344
Juvenile Diabetes Research Foundation: Mid-Ohio Chapter, 3320
Juvenile Diabetes Research Foundation: Min nesota Chapter, 3283
Juvenile Diabetes Research Foundation: Nevada Chapter, 3292
Juvenile Diabetes Research Foundation: New England/New Hampshire Chapter, 3295
Juvenile Diabetes Research Foundation: New York Chapter, 3308
Juvenile Diabetes Research Foundation: New England/Bay State Chapter, 3274, 3278
Juvenile Diabetes Research Foundation: Nor th Central CT and Western MA, 3237
Juvenile Diabetes Research Foundation: Nor th Florida Chapter, 3248
Juvenile Diabetes Research Foundation: Nor theast Wisconsin Chapter, 3309, 3366
Juvenile Diabetes Research Foundation: Nor thern Nevada Branch, 3228, 3262, 3293
Juvenile Diabetes Research Foundation: Nor thwestern Pennsylvania Chapter, 3333
Juvenile Diabetes Research Foundation: Northwest Arkansas Branch, 3222
Juvenile Diabetes Research Foundation: Oma ha Council Bluffs Chapter, 3290
Juvenile Diabetes Research Foundation: Ora nge County Chapter, 3229
Juvenile Diabetes Research Foundation: Ore gon/SW Washington Chapter, 3328
Juvenile Diabetes Research Foundation: Palmetto Chapter, 3338
Juvenile Diabetes Research Foundation: Phi ladelphia Chapter, 3334
Juvenile Diabetes Research Foundation: Phoenix Chapter, 3220
Juvenile Diabetes Research Foundation: Pie dmont Triad Chapter, 3315
Juvenile Diabetes Research Foundation: Roc hester Branch/Western New York Chapter, 3310
Juvenile Diabetes Research Foundation: Roc kland County/Northern New Jersey, 3300

Juvenile Diabetes Research Foundation: Roc ky Mountain Chapter, 3233
Juvenile Diabetes Research Foundation: San Diego Chapter, 3230
Juvenile Diabetes Research Foundation: Sea ttle Chapter, 3359
Juvenile Diabetes Research Foundation: Seattle Guild, 3358
Juvenile Diabetes Research Foundation: Shr eveport Chapter, 3272
Juvenile Diabetes Research Foundation: Sio ux Falls Chapter, 3340
Juvenile Diabetes Research Foundation: Sou th Florida Chapter, 3249
Juvenile Diabetes Research Foundation: South Central Texas Chapter, 3346
Juvenile Diabetes Research Foundation: South Jersey Chapter, 3297
Juvenile Diabetes Research Foundation: Southeastern Chapter, 3364
Juvenile Diabetes Research Foundation: Spo kane County Area Chapter, 3360
Juvenile Diabetes Research Foundation: St. Louis Chapter, 3286
Juvenile Diabetes Research Foundation: Tam pa Bay Chapter, 3250
Juvenile Diabetes Research Foundation: Tol edo/Northwest Ohio Chapter, 3323
Juvenile Diabetes Research Foundation: Triangle/Eastern North Carolina Chapter, 3313
Juvenile Diabetes Research Foundation: Tul sa Green County Chapter, 3326
Juvenile Diabetes Research Foundation: Wes t Michigan Chapter, 3281
Juvenile Diabetes Research Foundation: Wes t Texas Chapter, 3350
Juvenile Diabetes Research Foundation: Wes tchester County Chapter, 3311
Juvenile Diabetes Research Foundation: Wes tern Pennsylvania, 3335
Juvenile Scleroderma Network, 7357

K

Kaiser Foundation Research Institute, 374
Kalamazoo Center for Medical Studies Michigan State University, 3131
KALEIDOSCOPE, 6057
Kaleidoscope of Deaf America, 4532
Kanawha County Public Library, 9766
Kansas Association of the Deaf, 4344
Kansas City Association for the Blind, 9524
Kansas City Support Group: National Ataxia Foundation, 1548
Kansas City VA Medical Center, 10186
Kansas Department of Health & Environment: Bureau of Family Health, 8739
Kansas Department of Health & Environment: STI/HIV Section, 310
Kansas Industries for the Blind, 9500
Kansas Services for the Blind and Visually Impaired, 9808
Kansas State University Center on Aging, 125
Kansas State University: Terry C Johnson Center for Basic Cancer Research, 2310
Kansas University Medical Center: Cystic Fibrosis Center, 3115
Kathy's Hats: A Story of Hope, 2464
KDWB Family Resource Center, 10516
KDWB Variety Family Canter, 10517
Keep A Child Alive, 264
Keep it Simple, 8325
Keep Quit, 8324
Keeping the Balance, 5890
Kellogg Cancer Care Center Evanston Hospital, 2301
Kemo Shark, 2465
Kendall Demonstration Elementary School Curriculum Guides, 4533
Kennedy Krieger Institute, 3588
Kennedy Krieger Institute - Down Syndrome, 3598
Kennedy-Krieger Institute, 10273
Kent County Health Department, 8753
Kent County Library for the Blind, 9697
Kentucky Alliance for the Mentally Ill, 5962

Kentucky Association of the Deaf, 4345
Kentucky Cancer Program, 2312
Kentucky Hemophilia Foundation, 4979
Kentucky IMPACT, 6061
Kentucky Industries for the Blind, 9502
Kentucky Organ Donor Affiliates, 9193
Kentucky Talking Book Library, 9676
Kentucky University: Cystic Fibrosis Center, 3117
Keon Paschal Perry Sickle Cell Anemia Disease Awareness, 7625
Kernel Book Series, 9863
Kerrville VA Hospital South Texas Veterans Health Care System, 10247
Ketogenic Diet: A Treatment for Epilepsy, 7516
Kettering-Scott Magnetic Resonance Laboratory, 8211
Key Elements of Dementia Care, 1012
Keys for Networking: Kansas FFCMH, 5959
Keys to Parenting the Child with Autism, 1755
Keystone Blind Association, 9562
Kid, 5704
A Kid Again, 10653
Kid's 1st Cookbook: Delicious-Nutritious Treats to Make Yourself, 2466
Kid's Corner, 3498
Kid-Friendly Parenting with Deaf and Hard of Hearing Children, 4534
Kidd's Kids, 10668
Kidneeds, 5671
Kidney & Urology Foundation of America, 5629
Kidney Association of South Florida, 5598
Kidney Beginnings: A Patient's Guide to Li ving with Reduced Kidney Function, 5674
Kidney Cooking, 5675
Kidney Disease Institute, 5661
Kidney Disease: A Guide for Patients and Their Families, 5705
Kidney Transplant: A New Lease on Life, 5706
Kidneys for Kids, 5707
Kids and Alcohol: Get High on Life, 8442
Kids and Drugs: A Handbook for Parents & Professionals, 8574
Kids on the Block Arthritis Programs, 1258
Kids Wish Network, 10669
Kids with Food Allergies, 657
Kids with Heart National Association for Children's Heart Disorders, 2948
Kidscope, 2161
Kindey Beginnings: The Magazine, 5682
King County Crisis Clinic, 451
King James Bible: Large Print, 9864
King Midas, 4810
King Midas Videotape, 4811
King Midas With Selected Sentences in ASL, 4665
Kiss the Candy Days Good-bye, 3483
Kits for Adults with Epilepsy, 7536
Knollwoodpark Hospital Sleep Disorders Cen, 7772
Knollwoodpark Hospital Sleep Disorders Center, 7771
Knotholes are for Seeing: Therapy Through Poetry, Prose & Other Writings, 9865
Know Your Brain, 4242
Kosair Childrens Cystic Fibrosis Center, 3118
Krannert Institute of Cardiology, 4887
Kuakini Parkinson Disease (PD) Information & Referral, 6916
KY Partnership For Families and Children, 5961

L

Label Reading and Shopping, 3518
Laboratory of Dermatology Research Memorial Sloane-Kettering Cancer Center, 7668
Laboure College Library, 9692
LAC/USC Imaging Science Center, 4026
Lake City VA Medical Center North Florida/South Georgia, 10132
Lake County Public Library, 9668
Lancaster County Association for the Blind, 9563
Landon Center on Aging University of Kansas Medical Center, 126
Langley Porter Psychiatric Institute University of California, 6033

Language, Speech and Hearing Services in the Schools, 4713
Laparoscopy and Hysteroscopy, 5535
LaRabida Children's Hospital: Developmental Disabilities & Delays, 3589
Laradon Services for Children and Adults w ith Developmental Disabilities, 6051
Large Print American Heritage Dictionary, 9866
Large Print Loan Library Catalog, 9998
Las Vegas Clark County Library District, 9721
Last in Line, 6110
Late Onset Community Newsletter, 8985
Late Onset Tay-Sachs Disease Medical Bibliography, 8977
Late Onset Tay-Sachs Fact Sheet, 8987
Late Stage Care, 1050
Late-Deafened Adults: A Selected Annotated Bibliography, 4769
Latex Allergy, 708
Laugh at Your Muscles, 3883
LAUNCH Department of Special Education, 10387
Laurel's Kitchen Caring: Recipes for Everyday Home Caregiving, 10556
Lawyers Concerned for Lawyers, 8120, 8687
LD Alert Card, 9051
LD Awareness Packet, 9052
LD Child and the ADHD Child, 1623
LD: Diagnosis & Treatment, 9059
LD: Facts for Kids, 9060
Lead Line, 8467
Leaders Link, 1445
Leading Age, 33
Leading National Publications of and for Deaf People, 4770
Leading Self-Help Groups: Report on Workshop for Leaders of Groups, 2533
Learning Ally, 9430
Learning Among Children with Spina Bifida, 7937
Learning Disabilities and the Person with Spina Bifida, 7920
Learning Disabilities Association of America, 1607, 10388
Learning Disabilities in Children with Hydrocephalus, 5231
Learning Disability Quarterly, 10594
Learning How, 10389
Learning Problems & the Child with TS, 9116
Learning to be Independent and Responsible, 1789
Learning to Communicate: The First Three Years Videotape, 4812
Learning to Fall: the Blessings of an Imperfect Life, 1158
Learning to Hear Again, 4535
Learning to Live Drug Free: A Curriculum Model for Prevention, 8326
Learning to Live Well with Diabetes, 3449
Learning to Live with Neuromuscular Desease: A Message to Parents, 6554
Learning to Play, 9999
Learning to See: American Sign Language as a Second Language, 4536
Learning to Sign in my Neighborhood, 4666
Least Restrictive Environment: The Paradox of Inclusion, 4537
Lebanon VA Medical Center, 10229
Lee County Talking Books Library, 9637
Lee the Rabbit with Epilepsy, 7523
Legal and Ethical Aspects of Organ Transplantation, 9230
Legal and Financial Issues for Families, 4243
Legal Center for People with Disabilities, 10489
Legal Center for People with Disabilities and Older People, 10436
Legal Council for Health Justice, 62, 307, 10448
Legal Plans, 1051
Legal Rights for the Deaf and Hard of Hearing, 4538
Legal Rights of Hearing-Impaired People, 4539
Legislative Handbook for Parents, 9867
Lehigh Valley Chapter of the American Association of Kidney Patients, 5640
Lehigh Valley Sickle Cell Support Group, 7626
Les Turner Amyotrophic Lateral Sclerosis Foundation, 1152
Les Turner Research Laboratory Northwestern University Medical School, 1140

Lessons in Laughter: The Autobiography of a Deaf Actor, 4540

Let Community Employment Be the Goal for Individuals with Autism, 1756

Let Me Hear Your Voice A Family's Triumph Over Autism, 1757

Let's Be Friends, 4813

Let's Breathe Sarcoidosis Support Group, 7240

Let's Eat, 10000, 10038

Let's Learn About Deafness, 4541

Let's Solve the Smokeword Puzzle, 8575

Let's Talk, 8576

Let's Talk About Alcohol Abuse, 8327

Let's Talk About Depression, 6234

Let's Talk About Drug Abuse, 8443

Let's Talk About Having Asthma, 1432

Let's Talk About Having Lyme Disease, 9042

Let's Talk About When A Parent Dies, 10728

Let's Talk About When Someone You Love Has Alzheimer's Disease, 1026

Let's Talk Facts About Childhood Disorders, 6164

Lethal Secrets: The Psychology of Donor Insemination, 5469

Letter to a Friend Whose Child is Newly Diagnosed with Cancer, 2534

Letter to a Woman Alcoholic, 8577

Letting Go of the Need to Control, 8578

Leukemia & Lymphoma Society Chapter: New York City, 2209

Leukemia & Lymphoma Society: Orange, Riverside, And San Bernadino Counties, 2135

Leukemia & Lymphoma Society: Suncoast Chapter, 2155

Leukemia & Lymphoma Society: Tennessee Chapter, 2241

Leukemia & Lymphoma Society: Westchester/ Hudson Valley Chapter, 2210

Leukemia and Lymophoma Society: National Capital Area Chapter, 2250

Leukemia and Lymphoma Society, 2104, 2595

Leukemia and Lymphoma Society Chapter: New York City, 2211

Leukemia and Lymphoma Society: Southern Florida Chapter, 2156

Leukemia and Lymphoma Society: Alabama Chapter, 2115

Leukemia and Lymphoma Society: Central Florida Chapter, 2157

Leukemia and Lymphoma Society: Central New York Chapter, 2212

Leukemia and Lymphoma Society: Central Ohio Chapter, 2221

Leukemia and Lymphoma Society: Central Pennsylvania Chapter, 2231

Leukemia and Lymphoma Society: Connecticut Chapter, 2147

Leukemia and Lymphoma Society: Delaware Chapter, 2150

Leukemia and Lymphoma Society: Eastern North Carolina Chapter, 2217

Leukemia and Lymphoma Society: Eastern Pennsylvania Chapter, 2232

Leukemia and Lymphoma Society: Fairfield County Chapter, 2148

Leukemia and Lymphoma Society: Georgia Chapter, 2162

Leukemia and Lymphoma Society: Greater Los Angeles Chapter, 2138

Leukemia and Lymphoma Society: Greater Sacramento Area Chapter, 2137

Leukemia and Lymphoma Society: Illinois Chapter, 2166

Leukemia and Lymphoma Society: Indiana Chapter, 2168

Leukemia and Lymphoma Society: Kentucky Chapter, 2175

Leukemia and Lymphoma Society: Long Island Chapter, 2213

Leukemia and Lymphoma Society: Maryland Chapter, 2179

Leukemia and Lymphoma Society: Michigan Chapter, 2182

Leukemia and Lymphoma Society: Mid-America Chapter, 2172

Leukemia and Lymphoma Society: Minnesota Chapter, 2187

Leukemia and Lymphoma Society: Mississippi Chapter, 2189

Leukemia and Lymphoma Society: Mountain States Chapter, 2119, 2202

Leukemia and Lymphoma Society: Nebraska Chapter, 2193

Leukemia and Lymphoma Society: North Carolina Chapter, 2218

Leukemia and Lymphoma Society: North Texas Chapter, 2243

Leukemia and Lymphoma Society: Northern California Chapter, 2139

Leukemia and Lymphoma Society: Northern Florida Chapter, 2158

Leukemia and Lymphoma Society: Northern New Jersey Chapter, 2199

Leukemia and Lymphoma Society: Northern Ohio Chapter, 2222

Leukemia and Lymphoma Society: Oklahoma Chapter, 2225

Leukemia and Lymphoma Society: Orange, Riverside, And San Bernadino Counties, 2140

Leukemia and Lymphoma Society: Oregon Chapter, 2227

Leukemia and Lymphoma Society: Palm Beach Area Chapter, 2159

Leukemia and Lymphoma Society: Rhode Island Chapter, 2235

Leukemia and Lymphoma Society: San Diego/Hawaii Chapter, 2136

Leukemia and Lymphoma Society: South Carolina Chapter, 2237

Leukemia and Lymphoma Society: South/West, 2238

Leukemia and Lymphoma Society: South/West Texas Chapter, 2244

Leukemia and Lymphoma Society: Southern New Jersey Chapter, 2200

Leukemia and Lymphoma Society: Southern Ohio Chapter, 2223

Leukemia and Lymphoma Society: Texas Gulf Coast Chapter, 2245

Leukemia and Lymphoma Society: Tri-County Chapter, 2141

Leukemia and Lymphoma Society: Upstate New York Chapter, 2214

Leukemia and Lymphoma Society: Western New York & Finger Lakes Chapter, 2215

Leukemia and Lymphoma Society: Western Pennsylvania/West Virginia Chapter, 2233

Leukemia and Lymphoma Society: Wisconsin Chapter, 2255

Leukemia and Lymphona Society: Kansas Chapter, 2173

Leukemia Research Foundation, 2302

Lewis H Walker MD: Cystic Fibrosis Center, 3156

Lewiston Public Library, 9682

Lexington VA Health Care System, 10158

LIAFLine Newsletter, 1037

Library and Resource Center for the Blind and Physically Handicapped, 9611

Library for the Blind and Handicapped, Southwest, 9618

Library of Michigan Service for the Blind, 9698

Library Resources for the Blind and Physically Handicapped, 9868

Library Services to the Deaf Community, 4366

Library Users of America, 10069

Life After Brain Injury: Who am I, 4244

Life Connection of Ohio, 9210

Life Development Institute, 10390, 10501, 10638

Life of My Own: Daily Meditations on Hope and Acceptance, 8328

Life on Wheels: for the Active Wheelchair User, 1159

Life Planning and Down Syndrome, 3637

Life Share of the Carolinas, 9209

Life with Diabetes: A Series of Teaching Outlines, 3450

Life with Mic-Key, 3988

LifeBanc, 9211

LifeCenter Northwest, 9223

Lifeclinic.Com, 5292

Lifeline, 2642, 2980, 8986

Lifeline Letter, 3971

Lifeline of Ohio Organ Procurement Agency, Inc., 9212

Lifeline: The Action Guide to Adoption Search, 5470

Lifelines, 10595

LifeLink of Florida, 9184

LifeLink of Georgia, 9187

LifeLink of Southwest Florida, 9185

Lifelong Health and Fitness, 204

LifeNet, 9221

LifeSharing Community Organ & Tissue Donation, 9180

LifeSource, Upper Midwest Organ Procurement Organization, Inc., 9198

Lifetime of Freedom from Smoking: Maintenance Manual, 8579

Lifting of Canavan's Carrier Testing Facilities, 8978

Lighthouse for the Blind and Visually Impaired, 9472

Lighthouse for the Blind of Houston, 9583

Lighthouse for the Blind of Washington, 9595

Lighthouse Guild GuildCare, 9431

Lighthouse International, 10070

Lighthouse of the Blind of Fort Worth, 9584

Lilliput Families, 5379

Lincoln Cancer Center, 2332

LINK, 1163

LINK Directory Information, 5230

Linking Factor, 5095

Lion, 9933

Lion Who Had Asthma, 1433

Lions Industries for the Blind, 9543

Lions Quest, 10391

List of Agent Orange-Related Illnesses Recognized By the VA, 10304

List of Diseases Accepted by the VA for Presumptive Service-Connection, 10305

Listen to Me: Auditory Exercises for Adults, 4542

Listen Up, 9934

Listen with the Heart: Relationships and Hearing Loss, 4543

Listening, 4544

Listening & Talking, 4545

Listening and Spoken Knowledge Center, 4367

Listening and Spoken Language Knowledge Ce nter, 4319

Listening to Learn: A Handbook for Parents with Hearing-Impaired Children, 4546

Listening: Ways of Hearing in a Silent World, 4547

Literature Journal, 4548

Lithium and Manic Depression, 6235

Little Green Monsters, 4667

Little More About Alcohol, 8580

Little People of America, 4045

Little Red Book, 8329

Little Red Riding Hood, 4668

Little Star Foundation, 10687

Liver Cancer, 5776

Liver Disease in Children, 5777

Liver Function Tests, 5795

Liver Support, 5805

Liver Transplant Fund, 5796

Liver Transplantation, 5797

Liver Update, 5781

LiverLink, 5782

Living a Healthy Life with Chronic Conditions, 10557

Living and Loving: Information About Sexuality and Intimacy, 1331

Living Hell: The Real World of Chronic Fatigue Syndrome, 2893

Living in a Shelter?, 8582

Living on the Edge, 480

Living Positive, 265

Living Sober, 8330, 8581

Living Well in a Nursing Home, 173

Living Well with Diabetes, 3519

Living Well with Epilepsy, 7517

Living Well With HIV and AIDS, 479

Living Well, Despite Lupus!, 8952

Living with A Brain Tumor, 2061

Living with Allergies, 688

Living with ALS: Adapting to Breathing Changes/Use of Non Invasive Ventilation, 1172

Living with ALS: Adjusting to Swallowing Difficulties & Good Nutrition, 1173

Living with ALS: Communication Solutions & Symptom Management, 1174
Living with ALS: Mobility, Activities of Daily Living, Home Adaptions, 1175
Living with Arthritis, 1280
Living with Ataxia, 1567
Living with Blindness, 9899
Living with Brain Injury: A Guide for Families, 4201
Living with Cancer, 2467
Living with CFS: A Personal Story of the Struggle for Recovery, 2848
Living with Deafness, 4669
Living with Diabetes, 3484
Living with Gaucher Disease, 4031
Living with Hearing Loss, 4549
Living with Heart Disease, 4930
Living with Hepatitis C: Self Help Tips, 5177
Living with HIV: Talking with Your Child, 5115
Living with ME, 2849
Living with Mental Handicaps, 6111
Living with MS, 6472
Living with Multiple Sclerosis, 6443
Living with Multiple Sclerosis: A Wellness Approach, 6444
Living with Narcolepsy, 7823
Living with Osteoporosis, 6826
Living with Ovarian Cancer, 2583
Living with Parkinson's Disease, 6933
Living With Rheumatoid Arthritis, 1272
Living with Spinal Cord Injury, 8027
Living with Tourette Syndrome, 9088
Living Without Depression & Manic Depression: A Workbook, 6236
Local AIDS Sercices: The National Directory, 481
Loch Raven VA Community Living & Rehabilitation Center, 10165
LODAT: Brain Tumor Support Group, 2040
Lois Insolia ALS Center at Northwestern Memorial Hospital, 1105
Lois Remembers, 8331
Loma Linda University Sleep Disorders Clinic, 7773
Lone Star Chapter of the American Association of Kidney Patients, 5651
Lone Star Chapter of the National Hemophilia Foundation, 5004
Long Cane News, 9935
Long Island Alzheimers Foundation, 946, 967
Long Island Brain Tumor Support Group, 2002
Long Island Chapter of the American Association of Kidney Patients, 5630
Long-Awaited Stork: A Guide to Parenting After Infertility, 5471
LongTermCare.gov, 225
Look at Cross-Addiction, 8583
Look at Relapse, 8584
Look Good... Feel Better, 2406
Looking Back: A Reader on the History of Deaf Communities & Sign Language, 4550
Los Angeles Alliance Against Parkinson's Disease, 6875
Los Angeles Chapter of the American Association of Kidney Patients, 5586
Los Angeles Orthopaedic Hospital, 5039
Los Angeles Support Group: National Ataxia Foundation, 1528
Loss for Words, 4551
Lotsa Helping Hands, 226, 10639
Louis A. Johnson VA Medical Center, 10264
Louisiana Alliance for the Mentally Ill, 5963
Louisiana Association for the Blind, 9505
Louisiana Association of the Deaf, 4346
Louisiana Chapter of the National Hemophilia Foundation, 4980
Louisiana Comprehensive Hemophilia Care Center, 5040
Louisiana Department of Health: STD/HIV Program, 311
Louisiana Lupus Foundation, 8879
Louisiana Organ Procurement Agency, 9194
Louisiana State University Genetics Section of Pediatrics, 1841
Louisiana Support Group: National Ataxia Foundation, 1540
Louisville Talking Book Library for the Blind and Physically Handicapped, 9677

Love Cycles: The Science of Intimacy, 5472
Love Knot, 2443
Lovelace Medical Foundation, 5662
Lovelace Respiratory Research Institute, 5663
Loving Ben, 5212
Loving Journeys Guide to Adoption, 5473
Low Birthweight, 1886
Low Blood Sugar, 3510
Low Vision Questions and Answers, 10001
Low Vision: Reflections of the Past, Issues for the Future, 9869
Loyola University Medical Center: Department of Pediatrics, 3110
Loyola University of Chicago Cardiac Transplant Program, 4888
Loyola University of Children: Parmly Hearing Institute, 4380
LRC for Students with Disabilities, 9747
Luke Has Asthma Too!, 1434
Lung Cancer Alliance Support Group, 2407
Lung Disease, 5897
Lung Facts, 5874
Lupus Alliance of America LIQ Affiliate, 8895
Lupus Alliance of Upstate New York, 8896
Lupus Book, 8934
Lupus Eritematoso (Spanish Booklet), 8953
Lupus Erythematosus, 8954
Lupus Erythematosus: A Handbook for Physicians, Patients & Families, 8935
Lupus Foundation of America, 8853, 8962
Lupus Foundation of America Memphis Area Chapter Newsletter, 8914, 8944
Lupus Foundation of America Utah Chapter, 8921
Lupus Foundation of America: Alaska Chapter, 8854
Lupus Foundation of America: Arkansas Chapter, 8857
Lupus Foundation of America: Bronx Chapter, 8897
Lupus Foundation of America: California Chapter, 8859
Lupus Foundation of America: Central New York Chapter, 8898
Lupus Foundation of America: Central Pennsylvania Chapter, 8907
Lupus Foundation of America: Columbus Chapter, 8869
Lupus Foundation of America: Connecticut Chapter, 8861
Lupus Foundation of America: DC, Maryland and Central & Northern Virginia, 8881
Lupus Foundation of America: Delaware Chapter, 8862
Lupus Foundation of America: East Tennessee Chapter, 8915
Lupus Foundation of America: Eastern Virginia Chapter, 8923
Lupus Foundation of America: Genessee Valley Chapter, 8899
Lupus Foundation of America: Greater Arizona Chapter, 8855
Lupus Foundation of America: Greater Atlanta Chapter, 8870
Lupus Foundation of America: Greater Ohio Chapter, 8905
Lupus Foundation of America: Heartland Chapter, 8877
Lupus Foundation of America: Illinois Chapter, 8872
Lupus Foundation of America: Iowa Chapter, 8876
Lupus Foundation of America: Kansas City, 8886
Lupus Foundation of America: Massachusetts Chapter, 8882
Lupus Foundation of America: Michigan Lupus Foundation, 8883
Lupus Foundation of America: Mid-South Area Chapter, 8916
Lupus Foundation of America: Minnesota Chapter, 8884
Lupus Foundation of America: Mississippi Chapter, 8885
Lupus Foundation of America: Montana Chapter, 8888
Lupus Foundation of America: New Jersey Chapter, 8892
Lupus Foundation of America: New Mexico Chapter, 8894

Lupus Foundation of America: North Carolin a Chapter, 8904
Lupus Foundation of America: North Texas Chapter, 8917
Lupus Foundation of America: Northeast Florida Chapter, 8863
Lupus Foundation of America: Northeast Indiana Chapter, 8873
Lupus Foundation of America: Northeast Pennsylvania Chapter, 8908
Lupus Foundation of America: Northwest Florida Chapter, 8864
Lupus Foundation of America: Northwest Indiana Lupus Chapter, 8874
Lupus Foundation of America: Northwestern Pennsylvania Chapter, 8909
Lupus Foundation of America: Omaha Chapter, 8889
Lupus Foundation of America: Ozarks Chapter, 8887
Lupus Foundation of America: Pacific Northwest Chapter, 8924
Lupus Foundation of America: Rhode Island Chapter, 8912
Lupus Foundation of America: South Carolina Chapter, 8913
Lupus Foundation of America: South Central Texas Chapter, 8918
Lupus Foundation of America: South Jersey Chapter, 8893
Lupus Foundation of America: Southeast Florida Chapter, 8865
Lupus Foundation of America: Southern Arizona Chapter, 8856
Lupus Foundation of America: Suncoast Chapter, 8866
Lupus Foundation of America: Tampa Area Chapter, 8867
Lupus Foundation of America: Texas Gulf Coast Chapter, 8919
Lupus Foundation of America: Vermont Chapter, 8922
Lupus Foundation of America: West Texas Chapter, 8920
Lupus Foundation of America: Westchester, 8900
Lupus Foundation of America: Western Nebraska Chapter, 8890
Lupus Foundation of America: Western Pennsylvania Chapter, 8910
Lupus Foundation of America: Winston-Triad Lupus Chapter NCLF, 8903
Lupus Foundation of America: Wisconsin Chapter, 8925
Lupus Foundation of Colorado, 8860
Lupus Foundation of Florida, 8868
Lupus Foundation of Indiana, 8875
Lupus Foundation of Kentuckiana, 8878
Lupus Foundation of Mid and Northern New York, 8901
Lupus Foundation of Philadelphia, 8911
Lupus Group of Maine, 8880
Lupus Information Package, 8955
Lupus Informer, 8945
Lupus News, 8946
Lupus: Everything You Need to Know, 8936
Lutheran Library for the Blind, 9715
Lyme Alliance, 9033
Lyme Disease, 9043
Lyme Disease & Pets, 9053
Lyme Disease and Other Pest-Borne Illnesses, 9044
Lyme Disease Association, Inc., 9026
Lyme Disease Foundation, 9069
Lyme Disease Network, 9034
Lyme Disease Network of New Jersey, 9036
Lyme Disease Network of South Carolina, 9037
Lyme Disease Network Support Group of Alabama: Mobile Chapter, 9035
Lyme Disease: What You Should Know, 9061
Lymelight Newsletter, 9046
Lymphatic Research Foundation, 10392
Lymphatic Research Matters, 10596
Lynda Madaras Talks to Teens About AIDS, 482
Lyons Campus VA New Jersey Health Care System, 10195
Lysosomal Disease Center at the University of Pittsburgh, 3842

M

MA Report, 695, 1446
Macomb Library for the Blind and Physically Handicapped, 9699
Madness in the Streets, 6112
Madness of Usher's: Coping with Vision & Hearing Loss, 9870
Magazine of the National Institute of Hypertension Studies, 5274
MAGIC Foundation for Children's Growth, 4049
MAGIC Foundation for Children's Growth: Turner's Syndrome Division, 9373
Magic Moments, 10670
Magic of Humor in Caregiving, 5266, 8070
Magnifier, 10002
Magnifier Highlights, 10003
Maine Alliance for the Mentally Ill, 5964
Maine Alzheimer's Care Center, 835
Maine Center for the Blind and Visually Impaired, 9507
Maine Dept. of Health & Human Services: HIV, STD, & Viral Hepatitis Program, 312
Maine Hemophilia Treatment Center, 5041
Maine Medical Center: Cystic Fibrosis Clin, 3122
Maine Medical Center: Cystic Fibrosis Clinical Center, 3121
Maine SIDS Foundation, 8746
Maine SIDS Program Department Of Human Services, 8747
Maine State Library, 9683
Maine Support Group: National Ataxia Foundation, 1541
Maine VA Medical Center VA Maine Healthcare System, 10163
Mainstay, 10597
Mainstreaming & the American Dream: Soc. Logical Perspectives on Parental Coping, 9871
Mainstreaming Deaf and Hard of Hearing Students, 4552
Mainstreaming the Visually Impaired Child, 9872
Maintaining Good Nutrition with ALS, 1170
Make the Connection, 7152
Make-A-Wish Foundation of America, 10671
Making Child Welfare Work, 6113
Making Life More Livable: Adaptations for Living at Home After Vision Loss, 9873
Making New Friends, 4771
Making Peace with Food, 3751
Making the Most of Early Communication: Strategies for Supporting Communication, 10039
Making the Most of Your Next Doctor Visit, 1470
Malcom Randall VA Medical Center North Florida/South Georgia, 10133
Male Body, 5474
Male Infertility, 5536
Male Infertility and Vasectomy Reversal, 5537
Male Reproductive Function After Spinal Cord Injury, 8014
Male Sexual Dysfunction Clinic, 5303
Male Treatment Guide, 5314, 5317
Man Who Sang in the Dark, 9900
Man Without Words, 4553
Managed Mental Health Care, 6114
Management by Common Sense, 7537
Management of Acute Exacerbations of Chronic Obstructive Pulmonary Disease, 5878
Management of Autistic Behavior, 1758
Management of Hypertension, 5267
Managing Asthma in School: An Action Plan, 1498
Managing Attention Deficit Hyperactivity Disorder in Children:, 1624
Managing Childhood Asthma, 1499
Managing Cocaine Cravings, 8585
Managing Family & Friends, 5538
Managing Incontinence: a Guide to Living with Loss of Bladder Control, 5342
Managing Managed Care: A Mental Health Practitioner's Survival Guide, 6115
Managing Osteogenesis Imperfecta: A Medical Manual, 6788
Managing Post-Polio: A Guide for Polio Survivors and Their Families, 7016
Managing Post-Polio: A Guide to Living Well with Post-Polio Syndrome, 7017

Managing Seizure Disorder, 7518
Managing Type II Diabetes, 3451
Managing Your Activities, 1332
Managing Your Child's Crohn's Disease or Ulcerative Colitis, 3044
Managing Your Child's Eating Problems During Cancer Treatment, 2535
Managing Your Fatigue, 1333
Managing Your Gestational Diabetes, 3452
Managing Your Health Care, 1334
Managing Your Pain, 1335
Managing Your Psoriasis, 7681
Managing Your Stress, 1336
Manatee County Office Epilepsy Services of Southwest Florida, 7484
Manchester VA Medical Center VAMC Manchester, New Hampshire, 10193
Mandy, 4670
Manhattan Subregional Library of the Kansas Talking Books Service, 9671
Manhattan VA Medical Center VA NY Harbor Health Care System, 10203
Manic Depressive Illness, 6116
Manual of Pediatric Nutrition, 3453
Many Faces of Asthma, 1471
Many Shades of Lupus: Information for Multicultural Communities, 8956
Many Symptoms, One Disease, 6748
March is Chronic Fatigue Syndrome Awareness Month Tips, 2878
March of Dimes Canada, 8049
March of Dimes Foundation, 1835, 1896, 4050, 4069, 7912, 7947
Marcus Institute for Development and Learning, 3590
Margaret's Moves, 7931
MARGIN, 1574
Marijuana, 8332, 8586
Marijuana and Reproduction, 8335
Marijuana Anonymous World Services, 8121
Marijuana Smoking Prevention Program for Schools, 8333
Marijuana Today, 8334
Marin Institute, 8212
Marion Campus VA Northern Indiana Health Care System, 10152
Marion VA Medical Center, 10148
Marketing Booze to Blacks, 8336
Markings on the Journey, 8668
Martimer, 4554
Martinsburg VA Medical Center, 10265
Marty Lyons Foundation, Inc., 10672
Mary Margaret Walther Program Walther Cancer Institute, 2307
Maryland National Spinal Cord Injury Association Support Group Network, 7988
Maryland Psychiatric Research Center, 6259
Maryland SIDS Information & Counseling Program, 8749
Maryland State Alcohol and Drug Abuse Administration, 8160
Maryland State Library for the Blind and Physically Handicapped, 9689
Mask of Benevolence: Disabling the Deaf Community, 4555
Masqueraders of Sarcoidosis, 7274
Mass./New Hampshire Chapter of the Myasthenia Gravis Foundation of America, 6585, 6589
Massachusetts Alliance for the Mentally Ill, 5968
Massachusetts Alzheimers Disease Research Center, 968
Massachusetts Chapter of the ALS Association Newsletter, 1164
Massachusetts Commission for the Blind, 9512
Massachusetts Department of Public Health: Office Of HIV/AIDS, 313
Massachusetts Down Syndrome Congress, 3564
Massachusetts Eating Disorder Association, 3694
Massachusetts General Departments of Neurology and Neurosurgery, 8058
Massachusetts General Hospital, 3128
Massachusetts General Hospital: Harvard Cutaneous Biology Research Center, 7669
Massachusetts State Association of the Deaf, 4347
Massachusetts Sudden Infant Death Syndrome Boston City Hospital, 8809

Massachusetts Turner Syndrome Resource Group, 9350
Mastectomy: A Treatment for Breast Cancer, 2536
Matthew and the Tics, 9096
Matthew Pinkowski's Special Summer, 4671
Mature Health, 1031
Maximize Your Body Potential, 10558
Maximizing the Role of Nutrition in Diabetes Management, 3454
Maybe You Know My Kid: A Parent's Guide to Identifying ADHD, 1625
Mayo Clinic, 7083
Mayo Clinic and Foundation Mayo Foundation, 6517
Mayo Clinic and Foundation: Division of Allergic Diseases, 661
Mayo Clinic Health Oasis, 5293
Mayo Clinic Scottsdale Center for Scleroderma Care & Research, 7362
Mayo Clinic: Department of Neurology, 1141
Mayo Comprehensive Cancer Center, 2329
Mayo Comprehensive Hemophilia Center Mayo Clinic, 5042
Mayor Piscataway, NJ Proclamation: Sarcoidosis Awareness Day, 7275
McGruff's Surprise Party, 8444
MD/DC/Delaware Chapter of Myasthenia Gravis Foundation of America, 6576, 6577, 6584
MDA ALS Caregiver's Guide, 6525
MDA Camp: A Special Place, 6555
MDA Fact Sheet, 6556
MDA Services for the Individual, Family and Community, 6557
MDJunction, 7106
Me and My World Packet for Children, 7538
Meadowlands Chapter of the American Association of Kidney Patients, 5626
Meals Without Squeals Sense, 3752
Mealtime Notions - The 'Get Permission' Approach to Mealtimes and Oral Motor, 3989
MedEscort International ABE International Airport, 10393
Media Kit, 8587
Medical and Surgical Care for Children with Down Syndrome, 3616
Medical Center & Ambulatory Care Clinic Montana VA Health Care System, 10189
Medical Center Hospital of Vermont Cystic Fibrosis Center, 3175
Medical College of Georgia Alzheimers Research Center, 969
Medical College of Georgia: Sickle Cell Center, 7616
Medical College of Pennsylvania Center for the Mature Woman, 6814
Medical College of Pennsylvania: Eastern Psychiatric Institute, 6034
Medical College of Toledo: Cancer Research Division, 2356
Medical College of Wisconsin: Cystic Fibrosis Clinic, 3180
Medical Facilities and Resources for Ventilator Users, 8015
Medical Foundation of Buffalo Hauptman-Woodward Medical Research Insti, 2345
Medical Library Association, 266
Medical Management of Depression, 6217
Medical Management of Impotence, 5318
Medical Management of Pregnancy Complicated by Diabetes, 3455
Medical Management of Type I Diabetes, 3456
Medical Management of Type II Diabetes, 3457
Medical University of South Carolina, 1248
Medical University of South Carolina Center on Aging, 127
Medical University of South Carolina Health Services Administration, 430
Medical University of South Carolina Medical University of South Carolina, 7363
Medical University of South Carolina: Cystic Fibrosis Center, 3166
Medical University of South Carolina: Division of Rheumatology & Immunology, 1249
Medical Update Column, 7419
MedicAlert & Alzheimer's Association Safe Return, 1052
MedicAlert Foundation International, 10394

Medicare Health Plan Choices: Consumer Update, 211

Medicare Rx Consumer Workbook, 6117

Medications and Bone Loss, 6827

Medications for Attention Disorders and Related Medical Problems, 1626

MedicineNet, 17, 227, 617, 739, 1083, 1181, 1365, 1514, 1595, 1657, 1817, 1897, 2083, 2596, 2621, 2660, 2815, 2902, 2942, 2952, 2989

Medicines for Epilepsy, 7539

Medline Plus, 2953

MEDLINEplus Health Information, 1082

Medscape, 18, 228, 618, 740, 1084, 1182, 1366, 1515, 1596, 1658, 1818, 1898, 2084, 2597, 2661, 2816, 2903, 2943, 2990, 3077, 3205

Medstar Georgetown University Hospital Facility, 4889

Medsupport, 6335

Medtronic, 10642

Medulloblastoma, 2062

MedWebPlus, 1180

Meeting Halfway in ASL, 4556

Meeting the Challenge of Progressive Multiple Sclerosis, 6445

Meeting the Challenge: Employment Issues and Epilepsy, 7553

Meeting the Challenge: Hearing-Impaired Professionals in the Workplace, 4557

Melanoma Newsletter, 2489

Melanoma Research Foundation, 2293

Melanoma: Research Report, 2537

Melatonin: The Basic Facts, 7824

Melpomene Institute for Women's Health Research, 5436

Member's Eye View of Alcoholics Anonymous, 8588

Members in Relapse, 6749

Members of the Clergy Ask About Alcoholics Anonymous, 8589

Membership Directory, 6118

Memo to an Inmate Who May Be an Alcoholic, 8590

Memorial Miller Children's Hospital Cystic Fibrosis Center, 3095

Memorial Sloan-Kettering Cancer Center, 2346

Memphis Cystic Fibrosis Center LeBonheur Children's Medical Center, 3167

Memphis Regional Brain Tumor Survivors Group, 2026

Memphis VA Medical Center, 10240

Men Newcomer Packet, 8591

Men with Osteoporosis: In Their Own Words, 6828

Men's Work: How to Stop the Violence that Tears Our Lives Apart, 8669

Men, Women and Infertility, 5475

Mended Hearts, 4918

Meniere's Disease: Hearing Loss & Inner Ear Blood Flow, 4772

Meningioma, 2063

Meningioma/Benign Brain Tumor Support Group, 1973

Menninger Clinic: Department of Research, 6035

Menopause and Bladder Control, 5355

Menopause Without Medicine, 10559

Mental and Physical Disability Law Report, 6125

Mental Disability Law: A Primer, 6119

Mental Health America, 5913, 6197, 7107

Mental Health America (formerly NMHA) Information Center, 6185

Mental Health Association in Dutchess Coun ty, 6069

Mental Health Association in Orange County, 6070

Mental Health Association of Delaware, 5942

Mental Health Care in Prisons and Jails, 6120

Mental Health Concepts and Techniques for the Occupational Therapy Assistant, 6121

Mental Health Law News, 6157

Mental Health Law Reporter, 6122

Mental Health Matters, 7153

Mental Health Problems of Vietnam Veterans, 6165

Mental Health Services for Deaf People, 4558

Mental Health Services Training Center, 10395

Mental Health Today, 7154

Mental Health: Counseling Services, 6123

Mental Illness Research and Education Institute, 6036

Mental Illness-Opposing Viewpoints Series, 6124

Mental Retardation, 6152

MentalHelp.net, 7155

Mentally Ill Individuals, 6126

Mentally Ill Kids In Distress, 5926

Mentally Impaired Elderly, 174

MeritCare Children's Hospital Down Syndrome Outpatient Service, 3591

Merrimack Valley HPV Support Group Holy Family Hospital, 10457

Message Line Newsletter, 2053

Message to Correctional Facilities Administrators, 8592

Message to Teenagers, 8593

Messy Monsters, Jungle Joggers and Bubble Baths, 4672

Metabolic Research Institute, 3389

Metastatic Brain Tumors, 2064

Methodist Hospital Sleep Center Winona Memorial Hospital, 7774

Methotrexate, 1337

Methotrexate (MTX), 7709

Metropolitan DC Cystic Fibrosis Center Children s Hospital National Medical Cen, 3100

Meyer L Prentis Comprehensive Cancer Cente Barbara Ann Karmanos Cancer Institute, 2326

Meyer L Prentis Comprehensive Cancer Center of Metropolitan Detroit, 2325

MG Communicator, 6639

MGH Neurology, 6702

MGH Neurology WebForums, 7853, 9070

Miami Childrens Hospital Division of Pulmonology, 3102

Miami Comprehensive Hemophilia Center Jackson Medical Towers, 5043

Miami Dade Talking Book Library, 9638

Miami Project to Cure Paralysis, 7983, 8039

Miami VA Healthcare System, 10134

Miami Valley Ohio Chapter of the American Association of Kidney Patients, 5636

Michael E. DeBakey VA Medical Center, 10248

Michael J. Fox Foundation for Parkinson's Research, 6869

Michigan Alliance for the Mentally Ill, 5971

Michigan Alzheimer's Disease Research Center, 970

Michigan Deaf Association, 4348

Michigan Department of Health & Human Services, 8754

Michigan Department of Health & Human Services: Division of HIV & STD Programs, 315

Michigan Kidney Foundation, 5618

Michigan State University Hemophilia Comprehensive Care Clinic, 5044

Micrographia, 6968

Mid Missouri Support Group: National Ataxia Foundation, 1549

Mid-America Transplant Services, 9200

Mid-Illinois Talking Book Center, 9661

Mid-South Transplant Foundation, Inc. Tennessee, 9218

MidAtlantic AIDS Education and Training Center (MAAETC), 331, 426

Middle Georgia Subregional Library for the Blind and Physically Handicapped, 9651

Middle Tennessee Sarcoidosis Support Group, 7241

Midwest AIDS Education and Training Center (MATEC), 308, 397

MidWest Medical Center: Sleep Disorders Center, 7775

Midwest Transplant Network & Organ Bank, 9192

Midwestern Michigan Library Cooperative, 9700

Migraine and Coexisting Conditions: Other Illnesses That May Affect Migraine, 6318

Migraine and Other Headaches: Vascular Mechanisms, 6300

Migraine Awareness Group: A National Understanding for Migraineurs, 6291, 6336

Migraine: Fact Sheet, 6319

Migraine: The Complete Guide, 6301

Mild Brain Injury: Damage and Outcome, 4245

Mild Hemophilia, 5116

Mile High Down Syndrome Association, 3556

Miles City VA Clinic & Community Living Center, 10190

Miles to Go Before I Sleep, 7519

Military Packet, 8594

Milwaukee VA Medical Center (Zablocki), 10266

MindWise Innovations, 3678, 6198, 8122

Mine for Keeps, 2805

Minneapolis VA Health Care System, 10178

Minnesota AIDS Project AIDSLine, 452

Minnesota Alliance for the Mentally Ill, 5972

Minnesota Ambassador: National Ataxia Foundation, 1545

Minnesota Association for Children's Mental Health, 5973

Minnesota Department of Health, 316

Minnesota Disability Law Center, 10461

Minnesota Library for the Blind, 9709

Minnesota Obesity Center, 6717

Minnesota State Chapter of the Myasthenia Gravis Foundation of America, 6587

Minnesota Sudden Infant Death Center Minneapolis Children's Medical Center, 8757

Minority Advocacy Notebook, 6166

A Miracle to Believe In, 1729

Mirrored Lives, 175

Miscarriage, 5539

Miscarriage Women: Sharing from the Heart, 5476

Missed Conceptions: Overcoming Infertility, 5477

Missing Words: The Family Handbook on Adult Hearing Loss, 4559

Mississippi Alliance for the Mentally Ill, 5974

Mississippi Area Support Group: National Ataxia Foundation, 1547

Mississippi Client Assistance Program, 10462

Mississippi Families as Allies, 5975

Mississippi Hemophilia Foundation, 4985

Mississippi Industries for the Blind, 9521

Mississippi Library Commission, 9711

Mississippi Organ Recovery, 9199

Mississippi SIDS Alliance, 8758

Mississippi State Department of Health and Child Health Services, 8759

Mississippi State Department of Health: STD/HIV Office, 317

Missouri Coalition Alliance for the Mentally Ill, 5977

Missouri Department of Health & Senior Services: Bureau of HIV, STD & Hepatitis, 318

Missouri Division of Alcohol and Drug Abuse, 8167

Missouri Illinois Regional Hemophilia Comprehensive Treatment Center, 5045

Missouri Protection and Advocacy Services, 10463

Missouri Teratogen Information Service, 1855

Mistaken Beliefs About Relapse, 8337

Mitral Valve Prolapse Program of Cincinnati Support Group, 4919

Mitral Valve Prolapse Syndrome/Dysautonomia Survival Guide, 4931

MLA News, 552

MO-SPAN, 5976

MO-SPAN Southwest Region, 6064

Mobility: Issues Facing Stroke Survivors and Their Families, 5281, 8087

Modern Maturity, 192

Moisture Seekers Newsletter, 7644

Mom I Have a Staring Problem, 7540

Moment to Reflect on Codependency, 8595

Moment to Reflect on Self-Esteem, 8596

Mommy, Did I Grow in Your Tummy? Where Some Babies Come From, 5499

Monetary Allowance, Health Care and Vocational Training, 7938

Money Matters, 1053

Monmouth Medical Center: Cystic Fibrosis & Monmouth Medical Center, 3142

Monmouth Medical Center: Cystic Fibrosis & Pediatric Pulmonary Center, 3141

Monograph on Canavan's Disease, 8979

Monroe Institute Surgical Support Tapes, 3818

Montana Alliance for the Mentally Ill Mihelish's Residence, 5980

Montana Deptartment of Public Health & Human Services: HIV/STD/HepC Program, 319

Montana State Library, 9718

Montgomery County Association for the Blind, 9564

Month of Meals Set of 5, 3458

Montrose Campus: Franklin Delano Roosevelt VA Hudson Valley Health Care System, 10204

Mood and Anxiety Disorders Program of Emory University, 7090

Mood Apart, 6218

Mood Apart: Depression, Mania, and Other Afflictions of the Self, 6127

Moonrise: One Family, Genetic Identity, & Muscular Dystrophy, 6526

Morbus Fabry, 3852

MOSPAN Northwest Region, 6065

Most Frequently Asked Questions with Growth Hormone Deficiency, 4061

Mother Father Deaf: Living Between Sound and Silence, 4560

Mother Goose on Sign, 4673

Motherhood: A Feminist Perspective, 5478

Mothers Against Drunk Driving (MADD), 8123

Mothers of Thyme: Customs and Rituals of Infertility and Miscarriage, 5479

Motivating Moves for People with Parkinson's, 6996

Motivator, 6457

Motor Neuron Disease Clinic University of Connecticut Health Center, 1142

Motor Neuron Disease Program University of Michigan Health System, 1143

Mount Sinai Medical Center, 4890

Mount Sinai Medical Center Brain Tumor Support Group, 2003

Mount Sinai Sarcoidosis Support Group, 7242

Mount Sinai School of Medicine: Alzheimers Disease Research Center, 971

Mountain State Regional Hemophilia Center, 5046

Mountain State/Parents/Children/ Adolescents Network, 6020

Mountain West AIDS Education and Training Center (MWAETC), 296, 384

Mouth Magazine, 4214

Move with Me, 10004

Moving On! From Alateen to Al-Anon, 8597

Moving Toward the Standards, 4561

Moving with Multiple Sclerosis, 6473

MR Imaging in Parkinson's Disease, 6967

MS Connection, 6456

MS Toll-Free Information Line, 6435

MSRGSN Newsletter, 1575

MSWorld, 6436

Mt. Washington Pediatric Clinic, 3592

Multidisciplinary Clinico-Pathologic Conference, 7276

Multiple Sclerosis, 6446

Multiple Sclerosis Action Group, 6437

Multiple Sclerosis and Your Emotions, 6474

Multiple Sclerosis Association of America, 6342

Multiple Sclerosis Foundation, 6343, 6505

Multiple Sclerosis Quarterly Report, 6458

Multiple Sclerosis, The Questions you Have Answers You Need, 6447

Multiple Sclerosis: A Guide for Families, 6448

Multiple Sclerosis: A Guide for Patients and Their Families, 6449

Multiple Sclerosis: A Personal Exploration, 6450

Multiple Sclerosis: Your Legal Rights, 6451

Multipurpose Arthritis and Musculoskeletal Disease Center, 1250

Muscular Dystrophy, 6534, 6560

Muscular Dystrophy & Other Neuromuscular Diseases: Psychological Issues, 6527

Muscular Dystrophy Association, 6510, 6518, 6566

Muscular Dystrophy Canada, 6511

Muscular Dystrophy in Children: Guide for Families, 6528

Musculoskeletal Transplant Foundation, 9226

Music Appreciation, 2850

Music in Motion, 4562

Music Is for Everyone, 10005

Musical Mainstream, 9936

Muskegon County Library for the Blind, 9701

MVPS & Anxiety, 4939

My ABC Signs of Animal Friends, 4674

My Body is My House, 8445

My Book for Kids with Cancer, 2468

My Brother Matthew, 2806, 7541

My Fibromyalgia & Chronic Fatigue Syndrome, 3908

My First Book of Sign, 4675

My Friend Emily, 7542

My Mind is Out to Get Me: Humor and Wisdom in Recovery, 8338

My Name is Buddy, 2048

My Name is Caroline, 3753

My Prostate and Me: Dealing with Prostate Cancer, 2444

My Signing Book of Numbers, 4676

Myasthenia Gravis Foundation of America, 6572, 6648

Myasthenia Gravis Foundation: Geater South Texas, 6640

Myasthenia Gravis Foundation: Northwest Texas Chapter, 6641

Myasthenia Gravis Support Group of Ames, 6606

Myasthenia Gravis Support Group of Arizona Jim L. Walker Chapter, 6603

Myasthenia Gravis Support Group of Atlanta, 6605

Myasthenia Gravis Support Group of Central North Carolina, 6620

Myasthenia Gravis Support Group of Charlotte, 6619

Myasthenia Gravis Support Group of Columbu s, 6623

Myasthenia Gravis Support Group of Connect icut (Nutmeg Group), 6604

Myasthenia Gravis Support Group of Durham/ Chapel Hill, 6621

Myasthenia Gravis Support Group of Eastern Massachusetts and New Hampshire, 6609, 6614

Myasthenia Gravis Support Group of Fayette ville, 6622

Myasthenia Gravis Support Group of Fox Valley, 6632

Myasthenia Gravis Support Group of Louisia na, 6608

Myasthenia Gravis Support Group of Louisvi lle, 6607

Myasthenia Gravis Support Group of Low Country, 6627

Myasthenia Gravis Support Group of Manassa s, 6629

Myasthenia Gravis Support Group of Manhatt an, 6617

Myasthenia Gravis Support Group of Mid-Min n, 6611

Myasthenia Gravis Support Group of Milwauk ee, 6633

Myasthenia Gravis Support Group of New Mex ico, 6616

Myasthenia Gravis Support Group of Scranto n, 6626

Myasthenia Gravis Support Group of Seattle , Olympia and Poulsbo, 6630

Myasthenia Gravis Support Group of South East Minnesota, 6612

Myasthenia Gravis Support Group of Spokane, 6631

Myasthenia Gravis Support Group of Summit- Stark, 6624

Myasthenia Gravis Support Group of the Mountain and Up Country, 6628

Myasthenia Gravis Support Group of the Twin Cities, 6613

Myasthenia Gravis Support Group of Tulsa and Oklahoma City, 6625

Myasthenia Gravis Support Group of Upstate New York, 6618

Myasthenia Gravis Support Group of Western Massachusetts and New Hampshire, 6610, 6615

myFace, 1832

Myositis, .1338

Myositis Association of America, 1190

MyPTSD, 7156

Mystery of Contact Dermatitis, 7740

Myths & Facts, 5540

N

NAD Deaf Awareness Kit, 4563

Nadeene Brunini Comprehensive Hemophilia Care Center, 5047

NADF News, 12

NADmag, 4714

NAFC Fact Sheets, 5356

NAMES Project Foundation AIDS Memorial Quilt, 358

NAMI Arkansas, 5931

NAMI California, 5932

NAMI Indiana, 5956

NAMI Indiana - National Alliance on Mental Illness, 6059

NAMI Iowa: National Alliance on Mental Illness, 5958

NAMI Kansas: Kansas' Voice on Mental Illness, 5960

NAMI of Missouri, 5978

NAMI South Dakota, 6007

NAMI Washington (National Alliance for the Mentally Ill of Washington), 6018

NAMI West Virginia, 6021

NAMI-Oregon, 6001

NAMI-SC: National Alliance on Mental Illness: South Carolina, 6006

NAMI: The Local Affiliate of the National Alliance for the Mentally Ill, 5949

Nana Upstairs and Nana Downstairs, 10729

Naomi Berrie Diabetes Center at Columbia University Medical Center, 3373

Narcolepsy, 7839, 7845

Narcolepsy Institute/Montefiore Medical Center, 7817, 7834

Narcolepsy Network, 7759, 7818

Narcolepsy Primer, 7825

Narcolepsy Primer Package, 7826

Narcolepsy: Fanlight Productions, 7846

Narcotic and Drug Research, 8213

Narcotics Anonymous, 8339

Narcotics Anonymous World Services, 8124

Nashville VA Medical Center Tennessee Valley Healthcare System, 10241

NASPGHAN Foundation, 3935

NASS News, 7935

Nassau Library System, 9729

Natalie Warren Bryant Cancer Center St. Francis Hospital, 2360

Natioanl Multiple Sclerosis Society Desert Southwest Chapter, 6384

National Academy on an Aging Society, 128

National Adrenal Diseases Foundation, 8, 19

National Adult Day Services Association, 34

National AIDS Information Clearinghouse, 619

National AIDS Treatment Advocacy Project, 267

National Alliance for Autism Research, 1722, 1819

National Alliance for Caregiving, 35, 151, 10518

National Alliance for Hispanic Health, 5914

National Alliance for Research on Schizophrenia and Depression, 6260

National Alliance for the Mentally Ill, 6186, 6282

National Alliance for the Mentally Ill (NA MI) Alaska, 6049

National Alliance for the Mentally Ill of Colorado, 5936

National Alliance for the Mentally Ill of Connecticut, 5939

National Alliance for the Mentally Ill of Rhode Island (NAMI), 6005

National Alliance for the Mentally Ill: Maryland, 5966

National Alliance for the Mentally Ill: Nebraska (NAMI), 5981

National Alliance for the Mentally Ill: New Hampshire, 5984, 6067

National Alliance of Blind Students, 10073

National Alliance of Blind Students American Council of the Blind, 9432

National Alliance on Mental Illness, 6199

National Alliance on Mental Illness (NAMI), 5915, 6257, 7050

National Alliance on Mental Illness of Alabama: NAMI Alabama, 5924

National Alliance on Mental Illness of Alaska, 5925

National Alliance on Mental Illness of Arizona, 5927

National Alzheimer's Disease Institute, 757

National Anxiety Foundation, 6200, 6251

National Arthritis & Musculoskeletal & Skin Diseases Information Clearinghouse, 1367

National Association for Anorexia Nervosa and Associated Disorders, 3783

National Association for Children of Alcoholics (NACOA), 8125

National Association for Continence, 5332, 5371

National Association for Down Syndrome, 3545

National Association for Home Care, 10519

National Association for Home Care and Hospice, 10695

National Association for Parents of Children with Visual Impairments, 9433

National Association for Parents of the Visually Impaired, 9815
National Association of Alcoholism and Drug Abuse Counselors (NAADAC), 8126
National Association of Anorexia Nervosa and Associated Disorders, 3679, 3718, 3784
National Association of Blind Educators, 10074
National Association of Blind Lawyers, 9434, 10075
National Association of Blind Merchants, 9462
National Association of Blind Office Professionals, 9435
National Association of Blind Secretaries and Transcribers, 10076
National Association of Blind Students, 9436, 10077
National Association of Blind Teachers, 10078
National Association of Chronic Disease Directors, 6808
National Association of Councils on Developmental Disabilities, 10396
National Association of Epilepsy Centers, 7468
National Association of Guide Dog Users, 9437, 10079
National Association of Myofascial Trigger Point Therapists, 2916
National Association of Social Workers (NASW), 7051
National Association of Special Education Teachers, 2958
National Association of State Directors of Veterans Affairs, 10221
National Association of State Mental Health Program Directors, 5916
National Association of the Deaf, 4320, 4849
National Association on Drug Abuse Problems, 8127
National Association to Advance Fat Acceptance (NAAFA), 6710
National Association to Promote the Use of Braille, 9438
National Association to Promote the Use of Braille, 10080
National Ataxia Foundation, 1521, 1597
National Autism Hotline Autism Services Center, 1727
National Braille Association, 9439, 10081
National Braille Press, 9440
National Brain Tumor Foundation, 2085
National Brain Tumor Society, 1902
National Cancer Institute, 2105, 2408
National Cancer Institute Fact Book, 2445
National Capital Lyme Disease Association, 9027
National Captioning Institute, 4321, 4850
National Celiac Association, 2630, 2662
National Center for Complementary and Integrative Health, 639, 1382, 3680, 5736, 7052, 7469
National Center for Education in Maternal and Child Health, 8701, 8847
National Center for Family-Centered Care, 10397
National Center for Learning Disabilities, 1608
National Center for PTSD, 7071, 7082
National Center for Sight, 9816
National Center for the Prevention of SIDS, 8813
National Center for Victims of Crime, 7072
National Center for Voice and Speech: University of Iowa, 4322
National Center on Addiction and Substance Abuse, 8214
National Certification Board for Diabetes Educators, 3211
National CFIDS Foundation, 2831
National Children's Cancer Society, 2260
National Chronic Pain Outreach Association, 10398
National Clearinghouse for Alcohol and Drug Information, 8195, 8690
National Clearinghouse of Rehabilitation Training Materials, 10399, 10643
National Coalition for Cancer Survivorship, 2106
National Conference on Drug Abuse Researcg & Practice, 8340
National Consortium on Deaf-Blindness, 4323
National Council for Aging Care, 36, 229
National Council for Behavioral Health, 5917
National Council on Aging, 37, 230, 5333
National Council on Alcoholism and Drug Dependence, 8691
National Council on Disability, 10400, 10644

National Council on Independent Living, 10401
National Crime Prevention Council, 8128, 8692
National Diabetes Information Clearinghous e, 3374, 3533
National Digestive Diseases Information Clearinghouse, 2995, 3078, 3925, 4009, 10402, 10645
National Directory of Brain Injury Rehabilitatiom, 4202
National Directory of Drug Abuse and Alcoholism Treatment and Programs, 8341
National Directory of Head Injury Rehabilitation Services, 4203
National Down Syndrome Congress, 3546, 3600
National Down Syndrome Society, 3547, 3664
National Down Syndrome Society Hotline, 3601
National Down Syndrome Society Update, 3632
National Eating Disorder Information Centr e, 3681
National Eating Disorder Information Centr e Helpline, 3719
National Eating Disorders Association, 3682, 3785
National Eating Disorders Association Helpline, 3720
National Eczema Association, 640, 7663
National Endowment for the Arts: Office for Accessability, 10403
National Eye Health Education Program, 9817
National Eye Institute (NEI): National Institutes of Health (NIH), 9441
National Fabry Disease Foundation, 3840
National Families in Action (NFIA), 8129
National Family Association for Deaf-Blind, 4324
National Family Caregivers Association, 10520
National Federation of Families for Children's Mental Health, 1612, 5918
National Federation of the Blind, 9442, 10083
National Federation of the Blind in Computer Science, 9443, 10084
National Federation of the Blind: Alabama, 9464
National Federation of the Blind: Alaska, 9465
National Federation of the Blind: Arizona, 9468
National Federation of the Blind: Arkansas, 9471
National Federation of the Blind: Blind Merchants Division, 10085
National Federation of the Blind: Blind/Deaf Division, 10082
National Federation of the Blind: California, 9473
National Federation of the Blind: Colorado, 9476
National Federation of the Blind: Connecticut, 9477
National Federation of the Blind: DC, 9482
National Federation of the Blind: Deaf-Blind Division, 9444
National Federation of the Blind: Delaware, 9480
National Federation of the Blind: Florida, 9483
National Federation of the Blind: Georgia, 9487
National Federation of the Blind: Hawaii, 9491
National Federation of the Blind: Human Services Division, 9445, 10086
National Federation of the Blind: Idaho, 9492
National Federation of the Blind: Illinois, 9496
National Federation of the Blind: Indiana, 9498
National Federation of the Blind: Iowa, 9499
National Federation of the Blind: Kansas, 9501
National Federation of the Blind: Kentucky, 9503
National Federation of the Blind: Louisana, 9506
National Federation of the Blind: Maine, 9508
National Federation of the Blind: Maryland, 9510
National Federation of the Blind: Massachusetts, 9513
National Federation of the Blind: Michigan, 9518
National Federation of the Blind: Minnesota, 9520
National Federation of the Blind: Mississippi, 9522
National Federation of the Blind: Missouri, 9525
National Federation of the Blind: Montana, 9526
National Federation of the Blind: Music Division, 10087
National Federation of the Blind: Nebraska, 9527
National Federation of the Blind: Nevada, 9528
National Federation of the Blind: New Hampshire, 9530
National Federation of the Blind: New Jersey, 9532
National Federation of the Blind: New Mexico, 9533
National Federation of the Blind: New York, 9540
National Federation of the Blind: North Carolina, 9544
National Federation of the Blind: North Dakota, 9546

National Federation of the Blind: Ohio, 9550
National Federation of the Blind: Oklahoma, 9551
National Federation of the Blind: Oregon, 9554
National Federation of the Blind: Pennsylvania, 9565
National Federation of the Blind: Public Employees Division, 9446, 10088
National Federation of the Blind: Rhode Island, 9574
National Federation of the Blind: Science and Engineering Division, 9447, 10089
National Federation of the Blind: South Carolina, 9575
National Federation of the Blind: South Dakota, 9576
National Federation of the Blind: Tennessee, 9578
National Federation of the Blind: Texas, 9585
National Federation of the Blind: Utah, 9590
National Federation of the Blind: Vermont, 9592
National Federation of the Blind: Virginia, 9593
National Federation of the Blind: West Virginia, 9599
National Federation of the Blind: Wisconsin, 9600
National Federation of the Blind: Writers, 9601
National Federation of the Blind: Writers Division, 9448, 10090
National Federation of the Blind: Wyoming, 9603
National Fibromyalgia & Chronic Pain Association, 2917, 3862
National Fibromyalgia Association, 3863, 3909
National Fibromyalgia Partnership (NFP), 3864, 3910
National Forum, 2862
National Foundation for Cancer Research, 2261, 2319
National Foundation for Cancer Research Hotline, 2409
National Foundation for Depressive Illness, 6252
National Foundation for Transplants, 9169, 9250
National Gaucher Disease Foundation, 3843
National Gaucher Foundation, 4022, 5766
National Gaucher Foundation of Canada, 4023
National Headache Foundation, 6292, 6337, 7073
National Health Federation, 2142
National Health Information Center, 9, 152, 453, 672, 986, 1153, 1259, 1408, 1522, 1613, 1728, 1856, 1914, 2410, 2612, 2634, 2796, 2834, 2919, 2950, 2974
National Heart, Lung & Blood Institute, 4863, 5250, 5296, 5900, 8050, 8100
National Heart, Lung and Blood Institute, 4956
National Hemophilia Foundation, 359, 4963, 5012, 5136
National Hemophilia Foundation: Mary M. Gooley Hemophilia Center, 4991
National Hepatitis C Coalition, 5144
National Hospice & Palliative Care Organization (NHPCO), 38, 231, 268, 620, 2107, 2598, 10696, 10742
National Hospice Helpline, 2411, 10701
National Human Genome Research Institute, 641, 1383, 3548, 3683, 4325, 5737, 7053, 7470
National Hydrocephalus Foundation, 5198
National Hydrocephalus Foundation Newsletter, 5217
National Industries for the Blind, 9449
National Infertility Network Exchange, 5442
National Information Center on Deafness, 4851
National Information Center on Deafness Brochure, 4773
National Information Clearinghouse on Children Who are Deaf-Blind, 4852
National Institute for Jewish Hospice, 10697
National Institute for Occupational Safety and Health, 642, 1384, 3549, 3684, 5738, 7471
National Institute for People with Disabil ities, 10404
National Institute of Aging, 232
National Institute of Allergy and Infectious Diseases, 643, 1385, 2827, 7570, 9170, 9259
National Institute of Arthritis & Musculoskeletal & Skin Diseases, 1191, 1251, 2608, 2610, 7664, 7670
National Institute of Biomedical Imaging and Bioengineering, 644, 1386, 4326, 5739, 7472
National Institute of Child Health and Human Development, 3550, 4046, 6778, 7163, 8702, 8968, 10405
National Institute of Diabetes & Digestive & Kidney Diseases, 6, 2996, 3212, 4964, 5300, 5334, 5579, 5740, 9381
National Institute of Disability and Rehabilitation Research, 10406

National Institute of Environmental Health Sciences, 645, 1387, 3551, 3685, 4327, 5741, 7054, 7473

National Institute of Food and Agriculture, 646

National Institute of General Medical Sciences, 647, 1388, 3552, 5742, 7055, 7474

National Institute of Mental Health, 1820, 5919, 7056, 7094

National Institute of Neurological Disorders and Stroke, 1669, 1903, 2670, 3837, 6344, 6870, 7475, 7760, 8051, 8969, 9080

National Institute of Nursing Research, 1391

National Institute on Aging, 39, 758, 2108

National Institute on Alcohol Abuse and Alcoholism, 5753

National Institute on Deafness and Other Communication Disorders, 4853

National Institute on Deafness and other Communication Disorders, 4328

National Institute on Drug Abuse, 3563, 5754

National Institutes of Health, 5572

National Jewish Center for Immunology, 5870

National Jewish Center for Immunology and Respiratory Medicine, 662

National Jewish Division of Immunology, 1404

National Jewish Health, 5812

National Job Accommodation Network, 10407

National Kidney and Urologic Diseases Information Clearinghouse, 2109

National Kidney Foundation, 5580

National Kidney Foundation of Arkansas, 5584

National Kidney Foundation of Central New York, 5631

National Kidney Foundation of Colorado, Idaho, Montana, and Wyoming, 5606

National Kidney Foundation of Colorado/Idaho/Montana/Wyoming, 5622, 5660

National Kidney Foundation of Colorado: Idaho, Montana, and Wyoming, 5592

National Kidney Foundation of Connecticut, 5594

National Kidney Foundation of Delaware Valley, 5641

National Kidney Foundation of East Tennessee, 5646

National Kidney Foundation of Eastern Missouri and Metro East, 5621

National Kidney Foundation of Florida, 5599

National Kidney Foundation of Georgia, 5603

National Kidney Foundation of Hawaii, 5605

National Kidney Foundation of Illinois, 5608

National Kidney Foundation of Indiana, 5609

National Kidney Foundation of Kansas and Western Missouri, 5611

National Kidney Foundation of Kentucky, 5612

National Kidney Foundation of Louisiana, 5614

National Kidney Foundation of MA/RI/NH/VT, 5617, 5624, 5643, 5657

National Kidney Foundation of Maine, 5615

National Kidney Foundation of Maryland, 5616

National Kidney Foundation of Minnesota, 5619

National Kidney Foundation of Mississippi, 5620

National Kidney Foundation of New Mexico, 5628

National Kidney Foundation of North Carolina, 5635

National Kidney Foundation of North Texas, 5652

National Kidney Foundation of Northeast New York, 5632

National Kidney Foundation of Northern California, 5587

National Kidney Foundation of Ohio, 5637

National Kidney Foundation of Oklahoma, 5639

National Kidney Foundation of South Carolina, 5644

National Kidney Foundation of Southeast Texas, 5653

National Kidney Foundation of Southern California, 5588

National Kidney Foundation of Texas, 5654

National Kidney Foundation of the National Capital Area, 5596

National Kidney Foundation of the Texas Coastal Bend, 5655

National Kidney Foundation of Utah, 5656

National Kidney Foundation of Virginia, 5658

National Kidney Foundation of West Tennessee, 5647

National Kidney Foundation of West Texas, 5648

National Kidney Foundation of Western New York, 5633

National Kidney Foundation of Western Pennsylvania, 5642

National Kidney Foundation of Wisconsin, 5659

National Kidney Foundation Serving Minneso ta, Dakotas & Iowa Division Office, 5645

National Legal Center for the Medically Dependent & Disabled, 10408

National Library of Dermatologic Teaching Slides, 7741

National Library of Medicine, 362

National Library Service for the Blind, 10091

National Library Service for the Blind and Physically Handicapped, 9631

National Library Service for the Blind and Physically Handicapped, 9450

National Marrow Donor Program, 2110

National ME/FM Action Network, 2828, 3865

National Mental Health Consumer's Self-Help Clearinghouse, 6028

National Mental Health Consumers' Self- Help Clearinghouse, 6029

National Mental Health Services Knowledge Exchange Network, 6187

National MS Soceity: Western Ohio Chapter The Woolpert Building, 6402

National MS Society: Blue Ridge Chapter, 6422

National MS Society: Central New England Chapter, 6386

National MS Society: Central North Carolina Chapter, 6397

National MS Society: Central Pennsylvania Chapter, 6408

National MS Society: Central Virginia Chapter, 6423

National MS Society: Chicago, Greater Illinois Chapter, 6368

National MS Society: Colorado Chapter, 6357

National MS Society: Dakota Chapter, 6400

National MS Society: Delaware Chapter, 6359

National MS Society: Eastern North Carolina Chapter, 6398

National MS Society: Gateway Area Chapter, 6381

National MS Society: Georgia Chapter, 6365

National MS Society: Great Basin Sierra Chapter, 6385

National MS Society: Greater Connecticut Chapter, 6358

National MS Society: Greater Delaware Valley Chapter, 6409

National MS Society: Greater North Jersey Chapter, 6387

National MS Society: Greater Washington Chapter, 6425

National MS Society: Hampton Roads Chapter, 6424

National MS Society: Hawaii Chapter, 6366

National MS Society: Idaho Division, 6367

National MS Society: Indiana State Chapter, 6369

National MS Society: Inland Northwest Chapter, 6426

National MS Society: Iowa Chapter, 6370

National MS Society: Kentucky Chapter, 6373

National MS Society: Long Island Chapter, 6390

National MS Society: Maine Chapter, 6375

National MS Society: Maryland Chapter Hunt Valley Business Center, 6376

National MS Society: Massachusetts Chapter, 6377

National MS Society: Michigan Chapter, 6378

National MS Society: Mid-America Chapter, 6371

National MS Society: Mid-Jersey Chapter, 6388

National MS Society: Mid-South Chapter, 6413

National MS Society: Mid-South Chapter, Nashville Office, 6414

National MS Society: Midlands Chapter Community Health Plaza, 6383

National MS Society: Minnesota Chapter, 6379

National MS Society: Montana Division, 6382

National MS Society: National Capital Chapter, 6360

National MS Society: New York City Chapter, 6391

National MS Society: North Central Texas Chapter, 6415

National MS Society: Northeast Ohio Chapter, 6404

National MS Society: Northeastern New York Chapter, 6392

National MS Society: Northwest Ohio Chapter, 6405

National MS Society: Oklahoma Chapter, 6406

National MS Society: Oregon Chapter, 6407

National MS Society: Panhandle Chapter, 6416

National MS Society: Rhode Island Chapter, 6410

National MS Society: Rio Grande Division, 6389

National MS Society: South Carolina Branch, 6411

National MS Society: South Central & West Kansas Division, 6372

National MS Society: Southeast Tennessee/North Georgia Chapte, 6412

National MS Society: Southern New York Chapter, 6393

National MS Society: Southern Texas, 6417

National MS Society: Southwestern Ohio/Northern Kentucky, 6403

National MS Society: Upstate New York Chapter, 6394

National MS Society: Utah State Chapter, 6420

National MS Society: Vermont Division, 6421

National MS Society: West Texas Division, 6418

National MS Society: Western New York/ Northwestern Pennsylvania Chapter, 6395

National MS Society: Wisconsin Chapter, 6427

National MS Society: Wyoming Chapter, 6428

National MS Socisty: Southeast Texas Chapter, 6419

National Multiple Sclerosis Society, 6345, 6399, 6506

National Multiple Sclerosis Society Channel Islands Chapter, 6352

National Multiple Sclerosis Society Desert Southwest Chapter, 6348

National Multiple Sclerosis Society: Alaba ma-Mississippi Chapter, 6380

National Multiple Sclerosis Society: Alabama Chapter, 6346

National Multiple Sclerosis Society: Alaska Chapter, 6347

National Multiple Sclerosis Society: Allegheny District Chapter, 6459

National Multiple Sclerosis Society: Arkansas Chapter, 6349

National Multiple Sclerosis Society: Louisiana, 6374

National Multiple Sclerosis Society: North Florida Chapter, 6363

National Multiple Sclerosis Society: Silicon Valley Chapter, 6353

National Multiple Sclerosis Society: Southern California Chapter, 6351

National Multiple Sclerosis: Upstate New York Chapter, 6396

National Native American AIDS Prevention Center, 269

National Network of Learning Disabled Adults, 10409

National Networker, 10599

National NF Medical Resource Listing, 6695

National Organization for Hearing Research Foundation, 4329

National Organization for Rare Disorders, 3838, 3853, 4021, 4039, 8703, 8848, 8970, 9000, 10410, 10646

National Organization of Parents of Blind Children, 9451, 10092

National Organization of the Senior Blind, 10093

National Organization on Disability, 10411

National Organization on Fetal Alcohol Syndrome, 8130

National Osteoporosis Foundation, 6809, 6851

National Osteoporosis Foundation (NOF), 6819

National Ovarian Cancer Coalition, 2111, 2599

National Parent Network on Disabilities, 10412

National Parent to Parent Support and Information System, 10522

National Parkinson Foundation, 7004

National Parkinson Foundation Hotline, 6914

National Parkinson Foundation: California Office, 6876

National Parkinson Foundation: New York Office, 6897

National Parkinson Foundation: Orange County Chapter, 6877

National Parkinson Foundation:Cape Cod Chapter, 6893

National Plan for Research on Child and Adolescent Mental Disorders, 6128

National Prevention Resource Center CSAP Division of Communications Programs, 8215

National Psoriasis Foundation, 7665, 7753

National Public Policy Program to Conquer Alzheimer's Disease, 1054

National Rehabilitation Information Center, 2671, 2817, 10413
National Resource Library on Youth with Disabilities, 10508
National Reye's Syndrome Foundation, 5774
National Sarcoidosis Resource Center, 7235, 7277, 7322
National Science Foundation, 1395, 4356, 5763, 7064, 7488
National Scoliosis Foundation, 7399
National Seniors Council, 40
National Service Dog Center, 9819
National Sexual Violence Resource Center, 7074
National Sjogren's Syndrome Association, 7653
National Sleep Foundation, 7761, 7856
National Society for MVP and Dysautonomia, 4921
National Society of Genetic Counselors, 3854
National Spinal Cord Injury Association, 7973, 7977
National Spinal Cord Injury Association: Central Indiana Chapter, 7970
National Spinal Cord Injury Association: Connecticut Chapter, 7967
National Spinal Cord Injury Association: Derby City Area Chapter, 7971
National Spinal Cord Injury Association: Greater Boston Chapter, 7974
National Spinal Cord Injury Association: Los Angeles Chapter, 7966
National Spinal Cord Injury Association: Louisiana Chapter, 7972
National Spinal Cord Injury Association: San Diego County Chapter, 7965
National Spinal Cord Injury Statistical Center, 7957
National Spinal Cord Injury Support Goups, 7990
National Spinal Cord Injury Support Groups, 7992, 7993, 7994
National Stroke Association, 5251, 8101
National Tay-Sachs & Allied Diseases Association of Delaware Valley, 8973
National Tay-Sachs and Allied Diseases Association, 3839, 8971
National TaySachs & Allied Diseases Association, 8974
National Transplant Assistance Fund (NTAF), 9171, 9251
National Treatment Consortium for Alcohol and Other Drugs, 8216
National Tuberous Sclerosis Association, 9326, 9337
National Veterans Services Fund, 10277, 10318
National Volunteer Training Center for Sub CSAP Division of Communications Programs, 8218
National Volunteer Training Center for Substance Abuse Prevention, 8217
National Women's Health Network, 3796, 5380
Nationwide Survey of Sudden Infant Death Syndrome (SIDS) Service, 8829
Natural Attenuation for Groundwater Remediation, 10280
Navaho Nation K'E Project Children and Families Advocacy Corp, 5988
Navaho Nation K'E Project: Tuba City Children & Families Advocacy Corp, 5928
Navaho Nation K'E Project: Winslow Children & Families Advocacy Corp, 5929
Navajo Nation K'E Project: Shiprock Children & Families Advocacy Corp, 5989
Navajo Nation Office of Special Education & Rehabilitation Services (OSERS), 6050
Navajo Nation Office Special Education & R ehabilitation Services, 6068
NAVH UPDATE, 9937
Navigating the Social World: A Curriculum for Individuals with Asperger's Syndrome, 1759
NCOA Week, 205
ND FFCMH Region II, 6071
ND Region V FFCMH Chapter-Federation of Fa milies for Children's Mental Health, 6072
ND Region VII FFCMH-Federation of Families for Children's Mental Health, 6073
Nebraska Chapter of the National Hemophilia Foundation, 4987
Nebraska Department of Health Perinatal Child and Adolescent Health, 8764
Nebraska Information Service, 1857
Nebraska Kidney Association, 5623

Nebraska Library Commission Talking Book and Braille Services, 9719
Nebraska Organ Retrieval System, 9201
Nebraska SIDS Foundation University of Nebraska Medical Center, 8765
Need to Know, 9117
NEEDLE TIPS & the Hepatitis B Coalition News, 5159
Negotiating the Special Education Maze: A Guide for Parents and Teachers, 7921
Nemours Childrens Clinic, 3103
NERG News, 1576
Neuro-Oncology Information and Support Group, 1936
Neurobiology of Autism, 1760
Neurocognitive Aspects of CFS, 2894
Neurofibromatosis, 6685, 6690, 6696
Neurofibromatosis Association of Arizona, 6657
Neurofibromatosis Foundation: Colorado, 6686
Neurofibromatosis Kansas and Central Plains, 6673
Neurofibromatosis Network, 6654
Neurofibromatosis Society of Ontario, 6655
Neurofibromatosis Support Network, 6687
Neurofibromatosis Type 2: Information for Patients and Families, 6697
Neurofibromatosis: Mid-Atlantic, 6675
Neurofibromatosis: Minnesota, 6677
Neurofibromatosis: New England, 6676
Neurological Center of Iowa, 1969
Neurological Support Group of St. Luke's Hospital, 1985
Neurology Channel, 1085, 1183, 2622, 2818, 3911, 4279, 5247, 6338, 6507, 6649, 6705, 7005, 7565, 7857, 8102, 9073
Neurology of Down Syndrome, 3638
Neurology Research Center Helen Hayes Hospital, 7492
Neuromuscular and ALS Center The Clinical Academic Building, 1144
Neuromuscular Dis. of Infancy, Childhood & Adolesece: A Clinician's Approach, 6529
Neuromuscular Treatment Center: Univ. of Texas Southwestern Medical Center, 6433
Neuropsychological Assessment: What it Does & Does Not Do, 4265
Neuropsychological Performance in Adults with TS, 9118
Neuropsychological Rehabilitation Suggestions/Techniques, 2879
Neuropsychology and Parkinson's Disease, 6969
Neuropsychology of Attention and Memory, 4246
Neurosarcoidosis, 7278
Neurosarcoidosis or Multiple Sclerosis?, 7279
Neuroscience Institute at Mercy Hospital, 6688
Neuroscience Institute Brain Tumor Hotline, 1937
Neurosciences Institute of the Neurosciences Research Program, 972
Neurosurgical Service, 10458
Neurotrophic Factors in Parkinson's Disease, 6970
Nevada Alliance for the Mentally Ill, 5982
Nevada Department of Health & Human Services: Office Of HIV Prevention, 320
Nevada Donor Network, 9202
Nevada Kidney Disease & Hypertension Cente rs, 5664
Nevada PEP, 6066
Nevada State Health Division Bureau of Family Health Services, 8766
Nevada State Library and Archives, 9722
Never the Twain Shall Meet: The Communications Debate, 4564
Never to Be a Mother, 5480
New Beginnings: The Blind Children's Cente, 9798
New Beginnings: The Blind Children's Center, 9797
New Challenge: Responding to Families, 6167
A New Civil Right: Telecommunications Equality for Deaf and Hard of Hearing, 4419
New England AIDS Education and Training Center, 314, 409
New England Area Support Group: National Ataxia Foundation, 1543
New England Hemophilia Association, 4982
New England Hemophilia Association Newsletter, 5096
New England Medical Center: ALS Laboratory, 1145

New England Organ Bank Massachusetts, 9196
New England Region: Helen Keller National Center, 9514
New England Regional Genetics Group, 1842
New Expectations, 3651
New Eyes for the Needy, 9452
New Food Labels, 683
New Hampshire Cancer Pain Initiative, 2196
New Hampshire Chapter NSCIA, 7975
New Hampshire Cystic Fibrosis Care Teaching and Research Center, 3140
New Hampshire Department of Health and Human Services, 321
New Hampshire Lupus Foundation, 8891
New Hampshire SIDS Program, 8767
New Hampshire State Library, 9723
New Hope for Kids Wish Program, 10673
New Jersey AIDS Services, 322
New Jersey Alliance for the Mentally Ill, 5987
New Jersey Department of Health: Child Health Program, 8768
New Jersey Department of Health: Division of HIV, STD And TB Services, 323
New Jersey Institute of Technology Center for Biomedical Engineering, 4053
New Jersey Library for the Blind and Handicapped, 9725
New Jersey Medical School, 3143
New Jersey Parkinson's Disease Information Center, 6921
New Jersey Pregnancy Risk Information Service, 1858
New Jersey SIDS Alliance, 8769
New Jersey Turner Syndrome Resource Group, 9353
New Language of Toys: Teaching Communication Skills to Children..., 7922
New Mexico Alliance for the Mentally Ill, 5990
New Mexico Branch, 9293
New Mexico Department of Health: HIV Services Program, 324
New Mexico Donor Services, 9204
New Mexico Industries for the Blind, 9534
New Mexico SIDS Information and Counseling Program, 8771
New Mexico State Library for the Blind and Physically Handicapped, 9726
New Parents, 3639
New Set of Fears, a New Set of Hopes, 3652
New Sjogren's Syndrome Handbook, 7643
New Start News, 9241
New What Do You Do When You See a Blind Person?, 10040
New York Alliance for the Mentally Ill, 5993
New York Ambassador National Ataxia Foundation, 1551
New York Brain Tumor Support Group, 2004
New York Chapter of the American Association of Kidney Patients, 5634
New York Chapter of the Arthritis Foundation, 1239
New York City Center for SIDS, 8773
New York College of Osteopathic Medicine, 6923
New York Department of Health: AIDS Institute, 325
New York Male Reproductive Center: Sexual Dysfunction Unit, 5304
New York Obesity/Nutrition Research Center, 6718
New York Obesity/Nutrition Research Center (ONRC), 6770
New York Organ Donor Network, Inc, 9207
New York State Center for SIDS: School of Social Welfare, 8774
New York State Talking Book & Braille Library, New York State Library, DOE, 9730
New York University Cancer Institute New York University Medical Center, 2347
New York University General Clinical Research Center, 5257
New York University Medical Center Auxiliary of Tisch Hospital, 5218
New York University Medical Center Head Trauma Program, 4132
New York/New Jersey VA Health Care Network, 10205
Newcomer Asks, 8599
Newport News Public Library System, 9759
News & Notes, 6158

News & Review, 6943
News Across Our Horizons, 1295
News from the Border: A Mother's Memoir of Her
  Autistic Son, 1761
News Report, 5275
Newsletter of American Hearing Research, 4742
Newsletter of the Central Pennsylvania Chapter, 1296
Newsletter: SIDS, 8822
NewsLine, 1875
Newsline, 4743
Newsline for the Blind, 9941
Next Step, 4565
Next Step in Care, 233, 10647
NF Center: North Broward Medical Center
  Neurofibromatosis, 6665
NF Support Group of West Michigan, 6683
NFDI Newsletter, 6231
NHF Head Lines, 6306, 10598
Niagara Cerebral Palsy, 2751
Nick Joins In, 7923
Nick's Mission, 4677
Nicotine Addiction and Cigarettes, 8600
NIDA Capsules, 8598
Night Kites, 483, 504
Night Light: A Book of Nighttime Meditations, 8342
Night-Side: CFS and the Illness Experience, 2851
NIH Clinical Center, 6037
NIH Osteoporosis and Related Bone Disease, 6850
NIH Osteoporosis and Related Bone Diseases -
  National Resource Center, 6780, 6813
NIH Osteoporosis and Related Bone Diseases
  National Resource Center, 6777
NLS News, 9938
NLS Update, 9939
NMAC Update, 553
NNFF Alabama Affiliate, 6656
NNFF Arkansas Affilaite, 6658
NNFF Colorado Chapter, 6659
NNFF Connecticut Chapter, 6660
NNFF Florida Chapter, 6661
NNFF Georgia Affiliate, 6662
NNFF Idaho Chapter, 6663
NNFF Illinois Chapter: Chicago Area, 6666
NNFF Illinois Chapter: Silvis Area, 6667
NNFF Illinois Chapter: Springfield Area, 6668
NNFF Illinois Chapter:Peoria Region, 6669
NNFF Indiana Chapter, 6670
NNFF Iowa Chapter, 6671
NNFF Kansas Affiliate, 6672
NNFF Louisiana Chapter, 6674
NNFF Nevada Affiliate: Reno Area, 6678
NNFF Oregon Affiliate Kaiser Permanente
  Northwest, 6679
NNFF South Carolina Chapter, 6680
NNFF Wisconsin Chapter, 6681
No Fears, No Tears, 10608
No Fears, No Tears: 13 Years Later, 10609
No Less a Woman, 2446
No Longer Immune: A Counselor's Guide to AIDS,
  484
No Smoking Coloring Book, 8601
No Smoking: Lungs At Work, 8602
No Sound, 4566
No Walls of Stone: An Anthology of Literature by
  Deaf Writers, 4567
No-Hysterectomy Option, 5481
No. Colorado FFCMH, 5937
NOAH News, 9940
Nobody Knows!, 2807
Nocturnal Asthma, 1472
Noise Can Be Harmful to Your Health, 4774
Nolo's Guide to Soc. Security Disability: Getting and
  Keeping Your Benefits, 10560
Non Chew Cookbook, 1160
None So Deaf, 4568
Noninsulin-Dependent Diabetes, 3511
Noninvasive Mechanical Ventilation, 6530
Nonprofit Housing and Care Options for Older
  People, 212
Nonverbal Learning Disorder Syndrome, 5232
Norris Cotton Cancer Center Dartmouth-Hitchcock
  Medical Center, 2334
North American Association for the Study of Obesity,
  6771

North American Society for Pediatric
  Gastroenterology, Hepatology & Nutrition, 3926,
  3936, 4010, 10414, 10648
North Carolina Association of the Deaf, 4350
North Carolina Client Assistance Program, 10472
North Carolina Department of Health and Human
  Services, 327
North Carolina Library for the Blind, 9733
North Central Sight Services, 9566
North Dakota Alliance for the Mentally Ill, 5995
North Dakota Association of the Deaf, 4351
North Dakota Comprehensive Hemophilia Center,
  5048
North Dakota FFCMH, 5996
North Dakota Hemostasis and Thrombosis Treatment
  Center, 5049
North Dakota SIDS Alliance, 8778
North Dakota SIDS Management Program, 8779
North Dakota State Library Services for the Disabled,
  9734
North East Ohio Support Group National Ataxia
  Foundation, 1554
North Florida: HPV Support Group, 10443
North Las Vegas VA Medical Center VA Southern
  Nevada Healthcare System, 10191
North Platte Public Library, 9720
North Texas Comprehensive Pediatric Hemophilia
  Center, 5050
North Texas FFCMH, 6010
North Texas Support Group: National Ataxia
  Foundation, 1560
Northcentral West Virginia HPV Support Group,
  10496
Northeast Kansas Parkinson Association, 6889
Northeast Louisiana Sickle Cell Anemia Foundation,
  7609
Northeast Oklahoma Resource Group (Tulsa), 9354
NorthEast Organ Procurement Organization, 9183
Northeast Parkinson's and Caregivers, 6894
Northeast/Caribbean AIDS Education and Training
  Center (NECAAETC), 326, 419
Northeastern Association of the Blind of Albany,
  9541
Northern Arizona Branch:Phoenix Area, 9264
Northern California Association of Persian Gulf
  Veterans, 10114
Northern California Chapter National Multiple
  Sclerosis Society, 6354
Northern California Support Group: National Ataxia
  Foundation, 1529
Northern California Turner Syndrome Resource
  Group, 9344
Northern Illinois University Research and Training
  Center, 4381
Northern Kentucky Talking Book Library, 9678
Northern New Jersey Chapter of the American
  Association of Kidney Patients, 5627
Northern Ohio Chapter of the National Hemophilia
  Foundation, 4994
Northland Library Cooperative, 9702
Northport VA Medical Center, 10206
Northstate Parkinson's Chapter, 6878
Northwest Florida Panhandle Turner Syndrome
  Resource Group, 9346
Northwest Florida Support Group: National Ataxia
  Foundation, 1534
Northwest Georgia Parkinson Disease Association,
  6887
Northwest Kansas Library System, 9672
Northwest Ohio Hemophilia Association, 4995
Northwest Ohio Hemophilia Treatment Center, 5051
Northwest Ohio Sleep Disorders Center Toledo
  Hospital, 7776
Northwest Regional Training Center: Canine
  Companions for Independence, 9474
Northwest Texas Chapter of the Myasthenia Gravis
  Foundation of America, 6597
Northwestern Medicine Digestive Health Center,
  3927
Northwestern Region: Helen Keller National Center,
  9596
Northwestern University: Division of Allergy and
  Immunology, 1405
Not God: A History of Alcoholics Anonymous, 8343
Not Just a Cancer Patient, 2584

November Days, 5268, 8071
Now I Understand, 4678
Now What Do I Do for Fun?, 8603
Now, More Than Ever: Progress in Multiple Sclerosis
  Research, 6499
NSF Packets, 7420
NTID Focus, 4741
NTSA Perspective, 9331
Number and Letter Games, 4679
Nurse Practitioners in Women's Health, 6812
Nursery Rhymes from Mother Goose, 4680
Nursing Home and You: Partners in Caring, 177
Nursing Home and You: Partners in Caring for a
  Relative with Alzheimer's Disease, 1013
Nursing Home Information Services, 176
Nutrition & the Kidney, 5676
Nutrition Action Healthletter, 2490
Nutrition and Changing Kidney Function, 5708
Nutrition Care for Adolescents and Adults with PWS,
  7213
Nutrition Care for Children with PWS, Ages 3-9,
  7214
Nutrition Care for Children with PWS: Infants and
  Toddlers, 7206
Nutrition for Patients Receiving
  Chemotherapy/Radiation Treatment, 2538
Nutrition Guide to Food Allergies, 709
Nutrition in Clinical Practice, 3961, 4011
Nutrition Screening Initiative, 1055
NYS Center for Sudden Infant Death: Eastern
  Satellite Office, 8772

O

Oakland County Health Division: SIDS Project, 8755
Oakland County Library for the Visually and
  Physically Impaired, 9703
Obesity, 6727
Obesity Canada, 6711
Obesity Online, 6765
Obesity Research Center St. Luke's-Roosevelt
  Hospital, 6719
Obesity: Theory and Therapy, 3754
Occupational Asthma, 1473
Occupational Asthma: Lung Hazards on the Job, 1474
Occupational Safety & Health Administration
  (OSHA), 9260
Occupational Therapy Practice Guidelines for Adults
  with Low Back Pain, 2926
Occupational Therapy Practice Guidelines for Adults
  with Low Vision, 1014, 2613, 2801, 2927, 6129,
  6267, 7997, 8072, 8344, 9874
Oconee Regional Library for the Blind and Physically
  Handicapped, 9652
Odyssey of Hearing Loss: Tales of Triumph, 4569
Of Course You're Angry, 8345
Of Their Own: Person to Person Show, 7311
Office of Alcohol and Drug Abuse Prevention, 8140,
  8159, 8171
Office of Alcohol and Drug Abuse Programs, 8181
Office of Alcohol and Other Drug Abuse, 8193
Office of Alcohol and Substance Abuse Department
  of Health and Social Services, 8138
Office of Chronic Disease Prevention and Nutrition
  Services, 6722
Office of Civil Rights, 10415
Office of Human Services: Division of Alcohol and
  Drug Abuse, 8158
Office of Maternal, Child & Family Health, 8806
Office of Policy Planning and Legislation, 10416
Office of Protection and Advocacy for Persons with
  Disabilities, 10437
Office of Public Health, 8743
Office of Special Education and Rehabilitative
  Services, 10649
Office of Special Education Programs, 10417
Office of Substance Abuse Services Department of
  Public Health, 8162
Office of the Special Assistant for Gulf War Illnesses,
  10319
Office of Women's Health, 3686
Office of Women's Services Substance Abuse &
  Mental Health Services, 8131

Office of Womens And Childrens Health: Alabama Department of Health, 8709
Office on Smoking and Health, 8693, 10418
Office on Smoking and Health: Centers for Disease Control & Prevention, 8132
Official Journal of NAASO, 6735
Official Prevention Month Poster, 6829
Official Prevention Week Poster, 6830
Oh, I See, 10041
Ohio Alliance for the Mentally Ill, 5998
Ohio Ambassador: National Ataxia Foundation, 1555
Ohio County Public Library Services for the Blind and Physically Handicapped, 9767
Ohio Department of Health, 8781
Ohio Department of Health: HIV/AIDS Surveillance Program, 328
Ohio Regional Library for the Blind and Physically Handicapped, 9737
Ohio Sleep Medicine Institute, 7777
Ohio State University Clinical Pharmacology Division, 8219
Ohio State University Comprehensive Cancer Center, 2357
Ohio State University General Clinical Research Center, 2358
Ohio State University Laboratory of Psychobiology, 4133
Ohio State University Neuroscience Program, 973
Ohio State University Otological Research Laboratories, 4382
Ohio University Therapy Associates: Hearing, Speech and Language Clinic, 4383
Ohio Valley LifeCenter, 9213
OHSU Homepage Search, 4072
Okada Hearing Ear Guide, 4570
Okizu Foundation Camps, 10523
Oklahoma Alliance for the Mentally Ill, 5999
Oklahoma Ambassador: National Ataxia Foundation, 1556
Oklahoma Association of the Deaf, 4352
Oklahoma Chapter of the Myasthenia Gravis Foundation of America, 6593
Oklahoma Chapter of the National Hemophilia Foundation, 4997
Oklahoma City HPV Support Group: PP of Cen tral Oklahoma, 10479
Oklahoma City VA Health Care System, 10220
Oklahoma Comprehensive Hemophilia Diagnostic Treatment Center, 5052
Oklahoma Department of Health: HIV/STD Service, 329
Oklahoma Department of Mental Health and Substance Abuse Services, 8180
Oklahoma League for the Blind, 9552
Oklahoma Library for the Blind and Physically Handicapped, 9739
Oklahoma Lupus Association, 8906
Oklahoma Medical Research Foundation, 1252
Oklahoma Medical Research Foundation Immunobiolgy & Cancer Research, 2361
Oklahoma Medical Research Foundation: Cardiovascular Research Program, 4891
Oklahoma Organ Sharing Network, 9214
Oklahoma State Department of Health: Maternal and Child Health Services, 8783
Old Dominion Area Chapter: NSCIA, 7981
Older Adults After Treatment, 8604
Older Adults in Treatment, 8605
Older Americans Information Directory, 178
Oley Foundation, 3937, 4012
Oligodendroglioma and Mixed Glioma, 2065
Omaha HPV Support Group: PP of Omaha, 10466
OMIM: Fabry Disease, 3855
On Death & Dying, 10716
On Death and Dying, 10717
On My Own, 4571
On the Air: A Guide to Creating A Smoke-Free Workplace, 8606
On the Question of Pregnancy, 6475
On the Up with Down Syndrome, 3633
On Top of My Game: Living with Diabetes, 3520
On Your Behalf, 179
On: Alternative Therapies, 6476
On: Diagnosis...Putting the Pieces Together, 6477
On: Energy Management, 6478

On: Fatigue, 6479
On: Genes, 6480
On: Pain, 6481
Once a Year for a Lifetime, 2539
Once Upon a Time - Children's Classics Ret old in American Sign Language, 4814
Oncology Hematology Associates of Central Illinois, 2303
Oncology Times: The News Center for the Cancer Care Team, 2491
One Day at a Time, 6750
One Day at a Time in Al-Anon, 8346
1 in Every 10 Persons Has Scoliosis, 7413
One Legacy Transplant Donor Network, 9181
One Step at a Time Brochure, 6971
One Women's Passionate Quest to Complete Her Family, 5482
One, Two, Three, Zero: Infertility, 5555
1-800-BRAILLE, 9809
One-Hundred-Fifty Most Asked Questions About Osteoporosis, 6820
A One-Stop Shop for Parkinson's Informatio n, 6946
10 Warning Signs of Alzheimer's Disease, 1038
101 Tips for Improving Your Blood Sugar, 3410
14 Worst Myths About Recovered Mental Patients, 6159
1st Capital FFCMH, 5997
Online Sarcoidosis Newsletter, 7257
Ontario HIV Treatment Network, 270
Open Windows, 9942
Operation PAR, 8347
Opportunities to Grow, 3653
Option Institute, 2829, 2904, 3866, 3912, 5920, 6201, 10419
Options: New Directions in the War on Cancer, 2492
Options: Spinal Cord Injury and the Future, 7998
Oral Cancers: Research Report, 2540
Oral Interpreting Selections from Papers from Kirsten Gonzales, 4572
Oral Retinoid Therapy (Soriatane), 7710
Orange County Chapter National Multiple Sclerosis Society, 6355
Orange County Library System: Orlando Public Library, 9639
Orange County Support Group: National Ataxia Foundation, 1530
Oregon Association of the Deaf, 4353
Oregon Family Support Network, 6002
Oregon Health & Science University, 3160
Oregon Health Authority, 8784
Oregon Health Authority: HIV Prevention Program, 330
Oregon Health Sciences University, 6927
Oregon Health Sciences University Oregon Hearing Research Center Tinnitus Clinic, 4384
Oregon Health Sciences University: Elk's Children's Eye Clinic, 9799
Oregon State Library, 9741
Orentreich Foundation for the Advancement of Science, 7671
Organ Donor Center of Hawaii, 9188
Organ Donor Program, 5709
Organ Procurement and Transplantation Network (OPTN), 9172, 9252
Organ Procurement and Transplantation:, 9231
Organ Transplants from Executed Prisoners:, 9232
Organizing a Support Group, 2066
Organizing and Maintaining Support Groups for Parents, 2447
Orphan Disease Update, 10600
Orthopaedic Associates of Michigan, 2611
Orthopaedic Biomechanics Laboratory Shriners Hospital for Crippled Children, 2794
Orthopaedic Rehabilitation Association, 7011
Oscar G. Johnson VA Medical Center, 10175
OSERS News in Print: Office of Special Education & Rehabilitative Services, 10606
Osteoarthritis, 1339
Osteogenesis Imperfecta Foundation, 6779, 6784, 6801
Osteogenesis Imperfecta: A Guide for Medic al Professionals, Individuals & Families, 6792
Osteonecrosis, 1340
Osteoperosis: The Silent Disease, 6843

Osteoporosis and Related Bone Diseases: National Resource Center (NIGH), 6802
Osteoporosis Canada, 6810
Osteoporosis Center Memorial Hospital/Advanced Medical Diagn, 6815
Osteoporosis Education Kit, 6831
Osteoporosis Education Poster, 6832
Osteoporosis in Men Information Package, 6835
Osteoporosis Information Package, 6833
Osteoporosis International, 6834
Osteoporosis Report, 6823
Osteoporosis: Clinical Updates, 6836
Osteoporosis: The Silent Disease-Slide Lecture Presentation, 6837
Ostomy Book: Living Comfortably with Colostomies, Ileostomies and Urostomies, 3045, 10561
Ostomy Quarterly, 3972
Other Important STD's, 7590
Other Side of Silence, 4573
Otitis Media, 4775
Otoscope, 4744
Our Brother Has Down's Syndrome: An Introduction for Children, 3625
Our Forgotten Children, 4574
Our Forgotten Children: Hard of Hearing Pupils in the Schools, 4575
Our Immune System, 505, 593
Our Mom Has Cancer, 2469
Out of Left Field, 10042
Out of the Corner of My Eye, 9901
Out of the Storm, 7109
Outpatient Treatment of Asthma, 1475
OUTReach, 554
Outsiders in a Hearing World, 4576
Outsmarting Diabetes, 3459
Overcoming Depression, 6219
Overcoming Headaches & Migraines, 6302
Overcoming Infertility, 5483
Overcoming Rheumatoid Arthritis, 1341
Overeaters Anonymous, 6712, 6728
Overeaters Anonymous Cares, 6751
Overeaters Anonymous is Not a Diet Club, 6752
Overton Brooks VA Medical Center, 10161
Ovulation Detection, 5541
Ovulation Drugs, 5542
Ozarks Parkinson Support Group, 6920

P

PAACNOTES, 555
PACCT, 6082
PACCT of Roanoke Valley, 6083
PACE I, 1356
PACE II, 1357
PACER Center, 6063
Pacific AIDS Education and Training Center (PAETC), 293, 375
Pacific Health Research Institute, 2298
Pacific Northwest Chapter of the Myasthenia Gravis Foundation of America, 6573, 6580, 6581, 6588, 6594, 6599, 6601
Pacific NW Support Group, 7244
Pacific NW Transplant Bank, 9215
Paget Foundation for Paget's Disease of Bone & Related Disorders, 6864
Pain & Hope, 4032
Pain and Sleep, 7827
Pain Free Typing Techniques: Simple Solutions to Prevent Strain Injury, 2614
Pain Syndromes and Parkinson's Disease, 6972
PAL News, 1876
Palm Beach County Library Annex: Talking Books, 9640
PALS Support Groups, 1859
Pancreas, 2482, 3962
Pandora's Aquarium, 7113
Panel of Experts, 9142
Panic Disorder, 6237
Panic Disorder in the Medical Setting, 6220
Panic Survivor, 7114
Pap Test: It Can Save Your Life, 2541
Paralyzed Veterans of America, 7958
Paranoid Psychosis Due to Neurosarcoidosis, 7280
Parent Care News Brief, 8823

Parent Education Network (PEN) Project Health, 6053
Parent Education Program-HIV/AIDS: A Challenge to Us All, 485
Parent Education/Support Group, 1986
Parent Professional Advocacy League, 1831, 5921
Parent Project: Muscular Dystrophy, 6512, 6567
Parent Sign Video Series, 4815
Parent Support Network of Rhode Island, 6076
Parent to Parent of New York State, 10524
Parent Training is Prevention, 8348
A Parent's Guide to Asperger's Syndrome & High-Functioning Autism, 1730
Parent's Guide to Down Syndrome: Toward a Brighter Future, 3617
Parent's Perspective: Diplomacy in Action, 9143
Parenting Preschoolers: Raising Young Blind & Visually Impaired Child, 10006
Parents and Teachers: Partners in Language Development, 4577
Parents and the Grieving Process, 8830
Parents as Trainers of Legislators, Other Parents and Researchers, 1790
Parents Helping Parents A Family Resource Center, 8815
Parents Helping Parents: A Directory of Support Groups for ADD, 1627
Parents Information Network FFCMH, 6058
Parents Involved Network, 6003
Parents Newcomer Packet, 8607
Parents of Children with Brain Tumors PCBT, 1965
Parents of Children with Down Syndrome, 3603, 3618
Parents Resource Institute for Drug Education, 8196
Parents Supporting Parents of MD, 5967
Parents United Network: Parsons Child Family Center, 5994
Parents' Hyperactivity Handbook: Helping the Fidgety Child, 1628
Parkersburg and Wood County Public Library, 9768
Parkingson's: Lynda's Story, 6998
Parkinson Alliance, 6896
Parkinson Association of Greater Daytona Beach, 6883
Parkinson Association of Greater Kansas City, 6890
Parkinson Association of Minnesota, 6895
Parkinson Association of South Dakota, 6903
Parkinson Association of Southwest Florida, 6884
Parkinson Association of the Sacramento Valley, 6879
Parkinson Canada, 6871
Parkinson Chapter of Greater Pittsburgh, 6901
Parkinson Council, 6902
Parkinson Foundation of the Heartland Oklahoma Branch, 6899
Parkinson Foundation of the National Capitol Area, 6904
Parkinson Handbook: A Guide for Patients and Their Families, 6973
Parkinson Network of Mount Diablo, 6880
Parkinson Report, 6944
Parkinson Support Groups of America, 6918
Parkinson's - A Personal Story of Acceptance, 6934
Parkinson's Advocacy: The Keys to Empowerment, 6974
Parkinson's Disease & Movement Disorders, 6935
Parkinson's Disease and the Menstrual Cycle, 6977
Parkinson's Disease Association of San Die go (PDASD), 6912
Parkinson's Disease Foundation Newsletter, 6945
Parkinson's Disease Handbook, 6936, 6975
Parkinson's Disease Q&A: A Guide for Patients, 6976
Parkinson's Disease: A Guide for Patient and Family, 6937
Parkinson's Disease: The Patient Experience, 6978
Parkinson's Foundation, 6872
Parkinson's Institute and Clinical Center, 6873
Parkinson's Patient: What You and Your Family Should Know, 6979
Parkinson's Resource Organization, 6907
Parkinson's Support Group of Upstate New York, 6924
Parkinsonian Syndromes, 6938
Parkinsons Disease Foundation, 6906
Parkinsons Resources of Oregon, 6900

Parkinsons Wellness Group of Western New York, 6898
Parkside Medical Services Corporation, 8153
Participate, 5350
Participating in a Clinical Trial: Your Life, Your Choice, 5117
Partnering with Your Doctor: A Guide for Persons with Memory Problems, 1056
Partnership for Drug-Free Kids, 8133
Pass it On, 8349
Passages Through Recovery, 8350
Pastoral Care of Depression, 6221
Pathways to Better Living, 1358
Patient Advocates for Advanced Cancer Treatments (PAACT), 2266
Patient Education Sample Pack, 6838
Patient Education Video, 6844
Patient Information Package, 7281
Patient Information Series Publications, 5543
Patient Packet, 2649
Patient Perspectives on Parkinson's, 6980
Patient Services, 1938
Patient with Scoliosis, 7421
Patient's Guide to Everyday Life, 7543
Patient's Guide to Visual Aids and Illumination, 10007
Patients Rate Their Scoliosis Doctors, 7458
Paul, 3619
PDF Exercise Program, 6997
PDQ, 2412
Peach Lines, 1165
Peak Flow Meter: A Thermometer for Asthma, 1476
Pediatric Allergy & Pulmonary Division University of Iowa Healthcare, 3114
Pediatric Brain Tumor Foundation, 1906
Pediatric Brain Tumor Foundation of the US, 2086
Pediatric Brain Tumor Foundation: California Chapter, 1907
Pediatric Brain Tumor Foundation: Georgia Chapter, 1908
Pediatric Brain Tumor Support Group, 1915, 1949
Pediatric Cancer Foundation of the Lehigh Valley, 2018
Pediatric Cancer Research Laboratory Children's Hospital of Orange County, 2279
Pediatric Crohn's and Colitis Association, 3079
Pediatric Database: Fabry Disease, 3856
Pediatric Endocrine Society, 7
Pediatric Network Initiative - Crohn's & Colitis Foundation, 2997
Pediatric Neurology Georgetown University Hospital, 10420
Pediatric Psychology, 10525
Pediatric Pulmonary and Cystic Fibrosis Center, 3162
Pediatric Pulmonary Center The Children's Medical Center of Dayton, 3157
Pediatric Pulmonary Unit Massachusetts General Hospital, 8810
Peel HIV/AIDS Network, 272
Peer Pressure Reversal, 8351
Peer Problems in Tourette's Disorder, 9119
PEERS Alliance, 271
Pelvic Inflammatory Disease, 7591
Pelvic Pain, 5544
Pembroke Pines Parkinson Support Group, 6915
Pen-Pal Directory, 1589
Penicillamine, 1342
Peninsula Support & Education Group for Parents of Children with Brain Tumors, 1939
Penn Center for Sleep Disorders: Hospital of the University of Pennsylvania, 7778
Pennsylvania Alliance for the Mentally Ill, 6004
Pennsylvania Department of Health Bureau of Family Health, 8785
Pennsylvania Department of Health: Division Of HIV Disease, 332
Pennsylvania Educational Network for Eating Disorders, 3700
Pennsylvania Lupus News, 8947
Pennsylvania State University Artificial Heart Research Project, 4892
Pennsylvania Turner Syndrome Resource Group, 9355
Pensacola Brain Injury TBI/ABI Support Group, 4090

People Against Cancer, 2170
People Like Us, 5717
People Living Through Cancer Support Groups, 1999
People with AIDS Health Group, 621
People-to-People Committee for the Handicapped, 10421
People...Not Patients: Source Book for Living with Bowel Disease, 3046
Perigee Visual Dictionary of Signing, 4578
Perioperative Management of Parkinson's Disease, 6981
Peritoneal Dialysis, 5710
Perkins Activity and Resource Guide: A Handbook for Teachers, 9875
Perkins Braille and Talking Book Library, 9693
Perry Point VA Medical Center VA Maryland Health Care System, 10166
Persisting Problems After Mild Head Injury: A Review of the Syndrome, 4247
Person to Person, 6753
Personal Guide to Living Well with Fibromyalgia, 1273
Personal Reader Update, 9943
Personality-Guided Therapy for Posttraumatic Stress Disorder, 7127
Perspectives Folio: Mainstreaming, 4579
Perspectives Folio: Parent-Child, 4776
Perspectives in Education and Deafness, 4715
Perspectives on Deafness, 4580
Perspectives on Living with Scleroderma, 7379
Pervasive Developmental Disorders: Finding a Diagnosis and Getting Help, 1762
Pet Scans: A New Look at Parkinson's Disease, 6982
Peter Wegner Is Alive and Well and Living in Providence, 4266
Pharmacologic Therapy of Pediatric Asthma, 1500
Pharmacotherapy of TS and Associated Disorders, 9120
Phase 3: Dementia Care Practice Recommendations, 1057
Philadelphia Biomedical Research Institute, 7617
Philadelphia Department of Public Health: STD Control Program, 333
Phoenix Area Support Group: National Ataxi a Foundation, 1525
Phoenix Magazine, 3052, 3963, 9391
Phoenix Public Library: Special Needs Section, 9616
Phoenix VA Health Care System, 10109
Phoenix: Newsletter, 2493
Physical Activity and the Aging, 180
Physical Medicine & Rehabilitation, 6531
Physical Therapy in Hemophilia, 5118
Physician Listings, 7282
Physician Referral and Information Line, 1409
Physicians Guide to Type I Diabetes, 3521
Pinellas Talking Book Library for the Blind and Physically Handicapped, 9641
Pitch of Grief, 10736
Pittsburgh Vision Services, 9567
Pituitary Tumors, 2067
Pityriasis Rosea, 7712
PKD Foundation Polycystic Kidney Disease Foundation, 5665
PKD Patient's Manual, 5677
PKD Progress, 5685
PKU Quick Reference and Fact Sheet, 1887
Place of Their Own: Creating the Deaf Community in America, 4581
Plain Talk About Depression, 6238
Plain Talk About...Dealing with the Angry Child, 6169
Plain Talk About...Handling Stress, 6170
Plaintalk: A Booklet About MS for Families, 6482
Planning for Long-Term Care, 181
Planning for the Future, 4204
Playing Cure, 6130
Please Don't Say Hello, 1763
Pocket Guide for Continence Care, 5343
Podiatry and Parkinson's Disease, 6983
Points for Parents Perplexed About Drugs, 8608
Polio Experience Network, 7028
Polio Network News, 7018
Polio Survivors Association, 7012
Politics of Deafness, 4582
Pollen and Spores Around the World, 710

Pollen Times: By State, By Month, 684
Polyarteritis Nodosa and Wegener's Granulomatosis, 1343
Polycystic Kidney Research Foundation, 5725
Polymyalgia Rheumatica and Giant Cell Arthritis, 1344
Pool Exercise Program, 1359
Popsicles are Cold, 4681
Porphyria Cutanea Tarda, 3984
Portland Public Library, 9684
Portland VA Medical Center VA Portland Health Care System, 10222
Positive Interactions Program of Activities for People with Alzheimer's, 1015
Positive Living, 557
Positive Living British Columbia, 273
Positive Living Niagara, 274
Positive Outlook, 558
Positive Social Support Newsletter, 559
Positive Voice Newsletter, 560
Positive Woman, 561
Positive Women's Network - USA, 275
Positively Aware, 562
Possible Association of Rheumatoid Arthritis & Sarcoidosis, 7283
Possible Dream: Mainstream Experiences of Hearing-Impaired Students, 4583
Post Milan, 4584
Post-Polio Awareness & Support Society of British Columbia, 7013
Post-Polio Health, 7019
Post-Polio Health International, 7020
Post-Polio Syndrome: Identifying Best Practices in Diagnosis and Care, 7024
Post-Traumatic Headaches: Subtypes & Behavioral Treatments, 4248
PostPolio Health International, 7015
Posttraumatic Stress Disorder (PTSD) Alliance, 7057, 7075
Postural Hypotension, 6984
Postural Screening Program, 7422
POZ Magazine, 520
A Practical Guide to PTSD Treatment: Pharmacological&Psychotheraputic Aprch, 7122
Practical Pointers for Parkinson Patients, 6985
Practice Guidelines for Eating Disorders, 3755
Practice Parameters, 2483
Practice Recommendations for Home Care Professionals, 1058
Prader-Willi Arkansas Association Prader-Willi Syndrome Association, 7167
Prader-Willi California Foundation, 7168
Prader-Willi Colorado Association, 7169
Prader-Willi Connecticut Association, 7170
Prader-Willi Delaware Assocition, 7171
Prader-Willi Florida Assocition, 7172
Prader-Willi Georgia Association, 7173
Prader-Willi Hawaii Association, 7174
Prader-Willi Idaho Association, 7175
Prader-Willi Illinois Association, 7176
Prader-Willi Indiana Association, 7177
Prader-Willi Iowa Association, 7178
Prader-Willi Kentucky Association, 7179
Prader-Willi Michigan Association, 7181
Prader-Willi Minnesota Association, 7182
Prader-Willi Missouri Association, 7183
Prader-Willi Nebraska Association, 7184
Prader-Willi New England Association, 7180
Prader-Willi New Jersey Association, 7185
Prader-Willi New York Association, 7186
Prader-Willi North Carolina Association, 7187
Prader-Willi North Dakota Association, 7188
Prader-Willi Ohio Association, 7189
Prader-Willi Oklahoma Association, 7190
Prader-Willi Oregon Association, 7191
Prader-Willi Pennsylvania Association, 7192
Prader-Willi South Carolina Association, 7193
Prader-Willi Syndrome Arizona Association, 7166
Prader-Willi Syndrome Arizona Association: Phoenix Area, 7165
Prader-Willi Syndrome Association, 7164
Prader-Willi Syndrome: An Overview for Health Professionals, 7216
Prader-Willi Syndrome: the Early Years, 7217
Prader-Willi Tennessee Association, 7194

Prader-Willi Texas Association, 7195
Prader-Willi Utah Association, 7196
Prader-Willi Washington Association, 7197
Prader-Willi Wisconsin Association, 7198
PraderWilli Syndrome Association, 7200
Predicting AIDS and Other Epidemics, 486, 506
Pregnancy After a Loss, 10732
Pregnancy After Infertility, 5545
Pregnancy and Exposure to Alcohol and Other Drug Use, 8352
Pregnancy Healthline: Pennsylvania Hospital, 1860
Pregnancy Heartbreak: Unfulfilled Promises, 10733
Pregnancy Risk Line, 1861
Pregnancy Safety Hotline, 1862
Pregnancy, Childbirth, and Bladder Control, 5357
Premenstrual Syndrome (PMS), 5546
Prenatal Hydrocephalus: A Book for Parents, 5233
Preparing for the Drug-Free Years: A Family Activity Book, 8353
Preparing your Child for a Bone Marrow Transplant, 2542
Preparing Yourself for Spinal Surgery for Teenagers with Severe Scoliosis, 7442
PreReading Strategies, 4585
Presbyterian Hospital of Dallas, 6929
Presbyterian-University Hospital: Pulmonary Sleep Evaluation Center, 7779
Preschool Learning Activities for the Visually Impaired Child, 9876
Prescriptions for Independence: Working with Older People Who Are Visually Imp., 9877
Presence at the Center, 8354
President's Committee on the Employment of People with Disabilities, 10422
Presidential Proclamation - National Sarcoidosis Awareness Day, 7284
Preston Robert Tisch Brain Tumor Center at Duke, 2007
Prevent Blindness, 9453
Prevent Blindness America News, 9944
Prevent Blindness Tri-State, 9478
Preventing & Reversing Osteoporosis: Every Woman's Guide, 6821
Preventing and Managing Osteoporosis, 6822
Preventing Childhood Obesity: Health in the Balance, 6729
Preventing Epilepsy, 7544
Preventing Miscarriage: The Good News, 5484
Preventing Relapse, 8609
Prevention in Action, 8364
Prevention Plus II: Tools for Creating & Sustaining a Drug-Free Community, 8355
Prevention Plus III: Assessing Alcohol & Other Prevention Programs, 8356
Prevention Resource Guide: Alcohol and Other Drug Related Periodicals, 8357
Prevention Resource Guide: American Indian/Native Alaskans, 8358
Prevention Resource Guide: Asian and Pacific Islander Americans, 8359
Prevention Resource Guide: Elementary Youth, 8360
Prevention Resource Guide: Pregnant Postpartum Women and Their Infants, 8361
Prevention Resource Guide: Secondary School Students, 8362
Prevention Resource Guide: Women, 8363
Preventive Medicine Research Institute, 4893
Pridelines, 301
Primary Brain Cancer Support Group, 1967
Primer of Brain Tumors, 2068
Primer on the Rheumatic Diseases, 1274
Prince George's County Memorial Library: Talking Book Center, 9690
Princess Pooh, 7924
Problem Behaviors & TS, 9121
Problem of AIDS, 507
Procedure Coding for Hemophilia Treatment, 5078
Professional's Role in Sudden Infant Death Syndrome, 8820
Profiles in Aging and Vision, 10043
Program Booklet, 8610
Program for You, 8365
Program of Recovery, 6754
Progress, 5783
Progress in Dermatology, 7694

Progress in Research, 8005
Progress Notes, 6736
Project Eyes and Ears, 4417
Project Inform, 276
Project Inform Hiv Health InfoLine, 454
Promise of a New Day: A Book of Daily Meditations, 8366
Prospect Child And Family Center, 2752
Prostate Cancer Foundation, 2262
Prostate Cancer: A Survivor's Guide, 2448
Prostate Cancer: What Every Man and His Family Needs to Know, 2449
Prostate Health Workbook, 2450
Protect Yourself and Those You Love Against HBV, 5178
Protecting Against Latex Allergy, 7941
Protection & Advocacy Agency, 10445
Protection and Advocacy Program for the Mentally Ill, 6131
Protection and Advocacy System of Alburque rque, 10470
Providence VA Medical Center, 10232
Providing Services for People with Vision Loss: Multidisciplinary Perspective, 9878
Prozac Nation: Young & Depressed in America: A Memoir, 6222
Pseudoxanthoma Elasticum Fact Sheet, 1345
Psoriasis Advance, 7689
Psoriasis and Psoriatic Arthritis Pocket G uide, 7682
Psoriasis Forum, 7690
Psoriasis Newsletter, 7695
Psoriasis on Specific Skin Sites, 7713
Psoriasis Research Institute, 7672
Psoriasis: How It Makes You Feel, 7714
Psoriatic Arthritis, 7715
Psoriatic Arthritis Information Package, 1346
Psychguides.com, 7159
Psychodynamic Technique in the Treatment of the Eating Disorders, 3756
Psychoeducational Assessment of Hearing-Impaired Students, 4586
Psychoeducational Assessment of Visually Impaired Students, 9879
Psychoeducational Profile (PEP-3): TEACCH Individualized Psychoeducational Assessm, 1764
Psychological Assessment Of Adult Post Traumatic States:Phenomenolgy,Diag&Meas, 7128
Psychological Factors in Sarcoidosis, 7285
Psychological Management of Chronic Pain: A Treatment Manual, 10562
Psychology in the Service of National Security, 7129
Psychopharmacology Bulletin, 6153
Psychosocial Rehabilitation Journal, 6154
Psychotherapy of Severe and Mild Depression, 6223
Psychotherapy with Traumatized Vietnam Combatants, 6171
PTSD and the Family: Secondary Traumatization, 6168
PTSD Family Support Group, 7110
PTSD Hotline, 7111
PTSD Research Quarterly, 7138
PTSD Support Services, 7157
PTSD: A Guide for the Frontline, 7141
PTSDanonymous.org, 7112
PTSDinfo.org, 7158
Public Health Services of Louisiana, 8744
Public Law 102-94, 7286
Public Schools and Students with Autism: Components of a Defensible Program, 1806
Publications from the National Information Center on Deafness, 4777
Pubmed, 9074
Puget Sound Blood Center, 5053
Puget Sound Chapter Newsletter, 6642
Pull-thru Network, 3948, 4013
Pull-Thru Network News, 5351
Pull-thru Network News, 3973
Pulmonary Fibrosis Foundation, 5813
Pulmonary Hypertension Association, 4922
Pulmonary Hypertension Association (PHA), 4864, 5252, 5814
Pulmonary Sarcoidosis: Evaluation with High Resolution, 7287
Pulmonary Sarcoidosis: What We Are Learning, 7288

Pulomonolgy Morgan Stanley Children's Hospital, 3149
Pumping Insulin, 3460
Puppy Walker Brochure, 10008
Purdue Cancer Center Purdue University, 2267
Purdue University Center for AIDS Research, 398
Purdue University William A Hillenbrand Biomedical Engineering Center, 4894
Purdue University: Center for Research on Aging and the Life Course, 129
Pure Facts, 1639
Pushin On: RRTC on Secondary Conditions of Spinal, 7984
Pushing on: University of Alabama, 8006
Put on the Brakes Bulletin: Take a Look at College Drinking, 8611
PUVA (Psoralen Plus Ultraviolet Light A), 7711
PWA Rag, 556
PXE International, 9820

Q

Q and A: Hepatitis B Prevention, 5179
Q&A About Smoking and Health, 8612
Q&A on PKD, 5678
Q&A's About Arthritis and Rheumatic Disease, 1347
Q&A's About Psoriasis, 7683
Quad Cities Brain Tumor Support Group, 1970
Quality Care, 5352
Quest Magazine, 6535
Questionnaire Responses for Demographics and Symptoms from 1000 Patients, 7289
Questions & Answers About Depression & Its Treatment, 6224
Questions & Answers About Diet and Nutrition, 3064
Questions & Answers About Paget's Disease of Bone, 6858
Questions and Answers, 6755
Questions and Answers About Breast Lumps, 2543
Questions and Answers About Choosing a Mammography Facility, 2544
Questions and Answers About Complications, 3065
Questions and Answers About Crohn's Disease & Ulcerative Colitis, 3066
Questions and Answers About DES Exposure During Pregnancy and Before Birth, 2545
Questions and Answers About Emotional Factors in Ileitis and Colitis, 3067
Questions and Answers About Employment of Deaf People, 4778
Questions and Answers About Metastatic Cancer, 2546
Questions and Answers About Pain Control, 2547
Questions and Answers About Pregnancy in Ileitis and Colitis, 3068
Questions and Answers About Surgery, 3069
Questions and Answers on Hearing Loss, 4779
Questions Most Often Asked the NSF, 7423
Quick and Easy Meals and Menus, 3461
Quick and Healthy Recipes & Ideas, 3462
Quick and Hearty Main Dishes, 3463
Quick Guide to Lyme Disease, 9054
Quick List to Build Pride in Your Communities, 8613
Quick Start Diet Guide, 2650
A Quiet World: Living with Hearing Loss, 4420
Quit & Stay Quit: A Personal Program to Stop Smoking, 8367
Quit Smoking Manual, 8368

R

RADAR Network National Clearinghouse for Alcohol & Dru, 8220
Radiation Therapy and You: A Guide To Self-Help During Treatment, 2548
Radiation Therapy of Brain Tumors: A Basic Guide, 2069
Rainbow Alliance of the Deaf, 4330
Rainbow Connection, 10674
Rainbows for All God's Children, 10702
Raised Dot Computing Newsletter, 9946
Raising a Child with Autism: A Guide to Applied Behavior Analysis for Parents, 1765

Raising a Child with Diabetes: A Guide for Parents, 3464
Raising a Child with Spina Bifida: An Introduction, 7942
Ralph H. Johnson VA Medical Center, 10234
Rambaugh-Goodwin Institute for Cancer Research, 2294
Randolph-Sheppard Vendors of America, 9454, 10094
RAP* Time, 563
Rape, Abuse & Incest National Network, 7115
Rare Cancer Alliance, 9327
Raymond G. Murphy VA Medical Center New Mexico VA Health Care System, 10196
Raynaud's Association, 7223, 7326
Raynaud's Phenomenon, 7227, 7228
Reach Out for Youth with Ileitis and Colitis, Inc., 2998, 9382
Reach to Recovery, 2413
Reaching Out, 1166
Reaching Out: A Creative Access Guide for Designing Exhibits & Cultural Programs, 10044
Reaching the Autistic Child: A Parent Training Program, 1766
Reaching, Crawling, Walking-Let's Get Moving, 10009
Read Easy, 182
Read My Lips, 4816
Reader-Transcriber Registry National Braille Association, 9800
Reading and Deafness, 4587
Reading is for Everyone, 10010
Reading Resources on Spinal Cord Injury, 8016
Reading with Low Vision, 10011
Real Life Parenting of Kids with Diabetes, 3465
Real Lifestyles Manual, 5679
Realities in Coping with Progressive Neuromuscular Diseases, 1161
Rebecca and John Moores UCSD Cancer Center, 2280
Rebuilt: My Journey Back to the Hearing World, 4588
Recognizing and Treating Low Blood Sugar (Hypoglycemia), 3512
Recognizing the Signs of Childhood Seizures, 7545
Recognizing TS in the Classroom, 9122
Record Book for Individuals with Autism Spectrum Disorders, 1767
Recorded Periodicals, 9821, 9912
Recording for the Blind Helpline, 9822
Recovering From the Chronic Fatigue Syndrome: A Guide to Self-Empowerment, 2852
Recovery and Cognitive Retraining After Craniocerebral Trauma, 4249
Recovery from Bereavement, 10718
Recovery from Brain Damage in the Elderly, 4205
Recovery International, 7116
Recovery Journal for Exploring Who I Am, 8369
Recurrence: What Do I Do Now?, 2549
Recurrent Stroke, 5282, 8088
Redding Chapter of the American Association of Kidney Patients, 5589
Reducing the Health Risks of Secondhand Smoke, 8614
Reference and Information Services from NLS, 10012
Reflex Sympathetic Dystrophy Syndrome Association (RSDSA), 2918
Reflex Sympathetic Dystrophy Syndrome Fact Sheet, 1348
Region 1 of the National Association for Parents of the Visually Impaired, 9515
Region 6 of the National Association for Parents of the Visually Impaired, 9469
Region I Office Program: Consultants for Maternal and Child Health, 8750
Region II Office Program: Consultants for Maternal and Child Health, 8775
Region III Office Program: Consultants for Maternal and Child Health, 8721
Region IV Office Program Consultants for Maternal and Child Health, 8722
Region IX Office Program Consultants for Maternal and Child Health, 8723
Region VI Office Program Consultants for Maternal and Child Health, 8795

Region VII Office Program: Consultants for Maternal and Child Health, 8760
Region VIII Office Program Consultants for Maternal and Child Health, 8724
Region X Office Program Consultants for Maternal and Child Health, 8803
Regional Bone Center Helen Hayes Hospital, 6816
Regional Cancer Foundation, 2143
Regional Hemophilia Treatment Center Children's Hospital of Michigan, 5054
Regional HIV/AIDS Connection, 277
Regional Organ Bank of Illinois, Inc., 9189
Regional Resource Center on Deafness Western Oregon State College, 4385
Registry of Interpreters for the Deaf, 4331, 4854
Regular Kid, 1501
A Regular Kid That's Me: Inservice Film for Educators, 9134
Rehab Outlook, 6483
Rehabilitation Engineering on Hearing Enha ncement, 4386
Rehabilitation Institute of Chicago, 1253
Rehabilitation Institute of Michigan, 4134
Rehabilitation International, 10423
Rehabilitation Services Administration, 10424
Reiter's Syndrome, 1349
Relapse and the Addict, 8615
Relation of Soft-Tissue Sarcome, Malignant Lymphoma & Colon Cancer, 10306
Relationships Between Personality Disorders, 4250
Relaxation Tape, 2935, 6323
Releasing Anger, 8616
Remove Intoxicated Drivers (RID-USA), 8134
Removing House Dust and Other Allergic Irritants From Your Home, 711
Renal Recipes Quarterly, 5686
Renalife, 9237
Renfrew Center of Bryn Mawr, 3701
Renfrew Center of Connecticut, 3690
Renfrew Center of Miami, 3691
Renfrew Center of New York, 3697
Renfrew Center of Northern New Jersey, 3696
Renfrew Center of Philadelphia, 3702
Renfrew Center of South Florida, 3692
Report of the Panel on Alzheimer's Disease, 1059
Report of the Secretary's Task Force on Youth Suicide, Volume 1, 6225
Reproductive Hazards in the Workplace: Mending Jobs, Managing Pregnancies, 5485
Research & Practice, 1032
Research and Training Center for Persons Who are Deaf or Hard of Hearing, 4387
Research at Gallaudet, 4745
Research Center, 234
Research Chair in Obesity Universit, Laval, 6713
Research Chair on Obesity, 6772
Research Directions in Multiple Sclerosis, 6484
Research Institute of Palo Alto Medical Foundation, 663
Research Institute on Alcoholism State University of New York at Buffalo, 8221
Research on Drugs and the Workplace, 8617
Research Report: Adult Kidney Cancer and Wilms' Tumor, 2550
Research to Prevent Blindness, 9455
Reseau ACCESS Network, 278
RESOLVE, 5573
RESOLVE Affiliate of Central Florida, 5392
RESOLVE Affiliate of Iowa, 5399
RESOLVE Affiliate of Northwest Arkansas, 5384
RESOLVE Helpline, 3807
RESOLVE of Alabama, 5382
RESOLVE of Central Texas, 5423
RESOLVE of Colorado, 5388
RESOLVE of Dallas/Fort Worth, 5424
RESOLVE of Fairfield County, 5389
RESOLVE of Georgia, 5395
RESOLVE of Greater Hartford, 5390
RESOLVE of Greater Los Angeles, 5385
RESOLVE of Greater San Diego, 5386
RESOLVE of Hawaii, 5396
RESOLVE of Houston, 5425
RESOLVE of Illinois, 5397
RESOLVE of Indiana, 5398
RESOLVE of Kentucky, 5400

RESOLVE of Long Island, 5410
RESOLVE of Louisiana, 5401
RESOLVE of Michigan, 5403
RESOLVE of Minnesota, 5404
RESOLVE of Nevada, 5406
RESOLVE of New Hampshire, 5407
RESOLVE of New Jersey, 5408
RESOLVE of New Mexico, 5409
RESOLVE of New York City, 5411
RESOLVE of North Carolina, 5413
RESOLVE of North Florida, 5393
RESOLVE of Northern California, 5387
RESOLVE of Ohio, 5414
RESOLVE of Oklahoma, 5415
RESOLVE of Oregon, 5416
RESOLVE of Philadelphia, 5417
RESOLVE of Pittsburgh, 5418
RESOLVE of South Carolina, 5421
RESOLVE of South Florida, 5394
RESOLVE of South Texas, 5426
RESOLVE of Southcentral Pennsylvania, 5419
RESOLVE of St. Louis, Missouri, 5405
RESOLVE of Tennessee, 5422
RESOLVE of the Bay State, 5402, 5506
RESOLVE of the Capital District, 5412
RESOLVE of the Ocean State, 5420
RESOLVE of the Washington Metro Area, 5391
RESOLVE of Utah, 5427
RESOLVE of Valley of the Sun, 5383
RESOLVE of Vermont, 5428
RESOLVE of Wisconsin, 5429
RESOLVE: The National Infertility Association, 5381
Resolving Infertility, 5486
Resource and Activities Guide, 3466
Resource Guide, 5234
Resource Guide for Parents of Children with Brain
    and Spinal Cord Tumors, 2043
Resource Guide: Normal Pressure
    Hydrocephalus/Adult Onset, 5235
Resource Guide: Products and Services for
    Incontinence, 5344
Resource List for Persons with Low Vision, 10013
Resources Family Centered Intervention for Infants,
    Toddlers & Preschoolers, 9880
Resources for Elders with Disabilities, 183
Resources for Seniors and People with Disabilities,
    10480
Resources List of Organizations, 4251
Respite Care Guide, 1060
Rest of the Family, 7554
Rethink Breast Cancer, 2112
Rethinking Alzheimer's Care, 1016
Rethinking Attention Deficit Disorders, 1629
Return from Madness, 6268
Returning to Work: Strategies for Brain Tumor
    Patients, 2070
Review, 9913
Rheumatoid Arthritis Information Package, 1350
Rhode Island Association of the Deaf, 4354
Rhode Island Brain & Spine Tumor Foundation, 2020
Rhode Island Department of Health, 334, 8787
Rhode Island Department of State Library for the
    Blind and Physically Handicapped, 9744
Rhode Island Disability Law Center, 10482
Rhode Island Hemophilia Foundation, 5001
Rhode Island Hospital: Cystic Fibrosis Center, 3165
Rhode Island Scleroderma Support Group, 7374
Richland County HPV Support Group, 10476
Richland Memorial Comprehensive Pediatric
    Hemophilia Center, 5055
Richmond HPV Support Group: Fan Free Clini c,
    10492
Richmond Support Group, 3722
Rick Hansen Foundation, 7959
RID-USA Newsletter, 8471
Riddle of Autism: A Psychological Analysis, 1768
Right & Left Ventricular Function at Rest in Patients
    with Sarcoidosis, 7290
Right from the Start, 3467
Riley Hemophilia & Hemophilia Center Riley
    Hospital for Children, 5056
Rio Grande Chapter: NSCIA Rio Vista Rehabilitation
    Hospital, 7980
Risk Factor Card: Can It Happen to You?, 6839
Risky Business, 521

Risperidone as a Treatment for TS, 9123
RNtoBSN.org, 7076
Road Less Traveled, 4280
Roanoke City Public Library System, 9760
Roanoke Vet Center, 10256
Robert H Lurie Comprehensive Cancer Center of
    Northwestern University, 2304
Robert J. Dole VA Medical Center, 10157
Robley Rex VA Medical Center Louisville VA
    Medical Center, 10159
Robyn's Book: A True Diary, 3186
Rochester Institute of Technology: Nationa l
    Technical Institute for the Deaf, 4388
Rockefeller University Laboratory for Investigative
    Dermatology, 7673
Rockefeller University Laboratory of Biology, 8222
Rockefeller University Laboratory of Cardiac
    Physiology, 4895
Rockefeller University, Laboratory for Investigative
    Dermatology, 7674
Rockford Parkinson's Support Group, 6917
Rocky Mountain CFIDS/FMS Association, 3870
Roger Williams Clinical Cancer Research Center,
    2370
Roger's Story: For Cori, 602
Role of Magnetic Resonance Imaging in
    Neurosarcoidosis, 7291
Role of Physical Therapy in Parkinson's Disease,
    6986
Role of the Allergist & Clinical Immunologist in
    Patient Care, 712
Rolling Along with Goldilocks and the Three Bears,
    7932
Rome Georgia Chapter of the American Association
    of Kidney Patients, 5604
Rome Subregional Library for People with
    Disabilities, 9653
Rosacea, 7716
Rosalind Russell Medical Research Center for
    Arthritis at UCSF, 1254
Rose Kushner Breast Cancer Advisory Center, 2144
Roseburg VA Health Care System, 10223
Roswell Park Cancer Institute National Cancer
    Institute, 2348
Roswellness Magazine, 2484
Roy M and Phyllis Gough Huffington Center on
    Aging, 130
RP Messenger, 9945
RRTC on Aging with a Disability Los Amigos
    Research and Education Instit, 7985
RRTC on Community Integration of Persons with
    TBI, 4110
RSI Resources, 2623
Running on Empty, 2853
Rush University Multiple Sclerosis Center, 6434
Russell is Extra Special, 1782
Rutgers Global Tuberculosis Institute New Jersey
    Medical School, 9261
Rutgers University Center of Alcohol Studies, 8223
Rutgers University: Controlled Drug- Delivery
    Research Center, 8224
Ruth E Golding Clinical Pharmacokinetics
    Laboratory, 8225
Ryan: A Mother's Story of her TS/ADHD Child, 9089

S

Sacramento Valley Chapter of the American
    Association of Kidney Patients, 5590
Sacramento Veterans Center, 10115
Sad Story of Mary Wanna or How Marijuana Harms
    You, 8446
Safe Homes, 8694
Saint Francis Medical Center Peoria Pulmonary
    Association, 3111
Salem VA Medical Center, 10257
Salk Institute Cancer Center, 2281
Sammie's New Mask: A Coloring Book for Friends of
    Children with Cancer, 2470
Sammy's Mommy Has Cancer: For Children Who
    Have a Loved One with Cancer, 2471
Samuel Roberts Noble Foundation Biomedical
    Division, 2362
Samueli Institute, 7098

San Antonio Bexar County FFCMH, 6011
San Antonio Cancer Institute, 2376
San Diego Area Chapter National Multiple Sclerosis
    Society, 6356
San Diego Support Group: National Ataxia
    Foundation, 1531
San Francisco AIDS Foundation (SFAF), 294
San Francisco Clinical Research Center, 6294
San Francisco Community Health Center:
    HHOME/GTZ-ICM, 295
San Francisco Heart & Vascular Institute, 4896
San Francisco Public Library for the Blind and Print
    Disabled, 9623
San Francisco VA Medical Center, 10116
San Jose State University Library, 9624
Sanders-Brown Center on Aging University of
    Kentucky, 131
Sanford Center for Aging University Of Nevada,
    Reno, 132
Sansum Diabetes Research Institute, 3390
Santa Barbara Breast Cancer Institute, 2282
Santa Rosa Medical Center, 3593
Sarasota Area Brain Tumor Support Group, 1957
Sarcoidosis, 7292
Sarcoidosis and Lyme Disease, 7314
Sarcoidosis and Pregnancy: Clinical Observation,
    7296
Sarcoidosis and You: A Listing of Possible
    Symptoms, 7297
Sarcoidosis Center, 7237
Sarcoidosis Conference 2, 7312
Sarcoidosis Conference 3, 7313
Sarcoidosis Diagnosed in a Patient with Known HIV
    Infection, 7293
Sarcoidosis HelpNet, 7245
Sarcoidosis in India: A Review of 125 Biopsy-Proven
    Cases from India, 7298
Sarcoidosis Networking Association, 7236
Sarcoidosis of the Liver, 7299
Sarcoidosis Patient Questionnaire, 7294
Sarcoidosis Questionnaire: Demographics and
    Symptomatology-The Patients Respond, 7295
Sarcoidosis Research Institute (SRI), 7246
Sarcoidosis Resource Guide and Directory, 7256
Sarcoidosis Self-Help Group: New York, 7247
Sarcoidosis Self-Help Group: Virginia, 7248
Sarcoidosis Support Group Delaware, 7249
Sarcoidosis Support Group: New Jersey, 7250
Sarcoidosis Support Group: Washington DC, 7251
Sarcoidosis Treatment and Research Center Thomas
    Jefferson University Hospital, 7238
Sarcoidosis: A Multisystem Disease, 7300
Sarcoidosis: International Review, 7301
Sarcoidosis: Pleural Involvement Mimicking a Coin
    Lesson, 7302
Sarcoidosis: Usual and Unusual Manifestations, 7303
Sarcoidosis: What's That?, 7315
Savory Soups and Salads, 3468
Say That Again, Please, 4589
SBAA General Information Packet, 7925
SBTF Brain Tumor Support Group, 1962
Scabies, 7717
Scalp Psoriasis, 7718
Scarlet Letters, 487
SCENE, 9947
Schedules of Development for Hearing Impaired
    Infants and their Parents, 4590
Schizophrenia, 6275
Schizophrenia and Primitive Mental States, 6269
Schizophrenia Bulletin, 6273
Schizophrenia Research Branch: Division of Clinical
    and Treatment Research, 6261
Schizophrenia Therapy Online Resource Center, 6283
Schizophrenia: From Mind to Molecule, 6270
Schneeweiss Adult Congenital Heart Disease Center,
    2949
School Answers Back: Responding to Student Drug
    Use, 8370
School Information Packet, 1477
School Screening with Dr. Robert Keller, 7443
School's Guide for Students with CFS, 2880
Schulze Diabetes Institute, 3375
SCI and Lower Extremity Orthoses, 8028
SCI Life, 8003

Science and Babies: Private Decisions, Public Dilemmas, 5487
Science of Sound, 4591
Scleroderma Book, 7380
Scleroderma Clinical & Research Center State University of New York at Stonybro, 7364
Scleroderma Foundation, 7231, 7327, 7393
Scleroderma Foundation: Arizona Chapter, 7329
Scleroderma Foundation: Bluebonnet Chapter, 7353
Scleroderma Foundation: Colorado Chapter, 7333
Scleroderma Foundation: Evergreen Chapter, 7356
Scleroderma Foundation: Georgia Chapter Scleroderma Foundation, 7336
Scleroderma Foundation: Greater Chicago Chapter, 7337
Scleroderma Foundation: Greater San Diego Chapter, 7330
Scleroderma Foundation: Greater Washington DC Chapter, 7334, 7355
Scleroderma Foundation: Michigan Chapter, 7340
Scleroderma Foundation: Minnesota Chapter, 7341
Scleroderma Foundation: Missouri Chapter, 7342
Scleroderma Foundation: Nevada Chapter, 7343
Scleroderma Foundation: New England Chapter, 7338, 7339, 7344, 7350, 7354
Scleroderma Foundation: Northern California Chapter, 7331
Scleroderma Foundation: Ohio Chapter, 7347
Scleroderma Foundation: Oregon Chapter, 7348
Scleroderma Foundation: South Carolina Chapter, 7351
Scleroderma Foundation: Southeast Florida Chapter, 7335
Scleroderma Foundation: Southern California Chapter, 7332
Scleroderma Foundation: Tennessee Chapter, 7352
Scleroderma Foundation: Tri-State Chapter, 7345
Scleroderma Foundation: Western New York Chapter, 7346
Scleroderma Foundation: Western Pennsylvania Chapter, 7349
Scleroderma Research Foundation, 7365
Scleroderma Society of Ontario, 7328
Scleroderma Support Groups, 7375
Scleroderma Voice, 7384
Scleroderma: a New Role for Patients and Families, 7382
Scleroderma: an Overview, 7386
Scleroderma: Surviving a Seventeen-Year Itch, 7381
Scoliosis, 7424
Scoliosis and Kyphosis, 7429
Scoliosis Association, 7459
Scoliosis Patient Becomes a Model, 7425
Scoliosis Research Society, 7400
Scoliosis Road Map, 7426
Scoliosis Screening: The Carlsbad Program, 7427
Scoliosis Surgery, What's It All About?, 7428
Scoliosis, Me?, 7430
Scoliosis... Now it Can Be Treated in Adults as Well as Children, 7431
Scoliosis: An Adult Perspective, 7444
Scoliosis: Handbook for Patients, 7432
Scorpions, 1435
Scottish Rite Center for Childhood Language Disorders, 4389
Screening Procedure Guidelines for Spinal Deformity, 7433
Scripps Clinic and Research Foundation: Autoimmune Disease Center, 7675
Scripps Clinic Sleep Disorders Center Scripps Clinic, 7780
Scripps Research Institute, 664
SEARCH, 2054
Search for Serenity, 8371
Season of Change, 4682
Season of Secrets, 7524
Seasonal Clustering of Sarcoidosis, 7304
Seasons, 565
Seattle HPV Support Group, 10494
Seborrheic Dermatitis, 7719
Seborrheic Keratoses, 7720
Second Sense: Beyond Vision Loss, 9456
Secondhand Smoke, 8618
Secret in the Dorm Attic, 4684
Secret Life of the Brain, 8092

Secret Place of the Stairs, 3626
Secret Signing: A Sign Language Activity Book, 4683
Secret to a Satisfied Life: The Way You Encounter Life Can Bring Happiness..., 8670
See What I'm Saying, 4817
Seeds of Disquiet: One Deaf Woman's Experience, 4592
Seeing and Hearing Speech: Lessons in Lipreading and Listening, 4818
Seeing Eye, 9457
Seeing Eye to Eye: An Administrator's Guide, 10014
Seeing Voices: A Journey Into the World of the Deaf, 4593
Seizure First Aid, 7555
Seizure Recognition and First Aid, 7546
Selected Book on Sudden Infant Death Syndrome, 8834
Selected Resources for Children Grieving the Loss of Another Child, 8835
Selecting a Program, 10015
Self Help: Your Strategy for Living with COPD, 10563
Self-Caring Fatigue, 2854
Self-Control Games & Workbook, 1633
Self-Help (S-H) Program, 9055
Self-Help for Hard of Hearing People, 4855
Self-Starvation, 3757
Senior Center Self: Assessment & National Accreditation Manual, 184
Senior Citizens and the Law, 185
Senior Focus, 206
Senior Resource LLC, 41
Seniorresource.com, 235
A Sense of Belonging: Including Students with Autism in their School Community, 1794
Septo-Optic Dysplasia, 4062
SERGG, 1577
Services for the Visually Impaired, 9735
Services to Families, 8988
Sesame Street Sign Language ABC, 4685
Sesame Street Sign Language Fun, 4686
Seven Minute Lesson, 10045
Seven Reasons Not to Use Drugs and Alcohol, 8619
Seven Steps to a Smoke-Free Life, 5879
Severe Brain Injury, 4252
Sex, Sexuality, and the Autism Spectrum, 1791
Sexual and Bladder Difficulties in Parkinson's Disease, 6987
Sexual Health Network, 8040
Sexual Intimacy and the Alcoholic Relationship, 8620
Sexual Issues in Spina Bifida, 7939
Sexual Problems Your Doctor Didn't Mention, 6485
Sexuality After Spinal Cord Injury, 8017
Sexuality and the Person with Spina Bifida, 7926
Sexuality and the Person with Traumatic Brain Injury, 4206
Sexuality in Down Syndrome, 3640
Sexually Transmitted Diseases, 7576
Sexually Transmitted Diseases: Journal, 7581
SGNA News, 3974
Shame Faced, 8372
Shape Up America!, 6730
ShapeWalking, 10564
Share Pregnancy and Infant Loss Support, Inc., 8704, 10698, 10743
Sharing Network Organ Tissue Donation Services, 9203
Sharing Scoliosis: You're Not Alone, 7445
Shawnee Library System: Southern Illinois Talking Book Center, 9662
She'll Never Walk Alone, 9902
Shelley, the Hyperactive Turtle, 1634
Shepherd Center, 7968
Sheridan VA Medical Center, 10270
SHHH Journal, 4716
Shiloh Senior Center for the Hearing Impaired, 4340
Shira: A Legacy of Courage, 3485
Short and OK, 4057
Should Drugs Be Legalized?, 8447
Should Tobacco Advertising and Promotion Be Banned?, 8621
Show & Tell: Explaining Hearing Loss to Teachers, 4819
Show 'N' Tell Stories, 4820

Show Me How: Manual for Parents Preschool Visually Impaired & Blind Children, 9881
Show Me No Mercy, 3620
Shriners Hospital for Children, 7978
Shriners Hospital for Crippled Children Chicago Unit, 7401
Shriver Center University Affiliated Program, 10274
Siblings of Children with Autism: A Guide for Families, 1769
Sick and Tired of Feeling Sick and Tired, 8937
Sickle Cell Anemia Association of Austin: Marc Thomas Chapter, 7628
Sickle Cell Anemia Research Foundation, 7619
Sickle Cell Association of Ontario, 7605
Sickle Cell Association of the Texas Gulf Coast, 7620
Sickle Cell Disease, 7630
Sickle Cell Disease Association of America, 7606, 7637
Sickle Cell Disease Association of America Philadelphia/Delaware Valley Chapter, 7629
Sickle Cell Disease: Faces of Our Children, 5891
Sickle Cell Foundation of Georgia, 7610
Sickle Cell Foundation of Greater Montgomery, 7611
Sickle Cell Information Center, 7607
Sidran Institute, 7077
SIDS Alliance Of Northern California, 8712
SIDS Alliance of the Carolinas, 8777
SIDS Center of Indiana, 8736
SIDS Center of New Jersey, 8770
SIDS Foundation of Southern California, 8713
SIDS Foundation of Washington, 8804
SIDS Information & Counseling: Division of Public Health, 8718
SIDS Information and Counseling Program: Alaska Department of Health, 8707
SIDS Information and Referral Hotline, 8816
SIDS Information for the EMT, 8831
SIDS LEAD: Children's Special Health Care Services, 8756
SIDS Mid-Atlantic, 8800
SIDS Network of Kansas, 8740
SIDS Network of Kentucky, 8742
SIDS Network of Ohio, 8782
SIDS Northwest Regional Center, 8805
SIDS of Illinois, 8733
SIDS of Pennsylvania, 8786
SIDS Program: Connecticut Department of Health, 8717
SIDS Research: An Analysis in Three Parts, 8832
SIDS Resources, 8761
SIDS Support Group, 8817
SIDS: Toward Prevention and Improved Infant Health, 8833
Sign Communication: A Family Affair, 4594
Sign Language and the Deaf Community: Essays in Honor of William Stokoe, 4599
Sign Language Feelings, 4595
Sign Language Interpreters and Interpreting, 4596
Sign Language Made Simple, 4597
Sign Language Talk, 4598
Sign Numbers, 4687
Sign-Me-A-Story, 4821
Sign-Me-Fine, 4688
SIGNAL, 9015
Signed English Starter, 4600
Signed Language Coloring Books, 4689
Signing Exact English, 4601
Signing for Kids, 4690
Signing Illustrated, 4602
Signing Naturally: Teacher's Curriculum Guide-Level 1, 4603
Signs Everywhere, 4604
Signs for Computing Terminology, 4605
Signs for Me: Basic Vocabulary for Children, Parents and Teachers, 4691
Silent Alarm: On the Edge with a Deaf EMT, 4606
Silent Dances, 4692
Silent Garden: Raising Your Deaf Child, 4607, 4693
Silent News, 4717
Silent News Job Bulletin, 4718
Silent Observer, 4694
Silent Sorrow, 5488
Silver Kiss, 2472
Silver Linings: Living with Cancer, 2473
Simon Foundation for Continence, 5335, 5372

Simon Foundation Helpline for Incontinence Information, 5340
Simple & Complex: A Hemophilia Primer, 5119
Simple and Tasty Side Dishes, 3469
Simple Signs, 4695
Simultaneous Communication, ASL and Other Communication Modes, 4608
Since Owen, 3621
Sing Praise, 4609
Singing from the Soul, 2451
Sinusitis and Sinus Surgery, 725
Sioux Falls VA Health Care System, 10237
Six Phases of Infertility Treatment: Medical & Emotional Aspects, 5556
Sjogren's Syndrome, 7646
Sjogren's Syndrome Foundation, 7654
SjoGren's Syndrome Survival Guide, 7647
Sj"gren's Syndrome Foundation, 7641
Skeptic's Guide to the 12 Steps, 8373
Skin Cancer, 7721
Skin Cancer Foundation, 2263
Skin Cancer Foundation Journal, 2485
Skin Cancer: Preventable and Curable, 2585
Skin Cancer: The Undeclared Epidemic, 7742
Skin Cancers, Basal Cell and Squamous Cell Carcinomas: Research Report, 2551
Skin Care Under the Sun, 7743
Skin Conditions Related to AIDS, 7722
Skin Store, 7754
Skokie Accessible Library Services, 9663
SLE Foundation, 8902
SLE Lupus Foundation, 8926
Sleep Aids: Everything You Wanted To Know But Were Too Tired To Ask, 7828
Sleep Alertness Center: Lafayette Home Hospital, 7781
Sleep and Chronobiology Center: Western Psychiatric Institute and Clinic, 7810
Sleep Apnea, 7829
Sleep Center: Community General Hospital, 7782
Sleep Diary, 7840
Sleep Disorders Center at California: Paci, 7789
Sleep Disorders Center at California: Pacific Medical Center, 7788
Sleep Disorders Center Bethesda Oak Hospital, 7783
Sleep Disorders Center Columbia Presbyterian Medical Center, 7784
Sleep Disorders Center Dartmouth Hitchcock Medical Center, 7785
Sleep Disorders Center Lankenau Hospital, 7786
Sleep Disorders Center of Metropolitan Toronto, 7790
Sleep Disorders Center of Rochester: St. Mary's Hospital, 7791
Sleep Disorders Center of Western New York Millard Fillmore Hospital, 7792
Sleep Disorders Center Ohio State University Medical Center, 7787
Sleep Disorders Center: Cleveland Clinic Foundation, 7793
Sleep Disorders Center: Community Medical Center, 7794
Sleep Disorders Center: Crozer-Chester Medical Center, 7795
Sleep Disorders Center: Good Samaritan Medical Center, 7796
Sleep Disorders Center: Kettering Medical Center, 7797
Sleep Disorders Center: Medical College of Pennsylvania, 7798
Sleep Disorders Center: Newark Beth Israel Medical Center, 7799
Sleep Disorders Center: Rhode Island Hospital, 7800
Sleep Disorders Center: St. Vincent Medical Center, 7801
Sleep Disorders Center: University Hospital, SUNY at Stony Brook, 7802
Sleep Disorders Center: Winthrop, University Hospital, 7803
Sleep Disorders Unit Beth Israel Deaconess Medical Center, 7804
Sleep Laboratory St Joseph's Hospital, 7805
Sleep Laboratory, Maine Medical Center, 7806
Sleep Medicine Alert, 7835
Sleep Medicine Associates of Texas, 7807
Sleep Problems with Parkinson's Disease, 6988

Sleep Research Foundation, 7808
Sleep Research Society, 7858
Sleep Research Society American Academy of Sleep Medicine, 7762
Sleep Strategies for Shift Workers, 7841
Sleep Wake Disorders Center Montefiore Sleep Disorders Center, 7809
Sleep-Wake Disorders Center: New York Hospital-Cornell Medical Center, 7811
Sleep/Wake Disorders Center: Community Hospitals of Indianapolis, 7812
Sleep/Wake Disorders Center: Hampstead Hospital, 7813
Sleeping Beauty, 4696
Sleeping Beauty Videotape, 4822
Sleeping Beauty: With Selected Sentences in ASL, 4823
SleepMatters, 7832
Sleepnet, 2905
Smart & Strong, 622
Smith-Kettlewell Eye Research Institute, 9458, 9801
Smith-Kettlewell Technical File, 9948
Smoke Free Family Promotional Leaflet, 8622
Smokeless Tobacco: No Way, 8623
Smoking and Pregnancy, 8624
Smoking and Pregnancy Kit for Health Care Providers, 8374
Smoking and Sudden Infant Death Syndrome, 8821
Smoking Cessation: Be Smoke Free in 3 Minutes, 5283, 8089
Smoking, Drinking & Illicit Drug Use, 8375
Smoking-At Issues Series, 8448
Snoring and Sleep Apnea, 7830
So You Have Asthma Too!, 1436, 1502
So You Have Had an Ear Operation...What Next?, 4780
So You're Going to Adopt, 5557
So You've Reached Goal Weight, 6756
Sober But Stuck, 8376
Sobering Thoughts, 8472
Social Development and the Person with Spina Bifida, 7927
Social Policy Prevention Handbook, 8377
Social Security Administration, 7029
Social Security Administration Office of Public Inquiries, 10425
Social Security Disability Benefits Information, 2881
Social Security, Medicare and Government Pensions, 10565
Social Skills Development in Children with Hydrocephalus, 5236
Society For Post-Acute and Long-Term Care Medicine, 6811
Society for Surgery of the Alimentary Foundation, 3938
Society for Surgery of the Alimentary Tract, 3928, 4014
Society for the Study of Celiac Disease, 2631
Society for the Study of Reproduction, 5430
Society of American Gastrointestinal Endoscopic Surgeons, 3929, 4015
Society of Gastroenterology Nurses and Associates, 3930
Society of Hearing Impaired Physicians, 4332
Society of Mitral Valve Prolapse Syndrome, 4923
Sociolinguistics in Deaf Communities, 4610
Software to Go, 4611
Solomon Park Research Institute, 1146
Solution Starts with You, 5364
Solutions for Everyday Living for Older People with Visual Impairments, 10046
Solve ME/CFS Initiative, 2830
Solving Cognitive Problems, 6486
Solving the Puzzle of CFS, 2855
Somatization Disorder in the Medical Setting, 6132
Someone You Know Has Hepatitis B, 5180
Someone You Know Has MS: A Book for Families, 6487
Somerset County Blind Center, 9568
Something in the Air: Airborne Allergens, 713
Sometimes I'm Mad, Sometimes I'm Glad - A Sibling Booklet, 7207
Son Rise Program, 1821
Son-Rise Method, 1792
Song of Superman, 5128

Songs in Sign, 4697
Sound and Sign, Childhood Deafness and Mental Health, 4612
Sound Hearing, 4824
South Carolina Commission on Alcohol and Drug Abuse, 8184
South Carolina Department of Health & Environmental Control, 335
South Carolina Protection & Advocacy System for the Handicapped, 10483
South Carolina State Library, 9745
South Central AIDS Education and Training Center (SCAETC), 340, 434
South Central Kansas Library System, 9673
South Central VA Health Care Network, 10183
South Dakota Advocacy Services, 10485
South Dakota Department of Health, 8789
South Dakota State Library, 9746
South Florida Chapter National Multiple Sclerosis Society, 6364
South Florida Chapter of the American Association of Kidney Patients, 5600
South Palm Beach County Chapter of NFP, 6885
South Texas Brain Tumor Foundation Support Group, 2030
South Texas Chapter of the ALS Association Newsletter, 1167
South Texas Lighthouse for the Blind, 9586
Southeast AIDS Education and Training Center (SEAETC), 336, 432
Southeast Louisiana Veterans Health Care System, 10162
Southeast Parkinson Disease Association, 6886
Southeast Regional Center: Canine Companions for Independence, 9484
Southeastern Region: Helen Keller National Center, 9488
Southeastern Wisconsin Chapter of the Nati onal Spinal Cord Injury Association, 7982
Southern Arizona Brain Tumor Support Group, 1917
Southern Arizona Branch: Tucson Area, 9265
Southern Arizona VA Health Care System, 10110
Southern California Research Institute, 8226
Southern Indiana Support Group: National Ataxia Foundation, 1539
Southern Nevada Sightless, 9529
Southern Tier Association for the Visually Impaired, 9542
Southern Tier Hemophilia Center United Health Services-Wilson Hospital, 5058
Southwest Association for Education in Biomedical Research, 2271
Southwest Center For HIV/AIDS, 287
Southwest Foundation for Biomedical Research, 2377
Southwest Ohio Brain Tumor Support Group, 2009
Southwest Regional Training Center: Canine Companions for Independence, 9475
Southwest SIDS Research Institute, 8796
SouthWestern Medical Center, 5057
Southwestern Ohio Chapter of the National Hemophilia Foundation, 4996
Spark M. Matsunaga VA Medical Center VA Pacific Islands Health Care System, 10141
Speak to Me, 4613
Speaking Our Minds: Personal Reflections from Individuals with Alzheimer's, 1017
Special Celebrations and Parties Cookbook, 3470
Special Needs Library of Northeast Georgia, 9654
Special Wish Foundation, 10675
Specialized Center of Research in Ischemic Heart Disease, 4897
Specific Classroom Strategies and Techniques for Students with TS, 9124
Specific Forms of Psoriasis, 7723
Spectrum, 1297
Speech & Swallowing Problems for Parkinsonians, 6989
Speech and Deafness Newsletter, 4746
Speech and Language in Children and Adolescents with Down Syndrome, 3641
Speech and the Hearing-Impaired Child, 4614
Speech and Voice Impairment, 6991
Speech Problems & Swallowing Problems in Parkinson's Disease, 6990
Speech Simulation Research Foundation, 4390

Speechreading in Context, 4615
Speechreading: A Way to Improve Understand ing, 4616
Spellman Center for HIV Related Disease The Spellman Center, 421
Spider Veins, Varicose Vein Therapy, 7724
Spina Bifida & Hydrocephalus Association of Nova Scotia, 5199
Spina Bifida and Hydrocephalus Association of Canada, 7864
Spina Bifida and Hydrocephalus Association of Southwestern Michigan, 7885
Spina Bifida Association of Alabama, 7865
Spina Bifida Association of Albany/Capital District, 7891
Spina Bifida Association of America, 7863, 7950
Spina Bifida Association of America: Insights into Spina Bifida, 5211
Spina Bifida Association of Arizona, 7866
Spina Bifida Association of Austin, 7905
Spina Bifida Association of Canton, 7895
Spina Bifida Association of Central Indiana, 7876
Spina Bifida Association of Central Ohio, 7896
Spina Bifida Association of Central Pennsylvania, 7900
Spina Bifida Association of Cincinnati, 7897
Spina Bifida Association of Colorado, 7868
Spina Bifida Association of Connecticut, 7869
Spina Bifida Association of Dallas, 7906
Spina Bifida Association of Delaware, 7870
Spina Bifida Association of Delaware Valley, 7901
Spina Bifida Association of Florida Space Coast, 7871
Spina Bifida Association of Georgia, 7874
Spina Bifida Association of Grand Rapids, 7883
Spina Bifida Association of Greater Dayton, 7898
Spina Bifida Association of Greater New Orleans, 7879
Spina Bifida Association of Greater Pennsylvania, 7902
Spina Bifida Association of Greater Rochester, 7892
Spina Bifida Association of Greater San Diego, 7867
Spina Bifida Association of Greater St. Louis, 7887
Spina Bifida Association of Iowa, 7877
Spina Bifida Association of Jacksonville, 7872
Spina Bifida Association of Kentucky, 7878
Spina Bifida Association of Maryland, 7880
Spina Bifida Association of Massachusetts, 7882
Spina Bifida Association of Minnesota, 7886
Spina Bifida Association of Nassau County, 7893
Spina Bifida Association of Nebraska, 7888
Spina Bifida Association of New Mexico, 7890
Spina Bifida Association of North Carolina, 7894
Spina Bifida Association of Northern Wisconsin, 7909
Spina Bifida Association of Northwest Ohio, 7899
Spina Bifida Association of Rhode Island, 7903
Spina Bifida Association of Southeastern Wisconsin, 7910
Spina Bifida Association of Tampa, 7873
Spina Bifida Association of Tennessee, 7904
Spina Bifida Association of Texas, Gulf Coast, 7907
Spina Bifida Association of the Eastern Shore, 7881
Spina Bifida Association of the Greater Fox Valley, 7911
Spina Bifida Association of the Tri-State Region, 7889
Spina Bifida Association of Upper Peninsula Michigan, 7884
Spina Bifida Association of Washington State, 7908
Spina Bifida Benefits Guide, 10307
Spinal Column, 8004
Spinal Cord Injury Association of Illinois, 7969
Spinal Cord Injury Awareness, 8018
Spinal Cord Injury Home Care Manual, 7999
Spinal Cord Injury Information Network Center, 8041
Spinal Cord Injury Network International, 7960, 8042
Spinal Cord Injury Program at Harmarville Rehabilitation Center, 7979
Spinal Cord Injury Video Access, 8029
Spinal Cord Injury: Statistical Information, 8019
Spinal Cord Society, 7961
Spinal Cord Society Newsletter, 8007
Spinal Deformity: Congenital Scoliosis and Kyphosis, 7434

Spinal Deformity: Scoliosis and Kyphosis, 7435
Spinal Injury Slide Series, 8030
Spinal Network, 8000
Spinal Screening Program, 7446
Spokane VA Medical Center Mann-Grandstaff VA Medical Center, 10259
Spouses of Persons Who Are Brain Injured: Overlooked Victims, 4253
St. Agnes Hospital Medical: Health Science Library, 6429
St. Alexius Medical Heart and Lung Clinic, 3153
St. Clark County Library for the Blind and Physically Handicapped, 9704
St. John's Episcopal Hospital, 6925
St. Joseph Medical Center Cystic Fibrosis Care and Teaching Center, 3116
St. Joseph's Hemophilia Center, 5059
St. Joseph's Medical Center, 3693
St. Jude Children's Research Hospital, 2372
St. Paul Regional Office, 10179
Stadtlanders LifeTIMES, 9238
Stages of Parkinson's Disease, 6992
Stand Strong, 8449
Stand Up to Osteoporosis, 6840
Standards and Inclusion: Can We Have Both?, 1807
Standards for the Diagnosis and Care of Patients with Asthma, 1478
Standing on My Own Two Feet, 10016
Stanford Center for Research in Disease Prevention, 8227
Stanford Center on Longevity, 133
Stanford CF Center Packard Children's Hospital At Stanford, 3096
Stanford University Center for Narcolepsy Dept of Psychiatry & Behavioral Sciences, 7814
Stanford University General Clinical Research Center, 376
Stanford University National Cooperative Drug Discovery/AIDS Group, 377
Stanford University: Beckman Center for Molecular and Genetic Medicine, 2283
STAR Center for Family Health, 10526
Starlight Children's Foundation, 10676, 10688
Starting a Support Group, 8020
Starting Points, 9882
Starting Strong-Staying Strong: A Resource Guide for Educational Support Groups, 1440
Starving to Death in a Sea of Objects, 3758
State Library of Louisiana, 9679
State Library of Ohio Talking Book Program, 9738
State of New Mexico Commission for the Blind, 9535
State University College at Fredonia Youngerman Clinic, 4391
State University College at Plattsburgh Auditory Research Laboratory, 4392
State University of New York at Buffalo Toxicology Research Center, 8228
State University of New York At Stony Brook: Mental Health Research, 6038
State University of New York Health Science Center At Brooklyn, 2349
State University of New York Health Sciences Center, 1723
State University of New York: SUNY Stony HIV Treatment Development Center, 422
State University of NY Hospital: Upstate Medical Center, 3150
Statewide Services for Deaf and Hard of Hearing People, 4781
Statewide SIDS Program: Illinois Department of Public Health, 8734
Staunton Public Library: Talking Book Center, 9761
Staying Clean, 8378
Staying Sober, 8379
Staying Well: Advanced Pain Management for ACPA Members, 2928
Stein Institute for Research on Aging UC San Diego School of Medicine, 134
Stem Cell Research Program University of Wisconsin-Madison, 1147
STEP Perspective, 564
Step Perspective, 7582
Step Zero: Getting to Recovery, 8380
Stepping Stones, 3654

Steps to a Better Understanding of Lung Cancer: A Patient and Family Guide, 5888
Steps to Diagnosis, 1061
Steps to Enhancing Communication, 1062
Steps to Independence: Teaching Everyday Skills to Children with Special Needs, 7928
Stereotactic Radiosurgery, 2071
Stinging Insect Allergy, 726
Stools and Bottles, 8381
Stop It!... I Can't!, 9144
Stop Smoking, Stay Trim, 8625
Stop Smoking: A Guide to Your Options, 8626
Stopping Scoliosis, 7407
Stories of Lupus, 8958
Straight Back Home, 8627
Straight Talk: A Magazine for Teens About AIDS, 522
Strategies for Community Access: Braille & Raised Large Print Facility Signs, 10047
Strategies for Healing, 2077
Strategies for People with Osteoporosis, 6841
Strength Training for Seniors, 10566
Strengthening the Role of Families in States' Early Intervention Systems, 6133
Stress in Recovery, 8628
Stress Management Following Head Injury: Strategies for Families & Caregivers, 4207, 4254
Stretch and Relax Tape, 6324
Stroke Book, 8073
Stroke Clubs International, 8066
Stroke Connection, 8080
Stroke Research and Treatment Center UAB Medical Center, 8059
Stroke: A Clinical Approach, 8074
Stroke: A Guide for Patient and Family, 8075
Stroke: Hope Through Research, 8090
Stroke: Touching the Soul of Your Family, 5285, 8093
Stroke: Your Complete Exercise Guide, 8076
Student Advocate, 9949
Student Asthma Action Card, 1479
Student with Hemophilia: A Resource for the Educator, 5120
Students Against Destructive Decisions, 8135
Students with Cancer: A Resource for the Educator, 2552
Students with Friedreich's Ataxia, 1590
Students with Seizures: A Manual for School Nurses, 7520
Study of American Deaf Folklore, 4617
Sub Regional Talking Book Library, 9642
Subarachnoid Hemorrhage & Aneurysm, 4255
Subregional Library for the Blind and Physically Handicapped, 9655
Substance Abuse and Mental Health Services Administration, 8695
Substance Abuse and Mental Health Services Administration (SAMHSA), 8136
Substance Abuse and Physical Disability, 8382
Substance Abuse and Recovery: Empowerment of Deaf Persons, 4618
Substance Abuse Bureau, 8174
Substance Abuse Funding News, 8473
Substance Abuse Services Office of Virginia, 8190
Substance Abuse Task Force White Paper, 4256
Succeeding Against the Odds: Strategies and Insights from the Learning Disabled, 10567
Success Stories from Drug-Free Schools, 8383
Successful Models of Community Long Term Care Services for the Elderly, 186
Successful Treatment of Myocardial Sarcoidosis with Steriods, 7305
Sudden Infant Death Syndrome (SIDS) Network, 8705
Sudden Infant Death Syndrome and Risk Reduction, 8836
Sudden Infant Death Syndrome Institute of the University of Maryland, 8811
Suffolk Cooperative Library System, 9731
Suggested Exercise Program for People with Parkinson's Disease, 6993
Suicide is Not an Option, 2882
Suicide Prevention Resource Center, 7078
Suicide.org, 7117
Sulzberger Institute for Dermatologic Educ, 7677

Sulzberger Institute for Dermatologic Education, 7676
Summer of Sassy Jo, 8450
Sun & Water Therapy, 7725
Sun and Skin News, 2494
Sun and Your Skin, 7727
Sun Protection for Children, 7726
Sunlight, Ultraviolet Radiation and the Skin, 2553, 7728
Sunshine Chapter of the American Association of Kidney Patients, 5601
Sunshine Dreams for Kids, 10689
Sunshine Foundation National Headquarters, 10677
SUNY at Buffalo National Cooperative Drug Discovery Group for AIDS Treatment, 420
SUNY Health Science Center at Brooklyn Sickle Cell Center, 7618
Superstuff, 1480
Support for Asthmatic Youth, 1410
Support for People with Oral and Head and Neck Cancer (SPOHNC), 2113, 2495, 2600
Support Group Directory, 2044
Support Group for Caregivers of Brain Tumor Patients, 1940
Support Group for Parents of Children with Brain Tumors, 1945, 2010
Support Group Listing, 7306
Support Systems for Parents of Children with Cancer, 2554
Support-Group.Com: Fabry Disease, 3857
Support4Hope, 7118
Supporting Adults with Prader-Willi Syndro me in a Residential Setting, 7208
Surgery for Epilepsy, 7547
Surgery: Information to Consider, 1351
Surrogate Motherhood: The Legal and Human Issues, 5489
A Survey of Accredited and Other Rehabilitation Facilities, 4220
Survival Skills for Diabetic Children, 3522
Survival Skills for the Family Unit, 5237
Surviving an Eating Disorder: Perspectives & Strategies, 3759
Surviving Coma: The Journey Back, 4268
Surviving Infertility, 5490
Surviving Mental Illness, 6134
Surviving Pregnancy Loss: A Complete Sourcebook for Women & Their Families, 5491
Susan's Dad: A Child's Story of Head Injury, 4257
Sweet Grapes: How to Stop Being Infertile and Living Again, 5492
Syndrome Sentinel, 2863
Synergy Clinical Research Center, 7084
Syphilis, 7592
Syracuse University Institute for Sensory Research, 4393
Syracuse VA Medical Center, 10207

T

Tackling Alcohol Problems on Campus: Tools for Media Advocacy, 8384
Tacoma Vet Center, 10260
Tactic, 9914
Tactile Graphics, 9883
TAG Annual Patient/Family Conference Video, 2983
Take-Charge Guide to Type I Diabetes, 3471
Taking Care of Caregivers, 10568
Taking Care of Gestational Diabetes, 3513
Taking Care: A Guide for Well Partners, 6488
Taking Charge, 7929
Taking Charge of Fibromyalgia, 3884
Taking Control of Anxiety: Small Steps for Getting The Best Of Worry,Stress&Fear, 7130
Taking Control of Depression, 6244
Taking Control of TMJ: Your Total Wellness Program, 3885
Taking the HIV (AIDS) Test: How to Help Yourself, 594
Taking the Mystery Out of Spinal Deformities, 7447
Taking Time: Support for People with Cancer & People Who Care for Them, 2555
Talk to Me, 10017

Talk to Me II, 10018
Talk with Me, 4619
Talking About Death - A Dialog Between Parent and Child, 10719
Talking About Tourette Syndrome, 9147
Talking Book Library at Worcester Public Library, 9694
Talking Book Topics, 9950
Talking Books for Senior Adults, 10019
Talking Books Service, 9674
Talking to Your Doctor About Seizure Disorders, 7548
Talking to Your Health Care Team About Bladder Control, 5358
Talking with Your Child About Cancer, 2556
Tallahassee Memorial Diabetes Center, 3376
Taming Stress in Multiple Sclerosis, 6489
Tampa Bay Research Institute, 388
Tampa Lighthouse for the Blind, 9485
Tap the Best Resource, 6320
Targeting Autism: What We Know, Don't Know and Can Do to Help Young Children, 1771
Tarheel Talk, 9951
Tasks Galore for the Real World, 1772
Taub Institute for Research on Alzheimers Disease and the Aging Brain, 974
Tax Credits and Deductions, 1063
Tax Options and Strategies for People with Disabilities, 10569
Tay-Sachs Carrier Testing Directory, 8980
Tay-Sachs Information Sheet, 8989
Tay-Sachs is, 8990
Tay-Sachs: The Dreaded Inheritance, 8981
TB Skin Test, 9315
TB: What You Should Know, 9316
TBI Challenge!, 4219
TBI Help, 4281
TBI Tool Kit, 4208
TBI: Traumatic Brian Injury, 4081, 4282
TEACCH Transition Assessment Profile, 1770
Teach Me Language: A Language Manual for Children with Autism, 1773
Teacher's Guide to Crohn's Disease and Ulcerative Colitis, 3070
Teacher's Guide to Neuromuscular Disease, 6558
Teacher's Role, A Guide for School Personnel, 7549
Teachers Who Are Blind or Visually Impaired, 9884
Teaching Adults with Mental Handicaps, 6135
Teaching Children with Autism: Strategies to Enhance Communication and Socializing, 1774
Teaching Community Skills and Behaviors to Students with Autism or Related Problems, 1775
Teaching English to the Deaf as a Second Language, 4620
Teaching Persons with A Brain Injury: What to Expect, 4258
Teaching Social Skills to Youngsters with Disabilities, 1888
Teaching the Infant with Down Syndrome: A Guide for Parents & Professionals, 3622
Teaching the Tiger: An Educator's Guide to TS/OCD/ADHD, 9090
Team Up for Drug Prevention with America's Young Athletes, 8385
Tech Talk, 4747
Technology Resource Center, 10477
Ted R Montoya Hemophilia Program University of New Mexico, 5060
Ted's Stroke: The Caregiver's Story, 5269, 8077
Teeens, Sexually Transmitted Diseases & HIV/AIDS, 595
Teen Alcoholism-Teen Issues, 8451
Teen Guide to AIDS Prevention, 488, 508
Teen Guide to Pregnancy, Drugs and Smoking, 8452
Teen Guide to Safe Sex, 7580
Teens and Tourette Syndrome, 9130
Teens Face to Face with Chronic Illness, 10570
Teens Talk to Teens About Asthma, 1481
Telecoil: Plugging Into Sound, 4825
Telecoil: Plugging into Sound, 4826
Telecommunications for the Deaf, 4333
Tell it Like it is, 8002
Telling Stories, 4827
Temple University Clinical Research Center Office of Clinical Research, 427

Temple University FELS Institute for Cancer Research, 2367
Temple University Speech and Hearing Science Laboratories, 4394
Temple University: Section of Auditory Research, 4395
Ten Steps to Help Your Child Say No: A Parent's Guide, 8386
Ten Years to Live, 1568
Tendon Transfer Surgery, 8021
Tenessee Department of Health, 8790
Tennessee Alliance for the Mentally Ill, 6008
Tennessee Department of Health: HIV Prevention Services, 337
Tennessee Donor Services, 9219
Tennessee Hemophilia & Bleeding Disorder Foundation, 5003
Tennessee Hemophilia and Bleeding Disorder Foundation, 5061
Tennessee Kidney Foundation, 5649
Tennessee Library for the Blind and Physically Handicapped, 9748
Tennessee Neuropsychiatric Institute Middle Tennessee Mental Health Institute, 6262
Tennessee SIDS Alliance, 8791
Tennessee Voices for Children, 6078
Tension-Type Headache: Fact Sheet, 6321
Teratogen and Birth Defects Information Project, 1864
Teratogen Information Services, 1863
Teratologies: A Cultural Study of Cancer, 2452
Teratology OTIS, 1843
Terms & Tips: An Alzheimer Care Handbook, 1064
Terri Gotthelf Lupus Research Institute, 8929
Test Positive Aware Network (TPAN), 309
Testicular Cancer: Research Report, 2557
Testicular Self-Examination, 2558
Testing for HIV Infection, 597
Testing Positive for HIV, 596
Texas Alliance for the Mentally Ill, 6012
Texas Ambassador: National Ataxia Foundation, 1561
Texas Association of Retinitis Pigmentosa, 9587
Texas Association of the Deaf, 4355
Texas Association on Mental Retardation, 3570
Texas Central Chapter of the National Hemophilia Foundation, 5005
Texas Children's Allergy and Immunology Clinic, 665
Texas Childrens Cystic Fibrosis Care Center, 3172
Texas Commission on Alcohol and Drug Abuse Department Of State Health, 8187
Texas Department of State Health Services: HIV-STD Program, 341
Texas FFCMH, 6013
Texas Heart Institute St Lukes Episcopal Hospital, 4898
Texas Neurofibromatosis Foundation, 6689
Texas State Library, 9750
Texas State Library: Talking Book Program, 9751
Texas Tech University Tarbox Parkinson's Disease Institute, 6909
Textbook Catalog, 9885
Thanks Mom and Dad: Profiles of Patrick, 3655
That's Unacceptable: Surviving a Brain Tumor: My Personal Story, 2045
The AIDS Network, 279
The Alzheimer's Disease & Memory Disorders Center, 975
The ARC of the United States, 3553
The Autism Sourcebook, 1776
The Cancer Prevention Institute, 2359
The Center for Culture, Trauma and Mental Health Disparities, 7085
The Center on Aging and Work at Boston College, 135
The Challenge, 7943
The Coalition of Behavioral Health, 5922
The Comfort of Home for Alzheimer's Disease A Guide for Caregivers, 1018
The Comfort of Home for Parkinson Disease: A Guide for Caregivers, 6928
The Comfort of Home for Stroke: A Guide fo r Caregivers, 8078
The Comfort of Home Multiple Sclerosis Edi tion: A Guide for Caregivers, 6452

The Dana Foundation, 7097

The Emily Program Foundation (merged with Anna Westin Foundation), 3704

The Essential Guide to Brain Tumors, 2046

The Everything Parent's Guide to Children with Autism, 1777

The Gluten-Free Gourmet, 2638

The Inside Tract, 4016

The International Alliance of ALS/MND Associations, 1090

The Kidney Foundation of Canada, 5200

The Loop, 8948

The Macula Foundation Manhattan Eye, Ear & Throat Hospital, 9952

The Magic Foundation, 9341

The Metropolitan Washington Ear, Inc., 9459

The Mountain You've Climbed: A Parent's Guide to Childhood Cancer Survivorship, 2453

The Mountain You've Climbed: A Young Adult Guide to Childhood Cancer Survivorship, 2474

The National Forum, 2864

The New ADD in Adults Workbook, 1630

The Personal Care Attendant Guide: The Art of Finding, Keeping, or Being One, 10571

The Phoenix, 2496

The Pioneer Projects and Programs Periodic al, 9953

The Post-Traumatic Gazette, 7139

The Post-Traumatic Stress Disorder Relationship, 7140

The Reeve Foundation, 7962

The Riley Cystic Fibrosis Center, 3112

The Sam and Rose Stein Institute for Research on the Aging, 976

The Society of Federal Health Professionals (AMSUS), 7058

The Thyroid Gland, 9008

The Turner Syndrome Society: Central Texas, Dallas/Ft.Worth, Houston, 9356

The Turner Syndrome Society: Kansas City Chapter, 9349

The Turner Syndrome Society: Michigan Chapter, 9351

The Turner Syndrome Society: Minnesota Chapter, 9352

The University of Memphis: School of Commu nication Sciences and Disorders, 4396

The Vanderbilt Hemostasis Clinic, 5062

The Well Project, 280

The West Virginia Autism Training Center Marshall University, 1724

Therapeutic Interventions in Alzheimer's, 1019

Therapeutic Strategies: A Guide for Occupational & Physical Therapists, 6789

Therapy for Diabetes Mellitus and Related Disorders, 3472

Therapy of Moderate-to-Severe Psoriasis, 7684

There are Solutions for the Student with Asthma, 1482

There is Only One Child, 8982

There Was a Child, 10737

There's a Hearing Impaired Child in my Class, 4621

They Never Want to Tell You: Children Talk About Cancer, 2475

Things I Wish Someone Had Told Me, 6490

Things My Sponsors Taught Me, 8387

Think First..., 6757

Thinking About Tomorrow: A Career Guide for Teens with Arthritis, 1352

Third Party Reproduction (Donor Eggs, Donor Sperm, Donor Embryos, & Surrogacy), 5547

Thirteen Keys to A Successful High School Experience, 4622

This Is AA, 8629

This is Mr. TB Germ, 9317

Thomas E. Creek VA Medical Center Amarillo VA Health Care System, 10249

Thomas Jefferson University Hospital, 7366

Thomas Jefferson University Ischemia-Shock, 4136

Thomas Jefferson University Ischemia-Shock Research Center, 4135

Thomas Jefferson University: Sleep Disorders Center, 7815

Thomas Jefferson University: Cardenza Foundation for Hematologic Research, 5063

Thomas Jefferson University: Center for Research in Medical Education, 428

Thomas Jefferson University: Daniel Baugh Institute, 1844

Three Rivers Regional Library, 9656

Three Talks to Medical Societies, 8630

300 Tips for Making Life with Multiple Sclerosis Easier, 6440

36-Hour Day, 987

3rd Opinion: International Directory to Complementary Therapy Centers, 2417

Thresholds Psychiatric Rehabilitation, 6039

Through Tara's Eyes: Helping Children Cope with Alzheimer's Disease, 1027

THYROID, 9013

Thyroid Disease: The Facts, 9009

Thyroid Federation International, 9005, 9020

Thyroid Foundation of Canada, 9006, 9021

Thyroid Sourcebook, 9010

Tick Talk, 9062

Time for Alzheimer's: A True Story, 1020

Time for Healing: Relaxation for Mind and Body, 10572

Time Out!, 213

Time to Start Living, 8631

Tina's Story...Scoliosis and Me, 7410

Tinea Versicolor, 7729

Tinnitus Today, 4719

Tips on Coping with Chronic Hepatitis, 5181

Tips to Remember, 1483

Tips to Remember Brochures, 714, 1484

TLC (Tips for Living And Coping), 2055

TN Hemo & Bleeding Disorders Foundation Newsletter, 5097

To Give an Edge: A Guide for New Parents of Children with Down's Syndrome, 3623

To Live, 2984

To Love a Child, 5493

To Love This Life: Quotations by Helen Keller, 9886

To the Family, 6758

To the Man, 6759

To the Newcomer, 6760

To the Teen, 6761

To Your Health and Healthpoints, 3896

Today I Will Do One Thing: Daily Readings for Awareness & Hope, 8388

Today's Gift, 8389

Together...There Is Hope, 1591

Tomah VA Medical Center, 10267

Too Little, Too Late, 603

Too Many Young People Drink and Know Too Little About the Consequences, 8632

Too Young?, 8633

Tools of Recovery, 6762

Toothpick, 3187

Toronto People with AIDS Foundation, 360

Touch the Baby: Blind & Visually Impaired Children as Patients, 10020

Touched with Fire:- Manic Depressive Illness & the Artistic Temperment, 6226

Touchstones, 8390

ToughLove International, 8247

Tourette Association of America, 9081

Tourette Syndrome and Human Behavior, 9091

Tourette Syndrome and the School Nurse, 9131

Tourette Syndrome Association Newsletter, 9097

Tourette Syndrome Clinic Yale Child Study Center, 9084

Tourette Syndrome Foundation of Canada, 9082

Tourette Syndrome: Advances in Neurology, 9092

Tourette Syndrome: Guide to Diagnosis, 9148

Tourette: The Man and His Times, 9132

Toward Effective Public School Programs for Deaf Students, 4623

Toward Healthy Living: A Wellness Journal, 1275

Toxoplasmosis, 1889

Trace Center University of Wisconsin: Madison, 4397

Traditional Tibetan Healing, 6439

Transient Ischemic Attack, 5284, 8091

TransLife/Florida Hospital, 9186

Transplant Chronicles, 5687

Transplant Resource Center of Maryland, 9195

Transplantation Ethics, 9233

Transplantation Society of Michigan, 9197

Transweb: All About Transplantation and Donation, 9253

Trauma Center, 7079, 7096

Trauma Services for Women in Substance Abuse Treatment: An Integrated Approach, 7131

Trauma & Health: Physical Health Consequences Of Exposure To Extreme Stress, 7132

Trauma & Substance Abuse: Causes, Consequences and Treatment Of Comorbid Disorders, 7133

Traumatic Brain Injury, 4283

Traumatic Brain Injury Rehabilitation: Brain Injury Consortium Monograph Series, 4209

Traumatic Head Injury: Cause, Consequence and Challenge, 4210

Travel After Spinal Cord Injury, 8022

Travel Resources for Deaf and Hard of Hearing People, 4782

Traveling with Allergies: Prepare and Avoid Problems, 685

Travis Association for the Blind, 9588

Travis, I Got Lots of Neat Stuff Children Living with Muscular Dystrophy, 6559

Treasure, 4828

Treat Yourself to a Brighter Future - It's Time to Hit the Freedom Trail, 5129

Treating Bulimia: A Psychoeducational Approach, 3760

Treating IBD, 3047

Treating Nicotine Addiction, 8634

Treating PTSD With Cognitive-Behavioral Therapies: Interventions That Work, 7134

Treatment Guide for the Health Insurance Industry, 7685

Treatment Issues, 566

Treatment of Complicated Mourning, 10720

Treatment of Hemophilia: Current Orthopedic Management, 5121

Treatment of Parkinson's Disease with Carbidopa-Levodopa, 6994

Treatment Overview, 7730

Treatments for Alzheimer's Disease, 1065

Tri County HPV Support Group, 10484

Tri-County Association for the Blind, 9569

Tri-Services Military Cystic Fibrosis Center, 3173

Tri-State Area Support Group: National Ataxia Foundation, 1552

Triangle Area Sarcoidosis Support Group, 7252

Triggers of Asthma, 1485

Trim & Fit, 6737

Tripod, 4334

Triumph Over Fear, 6172

Troubled Journey, 6136

TS and Other Tic Disorders, 9125

TS and the School Nurse, 9126

TS and the School Psychologist, 9127

TS-The Parent's Perspective: Diplomacy in Action, 9145

TS: A Look at the Interface Between TS & the Law, 9128

TS: A Panel of Experts, 9146

TSA Medical Letters, 9129

Tubal Factor Infertility, 5548

Tuberous Sclerosis, 9330

Tuberous Sclerosis Complex International, 9328

Tucson Interfaith HIV/AIDS Network (TIHAN), 288

Tucson Support Group: National Ataxia Foundation, 1526

Tufts Medical Center, 5064

Tulane University Center For Aging, 136

Tulane University Pulmonary Diseases Critical Care and Enviromental Medicine, 2316

Tulane University: US-Japan Biomedical Research Laboratories, 4137

Tulsa City: County Library System, 9740

Tulsa Unified FFCMH, 6000

Turnabout, 8391

Turner Syndrome Colorado, 9345

Turner Syndrome Society of Canada, 9343

Turner Syndrome Society of the United States, 9342

Turner Syndrome Society Resource Center, 9358

Turner's Syndrome News, 9360

Turner's Syndrome Society of the United States, 9376

Turner's Syndrome Society Resource Bibliographies, 9365

Turner's Syndrome: A Guide for Families, 9366

Turner's Syndrome: A Personal Perspective, 9367
Turner's Syndrome: Hows and Whys of the Missing X Chromosome, 9368
Turning Awareness Into Action: What Your Community Can Do About Drug Use, 8392
Turning Point, 6137
Turning Point Society of Central Alberta, 281
Tuscaloosa Subregional Library for the Blind & Physically Handicapped, 9612
Twelve Step Sponsorship: How it Works, 8393
Twelve Steps and Traditions, 8394
Twelve Steps and Twelve Traditions, 8395
Twelve Steps and Twelve Traditions for Alateen, 8396
Twelve Steps for Everyone...Who Really Wants Them, 8397
Twelve Steps for Tobacco Users, 8636
Twelve Steps Illustrated, 8635
Twelve Steps of Alcoholics Anonymous, 8398
Twelve Traditions of Overeaters Anonymous, 6763
Twenty Four Hours a Day, 8399
Twenty Years at Hull House, 7408
Twice Dead: Organ Transplants and the Reinvention of Death, 9234
Twin Cities Area Support Group: National Ataxia Foundation, 1546
25 Ways to Promote Spoken Language in Your Child with a Hearing Loss, 4749
250 Tips for Making Life with Arthritis Easier, 1260
Type 2 Diabetes: Your Healthy Living Guide, 3473

U

U Special Kids, 10527
U.S. Department of Health and Human Services, 7061
U.S. Food and Drug Administration, 648, 1389, 3554, 3687, 4335, 5743, 7476
UCD Northern Central California Hemophilia Program, 5065
UCLA AIDS Clinical Research Center, 378
UCLA Anxiety Disorders Research Center, 7086
UCLA Neuropsychiatric Institute, 4138
UCSD Antiviral Research Center, 379
UCSD Comprehensive Hemophilia Treatment Center, 5066
UCSF Children's Hospital Health Library, 3594
Ulcerative Colitis, 9395
UM/Sylvester Comprehensive Cancer Center, 2295
UNC Cystic Fibrosis Center Department of Pediatrics, 3151
Understanding & Managing Scleroderma, 7383
Understanding Addiction, 10573
Understanding Allergic Reactions, 727
Understanding Alzheimer's Disease, 1021
Understanding Anaphylaxis, 692
Understanding and Coping with Your Child's Brain Tumor, 2047
Understanding and Infertility, 5494
Understanding Anemia, 10574
Understanding Asthma, 1423, 1486
Understanding Autism, 1808
Understanding Birth Defects, 1871
Understanding Bladder Problems in Multiple Sclerosis, 6491
Understanding Bowel Problems in MS, 6492
Understanding Braille Literacy, 10048
Understanding Brain Tumors: Glioblastoma Multiforme, 2072
Understanding Breast Cancer Genetics, 2454
Understanding Cancer Therapies, 2455
Understanding CFIDS, 2883
Understanding Child Sexual Abuse, 10575
Understanding Childhood Obesity, 6731
Understanding Chronic Pain, 2929
Understanding Colon Cancer, 2456
Understanding Cosmetic Laser Surgery, 10576
Understanding Crohn Disease and Ulcerative Colitis, 3048
Understanding Cystic Fibrosis, 3184
Understanding Deafness Socially, 4624
Understanding Dental Health, 10577
Understanding Depression, 6138
Understanding Depression and Addiction, 8637

Understanding Diabetes: A User's Guide to Novolin, 3523
Understanding Dietary Supplements, 10578
Understanding Down's Syndrome An Introduction for Parents, 3624
Understanding Drugs, 8453
Understanding Ear Infections, 4625
Understanding Emphysema, 5889
Understanding Gestational Diabetes, 3514
Understanding Helps, 7577
Understanding Hemophilia: A Young Person's Guide, 5083
Understanding Hepatitis, 5122, 5151
Understanding Herpes: Revised Second Edition, 7578
Understanding Immunology, 1487
Understanding Juvenile Rheumatoid Arthritis, 1276
Understanding Lyme Disease: Entendiendo Lyme Disease, 9056
Understanding Lysosomal Storage Diseases, 8991
Understanding Major Anxiety Disorders and Addiction, 8638
Understanding Mental Retardation, 6139
Understanding Migrain and Other Headaches, 6303
Understanding Multiple Sclerosis, 6453
Understanding Nephrotic Syndrome, 5711
Understanding Neurofibromatosis, 6698
Understanding Obesity: The Five Medical Causes, 6732
Understanding Ourselves and Alcoholism, 8639
Understanding Panic and Other Anxiety Disorders, 6140
Understanding Panic Disorder, 6239
Understanding Personality Problems and Addiction, 8640
Understanding Post-Traumatic Fibromyalgia, 3886
Understanding Post-Traumatic Stress Disorder and Addiction, 8641
Understanding Sarcoidosis Self-Help Group, 7253
Understanding Scoliosis, 7448
Understanding Seizure Disorders, 7556
Understanding Spinal Muscular Atrophy, 8023
Understanding Stuttering, 10579
Understanding the Emotions Surrounding CFS, 2884
Understanding the Nature of Autism A Guide to the Autism Spectrum Disorders, 1778
Understanding the Pollen and Mold Season, 715
Understanding Ticks and Lyme Disease, 9057
Understanding Your Child with Asthma, 1488
Understanding Your Child's Education Needs/Individualized Education Program, 5238
Understanding Your Learning Disability, 10580
Understanding: A Guide to Impaired Fertility for Family and Friends, 5549
Undetectable: The New Face of AIDS, 604
Unexplained Infertility, 5550
Unheard Voices, 4829
UNICEF USA, 282
United Advocates for Children of California, 5933
United Cerebral Palsy Association of Indiana, 2725
United Cerebral Palsy Associations, 2672, 2726, 2819
United Cerebral Palsy Central PA, 2770
United Cerebral Palsy Land of Lincoln, 2717
United Cerebral Palsy of Alabama, 2673
United Cerebral Palsy of Alaska/PARENTS, 2680
United Cerebral Palsy of Baton Rouge McMains Children's Developmental Center, 2729
United Cerebral Palsy of Beaver, Butler & Lawrence Counties, 2771
United Cerebral Palsy of Berkshire County, 2735
United Cerebral Palsy of Central Arizona, 2681
United Cerebral Palsy of Central Arkansas, 2683
United Cerebral Palsy of Central California, 2684
United Cerebral Palsy of Central Florida, 2704
United Cerebral Palsy of Central Maryland, 2732
United Cerebral Palsy of Central Minnesota, 2739
United Cerebral Palsy of Central Ohio, 2764
United Cerebral Palsy of Chemung County, 2753
United Cerebral Palsy of Cincinnati, 2765
United Cerebral Palsy of Colorado, 2697
United Cerebral Palsy of Delaware, 2701
United Cerebral Palsy of East Central Alabama, 2674
United Cerebral Palsy of East Central Florida, 2705
United Cerebral Palsy of East Central Illinois, 2718
United Cerebral Palsy of Eastern Connecticut, 2698
United Cerebral Palsy of Florida, 2706

United Cerebral Palsy of Fulton & Montgomery Counties, 2754
United Cerebral Palsy of Georgia, 2714
United Cerebral Palsy of Greater Birmingha m, 2675
United Cerebral Palsy of Greater Chicago, 2719
United Cerebral Palsy of Greater Cleveland, 2766
United Cerebral Palsy of Greater Dane, 2767
United Cerebral Palsy of Greater Dane County, 2790
United Cerebral Palsy of Greater Hartford, 2699
United Cerebral Palsy of Greater Houston, 2783
United Cerebral Palsy of Greater Kansas City, 2741
United Cerebral Palsy of Greater New Orleans, 2730
United Cerebral Palsy of Greater Sacrament o, 2685
United Cerebral Palsy of Greater St. Louis, 2742
United Cerebral Palsy of Greater Suffolk, 2755
United Cerebral Palsy of Hawaii, 2715
United Cerebral Palsy of Hudson County, 2746
United Cerebral Palsy of Huntsville & Tennessee Valley, 2676
United Cerebral Palsy of Idaho, 2716
United Cerebral Palsy of Illinois, 2720
United Cerebral Palsy of Kansas, 2728
United Cerebral Palsy of Los Angeles & Ventura Counties, 2686
United Cerebral Palsy of MetroBoston, 2736
United Cerebral Palsy of Metropolitan Dallas, 2784
United Cerebral Palsy of Metropolitan Detroit, 2737
United Cerebral Palsy of Michigan, 2738
United Cerebral Palsy of Middle Tennessee, 2781
United Cerebral Palsy of Minnesota, 2740
United Cerebral Palsy of Mobile, 2677
United Cerebral Palsy of Morris-Somerset, 2747
United Cerebral Palsy of Nassau County, 2756
United Cerebral Palsy of Nebraska, 2744
United Cerebral Palsy of New Jersey, 2748
United Cerebral Palsy of New York City, 2757
United Cerebral Palsy of North Central Wisconsin, 2791
United Cerebral Palsy of North Florida: Tender Loving Care, 2707
United Cerebral Palsy of Northeast Florida, 2708
United Cerebral Palsy of Northeastern Maine, 2731
United Cerebral Palsy of Northern Nevada, 2745
United Cerebral Palsy of Northwest Alabama, 2678
United Cerebral Palsy of Northwest Florida, 2709
United Cerebral Palsy of Northwest Missouri, 2743
United Cerebral Palsy of Northwestern Pennsylvania, 2772
United Cerebral Palsy of Oklahoma, 2768
United Cerebral Palsy of Orange County, 2687
United Cerebral Palsy of Oregon & SW Washington, 2769
United Cerebral Palsy of Pennsylvania, 2773
United Cerebral Palsy of Philadelphia Vicinity, 2774
United Cerebral Palsy of Pierce County, 2789
United Cerebral Palsy of Pittsburgh, 2775
United Cerebral Palsy of Prince Georges & Montgomery Counties, 2733
United Cerebral Palsy of Putnam & Southern Dutchess Counties, 2758
United Cerebral Palsy of Queens: Queens Centers for Progress, 2759
United Cerebral Palsy of Rhode Island, 2780
United Cerebral Palsy of San Diego County, 2688
United Cerebral Palsy of San Joaquin, Calaveras & Amador Counties, 2689
United Cerebral Palsy of San Luis Obispo, 2690
United Cerebral Palsy of Santa Barbara County, 2691
United Cerebral Palsy of Santa Clara & San Mateo Counties, 2692
United Cerebral Palsy of Sarasota-Manatee, 2710
United Cerebral Palsy of South Central Pennsylvania, 2776
United Cerebral Palsy of South Florida, 2711
United Cerebral Palsy of Southeastern Wisconsin, 2792
United Cerebral Palsy of Southern Alleghenies Region, 2777
United Cerebral Palsy of Southern Connecticut, 2700
United Cerebral Palsy of Southern Illinois, 2721
United Cerebral Palsy of Southern Maryland, 2734
United Cerebral Palsy of Southern Arizona, 2682
United Cerebral Palsy of Southwestern Pennsylvania, 2778
United Cerebral Palsy of Stanislaus County, 2693

United Cerebral Palsy of Tallahassee, 2712
United Cerebral Palsy of Tampa Bay, 2713
United Cerebral Palsy of Tarrant County, 2785
United Cerebral Palsy of Texas, 2786
United Cerebral Palsy of the Blackhawk Region, 2723
United Cerebral Palsy of the Golden Gate, 2694
United Cerebral Palsy of the Inland Empire, 2695
United Cerebral Palsy of the Mid-South, 2782
United Cerebral Palsy of the North Bay, 2696
United Cerebral Palsy of the North Country, 2762
United Cerebral Palsy of the Wabash Valley, 2727
United Cerebral Palsy of Utah, 2787
United Cerebral Palsy of Washington DC, 2702
United Cerebral Palsy of Washington DC & Northern
Virginia, 2703
United Cerebral Palsy of West Alabama, 2679
United Cerebral Palsy of Westchester County, 2760
United Cerebral Palsy of Western New York, 2761
United Cerebral Palsy of Western Pennsylvania, 2779
United Cerebral Palsy of Will County, 2722
United Cerebral Palsy of Wisconsin, 2793
United Cerebral Palsy: Eastern Seals, 2724
United Families for Children's Mental Health, 5965
United Network for Organ Sharing (UNOS), 9173,
9254
United Organ Transplant Association (UOTA), 9174,
9255
United Ostomy Associations of America Advocacy
Hotline, 2414
United Ostomy Associations of America, Inc, 2999,
3080, 3931, 4017, 9383, 9402
United Special Sportsman Alliance, 10690
United Spinal Association, 7963
United States 211 Information and Referral Systems,
7119
United States Association for Blind Athletes, 9460
United Virginia Chapter of the National Hemophilia
Foundation, 5008
Universe of Women's Health, 3830
University Alzheimer Center UHC: Case Western
Reserve University, 978
University Alzheimer Center University of Alabama
at Birmingham, 977
University Drive Campus VA Pittsburgh Healthcare
System, 10230
University Library Services, 9762
University Medical Center Hemophilia Program,
5067
University of Alabama At Birmingham
Comprehensive Cancer Center, 2270
University of Alabama at Birmingham Parkinsons
Disease Center, 6910
University of Alabama at Birmingham: Congenital
Heart Disease Center, 4899
University of Alabama at Birmingham: National
Cooperative Drug/AIDS, 365
University of Alabama Birmingham, 7367
University of Alabama Speech and Hearing Center,
4398
University of Alabama, (UAB), 8043
University of Arizona Cancer Center, 2272
University of California at San Francisco Women's
Continence Center, 5341
University of California Berkeley Cancer Research
Laboratory, 2285
University of California Liver Research Unit, 5768
University of California Northern Comprehensive
Sickle Cell Center, 7621
University of California San Diego General Clinical
Research Center, 4900
University of California San Francisco Center for
AIDS Prevention, 381
University of California, San Francisco Brain Tumor
Research Center, 1913
University of California: Cardiovascular Research
Laboratory, 4901
University of California: Davis Gastroenterology &
Nutrition Center, 3943
University of California: Institute of Health Policy
Studies, 382
University of California: Irvine Brain Imaging Center,
4139
University of California: Los Angeles Alcohol
Research Center, 8229

University of California: Los Angeles Bone Marrow
Transplantation Program, 2286
University of California: Los Angeles Center for
Ulcer Research, 3944
University of California: San Francisco Dermatology
Drug Research, 7678
University of California: San Francisco Laboratory
for Neurotrauma, 4140
University of California: UCLA Population Research
Center, 5437
University of Chicago Cancer Research Center, 2305
University of Chicago Center for Advanced Medicine
Duchossis Center, 7368
University of Chicago Committee on Virology, 7573
University of Chicago Dept of Neurology University
of Chicago Hospital, 979
University of Chicago: Clinical Nutrition Research
Unit, 2306
University of Chicago: Comprehensive Diabetes
Center, 3391
University of Chicago: Temporal Bone Laboratory for
Ear Research, 4399
University of Cincinnati Adult Hemophilia Treatment
Program, 5069
University of Cincinnati College of Medicine
Division of Pediatrics, 3158
University of Cincinnati Department of Pathology &
Laboratory Medicine, 4902
University of Colorado Cancer Center, 2289
University of Colorado: General Clinical Research
Center, Pediatric, 3392
University of Connecticut Center on Aging, 139
University of Connecticut Health Center, 3098
University of Connecticut Osteoporosis Center, 6817
University of Florida Institute on Aging, 140
University of Florida: General Clinical Research
Center, 666
University of Hawaii: Cancer Research Center, 2299
University of Illinois at Chicago Consultation Clinic
for Epilepsy, 7493
University of Illinois at Chicago Craniofacial Center,
1845
University of Illinois at Chicago Lions, 9310
University of Illinois at Chicago Lions of Illinois Eye
Research Institute, 9803
University of Illinois at Chicago Medical Center
Outpatient Clinical Center, 7369
University of Illinois at Chicago: Institute for
Tuberculosis Research, 9311
University of Illinois Eye and Ear Infirma ry, 9802
University of Illinois Health Services Research, 980
University of Iowa Birth Defects and Genetic
Disorders Unit, 1846
University of Iowa College of Medicine, 8060
University of Iowa Mental Health Clinical Research
Center, 6263
University of Iowa Teratogen Information Service,
1865
University of Iowa: Diabetes Research Center, 3393
University of Iowa: Holden Comprehensive Cancer
Center, 2309
University of Iowa: Iowa Cardiovascular Center, 4903
University of Kansas Allergy and Immunology
Clinic, 667
University of Kansas Cray Diabtetes Center, 3394
University of Kansas Kidney and Urology Research
Center, 5666
University of Kentucky: Children Cancer Study
Group, 2313
University of Kentucky: Lucille Parker Markey
Cancer Center, 2314
University of Maine: Communication Science s &
Disorders, 4400
University of Maryland Center for Research, Grants
& Contracts, 401
University of Maryland Center for Studies Family
Studies Depatrment, 402
University of Maryland Center for Studies of
Cerebrovascular Disease & Stroke, 8061
University of Maryland School of Public Health
Center on Aging, 141
University of Maryland: Department of Pediatrics,
3595
University of Maryland: Division of Infectious
Diseases, 981

University of Maryland: Medical Biotechnology
Center, 403
University of Massachusetts Memorial Medical
Center, 3129
University of Massachusetts: Diabetes and
Endocrinology Research Center, 3395
University of Memphis: Department of Psych ology,
4141
University of Miami School of Medicine Department
of Neurology, 8062
University of Miami: Bascom Palmer Eye Institute,
9804
University of Miami: Center on Aging Center on
Aging, 982
University of Miami: Diabetes Research Institute,
3396
University of Miami: Mailman Center for Child
Development, 1847
University of Michigan Communicative Disorders
Clinic, 4401
University of Michigan Hemophilia Center, 5070
University of Michigan Michigan Gastrointestinal
Peptide Research Ctr., 3945
University of Michigan Montgomery: John M.
Sheldon Allergy Society, 668
University of Michigan Nephrology Division, 5667
University of Michigan Pulmonary and Critical Care
Division, 4904
University of Michigan Reproductive Sciences
Program, 5438
University of Michigan: Alcohol Research Center,
8230
University of Michigan: Cancer Center Cancer
Research Committee, 2327
University of Michigan: Cardiovascular Med icine,
4905
University of Michigan: Cystic Fibrosis Center, 3132
University of Michigan: Division of Hypertension,
5258
University of Michigan: Kresge Hearing Research
Institute, 4402
University of Michigan: Mental Health Research
Institute, 6040
University of Michigan: National Cooperative
Drug/AIDS Group, 410
University of Michigan: Orthopaedic Research
Laboratories, 1255
University of Michigan: Psychiatric Center, 8231
University of Minnesota Department of Psychiatry,
6041
University of Minnesota Masonic Cancer Center,
2330
University of Minnesota: Cystic Fibrosis Center, 3133
University of Minnesota: Hypertensive Research
Group, 5259
University of Minnesota: Program on Alcohol/Drug
Control, 8232
University of Mississippi Medical Center, 3134
University of Missouri Columbia Cystic Fibrosis
Center, 3136
University of Missouri Columbia Division of
Cardiothoracic Surgery, 4906
University of Missouri: Columbia Missouri Institute
of Mental Health, 6042
University of Missouri: Kansas City Drug
Information Service, 8233
University of Nebraska at Omaha Eppley Institute for
Research in Cancer, 2333
University of Nebraska Medical Center Cystic
Fibrosis Center, 3138
University of Nebraska Medical Center Tera Togen
Project, 1866
University of Nebraska: Lincoln, 4403
University of New Mexico General Clinical Research
Center, 3397
University of New Mexico: Cancer Research and
Treatment Center, 2335
University of New Mexico: Center for Non-Invasive
Diagnosis, 2336
University of North Carolina at Chapel Hill Division
of Speech & Hearing, 4404
University of North Carolina Sarcoidosis Support
Group, 7254
University Of North Carolina School of Medicine
Center for Aging and Health, 137

University of North Carolina UNC Lineberger Comprehensive Cancer Center, 2353
University of Oklahoma: Cystic Fibrosis Center, 3159
University of Oklahoma: Health Sciences Ce nter, 4405
University of Pennsylvania Diabetes and Endocrinology Research Center, 3398
University of Pennsylvania Institute on Aging, 142
University of Pennsylvania Muscle Institut e, 4907
University of Pennsylvania: Depression Research Unit, 6202
University of Pennsylvania: Harrison Department of Surgical Research, 3946
University of Pennsylvania: Penn Lung Center, 3163
University of Pittsburgh, 6928, 7370
University of Pittsburgh Cancer Institute, 2368
University of Pittsburgh Cystic Fibrosis Center: Children's Hospital, 3164
University of Pittsburgh Obesity/Nutrition Research Center, 6773
University of Pittsburgh: Department of Molecular Genetics and Biochemistry, 3399
University of Pittsburgh: Human Energy Research Laboratory, 4908
University of Pittsburgh: Western Psychiatric Institute & Clinic, 6043
University of Rhode Island Tick Research Laboratory, 9075
University of Rochester, 6926
University of Rochester: Clinical Research Center, 4909
University of Rochester: James P Wilmot Cancer Center, 2350
University of Rochester: Nephrology Research Program, 5668
University of South Florida Center for HIV Education and Research, 389
University of Southern California: Comprehensive Sickle Cell Center, 7622
University of Southern California: Coronary Care Research, 4910
University of Southern California: Division of Nephrology, 5260
University of Tennessee Drug Information Center, 8234
University of Tennessee Medical Group, 7371
University of Tennessee Memphis: Cancer Center, 2373
University of Tennessee: Center for Neuroscience, 7494
University of Tennessee: Division of Cardiovascular Diseases, 4911
University of Tennessee: Division of Reproductive Endocrinology, 3804
University of Tennessee: General Clinical Research Center, 3400
University of Texas at Austin: Drug Synamics Institute, 8236
University of Texas at Dallas Callier Center for Communication Disorders, 4406
University of Texas General Clinical Research Center, 3401
University of Texas Health Science Center, 7372
University of Texas Health Science Center Neurophysiology Research Center, 8235
University of Texas HSC at San Antonio, 6930
University of Texas Mental Health Clinical Research Center, 6203
University of Texas Sleep/Wake Disorders Center, 7816
University of Texas Southwestern Medical, 5770
University of Texas Southwestern Medical Center, 5769
University of Texas Southwestern Medical Center at Dallas, 669, 4912
University of Texas Southwestern Medical Center/Sickle Cell Management, 7623
University of Texas: MD Anderson Cancer Center, 2378
University of Texas: Medical Branch at Galveston Cancer Center, 2379
University of Texas: Southwestern Medical Center at Dallas, Immunodermatology, 7679
University of Utah Intermountain Cystic Fibrosis Center, 3174

University of Utah Rocky Mountain Center for Occupational & Environmental Health, 5871
University of Utah Utah Genome Depot University of Utah, 6519
University of Utah: Artificial Heart Research Laboratory, 4913
University of Utah: Cardiovascular Genetic Research Clinic, 4914
University of Utah: Center for Human Toxicology, 8237
University of Vermont Cancer Center University of Vermont, 2382
University of Vermont Larner College of Medicine Center on Aging, 143
University of Vermont: Office of Health Promotion Research, 435
University of Virginia School of Medicine Cystic Fibrosis Center, 3177
University of Virginia: General Clinical Research Center, 1406
University of Virginia: Hypertension and Atherosclerosis Unit, 5261
University of Washington, 6931
University of Washington Department of Speech & Hearing Sciences, 4407
University of Washington Diabetes: Endocrinology Research Center, 3402
University of Washington: Cystic Fibrosis Center, 3178
University of Washington: Experimental Education Unit, 3596
University of Wisconsin Madison Neurophysiology Laboratory, 7495
University of Wisconsin Milwaukee Medicinal Chemistry Group, 8238
University of Wisconsin Organ Procurement Organization, 9224
University of Wisconsin Paul P Carbone Comprehensive Cancer Center, 2387
University of Wisconsin-Madison: Cystic Fibrosis/Pulmonary Center, 3181
University of Wisconsin: Asthma, Allergy and Pulmonary Research Center, 1407
University Of Wyoming Center on Aging, 138
University Treatment Center of University Hospitals of Cleveland, 5068
Unlocking Potential: College and Other Choices for People with LD and AD/HD, 7930
Unloving Care, 187
Unproven Methods in Diagnosing and Treating Allergies, 1489
Unpuffables Promotional Brochure, 8642
Unseen Injury: Minor Head Injury, 4259, 4267
Unseen Minority: Social History of Blindness in the US, 9887
Up Against Eating Disorders, 3688
Up Front Drug Information, 567
Update, 6857
Uplift, 6087
Upper Peninsula Library for the Blind and Physically Handicapped, 9705
Upstate New York Transplant Services, Inc., 9208
Upstate NY Chapter of the Myasthenia Gravis Foundation of America, 6591
Urban Cardiology Research Center, 4915
Urinary Incontinence in Women, 5359
Urinary Tract Infections, 5712
Urologic Care of the Child with Spina Bifida, 7940
Urology Care Foundation, 5301, 5336
US Administration on Aging, 42, 236
US Department of Justice, 10426
US Department of Transportation, 10427
US Department Of Veterans Affairs, 10125
US Environmental Protection Agency: Indoor Environments Division, 5815
US Office of Personnel Management, 10428
US Organ Procurement System: A Prescription for Reform, 9235
USA Deaf Sports Federation, 4336, 4720, 4748, 4856
USC Internal Medicine, 380
USC/Norris Comprehensive Cancer Center, 2284
USC: Neonatology Research Units, 8812
Use of Low Dose Methotrexate in Refractory Sarcoidosis, 7307
Use of Steroids for Asthma and Allergies, 716, 1490

Useful Information on Alzheimer's Disease, 1066
Useful Information on Phobias and Panic, 6240
Using A Medical Library, 2073
Using Insulin, 3474
Utah Alliance for the Mentally Ill, 6014
Utah Chapter of the National Hemophilia Foundation, 5006
Utah Department of Health, 8797
Utah Department of Health: Bureau of Epidemiology, 342
Utah Industries for the Blind, 9591
Utah SIDS Alliance, 8798
Utah State Library Division, 9752
Utah Support Group: National Ataxia Foundation, 1562
Uterine Artery Embolization, 5574
Uterine Fibroids, 5551

V

VA Ann Arbor Healthcare System, 10176
VA Austin Information Technology Center, 10104
VA Austin Outpatient Clinic, 10250
VA Capitol Health Care Network, 10167
VA Caregiver Support, 7160, 10320, 10650
VA Central California Health Care System, 10117
VA Central Iowa Health Care System, 10154
VA Great Lakes Health Care System, 10149
VA Greater Los Angeles Healthcare System, 10118
VA Healthcare System of Ohio, 10218
VA Heart of Texas Health Care Network Dallas VA Medical Center, 10251
VA Heartland Network, 10187
VA Illiana Health Care System, 10150
VA Loma Linda Healthcare System, 10119
VA MidSouth Healthcare Network (VISN 9), 10242
VA Northern California Health Care System, 10120
VA Palo Alto Health Care System, 10121
VA Puget Sound Health Care System, 10261
VA Sierra Nevada Health Care System, 10192
VA Southeast Network, 10140
VA St. Louis Health Care System John Cochran & Jefferson Barracks, 10188
VA Western Colorado Health Care System, 10122
VACCINATE ADULTS! Coalition News, 5160
Vaginal Infections, 7593
Valdosta Talking Book Library, 9657
Valley Brain Tumor Support Group, 2033
VALT Support Group (Vital Active Life After Trauma), 4164
Vanderbilt Children's Hospital, 3168
Vanderbilt Clinical Nutrition Research Unit (CNRU), 6774
Vanderbilt Kennedy Center, 6044
Vanderbilt University Diabetes Center, 3403
Vanderbilt University: Center for Fertility and Reproductive Research, 5439
Vascular Birthmarks, 7731
Vector Borne & Zoonotic Diseases, 9045
Ventilation: Decision Making Process, 1176
Ventilator-Assisted Living, 7021
Ventilator: Assisted Living, 7022
Vermont Alliance for the Mentally Ill, 6015
Vermont Department of Health: Health Surveillance Division, 343
Vermont Department of Health: SIDS Information and Counseling Program, 8799
Vermont Department of Libraries Special Services Unit, 9753
Vermont FFCMH, 6016, 6081
Vermont Pregnancy Risk Information Service, 1867
Vermont Regional Hemophilia Center, 5071
Very Special Sister, 4698
Veterans Administration Medical Center: Alabama, 10106
Veterans Affairs Medical Center: Research Service, 3404
Veterans Association Medical Center, 10107
Veterans Benefits Clearinghouse, 10275
Veterans Crisis Line, 7120
Veterans Medical Center: Mental Health Clinical Research Center, 6045
Vetwives Living With PTSD, 7121
VIABL Services of Northampton County, 9570

Victims of Dementia, 6141
Video on Narcolepsy, 7847
Vietnam and All Veterans of Brevard, 10135
Viewpoints on Deafness, 4626
Views from Our Shoes: Growing Up with a Brother or Sister with Special Needs, 7933
Village by the Sea, 4935
Violence and Drugs, 8454
Viral Hepatitis, 5798
Viral Hepatitis: Everybody's Problem?, 5182
Viral Hepatitis: Scientific Basis and Clinical Management, 5152
Virginia Alliance for the Mentally Ill, 6017
Virginia Association of the Deaf, 4357
Virginia Beach Public Library, 9763
Virginia Commonwealth University Virginia Center on Aging, 144
Virginia Commonwealth University: Massey Cancer Center, 2384
Virginia Commonwealth University: Rehab Research and Training Center, 4142
Virginia Department of Health: Division of Disease Prevention, 344
Virginia Industries for the Blind, 9594
Virginia Mason Brain Tumor Support Group, 2036
Virginia Mason Medical Center Neuroscience Institute, 1148
Virginia Office for Protection and Advocacy, 10493
Virginia SIDS Alliance, 8801
Virginia SIDS Program: Virginia Department of Health, 8802
Visible Speech, 4627
Vision and Aging: Crossroads for Service Delivery, 9888
Vision Use in Employment, 9823
Visiting Nurse Association of America, 10528
Visual Aids and Informational Material, 9889
Visual Handicaps and Learning, 9890
Visual Impairment: An Overview, 9891
Visually Impaired Center, 9805
Visually Impaired Data Processors International, 10095
Visually Impaired Piano Tuners International, 10096
Visually Impaired Veterans of America, 10097
Vital Aging Report, 207
Vital Options International, 1941
Vitiligo, 7732
Viva Vital News, 9954
VIVA!, 7991
Voice of Hope, 2497
Voice of the Diabetic, 3475, 3493, 9915
Voice of Vision, 9955
Voices for the Blind, 9724
Voices from the Workplace, 7557
Voices of Vision Talking Book Center, 9664
Volta Review, 4721
Volta Voices, 4722
Volunteer at Your Braille and Talking Book Library, 10021
Volunteer Voice, 1298
Von Willebrand Disease: A Guide for Patients and Families, 5123
Voyage to an Island, 4628
VSA Arts, 10601

W

W. G. (Bill) Hefner VA Medical Center, 10211
Wainwright House Cancer Support Programs, 2415
Waiting for Johnny Miracle, 2476
Waiting: A Diary of Loss and Hope in Pregnancy, 5496
Wake Forest University: Arteriosclerosis Research Center, 5262
Wake Forest University: Cerebrovascular Research Center, 8063
Wake Up! Brochure, 7842
Wake-Up Call, 7836
Walk in Dry Places, 8400
Walk Talk, 568
Walking Alone and Marching Together, 9892
Walking Tomorrow: University of Alabama, 8008
Wallace Memorial Library, 4368
Warning Signs of Kidney Disease, 5713

Warren Grant Magnuson Clinical Center, 670, 1256, 2320, 3405, 4916, 5669, 5872
Warren Grant Magnuson Clinical Center National Institute of Health, 9806
Washington Ambassador National Ataxia Foundation, 1563
Washington Connection, 9824
Washington DC Department of Health: HIV/AIDS, Hepatitis, STD and TB Admin., 299
Washington DC Metropolitan Area Brain Tumor Support Group, 1981
Washington DC Metropolitan Area Support Group, 1950
Washington DC VA Medical Center, 10126
Washington Department of Health: HIV Program, 345
Washington Department of Social and Health Services, Alcohol and Drug Prog., 8191
Washington FFCMH, 6019
Washington Leukemia and Lymphoma Society: Alaska Chapter, 2252
Washington Regional Transplant Consortium, 9222
Washington State Client Assistance Program, 10495
Washington State Department of Services for the Blind, 9597
Washington Talking Book & Braille Library, 9764
Washington Turner Syndrome Resource Group, 9357
Washington University Chromalloy American Kidney Center, 5670
Washington University School of Medicine, 8064
Washington University: Cystic Fibrosis Center, 3137
Washington University: Diabetes Research and Training Center, 3406
Washington Update, 523
Washington-Greene County Branch for the Pennsylvania Association for Blind, 9571
Washtenaw County Library for the Blind and Physically Disabled, 9706
Wasted Tales of a Gen X Drunk, 8401
Waterville Public Library, 9685
Way to Go: School Success for Children wit h Mental Health Care Needs, 6142
Wayne County Regional Library for the Blind and Physically Handicapped, 9707
Wayne State University Center for Health Research, 411
Wayne State University Center for Molecular Medicine and Genetics, 2328
Wayne State University: Comprehensive Sickle Cell Center, 7624
Wayne State University: CS Mott Center for Human Growth and Development, 1848
Wayne State University: Gurdjian-Lissner Biomechanics Laboratory, 4143
Wayne State University: University Women's Care, 5440
Ways & Means, 5098
We Are Not Alone: Learning to Live with Chronic Illness, 8938
We Are the Children's Hope/Support Group, 6085
We Can Do it Together: Mobility for Students with Multiple Disabilities, 10049
We Can Do It!, 3627
We Can: A Guide for Parents of Children with Arthritis, 1277
We Have AIDS, 489, 509
We Will Remember, 10738
Webhelp, 2602
WebMD, 20, 237, 623, 741, 1086, 1184, 1368, 1516, 1598, 1659, 1822, 1899, 2087, 2601, 2663, 2820, 2906, 2944, 2991, 3081, 3206
Webster Large Print Dictionary, 9893
Week the World Heard Gallaudet, 4629
Weight Management for Type II Diabetes, 3476
Weight-Control Information Network, 3689, 3705, 3787, 6714, 6715, 6775
Welcome Back, 6764
Well Spouse Association, 153, 10529
Wellness Community Cancer Support Groups, 1942
Wellness Community: Kentucky, 1974
Wellness Community: South Bay Cities, 1943
Wellness Community: West Los Angeles, 1944
Wenatchee Valley Brain Tumor Support Group, 2037
West Central FL Support Group: National Ataxia Foundation, 1535

West Central Ohio Hemophilia Center Childens Medical Center, 5072
West Florida Public Library: Talking Book Library, 9643
West Palm Beach Area Brain Tumor Support Group, 1958
West Palm Beach VA Medical Center, 10136
West Roxbury Division VA Boston Healthcare System, 10171
West Tennessee Sarcoidosis Support Group, 7255
West Texas Lighthouse for the Blind, 9589
West Virginia Advocates, 10497
West Virginia Department of Health & Human Resources: Division of STD and HIV, 346
West Virginia Division of Alcohol & Drug Abuse, 8192
West Virginia Library Commission, 9769
West Virginia School for the Blind, 9770
West Virginia University Cystic Fibrosis Center, 3179
West Virginia University: Mary Babb Randolph Cancer Center, 2386
Westchester Task Force on Eating Disorders/American Anorexia Bulimia, 3698
Western Michigan University School of Medi cine, 3152
Western Pennsylvania Chapter of the National Hemophilia Foundation, 5000
Western Region SIDS Resources, 8762
Western Slope Chapter of the American Association of Kidney Patients, 5593
Western WA Support Group: National Ataxia Foundation, 1564
WFS' New Life Program, 8248
What, 6143
What are Clinical Trials All About?, 2575
What Are the Signs of Alcoholism?, 8643
What are TTY's? TDDs? TTs?, 4783
What Can Baby See? Vision Tests & Intervention Strategies for Infants, 10050
What Causes Scleroderma?, 7387
What Do You Do When You See a Blind Person — and What Don't You Do?, 10022
What Educators Should Know About Prader-Willi Syndrome, 7215
What Every Family Should Know Sixth Edition, 8983
What Every Parent Should Know About SIDS, 8837
What Every Patient Should Know About Asthma & Allergy Medications, 717, 1491
What Every Woman Must Know About Heart Disease, 4932
What Everyone Should Know About Multiple Sclerosis, 6493
What Fair Housing Means for People with Disabilities, 6144
What Happened to Joe?, 8644
What Happens After Treatment?, 8645
What Health Care Workers Should Know About Hepatitis B, 5183
What Helped Me When My Loved One Died, 10721
What if You Need an Operation for Scoliosis?, 7437
What is a Physiatrist?, 8025
What is AA?, 8646
What Is AIDS?, 490
What is an Allergic Reaction?, 718
What is an Audiogram?, 4630
What is Anoxic Brain Injury?, 4260
What Is Autism, 1793
What is Canavan Disease?, 8992
What is Cooley's Anemia, 2976
What Is Hemophilia?, 5124
What Is Multiple Sclerosis?, 6494
What is NA?, 8647
What is SIDS?, 8838
What is Spinal Cord Injury?, 8024
What is Tay-Sachs? Russian Translation, 8993
What is Thalassemia Trait?, 2982
What is Thalassemia?, 2977
What Makes Ryan Tic?, 9093
What Museum Guides Need to Know: Access for Blind & Visually Impaired Visitors, 9894
What School Bus Drivers Need to Know About Students with Tourette Syndrome, 9133
What School Personnel Should Know About Asthma, 1503

What to Do When a Friend is Depressed: Guide for Students, 6241

What to Do When an Employee is Depressed: A Guide for Supervisors, 6242

What Women Should Know About HIV Infection AIDS and Hemophilia, 5125

What Works: Schools Without Drugs, 8402

What You Can Do About Drug Use in America, 8403

What You Need to Know About Bladder Cancer, 2559

What You Need to Know About Brain Tumors, 2074

What You Need to Know About Cancer, 2560

What You Need to Know About Cancer of The Colon and Rectum, 2561

What You Need to Know About Cervical Cancer, 2562

What You Need to Know About Esophagal Cancer, 2563

What You Need to Know About Kidney Cancer, 2564

What You Need to Know About Larynx Cancer, 2565

What You Need to Know About Lung Cancer, 2566

What You Need to Know About Oral Cancers, 2567

What You Need to Know About Ovarian Cancer, 2568

What You Need to Know About Pancreatic Cancer, 2569

What You Need to Know About Prostate Cancer, 2570

What You Need to Know About Skin Cancer, 2571

What You Need to Know About Testicular Cancer, 2572

What You Need to Know About Uterine Cancer, 2573

What You Need to Know About..., 2574

What You Should Know About Hemophilia, 5126

What Young People & Their Parents Need to Know About Scoliosis, 7436

What Young People and Parents Need to Know about Scoliosis, 7411

What Your Female Patients Want to Know About Bladder Control, 5360

What's a Virus, Anyway? The Kid's Book About AIDS, 510

What's Drunk Mama?, 8455

What's Line, 9956

What's New in Spinal Cord Injury Research?, 8026

What's that Pig Outdoors? A Memoir of Deafness, 4631

What's the Best Medicine for My Headaches?, 6322

What's This Thing Called Scoliosis, 7449

What's Wrong with Grandma? A Family Experience with Alzheimer's, 1028

What's Your Cigarette Smoking IQ?, 8648

Wheel Life News, 10602

Wheels Down: Adjusting to Life After Deployment, 7135

When a Parent Has Cancer: A Guide to Caring for Your Children, 2457

When a Parent Has MS: A Teenager's Guide, 6495

When Cancer Recurs: Meeting the Challenge Again, 2576

When Diabetes Complicates Your Life, 3477

When Food is Love, 3761

When Madness Comes Home, 6145

When Mom Gets Sick, 8941

When Snow Turns to Rain, 1779

When Someone in Your Family Has Cancer, 2577

When Someone You Love Has a Mental Illness, 6146

When Someone You Love Suffers from Depression, 6245

When Sudden Infant Death Syndrome Occurs in Childcare Settings, 8839

When the Bough Breaks, 10739

When the Mind Hears, 4633

When the Spine Curves, 7438

When We Become the Parent to Our Parents, 1022

When You Can't Sleep, 7843

When You Go Back to Work, 8649

When Your Child Goes to School After an Injury, 4261

When Your Child is Deaf: A Guide for Parents, 4632

When Your Child is Seriously Injured: The Emotional Impact on Families, 4262

When Your Child Returns to School, 2075

When Your Student Has Arthritis: A Guide for Teachers, 1353

When Your Teen is in Treatment, 8650

Where Do I Go from Here?, 8651

Where Is Spot?, 4699

Whiskers Says No to Drugs, 8456

White City VA Rehabilitation Center VA Southern Oregon, 10224

White Lung Association, 5816

White River Junction VA Medical Center, 10253

Whitman Walker Clinic AIDS/Medical Services Programs, 386

Whitney Library for the Blind: Assemblies of God, 9716

Who is This Person Who Helped Save My Life, 2578

WHO Laboratory Manual, 5495

Who Speaks for the Deaf Community?, 4634

Who Will Tell Them of Your Special Needs?, 5127

Whooo's Report, 2643

Why Am I Afraid to Tell You Who I Am?, 8404

Why Anonymity in Al-Anon?, 8652

Why Are You So Scared? A Child's Book About Parents With PTSD, 7136

Why Did it Happen on a School Day: My Family's Experience with Brain Injury, 4211

Why Do People Drink Alcohol?, 8457

Why Do People Smoke?, 8458

Why Do People Take Drugs?, 8459

Why Do You Smoke?, 2579

Why God Gave Me Pain, 2477

Why My Child, 1891

Why Won't My Child Pay Attention?, 1653

Wichita Medical Research & Education Foundation, 1849

Wichita Public Library, 9675

Wild Boy of Aveyron, 1783

Wilkes-Barre VA Medical Center, 10231

Willamette Valley Support Group: National Ataxia Foundation, 1557

William S. Middleton Memorial Veterans Hospital, 10268

William T Gossett Parkinson's Disease Center, 6911

Wilmington VA Medical Center, 10123

Wilson's Disease, 10327

Wilson's Disease Association, 5775, 10324

WIN Notes, 3770, 3975

Win-Win Approach to Reasonable Accommodations, 6496

Window of Time, 1029

Wings for the Future, 10023

Winning Over Asthma, 1437

Winning the Battle Against Drugs: Rehabilitation Programs, 8460

Winning the Fight Against Silent Killers, 5714

Winston-Salem Industries for the Blind, 9545

Winter Blues, 6227

Wired for Sound, 4635

Wisconsin AIDS Update, 569

Wisconsin Alliance for the Mentally Ill, 6022

Wisconsin Association of the Deaf, 4358

Wisconsin Chapter of the Myasthenia Gravis Foundation of America, 6600

Wisconsin Department of Health Services: Wisconsin HIV Program, 348

Wisconsin Family Ties, 6023

Wisconsin Parkinson Association, 6905

Wisconsin Regional Library for the Blind Talking Book Program, 9772

Wiscraft: Wisconsin Enterprises for the Blind, 9602

Wish Fulfillment Organizations, 2580

Wish Upon A Star, 10678

A Wish with Wings, Inc., 10654

Wishing Star Foundation, 10679

Wishing Well Foundation USA, Inc., 10680

Wisonsin Donor Network, 9225

With a Little Help from My Friends, 6174

Withering Child, 3762

Within Reach, 6794

Without Child, 5497

Without Sight and Sound, 10024

WM Krogman Center for Research in Child Growth and Development, 4054

WNYS Center for SIDS, 8776

Wolff's Headaches & Other Head Pain, 6304

Wolfner Memorial Library for the Blind, 9717

Woman's Perspective, 5315, 5319

Woman's Way Through the Twelve Steps, 8405

Women & AIDS, 491

Women Alive, 283

Women and AIDS: A Practical Guide for Those Who Help Others, 492

Women and Aids: Coping and Caring, 493

Women and Cancer: A Compassionate Reource for Patients and Their Families, 2458

Women and Depression, 6228

Women and Heart Disease, 4934

Women and Sleep, 7844

Women at Risk, 7579

Women in Your Life: Protect Yourself, Protect Your Family, 5270, 8079

Women Take Heart, 4933

Women Without Children, 5498

Women's Resource Center, 7080

Women's Suffrage for Prostate Cancer Awareness, 2416

Women, Sex, and HIV, 598

Women: Coming Out of the Shadows, 8671

Word Signs: A First Book of Sign Language, 4700

Workers at Risk: Drugs and Alcohol on the Job, 8653

Working After A Head Injury, 4263

Working After Brain Injury, 4212

Working Together, 3771

Working with Deaf People: Accessibility and Accommodation in the Workplace, 4636

Working with Deaf Persons in Sunday School, 4637

Worklife: A Publication of Employment and People with Disabilities, 10603

World Around You, 4723

World Association Sarcoidosi Other Granulatomous, 7308

World Endometriosis Society, 3797

World Federation for Mental Health, 5923, 6189

World Federation of Hemophilia, 4965

World Hypertension League, 5201

World Institute on Disability, 10429, 10652

A World of Genetic Societies, 3846

World of Sound, 4784

World Services for the Blind, 9461

World/Mundo, 570

Wound Ostomy and Continence Nurses Society, 3000

Writer's Workshop, 4638

Writing from Within, 10581

Wyoming Alliance for the Mentally Ill, 6024

Wyoming Department of Health, 8808

Wyoming Department of Health: Communicable Disease Unit, 349

Wyoming Protection & Advocacy System, 10499

Wyoming Services for the Visually Disabled, 9773

X

Xavier Society for the Blind, 9732

XIV International World Conference on Sarcoidosis: Patient Symposium, 7316

Y

Yale Child Study Center, 7087

Yale University Comprehensive Cancer Center, 2290

Yale University Cystic Fibrosis Research Center, 3099

Yale University: Behavioral Medicine Clinic, 6204

Yale University: Ribicoff Research Facilities/CT Mental Health Center, 6205

Yale University: Vision Research Center, 9807

Yale: Congenital Heart Disease, 2954

Yard Sale Coloring Book, 1281

Year it Rained, 6271

Yes, You Can, 10281

Yes, You Can!: Go Beyond Physical Adversity and Live Life to Its Fullest, 10582

Yeshiva University General Clinical Research Center, 4917

Yeshiva University Marion Bessin Liver Research Center, 5771

Yeshiva University: Institute of Communication Disorders, 4408

Yeshiva University: Resnick Gerontology Center, 983

Yeshiva University: Soundview-Throgs Neck Community Mental Health Center, 6046

Yesterday's Tomorrow, 6229

York Industries for the Blind: Division of York County Blind Center, 9572

You and Your Brace, 7439

You and Your Deaf Child, 4640

You Are Not Alone, 6795, 7450

You Are One of Us: Clergy/Church Connections to Alzheimer Families, 1067

You Can Help Your Community Get Rid of Drugs, 8654

You Don't Have to Hate Meetings: Try Computer-Assisted Notetaking Instead, 4785

You Don't LOOK Sick!: Living Well with Invisible Chronic Illness, 7831

You Don't Outgrow Down Syndrome, 3656

You Have HIV: A Day at a Time, 494

You Just Don't Understand, 4639

You Mean I'm Not Lazy, Stupid or Crazy?, 1631

You Seem Like a Regular Kid to Me, 10025

You're Bigger Than it, 9390

You're in Charge: Teens with Asthma, 1504

You're Not Alone, 2985

Young Children and Drugs: What Parents Can Do, 8655

Young People and AA, 8672

Young People and Psoriasis, 7733

Young People with Cancer: A Handbook for Parents, 2459, 2581

Young Person's Guide to the Twelve Steps, 8461

Young Teens: Who They Are and How to Talk to Them About Alcohol & Drugs, 8406

Young, Sober & Free, 8462

Your Body's Design for Bladder Control, 5361

Your Child and Asthma, 1492

Your Child, Your Family & ARPKD, 5680

Your Child, Your Family and Autosomal Recessive Polycystic Kidney Disease, 5681

Your Daily Bladder Diary, 5362

Your Diet & Psoriasis, 7734

Your Job and HIV: Are There Risks?, 599

Your Kidneys: Master Chemists of the Body, 5715

Your Life After Trauma, 7137

Your Liver Lets You Live, 5799

Your Medicines and Bladder Control, 5363

Your Pain is Real: Free Yourself from Chronic Pain, Breakthrough Med. Trtmnt., 2930

Your Personal Guide to Bladder Health, 5345

Your Sexuality & Health, 5311

Your Skin and Your Dermatologist, 7735

Your Thyroid: A Home Reference, 9011

Youth and the Alcoholic Parent, 8656

Z

Zink the Zebra, 10585

Alabama

AARP Alabama, 43
AIDS Alabama, 439
ALS Association: Alabama Chapter, 1091
Alabama Ambassador: National Ataxia Foundation, 1523
Alabama Chapter of the American Association of Kidney Patients, 5581
Alabama Chapter of the Arthritis Foundation, 1192
Alabama Council of the Blind, 9463
Alabama Department of Public Health, 284
Alabama Education of Homeless Children and Youth Program, 6048
Alabama Head Injury Foundation, 4082
Alabama Head Injury Foundation Helpline, 4145
Alabama Institute for Deaf and Blind, 4337
Alabama Organ Center, 9175
Alabama Radio Reading Service Network, 9607
Alabama Regional Library for the Blind and Physically Handicapped, 9608
Alzheimer's Association: North Alabama Chapter, 759
Alzheimer's Association: Southeast Alabama Chapter, 760
Alzheimer's Association: Southwest Alabama Chapter, 761
Alzheimer's Disease Center: University of Alabama at Birmingham, 956
American Cancer Society: Alabama, 2114
American Council on Addiction & Alcohol Problems, 8110
American Diabetes Association: Alabama, 3213
American Lung Association of Alabama, 5817
American Lung Association of Alabama, 9262
American Obesity Treatment Association, 6709
American Society for Reproductive Medicine, 3791
American Society for Reproductive Medicine, 5376
Arthritis and Musculoskeletal Center: UAB Shelby Interdisciplinary Biomedical Rese, 1241
Autism Society of Alabama, 1670
Birmingham Support Group: National Ataxia Foundation, 1524
Birmingham VA Medical Center: Research and Development, 2268
Breast Cancer Resource Foundation of Alabama, 2269
Bureau of Family Health Services: Alabama Department of Public Health, 8706
CCFA Alabama Chapter, 3001
Cardiovascular Research and Training Center University of Alabama, 4870
Center for Neuroimmunology: University of Alabama at Birmingham, 6431
Centers for AIDS Research: University of Alabama at Birmingham, 363
Civitan International Research Center, 4373
Diabetes Research and Training Center: University of Alabama at Birmingham, 3381
Division of Mental Illness and Substance Abuse Community Programs, 8137
Division of Rehabilitation: Montgomery, 10430
General Clinical Research Center: UAB, 364
Gulf War Veterans of Alabama, 10105
Hemophilia Clinic: Childrens' Rehabilitation Service, 5037
Hemophilia and Bleeding Disorders of Alaba ma, Inc., 4966
Horizons Schools, 10500
Houston Love Memorial Library, 9609
Huntsville Subregional Library for the Blind and Physically Handicapped, 9610
Juvenile Diabetes Research Foundation: Birmingham, 3214
Knollwoodpark Hospital Sleep Disorders Cen, 7772
Knollwoodpark Hospital Sleep Disorders Center, 7771
Leukemia and Lymphoma Society: Alabama Chapter, 2115
Library and Resource Center for the Blind and Physically Handicapped, 9611
Lyme Disease Network Support Group of Alabama: Mobile Chapter, 9035
Magic Moments, 10670
NNFF Alabama Affiliate, 6656

National Alliance on Mental Illness of Alabama: NAMI Alabama, 5924
National Federation of the Blind: Alabama, 9464
National Multiple Sclerosis Society: Alabama Chapter, 6346
National Society for MVP and Dysautonomia, 4921
National Spinal Cord Injury Statistical Center, 7957
National Spinal Cord Injury Support Groups, 7994
Pediatric Brain Tumor Support Group, 1915
Pull-thru Network, 3948
Pushin On: RRTC on Secondary Conditions of Spinal, 7984
Sickle Cell Foundation of Greater Montgomery, 7611
Specialized Center of Research in Ischemic Heart Disease, 4897
Spina Bifida Association of Alabama, 7865
Stroke Research and Treatment Center UAB Medical Center, 8059
Tuscaloosa Subregional Library for the Blind & Physically Handicapped, 9612
United Cerebral Palsy of Alabama, 2673
United Cerebral Palsy of East Central Alabama, 2674
United Cerebral Palsy of Greater Birmingha m, 2675
United Cerebral Palsy of Huntsville & Tennessee Valley, 2676
United Cerebral Palsy of Mobile, 2677
United Cerebral Palsy of Northwest Alabama, 2678
United Cerebral Palsy of West Alabama, 2679
University Alzheimer Center University of Alabama at Birmingham, 977
University of Alabama At Birmingham Comprehensive Cancer Center, 2270
University of Alabama Birmingham, 7367
University of Alabama Speech and Hearing Center, 4398
University of Alabama at Birmingham Parkinsons Disease Center, 6910
University of Alabama at Birmingham: Congenital Heart Disease Center, 4899
University of Alabama at Birmingham: National Cooperative Drug/AIDS, 365
Veterans Administration Medical Center: Alabama, 10106
Veterans Association Medical Center, 10107

Alaska

AARP Alaska, 44
Alaska Department of Health and Social Services: HIV/STD Program, 285
Alaska State Library Talking Book Center, 9613
Alaska VA Healthcare System, 10108
Alaskan Statewide AIDS Helpline, 443
Alzheimer's Disease Resource Agency of Alaska, 762
American Cancer Society: Alaska, 2116
American Diabetes Association: Alaska, 3215
American Lung Association of Alaska, 5818
American Lung Association of Alaska, 9263
Asthma and Allergy Foundation of America: Alaska Chapter, 649
Asthma and Allergy Foundation of America: Alaska Chapter, 1390
Client Assistance Program: Anchorage, 10431
Lupus Foundation of America: Alaska Chapter, 8854
National Alliance for the Mentally Ill (NA MI) Alaska, 6049
National Alliance on Mental Illness of Alaska, 5925
National Federation of the Blind: Alaska, 9465
National Multiple Sclerosis Society: Alaska Chapter, 6347
Office of Alcohol and Substance Abuse Department of Health and Social Services, 8138
SIDS Information and Counseling Program: Alaska Department of Health, 8707
United Cerebral Palsy of Alaska/PARENTS, 2680

Arizona

AARP Arizona, 45
ALS Association: Arizona Chapter, 1092
Alcoholism and Drug Abuse: Office of Community Behavioral Health, 8139

Alzheimer's Association: Desert Southwest Chapter, 763
Alzheimer's Association: Northern Arizona, 764
Alzheimer's Association: Northern Nevada, 765
Alzheimer's Association: Southern Arizona, 766
Alzheimer's Association: Southern Arizona Region, 767
American Cancer Society: Arizona, 2117
American Diabetes Association: Arizona, 3216
American Diabetes Association: Arizona, Border Area, 3217
American Diabetes Association: Atlanta Met, 3218
American Diabetes Association: Northern Arizona, 3219
American Fibromyalgia Syndrome Association, 2824
American Fibromyalgia Syndrome Association, 3860
American Liver Foundation Arizona Chapter, 5744
American Lung Association of Arizona, 5819
Arizona Association of the Deaf, 4338
Arizona Brain Tumor Support Group, 1916
Arizona Center for the Blind and Visually Impaired, 9466
Arizona Chapter of the National Parkinson Foundation, 6874
Arizona Department of Health Services: HIV Prevention Program, 286
Arizona Heart Institute, 4865
Arizona Industries for the Blind, 9467
Arizona Kidney Foundation, 5582
Arizona SIDS Founation, 8708
Arizona Spinal Cord Injury Association, 7964
Arizona State Braille and Talking Book Library, 9614
Arizona Telemedicine Program, 7225
Arthritis Foundation: Central Arizona Chapter, 1193
Autism Society of Southern Arizona, 1671
Brain Injury Association of Arizona, 4083
Brain Injury Association of Arizona, 4146
CCFA Southwest Chapter: Arizona, 3002
Center for Neurodevelopmental Studies, 1718
Central Arizona Chapter of the American Association of Kidney Patients, 5583
Child Help, 7103
Commission on Accreditation of Rehabilitation Facilities, 26
Cystic Fibrosis Center: Phoenix Childrens Hospital, 3088
Do it Now Foundation, 8202
Donor Network of Arizona, 9176
Eating Disorders Anonymous, 3674
Fibromyalgia Network, 3868
Flagstaff City Coconino County Public Library, 9615
HPV Support Groups: Arizona, 10432
International Holistic Center, 2118
Jim L Walker: Arizona Chapter of the Myasthenia Gravis Foundation of America, 6574
Juvenile Diabetes Research Foundation: Phoenix Chapter, 3220
Leukemia and Lymphoma Society: Mountain States Chapter, 2119
Life Development Institute, 10390
Life Development Institute, 10501
Lupus Foundation of America: Greater Arizona Chapter, 8855
Lupus Foundation of America: Southern Arizona Chapter, 8856
Make-A-Wish Foundation of America, 10671
Mayo Clinic, 7083
Mayo Clinic Scottsdale Center for Scleroderma Care & Research, 7362
Mentally Ill Kids In Distress, 5926
Mountain State Regional Hemophilia Center, 5046
Muscular Dystrophy Association, 6518
Myasthenia Gravis Support Group of Arizona Jim L. Walker Chapter, 6603
National Alliance on Mental Illness of Arizona, 5927
National Federation of the Blind: Arizona, 9468
National Multiple Sclerosis Society Desert Southwest Chapter, 6348
National Network of Learning Disabled Adults, 10409
Navaho Nation K'E Project: Tuba City Children & Families Advocacy Corp, 5928
Navaho Nation K'E Project: Winslow Children & Families Advocacy Corp, 5929

Navajo Nation Office of Special Education & Rehabilitation Services (OSERS), 6050
Neurofibromatosis Association of Arizona, 6657
Northern Arizona Branch:Phoenix Area, 9264
Office of Chronic Disease Prevention and Nutrition Services, 6722
Office of Womens And Childrens Health: Alabama Department of Health, 8709
Phoenix Area Support Group: National Ataxi a Foundation, 1525
Phoenix Public Library: Special Needs Section, 9616
Phoenix VA Health Care System, 10109
Prader-Willi Syndrome Arizona Association, 7166
Prader-Willi Syndrome Arizona Association: Phoenix Area, 7165
RESOLVE of Valley of the Sun, 5383
Rare Cancer Alliance, 9327
Ruth E Golding Clinical Pharmacokinetics Laboratory, 8225
Scleroderma Foundation: Arizona Chapter, 7329
Southern Arizona Brain Tumor Support Group, 1917
Southern Arizona Branch: Tucson Area, 9265
Southern Arizona VA Health Care System, 10110
Southwest Association for Education in Biomedical Research, 2271
Southwest Center For HIV/AIDS, 287
Spina Bifida Association of Arizona, 7866
St. Joseph's Hemophilia Center, 5059
Teratology OTIS, 1843
Tucson Interfaith HIV/AIDS Network (TIHAN), 288
Tucson Support Group: National Ataxia Foundation, 1526
United Cerebral Palsy of Central Arizona, 2681
United Cerebral Palsy of Southern Arizona, 2682
University of Arizona Cancer Center, 2272

Arkansas

AARP Arkansas, 46
ALS Association: Arkansas Chapter, 1093
Alzheimer's Arkansas Programs and Services, 768
Alzheimer's Association: Western Arkansas Chapter, 769
American Cancer Society: Arkansas, 2120
American Diabetes Association: Arkansas, 3221
American Lung Association of Arkansas, 5820
American Lung Association of Arkansas, 9266
Arkansas Association of the Deaf, 4339
Arkansas Cystic Fibrosis Center Arkansas Children's Hospital, 3089
Arkansas Department of Health: HIV Prevention Program, 289
Arkansas Department of Health: SIDS Information & Counseling Program, 8710
Arkansas FFCMH Jane Burgan, 5930
Arkansas Lighthouse for the Blind, 9470
Arkansas Regional Library for the Blind and Physically Handicapped, 9617
Arkansas Regional Organ Recovery Agency, 9177
Arthritis Foundation: Arkansas Chapter, 1194
Brain Injury Association of Arkansas, 4084
Brain Injury Association of Arkansas Helpl ine, 4147
Disability Rights Center of Arkansas, 10433
Eugene J. Towbin Healthcare Center Central Arkansas VA Healthcare System, 10111
Gulf War Veterans of Arkansas, 10112
Health Resource, 2121
Hemophilia Foundation of Arkansas, 4967
John L McClellan Memorial Veterans' Hospital Research Office, 4886
Juvenile Diabetes Research Foundation: Northwest Arkansas Branch, 3222
Library for the Blind and Handicapped, Southwest, 9618
Lupus Foundation of America: Arkansas Chapter, 8857
NAMI Arkansas, 5931
NNFF Arkansas Affiliate, 6658
National Federation of the Blind: Arkansas, 9471
National Kidney Foundation of Arkansas, 5584
National Multiple Sclerosis Society: Arkansas Chapter, 6349
Office of Alcohol and Drug Abuse Prevention, 8140

Prader-Willi Arkansas Association Prader-Willi Syndrome Association, 7167
RESOLVE Affiliate of Northwest Arkansas, 5384
Research and Training Center for Persons Who are Deaf or Hard of Hearing, 4387
United Cerebral Palsy of Central Arkansas, 2683
World Services for the Blind, 9461

California

1-800-BRAILLE, 9809
AAGL - Elevating Gynecologic Surgery, 3789
AARP California: Pasadena, 47
AARP California: Sacramento, 48
AEGIS AIDS Education Global Information System, 438
AIDS Clinical Trials Unit CARES Clinic, 366
AIDS Healthcare Foundation, 350
ALS Association Free Standing Support Groups, 1149
ALS Association: Golden West Chapter, 1094
ALS Association: Golden West Chapter - Greater Los Angeles Office, 1095
ALS Association: Golden West-Greater Bay, 1096
ALS Association: Greater Sacramento Chapte r, 1097
ALS Association: Greater San Diego Chapter, 1098
ALS Association: Orange County Chapter, 1099
ALS Center at UCSF, 1136
ASTHMA Hotline, 671
Adult Research Opportunities, 367
Advocates 4 Health: Tick-borne Disease Self-Help Group, 9031
Alcohol Drug Treatment Referral, 8240
Alcohol Research Group Public Health Institute, 8198
Alta Bates Summit Medical Center, 6026
Alzheimer's Association San Diego/Imperial Chapter, 770
Alzheimer's Association: California Central Chapter: Ventura County Office, 771
Alzheimer's Association: Greater North Valley Chapter, 773
Alzheimer's Association: Greater Sacramento, 772
Alzheimer's Association: Los Angeles Chapter, 774
Alzheimer's Association: Monterey County Chapter, 775
Alzheimer's Association: North Bay Chapter, 776
Alzheimer's Association: Orange County Chapter, 777
Alzheimer's Association: Riverside/San Bernardino Counties Chapter, 778
Alzheimer's Association: San Francisco Bay Area Chapter, 779
Alzheimer's Association: Santa Barbara Central Coast Chapter, 780
Alzheimer's Association: Santa Cruz County Chapter, 781
Alzheimer's Disease Center: University of California, Davis, 955
American Academy of Ophthalmology, 9406
American Association for Pediatric Ophthalmology And Strabismus, 6570
American Cancer Society Santa Clara County / Silicon Valley / Central Coast Region, 2122
American Cancer Society: Central Los Angeles, 2123
American Cancer Society: East Bay/Metro Region, 2124
American Cancer Society: Fresno/Madera Counties, 2125
American Cancer Society: Inland Empire, 2126
American Cancer Society: Orange County, 2127
American Cancer Society: Sacramento County, 2128
American Cancer Society: San Diego County, 2129
American Cancer Society: San Francisco County, 2130
American Cancer Society: San Jose Prostate Cancer Support Group, 2388
American Cancer Society: Santa Maria Valley, 2131
American Cancer Society: Sonoma County, 2132
American Chronic Pain Association, 252
American Chronic Pain Association, 1186
American Chronic Pain Association, 1518
American Chronic Pain Association, 2091
American Chronic Pain Association, 2605
American Chronic Pain Association, 2666

American Chronic Pain Association, 2823
American Chronic Pain Association, 2908
American Chronic Pain Association, 2993
American Chronic Pain Association, 3790
American Chronic Pain Association, 3859
American Chronic Pain Association, 4076
American Chronic Pain Association, 6191
American Chronic Pain Association, 6287
American Chronic Pain Association, 6341
American Chronic Pain Association, 6806
American Chronic Pain Association, 6854
American Chronic Pain Association, 7009
American Chronic Pain Association, 7036
American Chronic Pain Association, 7222
American Chronic Pain Association, 7233
American Chronic Pain Association, 7397
American Chronic Pain Association, 7603
American Chronic Pain Association, 7640
American Chronic Pain Association, 7757
American Chronic Pain Association, 7954
American Chronic Pain Association, 8109
American Chronic Pain Association, 9379
American Diabetes Association: California, 3223
American Head and Neck Society, 4077
American Liver Foundation Greater Los Angeles Chapter, 5745
American Liver Foundation Northern CA Chapter, 5746
American Liver Foundation San Diego Chapte r, 5747
American Lung Association of California, 5821
American Lung Association of California, 9267
Amyotrophic Lateral Sclerosis Toll Free Hotline, 1151
Archstone Foundation, 111
Arthritis Foundation: Northern California Chapter, 1195
Arthritis Foundation: San Diego Area Chapter, 1196
Arthritis Foundation: Southern California Chapter, 1197
Autism Society of California, 1672
Bay Area LE Foundation, 8858
Bees-Stealy Research Foundation, 4867
Bereavement Group for Children, 1918
Bereavement Group for Children, 10699
Blind Childrens Center, 9619
Braille Institute Desert Center, 9776
Braille Institute Library Services, 9620
Braille Institute Orange County Center, 9777
Braille Institute Santa Barbara Center Braille Institute of Los Angeles, 9778
Braille Institute Sight Center, 9779
Braille Institute Youth Center, 9780
Braille Institute of America, 9417
Brain Injury Association of California Hel pline, 4148
Brain Tumor Society, 1919
Brain Tumor Support Group: Fresno, 1921
Brain Tumor Support Group: Fullerton, 1922
Brain Tumor Support Group: Newport Beach, 1923
Brain Tumor Support Group: Orange, 1924
Brain Tumor Support Group: Redding, 1925
Brain Tumor Support Group: Sacramento, 1926
Brain Tumor Support Group: San Diego, 1927
Brain Tumor Support Group: San Francisco, 1928
Brain Tumor Support Group: Santa Barbara, 1929
Brain Tumor Support Group: Stanford, 1930
Brain Tumor Support Group: Westlake Village, 1931
Brain Tumor/Pituitary Patient Support Group, 1932
Breast Cancer Action, 2094
Burnham Institute Cancer Center The Burnham Institute for Medical Resear, 2273
CCFA California: Greater Los Angeles Chapter, 3003
California Ambassador: National Ataxia Foundation, 1527
California Association of Persian Gulf Veterans, 10113
California Collaborative Treatment Group, 290
California Department of Public Health: Office of AIDS, 291
California Institute for Medical Research, 6908
California Lyme Disease Association, 9028
California SIDS Program, 8711
California State Library Braille and Talking Book Library, 9621
California Teratogen Information Service UC San Diego School of Medicine Dept of, 1837

California Transplant Donor Network, 9178
California Women's Commission on Alcohol and
    Drug Dependencies, 8141
Cancer Control Society and Cancer Book House,
    2133
Cancer Federation, 2264
Cancer Prevention Institute of California, 2274
Cancer Support Community, 2392
Cancervive, 2393
Canine Companions for Independence, 9418
Celiac Disease Foundation, 2632
Celiac Disease Foundation, 2633
Center for AIDS Prevention Studies AIDS Research
    Institute University of C, 368
Center for Adaptive Learning, 10502
Center for Cancer Survival, 2394
Center for Interdisciplinary Research in Immunology
    and Diseases at UCLA, 369
Center for Reconstructive Urology, 5299
Centers for AIDS Research: North-Central California,
    370
Centers for AIDS Research: USCD Center for AIDS
    Research, 371
Centers for AIDS Research: University of California,
    Los Angeles, 372
Central California Chapter National Multiple
    Sclerosis Society, 6350
Central California Chapter of the National
    Hemophilia Foundation, 4968
Children Living with Illness, 1933
Children of Deaf Adults, 4411
Children's Gaucher Research Fund, 4024
Children's Hospital of Los Angeles, 3090
Children's Hospital of Orange County, 3087
Children's Liver Association for Support S ervices,
    5772
Childrens Hospital at Oakland, 3091
City of Hope Comprehensive Cancer Research
    Center, 2275
City of Hope National Medical Center Beckman
    Research Institute, 2134
City of Hope National Medical Center Drug
    Discover/AIDS Group, 373
Clearinghouse for Specialized Media and
    Translation, 9783
Cocaine Anonymous World Services, 8114
Collaborative Medicine Center, 2395
Commonwealth Cancer Help Program, 2396
Comprehensive Gaucher Treatment Center at Tower
    Hermatology Oncology, 4025
Cooley's Anemia Foundation (CAF): California, 2959
County of Los Angeles Public Health: Division of
    HIV And STD Programs, 292
Crime Survivors, 7104
Cystic Fibrosis Center: Cedars-Sinai Medical Center,
    3092
Cystic Fibrosis Center: University of California at
    San Francisco, 3093
Cystic Fibrosis Research, 3094
Department of Alcohol and Drug Programs, 8142
Departments of Neurology & Neurosurgery:
    University of California, San Francisco, 8056
Diabetes Control Program, 3369
Diabetes Society, 3408
Diabetes Society of Santa Clara Valley, 3224
Disability Rights California, 10434
Down Syndrome Association of Los Angeles, 3555
Dream Foundation, 10662
Drug Abuse Resistance Education of America, 8115
Enzymology Research Laboratory Dept. of Veterans
    Affairs Medical Center, 5869
Epilepsy Foundation of Northern California, 7477
Ernest Gallo Clinic and Research Center, 8204
Estate Planning for the Disabled, 10374
Extensions for Independence, 10375
Family Caregiver Alliance/National Center on
    Caregiving, 27
Family Caregiver Alliance/National Center on
    Caregiving, 4079
Foundation for Prader-Willi Research, 7162
Fresno County Public Library: Talking Book Library
    for the Blind, 9622
Friday Night Live, 8243
General Clinical Research Center: University of
    California at LA, 4880

Geraldine Brush Cancer Research Institute California
    Pacific Medical Center, 2276
Glaucoma Research Foundation, 9426
Glaucoma Research Foundation, 9605
Glaucoma Research Foundation, 9789
Glendale Adventist Medical Center Brain Tumor
    Support Group, 1934
Golden State Donor Services, 9179
Guide Dogs for the Blind, 9428
HIV/Hepatitis C in Prison (HIP) Committee, 5140
Harbor-South Bay Orange County Chapter of the
    American Assoc. of Kidney Patients, 5585
Heads Up!, 1935
Hear Center, 4378
Hearing Education and Awareness for Rocker s, 4310
Heart Research Foundation of Sacramento, 4884
Heart Touch Project™, 30
Heart Touch Project™, 261
Heart Touch Project™, 10384
Hemophilia Association of San Diego County, 4969
Hemophilia Center of the Huntington Hospital, 5036
Hemophilia Foundation of Northern California, 4970
Hemophilia Foundation of Southern California, 4971
House Ear Institute, 4315
HypoPARAthyroidism Association, 5
Ida and Joseph Friend Cancer Resource Center, 2277
Independence Center, 10503
Institute on Violence, Abuse and Trauma, 7070
International Association of Cancer Victors and
    Friends, 2404
International Skeletal Dysplasia Registry Medical
    Genetics Institute, 4052
Jane & Terry Semel Institute for Neuroscie nce &
    Human Behavior, 6032
Jodi House, 4149
John Douglas French Alzheimer's Foundation, 756
John Tracy Clinic, 4318
John Tracy Clinic on Deafness, 4415
Jonsson Comprehensive Cancer Center University of
    California At Los Angeles, 2278
Juvenile Diabetes Research Foundation: Bakersfield
    Chapter, 3225
Juvenile Diabetes Research Foundation: Inl and
    Empire Chapter, 3226
Juvenile Diabetes Research Foundation: Los Angeles
    Chapter, 3227
Juvenile Diabetes Research Foundation: Nor thern
    California Inland Chapter, 3228
Juvenile Diabetes Research Foundation: Ora nge
    County Chapter, 3229
Juvenile Diabetes Research Foundation: San Diego
    Chapter, 3230
Juvenile Scleroderma Network, 7357
Kaiser Foundation Research Institute, 374
LAC/USC Imaging Science Center, 4026
Langley Porter Psychiatric Institute University of
    California, 6033
Leukemia & Lymphoma Society: Orange, Riverside,
    And San Bernadino Counties, 2135
Leukemia and Lymphoma Society: Greater Los
    Angeles Chapter, 2138
Leukemia and Lymphoma Society: Greater
    Sacramento Area Chapter, 2137
Leukemia and Lymphoma Society: Northern
    California Chapter, 2139
Leukemia and Lymphoma Society: Orange, Riverside,
    And San Bernadino Counties, 2140
Leukemia and Lymphoma Society: San Diego/Hawaii
    Chapter, 2136
Leukemia and Lymphoma Society: Tri-County
    Chapter, 2141
LifeSharing Community Organ & Tissue Donation,
    9180
Lighthouse for the Blind and Visually Impaired, 9472
Lilliput Families, 5379
Little People of America, 4045
Loma Linda University Sleep Disorders Clinic, 7773
Los Angeles Alliance Against Parkinson's Disease,
    6875
Los Angeles Chapter of the American Association of
    Kidney Patients, 5586
Los Angeles Orthopaedic Hospital, 5039
Los Angeles Support Group: National Ataxia
    Foundation, 1528

Lupus Foundation of America: California Chapter,
    8859
Marijuana Anonymous World Services, 8121
Marin Institute, 8212
MedicAlert Foundation International, 10394
Memorial Miller Children's Hospital Cystic Fibrosis
    Center, 3095
NAMI California, 5932
Narcotics Anonymous World Services, 8124
National Association to Advance Fat Acceptance
    (NAAFA), 6710
National Eczema Association, 640
National Eczema Association, 7663
National Federation of the Blind in Computer
    Science, 9443
National Federation of the Blind: California, 9473
National Federation of the Blind: Science and
    Engineering Division, 9447
National Fibromyalgia Association, 3863
National Health Federation, 2142
National Hepatitis C Coalition, 5144
National Hydrocephalus Foundation, 5198
National Kidney Foundation of Northern California,
    5587
National Kidney Foundation of Southern California,
    5588
National Multiple Sclerosis Society Channel Islands
    Chapter, 6352
National Multiple Sclerosis Society: Silicon Valley
    Chapter, 6353
National Multiple Sclerosis Society: Southern
    California Chapter, 6351
National Parkinson Foundation: California Office,
    6876
National Parkinson Foundation: Orange County
    Chapter, 6877
National Spinal Cord Injury Association: Los Angeles
    Chapter, 7966
National Spinal Cord Injury Association: San Diego
    County Chapter, 7965
Neuro-Oncology Information and Support Group,
    1936
Neurofibromatosis Support Network, 6687
Neuroscience Institute Brain Tumor Hotline, 1937
Neurosciences Institute of the Neurosciences
    Research Program, 972
New Beginnings: The Blind Children's Cente, 9798
New Beginnings: The Blind Children's Center, 9797
Northern California Association of Persian Gulf
    Veterans, 10114
Northern California Chapter National Multiple
    Sclerosis Society, 6354
Northern California Support Group: National Ataxia
    Foundation, 1529
Northern California Turner Syndrome Resource
    Group, 9344
Northstate Parkinson's Chapter, 6878
Northwest Regional Training Center: Canine
    Companions for Independence, 9474
Okizu Foundation Camps, 10523
One Legacy Transplant Donor Network, 9181
Orange County Chapter National Multiple Sclerosis
    Society, 6355
Orange County Support Group: National Ataxia
    Foundation, 1530
Osteoporosis Center Memorial Hospital/Advanced
    Medical Diagn, 6815
Pacific AIDS Education and Training Center
    (PAETC), 293
Pacific AIDS Education and Training Center
    (PAETC), 375
Parents Helping Parents A Family Resource Center,
    8815
Parkinson Association of the Sacramento Valley, 6879
Parkinson Network of Mount Diablo, 6880
Parkinson's Disease Association of San Die go
    (PDASD), 6912
Parkinson's Institute and Clinical Center, 6873
Parkinson's Resource Organization, 6907
Patient Services, 1938
Pediatric Brain Tumor Foundation: California
    Chapter, 1907
Pediatric Cancer Research Laboratory Children's
    Hospital of Orange County, 2279

Peninsula Support & Education Group for Parents of Children with Brain Tumors, 1939
Polio Survivors Association, 7012
Positive Women's Network - USA, 275
Prader-Willi California Foundation, 7168
Preventive Medicine Research Institute, 4893
Project Inform, 276
Project Inform Hiv Health InfoLine, 454
Prostate Cancer Foundation, 2262
RESOLVE of Greater Los Angeles, 5385
RESOLVE of Greater San Diego, 5386
RESOLVE of Northern California, 5387
RRTC on Aging with a Disability Los Amigos Research and Education Instit, 7985
Rebecca and John Moores UCSD Cancer Center, 2280
Redding Chapter of the American Association of Kidney Patients, 5589
Region 6 of the National Association for Parents of the Visually Impaired, 9469
Regional Cancer Foundation, 2143
Research Institute of Palo Alto Medical Foundation, 663
Rosalind Russell Medical Research Center for Arthritis at UCSF, 1254
Rose Kushner Breast Cancer Advisory Center, 2144
SIDS Alliance Of Northern California, 8712
SIDS Foundation of Southern California, 8713
Sacramento Valley Chapter of the American Association of Kidney Patients, 5590
Sacramento Veterans Center, 10115
Salk Institute Cancer Center, 2281
San Diego Area Chapter National Multiple Sclerosis Society, 6356
San Diego Support Group: National Ataxia Foundation, 1531
San Francisco AIDS Foundation (SFAF), 294
San Francisco Clinical Research Center, 6294
San Francisco Community Health Center: HHOME/GTZ-ICM, 295
San Francisco Heart & Vascular Institute, 4896
San Francisco Public Library for the Blind and Print Disabled, 9623
San Francisco VA Medical Center, 10116
San Jose State University Library, 9624
Sansum Diabetes Research Institute, 3390
Santa Barbara Breast Cancer Institute, 2282
Scleroderma Foundation: Greater San Diego Chapter, 7330
Scleroderma Foundation: Northern California Chapter, 7331
Scleroderma Foundation: Southern California Chapter, 7332
Scleroderma Research Foundation, 7365
Scripps Clinic Sleep Disorders Center Scripps Clinic, 7780
Scripps Clinic and Research Foundation: Autoimmune Disease Center, 7675
Scripps Research Institute, 664
Sleep Disorders Center at California: Paci, 7789
Sleep Disorders Center at California: Pacific Medical Center, 7788
Sleep Disorders Center of Metropolitan Toronto, 7790
Smith-Kettlewell Eye Research Institute, 9458
Smith-Kettlewell Eye Research Institute, 9801
Society of American Gastrointestinal Endoscopic Surgeons, 3929
Society of Hearing Impaired Physicians, 4332
Solve ME/CFS Initiative, 2830
Southern California Research Institute, 8226
Southwest Regional Training Center: Canine Companions for Independence, 9475
Spina Bifida Association of Greater San Diego, 7867
Spinal Cord Injury Network International, 7960
Stanford CF Center Packard Children's Hospital At Stanford, 3096
Stanford Center for Research in Disease Prevention, 8227
Stanford Center on Longevity, 133
Stanford University Center for Narcolepsy Dept of Psychiatry & Behavioral Sciences, 7814
Stanford University General Clinical Research Center, 376
Stanford University National Cooperative Drug Discovery/AIDS Group, 377

Stanford University: Beckman Center for Molecular and Genetic Medicine, 2283
Starlight Children's Foundation, 10676
Starlight Children's Foundation, 10688
Stein Institute for Research on Aging UC San Diego School of Medicine, 134
Support Group for Caregivers of Brain Tumor Patients, 1940
Support Group for Parents of Children with Brain Tumors, 1945
Synergy Clinical Research Center, 7084
The Center for Culture, Trauma and Mental Health Disparities, 7085
The Sam and Rose Stein Institute for Research on the Aging, 976
Tripod, 4334
UCD Northern Central California Hemophilia Program, 5065
UCLA AIDS Clinical Research Center, 378
UCLA Anxiety Disorders Research Center, 7086
UCLA Neuropsychiatric Institute, 4138
UCSD Antiviral Research Center, 379
UCSD Comprehensive Hemophilia Treatment Center, 5066
UCSF Children's Hospital Health Library, 3594
USC Internal Medicine, 380
USC/Norris Comprehensive Cancer Center, 2284
USC: Neonatology Research Units, 8812
United Advocates for Children of California, 5933
United Cerebral Palsy of Central California, 2684
United Cerebral Palsy of Greater Sacramento, 2685
United Cerebral Palsy of Los Angeles & Ventura Counties, 2686
United Cerebral Palsy of Orange County, 2687
United Cerebral Palsy of San Diego County, 2688
United Cerebral Palsy of San Joaquin, Calaveras & Amador Counties, 2689
United Cerebral Palsy of San Luis Obispo, 2690
United Cerebral Palsy of Santa Barbara County, 2691
United Cerebral Palsy of Santa Clara & San Mateo Counties, 2692
United Cerebral Palsy of Stanislaus County, 2693
United Cerebral Palsy of the Golden Gate, 2694
United Cerebral Palsy of the Inland Empire, 2695
United Cerebral Palsy of the North Bay, 2696
United Organ Transplant Association (UOTA), 9174
University of California Berkeley Cancer Research Laboratory, 2285
University of California Liver Research Unit, 5768
University of California San Diego General Clinical Research Center, 4900
University of California San Francisco Center for AIDS Prevention, 381
University of California at San Francisco Women's Continence Center, 5341
University of California, San Francisco Brain Tumor Research Center, 1913
University of California: Cardiovascular Research Laboratory, 4901
University of California: Davis Gastroenterology & Nutrition Center, 3943
University of California: Institute of Health Policy Studies, 382
University of California: Irvine Brain Imaging Center, 4139
University of California: Los Angeles Alcohol Research Center, 8229
University of California: Los Angeles Bone Marrow Transplantation Program, 2286
University of California: Los Angeles Center for Ulcer Research, 3944
University of California: San Francisco Dermatology Drug Research, 7678
University of California: San Francisco Laboratory for Neurotrauma, 4140
University of California: UCLA Population Research Center, 5437
University of Southern California: Comprehensive Sickle Cell Center, 7622
University of Southern California: Coronary Care Research, 4910
University of Southern California: Division of Nephrology, 5260
VA Central California Health Care System, 10117
VA Greater Los Angeles Healthcare System, 10118

VA Loma Linda Healthcare System, 10119
VA Northern California Health Care System, 10120
VA Palo Alto Health Care System, 10121
Veterans Medical Center: Mental Health Clinical Research Center, 6045
Vital Options International, 1941
Wellness Community Cancer Support Groups, 1942
Wellness Community: South Bay Cities, 1943
Wellness Community: West Los Angeles, 1944
Wish Upon A Star, 10678
Women Alive, 283
Women's Suffrage for Prostate Cancer Awareness, 2416
World Institute on Disability, 10429

Canada

AIDS Coalition of Cape Breton, 239
AIDS Committee of Durham Region, 240
AIDS Committee of North Bay & Area, 241
AIDS Committee of Ottawa, 242
AIDS Committee of Toronto, 243
AIDS Committee of York Region, 244
AIDS New Brunswick, 245
ALEH Rehabilitation of Canada, 3574
ANKORS: Kootenay & Boundary HIV/AIDS and Hepatitis C Support Services, 248
Action Autonomie, 5903
Active Healthy Kids Canada, 6708
Alberta Reappraising AIDS Society, 250
Alzheimer Society of Alberta and Northwest Territories, 743
Alzheimer Society of B.C., 744
Alzheimer Society of Canada, 745
Alzheimer Society of Manitoba, 746
Alzheimer Society of New Brunswick, 747
Alzheimer Society of Newfoundland & Labrador, 748
Alzheimer Society of Nova Scotia, 749
Alzheimer Society of Ontario, 750
Alzheimer Society of Prince Edward Island, 751
Alzheimer Society of Saskatchewan, 752
Arthritis & Autoimmunity Research Centre, 1188
Asthma Canada, 632
Asthma Canada, 1377
Ataxia Canada - Claude St-Jean Foundation, 1520
Black Coalition for AIDS Prevention, 254
Brain Tumor Foundation of Canada, 1904
Breast Cancer Society of Canada, 2095
Bulimia Anorexia Nervosa Association, 3671
Canadian & American Spinal Research Organizations, 7861
Canadian ADHD Resource Alliance, 1601
Canadian Addison Society, 3
Canadian Adult Congenital Heart Network, 4861
Canadian Cancer Society, 2097
Canadian Celiac Association, 2627
Canadian Cerebral Palsy Sports Association, 2667
Canadian Dermatology Association, 7325
Canadian Down Syndrome Society, 3538
Canadian Fabry Association, 3834
Canadian Foundation for AIDS Research, 353
Canadian Hard of Hearing Association, 4300
Canadian National Seniors Council, 25
Canadian Pain Society, 2912
Canadian Society of Allergy and Clinical Immunology, 634
Canadian Society of Allergy and Clinical Immunology, 1379
Childhood Cancer Canada, 2100
Children's Heart Society, 4862
Children's Wish Foundation of Canada, 10683
Christian Horizons, 10367
Chronic Pain Association of Canada, 2913
Colorectal Cancer Canada, 2102
Cystic Fibrosis Canada, 3084
Elevate NWO, 258
Federation of Quebec Alzheimer Societies, 755
Fondation quebecoise du sida, 356
HIV West Yellowhead Services, 259
Heart and Stroke Foundation of Canada, 8048
Institute for Life Course and Aging, 31
Inter-Provincial Roof Consultants, Ltd., 5143
International Federation on Ageing, 32
Jessie's Legacy, 3677

Juvenile Diabetes Research Foundation Cana da, 3368
March of Dimes Canada, 8049
Muscular Dystrophy Canada, 6511
National Eating Disorder Information Centr e, 3681
National Eating Disorder Information Centr e Helpline, 3719
National Gaucher Foundation of Canada, 4023
National ME/FM Action Network, 2828
National ME/FM Action Network, 3865
Neurofibromatosis Society of Ontario, 6655
Obesity Canada, 6711
Ontario HIV Treatment Network, 270
PEERS Alliance, 271
Positive Living Niagara, 274
Post-Polio Awareness & Support Society of British Columbia, 7013
Regional HIV/AIDS Connection, 277
Reseau ACCESS Network, 278
Rethink Breast Cancer, 2112
Rick Hansen Foundation, 7959
Scleroderma Society of Ontario, 7328
Sickle Cell Association of Ontario, 7605
Spina Bifida and Hydrocephalus Association of Canada, 7864
Sunshine Dreams for Kids, 10689
Thyroid Federation International, 9005
Thyroid Foundation of Canada, 9006
Tourette Syndrome Foundation of Canada, 9082
Turner Syndrome Society of Canada, 9343
Turning Point Society of Central Alberta, 281
World Endometriosis Society, 3797
World Federation of Hemophilia, 4965

Colorado

AARP Colorado, 49
ALS Association: Rocky Mountain Chapter, 1100
AMC Cancer Research Center, 2287
Alcohol and Drug Abuse Division Department of Human Services, 8143
Alzheimer's Association: Greater Grand Junction Area Chapter, 782
Alzheimer's Association: Rocky Mountain Chapter, 783
American Cancer Society: Colorado, 2145
American Diabetes Association: Denver, 3231
American Homes for the Aging: Western, 784
American Liver Foundation Rocky Mountain Division, 5748
American Lung Association of Colorado, 5822
American Lung Association of Colorado, 9268
Americas Association for the Care of the Children, 2093
Americas Association for the Care of the Children, 10351
Arthritis Foundation: Rocky Mountain Chapter, 1198
Autism Society of Colorado, 1673
Barbara Davis Center for Childhood Diabetes, 3377
Boulder Public Library, 9625
Brain Injury Association of Colorado, 4085
Brain Injury Association of Colorado Helpline, 4150
Brain Tumor Resource and Vital Encouragement, 1946
CCFA Rocky Mountain Chapter, 3004
Centers for AIDS Research: University of Colorado Health Sciences Center, 383
Colorado Brain Tumor Support Group, 1947
Colorado Cancer Research Program, 2288
Colorado Chapter National Hemophilia Foun dation, 4972
Colorado Chapter of the American Association of Kidney Patients, 5591
Colorado FFCMH, 5934
Colorado Parkinson Foundation, 6881
Colorado SIDS Program, 8714
Colorado Talking Book Library, 9626
Colordao Department of Health and Environment, 8715
Denver Childrens Hospital, 3097
Denver Support Group: National Ataxia Foundation, 1532
Disability Careers, 10435
Donor Alliance, 9182

FFCMH: Denver/Aurora Chapter, 5935
Hands & Voices, 4307
International Hearing Dog, 4316
Jimmie Heuga Center, 6432
Juvenile Diabetes Research Foundation: Colorado Springs Chapter, 3232
Juvenile Diabetes Research Foundation: Roc ky Mountain Chapter, 3233
Laradon Services for Children and Adults w ith Developmental Disabilities, 6051
Legal Center for People with Disabilities and Older People, 10436
Little Star Foundation, 10687
Lung Facts, 5874
Lupus Foundation of Colorado, 8860
Mile High Down Syndrome Association, 3556
NNFF Colorado Chapter, 6659
National Alliance for the Mentally Ill of Colorado, 5936
National Association of Blind Lawyers, 9434
National Federation of the Blind: Colorado, 9476
National Jewish Center for Immunology, 5870
National Jewish Center for Immunology and Respiratory Medicine, 662
National Jewish Division of Immunology, 1404
National Jewish Health, 5812
National Kidney Foundation of Colorado, Idaho, Montana, and Wyoming, 5606
National Kidney Foundation of Colorado/Idaho/Montana/Wyoming, 5622
National Kidney Foundation of Colorado/Idaho/Montana/Wyoming, 5660
National Kidney Foundation of Colorado: Idaho, Montana, and Wyoming, 5592
National MS Society: Colorado Chapter, 6357
National Native American AIDS Prevention Center, 269
National Stroke Association, 5251
Neurofibromatosis Foundation: Colorado, 6686
No. Colorado FFCMH, 5937
Prader-Willi Colorado Association, 7169
RESOLVE of Colorado, 5388
Rocky Mountain CFIDS/FMS Association, 3870
Scleroderma Foundation: Colorado Chapter, 7333
Spina Bifida Association of Colorado, 7868
Turner Syndrome Colorado, 9345
United Cerebral Palsy of Colorado, 2697
United States Association for Blind Athletes, 9460
University of Colorado Cancer Center, 2289
University of Colorado: General Clinical Research Center, Pediatric, 3392
VA Western Colorado Health Care System, 10122
Western Slope Chapter of the American Association of Kidney Patients, 5593

Connecticut

AARP Connecticut, 50
ALS Association: Connecticut Chapter, 1101
Alzheimer's Association: Connecticut Chapter, 785
Alzheimer's Association: South Central Connecticut Chapter, 786
American Cancer Society: Connecticut, 2146
American Diabetes Association: Connecticut, 3234
American Liver Foundation: Connecticut Chapter, 5749
American Lung Association of Connecticut, 5823
American Lung Association of Connecticut, 9269
American Lyme Disease Foundation, 9023
American Lyme Disease Foundation, 9032
Arthritis Foundation: Southern New England Chapter, 1199
Arthritis Foundation: Southern New England Chapter, 1230
Brain Injury Association of Connecticut, 4086
Brain Injury Association of Connecticut Helpline, 4151
CCFA Central Connecticut Chapter, 3005
CCFA Northern Connecticut Affiliate Chapter, 3006
Chapel Haven, 10504
Connecticut Alcohol and Drug Abuse Commission, 8144
Connecticut Brain Tumor Support Group, 1948

Connecticut Chapter of the Myasthenia Gravis Foundation of America, 6575
Connecticut Chapter of the Myasthenia Gravis Foundation of America, 6583
Connecticut Chapter of the Myasthenia Gravis Foundation of America, 6595
Connecticut Chapter of the Myasthenia Gravis Foundation of America, 6598
Connecticut Department of Health Services AIDS Programs, 297
Connecticut Down Syndrome Congress, 3557
Connecticut Pregnancy Exposure Information Service, 1852
Connecticut SIDS Alliance, 8716
Connecticut State Library for the Blind and Physically Handicapped, 9627
Cornelia de Lange Syndrome Foundation, Inc, 1834
Exceptional Cancer Patients/ECaP, 2398
Families United For CMH, Inc., 5938
Favarh, 10376
Fidelco Guide Dog Foundation, 9423
First Candle, 8700
Global Lyme Alliance, 9024
HonorBound Foundation, 10103
International Lawyers in Alcoholics Anonymous, 8245
Juvenile Diabetes Research Foundation: Fai rfield County Chapter, 3236
Juvenile Diabetes Research Foundation: Greater New Haven Chapter, 3235
Juvenile Diabetes Research Foundation: Nor th Central CT and Western MA, 3237
Leukemia and Lymphoma Society: Connecticut Chapter, 2147
Leukemia and Lymphoma Society: Fairfield County Chapter, 2148
Lupus Foundation of America: Connecticut Chapter, 8861
Motor Neuron Disease Clinic University of Connecticut Health Center, 1142
Myasthenia Gravis Support Group of Connect icut (Nutmeg Group), 6604
NNFF Connecticut Chapter, 6660
National Alliance for the Mentally Ill of Connecticut, 5939
National Federation of the Blind: Connecticut, 9477
National Kidney Foundation of Connecticut, 5594
National MS Society: Greater Connecticut Chapter, 6358
National Organization for Rare Disorders, 3838
National Organization for Rare Disorders, 4021
National Organization for Rare Disorders, 8703
National Organization for Rare Disorders, 8970
National Organization for Rare Disorders, 10410
National Spinal Cord Injury Association: Connecticut Chapter, 7967
National Veterans Services Fund, 10277
NorthEast Organ Procurement Organization, 9183
Office of Protection and Advocacy for Persons with Disabilities, 10437
Prader-Willi Connecticut Association, 7170
Prevent Blindness Tri-State, 9478
RESOLVE of Fairfield County, 5389
RESOLVE of Greater Hartford, 5390
Raynaud's Association, 7223
Raynaud's Association, 7326
Reflex Sympathetic Dystrophy Syndrome Association (RSDSA), 2918
Renfrew Center of Connecticut, 3690
SIDS Program: Connecticut Department of Health, 8717
Spina Bifida Association of Connecticut, 7869
Sudden Infant Death Syndrome (SIDS) Network, 8705
Terri Gotthelf Lupus Research Institute, 8929
Tourette Syndrome Clinic Yale Child Study Center, 9084
United Cerebral Palsy of Eastern Connecticut, 2698
United Cerebral Palsy of Greater Hartford, 2699
United Cerebral Palsy of Southern Connecticut, 2700
University of Connecticut Center on Aging, 139
University of Connecticut Health Center, 3098
University of Connecticut Osteoporosis Center, 6817
Yale Child Study Center, 7087
Yale University Comprehensive Cancer Center, 2290

Yale University Cystic Fibrosis Research Center, 3099
Yale University: Behavioral Medicine Clinic, 6204
Yale University: Ribicoff Research Facilities/CT Mental Health Center, 6205
Yale University: Vision Research Center, 9807

Delaware

AARP Delaware, 51
Alliance for the Mentally Ill in Delaware (AMID), 5940
Alzheimer's Association: Delaware Chapter, 787
American Cancer Society: Delaware, 2149
American Diabetes Association: Delaware, 3238
American Lung Association of Delaware, 5824
American Lung Association of Delaware, 9270
Brain Injury Association of Delaware, 4087
Brain Injury Association of Delaware Helpl ine, 4152
Client Assistance Program: Delaware, 10438
Delaware Assocation for the Blind Department of Health & Social Services, 9479
Delaware Department of Health and Social: Services HIV Prevention Program, 298
Delaware Division of Alcoholism, Drug Abuse and Mental Health, 8145
Delaware Division of Libraries: Library for the Blind and Physically Handicapped, 9628
Delaware FFMCH, 5941
Juvenile Diabetes Research Foundation: Del aware, 3239
Leukemia and Lymphoma Society: Delaware Chapter, 2150
Lupus Foundation of America: Delaware Chapter, 8862
Mental Health Association of Delaware, 5942
National Federation of the Blind: Delaware, 9480
National MS Society: Delaware Chapter, 6359
Pediatric Brain Tumor Support Group, 1949
Prader-Willi Delaware Association, 7171
SIDS Information & Counseling: Division of Public Health, 8718
Sarcoidosis Support Group Delaware, 7249
Spina Bifida Association of Delaware, 7870
United Cerebral Palsy of Delaware, 2701
Wilmington VA Medical Center, 10123

District of Columbia

AAA Foundation for Traffic Safety, 8105
AARP Foundation, 108
AARP Washington DC, 52
ABA Commission on Law and Aging, 22
AIDS United, 246
ALS Association National Office, 1088
Academy for Gerontology in Higher Education, 23
Academy for Gerontology in Higher Education, 113
Administration for Children and Families, 1370
Administration for Children and Families, 3536
Administration for Children and Families, 3669
Administration for Children and Families, 4288
Administration for Children and Families, 5728
Administration for Children and Families, 7031
Administration for Children and Families, 7462
Administration for Community Living, 7059
Agent Orange Registry Department of Veterans Affairs, 10100
Alliance for Aging Research, 9405
Alzheimer's Association: Greater Washington DC Chapter, 788
American Academy of Child and Adolescent Psychiatry (AACAP), 5904
American Academy of Child and Adolescent Psychiatry (AACAP), 7035
American Association for the Advancement of Science, 10338
American Association of People with Disabilities, 10339
American Association of Retired Persons, 24
American Bar Association Commission on Mental and Physical Disability Law, 10341
American Cancer Society: District of Columbia, 2151

American Diabetes Association: District of Columbia, 3240
American Hellenic Educational Progressive Association, 2956
American Institute for Cancer Research, 2152
American Institute for Cancer Research, 2390
American Institutes for Research Center on Aging, 114
American Lung Association of Washington, 9271
American Lung Association of the District of Columbia, 5825
American Lung Association of the District of Columbia, 9272
American Psychiatric Association, 5906
American Psychiatric Association, 6193
American Psychiatric Association, 7038
American Psychological Association, 5907
American Psychological Association, 7039
American Public Health Association (APHA), 7040
American Red Cross Blood Services, 4959
American Red Cross Hemophilia Center, 5015
American Red Cross National Headquarters, 10348
American Sleep Apnea Association, 7758
American Society for Bone and Mineral Research, 6781
American Society of Hematology, 2957
American Tinnitus Association, 4298
Arthritis Foundation: Metropolitan Washington Chapter, 1200
Autism Society of District Columbia, 1674
Better Breather's Clubs, 7239
Brain Research Center Children s Hospital National Medical Cen, 1909
Caregiver Action Network, 147
Caregiver Action Network, 10512
Center for Mind-Body Medicine, 7088
Center for Science in the Public Interest, 2153
Children's AIDS Fund International, 256
Children's National Medical Center, 10366
Children's Rights Program, 4412
Clearinghouse on Disability Information Office of Special Education & Rehab Svcs, 10368
Client Assistance Program: District of Columbia, 10439
Columbia Lighthouse for the Blind, 9481
Council of Families with Visual Impairment, 9629
DC Department of Health Maternal and Family Health Administration, 8719
DC Public Library Adaptive Services Division, 9630
DC Threshold Alliance for the Mentally Ill, 5943
Department of Health and Human Services, 8720
Digestive Disease National Coalition, 3924
Disabled American Veterans Organization, 10124
Distance Education and Training Council, 10371
District of Columbia Public Library Librarian for the Deaf Community, 9606
ERIC Clearinghouse on Disabilities and Gifted Education, 10505
Eating Disorders Coalition for Research, Policy and Action, 3675
Elizabeth Glaser Pediatric AIDS Foundation, 355
Endocrine Society, 4
Equal Opportunity Employment Commission, 10373
Family Advocacy and Support Association, 5944
Federal Emergency Management Agency, 7060
Food Safety and Inspection Service, 638
Gallaudet University: Center for Auditory and Speech Sciences, 4377
Genetic Alliance, 1726
Genetic Alliance, 4043
Genetic Alliance, 10379
George Washington National Cooperative: Drug Discovery/AIDS Treatment, 385
George Washington University Center for Aging, Health and Humanities, 119
Georgetown University Center for Hypertension and Renal Disease Research, 5595
Georgetown University Child Development Center, 1840
Georgetown University Hospital Transplant Institute, 9227
Georgetown University Hospital: Department of Rheumatology, 7360
Georgetown University: Vincent T Lombardi Cancer Research Center, 2291

Gerontological Society of America, 28
HEATH Resource Center, 1610
HEATH Resource Center, 10381
Health Planning and Development, 8146
Hearing Industries Association, 4312
Hemophilia Treatment Center at Children's National Medical Center, 5038
Howard University Cancer Center, 2292
Howard University Center for Sickle Cell Disease, 7615
Information Protection & Advocacy Center for Handicapped Individuals, 10440
International Association for the Study of Pain, 2914
International Association for the Study of Pain, 10385
International Council on Disability, 10386
International Pelvic Pain Society, 2915
International Pelvic Pain Society, 3795
International Society for the Study of Trauma and Dissociation, 6256
International Society for the Study of Trauma and Dissociation, 7049
Juvenile Diabetes Research Foundation: Cap itol Chapter, 3241
Leading Age, 33
Library Services to the Deaf Community, 4366
Listening and Spoken Knowledge Center, 4367
Listening and Spoken Language Knowledge Ce nter, 4319
Lung Cancer Alliance Support Group, 2407
Lupus Foundation of America, 8853
Lupus Foundation of America: DC, Maryland and Central & Northern Virginia, 8881
Medstar Georgetown University Hospital Facility, 4889
Melanoma Research Foundation, 2293
Metropolitan DC Cystic Fibrosis Center Children s Hospital National Medical Cen, 3100
National Academy on an Aging Society, 128
National Alliance for Hispanic Health, 5914
National Association for Home Care, 10519
National Association for Home Care and Hospice, 10695
National Association of Councils on Developmental Disabilities, 10396
National Association of Epilepsy Centers, 7468
National Association of Social Workers (NASW), 7051
National Association of Special Education Teachers, 2958
National Center for Education in Maternal and Child Health, 8701
National Center for Learning Disabilities, 1608
National Center for Victims of Crime, 7072
National Council for Aging Care, 36
National Council for Behavioral Health, 5917
National Council on Disability, 10400
National Council on Independent Living, 10401
National Endowment for the Arts: Office for Accessability, 10403
National Fabry Disease Foundation, 3840
National Federation of the Blind: DC, 9482
National Institute for Occupational Safety and Health, 642
National Institute for Occupational Safety and Health, 1384
National Institute for Occupational Safety and Health, 3549
National Institute for Occupational Safety and Health, 3684
National Institute for Occupational Safety and Health, 5738
National Institute for Occupational Safety and Health, 7471
National Institute of Disability and Rehabilitation Research, 10406
National Institute of Food and Agriculture, 646
National Kidney Foundation of the National Capital Area, 5596
National Library Service for the Blind and Physically Handicapped, 9450
National Library Service for the Blind and Physically Handicapped, 9631
National MS Society: National Capital Chapter, 6360
National Organization on Fetal Alcohol Syndrome, 8130

National Osteoporosis Foundation (NOF), 6819
National Parent Network on Disabilities, 10412
National Sleep Foundation, 7761
National Treatment Consortium for Alcohol and Other Drugs, 8216
National Women's Health Network, 3796
National Women's Health Network, 5380
Nurse Practitioners in Women's Health, 6812
Occupational Safety & Health Administration (OSHA), 9260
Office of Civil Rights, 10415
Office of Policy Planning and Legislation, 10416
Office of Special Education Programs, 10417
Office of Women's Health, 3686
PXE International, 9820
Paralyzed Veterans of America, 7958
Pediatric Neurology Georgetown University Hospital, 10420
People-to-People Committee for the Handicapped, 10421
President's Committee on the Employment of People with Disabilities, 10422
Project Eyes and Ears, 4417
Rape, Abuse & Incest National Network, 7115
Region III Office Program: Consultants for Maternal and Child Health, 8721
Region IV Office Program Consultants for Maternal and Child Health, 8722
Region IX Office Program Consultants for Maternal and Child Health, 8723
Region VIII Office Program Consultants for Maternal and Child Health, 8724
Rehabilitation Engineering on Hearing Enhancement, 4386
Rehabilitation Services Administration, 10424
Sarcoidosis Support Group: Washington DC, 7251
Scottish Rite Center for Childhood Language Disorders, 4389
Shiloh Senior Center for the Hearing Impaired, 4340
Staunton Public Library: Talking Book Center, 9761
Students Against Destructive Decisions, 8135
The ARC of the United States, 3553
The International Alliance of ALS/MND Associations, 1090
U.S. Department of Health and Human Services, 7061
US Administration on Aging, 42
US Department Of Veterans Affairs, 10125
US Department of Justice, 10426
US Department of Transportation, 10427
US Environmental Protection Agency: Indoor Environments Division, 5815
US Office of Personnel Management, 10428
United Cerebral Palsy Associations, 2672
United Cerebral Palsy of Washington DC, 2702
United Cerebral Palsy of Washington DC & Northern Virginia, 2703
Visiting Nurse Association of America, 10528
Washington Connection, 9824
Washington DC Department of Health: HIV/AIDS, Hepatitis, STD and TB Admin., 299
Washington DC Metropolitan Area Support Group, 1950
Washington DC VA Medical Center, 10126
Whitman Walker Clinic AIDS/Medical Services Programs, 386

Florida

AARP Florida: Doral, 53
AARP Florida: St. Petersburg, 54
AARP Florida: Tallahassee, 55
ALS Association: Florida Chapter, 1103
Alcohol and Drug Abuse Program Department Of Children And Families, 8147
Alzheimer's Association: Broward County Chapter, 789
Alzheimer's Association: East Central Florida Chapter, 790
Alzheimer's Association: Florida Gulf Coast Chapter, 791
Alzheimer's Association: Greater Miami Chapter, 792
Alzheimer's Association: Greater Orlando Area Chapter, 793

Alzheimer's Association: Greater Palm Beach Area Chapter, 794
Alzheimer's Association: Northeast Florida, 795
Alzheimer's Association: Northern Central Florida Chapter, 796
Alzheimer's Association: Northwest Florida Chapter, 797
Alzheimer's Association: Southwest Florida Chapter, 798
Alzheimer's Association: Tampa Bay Chapter, 799
Alzheimer's Association: Volusia/Flagler Branch, 800
Alzheimer's Association: West Central Florida Chapter, 801
Alzheimer/Parkinson Association of Indian River County, 6882
American Association of Caregiving Youth, 146
American Association of Kidney Patients, 5577
American Association of Kidney Patients, 5597
American Cancer Society: Florida, 2154
American Diabetes Association: Northeast Florida/Southeast Georgia, 3242
American Diabetes Association: Seattle, 3243
American Diabetes Association: South Coast Regional/Central Florida, 3244
American Hemochromatosis Society, 3918
American Liver Foundation Gulf Coast Chapter, 5750
American Lung Association of Florida, 5826
American Lung Association of Florida, 9273
American SIDS Institute, 8698
American Society of Dermatology, 10350
Angels in the Sun Brain Tumor Support Group, 1951
Arthritis Foundation: Florida Chapter, Gulf Coast Branch, 1201
Autism Society of Florida, 1675
BASE Camp Children's Cancer Foundation, 10655
Bay Pines VA Healthcare System, 10127
Birth Defect Research for Children, Inc., 633
Birth Defect Research for Children, Inc., 1378
Birth Defect Research for Children, Inc., 1825
Brain Injury Association of Florida, 4088
Brain Injury Association of Florida, 4153
Brain Tumor Support Group, 1952
Brave Kids, 4027
Brevard County Libraries: Talking Books Library, 9632
Broward County Talking Book Library, 9633
CCFA Florida Chapter, 3007
Center for the Study of Emotion and Attention, 7089
Central Florida Chapter, 6361
Chef David's Kids, 10682
Children's Medical Services Program: Florida SIDS Program, 8725
Choices for Work Program Goodwill Industries-Suncoast, 4089
Coconut Creek Eating Disorders Support Group, 3713
Comprehensive Pediatric Hemophilia Center University of South Florida, 5022
Cystic Fibrosis Center: All Children's Hospital, 3101
Department of Epidemiology and Health Policy Research: University of Florida, 387
Desert Storm Justice Foundation: Florida, 10128
Desert Storm Veterans of Florida, Inc., 10129
Disability Rights: Florida, 10441
Dreams Come True, 10684
Endometriosis Research Center and Women's Hospital, 3802
Endometriosis Research Center, 3793
Endometriosis Research Center, 3803
Epilepsy Association of Big Bend, 7478
Epilepsy Foundation of South Florida, 7479
Epilepsy Services Foundation, 7480
Epilepsy Services of North Central Florida, 7481
Epilepsy Services of Northeast Florida, 7482
Epilepsy Services of Southwest Florida, 7483
Florida Alliance for the Mentally Ill, 5945
Florida Ambassador: National Ataxia Foundation, 1533
Florida Association of the Deaf, 4341
Florida Brain Tumor Association, 1953
Florida Brain Tumor Support Group, 1954
Florida Brain Tumor Support Group: Deerfield Beach, 1955
Florida Bureau of Braille and Talking Book Library Services, 9634

Florida Chapter of the Myasthenia Gravis Foundation of America, 6578
Florida Department of Health, 8726
Florida Department of Health: HIV/AIDS Section, 300
Florida Disabled Outdoor Association, 10378
Florida FFCMH: Tampa Chapter, 5946
Florida Gulf Coast Chapter National Multiple Sclerosis Society, 6362
Florida Heart Research Institute, 4877
Florida Hemophilia Association, 4973
Florida Institute for Family Involvement (FIFI), 6052
Florida Ophthalmic Institute, 9787
Florida SIDS Alliance, 8727
Gilda's Club: South Florida, 2402
Give Kids the World Village, 10664
Gold Coast Down Syndrome Organization, 3558
Goodwill Industries-Suncoast, 56
Goodwill Industries-Suncoast, 1609
Goodwill Industries-Suncoast, 1676
Goodwill Industries-Suncoast, 1833
Goodwill Industries-Suncoast, 3559
Goodwill Industries-Suncoast, 4047
Goodwill Industries-Suncoast, 5947
Goodwill Industries-Suncoast, 7062
Goodwill Industries-Suncoast, 9083
Goodwill Industries-Suncoast, 10130
Goodwill Industries-Suncoast, 10442
Greater Daytona Area Parkinson Support Group, 6913
HEALTHSOUTH Rehabilitation Hospital of Tallahassee, 7987
Hillsborough County Talking Book Library, 9635
Hollywood Area Brain Tumor Support Group, 1956
Jacksonville Public Library, 9636
James A. Haley Veterans' Hospital, 10131
Juvenile Diabetes Research Foundation: Central Florida Chapter, 3245
Juvenile Diabetes Research Foundation: Florida Sun Coast Chapter, 3246
Juvenile Diabetes Research Foundation: Greater Palm Beach County Chapter, 3247
Juvenile Diabetes Research Foundation: North Florida Chapter, 3248
Juvenile Diabetes Research Foundation: South Florida Chapter, 3249
Juvenile Diabetes Research Foundation: Tampa Bay Chapter, 3250
Kidney Association of South Florida, 5598
Kids Wish Network, 10669
Lake City VA Medical Center North Florida/South Georgia, 10132
Lee County Talking Books Library, 9637
Leukemia & Lymphoma Society: Suncoast Chapter, 2155
Leukemia and Lymphoma Society: Southern Florida Chapter, 2156
Leukemia and Lymphoma Society: Central Florida Chapter, 2157
Leukemia and Lymphoma Society: Northern Florida Chapter, 2158
Leukemia and Lymphoma Society: Palm Beach Area Chapter, 2159
LifeLink of Florida, 9184
LifeLink of Southwest Florida, 9185
Lupus Foundation of America: Northeast Florida Chapter, 8863
Lupus Foundation of America: Northwest Florida Chapter, 8864
Lupus Foundation of America: Southeast Florida Chapter, 8865
Lupus Foundation of America: Suncoast Chapter, 8866
Lupus Foundation of America: Tampa Area Chapter, 8867
Lupus Foundation of Florida, 8868
MSWorld, 6436
Malcom Randall VA Medical Center North Florida/South Georgia, 10133
Manattee County Office Epilepsy Services of Southwest Florida, 7484
Metabolic Research Institute, 3389
Miami Childrens Hospital Division of Pulmonology, 3102

Miami Comprehensive Hemophilia Center Jackson Medical Towers, 5043
Miami Dade Talking Book Library, 9638
Miami Project to Cure Paralysis, 7983
Miami VA Healthcare System, 10134
Mount Sinai Medical Center, 4890
Multiple Sclerosis Foundation, 6343
NNFF Florida Chapter, 6661
National Association of Guide Dog Users, 9437
National Federation of the Blind: Florida, 9483
National Kidney Foundation of Florida, 5599
National Multiple Sclerosis Society: North Florida Chapter, 6363
National Parkinson Foundation Hotline, 6914
National Spinal Cord Injury Support Goups, 7990
National Spinal Cord Injury Support Groups, 7993
Nemours Childrens Clinic, 3103
New Hope for Kids Wish Program, 10673
North Florida: HPV Support Group, 10443
Northwest Florida Panhandle Turner Syndrome Resource Group, 9346
Northwest Florida Support Group: National Ataxia Foundation, 1534
Orange County Library System: Orlando Public Library, 9639
Palm Beach County Library Annex: Talking Books, 9640
Parent Education Network (PEN) Project Health, 6053
Parkinson Association of Greater Daytona Beach, 6883
Parkinson Association of Southwest Florida, 6884
Parkinson's Foundation, 6872
Pembroke Pines Parkinson Support Group, 6915
Pensacola Brain Injury TBI/ABI Support Group, 4090
Pinellas Talking Book Library for the Blind and Physically Handicapped, 9641
Prader-Willi Florida Associton, 7172
Prader-Willi Syndrome Association, 7164
PraderWilli Syndrome Association, 7200
Pridelines, 301
RESOLVE Affiliate of Central Florida, 5392
RESOLVE of North Florida, 5393
RESOLVE of South Florida, 5394
Rambaugh-Goodwin Institute for Cancer Research, 2294
Renfrew Center of Miami, 3691
Renfrew Center of South Florida, 3692
Sarasota Area Brain Tumor Support Group, 1957
Scleroderma Foundation: Southeast Florida Chapter, 7335
South Florida Chapter National Multiple Sclerosis Society, 6364
South Florida Chapter of the American Association of Kidney Patients, 5600
South Palm Beach County Chapter of NFP, 6885
Southeast Parkinson Disease Association, 6886
Southeast Regional Center: Canine Companions for Independence, 9484
Spina Bifida Association of Florida Space Coast, 7871
Spina Bifida Association of Jacksonville, 7872
Spina Bifida Association of Tampa, 7873
Sub Regional Talking Book Library, 9642
Sunshine Chapter of the American Association of Kidney Patients, 5601
Tallahassee Memorial Diabetes Center, 3376
Tampa Bay Research Institute, 388
Tampa Lighthouse for the Blind, 9485
Teratogen Information Services, 1863
TransLife/Florida Hospital, 9186
UM/Sylvester Comprehensive Cancer Center, 2295
United Cerebral Palsy of Central Florida, 2704
United Cerebral Palsy of East Central Florida, 2705
United Cerebral Palsy of Florida, 2706
United Cerebral Palsy of North Florida: Tender Loving Care, 2707
United Cerebral Palsy of Northeast Florida, 2708
United Cerebral Palsy of Northwest Florida, 2709
United Cerebral Palsy of Sarasota-Manatee, 2710
United Cerebral Palsy of South Florida, 2711
United Cerebral Palsy of Tallahassee, 2712
United Cerebral Palsy of Tampa Bay, 2713
University of Florida Institute on Aging, 140

University of Florida: General Clinical Research Center, 666
University of Miami School of Medicine Department of Neurology, 8062
University of Miami: Bascom Palmer Eye Institute, 9804
University of Miami: Center on Aging Center on Aging, 982
University of Miami: Diabetes Research Institute, 3396
University of Miami: Mailman Center for Child Development, 1847
University of South Florida Center for HIV Education and Research, 389
Vietnam and All Veterans of Brevard, 10135
West Central FL Support Group: National Ataxia Foundation, 1535
West Florida Public Library: Talking Book Library, 9643
West Palm Beach Area Brain Tumor Support Group, 1958
West Palm Beach VA Medical Center, 10136

Georgia

AARP Georgia, 57
AIDS School Health Education Database Centers for Disease Control, 390
ALS Association: Georgia Chapter, 1104
Act Against AIDS, 249
Agency for Toxic Substances and Disease Registry, 627
Agency for Toxic Substances and Disease Registry, 1372
Agency for Toxic Substances and Disease Registry, 4290
Agency for Toxic Substances and Disease Registry, 5730
Agency for Toxic Substances and Disease Registry, 7034
Agency for Toxic Substances and Disease Registry, 7464
Albany Library for the Blind and Physically Handicapped, 9644
Alcohol and Drug Services Addictive Diseases Program, 8148
All Ages Support Group, 1959
Alzheimer's Association: Atlanta Chapter, 802
Alzheimer's Association: Augusta Chapter, 803
Alzheimer's Association: Central Georgia Chapter, 804
Alzheimer's Association: Greater Columbus Chapter, 805
Alzheimer's Association: Greater Georgia Chapter, 806
Alzheimer's Association: Southeast Georgia Chapter, 807
Alzheimer's Association: Southwest Georgia Chapter, 808
Alzheimer's Disease Center Emory University/VA Medical Center, 949
American Cancer Society, 2089
American Cancer Society: Georgia, 2160
American Diabetes Association: Atlanta Met ro, 3251
American Diabetes Association: Savannah, 3252
American Juvenile Arthritis Organization, 1187
American Juvenile Arthritis Organization, 8852
American Lung Association of Georgia, 5827
American Lung Association of Georgia, 9274
Arthritis Foundation, 1238
Arthritis Foundation, 6855
Arthritis Foundation, 7224
Arthritis Foundation Information Helpline, 1257
Arthritis Foundation: Georgia Chapter, 1202
Atlanta Georgia Chapter of the American Association of Kidney Patients, 5602
Atlanta Metro Subregional Library, 9645
Atlanta VA Medical Center Atlanta VA Health Care System, 10137
Augusta Regional Library Talking Book Center, 9646
Autism Society of Greater Georgia, 1677
Bainbridge Subregional Library for the Blind and Physically Handicapped, 9647
CCFA Georgia Chapter, 3008

CDC National Prevention Information Network, 255
CDC National Prevention Information Network, 391
Carl Vinson VA Medical Center Dublin VA Medical Center, 10138
Center for AIDS Research: Emory University Rollins School of Public Health, 392
Center for Chronic Disease Prevention and Centers for Disease Control, 10356
Center for Disease Control and Prevention, 10359
Centers for Disease Control, 10101
Centers for Disease Control & Prevention Hepatitis Branch, 5139
Centers for Disease Control & Prevention: Division of Adolescent & School Health, 635
Centers for Disease Control & Prevention: Division of Adolescent & School Health, 1380
Centers for Disease Control & Prevention: Division of Adolescent & School Health, 3540
Centers for Disease Control & Prevention: Division of Adolescent & School Health, 3672
Centers for Disease Control & Prevention: Division of Adolescent & School Health, 7569
Centers for Disease Control Division of Vector Borne Infectious Diseases, 9030
Centers for Disease Control and Prevention, 2832
Centers for Disease Control and Prevention, 9258
Charlie Norwood VA Medical Center, 10139
Children's Wish Foundation International, 10658
Columbus Library for Accessible Services (CLASS), 9648
Creative Community Services (CCS), 10506
Department of Pediatrics Medical College of Georgia, 3104
Division of Diabetes Translation, 3370
Division of Rehabilitation Service, 10444
Down Syndrome Association of Atlanta, 3560
Educational Materials Database Centers for Disease Control, 393
Emory Autism Resource Center, 1716
Emory Brain Tumor Support Group, 1960
Emory University: Cystic Fibrosis Center, 3105
Emory University: Georgia Center for Cancer Statistics, 2296
Emory University: Laboratory for Ophthalmic Research, 9786
Emory University: National Cooperative Drug Discovery for AIDS Treatment, 394
Emory University: Winship Cancer Institute, 2297
Fertility Clinic at the Shepherd Spinal Center, 5434
Funding Database Centers for Disease Control, 395
Georgia Alliance for the Mentally Ill, 5948
Georgia Association of the Deaf, 4342
Georgia Chapter of the Myasthenia Gravis Foundation of America, 6579
Georgia Department of Public Health: Center for Family Resource Planning, 8728
Georgia Department of Public Health: Infan t and Child Health, 8729
Georgia Department of Public Health: Office Of HIV/AIDS, 302
Georgia Industries for the Blind, 9486
Georgia Library for Accessible Services (GLASS), 9649
Georgia National Spinal Cord Injury Association Support Group Network, 7986
Georgia Parent Support Network (GPSN), 6054
Georgia SIDS Project, 8730
Georgia Support Group: National Ataxia Foundation, 1536
HIV/AIDS Prevention Program, 449
Hall County Library System: East Hall Branch and Special Needs Library, 9650
Hearts and Minds, 1961
Hemophilia Foundation of Georgia, 4974
I Can Cope, 2403
Immunization Division Centers for Disease Control, 450
International Association of Laryngectomees, 2103
Juvenile Diabetes Research Foundation: Geo rgia Chapter, 3253
Kids on the Block Arthritis Programs, 1258
Kidscope, 2161
Leukemia and Lymphoma Society: Georgia Chapter, 2162
LifeLink of Georgia, 9187

Look Good... Feel Better, 2406
Lupus Foundation of America: Columbus Chapter, 8869
Lupus Foundation of America: Greater Atlanta Chapter, 8870
Marcus Institute for Development and Learning, 3590
Medical College of Georgia Alzheimers Research Center, 969
Medical College of Georgia: Sickle Cell Center, 7616
Middle Georgia Subregional Library for the Blind and Physically Handicapped, 9651
Mood and Anxiety Disorders Program of Emory University, 7090
Myasthenia Gravis Support Group of Atlanta, 6605
NAMES Project Foundation AIDS Memorial Quilt, 358
NNFF Georgia Affiliate, 6662
National Association of Chronic Disease Directors, 6808
National Down Syndrome Congress, 3546
National Down Syndrome Congress, 3600
National Families in Action (NFIA), 8129
National Federation of the Blind: Georgia, 9487
National Gaucher Disease Foundation, 3843
National Kidney Foundation of Georgia, 5603
National MS Society: Georgia Chapter, 6365
National Parent to Parent Support and Information System, 10522
National Spinal Cord Injury Support Groups, 7992
Northwest Georgia Parkinson Disease Association, 6887
Oconee Regional Library for the Blind and Physically Handicapped, 9652
Office on Smoking and Health, 10418
Office on Smoking and Health: Centers for Disease Control & Prevention, 8132
Pediatric Brain Tumor Foundation: Georgia Chapter, 1908
Prader-Willi Georgia Association, 7173
RESOLVE of Georgia, 5395
Reach to Recovery, 2413
Rome Georgia Chapter of the American Association of Kidney Patients, 5604
Rome Subregional Library for People with Disabilities, 9653
SBTF Brain Tumor Support Group, 1962
Scleroderma Foundation: Georgia Chapter Scleroderma Foundation, 7336
Shepherd Center, 7968
Sickle Cell Foundation of Georgia, 7610
Sickle Cell Information Center, 7607
Southeastern Region: Helen Keller National Center, 9488
Special Needs Library of Northeast Georgia, 9654
Spina Bifida Association of Georgia, 7874
Subregional Library for the Blind and Physically Handicapped, 9655
Three Rivers Regional Library, 9656
United Cerebral Palsy of Georgia, 2714
VA Southeast Network, 10140
Valdosta Talking Book Library, 9657

Hawaii

AARP Hawaii, 58
Alcohol and Drug Abuse Division Department of Health, 8149
Alzheimer's Association: Honolulu Chapter, 809
Alzheimer's Association: West Hawaii Chapter, 810
American Cancer Society: Hawaii, 2163
American Diabetes Association: Hawaii, 3254
American Lung Association of Hawaii, 5828
American Lung Association of Hawaii, 9275
Autism Society of Hawaii, 1678
Brain Injury Association of Hawaii, 4091
Brain Injury Association of Hawaii, 4154
Division of Vocational Rehabilitation and Services for the Blind, 9489
Hawaii Department of Health: Family Health Division, 8731
Hawaii Department of Health: Harm Reduction Services Branch, 303
Hawaii Down Syndrome Congress, 3561
Hawaii Families As Allies (HFAA), 6055

Hawaii Lupus Foundation, 8871
Hawaii Parkinson Association Gwendolyn A Montibon President, 6888
Hawaii State Library for the Blind and Physically Handicapped, 9658
Hemophilia Foundation of Hawaii Kapiolani Medical Center, 4975
Ho'opono Workshop for the Blind, 9490
Juvenile Diabetes Research Foundation: Haw aii Chapter, 3255
Kuakini Parkinson Disease (PD) Information & Referral, 6916
NAMI: The Local Affiliate of the National Alliance for the Mentally Ill, 5949
National Federation of the Blind: Hawaii, 9491
National Kidney Foundation of Hawaii, 5605
National MS Society: Hawaii Chapter, 6366
Organ Donor Center of Hawaii, 9188
Pacific Health Research Institute, 2298
Prader-Willi Hawaii Association, 7174
Protection & Advocacy Agency, 10445
RESOLVE of Hawaii, 5396
Spark M. Matsunaga VA Medical Center VA Pacific Islands Health Care System, 10141
United Cerebral Palsy of Hawaii, 2715
University of Hawaii: Cancer Research Center, 2299

Idaho

AARP Idaho, 59
Alzheimer's Association: Greater Idaho Chapter, 811
Alzheimer's Association: Northern Idaho Chapter, 812
American Cancer Society: Idaho, 2164
American Lung Association of Idaho, 5829
Autism Society of Treasure Valley, 1679
Boise VA Medical Center, 10142
Brain Injury Association of Idaho, 4092
Co-Ad, 10446
Department of Health and Welfare Department Of Health And Welfare, 8150
FFCMH: Idaho Chapter, 5950
Hemophilia Foundation of Idaho, 4976
Idaho Alliance for the Mentally Ill, 5951
Idaho Commission for Libraries Talking Book Service, 9659
Idaho Department of Health and Welfare, 8732
Idaho Department of Health and Welfare: The STD/AIDS Program, 304
Idaho Persian Gulf Veterans, 10143
NNFF Idaho Chapter, 6663
National Federation of the Blind: Idaho, 9492
National MS Society: Idaho Division, 6367
Prader-Willi Idaho Association, 7175
United Cerebral Palsy of Idaho, 2716

Illinois

AARP Illinois: Chicago, 60
AARP Illinois: Springfield, 61
Academy of Nutrition & Dietetics, 625
Academy of Nutrition & Dietetics, 2625
Academy of Nutrition & Dietetics, 3668
Academy of Nutrition & Dietetics, 3915
Adult Down Syndrome Center of Lutheran General Hospital, 3575
Aid to the Aged, Blind or Disabled, 9493
Alzheimer's Association, 754
Alzheimer's Association: Central Illinois Chapter, 813
Alzheimer's Association: East Central Illinois Chapter, 814
Alzheimer's Association: Four Rivers Chapter, 815
Alzheimer's Association: Greater Illinois Chapter, 816
Alzheimer's Association: Greater Illinois Chapter: Carbondale Office, 817
Alzheimer's Association: Land of Lincoln Chapter, 818
American Academy of Dermatology, 7657
American Academy of Orthopaedic Surgeons, 2604
American Academy of Orthopaedic Surgeons, 7396
American Academy of Pediatrics, 10337

American Academy of Sleep Medicine, 2822
American Association of Diabetes Educators, 3208
American Brain Tumor Association, 1901
American Brain Tumor Association, 1963
American Brain Tumor Association, 4075
American Brain Tumor Association, 4155
American Cancer Society: Illinois, 2165
American College of Allergy, Asthma & Immunology, 631
American College of Allergy, Asthma & Immunology, 1375
American College of Allergy, Asthma & Immunology Foundation, 654
American College of Allergy, Asthma & Immunology Foundation, 1397
American Dental Association, 8111
American Diabetes Association: Greater Ill inois, 3256
American Diabetes Association: Northern Il linois, 3257
American Epilepsy Society, 7465
American Foundation for Surgery of the Hand, 2609
American Hearing Research Foundation, 4362
American Homes for the Aging: Midwest Regional Office, 819
American Liver Foundation Illinois Chapter, 5751
American Lung Association, 1376
American Lung Association, 5811
American Lung Association, 9257
American Lung Association HelpLine, 5873
American Lung Association of Illinois, 5830
American Lung Association of Illinois-Iowa, 9276
American Medical Association (AMA), 7037
American Osteopathic Association, 2909
American Pain Society, 2910
American Society for Dermatologic Surgery, 7659
American Society for Gastrointestinal Endoscopy, 3921
American Society for Surgery of the Hand, 2606
American Society of Colon and Rectal Surgeons, 2092
American Society of Plastic Surgeons, 7660
Arthritis Foundation: Greater Chicago Chapter, 1203
Arthritis Foundation: Greater Illinois Chapter, 1204
Arthritis Foundation: Northwestern Ohio Chapter, 1225
Association of Late-Deafened Adults, 4299
Association of Spinal Cord Injury Professionals, Inc., 7956
Autism Society of Illinois, 1680
Baxter Hyland Division, 4960
Brain Injury Association of Illinois, 4093
Brain Injury Association of Illinois Helpline, 4156
Brain Research Foundation, 1910
Brain Tumor Support Group, 1964
CANDU Parent Group, 6056
CCFA Illinois: Carol Fisher Chapter, 3009
Cancer and Leukemia Group B, 2300
Captain James A. Lovell Federal Health Care Center, 10144
Center for Narcolepsy Research at the University of Illinois at Chicago, 7765
Central Brain Tumor Registry of the US, 1912
Chicago Area Support Group: National Ataxia Foundation, 1537
Chicago Department of Public Health, 305
Chicago Lighthouse for People Who are Blind and Visually Impaired, 9494
Chicago Metro Support Group: National Ataxia Foundation, 1538
Chicagoland Chapter of the American Association of Kidney Patients, 5607
Clinical Research Center Northwestern Center for Clinical Researc, 396
Cognitive Neurology and Alzheimer's Disease Center, 960
Comer Children's Hospital at the Universit, 3107
Comer Children's Hospital at the University of Chicago, 3106
Compassionate Friends, 8699
Compassionate Friends, 10692
Cooley's Anemia Foundation (CAF): Illinois Oakbrook Towers, 2960
Cystic Fibrosis Center: Childrens Memorial Hospital, 3108

Cystic Fibrosis Center: Park Ridge Lutheran General Children's Hospital, 3109

David T Siegel Institute for Communicative Disorders, 4375

Department of Alcoholism and Substance Abuse, 8151

Department of Ophthalmology Information Line, 9813

Depression and Bipolar Support Alliance, 6206

Dermatology Foundation, 2259

Dermatology Foundation, 7661

Desert Storm Justice Foundation: Illinois, 10145

Division on Endocrinology Northwestern University Feinberg School, 3382

Dreams for Seniors Charity Inc, 10685

Easterseals, 1828

Easterseals, 2668

Easterseals, 7862

Edward Hines Jr. VA Hospital, 10146

Families Anonymous, Inc. Recovery Fellowship, 8117

Federation of Spine Associations, 7398

Gastro-Intestinal Research Foundation, 3933

Gastro-Intestinal Research Foundation, 3942

Green-Field Library-Alzheimer's Association, 947

Hands Organization: Advocacy Network for the Deaf and Hearing Impaired, 4308

Helen Keller National Center Regional Representatives, 9495

Hemophilia Foundation of Illinois, 4977

Illinois Alliance for the Mentally Ill, 5952

Illinois Association of the Deaf, 4343

Illinois Church Action on Alcohol Problems, 8152

Illinois Client Assistance Program, 10447

Illinois Department of Public Health: Division of Infectious Diseases, 306

Illinois Federation of Families, 5953

Illinois Midwest Neurofibromatosis, 6664

Illinois Spina Bifida Association, 7875

Illinois State Library Talking Book and Braille Service, 9660

Illinois Teratogen Information Service (IT IS), 1853

Illinois Turner Syndrome Resource Group, 9347

Inflammatory Bowel Disease Program, 2994

International Association of Eating Disorders Professionals Foundation, 3703

International Society for Traumatic Stress Studies, 7048

International Society for Traumatic Stress Studies, 7091

Jesse Brown VA Medical Center, 10147

Juvenile Diabetes Research Foundation: Gre ater Chicago Chapter, 3258

KALEIDOSCOPE, 6057

Kellogg Cancer Care Center Evanston Hospital, 2301

LaRabida Children's Hospital: Developmental Disabilities & Delays, 3589

Legal Council for Health Justice, 62

Legal Council for Health Justice, 307

Legal Council for Health Justice, 10448

Les Turner Amyotrophic Lateral Sclerosis Foundation, 1152

Les Turner Research Laboratory Northwestern University Medical School, 1140

Let's Breathe Sarcoidosis Support Group, 7240

Leukemia Research Foundation, 2302

Leukemia and Lymphoma Society: Illinois Chapter, 2166

Lions Quest, 10391

Lois Insolia ALS Center at Northwestern Memorial Hospital, 1105

Loyola University Medical Center: Department of Pediatrics, 3110

Loyola University of Chicago Cardiac Transplant Program, 4888

Loyola University of Children: Parmly Hearing Institute, 4380

Lupus Foundation of America: Illinois Chapter, 8872

MAGIC Foundation for Children's Growth, 4049

Male Sexual Dysfunction Clinic, 5303

Marion VA Medical Center, 10148

Medical Library Association, 266

Mid-Illinois Talking Book Center, 9661

Midwest AIDS Education and Training Center (MATEC), 308

Midwest AIDS Education and Training Center (MATEC), 397

Muscular Dystrophy Association, 6510

NF Center: North Broward Medical Center Neurofibromatosis, 6665

NNFF Illinois Chapter: Chicago Area, 6666

NNFF Illinois Chapter: Silvis Area, 6667

NNFF Illinois Chapter: Springfield Area, 6668

NNFF Illinois Chapter:Peoria Region, 6669

National Adrenal Diseases Foundation, 8

National Association for Down Syndrome, 3545

National Association of Anorexia Nervosa and Associated Disorders, 3679

National Association of Anorexia Nervosa and Associated Disorders Helpline, 3718

National Center for Sight, 9816

National Certification Board for Diabetes Educators, 3211

National Eye Health Education Program, 9817

National Federation of the Blind: Illinois, 9496

National Headache Foundation, 6292

National Headache Foundation, 7073

National Kidney Foundation of Illinois, 5608

National MS Society: Chicago, Greater Illinois Chapter, 6368

Neurofibromatosis Network, 6654

Nevada Kidney Disease & Hypertension Cente rs, 5664

Northern Illinois University Research and Training Center, 4381

Northwestern Medicine Digestive Health Center, 3927

Northwestern University: Division of Allergy and Immunology, 1405

Oncology Hematology Associates of Central Illinois, 2303

Parents Information Network FFCMH, 6058

Parents of Children with Brain Tumors PCBT, 1965

Parkside Medical Services Corporation, 8153

Prader-Willi Illinois Association, 7176

Prevent Blindess, 9453

Pulmonary Fibrosis Foundation, 5813

RESOLVE of Illinois, 5397

Rainbows for All God's Children, 10702

Recovery International, 7116

Regional Organ Bank of Illinois, Inc., 9189

Rehabilitation Institute of Chicago, 1253

Robert H Lurie Comprehensive Cancer Center of Northwestern University, 2304

Rockford Parkinson's Support Group, 6917

Rush University Multiple Sclerosis Center, 6434

SIDS of Illinois, 8733

Saint Francis Medical Center Peoria Pulmonary Association, 3111

Sarcoidosis Networking Association, 7236

Scleroderma Foundation: Greater Chicago Chapter, 7337

Second Sense: Beyond Vision Loss, 9456

Shawnee Library System: Southern Illinois Talking Book Center, 9662

Shriners Hospital for Crippled Children Chicago Unit, 7401

Simon Foundation Helpline for Incontinence Information, 5340

Simon Foundation for Continence, 5335

Skokie Accessible Library Services, 9663

Sleep Research Society American Academy of Sleep Medicine, 7762

Society for the Study of Celiac Disease, 2631

Society of Gastroenterology Nurses and Associates, 3930

Society of Mitral Valve Prolapse Syndrome, 4923

Spinal Cord Injury Association of Illinois, 7969

Statewide SIDS Program: Illinois Department of Public Health, 8734

Sulzberger Institute for Dermatologic Educ, 7677

Sulzberger Institute for Dermatologic Education, 7676

Test Positive Aware Network (TPAN), 309

The Magic Foundation, 9341

Thresholds Psychiatric Rehabilitation, 6039

United Cerebral Palsy Land of Lincoln, 2717

United Cerebral Palsy of East Central Illinois, 2718

United Cerebral Palsy of Greater Chicago, 2719

United Cerebral Palsy of Illinois, 2720

United Cerebral Palsy of Southern Illinois, 2721

United Cerebral Palsy of Will County, 2722

United Cerebral Palsy of the Blackhawk Region, 2723

United Cerebral Palsy: Eastern Seals, 2724

University of Chicago Cancer Research Center, 2305

University of Chicago Center for Advanced Medicine Duchossis Center, 7368

University of Chicago Committee on Virology, 7573

University of Chicago Dept of Neurology University of Chicago Hospital, 979

University of Chicago: Clinical Nutrition Research Unit, 2306

University of Chicago: Comprehensive Diabetes Center, 3391

University of Chicago: Temporal Bone Laboratory for Ear Research, 4399

University of Illinois Eye and Ear Infirma ry, 9802

University of Illinois Health Services Research, 980

University of Illinois at Chicago Consultation Clinic for Epilepsy, 7493

University of Illinois at Chicago Craniofacial Center, 1845

University of Illinois at Chicago Lions, 9310

University of Illinois at Chicago Lions of Illinois Eye Research Institute, 9803

University of Illinois at Chicago Medical Center Outpatient Clinical Center, 7369

University of Illinois at Chicago: Institute for Tuberculosis Research, 9311

VA Great Lakes Health Care System, 10149

VA Illiana Health Care System, 10150

Voices of Vision Talking Book Center, 9664

Indiana

AARP Indiana, 63

ALS Association: Indiana Chapter, 1106

Alzheimer's Association: Central Indiana Chapter, 820

Alzheimer's Association: Northern Indiana Chapter, 821

Alzheimer's Support Group, 985

American Camp Association, 10342

American Cancer Society: Indiana, 2167

American Diabetes Association: Northern In diana/Northern Ohio, 3259

American Liver Foundation Indiana Chapter, 5752

American Lung Association of Indiana, 5831

American Lung Association of Indiana: State Office & Support Office, 9277

Ann Whitehill Down Syndrome Program, 3576

Arthritis Foundation: Indiana Chapter, 1205

Autism Society of Indiana, 1681

Ball State University Public Health Entomology Laboratory, 9029

Bartholomew County Public Library, 9665

Bosma Industries for the Blind, 9497

Brain Injury Association of Indiana, 4094

Brain Injury Association of Indiana Helpli ne, 4157

Brain Tumor Support Group, 1966

Breaking New Ground Resource Center, 10354

CCFA Indiana Chapter, 3010

Children's Organ Transplant Association (COTA), 9165

Chronic Fatigue Syndrome & Fibromyalgia Support, 2833

Diabetes Youth Foundation of Indiana, 3260

Division of Addiction Services Department of Mental Health, 8154

Evansville-Vanderburgh County Public Library, 9666

FFCMH: Indiana Chapter, 5954

Family Action Network, 5955

Feingold Association of the US, 1605

Fort Wayne Campus VA Northern Indiana Health Care System, 10151

GoldPoint Clinical Research, 7092

Greater Indianapolis Chapter of the Myasthenia Gravis Foundation of America, 6582

Hemophilia Foundation of Indiana, 4978

Indiana Down Syndrome Foundation, 3562

Indiana Organ Procurement Organization,, 9190

Indiana Protection and Advocacy Services, 10449

Indiana Resource Center for Autism (IRCA), 1717

Indiana State Department of Health Maternal And Child Health Services, 8735
Indiana Talking Book & Braille Library, 9667
Indiana Teratogen Information Service, 1854
Indiana University Center for Aging Research, 964
Indiana University School of Medicine Center for Aging Research, 122
Indiana University: Area Health Education Center, 3384
Indiana University: Center for Diabetes Research, 3385
Indiana University: Human Genetics Center of Medical & Molecular Genetics, 965
Indiana University: Hypertension Research Center, 5256
Indiana University: Pharmacology Research Laboratory, 3386
Juvenile Diabetes Research Foundation: Ind iana State Chapter, 3261
Juvenile Diabetes Research Foundation: Nor thern Indiana Chapter, 3262
Krannert Institute of Cardiology, 4887
Lake County Public Library, 9668
Leukemia and Lymphoma Society: Indiana Chapter, 2168
Lupus Foundation of America: Northeast Indiana Chapter, 8873
Lupus Foundation of America: Northwest Indiana Lupus Chapter, 8874
Lupus Foundation of Indiana, 8875
Marion Campus VA Northern Indiana Health Care System, 10152
Mary Margaret Walther Program Walther Cancer Institute, 2307
MidWest Medical Center: Sleep Disorders Center, 7775
Multipurpose Arthritis and Musculoskeletal Disease Center, 1250
NAMI Indiana, 5956
NAMI Indiana - National Alliance on Mental Illness, 6059
NNFF Indiana Chapter, 6670
National Federation of the Blind: Indiana, 9498
National Kidney Foundation of Indiana, 5609
National Legal Center for the Medically Dependent & Disabled, 10408
National MS Society: Indiana State Chapter, 6369
National Spinal Cord Injury Association: Central Indiana Chapter, 7970
Prader-Willi Indiana Association, 7177
Primary Brain Cancer Support Group, 1967
Purdue Cancer Center Purdue University, 2267
Purdue University Center for AIDS Research, 398
Purdue University William A Hillenbrand Biomedical Engineering Center, 4894
Purdue University: Center for Research on Aging and the Life Course, 129
RESOLVE of Indiana, 5398
Riley Hemophilia & Hemophilia Center Riley Hospital for Children, 5056
SIDS Center of Indiana, 8736
Sleep Alertness Center: Lafayette Home Hospital, 7781
Sleep/Wake Disorders Center: Community Hospitals of Indianapolis, 7812
Southern Indiana Support Group: National Ataxia Foundation, 1539
Spina Bifida Association of Central Indiana, 7876
The Riley Cystic Fibrosis Center, 3112
United Cerebral Palsy Association of Indiana, 2725
United Cerebral Palsy Associations, 2726
United Cerebral Palsy of the Wabash Valley, 2727

Iowa

AARP Iowa, 64
Alzheimer's Association: Big Sioux Chapter, 822
Alzheimer's Association: East Central Iowa Chapter, 823
Alzheimer's Association: Greater Iowa Chapter, 824
Alzheimer's Association: Heart of Iowa Chapter, 825
American Cancer Society: Iowa, 2169
American Diabetes Association: Cedar Rapid s District, 3263

American Lung Association of Iowa, 5832
Arthritis Foundation: Iowa Chapter, 1206
Association for Glycogen Storage Disease, 5733
Autism Society of Iowa, 1682
Blank Childrens Hospital Pediatric Pulmonology Clinic, 3113
Brain Injury Alliance of Iowa Helpline, 4158
Brain Injury Association of Iowa, 4095
CCFA Iowa Chapter, 3011
Center for Disabilities and Development, 3578
Client Assistance Program: Iowa Division o n Persons with Disabilities, 10450
Department of Public Health: Division of Substance Abuse and Health, 8155
FFCMH: Iowa Chapter, 5957
Gilda's Club: Quad Cities, 2401
Great Plains Regional Hemophilia Center University of Iowa Hospitals, 5026
Greater Iowa Chapter Alzheimer's Association Quadcity Office, 826
Iowa Brain Tumor Support Group, 1968
Iowa Chapter of the Association of Kidney Patients, 5610
Iowa City VA Health Care System, 10153
Iowa Department for the Blind, 9669
Iowa Donor Network, 9191
Iowa Federaion of Families for Children's Mental Health (FFCMH), 6060
Iowa Oncology Research Association, 2308
Iowa SIDS Alliance, 8737
Iowa SIDS Program Iowa Department of Public Health, 8738
Iowa Turner Syndrome Resource Group, 9348
Juvenile Diabetes Research Foundation: Eas tern Iowa Chapter, 3264
Juvenile Diabetes Research Foundation: Gre ater Iowa Chapter, 3265
Kidneeds, 5671
Lupus Foundation of America: Iowa Chapter, 8876
Myasthenia Gravis Support Group of Ames, 6606
NAMI Iowa: National Alliance on Mental Illness, 5958
NNFF Iowa Chapter, 6671
National Center for Voice and Speech: Univ ersity of Iowa, 4322
National Federation of the Blind: Iowa, 9499
National MS Society: Iowa Chapter, 6370
Neurological Center of Iowa, 1969
Orthopaedic Biomechanics Laboratory Shriners Hospital for Crippled Children, 2794
Pediatric Allergy & Pulmonary Division University of Iowa Healthcare, 3114
People Against Cancer, 2170
Prader-Willi Iowa Association, 7178
Quad Cities Brain Tumor Support Group, 1970
RESOLVE Affiliate of Iowa, 5399
Spina Bifida Association of Iowa, 7877
University of Iowa Birth Defects and Genetic Disorders Unit, 1846
University of Iowa College of Medicine, 8060
University of Iowa Mental Health Clinical Research Center, 6263
University of Iowa Teratogen Information Service, 1865
University of Iowa: Diabetes Research Center, 3393
University of Iowa: Holden Comprehensive Cancer Center, 2309
University of Iowa: Iowa Cardiovascular Center, 4903
VA Central Iowa Health Care System, 10154

Kansas

AARP Kansas, 65
ALS Association: Mid America Chapter Centr al Kansas Office, 1108
ALS Association: Mid America Chapter Kansas City Metro Area, 1107
Alcohol and Drug Abuse Services, 8156
Alzheimer's Association: Heart of America Chapter, 827
Alzheimer's Association: Sunflower Chapter, 828
American Academy of Environmental Medicine, 630
American Cancer Society: Kansas City, 2171
American Diabetes Association: Kansas, 3266

American Lung Association of Kansas, 5833
American Lung Association of Kansas, 9278
American Lung Association of Missouri, 5842
American Organ Transplant Association, 10347
American Stroke Foundation, 8052
Arthritis Foundation: Kansas Chapter, 1207
Arthritis Foundation: Western Missouri, Greater Kansas City, 1215
Autism Society of Kansas Autism Society of America, 1683
Beach Center on Disability, 10353
Brain Injury Association of Kansas and Greater Kansas City, 4096
Brain Injury Association of Kansas and Greater Kansas City Helpline, 4159
CKLS Headquarters, 9670
Colmery-O'Neil VA Medical Center VA Eastern Kansas Health Care System, 10155
Council for Learning Disabilities (CLD), 10369
Disability Rights Center of Kansas, 10451
Dwight D. Eisenhower VA Medical Center VA Eastern Kansas Health Care System, 10156
Gray Matters Support: Kansas City, 1971
Headstrong Brain Tumor Support Group, 1972
Hospice and Homecare, 150
Hospice and Homecare, 10515
Kansas Association of the Deaf, 4344
Kansas Department of Health & Environment: Bureau of Family Health, 8739
Kansas Department of Health & Environment: STI/HIV Section, 310
Kansas Industries for the Blind, 9500
Kansas Services for the Blind and Visually Impaired, 9808
Kansas State University Center on Aging, 125
Kansas State University: Terry C Johnson Center for Basic Cancer Research, 2310
Kansas University Medical Center: Cystic Fibrosis Center, 3115
Keys for Networking: Kansas FFCMH, 5959
Landon Center on Aging University of Kansas Medical Center, 126
Leukemia and Lymphoma Society: Mid-America Chapter, 2172
Leukemia and Lymphona Society: Kansas Chapter, 2173
Lupus Foundation of America: Heartland Chapter, 8877
Manhattan Subregional Library of the Kansas Talking Books Service, 9671
Midwest Transplant Network & Organ Bank, 9192
NAMI Kansas: Kansas' Voice on Mental Illness, 5960
National Federation of the Blind: Kansas, 9501
National Kidney Foundation of Kansas and Western Missouri, 5611
National MS Society: Mid-America Chapter, 6371
National MS Society: South Central & West Kansas Division, 6372
Neurofibromatosis Kansas and Central Plains, 6673
Northeast Kansas Parkinson Association, 6889
Northwest Kansas Library System, 9672
Parkinson Association of Greater Kansas City, 6890
Region VII Office Program: Consultants for Maternal and Child Health, 8760
Robert J. Dole VA Medical Center, 10157
SIDS Network of Kansas, 8740
South Central Kansas Library System, 9673
St. Joseph Medical Center Cystic Fibrosis Care and Teaching Center, 3116
Talking Books Service, 9674
The Turner Syndrome Society: Kansas City Chapter, 9349
United Cerebral Palsy of Kansas, 2728
University of Kansas Allergy and Immunology Clinic, 667
University of Kansas Cray Diabetes Center, 3394
University of Kansas Kidney and Urology Research Center, 5666
Wichita Medical Research & Education Foundation, 1849
Wichita Public Library, 9675

Kentucky

AARP Kentucky, 66
ALS Association: Kentucky Chapter, 1109
Academy of Doctors of Audiology, 4286
Alzheimer's Association: Lexington/ Bluegrass Chapter, 829
Alzheimer's Association: Louisville Chapter, 830
Alzheimer's Disease Center Kentucky University, 950
American Association of Endocrine Surgeons, 2
American Cancer Society: Kentucky, 2174
American Deafness and Rehabilitation Association, 4295
American Diabetes Association: Kentucky, 3267
American Lung Association of Kentucky, 5834
American Lung Association of Kentucky, 9279
American Printing House for the Blind, 9412
Arthritis Foundation: Kentucky Chapter, 1208
Autism Chapter of Bluegrass Chapter, 1684
Autism Society of Western Kentucky, 1685
Brain Injury Alliance of Kentucky, 4160
Brain Injury Association of Kentucky, 4097
Client Assistance Program: Kentucky, 10452
Department of Public Health: Adult and Child Health Division, 8741
Division of Substance Abuse: Department of Mental Health, 8157
Dream Factory, Inc., 10661
Henry Vogt Cancer Research Institute James Graham Brown Cancer Center, 2311
Jewish Hospital Transplant Center KentuckyOne Health, 9168
Juvenile Diabetes Research Foundation: Kentuckiana Chapter, 3268
KY Partnership For Families and Children, 5961
Kentucky Alliance for the Mentally Ill, 5962
Kentucky Association of the Deaf, 4345
Kentucky Cancer Program, 2312
Kentucky Hemophilia Foundation, 4979
Kentucky IMPACT, 6061
Kentucky Industries for the Blind, 9502
Kentucky Organ Donor Affiliates, 9193
Kentucky Talking Book Library, 9676
Kentucky University: Cystic Fibrosis Center, 3117
Kosair Childrens Cystic Fibrosis Center, 3118
Leukemia and Lymphoma Society: Kentucky Chapter, 2175
Lexington VA Health Care System, 10158
Louisville Talking Book Library for the Blind and Physically Handicapped, 9677
Lovelace Respiratory Research Institute, 5663
Meningioma/Benign Brain Tumor Support Group, 1973
Myasthenia Gravis Support Group of Louisvi lle, 6607
National Anxiety Foundation, 6200
National Federation of the Blind: Kentucky, 9503
National Kidney Foundation of Kentucky, 5612
National MS Society: Kentucky Chapter, 6373
National Spinal Cord Injury Association: Derby City Area Chapter, 7971
Northern Kentucky Talking Book Library, 9678
Parents Resource Institute for Drug Education, 8196
Prader-Willi Kentucky Association, 7179
RESOLVE of Kentucky, 5400
Robley Rex VA Medical Center Louisville VA Medical Center, 10159
SIDS Network of Kentucky, 8742
Sanders-Brown Center on Aging University of Kentucky, 131
Spina Bifida Association of Kentucky, 7878
University of Kentucky: Children Cancer Study Group, 2313
University of Kentucky: Lucille Parker Markey Cancer Center, 2314
Wellness Community: Kentucky, 1974

Louisiana

AARP Louisiana: Baton Rouge, 67
AARP Louisiana: New Orleans, 68
Advocacy Center, 10453
Alexandria VA Healthcare System, 10160

Alzheimer's Association: Greater New Orleans Chapter, 832
Alzheimer's Association: Northeast/Central Louisiana Chapter, 831
Alzheimer's Services of the Capital Area, 833
American Cancer Society: Louisiana, 2176
American Celiac Society, 2626
American Diabetes Association: Louisana, 3269
American Lung Association of Louisiana, 5835
American Lung Association of Louisiana, 9280
Autism Society of Louisiana, 1686
Baton Rouge Regional Tumor Registry Mary Bird Perkins Cancer Center, 2315
Bayou Area Chapter of the American Association of Kidney Patients, 5613
Brain Injury Association of Louisiana Help line, 4161
Brain Tumor Support Group, 1975
CCFA Louisiana Chapter, 3013
Central Louisiana State Hospital Medical and Professional Library, 6027
Clinical Immunology, Allergy, and Rheumatology, 1401
Eljay Foundation for Parkinson Syndrome Awareness, 6891
Ernest N Morial Asthma, Allergy & Respiratory Disease Center, 3119
Industries for the Blind and Visually Impaired of Louisiana, 9504
Juvenile Diabetes Research Foundation: Bat on Rouge Chapter, 3270
Juvenile Diabetes Research Foundation: Lou isiana Chapter, 3271
Juvenile Diabetes Research Foundation: Shr eveport Chapter, 3272
Louisiana Alliance for the Mentally Ill, 5963
Louisiana Association for the Blind, 9505
Louisiana Association of the Deaf, 4346
Louisiana Chapter of the National Hemophilia Foundation, 4980
Louisiana Comprehensive Hemophilia Care Center, 5040
Louisiana Department of Health: STD/HIV Program, 311
Louisiana Lupus Foundation, 8879
Louisiana Organ Procurement Agency, 9194
Louisiana State University Genetics Section of Pediatrics, 1841
Louisiana Support Group: National Ataxia Foundation, 1540
Myasthenia Gravis Support Group of Louisia na, 6608
NNFF Louisiana Chapter, 6674
National Federation of the Blind: Louisiana, 9506
National Kidney Foundation of Louisiana, 5614
National Multiple Sclerosis Society: Louisiana, 6374
National Spinal Cord Injury Association: Louisiana Chapter, 7972
Northeast Louisiana Sickle Cell Anemia Foundation, 7609
Office of Human Services: Division of Alcohol and Drug Abuse, 8158
Office of Public Health, 8743
Overton Brooks VA Medical Center, 10161
Public Health Services of Louisiana, 8744
RESOLVE of Louisiana, 5401
Randolph-Sheppard Vendors of America, 9454
Southeast Louisiana Veterans Health Care System, 10162
Spina Bifida Association of Greater New Orleans, 7879
State Library of Louisiana, 9679
Tulane University Center For Aging, 136
Tulane University Pulmonary Diseases Critical Care and Enviromental Medicine, 2316
Tulane University: US-Japan Biomedical Research Laboratories, 4137
United Cerebral Palsy of Baton Rouge McMains Children's Developmental Center, 2729
United Cerebral Palsy of Greater New Orleans, 2730
Wishing Well Foundation USA, Inc., 10680

Maine

AARP Maine, 69

Alzheimer's Association: Maine Chapter, 834
American Cancer Society: Maine, 2177
American Diabetes Association: Maine, 3273
American Lung Association of Maine, 5836
American Lung Association of Maine, 9281
Autism Society of Maine, 1687
Bangor Public Library, 9680
Brain Injury Association of Maine, 4098
Brain Tumor Support Group of Maine, 1976
Cary Library, 9681
Central Maine Cystic Fibrosis Center, 3120
Department of Human Services, 8745
Disability Rights Center: Maine, 10454
Gift From Within, 7069
HOSPICELINK Hospice Education Institute, 10693
Juvenile Diabetes Research Foundation: New England/Maine Chapter, 3274
Lewiston Public Library, 9682
Lupus Group of Maine, 8880
Maine Alliance for the Mentally Ill, 5964
Maine Alzheimer's Care Center, 835
Maine Center for the Blind and Visually Impaired, 9507
Maine Dept. of Health & Human Services: HIV, STD, & Viral Hepatitis Program, 312
Maine Hemophilia Treatment Center, 5041
Maine Medical Center: Cystic Fibrosis Clin, 3122
Maine Medical Center: Cystic Fibrosis Clinical Center, 3121
Maine SIDS Foundation, 8746
Maine SIDS Program Department Of Human Services, 8747
Maine State Library, 9683
Maine Support Group: National Ataxia Foundation, 1541
Maine VA Medical Center VA Maine Healthcare System, 10163
National Federation of the Blind: Maine, 9508
National Kidney Foundation of Maine, 5615
National MS Society: Maine Chapter, 6375
Office of Alcohol and Drug Abuse Prevention, 8159
Portland Public Library, 9684
Sleep Laboratory, Maine Medical Center, 7806
United Cerebral Palsy of Northeastern Maine, 2731
United Families for Children's Mental Health, 5965
United Ostomy Associations of America, Inc, 2999
United Ostomy Associations of America, Inc, 3931
United Ostomy Associations of America, Inc, 9383
University of Maine: Communication Science s & Disorders, 4400
Waterville Public Library, 9685

Maryland

AARP Maryland, 70
ACG Institute for Clinical Research and Education, 3939
AIDSinfo, 247
AIDSinfo, 442
ALS Association: National Capital Area Chapter, 1102
Agency for Healthcare Research and Quality, 626
Agency for Healthcare Research and Quality, 1371
Agency for Healthcare Research and Quality, 3537
Agency for Healthcare Research and Quality, 3670
Agency for Healthcare Research and Quality, 4289
Agency for Healthcare Research and Quality, 5729
Agency for Healthcare Research and Quality, 7033
Agency for Healthcare Research and Quality, 7463
Alzheimer's & Related Dementias Education & Referral Center, 753
Alzheimer's Association: Central Maryland Chapter, 836
Alzheimer's Association: Eastern Shore Chapter, 837
Alzheimer's Association: Western Maryland Chapter, 838
Alzheimer's Disease Center: Johns Hopkins University School of Medicine, 954
American Action Fund for Blind Children and Adults, 9686
American Association of the Deaf-Blind, 9407
American Association on Intellectual and Developmental Disabilities, 5905
American Cancer Society: Maryland, 2178

American Childhood Cancer Organization, 2090
American College of Gastroenterology, 3916
American Diabetes Association: Maryland, 3275
American Foundation for Urologic Disease: Us Too Line, 2389
American Gastroenterological Association, 9380
American Gastroenterological Association National Office, 3917
American Kidney Fund, 5578
American Lung Association of Maryland, 5837
American Lung Association of Maryland, 9282
American Society for Deaf Children, 4296
American Society for Parenteral and Enteral Nutrition (ASPEN), 3922
American Society of Human Genetics, 1150
American Speech-Language-Hearing Association, 4297
Anxiety Disorders Association of America, 6194
Anxiety Disorders Association of America, 7042
Arthritis Foundation: Maryland Chapter, 1209
Asthma and Allergy Foundation of America, 655
Asthma and Allergy Foundation of America, 1398
Autism Society of America, 1663
Autism Society of America, 1725
Autism Society of Baltimore-Chesapeake, 1688
Baltimore Headache Institute, 6293
Baltimore VA Medical Center VA Maryland Health Care System, 10164
Believe In Tomorrow Children's Foundation, 10656
Blind Industries and Services of Maryland, 9509
Brain Injury Association of Maryland, 4099
Brain Injury Association of Maryland Helpl ine, 4162
Brain Tumor Networking Group, 1977
Brain Tumor Support Group: Maryland, 1978
Brainiacs, 1979
CCFA Maryland Chapter, 3014
Cancer Information Service, 2265
Captioned Films/Videos, 4363
Captioned Media Program, 4364
Center for AIDS Research: Johns Hopkins University School of Medicine, 399
Center for Mental Health Services, 7063
Center for Substance Abuse Prevention Substance Abuse & Mental Health Services, 8113
Center for the Study of Traumatic Stress, 7068
Center for the Study of Traumatic Stress, 7093
Centers for Medicare & Medicaid Services, 636
Centers for Medicare & Medicaid Services, 1381
Centers for Medicare & Medicaid Services, 3541
Centers for Medicare & Medicaid Services, 3673
Centers for Medicare & Medicaid Services, 4303
Centers for Medicare & Medicaid Services, 5734
Centers for Medicare & Medicaid Services, 7045
Centers for Medicare & Medicaid Services, 7466
Chesapeake Area Support Group: National Ataxia Foundation, 1542
Children & Adults with Attention Deficit /Hyperactivity Disorder, 1603
Client Assistance Program: Maryland, 10455
Clinical Focus on Primary Immune Deficiency Diseases, 354
Community Services for Autistic Adults & Children, 1665
Cooley's Anemia Foundation (CAF): Capital Area, 2961
Cystic Fibrosis Center: National Institute of Health NIDDK, 3123
Cystic Fibrosis Foundation, 3086
Cystic Fibrosis Foundation, 3124
Diabetes Action Network for the Blind, 3210
Diabetics Action Network, 9422
Digestive Disorders Associates Ridgely Oaks Professional Center, 3941
Disability Resource Center of Montgomery County Public Libraries, 9687
Drug Free Workplace Hotline, 8242
Epilepsy Foundation, 7467
Epilepsy Foundation of America Helpline, 7496
Family Service Foundation, Inc., 6025
First Candle, 8748
Foundation Fighting Blindness, 9425
Foundation Fighting Blindness, 9604
Frederick Cancer Research Center, 2317
Friends Medical Science Research Center, 8206
Friends of Libraries for Deaf Action USA, 4365

Genetic and Rare Diseases Information Center, 3835
Goodwill Industries International, Inc., 29
Goodwill Industries International, Inc., 1606
Goodwill Industries International, Inc., 1668
Goodwill Industries International, Inc., 1830
Goodwill Industries International, Inc., 3544
Goodwill Industries International, Inc., 4044
Goodwill Industries International, Inc., 5912
Goodwill Industries International, Inc., 7047
Goodwill Industries International, Inc., 9079
Goodwill Industries International, Inc., 10102
Goodwill Industries International, Inc., 10380
Health Resources and Services Administration (HRSA), 9167
Hearing Loss Association of America, 4313
Hemophilia Foundation of Maryland, 4981
Hepatitis Foundation International, 5141
Hydrocephalus Association, 5197
Hydrocephalus Association, 5202
Immune Deficiency Foundation, 357
Immune Deficiency Foundation, 656
Impotents Anonymous, 5306
Indian Health Service Federal Health Program, 8119
Institute of Psychiatry and Human Behavior: University of Maryland, 6031
International Association for Chronic Fati gue Syndrome/Myalgic Encephalomyelitis, 2826
International Braille and Technology Center for the Blind, 9688
International Foundation for Research and Education for Depression (iFred), 6196
International Society of Dermatology, 7662
Job Opportunities for the Blind, 9814
Johns Hopkins Brain Tumor Education Group, 1980
Johns Hopkins Center on Aging and Health, 124
Johns Hopkins University: Asthma and Allergy Center, 1403
Johns Hopkins University: Behavioral Pharmacology Research Unit, 8210
Johns Hopkins University: Center for Communication Programs, 400
Johns Hopkins University: Dana Center for Preventive Ophthalmology, 9796
Johns Hopkins University: Scleroderma Center, 7361
Johns Hopkins University: Sleep Disorders Francis Scott Key Medical Center, 7770
Johns Hopkins University: Sydney Kimmel Comprehensive Cancer Center, 2318
Joslin Center at University of Maryland Medicine, 3372
Juvenile Diabetes Research Foundation: Mar yland Chapter, 3276
Kennedy Krieger Institute, 3588
Kennedy Krieger Institute - Down Syndrome, 3598
Kennedy-Krieger Institute, 10273
Learning How, 10389
Leukemia and Lymphoma Society: Maryland Chapter, 2179
Loch Raven VA Community Living & Rehabilitation Center, 10165
MD/DC/Delaware Chapter of Myasthenia Gravis Foundation of America, 6576
MD/DC/Delaware Chapter of Myasthenia Gravis Foundation of America, 6577
MD/DC/Delaware Chapter of Myasthenia Gravis Foundation of America, 6584
Maryland National Spinal Cord Injury Association Support Group Network, 7988
Maryland Psychiatric Research Center, 6259
Maryland SIDS Information & Counseling Program, 8749
Maryland State Alcohol and Drug Abuse Administration, 8160
Maryland State Library for the Blind and Physically Handicapped, 9689
Mental Health Services Training Center, 10395
Mt. Washington Pediatric Clinic, 3592
NIH Clinical Center, 6037
NIH Osteoporosis and Related Bone Diseases - National Resource Center, 6780
NIH Osteoporosis and Related Bone Diseases - National Resource Center, 6813
NIH Osteoporosis and Related Bone Diseases National Resource Center, 6777
National Alliance for Caregiving, 35

National Alliance for Caregiving, 151
National Alliance for Caregiving, 10518
National Alliance for the Mentally Ill: Maryland, 5966
National Association for Children of Alcoholics (NACOA), 8125
National Association of the Deaf, 4320
National Cancer Institute, 2105
National Cancer Institute, 2408
National Center for Complementary and Integrative Health, 639
National Center for Complementary and Integrative Health, 1382
National Center for Complementary and Integrative Health, 3680
National Center for Complementary and Integrative Health, 5736
National Center for Complementary and Integrative Health, 7052
National Center for Complementary and Integrative Health, 7469
National Center for the Prevention of SIDS, 8813
National Clearinghouse for Alcohol and Drug Information, 8195
National Coalition for Cancer Survivorship, 2106
National Crime Prevention Council, 8128
National Diabetes Information Clearinghous e, 3374
National Digestive Diseases Information Clearinghouse, 2995
National Digestive Diseases Information Clearinghouse, 3925
National Digestive Diseases Information Clearinghouse, 10402
National Eye Institute (NEI): National Institutes of Health (NIH), 9441
National Family Caregivers Association, 10520
National Federation of Families for Children's Mental Health, 1612
National Federation of Families for Children's Mental Health, 5918
National Federation of the Blind, 9442
National Federation of the Blind: Maryland, 9510
National Foundation for Cancer Research, 2261
National Foundation for Cancer Research, 2319
National Foundation for Cancer Research Hotline, 2409
National Gaucher Foundation, 4022
National Gaucher Foundation, 5766
National Health Information Center, 9
National Health Information Center, 152
National Health Information Center, 453
National Health Information Center, 672
National Health Information Center, 986
National Health Information Center, 1153
National Health Information Center, 1259
National Health Information Center, 1408
National Health Information Center, 1522
National Health Information Center, 1613
National Health Information Center, 1728
National Health Information Center, 1856
National Health Information Center, 1914
National Health Information Center, 2410
National Health Information Center, 2612
National Health Information Center, 2634
National Health Information Center, 2796
National Health Information Center, 2834
National Health Information Center, 2919
National Health Information Center, 2950
National Health Information Center, 2974
National Health Information Center, 3042
National Health Information Center, 3182
National Health Information Center, 3409
National Health Information Center, 3602
National Health Information Center, 3721
National Health Information Center, 3806
National Health Information Center, 3845
National Health Information Center, 3869
National Health Information Center, 3947
National Health Information Center, 4028
National Health Information Center, 4055
National Health Information Center, 4144
National Health Information Center, 4416
National Health Information Center, 4920
National Health Information Center, 5073
National Health Information Center, 5149

National Health Information Center, 5209
National Health Information Center, 5263
National Health Information Center, 5307
National Health Information Center, 5339
National Health Information Center, 5441
National Health Information Center, 5672
National Health Information Center, 5773
National Health Information Center, 5875
National Health Information Center, 6047
National Health Information Center, 6207
National Health Information Center, 6264
National Health Information Center, 6295
National Health Information Center, 6438
National Health Information Center, 6521
National Health Information Center, 6602
National Health Information Center, 6684
National Health Information Center, 6721
National Health Information Center, 6783
National Health Information Center, 6818
National Health Information Center, 6856
National Health Information Center, 7014
National Health Information Center, 7108
National Health Information Center, 7199
National Health Information Center, 7226
National Health Information Center, 7243
National Health Information Center, 7373
National Health Information Center, 7402
National Health Information Center, 7497
National Health Information Center, 7574
National Health Information Center, 7627
National Health Information Center, 7642
National Health Information Center, 7680
National Health Information Center, 7819
National Health Information Center, 7913
National Health Information Center, 7989
National Health Information Center, 8065
National Health Information Center, 8246
National Health Information Center, 8814
National Health Information Center, 8930
National Health Information Center, 8972
National Health Information Center, 9007
National Health Information Center, 9038
National Health Information Center, 9085
National Health Information Center, 9228
National Health Information Center, 9312
National Health Information Center, 9329
National Health Information Center, 9359
National Health Information Center, 9385
National Health Information Center, 9818
National Health Information Center, 10276
National Health Information Center, 10326
National Health Information Center, 10521
National Heart, Lung & Blood Institute, 4863
National Heart, Lung & Blood Institute, 5250
National Heart, Lung & Blood Institute, 8050
National Human Genome Research Institute, 641
National Human Genome Research Institute, 1383
National Human Genome Research Institute, 3548
National Human Genome Research Institute, 3683
National Human Genome Research Institute, 4325
National Human Genome Research Institute, 5737
National Human Genome Research Institute, 7053
National Human Genome Research Institute, 7470
National Institute of Allergy and Infectious Diseases, 643
National Institute of Allergy and Infectious Diseases, 1385
National Institute of Allergy and Infectious Diseases, 2827
National Institute of Allergy and Infectious Diseases, 7570
National Institute of Allergy and Infectious Diseases, 9170
National Institute of Allergy and Infectious Diseases, 9259
National Institute of Arthritis & Musculoskeletal & Skin Diseases, 1191
National Institute of Arthritis & Musculoskeletal & Skin Diseases, 1251
National Institute of Arthritis & Musculoskeletal & Skin Diseases, 2608
National Institute of Arthritis & Musculoskeletal & Skin Diseases, 2610
National Institute of Arthritis & Musculoskeletal & Skin Diseases, 7664

National Institute of Arthritis & Musculoskeletal & Skin Diseases, 7670
National Institute of Biomedical Imaging and Bioengineering, 644
National Institute of Biomedical Imaging and Bioengineering, 1386
National Institute of Biomedical Imaging and Bioengineering, 4326
National Institute of Biomedical Imaging and Bioengineering, 5739
National Institute of Biomedical Imaging and Bioengineering, 7472
National Institute of Child Health and Human Development, 3550
National Institute of Child Health and Human Development, 4046
National Institute of Child Health and Human Development, 6778
National Institute of Child Health and Human Development, 7163
National Institute of Child Health and Human Development, 8702
National Institute of Child Health and Human Development, 8968
National Institute of Child Health and Human Development, 10405
National Institute of Diabetes & Digestive & Kidney Diseases, 6
National Institute of Diabetes & Digestive & Kidney Diseases, 2996
National Institute of Diabetes & Digestive & Kidney Diseases, 3212
National Institute of Diabetes & Digestive & Kidney Diseases, 4964
National Institute of Diabetes & Digestive & Kidney Diseases, 5300
National Institute of Diabetes & Digestive & Kidney Diseases, 5334
National Institute of Diabetes & Digestive & Kidney Diseases, 5579
National Institute of Diabetes & Digestive & Kidney Diseases, 5740
National Institute of Diabetes & Digestive & Kidney Diseases, 9381
National Institute of General Medical Sciences, 647
National Institute of General Medical Sciences, 1388
National Institute of General Medical Sciences, 3552
National Institute of General Medical Sciences, 5742
National Institute of General Medical Sciences, 7055
National Institute of General Medical Sciences, 7474
National Institute of Mental Health, 5919
National Institute of Mental Health, 7056
National Institute of Mental Health, 7094
National Institute of Neurological Disorders and Stroke, 1669
National Institute of Neurological Disorders and Stroke, 1903
National Institute of Neurological Disorders and Stroke, 2670
National Institute of Neurological Disorders and Stroke, 3837
National Institute of Neurological Disorders and Stroke, 6344
National Institute of Neurological Disorders and Stroke, 6870
National Institute of Neurological Disorders and Stroke, 7475
National Institute of Neurological Disorders and Stroke, 7760
National Institute of Neurological Disorders and Stroke, 8051
National Institute of Neurological Disorders and Stroke, 8969
National Institute of Neurological Disorders and Stroke, 9080
National Institute of Nursing Research, 1391
National Institute on Aging, 39
National Institute on Aging, 758
National Institute on Aging, 2108
National Institute on Alcohol Abuse and Alcoholism, 5753
National Institute on Deafness and other Communication Disorders, 4328
National Institute on Drug Abuse, 3563
National Institute on Drug Abuse, 5754

National Kidney Foundation of Maryland, 5616
National Kidney and Urologic Diseases Information Clearinghouse, 2109
National Library of Medicine, 362
National MS Society: Maryland Chapter Hunt Valley Business Center, 6376
National Organization of Parents of Blind Children, 9451
National Prevention Resource Center CSAP Division of Communications Programs, 8215
National Rehabilitation Information Center, 2671
National Rehabilitation Information Center, 10413
National Tuberous Sclerosis Association, 9326
National Volunteer Training Center for Sub CSAP Division of Communications Programs, 8218
National Volunteer Training Center for Substance Abuse Prevention, 8217
Neurofibromatosis, 6685
Neurofibromatosis: Mid-Atlantic, 6675
New York Obesity/Nutrition Research Center, 6718
Office of Women's Services Substance Abuse & Mental Health Services, 8131
Osteogenesis Imperfecta Foundation, 6779
Osteogenesis Imperfecta Foundation, 6784
PDQ, 2412
Parents Supporting Parents of MD, 5967
Parents of Children with Down Syndrome, 3603
Parkinson Support Groups of America, 6918
Perry Point VA Medical Center VA Maryland Health Care System, 10166
Prince George's County Memorial Library: Talking Book Center, 9690
Pulmonary Hypertension Association, 4922
Pulmonary Hypertension Association (PHA), 4864
Pulmonary Hypertension Association (PHA), 5252
Pulmonary Hypertension Association (PHA), 5814
RADAR Network National Clearinghouse for Alcohol & Dru, 8220
SIDS Information and Referral Hotline, 8816
Schizophrenia Research Branch: Division of Clinical and Treatment Research, 6261
Services for the Visually Impaired, 9735
Sickle Cell Disease Association of America, 7606
Sidran Institute, 7077
Social Security Administration Office of Public Inquiries, 10425
Society For Post-Acute and Long-Term Care Medicine, 6811
Spina Bifida Association of Maryland, 7880
Spina Bifida Association of the Eastern Shore, 7881
St. Joseph's Medical Center, 3693
Substance Abuse and Mental Health Services Administration (SAMHSA), 8136
Sudden Infant Death Syndrome Institute of the University of Maryland, 8811
Telecommunications for the Deaf, 4333
The Metropolitan Washington Ear, Inc., 9459
The Society of Federal Health Professionals (AMSUS), 7058
Transplant Resource Center of Maryland, 9195
Tuberous Sclerosis Complex International, 9328
U.S. Food and Drug Administration, 648
U.S. Food and Drug Administration, 1389
U.S. Food and Drug Administration, 3554
U.S. Food and Drug Administration, 3687
U.S. Food and Drug Administration, 4335
U.S. Food and Drug Administration, 5743
U.S. Food and Drug Administration, 7476
United Cerebral Palsy of Central Maryland, 2732
United Cerebral Palsy of Prince Georges & Montgomery Counties, 2733
United Cerebral Palsy of Southern Maryland, 2734
University of Maryland Center for Research, Grants & Contracts, 401
University of Maryland Center for Studies Family Studies Depatment, 402
University of Maryland Center for Studies of Cerebrovascular Disease & Stroke, 8061
University of Maryland School of Public Health Center on Aging, 141
University of Maryland: Department of Pediatrics, 3595
University of Maryland: Division of Infectious Diseases, 981

University of Maryland: Medical Biotechnology Center, 403
Urban Cardiology Research Center, 4915
Urology Care Foundation, 5301
Urology Care Foundation, 5336
VA Capitol Health Care Network, 10167
Warren Grant Magnuson Clinical Center, 670
Warren Grant Magnuson Clinical Center, 1256
Warren Grant Magnuson Clinical Center, 2320
Warren Grant Magnuson Clinical Center, 3405
Warren Grant Magnuson Clinical Center, 4916
Warren Grant Magnuson Clinical Center, 5669
Warren Grant Magnuson Clinical Center, 5872
Warren Grant Magnuson Clinical Center National Institute of Health, 9806
Washington DC Metropolitan Area Brain Tumor Support Group, 1981
Weight-Control Information Network, 3689
Weight-Control Information Network, 3705
Weight-Control Information Network, 6714
Weight-Control Information Network, 6715
White Lung Association, 5816

Massachusetts

AARP Massachusetts, 71
AIDS Support Group of Cape Cod, 441
ALS Association: Massachusetts Chapter, 1110
Affiliated Children's Arthritis Centers of New England, 1240
Alzheimer's Association: Massachusetts Chapter, 839
Alzheimer's Association: Western Regional Office: Massachusetts Chapter, 840
Alzheimer's Disease Center: Boston University, 953
American Cancer Society: Boston, 2180
American Cancer Society: Central New England Region-Weston MA, 2181
American Diabetes Association: Boston, 3277
American Lung Association of Massachusetts, 5838
American Lung Association of Massachusetts, 9283
American Macular Degeneration Foundation, 9410
Arthritis Foundation: Massachusetts Chapter, 1210
Association of Gastrointestinal Motility Disorders, 3712
Asthma and Allergy Foundation of America: New England Chapter, 650
Asthma and Allergy Foundation of America: New England Chapter, 1392
Attention Deficit Information Network, 1611
Autism Society of Massachusetts, 1689
Autism Treatment Center of America, 1664
Baystate Medical Center Wesson Memorial Unit, 3125
Berkshire Center, 10507
BermanGund Laboratory for the Study of Retinal Degenerations, 9775
Boston Hemophilia Center Fegan 5 Children's Hospital, 5016
Boston Sickle Cell Center Boston Medical Center, 7612
Boston University Arthritis Center, 1242
Boston University Cancer Research Center, 2321
Boston University Center for Human Genetics, 1836
Boston University Laboratory of Neuropsychology, 8199
Boston University Medical Campus General Clinical Research Center, 1243
Boston University University Medical Center, 7358
Boston University, Whitaker Cardiovascular Institute, 4869
Brain Injury Association of Massachusetts, 4100
Brain Injury Association of Massachusetts Helpline, 4163
Brain Tissue Resource Center McLean Hospital, 1911
Brain Tumor Patient and Caregiver Support Group, 1982
Brain Tumor Support Group: Duarte, 1920
Brain Tumor Support Group: Lahey, 1983
Brain Tumor Support Group: Worcester, 1984
Brigham and Women's Hospital: Center for Neurologic Diseases, 6430
Brigham and Women's Hospital: Rheumatology Immunology, and Allergy Division, 1399

Brigham and Women's Orthopedica and Arthritis Center, 1244
Brockton Division VA Boston Healthcare System, 10168
CCFA New England Chapter: Massachusetts, 3015
California Center for Population Research, 5433
Cape Cod Chapter National Parkinson Foundation, 6892
Caption Center, 9691
Carroll Center for the Blind, 9511
Carroll Center for the Blind, 9782
Carroll Center for the Blind, 9812
Center for AIDS Research: Harvard Medical School, Division of AIDS, 404
Center for Anxiety and Related Disorders at Boston University, 7095
Center for Blood Research Harvard Medical School/CBR, 405
Centers for AIDS Research: University of Massachusetts Medical School, 406
Childrens Hospital Immunology Division Children's Hospital, 1400
Childrens Hospital Medical Center Cystic Fibrosis Center, 3126
Client Assistance Program: Massachusetts, 10456
Committee of Ten Thousand, 257
Cooley's Anemia Foundation (CAF): Massachusetts Chapter, 2962
Cystic Fibrosis Worldwide, 3085
Cystic Firbrosis Center: Tufts New England Medical Center, 3127
Dana Farber Cancer Institute National Drug Discovery Group for AIDS Treatment, 407
Dana-Farber Institute: Department of Biostatistics and Computational Biology, 2322
David H. Koch Institute for Integrative Ca ncer Research, 2323
Developmental Medicine Center (DMC), 3583
Developmental Medicine Center Children's Hospital Boston, 408
Division of Substance Abuse, 8161
Eaton-Peabody Laboratory of Auditory Physiology, 4376
Edith Nourse Rogers Memorial Veterans Hospital: Bedford VA, 10169
Facioscapulohumeral Muscular Dystrophy Soc iety (FSH Society), 6520
Federation for Children with Special Needs, 1829
Federation for Children with Special Needs, 10377
Fertility and Women's Health Care Center, 5435
Framingham Heart Study, 4878
General Clinical Research Center at Beth Israel Hospital, 4879
Harris Center for Education and Advocacy in Eating Disorders, 3709
Harvard Clinical Nutrition Research Center, 6716
Harvard Cocaine Recovery Project, 8208
Harvard Throndike Laboratory Harvard Medical Center, 4882
Harvard University Howe Laboratory of Ophthalmology, 9790
Health Care For All, 10382
Jamaica Plain Division VA Boston Healthcare System, 10170
Jean Mayer USDA Human Nutrition Research Center on Aging at Tufts University, 123
Joslin Diabetes Center, 3388
Juvenile Diabetes Research Foundation: New England/Bay State Chapter, 3278
Laboure College Library, 9692
Lupus Foundation of America: Massachusetts Chapter, 8882
Mass./New Hampshire Chapter of the Myasthenia Gravis Foundation of America, 6585
Mass./New Hampshire Chapter of the Myasthenia Gravis Foundation of America, 6586
Massachusetts Alliance for the Mentally Ill, 5968
Massachusetts Alzheimers Disease Research Center, 968
Massachusetts Commission for the Blind, 9512
Massachusetts Department of Public Health: Office Of HIV/AIDS, 313
Massachusetts Down Syndrome Congress, 3564
Massachusetts Eating Disorder Association, 3694

Massachusetts General Departments of Neurology and Neurosurgery, 8058
Massachusetts General Hospital, 3128
Massachusetts General Hospital: Harvard Cutaneous Biology Research Center, 7669
Massachusetts State Association of the Deaf, 4347
Massachusetts Sudden Infant Death Syndrome Boston City Hospital, 8809
Massachusetts Turner Syndrome Resource Group, 9350
Merrimack Valley HPV Support Group Holy Family Hospital, 10457
MindWise Innovations, 3678
MindWise Innovations, 6198
MindWise Innovations, 8122
Myasthenia Gravis Support Group of Eastern Massachusetts and New Hampshire, 6609
Myasthenia Gravis Support Group of Eastern Massachusetts and New Hampshire, 6614
Myasthenia Gravis Support Group of Western Massachusetts and New Hampshire, 6610
Myasthenia Gravis Support Group of Western Massachusetts and New Hampshire, 6615
National Association for Parents of the Visually Impaired, 9815
National Braille Press, 9440
National Brain Tumor Society, 1902
National CFIDS Foundation, 2831
National Celiac Association, 2630
National Federation of the Blind: Massachusetts, 9513
National Kidney Foundation of MA/RI/NH/VT, 5617
National Kidney Foundation of MA/RI/NH/VT, 5624
National Kidney Foundation of MA/RI/NH/VT, 5643
National Kidney Foundation of MA/RI/NH/VT, 5657
National MS Society: Central New England Chapter, 6386
National MS Society: Massachusetts Chapter, 6377
National Parkinson Foundation:Cape Cod Chapter, 6893
National Scoliosis Foundation, 7399
National Spinal Cord Injury Association, 7973
National Spinal Cord Injury Association: Greater Boston Chapter, 7974
National Tay-Sachs and Allied Diseases Association, 3839
National Tay-Sachs and Allied Diseases Association, 8971
National TaySachs & Allied Diseases Association, 8974
Neurofibromatosis: New England, 6676
Neurological Support Group of St. Luke's Hospital, 1985
Neurosurgical Service, 10458
New England AIDS Education and Training Center, 314
New England AIDS Education and Training Center, 409
New England Area Support Group: National Ataxia Foundation, 1543
New England Hemophilia Association, 4982
New England Medical Center: ALS Laboratory, 1145
New England Organ Bank Massachusetts, 9196
New England Region: Helen Keller National Center, 9514
New England Regional Genetics Group, 1842
Northeast Parkinson's and Caregivers, 6894
Option Institute, 2829
Option Institute, 3866
Option Institute, 5920
Option Institute, 6201
Option Institute, 10419
PALS Support Groups, 1859
Parent Education/Support Group, 1986
Parent Professional Advocacy League, 1831
Parent Professional Advocacy League, 5921
Pediatric Pulmonary Unit Massachusetts General Hospital, 8810
Perkins Braille and Talking Book Library, 9693
Prader-Willi New England Association, 7180
RESOLVE of the Bay State, 5402
Region 1 of the National Association for Parents of the Visually Impaired, 9515
Region I Office Program: Consultants for Maternal and Child Health, 8750

Rhode Island Hemophilia Foundation, 5001
SIDS Support Group, 8817
Scleroderma Foundation, 7327
Scleroderma Foundation: New England Chapter, 7338
Scleroderma Foundation: New England Chapter, 7339
Scleroderma Foundation: New England Chapter, 7344
Scleroderma Foundation: New England Chapter, 7350
Scleroderma Foundation: New England Chapter, 7354
Scleroderma Support Groups, 7375
Shriver Center University Affiliated Program, 10274
Sleep Disorders Unit Beth Israel Deaconess Medical Center, 7804
Sleep Research Foundation, 7808
Society for Surgery of the Alimentary Foundation, 3938
Society for Surgery of the Alimentary Tract, 3928
Spina Bifida Association of Massachusetts, 7882
Suicide Prevention Resource Center, 7078
Talking Book Library at Worcester Public Library, 9694
The Center on Aging and Work at Boston College, 135
Traditional Tibetan Healing, 6439
Trauma Center, 7079
Trauma Center, 7096
Tufts Medical Center, 5064
United Cerebral Palsy of Berkshire County, 2735
United Cerebral Palsy of MetroBoston, 2736
University of Massachusetts Memorial Medical Center, 3129
University of Massachusetts: Diabetes and Endocrinology Research Center, 3395
VALT Support Group (Vital Active Life After Trauma), 4164
Veterans Benefits Clearinghouse, 10275
Vision Use in Employment, 9823
West Roxbury Division VA Boston Healthcare System, 10171

Michigan

AARP Michigan, 72
ALS Association: East Michigan Chapter, 1111
ALS Association: West Michigan Chapter, 1112
Aleda E. Lutz VA Medical Center: Saginaw, Michigan, 10172
Alzheimer's Association: East Central Michigan Chapter, 841
Alzheimer's Association: Greater Michigan Chapter, 842
Alzheimer's Association: Greater Michigan Chapter: Upper Peninsula Region, 843
Alzheimer's Association: Michigan Great Lakes Chapter: West Shore Region, 844
Alzheimer's Association: Mid-Michigan Chapter, 845
Alzheimer's Association: Northeast Michigan Chapter, 846
Alzheimer's Association: Northwest Michigan Chapter, 847
American Autoimmune Related Diseases Association, 251
American Autoimmune Related Diseases Association, 4859
American Autoimmune Related Diseases Association, 8851
American Autoimmune Related Diseases Association, 10340
American Diabetes Association: Michigan, 3279
American Institute for Preventive Medicine, 10345
American Institute for Preventive Medicine, 10346
American Liver Foundation Michigan Chapter, 5755
American Lung Association of Michigan, 5839
American Lung Association of Michigan, 9284
American Motility Society, 3919
Anxiety Resource Center, 7065
Apnea Identification Program Children's Ho spital of Michigan, 8751
Arthritis Foundation: Michigan Chapter Chapter and Metro Detroit, 1211
Association for Children's Mental Health, 5969
Association for the Blind & Visually Impaired, 9516
Asthma and Allergy Foundation of America: Michigan Chapter, 651

Asthma and Allergy Foundation of America: Michigan Chapter, 1393
Autism Society of Michigan, 1690
Battle Creek VA Medical Center, 10173
Brain Injury Association of Michigan, 4101
Brain Injury Association of Michigan Helpline, 4165
Brain Tumor Networking Club, 1987
Brain Tumor Support Group for Patients & Families, 1988
Brain Tumor Support Group: Ann Arbor, 1989
Brain Tumor Support Group: West Bloomfield, 1990
CCFA Michigan Chapter: Farmington Hills, 3016
Childhood Liver Disease Research Network, 3083
Client Assistance Program: Michigan, 10459
Commission for the Blind, 10460
Detroit Subregional Library for the Blind and Physically Handicapped, 9695
Detroit Support Group: National Ataxia Foundation, 1544
East Lansing Cystic Fibrosis Center Michigan State University, 3130
Eastern Michigan Hemophilia Center St. Joseph Hospital, 5023
Genesee County Health Department, 8752
Gershenson Radiation Oncology Center Barbara Ann Karmanos Cancer Institute, 2324
Gilda's Club: Grand Rapids, 2399
Glaucoma Laser Trabeculoplasty Study Sinai Hospital of Detroit, 9788
Grand Traverse Area Library for the Blind and Physically Handicapped, 9696
Great Lakes Chapter of the Myasthenia Gravis Foundation of America, 6586
Greater Detroit Agency for the Blind and Visually Impaired, 9517
Greater Grand Rapids Pediatric Hemophilia Program, 5027
Hemophilia Foundation of Michigan, 4983
Henry Ford Hospital: Hypertension and Vascular Research Division, 5255
Hydrocephalus Support Group of Michigan Children's Hospital of Michigan, 5203
International Hearing Society, 4317
International Hearing Society, 4414
JIMHO Affiliated Centers (Justice in Mental Health Organization), 5970
John D. Dingell VA Medical Center, 10174
Juvenile Diabetes Research Foundation: Metropolitan Detroit/SE Michigan, 3280
Juvenile Diabetes Research Foundation: Wes t Michigan Chapter, 3281
Kalamazoo Center for Medical Studies Michigan State University, 3131
Kent County Health Department, 8753
Kent County Library for the Blind, 9697
Leukemia and Lymphoma Society: Michigan Chapter, 2182
Library of Michigan Service for the Blind, 9698
Lupus Foundation of America: Michigan Lupus Foundation, 8883
Lyme Alliance, 9033
Macomb Library for the Blind and Physically Handicapped, 9699
Meyer L Prentis Comprehensive Cancer Cente Barbara Ann Karmanos Cancer Institute, 2326
Meyer L Prentis Comprehensive Cancer Center of Metropolitan Detroit, 2325
Michigan Alliance for the Mentally Ill, 5971
Michigan Alzheimer's Disease Research Center, 970
Michigan Deaf Association, 4348
Michigan Department of Health & Human Services, 8754
Michigan Department of Health & Human Services: Division of HIV & STD Programs, 315
Michigan Kidney Foundation, 5618
Michigan State University Hemophilia Comprehensive Care Clinic, 5044
Midwestern Michigan Library Cooperative, 9700
Motor Neuron Disease Program University of Michigan Health System, 1143
Muskegon County Library for the Blind, 9701
NF Support Group of West Michigan, 6683
National Federation of the Blind: Michigan, 9518
National MS Society: Michigan Chapter, 6378
Northland Library Cooperative, 9702

Oakland County Health Division: SIDS Project, 8755
Oakland County Library for the Visually and Physically Impaired, 9703
Office of Substance Abuse Services Department of Public Health, 8162
Orthopaedic Associates of Michigan, 2611
Oscar G Johnson VA Medical Center, 10175
Patient Advocates for Advanced Cancer Treatments (PAACT), 2266
Prader-Willi Michigan Association, 7181
RESOLVE of Michigan, 5403
Rainbow Connection, 10674
Regional Hemophilia Treatment Center Children's Hospital of Michigan, 5054
Rehabilitation Institute of Michigan, 4134
SIDS LEAD: Children's Special Health Care Services, 8756
Scleroderma Foundation: Michigan Chapter, 7340
Spina Bifida Association of Grand Rapids, 7883
Spina Bifida Association of Upper Peninsula Michigan, 7884
Spina Bifida and Hydrocephalus Association of Southwestern Michigan, 7885
St. Clark County Library for the Blind and Physically Handicapped, 9704
The Turner Syndrome Society: Michigan Chapter, 9351
Transplantation Society of Michigan, 9197
United Cerebral Palsy of Metropolitan Detroit, 2737
United Cerebral Palsy of Michigan, 2738
University of Michigan Communicative Disorders Clinic, 4401
University of Michigan Hemophilia Center, 5070
University of Michigan Michigan Gastrointestinal Peptide Research Ctr., 3945
University of Michigan Montgomery: John M. Sheldon Allergy Society, 668
University of Michigan Nephrology Division, 5667
University of Michigan Pulmonary and Critical Care Division, 4904
University of Michigan Reproductive Sciences Program, 5438
University of Michigan: Alcohol Research Center, 8230
University of Michigan: Cancer Center Cancer Research Committee, 2327
University of Michigan: Cardiovascular Med icine, 4905
University of Michigan: Cystic Fibrosis Center, 3132
University of Michigan: Division of Hypertension, 5258
University of Michigan: Kresge Hearing Research Institute, 4402
University of Michigan: Mental Health Research Institute, 6040
University of Michigan: National Cooperative Drug/AIDS Group, 410
University of Michigan: Orthopaedic Research Laboratories, 1255
University of Michigan: Psychiatric Center, 8231
Upper Peninsula Library for the Blind and Physically Handicapped, 9705
VA Ann Arbor Healthcare System, 10176
Visually Impaired Center, 9805
Washtenaw County Library for the Blind and Physically Disabled, 9706
Wayne County Regional Library for the Blind and Physically Handicapped, 9707
Wayne State University Center for Health Research, 411
Wayne State University Center for Molecular Medicine and Genetics, 2328
Wayne State University: CS Mott Center for Human Growth and Development, 1848
Wayne State University: Comprehensive Sickle Cell Center, 7624
Wayne State University: Gurdjian-Lissner Biomechanics Laboratory, 4143
Wayne State University: University Women's Care, 5440
William T Gossett Parkinson's Disease Center, 6911

Minnesota

AARP Minnesota, 73
ALS Association: Minnesota, South Dakota, North Dakota Chapter, 1113
African American Family Services, 8106
Alzheimer's Association: Minnesota/Dakotas, 848
Alzheimer's Disease Center Mayo Clinic Mayo Medical School, 951
American Academy of Neurology, 6286
American Academy of Neurology: Tourette Syndrome, 9078
American Association of Neuromuscular & Electrodiagnostic Medicine, 1089
American Association of Neuromuscular & Electrodiagnostic Medicine, 6571
American Association of Neuromuscular & Electrodiagnostic Medicine, 7008
American Cancer Society: Duluth, 2183
American Cancer Society: Mendota Heights Mendota Heights, 2184
American Cancer Society: Rochester, 2185
American Cancer Society: Saint Cloud, 2186
American Diabetes Association: Minnesota, 3282
American Liver Foundation Minnesota Chapte r, 5756
American Lung Association of Minnesota, 5840
American Lung Association of Minnesota, 9285
Arthritis Foundation: North Central Chapter, 1212
Autism Society of Minnesota, 1691
Behavioral Pediatrics Program, 10511
Brain Injury Alliance of Minnesota, 4166
Brain Injury Association of Minnesota, 4102
CCFA Minnesota Chapter, 3017
Center for Children with Chronic Illness and Disability, 10355
Chemical Dependency Program Division Department of Human Services, 8163
Dentists Concerned for Dentists, 8164
Desert Storm Justice Foundation: Minnesota, 10177
Down Syndrome Association of Minnesota, 3565
Duluth Lighthouse for the Blind, 9519
Duluth Public Library, 9708
Emotional Health Anonymous, 6062
Fairview-University Hemophilia & Thrombosis Center, 5025
Fetal Alcohol Network, 10513
Hazelden Betty Ford Foundation, 8118
Hear Now: Starkey Hearin Foundation, 4309
Hemophilia Foundation of Minnesota and the Dakotas, 4984
Immunization Action Coalition, 5142
Impotence Information Center, 5305
International Diabetes Center at Nicollet, 3387
Juvenile Diabetes Research Foundation: Min nesota Chapter, 3283
KDWB Family Resource Center, 10516
KDWB Variety Family Canter, 10517
Lawyers Concerned for Lawyers, 8120
Leukemia and Lymphoma Society: Minnesota Chapter, 2187
LifeSource, Upper Midwest Organ Procurement Organization, Inc., 9198
Lupus Foundation of America: Minnesota Chapter, 8884
Mayo Clinic and Foundation Mayo Foundation, 6517
Mayo Clinic and Foundation: Division of Allergic Diseases, 661
Mayo Clinic: Department of Neurology, 1141
Mayo Comprehensive Cancer Center, 2329
Mayo Comprehensive Hemophilia Center Mayo Clinic, 5042
Melpomene Institute for Women's Health Research, 5436
Minneapolis VA Health Care System, 10178
Minnesota AIDS Project AIDSLine, 452
Minnesota Alliance for the Mentally Ill, 5972
Minnesota Ambassador: National Ataxia Foundation, 1545
Minnesota Association for Children's Mental Health, 5973
Minnesota Department of Health, 316
Minnesota Disability Law Center, 10461
Minnesota Library for the Blind, 9709
Minnesota Obesity Center, 6717

Minnesota State Chapter of the Myasthenia Gravis Foundation of America, 6587
Minnesota Sudden Infant Death Center Minneapolis Children's Medical Center, 8757
Myasthenia Gravis Support Group of Mid-Min n, 6611
Myasthenia Gravis Support Group of South East Minnesota, 6612
Myasthenia Gravis Support Group of the Twin Cities, 6613
National Association to Promote the Use of Braille, 9438
National Ataxia Foundation, 1521
National Federation of the Blind: Minnesota, 9520
National Kidney Foundation Serving Minneso ta, Dakotas & Iowa Division Office, 5645
National Kidney Foundation of Minnesota, 5619
National MS Society: Minnesota Chapter, 6379
National Marrow Donor Program, 2110
National Resource Library on Youth with Disabilities, 10508
Neurofibromatosis: Minnesota, 6677
PACER Center, 6063
Parkinson Association of Minnesota, 6895
Pediatric Psychology, 10525
Prader-Willi Minnesota Association, 7182
RESOLVE of Minnesota, 5404
STAR Center for Family Health, 10526
Schulze Diabetes Institute, 3375
Scleroderma Foundation: Minnesota Chapter, 7341
Spina Bifida Association of Minnesota, 7886
Spinal Cord Society, 7961
St. Paul Regional Office, 10179
The Emily Program Foundation (merged with Anna Westin Foundation), 3704
The Turner Syndrome Society: Minnesota Chapter, 9352
Twin Cities Area Support Group: National Ataxia Foundation, 1546
U Special Kids, 10527
United Cerebral Palsy of Central Minnesota, 2739
United Cerebral Palsy of Minnesota, 2740
United Ostomy Associations of America Advocacy Hotline, 2414
University of Minnesota Department of Psychiatry, 6041
University of Minnesota Masonic Cancer Center, 2330
University of Minnesota: Cystic Fibrosis Center, 3133
University of Minnesota: Hypertensive Research Group, 5259
University of Minnesota: Program on Alcohol/Drug Control, 8232

Mississippi

AARP Mississippi, 74
Alzheimer's Association: Mississippi Chapter, 849
Alzheimer's Foundation of the South: Mississippi Division, 850
American Cancer Society: Jackson, 2188
American Diabetes Association: Mississippi, 3284
American Lung Association of Mississippi, 5841
American Lung Association of Mississippi, 9286
Arthritis Foundation: Mississippi Chapter, 1213
Brain Injury Association of Mississippi, 4103
Brain Injury Association of Mississippi Helpline, 4167
Christian Resource for People Who Are Blind, 9710
Division of Alcohol & Drug Abuse: Mississippi, 8165
Division of Alcohol & Drug Abuse: South Department of Mental Health, 8166
G.V. (Sonny) Montgomery VA Medical Center, 10180
Gulf Coast Veterans Health Care System, 10181
Jackson Regional Office, 10182
Leukemia and Lymphoma Society: Mississippi Chapter, 2189
Lupus Foundation of America: Mississippi Chapter, 8885
Mississippi Alliance for the Mentally Ill, 5974
Mississippi Area Support Group: National Ataxia Foundation, 1547
Mississippi Client Assistance Program, 10462

Mississippi Families as Allies, 5975
Mississippi Hemophilia Foundation, 4985
Mississippi Industries for the Blind, 9521
Mississippi Library Commission, 9711
Mississippi Organ Recovery, 9199
Mississippi SIDS Alliance, 8758
Mississippi State Department of Health and Child Health Services, 8759
Mississippi State Department of Health: STD/HIV Office, 317
National Federation of the Blind: Human Services Division, 9445
National Federation of the Blind: Mississippi, 9522
National Kidney Foundation of Mississippi, 5620
National Multiple Sclerosis Society: Alaba ma-Mississippi Chapter, 6380
South Central VA Health Care Network, 10183
University of Mississippi Medical Center, 3134

Missouri

AARP Missouri, 75
ALS Association: Mid America Chapter- Southern Missouri Office, 1114
ALS Association: St. Louis Regional Chapter, 1115
APDA Center for Advanced Parkinson Disease Research, 6919
Adriene Resource Center for Blind Children, 9712
Alphapointe Association for the Blind, 9523
Alzheimer's Association: Mid-Missouri Chapter, 851
Alzheimer's Association: Northwest Missouri-Chapter, 852
Alzheimer's Association: Southwest Missouri Chapter, 853
Alzheimer's Association: St. Louis Chapter, 854
Alzheimer's Disease Research Center Washington University School of Medicine, 958
American Cancer Society: Saint Louis, 2190
American Diabetes Association: Missouri, 3285
American Liver Foundation Greater Kansas City Chapter, 5757
American Lung Association of Eastern Missouri, 5843
American Lung Association of Missouri, 9287
American Lung Association: Kansas City Office, 5844
American Optometric Association, 9411
Arthritis Foundation: Eastern Missouri Chapter, 1214
Assemblies of God National Center for the Blind, 9713
Asthma and Allergy Foundation of America: St. Louis Chapter, 652
Asthma and Allergy Foundation of America: St. Louis Chapter, 1394
Autism Society of Gateway Chapter, 1692
Brain Cancer Support Group, 1991
Brain Injury Association of Missouri, 4104
Brain Injury Association of Missouri Helpline, 4168
Brain Tumor Support Group: Kansas City, 1992
Brain Tumor Support and Networking Group, 1993
CCFA Mid-America Chapter: Kansas, 3012
CCFA Mid-America Chapter: Missouri, 3018
Cancer Research Center, 2331
Central Institute for the Deaf, 4371
Central Missouri Regional Arthritis Center Stephen's College Campus, 1245
Children's Mercy Hospital Children's Mercy Hospitals & Clinics, 3135
Church of the Nazarene, 9714
Fabry Support & Information Group, 3844
Gateway Hemophilia Association, 4986
Guide Dog Users, Inc., 9427
Harry S. Truman Memorial Veterans' Hospital, 10184
Harvey A Friedman Center for Aging Washington University, 120
John J. Pershing VA Medical Center, 10185
Juvenile Diabetes Research Foundation: St. Louis Chapter, 3286
Kansas City Association for the Blind, 9524
Kansas City Support Group: National Ataxia Foundation, 1548
Kansas City VA Medical Center, 10186
Lupus Foundation of America: Kansas City, 8886
Lupus Foundation of America: Ozarks Chapter, 8887

Lutheran Library for the Blind, 9715
MO-SPAN, 5976
MO-SPAN Southwest Region, 6064
MOSPAN Northwest Region, 6065
Mid Missouri Support Group: National Ataxia
    Foundation, 1549
Mid-America Transplant Services, 9200
Missouri Coalition Alliance for the Mentally Ill, 5977
Missouri Department of Health & Senior Services:
    Bureau of HIV, STD & Hepatitis, 318
Missouri Division of Alcohol and Drug Abuse, 8167
Missouri Illinois Regional Hemophilia
    Comprehensive Treatment Center, 5045
Missouri Protection and Advocacy Services, 10463
Missouri Teratogen Information Service, 1855
NAMI of Missouri, 5978
NNFF Kansas Affiliate, 6672
National Children's Cancer Society, 2260
National Federation of the Blind: Missouri, 9525
National Kidney Foundation of Eastern Missouri and
    Metro East, 5621
National MS Society: Gateway Area Chapter, 6381
Ozarks Parkinson Support Group, 6920
PKD Foundation Polycystic Kidney Disease
    Foundation, 5665
PostPolio Health International, 7015
Prader-Willi Missouri Association, 7183
RESOLVE of St. Louis, Missouri, 5405
SIDS Resources, 8761
Scleroderma Foundation: Missouri Chapter, 7342
Share Pregnancy and Infant Loss Support, Inc., 8704
Share Pregnancy and Infant Loss Support, Inc., 10698
Spina Bifida Association of Greater St. Louis, 7887
United Cerebral Palsy of Greater Kansas City, 2741
United Cerebral Palsy of Greater St. Louis, 2742
United Cerebral Palsy of Northwest Missouri, 2743
University of Missouri Columbia Cystic Fibrosis
    Center, 3136
University of Missouri Columbia Division of
    Cardiothoracic Surgery, 4906
University of Missouri: Columbia Missouri Institute
    of Mental Health, 6042
University of Missouri: Kansas City Drug
    Information Service, 8233
VA Heartland Network, 10187
VA St. Louis Health Care System John Cochran &
    Jefferson Barracks, 10188
Washington University Chromalloy American Kidney
    Center, 5670
Washington University School of Medicine, 8064
Washington University: Cystic Fibrosis Center, 3137
Washington University: Diabetes Research and
    Training Center, 3406
Western Region SIDS Resources, 8762
Whitney Library for the Blind: Assemblies of God,
    9716
Wolfner Memorial Library for the Blind, 9717

Montana

AARP Montana, 76
Alzheimer's Association: Greater Billings Area
    Chapter, 855
American Cancer Society: Montana, 2191
American Diabetes Association: Montana, 3287
American Lung Association of Northern Rockies,
    5845
American Lung Association of the Northern Rockies:
    Montana and Wyoming, 9288
Brain Injury Alliance of Montana, 4169
Brain Injury Association of Montana, 4105
Cancer Patient/Caregiver Support Group, 1994
Department of Institutions, Alcohol and Drug Abuse
    Division, 8168
Department of Public Health and Human Services,
    8763
Disability Rights Montana, 10464
Family Support Network, 5979
Lupus Foundation of America: Montana Chapter,
    8888
Medical Center & Ambulatory Care Clinic Montana
    VA Health Care System, 10189
Miles City VA Clinic & Community Living Center,
    10190

Montana Alliance for the Mentally Ill Mihelish's
    Residence, 5980
Montana Deptartment of Public Health & Human
    Services: HIV/STD/HepC Program, 319
Montana State Library, 9718
National Federation of the Blind: Montana, 9526
National MS Society: Montana Division, 6382

Nebraska

AARP Nebraska: Lincoln, 77
AARP Nebraska: Omaha, 78
ALS Association: MidAmerica Chapter - Nebr aska
    Office, 1116
Alzheimer's Association: Great Plains Chap ter, 856
Alzheimer's Association: Lincoln/Greater Nebraska
    Chapter, 857
Alzheimer's Association: Omaha/Eastern Nebraska
    Chapter, 858
American Cancer Society: Nebraska, 2192
American Diabetes Association: Nebraska, 3288
American Lung Association of Nebraska, 5846
American Lung Association of Nebraska, 9289
Arthritis Foundation: Nebraska Chapter, 1216
Autism Society of Nebraska, 1693
Boys Town National Research Hospital, 4369
Caregiver Support Services, 148
Center for Hearing Loss in Children Boystown
    National Research Hospital, 4370
Client Assistance Program: Nebraska Division of
    Rehabilitative Services, 10465
Creighton University Allergic Disease Center, 659
Creighton University Cardiac Center, 4875
Creighton University Midwest Hypertension
    Research Center, 5253
Department of Public Instruction: Division of
    Alcoholism and Drug Abuse, 8169
Family Support Network, 2795
Home Instead Center for Successful Aging University
    of Nebraska Medical Center, 121
Juvenile Diabetes Research Foundation: Lin coln
    Chapter, 3289
Juvenile Diabetes Research Foundation: Oma ha
    Council Bluffs Chapter, 3290
Leukemia and Lymphoma Society: Nebraska Chapter,
    2193
Lincoln Cancer Center, 2332
Lupus Foundation of America: Omaha Chapter, 8889
Lupus Foundation of America: Western Nebraska
    Chapter, 8890
National Alliance for the Mentally Ill: Nebraska
    (NAMI), 5981
National Federation of the Blind: Nebraska, 9527
National MS Society: Midlands Chapter Community
    Health Plaza, 6383
Nebraska Chapter of the National Hemophilia
    Foundation, 4987
Nebraska Department of Health Perinatal Child and
    Adolescent Health, 8764
Nebraska Information Service, 1857
Nebraska Kidney Association, 5623
Nebraska Library Commission Talking Book and
    Braille Services, 9719
Nebraska Organ Retrieval System, 9201
Nebraska SIDS Foundation University of Nebraska
    Medical Center, 8765
North Platte Public Library, 9720
Omaha HPV Support Group: PP of Omaha, 10466
Prader-Willi Nebraska Association, 7184
Spina Bifida Association of Nebraska, 7888
United Cerebral Palsy of Nebraska, 2744
University of Nebraska Medical Center Cystic
    Fibrosis Center, 3138
University of Nebraska Medical Center Tera Togen
    Project, 1866
University of Nebraska at Omaha Eppley Institute for
    Research in Cancer, 2333
University of Nebraska: Lincoln, 4403

Nevada

AARP Nevada, 79

Alcohol and Drug Abuse Bureau: Department of
    Human Resources, 8170
Alzheimer's Association: Northern Nevada Chapter,
    859
Alzheimer's Association: Southern Nevada Chapter,
    860
American Cancer Society: Nevada, 2194
American Diabetes Association: Nevada, 3291
American Lung Association of Idaho/Nevada, 9290
American Lung Association of Nevada, 5847
Association of Halfway House Alcoholism Programs
    of North America (AHHAP), 8112
Autism Society of Northern Nevada, 1694
Children's Lung Specialists, 3139
Client Assistance Program: Nevada, 10467
Cure Our Children Foundation, 10659
Hemophilia Foundation of Nevada, 4988
Juvenile Diabetes Research Foundation: Nevada
    Chapter, 3292
Juvenile Diabetes Research Foundation: Nor thern
    Nevada Branch, 3293
Las Vegas Clark County Library District, 9721
NNFF Nevada Affiliate: Reno Area, 6678
Natioanl Multiple Sclerosis Society Desert Southwest
    Chapter, 6384
National Federation of the Blind: Nevada, 9528
National MS Society: Great Basin Sierra Chapter,
    6385
Nevada Alliance for the Mentally Ill, 5982
Nevada Department of Health & Human Services:
    Office Of HIV Prevention, 320
Nevada Donor Network, 9202
Nevada PEP, 6066
Nevada State Health Division Bureau of Family
    Health Services, 8766
Nevada State Library and Archives, 9722
North Las Vegas VA Medical Center VA Southern
    Nevada Healthcare System, 10191
RESOLVE of Nevada, 5406
Sanford Center for Aging University Of Nevada,
    Reno, 132
Scleroderma Foundation: Nevada Chapter, 7343
Southern Nevada Sightless, 9529
United Cerebral Palsy of Northern Nevada, 2745
University Medical Center Hemophilia Program,
    5067
VA Sierra Nevada Health Care System, 10192

New Hampshire

AARP New Hampshire, 80
ALS Association: Northern New England Chapter,
    1117
Alzheimer's Association of Vermont and New
    Hampshire, 861
American Cancer Society: New Hampshire Gail
    Singer Memorial Building, 2195
American Diabetes Association: New Hampshire,
    3294
American Lung Association of New Hampshire, 5848
American Lung Association of New Hampshire, 9291
Arthritis Foundation: Northern New England Chapter,
    1234
Autism Society of New Hampshire, 1695
Brain Injury Association of New Hampshire, 4106
Brain Injury Association of New Hampshire, 4170
Brain Injury/Brain Tumor Support Group, 1995
Camp Allen, 10509
Client Assistance Program: New Hampshire, 10468
Dartmouth Medical School: Microbiology
    Department, 3800
Dartmouth-Hitchcock Medical Center - Genetics and
    Development, 3581
Granite State FFCMH, 5983
High Hopes Foundation, 10665
Juvenile Diabetes Research Foundation: New
    England/New Hampshire Chapter, 3295
Manchester VA Medical Center VAMC Manchester,
    New Hampshire, 10193
National Alliance for the Mentally Ill: New
    Hampshire, 5984
National Alliance for the Mentally Ill: New
    Hampshire, 6067

National Federation of the Blind: New Hampshire, 9530
New Hampshire Cancer Pain Initiative, 2196
New Hampshire Chapter NSCIA, 7975
New Hampshire Cystic Fibrosis Care Teaching and Research Center, 3140
New Hampshire Department of Health and Human Services, 321
New Hampshire Lupus Foundation, 8891
New Hampshire SIDS Program, 8767
New Hampshire State Library, 9723
Norris Cotton Cancer Center Dartmouth-Hitchcock Medical Center, 2334
Office of Alcohol and Drug Abuse Prevention, 8171
RESOLVE of New Hampshire, 5407
Sleep Disorders Center Dartmouth Hitchcock Medical Center, 7785
Sleep/Wake Disorders Center: Hampstead Hospital, 7813
Voices for the Blind, 9724

New Jersey

AARP New Jersey, 81
Alcohol Disease Foundation, 8197
All Access Mental Health, 5985
Alzheimer's Association: Greater New Jersey Chapter, 862
Alzheimer's Association: South Jersey Chapter, 863
American Anorexia Bulimia Association: New Jersey Chapter, 3695
American Auditory Society, 4294
American Cancer Society: New Jersey, 2197
American Diabetes Association: New Jersey, 3296
American Headache Society, 6288
American Lung Association of New Jersey, 5849
American Lung Association of New Jersey, 9292
American Migraine Foundation, 6289
American Society of Transplantation (AST), 9163
Angelwish, Inc., 10681
Arthritis Foundation: New Jersey Chapter, 1217
Autism Society of Southwest New Jersey, 1696
Bestwork Industries for the Blind, 9531
Brain Injury Alliance of New Jersey, 4171
Brain Injury Association of New Jersey, 4107
Brain Tumor Support Group: New Jersey, 1996
Brain Tumor Support Group: Toms River, 1997
CCFA New Jersey Chapter, 3019
COPLINE, 7102
CanHelp, 2198
Center for Parent Information & Resources, 1602
Center for Parent Information & Resources, 3539
Center for Parent Information & Resources, 4301
Center for Parent Information & Resources, 10362
Central New Jersey Brain Tumor Support Group, 1998
Christ Hospital Hepatitis C Support Group, 5147
Community Mental Health Foundation, 5986
Cooley's Anemia Foundation (CAF): New Jersey Chapter, 2963
Department of Health, 8172
Disability Rights New Jersey, 10469
Division of Narcotic and Drug Abuse Control, 8173
East Orange Campus VA New Jersey Health Care System, 10194
Eating Disorders Association of New Jersey, 3715
Epilepsy Foundation of New Jersey, 7485
Friends Health Connection, 10514
Garden State Chapter of the Myasthenia Gravis Foundation of America, 6590
Garrett Mountain Chapter of the American Association of Kidney Patients, 5625
Greater New York Pull-Thru Network, 5338
HealthyWomen, 3794
HealthyWomen, 5377
HealthyWomen, 9004
HealthyWomen, 10383
Helping Other Parents in Normal Grief, 10694
Hopes & Dreams for Children, 10667
Huxley Insititute-American Schizophrenic Association, 6258
Hydrocephalus Parents Support Group, 5208
Institute of Ophthalmology and Visual Scie nce New Jersey Medical School, 9794

Jason's Dreams for Kids Foundation, Inc., 10686
Juvenile Diabetes Research Foundation: Cen tral Jersey Chapter, 3298
Juvenile Diabetes Research Foundation: Mid -Jersey Chapter, 3299
Juvenile Diabetes Research Foundation: Roc kland County/Northern New Jersey, 3300
Juvenile Diabetes Research Foundation: South Jersey Chapter, 3297
Learning Ally, 9430
Leukemia and Lymphoma Society: Northern New Jersey Chapter, 2199
Leukemia and Lymphoma Society: Southern New Jersey Chapter, 2200
Lupus Foundation of America: New Jersey Chapter, 8892
Lupus Foundation of America: South Jersey Chapter, 8893
Lyme Disease Association, Inc., 9026
Lyme Disease Network, 9034
Lyme Disease Network of New Jersey, 9036
Lyons Campus VA New Jersey Health Care System, 10195
Meadowlands Chapter of the American Association of Kidney Patients, 5626
Monmouth Medical Center: Cystic Fibrosis & Monmouth Medical Center, 3142
Monmouth Medical Center: Cystic Fibrosis & Pediatric Pulmonary Center, 3141
Multiple Sclerosis Association of America, 6342
Musculoskeletal Transplant Foundation, 9226
Nadeene Brunini Comprehensive Hemophilia Care Center, 5047
National Federation of the Blind: Deaf-Blind Division, 9444
National Federation of the Blind: New Jersey, 9532
National MS Society: Greater North Jersey Chapter, 6387
National MS Society: Mid-Jersey Chapter, 6388
National Sarcoidosis Resource Center, 7235
Neuromuscular and ALS Center The Clinical Academic Building, 1144
New Eyes for the Needy, 9452
New Jersey AIDS Services, 322
New Jersey Alliance for the Mentally Ill, 5987
New Jersey Department of Health: Child Health Program, 8768
New Jersey Department of Health: Division of HIV, STD And TB Services, 323
New Jersey Institute of Technology Center for Biomedical Engineering, 4053
New Jersey Library for the Blind and Handicapped, 9725
New Jersey Medical School, 3143
New Jersey Parkinson's Disease Information Center, 6921
New Jersey Pregnancy Risk Information Service, 1858
New Jersey SIDS Alliance, 8769
New Jersey Turner Syndrome Resource Group, 9353
Northern New Jersey Chapter of the American Association of Kidney Patients, 5627
Orthopaedic Rehabilitation Association, 7011
Parent Project: Muscular Dystrophy, 6512
Parkinson Alliance, 6896
Prader-Willi New Jersey Association, 7185
RESOLVE of New Jersey, 5408
Recording for the Blind Helpline, 9822
Renfrew Center of Northern New Jersey, 3696
Rutgers Global Tuberculosis Institute New Jersey Medical School, 9261
Rutgers University Center of Alcohol Studies, 8223
Rutgers University: Controlled Drug- Delivery Research Center, 8224
SIDS Center of New Jersey, 8770
Sarcoidosis Support Group: New Jersey, 7250
Seeing Eye, 9457
Sharing Network Organ Tissue Donation Services, 9203
Sleep Disorders Center: Newark Beth Israel Medical Center, 7799
Spina Bifida Association of the Tri-State Region, 7889
The Reeve Foundation, 7962
United Cerebral Palsy of Hudson County, 2746

United Cerebral Palsy of Morris-Somerset, 2747
United Cerebral Palsy of New Jersey, 2748
Well Spouse Association, 153
Well Spouse Association, 10529
Wound Ostomy and Continence Nurses Society, 3000

New Mexico

AARP New Mexico, 82
ALS Association: New Mexico Chapter, 1118
Alzheimer's Association: New Mexico Chapter, 864
American Cancer Society: New Mexico, 2201
American Diabetes Association: New Mexico, 3301
American Lung Association of New Mexico, 5850
Autism Society of New Mexico, 1697
Brain Injury Alliance of New Mexico, 4172
Brain Injury Association of New Mexico, 4108
Hemophilia Foundation of New Mexico, 4989
Juvenile Diabetes Research Foundation: Albuquerque, 3302
Leukemia and Lymphoma Society: Mountain States Chapter, 2202
Lovelace Medical Foundation, 5662
Lupus Foundation of America: New Mexico Chapter, 8894
Myasthenia Gravis Support Group of New Mex ico, 6616
National Federation of the Blind: New Mexico, 9533
National Kidney Foundation of New Mexico, 5628
National MS Society: Rio Grande Division, 6389
Navaho Nation K'E Project Children and Families Advocacy Corp, 5988
Navajo Nation K'E Project: Shiprock Children & Families Advocacy Corp, 5989
Navajo Nation Office Special Education & R ehabilitation Services, 6068
New Mexico Alliance for the Mentally Ill, 5990
New Mexico Branch, 9293
New Mexico Department of Health: HIV Services Program, 324
New Mexico Donor Services, 9204
New Mexico Industries for the Blind, 9534
New Mexico SIDS Information and Counseling Program, 8771
New Mexico State Library for the Blind and Physically Handicapped, 9726
Overeaters Anonymous, 6712
People Living Through Cancer Support Groups, 1999
Protection and Advocacy System of Alburque rque, 10470
RESOLVE of New Mexico, 5409
Raymond G. Murphy VA Medical Center New Mexico VA Health Care System, 10196
Spina Bifida Association of New Mexico, 7890
State of New Mexico Commission for the Blind, 9535
Substance Abuse Bureau, 8174
Ted R Montoya Hemophilia Program University of New Mexico, 5060
USA Deaf Sports Federation, 4336
University of New Mexico General Clinical Research Center, 3397
University of New Mexico: Cancer Research and Treatment Center, 2335
University of New Mexico: Center for Non-Invasive Diagnosis, 2336

New York

AARP New York: Albany, 83
AARP New York: New York City, 84
AARP New York: Rochester, 85
ACLU National Prison Project, 10334
AFB Toll-Free Hotline, 9810
AIDS Hotline of Central New York, 440
ALEH Israel Foundation, 3573
ALS Association: Greater New York Chapter, 1119
ALS Association: Upstate New York Chapter, 1120
Aaron Diamond AIDS Research Center, 412
Access Unlimited, 10336
Ackerman Institute for the Family, 2337
Aging In America, 109
Albany Medical College Joint Center for Cancer and Blood Disorders, 2338

Albany Medical College Pediatric Pulmonary & Cystic Fibrosis Center, 3144
Albany Medican Center, 5013
Albany Stratton VA Medical Center, 10197
Albert Einstein Cancer Center Albert Einstein College of Medicine, 2339
Alcoholics Anonymous, 8108
Alcoholics Anonymous World Services, 8241
Alliance for Lupus Research, 8927
Alzheimer's Association: Central New York Chapter, 866
Alzheimer's Association: Hudson Valley/ Rockland/Westchester NY Chapter, 867
Alzheimer's Association: Long Island Chapter, 868
Alzheimer's Association: New York City Chapter, 869
Alzheimer's Association: Northeastern New York Chapter, 870
Alzheimer's Association: Putnam County Chapter, 871
Alzheimer's Association: Rochester Chapter, 872
Alzheimer's Association: Southern Tier Chapter, 873
Alzheimer's Association: Sullivan/Delaware Chapter, 865
Alzheimer's Association: Western New York Chapter, 874
Alzheimer's Foundation of Staten Island, 875
American Association of Spinal Cord Injury Nurses (AASCIN), 7953
American Cancer Society: Central New York Region/East Syracuse, 2203
American Cancer Society: Long Island, 2204
American Cancer Society: New York City, 2205
American Cancer Society: Queens Region / Rego Park, 2206
American Cancer Society: Westchester Region/White Plains, 2207
American Civil Liberties Union LGBT & AIDS Project, 253
American Diabetes Association: New York, 3303
American Federation for Aging Research, 110
American Foundation for AIDS Research, 351
American Foundation for The Blind, 10344
American Liver Foundation, 5732
American Liver Foundation, 10323
American Liver Foundation Greater New York Chapter, 5758
American Liver Foundation Western New York Chapter, 5759
American Lung Association of Mid New York, 9294
American Lung Association of New York State, 5851
American Parkinson Disease Association (APDA), 6867
American Parkinson Disease Association Hotline, 6922
American Skin Association, 7658
Armond V Mascia Cystic Fibrosis Center NY Medical College, 3145
Arthritis Foundation: Central New York Chapter, 1218
Arthritis Foundation: Long Island Chapter, 1219
Arthritis Foundation: New York Chapter, 1220
Arthritis Foundation: Rockland/Orange Unit, 1221
Association for Behavioral and Cognitive Therapies, 7043
Association for Children with Down Syndrome, 3566
Association for Macular Diseases, 9415
Association for Research of Childhood Cancer, 2340
Association for the Blind & Visually Impaired of Greater Rochester, 9536
Aurora of Central New York, 4409
Aurora of Central New York, 9811
Autism Society of Albany, 1698
Bassett Research Institute, 2341
Batavia VA Medical Center VA Western New York Healthcare System, 10198
Bath VA Medical Center, 10199
Blind Association of Western New York, 9537
Blind Work Association, 9538
Bone Marrow & Cancer Foundation, 2257
Brady Institute Jamaica Hospital Medical Center, 4129
Braille Textbook Assignment Service National Braille Association, 9781
Brain & Behavior Research Foundation, 6195

Brain & Behavior Research Foundation, 6255
Brain Injury Association of New York State, 4109
Brain Injury Association of New York State Helpline, 4173
Brain Trauma Foundation, 4128
Brain Tumor Support Group for Patients and Families, 2000
Brain Tumor Support Group: Long Island, 2001
Brooklyn Campus VA NY Harbor Health Care System, 10200
Buffalo VA Medical Center VA Western New York Healthcare System, 10201
CCFA Greater New York Chapter: National Headquarters, 3020
CCFA Long Island Chapter, 3021
CCFA Rochester/Southern Tier Chapter, 3022
CCFA Upstate/Northeastern New York Chapter, 3023
CCFA Western New York Chapter, 3024
CF & Pediatric Pulmonary Care Center, 3146
COMPASS Program, 445
COPIN Foundation, 10272
CUNY: Teratogen Information Service, 1851
Cafe Plus, 4174
Camp Good Days, 10657
Canandaigua VA Medical Center VA Health Care Upstate New York, 10202
Cancer Institute of Brooklyn, 2342
Cancer Research Institute: New York, 2343
CancerCare, 2099
Canine Helpers for the Handicapped, Inc., 9419
Capital Regional Sleep-Wake Disorders Center, 7764
Center for Donation & Transplantation, 9205
Center for Hearing and Communication, 4349
Center for Medical Consumers, 10361
Center for Medical Consumers, 10510
Center for Rheumatology, 7359
Center for Sleep Medicine of the Mount Sinai Medical Center, 7768
Center for the Disabled, 2749
Center for the Study of Anorexia and Bulimia, 3707
Center on Employment: Rochester Institute of Technology, 4302
Centers for AIDS Research: Albert Einstein College of Medicine, 413
Centers for AIDS Research: Columbia University College of Physicians, 414
Centers for AIDS Research: NYU School of Medicine, 415
Central Association for the Blind and Visually Impaired, 9539
Central NY Area Support Group: National Ataxia Foundation, 1550
Central New York Male Sexual Dysfunction Center, 5302
Central Texas Brain Tumor Support Group, 2028
Cerebral Palsy Associations of New York State, 2750
Chemotherapy Foundation, 2258
Children's Brain Tumor Foundation, 1905
Children's Mental Health Coalition of WNY, Inc., 5991
Children's Tumor Foundation, 6653
Children's Tumor Foundation, 6682
Childrens Lung and Cystic Fibrosis Center, 3147
Choice Magazine Listening, 9727
Chronic Syndrome Sufferers Association, 7010
City University of New York Center for Research in Speech and Hearing, 4372
Client Assistance Program: NY State Commission of Quality of Care, 10471
Columbia Presbyterian Medical Center Neurological Institute, 6514
Columbia University Clinical Research Center for Muscular Dystrophy, 6515
Columbia University Comprehensive Cancer Center, 2344
Columbia University Irving Center for Clinical Research Adult Unit, 4873
Columbia University Robert N. Butler Aging Center, 117
Columbia University: Comprehensive Sickle Cell Center, 7613
Community Access, Inc., 5911
Cooley's Anemia Foundation, 2972
Cooley's Anemia Foundation (CAF): Buffalo, 2965

Cooley's Anemia Foundation (CAF): Long Island, 2966
Cooley's Anemia Foundation (CAF): Queens, 2967
Cooley's Anemia Foundation (CAF): Staten Island, 2968
Cooley's Anemia Foundation (CAF): Suffolk Chapter Office, 2969
Cooley's Anemia Foundation (CAF): Westches ter/Rockland Chapter, 2970
Cornell University: Winifred Masterson Burke Medical Research-Dementia, 961
Cornerstone Medical Arts Center Hospital, 8201
Corporate Angel Network, 2397
Crohn's & Colitis Foundation, 3039
Crohn's & Colitis Foundation, 9384
Cystic Fibrosis Center St. Vincent's Hospital & Medical Center, 3148
Dana Alliance for Brain Initiatives, 4130
Developmental Evaluation Clinic, 3582
Disabled & Alone: Life Services for the Handicapped, 10370
Division of Digestive & Liver Diseases of Cloumbia University, 3708
Division of Substance Abuse Services, 8175
Eating Disorder Resource Center, 3714
Educational Equity Center at The Academy for Educational Development, 10372
Endocrinology Research Laboratory Cabrini Medical Center, 3383
Epilepsy Foundation of Long Island, 7486
Facing Addiction with NCADD, 8116
Families Together in New York State, 5992
Fertility Research Foundation, 3798
Fertility Research Foundation, 5431
Fibromyalgia Resources Group, 3867
Fight for Sight, 9424
Finger Lakes Donor Recovery Network, 9206
First Presbyterian Church in the City of New York Support Groups, 3716
Foundation for Advancement in Cancer Therapy, 2208
Freedom From Fear, 7046
Friends of Karen, 10663
General Clinical Research Center Mount Sinai School of Medicine, 416
Gilda's Club: New York City, 2400
Greater New York Metro Intergroup of Overeaters Anonymous, 6720
Greater Rochester Area Chapter NSCIA, 7976
HEAL, 448
HIV Center for Clinical and Behavioral Studies, 417
Hearing Health Foundation, 4311
Heart Disease Research Foundation, 4883
Helen Keller International, 9791
Helen Keller National Center for Deaf-Blind Youths and Adults, 9429
Helen Keller National Center for Deaf/Blind Youth and Adults, 4314
Helen Keller National Center for Deaf/Blind Youths and Adults, 9792
Hemophilia Center of Western New York, 4990
Hemophilia Center of Western New York Erie County Medical Center, 5035
Holliswood Hospital Psychiatric Care, Serv ices and Self-Help/Support Groups, 3717
Housing Works, 262
Human Growth Foundation, 4048
Human Growth Foundation, 9340
Hy Feinstein Clubhouse, 4175
Images Within: A Child's View of Parental Alcoholism, 8244
Institute for Basic Research in Developmental Disabilities, 966
Institute for Basic Research in Developmental Disabilities, 1720
Institute for Basic Research in Developmental Disabilities, 3597
Institute for Clinical Research Weill Cornell Medical College, 418
Institute for Visual Sciences, 9793
Institute on Communication and Inclusion at Syracuse University, 1721
International Center for Fabry Disease, 3836
International Center for Fabry Disease, 3841
International Union Against Venereal Diseases, 7572

JGB Cassette Library International, 9728
Jerusalem Center for Multi-Handicapped Blind Children, 9795
Jewish Genetics Disaese Center, 4020
Jewish Genetics Disease Center, 8967
John A. Hartford Foundation, 112
Juvenile Diabetes Research Foundation, 3304
Juvenile Diabetes Research Foundation International, 3367
Juvenile Diabetes Research Foundation: Buf falo/Western New York Chapter, 3306
Juvenile Diabetes Research Foundation: Hud son Valley Chapter, 3307
Juvenile Diabetes Research Foundation: Long Island/South Shore Chapter, 3305
Juvenile Diabetes Research Foundation: New York Chapter, 3308
Juvenile Diabetes Research Foundation: Nor theastern New York, 3309
Juvenile Diabetes Research Foundation: Roc hester Branch/Western New York Chapter, 3310
Juvenile Diabetes Research Foundation: Wes tchester County Chapter, 3311
Keep A Child Alive, 264
Kidney & Urology Foundation of America, 5629
Kidney Disease Institute, 5661
Laboratory of Dermatology Research Memorial Sloane-Kettering Cancer Center, 7668
Leukemia & Lymphoma Society Chapter: New York City, 2209
Leukemia & Lymphoma Society: Westchester/ Hudson Valley Chapter, 2210
Leukemia and Lymphoma Society, 2104
Leukemia and Lymphoma Society Chapter: New York City, 2211
Leukemia and Lymphoma Society: Central New York Chapter, 2212
Leukemia and Lymphoma Society: Long Island Chapter, 2213
Leukemia and Lymphoma Society: Upstate New York Chapter, 2214
Leukemia and Lymphoma Society: Western New York & Finger Lakes Chapter, 2215
Lighthouse Guild GuildCare, 9431
Long Island Alzheimers Foundation, 946
Long Island Alzheimers Foundation, 967
Long Island Brain Tumor Support Group, 2002
Long Island Chapter of the American Association of Kidney Patients, 5630
Lupus Alliance of America LIQ Affiliate, 8895
Lupus Alliance of Upstate New York, 8896
Lupus Foundation of America: Bronx Chapter, 8897
Lupus Foundation of America: Central New York Chapter, 8898
Lupus Foundation of America: Genessee Valley Chapter, 8899
Lupus Foundation of America: Westchester, 8900
Lupus Foundation of Mid and Northern New York, 8901
Lymphatic Research Foundation, 10392
MS Toll-Free Information Line, 6435
Manhattan VA Medical Center VA NY Harbor Health Care System, 10203
Marty Lyons Foundation, Inc., 10672
Medical Foundation of Buffalo Hauptman-Woodward Medical Research Insti, 2345
Memorial Sloan-Kettering Cancer Center, 2346
Mental Health Association in Dutchess Coun ty, 6069
Mental Health Association in Orange County, 6070
Michael J. Fox Foundation for Parkinson's Research, 6869
Montrose Campus: Franklin Delano Roosevelt VA Hudson Valley Health Care System, 10204
Mount Sinai Medical Center Brain Tumor Support Group, 2003
Mount Sinai Sarcoidosis Support Group, 7242
Mount Sinai School of Medicine: Alzheimers Disease Research Center, 971
Multiple Sclerosis Action Group, 6437
Myasthenia Gravis Foundation of America, 6572
Myasthenia Gravis Support Group of Manhatt an, 6617
Myasthenia Gravis Support Group of Upstate New York, 6618

NYS Center for Sudden Infant Death: Eastern Satellite Office, 8772
Naomi Berrie Diabetes Center at Columbia University Medical Center, 3373
Narcolepsy Institute/Montefiore Medical Center, 7817
Narcotic and Drug Research, 8213
Nassau Library System, 9729
National AIDS Treatment Advocacy Project, 267
National Alliance for Autism Research, 1722
National Alliance for Research on Schizophrenia and Depression, 6260
National Association for Parents of Children with Visual Impairments, 9433
National Association on Drug Abuse Problems, 8127
National Braille Association, 9439
National Center for Family-Centered Care, 10397
National Center on Addiction and Substance Abuse, 8214
National Down Syndrome Society, 3547
National Down Syndrome Society Hotline, 3601
National Eating Disorders Association, 3682
National Eating Disorders Association Helpline, 3720
National Family Association for Deaf-Blind, 4324
National Federation of the Blind: New York, 9540
National Hemophilia Foundation, 359
National Hemophilia Foundation, 4963
National Hemophilia Foundation, 5012
National Hemophilia Foundation: Mary M. Gooley Hemophilia Center, 4991
National Infertility Network Exchange, 5442
National Institute for Jewish Hospice, 10697
National Institute for People with Disabil ities, 10404
National Kidney Foundation, 5580
National Kidney Foundation of Central New York, 5631
National Kidney Foundation of Northeast New York, 5632
National Kidney Foundation of Western New York, 5633
National MS Society: Long Island Chapter, 6390
National MS Society: New York City Chapter, 6391
National MS Society: Northeastern New York Chapter, 6392
National MS Society: Southern New York Chapter, 6393
National MS Society: Upstate New York Chapter, 6394
National MS Society: Western New York/ Northwestern Pennsylvania Chapter, 6395
National Multiple Sclerosis Society, 6345
National Multiple Sclerosis: Upstate New York Chapter, 6396
National Organization on Disability, 10411
National Parkinson Foundation: New York Office, 6897
National Spinal Cord Injury Association, 7977
Neurology Research Center Helen Hayes Hospital, 7492
New York Alliance for the Mentally Ill, 5993
New York Ambassador National Ataxia Foundation, 1551
New York Brain Tumor Support Group, 2004
New York Chapter of the American Association of Kidney Patients, 5634
New York Chapter of the Arthritis Foundation, 1239
New York City Center for SIDS, 8773
New York College of Osteopathic Medicine, 6923
New York Department of Health: AIDS Institute, 325
New York Male Reproductive Center: Sexual Dysfunction Unit, 5304
New York Organ Donor Network, Inc, 9207
New York State Center for SIDS: School of Social Welfare, 8774
New York State Talking Book & Braille Library, New York State Library, DOE, 9730
New York University Cancer Institute New York University Medical Center, 2347
New York University General Clinical Research Center, 5257
New York University Medical Center Head Trauma Program, 4132
New York/New Jersey VA Health Care Network, 10205
Niagara Cerebral Palsy, 2751

Northeast/Caribbean AIDS Education and Training Center (NECAAETC), 326
Northeast/Caribbean AIDS Education and Training Center (NECAAETC), 419
Northeastern Association of the Blind of Albany, 9541
Northport VA Medical Center, 10206
Obesity Research Center St. Luke's-Roosevelt Hospital, 6719
Oley Foundation, 3937
Orentreich Foundation for the Advancement of Science, 7671
Parent to Parent of New York State, 10524
Parents United Network: Parsons Child Family Center, 5994
Parkinson's Support Group of Upstate New York, 6924
Parkinsons Disease Foundation, 6906
Parkinsons Wellness Group of Western New York, 6898
Partnership for Drug-Free Kids, 8133
Pediatric Network Initiative - Crohn's & Colitis Foundation, 2997
Prader-Willi New York Association, 7186
Prospect Child And Family Center, 2752
Pulomonolgy Morgan Stanley Children's Hospital, 3149
RESOLVE of Long Island, 5410
RESOLVE of New York City, 5411
RESOLVE of the Capital District, 5412
Reach Out for Youth with Ileitis and Colitis, Inc., 2998
Reach Out for Youth with Ileitis and Colitis, Inc., 9382
Reader-Transcriber Registry National Braille Association, 9800
Region II Office Program: Consultants for Maternal and Child Health, 8775
Regional Bone Center Helen Hayes Hospital, 6816
Rehabilitation International, 10423
Remove Intoxicated Drivers (RID-USA), 8134
Renfrew Center of New York, 3697
Research Institute on Alcoholism State University of New York at Buffalo, 8221
Research to Prevent Blindness, 9455
Rochester Institute of Technology: Nationa l Technical Institute for the Deaf, 4388
Rockefeller University Laboratory for Investigative Dermatology, 7673
Rockefeller University Laboratory of Biology, 8222
Rockefeller University Laboratory of Cardiac Physiology, 4895
Rockefeller University, Laboratory for Investigative Dermatology, 7674
Roswell Park Cancer Institute National Cancer Institute, 2348
SLE Foundation, 8902
SLE Lupus Foundation, 8926
SUNY Health Science Center at Brooklyn Sickle Cell Center, 7618
SUNY at Buffalo National Cooperative Drug Discovery Group for AIDS Treatment, 420
Sarcoidosis HelpNet, 7245
Sarcoidosis Self-Help Group: New York, 7247
Schneeweiss Adult Congenital Heart Disease Center, 2949
Scleroderma Clinical & Research Center State University of New York at Stonybro, 7364
Scleroderma Foundation: Tri-State Chapter, 7345
Scleroderma Foundation: Western New York Chapter, 7346
Skin Cancer Foundation, 2263
Sleep Center: Community General Hospital, 7782
Sleep Disorders Center Columbia Presbyterian Medical Center, 7784
Sleep Disorders Center of Rochester: St. Mary's Hospital, 7791
Sleep Disorders Center of Western New York Millard Fillmore Hospital, 7792
Sleep Disorders Center: University Hospital, SUNY at Stony Brook, 7802
Sleep Disorders Center: Winthrop, University Hospital, 7803
Sleep Laboratory St Joseph's Hospital, 7805

Sleep Wake Disorders Center Montefiore Sleep Disorders Center, 7809
Sleep-Wake Disorders Center: New York Hospital-Cornell Medical Center, 7811
Southern Tier Association for the Visually Impaired, 9542
Southern Tier Hemophilia Center United Health Services-Wilson Hospital, 5058
Spellman Center for HIV Related Disease The Spellman Center, 421
Spina Bifida Association of Albany/Capital District, 7891
Spina Bifida Association of Greater Rochester, 7892
Spina Bifida Association of Nassau County, 7893
St. Agnes Hospital Medical: Health Science Library, 6429
St. John's Episcopal Hospital, 6925
State University College at Fredonia Youngerman Clinic, 4391
State University College at Plattsburgh Auditory Research Laboratory, 4392
State University of NY Hospital: Upstate Medical Center, 3150
State University of New York At Stony Brook: Mental Health Research, 6038
State University of New York Health Science Center At Brooklyn, 2349
State University of New York Health Sciences Center, 1723
State University of New York at Buffalo Toxicology Research Center, 8228
State University of New York: SUNY Stony HIV Treatment Development Center, 422
Suffolk Cooperative Library System, 9731
Support for Asthmatic Youth, 1410
Support for People with Oral and Head and Neck Cancer (SPOHNC), 2113
Syracuse University Institute for Sensory Research, 4393
Syracuse VA Medical Center, 10207
Taub Institute for Research on Alzheimers Disease and the Aging Brain, 974
The Coalition of Behavioral Health, 5922
The Dana Foundation, 7097
Tourette Association of America, 9081
Tri-State Area Support Group: National Ataxia Foundation, 1552
UNICEF USA, 282
United Cerebral Palsy of Chemung County, 2753
United Cerebral Palsy of Fulton & Montgomery Counties, 2754
United Cerebral Palsy of Greater Suffolk, 2755
United Cerebral Palsy of Nassau County, 2756
United Cerebral Palsy of New York City, 2757
United Cerebral Palsy of Putnam & Southern Dutchess Counties, 2758
United Cerebral Palsy of Queens: Queens Centers for Progress, 2759
United Cerebral Palsy of Westchester County, 2760
United Cerebral Palsy of Western New York, 2761
United Cerebral Palsy of the North Country, 2762
United Spinal Association, 7963
University of Rochester, 6926
University of Rochester: Clinical Research Center, 4909
University of Rochester: James P Wilmot Cancer Center, 2350
University of Rochester: Nephrology Research Program, 5668
Upstate NY Chapter of the Myasthenia Gravis Foundation of America, 6591
Upstate New York Transplant Services, Inc., 9208
WNYS Center for SIDS, 8776
Wainwright House Cancer Support Programs, 2415
Wallace Memorial Library, 4368
Westchester Task Force on Eating Disorders/American Anorexia Bulimia, 3698
Wilson's Disease Association, 10324
Xavier Society for the Blind, 9732
Yeshiva University General Clinical Research Center, 4917
Yeshiva University Marion Bessin Liver Research Center, 5771
Yeshiva University: Institute of Communication Disorders, 4408

Yeshiva University: Resnick Gerontology Center, 983
Yeshiva University: Soundview-Throgs Neck Community Mental Health Center, 6046
myFace, 1832

North Carolina

AARP North Carolina, 86
ACPA Family Services, 1850
Alcohol and Drug Abuse Section, 8176
Alzheimer's Association: Eastern North Carolina Chapter, 876
Alzheimer's Association: Western North Carolina Chapter, 877
Alzheimer's Disease Research Center Duke University, 959
American Cancer Society: North Carolina, 2216
American Cleft Palate - Craniofacial Association, 1824
American Diabetes Association: North Carolina, 3312
American Lung Association of North Carolina, 5852
American Lung Association of North Carolina, 9295
American Sexual Health Association (ASHA), 7568
Arthritis Foundation: Carolinas Chapter, 1222
Autism Society of North Carolina, 1699
Beginnings for Parents of Children Who are Deaf or Hard of Hearing, 4410
Bowman Gray School of Medicine, 8053
Bowman Grey School of Medicine: Hemophilia Diagnostic Center, 5017
Brain Injury Association of North Carolina, 4111
Brain Injury Association of North Carolina Helpline, 4176
Brain Tumor Support Group: Raleigh Area, 2005
CCFA Carolinas Chapter, 3025
CCFA South Carolina Chapter, 3026
Cancer Center of Wake Forest University at Bowman Gray School of Medicine, 2351
Carolinas Chapter of the Myasthenia Gravis Foundation of America, 6592
Carolinas Chapter of the Myasthenia Gravis Foundation of America, 6596
Center for Universal Design North Carolina State University, 10363
Centers for AIDS Research: Univeristy of North Carolina at Chapel Hill, 423
Charles George VA Medical Center, 10208
Comprehensive Hemophilia Diagnostic and Treatment Center, 5021
Department of Pediatrics, Division of Rheumatology, 1246
Division TEACCH University of North Carolina at Chapel H, 1719
Dorothea Dix Hospital Clinical Research Unit, 8203
Duke Asthma, Allergy and Airway Center, 1402
Duke Comprehensive Cancer Center, 2352
Duke Pediatric Brain Tumor Family Support Program, 2006
Duke University Center for the Advanced Study of Epilepsy, 7491
Duke University Center for the Study of Aging and Human Development, 118
Duke University Center for the Study of Aging and Human Development, 962
Duke University Clinical Research Institute, 963
Duke University Pediatric Cardiac Catheterization Laboratory, 4876
Duke University Plastic Surgery Research Laboratories, 7667
Durham VA Health Care System, 10209
Early Childhood Technical Assistance Center, 1827
Early Childhood Technical Assistance Center, 3543
Easterseals UCP North Carolina & Virginia, 2763
Families in Action National Drug Abuse Center, 8205
Fayetteville VA Medical Center, 10210
Hemophilia Foundation of North Carolina, 4992
Herpes Resource Center, 7571
International Society for Adult Congenital Heart Disease (ISACHD), 2947
Juvenile Diabetes Research Foundation: Charlotte Chapter, 3314
Juvenile Diabetes Research Foundation: Piedmont Triad Chapter, 3315

Juvenile Diabetes Research Foundation: Triangle/Eastern North Carolina Chapter, 3313
Leukemia and Lymphoma Society: Eastern North Carolina Chapter, 2217
Leukemia and Lymphoma Society: North Carolina Chapter, 2218
Life Share of the Carolinas, 9209
Lions Industries for the Blind, 9543
Lupus Foundation of America: North Carolina Chapter, 8904
Lupus Foundation of America: Winston-Triad Lupus Chapter NCLF, 8903
Myasthenia Gravis Support Group of Central North Carolina, 6620
Myasthenia Gravis Support Group of Charlotte, 6619
Myasthenia Gravis Support Group of Durham/ Chapel Hill, 6621
Myasthenia Gravis Support Group of Fayetteville, 6622
National Association of Blind Students, 9436
National Federation of the Blind: North Carolina, 9544
National Institute of Environmental Health Sciences, 645
National Institute of Environmental Health Sciences, 1387
National Institute of Environmental Health Sciences, 3551
National Institute of Environmental Health Sciences, 3685
National Institute of Environmental Health Sciences, 4327
National Institute of Environmental Health Sciences, 5741
National Institute of Environmental Health Sciences, 7054
National Institute of Environmental Health Sciences, 7473
National Kidney Foundation of North Carolina, 5635
National MS Society: Central North Carolina Chapter, 6397
National MS Society: Eastern North Carolina Chapter, 6398
National Multiple Sclerosis Society, 6399
North Carolina Association of the Deaf, 4350
North Carolina Client Assistance Program, 10472
North Carolina Department of Health and Human Services, 327
North Carolina Library for the Blind, 9733
Pediatric Brain Tumor Foundation, 1906
Prader-Willi North Carolina Association, 7187
Preston Robert Tisch Brain Tumor Center at Duke, 2007
RESOLVE of North Carolina, 5413
SIDS Alliance of the Carolinas, 8777
Spina Bifida Association of North Carolina, 7894
Triangle Area Sarcoidosis Support Group, 7252
UNC Cystic Fibrosis Center Department of Pediatrics, 3151
University Of North Carolina School of Medicine Center for Aging and Health, 137
University of North Carolina Sarcoidosis Support Group, 7254
University of North Carolina UNC Lineberger Comprehensive Cancer Center, 2353
University of North Carolina at Chapel Hill Division of Speech & Hearing, 4404
W. G. (Bill) Hefner VA Medical Center, 10211
Wake Forest University: Arteriosclerosis Research Center, 5262
Wake Forest University: Cerebrovascular Research Center, 8063
Western Michigan University School of Medicine, 3152
Winston-Salem Industries for the Blind, 9545

North Dakota

AARP North Dakota, 87
Alzheimer's Association: Fargo/Moorhead Regional Center, 878
American Cancer Society: North Dakota, 2219
American Diabetes Association: Nashville, 3316
American Diabetes Association: North Dakota, 3317

American Lung Association of North Dakota, 5853
American Lung Association of North Dakota, 9296
Autism Society of North Dakota, 1700
Brain Injury Association of North Dakota, 4177
Client Assistance Program: North Dakota, 10473
Division of Alcoholism & Drug Abuse: Department of Human Services, 8177
Fargo VA Health Care System, 10212
Healthy Weight Network, 3676
MeritCare Children's Hospital Down Syndrome Outpatient Service, 3591
ND FFCMH Region II, 6071
ND Region V FFCMH Chapter-Federation of Fa milies for Children's Mental Health, 6072
ND Region VII FFCMH-Federation of Families for Children's Mental Health, 6073
National Federation of the Blind: North Dakota, 9546
National MS Society: Dakota Chapter, 6400
North Dakota Alliance for the Mentally Ill, 5995
North Dakota Association of the Deaf, 4351
North Dakota Comprehensive Hemophilia Center, 5048
North Dakota FFCMH, 5996
North Dakota Hemostasis and Thrombosis Treatment Center, 5049
North Dakota SIDS Alliance, 8778
North Dakota SIDS Management Program, 8779
North Dakota State Library Services for the Disabled, 9734
Prader-Willi North Dakota Association, 7188
St. Alexius Medical Heart and Lung Clinic, 3153

Ohio

1st Capital FFCMH, 5997
A Kid Again, 10653
AARP Ohio, 88
ALS Association: Central & Southern Ohio Chapter, 1121
ALS Association: Northern Ohio Chapter, 1122
Alzheimer's Association: Canton Chapter, 879
Alzheimer's Association: Central Ohio Chapter, 880
Alzheimer's Association: Clark/Champaign, Miami Valley Chapter, 881
Alzheimer's Association: Cleveland Area Chapter, 882
Alzheimer's Association: Greater Cincinnati Chapter, 883
Alzheimer's Association: Greater East Ohio Chapter: Greater Youngstown Office, 884
Alzheimer's Association: Miami Valley Chapter, 885
Alzheimer's Association: Northwest Ohio Chapter, 886
Alzheimer's Association: West Central Ohio Chapter, 887
American Cancer Society: Ohio, 2220
American Diabetes Association: Ohio, 3318
American Lung Association of Ohio, 5854
American Lung Association of Ohio, 9297
American Sickle Cell Anemia Association, 7604
Arthritis Foundation: Central Ohio Chapter, 1223
Arthritis Foundation: Northeastern Ohio Chapter, 1224
Arthritis Foundation: Ohio River Valley Chapter, 1226
Arthritis Foundation; Great Lakes Region, Northeastern Ohio, 1227
Association for Neuro-Metabolic Disorders, 3833
Autism Society of Greater Cincinnati, 1701
Autism Society of Ohio Tri-County Chapter, 1702
Blick Clinic for Developmental Disabilities, 3577
Brain Injury Association of Ohio, 4112
Brain Injury Association of Ohio, 4178
Brain Tumor Support Group: Cincinnati, 2008
Bureau on Alcohol Abuse and Recovery Ohio Department of Health, 8178
Bureau on Drug Abuse: Ohio Department of Health, 8179
CCFA Central Ohio Chapter, 3027
CCFA Northeast Ohio Chapter, 3028
CCFA Southwest Ohio Chapter, 3029
Case Western Reserve University, 9736
Case Western Reserve University: Bolton Brush Growth Study Center, 4051

Case Western Reserve University: Center on Aging and Health, 115
Case Western Reserve University: Cystic Fibrosis Center, 3154
Case Western Reserve University: Ireland Cancer Center, 2354
Center for ALS and Related Diorders The Cleveland Clinic DepartmentOf Neurol, 1139
Center for Research in Sleep Disorders Affiliated with Mercy Hospital, 7766
Center for Sleep & Wake Disorders: Miami Valley Hospital, 7767
Centers for AIDS Research: Case Western University, 424
Central Ohio Chapter of the National Hemophilia Foundation, 4993
Central Ohio Support Group: National Ataxia Foundation, 1553
Chalmers P. Wylie Ambulatory Care Center VA Central Ohio Healthcare System, 10213
Child & Adolescent Behavioral Health, 6074
Children's Hospital Hemophilia Treatment Center, 5018
Children's Hospital Research Foundation, 2355
Chillicothe VA Medical Center, 10214
Cincinnati Association for the Blind, 9547
Cincinnati HPV Support Group: PP of Cincin nati, 10474
Cincinnati VA Medical Center, 10215
Cleveland Clinic Lerner Research Institute, 4872
Cleveland Hearing and Speech Center, 4374
Cleveland Sight Center, 9548
Cleveland Skilled Industries, 9549
Cleveland VA Medical Center VA Northeast Ohio Healthcare System, 10216
Clinical Research Center: Pediatrics Children's Hospital Research Foundation, 5767
Clovernook Center for the Blind and Visually Impaired, 9784
Columbus Center of the National Multiple Sclerosis Society, 6401
Columbus Children's Hospital: Cystic Fibrosis Center, 3155
Columbus Children's Research Institute, 658
Comprehensive Sickle Cell Center Children's Hospital Research Foundation, 7614
Congenital Heart Disease Anomalies Support, Education & Resources CHASER, 4874
Dayton VA Medical Center, 10217
Disability Rights Center at Ohio Legal Rights Service, 10475
District Board of Health: Mahoning County, 8780
Division Of Developmental and Behavioral Pediatrics, 1839
Down Syndrome Association of Greater Cinci nnati, 3567
Down Syndrome Association of Greater Cinci nnati, 3599
First Ohio Chapter: FFCMH, 6075
JamesCare For Life Support Groups & Services, 2405
Jane and Richard Thomas Center for Down Syndrome, 3587
Juvenile Diabetes Research Foundation/JDRF, 3319
Juvenile Diabetes Research Foundation: Akr on/Canton Chapter, 3321
Juvenile Diabetes Research Foundation: Gre ater Cincinnati Chapter, 3322
Juvenile Diabetes Research Foundation: Mid-Ohio Chapter, 3320
Juvenile Diabetes Research Foundation: Tol edo/Northwest Ohio Chapter, 3323
Kettering-Scott Magnetic Resonance Laboratory, 8211
Leukemia and Lymphoma Society: Central Ohio Chapter, 2221
Leukemia and Lymphoma Society: Northern Ohio Chapter, 2222
Leukemia and Lymphoma Society: Southern Ohio Chapter, 2223
Lewis H Walker MD: Cystic Fibrosis Center, 3156
Life Connection of Ohio, 9210
LifeBanc, 9211
Lifeline of Ohio Organ Procurement Agency, Inc., 9212

Lupus Foundation of America: Greater Ohio Chapter, 8905
Medical College of Toledo: Cancer Research Division, 2356
Miami Valley Ohio Chapter of the American Association of Kidney Patients, 5636
Mitral Valve Prolapse Program of Cincinnati Support Group, 4919
Myasthenia Gravis Support Group of Columbu s, 6623
Myasthenia Gravis Support Group of Summit- Stark, 6624
National Association of Blind Office Professionals, 9435
National Federation of the Blind: Ohio, 9550
National Kidney Foundation of Ohio, 5637
National MS Sceity: Western Ohio Chapter The Woolpert Building, 6402
National MS Society: Northeast Ohio Chapter, 6404
National MS Society: Northwest Ohio Chapter, 6405
National MS Society: Southwestern Ohio/Northern Kentucky, 6403
National Reye's Syndrome Foundation, 5774
North East Ohio Support Group National Ataxia Foundation, 1554
Northern Ohio Chapter of the National Hemophilia Foundation, 4994
Northwest Ohio Hemophilia Association, 4995
Northwest Ohio Hemophilia Treatment Center, 5051
Northwest Ohio Sleep Disorders Center Toledo Hospital, 7776
Ohio Alliance for the Mentally Ill, 5998
Ohio Ambassador: National Ataxia Foundation, 1555
Ohio Department of Health, 8781
Ohio Department of Health: HIV/AIDS Surveillance Program, 328
Ohio Regional Library for the Blind and Physically Handicapped, 9737
Ohio Sleep Medicine Institute, 7777
Ohio State University Clinical Pharmacology Division, 8219
Ohio State University Comprehensive Cancer Center, 2357
Ohio State University General Clinical Research Center, 2358
Ohio State University Laboratory of Psychobiology, 4133
Ohio State University Neuroscience Program, 973
Ohio State University Otological Research Laboratories, 4382
Ohio University Therapy Associates: Hearing, Speech and Language Clinic, 4383
Ohio Valley LifeCenter, 9213
Pediatric Pulmonary Center The Children's Medical Center of Dayton, 3157
Prader-Willi Ohio Association, 7189
RESOLVE of Ohio, 5414
Richland County HPV Support Group, 10476
SIDS Network of Ohio, 8782
Scleroderma Foundation: Ohio Chapter, 7347
Sleep Disorders Center Bethesda Oak Hospital, 7783
Sleep Disorders Center Ohio State University Medical Center, 7787
Sleep Disorders Center: Cleveland Clinic Foundation, 7793
Sleep Disorders Center: Kettering Medical Center, 7797
Sleep Disorders Center: St. Vincent Medical Center, 7801
Southwest Ohio Brain Tumor Support Group, 2009
Southwestern Ohio Chapter of the National Hemophilia Foundation, 4996
Special Wish Foundation, 10675
Spina Bifida Association of Canton, 7895
Spina Bifida Association of Central Ohio, 7896
Spina Bifida Association of Cincinnati, 7897
Spina Bifida Association of Greater Dayton, 7898
Spina Bifida Association of Northwest Ohio, 7899
State Library of Ohio Talking Book Program, 9738
Support Group for Parents of Children with Brain Tumors, 2010
Technology Resource Center, 10477
The Cancer Prevention Institute, 2359
United Cerebral Palsy of Central Ohio, 2764
United Cerebral Palsy of Cincinnati, 2765

United Cerebral Palsy of Greater Cleveland, 2766
United Cerebral Palsy of Greater Dane, 2767
University Alzheimer Center UHC: Case Western Reserve University, 978
University Treatment Center of University Hospitals of Cleveland, 5068
University of Cincinnati Adult Hemophilia Treatment Program, 5069
University of Cincinnati College of Medicine Division of Pediatrics, 3158
University of Cincinnati Department of Pathology & Laboratory Medicine, 4902
VA Healthcare System of Ohio, 10218
West Central Ohio Hemophilia Center Childens Medical Center, 5072

Oklahoma

AARP Oklahoma, 89
Alzheimer's Association: Oklahoma Chapter, 888
American Association of Kidney Patients: Tulsa Chapter, 5638
American Cancer Society: Oklahoma, 2224
American Diabetes Association: Oklahoma, 3324
American Lung Association of Oklahoma, 5855
American Lung Association of Oklahoma, 9298
Arthritis Foundation: Oklahoma Chapter, 1228
Autism Society of Central Oklahoma, 1703
Brain Injury Association of Oklahoma, 4113
Brain Injury Association of Oklahoma Helpl ine, 4179
CCFA Oklahoma Chapter, 3030
Client Assistance Program: Oklahoma Office of Handicapped Concerns, 10478
Dean A McGee Eye Institute, 9785
Jack C. Montgomery VA Medical Center Eastern Oklahoma VA Health Care System, 10219
Juvenile Diabetes Research Foundation: Cen tral Oklahoma Chapter, 3325
Juvenile Diabetes Research Foundation: Tul sa Green County Chapter, 3326
Leukemia and Lymphoma Society: Oklahoma Chapter, 2225
Myasthenia Gravis Support Group of Tulsa and Oklahoma City, 6625
Natalie Warren Bryant Cancer Center St. Francis Hospital, 2360
National Federation of the Blind: Oklahoma, 9551
National Kidney Foundation of Oklahoma, 5639
National MS Society: Oklahoma Chapter, 6406
Neuroscience Institute at Mercy Hospital, 6688
Northeast Oklahoma Resource Group (Tulsa), 9354
Oklahoma Alliance for the Mentally Ill, 5999
Oklahoma Ambassador: National Ataxia Foundation, 1556
Oklahoma Association of the Deaf, 4352
Oklahoma Chapter of the Myasthenia Gravis Foundation of America, 6593
Oklahoma Chapter of the National Hemophilia Foundation, 4997
Oklahoma City HPV Support Group: PP of Cen tral Oklahoma, 10479
Oklahoma City VA Health Care System, 10220
Oklahoma Comprehensive Hemophilia Diagnostic Treatment Center, 5052
Oklahoma Department of Health: HIV/STD Service, 329
Oklahoma Department of Mental Health and Substance Abuse Services, 8180
Oklahoma League for the Blind, 9552
Oklahoma Library for the Blind and Physically Handicapped, 9739
Oklahoma Lupus Association, 8906
Oklahoma Medical Research Foundation, 1252
Oklahoma Medical Research Foundation Immunobiolgy & Cancer Research, 2361
Oklahoma Medical Research Foundation: Cardiovascular Research Program, 4891
Oklahoma Organ Sharing Network, 9214
Oklahoma State Department of Health: Maternal and Child Health Services, 8783
Parkinson Foundation of the Heartland Oklahoma Branch, 6899
Prader-Willi Oklahoma Association, 7190

RESOLVE of Oklahoma, 5415
Samuel Roberts Noble Foundation Biomedical Division, 2362
Tulsa City: County Library System, 9740
Tulsa Unified FFCMH, 6000
United Cerebral Palsy of Oklahoma, 2768
University of California Northern Comprehensive Sickle Cell Center, 7621
University of Oklahoma: Cystic Fibrosis Center, 3159
University of Oklahoma: Health Sciences Ce nter, 4405

Oregon

AARP Oregon, 90
ALS Association: Oregon & SW Washington Chapter, 1123
ALS Association: Oregon & SW Washington Chapter, 1134
Aging and Alzheimer's Disease Center Oregon Health Sciences University, 948
Alzheimer's Association: Cascade/Coast Chapter, 890
Alzheimer's Association: Columbia-Willamet Chapter, 889
Alzheimer's Association: Mary's Peak Chapter, 891
Alzheimer's Association: Mid-Willamette Chapter, 892
American Cancer Society: Oregon, 2226
American Diabetes Association: Oregon, 3327
American Lung Association of Oregon, 5856
American Lung Association of Oregon, 9299
Autism Society of Oregon, 1704
Blind Enterprises of Oregon, 9553
Brain Injury Alliance of Oregon, 4180
Brain Injury Association of Oregon, 4114
Brain Tumor Education & Support Group, 2011
Cascade AIDS Project Hotline, 446
Center for Health Research, 10360
Central Oregon Brain Tumor Support Group, 2012
Child Center, 10364
Comprehensive Stroke Center of Oregon University of Oregon Health Sciences Cen, 8055
Dogs for Better Lives, 1667
Dogs for Better Lives, 4305
Fanconi Anemia Research Fund, 2973
Hemophilia Foundation of Oregon, 4998
Juvenile Diabetes Research Foundation: Ore gon/SW Washington Chapter, 3328
Leukemia and Lymphoma Society: Oregon Chapter, 2227
NAMI-Oregon, 6001
NNFF Oregon Affiliate Kaiser Permanente Northwest, 6679
National Association of State Directors of Veterans Affairs, 10221
National Consortium on Deaf-Blindness, 4323
National Federation of the Blind: Oregon, 9554
National MS Society: Oregon Chapter, 6407
National Psoriasis Foundation, 7665
Office of Alcohol and Drug Abuse Programs, 8181
Oregon Association of the Deaf, 4353
Oregon Family Support Network, 6002
Oregon Health & Science University, 3160
Oregon Health Authority, 8784
Oregon Health Authority: HIV Prevention Program, 330
Oregon Health Sciences University, 6927
Oregon Health Sciences University Oregon Hearing Research Center Tinnitus Clinic, 4384
Oregon Health Sciences University: Elk's Children's Eye Clinic, 9799
Oregon State Library, 9741
Pacific NW Transplant Bank, 9215
Parkinsons Resources of Oregon, 6900
Portland VA Medical Center VA Portland Health Care System, 10222
Prader-Willi Oregon Association, 7191
Psoriasis Research Institute, 7672
RESOLVE of Oregon, 5416
Regional Resource Center on Deafness Western Oregon State College, 4385
Resources for Seniors and People with Disabilities, 10480
Roseburg VA Health Care System, 10223

Scleroderma Foundation: Oregon Chapter, 7348
United Cerebral Palsy of Oregon & SW Washington, 2769
White City VA Rehabilitation Center VA Southern Oregon, 10224
Willamette Valley Support Group: National Ataxia Foundation, 1557

Pennsylvania

AARP Pennsylvania: Harrisburg, 91
AARP Pennsylvania: Philadelphia, 92
AIDS Library of Philadelphia, 361
ALS Association: Greater Philadelphia Chapter, 1124
ALS Association: Western Pennsylvania Chapter, 1125
ALS Clinic at Penn Neurological Institute ALS Association Greater Philadelphia Cha, 1137
Abramson Cancer Center of the University of Pennsylvania, 2363
Adult Congenital Heart Association, 2946
Albert Einstein Medical Center Hemophilia Program, 5014
Allegheny Singer Research Institute West Penn Allegheny Health System, 2364
Alzheimer's Association: Delaware Valley Chapter, 893
Alzheimer's Association: Greater Mid-Ohio, 895
Alzheimer's Association: Greater Pennsylvania Chapter: SW Regional Office, 894
Alzheimer's Association: Laurel Mountains Chapter, 896
Alzheimer's Association: Northeast Pennsylvania Chapter, 897
Alzheimer's Association: Northwest Pennsylvania Chapter, 898
Alzheimer's Association: South Central Pennsylvania Chapter, 899
Alzheimer's Disease Center Pennsylvania University School of Medicine, 952
American Anorexia Bulimia Association of Philadelphia, 3699
American Cancer Society: Harrisburg Capital Area Unit, 2228
American Cancer Society: Philadelphia, 2229
American Cancer Society: Pittsburgh, 2230
American Diabetes Association: Pennsylvania, 3329
American Diabetes Association: Western Pennsylvania, 3330
American Foundation for Children with AIDS, 352
American Liver Foundation Delaware Valley Chapter, 5760
American Liver Foundation Western Pennsylv ania, 5761
American Lung Association of Pennsylvania, 9300
American Respiratory Alliance of Western Pennsylvania, 5857
Arthritis Foundation: Central Pennsylvania Chapter, 1229
Associated Services for the Blind & Visually Impaired, 9413
Association for the Blind & Visually Impaired of Lehigh County, 9555
Autism Society of Greater Harrisburg, 1705
Beaver County Association for the Blind, 9556
Bockus Research Institute Graduate Hospital, 4868
Brain Injury Association of Pennsylvania, 4115
Brain Tumor Community Group, 2013
Brain Tumor Support Group: Johnstown, 2014
Brain Tumor Support Group: Philadelphia, 2015
Brain Tumor Support Group: Pittsburgh, 2016
Breathe Pennsylvania, 5858
CCFA Philadelphia/Delaware Valley Chapter, 3031
CCFA Western Pennsylvania/West Virginia Chapter, 3032
Cambria County Association for the Blind and Handicapped, 9557
Cancer Caring Center, 2098
Carnegie Library of Pittsburgh, 9742
Center for Organ Recovery & Education, 9216
Centers for AIDS Research: University of Pennsylvania, 425
Chester County Association for the Blind, 9558
Children of Aging Parents, 149

Children's Hospital of Philadelphia, 3579
Children's Liver Association For Support Services (CLASS), 5735
Childrens Hospital of Philadelphia Hemophilia Program, 5019
Client Assistance Program: Philadelphia, 10481
Coatesville VA Medical Center, 10225
Corporal Michael J. Crescenz VA Medical Center, 10226
Cystic Fibrosis Center: Polyclinic Medical Center, 3161
Delaware County Branch of the Pennsylvania Association for the Blind, 9559
Delaware Valley Chapter of the National Hemophilia Foundation, 4999
Delware Valley Brain Tumor Support Group at Jefferson, 2017
Department of Reproductive Genetics: Magee Women's Hospital, 1838
Diabetes Education and Research Center The Franklin House, 3380
Dial-a-Hearing Screening Test, 4413
Down Syndrome Center of Western Pennsylvania, 3584
Dr. Gertrude A Barber National Institute, 3586
Dream Come True, 10660
Drug and Alcohol Programs Department Of Health, 8182
Eastern Cooperative Oncology Group, 2365
Epilepsy Foundation of Western Pennsylvania, 7487
Erie VA Medical Center, 10227
Fox Chase Cancer Center, 2366
Free Library of Philadelphia, 9743
Geisinger Wyoming Valley Medical Center: Sleep Disorders Center, 7769
Gift of Life Donor Program Pennsylvania, 9217
Greater Wilkes-Barre Association for the Blind, 9560
H.J. Heinz Campus VA Pittsburgh Healthcare System, 10228
Hahnemann University Hospital, Orthopedic Wellness Center, 1247
Hahnemann University Laboratory of Human Pharmacology, 8207
Hahnemann University Likoff Cardiovascular Institute, 4881
Hahnemann University Lupus Study Center Hahnemann University Medical Center, 8928
Hahnemann University, Krancer Center for Inflammatory Bowel Disease Research, 3041
Hahnemann University: Division of Surgical Research, 5254
Hemophilia Center of Central Pennsylvania Penn State Milton S Hershey Medical Cent, 5032
Hepatitis B Foundation, 5145
Hepatitis B Foundation, 10325
Hopes & Dreams Foundation, Inc., 10666
Hospital of the University of Pennsylvania, 8057
Hospital of the University of Pennsylvania University of Pennsylvania, 6516
Hydrocephalus Association of Philadelphia, 5204
Indiana County Association for the Blind, 9561
Juvenile Diabetes Research Foundation: Ber ks County Chapter, 3332
Juvenile Diabetes Research Foundation: Central Pennsylvania Chapter, 3331
Juvenile Diabetes Research Foundation: Nor thwestern Pennsylvania Chapter, 3333
Juvenile Diabetes Research Foundation: Phi ladelphia Chapter, 3334
Juvenile Diabetes Research Foundation: Wes tern Pennsylvania, 3335
Keystone Blind Association, 9562
Kids with Food Allergies, 657
Lancaster County Association for the Blind, 9563
Learning Disabilities Association of America, 1607
Learning Disabilities Association of America, 10388
Lebanon VA Medical Center, 10229
Lehigh Valley Chapter of the American Association of Kidney Patients, 5640
Lehigh Valley Sickle Cell Support Group, 7626
Leukemia and Lymphoma Society: Central Pennsylvania Chapter, 2231
Leukemia and Lymphoma Society: Eastern Pennsylvania Chapter, 2232

Leukemia and Lymphoma Society: Western Pennsylvania/West Virginia Chapter, 2233
Lupus Foundation of America: Central Pennsylvania Chapter, 8907
Lupus Foundation of America: Northeast Pennsylvania Chapter, 8908
Lupus Foundation of America: Northwestern Pennsylvania Chapter, 8909
Lupus Foundation of America: Western Pennsylvania Chapter, 8910
Lupus Foundation of Philadelphia, 8911
Lysosomal Disease Center at the University of Pittsburgh, 3842
MedEscort International ABE International Airport, 10393
Medical College of Pennsylvania Center for the Mature Woman, 6814
Medical College of Pennsylvania: Eastern Psychiatric Institute, 6034
MidAtlantic AIDS Education and Training Center (MAAETC), 331
MidAtlantic AIDS Education and Training Center (MAAETC), 426
Montgomery County Association for the Blind, 9564
Myasthenia Gravis Support Group of Scranto n, 6626
NASPGHAN Foundation, 3935
National Federation of the Blind: Pennsylvania, 9565
National Kidney Foundation of Delaware Valley, 5641
National Kidney Foundation of Western Pennsylvania, 5642
National MS Society: Central Pennsylvania Chapter, 6408
National MS Society: Greater Delaware Valley Chapter, 6409
National Mental Health Consumer's Self-Help Clearinghouse, 6028
National Mental Health Consumers' Self- Help Clearinghouse, 6029
National Organization for Hearing Research Foundation, 4329
National Sexual Violence Resource Center, 7074
National Tay-Sachs & Allied Diseases Association of Delaware Valley, 8973
National Transplant Assistance Fund (NTAF), 9171
North American Society for Pediatric Gastroenterology, Hepatology & Nutrition, 3926
North American Society for Pediatric Gastroenterology, Hepatology & Nutrition, 3936
North American Society for Pediatric Gastroenterology, Hepatology & Nutrition, 10414
North Central Sight Services, 9566
Parents Involved Network, 6003
Parkinson Chapter of Greater Pittsburgh, 6901
Parkinson Council, 6902
Pediatric Cancer Foundation of the Lehigh Valley, 2018
Pediatric Pulmonary and Cystic Fibrosis Center, 3162
Penn Center for Sleep Disorders: Hospital of the University of Pennsylvania, 7778
Pennsylvania Alliance for the Mentally Ill, 6004
Pennsylvania Department of Health Bureau of Family Health, 8785
Pennsylvania Department of Health: Division Of HIV Disease, 332
Pennsylvania Educational Network for Eating Disorders, 3700
Pennsylvania State University Artificial Heart Research Project, 4892
Pennsylvania Turner Syndrome Resource Group, 9355
Philadelphia Biomedical Research Institute, 7617
Philadelphia Department of Public Health: STD Control Program, 333
Pittsburgh Vision Services, 9567
Prader-Willi Pennsylvania Association, 7192
Pregnancy Healthline: Pennsylvania Hospital, 1860
Pregnancy Safety Hotline, 1862
Presbyterian-University Hospital: Pulmonary Sleep Evaluation Center, 7779
RESOLVE of Philadelphia, 5417
RESOLVE of Pittsburgh, 5418
RESOLVE of Southcentral Pennsylvania, 5419
Recorded Periodicals, 9821
Renfrew Center of Bryn Mawr, 3701

Renfrew Center of Philadelphia, 3702
SIDS of Pennsylvania, 8786
Sarcoidosis Treatment and Research Center Thomas Jefferson University Hospital, 7238
Scleroderma Foundation: Western Pennsylvania Chapter, 7349
Shriners Hospital for Children, 7978
Sickle Cell Disease Association of America Philadelphia/Delaware Valley Chapter, 7629
Sleep Disorders Center Lankenau Hospital, 7786
Sleep Disorders Center: Community Medical Center, 7794
Sleep Disorders Center: Crozer-Chester Medical Center, 7795
Sleep Disorders Center: Good Samaritan Medical Center, 7796
Sleep Disorders Center: Medical College of Pennsylvania, 7798
Sleep and Chronobiology Center: Western Psychiatric Institute and Clinic, 7810
Somerset County Blind Center, 9568
Spina Bifida Association of Central Pennsylvania, 7900
Spina Bifida Association of Delaware Valley, 7901
Spina Bifida Association of Greater Pennsylvania, 7902
Spinal Cord Injury Program at Harmarville Rehabilitation Center, 7979
Sunshine Foundation National Headquarters, 10677
Temple University Clinical Research Center Office of Clinical Research, 427
Temple University FELS Institute for Cancer Research, 2367
Temple University Speech and Hearing Science Laboratories, 4394
Temple University: Section of Auditory Research, 4395
Thomas Jefferson University Hospital, 7366
Thomas Jefferson University Ischemia-Shock, 4136
Thomas Jefferson University Ischemia-Shock Research Center, 4135
Thomas Jefferson University: Sleep Disorders Center, 7815
Thomas Jefferson University: Cardenza Foundation for Hematologic Research, 5063
Thomas Jefferson University: Center for Research in Medical Education, 428
Thomas Jefferson University: Daniel Baugh Institute, 1844
ToughLove International, 8247
Tri-County Association for the Blind, 9569
Understanding Sarcoidosis Self-Help Group, 7253
United Cerebral Palsy Central PA, 2770
United Cerebral Palsy of Beaver, Butler & Lawrence Counties, 2771
United Cerebral Palsy of Northwestern Pennsylvania, 2772
United Cerebral Palsy of Pennsylvania, 2773
United Cerebral Palsy of Philadelphia Vicinity, 2774
United Cerebral Palsy of Pittsburgh, 2775
United Cerebral Palsy of South Central Pennsylvania, 2776
United Cerebral Palsy of Southern Alleghenies Region, 2777
United Cerebral Palsy of Southwestern Pennsylvania, 2778
United Cerebral Palsy of Western Pennsylvania, 2779
University Drive Campus VA Pittsburgh Healthcare System, 10230
University of Pennsylvania Diabetes and Endocrinology Research Center, 3398
University of Pennsylvania Institute on Aging, 142
University of Pennsylvania Muscle Institut e, 4907
University of Pennsylvania: Depression Research Unit, 6202
University of Pennsylvania: Harrison Department of Surgical Research, 3946
University of Pennsylvania: Penn Lung Center, 3163
University of Pittsburgh, 6928
University of Pittsburgh, 7370
University of Pittsburgh Cancer Institute, 2368
University of Pittsburgh Cystic Fibrosis Center: Children's Hospital, 3164
University of Pittsburgh: Department of Molecular Genetics and Biochemistry, 3399

University of Pittsburgh: Human Energy Research Laboratory, 4908
University of Pittsburgh: Western Psychiatric Institute & Clinic, 6043
VIABL Services of Northampton County, 9570
WFS' New Life Program, 8248
WM Krogman Center for Research in Child Growth and Development, 4054
Washington-Greene County Branch for the Pennsylvania Association for Blind, 9571
Western Pennsylvania Chapter of the National Hemophilia Foundation, 5000
Wilkes-Barre VA Medical Center, 10231
Women's Resource Center, 7080
York Industries for the Blind: Division of York County Blind Center, 9572

Rhode Island

AARP Rhode Island, 93
Alzheimer's Association: Rhode Island Chapter, 900
American Cancer Society: Rhode Island, 2234
American Diabetes Association: Rhode Island, 3336
American Lung Association of Rhode Island, 5859
Autism Society of Rhode Island, 1706
Brain Injury Association of Rhode Island, 4116
Brain Injury Association of Rhode Island H elpline, 4181
Brain Tumor Support Group: Providence, 2019
Brown University Division of Biology and Medicine, 2369
Center for Alcohol & Addiction Studies Brown University, 8200
Centers for AIDS Research: Brown University, 429
Children's Neurodevelopment Center, 3580
Division of Substance Abuse: Department of Mental Health and Hospitals, 8183
Hemophilia Center of Rhode Island Rhode Island Hospital, 5033
Hydrocephalus Association of Rhode Island, 5205
IN-SIGHT, 9573
Leukemia and Lymphoma Society: Rhode Island Chapter, 2235
Lupus Foundation of America: Rhode Island Chapter, 8912
Narcolepsy Network, 7818
National Alliance for the Mentally Ill of Rhode Island (NAMI), 6005
National Federation of the Blind: Rhode Island, 9574
National MS Society: Rhode Island Chapter, 6410
Parent Support Network of Rhode Island, 6076
Providence VA Medical Center, 10232
RESOLVE of the Ocean State, 5420
Rhode Island Association of the Deaf, 4354
Rhode Island Brain & Spine Tumor Foundation, 2020
Rhode Island Department of Health, 334
Rhode Island Department of Health, 8787
Rhode Island Department of State Library for the Blind and Physically Handicapped, 9744
Rhode Island Disability Law Center, 10482
Rhode Island Hospital: Cystic Fibrosis Center, 3165
Rhode Island Scleroderma Support Group, 7374
Roger Williams Clinical Cancer Research Center, 2370
Sleep Disorders Center: Rhode Island Hospital, 7800
Spina Bifida Association of Rhode Island, 7903
United Cerebral Palsy of Rhode Island, 2780

South Carolina

AARP South Carolina, 94
ALS Association: South Carolina Chapter, 1126
Agromedicine Program Medical University of South Carolina, 7666
Alzheimer's Association: Low Country Chapter, 901
Alzheimer's Association: Mid-State South Carolina Chapter, 902
Alzheimer's Association: Upstate South Carolina Chapter, 903
American Cancer Society: South Carolina, 2236
American Diabetes Association: South Carolina, 3337
American Lung Association of South Carolina, 5860
American Lung Association of South Carolina, 9301

Association for Traumatic Stress Specialists, 7044
Autism Society of South Carolina, 1707
Brain Injury Association of South Carolina, 4117
Brain Tumor Support Group: Charleston, 2021
Brain Tumor Support Group: Florence, 2022
Carolinas Support Group: National Ataxia National Ataxia Foundation, 1558
Center for Developmental Disabilities University of South Carolina, 10357
Center for Disability Resources, 10358
Children's Center for Cancer and Blood Disorders, 2371
Columbia VA Health Care System, 10233
Division of Perinatal Systems Mills Jarret Complex, 8788
Federation of Families of South Carolina, 6077
Hemophilia Association of South Carolina, 5002
Interdisciplinary Program in Cell and Molecular Pharmacology, 8209
James R Clark Memorial Sickle Cell Foundation, 7608
Juvenile Diabetes Research Foundation: Low Country Chapter, 3339
Juvenile Diabetes Research Foundation: Palmetto Chapter, 3338
Leukemia and Lymphoma Society: South Carolina Chapter, 2237
Leukemia and Lymphoma Society: South/West, 2238
Lupus Foundation of America: South Carolina Chapter, 8913
Lyme Disease Network of South Carolina, 9037
Medical University of South Carolina, 1248
Medical University of South Carolina Center on Aging, 127
Medical University of South Carolina Health Services Administration, 430
Medical University of South Carolina Medical University of South Carolina, 7363
Medical University of South Carolina: Cystic Fibrosis Center, 3166
Medical University of South Carolina: Division of Rheumatology & Immunology, 1249
Myasthenia Gravis Support Group of Low Country, 6627
Myasthenia Gravis Support Group of the Mountain and Up Country, 6628
NAMI-SC: National Alliance on Mental Illness: South Carolina, 6006
NNFF South Carolina Chapter, 6680
National Association for Continence, 5332
National Federation of the Blind: South Carolina, 9575
National Kidney Foundation of South Carolina, 5644
National MS Society: South Carolina Branch, 6411
Prader-Willi South Carolina Association, 7193
RESOLVE of South Carolina, 5421
Ralph H. Johnson VA Medical Center, 10234
Richland Memorial Comprehensive Pediatric Hemophilia Center, 5055
Scleroderma Foundation: South Carolina Chapter, 7351
South Carolina Commission on Alcohol and Drug Abuse, 8184
South Carolina Department of Health & Environmental Control, 335
South Carolina Protection & Advocacy System for the Handicapped, 10483
South Carolina State Library, 9745
Tri County HPV Support Group, 10484

South Dakota

AARP South Dakota, 95
ALS Association: Minnesota, South Dakota, North Dakota Chapter, 1127
American Cancer Society: South Dakota, 2239
American Lung Association of South Dakota, 5861
American Lung Association of South Dakota, 9302
Autism Society of Black Hills, 1708
Cancer Support Group, 2023
Division of Alcohol & Drug Abuse: South Dakota, 8185
Fort Meade Campus VA Black Hills Health Care System, 10235

Hot Springs Campus VA Black Hills Health Care System, 10236
Juvenile Diabetes Research Foundation: Sio ux Falls Chapter, 3340
NAMI South Dakota, 6007
National Federation of the Blind: South Dakota, 9576
Parkinson Association of South Dakota, 6903
Sioux Falls VA Health Care System, 10237
South Dakota Advocacy Services, 10485
South Dakota Department of Health, 8789
South Dakota State Library, 9746
Teratogen and Birth Defects Information Project, 1864

Tennessee

AARP Tennessee, 96
ALS Association: Tennessee Chapter, 1128
Alvin C. York VA Medical Center Tennessee Valley Healthcare System, 10238
Alzheimer's Association: Eastern Tennessee Chapter, 904
Alzheimer's Association: Highland Rim Chapter, 905
Alzheimer's Association: Memphis Area Office, 906
Alzheimer's Association: Middle Tennessee Chapter, 907
Alzheimer's Association: Northeast Tennessee Chapter, 908
Alzheimer's Association: Southeast Tennessee Chapter, 909
American Cancer Society: Tennessee, 2240
American Diabetes Association: Nashville, 3341
American Diabetes Association: Tennessee, 3342
American Liver Foundation Midsouth Chapter, 5762
American Lung Association of Tennesse, 9303
American Lung Association of Tennessee, 5862
Arthritis Foundation: Southeast Region, 1231
Arthritis Trust of America, 2607
Autism Society of East Tennessee, 1709
Brain Injury Association of Tennessee, 4118
Brain Injury Association of Tennessee Help line, 4182
CCFA Tennessee Chapter, 3033
Cancer Support Group: Knoxville, 2024
Cancer Support Group: Nashville, 2025
Centers for AIDS Research: Vanderbilt University Medical Center, 431
Coalition for Advanced Cancer Treatment and Prevention, 2101
Council of Citizens with Low Vision International, 9421
Department of Mental Health and Mental Retardation, Alcohol & Drug Service, 8186
Disability Law & Advocacy Center of Tennessee, 10486
Down Syndrome Association of Middle Tennessee, 3568
EAR Foundation, 4306
Ed Lindsey Industries of the Blind, 9577
Endometriosis Association Research Program : Vanderbuilt University, 3801
Hemophilia Health Services, 4962
James H. Quillen VA Healthcare System Mountain Home VA Healthcare System, 10239
Juvenile Diabetes Research Foundation: East Tennessee Chapter, 3343
Juvenile Diabetes Research Foundation: Mid dle Tennessee Chapter, 3344
LRC for Students with Disabilities, 9747
Leukemia & Lymphoma Society: Tennessee Chapter, 2241
Lupus Foundation of America Memphis Area Chapter, 8914
Lupus Foundation of America: East Tennessee Chapter, 8915
Lupus Foundation of America: Mid-South Area Chapter, 8916
Lupus Foundation of Kentuckiana, 8878
Memphis Cystic Fibrosis Center LeBonheur Children's Medical Center, 3167
Memphis Regional Brain Tumor Survivors Group, 2026
Memphis VA Medical Center, 10240
Mid-South Transplant Foundation, Inc. Tennessee, 9218

Middle Tennessee Sarcoidosis Support Group, 7241
Nashville VA Medical Center Tennessee Valley
    Healthcare System, 10241
National Alzheimer's Disease Institute, 757
National Association of Blind Merchants, 9462
National Federation of the Blind: Tennessee, 9578
National Foundation for Transplants, 9169
National Kidney Foundation of East Tennessee, 5646
National Kidney Foundation of West Tennessee, 5647
National MS Society: Mid-South Chapter, 6413
National MS Society: Mid-South Chapter, Nashville
    Office, 6414
National MS Society: Southeast Tennessee/North
    Georgia Chapte, 6412
Prader-Willi Tennessee Association, 7194
RESOLVE of Tennessee, 5422
Sarcoidosis Center, 7237
Sarcoidosis Research Institute (SRI), 7246
Scleroderma Foundation: Tennessee Chapter, 7352
Southeast AIDS Education and Training Center
    (SEAETC), 336
Southeast AIDS Education and Training Center
    (SEAETC), 432
Spina Bifida Association of Tennessee, 7904
St. Jude Children's Research Hospital, 2372
Support4Hope, 7118
Tenessee Department of Health, 8790
Tennessee Alliance for the Mentally Ill, 6008
Tennessee Department of Health: HIV Prevention
    Services, 337
Tennessee Donor Services, 9219
Tennessee Hemophilia & Bleeding Disorder
    Foundation, 5003
Tennessee Hemophilia and Bleeding Disorder
    Foundation, 5061
Tennessee Kidney Foundation, 5649
Tennessee Library for the Blind and Physically
    Handicapped, 9748
Tennessee Neuropsychiatric Institute Middle
    Tennessee Mental Health Institute, 6262
Tennessee SIDS Alliance, 8791
Tennessee Voices for Children, 6078
The University of Memphis: School of Commu
    nication Sciences and Disorders, 4396
The Vanderbilt Hemostasis Clinic, 5062
United Cerebral Palsy of Middle Tennessee, 2781
United Cerebral Palsy of the Mid-South, 2782
University of Memphis: Department of Psych ology,
    4141
University of Tennessee Drug Information Center,
    8234
University of Tennessee Medical Group, 7371
University of Tennessee Memphis: Cancer Center,
    2373
University of Tennessee: Center for Neuroscience,
    7494
University of Tennessee: Division of Cardiovascular
    Diseases, 4911
University of Tennessee: Division of Reproductive
    Endocrinology, 3804
University of Tennessee: General Clinical Research
    Center, 3400
VA MidSouth Healthcare Network (VISN 9), 10242
Vanderbilt Children's Hospital, 3168
Vanderbilt Kennedy Center, 6044
Vanderbilt University Diabetes Center, 3403
Vanderbilt University: Center for Fertility and
    Reproductive Research, 5439
West Tennessee Sarcoidosis Support Group, 7255

Texas

A Wish with Wings, Inc., 10654
AARP Texas: Austin, 97
AARP Texas: Dallas, 98
AARP Texas: Houston, 99
AARP Texas: San Antonio, 100
AIDS Outreach Center (AOC), 338
ALS Association: Greater Houston Office, 1129
ALS Association: South Texas Chapter, 1130
ALS Association: Texas Chapter - Austin, 1131
ALS Association: Texas Chapter - Dallas, 1132
Alzheimer's Alliance: Texarkana Area, 910

Alzheimer's Association: Capital of Texas Chapter,
    911
Alzheimer's Association: El Paso Chapter, 912
Alzheimer's Association: Greater Beaumont Area
    Chapter, 913
Alzheimer's Association: Greater Dallas Chapter, 914
Alzheimer's Association: Greater East Texas Chapter,
    915
Alzheimer's Association: Greater Wichita Falls
    Chapter, 916
Alzheimer's Association: Houston and Southeast
    Texas Chapter, 917
Alzheimer's Association: Northeast Texas Chapter,
    918
Alzheimer's Association: Rio Grande Valley Region,
    919
Alzheimer's Association: STAR Chapter, Midland
    Region, 920
Alzheimer's Association: South Central Texas, 921
Alzheimer's Association: Tarrant County Chapter,
    922
American Association for Respiratory Care, 5810
American Association of Kidney Patients: Piney
    Woods Chapter, 5650
American Association of the Deaf-Blind, 4293
American Cancer Society: Texas, 2242
American Diabetes Association: Texas, 3345
American Foundation for the Blind, 9579
American GI Forum NVOP, 10271
American Heart Association, 4860
American Heart Association, 8046
American Lung Association of Texas, 5863
American Lung Association of Texas, 9304
American Porphyria Foundation, 3932
American Pregnancy Association, 5375
American Stroke Association, 8047
Arthritis Foundation: North Texas Chapter, 1232
Audie L. Murphy Memorial VA Hospital South Texas
    Veterans Health Care System, 10243
Autism Society of Dallas, 1710
Baylor College of Medicine: Children's General
    Clinical Research Center, 3378
Baylor College of Medicine: Cullen Eye Institute,
    9774
Baylor College of Medicine: Debakey Heart Center,
    4866
Baylor College of Medicine: Epilepsy Research
    Center, 7490
Baylor College of Medicine: General Clinical
    Research Center for Adults, 3940
Baylor College of Medicine: Jerry Lewis
    Neuromuscular Disease Research, 6513
Baylor College of Medicine: Sleep Disorder and
    Research Center, 7763
Baylor University Bone Marrow Transplantation
    Research Center, 2374
Brain Injury Association of Texas, 4119
Brain Tumor Support Group: El Paso, 2027
CCFA Houston Gulf Coast/South Texas Chapter,
    3034
CCFA North Texas Chapter, 3035
Cancer Therapy and Research Center, 2375
Centers for AIDS Research: Baylor College of
    Medicine, 433
Central Texas FFCMH, 6009
Central Texas Veterans Health Care System, 10244
Cerebral Blood Flow Laboratories Veterans
    Administration Medical Center, 8054
Children's Heart Institute of Texas, 4871
Christus Santa Rosa Health System, 5020
Convention of American Instructors of the Deaf, 4304
Cook Children's Medical Center: Cystic Fibrosis
    Clinic, 3169
Cooley's Anemia Foundation (CAF): Texas, 2971
Cystic Fibrosis Care and Teaching Center Children's
    Medical Center, 3170
Cystic Fibrosis-Lung Disease Center: Santa Rosa
    Children's Hospital, 3171
Dallas Lighthouse for the Blind, 9580
Dallas/Ft.Worth Metroplex HPV Support Group,
    10487
Department of State Health Offices, 8792
Disability Rights Texas, 10488
Down Syndrome Clinic of Houston, 3585
Down Syndrome Guild of Dallas, 3569

East Texas Lighthouse for the Blind, 9581
El Paso Lighthouse for the Blind, 9582
El Paso VA Health Care Center, 10245
George H. O'Brien, Jr. VA Medical Center West
    Texas VA Health Care System, 10246
Greater Houston Chapter SIDS Alliance, 8793
Gulf States Hemophilia Diagnostic and Treatment
    Center, 5028
Harris County FFCMH, 6079
Harris County Public Health and Environmental
    Services, 8794
Houston Area Brain Tumor Network, 2029
Houston Ear Research Foundation, 4379
Houston Health Department: HIV-STD Viral
    Hepatitis Prevention, 339
Houston Public Library Access Center, 9749
Houston Support Group: National Ataxia Foundation,
    1559
Hydrocephalus Association of North Texas, 5206
Independent Living Research Utilization Project,
    2669
Institute for Rehabilitation and Research, 660
Institute for Rehabilitation and Research, 4131
Juvenile Diabetes Research Foundation: Dal las
    Chapter, 3347
Juvenile Diabetes Research Foundation: Gre ater Fort
    Worth/ Arlington Chapter, 3348
Juvenile Diabetes Research Foundation: Hou
    ston/Gulf Coast Chapter, 3349
Juvenile Diabetes Research Foundation: South
    Central Texas Chapter, 3346
Juvenile Diabetes Research Foundation: Wes t Texas
    Chapter, 3350
Kerrville VA Hospital South Texas Veterans Health
    Care System, 10247
Kidd's Kids, 10668
LAUNCH Department of Special Education, 10387
Leukemia and Lymphoma Society: North Texas
    Chapter, 2243
Leukemia and Lymphoma Society: South/West Texas
    Chapter, 2244
Leukemia and Lymphoma Society: Texas Gulf Coast
    Chapter, 2245
Lighthouse for the Blind of Houston, 9583
Lighthouse of the Blind of Fort Worth, 9584
Lone Star Chapter of the American Association of
    Kidney Patients, 5651
Lone Star Chapter of the National Hemophilia
    Foundation, 5004
Lupus Foundation of America: North Texas Chapter,
    8917
Lupus Foundation of America: South Central Texas
    Chapter, 8918
Lupus Foundation of America: Texas Gulf Coast
    Chapter, 8919
Lupus Foundation of America: West Texas Chapter,
    8920
Mended Hearts, 4918
Menninger Clinic: Department of Research, 6035
Methodist Hospital Sleep Center Winona Memorial
    Hospital, 7774
Michael E. DeBakey VA Medical Center, 10248
Mothers Against Drunk Driving (MADD), 8123
National Federation of the Blind: Texas, 9585
National Kidney Foundation of North Texas, 5652
National Kidney Foundation of Southeast Texas, 5653
National Kidney Foundation of Texas, 5654
National Kidney Foundation of West Texas, 5648
National Kidney Foundation of the Texas Coastal
    Bend, 5655
National MS Society: North Central Texas Chapter,
    6415
National MS Society: Panhandle Chapter, 6416
National MS Society: Southern Texas, 6417
National MS Society: West Texas Division, 6418
National MS Socisty: Southeast Texas Chapter, 6419
National Ovarian Cancer Coalition, 2111
Neuromuscular Treatment Center: Univ. of Texas
    Southwestern Medical Center, 6433
North Texas Comprehensive Pediatric Hemophilia
    Center, 5050
North Texas FFCMH, 6010
North Texas Support Group: National Ataxia
    Foundation, 1560

Northwest Texas Chapter of the Myasthenia Gravis Foundation of America, 6597
Prader-Willi Texas Association, 7195
Presbyterian Hospital of Dallas, 6929
RESOLVE of Central Texas, 5423
RESOLVE of Dallas/Fort Worth, 5424
RESOLVE of Houston, 5425
RESOLVE of South Texas, 5426
RNtoBSN.org, 7076
RRTC on Community Integration of Persons with TBI, 4110
Region VI Office Program Consultants for Maternal and Child Health, 8795
Rio Grande Chapter: NSCIA Rio Vista Rehabilitation Hospital, 7980
Roy M and Phyllis Gough Huffington Center on Aging, 130
San Antonio Bexar County FFCMH, 6011
San Antonio Cancer Institute, 2376
Santa Rosa Medical Center, 3593
Scleroderma Foundation: Bluebonnet Chapter, 7353
Sickle Cell Anemia Association of Austin: Marc Thomas Chapter, 7628
Sickle Cell Association of the Texas Gulf Coast, 7620
Sleep Medicine Associates of Texas, 7807
South Central AIDS Education and Training Center (SCAETC), 340
South Central AIDS Education and Training Center (SCAETC), 434
South Texas Brain Tumor Foundation Support Group, 2030
South Texas Lighthouse for the Blind, 9586
SouthWestern Medical Center, 5057
Southwest Foundation for Biomedical Research, 2377
Southwest SIDS Research Institute, 8796
Spina Bifida Association of Austin, 7905
Spina Bifida Association of Dallas, 7906
Spina Bifida Association of Texas, Gulf Coast, 7907
Stroke Clubs International, 8066
Texas Alliance for the Mentally Ill, 6012
Texas Ambassador: National Ataxia Foundation, 1561
Texas Association of Retinitis Pigmentosa, 9587
Texas Association of the Deaf, 4355
Texas Association on Mental Retardation, 3570
Texas Central Chapter of the National Hemophilia Foundation, 5005
Texas Children's Allergy and Immunology Clinic, 665
Texas Childrens Cystic Fibrosis Care Center, 3172
Texas Commission on Alcohol and Drug Abuse Department Of State Health, 8187
Texas Department of State Health Services: HIV-STD Program, 341
Texas FFCMH, 6013
Texas Heart Institute St Lukes Episcopal Hospital, 4898
Texas Neurofibromatosis Foundation, 6689
Texas State Library, 9750
Texas State Library: Talking Book Program, 9751
Texas Tech University Tarbox Parkinson's Disease Institute, 6909
The Alzheimer's Disease & Memory Disorders Center, 975
The Turner Syndrome Society: Central Texas, Dallas/Ft.Worth, Houston, 9356
Thomas E. Creek VA Medical Center Amarillo VA Health Care System, 10249
Travis Association for the Blind, 9588
Tri-Services Military Cystic Fibrosis Center, 3173
Turner Syndrome Society Resource Center, 9358
Turner Syndrome Society of the United States, 9342
United Cerebral Palsy of Greater Houston, 2783
United Cerebral Palsy of Metropolitan Dallas, 2784
United Cerebral Palsy of Tarrant County, 2785
United Cerebral Palsy of Texas, 2786
University of Texas General Clinical Research Center, 3401
University of Texas HSC at San Antonio, 6930
University of Texas Health Science Center, 7372
University of Texas Health Science Center Neurophysiology Research Center, 8235
University of Texas Mental Health Clinical Research Center, 6203
University of Texas Sleep/Wake Disorders Center, 7816

University of Texas Southwestern Medical, 5770
University of Texas Southwestern Medical Center, 5769
University of Texas Southwestern Medical Center at Dallas, 669
University of Texas Southwestern Medical Center at Dallas, 4912
University of Texas Southwestern Medical Center/Sickle Cell Management, 7623
University of Texas at Austin: Drug Synamics Institute, 8236
University of Texas at Dallas Callier Center for Communication Disorders, 4406
University of Texas: MD Anderson Cancer Center, 2378
University of Texas: Medical Branch at Galveston Cancer Center, 2379
University of Texas: Southwestern Medical Center at Dallas, Immunodermatology, 7679
VA Austin Information Technology Center, 10104
VA Austin Outpatient Clinic, 10250
VA Heart of Texas Health Care Network Dallas VA Medical Center, 10251
VIVA!, 7991
West Texas Lighthouse for the Blind, 9589

Utah

AARP Utah, 101
Allies with Families, 6080
Alzheimer's Association: Utah Chapter, 923
American Cancer Society: Utah, 2246
American Diabetes Association: Utah, 3351
American Lung Association of Utah, 5864
American Lung Association of Utah, 9305
Arthritis Foundation: Utah/Idaho Chapter, 1233
Brain Injury Alliance of Utah, 4183
Brain Injury Association of Utah, 4120
Brigham Young University Cancer Research Center, 2380
Cancer Wellness House, 2031
Department of Social Services: Division of Substance Abuse, 8188
George E. Wahlen Medical Center VA Salt Lake City Health Care System, 10252
Huntsman Cancer Institute University of Utah School of Medicine, 2381
Intermountain Donor Services, 9220
Legal Center for People with Disabilities, 10489
Lupus Foundation of America Utah Chapter, 8921
National Clearinghouse of Rehabilitation Training Materials, 10399
National Federation of the Blind: Utah, 9590
National Fibromyalgia & Chronic Pain Association, 2917
National Fibromyalgia & Chronic Pain Association, 3862
National Kidney Foundation of Utah, 5656
National MS Society: Utah State Chapter, 6420
Prader-Willi Utah Association, 7196
Pregnancy Risk Line, 1861
RESOLVE of Utah, 5427
United Cerebral Palsy of Utah, 2787
University of Utah Intermountain Cystic Fibrosis Center, 3174
University of Utah Rocky Mountain Center for Occupational & Environmental Health, 5871
University of Utah Utah Genome Depot University of Utah, 6519
University of Utah: Artificial Heart Research Laboratory, 4913
University of Utah: Cardiovascular Genetic Research Clinic, 4914
University of Utah: Center for Human Toxicology, 8237
Utah Alliance for the Mentally Ill, 6014
Utah Chapter of the National Hemophilia Foundation, 5006
Utah Department of Health, 8797
Utah Department of Health: Bureau of Epidemiology, 342
Utah Industries for the Blind, 9591
Utah SIDS Alliance, 8798
Utah State Library Division, 9752

Utah Support Group: National Ataxia Foundation, 1562
Veterans Affairs Medical Center: Research Service, 3404

Vermont

AARP Vermont, 102
ALS Clinical Department of Neurology, 1138
Alcohol and Drug Abuse Programs of Vermont Department Of Health, 8189
Alzheimer's Association: Vermont Chapter, 924
American Cancer Society: Vermont, 2247
American Diabetes Association: Vermont, 3352
American Lung Association of Vermont, 9306
Autism Society of Vermont Autism Society of America, 1711
Brain Injury Association of Vermont, 4121
Brain Injury Association of Vermont Helpli ne, 4184
Citizen Advocacy of Burlington, 10490
Client Assistance Program: Vermont Ladd Hall, 10491
Lupus Foundation of America: Vermont Chapter, 8922
Medical Center Hospital of Vermont Cystic Fibrosis Center, 3175
National Federation of the Blind: Vermont, 9592
National MS Society: Vermont Division, 6421
RESOLVE of Vermont, 5428
University of Vermont Cancer Center University of Vermont, 2382
University of Vermont Larner College of Medicine Center on Aging, 143
University of Vermont: Office of Health Promotion Research, 435
Vermont Alliance for the Mentally Ill, 6015
Vermont Department of Health: Health Surveillance Division, 343
Vermont Department of Health: SIDS Information and Counseling Program, 8799
Vermont Department of Libraries Special Services Unit, 9753
Vermont FFCMH, 6016
Vermont FFCMH, 6081
Vermont Pregnancy Risk Information Service, 1867
Vermont Regional Hemophilia Center, 5071
White River Junction VA Medical Center, 10253

Virginia

AABA Support Group, 3710
AAO-HNS Foundation, 4360
AARP Virginia, 103
AbleData, 4285
AbleData, 10335
Academy for Eating Disorders, 3667
Academy for Eating Disorders, 3706
Al-Anon Alateen Family Group Hotline, 8239
Al-Anon Family Group Headquarters, 8107
Allergy & Asthma Network, 628
Allergy & Asthma Network, 1373
Alzheimer's Association: Central Virginia Chapter, 925
Alzheimer's Association: Greater Richmond Chapter, 926
Alzheimer's Association: National Capital Area Chapter, 927
Alzheimer's Association: Piedmont-Valley Area Chapter, 928
Alzheimer's Association: Roanoke Salem Chapter, 929
Alzheimer's Association: Southeastern Virginia Chapter, 930
Alzheimer's Association: Southside Virginia Chapter, 931
American Academy of Audiology, 4291
American Academy of Audiology Foundation, 4361
American Academy of Otolaryngology - Head and Neck Surgery, 4292
American Association for the Study of Liver Diseases, 5731
American Cancer Society: Virginia, 2248
American Council of the Blind, 9408

American Counseling Association, 6192
American Counseling Association, 10343
American Diabetes Association, 3209
American Diabetes Association, 3407
American Diabetes Association: Richmond, 3353
American Diabetes Association: Virginia, 3354
American Foundation for the Blind, 9409
American Lung Association of Virginia, 5865
American Lung Association of Virginia, 9307
American Physical Therapy Association, 2911
American Physical Therapy Association, 6807
American Rehabilitation Counseling Association, 10349
American Spinal Injury Association (ASIA), 7955
American Thyroid Association, 9003
American Trauma Society (ATS), 7041
Arlin J Brown Information Center, 2249
Arlington County Department of Libraries, 9754
Arthritis Foundation: Virginia Chapter, 1235
Asbestos Information Association/North America, 10352
Association for Education & Rehabilitation of the Blind & Visually Impaired, 9414
Association of Organ Procurement Organizations (AOPO), 9164
Autism Society of Northern Virginia, 1712
Blinded Veterans Association, 9416
Brain Injury Association of America, 4078
Brain Injury Association of America's National Family Helpline, 4122
Brain Injury Association of Virginia, 4123
Brain Injury Association of Virginia Helpline, 4185
Brain Tumor Support Group: Richmond, 2032
BrainLine.org, 7067
CCFA Greater Washington DC/Virginia Chapter, 3036
Cancer Research Foundation of America, 2383
Central Rappahannock Regional Library, 9755
Cerebral Palsy of Virginia, 2788
Children's Hospice International, 10365
Children's Hospice International, 10691
Council for Exceptional Children, 1604
Council for Exceptional Children, 1666
Council for Exceptional Children, 1826
Council for Exceptional Children, 3542
Council for Exceptional Children, 9420
Division for the Visually Handicapped, 9756
Donate Life America, 9166
Down Syndrome Association of Hampton Roads, 3571
Eastern Virginia Medical School Children's Hospital of The King's Daught, 3176
Fairfax County Public Library, 9757
Food Allergy Research & Education, 637
Hampton Subregional Library for the Blind, 9758
Hampton VA Medical Center, 10254
Hemophilia Association of the Capital Area, 5007
Hunter Holmes McGuire VA Medical Center, 10255
Infectious Diseases Society of America, 9025
International Brain Injury Association, 4080
International Council on Infertility Information Dissemination, 5378
Juvenile Diabetes Research Foundation: Gre ater Blue Ridge Chapter, 3355
Keon Paschal Perry Sickle Cell Anemia Disease Awareness, 7625
Leukemia and Lymphoma Society: National Capital Area Chapter, 2250
LifeNet, 9221
Lupus Foundation of America: Eastern Virginia Chapter, 8923
March of Dimes Foundation, 1835
March of Dimes Foundation, 4050
March of Dimes Foundation, 7912
Mental Health America, 5913
Mental Health America, 6197
Mental Health America, 7107
Migraine Awareness Group: A National Understanding for Migraineurs (MAGNUM), 6291
Myasthenia Gravis Support Group of Manassa s, 6629
Myositis Association of America, 1190
National Adult Day Services Association, 34
National Alliance of Blind Students American Council of the Blind, 9432

National Alliance on Mental Illness, 6199
National Alliance on Mental Illness (NAMI), 5915
National Alliance on Mental Illness (NAMI), 6257
National Alliance on Mental Illness (NAMI), 7050
National Association of Alcoholism and Drug Abuse Counselors (NAADAC), 8126
National Association of State Mental Health Program Directors, 5916
National Capital Lyme Disease Association, 9027
National Captioning Institute, 4321
National Chronic Pain Outreach Association, 10398
National Council on Aging, 37
National Council on Aging, 5333
National Federation of the Blind: Virginia, 9593
National Fibromyalgia Partnership (NFP), 3864
National Hospice & Palliative Care Organization (NHPCO), 38
National Hospice & Palliative Care Organization (NHPCO), 268
National Hospice & Palliative Care Organization (NHPCO), 2107
National Hospice & Palliative Care Organization (NHPCO), 10696
National Hospice Helpline, 2411
National Hospice Helpline, 10701
National Industries for the Blind, 9449
National Kidney Foundation of Virginia, 5658
National MS Society: Blue Ridge Chapter, 6422
National MS Society: Central Virginia Chapter, 6423
National MS Society: Hampton Roads Chapter, 6424
National Osteoporosis Foundation, 6809
National Science Foundation, 1395
National Science Foundation, 4356
National Science Foundation, 5763
National Science Foundation, 7064
National Science Foundation, 7488
National Seniors Council, 40
Newport News Public Library System, 9759
Old Dominion Area Chapter: NSCIA, 7981
Organ Procurement and Transplantation Network (OPTN), 9172
PACCT, 6082
PACCT of Roanoke Valley, 6083
PTSD Family Support Group, 7110
Parkinson Foundation of the National Capitol Area, 6904
Pediatric Endocrine Society, 7
RESOLVE Helpline, 3807
RESOLVE of Alabama, 5382
RESOLVE of the Washington Metro Area, 5391
RESOLVE: The National Infertility Association, 5381
Registry of Interpreters for the Deaf, 4331
Richmond HPV Support Group: Fan Free Clini c, 10492
Richmond Support Group, 3722
Roanoke City Public Library System, 9760
Roanoke Vet Center, 10256
SIDS Mid-Atlantic, 8800
Salem VA Medical Center, 10257
Samueli Institute, 7098
Sarcoidosis Self-Help Group: Virginia, 7248
Scleroderma Foundation: Greater Washington DC Chapter, 7334
Scleroderma Foundation: Greater Washington DC Chapter, 7355
Sickle Cell Anemia Research Foundation, 7619
Sj"gren's Syndrome Foundation, 7641
Speech Simulation Research Foundation, 4390
Spina Bifida Association of America, 7863
Substance Abuse Services Office of Virginia, 8190
United Network for Organ Sharing (UNOS), 9173
United Virginia Chapter of the National Hemophilia Foundation, 5008
University Library Services, 9762
University of Virginia School of Medicine Cystic Fibrosis Center, 3177
University of Virginia: General Clinical Research Center, 1406
University of Virginia: Hypertension and Atherosclerosis Unit, 5261
Valley Brain Tumor Support Group, 2033
Virginia Alliance for the Mentally Ill, 6017
Virginia Association of the Deaf, 4357
Virginia Beach Public Library, 9763

Virginia Commonwealth University Virginia Center on Aging, 144
Virginia Commonwealth University: Massey Cancer Center, 2384
Virginia Commonwealth University: Rehab Research and Training Center, 4142
Virginia Department of Health: Division of Disease Prevention, 344
Virginia Industries for the Blind, 9594
Virginia Office for Protection and Advocacy, 10493
Virginia SIDS Alliance, 8801
Virginia SIDS Program: Virginia Department of Health, 8802
Washington Regional Transplant Consortium, 9222
World Federation for Mental Health, 5923

Washington

AARP Washington, 104
ALS Association: Evergreen Chapter, 1133
African American Post Traumatic Stress Disorder Association, 7032
Alzheimer's Association Autopsy Assistance Network, 984
Alzheimer's Association: Inland Northwest Chapter, 932
Alzheimer's Association: Western & Central Washington Chapter, 933
Alzheimer's Disease Center: Washington University, 957
American Cancer Society: Washington, 2251
American Diabetes Association: Seattle, 3356
American Diabetes Association: Washington, 3357
American Liver Foundation Pacific Northwest Chapter, 5764
American Lung Association of Washington, 5866
Arthritis Foundation: Washington/Alaska Chapter, 1236
Autism Society of Washington, 1713
BABES Network-YWCA, 444
Benaroya Research Institute Virginia Mason Medical Center, 3379
Bleeding Disorder Foundation of Washington, 5009
Brain Cancer Support Group: Port Orchard, 2034
Brain Cancer Support Group: Seattle, 2035
Brain Injury Association of Washington, 4124
Brain Injury Association of Washington Hel pline, 4186
Brain Injury Resource Center, 4187
Brain Injury Resource Center, 7066
CCFA Washington State Chapter, 3037
Cancer Information Service, 2391
Center for Anxiety and Traumatic Stress, 7099
Centers for AIDS Research: University of Washington, Harborview Medical Center, 436
Children's Hydrocephalus Support Group, 5207
Common Voice for Pierce County Parents, 6084
Dunshee House, 447
Epilepsy Foundation of North West Washington, 7489
Fred Hutchinson Cancer Research Center, 2385
Gluten Intolerance Group, 2629
HIV Prevention Trials Unit University of Washington/Seattle HPTU Si, 437
Health Information Network, 260
Hepatitis Education Project, 5146
Hepatitis Education Project, 5148
Hope Heart Institute, 4885
Inland Empire Bleeding Disorders, 5010
International Myopain Society, 3861
Jonathan M. Wainwright Memorial VA MC Walla Walla VA Medical Center, 10258
Juvenile Diabetes Research Foundation: Sea ttle Chapter, 3359
Juvenile Diabetes Research Foundation: Seattle Guild, 3358
Juvenile Diabetes Research Foundation: Spo kane County Area Chapter, 3360
King County Crisis Clinic, 451
LifeCenter Northwest, 9223
Lighthouse for the Blind of Washington, 9595
Lupus Foundation of America: Pacific Northwest Chapter, 8924
Mental Illness Research and Education Institute, 6036

Mountain West AIDS Education and Training Center (MWAETC), 296
Mountain West AIDS Education and Training Center (MWAETC), 384
Myasthenia Gravis Support Group of Seattle , Olympia and Poulsbo, 6630
Myasthenia Gravis Support Group of Spokane, 6631
NAMI Washington (National Alliance for the Mentally Ill of Washington), 6018
Narcolepsy Network, 7759
National Federation of the Blind: Public Employees Division, 9446
National MS Society: Greater Washington Chapter, 6425
National MS Society: Inland Northwest Chapter, 6426
National Service Dog Center, 9819
Northwestern Region: Helen Keller National Center, 9596
Pacific NW Support Group, 7244
Pacific Northwest Chapter of the Myasthenia Gravis Foundation of America, 6573
Pacific Northwest Chapter of the Myasthenia Gravis Foundation of America, 6580
Pacific Northwest Chapter of the Myasthenia Gravis Foundation of America, 6581
Pacific Northwest Chapter of the Myasthenia Gravis Foundation of America, 6588
Pacific Northwest Chapter of the Myasthenia Gravis Foundation of America, 6594
Pacific Northwest Chapter of the Myasthenia Gravis Foundation of America, 6599
Pacific Northwest Chapter of the Myasthenia Gravis Foundation of America, 6601
Prader-Willi Washington Association, 7197
Puget Sound Blood Center, 5053
Rainbow Alliance of the Deaf, 4330
Region X Office Program Consultants for Maternal and Child Health, 8803
SIDS Foundation of Washington, 8804
SIDS Northwest Regional Center, 8805
Scleroderma Foundation: Evergreen Chapter, 7356
Seattle HPV Support Group, 10494
Solomon Park Research Institute, 1146
Spina Bifida Association of Washington State, 7908
Spokane VA Medical Center Mann-Grandstaff VA Medical Center, 10259
Tacoma Vet Center, 10260
United Cerebral Palsy of Pierce County, 2789
University of Washington, 6931
University of Washington Department of Speech & Hearing Sciences, 4407
University of Washington Diabetes: Endocrinology Research Center, 3402
University of Washington: Cystic Fibrosis Center, 3178
University of Washington: Experimental Education Unit, 3596
VA Puget Sound Health Care System, 10261
Virginia Mason Brain Tumor Support Group, 2036
Virginia Mason Medical Center Neuroscience Institute, 1148
Washington Ambassador National Ataxia Foundation, 1563
Washington Department of Health: HIV Program, 345
Washington Department of Social and Health Services, Alcohol and Drug Prog., 8191
Washington FFCMH, 6019
Washington Leukemia and Lymphoma Society: Alaska Chapter, 2252
Washington State Client Assistance Program, 10495
Washington State Department of Services for the Blind, 9597
Washington Talking Book & Braille Library, 9764
Washington Turner Syndrome Resource Group, 9357
Wenatchee Valley Brain Tumor Support Group, 2037
Western WA Support Group: National Ataxia Foundation, 1564
Wishing Star Foundation, 10679
de Tornyay Center For Healthy Aging at University of Washington, 145

West Virginia

AARP West Virginia, 105
AFB Technology & Employment Center, 9598
Alzheimer's Association: Greater Mid-Ohio Valley Chapter, 934
Alzheimer's Association: N Central West Virginia Chapter, 935
Alzheimer's Association: South West Virginia Chapter, 936
American Cancer Society: West Virginia, 2253
American Diabetes Association: West Virginia, 3361
American Lung Association of West Virginia, 5867
American Lung Association of West Virginia, 9308
Autism Services Center, 1662
Autism Socity of West Virginia, 1714
Beckley VA Medical Center, 10262
Brain Injury Association of West Virginia, 4125
Brain Injury Association of West Virginia Helpline, 4188
Brain Tumor Support Group: Southern West Virginia, 2038
Cabell County Public Library, 9765
Health Science Library, 3371
Hemophilia Association of the Huntington Area, 5031
Hemophilia Center of West Virginia University Health Sciences Center, 5034
Hershel Woody Williams VA Medical Center, 10263
Juvenile Diabetes Research Foundation: Hun tington Chapter, 3362
Kanawha County Public Library, 9766
Louis A. Johnson VA Medical Center, 10264
Martinsburg VA Medical Center, 10265
Mountain State/Parents/Children/ Adolescents Network, 6020
NAMI West Virginia, 6021
National Autism Hotline Autism Services Center, 1727
National Federation of the Blind: West Virginia, 9599
National Job Accommodation Network, 10407
Northcentral West Virginia HPV Support Group, 10496
Office of Maternal, Child & Family Health, 8806
Ohio County Public Library Services for the Blind and Physically Handicapped, 9767
Parkersburg and Wood County Public Library, 9768
The West Virginia Autism Training Center Marshall University, 1724
West Virginia Advocates, 10497
West Virginia Department of Health & Human Resources: Division of STD and HIV, 346
West Virginia Division of Alcohol & Drug Abuse, 8192
West Virginia Library Commission, 9769
West Virginia School for the Blind, 9770
West Virginia University Cystic Fibrosis Center, 3179
West Virginia University: Mary Babb Randolph Cancer Center, 2386

Wisconsin

AARP Wisconsin, 106
ABCD: After Breast Cancer Diagnosis, 2088
AIDS Resource Center of Wisconsin, 347
ALS Association: Southeast Wisconsin Chapter, 1135
About Kids GI Disorders, 3711
Alzheimer's Association: Greater Wisconsin Chapter, 937
Alzheimer's Association: Indianhead Chapter, 938
Alzheimer's Association: Lake Superior Chapter, 939
Alzheimer's Association: Midstate Wisconsin Chapter, 940
Alzheimer's Association: North Central Wisconsin Chapter, 941
Alzheimer's Association: Northeast Wisconsin Chapter, 942
Alzheimer's Association: South Central Wisconsin Chapter, 943
Alzheimer's Association: Southeast Wisconsin Chapter, 944
American Academy for Cerebral Palsy and Developmental Medicine, 2665

American Academy of Allergy, Asthma & Immunology, 629
American Academy of Allergy, Asthma & Immunology, 1374
American Academy of Allergy, Asthma & Immunology Foundation, 653
American Academy of Allergy, Asthma & Immunology Foundation, 1396
American Cancer Society: Wisconsin, 2254
American Diabetes Association: Wisconsin, 3363
American Liver Foundation Wisconsin Chapter, 5765
American Lung Association of Wisconsin, 5868
American Lung Association of Wisconsin, 9309
Anxiety Disorders Center University of Wisconsin, 6030
Arthritis Foundation: Wisconsin Chapter Foundation, 1237
Association of Children's Residential Centers, 5908
Autism Society of Wisconsin, 1715
Brain Injury Alliance of Wisconsin, 4189
Brain Injury Association of Wisconsin, 4126
Brain Tumor Support Group: John Sierzant Lutheran Hospital, Gunderson Clinic, 2039
Brown County Library, 9771
CCFA Wisconsin Chapter, 3038
Center for Aging Research and Education at the UW-Madison School of Nursing, 116
Children's Brittle Bone Foundation, 6782
Cyclic Vomiting Syndrome Association, 3923
Down Syndrome Association of Wisconsin, 3572
Eau Claire Hemophilia Center, 5024
Endometriosis Association International, 3792
Endometriosis Association International, 3805
Governor's Committee for People with Disabilities, 10498
Great Lakes Hemophilia Foundation, 5011
Grief & Loss Support Group, 10700
Gundersen Clinic Comprehensive Hemophilia Treatment Center, 5029
Hematology Treatment Center of the Great Lakes Hemophilia Foundation, 5030
Infant Death Center of Wisconsin, 8807
Injury Research Center, 7100
International Foundation for Functional Gastrointestinal Disorders (IFFGD), 3040
International Foundation for Functional Gastrointestinal Disorders (IFFGD), 3934
International Foundation for Functional Gastrointestinal Disorders (IFFGD), 5337
International Parkinson and Movement Disorder Society, 1519
International Parkinson and Movement Disorder Society, 6868
Juvenile Diabetes Research Foundation: Gre ater Madison Chapter, 3365
Juvenile Diabetes Research Foundation: Nor theast Wisconsin Chapter, 3366
Juvenile Diabetes Research Foundation: Southeastern Chapter, 3364
LODAT: Brain Tumor Support Group, 2040
Leukemia and Lymphoma Society: Wisconsin Chapter, 2255
Lupus Foundation of America: Wisconsin Chapter, 8925
Medical College of Wisconsin: Cystic Fibrosis Clinic, 3180
Milwaukee VA Medical Center (Zablocki), 10266
Myasthenia Gravis Support Group of Fox Valley, 6632
Myasthenia Gravis Support Group of Milwauk ee, 6633
NNFF Wisconsin Chapter, 6681
National Federation of the Blind: Wisconsin, 9600
National Federation of the Blind: Writers, 9601
National Kidney Foundation of Wisconsin, 5659
National MS Society: Wisconsin Chapter, 6427
Office of Alcohol and Other Drug Abuse, 8193
Physician Referral and Information Line, 1409
Prader-Willi Wisconsin Association, 7198
RESOLVE of Wisconsin, 5429
Scoliosis Research Society, 7400
Society for the Study of Reproduction, 5430
Southeastern Wisconsin Chapter of the Nati onal Spinal Cord Injury Association, 7982

Spina Bifida Association of Northern Wisconsin, 7909

Spina Bifida Association of Southeastern Wisconsin, 7910

Spina Bifida Association of the Greater Fox Valley, 7911

Stem Cell Research Program University of Wisconsin-Madison, 1147

Tomah VA Medical Center, 10267

Trace Center University of Wisconsin: Madison, 4397

United Cerebral Palsy of Greater Dane County, 2790

United Cerebral Palsy of North Central Wisconsin, 2791

United Cerebral Palsy of Southeastern Wisconsin, 2792

United Cerebral Palsy of Wisconsin, 2793

United Special Sportsman Alliance, 10690

University of Wisconsin Madison Neurophysiology Laboratory, 7495

University of Wisconsin Milwaukee Medicinal Chemistry Group, 8238

University of Wisconsin Organ Procurement Organization, 9224

University of Wisconsin Paul P Carbone Comprehensive Cancer Center, 2387

University of Wisconsin-Madison: Cystic Fibrosis/Pulmonary Center, 3181

University of Wisconsin: Asthma, Allergy and Pulmonary Research Center, 1407

We Are the Children's Hope/Support Group, 6085

William S. Middleton Memorial Veterans Hospital, 10268

Wilson's Disease Association, 5775

Wisconsin Alliance for the Mentally Ill, 6022

Wisconsin Association of the Deaf, 4358

Wisconsin Chapter of the Myasthenia Gravis Foundation of America, 6600

Wisconsin Department of Health Services: Wisconsin HIV Program, 348

Wisconsin Family Ties, 6023

Wisconsin Parkinson Association, 6905

Wisconsin Regional Library for the Blind Talking Book Program, 9772

Wiscraft: Wisconsin Enterprises for the Blind, 9602

Wisonsin Donor Network, 9225

Wyoming

AARP Wyoming, 107

Alcohol & Drug Abuse Programs of Wyoming Department Of Health, 8194

Alzheimer's Wyoming, 945

American Cancer Society: Wyoming, 2256

Brain Injury Alliance of Wyoming, 4190

Brain Injury Association of Wyoming, 4127

Cheyenne VA Medical Center, 10269

Concerned Parent Coalition, 6086

Deaf Association of Wyoming, 4359

National Federation of the Blind: Wyoming, 9603

National MS Society: Wyoming Chapter, 6428

Sheridan VA Medical Center, 10270

University Of Wyoming Center on Aging, 138

Uplift, 6087

Wyoming Alliance for the Mentally Ill, 6024

Wyoming Department of Health, 8808

Wyoming Department of Health: Communicable Disease Unit, 349

Wyoming Protection & Advocacy System, 10499

Wyoming Services for the Visually Disabled, 9773

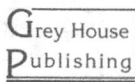
Grey House Publishing

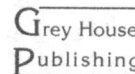
Grey House Publishing

2019 Title List
Visit www.GreyHouse.com for Product Information, Table of Contents, and Sample Pages.

General Reference
America's College Museums
American Environmental Leaders: From Colonial Times to the Present
Encyclopedia of African-American Writing
Encyclopedia of Constitutional Amendments
Encyclopedia of Human Rights and the United States
Encyclopedia of Invasions & Conquests
Encyclopedia of Prisoners of War & Internment
Encyclopedia of Religion & Law in America
Encyclopedia of Rural America
Encyclopedia of the Continental Congress
Encyclopedia of the United States Cabinet, 1789-2010
Encyclopedia of War Journalism
Encyclopedia of Warrior Peoples & Fighting Groups
The Environmental Debate: A Documentary History
The Evolution Wars: A Guide to the Debates
From Suffrage to the Senate: America's Political Women
Gun Debate: An Encyclopedia of Gun Rights & Gun Control in the U.S.
Opinions throughout History: National Security vs. Civil and Privacy Rights
Opinions throughout History: Immigration
Opinions throughout History: Drug Use & Abuse
Opinions throughout History: Gender: Roles & Rights
Opinions throughout History: The Environment
Opinions throughout History: Social Media Issues
Opinions throughout History: The Death Penalty
Opinions throughout History: Voters' Rights
Political Corruption in America
Privacy Rights in the Digital Age
The Religious Right: A Reference Handbook
Speakers of the House of Representatives, 1789-2009
This is Who We Were: 1880-1900
This is Who We Were: A Companion to the 1940 Census
This is Who We Were: In Colonial America
This is Who We Were: In the 1900s
This is Who We Were: In the 1910s
This is Who We Were: In the 1920s
This is Who We Were: In the 1940s
This is Who We Were: In the 1950s
This is Who We Were: In the 1960s
This is Who We Were: In the 1970s
This is Who We Were: In the 1980s
This is Who We Were: In the 1990s
This is Who We Were: In the 2000s
U.S. Land & Natural Resource Policy
The Value of a Dollar 1600-1865: Colonial Era to the Civil War
The Value of a Dollar: 1860-2019
Working Americans 1880-1999 Vol. I: The Working Class
Working Americans 1880-1999 Vol. II: The Middle Class
Working Americans 1880-1999 Vol. III: The Upper Class
Working Americans 1880-1999 Vol. IV: Their Children
Working Americans 1880-2015 Vol. V: Americans At War
Working Americans 1880-2005 Vol. VI: Women at Work
Working Americans 1880-2006 Vol. VII: Social Movements
Working Americans 1880-2007 Vol. VIII: Immigrants
Working Americans 1770-1869 Vol. IX: Revolutionary War to the Civil War
Working Americans 1880-2009 Vol. X: Sports & Recreation
Working Americans 1880-2010 Vol. XI: Inventors & Entrepreneurs
Working Americans 1880-2011 Vol. XII: Our History through Music
Working Americans 1880-2012 Vol. XIII: Education & Educators
Working Americans 1880-2016 Vol. XIV: Industry Through the Ages
Working Americans 1880-2017 Vol. XV: Politics & Politicians
World Cultural Leaders of the 20th & 21st Centuries

Education Information
Charter School Movement
The Comparative Guide to American Elementary & Secondary Schools
Complete Learning Disabilities Resource Guide
Educators Resource Guide
Special Education: A Reference Book for Policy and Curriculum
   Development

Health Information
Comparative Guide to American Hospitals
Complete Resource Guide for Pediatric Disorders
Complete Resource Guide for People with Chronic Illness
Complete Resource Guide for People with Disabilities
Complete Mental Health Resource Guide
Diabetes in America: Analysis of an Epidemic
Guide to Health Care Group Purchasing Organizations
Guide to U.S. HMO's & PPO's
Medical Device Market Place
Older Americans Information Resource

Business Information
Complete Television, Radio & Cable Industry Guide
Business Information Resources
Directory of Mail Order Catalogs
Guide to Venture Capital & Private Equity Firms
Environmental Resource Handbook
Financial Literacy Starter Kit
Food & Beverage Market Place
The Grey House Homeland Security Directory
The Grey House Performing Arts Industry Guide
The Grey House Safety & Security Directory
Hudson's Washington News Media Contacts Directory
New York State Directory
Sports Market Place

Statistics & Demographics
American Tally
America's Top-Rated Cities
America's Top-Rated Smaller Cities
Ancestry & Ethnicity in America
The Asian Databook
The Comparative Guide to American Suburbs
The Hispanic Databook
Nations of the World
Profiles of America
"Profiles of" Series – State Handbooks
Weather America

Financial Ratings Series
Financial Literacy Basics
TheStreet Ratings' Ultimate Guided Tour of Stock Investing
Weiss Ratings' Investment Research Guide to Bond & Money Market
   Mutual Funds
Weiss Ratings' Investment Research Guide to Stocks
Weiss Ratings' Investment Research Guide to Exchange-Traded Funds
Weiss Ratings' Investment Research Guide to Stock Mutual Funds
Weiss Ratings' Consumer Guides
Weiss Ratings' Financial Literary Basic Guides
Weiss Ratings' Guide to Banks
Weiss Ratings' Guide to Credit Unions
Weiss Ratings' Guide to Health Insurers
Weiss Ratings' Guide to Life & Annuity Insurers
Weiss Ratings' Guide to Property & Casualty Insurers

Bowker's Books In Print® Titles
American Book Publishing Record® Annual
American Book Publishing Record® Monthly
Books In Print®
Books In Print® Supplement
Books Out Loud™
Bowker's Complete Video Directory™
Children's Books In Print®
El-Hi Textbooks & Serials In Print®
Forthcoming Books®
Law Books & Serials In Print™
Medical & Health Care Books In Print™
Publishers, Distributors & Wholesalers of the US™
Subject Guide to Books In Print®
Subject Guide to Children's Books In Print®

Grey House Publishing | Salem Press | H.W. Wilson | 4919 Route, 22 PO Box 56, Amenia NY 12501-0056

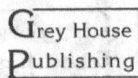

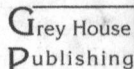

2019 Title List

Visit **www.GreyHouse.com** for Product Information, Table of Contents, and Sample Pages.

Canadian General Reference

Associations Canada
Canadian Almanac & Directory
Canadian Environmental Resource Guide
Canadian Parliamentary Guide
Canadian Venture Capital & Private Equity Firms
Canadian Who's Who
Financial Post Bonds
Financial Post Directory of Directors
Financial Post Equities
Financial Post Survey
Financial Services Canada
Government Canada
Health Guide Canada
The History of Canada
Libraries Canada
Major Canadian Cities

2019 Title List

Visit www.SalemPress.com for Product Information, Table of Contents, and Sample Pages.

Science, Careers & Mathematics

Ancient Creatures
Applied Science
Applied Science: Engineering & Mathematics
Applied Science: Science & Medicine
Applied Science: Technology
Biomes and Ecosystems
Careers in the Arts: Fine, Performing & Visual
Careers in Building Construction
Careers in Business
Careers in Chemistry
Careers in Communications & Media
Careers in Environment & Conservation
Careers in Financial Services
Careers in Green Energy
Careers in Healthcare
Careers in Hospitality & Tourism
Careers in Human Services
Careers in Law, Criminal Justice & Emergency Services
Careers in Manufacturing
Careers in Nursing
Careers Outdoors
Careers Overseas
Careers in Physics
Careers in Protective Services
Careers in Psychology
Careers in Sales, Insurance & Real Estate
Careers in Science & Engineering
Careers in Social Media
Careers in Sports & Fitness
Careers in Sports Medicine & Training
Careers in Technology Services & Equipment Repair
Careers in Transportation
Computer Technology Innovators
Contemporary Biographies in Business
Contemporary Biographies in Chemistry
Contemporary Biographies in Communications & Media
Contemporary Biographies in Environment & Conservation
Contemporary Biographies in Healthcare
Contemporary Biographies in Hospitality & Tourism
Contemporary Biographies in Law & Criminal Justice
Contemporary Biographies in Physics
Earth Science
Earth Science: Earth Materials & Resources
Earth Science: Earth's Surface and History
Earth Science: Physics & Chemistry of the Earth
Earth Science: Weather, Water & Atmosphere
Encyclopedia of Energy
Encyclopedia of Environmental Issues
Encyclopedia of Environmental Issues: Atmosphere and Air Pollution
Encyclopedia of Environmental Issues: Ecology and Ecosystems
Encyclopedia of Environmental Issues: Energy and Energy Use
Encyclopedia of Environmental Issues: Policy and Activism
Encyclopedia of Environmental Issues: Preservation/Wilderness Issues
Encyclopedia of Environmental Issues: Water and Water Pollution
Encyclopedia of Global Resources
Encyclopedia of Global Warming
Encyclopedia of Mathematics & Society
Encyclopedia of Mathematics & Society: Engineering, Tech, Medicine
Encyclopedia of Mathematics & Society: Great Mathematicians
Encyclopedia of Mathematics & Society: Math & Social Sciences
Encyclopedia of Mathematics & Society: Math Development/Concepts
Encyclopedia of Mathematics & Society: Math in Culture & Society
Encyclopedia of Mathematics & Society: Space, Science, Environment
Encyclopedia of the Ancient World
Forensic Science
Geography Basics
Internet Innovators
Inventions and Inventors
Magill's Encyclopedia of Science: Animal Life
Magill's Encyclopedia of Science: Plant life
Notable Natural Disasters

Principles of Artificial Intelligence & Robotics
Principles of Astronomy
Principles of Biology
Principles of Biotechnology
Principles of Business: Accounting
Principles of Business: Economics
Principles of Business: Entrepreneurship
Principles of Business: Finance
Principles of Business: Globalization
Principles of Business: Leadership
Principles of Business: Management
Principles of Business: Marketing
Principles of Chemistry
Principles of Climatology
Principles of Ecology
Principles of Modern Agriculture
Principles of Pharmacology
Principles of Physical Science
Principles of Physics
Principles of Programming & Coding
Principles of Research Methods
Principles of Sociology: Group Relationships & Behavior
Principles of Sociology: Personal Relationships & Behavior
Principles of Sociology: Societal Issues & Behavior
Principles of Sustainability
Science and Scientists
Solar System
Solar System: Great Astronomers
Solar System: Study of the Universe
Solar System: The Inner Planets
Solar System: The Moon and Other Small Bodies
Solar System: The Outer Planets
Solar System: The Sun and Other Stars
USA in Space
World Geography

Literature

American Ethnic Writers
Classics of Science Fiction & Fantasy Literature
Critical Approaches to Literature
Critical Insights: Authors
Critical Insights: Film
Critical Insights: Literary Collection Bundles
Critical Insights: Themes
Critical Insights: Works
Critical Survey of Drama
Critical Survey of Graphic Novels: Heroes & Superheroes
Critical Survey of Graphic Novels: History, Theme & Technique
Critical Survey of Graphic Novels: Independents/Underground Classics
Critical Survey of Graphic Novels: Manga
Critical Survey of Long Fiction
Critical Survey of Mystery & Detective Fiction
Critical Survey of Mythology and Folklore: Gods & Goddesses
Critical Survey of Mythology and Folklore: Heroes & Heroines
Critical Survey of Mythology and Folklore: Love, Sexuality & Desire
Critical Survey of Mythology and Folklore: World Mythology
Critical Survey of Poetry
Critical Survey of Poetry: American Poets
Critical Survey of Poetry: British, Irish & Commonwealth Poets
Critical Survey of Poetry: Cumulative Index
Critical Survey of Poetry: European Poets
Critical Survey of Poetry: Topical Essays
Critical Survey of Poetry: World Poets
Critical Survey of Science Fiction & Fantasy Literature
Critical Survey of Shakespeare's Plays
Critical Survey of Shakespeare's Sonnets
Critical Survey of Short Fiction
Critical Survey of Short Fiction: American Writers
Critical Survey of Short Fiction: British, Irish, Commonwealth Writers
Critical Survey of Short Fiction: Cumulative Index
Critical Survey of Short Fiction: European Writers
Critical Survey of Short Fiction: Topical Essays

2019 Title List

Visit www.SalemPress.com for Product Information, Table of Contents, and Sample Pages.

Critical Survey of Short Fiction: World Writers
Critical Survey of World Literature
Critical Survey of Young Adult Literature
Cyclopedia of Literary Characters
Cyclopedia of Literary Places
Holocaust Literature
Introduction to Literary Context: American Poetry of the 20th Century
Introduction to Literary Context: American Post-Modernist Novels
Introduction to Literary Context: American Short Fiction
Introduction to Literary Context: English Literature
Introduction to Literary Context: Plays
Introduction to Literary Context: World Literature
Magill's Literary Annual
Magill's Survey of American Literature
Magill's Survey of World Literature
Masterplots
Masterplots, 2002-2018 Supplement
Masterplots II: African American Literature
Masterplots II: American Fiction Series
Masterplots II: British & Commonwealth Fiction Series
Masterplots II: Christian Literature
Masterplots II: Drama Series
Masterplots II: Juvenile & Young Adult Literature, Supplement
Masterplots II: Nonfiction Series
Masterplots II: Poetry Series
Masterplots II: Short Story Series
Masterplots II: Women's Literature Series
Notable African American Writers
Notable American Novelists
Notable Playwrights
Notable Poets
Novels into Film: Adaptations & Interpretation
Recommended Reading: 600 Classics Reviewed
Short Story Writers

History and Social Science
The 1910s in America
The 2000s in America
50 States
African American History
Agriculture in History
American First Ladies
American Heroes
American Indian Culture
American Indian History
American Indian Tribes
American Presidents
American Villains
America's Historic Sites
Ancient Greece
The Bill of Rights
The Civil Rights Movement
The Cold War
Countries: Their Wars & Conflicts: A World Survey
Countries, Peoples & Cultures
Countries, Peoples & Cultures: Central & South America
Countries, Peoples & Cultures: Central, South & Southeast Asia
Countries, Peoples & Cultures: East & South Africa
Countries, Peoples & Cultures: East Asia & the Pacific
Countries, Peoples & Cultures: Eastern Europe
Countries, Peoples & Cultures: Middle East & North Africa
Countries, Peoples & Cultures: North America & the Caribbean
Countries, Peoples & Cultures: West & Central Africa
Countries, Peoples & Cultures: Western Europe
Defining Documents: American Revolution
The Criminal Justice System
Defining Documents: American West
Defining Documents: Ancient World
Defining Documents: Asia
Defining Documents: Business Ethics
Defining Documents: Capital Punishment
Defining Documents: Civil Rights

Defining Documents: Civil War
Defining Documents: Court Cases
Defining Documents: Dissent & Protest
Defining Documents: Emergence of Modern America
Defining Documents: Exploration & Colonial America
Defining Documents: The Free Press
Defining Documents: The Gun Debate
Defining Documents: Immigration & Immigrant Communities
Defining Documents: The Legacy of 9/11
Defining Documents: LGBTQ+
Defining Documents: Manifest Destiny
Defining Documents: Middle Ages
Defining Documents: Middle East
Defining Documents: Nationalism & Populism
Defining Documents: Native Americans
Defining Documents: Political Campaigns, Candidates & Debates
Defining Documents: Postwar 1940s
Defining Documents: Prison Reform
Defining Documents: Reconstruction
Defining Documents: Renaissance & Early Modern Era
Defining Documents: Secrets, Leaks & Scandals
Defining Documents: Slavery
Defining Documents: Supreme Court Decisions
Defining Documents: 1920s
Defining Documents: 1930s
Defining Documents: 1950s
Defining Documents: 1960s
Defining Documents: 1970s
Defining Documents: The 17th Century
Defining Documents: The 18th Century
Defining Documents: The 19th Century
Defining Documents: The 20th Century: 1900-1950
Defining Documents: Vietnam War
Defining Documents: Women's Rights
Defining Documents: World War I
Defining Documents: World War II
Education Today
The Eighties in America
Encyclopedia of American Immigration
Encyclopedia of Flight
Encyclopedia of the Ancient World
Ethics: Questions & Morality of Human Actions
Fashion Innovators
The Fifties in America
The Forties in America
Great Athletes
Great Athletes: Baseball
Great Athletes: Basketball
Great Athletes: Boxing & Soccer
Great Athletes: Cumulative Index
Great Athletes: Football
Great Athletes: Golf & Tennis
Great Athletes: Olympics
Great Athletes: Racing & Individual Sports
Great Contemporary Athletes
Great Events from History: 17th Century
Great Events from History: 18th Century
Great Events from History: 19th Century
Great Events from History: 20th Century (1901-1940)
Great Events from History: 20th Century (1941-1970)
Great Events from History: 20th Century (1971-2000)
Great Events from History: 21st Century (2000-2016)
Great Events from History: African American History
Great Events from History: Cumulative Indexes
Great Events from History: Human Rights
Great Events from History: LGBTQ Events
Great Events from History: Middle Ages
Great Events from History: Modern Scandals
Great Events from History: Secrets, Leaks & Scandals
Great Events from History: Renaissance & Early Modern Era
Great Lives from History: 17th Century
Great Lives from History: 18th Century

2019 Title List

Visit **www.SalemPress.com** for Product Information, Table of Contents, and Sample Pages.

Great Lives from History: 19th Century
Great Lives from History: 20th Century
Great Lives from History: 21st Century (2000-2017)
Great Lives from History: American Heroes
Great Lives from History: American Women
Great Lives from History: Ancient World
Great Lives from History: Asian & Pacific Islander Americans
Great Lives from History: Cumulative Indexes
Great Lives from History: Incredibly Wealthy
Great Lives from History: Inventors & Inventions
Great Lives from History: Jewish Americans
Great Lives from History: Latinos
Great Lives from History: Renaissance & Early Modern Era
Great Lives from History: Scientists & Science
Historical Encyclopedia of American Business
Issues in U.S. Immigration
Magill's Guide to Military History
Milestone Documents in African American History
Milestone Documents in American History
Milestone Documents in World History
Milestone Documents of American Leaders
Milestone Documents of World Religions
Music Innovators
Musicians & Composers 20th Century
The Nineties in America
The Seventies in America
The Sixties in America

Sociology Today
Survey of American Industry and Careers
The Thirties in America
The Twenties in America
United States at War
U.S. Court Cases
U.S. Government Leaders
U.S. Laws, Acts, and Treaties
U.S. Legal System
U.S. Supreme Court
Weapons and Warfare
World Conflicts: Asia and the Middle East

Health
Addictions, Substance Abuse & Alcoholism
Adolescent Health & Wellness
Aging
Cancer
Complementary & Alternative Medicine
Community & Family Health Issues
Genetics & Inherited Conditions
Infectious Diseases & Conditions
Magill's Medical Guide
Nutrition
Psychology & Behavioral Health
Psychology Basics
Women's Health

Grey House Publishing | Salem Press | H.W. Wilson | 4919 Route, 22 PO Box 56, Amenia NY 12501-0056

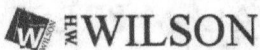
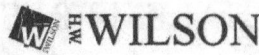

2019 Title List
Visit www.HWWilsonInPrint.com for Product Information, Table of Contents and Sample Pages.

Current Biography
Current Biography Cumulative Index 1946-2013
Current Biography Monthly Magazine
Current Biography Yearbook: 2003
Current Biography Yearbook: 2004
Current Biography Yearbook: 2005
Current Biography Yearbook: 2006
Current Biography Yearbook: 2007
Current Biography Yearbook: 2008
Current Biography Yearbook: 2009
Current Biography Yearbook: 2010
Current Biography Yearbook: 2011
Current Biography Yearbook: 2012
Current Biography Yearbook: 2013
Current Biography Yearbook: 2014
Current Biography Yearbook: 2015
Current Biography Yearbook: 2016
Current Biography Yearbook: 2017
Current Biography Yearbook: 2018

Core Collections
Children's Core Collection
Fiction Core Collection
Graphic Novels Core Collection
Middle & Junior High School Core
Public Library Core Collection: Nonfiction
Senior High Core Collection
Young Adult Fiction Core Collection

The Reference Shelf
Affordable Housing
Aging in America
Alternative Facts: Post Truth & the Information War
The American Dream
American Military Presence Overseas
The Arab Spring
Artificial Intelligence
The Brain
The Business of Food
Campaign Trends & Election Law
Conspiracy Theories
Democracy Evolving
The Digital Age
Dinosaurs
Embracing New Paradigms in Education
Faith & Science
Families: Traditional and New Structures
The Future of U.S. Economic Relations: Mexico, Cuba, and Venezuela
Global Climate Change
Graphic Novels and Comic Books
Guns in America
Immigration
Immigration in the U.S.
Internet Abuses & Privacy Rights
Internet Safety
LGBTQ in the 21st Century
Marijuana Reform
New Frontiers in Space
The News and its Future
The Paranormal
Politics of the Ocean
Prescription Drug Abuse
Racial Tension in a "Postracial" Age
Reality Television
Representative American Speeches: 2008-2009
Representative American Speeches: 2009-2010
Representative American Speeches: 2010-2011
Representative American Speeches: 2011-2012
Representative American Speeches: 2012-2013
Representative American Speeches: 2013-2014

Representative American Speeches: 2014-2015
Representative American Speeches: 2015-2016
Representative American Speeches: 2016-2017
Representative American Speeches: 2017-2018
Representative American Speeches: 2018-2019
Rethinking Work
Revisiting Gender
Robotics
Russia
Social Networking
Social Services for the Poor
The South China Seas Conflict
Space Exploration & Development
Sports in America
The Supreme Court
The Transformation of American Cities
The Two Koreas
U.S. Infrastructure
U.S. National Debate Topic: Educational Reform
U.S. National Debate Topic: Surveillance
U.S. National Debate Topic: The Ocean
U.S. National Debate Topic: Transportation Infrastructure
Whistleblowers

Readers' Guide
Abridged Readers' Guide to Periodical Literature
Readers' Guide to Periodical Literature

Indexes
Index to Legal Periodicals & Books
Short Story Index
Book Review Digest

Sears List
Sears List of Subject Headings
Sears: Lista de Encabezamientos de Materia

Facts About Series
Facts About American Immigration
Facts About China
Facts About the 20th Century
Facts About the Presidents
Facts About the World's Languages

Nobel Prize Winners
Nobel Prize Winners: 1901-1986
Nobel Prize Winners: 1987-1991
Nobel Prize Winners: 1992-1996
Nobel Prize Winners: 1997-2001
Nobel Prize Winners: 2002-2018

World Authors
World Authors: 1995-2000
World Authors: 2000-2005

Famous First Facts
Famous First Facts
Famous First Facts About American Politics
Famous First Facts About Sports
Famous First Facts About the Environment
Famous First Facts: International Edition

American Book of Days
The American Book of Days
The International Book of Days

Monographs
American Game Changers
American Reformers

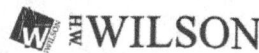

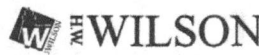

2019 Title List

Visit **www.HWWilsonInPrint.com** for Product Information, Table of Contents and Sample Pages.

The Barnhart Dictionary of Etymology
Celebrate the World
Guide to the Ancient World
Indexing from A to Z
Nobel Prize Winners
The Poetry Break
Radical Change: Books for Youth in a Digital Age
Speeches of American Presidents

Wilson Chronology

Wilson Chronology of Asia and the Pacific
Wilson Chronology of Human Rights
Wilson Chronology of Ideas
Wilson Chronology of the Arts
Wilson Chronology of the World's Religions
Wilson Chronology of Women's Achievements

Grey House Publishing | Salem Press | H.W. Wilson | 4919 Route, 22 PO Box 56, Amenia NY 12501-0056